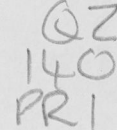

Pathophysiology

CLINICAL CONCEPTS
OF
DISEASE PROCESSES

CONGRATULATIONS

You now have access to a Bonus Online Package!

visit us at:

http://www.mosby.com/MERLIN/PriceWilson/

A website just for you as you learn pathophysiology with the new sixth edition of
Pathophysiology: Clinical Concepts of Disease Processes

for students:

Online access means traveling light, without extra workbooks. Student review and study resources available through the website include:

- More than 2000 additional Study Questions, with immediate access to answers and detailed rationales. Print them out or complete them online!
- Learning Objectives for each chapter
- A Glossary, with definitions of more than 3000 key terms

plus: 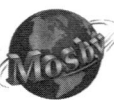 WebLinks

An exciting resource that lets you link to hundreds of websites carefully chosen to supplement the content of your textbook. The WebLinks are regularly updated, with news ones added as they develop.

for instructors:

State-of-the-art security protects valuable online teaching tools.
A unique passcode is your key to web-based materials that include:

A complete Instructor's Manual with:
- A Test Bank of more than 3000 multiple choice questions
- Approximately 30 Case Studies, with complete answers to the questions posed

These same instructor materials are available on CD-ROM (0-323-02299-5) from your sales representative.

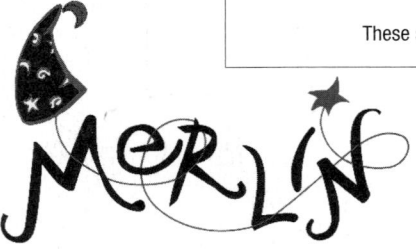

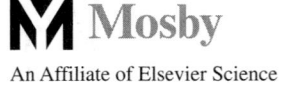
An Affiliate of Elsevier Science

SIXTH EDITION

Pathophysiology

CLINICAL CONCEPTS OF DISEASE PROCESSES

Sylvia Anderson Price, RN, PhD

Professor (Retired)
College of Nursing
The University of Tennessee Health Science Center
Memphis, Tennessee

Lorraine McCarty Wilson, RN, PhD

Professor
Pathophysiology Instructor
Eastern Michigan University
Ypsilanti, Michigan

Illustrations by
Margaret Croup Brudon

Includes 70 color plates

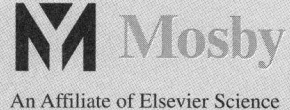

Mosby

An Affiliate of Elsevier Science

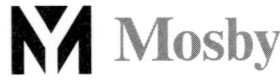

An Affiliate of Elsevier Science

11830 Westline Industrial Drive
St. Louis, Missouri 63146

Previous editions copyrighted 1997, 1992, 1986, 1982, and 1978.

International Standard Book Number 0-323-01455-0

Vice President, Publishing Director: Sally Schrefer
Executive Editor: Darlene Como
Developmental Editor: Laura M. Selkirk
Publishing Services Manager: Catherine Albright Jackson
Project Manager: Clay S. Broeker
Designer: Teresa Breckwoldt

GW/KPT

Printed in the United States of America

Last digit is the print number: 9 8 7 6 5 4 3 2 1

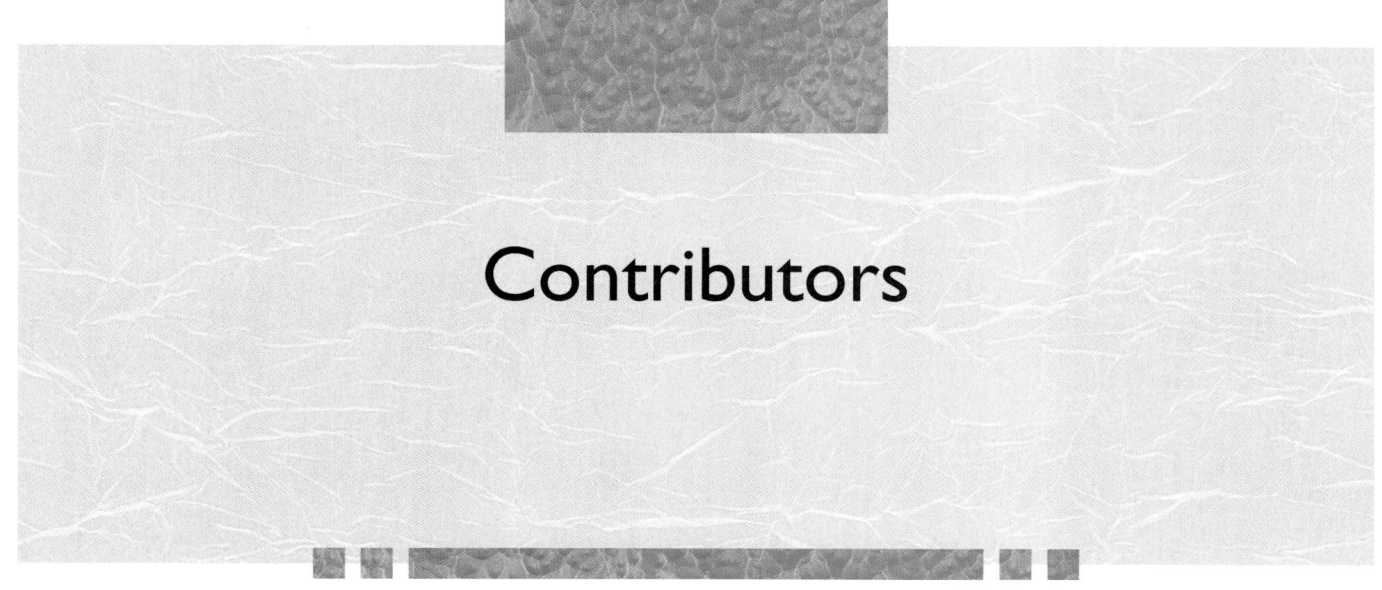

Contributors

CATHERINE M. BALDY, RN, MS, OCN
Clinical Nurse Specialist in Hematology
Henry Ford Hospital
Detroit, Michigan

MARJORIE A. BOLDT, RN, MS, JD
Former Head Nurse
Coronary Care Unit
Beth Israel Hospital
Boston, Massachusetts

CAROL T. BROWN, MN, RN, CS, ANP
Adult Nurse Practitioner in Cardiology
Massachusetts General Hospital
Boston, Massachusetts

MARGARET CROUP BRUDON, BS
Former President
Association of Medical Illustrators
Staff Medical Illustrator and Assistant Professor of
    Medical and Biological Illustrations
University of Michigan
Ann Arbor, Michigan

PENNY FORD CARLETON, RN, MS, MPA
Cardiovascular Clinical Nurse Specialist
Anesthesia Bioengineering Unit
Massachusetts General Hospital
Research Associate
Harvard Medical Center
Boston, Massachusetts

MICHAEL A. CARTER, DNSc, FAAN
University Distinguished Professor
College of Nursing
The University of Tennessee Health Science Center
Memphis, Tennessee

LINDA COUGHLIN DeBEASI, MS, RN, CCRN
Cardiac Clinical Nurse Specialist
Milford, Massachusetts

LINDA J. DENEKAMP, MS, RN, CS
Nurse Manager, Vascular Unit
Beth Israel Deaconess Medical Center
Boston, Massachusetts

SUSAN T. DiMATTIA, MSN, RN, NP
Cardiovascular Nurse Practitioner
Beth Israel Deaconess Medical Center
Boston, Massachusetts

PATRICIA HENRY FOLCARELLI, RN,
    PhC, MA
Vascular Unit
Beth Israel Deaconess Medical Center
Instructor in Surgery
Harvard Medical School
Boston, Massachusetts

BETTY B. GALLUCCI, PhD, RN
Professor
Biobehavioral Nursing and Health Systems
School of Nursing
University of Washington
Seattle, Washington

REBECCA HARMSEN, RN, MN
Clinical Research Nurse
Westat
Rockville, Maryland

MARY S. HARTWIG, RN, APN, PhD
Director of Nursing Education
Area Health Educational Center—Northeast
University of Arkansas for Medical Sciences
Jonesboro, Arkansas

KATHLEEN BRANSON HILLEGAS, RN,
    MS, PhD
Associate Professor
Maternal and Child Health
Eastern Michigan University
Ypsilanti, Michigan

VIRGINIA MACEDA LAN, RN, PhD
Associate Professor
Eastern Michigan University
Ypsilanti, Michigan

GLENDA N. LINDSETH, RN, PhD
Professor and Director of Research
College of Nursing
University of North Dakota
Grand Forks, North Dakota

MARY CARTER LOMBARDO, RN, MSN, CEN
Clinical Nurse Specialist, Neurology
Howard County General Hospital
Columbia, Maryland

MADELINE M. O'DONNELL, RN, MS
Cardiac Clinical Specialist
Intensive Care Nursing Service
Massachusetts General Hospital
Boston, Massachusetts

NANCY A. PRINCE, RN, MSN, WHNP, FNP
Extensive practice experience in Family Planning and
    Sexually Transmitted Disease clinics
Assistant Professor
Eastern Michigan University
Ypsilanti, Michigan

DAVID E. SCHTEINGART, MD
Professor of Internal Medicine
University of Michigan
Medical Center
Ann Arbor, Michigan

WILLIAM R. SOLOMON, MD
Professor of Internal Medicine
University of Michigan
Medical Center
Ann Arbor, Michigan

MARILYN SAWYER SOMMERS, RN,
    PhD, FAAN
Professor and Associate Dean
College of Nursing
University of Cincinnati
Cincinnati, Ohio

MAREK A. STAWISKI, MD
Associate Clinical Professor of Internal Medicine
Michigan State University
East Lansing, Michigan

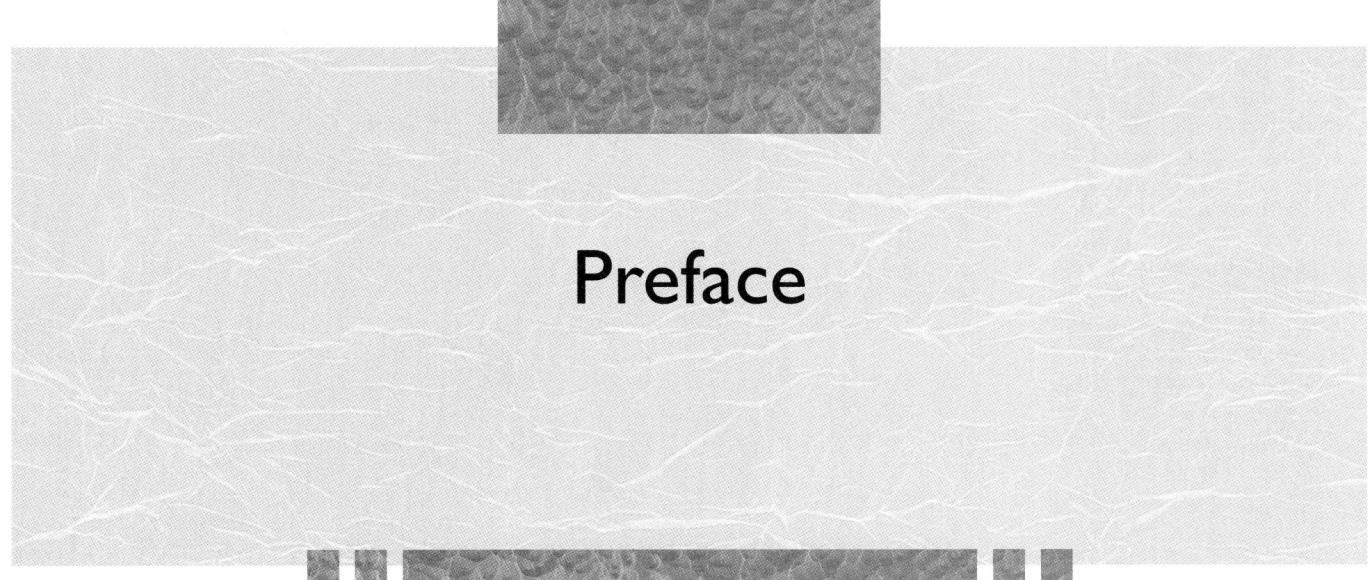

Preface

Pathophysiology deals with the *dynamic* aspects of disease processes. It is the study of altered or disordered functions—the physiologic mechanisms altered by disease in the living organism. Pathophysiology provides the basic link between clinical practice and the scientific realm of anatomy, physiology, and biochemistry. The study of pathophysiology is essential to understand the rationale for diagnosis and therapeutic intervention in disease conditions.

The sixth edition of *Pathophysiology: Clinical Concepts of Disease Processes* retains the same philosophy and organizational framework as the five previous editions. Our focus is on alterations in disease processes that affect the body's dynamic equilibrium, or *homeostasis*, a conceptual approach designed to integrate knowledge from the basic and clinical sciences.

The conceptual framework is designed to first present the general concepts of disease processes. The various dysfunctions of an organ or organ system are then examined. Emphasis is on understanding the etiology and pathogenesis of a given disorder, which is an essential factor in the development of clinical insight.

Throughout this sixth edition, we (and our many expert contributors) have incorporated recent research findings, new diagnostic procedures, current treatment measures, and preventative measures. Many updates and revisions incorporate significant changes suggested by instructors, students, and practitioners.

The hallmark features of the textbook have been retained in this edition, with some new features added, including **key concepts at the end of every chapter** and a **new website:** *www.mosby.com/MERLIN/PriceWilson/*

Hallmark Features

- Students usually find pathophysiology to be a very complex and intimidating subject, so **short, clearly focused chapters** are offered to make the content easier to read and synthesize. The textbook is divided into 13 parts, with the first part dealing with general pathophysiologic principles and the remaining 12 parts divided according to the traditional body systems approach. It is further divided into 82 concise chapters that present the challenging concepts of pathophysiology to students in manageable increments.
- A **focused illustration program,** with more than 725 photographs and drawings throughout the textbook, serves to **clarify the more difficult concepts** and demonstrate normal processes as well as disease processes.
- The **color plates** clearly depict certain disease manifestations and enhance the content for students. The plates are grouped together and appear in the front section of the text for easy access. Students can quickly turn to the plates for reference as they read the related content in the textbook.
- The **chapter outlines** and **end-of-chapter study questions** have always been a popular feature with students and instructors. No other text offers a "built-in study guide" like this one, with more than 3000 study questions. About 1000 short answer, matching, true/false, fill-in-the-blank, and multiple choice questions can be found at the end of the chapters in the textbook, while about 2000 of these study questions can be found on the new website at *www.mosby.com/MERLIN/PriceWilson/*

New Content

- **Genetic factors in disease pathogenesis** have been incorporated throughout the book, including the new understanding of the genetic basis of carcinogenesis.
- **Up-to-date research findings, diagnostic procedures and preventive measures,** and **current treatments** are integrated throughout to demonstrate clinical application of knowledge.
- **Completely revised chapters,** including Heredity, Environment, and Disease: Interaction of Heredity and Environment (Chapter 2), Cerebrovascular Disease (Chapter 53), Adrenal Insufficiency (Chapter 62), and Infections of the Genital Tract (Chapter 66), and **extensive chapter rewrites,** including White Blood Cell and Plasma Cell Disorders (Chapter 18), Anatomy of the Cardiovascular System (Chapter 28), Physiology of the Cardiovascular System (Chapter 29), Cardiac Mechanical Dysfunction and Circulatory Support (Chapter 33), Seizure Disorders (Chapter 55), Pancreas: Glucose

Metabolism and Diabetes Mellitus (Chapter 63), and Female Reproductive System Disorders (Chapter 64), reflect advances in scientific knowledge.

- **Twenty-eight new color plates**, including such illustrations as acute hemorrhagic gastritis (stress ulcer), appendicitis, acute pancreatitis, primary and secondary syphilis, and primary herpes have been added to the textbook. The color plates section includes a **total of 70 color photographs**.
- **More than 40 new two-color line illustrations** have been added, updated, or replaced to augment the text description of pathophysiologic concepts and processes.

New Features

- **Comprehensive key concepts reviews** at the end of each chapter help students review material.
- **Numbered boxes** help students find information quicker and easier.
- The **new website** at *www.mosby.com/MERLIN/PriceWilson/* contains additional study questions, learning objectives, select key terms with definitions, and WebLinks for the student. The online study questions, a self-paced tool that provides **immediate feedback**, enables the student to actively participate in the learning process by reading, reasoning, and demonstrating his or her mastery of the concepts.

This textbook provides the reader with a comprehensive presentation of pathophysiologic mechanisms in disease processes. We have emphasized relevant concepts that will enable the practitioner to function effectively in the health care delivery system. Our intent is to offer a textbook that not only is informative, but will also challenge and broaden the horizons of the health care professional.

This textbook of pathophysiology is designed to meet the more sophisticated needs of health care consumers and health professionals alike. Changes in the pattern of health care delivery have made it ever more important to better understand the reasoning behind the care given. Rapid advances in biomedical sciences, coupled with changes in health care delivery and its effect on consumerism, have made nurses and other health care professionals accountable for creating an environment that promotes high-quality, patient-centered care. The role of the practitioner in the health care system, as well as the role of the consumer, continue to change. Nurses are functioning as independent practitioners in a variety of health care settings, such as in primary health care, and are responsible for managing the holistic health care of patients. They cooperate with professionals from other disciplines to provide the best possible care to meet patients' needs. It is essential that these professionals synthesize pathophysiologic concepts to understand the ra-

tionale for preventive measures and therapeutic interventions. It is also becoming more incumbent on those who receive the health care to take an active role in maintaining or improving their health.

For the Instructor

The **new website** at *www.mosby.com/MERLIN/PriceWilson/* allows instructors to access the *Instructor's Manual* and *Test Bank* via a **secure passcode**.

The *Instructor's Manual* provides additional teaching and learning devices to help instructors teach. Divided into chapters to correspond with the textbook, each chapter of the *Instructor's Manual* includes a complete chapter outline with page numbers for easy reference, key terms with definitions, and a list of learning objectives for that particular chapter. A selection of case studies also is included in the *Instructor's Manual* to help instructors teach clinical application of the content. These case studies cover each of the body systems and include answers to the questions posed.

The *Test Bank* is extremely comprehensive and complete, offering instructors a wide array of test questions to include in their examinations. The *Test Bank* includes approximately 3000 questions. All of the questions are multiple choice, and all are keyed to the learning objectives for each chapter.

The *Instructor's Manual* and *Test Bank* are also available on CD-ROM for those instructors who do not wish to access them online.

ACKNOWLEDGMENTS

Our sincere appreciation to Darlene Como, Executive Editor, for her valuable contributions during the planning and execution of this revision; to Laura Selkirk, Developmental Editor, for the excellent quality of her editorial assistance; to Marc Syp, Project Manager, for his meticulous attention to detail; to Marjorie Boldt for her coordination and contributions to the cardiovascular section; and to Margaret Croup Brudon for the creative illustrations that she prepared for this and all previous editions of the book. We wish to thank Gerald D. Abrams, MD, Professor of Pathology and exemplary teacher at the University of Michigan, for his encouragement with this textbook. Dr. Abrams was the author of the first eight chapters (covering pathophysiologic principles) for the first five editions. Finally, we also appreciate the comprehensive reviews and suggestions for changes in the manuscript offered by the many reviewers.

LORRAINE MCCARTY WILSON
SYLVIA ANDERSON PRICE

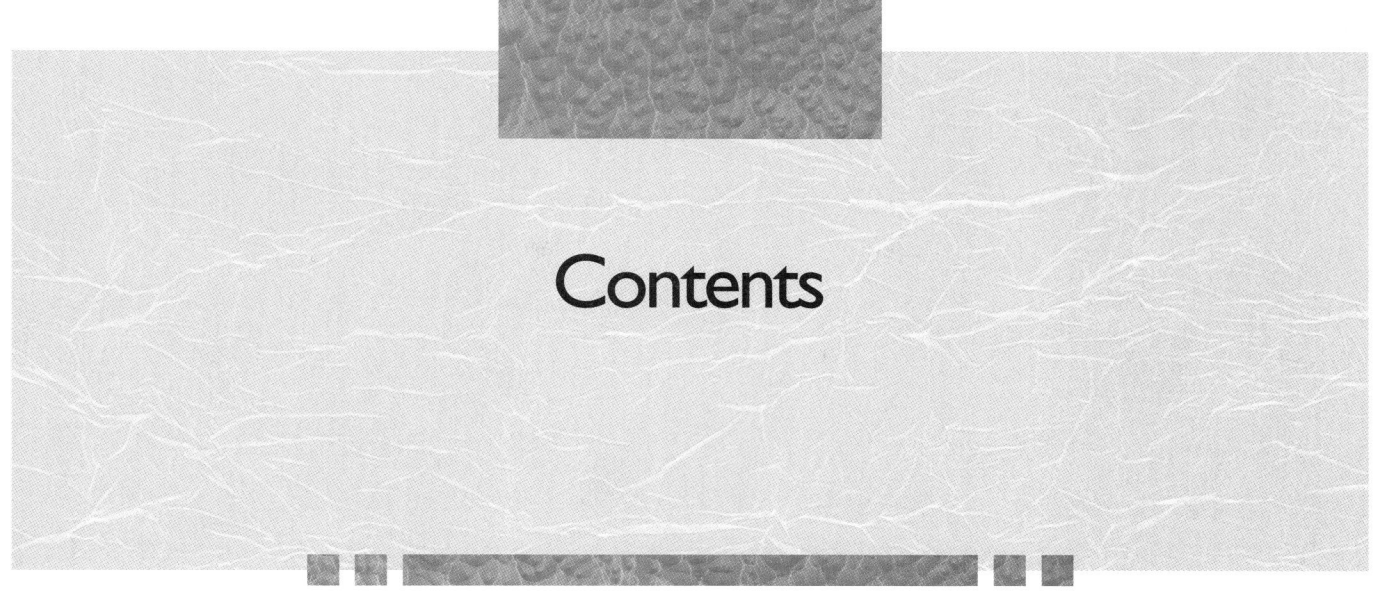

Contents

COLOR PLATES

Color Plate Credits

Plates 1, 2, 3, 4, 5, 6, 7, and 8 from Grimes DE, Grimes RM: *AIDS and HIV infection*, St Louis, 1994, Mosby; courtesy The Centers for Disease Control and Prevention.

Plates 9, 10, 11, 14, 15, 16, 17, 18, 19, 20, 21, 23, and 26 courtesy Herminia Bigornia, MT, and Muhammad S. Shurafa, MD, Division of Hematology/Oncology, Henry Ford Hospital, Detroit, Michigan.

Plates 12, 22, and 24 courtesy Kolichi Maeda, MD, Division of Hematology/Oncology, Henry Ford Hospital, Detroit, Michigan.

Plates 13 and 25 courtesy Sheikh Saeed, MD, Division Head of Hematopathology, Henry Ford Hospital, Detroit, Michigan.

Plate 27, 29, 34, and 36 courtesy Gerald D. Abrams, MD, Department of Pathology, University of Michigan, Ann Arbor, Michigan.

Plate 28 from Cotran RS, Kumar V, Collins T: *Robbins pathologic basis of disease*, ed 6, Philadelphia, 1999, WB Saunders; courtesy Dr. James Gulizia, Brigham and Women's Hospital, Boston, Massachusetts.

Plates 30, 33, 35, and 37 from Damjanov I, Linder J: *Pathology: a color atlas*, St Louis, 2000, Mosby.

Plate 31 from Doughty D: *Gastrointestinal disorders*, St Louis, 1993, Mosby.

Plates 32 and 38 from Hill M: *Skin disorders*, St Louis, 1994, Mosby.

Plates 39, 41, 43, 44, and 45 from Centers for Disease Control and Prevention: *Sexually transmitted disease*, Centers for Disease Control and Prevention, Atlanta, Georgia.

Plates 40, 42, 46, 55, 57, 58, 59, 60, 61, 62, 63, 66, 68, and 70 from Habif TP et al: *Skin disease: diagnosis and treatment*, St Louis, 2001, Mosby.

Plates 47, 48, 49, 50, 51, 52, 53, 54, 56, 64, 65, 67, and 69 courtesy Marek A. Stawiski, MD, Associate Clinical Professor of Internal Medicine, Michigan State University, East Lansing, Michigan.

Color Plates

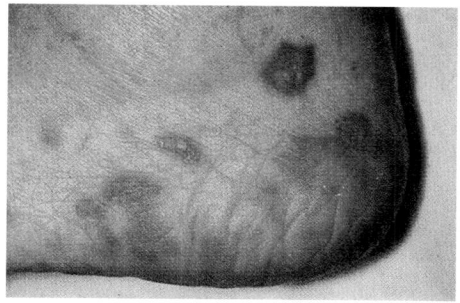

1   **Kaposi's sarcoma** of heel and lateral foot.

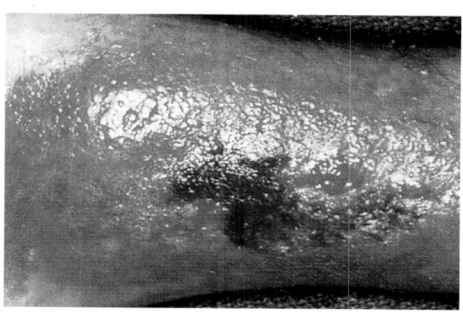

2   **Kaposi's sarcoma** of distal leg and ankle.

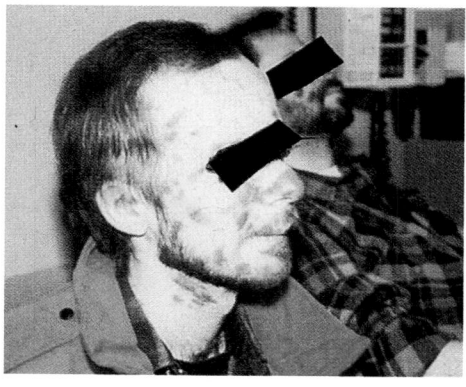

3   **Kaposi's sarcoma** of face.

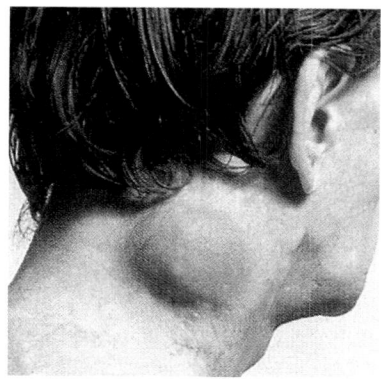

4   **Lymphoma** on neck.

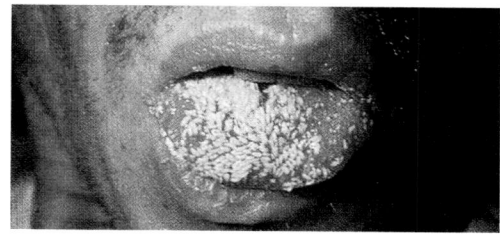

5   **Severe pseudomembranous candidiasis of tongue** in patient with AIDS.

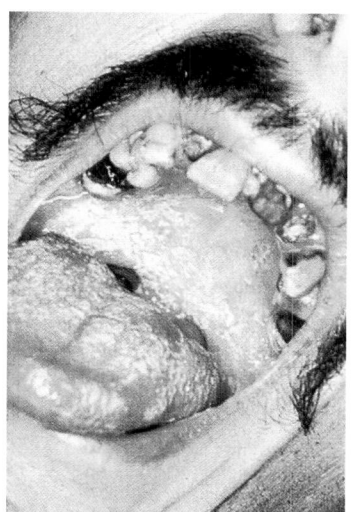

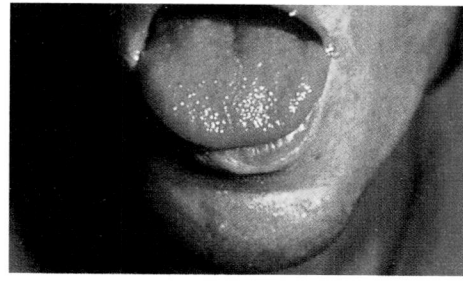

7   **Candidiasis of tongue** in AIDS patient resistant to fluconazole.

6   **Candidiasis of tongue** in patient shown in Plate 5 after 48 hours of treatment with fluconazole.

For color plate credits, see p. xvi.

Color Plates

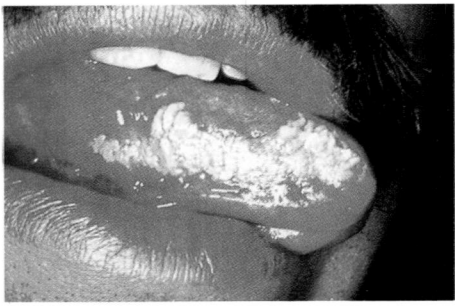

8 **Oral hairy leukoplakia** often presents as white plaques on lateral tongue and is associated with Epstein-Barr virus infection.

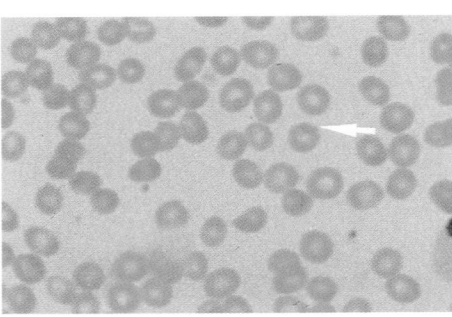

9 **Normal red blood cells (RBCs)** are round, possess an area of central pallor, appear slightly smaller than nucleus of mature lymphocyte *(lower right)*, and vary little in size or shape.

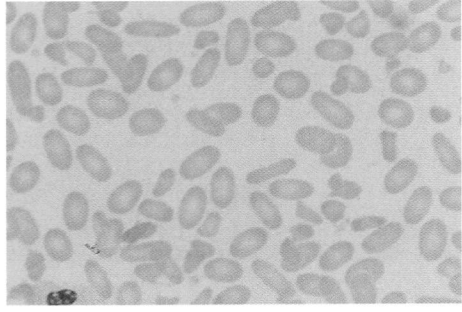

10 **Anisocytosis and poikilocytosis,** or RBCs that vary in size and shape, respectively.

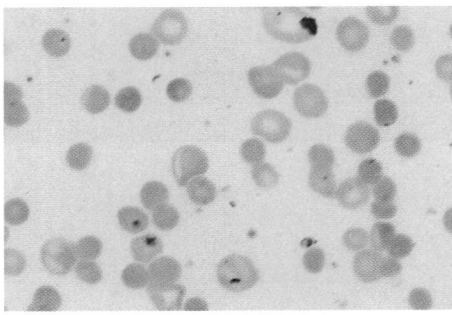

11 **Spherocytes** are smaller than normal RBCs, do not have central pallor, stain deeper, and tend to hemolyze readily.

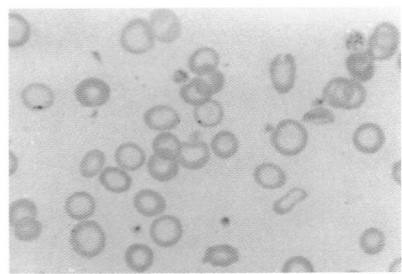

12 Hypochromic, microcytic RBCs characteristic of **iron deficiency anemia**. Poikilocytosis is seen.

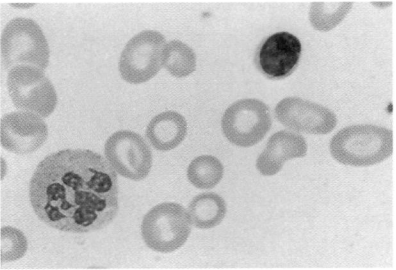

13 Peripheral blood findings seen in **megaloblastic (macrocytic) anemia**. Hypersegmented neutrophil and ovalocytes (large, oval-shaped RBCs) are evident.

For color plate credits, see p. xvi.

Color Plates

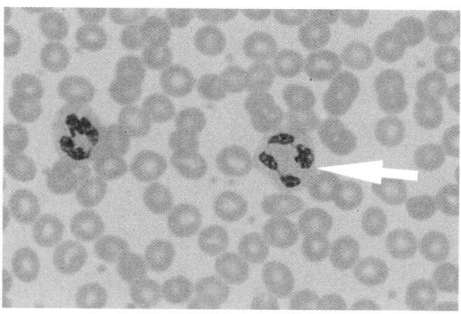

14 Normal mature **neutrophil (PMN).** PMN has segmented nucleus (two to five lobes) with heavy, clumped chromatin; fine, neutrophilic (lilac-colored) granules are dispersed throughout its cytoplasm.

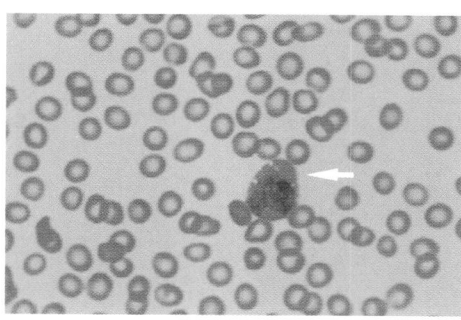

15 Normal **eosinophil.** Nucleus is bilobed, and cytoplasm contains purplish red granules.

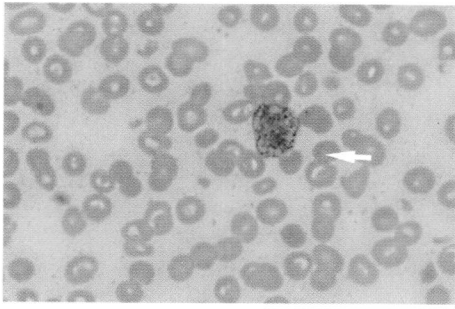

16 Normal **basophil** contains large, dark-blue granules that fill cell and obscure nucleus.

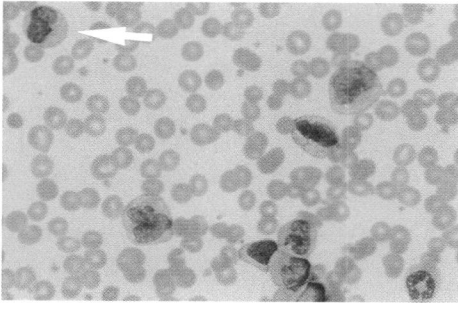

17 Normal **monocyte** is large cell with indented or folded nucleus containing loose, strandlike chromatin; cytoplasm has blue-gray color and usually contains fine, azurophilic granules.

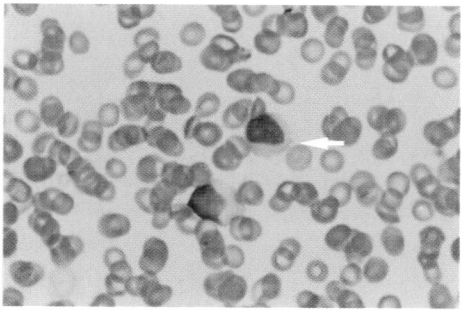

18 Normal **lymphocytes** have small, round or slightly indented nucleus with abundant, dark-staining condensed chromatin. Only thin external rim of slightly basophilic cytoplasm is visible.

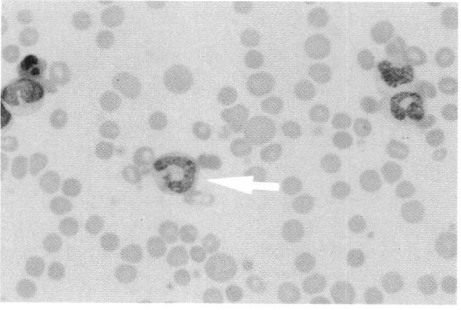

19 **Band neutrophil** is slightly immature neutrophil with band-like nucleus, usually shaped like a horseshoe. Numbers rise in acute bacterial infections.

For color plate credits, see p. xvi.

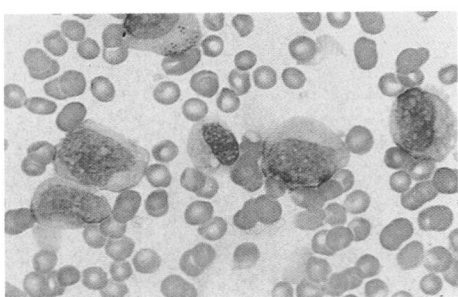

20 Myeloblasts in acute myelogenous leukemia. Cells have large nucleus with fine nuclear chromatin, very little cytoplasm, and usually two to five nucleoli.

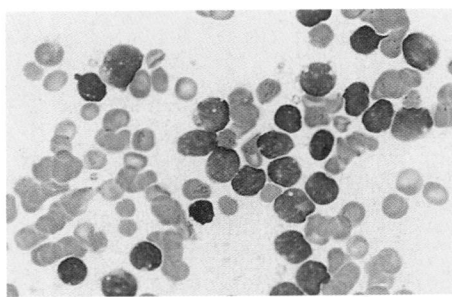

21 Lymphoblast in acute lymphocytic leukemia. Cells have fine chromatin nuclei with minimal cytoplasm and usually one or two nucleoli.

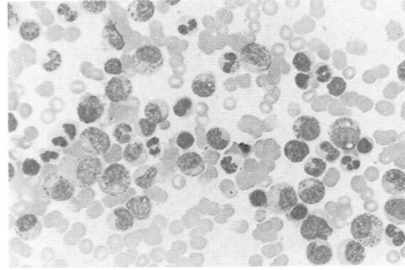

22 Bone marrow characteristic of **chronic granulocytic leukemia.** Marrow is hypercellular with an increase in granulocytic line.

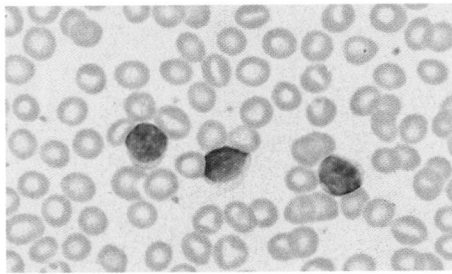

23 Chronic lymphocytic leukemia. Mature lymphocytes with coarse nuclear chromatin and thin cytoplasm.

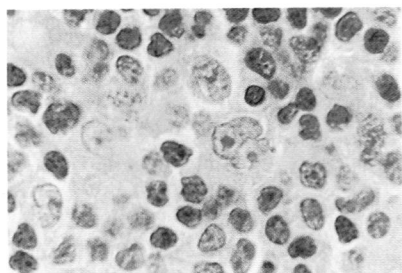

24 Reed-Sternberg cell. Giant binucleated cell *(center)* typically seen in Hodgkin's disease. Small, mature lymphocytes are seen in background. To left of Reed-Sternberg cell is eosinophil containing red-orange cytoplasmic granules.

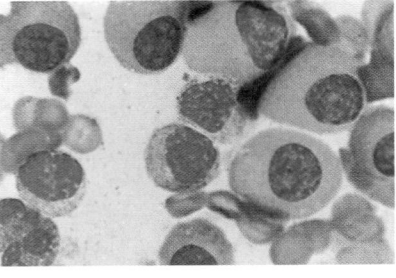

25 Bone marrow aspirate depicting cells seen in **multiple myeloma.**

26 Platelets (thrombocytes) lack a nucleus because they are derived from cytoplasmic fragments of megakaryocytes. Platelets show central granular region with prominent purple-staining granules and nongranular periphery that stains pale transparent blue.

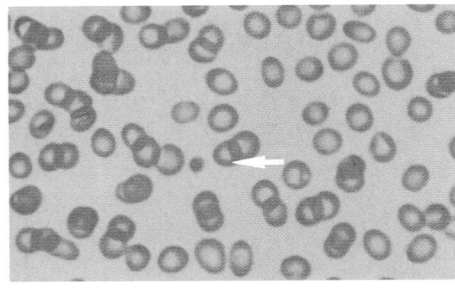

For color plate credits, see p. xvi.

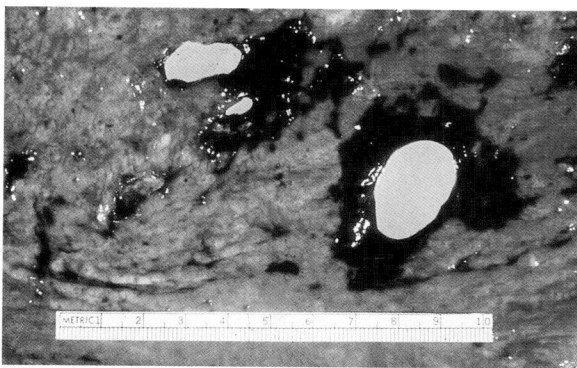

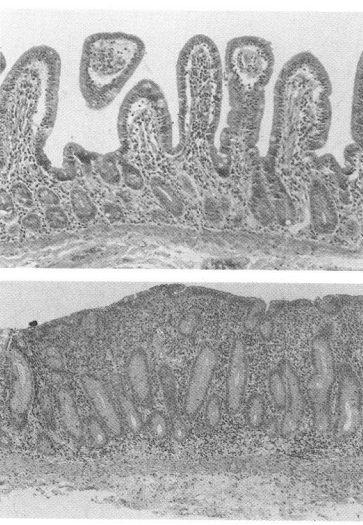

27 **Acute hemorrhagic gastritis (stress ulcer)** complicated by complete perforation through the gastric wall. This stress ulcer was induced by an acute alcoholic bout and aspirin ingestion in a university student.

28 **Celiac sprue** (gluten-sensitive enteropathy) (*bottom*) compared with normal jejunum (*top*). In sprue there is diffuse sever atrophy and blunting of villi, with a chronic inflammatory infiltrate of the lamina propria.

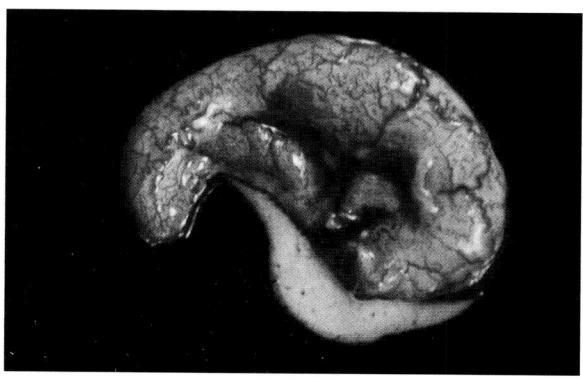

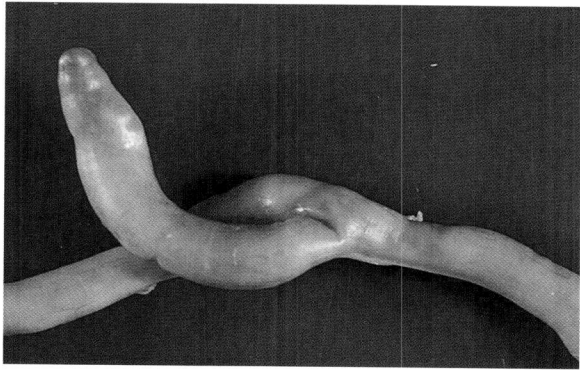

29 **Appendicitis**. This appendix is inflamed and distended with yellowish pus.

30 **Meckel's diverticulum.** This blind intestinal loop of the ileus, about 2 inches long, is found in about 2% of the population. It may become ulcerated, bleed, and cause symptoms similar to those of acute appendicitis in 2% of those who have it.

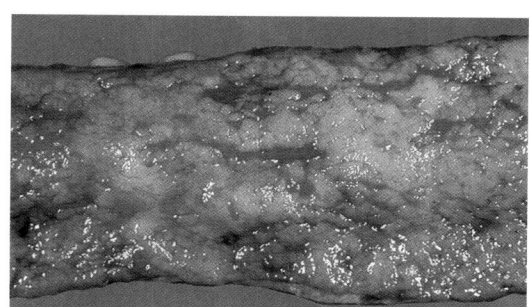

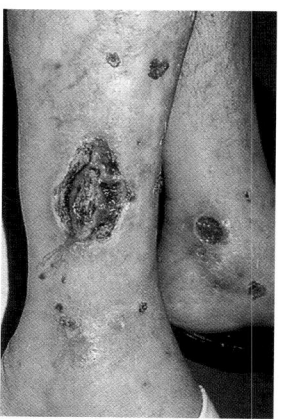

31 **Ulcerative colitis** showing severe mucosal edema and inflammation with ulcerations and bleeding.

32 **Pyoderma gangrenosum** of legs in patient with ulcerative colitis.

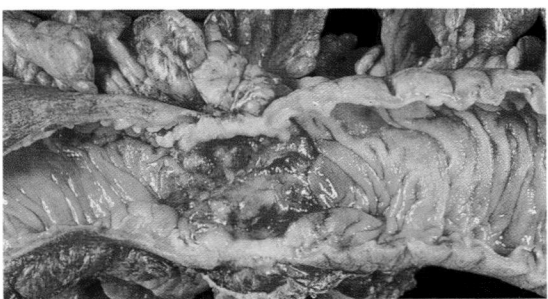

33 **Adenocarcinoma of the sigmoid colon,** forming a circumferential mass and narrowing the intestinal lumen.

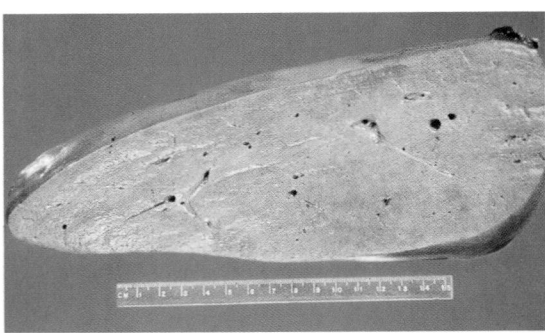

34 **Fatty infiltration of the liver**. Lipid infiltration within the cells causes liver to appear yellow-brown in color rather than the normal dark brown; liver is enlarged and cut surface feels greasy.

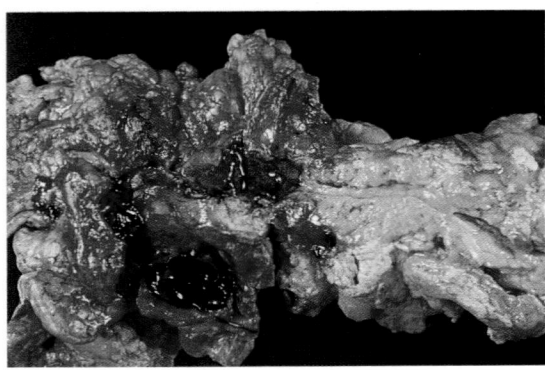

35 **Acute hemorrhagic pancreatitis**. Hemorrhage, fat necrosis, and a pseudocyst filled with blood are seen on cross-section.

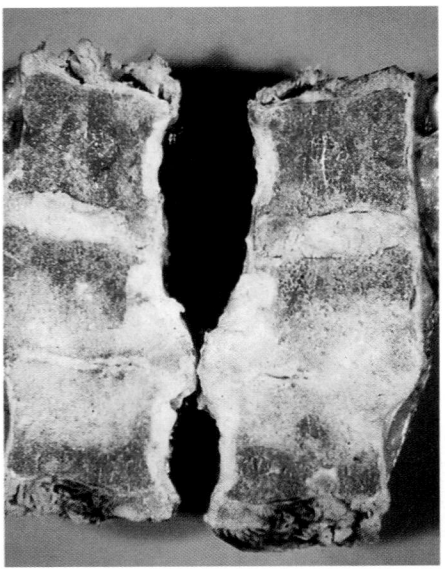

36 **Cancer metastasis to the spine,** originating from the lung and spread via the bloodstream. Whitish tissue is the cancer eroding vertebrae, which may result in compression fracture.

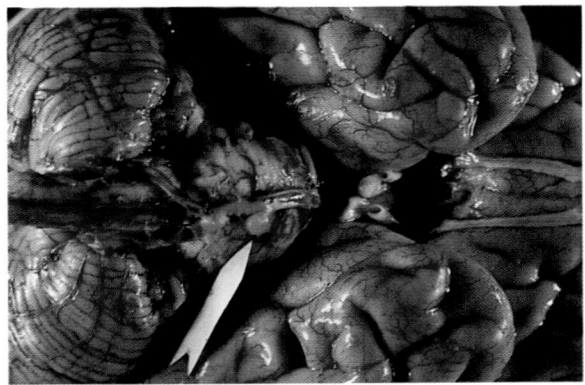

37 **Berry aneurysm** of the circle of Willis (arrow).

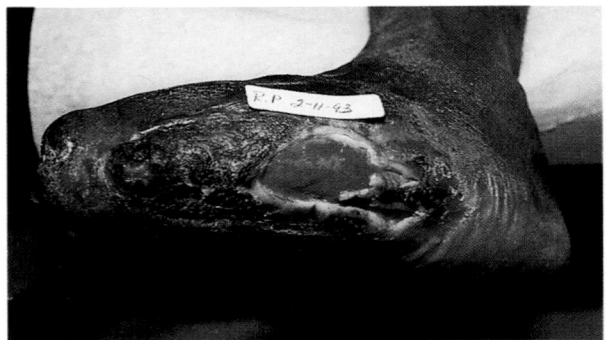

38 **Diabetic foot ulcer** caused by abnormal pressure distribution secondary to diabetic neuropathy. Vascular disease with diminished blood supply also contributes to development of the lesion, and infection is common.

Color Plates

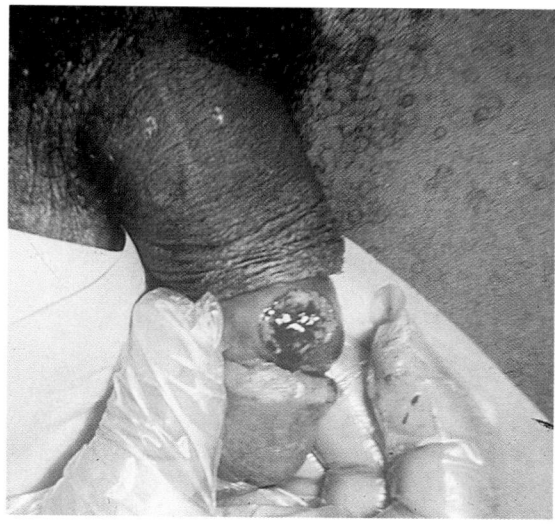

39 **Primary syphilis**. Chancre (painless hard ulcer) on the penis.

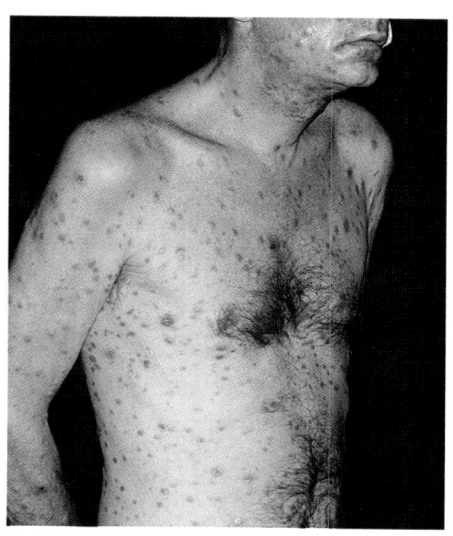

40 **Secondary syphilis**. Papulosquamous rash.

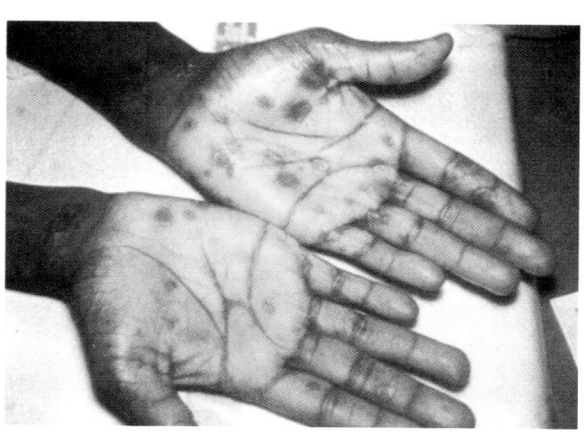

41 **Secondary syphilis**. Lesions on hands.

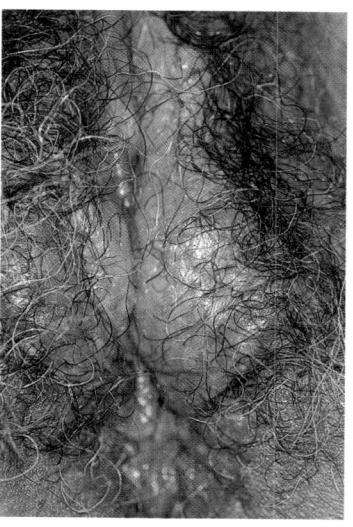

42 **Primary herpes.** Grouped painful vesicles on female genitalia.

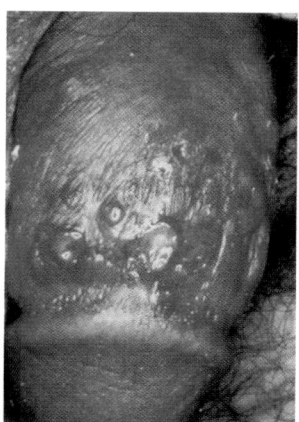

43 **Primary herpes.** Male.

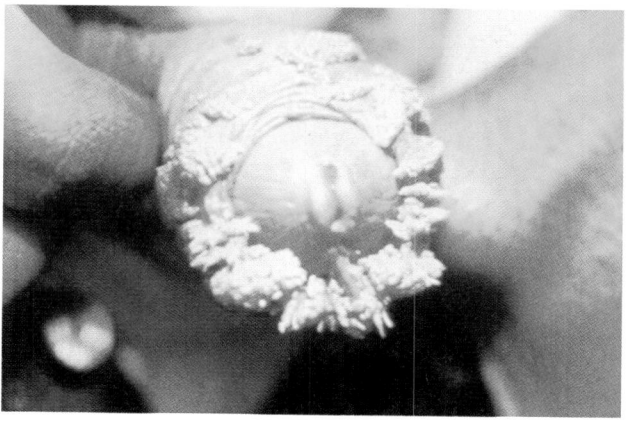

44 **Condyloma acuminata**. Verrucous (wart-like), moist nodules on the penis.

Color Plates

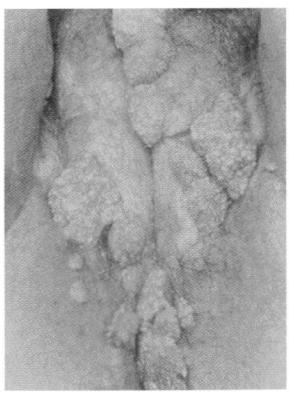

45 **Condyloma acuminata**. Vulva.

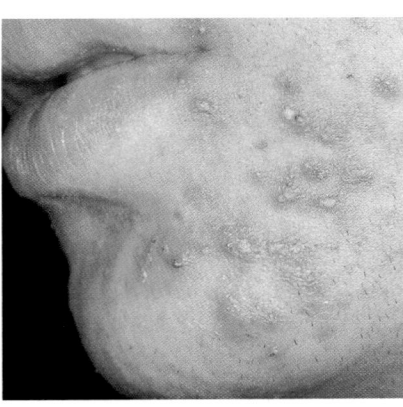

46 **Pustular acne**. Classic inflamed acne lesion. Scarring is possible. Topical medications and oral antibiotics are the treatments of first choice.

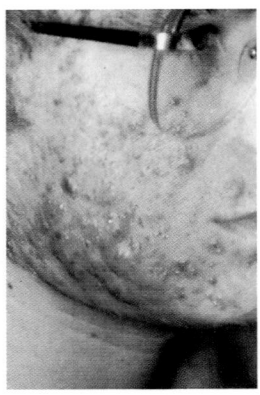

47 **Acne grade IV**. Conglobate, cysts, and scars.

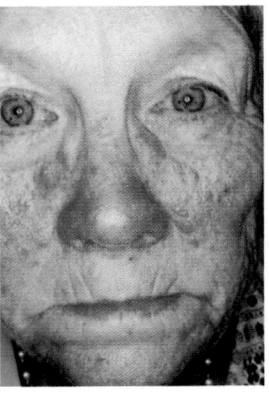

48 **Acne rosacea**. Central facial erythema and pustules.

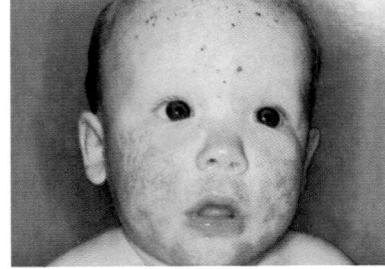

49 **Infantile eczema**. Weeping, erythematous patches.

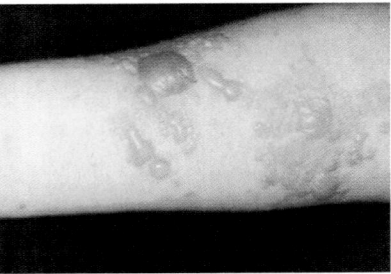

50 **Poison ivy**. Vesicles in linear and grouped configuration.

Color Plates

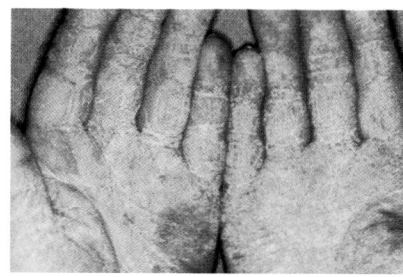

51 Hand eczema. Scaliness and fissures.

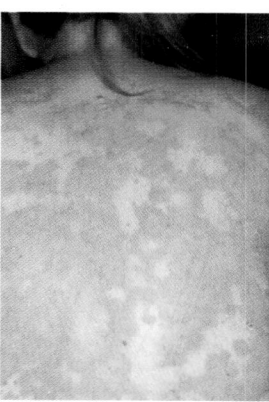

52 Urticaria (hives). Annular and arciform wheals.

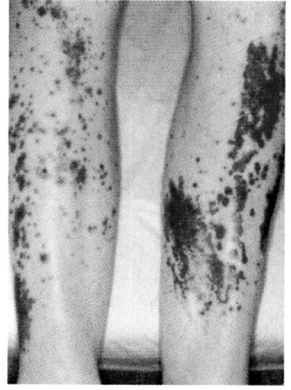

53 Vasculitis. Hemorrhagic, necrotic patches and papules.

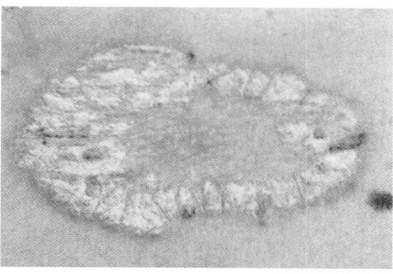

54 Psoriasis. Sharply marginated plaque with thick, white scale.

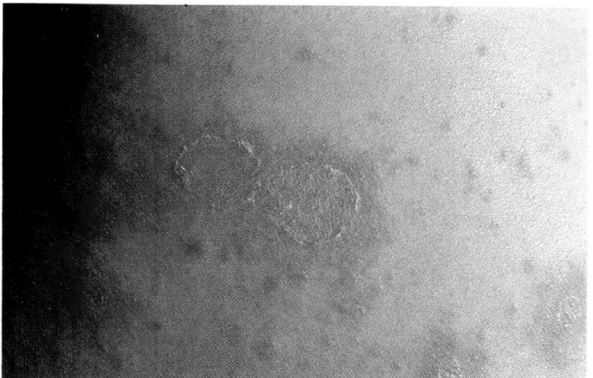

55 Pityriasis rosea. A ring of tissue-like scale remains attached within the border of the red oval-shaped patches on the trunk

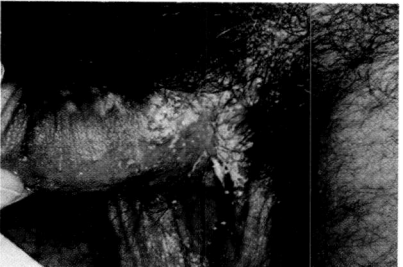

56 Chronic herpes simplex in AIDS patient. Chronic ulceration 3 months in duration with positive herpetic culture.

For color plate credits, see p. xvi.

Color Plates

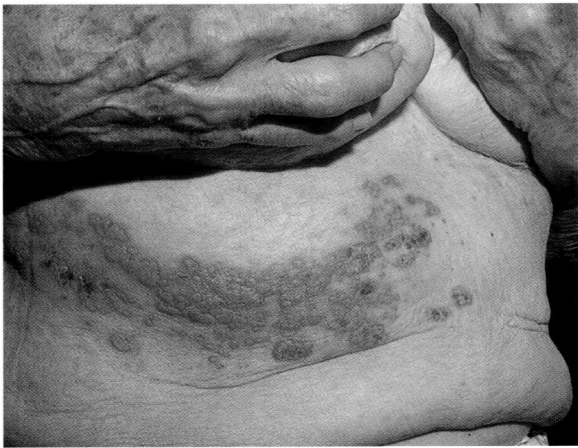

57 **Herpes zoster**. Linear vesicles on erythematous base along one dermatome. Elderly or debilitated patients may have a prolonged and difficult course.

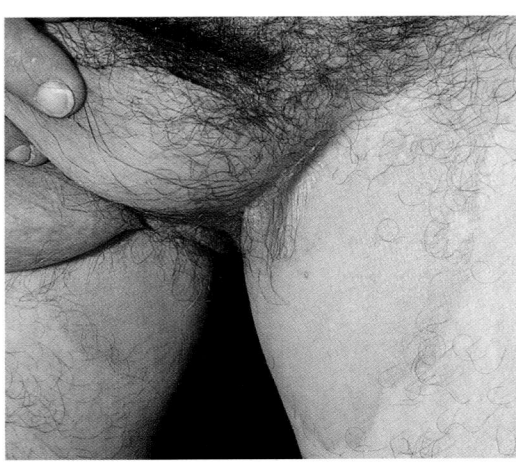

58 **Tinea cruris (jock itch)**. Tinea of the groin, a dermatophyte infection, begins in the crural fold and extends peripherally but does not usually involve the scrotum.

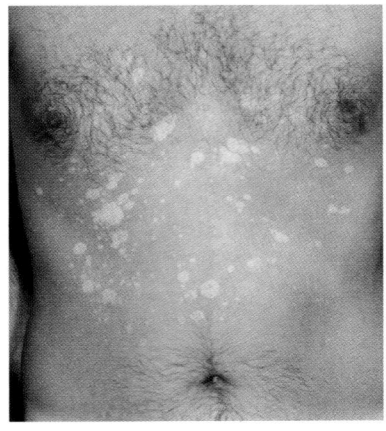

59 **Tinea versicolor**. Whitish, scaly, confluent macules.

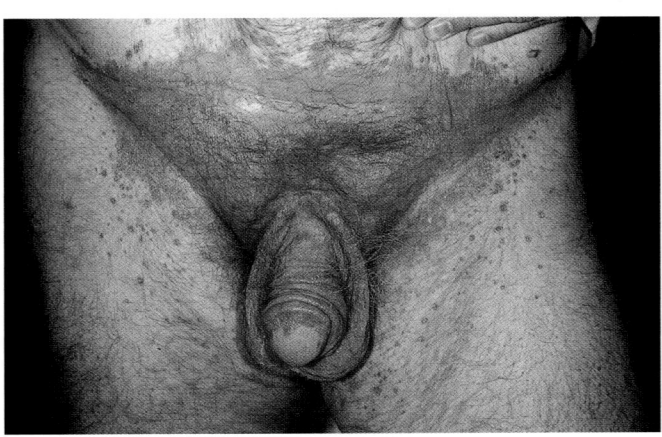

60 **Intertriginous candidiasis**. A red plaque extends to the border of all apposing skinfolds with satellite pustules.

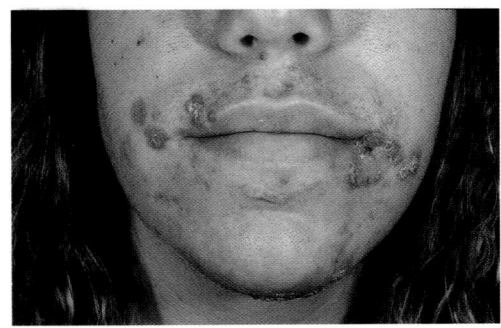

61 **Impetigo** occurs most often on the face. Here lesions are in all stages of development. Note the thick, honey-yellow adherent crusts.

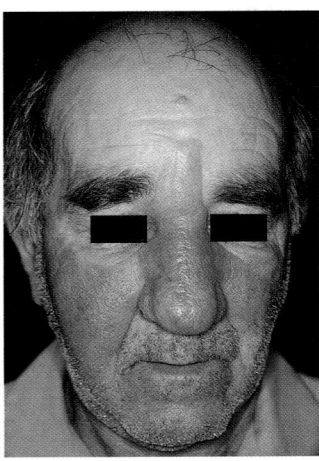

62 **Facial erysipelas**. Bright-red, sharply marginated, painful, hot lesion.

For color plate credits, see p. xvi.

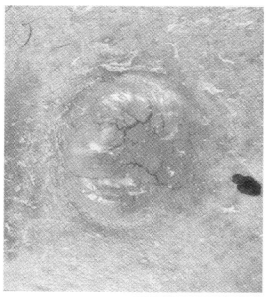

63 **Basil cell carcinoma**.

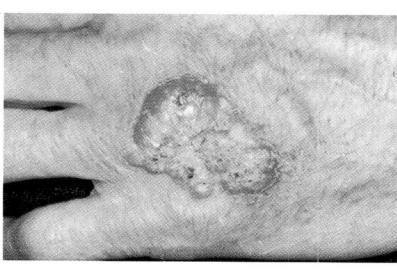

64 **Early squamous cell carcinoma**. Erythematous, infiltrating, ulcerated tumor on sun-exposed area.

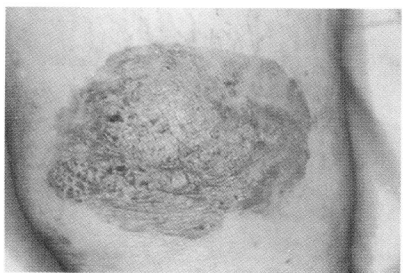

65 **Bowen's disease**. Erythematous, scaly patch with irregular configuration on sun-exposed area.

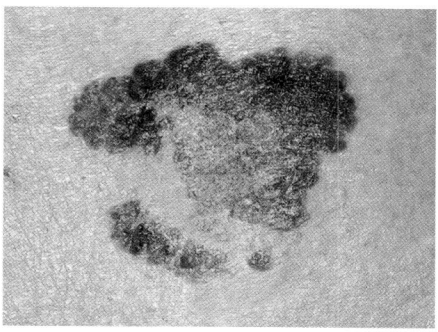

66 **Superficial spreading melanoma**. Variegated colors and infiltration of surrounding skin with diffusion of pigment.

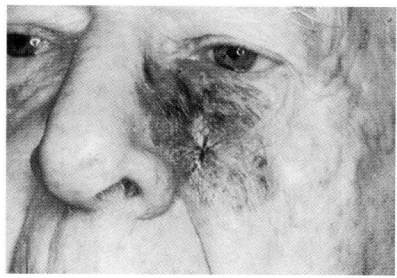

67 **Lentigo maligna melanoma**. Brown-black patch with central black nodule of melanoma arising.

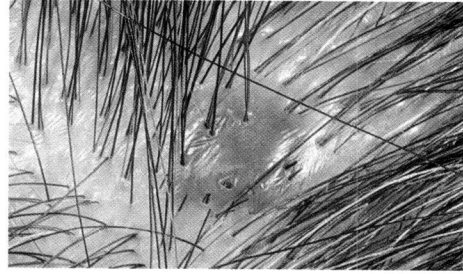

68 **Blue nevus**. Blue uniform color of a benign nevus most commonly found on the head, neck, or buttocks. Coloration is attributed to intensely pigmented melanocytes in the deep dermis.

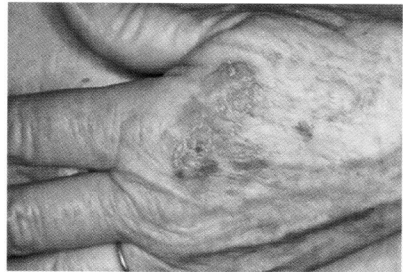

69 **Actinic keratosis**. Erythematous, scaly, firm papulation on plaque.

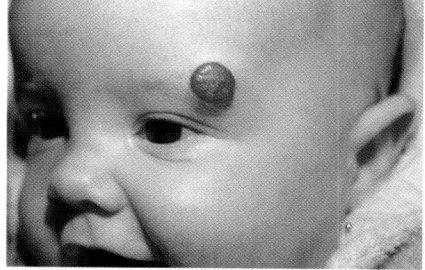

70 **Strawberry hemangioma**. Most are small, harmless birthmarks that proliferate for 8 to 18 months and then slowly regress over the next 5 to 8 months.

INTRODUCTION TO GENERAL PATHOLOGY: MECHANISMS OF DISEASE

*P*art One of this book provides the background for understanding the disease process. The number and variety of human illnesses are immense, because every organ or system within the body is subject to disease. However, the basic ways in which an organ can become diseased are quite limited, and the large and bewildering array of diseases represents different combinations and permutations of a smaller number of basic biologic processes that lead to the alterations of structure and function. This first section focuses on these basic biologic processes.

Pathology is the science or study of disease. In its broadest sense, pathology is literally abnormal biology, the study of biologic processes gone awry, or the study of individuals who are ill or disordered. As a basic biologic science, pathology includes fields such as plant pathology, insect pathology, and veterinary and comparative pathology, as well as human pathology.

Pathology, in the context of human medicine, is not only a basic or theoretic science but also a clinical medical specialty. Pathologists are physicians who specialize in laboratory medicine; they consult with other physicians, thereby assisting in the diagnosis and treatment of disease. The scope of laboratory medicine includes all the studies performed on patient samples, including samples of tissue, blood, and other body fluids. Laboratory studies involving *anatomic pathology* examine and assess morphologic alterations in cells and tissues. Surgical pathology, cytopathology, and autopsy pathology are included in this category. Many studies are performed using other means. These areas of *clinical pathology* include clinical chemistry, microbiology, hematology, immunology, and immunohematology. *Pathophysiology* deals with the dynamic aspects of the disease process; it is the study of disordered or altered functions, for example, the physiologic changes resulting from disease in a living organism.

Fundamental disease processes, such as inflammation, neoplasia, and immunologic injury, are described in this part of the textbook. The details of specific illnesses are addressed in later parts of the text.

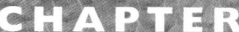

CHAPTER

I

General Concepts of Disease

Health Versus Disease

LORRAINE M. WILSON

CHAPTER OUTLINE

CONCEPT OF NORMALCY

Most people have some notion of *normal* and would define disease or illness as a deviation from or an absence of that normal state. However, on closer scrutiny, the concept of normalcy turns out to be complex and cannot be defined succinctly. Correspondingly, the concept of disease is far from simple.

Any parameter of measurement applied to an individual or group of individuals has some sort of average value that is considered normal. Average values for height, weight, and blood pressure are derived from observation of many individuals and include a certain amount of variation.

Variations in normal values occur for several reasons. First, individuals differ from one another in their genetic makeup. Thus no two individuals in the world, except those derived from the same fertilized ovum, have exactly the same genes. Second, individuals differ in their life experiences and in their interaction with the environment. Third, in every individual, variations in physiologic parameters exist because of the way in which the control mechanisms of the body function. For instance, blood glucose concentrations in a healthy person vary significantly at different times during the day, depending on food intake, activities of the individual, and so forth. These variations generally occur within a certain range. The situation is somewhat analogous to a ther-

mostatically controlled room. The temperature may dip slightly below the desired level before the thermostat senses such a drop. The corrective action triggered by the thermostat may, in turn, overshoot the ideal slightly before the heat input is halted. Indeed, such variations in body temperature, even in the normal state, occur in all individuals. Finally, for physiologic parameters measured by fairly intricate means, a significant amount of variation in observed values may result from error or imprecision that is inherent in the measurement process itself.

Because of these considerations, determining a normal range of variation from an average value is a complex matter. This complexity includes knowing the degree of physiologic oscillation of a particular measurement, accounting for the degree of variation among normal individuals even under baseline conditions, and evaluating the precision of the measurement method. Finally, the biologic significance of the measurement must be estimated. Single measurements, observations, or laboratory results that appear to indicate abnormality must always be judged in the context of the entire situation of the individual. A single reading of elevated blood pressure does not make an individual hypertensive; a single slightly elevated blood glucose level does not mean that the individual is diabetic; and a single hemoglobin value lower than average does not necessarily indicate anemia.

To place such considerations in perspective, concepts of normalcy and even of disease are, to an extent, arbitrary and influenced by cultural values and by biologic realities. For example, in our culture, a defect of a central nervous system function may produce a significant reading disability and would be an abnormality, whereas the same defect might never be noted in a culture in which reading is not an important aspect of everyday life. Furthermore, a trait that might be average and thus normal in one population might be considered distinctly abnormal in another. It might be considered, for instance, how a "normal" person from our population would be viewed by a group of central African pygmies, or conversely, how an infant from a less developed area, in which chronic diarrhea and relatively low weight gain are "normal" for that population, might be viewed in one of our well-baby clinics.

CONCEPT OF DISEASE

Disease can be defined as changes in individuals that cause their health parameters to fall outside the range of normal. The most useful biologic yardstick for normalcy relates to the individual's ability to meet the demands placed on the body and to adapt to these demands or changes in the external environment so as to maintain reasonable constancy of the internal environment. All cells in the body need a certain amount of oxygen and nutrients for their continuing survival and function, and they also require an environment that provides narrow ranges of temperature, water content, acidity, and salt concentration. Thus the maintenance of internal conditions within fairly narrow limits is an essential feature of the normal body. When some of the structures and functions of the body deviate from the norm to the point at which the ability to maintain homeostasis is destroyed or threatened or at which the individual can no longer meet environmental challenges, disease is said to exist. A person's subjective perception of disease is related to impairment of the ability to carry on daily activities comfortably.

Disease does not involve the development of a completely new form of life, but rather, is an extension or distortion of the normal life processes present in the individual. Even in the case of an obviously infectious disease, during which the body is literally invaded, the infectious agent itself does not constitute the disease but only evokes the changes that ultimately are manifested as disease. Thus disease is actually the sum of the physiologic processes that have been distorted. To understand and treat the disease adequately, the identity of the normal processes interfered with, the character of the disturbances, and the secondary effects of such disturbances on other vital processes must be taken into account.

Historically, it was believed that disease is actually a new form of life, a sort of possession of the body by an outside agent. From this notion, it would follow that some form of "exorcism" to drive out the disease agent is proper therapy. However, even in the instance of an invasive infectious agent, attempted treatment with antibiotics alone may not cure the patient if proper attention is not directed toward the intrinsic body processes that have become deranged.

A recurring theme, with variations, throughout this volume is that, above all, disease is "part and parcel" of the patient. *Normal and abnormal processes represent different points on the same continuous spectrum.* In fact, the seeds of disease often lie within the adaptive mechanisms of the body itself, mechanisms that constitute a potential two-edged sword. For example, the leukocytes, which are essential in responding to microbial invaders, may themselves become agents of tissue injury. The mechanisms that allow a person to become immune to certain infections also form the basis for allergic reactions, such as hay fever and asthma. Similarly, the mechanism of cellular proliferation that allows individuals to repair wounds and constantly renew cell populations in various tissues may run amok, giving rise to cancer.

DEVELOPMENT OF DISEASE

Etiology

Etiology, in its most general definition, is the assignment of causes or reasons for phenomena. A description of the cause of a disease includes the identification of those factors that provoke the particular disease. Thus the tubercle bacillus is designated as the etiologic agent of tuberculosis. Other etiologic factors in the development of tuberculosis include the age, nutritional status, and even the occupation of the individual. Even in the case of an infectious disease, such as tuberculosis, the agent itself does not constitute the disease. Rather, all the resulting responses to that agent, all the perversions of biologic processes taken together, constitute the disease. In the etiology of a particular disease, therefore, a range of extrinsic or exogenous factors in the environment must be considered along with a variety of intrinsic or endogenous characteristics of the individual.

Pathogenesis

Pathogenesis of a disease refers to the development or evolution of the disease. To continue with the previous example, the pathogenesis of tuberculosis would include the mechanisms whereby the invasion of the body by the tubercle bacillus ultimately leads to the observed abnormalities.

Such an analysis would relate the proliferation and spread of tubercle bacilli to the evolving inflammatory responses, the immunologic defenses of the body, and the destruction of cells and tissues. The pattern and extent of the tissue damage would ultimately be related to the overt manifestations of clinical disease. Pathogenesis also takes into account the sequential occurrence of certain phenomena and the temporal aspects of the evolving disease. A given disease is not static; it is a dynamic phenomenon with a rhythm and pattern of its own. Thus each disease has a characteristic *natural history*—a typical pattern of evolution, effect, and duration that is observed unless some intervention successfully modifies the disease. In the diagnostic evaluation of patients and the assessment of therapy, this concept of natural history and the range of variation among different diseases with regard to their natural history is essential to keep in mind. Some diseases characteristically have a rapid response, whereas others have a long prodrome. Some diseases are self-limited; that is, they resolve spontaneously in a brief time. Others become chronic, and still others are subject to frequent remissions and exacerbations.

Manifestations

Early in the development of a disease, the etiologic agent or agents may provoke a number of changes in biologic processes that laboratory analysis can detect, even though the patient has no subjective symptoms. Thus many diseases have a *subclinical stage,* during which the patient functions normally, even though the disease processes are well established. The structure and function of many organs provide a large reserve or safety margin, and functional impairment may become evident only when the disease has become quite advanced. For example, chronic renal disease might destroy one kidney and partly affect the other before any symptoms related to decreased renal function would be perceived. However, some diseases appear to begin as functional derangements and actually become clinically evident although no anatomic abnormalities can be detected at the time. Such functional illnesses may lead to secondary structural abnormalities.

As certain biologic processes are encroached on, the patient begins to believe subjectively that something is wrong. These subjective feelings are called symptoms of disease. By definition, *symptoms* are subjective and can be reported only by the patient to an observer. However, when an observer can objectively identify manifestations of the disease, these are termed *signs* of the disease. Nausea, malaise, and pain are symptoms, whereas fever, reddening of the skin, and a palpable mass are signs of disease. A demonstrable structural change produced in the course of a disease is referred to as a *lesion*. Lesions may be evident at a gross level, a microscopic level, or both. The outcome of a disease is sometimes referred to as a *sequela* (plural, *sequelae*). For example, the sequela to an inflammatory process in a given tissue might be a scar in that tissue. The sequela to acute rheumatic inflammation of the heart might be scarred, deformed cardiac valves. A *complication* of a disease is a new or separate process that may arise secondarily because of some change that the original entity produces. For example, bacterial pneumonia may be a complication of viral infection of the respiratory tract. Fortunately, many diseases can also undergo what is termed *resolution*, and the host returns to a completely normal state, without sequelae or complications. Resolution can occur spontaneously, that is, resulting from body defenses, or it can result from successful therapy.

Finally, that disease is dynamic rather than static is essential to reemphasize. The manifestations of disease in a given patient may change from day to day as biologic equilibria shift and as compensatory mechanisms are brought into play. Environmental influences brought to bear on the patient also affect the disease. Therefore every disease has a range of manifestations and a spectrum of expressions that may vary from patient to patient.

CLASSIFICATION OF DISEASE

Many strategies exist for classifying disease. Each strategy has its own rationale and individual appeal. Among clinical specialists, diseases are traditionally grouped according to the organ system affected, and this plan will be followed in this text. This scheme may mislead one into thinking that disease is restricted to compartments within the body, when in actuality a disturbance in one organ system tends to provoke imbalances elsewhere in the body. Furthermore, despite their origin in the same organ system, diseases such as pneumonia, tuberculosis, and bronchogenic carcinoma have distinctly different pathologic aspects with different causes.

In addition to classification according to organ system, patterns of disease may also be classified according to causes (Table 1-1). However, numerous interrelationships exist among these broad categories, a point that cannot be overemphasized. Some diseases fall into multiple categories and the origin of many diseases is unknown. A brief explanation is provided for each of these etiologic categories; more detailed information will be included in the subsequent chapters of this text.

TABLE 1-1

Etiologic Classification of Disease

Inherited or familial disease	Caused by faults inherent in the chromosomes or genes of one or both parents that is transmitted to the offspring. The altered chromosome or gene can cause an abnormal protein to be produced resulting in the disruption of an essential body function. An example of a chromosomal disorder is Down syndrome caused by an abnormal chromosome number in the 21 position. Hemophilia is an example of a coagulation disorder caused by recessive genes resulting in a deficiency of Factor VIII. *Not all familial diseases (running in a family) are inherited;* some may be caused by environmental influences to which the family is exposed (e.g., a nutritional deficiency) while others may result from a new gene mutation in the offspring.
Congenital disease	Present at birth; some are inherited while others may be caused by a developmental defect of known or unknown origin. *Not all hereditary disease is congenital (present at birth) and not all congenital disease is hereditary.* For example, Huntington's disease is hereditary but does not become manifested until middle age. Fetal alcohol syndrome is congenital but results from a pregnant mother ingesting alcohol.
Toxic disease	Caused by ingestion of a poison. Example: inhalation of carbon monoxide from an automobile exhaust in an enclosed garage may cause tissue hypoxia and death. Carbon monoxide is rapidly absorbed through the lungs and binds to hemoglobin (forming carboxyhemoglobin) with an affinity more than 200 times that of oxygen. This limits the oxygen-carrying capacity of hemoglobin.
Infectious disease	Resulting from an invasion of living pathogenic organisms (e.g., bacteria, viruses, fungi, protozoa, blood flukes, helminths).
Traumatic disease	Caused by physical injury. Violent mechanical injury, extreme heat or cold, electricity, and radiation are examples of physical agents that may cause trauma to the body. Trauma resulting from motor vehicle accidents is a major cause of disability and death in the United States.
Degenerative disease	The primary abnormality is degeneration of various parts of the body. Degenerative diseases are associated with the normal aging process and increasingly common with the increased life span in the United States. In many cases, degenerative lesions are more advanced or occur sooner than would be expected if they were age related. Common examples of degenerative diseases include osteoarthritis and arteriosclerosis.

Continued

TABLE 1-1 ▪▪▪

Etiologic Classification of Disease—cont'd

Immunologic disease	The immune system normally reacts protectively against the invasion of foreign antigens and cancer. Hypersensitivity (allergy), autoimmunity, and immunodeficiency represent three types of immune reaction with harmful effects on the host. Anaphylactic immune responses to allergens (e.g., bee venom) may be lethal in hypersensitive individuals. Autoimmunity involves loss of tolerance to self-antigens such that an immune reaction is mounted against the self. Many diseases, such as systemic lupus erythematosus, myasthenia gravis, and glomerulonephritis, are believed to involve autoimmunity. Immunodeficiency may be inherited or acquired (e.g., acquired immunodeficiency syndrome) causing the host to become vulnerable to opportunistic infections and malignancies.
Neoplastic disease	Neoplastic diseases are characterized by abnormal cell growth that leads to various types of benign and malignant tumors. Malignancies are a major cause of morbidity and mortality, affecting more than 20% of the population in the United States.
Nutritional disease	Deficiency of protein, calories, or vitamins is responsible for many diseases, particularly in developing countries. Malnutrition and infectious disease are common causes of death in these countries. Deficiency of a specific nutrient, such as vitamin C causing scurvy or iodine causing goiter, are uncommon in the industrialized world because of our improved knowledge of nutrition.
Metabolic disease	Resulting from a disturbance in some important metabolic process in the body. For example the thyroid may not properly regulate the rate of cell metabolism or the cells may not utilize glucose normally. Fluid and electrolyte imbalances, diabetes mellitus, and other endocrine disturbances are examples of metabolic disease.
Molecular disease	Resulting from a defect in a single molecule causing the molecular product of cellular activity to be abnormal. Many of these diseases are genetic. For example, sickle cell anemia involves a wrong sequence of two amino acids in the hemoglobin molecule causing the abnormal (sickle) shape of the red blood cell characteristic of the disease.
Psychogenic disease	Originating in the mind, having an emotional or psychologic origin in relation to a symptom. Example: schizophrenia, various types of dementia. Emotional factors contribute to many organic diseases.
Iatrogenic disease	A disease or disorder produced inadvertently as a result of treatment by a health care professional for some other disorder. The term implies that such effects might have been avoided by proper and judicious care. For example, a known side effect of thiazide diuretics is hypokalemia, which, in turn, can cause a serious cardiac dysrhythmia. Careful monitoring of serum potassium levels and offering foods high in potassium or administering potassium supplements when indicated can avoid this adverse effect. The health care professional can avert many hospital-acquired wound infections through proper attention to aseptic and sterile techniques.
Idiopathic disease	Disease of unknown cause. The cause of many diseases is unknown. In more than 90% of the cases of hypertension, the cause is unknown; it is therefore called essential or idiopathic hypertension.

*K*EY CONCEPTS

- *Pathology* is the science or study of disease. It is also a clinical specialty in human medicine.
- The two broad divisions of pathology are *anatomic pathology* (surgical, cytology, necropsy) and *clinical pathology* (clinical chemistry, clinical microbiology, hematology, blood bank, immunology).
- Pathology emphasizes the measurable aspects of disease such as altered structure of cells, tissues, and organs (gross and microscopic) and laboratory findings.
- *Pathophysiology* is the study of disordered functions or functions altered by the disease process.
- Pathophysiology is an integrative science that draws on concepts from many basic and clinical sciences, including anatomy, physiology, biochemistry, cell and molecular biology, genetics, pharmacology, and pathology.
- Pathophysiology differs from the other biomedical sciences in that it focuses on the *mechanisms of disease,* or the *dynamic processes* that give rise to the signs and symptoms. Understanding the mechanisms of disease is essential to the health care practitioner because interpretation of signs and symptoms,

appropriate treatment, and prevention are logically related to this knowledge.
- Concepts of normal and disease are complex and to an extent arbitrary and influenced by cultural values, as well as biologic factors.
- *Disease* may be defined as a failure of the organism to adapt or to maintain homeostasis; it is actually the sum of the physiologic processes that have been distorted.
- The seeds of disease often lie within the adaptive mechanisms of the body that have the potential to result in a good or bad outcome. Examples: the combination of genes from sexual reproduction enhances genetic variability and survival of the species but may also result in genetic disease; immune response mechanisms protect the body from invasion from foreign antigens but may also give rise to immunologic disease such as allergy or autoimmune disease. The body has only a limited number of response mechanisms, which when put together in various combinations give rise to a host of diseases. Thus if several basic response mecha-

nisms are understood, understanding the disease comes easily.

■ *Etiology* is the study of causes or reasons for phenomena. Etiology is a complex concept because most diseases are multifactorial and result from an interaction of intrinsic or genetic and environmental factors. Knowing causes is important; without knowledge of cause, prevention would be difficult.

■ *Pathogenesis* refers to the sequence of events in the development of a disease from its earliest beginnings, including factors influencing its development.

■ The *natural history of a disease* refers its usual course from beginning to end without treatment. The health practitioner must be familiar with the natural history of a disease for proper assessment and evaluation of treatment.

■ A *lesion* is a demonstrable structural change in the tissues produced by disease that is evident at a gross (visible to the naked eye) or microscopic level.

■ *Signs* are observable (objective) clinical manifestations of disease, such as a heart murmur, hypertension, fever, or a palpable mass.

■ *Symptoms* are subjective feelings that something is wrong and can be reported only by the patient to an observer. Examples of symptoms are pain, nausea, vertigo, or lethargy.

■ *Sequela* (plural, sequelae) refers to the outcome or aftereffect of a disease or injury. The sequela of acute rheumatic fever might be scarred and deformed heart valves.

■ A *complication of a disease* is an accidental condition or second disease occurring in the course of a primary process. An example would be peritonitis resulting from the rupture of an inflamed appendix.

■ *Resolution* refers to the subsidence of a disease process, as inflammation, and the return to normal of affected tissues.

■ Disease may be classified according to organ system or by etiologic categories. Neither of these systems of classifications is completely comprehensive, and diseases may include more than one category at a time.

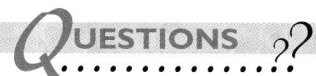

QUESTIONS ??

A sampling of review questions for this chapter appears here. Visit http://www.mosby.com/MERLIN/PriceWilson/ for additional questions. MERLIN

Answer the following on a separate sheet of paper.

1. Formulate definitions for pathology and pathophysiology.

2. Explain the difference between anatomic and clinical pathology. List at least three examples of types of studies included under each of these categories.

3. What is meant by pathogenesis of a disease?

4. Describe the complex factors associated with the concept of normalcy.

5. Explain why a given disease is not a static phenomenon.

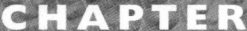

CHAPTER

2

Heredity, Environment, and Disease

Interaction of Heredity and Environment

REBECCA HARMSEN AND BETTY B. GALLUCCI

*T*his chapter contains a brief review of molecular genetics and an introduction to human genetics, including patterns of inheritance with respect to human disease. Both intrinsic and extrinsic contributors to disease are explored. Although the general concepts of genetic illness are discussed, some of these illnesses are explored in greater detail in other chapters. This chapter is not meant to provide an exhaustive review of molecular genetics. The reader desiring additional detail about any of the topics presented should consult molecular genetics and nursing genetics texts. This chapter provides a framework for understanding human disease, which is an important tool to aid the clinician in the diagnosis, treatment, and counseling of afflicted individuals and their families.

EXTRINSIC AND INTRINSIC FACTORS

A myriad of factors cause human disease. These factors are found in the environment and in each individual. Few disease conditions can be attributed exclusively to one or the other. An understanding of the characteristics of these factors aids in the treatment and prevention of human disease.

Extrinsic Factors

Extrinsic or external factors are those that are found *outside* the individual. For example, factors such as cigarette smoke, diet regimens, medications, and exposure to pollutants are all known contributors to disease. The degree to which an individual has control over these factors varies, ranging from possible complete control over diet to minimal control over pollutants found in the water supply. Additionally, the degree to which each factor contributes to disease development and progression varies. For example, eating a low-fat diet aids in the prevention of heart disease; but diet alone is not the only predictor of disease development, and eating a low-fat diet alone will not prevent every case of heart disease. Clearly, each individual will respond differently to this type of diet, depending on his or her intrinsic contribution.

Intrinsic Factors

Intrinsic or internal factors are those that are found within each person and are seldom under the control of the individual. These factors include age, gender, and height. Similar to extrinsic factors, the contribution of any of these varies. Perhaps the most significant intrinsic factor is the genetic makeup of each individual. The "gene pool" received at conception exerts a powerful influence on human growth and development. Although not all disease is genetic *per se*, at some level, all human disease is influenced by the genome. For example, an individual may be ill from an airborne infection (extrinsic factor) that is seemingly not a genetic disorder. Yet, the genetic makeup of that individual will largely determine the immune response to that threat.

Interaction between Extrinsic and Intrinsic Factors

Knowing the definition of a few key terms relating to disease is necessary. *Congenital* refers to a disease condition or anomaly that is present at birth; *inherited disease* refers to disease conditions that are genetically inherited from a parent; and *familial diseases* are those that affect members of the same family without necessarily being inherited.

With the exception of incidents such as motor vehicle accidents, the majority of human disease is caused by an interaction of both extrinsic and intrinsic factors. This interaction falls along a continuum, with some conditions mostly the result of extrinsic factors and vice versa. For example, although the genetic contribution to lung cancer is unclear at this point, cigarette smoking is a known predictor and risk factor for this disease process. Conversely, although extrinsic factors may influence the severity of trisomy 21 (Down syndrome), it is caused by the presence of an extra chromosome 21. The contribution of genetic makeup is referred to as the *heritability* of a disease. Understanding the relationship and contribution of these factors allows for an appropriate treatment and prevention strategy. However, a great deal remains unknown about the relative contribution of these factors to the majority of diseases. The interaction of these factors highlights the need for the clinician to obtain an accurate and a complete family health history, as well as an accurate detailing of social and environmental activities or history.

BASICS

Humans have approximately 30,000 to 70,000 genes. A gene is the basic unit of heredity and is composed of deoxyribonucleic acid (DNA). *The central dogma of genetics is that DNA is transcribed into ribonucleic acid (RNA), which is translated into an amino acid chain (protein).* DNA serves as the template that guides all human development and physiologic processes. An understanding of genetics requires a basic knowledge of three molecules: DNA, RNA, and proteins.

DNA

DNA is found in the nucleus of all cells and is composed of a five-carbon sugar (deoxyribose), a phosphate group, and one of four types of nitrogenous bases. Each unit is referred to as a nucleotide. The nitrogenous bases fall into two categories: pyrimidines and purines. Pyrimidines consist of a single carbon ring, and purines consist of a double carbon ring. Both *cytosine* (C) and *thymine* (T) are pyrimidine bases; *adenine* (A) and *guanine* (G) are purine bases.

DNA is organized into a chain that is held together by phosphodiester bonds. This bond joins the 5'-carbon of one DNA molecule to the 3'-carbon of another DNA molecule. Thus in such a long chain, one 5'-carbon and one 3'-carbon are always unattached. Using this orientation, DNA is read in a 3'-to-5' direction (Fig. 2-1).

In 1953 James Watson and Frances Crick determined that the basic structure of DNA is a double helix. A single DNA strand is rarely found in humans; DNA is normally a double-stranded unit. Each DNA chain or strand has a complementary strand to which it is attached. These strands are aligned in the opposite 5'-to-3' direction. Additionally, these strands are held together by hydrogen bonding of their complementary nitrogenous bases: adenine always pairs with thymine, and guanine always pairs with cytosine. A pyrimidine and purine are paired, maintaining the structure of the double helix. Each strand contains the same information because of this strict pairing, but one strand has the information in the "antisense" form, similar to a negative of a photograph.

RNA

RNA is similar to DNA in that it is composed of a sugar, phosphate group and a nitrogenous base. However, RNA differs from DNA in that its sugar group is ribose rather than deoxyribose. RNA also has the nitrogenous base of *uracil* (U) rather than thymine. Unlike DNA, RNA is usually single stranded. The RNA strand is held together in the same manner as is DNA, through phosphodiester bonding between the 5'-carbon of one nucleotide and the 3'-carbon of another.

Proteins

Proteins consist of amino acids connected by polypeptide bonds. The carboxyl group of one amino acid is bonded to the amino group of another amino acid. Thus proteins have a free carboxyl terminus (C-) and an amino terminus (N-). The resultant protein is determined by its amino acid sequence. The structural properties of proteins are also determined to some degree by its amino acid sequence. Structural folding of protein is critical for its functioning. Primary protein structures include alpha-helix and beta-pleated sheets. These primary structures form larger more complex functioning units by combining with other proteins. Proteins serve many functions, including structural components of cells, enzymes that catalyze chemical reactions, or regulatory molecules that alter the site of DNA transcription.

To function as the building block of life, DNA must be faithfully copied and transmitted to daughter cells, and the information contained in DNA must be expressed.

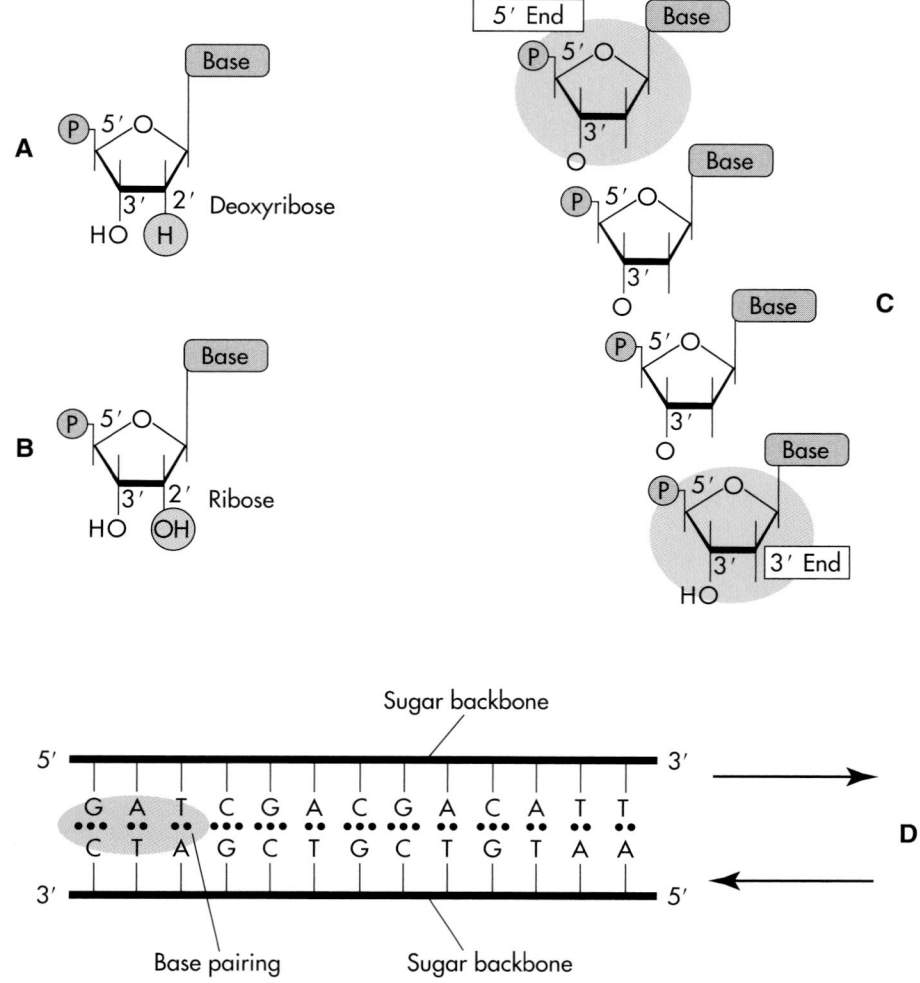

FIG. 2-1   Nucleic acids. **A**, Deoxyribonucleotide. **B**, Ribonucleotide. **C**, Polymer of deoxyribonucleotides joined by phosphodiester bonds. **D**, Double-stranded deoxyribonucleic acid (DNA) held together by hydrogen bonding between complementary base pairs.

The process by which DNA is eventually translated into protein is complicated. DNA and RNA are written in the same language: nucleic acids. Therefore the process of going from DNA to RNA is called *transcription*, such as going from the handwritten word to the typed word in the same language. Whereas going from RNA to protein is similar to going from one language to another; nucleic acids are coded for or *translated* to amino acids, the building blocks of protein. This section discusses the basic characteristics of DNA replication, transcription, and translation.

DNA Replication

The notion that a single cell can divide into a fully functional human being with the same genetic material in each cell indicates the accuracy and fidelity with which DNA is replicated from parent cell to daughter cell.

DNA replication is accomplished in the nucleus of the cell. Initially, enzymes, allowing each strand to serve as a template for replication, must break the hydrogen bond holding the double-stranded DNA together. The enzyme *DNA polymerase* is responsible for the formation of the new strand. As this enzyme moves along the template

strand in a 3'-to-5' direction, free complementary nucleotides are added to the new, developing strand of DNA. This new strand is formed in the 5'-to-3' direction, meaning that the free nucleotides are added to the 3' end of the developing strand. Because of the length of the human genome, replication is simultaneously initiated at thousands of sites (Fig. 2-2).

The strictness of complementary base pairing ensures that each nucleotide in each strand will only attract the correct complementary base. DNA polymerase also has a role in maintaining the accuracy of DNA replication. This enzyme, in a sense, "proofs" the new strand. If an incorrect nucleotide is found, then it is excised and replaced with the correct, complementary nucleotide. Replication errors are made at a rate of less than one per one million nucleotides. These errors, although rare, introduce mutations into the DNA strand. DNA mutations are one source of genetic disorders. Mutations are discussed in greater detail at another point in the chapter.

Transcription

Using one DNA strand as a template, DNA is transcribed into a single strand of RNA. Enzymes known as *RNA poly-*

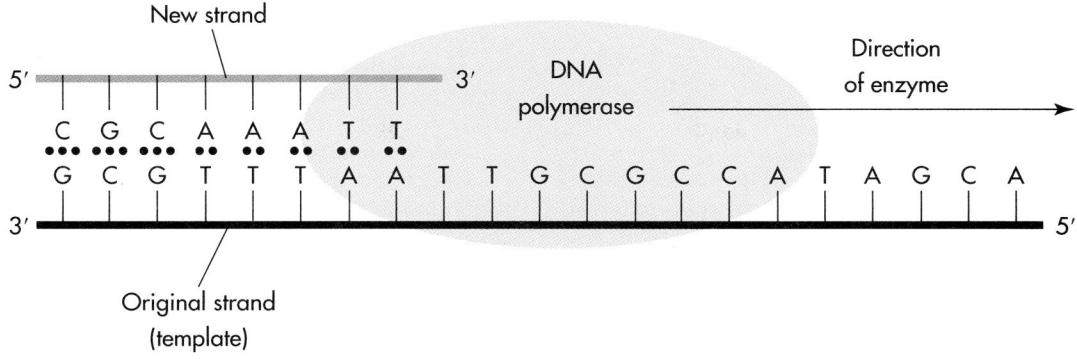

FIG. 2-2   DNA polymerase replicating DNA.

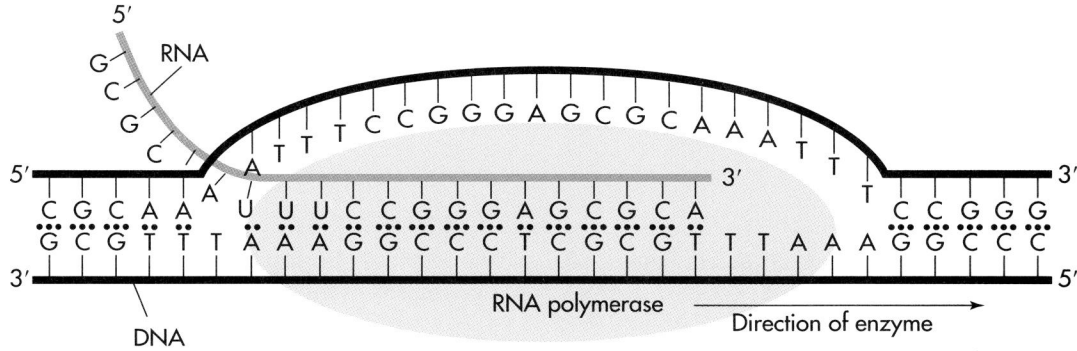

FIG. 2-3   Ribonucleic acid (RNA) polymerase forming RNA by transcribing a DNA template.

merases carry out this process. These enzymes bind to the DNA template strand at the *promoter* site and release at the *terminator* site. Although both strands of the double-stranded DNA can serve as the template, only one strand is used. Enzymes pull apart or separate a section of the double-stranded complex, allowing one exposed DNA strand to serve as a template for the emerging RNA strand. Enzymes move along the DNA template strand in a 3'-to-5' direction, with the resultant primary RNA transcript formed in a 5'-to-3' direction (Fig. 2-3). As stated, RNA substitutes the nitrogenous base uracil for thymine, which enables an adenine DNA nucleotide to bind with a uracil RNA nucleotide. Primary RNA is also flanked with additional nucleotides: a guanine molecule on the 5' end (guanine cap) and several adenine molecules on the 3' end (poly-A tail) of the primary transcript. These additions serve to add stability to the primary transcript as it moves to the cytoplasm. The poly-A tail is eventually degraded.

The initial transcript (heteronuclear RNA) is formed in the nucleus of the cell and is not the final form of RNA. Protein is formed in the cytoplasm, requiring the RNA to travel from the nucleus. This process involves many key steps, one of which is known as *splicing*. In most structural genes, this action involves the process of excising RNA stretches known as *introns* (intervening sequences) and the joining of the remaining *exons* (expressed sequences). Messenger RNA or mRNA is the result of splicing and other processing events. This splicing process is highly regulated, thus enabling different exons to remain in the final mRNA and allowing for different protein products to result from the same gene (Fig. 2-4).

The mature RNA is then able to leave the nucleus and travel to the cytoplasm.

Translation

Once in the cytoplasm, the mRNA serves as a template for the formation of an amino acid chain. However, mRNA is unable to bind directly with amino acids. Therefore, translation occurs on a specialized organelle called the ribosome. Ribosomal RNA (rRNA) and proteins form a complex with mRNA and transfer RNA (tRNA). tRNA picks up a specific amino acid and transports it to the ribosome. As the ribosome moves along the mRNA, it "reads" the transcript in groups of three nucleotide bases. The three-base sequence is called a *codon*. The three-base sequence in mRNA and tRNA bind in a complementary fashion. As the sequence is read, the amino acids at the end of the tRNAs are hooked together to form a growing amino acid chain. The chain is released from the ribosome at the *stop codon*. The correspondence of a codon to a specific amino acid is known as the genetic code. Twenty different amino acids exist, with 64 possible nucleotide combinations ($4 \times 4 \times 4$). Obviously, more than one codon can code for a specific amino acid. For example, GCC and GCU both code for the amino acid alanine. The genetic code displays redundancy, minimizing the possibility that an amino acid change or substitution will cause a functional deficit. Three codons do not code for amino acids but are considered *stop codons*: UAA, UGA, and UAG. AUG, which codes for the amino acid methionine, also serves as the *start codon*. The resultant protein is determined by the order of amino acids.

Regulation

Regulating which genes are expressed in each cell at any given time is essential for an organism. Regulation determines which genes are turned on (expressed) in a cell and which genes are turned off. For instance, a muscle cell must manufacture the protein actin, but it does not manufacture hemoglobin. Regulation may affect any part of this process, from the initiation of transcription to posttranslational modification. Transcription factors are proteins that bind to DNA to signal the binding of polymerase to begin transcription. Other proteins may also bind to enhancer sites, which increases the expression of a gene. Conversely, the binding of other sites known as silencers decreases transcription. The combined effects of enhancers and silencers control the timing and specificity of most gene expression. The abnormal regulation of a gene can affect an organism as profoundly as an abnormal gene.

Genes and Genetic Terminology

The human genome is composed of 3 billion nucleotides per cell. A gene is a transcriptional unit, a region of DNA that will be transcribed to form RNA. Most RNA transcripts are translated into proteins. Genes that are eventually translated into proteins are referred to as functional genes.

To understand clinical genetics, the reader must be familiar with a few key terms. The term *locus* refers to the location of a gene on a chromosome. For all individuals, a gene is normally found at the same locus of a given chromosome. However, comparing genes from individuals, copies of a particular gene are likely to have a slightly different nucleotide sequence. These different

sequences are referred to as *alleles.* A polymorphism is defined as a common allele that occurs in 1% or more of the population. When an individual has the same allele on a pair of chromosomes, he or she is a *homozygote,* and an individual with a different allele on each chromosome is a *heterozygote.*

A *genotype* is the actual allelic representation for an individual, either at a particular locus or for the entire genome. The *phenotype* refers to the characteristics that are actually observed as a result of a genotype. For example, a patient has two allelic variants at a particular locus on a particular chromosome: the allele "B" on one chromosome in the pair and the allele "b" on the other. This individual's genotype for this particular locus is Bb. He or she is a heterozygote at this particular locus. Supposing, for example, that "B" confers brown eyes and "b" confers blue eyes and that "B" is the dominant allele, this individual would phenotypically express the dominant physical property of brown eyes, even though the genotype contains one blue eye allele ("b"). This example illustrates the fact that genotypes do not always correspond to phenotypes.

Chromosomes
Structure and Characteristics

The double-stranded DNA, or double helix, constructs what is known as a chromosome (*chroma* = color; *soma* = body). The structure of a chromosome, however, goes beyond this double helix. Stretched out, DNA within a cell would be nearly 2 meters long. To package DNA within the nucleus, DNA is coiled around proteins known as *histones* to form nucleosomes. *Chromatin* is a term used to describe the combination of nucleic acids and associated proteins as seen by light microscopy.

Chromosomes are only apparent as discrete structures in dividing cells as the chromatin condenses. This discrete structure is often thought of as a chromosome. Clin-

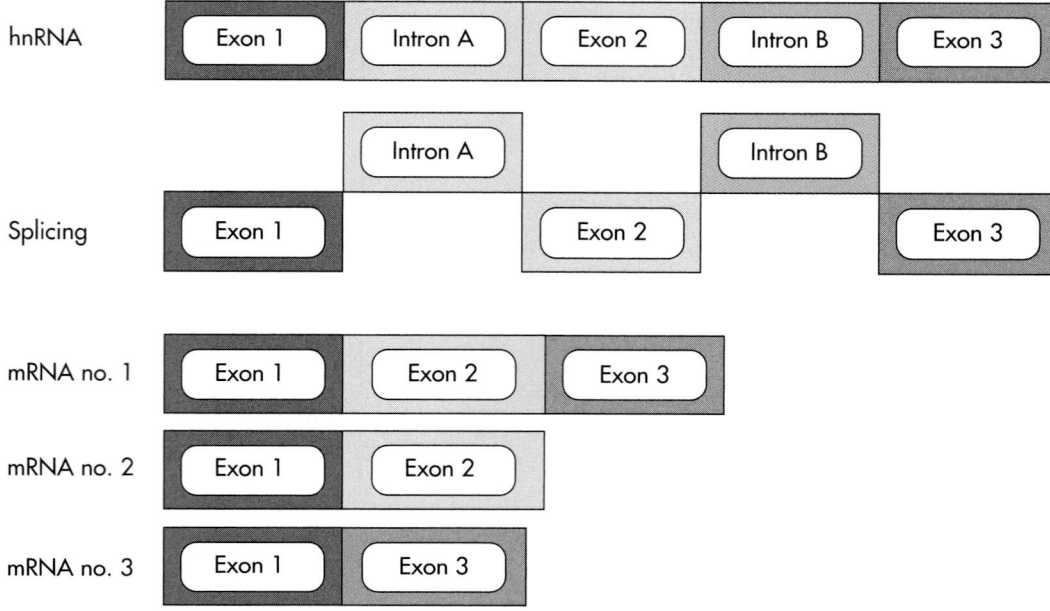

FIG. 2-4 Splicing removes introns in the conversion of heteronuclear RNA into mRNA (see text).

ically, these chromosomes are used to identify chromosome number and type in genetic analysis.

With the exception of the *gametes* (sperm and ova), each normal human somatic cell (nongamete cell) contains 46 total chromosomes. Forty-four of these chromosomes are known as *autosomes*, which are organized into homologous pairs. Each cell has two copies of chromosome 1 and so on. Each chromosome within the pair contains the same genes. Additionally, human cells contain two sex chromosomes. Females have two X chromosomes, with each chromosome containing the same genes. Males, on the other hand, have one X and one Y chromosome and thus the genes on these sex chromosomes differ. In chromosomal nomenclature, *haploid* refers to cells with one copy of each chromosome; *diploid* refers to two copies of a chromosome within a cell. Normal somatic cells are diploid (2N = 46 chromosomes).

In the dividing cell, each chromosome consists of two *chromatids* (identical pieces of DNA). These chromatids are joined at a centromere (Fig. 2-5). The centromere is a key structure in the separation of chromatin during cell division. For example, trisomy 21 (Down syndrome) is commonly a result of *nondisjunction* of chromosome 21;

that is, during cell division, the chromatin failed to separate properly, resulting in an additional chromosome 21. The centromere is also the location within a chromosome that separates its two arms: the short arm (p) and the long arm (q).

DNA therefore has many levels of organization. At its simplest level, DNA is a single, linear chain of nucleotides. Most single gene defects are now understood to result from discrete changes in the specific nucleotide order. At the next level, DNA is a linear, double-stranded molecule consisting of complementary bases, spatially aligned in a double helix. At a higher level, DNA is complexed with proteins to constitute chromatin. Chromosomal disorders (e.g., Down syndrome) are frequently diagnosed by changes in the gross chromosomal number or breaks and rearrangements.

A *karyotype* constitutes the complete set of chromosomes within a somatic cell. Living tissue (e.g., blood) is treated with a stain to visualize chromosomes during cell division (metaphase). Pairs of chromosomes are ordered by height, from largest to smallest (Fig. 2-6). Therefore chromosome 1 is the largest, and chromosome 22 is the smallest. Each chromosome is distinguished by its size and specific banding pattern when stained. This tool allows for the observation of chromosomes at metaphase to determine whether any chromosome is absent or present in excessive amount. The karyotype can also be illustrated as a written expression. For example, a normal female would have a karyotype of 46, XX, indicating that this individual has 46 total chromosomes, and two Xs as her sex chromosomes. Similarly, a normal male karyotype is expressed as 46, XY. Being able to interpret this written expression is a clinically valuable tool, because many genetic disorders are the result of alterations in the number of chromosomes. In the example of trisomy previously illustrated, a person with this condition would have a karyotype of 47, XX +21, indicating that this individual is a female and has 47 chromosomes resulting from the addition of an extra chromosome 21.

Cell Division

Cells undergo two types of division: *mitosis* and *meiosis*. Before cell division, the genetic material within a cell

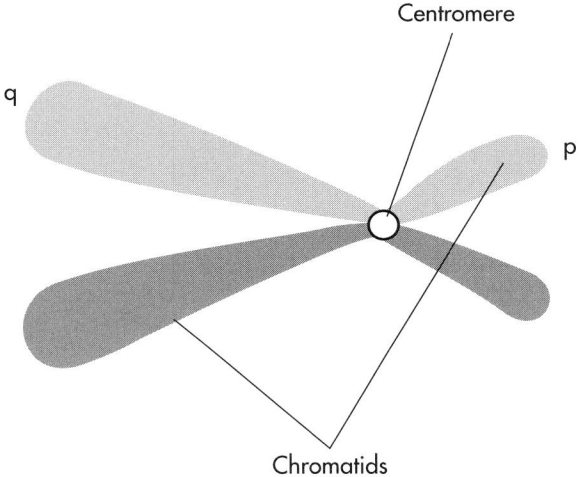

FIG. 2-5   Chromosome structure.

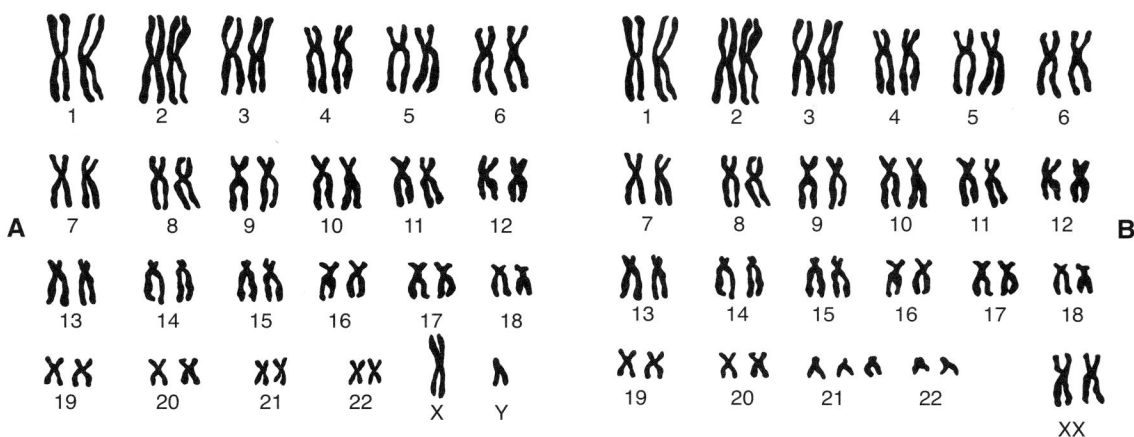

FIG. 2-6   **A,** Example of a karyotype of a normal male displayed in the standard format. **B,** Karyotype of a female with Down syndrome. In the position conventionally designated as 21, three chromosomes exist instead of two (trisomy 21).

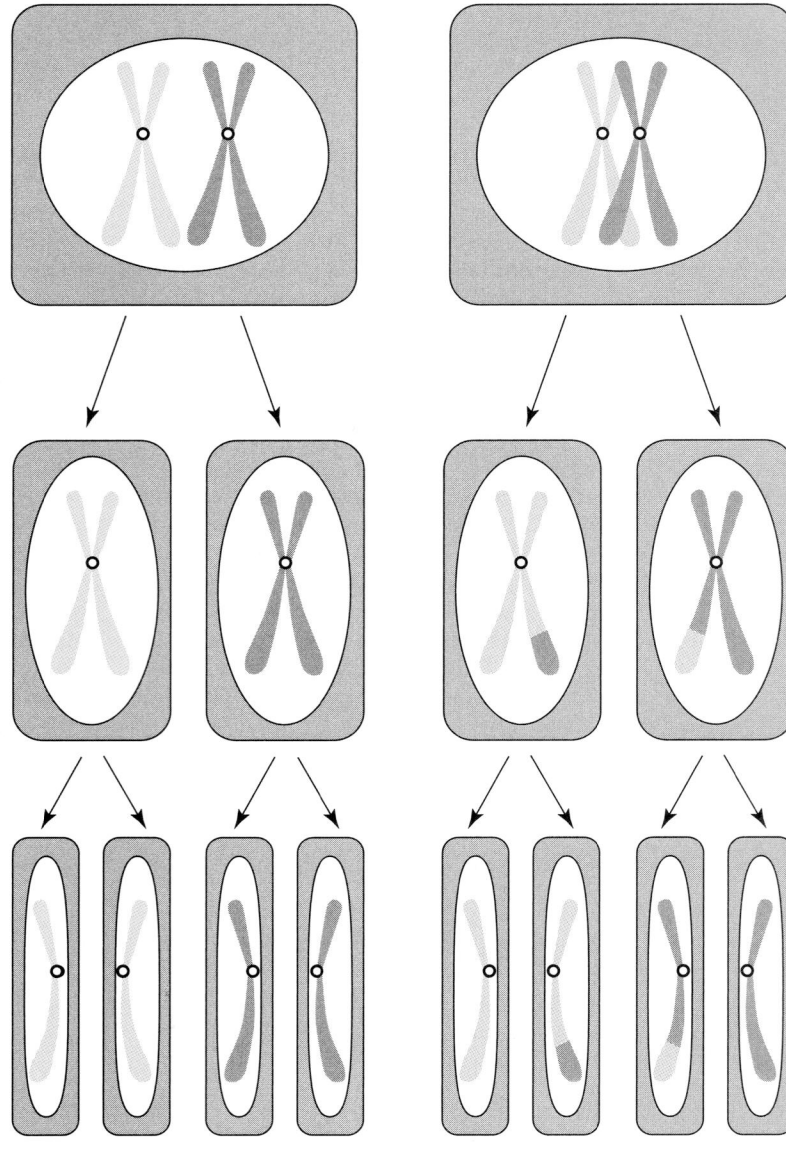

FIG. 2-7 Chromosomal and chromatid segregation during meiosis. **A**, Simple segregation of chromosomes into daughter cells. **B**, Segregation and meiotic recombination.

A   B

has been duplicated, thus each cell contains two identical copies of each chromosome, referred to as sister chromatids.

All somatic cells experience mitotic division. In mitosis, the two sets of sister chromatids separate into daughter cells that contain the identical genetic information as the parent cell; that is, the chromatids are equally distributed among the daughter cells.

Germline cells (sperm and ova) undergo meiosis. Sperm and ovum DNA are combined to form one cell during conception. If no meiosis takes place, then each of these cells would contain 46 chromosomes, and the zygote would then have 92 chromosomes! Meiosis is the process by which the DNA in these germline cells is reduced by one half, resulting in daughter cells with 23 chromosomes each. Meiosis is accomplished in two phases. The first phase results in each daughter cell receiving one of each chromosome set (two chromatids) from the parent cell. This phase is called the *reduction division phase*. The second phase is called *equational division* because the sister chromatids of each chromosome are separated, and each of the two daughter cells receive the

same genetic information. Thus sperm and ova each contain 23 chromosomes and unite to form 46 chromosomes (Fig. 2-7).

One key element of meiosis is crossing over. Homologous chromosomes line up and exchange genetic information during the first phase of meiosis. For instance, the maternal chromosome 4 receives some genes from the paternal chromosome 4 and vice versa. This action results in chromosomes that have original and "new" genetic information, which is subsequently passed on to all daughter cells. This mechanism greatly increases genetic diversity within offspring. For example, with the exception of twins, some physical characteristics differ from family members. Crossing over is one means for increasing the diversity of human traits.

Genetic Variation

A considerable degree of genetic variation exists. This dissimilarity is obvious by simply observing individuals and noting various and unique physical features. With the

Single Base–Pair Mutations

Original mRNA transcript:	5' -	AUG	CCA	AAA	GUG	UAG	- 3'
Amino acid chain		met	pro	lys	val	stop	
Nonsense mutation:	5' -	AUG	CCA	UAA	GUG	UAG	- 3'
Amino acid chain		met	pro	stop			
Missense mutation:	5' -	AUG	GCA	AAA	GUG	UAG	- 3'
Amino acid chain		met	ala	lys	val	stop	
Frameshift mutation:	5' -	AUG	GCC	AAA	AGU	GUA	G — 3'
Amino acid chain		met	ala	lys	ser	val	+ additional G

exception of identical twins, no two humans are exactly the same; that is, no two humans share an identical genome. This genetic variation can have benign results, such as variance in hair color, or detrimental consequences, such as human disease. Variation is the result of changes in the DNA, a phenomenon known as *mutation.* Mutations are rare and occur in less than 1% of the population. Mutations generally alter the expression of a gene.

It is estimated that a mutation is generated at a rate of one per cell per cell division. Both somatic and germline cells can be affected. Mutations can affect the entire genome, a particular chromosome, or a single gene. Trisomy 21 is an example of a mutation that affects the entire genome. As a result of nondisjunction of chromosome 21 during cell division, nearly every cell in the body has an additional chromosome 21 (47 chromosomes in each cell). Cells that do not have a multiple of 23 chromosomes display *aneuploidy.* Monosomy (absence of a single chromosome) and trisomy (addition of an extra chromosome) are aneuploid conditions. A chromosome can also exchange some genetic material with another chromosome that is not its paired chromosome (nonhomologous). This exchange is known as *translocation.* One common example of translocation involves chromosomes 9 and 22, known as the Philadelphia chromosome (Ph1), in which some of chromosome 9 moves to chromosome 22, and vice versa. This translocated chromosome is associated with leukemias. Approximately 70% to 90% of individuals with chronic myelogenous leukemia (CML) have this translocation.

Genetic information can be added to a chromosome (*insertion*), excised from a chromosome (*deletion*), and rearranged (*inversion*). A single gene can also have mutations. Another nucleotide can replace a single base pair. The significance of a mutation is largely determined by its effect on the resultant protein product. For example, consider the mRNA transcript (Box 2-1):

5' – AUG CCA AAA GUG UAG – 3'

The resultant amino acid sequence from the original mRNA transcript is methionine-proline-lysine-valine-STOP. A single base pair substitution can result in a *nonsense mutation:* a premature stop codon or the removal of a stop codon. In this example, the amino acid sequence is stopped too early and the protein has been truncated. A single base pair substitution can also change one amino acid to another. A *missense mutation* refers to a mutation that alters the intended amino acid sequence. The term *point mutation* refers to all these single base pair substitutions. The significance of such a mutation depends on the way in which the protein is affected. Altering the amino acid sequence without any significant effect is possible if the amino acid of interest is not critical to the shape or function of the protein.

When a nucleotide is added or deleted, it causes a shifting of the codons. Referring to Box 2-1, a *frameshift mutation* occurs any time that an insertion or deletion occurs that is not in a multiple of three. In the example in Box 2-1, a G nucleotide is added to the original strand in the fourth nucleotide position. The amino acid sequence differs from the original sequence, as though the reading of the transcript has shifted by one or two nucleotides. Frameshift mutations are almost always clinically significant because the entire protein is altered.

Many other types of mutations exist. Some examples include entire gene duplication and an expanded number of nucleotide repeats within the gene. Mutations arise from a number of mechanisms, from uncorrected errors in DNA replication to exogenous (external) influences such as smoking, ultraviolet light, or viral infection.

Mendelian Concepts

Gregor Mendel (1822-1884) is referred to as the father of genetics. Although he experimented with garden peas, many of the principles he observed apply to human genes as well:

1. *Principle of Segregation.* Organisms that are capable of reproduction have a pair of chromosomes and thus two of each gene, one maternal and one paternal contribution. During reproduction, only one of the two genes is passed to each offspring.
2. *Principle of Independent Assortment.* Genes at two different loci are distributed to their offspring independently of one another.

Clinically, these principles suggest that each parent passes on one chromosome from each pair to their offspring, and which chromosome is received by the offspring is random and independent. This random segregation of genes can be predicted and expressed as probabilities and can be visually appreciated with the use of *Punnett squares* (Fig. 2-8). If the assumption were that a gene has two different alleles, *A* and *a,* and if an individual is homozygous for *A* (AA), then all of that individual's gametes will receive this *A* allele. Another individual who is homozygous for the *a* (aa) allele will produce gametes with the *a* allele only. If these two individuals mate, with each individual contributing one allele for this particular gene, all of the union's progeny will then be heterozygous (Aa) for this gene. In another situation, when two heterozygotes (Aa) for the same gene mate, looking at the Punnett square, both individuals can evidently contribute both the *A* and an *a* allele. Figure 2-8, *C* shows the Punnett square of this type of union. In this instance, one quarter of the offspring will be homozygous for the *A* allele (AA), another one quarter will be homozygous for the *a* allele (aa), and one half of the progeny will be heterozygotes

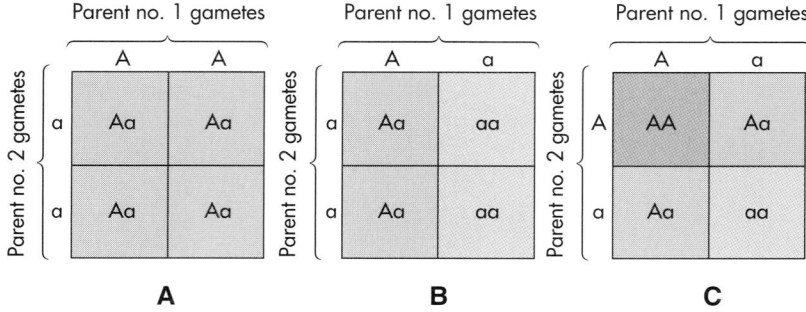

FIG. 2-8 Examples of Punnet squares. **A**, Parents homozygous with different alleles (*AA* and *aa*) will produce only heterozygous progeny (*Aa*). **B**, Heterozygous parent (*Aa*) and homozygous parent (*aa*) will produce homozygous progeny (*aa*) half the time and heterozygous progeny (*Aa*) half the time. **C**, Heterozygous (*Aa*) parents will produce homozygous progeny (*AA* or *aa*) half the time and heterozygous progeny (*Aa*) half the time.

(*Aa*). Thus the probability that a heterozygous union will produce a heterozygous offspring is two out of four, or 50%.

Punnett squares can also be used to predict the probabilities of segregation for those genes located on the X chromosome. Recalling that females have two X chromosomes (XX), whereas males have only one (XY), the Y chromosome acts as a homologous chromosome to the X during cell division. If a gene on the X chromosome has two alleles, *B* and *b*, then the female can be either homozygous or heterozygous for this allele, whereas the male will be *hemizygous* (a single copy of a gene) because he has only one X chromosome. If a female who is heterozygous for this gene ($X^B X^b$) mates with a male who has a single copy of the recessive gene ($X^b Y$), the female can then donate either the *B* or *b* allele to each offspring. The male can only donate the *b* allele if he passes on the X chromosome, or he can donate the Y chromosome. Female offspring can be either homozygous for the *b* gene ($X^b X^b$) or heterozygous ($X^B X^b$). The male offspring can receive either the *B* or *b* allele from their mother and will be $X^B Y$ or $X^b Y$. A male's phenotype will correspond to his X-chromosomal genotype because of hemizygosity. For this reason, males are more often affected by X-linked genetic disorders.

As illustrated in the Punnett squares, allelic variants can be dominant one to the other phenotypically. The allele that is expressed whenever it is present in the genotype, even when only one copy is present, is considered the *dominant* allele and is generally denoted by a capital letter. Most dominant alleles usually code for or confer a positive attribute. Traits can also exhibit *codominance*, as is the case for the ABO blood group, in which case the *A* and *B* alleles are both expressed in the phenotype. *Recessive* alleles, on the other hand, are not expressed in the presence of a dominant allele. Heterozygotes for recessive conditions are termed *carriers* because they carry the mutation without expressing it. Both copies of the recessive allele must exist for the mutation to be expressed. Lowercase letters generally denote recessive alleles. In the previous example, an individual with the genotype *AA* obviously expresses the dominant phenotype. A heterozygote (*Aa*) will as well because of the presence of one dominant allele. Only individuals with the *aa* genotype will express the recessive trait (aa).

This principle applies to physical human traits, as well as diseases. Before exploring the characteristics of autoso-

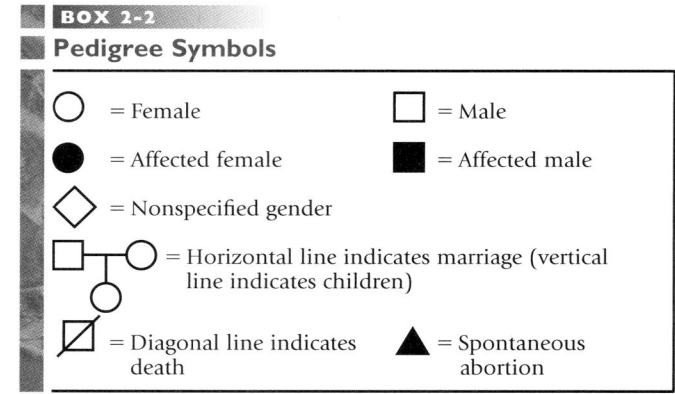

BOX 2-2
Pedigree Symbols

○ = Female   □ = Male

● = Affected female   ■ = Affected male

◇ = Nonspecified gender

□—○ = Horizontal line indicates marriage (vertical line indicates children)

⌀ = Diagonal line indicates death   ▲ = Spontaneous abortion

mal and X-linked diseases, the reader must be familiar with the use and meaning of a pedigree.

A *pedigree* is a visual tool to explore the relationship of a particular disease or trait among family members. This commonly used tool is a visual representation of a family medical history and represents the phenotype of multiple family members. The basic pedigree notations are located in Box 2-2. The observation of a pedigree is a key tool in determining the way in which a particular trait or disease is inherited. Being comfortable with writing and reading pedigrees is a useful clinical tool for nurses.

Cautions with Mendelian Inheritance

Although the concepts of Mendelian inheritance explain a variety of human conditions, an exception to the rule always occurs. Inheritance is not always straightforward. The term *penetrance* refers to the proportion of people with a particular disease genotype that actually expresses the disease phenotype. Frequently, genetic disorders display reduced penetrance; individuals may not express the expected phenotype given their genotype. Importantly, even though an individual may show reduced penetrance for a disease, he or she is still capable of transmitting the disease allele.

Genetic conditions can also show *variable expressivity*, in which the penetrance of a genetic disease may be complete, but the actual clinical expression of that disease varies in severity from individual to individual. Cystic fibrosis displays variable expressivity. Symptoms range in these patients from mild to severe, although all the

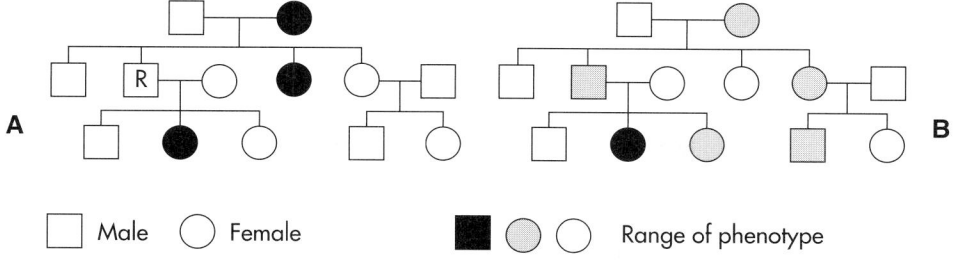

□ Male   ○ Female   ■ ● ○ Range of phenotype

FIG. 2-9   Typical pedigrees for a dominant allele with reduced penetrance (male R) **(A)** and a dominant allele with variable expressivity **(B)**.

patients have a defect in the gene of interest (Fig. 2-9). Environment may play a significant role in variable expressivity. In addition, genetic disorders may also display a *delayed age of onset*. Some genetic disorders are typically adult onset (i.e., Huntington's disease).

GENETIC DISORDERS

Single Gene Disorders

Currently, more than 3000 different single gene disorders have been identified. All tissues and organ systems are affected by single gene disorders and are present in approximately 1% of live births. As a consequence, health care providers in every specialty will encounter single gene disorders, requiring familiarity with the concepts and principles of these disorders. Box 2-3 lists a few single gene disorders, some of which are described in this section. An overview of treatment options for genetic conditions is provided at another point in this chapter.

Autosomal Dominant Disorders

Autosomal dominant disorders are expressed by both heterozygotes and homozygotes. Individuals homozygous for the mutated allele generally have a more extreme phenotype. Autosomal dominant disorders generally display variable expressivity in the severity of the phenotype. Box 2-4 lists the characteristics associated with autosomal dominant inheritance.

Males and females are equally capable of having and passing on a particular autosomal dominant allele. Generations are not skipped; that is, if an individual has an autosomal dominant trait, then one of his parents must also have the same trait, except in the case of reduced penetrance. Vertical transmission is also evident, from parent to child. Another important general characteristic of autosomal dominant inheritance is that all the offspring of an affected individual with an autosomal dominant disorder will have a 50% probability of also having the same disorder (Fig. 2-10). For example, a particular gene has two alleles, D and d, for which d is the normal allele and D is the mutated allele conferring a disease trait. Two individuals mate, with the genotypes of Dd and dd. Using the Punnett square, their offspring will have the possibility of receiving two genotypes: Dd or dd. Each genotype is equally likely to occur; thus an autosomal dominant trait has a recurrence probability of 50%. Autosomal dominant disorders are often adult onset; those that are evident early in life are often the result of new mutations.

BOX 2-3
Examples of Single Gene Disorders

AUTOSOMAL DOMINANT
Achondroplasia
Familial hypercholesterolemia
Hereditary spherocytosis
Huntington's disease
Marfan's syndrome
Neurofibromatosis type 1
Osteogenesis imperfecta
Adult polycystic kidney disease
von Willebrand's disease

AUTOSOMAL RECESSIVE
Albinism
Color blindness
Cystic fibrosis
Galactosemia
Glycogen storage disease
Mucopolysaccharidosis
Phenylketonuria (PKU)
Sickle cell anemia
Tay-Sachs disease

X-LINKED
Duchenne's muscular dystrophy
Hemophilia A and B
Glucose-6-phosphate dehydrogenase deficiency
Bruton's hypogammaglobulinemia

Y-LINKED
Gonadal dysgenesis, XY type

MITOCHONDRIAL
Leber's hereditary optic neuropathy
Kearns-Sayre syndrome

Estimates indicate that 1 out of every 200 individuals has an autosomal dominant disorder, although each individual disorder itself is relatively rare in general populations.

Neurofibromatosis 1 (NF1) affects approximately 1 in 3000 to 1 in 5000 individuals and is one of the most common autosomal dominant disorders. Although this disorder is thought to have nearly 100% penetrance (the gene is phenotypically evident in all individuals who carry it), a great deal of variable expressivity is present. The *NF1* gene is located on chromosome 17 and codes for a protein (neurofibromin) that acts to suppress tumors. This gene is extremely large and, as such, displays a high mutation rate. Although this disorder is inherited according to the Mendelian principles, it also develops as a new mutation; that is, the individual develops a mutation in his or her *NF1* gene, even though the parents do not have the mutated gene. Clinical manifestations of *NF1* include *café-au-lait* spots (hyperpigmented skin patches), benign nodules on the iris (Lisch nodules), neurofibromas (benign peripheral tumors of the nerves), optic gliomas, hypertension, and even malignant tumors. Again, this condition is highly variable in its expression.

Marfan's syndrome affects approximately 1 in 10,000 North Americans and is caused by a mutation on chromosome 15, in a gene encoding for a connective tissue protein, fibrillin. This protein is found in the lens, periosteum, and aorta. Over 100 mutations in this gene have been identified to date and include missense, nonsense, and frameshift alterations. The clinical presenta-

tion of this disorder includes skeletal, ocular, and cardiovascular alterations. Physical characteristics include unusually slender and long arms and legs, scoliosis, pectus carinatum ("pigeon chest"), and long and thin fingers. Periosteum is a fibrous connective tissue that covers bones. In these individuals, the periosteum is more elastic than it should be, resulting in increased bone growth. In the ocular system, most patients will have myopia, and many will have a detached lens. Of most critical importance, the majority of these individuals (90%) experience dilation of the aorta. With increased dilation, the aorta is susceptible to rupture, particularly during periods of high cardiac output, such as strenuous exercise. Cardiomyopathy is a cardiac finding associated with aortic dilation. Some patients also show mitral prolapse, allowing regurgitation of blood from the left ventricle to the left atrium.

Huntington's disease, an autosomal dominant disorder, is the result of an expansion of triplet nucleotide repeats and is addressed at another point in the chapter.

Autosomal Recessive Disorders

Autosomal recessive disorders are generally apparent in individuals who are homozygous for the mutated allele, whereas heterozygotes rarely display the disease phenotype. Autosomal recessive inheritance shares some similarities with autosomal dominant inheritance; namely, males and females are generally affected equally. However, differences exist between these two types of inheritance. For example, when two individuals, both heterozygotes (Cc) for a particular gene, mate, they do not express the recessive trait but serve as carriers of the recessive allele. The progeny can be CC, Cc, or cc. The recurrence risk for cc is then 25% or one-fourth probability. Heterozygotes for a particular recessive disease gene are far more common in the population than are affected homozygous individuals. Thus looking at a pedigree for an autosomal recessive trait reveals *horizontal* transmission. Affected individuals rarely have affected parents, although both of the parents of an affected individual must be heterozygotes for the gene of interest. The pedigree will rarely show parent-to-child transmission, although multiple siblings may be affected (Fig. 2-11). Autosomal recessive disorders are often the result of mating between blood relatives (consanguinity). Box 2-5 highlights the characteristics of autosomal recessive transmission.

Most autosomal recessive disorders are rare in the general population, whereas others occur at a higher fre-

BOX 2-4

Characteristics of Autosomal Dominant Inheritance

- Gene is on an autosome.
- Expressed in both heterozygotes (Aa) and homozygotes (AA).
- Males and females are equally affected.
- Vertical family history appears on pedigree chart (appears in every generation).
- From a normal parent and a heterozygous parent, each offspring has a 50% probability of being affected.
- Delayed age onset of disease is common.
- Wide variety in clinical expression is observed.
- Penetrance may be incomplete.
- Structural protein defect (membrane receptor, collagen) is often involved.
- New gene mutation is common.
- Tends to be less severe than recessive disorders.

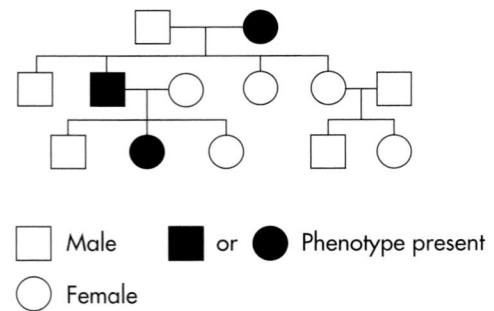

☐ Male ■ or ● Phenotype present
○ Female

FIG. 2-10 Typical pedigree for dominant allele.

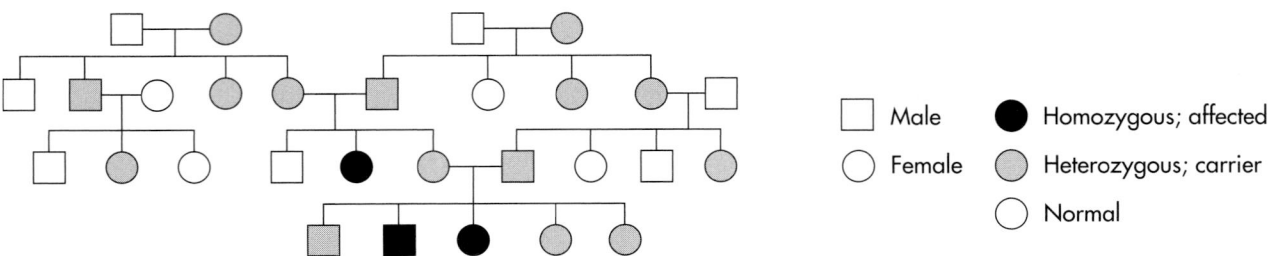

☐ Male ● Homozygous; affected
○ Female ◉ Heterozygous; carrier
○ Normal

FIG. 2-11 Typical pedigree for a recessive allele.

quency in a given population, such as sickle cell disease. *Cystic fibrosis (CF)* is one of the most common genetic diseases in Caucasian populations, affecting approximately 1 in 3300 individuals. The carrier frequency for this disorder is significantly higher, approximately 1 in 25. CF is a disease of defective chloride ion transport across cell membranes, resulting in thickened, more viscous secretions. This condition is typically diagnosed within the first year of life. However, the presentation of the disease varies considerably. The cystic fibrosis transmembrane conductance regulator (CFTR) gene, located on chromosome 7, cloned in 1989, is involved in the regulation of chloride channel activity. Over 700 mutations in this gene have been identified in individuals with CF. The pathophysiology, clinical manifestations, and treatment of this condition is described in Chapter 38.

Sickle cell anemia (SCA) is a major disease affecting hemoglobin and affects approximately 1 in 400 to 1 in 600 African Americans. The sheer prevalence of this disorder highlights its clinical significance. Homozygosity for the mutant allele confers the sickle cell disease, and heterozygosity confers the *sickle cell trait*. Making this distinction is critically important. Individuals with sickle cell trait are carriers of one mutated allele and are capable of transmitting this allele to their offspring, but they do not have sickle cell disease. The history of associating sickle cell trait with sickle cell disease produced a great deal of discrimination in this patient population. Vigilance is needed to prevent any future discrimination. A single-point mutation in the beta-globin gene causes sickle cell anemia. This gene is located on chromosome 11. In the formation of hemoglobin, globin chains combine with heme chains. Hemoglobin is the molecule responsible for transporting oxygen throughout the body. The mutation in this gene alters the shape of the hemoglobin molecule, resulting in a sickle cell–shaped erythrocyte. Sickling of cells reduces flexibility, and these cells are unable to squeeze through capillaries, denying needed oxygen to tissues. Additionally, sickled cells are prematurely destroyed, leading to an anemic state. Clinical manifestations of SCA include anemia, failure to thrive in the infant, pain in the extremities resulting from occlusion of capillaries, splenomegaly, and recurrent infections. Chapter 17 contains additional details on SCA.

Phenylketonuria (PKU) affects approximately 1 in 10,000 Caucasian individuals. PKU is considered an inborn error of metabolism. Phenylalanine is an essential amino acid necessary for normal growth and development. Phenylalanine is broken down by the enzyme *phenylalanine hydroxylase (PAH)*. This process is critical because an elevated level of phenylalanine in the blood is neurologically damaging. Individuals with PKU have a mutation in the PAH gene, resulting in dangerously elevated levels of phenylalanine. If not immediately corrected, these high levels can then result in severe mental retardation. Newborn population screening in many western societies presently diagnoses PKU. When screening tests identify the newborn as having PKU, treatment consists of immediate dietary modification and management.

Sex-Linked Disorders

Disorders encoded on the X chromosome are termed *X-linked*, and those encoded on the Y chromosome are termed *Y-linked*. The principles guiding sex-linked inheritance are different from those of autosomal inheritance. All normal females have two X chromosomes, and normal males have one X and one Y chromosome. As such, the Y chromosome, containing few genes, encodes only for traits unique to males and cannot encode for any functions required for viability. Females receive one X chromosome from both parents and are equally likely to donate either X chromosome to their offspring. Males can receive only their X chromosome from their mothers and can donate it only to their daughters.

One consequence of male hemizygosity is that any allele on the X chromosome will be expressed in males as if it were dominant. Females possess two X chromosomes and can express a dominant or recessive phenotype accordingly. As such, X-linked disorders are expressed at a much higher rate in males than they are in females, although in the case of X-linked dominant disorders, females can express the disorder as frequently as do males.

X-linked recessive disorders are more common compared with X-linked dominant disorders. Females require homozygous alleles for the disorder to be expressed. In this manner, X-linked–recessive inheritance in females is similar to autosomal recessive inheritance. Males inherit an X-linked trait from their mothers, who are usually asymptomatic carriers. Affected males can transmit their X chromosome only to their daughters; as such, no father-to-son transmission is evident in X-linked recessive disorders. An affected male will pass on his mutated X chromosome to all of his daughters (Fig. 2-12). Box 2-6 highlights some characteristics of X-linked recessive inheritance.

X-linked disorders display variable expressivity, particularly in females because of the phenomenon known as *X-inactivation*. When females have two copies of the X chromosome and males have only one, do females have more protein product than males? The answer to that question is no; males and females carry the same amount of protein product resulting from the X chromosome. How is this

---

BOX 2-5

Characteristics of Autosomal Recessive Inheritance

- Gene is on an autosome.
- Expressed only in homozygotes (aa); heterozygotes (Aa) are phenotypically normal carriers.
- Males and females are equally affected.
- Horizontal inheritance pattern appears on the pedigree chart (appears in siblings but not usually in parents)
- Consanguinity of heterozygote parents, who are carriers, is often present.
- When both parents are carriers, each offspring has a 50% probability of being a carrier, a 25% probability of having the disease, and a 25% probability of being a (normal) non-carrier.
- Early age onset of disease is common
- Gene defect often results in enzyme deficiency (inborn error of metabolism).
- New gene mutation is rare.

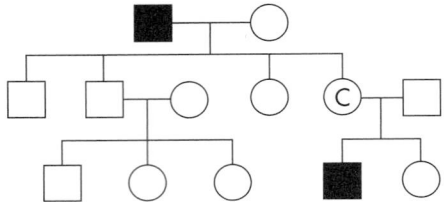

FIG. 2-12 Typical X-linked pedigree for a recessive allele. Female *C* is an asymptomatic carrier.

possible? In the 1960s, Mary Lyon offered a hypothesis (*Lyon hypothesis*) suggesting that in females, one of the X chromosomes in somatic cells is inactivated, leaving only one X chromosome active. This X-inactivation leads to dose equalization for X-linked genes in males and females. *X-inactivation* occurs early in embryonic development, and in any cell, the inactive X may be contributed at random from the mother or the father. After a cell has had an X chromosome inactivated, all resulting daughter cells will have the same X chromosome (either maternal or paternal) inactivated. The inactivated X becomes condensed and appears at the periphery of the cell nucleus as sex chromatin or *Barr body*.

Duchenne's muscular dystrophy (DMD), the most severe form of muscular dystrophy and affecting approximately 1 in every 3500 males, is characterized by a progressive loss of skeletal muscle. The DMD gene, located on the X chromosome, is the largest known gene, covering more than 2 million base pairs. The gene product, *dystrophin*, is involved in maintaining the muscle cell's structural integrity. When muscle cells lack dystrophin, they gradually die when they are stressed, such as during muscle contractions. Skeletal muscle deterioration begins early in life, and most patients with DMD are wheelchair bound by 11 years of age. These individuals also develop cardiomyopathy and respiratory complications, requiring the eventual use of mechanical ventilation because they lack the muscle strength and ability to breath on their own. Death is usually the result of respiratory or cardiac failure and usually occurs before the age of 25. No effective treatment for this condition is available at present, although research into gene therapy for this population is an active and ongoing process. Gene therapy is discussed later in this chapter.

Another X-linked recessive disorder, *hemophilia A*, affects up to 1 in 10,000 males globally. Hemophilia A is characterized by a deficiency of factor VIII, a critical protein within the clotting cascade. These individuals exhibit prolonged bleeding time. The gene encoding for factor VIII is located on the distal arm of the X chromosome. A variety of mutations have been identified, and the nature of the mutation frequently confers severity of the disease. For example, nonsense mutations produce a more severe phenotype than do missense mutations, owing to the truncation of the protein. The severity of disease is correlated with the amount of factor VIII level that each individual possesses. The variety within genotype-phenotype correlation is clinically apparent, from mild infrequent bleeding episodes to severe frequent episodes. Clinical manifestations of hemophilia A include bruising and hemarthrosis, a painful condition of bleeding into the joints (see Chapter 19).

Characteristics of X-Linked Recessive Inheritance

- The mutant gene is on an X chromosome.
- Males are more commonly affected than are females; only one copy of the mutant gene is needed for expression in males (hemizygous); two copies of the mutant gene are needed for expression in females.
- An unequal X-inactivation can lead to disease symptoms in females.
- A carrier mother and a normal father will produce sons with a 50% probability for having the disease and daughters with a 50% probability for being carriers (on average).
- All daughters of an affected father and a normal mother will be carriers.
- No father-to-son transmission exists.

Non-Mendelian Patterns of Inheritance
Mitochondrial Inheritance
The nucleus is not the only organelle in the body that contains DNA. Mitochondria contain a circular chromosome composed of mitochondrial DNA (mtDNA). Each cell contains several copies of this chromosome per mitochondrion. A small number of genes reside in mtDNA. Mitochondrial genetic disorders are quite rare, although they have a population impact. *Leber's disease* (Leber's hereditary optic neuropathy) is a mitochondrial disorder characterized by bilateral central vision loss resulting from optic nerve death. This disorder is diagnosed in young adults and is usually irreversible. Another mitochondrial disease is *Kearns-Sayre syndrome*, which is discernible by retinal degeneration, heart block, and muscle weakness. Pedigrees of mitochondrial genetic disorders show exclusively maternal transmission. Sperm cells contain few mtDNA molecules, thus mtDNA in offspring is inherited from the mother. Females can pass the mitochondrial disorders to both sons and daughters, although only daughters can, in turn, transmit the disorder.

Genomic Imprinting
Genomic imprinting is defined as the expression of an allele, depending on the parent from which the allele was inherited. *Angelman's syndrome* and *Prader-Willi syndrome* are examples of genomic imprinting. Severe mental retardation; an absence of speech; seizures; and a jerky, unstable gait characterize Angelman's syndrome. By contrast, mild-to-moderate mental retardation, short stature, obesity, and small hands and feet characterize Prader-Willi syndrome. Interestingly, both disorders are caused by a deletion of the same region on chromosome 15. The determination between these two disorders depends on the parent from whom the deletion was inherited. Paternal inheritance of the deletion confers Prader-Willi syndrome, whereas maternal inheritance of the deletion results in Angelman's syndrome.

Triplet Repeat Expansion
Another category of genetic diseases is characterized by an expanded number of nucleotide triplet repeats. *Huntington's disease* (HD) is a neurodegenerative disease characterized by triplet repeat expansion. HD affects approxi-

mately 1 in 20,000 individuals. The HD gene is located on chromosome 4. Mutation in this gene shows an expanded number of CAG repeats. Unaffected individuals have 11 to 35 CAG repeats, whereas individuals with HD have more than 36 CAG repeats, occasionally with more than 100 repeats. Earlier age of disease onset and greater severity is generally positively correlated with a higher number of repeats. The mutation is transmitted in an autosomal dominant manner.

HD is an adult-onset disease, with an average age of onset of approximately 40 years, although there is a wide range of age of onset. Symptoms of HD include choreic movements (spasmodic, involuntary movements), loss of memory, and loss of neurons within the brain. These symptoms are progressive in nature; that is, they worsen over time. The average interval from diagnosis to death is approximately 15 years. Death is usually the result of aspiration pneumonia. No curative treatment is available for HD. Current treatment protocols are aimed at symptom management.

HD differs from other autosomal dominant disorders in that it shows nearly 100% penetrance, meaning that nearly 100% of individuals with the mutation will develop HD. Most genetic disorders are not 100% penetrant. Predictive genetic testing is available for individuals with a family history of HD. Predictive and presymptomatic testing for a nearly completely penetrant, fatal disease without any known treatment is laden with significant issues. For example, individuals who test positive for the mutation will often feel a great deal of guilt, considering the 50% likelihood that they passed on the mutation to their children. Similarly, noncarriers often report guilt for not having the mutation when other family members may not be as fortunate. The complexity surrounding presymptomatic testing highlights the need for comprehensive and supportive genetic counseling, before and after genetic testing.

Chromosomal Abnormalities

Chromosomal abnormalities constitute a significant portion of genetic disorders, occurring in as many as 1 in every 150 live births. In fact, chromosomal abnormalities are the leading cause of spontaneous abortions (miscarriages). Chromosomal abnormalities can be either structural or numerical. *Structural abnormalities*, such as Robertsonian translocations, involve deletions, duplications, insertions, or translocations of a portion of one or more chromosomes. *Numerical abnormalities* are *aneuploid* conditions.

The most common cause of aneuploidy is nondisjunction (abnormality of chromosome segregation) during meiosis or after fertilization during mitosis. Nondisjunction can involve the autosomes or sex chromosomes. Nondisjunction during meiosis gives rise to haploid gametes that contain an abnormal chromosome complement. If the gamete is then fertilized, all daughter cells will be affected and have the same chromosomal abnormality (commonly giving rise to monosomies and trisomies). Many of these abnormal gametes are incapable of participating in fertilization, and if fertilization does occur, the fetus dies *in utero* and is spontaneously aborted.

BOX 2-7
Chromosomal Abnormalities

- Trisomy 21 (Down syndrome)
- Trisomy 13 (Patau's syndrome)
- Trisomy 18 (Edwards' syndrome)
- Monosomy of the X chromosome; 46, X0 (Turner's syndrome)
- 47, XXY (Klinefelter's syndrome)
- Philadelphia chromosome (translocation 9; 22)
- *Cri du chat* (deletion in 5p)

A problem in chromosome separation that originates in the embryo after fertilization during mitosis is transmitted only to daughter cells formed after the defect has occurred. The resulting embryo therefore contains at least two cell lines and is described as a *mosaic*. Mosaicism may involve abnormalities in the autosomes (e.g., Down syndrome) or the sex chromosomes (e.g., Turner's syndrome). Mosaicism is a common finding in chromosomal syndromes, and the degree to which a person is clinically affected depends on the percentage of cells with the abnormal chromosomal makeup. Box 2-7 lists a few chromosomal abnormalities.

Numerical Abnormalities (Aneuploidy)
Down Syndrome
Down syndrome (DS) or *trisomy 21* (47, XX, +21 or 47, XY, +21) is the most common chromosomal disorder in live births. Approximately 1 in 800 to 1 in 900 live births are affected with DS. Nondisjunction of chromosome 21 during meiosis is the cause of DS 95% of the time. Of these cases, 95% of the additional chromosome 21 originates from the mother. Maternal age is a strong risk factor for DS. For example, women under 30 years of age have a 1 in 1000 risk of having a fetus with trisomy 21 compared with women who are 40 years of age, whose risk rises to 1 in 100. One hypothesis to explain this phenomenon is the fact that all of a female's oocytes are formed before birth. These cells remain suspended in meiosis until ovulation, at which point they complete meiotic division. The increased age of oocytes may contribute to nondisjunction.

Individuals with DS display characteristic facial features, including upward slanting of the eyes, flattened face, epicanthal folds, and an enlarged tongue. This population displays varying degrees of growth and mental retardation. Persons with DS are also at an increased risk for other significant medical conditions, such as congenital heart defects, hearing loss, duodenal stenosis, and increased susceptibility to infection.

Turner Syndrome
Turner syndrome (45, X or 45, X0) affects approximately 1 in 5000 liveborn females; however, it has been suggested that the majority (up to 99%) of fetuses with this karyotype are spontaneously aborted. About half have the 45, X karyotype, 25% have mosaicism (46, XX/45, X), and the remainder have a structurally abnormal X chromosome with or without mosaicism. In individuals with mosaicism or structural abnormalities of the X chromosome, phenotypes on average are intermediate in severity between the 45, X variety and the normal. Paternal

nondisjunction during spermatogenesis is the cause of approximately 80% of Turner's syndrome cases, meaning that these individuals do not receive any sex chromosome from the father.

Individuals with Turner's syndrome are short in stature, have a triangle-shaped face, and a webbed neck but generally are not mentally retarded; they often have congenital heart defects. Additionally, these females often do not have ovaries, do not develop secondary sexual characteristics, and are infertile.

Klinefelter's Syndrome

The incidence of *Klinefelter's syndrome* (47, XXY) is about 1 in 500 live male births, making it one of the most frequent abnormalities of sex differentiation. The common karyotype is the classic 47, XXY chromosomal pattern or 46, XY/47, XXY mosaicism. The classic form is caused by meiotic nondisjunction during gametogenesis—about 60% of the time during oogenesis and 40% of the time during spermatogenesis. The mosaic form is believed to result from chromosomal mitotic nondisjunction after fertilization in the zygote and can take place in either a 46, XY zygote or 47, XXY zygote.

Klinefelter's syndrome is rarely diagnosed before puberty when incomplete development of secondary sex characteristics becomes apparent—small testes and sparse body hair. Other characteristics include elevated luteinizing hormone (LH) and follicle stimulating hormone (FSH), gynecomastia (enlarged breasts), azoospermia and infertility, mild mental deficiency, increased mean body height (from longer arms and legs), and a somewhat effeminate body contour. These characteristics result from a deficit of testosterone. Signs and symptoms are usually milder in the mosaic form of Klinefelter's syndrome with gynecomastia and infertility being less common than in the classical 47, XXY form. The risk of breast cancer is 20 times higher in patients with Klinefelter's syndrome than in other males. This condition may be treated with testosterone and the gynecomastia is treated surgically.

Structural Chromosomal Abnormalities

The *Philadelphia chromosome* represents a structural chromosomal disorder caused by a translocation between chromosomes 9 and 22, noted as t(9;22). It is present in up to 90% of patients with chronic myelogenous leukemia. The t(9;22) is also seen in 15% of the cases of acute lymphocytic leukemia (ALL) and in 5% of the cases of acute non-lymphocytic leukemia.

The *cri du chat syndrome* is an example of an uncommon structural chromosomal abnormality caused by deletion of part of short arm of chromosome 5, noted as 46, XY, del(5p) in a male child or 46, XX, del(5p) in a female child. *Cri du chat* is characterized by microcephaly, muscular hypotonia, severe mental retardation, and a shrill cry arising from maldevelopment of the posterior vocal cords. Hence the French name, *cri du chat*, meaning "cry of the cat." The average life expectancy of these infants is only a few weeks after birth.

Multifactorial Inheritance

Most genetic disorders and human disease do not appear to follow any of the patterns of inheritance or

---

BOX 2-8

Multifactorial Disorders

- Alcoholism
- Alzheimer's disease
- Cancer (all types)
- Cleft lip and palate
- Coronary heart disease
- Diabetes (types 1 and 2)
- Hypertension
- Migraine headaches
- Neural tube defects
- Obesity
- Osteoporosis
- Parkinson's disease
- Schizophrenia

---

structural abnormality as described in this chapter. Diseases such as coronary heart disease, breast cancer, neural tube defects, and schizophrenia tend to run in families, although they generally lack any specific pattern. This obscurity most likely represents the strong influence of extrinsic factors on the development of the disease, as well as the *polygenic* (many genes) requirements underlying these disorders. Multiple genes may be required to contribute to the final phenotype. Because these genes may lie on different chromosomes, their conjunction in any individual is unpredictable. Furthermore, multifactorial diseases may also require a specific environmental trigger or influence, thus they are only expressed after a given exposure.

The risk for multifactorial conditions varies from family to family. Within a family, the risk increases as the number of affected family members increases. Similarly, the risk afforded relatives of an affected individual increases in proportion to the severity of the condition. Additionally, if one child is affected with a particular condition, the risk of a sibling being affected then rises to 3% to 5%. Given these variables, predicting the occurrence of these disorders and appreciating the underlying genetic contribution are problematic. However, many if not most of the common disorders are indeed multifactorial in nature. Box 2-8 presents some multifactorial conditions.

Neural tube defects (NTD) are characterized by failure of the neural tube to effectively close during embryonic development. Types of NTD include *anencephaly* (partial absence of the brain), *encephalocele* (a congenital gap in the skull and herniation of brain tissue), and *spina bifida* (failure of the vertebral arches to close). The severity of clinical manifestations depends largely on the extent of defect and the subsequent damage to tissue of the central nervous system.

In the United States NTD affects approximately 1 in 1000 individuals. The risk of having a child with NTD in the general population is fairly low. However, the risk of having additional affected children increases to 2% to 5% with one affected child and up to 10% with two affected children. The familial relationship implies a certain degree of genetic cause, although it certainly is not the only contributor to NTD development. Folic acid deficiency is also a known contributor to the development of NTD, implying an extrinsic contribution to disease.

The search to understand multifactorial disorders is extraordinarily important. Because these disorders represent a significant number of common illnesses, advances in the diagnosis and treatment of these disorders will affect the health care system and the overall health of a population. Identification of the intrinsic factors underlying a disease will provide the diagnostic tools to promote behavior, lifestyle changes, and other interventions that may prevent or delay disease development.

Environmentally Induced Congenital Disorders

The majority of this chapter has been focused on the underlying genetic basis of human disease. However, certain subsets of congenital anomalies are a result of extrinsic factors.

The term *congenital* is defined as existing at birth. Therefore a congenital anomaly is a developmental disorder present at birth. Congenital anomalies can be structural or functional and are a result of both genetic (intrinsic) causes and environmentally induced (extrinsic) causes. These anomalies can be divided into four clinically significant subtypes: malformation, dysplasia, deformation, and disruption.

- *Malformation* is a morphologic defect of an organ or a larger portion of the body as a result of an intrinsically abnormal developmental process, such as a chromosomal abnormality.
- *Dysplasia* is defined as an abnormal arrangement or organization of cells.
- *Deformation* is an abnormal shape or position of a body part resulting from mechanical forces, such as intrauterine compression.
- *Disruption* is a morphologic defect of an organ or a larger portion of the body caused by extrinsic interference with normal growth and development. Disruptions are the result of environmental exposures and are the focus of this section.

The World Health Organization defines *teratogen* as a substance, organism, physical agent, or deficiency state present during gestation capable of causing adverse effects. An estimated 7% to 10% of all congenital anomalies are a result of environmental teratogens. Teratogens encompass drugs (including alcohol), chemical agents, infectious processes in the mother, radiation, and even maternal nutrition and disease states. Although exposure to a known teratogen is linked to congenital defects, not all exposed fetuses are affected (Box 2-9).

Teratogenicity is critically linked to the timing of exposure. Critical periods in fetal development are centered on tissue and organ development, and each organ system has its own critical period. For example, the critical period for limb formation is approximately $3^{1}/_{2}$ to 5 weeks. Exposure to teratogens during this critical period may produce limb malformations, such as the case with thalidomide exposure.

Drugs, Alcohol, and Chemical Agents

Approximately 2% of congenital anomalies are a result of drugs and chemical agents. A few drugs are definitely known teratogens, although considerable variability exists in their effects. Much of their teratogenic effects are caused by amount and timing of exposure. One such drug is thalidomide, a tranquilizer and sedative that produces limb malformations and other organ anomalies. Retinoic acid, or vitamin A, is another example of a teratogen. Maternal exposure to this agent produces spontaneous abortion, cleft palate, and other anomalies. Acne medications, such as Accutane, contain large amounts of retinol,

---

BOX 2-9

Known Teratogens

DRUGS
- Alcohol
- Cocaine
- Phenytoin
- Retinoic acid
- Thalidomide
- Warfarin

CHEMICALS
- Methylmercury

INFECTIONS
- Cytomegalovirus
- Epstein-Barr virus
- Herpes simplex virus
- Human immunodeficiency virus
- Rubella
- Toxoplasmosis
- Varicella

MATERNAL PROCESSES
- Diabetes mellitus
- Hypertension
- Phenylketonuria

---

and exposure to these medications in recent years has been one source of congenital defects. Vitamin A is a critical nutrient during pregnancy, although large doses are teratogenic. Cigarette smoking is well linked to *intrauterine growth retardation (IUGR)*, resulting in low birth weight. *Fetal alcohol syndrome (FAS)* is the result of maternal alcohol consumption and is characterized by mental retardation and other anomalies. The severity of FAS is proportional to the amount of alcohol intake. FAS is thought to be one of the leading causes of mental retardation.

Infectious Processes

Organisms infecting a mother can cross the placenta and subsequently infect the fetus. Many microorganisms produce teratogenic effects. One such microorganism is rubella, otherwise known as the German measles. As a result of cross-placental transmission, the fetus develops congenital rubella syndrome, which is characterized by cardiac defects, deafness, cataracts, and frequently mental deficits. Timing of exposure is critical with infectious processes, and in the case of congenital rubella syndrome, anomalies are observed when the fetus is infected within 5 weeks after fertilization. Defects can also occur with exposure later in pregnancy.

Exposure to infectious agents early in pregnancy is associated with cardiac, neurologic, and hearing defects; late exposure can lead to neurosensory defects. The severity of defects and the number of affected infants decreases as the gestational age at exposure increases. **TORCH** is a useful acronym to remember infectious teratogens:

T—toxoplasmosis
O—others (i.e., hepatitis B, mumps, human immunodeficiency virus)
R—rubella
C—cytomegalovirus
H—herpes simplex

Radiation

High levels of radiation exposure may result in a decrease in the physical growth of the fetus, mental retardation, and leukemia.

Maternal Processes

Many maternal health conditions can serve as teratogens. For example, uncontrolled maternal phenylalanine levels in women with phenylketonuria can produce *microcephaly* (small head), mental retardation, and even cardiac defects in the fetus.

DIAGNOSTIC TESTING

Progress in understanding human molecular genetics will shift health care from treatment of symptomatic disease states to disease prediction and prevention. Available technologies allow for early diagnosis in adults and prenatal screening to detect potential problems in the fetus. Prenatal diagnosis affords parents the opportunity to discuss abortion, plan for management of the newborn with impending disease, or even plan for lifestyle changes to alleviate or minimize the symptoms of a genetic illness in the newborn. Additionally, diagnostic testing of potential parents is available to provide risk information for future pregnancies.

Phenotypic Screening

Many genetic disorders can be diagnosed by the phenotype they generate (i.e., the clinical manifestations of the disease). Cystic fibrosis is diagnosable using the chloride sweat test (genetic confirmation of a mutated CFTR gene is also done), and phenylketonuria is diagnosable by determining the phenylalanine concentration in the neonate's blood.

Some disorders can be diagnosed prenatally. For example, neural tube defects often lead to an elevation of alphafetoprotein (AFP) levels. AFP is a protein found only in fetal tissues. Neural tube defects allow the fetal internal organs to come into close proximity with the amniotic fluid, resulting in an increased level of this protein. Normally, AFP levels increase within the amniotic fluid through approximately 14 weeks of gestation, after which the level sharply declines. AFP diffuses across the placenta to the serum of the mother; as such, AFP and *maternal serum AFP (MSAFP)* levels are proportional. Therefore MSAFP can be measured to determine the status of the fetus with minimal invasiveness as compared with sampling of the amniotic fluid.

The positive predictive value of MSAFP is low, meaning that an elevated level is not entirely 100% accurate in diagnosing neural tube defects. MSAFP can be elevated for other reasons, including twins, fetal demise, trisomy 13, and other chromosomal abnormalities. Conversely, MSAFP is often low in patients with Down syndrome.

Ultrasound is another method used to visualize developmental abnormalities. Many structural disorders, such as *anencephaly* (absence of a brain) and congenital heart defects, can generally be visualized by the second trimester.

Fetal Cell Sampling

One of the several methods available for prenatal diagnosis is amniocentesis. *Amniocentesis* involves using a needle to aspirate (withdraw) approximately 20 to 30 ml of fluid from the amniotic sac of a pregnant woman, usually in the second trimester. Amniotic fluid contains cells shed by the fetus and fetal urine. *Cytogenetic studies* (i.e., karyotyping) are carried out on these cells and take approximately 2 to 3 weeks to obtain results. Amniocentesis is recommended for pregnant women over 35 years of age, women who have given birth previously to a child with chromosomal abnormalities and women who have a family history of a genetic defect. Amniocentesis is not without risks, posing a fetal loss rate of approximately 0.5%.

Chorionic villus sampling (CVS) involves the direct acquisition of fetal trophoblastic cells (chorionic villi of the placental bed). CVS is performed late in the first trimester and can therefore provide a diagnosis earlier in pregnancy compared with amniocentesis. CVS is performed by inserting a needle transabdominally or a catheter transcervically. Cells obtained from CVS are rapidly dividing, and a karyotype can be accomplished in as few as 48 hours in some cases and up to 2 weeks in other cases. CVS has a higher fetal loss rate than does amniocentesis, at 1% to 1.5%.

Percutaneous umbilical blood sampling (PUBS) is a method to access the blood supply of the fetus. Fetal blood is withdrawn from the umbilical cord under ultrasound guidance. PUBS is performed after the sixteenth week of gestation and is used to rapidly analyze the cytogenetics of a fetus. Results are available within 2 to 3 days.

A still largely experimental technique is preimplantation embryo analysis. In this technique, a few cells are removed from an eight-cell embryo generated by in vitro fertilization. These cells are analyzed for genetic defects, including single-gene disorders and aneuploidy. If a cell is found free of genetic defects, it is then implanted into the female's uterus, and the fetus develops.

Molecular Genetic Analysis
Polymerase Chain Reaction

Although the chemical analysis of fluid and tissue samples has allowed for important gains in prenatal analysis, the diagnostic strategies that are evolving most rapidly and hold the greatest promise are based on molecular genetics. *Polymerase chain reaction (PCR)* amplifies DNA obtained from blood or other tissues and is the initial step for many other molecular genetic tests. This laboratory procedure mimics the way the cell copies DNA. The double-stranded DNA is separated, and each strand is copied, making two new strands. These steps are repeated up to 30 times, resulting in an exponential amplification of DNA (Fig. 2-13). Two strands make 4 strands, 4 strands make 16 strands, and so forth. PCR amplifies a small amount of DNA to detectable amounts, producing nearly unlimited copies of the original DNA. Duchenne muscular dystrophy is detected using PCR.

Direct sequencing of a known gene is the gold standard for molecular genetic analysis, during which the first to the last nucleotide of the gene is identified. For instance,

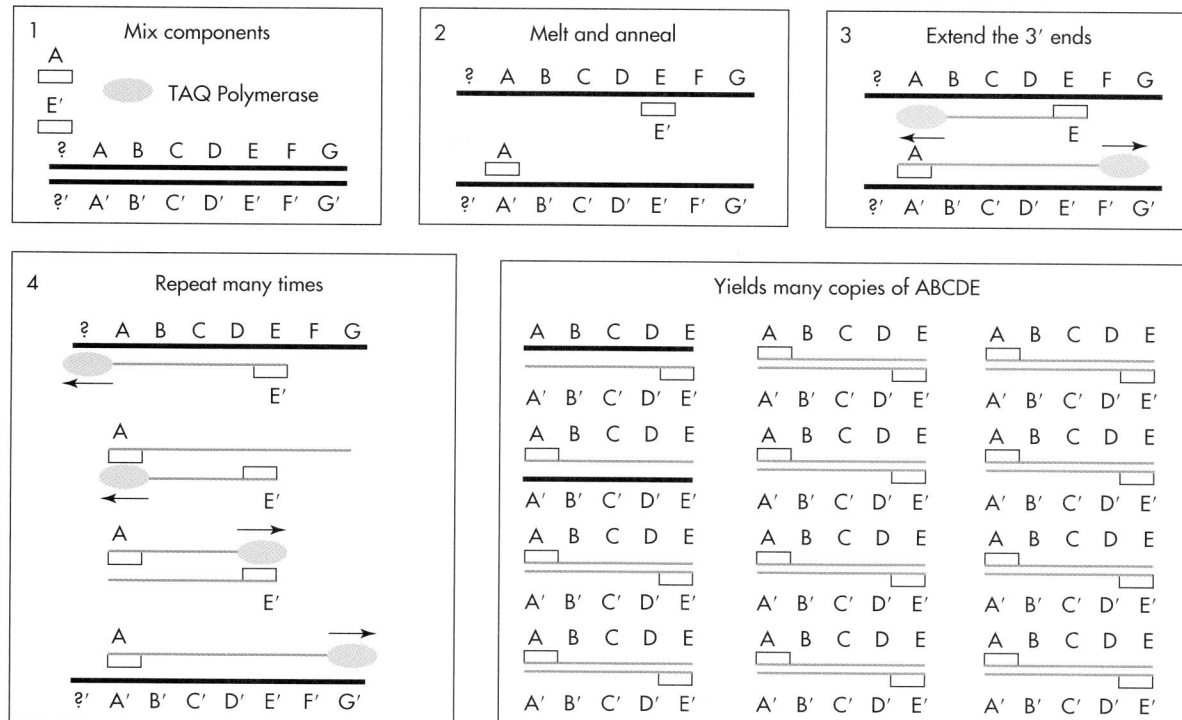

FIG. 2-13   Amplification of DNA by the polymerase chain reaction (PCR).

the BRCA1 gene, responsible for about one half of hereditary breast cancers, is approximately 5600 base pairs long. Direct sequencing will identify which nucleotide is present in each position along the gene. This process is expensive and time consuming.

Interpretation of direct sequencing results is straightforward when the gene is normal or when the gene has one or two of the known mutations that interrupts its protein function. Interpretation is more problematic when a rare mutation or polymorphism is found for which little or no available data exist linking that particular genetic change to breast cancer.

To ensure more definitive results, the gene is sequenced first in a family member that already has the disease to determine the family mutation. Other family members and relatives at risk desiring genetic testing can then be tested for the family mutation.

Protein truncation tests evaluate the size of a protein rather than nucleotide changes. If a mutation causes a protein to be shorter than a nonmutated protein would be (nonsense mutation), it exhibits different chemical characteristics. Length of the chain is determined via gel electrophoresis, in which the proteins are isolated and placed on a gel to which electric current is applied. The smaller fragments travel farther than do larger fragments. This test can be used when the exact mutation is unknown; however, this technology cannot detect nontruncating mutations, such as missense mutations.

Restriction Fragment Length Polymorphism

When direct sequencing is not reasonable, genetic markers linked to a particular gene of interest are useful tools.

Genetic markers are polymorphisms that are scattered throughout the genome. The utility of genetic markers is based on the principle of segregation. When a marker and a gene are located closely together on a chromosome, there is an increased probability that they will segregate together and thus be inherited together or "linked." When a marker is associated with a particular disease phenotype, it can be used as a marker for disease susceptibility.

Restriction fragment length polymorphism (RFLP) is one of the most common techniques used for detecting linkage, although it is being replaced with newer technologies. RFLP uses a class of enzymes known as restriction endonucleases that cut DNA at specific intervals based on DNA sequence. When a mutation occurs, often the enzyme cannot cut the strand in the same place as it does in the normal DNA strand, thus different sizes of fragments arise. DNA fragments are sorted according to size using gel electrophoresis.

Single Nucleotide Polymorphisms

Single nucleotide polymorphism (SNP, pronounced *snip*) is similar in theory to RFLP. However, rather than using enzymes to fragment DNA, this technology directly identifies the many polymorphisms within the human genome. Variety in the nucleotide sequence of the human genome is approximately 1 in 1250 nucleotides. Because 3 billion nucleotides are present in the entire genome, several million single nucleotide differences exist in a population. Some of these differences or DNA variants might be markers for disease or reside within a particular gene, contributing to disease development.

This premise is called the *common disease variant hypothesis*. A particular variant such as the apolipoprotein E4 (Apo E4) allele (4 variant or polymorphism of the apolipoprotein enzyme) is associated with Alzheimer's disease. The nucleotide variant changes the amino acid sequence in the protein and possibly modifies the function of the protein.

DNA microarrays, or DNA chips, are currently being used to detect SNPs or polymorphisms. On any given array, known gene or nucleotide sequences are laid down. Enough of the sequence is present to identify the gene, the mutation, or the polymorphism. The DNA fragments on the chip bind only to DNA strands from the patient that are complementary to the known sequence. Each DNA chip can identify hundreds to thousands of polymorphisms and genes yet is only the size of a postage stamp.

This technology holds great promise to detect diseases and will be increasingly used to detect risk factors for multifactorial and multigenic disease, such as cardiovascular disease and cancer.

OVERVIEW OF TREATMENT FOR GENETIC DISORDERS

Many therapeutic modalities exist for the treatment of genetic disorders or the resultant symptoms, from surveillance to gene therapy. Management of genetic disorders depends on the individual disorder; no universal treatment exists to comprehensively manage all disorders. Modification of both extrinsic and intrinsic factors is used in disease management. Some methods of therapeutic management are presented in this section.

Management of Phenotype

The manifestations of a genetic disorder are often treated rather than treating the underlying condition. For many genetic disorders, the only treatment available is management of disease phenotype. Individuals with CF experience numerous respiratory infections and are managed with antibiotic therapy. Postural drainage and physical therapy decreases the viscosity of secretions, and pancreatic enzymes manage pancreatic insufficiency in patients with cystic fibrosis. In another scenario, surgical intervention may be performed to treat congenital anomalies, such as cleft palate and congenital heart defects.

Dietary Modification

For some genetic disorders that result in the buildup of unmetabolized metabolic components, the treatment is based on dietary modification. Phenylketonuria (PKU) is one such condition. Individuals with PKU are treated with a strict low-phenylalanine diet to maintain an appropriate level of phenylalanine in the body. Insufficient phenylalanine inhibits normal growth and development; excessive amounts lead to mental retardation. Dietary modification is instituted immediately on diagnosis, usually within weeks of birth, and is continued throughout life. Although this treatment modality is effective, it is not without its costs, financially and emotionally.

Replacement

Genetic disorders resulting in absent or diminished protein products are treated by replacing the product. For example, individuals with hemophilia A lack factor VIII to varying degrees. Factor VIII can be transfused to the patient using donor plasma or recombinant factor VIII.

Surveillance

Presymptomatic genetic testing for a number of disorders provides individuals with an awareness of their risk for a particular disease. Intervention in this situation is not treatment *per se*; rather, conscientious surveillance is used to detect the disease at its earliest stage and to subsequently treat the disease from the onset. Unaffected individuals with BRCA1 (breast cancer gene 1) mutation should be under increased surveillance. Because their risk for developing breast cancer is greater than in the general population, surveillance is started at an earlier age. For example, if breast cancer occurred in a BRCA1 family at the age of 35, surveillance (including mammograms, clinical and self breast examinations) should then start at the age of 25 for unaffected family members who have the BRCA1 mutation. Some genetic conditions for which presymptomatic testing is available are without known medical treatments, such as HD. Nonetheless, vigilant monitoring for the presence of symptom manifestation aids in the institution of palliative measures.

Prophylactic Surgery

Unaffected individuals that are at elevated risk for developing a particular illness may also be treated prophylactically to minimize the chance of developing a particular disease. *Familial adenopolyposis (FAP)* is a genetic condition characterized by diffuse and numerous colonic growths, known as polyps. These individuals are at a significantly increased risk for developing colon cancer compared with the general population. Standard treatment in this instance includes the surgical removal of the colon (colectomy) to reduce or prevent the development of colon cancer. This modality is also available for other known genetic cancers, including breast cancer (surgical removal of breasts or ovaries or both) and hereditary nonpolyposis colorectal cancer (colectomy), although as a general rule, surgery does not reduce the disease risk by 100%.

All of these modalities are similar in that the effects of the disease are managed or prevented, but the genetic defect is not corrected. Extrinsic factors have been modulated or manipulated to treat the condition. Gene therapy is the attempt to correct the defect at the genetic level, to modify the intrinsic contribution to disease.

Gene Therapy

In *human gene therapy (HGT)*, a functional gene or set of genes are inserted into somatic cells to elicit a therapeutic response. The aim of HGT is to replace a mutated or absent gene in a cell with a corrected gene, as well as to alter cell function. Because therapy of germline cells may potentially alter the entire genetic makeup of an individual and his or her posterity, germline therapy is

TABLE 2-1

Examples of Target Sites for Gene Therapy in Selected Diseases

Disease	Target Gene	Target Cells
Cystic fibrosis	Cystic fibrosis transmembrane conductance regulator (CFTR) gene	Lung cells
Familial hypercholesterolemia	Low-density lipoprotein receptor gene	Liver cells
Sickle cell anemia	Beta-globin gene	Hematopoietic stem cells
Adenosine deaminase deficiency (immunodeficiency)	Adenosine deaminase (ADA) gene	Lymphocytes

not approved at this time. HGT using somatic cells does not alter the entire genetic makeup of an individual, only the cells of interest. The obvious advantage of HGT over other modalities mentioned is the specific targeting of the genetic root of the disease. HGT is still an experimental treatment and is being studied actively for use in cancer, cardiovascular disease, immunodeficiency disorders, and acquired immunodeficiency syndrome (AIDS), among other conditions.

Successful HGT depends on locating the suitable gene, having a favorable delivery system, and maintaining safety. No one universal form of gene therapy exists. HGT is accomplished through introducing a correct gene into the human genome. This initial step can be accomplished in two ways: *ex vivo*, in which proliferating cells are removed from the patient and cultured in the laboratory, injected with the gene of interest, and returned to the patient via standard IV infusion; or *in vivo*, in which the gene is delivered directly into the patient using a vector to deliver the gene to its target.

The first issue in gene therapy is to deliver the gene inside the cell. Delivery of the gene depends on vectors, including viral and nonviral forms. Viruses, such as retroviruses and adenoviruses, are often used because of their properties. A virus is capable of effectively entering a cell, integrating itself into the host's genome, and using the host's machinery to replicate. Viruses provide a means to insert a gene into a host cell and to allow for its expression. However, viruses are not perfect vectors. Concerns have been raised that using a viral vector to insert a gene in a cell nucleus may result in a viral infection, although the virus is altered to prevent it from causing disease.

Stem cells are often used as targets for gene therapy because of their proliferating nature. Tumor, muscle, and liver cells are also possible sites for HGT (Table 2-1).

After the gene is inserted into the cell, it must be integrated into the host genome, and normal expression of the gene must occur. Clinical trials to date have not provided conclusive evidence of HGT's efficacy. The application of gene therapy is not straightforward and is constrained by many limitations. For example, one infusion of the corrected gene product may not last indefinitely, and repeated dosing is required. Similarly, the reliability of introducing the corrected gene into the genome of the host cell is much less than 100%, leading to a low expression of the gene product.

Safety issues are also of concern. Although the overall safety profile of HGT has been favorable, some deaths have been attributed to gene therapy. Other risks of gene therapy include the overexpression of the transferred gene, resulting in harm to the patient, an inflammation and immune reaction as a response to the introduction of a virus, and the insertion of the correct gene into the incorrect place in the host genome, possibly leading to cancer.

The first clinical trials involving HGT and the first disease approved for HGT treatment is adenosine deaminase deficiency (ADA), which results in immunodeficiency syndrome. The first trial began in 1990, during which two children with ADA were treated with gene therapy. The corrected gene was introduced into the patient's lymphocytes (*ex vivo*), and these lymphocytes were infused back into the patient (Fig. 2-14). The subjects' immune function responded, although the duration of effect was short, requiring additional administration of the therapy. Even though HGT was given, the need for supplemental medication to control their disease was not negated. The participants had to continue to take medication to control the disease, although at much smaller doses.

The promise of gene therapy is vast, although its practical use, efficacy, and application is not yet realized.

PHARMACOGENETICS

Pharmacogenetics is an exciting area of research with potential for immense clinical application. Pharmacogenetics is the study of the way in which individual genetic differences influence response to medications. A wide spectrum of patient responses to a particular medication is often observed. The variety of responses may largely be caused by polymorphisms within genes that are involved in the absorption, metabolism, and elimination of a medication. Pharmacogenetics does not inform the clinician about the state of disease; rather, it predicts an individual's responsiveness to a particular drug.

The cytochrome p450 gene family is involved in the metabolism of a majority of medications. One gene within this family, CYP2D6, is responsible for the metabolism of antidepressants, morphine derivatives, and some cardiovascular drugs. Although the majority of the population has no problem with the metabolism of these drugs, a subpopulation exists that are considered "poor metabolizers" because of a polymorphism in the CYP2D6 gene. Poor metabolizers do not break down the drug as rapidly as do individuals with the more common variant of the

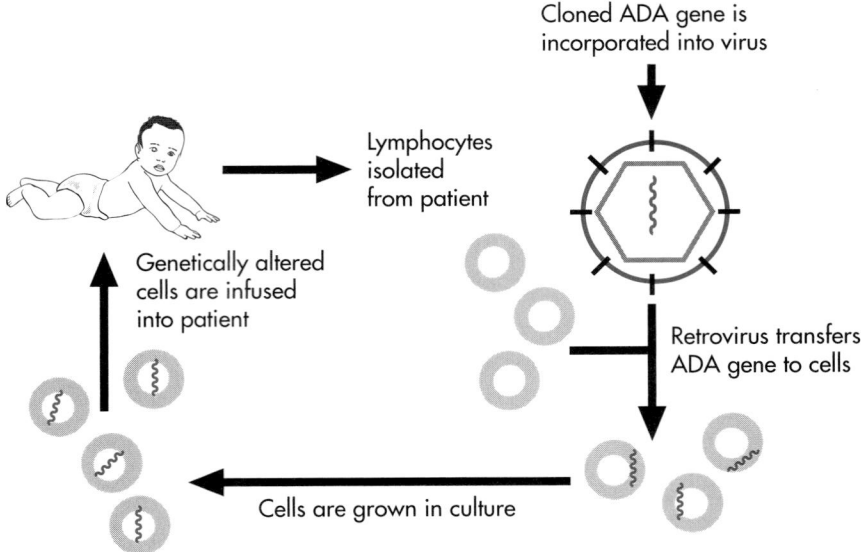

FIG. 2-14 The ADA gene is inserted into a viral vector, after which the virus infects white blood cells that have been removed from the patient. White blood cells are grown in culture to achieve adequate numbers of infected cells. Once this point is reached, the cells are reimplanted in the patient via IV fusion. (Modified from Klug WS, Cummings MR: *Essentials of genetics,* ed 4, New Jersey, 2000, Prentice Hall).

gene. These individuals will exhibit increased adverse drug reactions with standard doses of these medications as a result of decreased clearance time.

In contrast, other variations may have the opposite effect. For example, certain individuals might receive codeine for pain control. If these individuals have a particular polymorphism in the CYP2D6 gene, then they cannot convert codeine to its active form and will therefore not experience pain control. Although nurses may interpret this response as drug-seeking behavior, in fact, it may be the result of underlying genetic variation.

The clinical utility of pharmacogenetics is the ability to predict an individual's response to a medication and to treat accordingly; the goal is to prescribe the right drug at the right dose at the right time. DNA microarray, or DNA chip technology provides a useful tool to identify individual polymorphisms from which an individualized medication plan can be devised.

The nurse's responsibility in the emerging role of pharmacogenetics includes patient education of the rationale behind pharmaceutical selection, dosage, and timing determination and to anticipate potential alterations in drug metabolism within a particular patient population.

HUMAN GENOME PROJECT

Genetics touch and affect all human disease to some degree. Much of the interest and excitement about genetics is derived from the *Human Genome Project (HGP)*. This international undertaking began in 1990 with goals that included the construction of a physical map of all human genes, the complete sequencing of the human genome, and the development of new technologies.

In February 2001 the announcement was made that the human genome was sequenced. What does this mean? The order of nucleotides for the entire human genome has been determined. Although this is an enormous accomplishment in itself, a great deal of work remains. DNA sequences may be known, but the significance and functionality of much of the genome remains elusive.

One aspect of the HGP is the creation of a program known as ELSI: Ethical, Legal, and Social Issues related to genetics. The purpose of ELSI is to examine the impact of the HGP and increasing genetic knowledge in the context of ethics, law, and society. Genetic testing raises many questions and issues in this venue.

Genetic information is unique from other medical information in that it has important implications for the family, not only for the individual. One tenant of Western medical practice is patient confidentiality and patient autonomy. This ethical principle is challenged with genetic testing. The following example illustrates the point:

Samantha is an adult woman who was recently discovered as having a mutation in the BRCA1 gene, associated with an increased risk for breast cancer. She has siblings and children of her own that are also at risk for this heritable mutation. Samantha does not want any of her family members to know her genetic test results. Is the duty of the health care provider to maintain Samantha's autonomous decision and confidentiality or to warn other family members? What about determining the BRCA1 status of her minor child when the disease is not expected to manifest until the child reaches adulthood? In this case, testing of children would not be recommended until they become legal adults, whereas children in a familial adenopolyposis family may be tested at an early age because polyps can develop in the adolescent years. The risk of labeling a child with a mutation must be weighed against the benefit of available intervention and monitoring.

Other complex issues, such as disclosure of genetic test results, and genetic discrimination, such as potential employment or insurance discrimination, are common issues facing individuals and families confronted with the possibility of genetic testing. The nurse may advise the individual at risk for a mutation to have health, life, and disability insurance in place before initiating the process of genetic testing.

This complexity highlights the need for health care providers to be able to anticipate and discuss these issues before genetic testing, as well as the necessity for referral to genetic counseling. Genetic counseling is a nondirective approach that provides information and support for individuals and families undergoing genetic testing.

Counseling is performed by certified genetic counselors and advanced practice genetics nurses.

Nurses play a key role within an interdisciplinary team in disseminating genetic information to patients and their families. From answering patients' questions about the HGP to treating genetic illnesses, nurses are required to have knowledge of genetics and an awareness of issues surrounding this genetic revolution.

Genetic information is increasing at a rapid rate. As such, on-line genetic sources provide the most current and up-to-date information:
National Human Genome Research Institute
http://www.nhgri.nih.gov/
Gene Clinics
http://www.geneclinics.com/
Online Mendelian Inheritance in Man
http://www.ncbi.nlm.nih.gov/Omim/

KEY CONCEPTS

- Both intrinsic (within the individual) factors and extrinsic (environmental) factors *alone* are an incomplete explanation of disease. *Disease nearly always results from an interaction between heredity and environment.*
- The spectrum of diseases or disorders falls along a continuum representing interaction between heredity and environment. At the extremes are those largely determined by genetic factors (e.g., Down syndrome) or by environmental factors (e.g., being hit by a truck).
- *DNA,* the primary genetic material, is found in the nucleus of all cells; DNA is composed of subunits called *nucleotides* combined into a double helix (spiral staircase).
- *Nucleotides* are composed of three basic molecules: deoxyribose, phosphate, and nitrogenous bases. The two purine bases include adenine and guanine. The two pyrimidine bases are thymine and cytosine.
- The *structure of DNA* is similar to that of a spiral staircase, with chemical bonds as the steps. The two railings are constructed of deoxyribose and phosphate molecules. Each step is made of two halves consisting of any of the four bases joined by a hydrogen bond, whichever it happens to be; A always pairs with T and G with C. This structure is the secret of precise *replication of DNA.* When a cell divides, its DNA staircase unwinds and divides down the middle of each step. From these two halves, the cell produces two complete staircases that are identical to the original. Pairing of the bases is then proofread and corrected as needed. Replication takes place within the cell nucleus.
- *DNA polymerase* is an important enzyme involved in DNA replication; it travels along the DNA strand, adding the correct nucleotides to the free end of the new strand and proofreads it.
- A *gene* is the basic unit of heredity located on the chromosomes. Genes are composed of a sequence of DNA containing information necessary for controlling functional products, such as RNA or polypeptides (proteins).
- *Genes control not only inheritance, but also the day-to-day functions of cells.* Each gene provides instruction for the synthesis of a protein: enzymes, hormones, antigens, and receptors on cell membranes. Through the control of protein synthesis, the cellular activities of the body are controlled.
- *The central dogma of molecular genetics is that DNA makes RNA, which makes protein.*
- Basically, *protein synthesis* is the process by which the sequence of bases in DNA result in corresponding sequences of amino acids in the polypeptide chain produced. A sequence of three bases in the DNA, a *codon,* specifies an amino acid.
- *DNA-directed protein synthesis* takes place by means of two processes: transcription in the nucleus and translation in the cytoplasm.
- *Transcription* is the process by which complementary mRNA is synthesized from a DNA template thus transmitting the genetic code for protein synthesis from DNA to mRNA, assisted by RNA polymerases.
- *RNA* is chemically similar to DNA except that it is single stranded (rather than double stranded), has a ribose sugar molecule (rather than deoxyribose), and has uracil (rather than thymine) as one of its four bases.
- *Translation* is the process by which the amino acids in a given polypeptide are synthesized from the mRNA template, with amino acids placed in an ordered sequence as determined by the base sequence in mRNA. Assembly of the polypeptide (protein) takes place in the ribosomes with the assistance of ribosomal RNA (rRNA) and transfer RNA (tRNA).
- Although all cell nuclei carry the same genetic code, only some of these genes are expressed at a given time. *Regulatory genes* determine which genes are turned on (expressed) and which ones are silenced. Thus a muscle cell may synthesize the protein actin but not insulin.
- Within the cell nucleus, DNA is tightly wound around a rodlike protein (histone) to form a *chromosome.*

- *Gametes* (ova or sperm) have 23 chromosomes, the *haploid number* (N = 23) produced by a type of cell division called *meiosis*. Combination of the ova and sperm in reproduction results in the *diploid number* (2N = 46) of chromosomes.
- Humans have 46 chromosomes (23 pairs) in all somatic body cells. One member of each pair is inherited from the mother and the other from the father. Twenty-two pairs are *autosomes* and the remaining pair is the *sex chromosomes* conferring femaleness (XX) or maleness (XY).
- *Locus* refers to the site at which a particular gene (a transcriptional unit of DNA) is located on a chromosome. A gene is normally found at the same locus of a given chromosome.
- An *allele* is any one of two or more alternate forms of a gene located at the same locus. A single allele for each locus is inherited from each parent.
- A *homozygote* is an individual who has two identical alleles at a given locus on a pair of homologous chromosomes.
- A *heterozygote* is an individual who has two different alleles at a given locus on a pair of homologous chromosomes.
- The *genotype* is the actual allelic representation for an individual, either at a particular locus or for the entire genome.
- The *phenotype* is the observable characteristics of an individual, the expression of the genotype.
- A *chromosome* consists of two chromatids (identical pieces of DNA) joined at the center by the centromere, which separates its short arms (p) and long arms (q).
- A *karyotype* is the photomicrograph arrangement of an individual's chromosome pairs according to centromere position and length (largest to smallest). The normal female karyotype is written 46, XX and a normal male as 46, XY. A karyotype is helpful in revealing chromosomal abnormalities that are symptomatic of various disorders.
- A *mutation* may be defined as a permanent change in the DNA. Mutations that occur in the gametes are transmitted to the progeny and may give rise to inherited diseases; those that arise in somatic cells are important in the genesis of cancers and some congenital malformations.
- *Mutations* may be classified into three categories, based on the extent of genetic change: (1) *genome mutations*, involving the loss or gain of whole chromosomes giving rise to monosomy or trisomy; (2) *chromosomal mutations*, resulting from the rearrangement of genetic material giving rise to visible structural changes in the chromosome; and (3) *gene mutations*, *point mutations* (single-base substitution), and *frameshift mutations* from small deletions or insertions involving the coding sequence.
- Genetic disorders are generally of three types: single-gene disorders transmitted by Mendelian inheritance, multifactorial disorders, and chromosomal aberrations.
- *Pedigree charts* and *Punnett squares* are genetic analytic tools used to demonstrate or predict patterns of inheritance in families.

- Single-gene defect diseases are of varied Mendelian patterns and can be classified as to whether the abnormal gene is located on one of the 22 autosomes (*autosomal*) or on the sex chromosome (*sex-linked*).
- An *autosomal recessive disease* is expressed only in the homozygote (two copies of the abnormal gene [aa], one on each of the chromosomal pair). A heterozygote with only one copy of the abnormal gene is called a *carrier* (Aa) and can transmit the disease to offspring but does not express the disease.
- An *autosomal dominant disease* can occur in a *heterozygote* (one copy of the abnormal gene [Aa] on the chromosome pair, whereas the other gene is normal) or in a *homozygote* (two copies of the abnormal gene [AA], one on each chromosome).
- *Penetrance* refers to the proportion of people with a particular disease genotype that actually expresses the disease phenotype. Reduced penetrance means that individuals who harbor a mutation do not always physically express the mutant phenotype.
- *Expressivity* is the extent to which a gene's characteristic is present in an individual. If a gene is to have variable expressivity, then the trait may vary from mild to severe.
- *Characteristics of autosomal dominant disorders* include the following: (1) expressed in both heterozygotes (common) or homozygotes (rare); (2) males and females are equally affected; (3) vertical family history on pedigree chart is common (appears in every generation); (4) each offspring of a normal parent and an affected heterozygote has a 50% probability of being affected; (5) delayed age onset of the disease is common; (6) wide variety in clinical expression is observed; (7) penetrance may be incomplete; (8) structural protein defect is often involved (e.g., membrane receptor, key structural protein such as collagen); (9) new gene mutation is common; and (10) there is tendency to be less severe than recessive disorders.
- *Examples of autosomal dominant disorders* include familial hypercholesterolemia, adult polycystic kidney disease, von Willebrand's disease, neurofibromatosis, retinoblastoma, and Marfan's syndrome.
- *Characteristics of autosomal recessive disorders* include the following: (1) expressed only in the homozygote (aa); (2) heterozygotes (Aa) are phenotypically normal carriers; (3) males and females are equally affected; (4) horizontal pattern of inheritance is observed (present in siblings but not usually in parents); (5) consanguinity of parents who are carriers is often present; (6) when both parents are carriers, each offspring has a 50% probability of being a carrier, a 25% probability of having the disease, and a 25% probability of being unaffected; (7) early age onset of the disease is common; (8) mutant gene often results in an enzyme deficiency (inborn error of metabolism); and (9) new gene mutation is rare.
- *Examples of autosomal recessive disorders* include albinism, cystic fibrosis, phenylketonuria, albinism, sickle cell disease, Tay-Sachs disease, glycogen storage disease, and color blindness.

- *Characteristics of sex-linked recessive disorders* include the following: (1) mutant gene is on the X chromosome; (2) males are more commonly affected than females; (3) only one copy of the mutant gene is needed for expression in males (hemizygous); (4) two copies of the mutant gene are usually needed for expression in females; (5) unequal X-inactivation can lead to expression in carrier females; (6) a carrier mother and a normal father will produce sons with a 50% probability of being affected and daughters with a 50% probability of being carriers; (7) all daughters of affected fathers and normal mothers will be carriers; and (8) no father-to-son transmission occurs.
- *Examples of sex-linked recessive disorders* include Duchenne muscular dystrophy, hemophilia A and B, glucose-6-phosphate dehydrogenase (G6PD) deficiency, and Bruton's hypogammaglobulinemia.
- Some single-gene disorders have unusual *non-Mendelian transmission patterns*, including mtDNA mutation, genomic imprinting, and triplet repeat expansions.
- Although most genetic material is located in the cell nucleus, DNA is also found in the mitochondria. *mitochondrial DNA (mtDNA)* is transmitted to male and female offspring only through *maternal inheritance* (because mitochondria in the embryo are derived from the ovum). *Leber's disease* and *Kearns-Sayre syndrome*, which causes visual disturbances, are mitochondrial diseases inherited from the mother.
- *Genomic imprinting* is the differential expression of a gene in a child, depending on the parent from which the allele was inherited. *Prader-Willi syndrome* and *Angelman's syndrome* both result from a deletion on chromosome 15. The former disease is expressed when inherited from the father; the latter disease when inherited from the mother.
- *Huntington's disease* is an example of a genetic disorder known to be the result of inserts of multiple triplet repeats and transmitted in an autosomal dominant manner.
- The two principal types of abnormalities of chromosomes using cytogenetic analysis include *aneuploidy* or abnormality of the number of individual chromosomes and *structural abnormalities* in individual chromosomes.
- A normal haploid gamete (ova or sperm) has 22 autosomes and one sex chromosome. However, abnormal chromosome separation during meiosis may result in deletion, nondisjunction, or translocation of chromosomal material in either autosomes or sex chromosomes.
- The most important abnormalities of chromosomal number are the *trisomies*. In *Down syndrome* (trisomy 21), the additional chromosome 21 is usually the result of nondisjunction during formation of the haploid maternal ovum.
- *Disorders of sex chromosome number* arise by nondisjunction. Important syndromes are Turner's syndrome (46, X0) and Klinefelter's syndrome (47, XXY).
- Breaking and rejoining of chromosomal material (deletion, translocation, inversion) leads to *structural chromosomal abnormalities*. *Cri du chat* is one of the most common deletion syndromes caused by deletion of part of chromosome 5.
- *Multifactorial disorders* are common and thought to involve two or more mutant genes, as well as environmental triggers; examples are hypertension, diabetes, cancer, and Alzheimer's disease.
- Factors that induce abnormal embryologic development are known as *teratogens*. The most important teratogenic factors include drugs and chemicals (e.g., thalidomide, alcohol), ionizing radiation (e.g., x-ray exposure), and maternal infections (e.g., rubella).
- *Ultrasound, amniocentesis,* and *chorionic villous sampling* are the primary methods of prenatal assessment for genetic disorders.
- Genetic disorders are now identifiable by *molecular genetic techniques*, including polymerase chain reaction (PCR), restriction fragment length polymorphisim (RFLP), and single nucleotide polymorphism (SNP).
- *Gene therapy* is the treatment of genetic disorders whereby defective genes are replaced with normal genes.
- *The Human Genome Project*, which is the mapping and sequencing of the entire human genome, offers promise for the advancement of gene replacement therapy for a variety of genetic diseases, advancement in the field of pharmacogenetics, and a greater understanding of the genetic basis of many diseases.

QUESTIONS ??

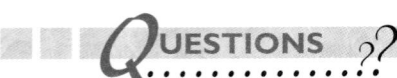

A sampling of review questions for this chapter appears here. Visit http://www.mosby.com/MERLIN/PriceWilson/ for additional questions.

Answer the following on a separate sheet of paper.

1. Describe the flow of genetic information from mother cell to daughter cells at the molecular (replication) and cellular (meiosis and mitosis) levels.
2. Describe the flow of genetic information from DNA to RNA (transcription) and protein (translation), including key enzymes, specific sites, and regulators.

3. What determines whether an allele is dominant or recessive?
4. Construct a Punnett square for the mating of two heterozygotes (Bb with Bb), where B is the normal allele and b is a recessive mutant allele. What is the probability that a progeny would have the mutant phenotype?
5. How does X-chromosome inactivation contribute to variable expressivity for females?

6. Why are translocations often associated with hematologic cancers?
7. What are the advantages and disadvantages of chorionic villus sampling (CVS) compared with amniocentesis?
8. How can antisense genes be used to correct dominant disorders?

Match the genetic disorder in column A with the type of defect in column B.

Column A
9. _____ Leber's hereditary optic neuropathy
10. _____ Klinefelter's syndrome
11. _____ Leukemia
12. _____ Down syndrome
13. _____ Prader-Willi syndrome
14. _____ Angelman's syndrome

Column B
a. Translocations
b. Mitochondrial
c. Genomic imprinting
d. Aneuploidy

Match the genetic condition in column A with the type of inheritance in column B.

Column A
15. _____ Phenylketonuria
16. _____ ABO blood group
17. _____ Sickle cell anemia
18. _____ Cystic fibrosis
19. _____ Neurofibromatosis type 1
20. _____ Duchenne muscular dystrophy

Column B
a. X-linked
b. Autosomal dominant
c. Autosomal recessive
d. Codominant

Cellular Injury and Death

LORRAINE M. WILSON

CELLULAR ORGANIZATION

Although the body contains many different types of cells with highly specialized functions, all cells, to a large extent, have similar lifestyles and similar structural elements. These cells have parallel requirements for oxygen and nutrient supplies, for a constant temperature, for water supply, and for a means of waste disposal. The cell is literally the unit of life, the smallest entity that manifests the various phenomena associated with living. Therefore the cell is also the basic unit of disease.

The organization of a hypothetic "typical" cell is diagramed in Fig. 3-1. The cell is bounded by a cell membrane, which gives the cell its shape and attaches it to other cells. The cell membrane is the gateway to and from the cell, allowing only certain substances to pass in either direction and even actively transporting some matter in a selective fashion. The cell membrane also

receives many of the control signals from around the body and transmits these signals to the interior of the cell.

Within the cell is the *nucleus,* which serves as the control center because the deoxyribonucleic acid (DNA) is concentrated within it. The instructions coded within the nuclear DNA are actually executed within the *cytoplasm,* the portion of the cell outside the nucleus. The cytoplasm is a watery medium that contains many structures so small that they can be observed only with an electron microscope. These ultramicroscopic organs are called *organelles* and are highly specialized as to function even within the confines of a single cell.

The *mitochondria* are organelles devoted to energy production within the cell; they are the power plant of the cell. Within them, various foodstuffs are oxidized to produce the driving force for other cellular activities. The *endoplasmic reticulum* and *Golgi apparatus* constitute a sort of manufacturing, processing, and plumbing system within the cytoplasm. The endoplasmic reticulum is a network of interconnecting tubules and cisterns, and the Golgi complex is a closely related array of flattened cisterns and associated vesicles. Protein synthesis is carried out along the endoplasmic reticulum under control of ribonucleic acid (RNA) in the *ribosomes.* Nuclear DNA produce and direct the cytoplasmic RNA to act as a sort of assembly team in relation to the executive role of the DNA. The ribosomes carry out protein synthesis by assembling amino acids into complex molecules according to the directions supplied by the DNA. The Golgi apparatus is a packaging device that wraps the cell products for export (secretion) or for storage within the cell. Certain glycoprotein complexes are also elaborated within the Golgi apparatus. The *lysosomes* are membrane-bound packages of digestive enzymes prepared by the cell and held inactive until needed. Still other organelles not shown in Fig. 3-1 account for additional special functions within the cell, such as providing rigidity and movement in the manner of a musculoskeletal system. The various organelles represent a total organism in microcosm, and their activity must be closely coordinated and controlled to preserve cellular integrity.

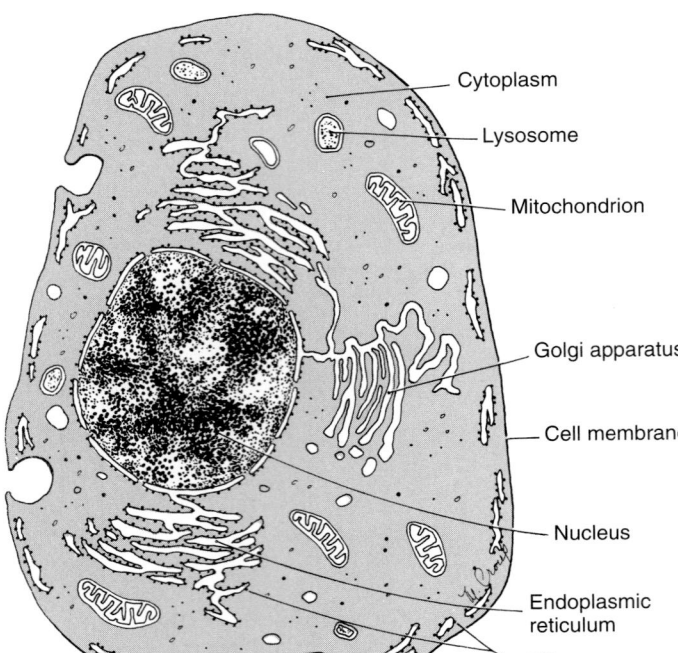

FIG. 3-1 Diagram of a hypothetic typical cell. The structural basis for division of labor within the cell is shown. It should be noted that in the living body, the cell membrane not only bounds the cell and controls access to the interior but also joins the cell with others to form tissues.

Individual cells relate to one another in a variety of ways as they assemble into tissues and organs. Some tissues, such as lining or covering epithelia, consist of densely packed cells directly and tightly adherent to one another with little intervening space. Groups of cells of this type are soft and pliable and cannot maintain the form of various organs or the strength of the entire body. Connective tissue actually holds the body together because of its *intercellular substance*—literally, material between the cells. This substance includes *collagen*, which is a protein produced in the form of extremely tough fibers (similar to those in tendons and ligaments), and *elastin*, which is also a protein assembled into fibers, but which also has elastic properties. Between these fibers is a gelatinous matrix, or *ground substance*. The combination of tough and elastic fibers and the matrix gives the body its strength, form, and resiliency. In the skeleton the intercellular substance is impregnated with calcium salts, producing the rigid bony support of the body.

MODALITIES OF CELLULAR INJURY

Cells can be injured or killed in many ways, but important types of injury tend to fall into only a few categories. One of the most common factors in cellular injury is a *deficiency of oxygen or other critical nutrient material*. Cells depend on a continuous supply of oxygen, because it is the energy of oxidative chemical reactions that drives the machinery of the cell and maintains the integrity of the various components of the cell. Therefore without oxy-gen the various maintenance and synthesizing activities of cells quickly come to a halt.

A second type of injury is *physical*, which involves actual disruption of cells or at least disturbance of the usual spatial relationships among the various organelles or of the structural integrity of one or more types of organelles. Thus mechanical and thermal means of injury are significant causes of human disease. Sudden changes in pressure, radiation, and electric shock are less common modes of physical injury.

Living *infectious agents* constitute a third means of cellular injury, and particular organisms injure cells in a variety of ways. *Immunologic reactions* are a fourth means of cellular injury. Although the immune system normally serves as a defense against foreign antigens, immune reactions may also cause cell injury. The anaphylactic reaction to a bee sting or a drug is a prime example (see Chapter 9).

Finally, *chemical agents* are a common means of cellular injury. Not only do toxic substances find their way into cells from the environment but also accumulation of endogenous substances (such as with genetically determined metabolic "errors") may injure cells.

THE CELL UNDER ATTACK

When an injurious stimulus is applied to a cell, the first important effect is a *biochemical lesion*. This process involves a change in the chemistry of one or more metabolic reactions within the cell. Few types of injury are actually understood at this initial level. Although biochemical changes can be noted in injured cells, the abnormalities noted are often second- or third-order effects rather than evidence of the primary biochemical lesion. When a biochemical lesion is established, the cell may or may not manifest a functional abnormality. In the case of many injuries, the cell possesses sufficient reserve to perform without significant functional impairment; in other instances, a failure of contraction, secretion, or other activities of the cell can occur. Particularly important determinants in this regard are the extent of impairment of energy production (with adenosine triphosphate [ATP] depletion) and the extent of impairment of cell membrane functions.

A cell with biochemical and functional abnormalities may or may not display a detectable morphologic change. The limitation in this instance is one of technique. Changes that are evident on routine microscopic examination are generally late changes, because many biochemical and functional abnormalities may have occurred before the anatomic abnormality became evident. With the advent of electron microscopy, increasingly earlier detection of microscopic lesions of the various organelles is becoming possible. However, with presently available techniques, many functionally impaired cells may yield no evidence of their impairment in morphologic terms.

The result of an attack on a cell is not always impairment of function. In fact, cellular mechanisms of adaptation exist to various kinds of adversity. For example, a common reaction of a muscle cell placed under abnormal stress is to increase strength by enlargement, a process called *hypertrophy*. Thus the heart muscle cells of an individual with high blood pressure will enlarge to cope with the strain of pumping against increased resistance. A similar type of adaptation occurs with regard to certain chemical challenges. Barbiturates and certain other substances are usually metabolized in liver cells, under the influence of enzyme systems found within these cells in association with the endoplasmic reticulum. An individual who is taking barbiturates often has a striking increase in the amount of endoplasmic reticulum within liver cells, which is associated with an increased enzyme content in these cells and an increased ability to metabolize the drug.

MORPHOLOGIC CHANGES IN SUBLETHALLY INJURED CELLS

When cells are injured but not killed, they often manifest easily identifiable morphologic changes. These sublethal changes are at least potentially reversible. That is, if the injurious stimulus can be withdrawn, the cells return to their previous state of health. On the other hand, these changes may be a step toward cell death if the noxious influence cannot be corrected. Sublethal changes in cells are traditionally called *degenerations* or *degenerative changes*. Although any cells of the body may manifest such changes, metabolically active cells such as those in the liver, kidney, and heart are typically involved. Degenerative changes tend to involve the cytoplasm of cells, whereas nuclei maintain their integrity as long as the cell is not lethally injured. Although an extremely large number of injurious agents or specific ways of attacking cells exist, the repertory of morphologic expression of injury is actually quite limited.

The most common form of cellular degenerative change involves the *accumulation of water* within the affected cells. In effect, the injury causes loss of volume control on the part of the cells. To maintain constancy of its internal environment, a cell must expend metabolic energy to pump sodium ions out of the cell. This process occurs at the level of the cell membrane. Anything that disturbs energy metabolism in the cell or slightly injures the cell membrane may render the cell unable to pump out a sufficient amount of sodium ions. The natural osmotic result of increased intracellular concentration of sodium is an influx of water into the cell. The result is a morphologic change termed *cellular swelling*. A previous name for this change was cloudy swelling, because an organ whose cells suffered this change acquired a peculiar parboiled appearance grossly, and the affected cells acquired an unusual granular appearance of the cytoplasm microscopically. When water accumulates within the cytoplasm, the cytoplasmic organelles also absorb it, causing mitochondrial swelling, dilation of the endoplasmic reticulum, and so forth.

Microscopically, the changes of cellular swelling are quite subtle and involve simply an enlargement of the cell and a slight change in its texture. The gross counterpart of this change is the enlargement of the affected tissue or organ, which is usually detectable by a moderate increase in weight. If the noxious influence that produces cellular swelling can be removed, after a time the cells

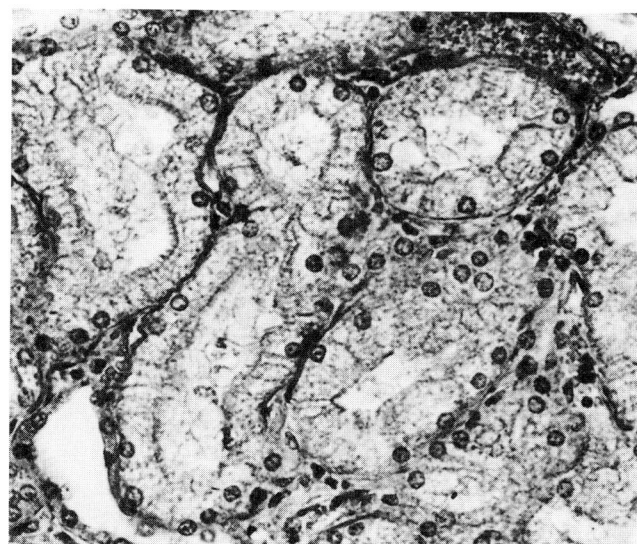

FIG. 3-2 Hydropic change in renal tubular epithelium. The epithelial cells lining these convoluted tubules are enlarged and have vacuolated, lacy-appearing cytoplasm because of intracellular accumulation of water. (Photomicrograph, × 500.)

usually begin to extrude sodium, and along with it water, and the volume returns to normal. This change is only a slight perturbation in the normal state of affairs.

When a severe influx of water occurs, some of the cytoplasmic organelles, such as the endoplasmic reticulum, may be converted into water-filled sacs. When examined under a microscope, the cytoplasm of the cell is observed to be vacuolated (Fig. 3-2). This condition is termed *hydropic change* or sometimes vacuolar change. The gross appearance of affected organs and the significance of the change are identical to those of cellular swelling.

A more significant change than simple cellular swelling involves the intracellular accumulation of lipid within affected cells. This type of change usually involves the kidneys, heart muscle, and liver, particularly the liver. Microscopically, the cytoplasm of the affected cells appears vacuolated in a manner similar to that observed in hydropic change, but the content of the vacuoles is lipid rather than water. In the case of the liver, the amount of lipid accumulating within a cell is often relatively large, thus the nucleus of the cell is pushed to one side and the cytoplasm of the cell is occupied by one lipid-containing vacuole (Fig. 3-3). The counterpart of these changes with respect to the gross appearance of affected tissues involves swelling of the tissues, increase in weight of the affected organ, and often a distinct yellowish cast to the tissue resulting from the contained lipid. Severely affected livers are often bright yellow and greasy to the touch. This type of change is called *fatty change* or *steatosis* (or sometimes fatty degeneration or fatty infiltration).

Steatosis occurs often because it can be produced by many different mechanisms, particularly in the liver. Hepatocytes (and other types of cells) are normally involved in an active metabolic exchange of lipids. These substances are constantly mobilized from adipose tissue into the bloodstream, from which they are extracted by the liver cells. Some of the lipid absorbed by the cell is oxidized, whereas some of it is combined with protein synthesized by the cell and then exported from the cell (i.e., into the bloodstream) in the form of lipoprotein.

Interfering with the usual exchange processes at any of several points can produce accumulation of fat within the cell. For example, when an excess of lipid is presented to the liver cell, the metabolic and synthetic capabilities of the cell may be exceeded, and the lipid will accumulate intracellularly. On the other hand, when normal amounts of lipid reach the cell but oxidation is impaired by some cellular injury, lipid will accumulate. Finally, when the process of lipoprotein synthesis and export is interfered with at any of several points, lipid will also accumulate. For these reasons, a fatty liver may be encountered in diverse situations, ranging from malnutrition, which impairs protein synthesis, to overfeeding, which swamps the liver with lipids. Hypoxia sufficiently impairs cellular metabolism to produce fatty accumulation, and numerous toxic substances from the environment affect the cells in such a manner as to promote lipid accumulation. One of the most potent and widespread toxins in the environment that produce fatty livers is alcohol. This substance is directly toxic to liver cells, as well as being indirectly injurious to individuals whose alcohol intake is extreme, primarily because this often leads to malnutrition. Fatty change is potentially reversible but frequently reflects a severe injury to the cell and thus is a step on the way to cell death.

Another response of cells under attack is to undergo a reduction in mass, literally, shrinkage. This acquired reduction in the size of a cell, a tissue, or an organ is referred to as *atrophy*. The atrophic cell or tissue appears to be able to achieve equilibrium under the adverse conditions imposed on it by reducing the total demand it must meet. Grossly, atrophic tissues or organs are smaller than normal.

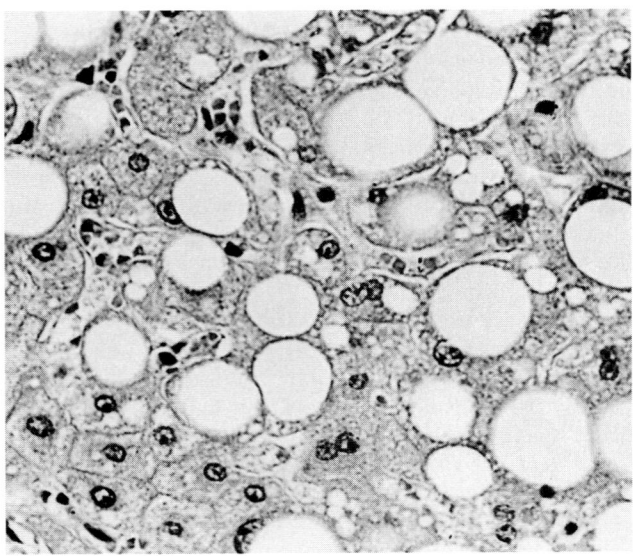

FIG. 3-3 Fatty change in liver. Many liver cells have several small "holes" in their cytoplasm or a single huge vacuole that distorts the entire cell. These apparently empty spaces once contained abundant lipid, which was dissolved during histologic preparation. The liver cells at the lower left are virtually normal. (Photomicrograph, ×500.)

In the course of becoming atrophic, the cell must absorb some of its constituent parts. This involves *autophagocytosis* or *autophagy*, literally a self-eating process, during which enzymes digest portions of the cell contained within cytoplasmic vacuoles. This same process occurs not only in the cell undergoing atrophy but also in the "wear and tear" of everyday cellular existence. When cytoplasmic organelles become damaged, they are sequestered within cytoplasmic vacuoles and digested enzymatically. The digestion process tends to leave traces of residual indigestible material, which gradually accumulates within the cells. This material is derived for the most part from membranous structures within the cells and generally has a dark-brown color. As cells age, they accumulate more and more of this intracytoplasmic pigment, referred to as *lipofuscin, aging pigment*, or *wear-and-tear pigment*. As cells become atrophic, lipofuscin may become even more concentrated because of increased autophagocytic activity. Occasionally, the atrophic tissue is pigmented, even grossly; the process responsible is called *brown atrophy*. Insoluble residual material may also accumulate as the result of *heterophagocytosis* or *heterophagy*, which is the cellular uptake of materials from outside the cell.

A discussion of degenerative changes must inevitably focus on the topic of aging. Clearly, the process of aging or senescence is exceedingly complex and involves many genetic, endocrine, immunologic, and environmental factors. The process is poorly understood at all levels, that is, from the level of the whole individual down to the level of single cells. Theories suggest that aging may result from an actual genetic limitation on the replicative ability of cells, coupled with the progressive accumulation of small injuries in cells that no longer proliferate. However, identifying any cellular features specific to the process of aging is not yet possible, and the true functional implications of even the nonspecific changes are unknown.

CELLULAR DEATH

If a noxious influence on a cell is severe enough or continued long enough, the cell will reach a point at which it can no longer compensate and cannot carry on metabolically. At some hypothetic point of no return, the processes become irreversible and the cell is in effect dead. At this hypothetic instant of death, when the cell simply reaches the point of no return, it may be impossible to recognize morphologically that the cell is irreversibly dead. However, if a group of cells that has reached this state remains in the living host for even a few hours, additional events occur that permit the recognition of the cells or the tissue as being dead. All cells have within them a variety of enzymes, many of them lytic. While the cell is alive, these enzymes do no damage to the cell, but they are released when the cell dies and begin to dissolve various cellular constituents. Additionally, as the dead cells change chemically, the living tissues immediately adjacent respond to the changes and mount an acute inflammatory reaction (see Chapter 4). Part of this latter reaction is the delivery of many leukocytes or white blood cells to the area, and these cells assist in the digestion of the dead cells. Thus, from their own digestive enzymes or as a result of the inflammatory process, the cells that have reached the point of no return begin to undergo discernible morphologic changes.

When a cell, a group of cells, or tissue in a living host is recognizably dead, it is referred to as *necrotic*. Necrosis therefore represents local cell death.

Morphologic Changes of Necrosis

Generally, although the lytic changes in necrotic tissue may involve the cytoplasm of cells, the nuclei manifest the changes most clearly, indicative of cell death. Typically, the nucleus of the dead cell shrinks, develops an irregular outline, and stains densely with the usual dyes that pathologists use. This process is referred to as *pyknosis*, and the nuclei are said to be *pyknotic*. Alternatively, nuclei may crumble, leaving scattered fragments of chromatin material within the cell. This process is referred to as *karyorrhexis*. Finally, in some instances, the nuclei of dead cells lose their staining ability and simply disappear, the process being referred to as *karyolysis* (Fig. 3-4).

The morphologic appearance of necrotic tissue varies, depending on the results of lytic activities within the dead tissue. When the activity of lytic enzymes is inhibited somewhat by local conditions, the necrotic cells will maintain their outline and the tissue will maintain its architectural features for some time. This type of necrosis is called *coagulative necrosis* and is particularly common when deprivation of blood supply causes the necrosis (Fig. 3-5). Generally, coagulative necrosis is the most frequently encountered type of necrosis. In some instances, the necrotic tissue gradually liquefies through enzymatic action; the process is called *liquefactive necrosis*. This condition is likely to occur in an area of necrotic brain, and the result is literally a hole in the brain filled with fluid (Fig. 3-6). In other situations, the necrotic cells disintegrate, but the finely divided cellular fragments remain in the area for months or even years, virtually undigested. This type of necrosis is referred to as *caseous necrosis* because the affected area has the appearance of crumbly cheese when viewed grossly (Fig. 3-7). A

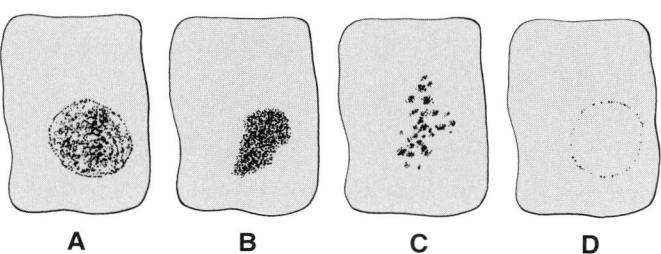

FIG. 3-4   Nuclear changes in cell death. The morphologic changes most clearly indicative of cell death involve the nucleus. **A**, Normal nucleus; **B**, pyknotic nucleus; **C**, karyorrhectic nucleus; and **D**, nucleus that has undergone karyolysis.

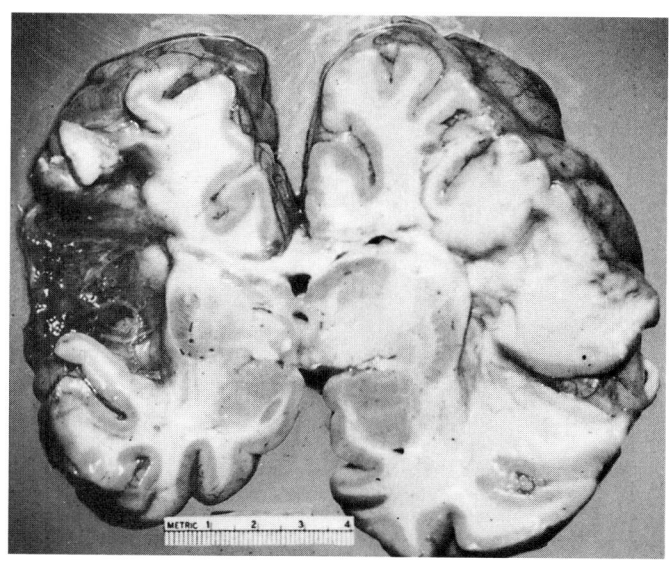

FIG. 3-6   Liquefactive necrosis. A large defect is seen at the left in this section of the brain. The brain substance in this area became necrotic because of deprivation in the blood supply. As is generally true in this organ, the necrotic tissue gradually softened, then liquefied, leaving a permanent defect.

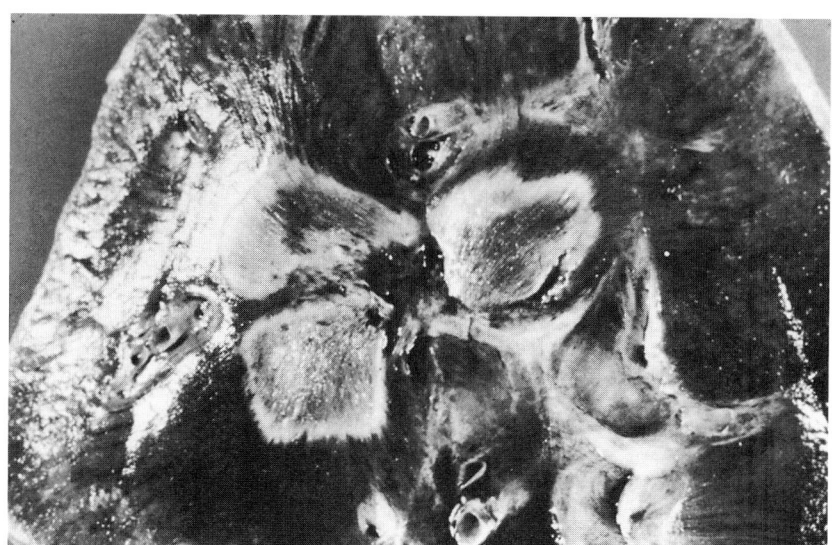

FIG. 3-5   Coagulative necrosis. In this close-up of the cut surface of a kidney, three pale areas of necrosis can be seen approximately in the center of the field. The architectural outlines are obviously maintained in the dead tissue, hence the designation of coagulative necrosis. (Because the renal papillae are involved, this condition is specifically termed *renal papillary necrosis*.)

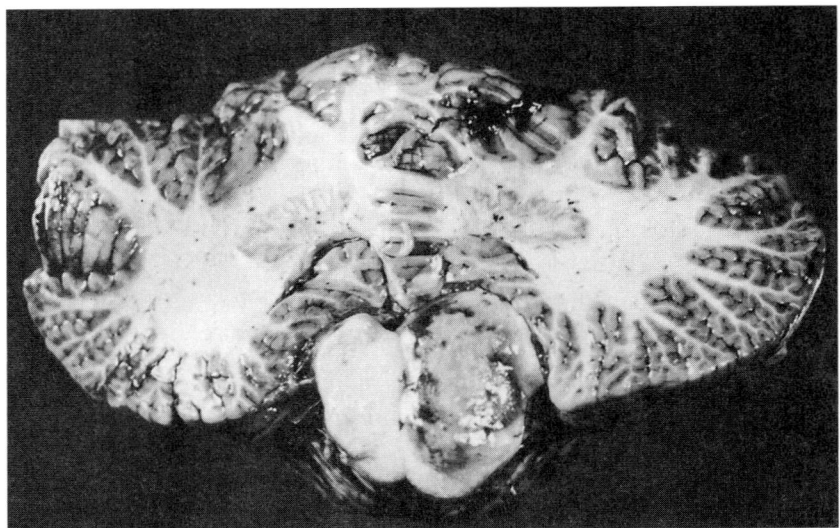

FIG. 3-7 Caseous necrosis. A large necrotic area is evident in the brainstem at the right of center. In this instance the dead tissue crumbled but did not liquefy. Because of an apparent gross resemblance to cheese, this type of necrosis is termed *caseous*. (This particular lesion was the result of tuberculosis, one of many causes of caseation.)

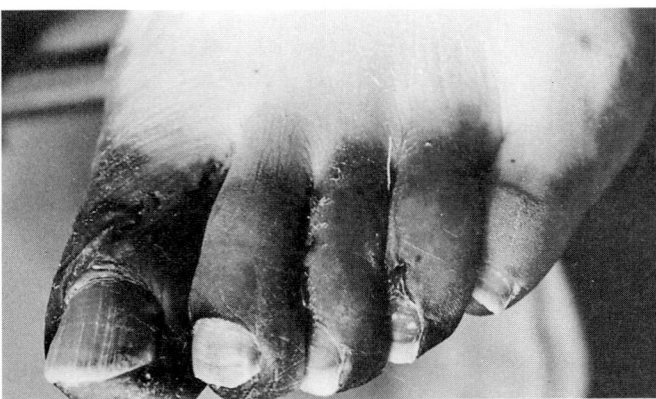

FIG. 3-8 Gangrene. The toes of this foot have become necrotic because of poor blood supply. Saprophytic microorganisms are growing in the blackened dead tissue. On the extremities, gangrene of this type is frequently termed *dry*.

standard situation that gives rise to caseous necrosis is tuberculosis, although this type of necrosis can arise in many other situations.

Certain special local conditions produce other variants of necrosis. *Gangrene* is defined as coagulative necrosis, usually resulting from a deprivation of blood supply, with superimposed growth of saprophytic bacteria. Gangrene occurs in necrotic tissues that are exposed to living bacteria. This condition is common in the extremities (Fig. 3-8) or in a segment of bowel that becomes necrotic (Fig. 3-9). The shriveled, blackened tissue of a gangrenous area on an extremity is often described as being the seat of *dry gangrene,* whereas on an internal area that cannot become desiccated, it is designated as *moist gangrene.* In either situation, the process involves the growth of saprophytic bacteria superimposed on necrotic tissue.

Necrotic adipose tissue constitutes another special case. When the duct system of the pancreas is ruptured, either by trauma or in the course of spontaneous disease of the pancreas, the pancreatic enzymes ordinarily carried within the duct may be spilled into the surrounding tissues. The secretions of the pancreas contain many powerful hydrolytic enzymes, including lipases that cleave

the lipids of adipose tissue. When this cleavage occurs, free fatty acids are formed by enzymatic action and these are rapidly combined with cations (e.g., calcium ions) in the area, producing deposits of soaps. This *enzymatic* (or pancreatic) *fat necrosis* is largely restricted to the abdominal cavity, because this is the area exposed to leaking pancreatic enzymes. When adipose tissue elsewhere becomes necrotic, spillage of lipid from the dead cells may evoke an inflammatory response, but no formation of the yellow, chalky deposits characteristic of enzymatic fat necrosis occurs.

Apoptosis: Programmed Cell Death

In recent years, another pattern of cell death referred to as *apoptosis* has been recognized. This form of cell death is actually programmed by genetic information already within the cell; that is, gene activation or release of some process from normal inhibition triggers the events that lead to cell death. A variety of extrinsic injurious stimuli can trigger apoptosis, but it can also be part of the physiologic relationship of cell populations. The process usually involves single cells or groups of a few cells, and as the cells die, they fragment into membrane-bound pieces that are rapidly phagocytosed by adjacent cells or macrophages. The process is morphologically subtle, with little or none of the obvious inflammatory response observed in conjunction with various patterns of necrosis.

Programmed cell death or apoptosis is needed for proper development as much as is mitosis. Examples include the following: (1) the formation of the fingers and toes of the fetus requires the removal, by apoptosis, of the tissue between them; (2) the sloughing of the endometrium at the start of menstruation occurs by apoptosis; and (3) the formation of the proper connections (synapses) between neurons in the brain requires that surplus cells be eliminated by apoptosis.

Programmed cell death is also needed to destroy cells that represent a threat to the integrity of the organism, such as the following: (1) cells infected with viruses; (2) cells of the immune system; (3) cells with DNA damage; and (4) cancer cells. One of the methods by which cytotoxic T cells kill virus-infected cells is by inducing apoptosis

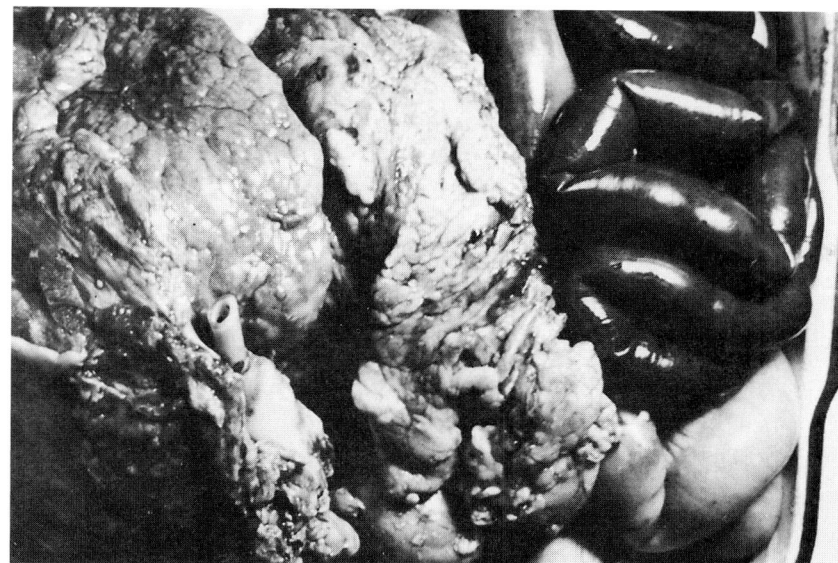

FIG. 3-9   Gangrene. In this instance a major portion of small intestine has been deprived of its blood supply. The gangrenous loops of intestine at the upper right contrast with the viable ones at the lower right. Saprophytes flourish in the necrotic tissue. Internal gangrene of this type is inevitably *moist* as contrasted to that on the extremities.

(see Chapter 5). Some viruses also mount countermeasures to thwart apoptosis. As cell-mediated immune responses wane, cytotoxic T cells induce apoptosis in each other and even in themselves to avert attack on body constituents. Apoptosis appears to be the mechanism responsible for the progressive depletion of CD4+ cells (T helper lymphocytes) in human immunodeficiency virus (HIV) infection and acquired immunodeficiency syndrome (AIDS) (see Chapter 15). Defects in the apoptotic machinery are associated with autoimmune diseases such as lupus erythematosus and rheumatoid arthritis. Damage to the DNA of a cell can cause the cell to disrupt proper embryonic development or to become cancerous. Cells normally increase their production of p53, a potent inducer of apoptosis, as a response to DNA damage. Not suprisingly, mutations in the p53 gene, producing a defective protein, are often found in cancer cells that represent a lethal threat to the organism if permitted to live. In other words, apoptosis fails to occur in the cell with damaged DNA and the cell becomes malignant.

The molecular mechanisms leading to apoptosis are currently the focus of intense research. That cell death is a normal part of normal biologic processes is increasingly clear. This fact has not been appreciated until recently, and an understanding of such death and an ability to manipulate it may allow therapeutic intervention in major diseases such as cancer, autoimmunity, AIDS, degenerative diseases, and others.

Effects of Necrosis

The most obvious effect of necrosis is loss of function in the dead area. If the necrotic tissue represents a small fraction of an organ with a large reserve (e.g., the kidney), then no functional effect on the body occurs, whereas if the area of necrosis is in a portion of brain, then a severe neurologic deficit or even death may result. Additionally, the necrotic area in some instances can become a focus of infection, representing an excellent culture medium for the growth of certain organisms that may then spread elsewhere in the body. Even without becoming infected, the presence of necrotic tissue within the body may evoke

certain systemic changes (e.g., fever), increased numbers of leukocytes within the circulating blood, and a variety of subjective symptoms. Finally, the necrotic tissue often leaks its constituent enzymes into the bloodstream as the cells die, and the permeability of cell membranes increases. Analyzing a specimen of blood and determining the level of various enzymes, such as creatine phosphokinase (CPK), lactic dehydrogenase (LDH), or aspartate aminotransferase (AST), is possible. Then an increased level of one or another enzyme may indicate that the patient has an area of necrosis hidden deep in some tissue. This principle has given rise to an important diagnostic field, *clinical enzymology*.

FATE OF NECROTIC TISSUE

When an area of tissue becomes necrotic, the event usually evokes an *inflammatory response* from the adjacent tissues (see Chapter 4). As a result of this inflammatory response, the dead tissue is ultimately demolished and removed, making way for the reparative process that replaces the necrotic area with regenerating cells of the sort that are lost or, in many instances, with scar tissue. When the necrotic tissue is located on a body surface (e.g., along the lining of the gastrointestinal tract), it may slough off, leaving a gap in the continuity of the surface, which is referred to as an *ulcer*. Finally, when the necrotic area is neither demolished nor cast off, it is often encapsulated by fibrous connective tissue and is ultimately impregnated with calcium salts precipitated from the circulating blood in the area of necrosis. This process of calcification may lead to the necrotic area becoming stony hard and remaining so for the life of the individual.

PATHOLOGIC CALCIFICATION

The deposition of insoluble calcium salts from the bloodstream, which renders tissues rigid and hard, is perfectly normal in the formation of bones and teeth. When this phenomenon occurs elsewhere, it is abnormal and is referred to as *pathologic calcification* or *heterotopic calcification*. This condition may occur in several situations.

Dystrophic Calcification

Frequently, as described earlier, injured tissue or necrotic tissue that is not quickly demolished may become a site of calcification. This particular form of calcification is referred to as *dystrophic*. Because an area of caseous necrosis by its very nature remains undigested for long periods, it typically becomes calcified. Thus, because tiny foci of tuberculosis or other infections occur in the lung and in the lymph nodes draining the lung, small foci of dystrophic calcification often appear in these areas. These foci are not particularly important biologically, but they often appear on radiographs because of the opacity of the dense deposits of calcium salts. Another common site of dystrophic calcification is in the wall of arteries that have become atherosclerotic (see Chapter 7). In fact, the texture of this "hardening of the arteries" is caused by the calcium deposition. Calcium salts also tend to deposit, with advancing age, in previously cartilaginous areas such as the rib cartilages. Ultimately, dystrophic calcific deposits in any location may undergo actual conversion to bone; the process is called *heterotopic ossification*.

Metastatic Calcification

Calcium salts may also be deposited in the soft tissues of the body in the absence of prior tissue damage or necrosis. This type of calcification is referred to as *metastatic calcification*. This process occurs not because of an abnormality of tissues, but because an abnormal concentration of calcium and phosphorus salts exists within the circulating blood. Specifically, when the concentration of these substances rises beyond a certain critical level, their solubility product is exceeded and precipitation occurs in a variety of tissues, especially lung, kidney, stomach, and the walls of blood vessels. Activity of the parathyroid glands, renal function, intake of calcium and vitamin D in the diet, and the integrity of the skeleton can affect the concentrations of calcium and phosphates in the blood. Thus metastatic calcification may be seen with hyperparathyroidism, decreased renal function, abnormal diet, and destructive lesions of the skeletal system that liberate large quantities of calcium salts from the bones.

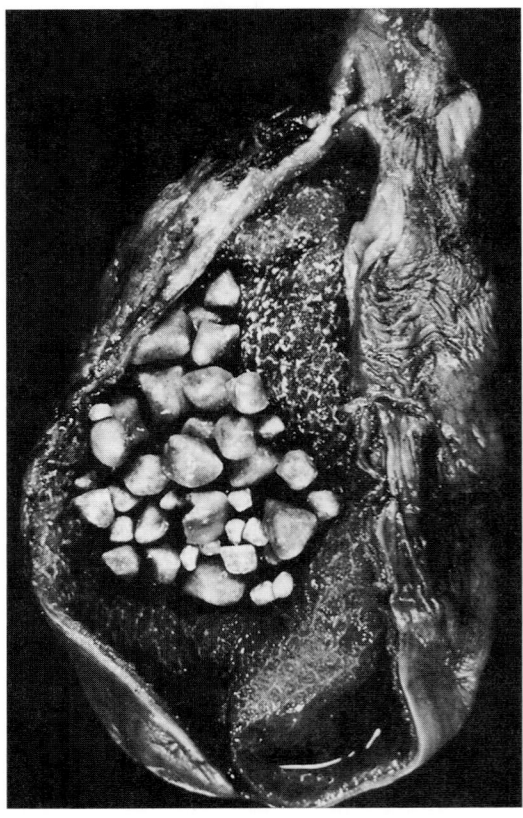

FIG. 3-10 Gallstones within the gallbladder. Calculi of this type are composed largely of bile pigments and cholesterol. It is apparent that stones of this size may be propelled into the common bile duct, where they can obstruct the flow of bile.

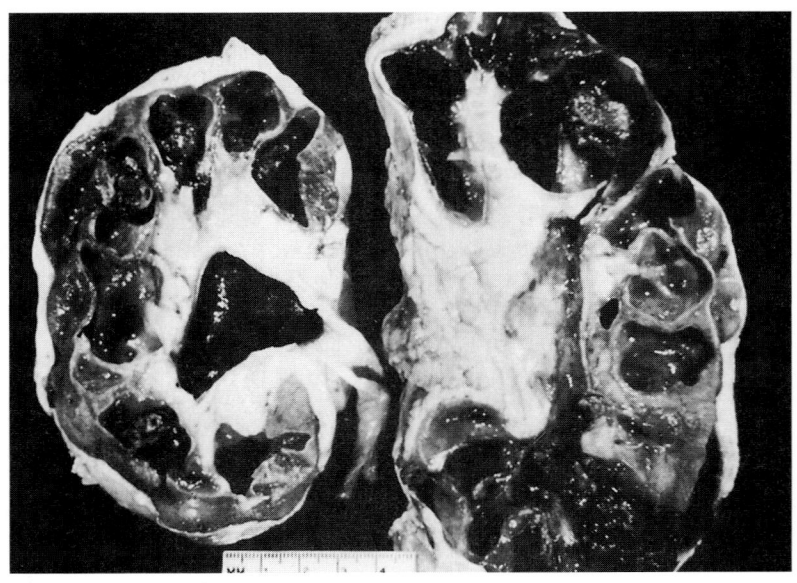

FIG. 3-11 Renal calculi. Numerous large stones are present within the calyces and pelvis of these hemisected kidneys. The associated obstruction of urine flow and infection have led to marked loss of renal parenchyma.

Stone Formation

Calcium salts may also be deposited in the form of stones, or *calculi,* within the duct systems of a variety of organs. Calculi may be formed from calcium or from a variety of other locally available substances within the secretions of the particular organ. Thus, although they frequently contain calcium as one constituent, many calculi are not primarily calcific. Some calculi form as a result of encrustation of necrotic debris within a duct, whereas others form because of an imbalance in the constituents of a particular secretion such that precipitation occurs from what is ordinarily a dissolved state. For a variety of reasons therefore, calculi are often encountered in the biliary tract (Fig. 3-10), the pancreas, the salivary glands, the prostate, and the urinary system.

Although calculi are often silent and discovered incidentally, if at all, many move along the duct system of the particular organ and cause pain and bleeding. Calculi may lodge in the narrow part of the duct system and produce obstruction of the outflow of the particular secretion, which frequently causes infection of the obstructed organ and atrophy of the parenchyma (Fig. 3-11).

SOMATIC DEATH

Death of the entire individual, as contrasted to localized death or necrosis, is referred to as *somatic death.* In the past the definition of somatic death was a relatively simple matter. An individual was declared dead when "vital functions" such as heart action and respiration ceased beyond any chance of reversal. Thus when an individual stopped breathing and could not be resuscitated, the heart rather quickly stopped beating as a result of anoxia, and the individual was indisputably dead. Today, with technologic advances, a patient can be attached to a mechanical ventilator when breathing stops. If the patient's heart begins to falter, then an electronic pacemaker may be put in place. With such "life-sustaining" machinery available, the definition of death becomes a different matter. In fact, not all cells of the body die at once. Living tissue cultures have been established from tissues removed from corpses. In hospitals today, a common definition of somatic death concerns the activity of the central nervous system, specifically the brain. Clearly, when the brain is actually dead, no chance exists for the subject to regain a conscious state. Such "brain death" involves irreversible loss of responsivity, including certain key reflexes, and irreversible loss of electrical activity, as indicated by an isoelectric or "flat" electroencephalogram (EEG) reading. When the absence of electrical activity has been demonstrated for a predetermined period under rigidly defined circumstances, medical authorities consider the patient dead, despite the fact that heart and lung actions may be artificially continued for some time.

Postmortem Changes

After death, certain so-called postmortem changes ensue. Because of a chemical reaction in the muscles of the dead subject, a stiffness called *rigor mortis* develops. The phrase *algor mortis* refers to the inevitable cooling of a dead subject as the body temperature approaches environmental temperature. Another set of changes is referred to as *livor mortis* or postmortem lividity. Generally, this lividity results because when the circulation stops, the blood within the vessels settles according to the pull of gravity, and the tissues lowermost in the body develop a purple discoloration because of their increased content of blood. At a microscopic level, as the individual tissues within the corpse die, their enzymes are released locally, and lytic reactions begin. These reactions, termed *postmortem autolysis* (literally self-dissolution), are similar to the changes observed in necrotic tissue but, of course, are not accompanied by an inflammatory reaction. Finally, unless prevented by special measures (e.g., embalming), massive bacterial overgrowth and putrefaction will occur. The speed of onset of various postmortem changes is extremely variable, depending on individual and associated environmental characteristics. Thus the amazingly accurate pinpointing of the time of death by medical authorities in detective fiction is largely just that—fiction.

KEY CONCEPTS

- A typical human cell is bounded by a cell membrane with an internal aqueous cytoplasm that contains a nucleus and various organelles.
- The *cell membrane* gives the cell its shape and attaches it to other cells. The cell membrane functions as a gateway, which allows for selective transport of nutrients and waste products into and out of the cell, generates membrane potentials, and serves as a communication channel for control signals from around the body.
- The *nucleus* contains the genomic DNA, which codes for the synthesis of proteins.
- The *endoplasmic reticulum* and the *Golgi apparatus* function together to synthesize proteins under the control of RNA in the ribosomes according to the directions of DNA.
- *Mitochondria* are organelles involved in the production of ATP, the energy currency of the cell.
- *Lysosomes* are membrane-bound packages of digestive enzymes that degrade intracellular debris and phagocytized materials.
- *Modes of injury to the cell* include deprivation of oxygen (hypoxia) or essential nutrients, physical agents (e.g., mechanical trauma, extremes of heat or cold, radiation, electric shock), chemical agents and drugs, infectious agents, immunologic reactions, and genetic derangements (e.g., the many inborn errors of metabolism arising from enzymatic abnormalities).
- The *order of changes in an injured cell* is, at first, biochemical, then functional, and finally morphologic changes (lesion).
- *Sublethal or reversible morphologic changes in injured cells* include cellular swelling and hydropic change (water droplets) in the cytoplasm caused by failure of the Na+/K+ pump in the cell membrane. Fat

- may also accumulate in the cell (fatty infiltration or degeneration) in conditions of overfeeding, starvation, or alcoholism.

- *Necrosis* is a type of irreversible cell death that occurs when an injury is severe or prolonged to the extent that the cell cannot adapt or repair itself. The cell nucleus undergoes progressive destruction known as *pyknosis, karyorrhexis,* and finally *karyolysis.*

- Different tissues typically exhibit different morphological *patterns of necrosis:* coagulative (heart, kidney, spleen); liquefactive (brain and spinal cord); caseous (lung); dry gangrene (extremities); wet gangrene (intestines); and enzymatic fat necrosis (pancreas).

- Local and systemic indicators of necrosis include loss of organ function (if sufficiently extensive), inflammation surrounding the area of necrosis, fever, malaise, leukocytosis, and elevated serum enzymes.

- Three major types of pathologic calcification have been identified: *dystrophic calcification* occurs in an area of necrosis despite normal serum calcium and in the absence of derangements in calcium metabolism; *metastatic calcification* consists of the deposition of calcium salts in the soft tissues of the body and almost always occurs in the presence of a disturbance in calcium metabolism (e.g., hyperparathy-

roidism); and *calculi* are stones, usually containing calcium, that form in the duct system of an organ.

- *Apoptosis* (pronounced ap-a-tow′-sis) is a genetically mediated type of *programmed cell death or suicide* that is a central part of normal development, in contrast to necrosis, which is not observed in normal development and is invariably a response to injury or toxic damage. Apoptosis characteristically affects scattered individual cells and does not result in inflammation, in contrast to necrosis, which usually involves tracts of contiguous cells with an area of surrounding inflammation.

- Apoptosis is involved in organogenesis; tissue homeostasis such as destruction of cells infected by a virus, cancer cells, or DNA damage; and the editing of the immune system to remove autoreactive clones.

- *Criteria for somatic death* include irreversible cessation of circulatory function (heartbeat), pulmonary function (breathing), and brain function (all signs of responsivity absent, including brainstem reflexes and an isoelectric [flat] electroencephalogram).

- Postmortem changes include *rigor mortis* (stiffening), *livor mortis* (bluish-purple color), *algor mortis* (cooling), and autolysis (self-dissolution).

- Precise fixing of the time of death by medical authorities is largely fiction.

QUESTIONS ??

A sampling of review questions for this chapter appears here. Visit http://www.mosby.com/MERLIN/PriceWilson/ for additional questions.

Fill in the blanks with the correct words.

1. The sequence of events involved in cellular degeneration includes
   _____, _____, and finally
   _____ alterations.
2. Somatic death concerns the activity of the _____ system, especially
   the _____.
3. Two major categories of pathologic calcification are _____ and
   _____.
4. After death, a chemical reaction in the muscles causing them to stiffen produces
   _____.

— · — · — · — · — · — · — · — · —

Match the type of necrosis in column A with its characteristic manifestation or description in column B.

Column A	**Column B**
5. _____ Coagulative necrosis	a. Massive necrosis with superimposed bacterial growth
6. _____ Liquefactive necrosis	b. Characteristic of tuberculosis or fungal infections
7. _____ Caseation	c. Events leading to cell death triggered by gene activation
8. _____ Enzymatic fat necrosis	d. Characteristic necrosis of heart and kidney resulting from ischemia
9. _____ Gangrene	e. Related to rupture of the pancreatic duct system
10. _____ Apoptosis	f. Characteristic of brain

— · — · — · — · — · — · — · — · —

Match the type of cell death in column B to its characteristics in column A.

Column A	**Column B**
11. _____ Genetically programmed cell death	a. Necrosis
12. _____ Induced by mechanical or toxic injury	b. Apoptosis
13. _____ Only a few scattered cells involved	
14. _____ Surrounding inflammatory response	
15. _____ Little or no inflammation	
16. _____ Part of normal physiologic cell relations	
17. _____ Large areas of contiguous cells involved	

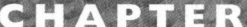

CHAPTER

4

Response of the Body to Injury

Inflammation and Repair

LORRAINE M. WILSON

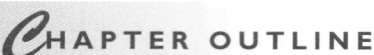HAPTER OUTLINE

▥ INFLAMMATORY REACTION

Whenever cells or tissues of the body are injured or killed, as long as the host survives, the surviving adjacent tissues make a striking response called *inflammation*. More specifically, inflammation is a vascular reaction during which the net result is the delivery of fluid, dissolved substances, and cells from the circulating blood into the interstitial tissues in an area of injury or necrosis.

The natural tendency is to view inflammation as something undesirable, because an inflamed throat, skin, or soft tissue can cause considerable discomfort. However, inflammation is actually a beneficial and defensive phenomenon. The net result is the neutralization and elimination of an offending agent, the demolition of necrotic tissue, and the establishment of conditions necessary for repair and restitution. The events that occur when the body cannot produce a needed inflammatory reaction dramatically demonstrates the beneficial character of the inflammatory reaction, for example, when it becomes necessary to administer high doses of drugs that also suppress such reactions. Under these conditions, ordinarily harmless microorganisms can cause a high incidence of extremely severe, rapidly spreading, or even lethal infections.

The inflammatory reaction is actually a dynamic and continuous succession of well-coordinated events. To manifest an inflammatory reaction, a tissue must be alive and, in particular, must possess a functional microcirculation. If an area of tissue necrosis is extensive, then the inflammatory reaction will be found not in its midst, but rather at its edges, that is, at the interface between the dead tissue and living tissue with an intact circulation. Additionally, when a particular injury kills the host instantly, no evidence exists of an associated inflammatory reaction, because the response would take time to develop.

The causes of inflammation are numerous and varied, and understanding that *inflammation and infection are not synonymous* is essential. Thus *infection* (the presence of living microorganisms within the tissue) is simply one cause of inflammation. Inflammation can easily occur under conditions of perfect sterility, such as when a portion of tissue dies because of deprivation of blood supply. Because of the broad range of situations that result in inflammation, an understanding of the process is basic to much of biology and health care. Without an understanding of the process, comprehending the principles of infectious disease; the principles of surgery, wound healing, and the response to a variety of trauma; or the principles of how the body copes with catastrophes of tissue death such as cerebrovascular accidents (CVAs, strokes), "heart attacks," and the like is impossible.

Despite the numerous causes of inflammation and the variety of situations in which it appears, the events set in motion generally tend to be the same, with various types of inflammation differing in their quantitative detail. Therefore the inflammatory reaction can be studied as a general phenomenon, and the quantitative variations can be dealt with secondarily.

GROSS FEATURES OF ACUTE INFLAMMATION

Acute inflammation is the immediate response of the body to injury or cell death. The gross features were described some 2000 years ago and are still known as *cardinal signs of inflammation;* these include redness, warmth, pain, and swelling, or in the classic Latin, *rubor, calor, dolor,* and *tumor.* A fifth cardinal sign, altered function, or *functio laesa,* was added in the last century.

Rubor (Redness)

Rubor, or redness, is usually the first thing to be noted in an area becoming inflamed. As the inflammatory reaction begins, the arterioles supplying the area dilate thus allowing more blood into the local microcirculation. Capillaries that were previously empty, or perhaps only partly distended, quickly become packed with blood (Fig. 4-1). This condition, termed *hyperemia* or *congestion,* accounts for the local blush of acute inflammation. The body controls the production of hyperemia at the start of an inflammatory reaction, both neurologically and chemically, via the release of substances such as histamine.

Calor (Heat)

Calor, or heat, parallels the redness of an acute inflammatory reaction. Actually, heat is a characteristic only of inflammatory reactions at the body surface, which is normally cooler than the 37° C core temperature. An area of cutaneous inflammation becomes warmer than its surroundings because more blood (at 37° C) is being conducted from the inside of the body to the surface in the affected area compared with a normal area. This phenomenon of local warmth is not observed in inflamed areas deep within the body, because such tissues are already at the core temperature of 37° C and local hyperemia would make no difference.

Dolor (Pain)

The dolor, or pain, of an inflammatory reaction is likely produced in a variety of ways. Change in local pH or in

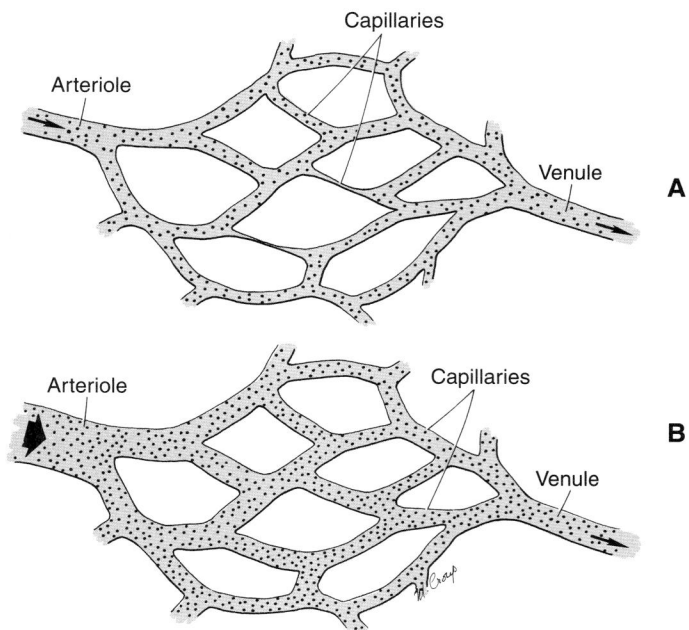

FIG. 4-1 Mechanism of hyperemia in acute inflammation. The caliber of the arteriole controls the volume flow of blood into a capillary bed. In the normal state, **A,** the flow is such that some capillaries appear collapsed and others extremely narrow. With arteriolar dilation, **B,** the increased volume of blood flowing into the capillaries distends them and produces the gross red-purple discoloration of tissue from increased blood content.

the local concentration of certain ions can stimulate nerve endings. Similarly, the release of certain chemicals, such as histamine or other bioactive chemicals, can stimulate the nerves. Additionally, swelling of inflamed tissues leading to increased local pressure can undoubtedly produce pain.

Tumor (Swelling)

Perhaps the most striking aspect of acute inflammation is the tumor, or local swelling produced by fluid and cells transferred from the bloodstream to the interstitial tissues. This mixture of fluid and cells that accumulates in an area of inflammation is called an *exudate.* Early in the course of inflammatory reactions, most of the exudate is fluid, such as that which appears quickly within a blister after a minor burn of the skin. Somewhat later, white blood cells, or leukocytes, leave the bloodstream and accumulate as part of the exudate.

Functio Laesa (Altered Function)

Functio laesa, or altered function, is a familiar part of the inflammatory reaction. In a superficial way, the means by which a swollen, painful part with an abnormal circulation and abnormal local chemical environment should function abnormally is easy to understand. However, the means whereby function of an inflamed tissue is impaired is not understood in detail.

FLUID ASPECTS OF INFLAMMATION

Exudation

To understand the rapid flux of fluid across vessel walls into inflamed tissue, recalling the principles governing normal fluid transport becomes necessary. Ordinarily, the walls of the smallest vascular channels (e.g., capillaries, venules) allow small molecules to pass but retain large molecules, such as plasma proteins, within the vascular lumen. The semipermeable character of the vessels produces an osmotic force that tends to keep fluid within the vasculature. This event is counterbalanced by the outward thrust of hydrostatic pressure within the vessels. A simplified diagram of the balance of forces is shown in Fig. 4-2. The lymphatics siphon off fluid that reaches the interstices of the tissue, and equilibrium is thus normally maintained.

Shifts of fluid in the evolving inflammatory reaction are exceedingly rapid, as illustrated by the previously cited example of a blister following thermal injury. Such inflammatory exudates contain significant amounts of plasma protein. Thus a key event in acute inflammation is the alteration of permeability of the tiny vessels in the area, which leads to protein leakage. This process is fol-lowed by a shift in osmotic balance, and water follows the protein, producing swelling of the tissues. The arteriolar dilation that produces local hyperemia and redness also results in an increase in intravascular pressure locally as vessels become engorged. This action, too, augments the fluid shift (see Fig. 4-2). The major factor, however, is the increase in vascular permeability to protein.

The endothelial cells that line the small vessels are responsible for the usual semipermeable character of the vessels, and it is these cells that change their relationship to one another in acute inflammation, producing the leakage of protein and fluid. In the normal small vessel (Fig. 4-3, A), the endothelial lining cells are joined tightly to one another. The dots in the lumen represent large molecules, such as those of serum proteins or of large marker particles injected experimentally to simulate protein molecules. Ordinarily, these large molecules or particles cannot penetrate the intercellular junctions. However, when an inflammatory reaction occurs locally, an actual separation between contiguous endothelial cells develops in the area and the marker particles (and presumably the protein molecules) exit from the lumen (Fig. 4-3, B). If a pigmented marker particle is used for such an experiment, entire vessels become discolored

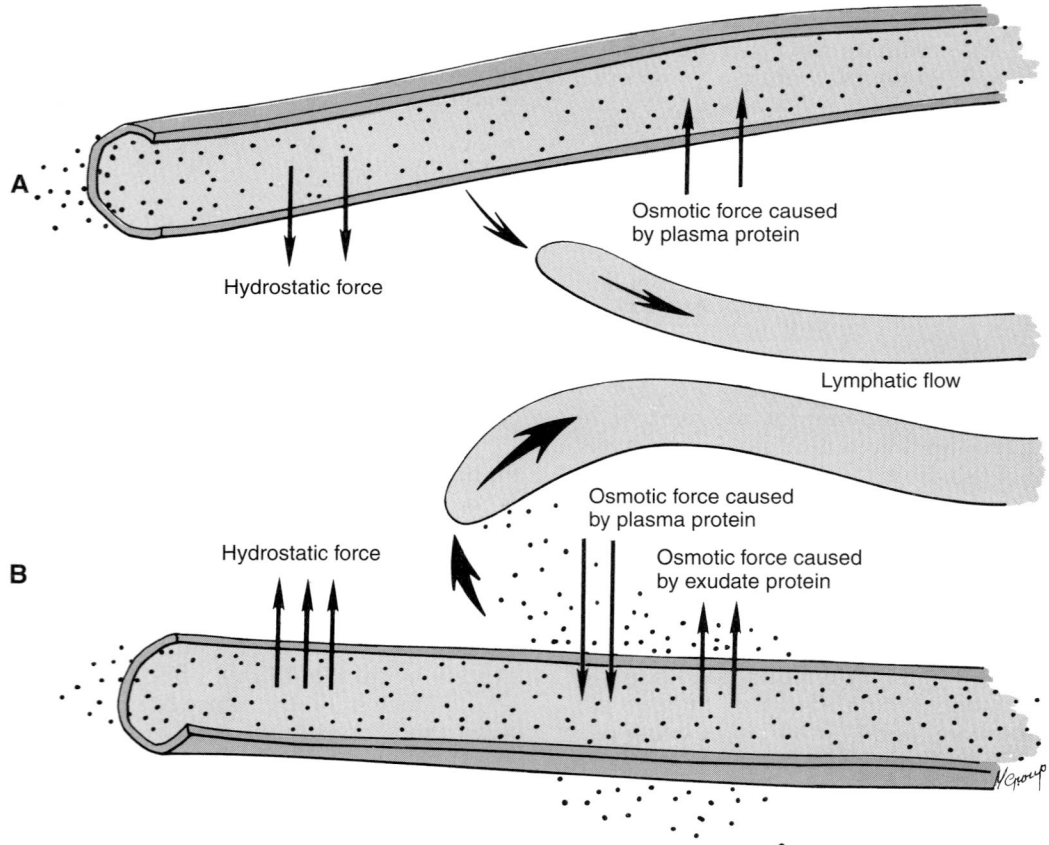

FIG. 4-2 Factors involved in fluid exchange between blood vessels and tissues. In the normal or resting state, **A**, hydrostatic forces tend to push fluid into the interstitial spaces. This is largely balanced by the osmotic force exerted by plasma proteins *(dots)* that ordinarily do not pass through vessel walls. The fluid that does pass into the interstices drains via the lymphatics. In acute inflammation, **B**, protein escapes from the vessels as permeability increases. This, along with a smaller contribution from the increased hydrostatic pressure related to hyperemia, accounts for a significant fluid flux. Lymphatic flow is correspondingly increased.

and observing which part of the microcirculation is actually leaking in the course of inflammation becomes possible. In most instances studied in this fashion, the leak appears to occur chiefly at the venular end of the microcirculation rather than within the true capillaries (Fig. 4-3, *C*).

Lymphatics and Flow of Lymph

Events in the lymphatic system parallel those in the blood vascular system in the acute inflammatory reaction. Ordinarily, interstitial fluid slowly percolates into lymphatic channels and the lymph is carried centrally in the body, ultimately to rejoin venous blood. As an area becomes inflamed, a striking increase usually occurs in the flow of lymph draining from the area. In the course of acute inflammation, the contiguous lining cells of the smallest lymphatics separate somewhat, just as they do within the venules, allowing more ready access to material from the interstices of tissues into the lymphatics. Lymphatic channels are likely maintained in an open position as a tissue swells by a system of connective tissue fibers anchored to the walls of the lymphatics. In any event, not only does the flow of lymph increase but also the protein and cell content of the lymph likewise increases during acute inflammation.

On the one hand, this increased flow of material through lymphatics is beneficial, because it tends to minimize the swelling of the inflamed tissue by draining off a portion of the exudate. However, lymphatics can carry potentially injurious agents from a primary site of inflammation to distant points in the body. By such means, infectious agents may spread. However, the filter-ing action of regional lymph nodes through which the lymph flows often limits this spread, but agents or materials carried within the lymph may pass through the nodes and eventually reach the bloodstream.

For these reasons, the possible involvement of the lymphatic system must always be considered in inflammation of any cause. *Lymphangitis* is the inflammation of a lymphatic vessel; *lymphadenitis* is the inflammation of a lymph node. Regional lymphadenitis often accompanies inflammation. One familiar example is the enlarged, tender cervical lymph nodes observed with tonsillitis. The more general term *lymphadenopathy* is used to describe virtually any abnormality of lymph nodes. In practice, the term refers not only to lymphadenitis but also to any enlargement of lymph nodes, because most nodal reactions are accompanied by enlargement.

CELLULAR ASPECTS OF INFLAMMATION

Margination and Emigration

As arterioles dilate early in acute inflammation, the flow of blood into the inflamed area increases. However, the character of the blood flow soon changes. As fluid leaks out of the microcirculation with its increased permeability, large numbers of formed elements (red blood cells, platelets, white blood cells) remain behind and the viscosity of the blood increases. The circulation within the affected area then slows, leading to some important consequences. Normally, the flow of blood is more or less streamlined (Fig. 4-4, *A*) and the formed

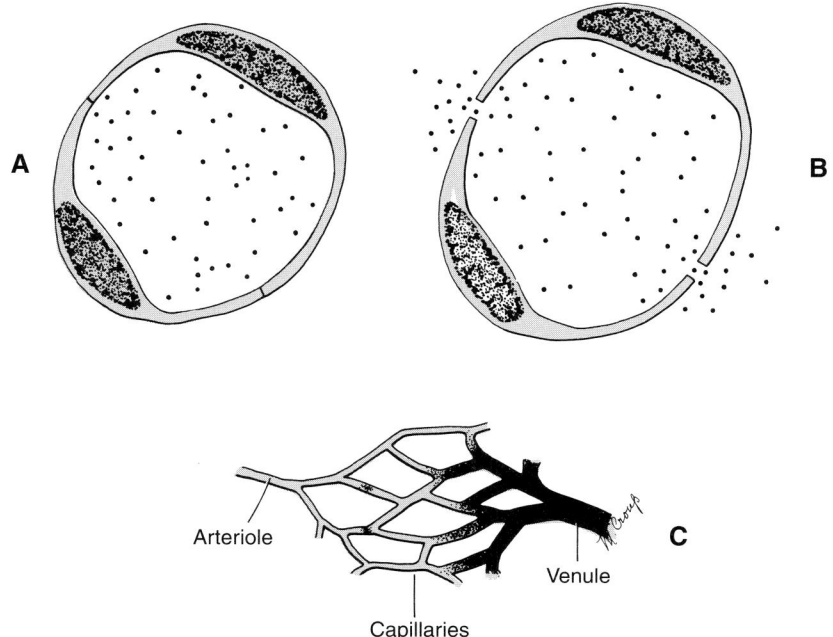

FIG. 4-3 Mechanism of increased vascular permeability in acute inflammation. In normal vessels, **A**, the junctions between endothelial lining cells are sufficiently tight to keep large molecules *(dots)* within the lumen. In acute inflammation, **B**, contraction of endothelial cells creates gaps that allow leakage of macromolecules. As shown in **C**, the permeability change is at the venular side of the microcirculatory bed.

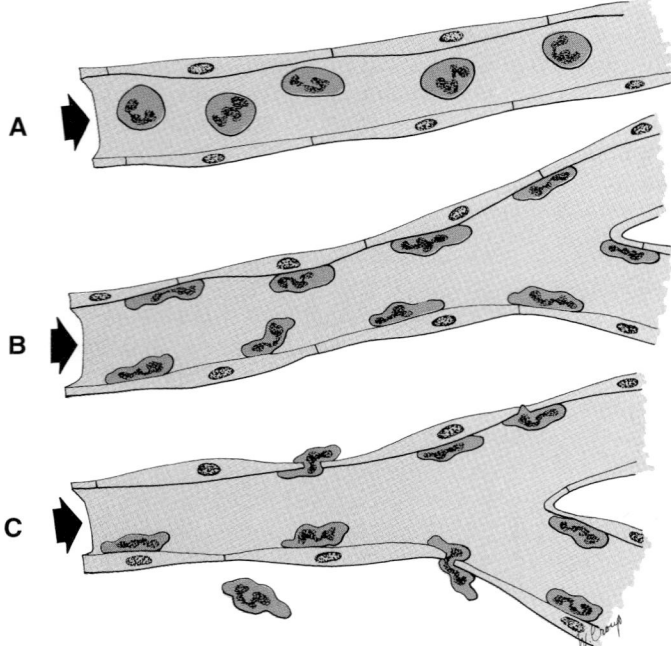

FIG. 4-4 Blood flow and cellular phenomena in acute inflammation. Normally, **A**, formed elements of the blood, especially the leukocytes shown, are carried in the main stream. As the circulation slows, **B**, margination of leukocytes occurs. This is a prelude to emigration of leukocytes between endothelial cells, **C**.

elements do not bump against the sides of the vessel appreciably. As the viscosity of the blood increases and the flow slows, the leukocytes begin to *marginate;* that is, they move to the periphery of the stream, along the lining of the vessel (Fig. 4-4, *B*). As the phenomenon progresses, the marginated leukocytes begin to adhere to the endothelium, producing an appearance reminiscent of a cobblestone street, thus giving rise to the term *pavementing.* Margination and pavementing are preludes to the emigration of leukocytes from the blood vessels to the surrounding tissue.

Leukocytes move in an ameboid fashion(Fig. 4-4, *C*); they appear to have the ability to extend a pseudopod into the potential space between two endothelial cells and then gradually push through to appear on the other side, a process—called *emigration* or *diapedesis*—requiring a matter of minutes. The result, because this event is repeated in innumerable venules and because more and more leukocytes are delivered into the area via the circulating blood, is that tremendous numbers of cells are delivered into the area of inflammation in a relatively short time. Literally millions of cells emigrate to even a small area of inflammation within several hours.

Chemotaxis

The movement of the leukocytes in the interstices of inflamed tissues after they emigrate is apparently not random but is directionally oriented by a variety of chemical "signals." This phenomenon is referred to as *chemotaxis.* Various agents may provide a chemotactic signal to attract leukocytes, including infectious agents, damaged

tissues, and substances activated within the protein fraction of plasma leaking from the bloodstream. Thus a smooth combination of increased delivery of leukocytes to the area (as a result of hyperemia), changes in blood flow resulting in margination and pavementing, and chemotactic orientation of leukocyte motion results in the rapid accumulation of a significant leukocytic component in the exudate.

MEDIATION OF INFLAMMATION

The dramatic vascular, fluid, and cellular phenomena of inflammation are obviously under meticulous control. Although some injuries directly damage vascular endothelium and by themselves lead to leakage of protein and fluid in the zone of injury, in most cases injury triggers the formation and/or release of chemical substances within the body, and these mediators elicit the phenomena of inflammation. Many types of injuries can activate the same endogenous mediators, which might explain the stereotyped character of the inflammatory response to diverse stimuli. The period of latency between the injurious stimulus and the development of inflammatory response also points to the role of mediators; the ability to circumvent certain aspects of the reaction with pharmacologic blocking agents emphasizes the importance of mediators.

Many endogenously released substances have been identified as mediators of the inflammatory response. This sort of knowledge has, on the one hand, led to a better understanding of deficiencies and perturbations of the inflammatory response and, on the other hand, suggested the means of suppressing unwanted inflammation when dictated by the clinical setting. Although the list of proposed mediators is long and complex, the better recognized mediators fall into the following classes:

1. Vasoactive amines
2. Substances produced by plasma enzyme systems
3. Arachidonic acid metabolites
4. Miscellaneous cell products

Histamine

The most important vasoactive amine is histamine, which is capable of producing vasodilation and increased vascular permeability. Large amounts of histamine are stored within the granules of connective tissue cells known as *mast cells,* which are widely distributed in the body (histamine is also present in blood basophils and platelets). The stored histamine is inactive and exerts its vascular effects only when released. Many physical injuries cause mast cell degranulation and histamine release. Some injuries first trigger activation of the serum complement system (described later and in Chapter 5), certain components of which then lead to histamine release. Some immunologic reactions (detailed in Chapter 5) also trigger release of this mediator from mast cells. Histamine is particularly important early in inflammation and is a prime mediator in some common allergic reactions. Antihistamines are drugs designed to block the mediator effects of histamine.

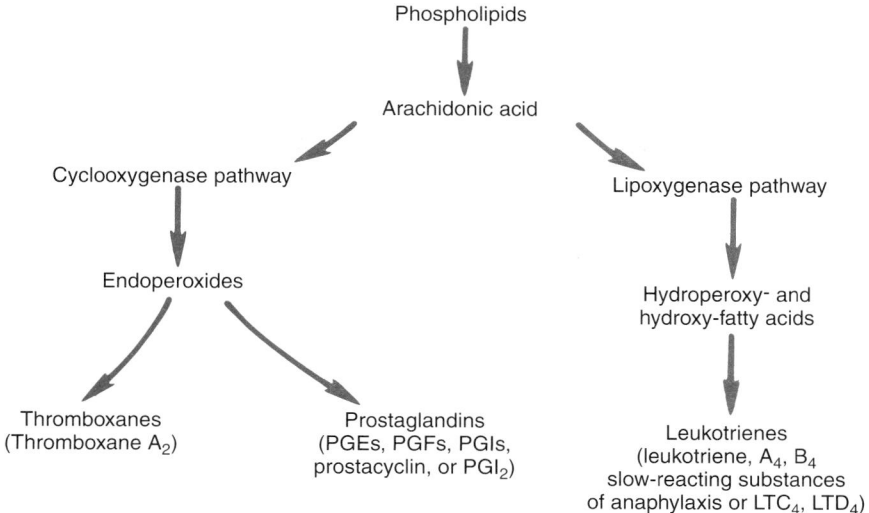

FIG. 4-5   Arachidonic acid metabolism and inflammatory mediators.

Plasma Factors

Blood plasma is a rich source of a number of important mediators. These are formed through the action of certain proteolytic enzymes that make up a sort of interconnected defensive system. The key agent coordinating these systems is the *Hageman factor (factor XII)*, which is present in the plasma in an inactive form and which can be activated by a variety of injuries. Activated Hageman factor triggers the clotting cascade, leading to the formation of fibrin (see Chapter 19). Clotting, per se, is an important defensive reaction to injury, but certain products derived from fibrin also act as vasoactive mediators in inflammation. Hageman factor also activates the plasminogen system, liberating plasmin or fibrinolysin. This protease not only splits fibrin but also activates the complement system. Several components of the complement system function as important inflammatory mediators. For example, derivatives of the third and fifth components, the *anaphylatoxins*, release histamine and affect vascular permeability. A derivative of the fifth component and a complex of the fifth, sixth, and seventh components are potent chemotactic agents when activated in tissues. These effects are important in many examples of inflammation, not only in immunologically provoked reactions (although, as described in Chapter 5, union of antigen and certain antibodies is a potent activator of the complement system). Activated Hageman factor also converts *prekallikrein* (an inactive substance in plasma) to *kallikrein* (a proteolytic enzyme), which, in turn, acts on plasma kininogen to liberate *bradykinin*, a peptide that dilates blood vessels and increases permeability.

Arachidonic Acid Metabolites

In recent years, attention has been directed to arachidonic acid metabolites as important inflammatory mediators. Arachidonic acid is derived from the phospholipid of many cell membranes when phospholipases are activated by injury (or by other mediators). Subsequently, two different pathways can metabolize arachidonic acid:

the *cyclooxygenase pathway* and the *lipoxygenase pathway*, yielding a variety of prostaglandins, thromboxanes, and leukotrienes (Fig. 4-5). These substances show a broad range of vascular and chemotactic effects in inflammation, and some are important in hemostasis as well. Aspirin and many nonsteroidal antiinflammatory drugs are now recognized as inhibiting the cyclooxygenase pathway.

Miscellaneous Cell Products

In addition to the mediators mentioned, a variety of cell-derived substances have properties that may also be important in inflammation. A partial list would include oxygen metabolites produced by neutrophils and macrophages, lysosomal contents of these cells (following discussion), and cytokines released by a variety of cells, particularly activated lymphocytes and macrophages. Cytokines that have an important role in mediating inflammation include *interleukins 1 and 8* (IL-1, IL-8) and *tumor necrosis factor (TNF)*. *Nitric oxide (NO)* is another cell-derived mediator discovered within recent years. This substance, produced by macrophages, endothelial cells, and other cells, can have important vasomotor effects, affect platelet function, and even act as a cytotoxic free radical. Finally, the mediation of leukocyte adhesion and transmigration has been shown to involve the binding of complementary adhesion molecules on the surfaces of endothelial cells and leukocytes. These molecules include *selectins, endothelial adhesion molecules,* and *integrins.* Certain mediators such as histamine and certain cytokines can stimulate the expression of selectins and other adhesion molecules (e.g., intercellular adhesion molecule 1 [ICAM-1], vascular cell adhesion molecule 1 [VCAM-1]) on endothelial surfaces. Then, as leukocytes are activated, integrins on their surfaces interact with the endothelial adhesion molecules, and the ultimate result is leukocyte extravasation.

Thus the total list of proposed mediators of inflammation is extensive, and knowledge of which substances are significantly involved in a given reaction is still quite limited. Considerable overlap and redundancy appear to be involved in effectively blocking inflammatory reactions.

TYPES OF LEUKOCYTES AND THEIR FUNCTIONS

Leukocytes that circulate in the bloodstream and emigrate into inflammatory exudates originate in the bone marrow, where red blood cells and platelets are also continuously produced (see Chapter 16). Normally within the bone marrow, large numbers of immature leukocytes of various types may be found, and a "pool" of mature leukocytes is held in reserve for release into the circulating blood. The numbers of each type of leukocyte circulating in the peripheral blood are closely limited (see Chapter 18) but are altered "on demand" when an inflammatory process arises. That is, with the instigation of an inflammatory response, feedback signals to the bone marrow alter the rate of production and release of one or more kinds of leukocytes into the bloodstream.

Granulocytes

Granulocytes, a class of leukocytes including neutrophils, eosinophils, and basophils, are so named because of the granules within the cytoplasm visible after the application of certain dyes. Two other types of leukocytes, monocytes and lymphocytes, do not contain the numerous cytoplasmic granules that characterize the previously listed cells. Although each of the types of cells listed is available in the circulating blood, leukocytes do not randomly appear within exudates, but likely as a result of specific chemotactic signals arising in the evolution of the inflammatory process.

The first cells to appear in large numbers within exudates in the early hours of inflammation are neutrophils. The nuclei of these cells are irregularly lobed or polymorphous (Fig. 4-6). These cells are therefore called *polymorphonuclear neutrophils, PMNs,* or *"polys."* These cells have a developmental sequence within the bone marrow that requires approximately 2 weeks for completion. When they are released into the circulating blood, their circulatory half-life is 6 hours or so. Approximately 5000 neutrophils per cubic millimeter of blood are in circulation at any given time, with approximately 100 times this number being held in reserve as mature cells within the bone marrow, ready to be released on signal. Although bone marrow replaces literally billions of neutrophils per day, their production and release are quite rigidly controlled.

When released into the bloodstream, PMNs are usually incapable of further cell division or significant synthesis of cellular enzymes. The numerous granules visible within the cytoplasm of the neutrophils, however, actually represent membrane-bound packets of enzymes *(lysosomes)* produced during maturation of the cells. These enzymes include a variety of hydrolases, including proteases, lipases, and phosphatases. Additionally, associated with the granules are a variety of antimicrobial substances. Thus, in effect, the mature PMN is a suitcase of enzyme-loaded and antimicrobial particles.

PMNs are capable of active ameboid motion and are able to engulf a variety of materials through a process called *phagocytosis.* As illustrated in Fig. 4-7, the neutrophil approaches the particle (e.g., a bacterium) to be phagocytosed, flows its cytoplasm around the particle, and eventually takes the particle into the cytoplasm enveloped in a membrane-bound vesicle that pinches off from the cell membrane of the neutrophil. Certain substances that coat the object to be ingested and render it more easily internalized by the leukocyte aid this phago-

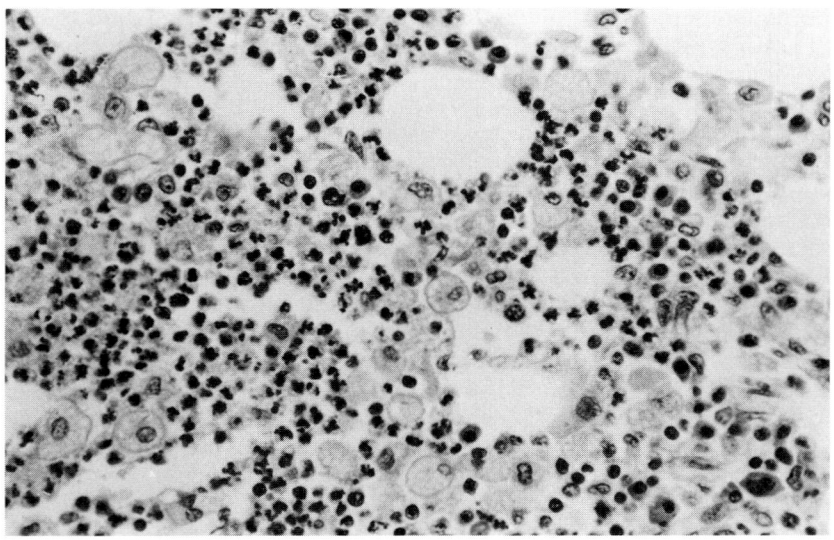

FIG. 4-6 Macrophages and neutrophils in connective tissue. These cells are part of a voluminous exudate that is formed, in this instance in response to bacterial infection. Most of the cells shown are neutrophils. Their cytoplasmic granules cannot be seen at this magnification, but their irregularly lobed (polymorphous) nuclei are evident. The macrophages are several-fold larger and, in this particular exudate, have a bubbly appearing cytoplasm. They are scattered but are prominent in the lower center and lower left of the field. (Photomicrograph, ×500.)

cytic process. These kinds of leukocytosis-promoting substances, called *opsonins*, include immunoglobulins (antibodies) and components of the complement system (see Chapter 5). Having ingested a particle and incorporated it into the cytoplasm in a *phagocytic vacuole* or *phagosome*, the leukocyte's next task is to kill the particle, if it is a living microbial agent, and to digest it. Living agents may be killed in a variety of ways, including altering the intracellular pH after phagocytosis, releasing antibacterial substances into the phagocytic vacuole, and producing antibacterial substances such as hydrogen peroxide (and other highly reactive oxygen metabolites) as a result of cellular metabolic processes initiated after the phagocytic event. The phagocytosed particles are generally digested within the vacuoles formed by fusion of lysosomes with phagosomes. The previously inactive digestive enzymes are now activated within these *phagolysosomes*, resulting in the enzymatic digestion of the objects.

Under certain circumstances, digestive enzymes and oxygen metabolites of the neutrophils may be released into the host tissues rather than into intracellular phagolysosomes. When this occurs, the neutrophils become potent agents of tissue injury. This extracellular release occurs with death and disintegration of neutrophils; it occurs after phagocytosis by neutrophils of certain crystals, such as urates (because phagocytosis of these crystals is followed by rupture of phagolysosomes); it also occurs when neutrophils attempt to ingest immune complexes under certain circumstances. These types of situations are described more fully in Chapters 5 and 12.

The *eosinophil* is another type of granulocyte that may appear in inflammatory exudates, although usually in relatively small quantities. Eosinophils have irregular nuclei similar to neutrophils, but the cytoplasmic granules stain a bright red when dyed with eosin and are much more prominent than are the lavender-colored granules of neutrophils. The granules of eosinophils are packets of enzymes quite similar to those of neutrophils. In fact, eosinophils have many of the same functions: they respond to chemotactic stimuli; they phagocytose various kinds of particles; and they even kill certain microorganisms. What appears to be distinctive about eosinophils, however, is that they respond to certain unique chemotactic stimuli generated in the course of allergic reactions and they contain substances toxic to certain parasites and substances that may mediate inflammatory reactions. Additionally, eosinophils tend to accumulate in significant concentrations at the site of parasitic infestation and allergic reactions.

The third type of granulocyte is the *basophil*, the cytoplasm of which is crowded with large granules that stain a deep blue with basic dyes. Although these cells come from the bone marrow as do other granulocytes, they have many features in common with certain cells of the connective tissues called *mast cells* or *tissue basophils*. The granules of both of these types of cells contain a variety of enzymes, heparin, and histamine. *Blood basophils* appear to respond to chemotactic signals released in the course of certain immunologic reactions and are ordinarily present in small numbers in exudates. Blood basophils and tissue mast cells are stimulated to release the contents of their granules into the surroundings in a variety of injurious circumstances, including both immunologic and nonspecific reactions. The mast cells are a major source of histamine early in any acute inflammatory reaction. The immunologic means of stimulating granule release by mast cells or basophils is discussed in Chapter 5.

Monocytes and Macrophages

The *monocyte* is a form of leukocyte that differs from the granulocyte because of its nuclear morphology and its relatively agranular cytoplasm (see Fig. 4-6). The monocyte also originates within the bone marrow, but its circulatory life is three to four times longer than that of granulocytes. In the course of acute inflammatory reactions, monocytes begin to emigrate at approximately the same time as do neutrophils, but they do so in much smaller numbers and at a slower rate. Consequently, in the early hours of inflammation, relatively few such cells are within exudate. However, as exudates age, the percentage of these cells usually increases. The same cell that is called a monocyte in the circulating blood is called a *macrophage* when it appears within exudates. In fact, the same type of cell is found wandering in small numbers through the connective tissues of the body, even in the absence of overt inflammation. These wandering macrophages in the connective tissues are known as *histiocytes*.

Macrophages have functions similar to those of PMNs in that macrophages are actively motile cells that respond to chemotactic stimuli, are actively phagocytic, and are able to kill and digest a variety of agents. Several important differences between macrophages and PMNs exist. First, macrophages may survive weeks or even months within the tissues, in contrast to the short-lived PMNs.

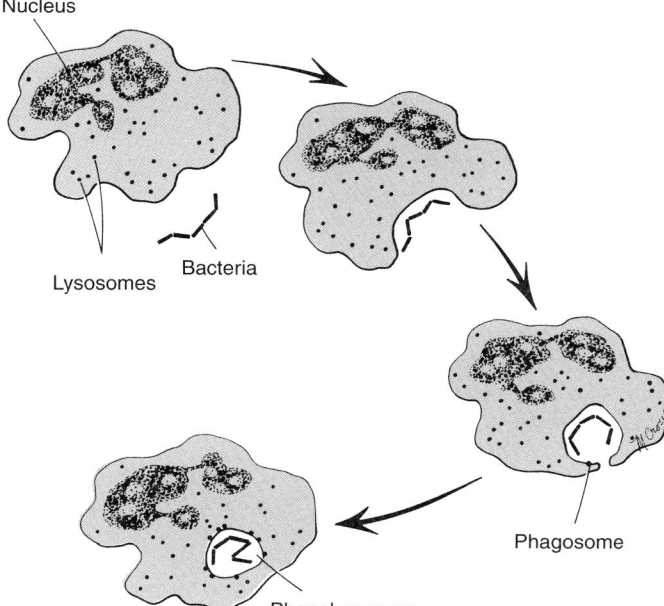

Nucleus

Lysosomes   Bacteria

Phagosome

Phagolysosome

FIG. 4-7   Diagram of phagocytosis. Neutrophils and monocytes ingest particles by flowing their cytoplasm around the objects and internalizing them in an envelope of cell membrane, the phagosome. The digestive enzymes of the lysosomes are then released into the phagolysosomes.

Second, when the monocyte leaves the bone marrow, enters the bloodstream, and then passes into the tissues, the cell is not fully mature in the same sense as is the neutrophil. Third, PMNs are incapable of further division and are also incapable of active synthesis of digestive enzymes. Monocytes, on the other hand, can be stimulated under some circumstances to divide within the tissues, and they are capable of synthesizing a variety of intracellular enzymes, thereby responding to local conditions. This ability to undergo "on-the-job training" is a vital property of macrophages, particularly in certain immunologic reactions where they are trained by lymphocytes. In such circumstances, macrophages increase their metabolic activities, become more effective in phagocytosis, and become more efficient in killing and digesting certain microbes. Macrophages may also alter their form as they undergo such changes, giving rise to cells known as *epithelioid cells*. Macrophages are also able to fuse together to form multinucleated *giant cells*. These forms are illustrated in Figs. 4-13 and 4-14.

Although macrophages are significant components of various exudates, they are also widely distributed in the body under normal conditions. This fact was recognized many years ago, and the term *reticuloendothelial system (RES)* was coined to denote mononuclear cells sharing the same property, namely, phagocytosis. *Monocyte-macrophage system* is the current name applied to the RES because the term is actually more descriptive. As typically conceived, the RES, or monocyte-macrophage system, includes not only the blood monocytes and tissue histiocytes, or wandering macrophages, but also a large population of more or less fixed mononuclear phagocytic cells closely related to the more mobile members of the system. This population of less mobile cells includes lining cells along blood channels within the spleen, the liver (where the cells are known as *Kupffer's cells*), and the bone marrow. Similar fixed macrophages are present along many of the lymphatic channels within the lymph nodes of the body. Additionally, many macrophages are present within the serosal cavities of the body, within the lungs (alveolar macrophages), and even within the central nervous system (microglial cells).

The important functions of this system involve the vigorous phagocytic activities of the component cells. These cells clean the blood, the lymph, and the interstitial spaces of foreign material thus performing a vital defensive function. Even when millions of microorganisms are injected into the circulating blood, many millions of macrophages located strategically around the body would remove the microorganisms within a matter of a few hours. This characteristic is exceedingly important, because at least a few microorganisms may be released into the circulating fluids of the body with vigorous brushing of the teeth, with defecation, or with certain medical or dental manipulations. Because of the phagocytic activities of the macrophage system, such episodes of bacteremia are transient and trivial. The macrophages in the body cavities and connective tissues perform a similar police function. Additionally, the uptake of foreign material by macrophages is an essential first step in the chain of events that leads to the induction of an immune response (see Chapter 5).

An important everyday function of the monocyte-macrophage system involves the processing of the hemoglobin of red blood cells that have reached the end of their life span. Macrophages trap and recycle the components of this essential substance by splitting hemoglobin into an iron-containing portion and a non–iron-containing portion. The iron is recycled for the building of other red blood cells in the bone marrow; the non–iron-containing portion is further processed, liberating a substance known as *bilirubin*, which is carried in the bloodstream to the liver, where the hepatocytes extract it and secrete it as part of the bile.

Lymphocytes

One type of leukocyte, the lymphocyte, has not yet been mentioned. *Lymphocytes* are generally present in exudates only in small numbers until the exudates are quite old, that is, until the inflammatory reactions have become chronic. Because the known functions of lymphocytes are all within the immunologic realm, these cells are more fully described in Chapter 5.

Each component of the inflammatory response has a unique importance. Vasodilation early in acute inflammation brings to the area the "raw materials" for the reaction. When the arteriolar dilation and increased blood flow are circumvented by local conditions or by the administration of certain drugs, later aspects of the inflammatory reaction are significantly frustrated. The increased vascular permeability not only accomplishes the outpouring of fluid, which may dilute noxious agents, but also transfers important protein substances such as opsonins or other antibodies to the "battleground." Furthermore, one of the proteins that leaks into the area of inflammation is *fibrinogen*, which is quickly converted to form *fibrin*, which may act as kind of a sealer or "glue" in wounds. Because of its fibrillar character, fibrin may act as a scaffold for the migration of phagocytic leukocytes and ultimately for the cells that form scar tissue in the reparative phase. Mobilized leukocytes not only apprehend invading microbes but also demolish tissue debris thus repair processes can begin.

PATTERNS OF INFLAMMATION

Although the inflammatory reaction tends to follow the mechanisms described earlier, various patterns of inflammation can emerge based on the type of exudate that is formed, the particular organ or tissue involved, and the duration of the inflammatory process. The nomenclature of inflammatory processes takes into account each of these variables. Different types of exudates are given descriptive names. The duration of the inflammatory response is designated as *acute* during the phase of active exudation, as *chronic* when evidence of advanced repair exists along with the exudation, and as *subacute* when only early evidence of repair exists along with the exudation. The location of the inflammatory reaction is designated by the organ or tissue name, to which is appended the suffix *-itis* (e.g., appendicitis, tonsillitis, arthritis).

Noncellular Exudates

Serous Exudate

In some instances of inflammation, the exudate consists almost entirely of fluid and dissolved substances with few leukocytes. The simplest type of noncellular exudate is a *serous exudate*, which consists basically of the protein that leaks from permeable blood vessels in an area of inflammation along with the accompanying fluid. The most familiar example of serous exudate is blister fluid. Similar accumulations of serous exudate are common within body cavities, such as the pleural cavity or the peritoneal cavity, and although not as striking, serous exudates often spread through connective tissues.

Sometimes collections of fluid occur in body cavities for reasons other than inflammation, usually increased hydrostatic pressure or depletion of plasma protein. Such noninflammatory collections are termed *transudates* and are protein poor and cell poor compared with exudates.

Fibrinous Exudate

A second type of noncellular exudate is *fibrinous exudate*, which forms when the protein extravasated in an area of inflammation contains abundant fibrinogen. This fibrinogen is converted to fibrin, a sticky, elastic meshwork (perhaps more familiar as the backbone of a blood clot). Fibrinous exudates are often encountered on inflamed serosal surfaces such as the pleura and the pericardium, where the precipitated fibrin compacts to a shaggy layer on the involved membrane (Fig. 4-8). When such a shaggy layer of fibrin accumulates on serosal surfaces, it is frequently accompanied by pain when one surface rubs against another. Thus, for instance, the patient with pleu-

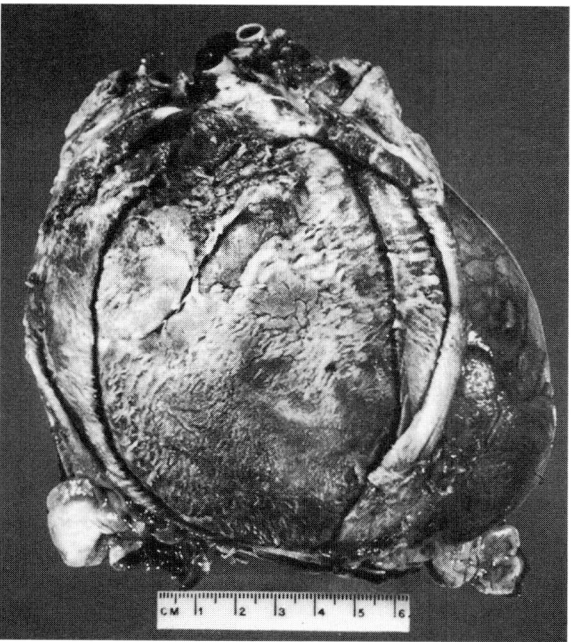

FIG. 4-8 Fibrinous exudate on the surface of the heart. The pericardium has been opened, and instead of the normally smooth epicardial surface, a shaggy layer of fibrin is evident. This has formed from fibrinogen exuded from underlying vessels. Classically, this condition has been termed "bread-and-butter heart."

ritis feels pain on respiration when the roughened surfaces rub together during inspiration. This rubbing of shaggy surfaces also produces a sign called *friction rub*, which is audible through the stethoscope over the affected area, whether it is the pleura, pericardium, or similar structure.

Mucinous Exudate

Another noncellular exudate is the *mucinous* or *catarrhal* exudate. This type of exudate forms only on the surface of a mucous membrane, on which cells are capable of secreting mucin. This type of exudate differs from others in that it represents a cellular secretion rather than something that escapes from the bloodstream. Mucin secretion is a normal property of mucous membranes, and mucinous exudate represents nothing more than an acceleration of a basic physiologic process. The most familiar example of a mucinous exudate is the runny nose that accompanies many upper respiratory infections.

Cellular Exudates

Neutrophilic Exudate

The most common exudates consist predominantly of PMNs, in such numbers as to overshadow the fluid and proteinaceous parts of exudate. Such neutrophilic exudates are referred to as *purulent*. Purulent exudates (Fig. 4-9) are usually formed in response to bacterial infection; they are also present in response to many aseptic injuries and are prominent nearly anywhere in the body where tissues have become necrotic.

Bacterial infection often causes extremely high concentrations of PMNs to accumulate in a tissue, and many of these cells die and liberate their powerful hydrolytic enzymes into the surroundings. Under such circumstances, the enzymes of the PMNs literally digest the underlying tissue and liquefy it. This combination of neutrophil aggregation and liquefaction of underlying tissues is referred to as *suppuration*, and the exudate thus formed is called *suppurative exudate*, or more commonly, *pus*. Therefore pus consists of living, dying, and disintegrated PMNs; liquefied, digested underlying tissue; fluid exudate of the inflammatory process; and often the inciting bacteria. The significant difference between suppurative and purulent inflammation is that with suppuration, liquefactive necrosis of underlying tissue occurs (Fig. 4-10). (Although a significant difference exists between purulent and suppurative inflammation, many unfortunately use the terms interchangeably.)

When localized suppuration occurs within a solid tissue, the resulting lesion is termed an *abscess*. An abscess is quite literally a hole filled with pus in the involved tissue (see Fig. 4-10). Abscesses are difficult lesions for the body to handle because of their tendency to expand with the liquefaction of more tissue, their tendency to burrow, and their resistance to healing. When an abscess forms, delivering therapeutic agents such as antibiotics into the abscess via the bloodstream is difficult. Generally, the handling of abscesses by the body is greatly aided through the process of draining them surgically, thus allowing the closed space previously filled with pus to collapse and heal. If pathways chosen by the surgeon do not surgically drain abscesses, they tend to expand, destroying additional structures in their path. An abscess in a lung might burrow until it communicates with the pleural cavity, and if the contents are discharged into the pleural cavity and infection spreads, the result might be *empyema,* which is a purulent inflammatory process involving the entire pleural cavity. Occasionally, an abscess ruptures onto a surface

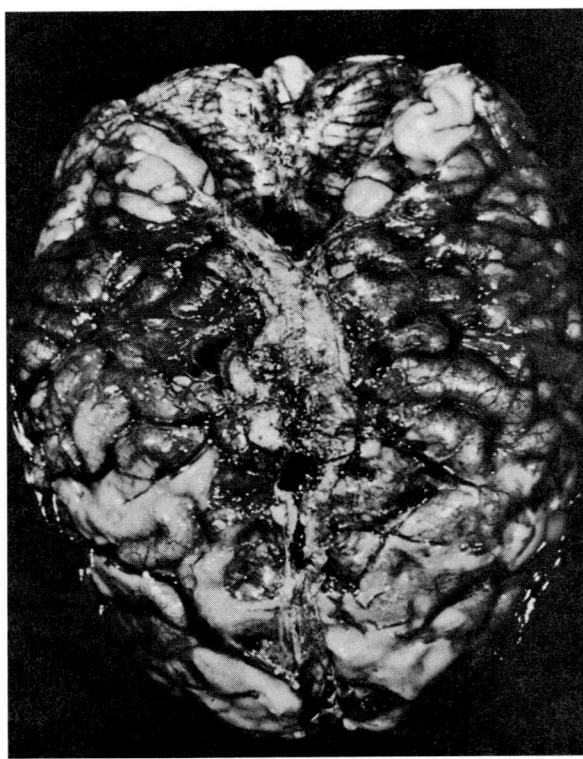

FIG. 4-9 Purulent exudate within the cerebral meninges. The membranes covering the brain contain literally millions of neutrophils forming a purulent exudate. The creamy patches of exudate are especially prominent at the bottom. The gyri in the center of the photograph are dark because of intense vascular congestion, part of the inflammatory response. (This is pneumococcal meningitis.)

and produces a draining tract that ends blindly in the space of the abscess. Any such blind tract communicating with a surface is referred to as a *sinus.* When, on the other hand, an abscess extends to two separate surfaces, it might result in an abnormal tract connecting two organs or connecting the lumen of a hollow organ and the body surface. Such an abnormal connection is referred to as a *fistula.* (Fistulas are named according to their communications [e.g., gastrocolic, bronchopleural, colocutaneous].)

Another common example of suppurative inflammation is the *furuncle,* or boil, which is a cutaneous abscess forming in a hair follicle as a result of bacterial infection. A *carbuncle* is a more deep-seated area of suppuration involving the subcutaneous tissue, with multiple areas of discharge onto the skin surface.

When purulent inflammation extends diffusely through a tissue, the process is referred to as phlegmonous; more often, the term *cellulitis* is used clinically to describe an area of phlegmonous inflammation. Such a spreading purulent process is usually observed as a result of bacterial infection when the particular agent is capable of spreading rapidly through the loose connective tissue of the body.

Mixed Exudates

As one might expect, mixtures of noncellular and cellular exudates are frequently present, and these are named accordingly. These mixtures include *fibrinopurulent* exudates, which consist of fibrin and PMNs; *mucopurulent* exudates consisting of mucin and PMNs; *serofibrinous* exudates; and so forth. Certain exudates, such as mucinous and mucopurulent, are unique to mucous membranes.

Occasionally, in association with damage to mucous membranes, a necrotic area may actually slough off, leaving a gap in the continuity of the mucosal surface. Such a defect is termed an *ulcer.* Most often, fibrinopurulent exudate emanating from the underlying blood vessels forms the surface of an ulcer bed (Fig. 4-11). Occasionally, broad areas of mucous membrane will become necrotic and the dead cells may become enmeshed in a web of fibrinopurulent exudate, which coats the mucosal surface. Such an area grossly resembles a ragged mucous membrane, and hence this type of process is referred to

FIG. 4-10 Brain abscess. As a result of bacterial infection in the cerebral hemisphere on the right, large numbers of neutrophils emigrated into the region. Liquefaction of the regional tissue by lysosomal enzymes of the neutrophils produced the defect illustrated.

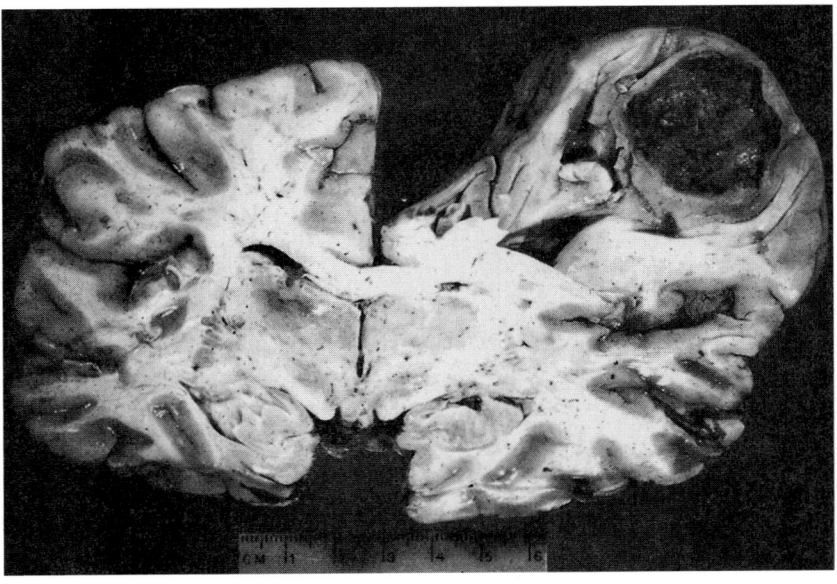

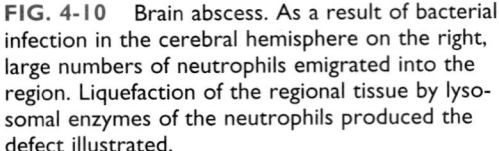

as *pseudomembranous inflammation* (Fig. 4-12). The classic example of pseudomembranous inflammation in the past was the pseudomembrane of diphtheria within the respiratory tract. Thus such membranes are occasionally referred to as *diphtheritic*. Pseudomembranous inflammation may be observed within the gastrointestinal tract, particularly the colon, as the result of an upset in the microbial ecology of the tract, usually a result of the administration of antibiotics.

Granulomatous Inflammation

A unique and distinctive pattern of inflammation that can occur virtually anywhere is granulomatous inflam- mation. The massing of large numbers of macrophages and their aggregation into nodular clumps referred to as *granulomas* are characteristics of this type of inflammation. Although many inflammatory exudates contain appreciable quantities of macrophages, in granulomatous inflammation, sheets of these cells or their derivatives, such as epithelioid cells or multinucleated giant cells, dominate the field. Granulomas take time to evolve and generally pass through rather nondescript acute stages whereby exudation of fluid, neutrophils, and protein takes place. The continued emigration of monocytes and the local proliferation of these cells lead to their massing as a granuloma. Granulomas usually form because of the persistence within the tissues of some

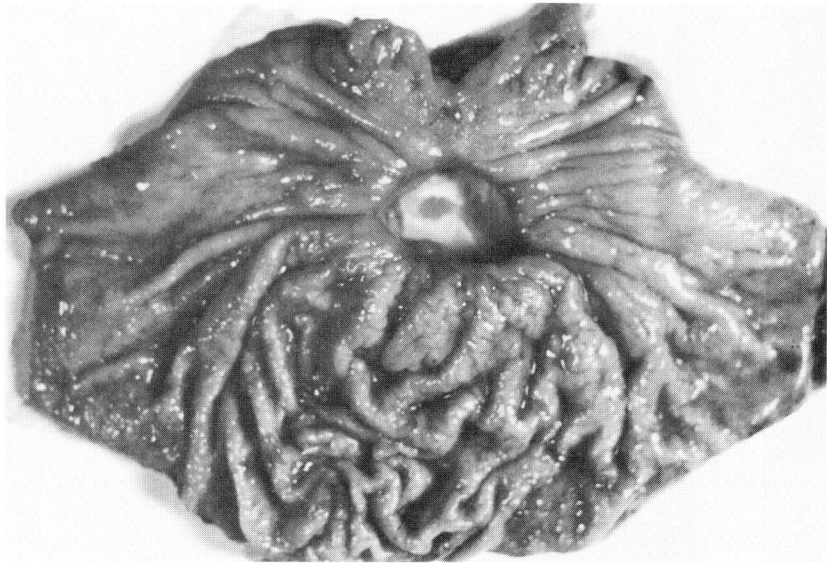

FIG. 4-11   Gastric ulcer. This type of gap in the continuity of a surface is termed an *ulcer*. An inflammatory reaction is invariably present in the base. Blood vessels may be eroded, giving rise to hemorrhage, or the full thickness of the wall may be perforated.

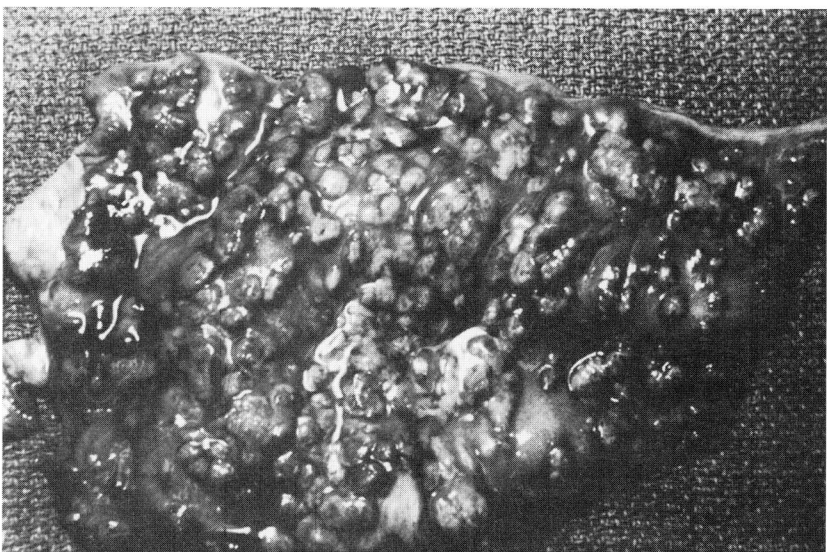

FIG. 4-12   Pseudomembranous colitis. The many plaquelike lesions on the colonic mucosal sur- face are patches of *pseudomembrane* consisting of fibrinopurulent exudate and necrotic epithelial debris.

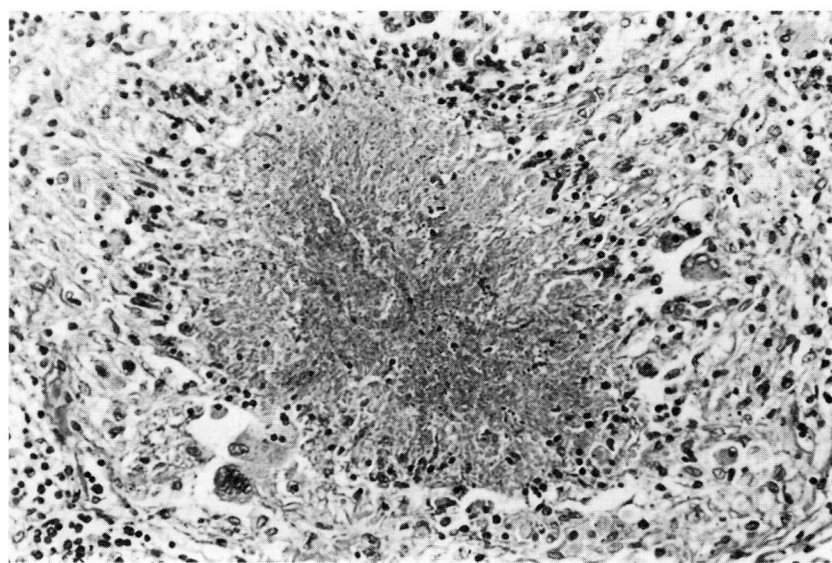

FIG. 4-13 Epithelioid tubercle. A tubercle is a mass of macrophages that have acquired an epithelioid appearance. The zone of poorly defined, light-staining cells at the periphery of the field (outer third) consists of epithelioid macrophages and multinucleated giant cells (3 o'clock and 7 o'clock). The center of the tubercle has undergone caseous necrosis. The small, dark cells are lymphocytes. (Photomicrograph, ×315.)

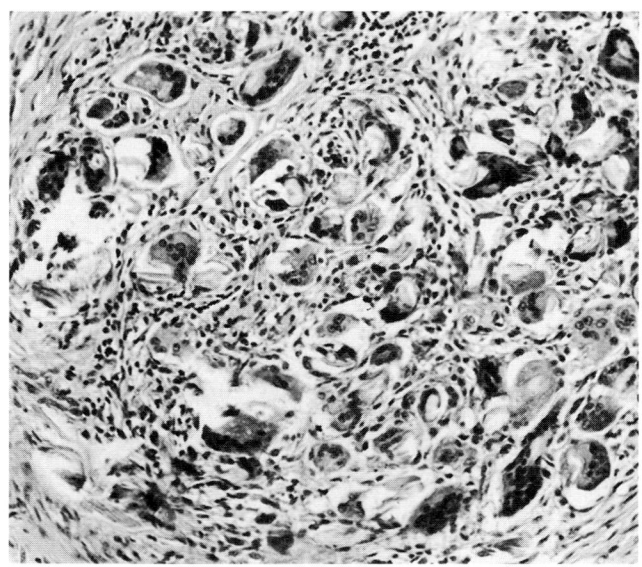

FIG. 4-14 Foreign body granuloma. In this instance the granuloma is a mass of macrophages that have fused to form many giant cells. Many of these have engulfed fibrils, which represent fragments of suture material. (Photomicrograph, ×200.)

offensive agent that is resistant to the efforts of the body to dispose of it. Such agents can include insoluble but sterile materials or particularly resistant microorganisms. The prototypical microorganism that evokes the formation of granulomas is the *Mycobacterium tuberculosis*, or tubercle bacillus. The response to this organism is characteristically granulomatous, and the macrophages usually mass in nodular aggregates of epithelioid cells and giant cells. This type of a nodular mass of epithelioid cells is referred to as a *tubercle* (Fig. 4-13). Granulomas also form in response to foreign bodies such as suture materi-

als (Fig. 4-14). Generally, the presence of a granuloma is the hallmark of "tissue indigestion." As the granuloma evolves in some instances, the macrophages acquire increasing ability to handle the offensive agent, in which case it is eliminated. In other instances, the agent remains refractory, and the net effect of the granuloma formation is to wall off that agent from the remainder of the body.

FATE OF THE INFLAMMATORY REACTION

Given the presence of an inflammatory reaction, the best result that can be obtained occurs when little or no destruction of underlying tissue has taken place. In such instances, when the offending agent has been neutralized and removed, the stimulus for continuing exudation of fluid and cells gradually disappears. The small blood vessels in the area regain their usual semipermeability, fluid flux ceases, and emigration of leukocytes likewise stops. The fluid that has been exuded is gradually absorbed by the lymphatics, and the cells of the exudate disintegrate, wander off via the lymphatics, or are actually eliminated from the body (e.g., lung exudates being coughed up). The net result of this process is that the previously inflamed tissue is left precisely as it was before the reaction started. This phenomenon is called *resolution*.

In contrast, when significant amounts of tissue have been destroyed, resolution cannot occur. The destroyed tissue must be repaired by proliferation of adjacent surviving host cells. Repair actually involves two separate but coordinated components. The first, *regeneration*, actually involves proliferation of parenchymal elements identical to those lost, the net result being replacement of those lost elements by the same type of cells. The second component of repair involves the proliferation of con-

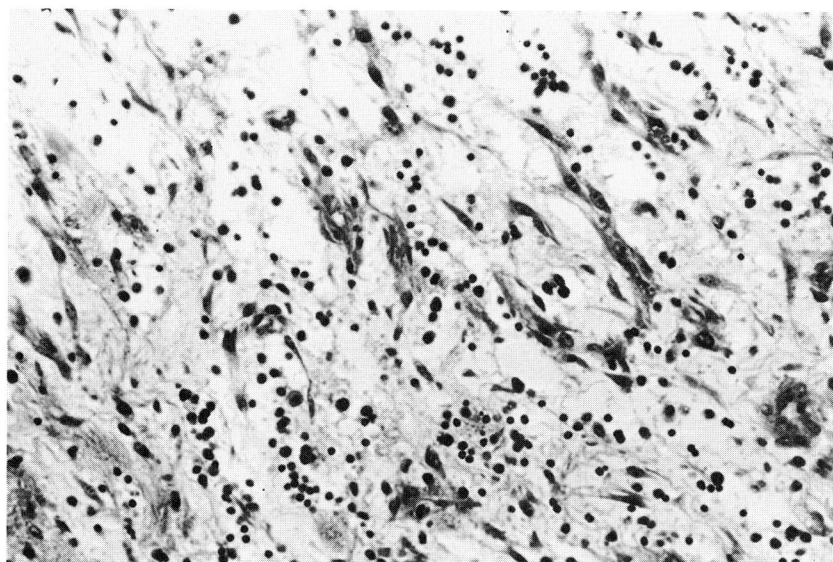

FIG. 4-15   Early organization. The field depicts granulation tissue growing into an area of repair. The elongated, spindle-shaped cells are fibroblasts. Capillary sprouts are recognized as tubular structures, round in cross section (as at the lower right). The small, dark cells are leukocytes, and the interstitial spaces contain exudate fluid and connective tissue ground substance. Compare with Fig. 4-16. (Photomicrograph, ×315.)

nective tissue elements, leading to the formation of *scar tissue*. In most tissues, a combination of these two activities occurs.

Various cells and tissues differ widely in their ability to regenerate. Most epithelial tissues, such as the covering of the skin and the lining of the mouth, pharynx, and gastrointestinal tract, regenerate easily after a portion of the tissue has been lost. Other epithelial cells, such as those of the liver parenchyma, renal tubules, or the secretory elements of certain glands, regenerate well, provided the outlines of the tissue are maintained without extensive collapse during the inflammatory process. Complex specialized structures such as renal glomeruli do not regenerate if destroyed. Some types of cells regenerate very poorly or not at all. Useful regeneration is extremely limited in involuntary and voluntary muscle if restoration is present at all, and no regeneration occurs in heart muscle, which is unfortunate given the frequency of necrosis of portions of myocardium. Finally and importantly, no regeneration of neurons or nerve cells occurs within the central nervous system. When these cells are lost, the loss is permanent.

Repair by formation of scar tissue is an efficient process in virtually any tissue of the body. Formation of scar tissue involves proliferating connective tissue from areas adjoining the necrotic tissue extending into the area as the tissue is demolished by the inflammatory reaction. Such ingrowth of a proliferating young connective tissue into an area of inflammation is referred to as *organization*, and the connective tissue itself is referred to as *granulation tissue*. The components of granulation tissue actually include proliferating fibroblasts, proliferating capillary sprouts (the endothelial cells are sometimes referred to as *angioblasts*), various leukocytes of the inflammatory process, fluid portions of the exudate, and a loose semifluid connective tissue ground substance. Organization

occurs when abundant tissue has become necrotic, when inflammatory exudates persist and do not resolve, and when masses of blood (hematomas) or blood clots do not resolve quickly. The fibroblasts and angioblasts of granulation tissue originate from preexisting fibroblasts and capillaries in the surroundings, and their migration is somehow oriented such that this tissue gradually extends into the appropriate area (Fig. 4-15).

The earliest evidence of organization usually occurs several days after the start of the inflammatory reaction. After approximately a week, the granulation tissue is still quite loose and cellular. At this point, the fibroblasts of the granulation tissue gradually begin to secrete the soluble precursors of the protein collagen, which gradually precipitates as fibrils in the interstices of the granulation tissue. Over time, more and more collagen is deposited in the granulation tissue, which is now gradually maturing to a rather dense collagenous connective tissue or scar (Fig. 4-16). Although the scar achieves much of its strength after approximately 2 weeks, a continuing remodeling process and increase in the density and strength of the scar occur over the ensuing weeks. The granulation tissue, which at first was quite cellular and vascular, gradually becomes less cellular and less vascular and more densely collagenous. The gross counterpart of this evolution is familiar in the appearance of healing incisions, whereby the resulting scar is at first somewhat loose and quite pink because of the vascularity, ultimately becoming denser and paler as the blood vessels regress.

Wound Healing

The coordination of scar formation and regeneration is perhaps most easily illustrated through the healing of cutaneous wounds. The simplest type of healing is that observed in the body's handling of wounds such as

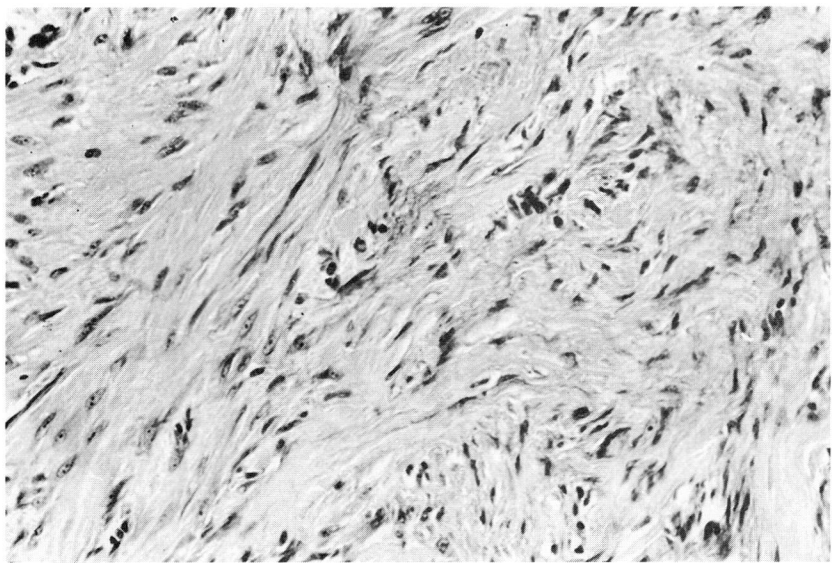

FIG. 4-16 Maturing scar. As granulation tissue matures, the fibroblasts synthesize collagen, which forms the tough scar. In this field the interstitial material has a "stringy" appearance because of abundant collagen in fibrillar form. As the scar ages, it becomes less cellular and more densely collagenous. (Photomicrograph, ×315.)

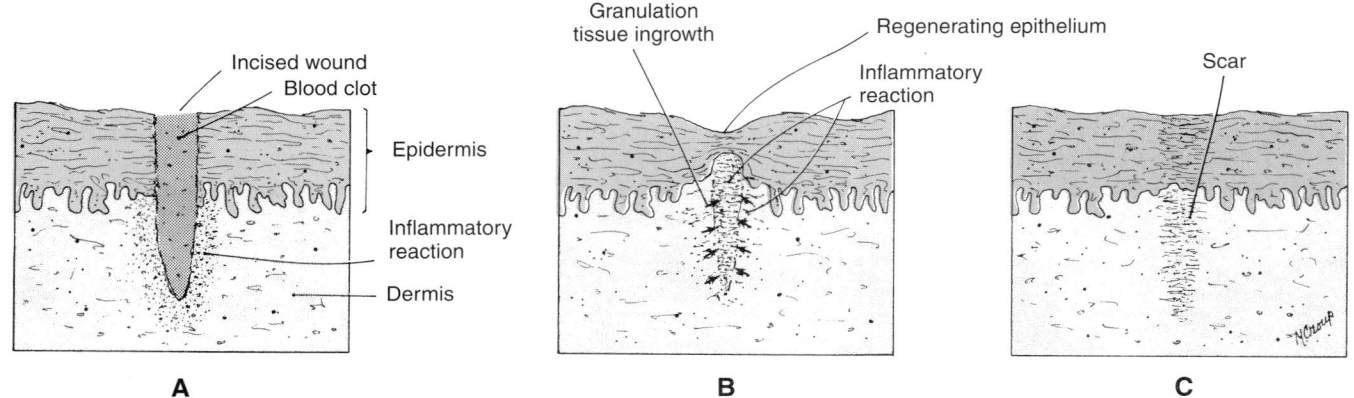

FIG. 4-17 Healing of an incised, primarily closed wound. The wound edges are initially held together by a blood clot, **A**, and perhaps also by sutures. An acute inflammatory response is mounted in the adjacent tissue, which leads to ingrowth of granulation tissue after several days, **B**. At this stage, epidermal regeneration is under way. The usual result is complete epidermal regeneration and a compact dermal scar, which forms as the granulation tissue matures, **C**.

surgical incisions, whereby the wound edges can be brought together for the healing process to begin. Such healing is referred to as *primary healing* or *healing by first intention*. Immediately after wounding, the wound edges are bound together by part of a blood clot, the fibrin of which acts somewhat as a glue (Fig. 4-17, *A,*). Immediately thereafter, an acute inflammatory reaction develops at the edges of the wound, and the inflammatory cells, particularly macrophages, enter the blood clot and begin to demolish it. After this exudative inflammatory reaction, the ingrowth of granulation tissue into the area formerly occupied by the clot begins. Thus over several days, the wound is bridged by granulation tissue destined to mature to a scar. While this is occurring (Fig. 4-17, *B*), the surface epithelium at the edges begins to regenerate, and within a few days a thin layer of epithelium migrates across the wound surface. As the scar beneath matures, this epithelium also thickens and matures, thus it comes to resemble the adjacent skin. The result (Fig. 4-17, *C*) is a reconstituted skin surface and an underlying scar that may be virtually invisible or barely visible as a thickened line. Many skin wounds heal in this manner with no medical attention. In others, sutures are placed to hold the wound edges in apposition until healing occurs. Sutures can be removed when organization and epithelial regeneration have progressed to the point at which the edges will not gape when the sutures are removed. Thus in an area of skin with relatively little tension, sutures can be removed in several days, long before maximal strength of the scar has been achieved and before appreciable amounts of collagen have been deposited. In areas under stress,

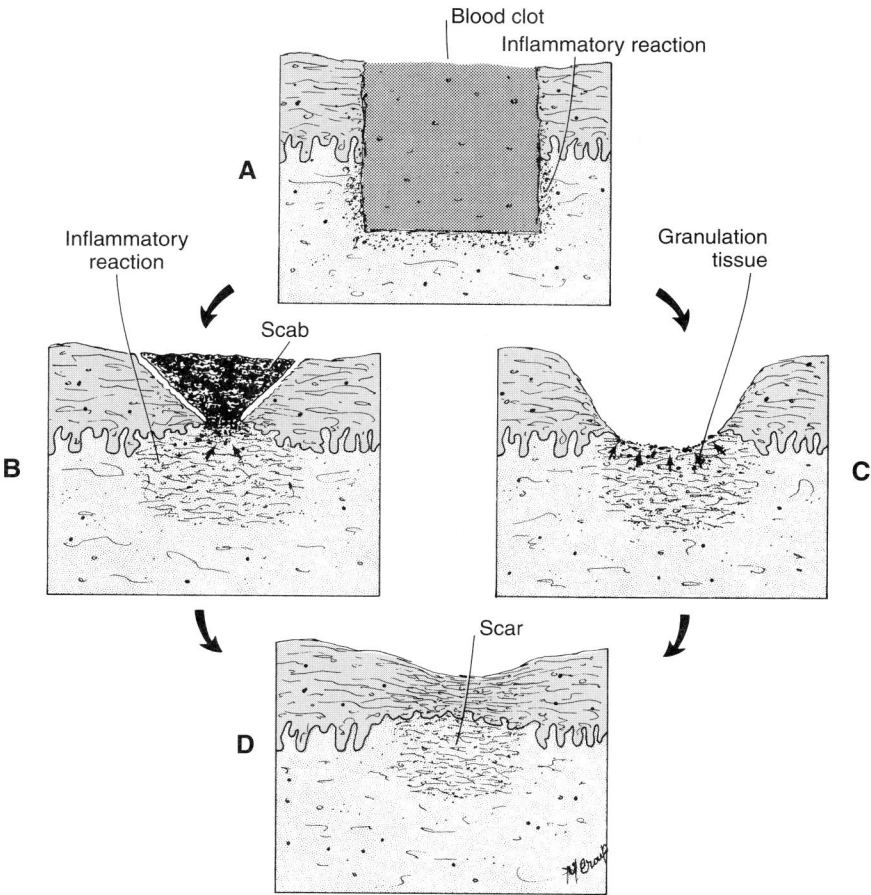

FIG. 4-18 Healing of an open wound by second intention. The process is qualitatively similar to that shown in Fig. 4-17 but involves more extensive epithelial regeneration and formation of more abundant scar. **A**, The situation shortly after wounding; **B**, healing under a scab; **C**, an open wound with visible granulation tissue. **D**, The end result involves a large scar and often a thin area of "new" epidermis devoid of hair and other appendages.

sutures must be left in place longer to hold the tissue together until a tough scar can form.

A second pattern of healing occurs when the wounding of skin is such that the edges cannot be brought together during the healing process. This is referred to as *healing by second intention* or sometimes *healing by granulation* (Fig. 4-18). This type of healing is qualitatively identical to that previously described. The difference lies only in that more granulation tissue is formed, more epithelial regeneration is necessary, and usually a larger scar is formed. The entire process, of course, takes longer than healing by primary intention. Often in such large open wounds, granulation tissue can be observed covering the floor of the wound as a delicate nappy carpet that bleeds easily on touch. In other situations, the granulation tissue actually grows beneath a scab and epithelial regeneration likewise occurs beneath the scab. Ultimately in such circumstances, the scab is cast off when healing is complete. Most can recall having impatiently removed a scab in the approximate stage shown in Fig. 4-18, *B*, to reveal a central pinpoint of bleeding granulation tissue where epithelial regeneration was not yet total. Although identical in many ways to healing by primary intention, secondary healing is less desirable (not that a choice is often available) because of the time

involved and the termination in a larger and potentially disfiguring scar.

Healing in virtually any tissue of the body occurs by a process paralleling that described for the skin, with local variations, depending on the ability of the tissues to regenerate and so forth.

The designation of an inflammatory process as acute, subacute, or chronic reflects the duration in terms of the extent of repair. *Acute* inflammation, by definition, has no reparative aspects; it consists only of the exudative phenomena of inflammation. In *subacute* inflammation, beginning granulation tissue ingrowth and perhaps beginning regeneration takes place. In *chronic* inflammation, evidence of advanced repair side by side with continuing exudation occurs. Evidence of advanced repair includes extensive regenerative proliferation and extensive formation of scar with abundant collagen.

FACTORS AFFECTING INFLAMMATION AND HEALING

In some situations, the inflammatory process may be impaired from the beginning, that is, in its exudative stages. The entire inflammatory process depends on intact circulation to the affected area. Thus, when blood supply to an area is deficient, the result may be sluggish inflammatory processes, persistent infections, and poor healing. Another requisite for efficient exudative inflammation is a liberal supply of leukocytes in the circulating blood. Patients with destroyed or depressed marrow (e.g., from malignant disease or adverse reaction to drugs) are unable to produce cellular exudates with normal function and as a result are susceptible to severe infections. More rarely, the functions of leukocytes, even when they are present in normal numbers, may be impaired (e.g., abnormal chemotaxis, abnormal phagocytosis, abnormal intracellular killing and digestion), and the patient is rendered similarly susceptible to aggressive infections. Because certain antibodies assist leukocyte function (see Chapter 5), the inflammatory reaction is also less than normally effective in immunodeficient patients. Finally, certain drugs in sufficiently high doses are capable of inhibiting essential aspects of the inflammatory response. For example, when a patient receives high doses of corticosteroids or other antiinflammatory drugs, inflammation and healing may be impaired.

Many factors can affect the healing of wounds or other areas of tissue injury and inflammation. The healing process, because of its dependence on cellular proliferation and synthetic activity, is particularly sensitive to local deficiencies of blood supply (with attendant impairment of raw material delivery) and is also sensitive to the patient's nutritional state. Patients who are extremely malnourished do not optimally heal wounds. The presence of foreign material or necrotic tissue in the wound, the presence of wound infection, and incomplete immobilization and apposition of wound edges also adversely affect the healing of wounds. In extreme cases, with failure of healing, a surgical wound might even undergo *dehiscence*, or breaking open.

Complications of Healing

Even when healing proceeds adequately on a cellular level, complications occasionally occur as a result. The nature of scar tissue is to shorten and to become more dense and compact over time. Occasionally, the result is *contracture*, which may disfigure an area or limit motion at a joint. When the scar tissue encircles a tubular structure (e.g., the urethra), the result may be a *stricture*, which narrows the structure in question and may produce serious difficulty. When serosal surfaces are inflamed and the exudate does not resolve, granulation tissue and scar tissue may eventually bind serosal surfaces, forming *adhesions*. In many areas, such as the pleura or the pericardium, adhesions generally have a negligible effect on organ function. Within the peritoneal cavity, however, adhesions, whether between loops of bowel or between abdominal viscera and the body wall, may produce webs that can constrict portions of the gastrointestinal tract or

can actually entrap them, forming *internal hernias* that may strangulate and become gangrenous. Another complication that is occasionally observed in healing wounds of the body wall is the *incisional hernia*. In this situation, the granulation tissue and scar that bridge the surgical defect in the body wall gradually yield to intraperitoneal pressure and a bulging sac in the incision is formed. Another minor local complication of healing is the protrusion of a piece of granulation tissue above the surface of the healing wound, forming what is sometimes called "proud flesh." Healing generally proceeds well when such excrescences are cauterized or nipped off. A complication of healing occasionally encountered is the *amputation*, or *traumatic*, *neuroma*, which simply represents regenerative proliferation of nerve fibers into the area of healing, where they become entrapped in dense scar. Such a neuroma may constitute an unsightly or even painful lump within a scar. Finally, some individuals, apparently on a genetic basis, handle the production and/or remodeling of collagen in a healing wound abnormally such that excess collagen is formed, leading to a protrusion called a *keloid*. These wounds are somewhat more common in African Americans and Asians and in younger patients. Keloids are biologically trivial but cosmetically may assume great importance.

SYSTEMIC ASPECTS OF INFLAMMATION

The emphasis of the previous discussion is on the local aspects of the response to injury. Noteworthy, however, are the important and prominent systemic effects that accompany local inflammatory reactions. These *acute-phase reactions* are apparently mediated by cytokines produced by leukocytes participating in the inflammatory reactions. One familiar reaction is *fever*, which is produced by cytokine action on hypothalamic temperature-regulating centers. *Leukocytosis*, an increase in the number of circulating leukocytes, results from cytokine-medicated stimulation of leukocyte maturation and release from the bone marrow. Other acute-phase reactions include increased hepatic synthesis of "acute-phase proteins," such as C-reactive protein and serum amyloid-associated (SAA) protein, and components of the coagulation and complement system. The increase in some proteins is associated with an increased erythrocyte sedimentation rate (ESR), giving rise to a blood test for the presence of inflammation that is sometimes useful clinically. Severe injuries can cause striking metabolic and endocrine changes. Local inflammatory reactions are accompanied by a variety of poorly defined "constitutional symptoms," including malaise, anorexia or loss of appetite, and varying degrees of disability or even prostration. Presumably, substances released from the areas of inflammation also mediate these symptoms.

KEY CONCEPTS

- *Inflammation* is a local reaction of the vascular and supporting elements of a tissue to injury resulting in the formation of a protein-rich exudate; it is a protective response of the nonspecific immune system that serves to localize, neutralize, or destroy an injurious agent in preparation for the process of healing.
- The cardinal signs of inflammation are *rubor* (redness), *calor* (heat), *dolor* (pain), *tumor* (swelling), and *functio laesa* (loss of function).
- Causes of inflammation include physical agents, chemical agents, immunologic reactions, and infection by pathogenic organisms. *Note that infection is not synonymous with inflammation and is but one cause of inflammation.*
- *Starling's Law of the Capillaries* governs the normal movement of fluid between the semipermeable capillary endothelium and the tissue spaces. The direction of net diffusion is determined by the hydrostatic pressure of the blood tending to push fluid out, opposed by the osmotic force of the protein molecules tending to hold the fluid within the capillaries. The balance of these forces normally favors fluid exudation at the arterial end and fluid reabsorption at the venous end of the capillary to allow provision of nutrients to the cells and removal of waste products from the cells. The lymphatic system removes any excess fluid remaining in the interstitial spaces.
- *Vascular phase alterations in acute inflammation* include transient vasoconstriction in response to the injury, followed by vasodilation and an increase in blood flow to the injured area (resulting in redness and heat). The release of histamine from mast cells causes an increase in permeability of the capillaries, allowing protein-rich fluid to leak out into the area of injury (resulting in tissue swelling and pain). Lymphatic flow increases in parallel with the increased blood flow.
- *Cellular phase alterations in acute inflammation* include margination of leukocytes (pavementing) along the capillary wall as blood flow slows (fluid and protein move out, causing blood sludging). Leukocytes emigrate out of the blood vessel *(diapedesis)* by forming pseudopods and are directionally attracted to the area of inflammation *(chemotaxis)*.
- The cells involved in the inflammatory process include phagocytic leukocytes (*neutrophils or PMNs*, macrophages, or eosinophils), platelets, and lymphocytes.
- Egress of cells from vascular channels in acute inflammation takes place in two stages: neutrophils or PMNs predominate in the early exudate and later the *macrophage* (monocyte that has emigrated out of the blood vessel) predominates. Lymphocytes and plasma cells (activated B lymphocytes) are found in chronic inflammation.
- Phagocytic cells ingest particles by flowing their cytoplasm around the objects and internalizing them in an envelope of cell membrane (the *phago-*

some). The digestive enzymes of the *lysosome* are then released into the *phagolysosome*, killing the particle if it is a living microorganism.
- Macrophages are longer-lived and more potent phagocytes than are PMNs, which are short-lived and die after phagocytosis.
- The progress of the acute inflammatory response is under the control of a group of molecular systems known as chemical mediators, which act locally. *Histamine*, the most important vasoactive amine released early in inflammation, increases vascular permeability. The *Hageman factor* initiates the intrinsic coagulation mechanism leading to a fibrin blood clot; it also activates the *fibrinolysin system* (dissolving the clot) and activates the *kallikrein-kinin system*, causing the release of *bradykinin* (which dilates blood vessels and increases permeability). Some components of the *complement system* act as chemotactic agents, *opsonins* (promoting phagocytosis), or as *anaphylatoxins* (causing histamine release). Arachidonic acid chemical mediators include prostaglandins, thromboxanes, and leukotrienes. Cytokines are released by a variety of cells that have an important role in inflammation including TNF, IL-1, and IL-8.
- Patterns of acute inflammation are characterized by the type of exudate. Noncellular exudates may be *serous* (e.g., blister), *fibrinous* (i.e., high in fibrinogen) or *mucinous* (e.g., runny nose accompanying a cold). Purulent exudates are usually formed in response to bacterial infections and contain pus. *Pus* is composed of water and solutes, dead and dying PMNs, necrotic tissue, and tissue debris. The combination of the accumulation of PMNs and liquefaction of underlying tissues is called *suppuration*. Purulent inflammation that extends diffusely through tissue is called phlegmonous or *cellulitis*. Hemorrhagic exudates contain red blood cells.
- The accumulation of pus in a pocket within soft tissue is called an *abscess*, and a tract leading from the abscess to the skin surface is called a *sinus tract*. A *fistula* is a tract leading from a normal cavity or tube to a body surface or to another cavity; they are named according to their communications (e.g., recto-vaginal, colocutaneous). A *furuncle* or *boil* is a cutaneous abscess. An abscess that is more deeply seated with multiple areas of discharge is called a *carbuncle*.
- Local manifestations of acute inflammation include the cardinal signs of inflammation, variation in the type of exudate and lesion, and enlargement of the regional lymph nodes (*lymphadenopathy*) in severe cases. Systemic manifestations include malaise, anorexia, fever, leukocytosis, elevations of certain serum proteins (such as C-reactive protein and gamma globulin) and the ESR.
- *Chronic inflammation* occurs when the injurious stimulus persists and is characterized by a lesion with partial healing and evidence of fibrous repair (scar),

a greater number of macrophages and lymphocytes, and persistent inflammation (e.g., base of a chronic gastric ulcer).

- *Granulomatous inflammation* is a process based on the action of the cellular immune system and involves a process fundamentally different from acute and chronic inflammation, characterized by the formation of sheets of *epithelioid cells* (aggregates of macrophages that have lost their phagocytic ability) and multinucleated *giant cells* (fused macrophages) called granulomas. Granulomas usually form in response to the persistence of some offensive agent resistant to disposal (e.g., tubercle of tuberculosis, nonabsorbable surgical suture).

- *Resolution* is the healing process by which tissue returns to normal following acute inflammation with little or no destruction of underlying tissue. When more extensive destruction of tissue occurs, the tissue may be repaired by replacement with cells of the same type (regeneration) or replacement by scar tissue, or both.

- The regenerative potential of tissues varies. *Labile cells* such as in epithelium, bone marrow, and lymphoid tissue reproduce readily as part of their normal activity. *Stable cells* such as liver cells, renal tubular epithelium, and bone can regenerate, provided their outlines are preserved. *Permanent cells* such as in heart muscle (and most other muscle), renal glomerulus, or central nervous system neurons do not have the ability to regenerate if destroyed, thus they must be repaired by scar tissue formation.

- The healing of a surgical incision wound with closely apposed edges is said to take place by *primary intention;* scar formation is minimal. In contrast, a jagged, gaping wound with much tissue destruction (e.g., a skin ulcer) results in a slower healing process with much more scar formation and is called *healing by second intention* or healing by granulation.

- Wound healing takes place in a series of sequential steps best followed in the repair of a simple, incisional wound of soft tissue: (1) incisional wound; (2) bleeding, hemostasis, clot formation—surface becomes desiccated, forming a scab; (3) acute inflammatory response; (4) contraction of wound edges; (5) débridement—clearance of blood and other debris by phagocytes; (6) organization or proliferation stage, forming granulation tissue to fill in the wound (formation of capillary buds from angioblasts, collagen from fibroblasts, and migration of epithelial cells from the wound edges under the scab to the wound center); (7) collagen maturation and scar contraction; and (8) scar remodeling.

- *Factors promoting wound healing* include a good blood supply to the area of injury, youth (children heal faster), good nutrition (adequate protein, vitamin C, zinc), good apposition of wound edges, and normal functioning leukocytes and inflammatory response. Wound healing may be impaired or retarded if corticosteroids (antiinflammatory drugs) are administered or in the presence of foreign material, necrotic tissue or infection of the wound; this is the reason for which incision and drainage of an abscess or wound débridement is often necessary to promote healing.

- Complications of wound healing include *proud flesh* (scar tissue protruding above the wound surface), *keloid* formation (scar tissue extending beyond the bounds of the original wound), *excessive wound contracture* interfering with mobility if over a joint, and stenosis or constriction whereby scar forms around a tubular structure such as a fallopian tube or ureter. Fibrous bands (resembling spider webs) may form on serous surfaces (*adhesions*) in the peritoneal cavity when the exudate is not cleared properly and may result in bowel obstruction. Peripheral nerve fibers that regenerate and become enmeshed in scar tissue following limb amputation is called a *traumatic neuroma. Dehiscence* is the bursting open of a surgical wound. *Evisceration* is the breaking open of an abdominal wound with the extrusion of the intestines and is a serious emergency. Finally, excessive intraabdominal pressure may cause an *incisional hernia* of bulging scar tissue to develop in the abdominal wall.

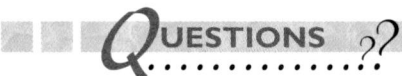

QUESTIONS ??

A sampling of review questions for this chapter appears here. Visit http://www.mosby.com/MERLIN/PriceWilson/ for additional questions.

Match the following types of exudates in column A with the statements in column B.

Column A
1. _____ Catarrhal
2. _____ Suppurative
3. _____ Phlegmonous (cellulitis)
4. _____ Serous
5. _____ Pseudomembranous

Column B
a. Poorly limited spreading or diffuse inflammation
b. Occurs only on mucous membranes and contains mucin
c. Includes a web of fibrinopurulent exudate coating the necrotic mucosal surface
d. Contains very few cells (e.g., blister fluid)
e. Contains many living and dead neutrophils and debris liquefied by enzymes released from the dead neutrophils

Fill in the blanks with the correct words.

6. A(n) _____ is a lesion within solid tissue and contains dead cells, liquefied tissue, neutrophils, and often bacteria.
7. A(n) _____ is a local gap in the continuity of the mucosal surface.
8. The accumulation of pus in the pleural cavity is called _____.
9. An abnormal communication tract between two organs or the lumen of a hollow organ and the body surface is called a(n) _____.
10. The suffix for inflammation is _____.
11. _____ is the term used to describe the movement of leukocytes from the axial stream to the periphery of the blood vessel lumen.
12. _____ is the term used to describe leukocytes inserting pseudopodia in intercellular junctions and sliding and wriggling through to the extravascular spaces.
13. The resorption of exudate with return of the area to normal is called _____.
14. _____ is the replacement of dead or injured tissues by new cells of parenchymal or stromal origin.
15. Inflammation of the lymph nodes is termed _____.
16. The correct sequence of the following events as they occur in an inflammatory reaction is _____.
   a. Tissue injury
   b. Increased local blood flow, leading to heat and redness
   c. Emigration of leukocytes
   d. Slowing of blood flow; margination of leukocytes
   e. Increased vascular permeability

Response of the Body to Immunologic Challenge

MARILYN SAWYER SOMMERS

*T*he function of the immune system in the human body is to differentiate "self" from "nonself." All organisms are a delicate integration of cells, tissues, and organs, with each being necessary for the sustenance of life. To support life, an organism must be able to protect itself against threats to its individuality. These threats can exist externally (e.g., a splinter stuck beneath the skin, a virus or bacterium ingested or inhaled) or internally (e.g., a neoplasm or tumor derived from the body's own cells).

IMMUNITY: OVERVIEW AND DEFINITIONS

To protect itself against threats to individuality, the human body has developed cellular defense reactions that are labeled the *immune response*. The terms *immunology* and *immunity* are derived from the Latin word *immunitas*, which was used in Roman times to describe the protection from civic duties and legal prosecution that Roman senators received during their terms in office. Historically, the terms have come to describe protection from infectious disease. As a means of protection, the body requires mechanisms to differentiate its own cells (self) from invading agents (nonself).

These mechanisms can be described as the body's *immunity*, a state of protection (primarily against infectious agents) that is characterized by memory and specificity. *Memory* is the heightened ability of an organism to respond to an *antigen* (a cell or molecule that promotes an immune response, also known as an *immunogen*) because of previous exposure to the antigen. *Specificity* is the property that immune system cells demonstrate as having the ability to react with one and only one antigenic determinant. Immunity has three primary functions: (1) its role in *defense* is to provide resistance to invaders such as microorganisms; (2) its role in *surveillance* is to identify and destroy the body's own cells that mutate and have the potential to form neoplasms (tumors); and (3) its role in *homeostasis* is to remove cellular debris and waste such that cell types remain uniform and unchanged.

Self Versus Nonself

An important key to the body's ability to distinguish self from nonself is the *major histocompatibility complex* (MHC), a single gene cluster on the short arm of the sixth chromosome. The MHC gene cluster controls the production of one particular set of molecules that serve as cellular antigens, "self-markers," to indicate that all cells belong to one particular organism. These surface antigens are inherited and unique to each person, and they serve as cellular labels; recognition of the MHC antigen by the body's immune system causes the development of *self-tolerance* (the body's ability to restrain from attacking native cells). In humans, MHC antigens are often called the *human leukocyte antigens* (HLAs) because they were first detected on white blood cells (WBCs).

MHC molecules are found on the surface of virtually all nucleated cells and are divided into three classes. Two will be discussed here briefly and a third under the section on Complement. Class I MHC molecules, which are found on the surface of all nucleated cells and platelets (except spermatozoa and ova), interact with virally infected cells. When a cell becomes virally infected, Class I molecules interact with microorganisms that are replicated intracellularly and help to cause destruction of the infected cell. The Class II MHC molecule is involved in types of cellular reactions originating from pathogens that replicate outside the cell, such as bacteria. Class II MHC molecules are found on monocytes, macrophages, and other immune system cells and are active during the process of phagocytosis. The functions of Class I, Class II, Class III MHC molecules and phagocytosis are discussed in greater detail later in the chapter.

The human body's system of determining self versus nonself includes numerous mechanisms, some of which are carried out by the lymphoid system. The lymphoid system defends against invaders through two arms: cell-mediated immunity and antibody-mediated (humoral) immunity. Cell-mediated immunity is the immune response primarily carried out by T lymphocytes, or T cells. When the body is exposed to a pathogen, the T cells proliferate, and direct cellular interactions occur specific to the antigen that triggers the response. An epitope (antigenic determinant) is a small chemical group, usually five amino acids or sugars, on the antigen that can elicit and react with an immunoglobulin (antibody). Antibody-mediated immunity, on the other hand, is specific immunity mediated by the production of immunoglobulins by B lymphocytes in response to an epitope.

Role of Antigens (Immunogens)

Although the terms *antigen* and *immunogen* are often used interchangeably, they have subtle differences. An antigen is a molecule or cell that reacts with *antibodies* (also known as *immunoglobulins*, which are plasma glycoproteins secreted by activated B lymphocytes). Immunoglobulins are capable of binding with the specific antigen that stimulated their production. An immunogen is a molecule or cell that induces an immune response. For the most part, either term (antigen or immunogen) is appropriate unless the molecule involved is a *hapten* (an antigen that is not an immunogen unless it is bound to a larger carrier molecule). A hapten therefore cannot initi-

ate an immunogenic response by itself; it is an antigen but not an immunogen. Penicillin G is an example of a medication that serves as a hapten and results in a severe allergic reaction in some people. Other haptens include toxins and certain hormones. Although most haptens are small molecules, some high-molecular-weight nucleic acids are also haptens.

Several features of molecules determine their potential ability to evoke an immune response. Molecules that are nonself are distinctly different from body cells. The *foreignness* of molecules therefore is an essential characteristic of molecules that elicit an immune response. The *size* of molecules is also important. The strongest immunogens are proteins with a molecular weight greater than 100,000 daltons. Molecules with a low molecular weight of less than 10,000 daltons are weakly immunogenic, and extremely small molecules such as haptens need a carrier protein to become immunogenic. The *chemical complexity* is also an important consideration. Complex molecules such as polymers (matter formed by a combination of two or more molecules of the same substance) are more immunogenic than is a single amino acid. Additionally, the *concentration* of an immunogen has to be of sufficient quantity to elicit an immune response.

A final important feature of immunogens is the presence of *epitopes* (some authors refer to an epitope as an *antigenic determinant*). An epitope is a small chemical group on the immunogen that can elicit an immune response and can react with an immunoglobulin (Fig. 5-1). Most immunogens have more than one type of epitope and are considered "multivalent" (i.e., able to react with more than one type of binding site). Other immunogens have repeated epitopes. Usually an epitope is about five

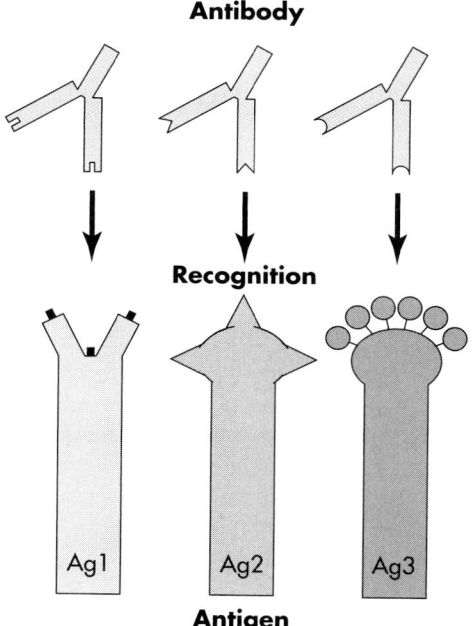

FIG. 5-1 Antigens, molecules that generate an immune response, each have a set of epitopes (antigenic determinants). The epitopes on one antigen (*Ag1, Ag2*) are usually different than those on another, although antigens such as *Ag3* may have repeated epitopes. Epitopes are molecular shapes recognized by the antibodies and T cell receptors of the adaptive immune system.

amino acids or sugars in size. The specificity of the immune response depends on the response to epitopes. Immunoglobulins are produced that are specific for the epitope rather than the whole immunogen cell or molecule. The immunoglobulin therefore does not bind to an entire cell or molecule but rather to the epitopes on the surface of the immunogen.

Common foreign immunogens include microorganisms such as bacteria, viruses, and fungi and organic substances such as pollen or house dust. When organs, tissues, cells, or molecules from other humans or even other species are introduced into a person through transplant surgery, blood transfusion, or vaccination, they also serve as immunogens. Native immunogens can also evoke an immune response, particularly when body cells mutate and become cancer cells.

OVERVIEW OF THE IMMUNE SYSTEM

The human body's lymphoid system works together with the monocyte-macrophage system (defense-related phagocytosis; see Chapter 4) to discriminate self from nonself. The lymphoid system defends the body against invaders through the use of two immune responses: cell-mediated immunity and humoral immunity. *Cell-mediated immunity*, or cellular immune response, is the immune response carried out by T lymphocytes. When the body is exposed to an immunogen, the T cells proliferate and direct a host of cellular and subcellular interactions to react to the specific epitope. Immunoglobulins and T cells can recognize the epitopes. *Humoral immunity*, or antibody-mediated immunity, is specific immunity mediated by the production of immunoglobulins (antibodies) by stimulated B lymphocytes, or *plasma cells*, in response to an epitope. Humoral immunity is also assisted by the *complement system*, an amplification system that completes the action of immunoglobulins to kill nonself immunogens and leads to lysis of certain pathogens and cells.

Lymphoid (Immune) System

The *lymphoid (immune) system* is composed of cells, tissues, and organs in which lymphocyte precursors and derivatives originate, differentiate, mature, and lodge. All blood cells originate from the common precursor, the pluripotential stem cell. *Pluripotential stem cells* are embryonic cells that can form different kinds of hematopoietic cells and are self-replicating. These cells are found in the bone marrow and other hematopoietic tissues and give rise to all the blood components (e.g., erythrocytes, platelets, granulocytes, monocytes, lymphocytes) (see Chapter 16). Stem cells differentiate and

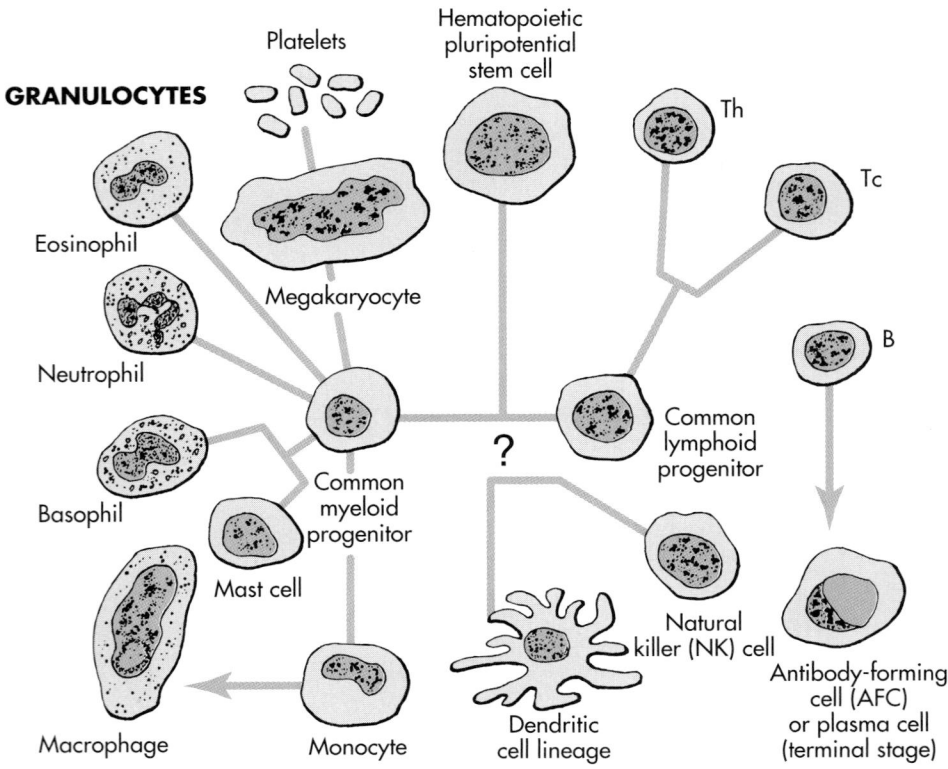

FIG. 5-2 All the cells involved in the immune system response are derived from hematopoietic pluripotential stem cells in the bone marrow. The stem cells give rise to two main lineages: lymphoid cells and myeloid cells. The common lymphoid progenitor differentiates into either a T cell or a B cell; the myeloid progenitor differentiates into the committed cells shown on the left. The term *granulocyte* is sometimes used for neutrophils, eosinophils, and basophils. Note: Pluripotential stem cells are embryonic cells that can form different kinds of hematopoietic cells. Progenitor cells are parent cells, or ancestors. (*Th*, helper T cell; *Tc*, cytotoxic T cell; *NK*, natural killer cell.)

mature into specific blood cells (Fig. 5-2) under the direction of a variety of *colony-stimulating factors* (group of substances that increase the production of various types of hematologic cells) and additional cell-derived growth factors. Three types of lymphocytes are derived from stem cells: *T lymphocytes* (known as T cells), *B lymphocytes* (known as B cells), and *natural killer* (NK) *cells* (Table 5-1). NK cells are sometimes classified as a type of T cell because they share some characteristics with T cells and have other individual characteristics. Protein markers on their cell surfaces called *clusters of differentiation* (CD) help differentiate these three cell types. CD proteins are used to differentiate T cells, NK cells, and B cells from each other and are also useful markers to identify subsets of T cells.

Primary Lymphoid Organs

Although lymphocytes exist in all parts of the body, they tend to be highly concentrated in several lymphoid organs, including the bone marrow, the thymus, the spleen, the lymph nodes, and in the organ-associated lymphoid tissues (Fig. 5-3). The bone marrow and thymus are considered the *primary lymphoid organs*. In the initial stages of lymphocyte development from stem cells in the bone marrow, lymphocytes do not produce receptors for reaction with immunogens. As they mature under the control of colony-stimulating factors, lympho-

cytes begin to express (i.e., present on their cell surface) immunogen receptors and become responsive to immunogenic stimulation; they also develop into the three different subclasses. T cells migrate from the bone marrow to the thymus gland for further maturation and are considered "thymus-dependent" lymphocytes. B cells likely remain in the bone marrow and are considered "thymus-independent" lymphocytes. NK cells are lymphocytes with some T cell markers. A primary difference between NK cells and T cells, however, is that NK cells are "prethymic"; that is, they do not pass through the thymus to mature.

The *thymus* is a two-lobed organ located in the mediastinum anterior to and above the heart. At birth, the thymus weighs 10 to 15 g and increases in size to its maximum at puberty, when it weighs as much as 40 g. During adulthood and older age, the thymus undergoes involution until it weighs less than 15% of its size at puberty. The thymus is a highly vascular organ with many lymphatic vessels that drain into the mediastinal lymph nodes. The thymus has both an outer cortex and an inner medulla (Fig. 5-4). The cortex contains a heavy concentration of *thymocytes* (T lymphocytes found in the thymus), whereas the medulla is more sparsely populated in comparison. *Hassall's corpuscles*, groups of tightly packed epithelial cells that may be areas of cell degeneration, are found in the medulla. The thymocytes are T lymphocytes that have arrived from the bone

TABLE 5-1

Types of Lymphocytes

Characteristics	T Cells	B Cells	NK cells
Origin	Stem cell	Stem cell	Stem Cell
Maturation	Thymus	? Bone marrow	? Bloodstream
Peripheral sites	Lymph nodes (paracortical area) Spleen (white pulp) GALT or Peyer's patches BALT	Lymph nodes (cortex) Spleen (white and red pulp) GALT, BALT	Bloodstream
Percentage of total blood lymphocytes	65-80	20-30	5-15
Type of immunity	Cell mediated	Humoral	Nonspecific
Subpopulations	CD4 (helper) CD8 (cytotoxic) CD8 (suppressor) Memory T cells	Plasma cells Memory B cells	None
Products	Lymphokines IL-2, IL-3, IL-4, IL-5, IL-6, IL-9, IL-10 Gamma interferon Colony-stimulating factors TNF Perforins	Immunoglobulins Lymphokines: IL-6	Perforins (chemicals that cause perforation of cells)
Protection against	Viruses (intracellular) Fungi Parasites Tumor cells Allografts (transplanted tissue)	Bacteria Viruses	Viruses (extracellular) Tumor cells Allografts
Other characteristics			
Surface immunogen receptors	Yes	Yes	No
Memory	Yes	Yes	No
CD proteins on surface	Yes: CD3 and others	No	Yes: CD2 and CD16
Immunoglobulins on surface	No	Yes	No

BALT, Bronchus-associated lymphoid tissue; *GALT,* gut-associated lymphoid tissue; *IL,* interleukin; *NK,* natural killer; *TNF,* tumor necrosis factor.

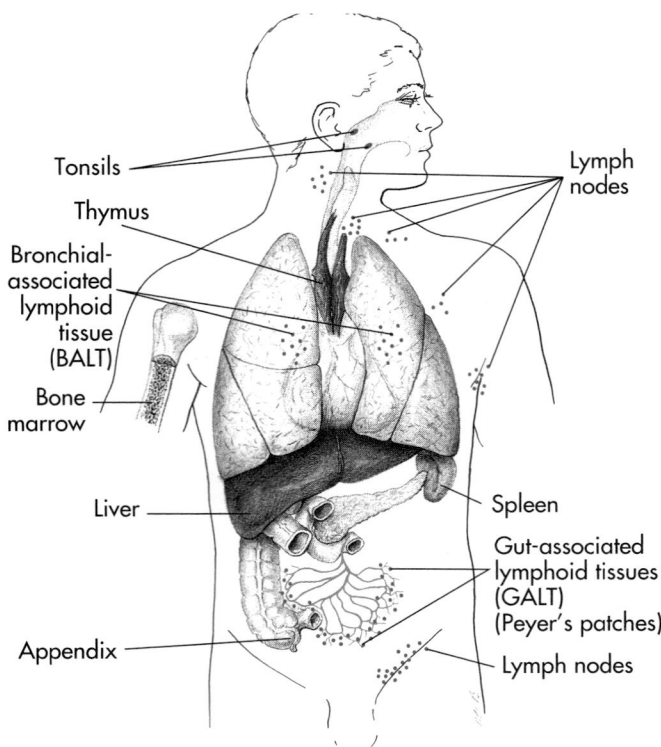

FIG. 5-3 Primary and secondary lymphoid organs and tissues.

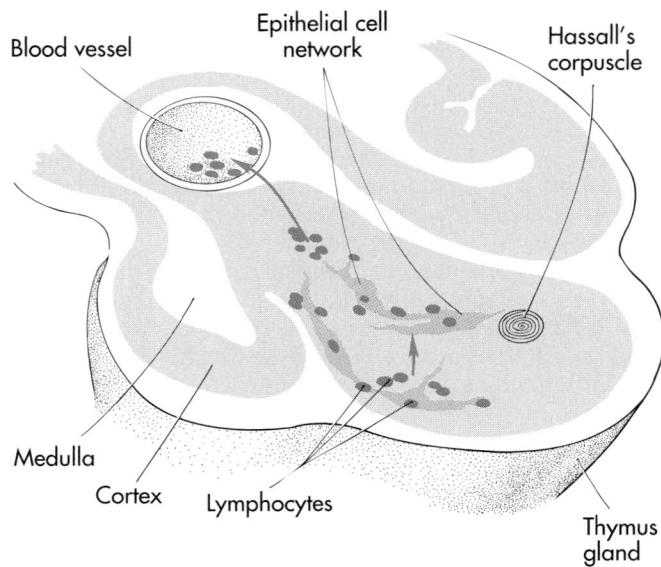

FIG. 5-4 Diagram of a portion of a lobe of the thymus gland. Lymphocytes divide in the cortex; migrate to the medulla, where they differentiate and mature; and finally enter the circulation.

marrow via the bloodstream and are at various stages of maturation.

Secondary Lymphoid Organs

The *secondary lymphoid organs* include the spleen, the lymph nodes, and nonencapsulated (without a capsule) tissue. Examples of nonencapsulated tissue are the tonsils, adenoids, and patches of lymphoid tissue in the lamina propria (fibrous connective tissue that lies directly beneath surface epithelium of a mucous membrane) and in the submucosa of the gastrointestinal (GI), respiratory, and genitourinary (GU) tracts. The *spleen* weighs approximately 150 g in adults and is located in the left upper quadrant of the abdomen behind the stomach. Blood supply arrives via the splenic artery, which divides into progressively smaller branches. When the branches divide into arterioles, they drain into vascular sinusoids that then drain into the venous system. The highly vascular design of the spleen provides a close association of the blood and splenic tissues to allow for a close interaction between blood-borne immunogens and the cells of the immune system. Essentially, blood percolates through the spleen and comes in contact with a larger number of macrophages (phagocytic WBCs) and lymphocytes, which initiate the immune response. The spleen contains two primary types of tissues: *red pulp* and *white pulp*. The red pulp is concerned mainly with destruction of worn-out erythrocytes (red blood cells [RBCs]) but also contains macrophages, platelets, and lymphocytes (B cells in particular). The white pulp of the spleen is dense, lymphoid tissue arranged around a central arteriole. This arrangement is often called the *periarteriolar lymphoid sheath* (PALS) (Fig. 5-5). The PALS con-

tains cell areas with both T and B cells, which are organized into follicles or aggregates of cells.

The spleen is the major site of immune responses to blood-borne immunogens, whereas the *lymph nodes* are responsible for processing immunogens in the lymph derived from regional tissues. Lymph nodes form a network that is responsible for filtering immunogens from the lymph and from fluid draining from the interstitial space (space between the cells). Lymph nodes, which are small and round or kidney-shaped structures 1 to 20 mm in diameter, generally occur at branches of lymphatic vessels. Lymph node clusters are found in the neck, axillae, groin, mediastinum, and abdominal cavity (Fig. 5-6). Lymph flows into the lymph nodes through afferent (inflowing) lymphatics into the subcapsular sinuses (Fig. 5-7). The lymph then flows toward the hilus (a central terminus for blood and lymph) and then exits through the efferent (outflowing) lymphatics.

Lymph nodes are surrounded by a connective tissue capsule and are organized into three main areas: the cortex, the paracortex, and the medulla. The *cortex* contains clusters of B cells called *lymphoid follicles* (primary follicles). When the body is exposed to an immunogen, B cells in this area form *germinal centers* (secondary follicles). Within these active centers, B cells divide, proliferate, and mature rapidly into immunoglobulin-producing cells. Primarily T cells and macrophages populate the *paracortex*, or inner cortex. Macrophages, other phagocytic cells, and B cells are also known as *antigen-presenting cells* (APCs) because they engulf and degrade immunogens and present epitopes on the cell surface to activate T lymphocytes. The paracortex is an important area where immunogens are presented on the macrophage, and T cells become activated as a result. The *medulla*, the smallest portion of lymph nodes, contains both T cells and B cells. Medullary sinuses drain into terminal sinuses to provide a mechanism for the lymph to drain out of the lymph node into the general lymphatic circulation.

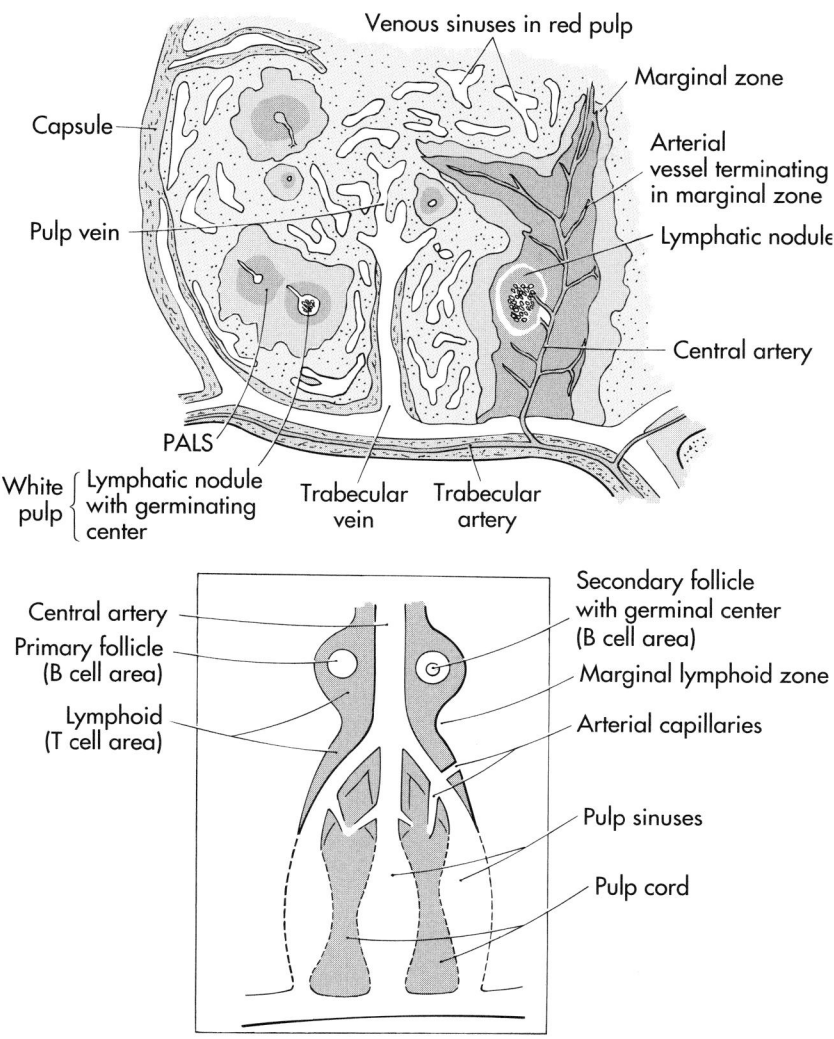

FIG. 5-5 Structure of the spleen. **A**, The white pulp is composed of periarteriolar lymphoid sheaths *(PALS)*, which contain germinal centers with mantle zones. The red pulp contains venous sinuses separated by splenic cords. **B**, In white pulp, B cell areas are primary and secondary follicles and the marginal lymphoid zone, whereas T cell areas are lymphoid cells around the follicles and arterial capillaries. (**B** redrawn from Videback A et al: *The spleen in health and disease,* Chicago, 1982, Mosby.)

Several areas of nonencapsulated lymphoid tissue exist in body systems. This tissue, often described as *mucosa-associated lymphoid tissue (MALT),* is organized into diffuse clumps of cells or nodules containing germinal centers (secondary follicles) similar to those in the spleen. MALT acts as a guard to protect the body at several submucosal entry sites in the GI, respiratory, and GU tracts and the skin. MALT is further divided into subclassifications organized by their location. *Gut-associated lymphoid tissue (GALT)* includes the tonsils, which are strategically positioned to intercept airborne and ingested immunogens. Peyer's patches (nodules of lymphoid tissue on the outer wall of the intestine) and the appendix have T and B cell areas and can also respond to alimentary immunogens. Immunoglobulins produced in GALT migrate to the GI tract, tear ducts, and salivary glands to defend against nonself penetration of epithelial surfaces. *Bronchus-associated lymphoid tissue (BALT)* resembles GALT and is found at the bifurcations of larger branches of the respiratory tree. *Skin-associated lymphoid tissue (SALT)* is found in the epidermis of the skin, where lymphocytes identify foreign invaders in the epidermis and transport the epitopes to a regional lymph node for processing (see Fig. 5-3).

Lymphocytic Traffic within the Body

The various components of the lymphoid system are joined by a sort of "double-plumbing" system—the blood vascular system and the lymphatic system (Fig. 5-8). At any given time, millions of lymphocytes are moving within the blood and the lymph. The various lymphatic channels in the body drain fluid from the interstices of organs and tissues. The lymph is conducted into large central channels that join and enter the bloodstream via the thoracic duct. A constant flow of lymph back into the blood and a constant formation of lymph by the movement of fluid from the blood into the tissues

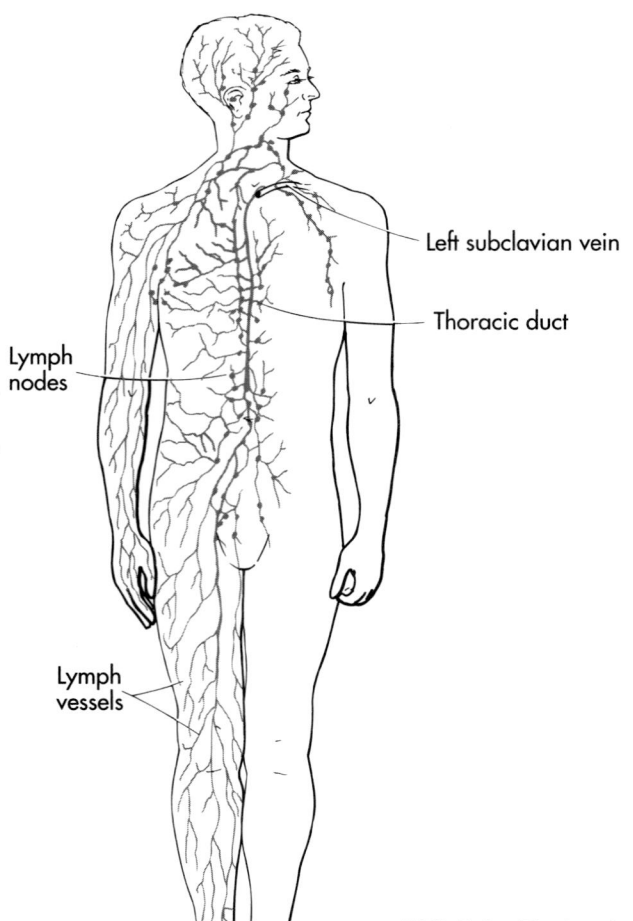

Left subclavian vein

Thoracic duct

Lymph nodes

Lymph vessels

therefore occur. Similarly, lymphocytes are constantly recirculated. The lymph within the thoracic duct contains many lymphocytes. Sufficient numbers of lymphocytes flow through the thoracic duct to replace the total number in circulation in the bloodstream several times per day.

Most lymphocytes flowing in the thoracic duct are being "recycled." Lymphocytes leave the bloodstream by specialized venules within lymphoid tissues, spend variable lengths of time within the lymphoid tissues, and then circulate via the lymph to rejoin the lymphocytes in the circulating blood. Lymphocytes differ from one another with respect to their movements around the body. Some lymphocytes are remarkably long-lived (many months or even years) and travel and recycle extensively. Other lymphocytes are relatively short-lived and do not move around quite as freely. Certain groups of lymphocytes also appear to have preferential "homing" patterns with respect to various parts of the lymphoid system. The key point is that a provision exists within the lymphoid system for moving lymphocytes from one area to another. The biologic importance of this fact is that members of a particular clone of lymphocytes that initially proliferate in one given location may circulate throughout the body and be available for interaction with immunogens at many locations.

Cell-Mediated Immunity

The role of T cells can be divided into two major functions: the regulator functions and the effector functions.

FIG. 5-6   The lymphatic system. Lymph nodes are found at junctures of lymphatic vessels and form a complete network, draining and filtering lymph derived from the tissue spaces. They are either superficial or visceral, draining the skin or deep tissues and internal organs of the body. The lymph eventually reaches the thoracic duct, which drains into the left subclavian vein and thus back into the circulation.

FIG. 5-7   Structure of a lymph node. Lymph nodes are organized into three main areas: the outer cortex, where B cells proliferate and mature; the deeper paracortex, populated mainly by macrophages and T cells; and the inner medulla, containing both B cells and T cells. Macrophages, B cells, and T cells interact with each other, often in the presence of antigen percolating through the node, resulting in the inductive phase of the immune response.

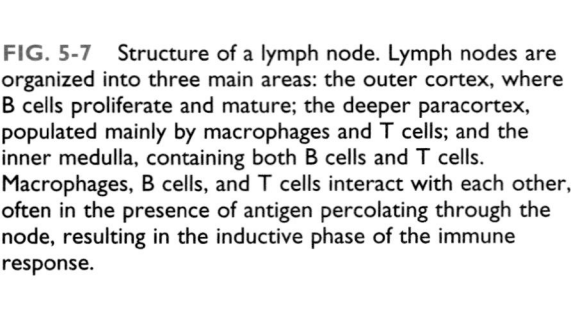

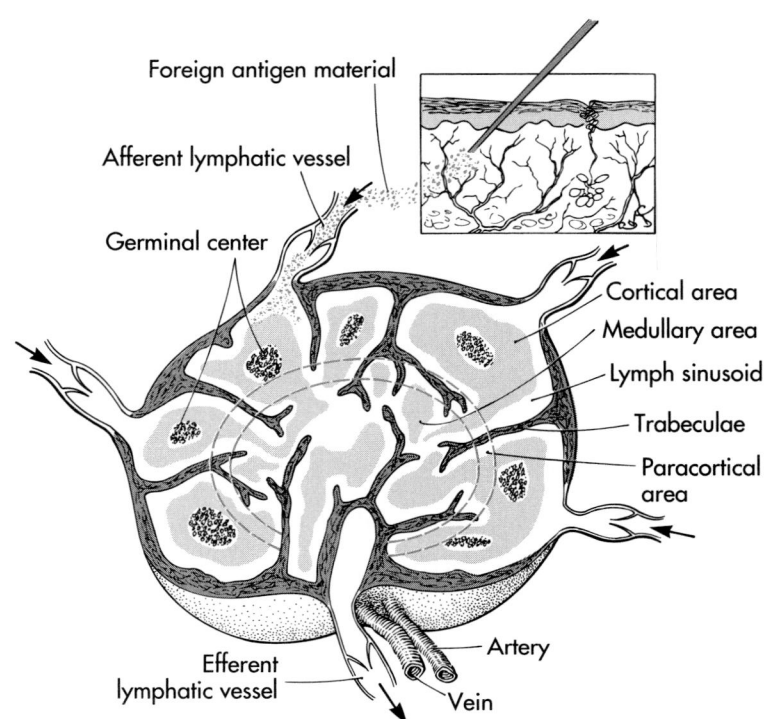

Foreign antigen material

Afferent lymphatic vessel

Germinal center

Cortical area

Medullary area

Lymph sinusoid

Trabeculae

Paracortical area

Efferent lymphatic vessel

Artery

Vein

The *regulator functions* are primarily performed by one subset of T cells, the *helper T cells* (also known as CD4 cells because the cluster of differentiation marker on the cell surface has been assigned the number 4). The CD4 cells release molecules known as *cytokines* (small molecular-weight proteins secreted by cells of the immune system), thereby performing their regulator function. Cytokines from CD4 cells regulate immune processes such as the production of immunoglobulins by B cells, the activation of other T cells, and the activation of macrophages. The *effector functions* are performed by *cytotoxic T cells* (formerly known as killer T cells but not to be confused with NK cells; currently known also as CD8 cells because the cluster of differentiation has been assigned the number 8). CD8 cells are able to kill virus-infected cells, tumor cells, and transplanted tissues by injecting chemicals called *perforins* into the "foreign" target.

Thymic Education

Both CD4 and CD8 cells undergo "thymic education" in the thymus gland so as to learn their functions. The *theory of clonal deletion* provides one explanation of the way in which T cells learn their functions. When immature T cells reach the thymus, they have no epitope-binding receptor and no CD4 or CD8 protein. The role of an epitope receptor in a mature T cell is to bind an antigenic epitope. The role of the CD4 or CD8 proteins associated with a mature T cell is to stabilize the interaction between a T cell and other cells (Fig. 5-9). A mature T cell leaving the thymus therefore has a receptor to bind with an epitope and either a CD4 protein (making the cell a *CD4 T cell*, also known as a *helper T cell*) or a CD8 protein (making the cell a *CD8 T cell*, also known as a *cytotoxic* or *suppressor T cell*).

If the T cell is to be ready to perform its functions when it leaves the thymus therefore, then it needs first to recognize nonself epitopes and second to have functioning CD4 or CD8 protein. Successful thymic education thus produces either CD4 or CD8 T cells with the following functions: (1) cells that recognize other self cells from the MHC antigen and do not bind with them (i.e., the T cell protein receptor will not have a good "fit" with other self cells); (2) cells that recognize nonself cells as invaders; and (3) cells that can bind with nonself cells with a functioning CD4 or CD8 protein to stabilize the interaction between the two cells (see Fig. 5-9). Cells potentially reactive with self-antigens *and* MHC components are probably also produced but are deleted within the thymus; they may be either killed by other cells or made to undergo *apoptosis* (programmed death).

Regulator Functions of CD4 Cells

The CD4 cells are found primarily in the medulla of the thymus, tonsils, and blood, making up approximately 65% of the total circulating T lymphocytes. CD4 cells have four primary functions: (1) CD4 cells have a regulatory function linking the monocyte-macrophage system to the lymphoid system, (2) CD4 cells interact with the APC to regulate immunoglobulin production, (3) CD4 cells produce cytokines to allow for growth of CD4 and CD8 cells, and (4) CD4 cells develop into memory cells.

One essential regulatory function of CD4 cells is their role in linking the *monocyte-macrophage system* (system containing defense-related phagocytic WBCs such as monocytes and macrophages) to the lymphoid system. When a macrophage ingests an immunogen such as a bacterium, it degrades the immunogen by the processes described in Chapter 4. The bacteria's epitopes are one of the products of bacterial destruction. An epitope binds with the macrophage's MHC antigen (MHC class II), which raises the MHC-epitope complex "as a flag" on the macrophage's cell surface. This "flag" activates CD4 cells, whose antigen receptor also binds with the epitope-MHC

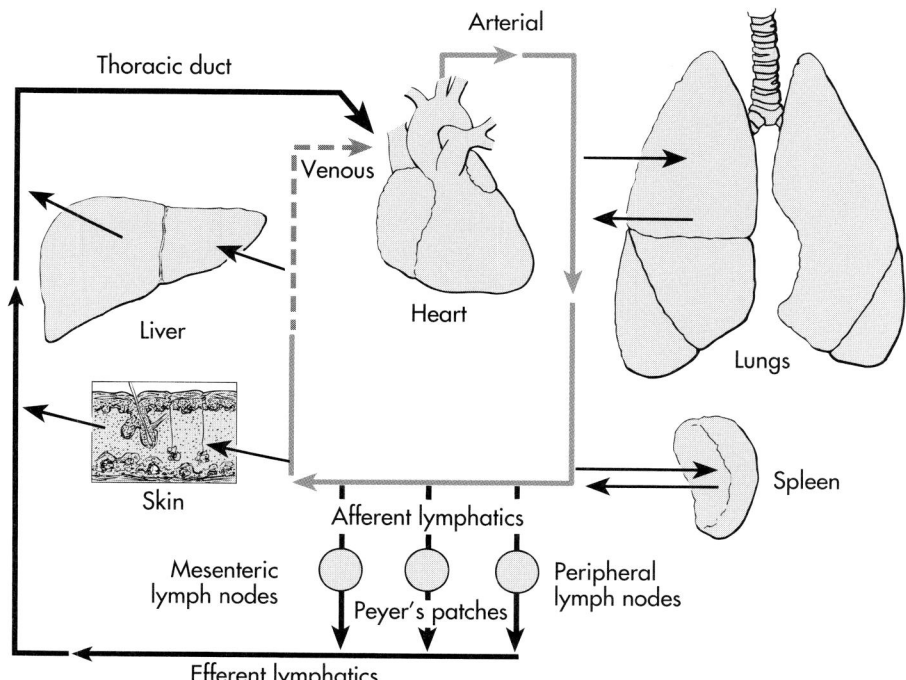

FIG. 5-8   Lymphocyte traffic in the body. (Modified from Mudge-Grout CL: *Immunologic disorders,* St Louis, 1992, Mosby.)

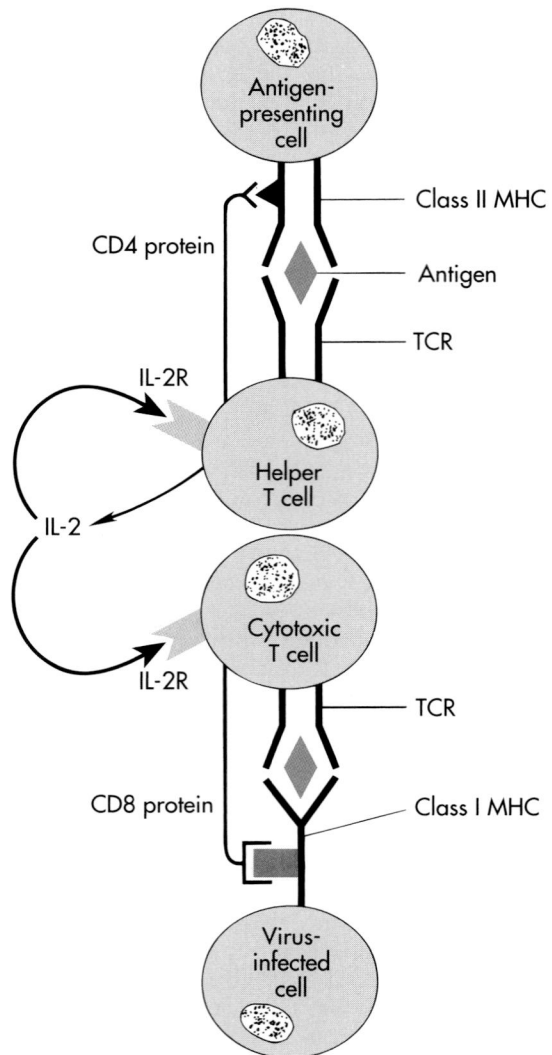

FIG. 5-9 Activation of T cells against a virally-infected cell. The antigen-presenting cell (APC) presents the antigen by means of class II MHC to the helper T cell. The reaction is stabilized by the CD4 protein. The helper T cell is activated to produce interleukin-2 (IL-2), which binds to the receptors and further activates the cells. The virally infected cell presents the antigen by means of class I MHC to the cytotoxic T cell, and in conjunction with IL-2 produced by the helper T cell, the cytotoxic T cell is activated to destroy the virally infected cell. The reaction is stabilized by the CD8 protein. (TCR, T cell receptor.)

complex. This interaction between phagocytic cells and the lymphoid cells is an essential link that allows the body to defend against invaders. The interaction between phagocytic and lymphoid cells unites two powerful body systems, the monocyte-macrophage system and the lymphoid system, into a defense system that protects self from nonself throughout the person's life. The interaction between the APC and the CD4 cells leads to an additional regulator function. CD4 cells in this reaction release gamma-(γ)-interferon (a cytokine) after the APC and the CD4 cell are bound. The release of γ-interferon by the CD4 cell attracts other macrophages into the area, activates them, and amplifies the tissue reaction to the foreign antigen.

The CD4 cell has other important regulatory functions, particularly those involved with immunoglobulin production. When an APC presents an epitope, the APC interacts with a CD4 cell and activates it. The activated CD4 cell produces chemicals or lymphokines such as interleukins 2, 4, and 5 (IL-2, IL-4, IL-5). These cytokines and other interactions stimulate B cells to divide and differentiate into *plasma cells*, the mature B cells that are capable of producing immunoglobulins. CD4 cells are essential therefore to stimulate B cells to produce immunoglobulins. Furthermore, the pattern of cytokines to which B cells are exposed affects gene rearrangements that determine the type of antibody to be secreted.

CD4 cells have other regulator functions. For example, when they interact with an APC, IL-2 production is also important for the growth of other CD4 and CD8 cells; this role promotes cell-mediated immunity. Additionally, some T cells will develop into *memory T cells*, which are capable of rapid activation on exposure to the epitope at a later time.

Controversy exists as to whether a distinct subset exists of CD8 cells that have a regulatory function in the body. Some immunologists suggest that certain CD8 cells have a suppressor function that modulates or "turns off" the action of helper (CD4) and cytotoxic (CD8) T cells, thus they do not cause harmful responses. At present, however, immunologists are unable to identify a specific subset of suppressor CD8 cells that have this "moderating" role. Although CD8 cells do have suppressor function, current thinking is that suppressor CD8 cells and cytotoxic CD8 cells are indistinguishable.

Effector Functions of CD8 Cells

CD8 lymphocytes, which are found primarily in human bone marrow and GALT, make up approximately 35% of all circulating T lymphocytes. The CD8 cells perform two primary effector functions: delayed hypersensitivity and cytotoxicity. *Delayed hypersensitivity* occurs when immunogens of intracellular organisms such as fungi or mycobacteria cause an allergic response.

Cytotoxicity is concerned primarily with destruction of virus-infected cells, graft rejection, and destruction of tumor cells. All cells of the body contain one type of MHC antigens (MHC Class I) that can display a viral epitope on the cell surface. CD8 cells recognize that MHC-epitope complex and, with the help of CD4 cells, develop a clone of CD8 cells specific to the viral epitope. The CD8 cells then release *perforins*, (toxic chemicals that damage the infected cell's outer membrane) and granzymes (protease enzymes). Perforins form a channel through the cell membrane, allowing extracellular fluid to enter the cell. Additionally, DNA of the cell is degraded, triggering apoptosis, or programmed cell death (Fig. 5-10). When the virus-infected cell dies, the CD8 cell is unharmed and continues to kill other cells infected with the same virus.

When a foreign organ or tissue is transplanted, the recipient's CD8 cells recognize that the MHC antigens on the transplanted cells' surface are not self. With the help of CD4 cells, the CD8 cells develop a clone of cells that are specific to the destruction of the nonself epitopes on the transplanted cells' surface. The CD8 cells kill the cells in the foreign tissue by the release of perforins. A similar

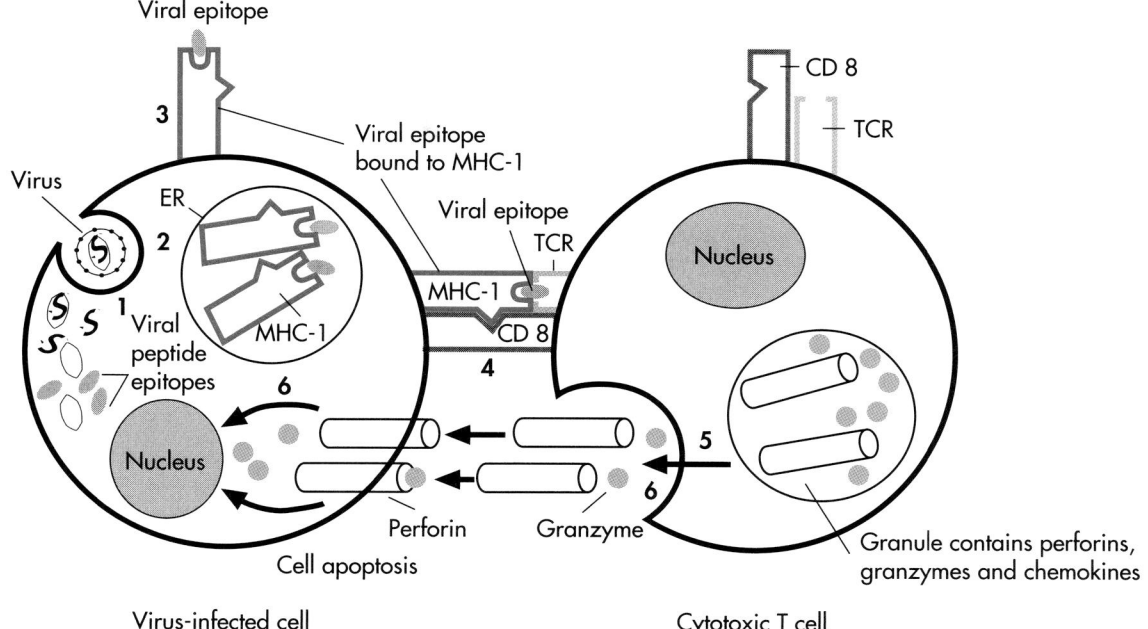

FIG. 5-10   Mechanism of virally-infected target cell destruction by the cytotoxic (killer) T cell (Tc). (1) As a virus replicates within a host cell, proteosomes degrade some of the viral proteins into peptide epitopes; (2) the viral epitopes then enter the endoplasmic reticulum (ER) where they bind to MHC-I molecules; (3) the MHC-I molecules with bound viral epitope are then transported to the surface of the host cell membrane; (4) the activated Tc cell binds to the MHC-I molecule with bound viral epitope with its CD8-TCR molecules; (5) binding of the Tc cell to the infected cell triggers the Tc cell to release perforins (pore-forming proteins) and proteolytic enzymes called granzymes; (6) granzymes pass through the pores and activate the enzymes that lead to apoptosis (programmed cell death or suicide) of the infected cell by means of destruction of its structural cytoskeleton and by chromosomal degradation. As a result the cell breaks into fragments that are subsequently removed by phagocytes. (*TCR*, T cell receptor, *CD8*, marker on cytotoxic T cell.)

process occurs with tumor cells. As tumors grow, they often develop new immunogens (different from the self components on normal body cells) on their surface. Relevant epitopes are recognized by CD8 cells, which form a clone to serve as tumor surveillance, ideally to kill neoplasms as they develop.

Major Functions of Cell-Mediated Immunity

In summary, cell-mediated immunity has four frequently cited functions:

1. CD8 T cells have a *cytotoxic* function. CD8 cells cause direct cell death of target cells such as virally infected cells or tumor cells. The CD8 cells perform this function by binding with the virally infected cell, or tumor cell, and releasing perforins to cause cell death.
2. T cells also cause *delayed hypersensitivity reactions* when they produce lymphokines that lead to inflammation. The lymphokines not only directly affect tissues, but also activate other cells such as APCs.
3. T cells have the capability to provide *memory*. Memory T cells allow for an accelerated immune response the second time the body is exposed to an immunogen and often long after the initial immunizing exposure.
4. T cells also have an important role in *regulation* or control. CD4 and CD8 cells facilitate or suppress (or both) cell-mediated and humoral immune responses.

Natural Killer Cells

Although NK cells are not truly T cells, they also perform important effector functions. NK cells specialize in destroying virus-infected cells and neoplasms by secreting perforins similar to those produced by CD8 cells. "Natural killer" cells are so named because they are active without prior exposure to a "sensitizing" epitope; they recognize nonself cells by nonimmunologic means such as unusual electrical charges on the cell surface. The primary differences between CD8 cells and NK cells are that they are not specific for the epitope and are not enhanced by the earlier exposure. The NK cells, however, perform an important function; they are always available to attack cells displaying "foreign" markers without prior sensitization and likely kill these nonself cells before cell-mediated immunity is fully activated.

Approximately 5% to 15% of all circulating lymphocytes are NK cells. Although these lymphocytes have some T cell markers, they do not pass through the thymus to mature, they have no immunologic memory, and they have no T cell receptor.

Humoral Immunity

B cells have two essential functions: (1) they differentiate into plasma cells that produce immunoglobulins, and

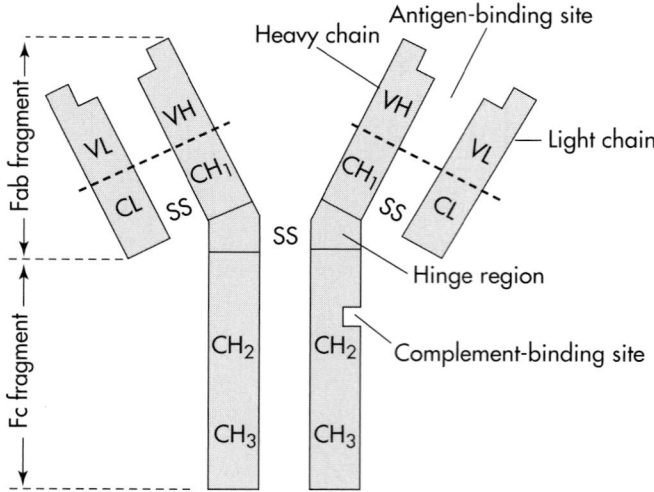

FIG. 5-11 Molecular structure of an antibody showing two light *(L)* and two heavy *(H)* polypeptide chains held together by disulfide bonds *(SS)*. The molecules have a variable *(V)* portion, constant *(C)* portion, and flexible hinge region, which can be cleaved at this site by the enzyme papain in experimental studies. The variable portion or antibody-binding *(Fab)* region of the molecule binds with the antigen epitope. It is also called the N-terminal end of the immunoglobulin. The constant region or C-terminal end of the immunoglobulin is called the Fc fragment and functions as the site for various nonspecific interactions, such as complement fixation and cell receptor binding.

(2) they are one group of APCs. In fetal life, B cell precursors are first found in the liver and then migrate into the bone marrow. B cells mature in two stages but unlike T cells do not mature in the thymus. The first phase of B cell maturation is *antigen-independent*. In this phase, which probably takes place in the bone marrow, stem cells mature first to pre-B cells and then to B cells that express immunoglobulin M (IgM) on their surface. Surface IgM production is independent of an immunogen (i.e., it is not a result of a reaction with an epitope). Both IgM and immunoglobulin D (IgD) can be epitope receptors on the surface of B cells.

In the second, *antigen-dependent,* phase, B cells interact with an immunogen, become activated, and form plasma cells capable of secreting immunoglobulins. *Clonal selection* is a theory that explains how immunoglobulins are produced. Each person has a pool of approximately 10^7 B cells, each of which has IgM or IgD on its surface that can react to one immunogen (or a closely related group of immunogens). An immunogen interacts with the B cell that shows the best "fit" with the immunoglobulin on its surface. When the B cell is activated by this reaction, it is stimulated to proliferate and form a clone of cells. These clone cells mature into plasma cells, which secrete an immunoglobulin specific for the immunogen that initiated this sequence. In the second, antigen-dependent, phase, B cells interact with an immunogen, become activated, and form plasma cells capable of secreting immunoglobulins.

FIG. 5-12 Structure of the five classes of immunoglobulins. IgG, IgD, and IgE are monomers. As a pentamer joined by a J chain, IgM is the largest immunoglobulin. IgA has several forms. Serum IgA is a monomer, but the IgA found in secretions *(secretory IgA)* can be a dimer or trimer joined by a J chain. The secretory piece wound around the IgA dimer facilitates its transport into secretions and protects it from proteolytic attack.

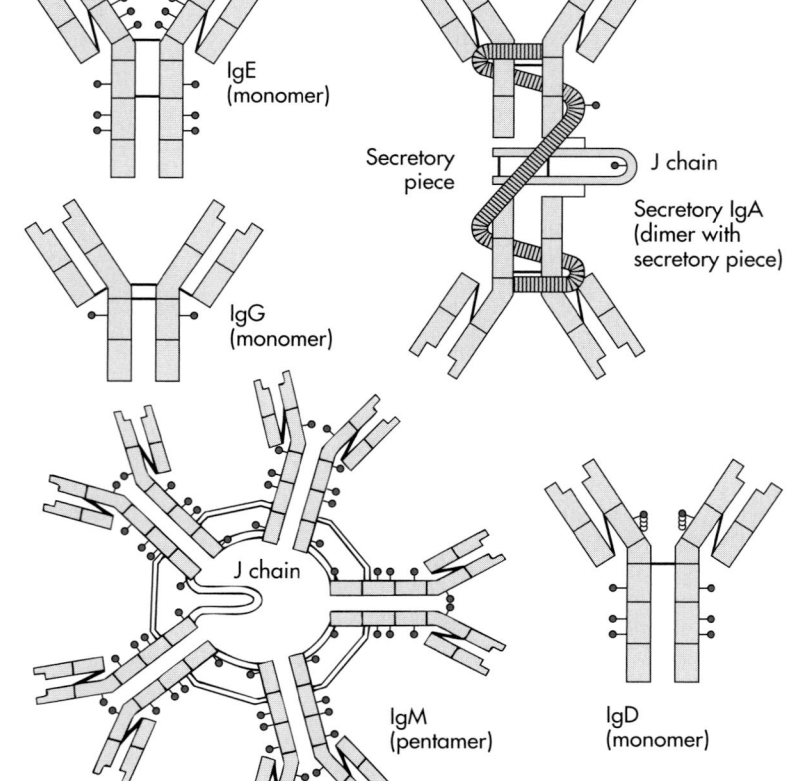

The B cell surface immunoglobulin-immunogen complex can also undergo *endocytosis* (ingestion of a foreign substance by a cell). The B cell then presents the epitope on its surface in the binding cleft of an MHC antigen. The epitope-MHC complex is recognized by a CD4 T cell (helper T), which produces interleukins that stimulate growth and differentiation of the B cell. A clone of B cells forms and produces immunoglobulins specific to the epitope. Additionally, some activated B cells become memory B cells, which stay inactive for months or years until reexposure to the immunogen a second time. Most B cell responses require T cell help.

Immunoglobulins

Immunoglobulins (antibodies), which make up approximately 20% of the protein in blood plasma, are the primary product of plasma cells. In addition to blood plasma, immunoglobulins are found in tears; saliva; mucosal secretions of the respiratory, GI, and GU tracts; and colostrum. A host of epitope-specific immunoglobulins are needed by the body to combine with a host of different epitopes; therefore different immunoglobulins with many different variable portions have to be produced to bind with millions of different epitopes. Immunoglobulins react with specific immunogens that stimulate their production. Although immunoglobulins of all classes do not have the exact same structure, many have a basic structure similar to that shown in Fig. 5-11, with a characteristic Y shape. Immunoglobulins are composed of light-molecular-weight (L) and heavy-molecular-weight (H) polypeptide chains. Although some differences exist, immunoglobulins have two H chains and two L chains variably linked by disulfide bonds. The L chains usually have one variable portion and one constant portion; the H chains usually have one variable portion and three constant portions. Table 5-2 summarizes the characteristics and functions of the five classes of immunoglobulins, and Fig. 5-12 depicts their structure.

The variable portion of the structure (at the "top" of the Y structure) is composed of distinctive amino acid

TABLE 5-2 ■ ■ ■

Classification of Immunoglobulins

Class	Percentage in Serum; Serum Concentration	Location	Description	Function
IgM	5%-10%; 80-170 mg/dl	Serum Surface of B cells	Most primitive and largest Ig with short half-life Circulates as pentamer (group of five) First to form in response to bacterial or viral infection First Ig formed by fetus	Responsible for primary response Most efficient Ig in agglutination and complement fixation Binds with immunogen on B cell surface Forms Ig against immunogens on foreign red blood cell (transfusion reactions)
IgG	75%-80%; 700-1700 mg/dl	Serum Interstitial fluid	Most abundant Ig in blood Only Ig that crosses placenta Has four subclasses	Responsible for secondary response Provides passive immunity for newborn Important in opsonization, precipitation, and agglutination Fixes complement
IgA	10%-15%; 170-280 mg/dl	Main Ig in secretions; colostrum, saliva, tears, and secretions of respiratory, GI, and GU tracts Serum	Monomer in serum (single Y) but dimer (double) or trimer (triple) forms present in secretions Complexed with secretory piece from epithelial cells to pass between epithelial cells into serosal fluids Synthesized by lymphoid tissues near mucous membranes	Neutralizes toxins in blood Primary defense against invasion of mucous membranes; prevents attachment of bacteria and virus to mucous membranes Coupled with a polypeptide for passage to mucosal surfaces
IgD	< 1% < 1 mg/dl	Serum Surface of B cells	Found in very low concentrations in blood	Function uncertain; may function as an immunogen receptor or in B cell differentiation
IgE	< 1 % < 1 mg/dl	Serum Interstitial fluid Exocrine secretions	Able to fix to receptors on mast cells and basophils	Acts as receptor for allergen when body triggers allergic response; triggers release of histamine and other mediators during allergic response Involved in type I hypersensitivity reactions Defense of parasitic infections

GI, Gastrointestinal; *GU,* genitourinary; *Ig,* immunoglobulin.

sequences that form the epitope-binding site. This portion has molecular variability because of the immune system's specificity. A host of epitope-specific immunoglobulins are needed by the body to combine with a host of different epitopes; therefore different immunoglobulins with many different variable portions have to be produced to bind with millions of different epitopes. The variable portion of immunoglobulins provides one aspect of the immune system's specificity through the large variation in amino acid sequence. The constant portion has an amino acid sequence that remains consistent among antibodies of different binding specificity. The variable and constant portions that make up each arm of the Y shape are called the *Fab fragment,* whose function is epitope binding.

The lower portion of the immunoglobulin is important for various biologic functions, such as cell receptor binding and complement fixation. The base of the Y is called the *Fc fragment* and is made up of four constant portions. A *flexible hinge region* (Hi region) lies at the intersection of the Fab and Fc fragments and gives the immunoglobulin great physical flexibility. The arms of the immunoglobulin can reach out as much as 180 degrees to bind an immunogen.

Functions of Imunoglobulins

Immunoglobulins have five primary effector functions:
1. Immunoglobulins lead to antibody-dependent cell-mediated cytotoxicity (ADCC).
2. Immunoglobulins allow for passive immunization (acquisition of immunity by receipt of preformed immunoglobulins).
3. Immunoglobulins promote opsonization (deposits of complement on an antigen, promoting stable adhesive contact with a phagocytic cell).
4. Immunoglobulins activate complement (collection of serum glycoproteins).
5. Immunoglobulins can also activate anaphylaxis.

The linking of immunoglobulins to target cells such as virally infected cells with receptors of the NK cells can kill the cell in the process of ADCC. In the process, the NK cell causes death by apoptosis. Passive immunity is relative resistance that depends on the production of immunoglobulins by another person or host. Passive immunity can occur naturally as maternal IgG is passed to the fetus or the newborn receives IgA in colostrum.

Other processes that occur in the presence of immunoglobulins include agglutination, neutralization, and lysis. *Agglutination* is the process that causes immunoglobulins and immunogens to clump together. Immunoglobulins can directly attack immunogens by agglutination, a process that may lead to neutralization (inactivation) and lysis of the immunogen. Immunoglobulins can also cause *neutralization* of toxins (poisons) released from bacteria by binding with them. The toxin and the immunoglobulins bind, a process that does not allow the toxins to bind to tissue cells and exert harmful effects. When the complexes are formed, they undergo *precipita-*

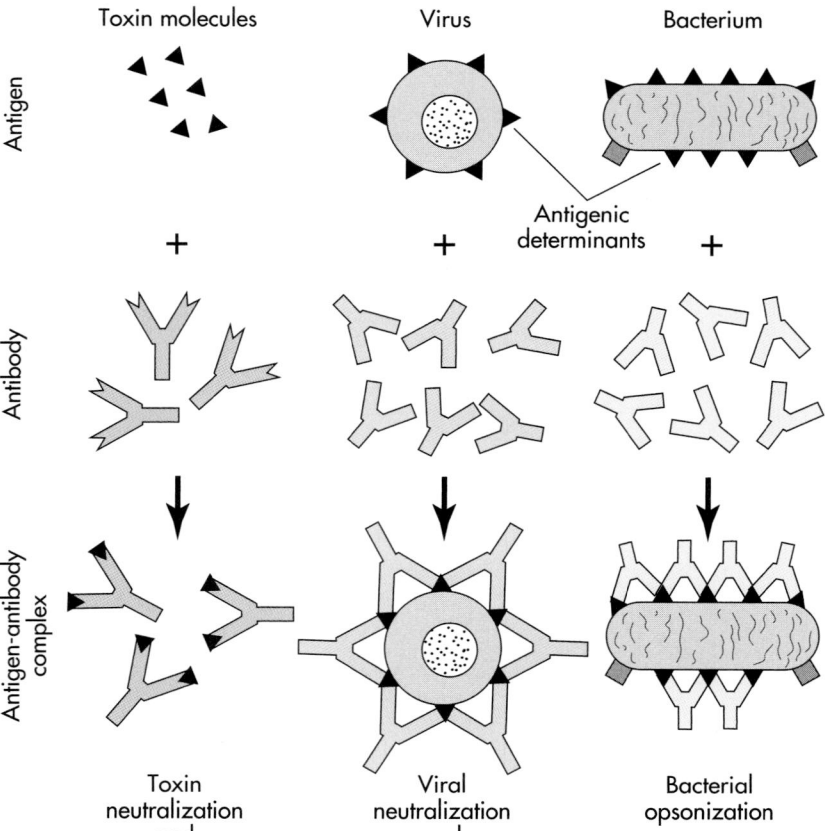

FIG. 5-13 Methods of invader destruction. Antibodies can neutralize bacterial exotoxins, neutralize viruses, and lead to opsonization of bacteria.

tion (a process that causes the complexes to fall out of solution). Phagocytic cells destroy the products of all these processes, and immunoglobulin binding promotes this degradation.

The process of *opsonization* is another important function of immunoglobulins. An *opsonin* is a substance that makes the bacteria more "tasty" to phagocytic cells, which often have surface receptors that bind IgG. When immunoglobulins (IgG in particular) coat the exterior surface of an immunogen by binding with surface epitopes, the phagocyte easily ingests the immunogen. Immunoglobulins can also activate the *complement (C) cascade*. Methods of antigen destruction by immunoglobulins are depicted in Fig. 5-13.

Immunoglobulins can activate anaphylaxis (systemic allergic reaction in a previously sensitized individual) by releasing histamine and other proinflammatory mediators into surrounding tissue fluid and the blood after exposure to an immunogen. The reintroduction of a sensitizer also may induce more limited forms of hypersensitivity reaction. This reaction causes the release of mediators from mast cells and basophils when the person is exposed to an allergen. Phagocytic cells ingest and readily degrade the immunoglobulin-immunogen com-

plexes with or without a recognizable hypersensitivity response.

Structure and Function of Complement

The *complement (C) system* consists of approximately 20 proteins that are found in human serum and tissue fluids. Initially, Paul Ehrlich coined the term *complement* to describe the ability of these proteins to complete or augment the actions of immunoglobulins during bacterial destruction. Most complement proteins are produced in the liver. The C system has three major biologic roles: (1) to cause lysis of immunogens such as bacteria, allografts (transplant tissue from the same species), and tumor cells; (2) to produce mediators or protein fragments that modulate the immune and inflammatory responses of the body; and (3) to cause opsonization, which is additive to that produced by immunoglobulins. The overall role of the C system is to act as an amplifier of all the immune reactions occurring in response to a nonself invader.

Complement Functions

A major function of the C system is cell *lysis;* its role in bacterial lysis occurs because of the activation of the C cascade. As C components are sequentially activated (Fig. 5-14), they interact with each other to build a *membrane attack complex (MAC)* on the surface of a target cell. The MAC inserts pore-forming molecules into the cell membrane of the immunogen. The cell membrane becomes disrupted, water and electrolytes enter the cell, and the target cell ruptures and dies.

A second function of complement, the *production of immune mediators*, contributes importantly to immune inflammation. The proteins of the C system lead to vasodilation at the site of inflammation. When tissues vasodilate, more blood and immune cells can circulate to the area. Additionally, C fragments (particularly C5a and the complex C567) attract neutrophils and macrophages to the area to contribute to phagocytosis. This process of attracting phagocytic cells to areas of inflammation is termed *chemotaxis*. Several fragments (C3a, C4a, C5a) cause *degranulation* (emptying out of vesicles containing histamine) of mast cells and basophils. The histamine that is released causes increased vascular permeability and smooth muscle contraction. Because these changes resemble the tissue effects following IgE-dependent reactions such as anaphylaxis, responsible C fragments are often called *anaphylatoxins*.

A third function of the C system is *opsonization*. Phagocytic cells are often able to ingest materials more easily if these immunogens are coated with complement (particularly C3b). Many phagocytic cells have C3b receptors on their surface. When the immunogen is coated with complement, the phagocytic cell receptors for complement are bound and phagocytosis proceeds rapidly.

Complement Activation

The C system becomes activated in one of two ways. Activation can occur because of the formation of immunogen-immunoglobulin complexes of IgG or IgM (*classic pathway*) or by a variety of molecules (*alternative pathway*), such as endotoxins (gram-negative bacterial

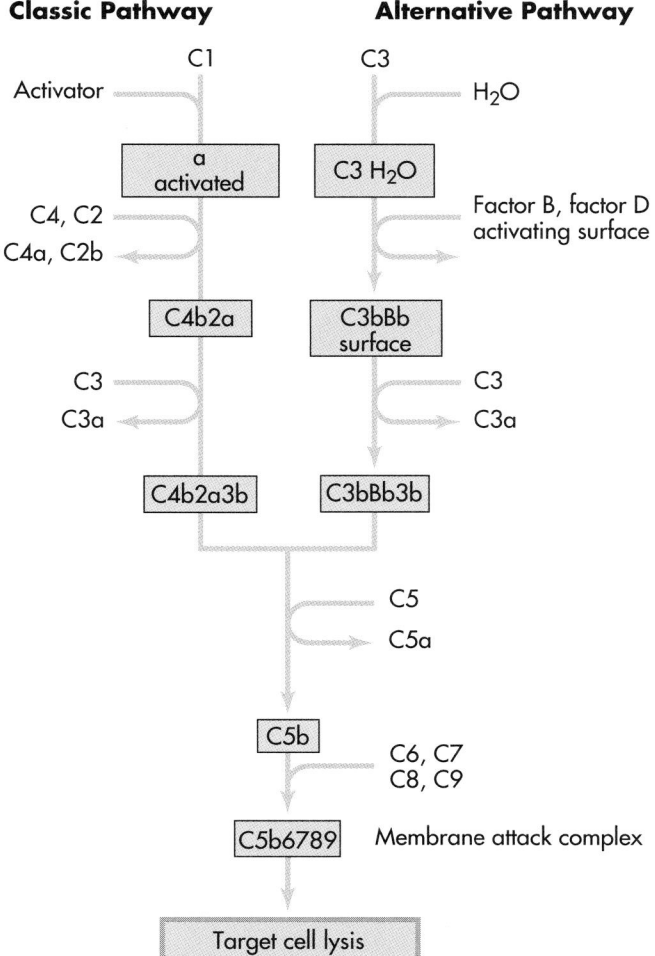

FIG. 5-14 The classic and alternative pathways of the complement cascade.

lipopolysaccharides), fungal cell walls, and viral outer envelopes. Of the two pathways, the alternative pathway is more important to host defense the first time a person is infected because the immunoglobulin necessary to trigger the classic pathway is not present. Both the classic and the alternative pathways lead to the formation of the central C molecule, C3b, which has two important functions: opsonization and formation of the MAC.

MAJOR HISTOCOMPATIBILITY COMPLEX

The MHC, also known as HLA complex, depends on a region on the short arm of human chromosome 6 (Fig. 5-15). Each person has two sets of these genes (haplotypes): one from the mother's chromosomes and one from the father's. This group of genes is responsible for producing *alloantigens* (antigens that differ among individual organisms of the same species), some of which are found on the surface of all nucleated cells. These alloantigens identify every nucleated cell in an individual as self cells.

Classes of MHC Antigens

The proteins encoded by the MHC are generally divided into three classes: class I, class II, and class III MHC antigens. *Class I MHC antigens* are found on the surface of all nucleated cells and platelets except spermatozoa. When any cell becomes infected with a virus, the viral epitope is presented on the surface of the cell by class I MHC molecules. In this complex, a CD8 T cell (cytotoxic T cell) bearing an appropriate T cell receptor (TCR) recognizes the epitope (Fig. 5-16). The CD8 protein on the CD8 cell stabilizes the interaction, and the CD8 cell becomes activated to continue the immune response.

Class II MHC molecules are involved in types of cellular reactions different from those of class I MHC components. When an APC such as a macrophage presents a processed epitope onto its surface, it is bound to the class

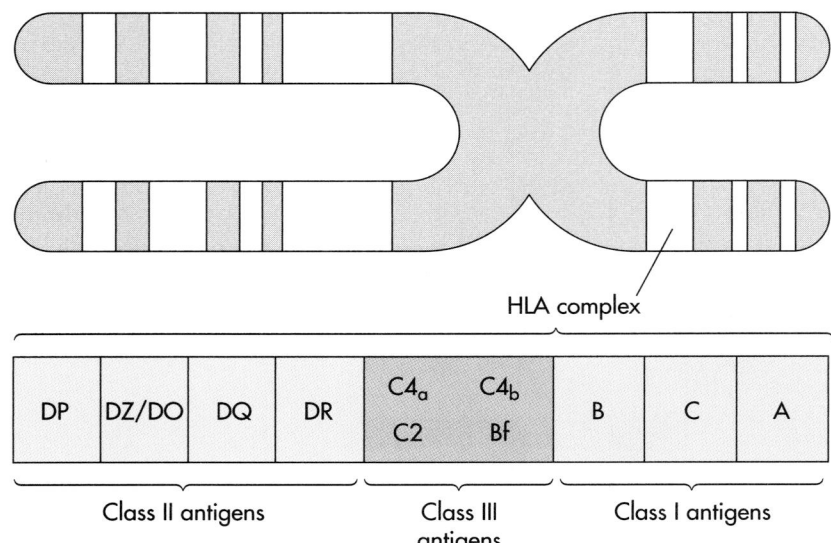

FIG. 5-15 The major histocompatibility complex (MHC), or human leukocyte antigen (HLA) complex, is located on the short arm of chromosome 6. It is the site of genes that encode HLA antigens. This gene complex is important for immune recognition, cell-cell interaction, and the coding of cell surface histocompatibility antigens that are essential for evoking an immune response. HLA complex antigens are divided into three groups. Class I antigens (loci: HLA A, B, and C) are found on the surface of most cells in the body and are important in immune recognition, tissue graph rejection, and elimination of virally infected cells. Class II antigens are found on immunocompetent cells (B cells, T cells, macrophages, monocytes) and are important in providing regulatory communication between these cells. Class III antigens are involved in both classic and alternative pathways of the complement system.

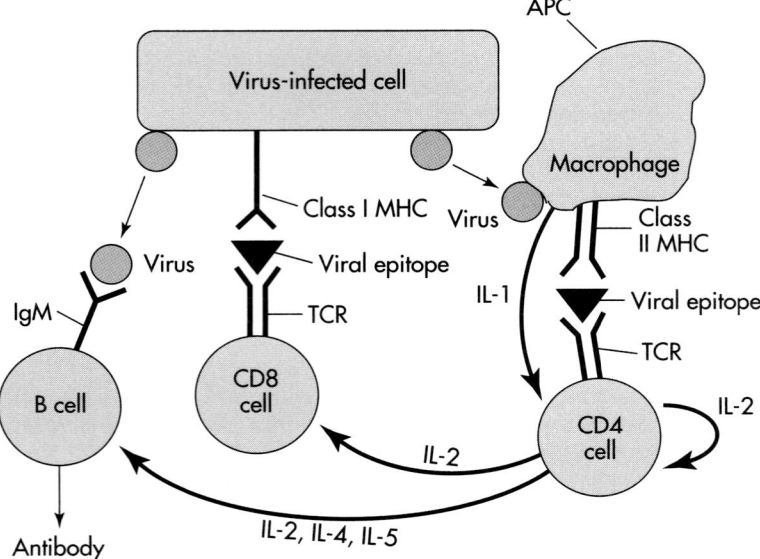

FIG. 5-16 Sequence of cell-mediated immunity and action of antibody against a viral infection. Virus released by the infected cell is ingested and processed by an antigen-presenting cell (APC) (e.g., a macrophage). The viral epitope is presented in association with a class II MHC protein to the virus-specific T cell receptor (TCR) on the CD4 cell. The macrophage makes IL-1, which helps to activate the CD4 cell. The activated CD4 cell makes interleukins (e.g., IL-2, which activates the CD8 cell to attack the virus-infected cell, and IL-4 and IL-5, which activate the B cell to produce antibody). The specificity of the cytotoxic response mounted by the CD8 cell is provided by its TCR, which recognizes the viral epitope presented by the virus-infected cell in association with the class I MHC protein.

II MHC antigen. A CD4 T cell (helper T cell) recognizes the epitope and binds to the immunogen-MHC complex with its TCR complex. The CD4 protein from the CD4 T cell stabilizes the interaction, and the CD4 cell becomes activated to continue the immune response. All nucleated cells have class I MHC antigens. When cells are infected with viruses therefore, the class I MHC antigen presents the viral immunogen on its surface to activate CD8 cells. The class II MHC antigens, however, are associated with APCs such as macrophages, monocytes, and B cells. When an antigen is presented on the APC by a class II MHC antigen, CD4 cells are activated.

Class III MHC antigens are actually part of the C cascade (C2 and C4) and are involved in both the alternative and the classic pathways of the C system. Two mediators, *tumor necrosis factor (TNF)* and *lymphotoxin*, as well as some apparently unrelated substances, are also coded in the class III MHC region.

Role of MHC Antigens in Transplants and Autoimmunity

Each person has two MHC *haplotypes* (the combination of several alleles in a gene cluster; *alleles* are one of two or more different genes containing the specific inheritable characteristics that occupy corresponding positions on a pair of chromosomes). Each parent passes his or her own haplotype to the offspring, who shares one haplotype with each parent. The more similar two persons are in their MHC makeup, the more likely that an organ or tissue transplant between them will be successful. *Tissue typing*, a process used in paternity testing and selection of donors for tissue transplantation, is the mechanism used to identify individual cellular specificities on the MHC (see Chapter 48).

Autoimmunity is defined as a condition in which structural or functional cellular damage may be caused by the reaction of lymphocytes or immunoglobulins with apparently normal components of the body. Many autoimmune diseases occur with increased frequency in people who carry certain MHC genes. The cause of these frequently strong associations is not completely clear. However, certain MHC gene products and not others can apparently present immunogens (including self antigens) for a possible immunologic response.

A person is usually tolerant to tissue immunogens that are recognized as self. In certain situations, however, tolerance to self may be lost and immune reactions may develop to self immunogens. Bacteria, viruses, and medications have all been implicated as the source of tissue changes that trigger activation of T cells and B cells to attack self cells.

The term *molecular mimicry* is used to explain this situation. The trigger bacteria or virus resemble a component of the body with sufficient similarity that an immune attack is directed against the body components rather than the trigger. Many autoimmune diseases have a marked family incidence *(genetic predisposition)* that can be linked to the MHC antigen. Autoimmune diseases that may be caused by molecular mimicry include rheumatic heart disease, systemic lupus erythematosus, rheumatoid arthritis, type 1 diabetes mellitus, myasthenia gravis, multiple sclerosis, and Graves' disease. Chapter 12 discusses additional mechanisms possibly initiating autoimmunity.

PUTTING IT ALL TOGETHER: THE IMMUNE RESPONSE

The immune response is a complex interaction (Fig. 5-17) between APCs, the cells of the immune system, and other proteins such as the C system and a host of cytokines (small-molecular-weight proteins that are secreted by cells participating in the immune response). The body has several mechanisms to encourage phagocytosis of nonself immunogens. Although APCs can ingest bacteria and viruses without opsonization, when an immunogen is coated with complement or immunoglobulins, the process of phagocytosis is amplified. When either an APC or a virally infected cell presents an epitope on the cell surface, T cells bind with the epitope and T cell activation occurs. The class I and class II MHC antigens are essential to present the immunogenic epitope and stabilize the cell-to-cell interaction, which leads to a clone of either CD8 or CD4 T cells. The class I MHC antigens stabilize reactions with virus-infected cells and CD8 (cytotoxic) T cells, whereas the class II MHC antigens stabilize reactions with APCs and CD4 (helper) T cells. The APC produces IL-1 to help the T cells activate, and the T cells, in turn, produce other interleukins to cause T cell differentiation and proliferation. Interleukins also stimulate B cells to produce immunoglobulins and affect the type of immunoglobulin produced.

Complement amplifies the response to aid in immunogen lysis and destruction. The "invading" immunogen is destroyed because of direct cytotoxic action by the CD8 T cells. Destruction and neutralization may also reflect immunoglobulin-mediated reactions that result in agglutination, precipitation, neutralization, opsonization, and activation of C enzymes and cell lysis. Memory T cells and B cells are developed to provide a more rapid response to the immunogen when it is next encountered.

Afferent and Efferent Limbs of the Immune Response

The immune response can be described in two phases: the afferent limb and the efferent limb. The *afferent limb*, also known as the *induction phase*, is the part of the immune response that leads to immunogen recognition and generation of responsive elements. The cells responsible for this aspect of the immune response are the lymphocytes (both T and B cells) and APCs, which proliferate during the afferent limb. The *efferent limb*, also known as the *effector phase*, occurs when immunocompetent lymphocytes and reactive antibodies are widely spread throughout the body. The role of these fixed and circulating components in the immune response is to react with the immunogen and render it inactive. The effector cells or immunoglobulin molecules participate in the efferent limb virtually anywhere in the body.

Primary and Secondary Immune Responses

A final important distinction in the immune response is the number of times the body has "seen" the immunogen. When the body first encounters an immunogen, immunologic events termed the *primary response* occur. Appearance of a specific antibody usually occurs within 7 to 10 days, reflecting production by a clone of B cells

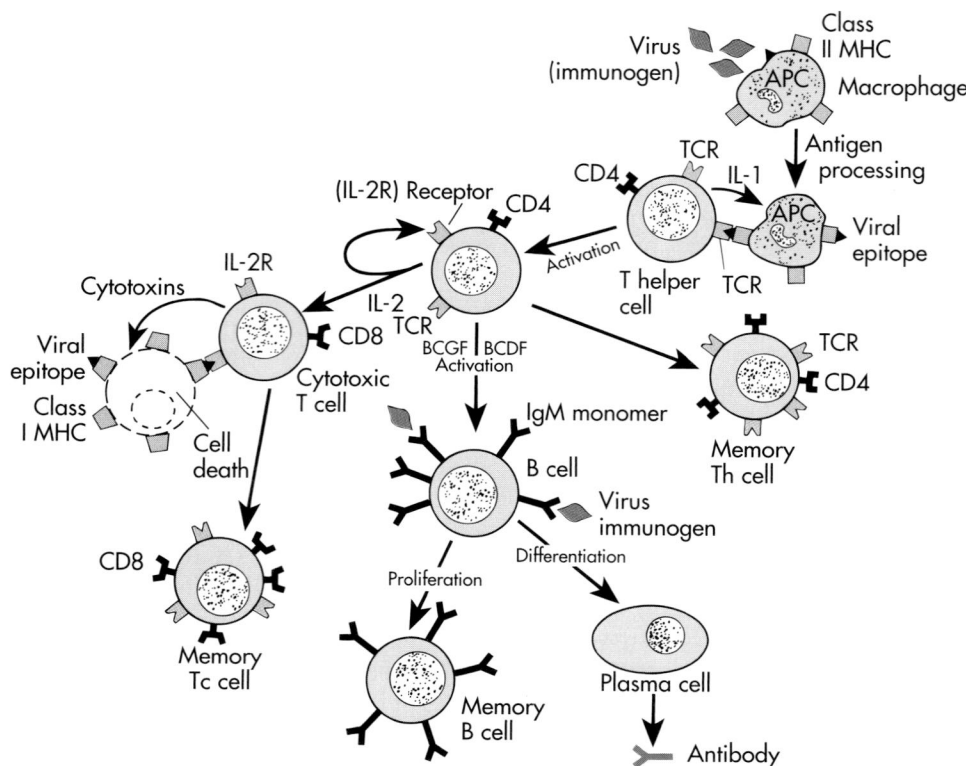

FIG. 5-17 Overview of the process by which the cell-mediated immune response and the humoral immune response are induced.

and plasma cells for the particular immunogen. Specific serum immunoglobulin level continues to increase for approximately 4 weeks and then decreases gradually. The first immunoglobulins to appear are IgM, followed by IgG and IgA (Fig. 5-18).

Months or even years after the person is exposed to the immunogen, when a second exposure occurs, the person has a *secondary response*. The secondary response is more rapid than the primary response because of the presence of the memory cells from the first contact with the immunogen. The memory cells proliferate to form a large clone of cells capable of producing IgM as during the primary response. However, the production of IgG is much larger than it is during the primary response, and levels tend to persist much longer than they do during the first contact with the immunogen. Additionally, the immunoglobulins tend to bind with the immunogen more tightly and inactivate or clear it from the body more effectively when compared with first contact.

TYPES OF IMMUNITY

Several types of immunity occur in individuals during the life span, depending on age and disease management. *Natural immunity* (native immunity, innate resistance) is the potential for resistance to a foreign "agent" without prior contact. Natural immunity is considered "nonspecific" because it is maintained by NK cells, the C cascade, the interferons, and the skin and mucous membranes without depending on specific immune mechanisms. Body processes such as phagocytosis and inflammation

also contribute to natural immunity. Species-dependent immunity is one aspect of natural immunity. Humans do not contract diseases specific to other species, such as cows, pigs, and horses.

Acquired immunity occurs after an exposure to an immunogen after birth. Acquired immunity can be either active or passive. *Active immunity* is resistance to an immunogen that occurs as a result of contact with the foreign immunogen. Contact may occur from an infection, immunization with live or killed immunogen, exposure to bacterial products such as endotoxin or toxoids, or transplantation of foreign cells or organs. In active immunity, the individual actively produces immunoglobulins or sensitized lymphocytes or both in response to the specific immunogen. The main advantage to active immunity is that resistance is longterm; its main disadvantage is that active immunity has a relatively slow onset. Active immunity occurs when a person comes in contact with a virus such as the one that causes chickenpox; the virus stimulates a response that makes the person resistant or immune during reexposure. Whole or parts of killed or weakened viruses, their toxic products, or genetically engineered antigens such as the hepatitis B surface antigen can also confer active immunity from vaccinations.

Passive immunity is relative resistance that depends on the production of immunoglobulins by another person or host. Passive immunity can occur naturally as maternal IgG is passed to the fetus or the newborn receives IgA in colostrum. Passive immunity can also be induced artificially as treatment with an immune serum to prevent or treat infections (e.g., smallpox, rabies, measles) or to

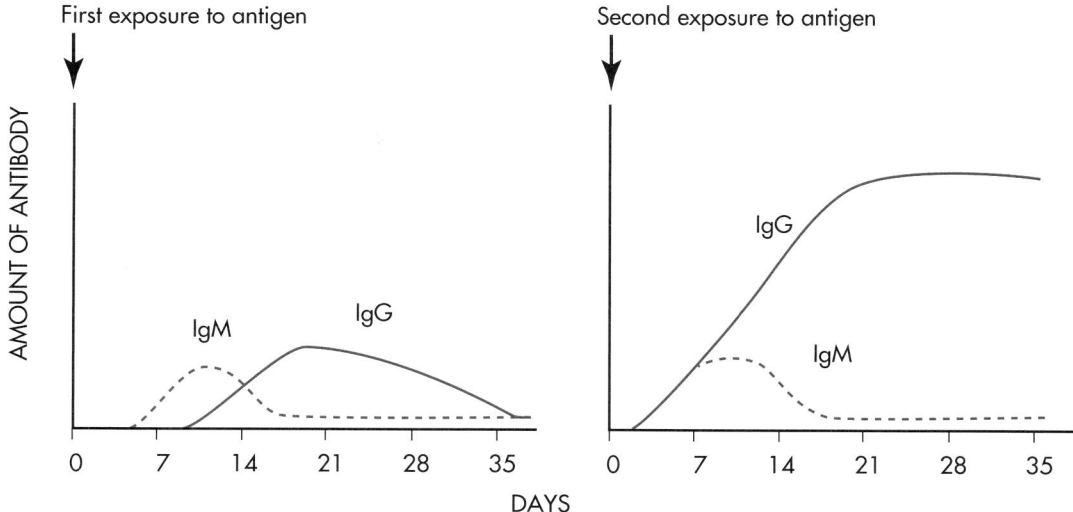

FIG. 5-18   Primary and secondary immune responses. The introduction of antigen induces a response dominated by two classes of antibodies, IgM and IgG. IgM predominates and is the first to appear in the primary response, with some IgG appearing later. After the host's immune system is primed, exposure to the same antigen induces the secondary response, in which some IgM and large amounts of IgG are produced.

neutralize toxins (e.g., diphtheria, tetanus, botulism, snake venoms). The primary advantage of passive immunity is that it is promptly available with large amounts of immunoglobulin. The major disadvantages are that passive immunization has a short life span and may produce an allergic reaction, especially when derived from "nonhuman" sources.

PHYSIOLOGY OF HYPERSENSITIVITY REACTIONS

Humoral and cell-mediated immunity clearly have an adaptive value to the body. The term *immunity* generally refers to such beneficial phenomena mediated by the immune system. However, the price humans pay for having adaptive immune machinery is that the interaction of immunoglobulins or T cells with immunogens may occasionally result in injury to the body. These injurious reactions are referred to as *hypersensitivity reactions*. The term *allergy* is also used to describe certain frequently observed hypersensitivity reactions in humans.

In the past, hypersensitivity reactions mediated by immunoglobulins were called *immediate-type* (or *humoral*) hypersensitivity reactions, whereas those mediated by cellular immune mechanisms were called *delayed* (or *cell-mediated*) hypersensitivity reactions. Although this terminology is still used today, considerable overlapping in the appearance rates of the various reactions deprives these terms of precision. A more useful classification of immunologic injuries developed by Gel and Coombs is used to classify them as types I, II, III, and IV reactions (Table 5-3).

Type I (Anaphylactic) Reactions

In *type I reactions* (anaphylactic-type reactions, immediate hypersensitivity reactions), the individual is sensitized to a particular immunogen by a previous exposure. During

the initial contact, IgE is produced, circulates throughout the body, and becomes fixed to the surface of mast cells and basophils. When the immunogen is reintroduced, its interaction with mast cell-fixed antibody results in the explosive release of proinflammatory substances such as histamine contained within these cells. When the amount of immunogen introduced to the person is small and in a well-defined, local area, the mediator release is local as well. In this situation, the result is a small area of vasodilation with increased permeability and some local swelling. This reaction is also the basis for skin testing by the allergist. However, when a larger amount of immunogen is introduced intravenously into the sensitized person, the release of mediators may be massive and widespread, producing an anaphylactic reaction. Common causes of type I reactivity are insect venoms, pollens, animal allergens, fungi, medications, and foods.

A classic example of this type of generalized anaphylactic reaction occurs when a previously sensitized person receives an intravenous infusion of an allergen such as penicillin. Signs of distress appear within a few minutes or less, and the person may die quickly after a period of agitation, seizures, bronchospasm, or circulatory collapse. An anaphylactic reaction such as this occurs because of bronchial obstruction, which leads to trapping of inspired air within the lungs, ventilatory failure, and oxygen deficit or to factors such as severe hypotension, laryngeal swelling, or cardiac rhythm disturbances. The chain of events is the result of the release of mediator substances from mast cells that target airway and vascular smooth muscle. Less severe reactions include allergic rhinitis (hay fever), angioedema, and urticaria (hives).

Type II (Cytotoxic) Reactions

Type II reactions are cytotoxic in nature. Circulating IgG or IgM unites with epitopes on the surface of the immunogen or MHC antigens presented on the cell surface. The

TABLE 5-3

Summary of Hypersensitivity Reactions

Type	Mechanism	Examples
Type I: Anaphylactic	Antigen reacts with IgE antibody bound to surface of mast cells; results in mediator release and medicator effects	Positive allergy scratch test Anaphylaxis Respiratory allergies Insect venom
Type II: Cytotoxic	Antibody unites with antigen that is part of body's cell or tissue; leads to complement activation, lysis, or phagocytosis of target cell and possibly antibody-dependent, cell-mediated cytotoxicity	Immune hemolytic anemias Goodpasture's syndrome
Type III: Immune complex	Union of antigen and antibody forms a complex that activates complement, attracting leukocytes and leading to tissue damage from leukocyte products	Serum sickness Some forms of glomerulonephritis Lesions of systemic lupus erythematosus
Type IV: Cell mediated	Reaction of T lymphocytes with antigen leads to lymphokine release, direct cytotoxicity, and recruitment of reactive cells	Allergic contact dermatitis Allograft rejection Tuberculosis lesions/skin test

IgE, Immunoglobulin E.

result of the interaction might be accelerated phagocytosis of the target cell or actual lysis of the target cell after activation of the C system. When the target cell is a foreign invader, such as a bacterium, the outcome of this reaction is beneficial. When the target cell is one of the body's own cells, such as an erythrocyte, the result may be a form of hemolytic anemia. Another kind of type II reaction is antigen-dependent cell-mediated cytotoxicity (ADCC). In this type of reaction, immunoglobulin directed against surface antigens of a cell binds to that cell. Leukocytes such as neutrophils and macrophages having receptors for a particular portion (the Fc portion) of the immunoglobulin molecules then bind to the cell and destroy it. Common examples of type II reactions include erythrocyte destruction during ABO-incompatible blood transfusions, myasthenia gravis, and Goodpasture's syndrome (attack on renal and lung basement membranes).

Type III (Immune Complex) Reactions

Type III reactions take a number of forms but are mediated ultimately by immune complexes (complexes of immunogen with immunoglobulin, usually IgG) that are deposited in tissues, arteries, and veins. A well-studied example of this type of reaction is the *Arthus reaction.* Classically, this reaction is elicited by first sensitizing a person to a foreign protein. Then the person is challenged by an intradermal injection of the same immunogen. The reaction evolves over several hours, when the area initially becomes swollen and red and eventually becomes necrotic and hemorrhagic in severe situations.

The basic mechanisms for these changes involve the formation of immunogen-immunoglobulin complexes in vessel walls. A key element in the reaction is activation of the C cascade by the immune complexes deposited within the vascular walls, although the vascular cells are not the source of the immunogen; rather, the immunogen diffuses into the walls from the blood. C activation results in the formation of chemotactic factors that attract neutrophils from the circulation. Vessel damage continues as neutrophils degranulate (release lytic enzymes)

into surrounding areas. Damage to surrounding tissue includes microthrombi, increased vascular permeability, and enzyme release leading to inflammation, tissue damage, and even tissue death. Type III reactions differ from type II reactions. Cell destruction during type II reactions is localized to a certain type of cell that is a specific "target," whereas type III reactions destroy tissue or organs anywhere the immune complexes are deposited. For example, glomerulonephritis can result when immune complexes are deposited in the kidneys, and systemic lupus erythematosus and arthritis can result when immune complexes are deposited in the skin and joints. Another example of a type III reaction is serum sickness, which develops 1 to 2 weeks after a person is injected with a foreign serum. Immune complexes are deposited on vessel walls, leading to complement activation and the resulting edema, fever, and inflammation.

Type IV (Cell-Mediated) Reactions

Type IV reactions (cell-mediated reactions, delayed hypersensitivity reactions) are mediated by the contact of sensitized T cells with the corresponding immunogen. These reactions tend to occur 12 to 24 hours after the initial exposure to the immunogen. CD4 cells (helper T cells) release cytokines that attract and stimulate macrophages to release inflammatory mediators. If the immunogen persists, then tissue damage caused by this process may develop into a chronic granulomatous reaction such as a collection of mononuclear cells in an area of damaged tissue.

A variety of immunogens, such as viruses, bacteria, fungi, haptens, and medications, can initiate a type IV reaction. The tubercle bacillus appears to cause a cell-mediated response leading to lymphotoxicity. Poison ivy, detergents, and perfumes can also cause a cell-mediated allergic dermatitis. Type IV reactions are also a principal source of rejection that occurs with some transplanted organs. When living tissue from one individual is grafted into another, whether it is a patch of skin or an entire organ, unless the donor and recipient are genetically identical, the graft tissue is sensed by the recipient's immune system as being foreign and nonself. After a brief induction phase, lymphocytes specifically sensitized to the MHC antigens from the donor invade the graft. These lymphocytes lead to graft destruction or rejection by a number of mechanisms involving either direct lymphocytoxicity or involvement of macrophages. Although T cells play a major role in graft rejection, under some circumstances, immunoglobulins play a significant parallel role. These types of rejection reactions limit the ability to replace defective organs in one individual with organs taken from another.

IMMUNODEFICIENCY

The existence of a competent immune system is essential to defend the individual from foreign antigens. Therefore an individual may develop disease because of a deficiency in any of the components of the immune system. These diseases are manifested clinically as an unusual susceptibility to infections, which may be so severe as to be lethal. The pattern of infection depends on the precise type of deficiency.

Immunologic deficiencies may be primary or secondary. *Primary immunologic deficiencies* have a genetic basis, and various parts of the immune system may be involved. An example of a defect in humoral immunity is *X-linked agammaglobulinemia* resulting from a deficiency of B cells. This condition results in almost total absence of immunoglobulin production, with consequent recurrent or chronic infections most often caused by pyrogenic bacteria such as *Haemophilus influenzae, Streptococcus pneumoniae,* and staphylococci. Humoral immunodeficiency can be of one particular immunoglobulin, such as *isolated IgA deficiency;* individuals with this condition have an increased number of respiratory and GI infections and may have severe anaphylactic reactions when transfused with normal blood (because they may develop significant levels of antibodies to IgA). Primary deficiencies of the T cell system (e.g., *DiGeorge syndrome*) or even *severe combined immunodeficiency disease (SCID)* may also occur. SCID involves functional impairment of both humoral and cell-mediated immunity. Infants with this condition are susceptible to devastating bacterial, fungal, and viral infections and often die within the first year of life. Complement abnormalities are another category of immunodeficiency (some of the primary immunodeficiency disorders are discussed in Chapter 14).

LIFE SPAN CONSIDERATIONS

The ability to maintain a functioning immune system is impaired at both the beginning and the end of the life span. Although questions exist about the relatively poor immune response in newborns, T cell function appears to be adequate. The newborn relies primarily on passive immunity to remain healthy. Antibodies are primarily supplied by the transfer of maternal IgG across the placenta before birth. Another protective mechanism for newborns is the high quantity of IgA in colostrum, which protects the newborn from respiratory and GI infections. By 3 to 6 months, however, little maternal IgG remains, and the risk of infection increases. Fetuses and newborns do have the capability for immunoglobulin production. The fetus can produce IgM in response to certain immunogens, such as the organisms that cause congenital syphilis. Shortly after birth, the newborn also begins to produce IgG and IgA, and levels of these immunoglobulins rise progressively after 4 to 6 months.

In elderly persons, the ability to mount an immune response generally diminishes from uncertain causes. The thymus, which reaches maximum size at sexual maturity, undergoes involution and by age 50, is only 15% of maximal size. Thymic hormone levels drop as well, and the thymus is unable to mediate T cell differentiation. In addition to involution of the thymus, elderly individuals have a decreased ability to produce IgG in response to immunogens; they also have fewer T cells and a delayed and diminished hypersensitivity response. Research suggests that vaccination is less effective in older adults. To complicate matters, older individuals have an increased level of circulating immunoglobulins against self (autoantibodies).

Older adults also have a decrease in the surveillance function of the immune system. When T cells and NK cells are less able to identify and destroy mutating cells, tumor cells may proliferate and the risk of cancer increases. For these reasons, infections in both newborns and older individuals have increased in both frequency and severity. Older adults are also at higher risk for the emergence of malignancies and neoplasms than in other periods during the life span.

*K*EY CONCEPTS

- To support life, an organism must be able to protect itself against threats to its individuality and recognize the difference between self and nonself. The key to the body's ability to distinguish self from nonself is the *major histocompatibility complex (MHC)*, a gene cluster on the short arm of chromosome 6 that controls the production of a particular set of molecules that serve as cellular antigens, or self-markers.

- Three functions of the immune system are: (1) defense (destruction of nonself agents such as viruses or bacteria, to prevent infection by foreign pathogens); (2) homeostasis (ridding the body of dysfunctional self-materials such as damaged cells, preventing cellular debris from posing a threat); and (3) surveillance (recognition and destruction of mutated cells, such as cancer cells).

- An *antigen* or *immunogen* is a molecule or cell that is capable of stimulating the immune response. Characteristics of substances that can serve as antigens include: (1) must be sufficiently large, complex, and foreign to the host; (2) present in sufficient quantities; (3) its epitope sites must be accessible; and (4) it is usually a protein with a molecular weight >10,000 daltons. *Haptens* are antigens that are too small to evoke an immune response alone and so must unite with a body protein to evoke an immune reaction.

- Antibodies (or immunoglobulins) are plasma glycoproteins secreted by activated B lymphocytes (plasma cells) that react with foreign antigens.

- All blood cells originate from the pluripotential stem cell. *Pluripotential stem cells* are embryonic cells that can form different kinds of hematopoietic cells and are self-replicating. Pluripotential stem cells are found in the bone marrow and other hematopoietic tissues and give rise to all blood components.

- The lymphoid system defends the body against invaders through the use of two immune responses: cell-mediated immunity and humoral immunity.

- The *primary lymphoid organs* are the bone marrow where development of B cells is completed and the thymus where the development of T cells is completed.

- *Secondary lymphoid tissue* includes lymph nodes, tonsils, spleen, and mucosal-associated tissue in the skin, respiratory, GI, and GU tracts. Adaptive immune responses are generated in the lymph nodes, spleen, and mucosa-associated lymphoid tissue. In the spleen and lymph nodes, the activation of lymphocytes by antigen occurs in distinctive B and T cell compartments of lymphoid tissue.

- *Cell-mediated immunity*, or cellular immune response, is the immune response carried out by T lymphocytes.

- The role of T cells can be divided into two major functions: the regulator functions and the effector functions.

- The regulator functions are primarily performed by one subset of T cells, the *helper T cells* (also known as *CD4 cells* because the CD marker on the cell surface has been assigned the number 4).

- CD4 cells have four primary functions: (1) CD4 cells have a regulator function, linking the monocyte-macrophage system to the lymphoid system; (2) CD4 cells interact with the antigen-presenting cell (APC) to regulate immunoglobulin production; (3) CD4 cells produce cytokines to allow for growth of CD4 and CD8 cells; and (4) CD4 cells develop into memory cells.

- The effector functions of cell-mediated immunity are performed by cytotoxic (killer) T cells (also known as CD8 cells because the cluster of differentiation has been assigned the number 8). CD8 cells are able to kill virus-infected cells, tumor cells, and transplanted tissue by injecting *perforins* (pore forming chemicals) into the "foreign" target and injecting *granzymes* (proteolytic enzymes) through the "pores" to cause *apoptosis* (programmed cell death or suicide) in the target cell.

- Cell-mediated immunity has four frequently cited functions: (1) CD8 T cells cause direct cell death of target cells such as virally infected cells or tumor cells. The CD8 T cells perform this function by binding with the target cell and releasing perforins to cause cell death by apoptosis. (2) T cells also cause delayed hypersensitivity reactions when they produce cytokines that lead to inflammation. The cytokines not only directly affect tissues but also activate other cells such as APCs. (3) T cells have the ability to provide memory. Memory T cells allow for an accelerated immune response the second time the body is exposed to an immunogen and often long after the initial immunizing exposure. (4) T cells also have an important role in regulation or control. CD4 and CD8 cells facilitate and/or suppress cell-mediated and humoral immune responses.

- *Natural killer (NK)* cells specialize in destroying virus-infected cells and neoplasms by secreting perforins similar to those produced by CD8 cells. The primary differences between CD8 cells and NK cells are that the latter are not specific for the epitope and are not enhanced by an earlier exposure.

- *Cytotoxic T cells* (CD8 cells) can recognize antigen only in conjunction with class I MHC molecules.

- *Helper T cells* (CD4 cells) can recognize antigen only in conjunction with class II MHC molecules.

- The humoral immune response is indirect and is effected by specific immunoglobulins (antibodies) produced by activated B cells (plasma cells).
- The basic structure of an immunoglobulin has a characteristic Y shape (two heavy chain and two light chain polypeptides joined by disulfide bridges). The variable or antibody-binding Fab region on the tips of the Y binds with the antigen epitope. The constant region or Fc fragment on the stem of the Y is important for complement fixation and is the site where IgE binds to basophils or mast cells.
- IgG (gamma globulin) is the most abundant immunoglobulin and is abundant in the plasma. IgG is the only Ig that crosses the placenta and is important in protection against bacterial infection.
- IgM is the largest of the immunoglobulins, circulates as a pentamer, and is responsible for the primary immune response.
- Humoral immunity involving IgG or IgM may be assisted by the complement system, an amplification system that completes the action of immunoglobulins and leads to lysis of certain pathogens and cells.
- *Complement* is a group of nine or more proteins that normally circulate in the blood as inactive precursors. When activated they can cause an inflammatory response. The complement cascade may be activated by the classic pathway (IgG or IgM) or the alternate pathway.
- Some actions of the complement components include chemotaxis (C5a; C5b67); anaphylatoxin or histamine release (C3a; C5a, C4a); opsonization (C3b); cytolysis of target cell by *membrane attack complex* (C5-C9).
- IgA may exist as a monomer, dimer, or trimer and has a secretory piece. IgA is present primarily in body secretions: colostrum, tears, saliva, and in secretions of the respiratory, GI, and GU tracts. The primary function of IgA is to defend the mucosal surfaces against invasion by bacteria and viruses.
- IgE is a cytophilic Ig and is primarily found affixed to mast cells and basophils. IgE is involved in type I hypersensitivity reactions.
- Immunoglobulins have five primary effector functions: (1) immunoglobulins lead to ADCC; (2) immunoglobulins allow for passive immunization (acquisition of immunity by receipt of preformed immunoglobulins); (3) immunoglobulins promote opsonization (deposits of complement on an antigen, promoting stable adhesive contact with a phagocytic cell); (4) immunoglobulins activate complement (collection

of serum glycoproteins); and (5) immunoglobulins can also activate anaphylaxis.
- The MHC or HLA complex is a group of genes located on the short arm of chromosome 6 that encode HLA antigens. HLA antigens are divided into three groups: Class I antigens (HLA loci: A, B, and C) are found on the surface of most cells in the body; Class II antigens (loci: DR, DQ, DP) are found chiefly on the surfaces of immunocompetent cells, including monocytes, macrophages, B cells, and T cells. Class I and II antigens are important in determining compatibility of transplanted tissue. Class III antigens are involved in the classic and alternative pathways of the complement system.
- The primary immune response occurs after the initial exposure to an antigen; the response is slow and initially IgM predominates followed by a small surge in IgG. On second exposure to the same antigen, the plasma cell mainly produces IgG and the response is much stronger and more rapid compared with the first exposure because memory B cells exist.
- There are two broad classes of acquired immunity:
  1. Naturally acquired immunity: (a) active: antibodies produced by contraction and recovery from the disease (e.g., chicken pox) or (b) passive: ready-made antibodies for infant borrowed through transfer from mother across placenta or in colostrum.
  2. Artificially acquired immunity: (a) active: active production of antibodies by the individual after vaccination (e.g., live weakened organisms, such as rabies, measles, mumps; killed organisms, such as typhoid, pertussis, Salk polio vaccine; a modified exotoxin, such as tetanus toxoid); or (b) passive: ready-made borrowed immunity and immune serum injected (e.g., tetanus antitoxin). Active immunity is slow and takes weeks to develop but is long lasting (but may need a "booster"); passive immunity is immediate but temporary, lasting only months.
- Immunologic disorders can be divided into three classes: (1) immunodeficiency disorders: primary or secondary (e.g., acquired immunodeficiency syndrome); (2) hypersensitivity disorders (e.g., allergies); and (3) autoimmune disease (e.g., systemic lupus erythematosus).
- Hypersensitivity disorders are divided into four types: type I (anaphylactic) reactions; type II (cytotoxic) reactions; type III (immune complex) reactions; and type IV (cell-mediated) reactions.

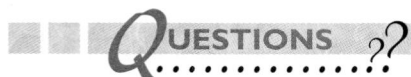

QUESTIONS ??

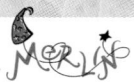

A sampling of review questions for this chapter appears here. Visit http://www.mosby.com/MERLIN/PriceWilson/ for additional questions.

Match the term in column A related to the basic structures of an immunoglobulin and the complement system with its description in column B.

Column A
1. _____ Fab region
2. _____ Fc region of IgE
3. _____ Classic pathway of complement activation
4. _____ Alternate pathway of complement activation

Column B
a. Only activated by immune complexes with IgG and IgM
b. Does not require an antigen-antibody reaction for activation (e.g., may be activated by a bacterial endotoxin)
c. Antigen binding site in antigen-antibody interactions
d. Cell membrane receptors are on the mast cell or blood basophil

Match the immunoglobulin (Ig) in column A with its description in column B.

Column A
5. _____ IgA
6. _____ IgD
7. _____ IgE
8. _____ IgG
9. _____ IgM

Column B
a. Most primitive and largest Ig; responsible for the primary immune response
b. Mediates anaphylaxis
c. Function uncertain
d. Most abundant Ig in blood; responsible for secondary immune response
e. Main Ig in secretions such as tears, saliva, and GI and GU secretions

Answer the following on a separate sheet of paper.

10. Name and describe the components and responses of the immune system, and name three functions.
11. State the purpose of immunoglobulins (antibodies). Name the five types and their specific functions.
12. Compare at least five differences between the humoral and cellular immune systems.
13. State the three classes of immunologic disorders.
14. Name the four types of hypersensitivity reactions, the immune system involved, the likely immune mechanism mediating the reaction, and an example of a prototype disease or disorder for each.

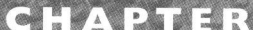

CHAPTER

6

Response of the Body to Infectious Agents

LORRAINE M. WILSON

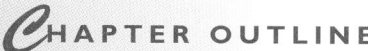
*I*nfection is a universal aspect of life. Plants and animals of all sizes and descriptions are infested with a variety of living microbes, and humans are no exception. The purpose of the following discussion is not to catalog the many specific infections to which human beings fall victim; rather, the purpose is to discuss in a general way the biologic principles that govern the interaction between host and infectious agents. Particularly, a goal of this chapter is to provide a proper perspective of the universe of infection, that is, to establish firmly the view that infectious disease is only an occasional outcome of the interaction between the host and the microbe.

HOST DETERMINANTS OF INFECTION

A requirement for the production of any infection is that the infectious organism must be able to *adhere to,* *colonize,* or *invade* the host and proliferate at least to

some extent. Not surprisingly therefore, animal species, including humans, have evolved certain elaborate defense mechanisms at the various interfaces with the environment.

Skin and Oropharyngeal Mucosa

A major interface between the environment and the human body is the skin. Fig. 6-1 shows the structure of a typical area of human skin. Clearly the intact skin, with its keratinized or horny layer at the outer surface and multilayered epithelium beneath, constitutes an excellent mechanical barrier to infection. Ordinarily, for any microorganism to breach this mechanical barrier is exceedingly difficult. However, cuts, abrasions, or areas of maceration (e.g., those folds of the body that are kept constantly moist) may allow infectious agents to enter. In addition to being a simple mechanical barrier, the skin also has a certain ability to decontaminate itself. Thus organisms that adhere to the outer layers of skin (assuming they do not simply die as they dry out) are shed as the outer flakes of skin fall off. In addition to this physical type of decontamination, a chemical decontamination is attributable to the properties of sweat and sebaceous secretions that bathe the surface of the skin. Finally, associated with the skin is the normal flora (described more fully later in this chapter), which may exert a type of biologic decontaminative effect by inhibiting the multiplication of organisms that land on the cutaneous surface.

The lining of the mouth and much of the pharynx is similar to that of the skin in that it has a surface with a multilayered epithelium that constitutes a formidable mechanical barrier to microbial invasion. This mechanical barrier, however, may be breached along gingival margins and in the region of the tonsils. The oropharyngeal mucosa is also decontaminated by the flow of saliva, which simply washes many particles away. Additionally, substances in the saliva inhibit certain microorganisms. Finally, a rich microbial flora within the mouth and pharynx may also impair the growth of some potential invaders.

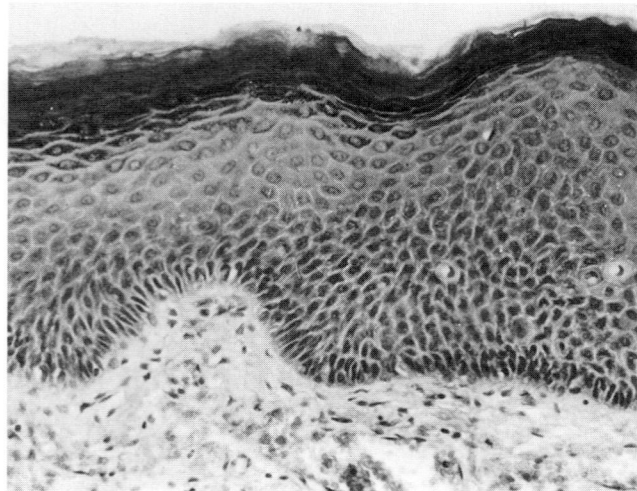

FIG. 6-1 Skin. The epidermis *(upper two thirds of field)* consists of multiple layers of cells, the most superficial of which are flattened, keratinized, and without nuclei. These layers constitute a formidable mechanical barrier. (Photomicrograph, ×300.)

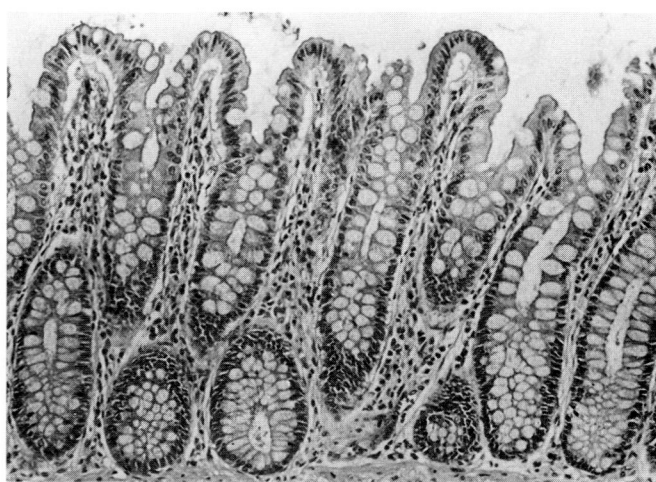

FIG. 6-3 Colon. This epithelium contains many mucus-secreting cells. During life the surface is bathed in a layer of mucus, but after tissue processing, only wisps remain *(upper right)*. The rich microbial flora that "defends" the colon is not visible in this preparation. (Photomicrograph, ×315.)

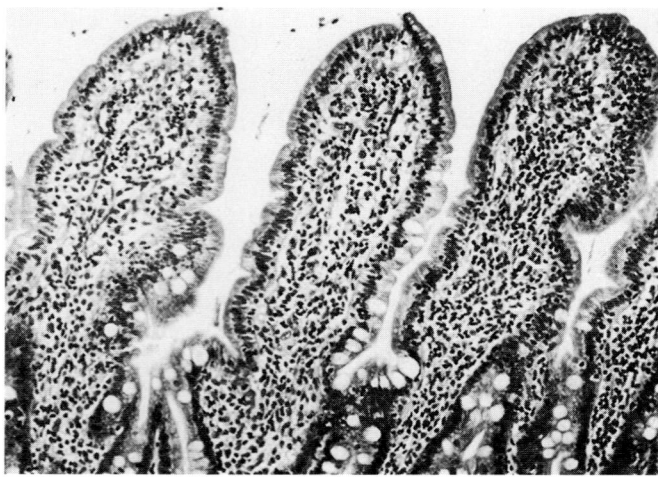

FIG. 6-2 Small intestine. The epithelium separating bowel contents from underlying tissue is actually quite delicate and is not a particularly good mechanical barrier. The surface is protected by mucus secreted by the light-staining "goblet cells," by antibody produced by the underlying lymphoid tissues, and by peristaltic emptying. (Photomicrograph, ×200.)

Gastrointestinal Tract

The gastric mucosa is of a glandular type and is not a particularly impressive mechanical barrier. Typically, small defects or erosions of the gastric lining occur, but these are of no consequence in relation to infection, because the gastric environment is extremely hostile to many microorganisms, largely because of the pronounced acidity of gastric secretions. Additionally, the stomach tends to empty its contents relatively rapidly into the small intestine. The lining of the small intestine (Fig. 6-2) is likewise not particularly tough mechanically, and many bacteria may easily penetrate the small intestine. However, peristaltic propulsion of the intestinal contents is extremely rapid in the small intestine, and bacterial pop-

ulations are kept quite sparse within the lumen. When intestinal motility is impaired, microbial counts are sharply elevated within the small intestine, and invasion of the mucosa may then occur. Several other features of the small intestine assist in the rapid propulsion of organisms through the tract. Intestinal lining cells constantly secrete abundant mucus, forming a viscous blanket over the intestinal surface, trapping bacteria, and propelling them distally by peristalsis. Additionally, the presence of antibodies within the intestinal secretions inhibits adhesion of bacteria to the mucosal surface. In the large intestine (Fig. 6-3) the lining is similarly not particularly tough mechanically. In this location, propulsion is not especially rapid, and intestinal contents are relatively stagnant. Here, the major defense against establishment of invading microbes is the presence of astronomic numbers of "normal" microbial inhabitants that coexist peacefully with the host. This mass of normal bacteria has many ecologic ways of discouraging invaders either by competing for foodstuffs or by actually secreting antibacterial (antibiotic) substances.

Respiratory Tract

Fig. 6-4 presents a microscopic view of the mucosal surface typical of conducting portions of the respiratory tract, for example, the lining of the nose, the nasopharynx, the trachea, and the bronchi. The epithelium consists of tall cells, some of which are mucus-secreting cells, but most of which are equipped with cilia at their luminal surfaces. These tiny projections beat as whips, with the action stroke directed upward toward the mouth, nose, and exterior of the body. The mucus-secreting cells produce a sticky blanket that rides on top of the cilia and glides continuously upward. When microbes are inhaled, they tend to impinge on the mucous blanket, to be moved outward and either expectorated or swallowed. The presence of antibodies within the secretions enhances this protective action. If some agents elude

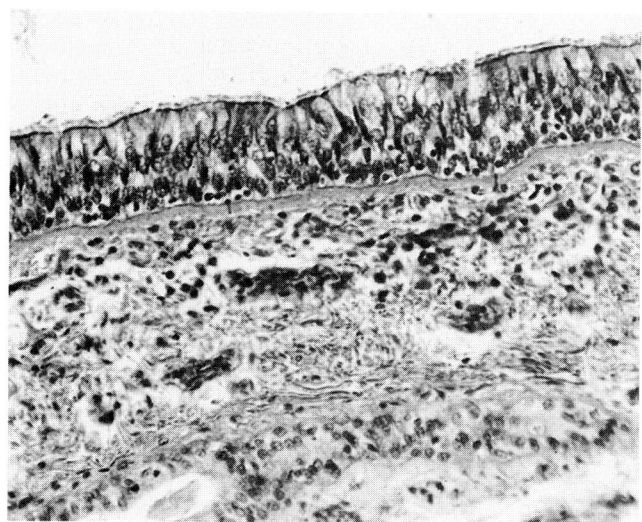

FIG. 6-4 Trachea. This type of epithelium is equipped with cilia, visible as a fringe along the upper surface. These are responsible for propelling a protective mucous blanket over the exposed surface of the air passages. (Photomicrograph, ×315.)

these defenses and reach the air spaces in the lung itself, then the ever-present macrophages provide another line of defense.

Other Defensive Barriers

Other surfaces in the body are similarly equipped with defensive mechanisms. Within the urinary tract, the lining is a multilayered epithelium that provides a mechanical barrier, but one of the main antimicrobial defenses is the flushing action of urine flow. Anything that interferes with the normal flow of urine will promote infection, whether obstruction of a ureter or simply bad habits of long-delayed micturition. Similarly, the ocular conjunctiva is defended in part mechanically and in part by the flow of tears. The vaginal mucosa is a tough, multilayered epithelium, the mechanical properties of which are augmented by a rich resident flora and by mucous secretions.

Inflammation as a Defense

If an infectious agent manages to penetrate one or another of the barriers of the body and enters the tissues, the next line of defense is the *acute inflammatory reaction*. From the discussion in Chapter 4, the value of the inflammatory reaction should be evident. The inflammatory reaction is an arena in which humoral (antibody) and cellular aspects of body defense converge. The opsonizing effects of antibodies and complement components, for instance, augment the antimicrobial activities of the phagocytes. As another example, cellular immune mechanisms may enhance the defensive properties of macrophages (see Chapter 5).

When the acute inflammatory reaction is not sufficient to handle the invader, the infection may spread elsewhere in the body. The usual means of spread is largely passive with regard to microbial action and usually involves currents of body fluid carrying the organisms. Locally, even the outpouring of exudate fluid may move the organisms about, and a phagocyte may actually be an agent of spread if it does not kill the ingested organism but wanders to another location. Spread tends to occur across natural spaces. For example, if something perforates part of the gastrointestinal (GI) tract and the contained microorganisms enter the peritoneal cavity, they may spread along the entire peritoneal surface. If some agent reaches a connective tissue plane, such as that along a muscle, it may then spread rapidly along that plane. When infectious organisms gain access to the meninges (the coverings around the central nervous system), they may rapidly spread along the entire cerebrospinal axis.

Lymphatics in Infection

For reasons outlined in Chapter 4, the flow of lymph is accelerated in acute inflammation. This means, unfortunately, that infectious agents may also occasionally spread quite rapidly along the course of lymphatics with the flowing lymph. Sometimes, lymphangitis is the result, but more often the infectious agents are carried directly to the lymph nodes, where they are rapidly phagocytosed by macrophages. In such instances, the effluent lymph moving centrally beyond a lymph node may be free of living organisms.

The Final Defenses

If spreading infectious agents are not arrested within lymph nodes or if such agents directly invade venous channels at the primary site, the bloodstream itself may then be infected. Bursts of bacteria in the bloodstream do occur, and these episodes of bacteremia are usually handled quickly and effectively by the macrophages of the monocyte-macrophage system. If large numbers of organisms are fed into the bloodstream and if these organisms are sufficiently resistant, the macrophage system may then be overwhelmed, which will result in persistence of organisms in circulation, with associated symptoms of malaise, prostration, and signs of fever, chills, and so forth. This condition is called *septicemia* or *sepsis*, often referred to by laypersons as "blood poisoning." Finally, in some instances, organisms reach such high numbers that they are circulating in clumps, lodging in many organs, and producing myriads of microabscesses (Fig. 6-5). This overwhelming situation is called *septicopyemia*, or simply *pyemia*.

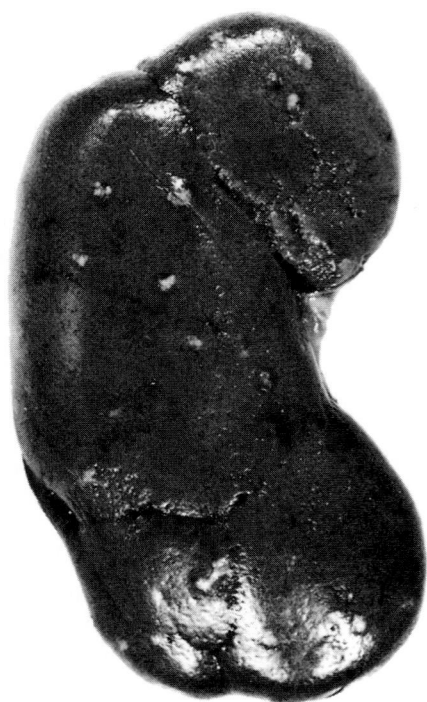

FIG. 6-5 Kidney in septicopyemia. The light-colored lesions scattered over the cortical surface are actually small abscesses formed as a result of lodgement of blood-borne bacteria.

MICROBIAL DETERMINANTS OF INFECTION

Transmissibility

An obviously essential feature in the production of infection is the transport of the living infectious agent to the body. Perhaps the most obvious means of transmission of infection is directly from person to person, for example, by coughing, sneezing, and kissing.

Organisms are transmitted indirectly in a variety of ways. Infected individuals shed organisms into the environment, and these are deposited on various surfaces and can be resuspended in air at a later time, thus spreading indirectly to others. Similarly, organisms can get into the soil, the water, the food, or other chains of indirect transmission. In hospitals, infection can also be spread via exudates and excreta. Blood transfusions may also be a means of spreading infection, as in the case of viral hepatitis. More complex types of indirect transmission involve vectors such as insects. These vectors may act in a strictly mechanical fashion, carrying the microbial agents from one place to another, or they may act in a biologic fashion, that is, by serving as intermediate hosts in some essential part of a life cycle of the infectious agent.

Certain intrinsic characteristics of microorganisms sharply influence their transmissibility or communicability. Organisms that are highly resistant to drying, such as spore-forming organisms, are readily transmissible through the environment. On the other hand, some organisms such as the spirochetes of syphilis are extremely sensitive to drying and temperature change, factors that sharply limit the mode of this transmission. Another natural selective factor that influences the communica-

bility of microbial agents is their resistance to antibiotics. Finding antibiotic-resistant strains of microorganisms emerging and then being communicated relatively freely in the hospital environment is distressingly common. A concern exists that antibiotic-resistant strains may also arise and spread in the community setting, especially with the use of suboptimal treatment regimens that permit such emergence.

Invasiveness

Once communicated to a new host, the microbial agent must establish itself on or in the body to produce infection. Great variability exists in the means adopted by various infectious agents for becoming established on or in the individual. Cholera, for instance, is caused by an organism that never invades the tissues but only colonizes the lining of the intestine, apparently by being able to adhere to some component of the surface and thus avoid being washed away. Some other organisms, such as those that produce bacillary dysentery, invade only the superficial lining of the bowel but never go any farther into the body. Still other organisms, such as the causative agent of typhoid, not only invade the superficial lining of the bowel, but they also eventually reach the bloodstream and disseminate throughout the body. Another efficient spreader is the spirochete of syphilis, which penetrates mucous membrane or skin at the portal of entry and is disseminated via the bloodstream with great rapidity.

Some organisms, after gaining access to the tissues and becoming established, never spread to any extent. The organisms that produce tetanus, for instance, do not actually spread throughout the body. When these organisms grow locally, they secrete a toxin that is carried via the bloodstream to produce the widespread effects that characterize the disease. The reasons for these differences in invasiveness of various organisms are not clearly understood, but they undoubtedly are related to specific chemical requirements of the organism and the extent to which these requirements can be met in various locales.

Microorganisms have evolved certain ways of breaching host barriers or eluding defense mechanisms. For example, some organisms develop a slimy capsule, thus the phagocytic cells of the host cannot ingest them efficiently. Other organisms have developed the enzymatic means of spreading through the ground substance of connective tissue by a chemical digestive process. Yet, other organisms secrete toxins that kill leukocytes, thus eluding capture. Some organisms have even evolved a resistance to the intracellular environment within phagocytes, and these organisms (e.g., the tubercle bacillus) tend to persist as intracellular parasites.

Ability to Produce Disease

Our knowledge of the chemical or molecular way an infectious agent produces disease has been relatively meager and is only now growing. Best understood are those situations in which the infectious agent actually secretes a soluble exotoxin, which then circulates and produces well-defined physiologic changes through action on specific cells. Thus the chemical mechanisms of disease production in tetanus and in diphtheria are relatively well understood.

Many other microorganisms, such as the gram-negative bacteria, contain endotoxin as part of their structure, a complex that is released with lysis of the microorganism. Although the biologic role of such endotoxins is far from completely understood, it is known that the release of endotoxin can be associated with the production of fever and, under more extreme circumstances, such as gram-negative septicemias, with the production of a shock syndrome.

Some organisms actually injure the host, largely by immunologic means. The tubercle bacillus, for instance, appears to have no direct toxin of its own. Rather, the patient becomes allergic to the tubercle bacillus (cell-mediated immune mechanism) and the caseous necrosis typical of the disease is produced on an immunologic basis. Similarly, some organisms affect the body by contributing to the formation of antigen-antibody complexes that may subsequently be injurious, such as via the development of immune complex glomerulonephritis.

At the far end of the spectrum are viruses that are obligate intracellular parasites. In effect, viruses are simply chunks of genetic material (deoxyribonucleic [DNA] and ribonucleic [RNA] acids) equipped to insert themselves into host cells. The cells are subsequently injured (if at all) by the new genetic information being expressed in altered cell function. One expression of such added genetic information is the replication of additional infectious virus, which may be accompanied by lysis of the affected cell. The cell may also be altered without actually becoming necrotic. In fact, the cell may even be stimulated to proliferate, as in the case of virally induced tumors. Viruses may also injure the host by evoking a variety of immunologic reactions in which part of the virus or the virus-infected cell behaves as an antigen.

INTERACTION OF HOST AND MICROBE

The interaction between a host and an infectious agent is usually viewed in terms of all-out war or a "fight to the death." The great tendency is to view infectious agents as intrinsically "bad" things, designed to produce disease. However, the real "business," biologically speaking, of any living agent is not to produce disease, but to produce more of the same kind of agent. In effect, a given microbial agent "could not care less" about producing disease in the host individual. In fact, an ideal infectious agent would simply reproduce within a given host (who constitutes a food supply) and not harm the host or otherwise "rock the boat."

Thinking in evolutionary terms, if a particular infectious agent were to be so effective in producing disease that it would be lethal to each host it entered, the organism would then rapidly run out of a food supply and quickly become extinct. The other side of the coin is that if a particular host species is to survive in the course of evolution, infectious agents within the environment must then be successfully controlled. Natural selection obviously would favor the hardier hosts. Therefore, in the course of evolution, more resistant hosts and less lethal infectious agents tend to be developed. Thus the dictates

of evolution are such that most interactions between host and infectious agent should turn out eventually to be rather "happy" ones, producing significant harm to neither party. When a relationship between host and infectious agent is inoffensive to either species, that type of interaction is referred to as *commensalism*. When the interaction affords both parties some benefit, the interaction is referred to as *mutualism*. Commensalism and mutualism are the most frequent outcomes of infectious interactions in nature, and the production of infectious disease is in an evolutionary sense (and numerically) an aberrant circumstance.

By this line of reasoning, most infectious diseases, predictably, should be mild or even most infections should be unaccompanied by disease. For most microbial "pathogens," the presence of the organism on or in the host is most usually trivial or inapparent and only as the exception is significant disease produced. Thus for every individual with an infectious disease of a particular type, several individuals in the population probably are infected with the same organism and are not sick. Pneumococci, staphylococci, meningococci, and many other pathogens can be recovered easily from perfectly healthy individuals in the population.

Certainly, exceptions to the principle exist that infection is most often mild or even inapparent. These exceptions can usually be explained on evolutionary grounds. Rabies, for instance, is almost 100% fatal to humans. The human species has not evolved with the virus but is only accidentally inserted into the chain of infection, which usually involves other mammalian species better adapted to the infection. The same is true of many other animal diseases in which humans "get in the way"; they become much more ill than the particular animal species adapted to that infection. Another sort of evolutionary exception is seen when "new" organisms are introduced into previously isolated human populations. Thus when individuals from the outside world suddenly invade isolated populations, or when island populations are exposed to agents that are commonplace in human experience (e.g., measles), the attack and fatality rates may be striking. This same evolutionary principle is involved in the spread of certain strains of influenza virus around the world. In this latter instance, the virus behaves as though it were "new" because of the development of antigenic traits that are unknown to the population at risk.

Simply knowing the line of transmission of an infectious agent from host to host does not explain fully the incidence of an infectious disease. To understand the epidemiology of such a disease completely, one must understand those aspects of the interaction between host and microbe that convert an ordinarily innocuous or inapparent infection into a clinically significant infectious disease.

OPPORTUNISTIC INFECTION

The concept of opportunistic infection reflects the fact that many organisms are not regarded as doing much to a healthy individual but, given the right circumstances, will take over and produce an infectious disease. These organisms are referred to as *opportunists* because they seemingly take advantage of the special circumstances of the host. Many opportunists are organisms that reside constantly within the body, and these are occasionally referred to as *endogenous infectious agents*. Some exogenous agents are similarly opportunistic in their behavior.

Opportunistic infections emerge when some factor or set of factors has compromised intrinsic defense mechanisms of the body or has in some way altered the ecology of the normal resident microbes (see later discussion). Many opportunistic infections are present in hospital patients who have been significantly debilitated by diseases that impair their nutrition, their immunologic reactions, or their ability to produce effectively functioning leukocytes. Leukemias and other forms of cancer are high on the list of such diseases associated with opportunistic infections. Similarly, pharmacologic agents used to treat certain diseases may have as an undesirable side effect the suppression of immunologic or inflammatory reactions, thus paving the way for opportunistic infections. Adrenal corticosteroids, which behave in many ways as antiinflammatory agents, are high on this list, as are cytotoxic agents given in the course of cancer chemotherapy or immunosuppressive therapy. Antimicrobial therapy occasionally leads to opportunistic infection, apparently via suppression of part of the normal microbial flora; it may alter the critical ecologic balance enabling another member of the flora to emerge and grow out of all proportion, thus producing disease. Antimicrobial therapy may also render the body more susceptible to some agent that ordinarily could not get a foothold because of the normal microbial flora.

Many other things happen to hospitalized patients that tend to favor an infectious organism, including certain phenomena associated with anesthesia, shock, and burns. Many diseases predispose individuals to the occurrence of infectious diseases. For example, certain cancers that involve the lymphoid tissues of the body result in defective cellular immune reactions. Individuals with these deficiencies develop infectious diseases caused by agents ordinarily controlled by the lymphocyte-macrophage system. Finally, one infectious disease may predispose to another. For example, an individual may develop a viral "cold" and thereby become likely to develop bacterial pneumonia as a complication.

Numerous environmental factors in the community at large favor a particular organism rather than the host. An example of an environmental factor involving a single individual would be occupational exposure, such as exposure to silica dust predisposing to tuberculosis. Entire populations of individuals may be involved at one time, as in famine conditions, during which depression of host response results in virtual epidemics of diseases such as tuberculosis. Finally, meteorologic changes may also influence the incidence of infectious disease as compared with infection. A variety of studies have indicated that certain infectious agents can be found within human populations year-round, but symptomatic infections with those agents have a seasonal incidence, perhaps related to the weather.

None of the previous discussion is intended to belittle the importance of germs in disease or to discourage attempts at interrupting the cycle of transmission of infectious agents among individuals. Importantly, however, a given organism may be a necessary condition for the production of a particular disease without being a sufficient condition. The complex interaction of many host and environmental factors ultimately determines the precise outcome in a given instance of infection. For these reasons, considering the "virulence" or the "pathogenicity" of a particular microorganism must be done in relation to the status of the given host at that time.

NORMAL MICROBIAL FLORA

The previous discussion mentioned the normal or indigenous microbial flora. That the host together with this microbial flora constitutes a sort of ecosystem whose equilibria are an essential part of what is considered to be health should be emphasized.

Quantitatively, the normal microbial flora of animal hosts (including humans) represents a staggering load. For example, a significant fraction of the dry weight of feces actually consists of bacterial carcasses. Humans excrete trillions of organisms each day from the GI tract. The skin also has a large resident flora, estimated to be in concentration of greater than 10,000 organisms per square centimeter of skin. These organisms do not simply adhere to dirty skin, but rather live deep within the various epithelial structures of the skin (and in fact are shed in larger numbers with scrubbing). Astronomic numbers of organisms also live within the mouth. Scrapings taken from the surfaces of teeth or gums may contain millions of organisms per milligram of material, and saliva may contain as many as 100 million organisms per milliliter.

This impressive microbial flora is not a random population. Of the many species of microbes encountered within the environment as humans move about each day, only relatively few have become adapted in the course of their own evolution to the particular environments that humans afford in various tissues. Therefore, within certain limits the flora of a given animal species is predictable and within a given species, such as humans, the flora of particular tissues is quite predictable. In most tissues that have been studied carefully, the anaerobic bacteria appear to outnumber the aerobic bacteria. This fact is especially true in the bowel, where the ratio is as high as 1000:1.

Biologists have known of the existence of the normal microbial flora for many decades, but opinions concerning the significance of the flora have varied tremendously through the years. In the early years of the twentieth century, some authorities had a dim view of the flora, judging it to be, at best, a neutral mass and, at worst, a cause of the degenerative diseases of aging. Gradually, this view has been replaced with the increasing recognition that no animal species would evolve with a particular flora in a disadvantageous relationship. To the contrary, it would be predicted that a mutually advantageous relationship should evolve.

Clearly, indigenous microbes perform many good actions for humans. Many chemical reactions within the lumen of the bowel, for instance, are actually carried out by the resident microbes. The ecologic functions of such microbes in repelling potential invaders have been discussed. Many traits of humans have evolved as they did partly as a result of the presence of the microbial associates, which means that a number of anatomic and physiologic traits considered normal and innate actually developed as a response to the presence of the flora. In other words, to a significant extent, the body depends for normalcy on the microbial flora. For example, the structure and function of the lining of the GI tract are influenced by the presence of the flora, the motility of the tract is influenced by the flora, and many of the reactions of the tract to challenge are similarly conditioned by the flora.

Although such considerations are perhaps more obvious within the GI tract, the direct and indirect effects of the indigenous flora are not limited to that area. There is reason to believe that flora even influences immunologic function and leukocyte function.

The actual means by which the microbial flora acts on the body are not well understood. In fact, even the identity of some components of the flora in humans is far from clear. Only now are health care professionals beginning to learn what controls the usual ecologic balance of the flora itself: a combination of factors involving microbe-to-microbe and host-to-microbe interactions. What is evident at this point, however, is that when one disrupts the normal ecology of the microbial flora, it is done at significant risk to the host.

KEY CONCEPTS

- *Infection* is said to be present when some microbial agent has been able to adhere to some body surface or to invade and colonize the tissues of a host and then grow and multiply. Infection is a common event, usually asymptomatic, and the production of a specific disease is uncommon.
- The *first line of defense* against invasion by infectious agents that might potentially cause disease are the *physical, chemical, and biologic barriers of the body.*
- The epithelium, dry keratin layer, and shedding of skin cells provide a mechanical barrier to infection. The chemical properties of sweat and the sebaceous glands have a mild bacteriocidal effect, and the normal flora of the skin provides a biologic barrier.
- The alimentary canal, lined with mucous membrane and a protective layer of mucus, provides a mechanical barrier to invasion by microbes. The flow of saliva washes away many microbes mechanically. Rapid peristalsis of the stomach and small intestine provides another mechanical barrier. The high acidity of the stomach provides a chemical barrier. Finally, the normal flora of the mouth, throat, and large intestine provides a biologic barrier to microbial proliferation. The GI mucus contains antibodies that provide immunologic defense.
- The mucociliary escalator of the respiratory tract provides a mechanical barrier to infection. The motile alveolar macrophages and antibody present in respiratory secretions are able to destroy microbes.
- The multilayered epithelium and the flushing action of urine flow provide defense against infection in the urinary tract.
- The flow of tears from the eyes is a defense against infection, as well as the antibodies present in tears.

- The *second line of defense* against microbial infection is the *inflammatory reaction*, which acts to localize, neutralize, and destroy invading organisms.
- When an infectious agent is not contained locally by the inflammatory response or the regional lymph nodes, the microorganisms may enter the blood (septicemia or sepsis) and possibly spread throughout the body. The phagocytic cells of the *monocyte-macrophage system and specific immunity*, chiefly in the liver and spleen, provide the *final line of defense* in eliminating the microorganisms.
- Modes of infection include surface contact (skin or mucous membranes) and the inhalation or ingestion of microorganisms. These modes include direct person-to-person transmission or indirect transmission through contact with contaminated objects, water, food, soil, or vectors.
- Whether a specific disease results from the invasion of pathogenic organisms depends on the interaction of the characteristics of the organism, its virulence and ability to produce disease, and the tissue and humoral defenses and general state of health of the host. Many people harbor pneumococci, meningococci, and other pathogens but are perfectly healthy. *Thus infection is a necessary but insufficient condition for causing an infectious disease.*
- *Opportunistic infections* occur as a result of the opportunity afforded by the altered physiologic state of the host. Thus when certain antibiotics or corticosteroids are given for long periods, certain microorganisms that would otherwise be nonpathogenic become pathogenic because of the suppression of the normal flora or the immune defenses. Opportunistic infection is especially likely to occur in patients with acquired immunodeficiency syndrome (AIDS).

 **QUESTIONS** ??

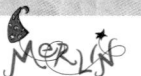

A sampling of review questions for this chapter appears here. Visit http://www.mosby.com/MERLIN/PriceWilson/ for additional questions.

Answer the following on a separate sheet of paper.

1. What are the criteria used to determine whether a body is infected? Does an infected individual necessarily have an infectious disease?
2. Name at least five portals of entry of infectious agents into the body. Describe the characteristics of the defenses at each of these portals.

3. Briefly describe what can occur when an acute inflammatory reaction is unable to contain an invading microorganism locally.
4. What is the final line of defense against widespread dissemination of an infectious agent throughout the body?
5. What is meant by an opportunistic infection?
6. What are some situations that can change an inapparent infection into an infectious disease?

7. Briefly discuss the interaction of the human host and the bacteria forming the normal flora on body surfaces. What value does this relationship provide for the host?
8. List several known mechanisms causing tissue injury by infectious agents.

Match the organisms listed in column A with their specific invasive characteristic in column B.

Column A
9. _____ *Vibrio cholerae*
10. _____ Typhoid bacillus
11. _____ Syphilis spirochete
12. _____ Tetanus bacillus

Column B
a. Penetrates the mucous membrane or skin and enters the bloodstream; disseminated widely in body
b. Invades the lining of the bowel and enters the bloodstream
c. Colonizes bowel lumen; never invades
d. Remains local but secretes a toxin that is carried in the bloodstream

Match the terms in column A, which indicate the type of relationship between two dissimilar organisms living in close association (e.g., human and microorganism), with their correct interpretation in column B.

Column A
13. _____ Commensalism
14. _____ Parasitism
15. _____ Mutualism

Column B
a. The association is beneficial to one but detrimental to the other.
b. The association is without injury to either organism.
c. The association is beneficial to both.

Disturbances in Circulation

LORRAINE M. WILSON

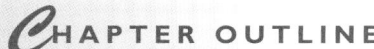
CONGESTION (HYPEREMIA)

Congestion is an overabundance of blood within the vessels in a given region. Another word for congestion is *hyperemia*. When observed grossly, an area of tissue or an organ that is congested has a deeper red (or purplish) color than is usual because of the increase in blood within the tissue. Microscopically, the capillaries in a hyperemic tissue are dilated and engorged with blood. Basical-

ly, congestion may be produced by two mechanisms: (1) an increase in the amount of blood flowing into an area and (2) a decrease in the amount of blood draining from an area.

Active Congestion

When the flow of blood into an area is increased and produces congestion, the phenomenon is called *active congestion*, in that more blood than usual is actively flowing into the area. Dilation of arterioles, which behave as valves governing the flow into the local microcirculation, causes this increase in local blood flow. One common example of active congestion is the hyperemia accompanying acute inflammation; this accounts for the redness described in Chapter 4 (see Fig. 4-1). Another example of active congestion is a blush, which is basically a matter of vasodilation produced in response to a neurogenic stimulus. A physiologic example of active congestion is the delivery of more blood on "demand" of a working tissue, such as an actively contracting muscle, which is called *functional hyperemia*. By its very nature, active congestion is often short-lived. As the stimulus to arteriolar dilation is withdrawn, the flow of blood to the affected area is decreased, and the situation returns to normal.

Passive Congestion

As the name suggests, *passive congestion* does not involve an increase in the amount of blood flowing into an area; rather; it is an impairment in drainage of blood from the area. Anything that compresses the venules and veins that drain a tissue may produce passive congestion. When an elastic tourniquet is placed around the arm before drawing blood from a vein, an artificial form of passive congestion is induced. A similar and more significant change can be produced, for instance, by a tumor that compresses the local venous drainage from an area. In addition to such local causes of passive congestion, central or systemic reasons exist for impaired venous drainage. Occasionally, the heart fails in its pumping action (see Part Six), which leads to impaired venous drainage. For

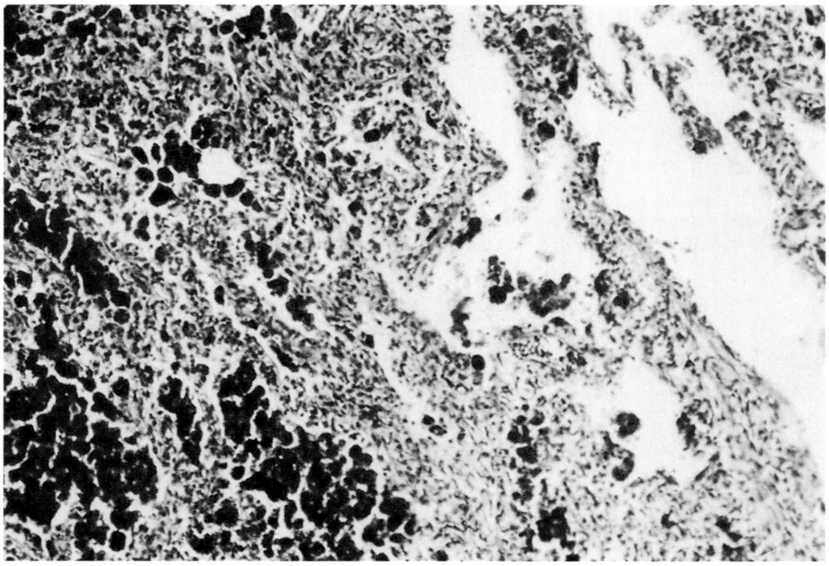

FIG. 7-1 Chronic passive congestion of lung. Alveolar septa are thickened *(evident at the right),* and many air spaces contain deeply pigmented macrophages containing hemosiderin. (Photomicrograph, ×200.)

instance, when the left side of the heart fails in its pumping action, the flow of blood returning to the heart from the lung is somewhat impaired. Under these circumstances, blood is dammed back into the lung, producing passive congestion of the pulmonary vasculature. Similarly, when the right side of the heart fails, the damming of blood affects systemic venous return, and many tissues throughout the body become passively congested. Patients typically have simultaneous right-sided and left-sided cardiac failure.

Passive congestion may be relatively short-lived, in which case it is called *acute passive congestion,* or it may be longstanding, in which case it is called *chronic passive congestion.* When the passive congestion is short-lived, the involved tissue is unaffected. Chronic passive congestion, however, may cause permanent changes in the tissues. These changes generally take place in a passively congested area, and when the change in blood flow is severe enough, tissue hypoxia may lead to shrinkage or even loss of cells of the involved tissue. In certain organs, this condition also leads to an increase in the amount of fibrous connective tissue. In many areas, evidence also exists of local breakdown of red blood cells (RBCs), which results in the deposition of hemoglobin-derived pigments within the tissues.

The effects of chronic passive congestion are particularly notable in the lungs and the liver. In the lungs (Fig. 7-1) the walls of air spaces tend to become thickened, and numerous macrophages are found to contain hemosiderin pigment, a product of the breakdown of hemoglobin from RBCs that escape the congested vessels into the air spaces. These hemosiderin-containing macrophages are called *heart failure cells* and can be found in the sputum of patients with chronic left-sided cardiac failure. In the liver, chronic passive congestion leads to marked dilation of the blood channels in the center of each hepatic lobule, with shrinkage of liver cells in this area. The result of this action is a striking gross appear-

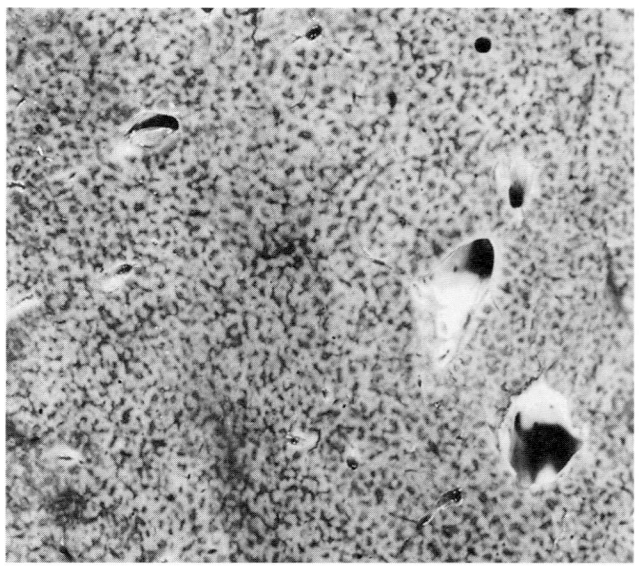

FIG. 7-2 Chronic passive congestion of liver. Dark areas on this cut surface are hyperemic centrilobular zones, and light areas are less affected peripheral zones. The result is this typical "nutmeg" pattern.

ance of the liver (Fig. 7-2) produced by the hyperemic centrilobular zone alternating with the less affected peripheral areas of each lobule. This gross appearance is occasionally referred to as "nutmeg liver" because of the fancied resemblance of the cut surface of such a liver to the cut surface of a nutmeg.

Another effect of chronic passive congestion is dilation of the veins in the affected area. As the walls of affected veins are chronically stretched, they become somewhat fibrotic, and the veins also tend to lengthen. Because veins are fixed at various points along their length, they necessarily become tortuous as they lengthen; that is, they twist back and forth between points of fixation. Dilated, somewhat tortuous, thick-walled veins are referred to as *varicose veins* or *varices*. Varicose veins in the legs are a familiar sight. Also common are *hemorrhoids*, which are actually varicose veins of the anus (in the hemorrhoidal plexus of veins). More important are the venous varices that often form in the lower esophagus in cases of chronic liver disease (see Chapters 23 and 27), and rupture of such congested varices that may lead to fatal hemorrhage.

EDEMA

Edema is an accumulation of excess fluid between the cells of the body or within the various body cavities. (Some authors also include in the definition the accumulation of excess fluids intracellularly.) Fluid that accumulates in a cavity is usually called an *effusion*, such as pericardial effusion and pleural effusion. An accumulation of fluid in the peritoneal cavity is usually called *ascites*. Massive generalized edema is typically referred to as *anasarca*. Hydrops and dropsy are older terms also referring to edema.

Etiology and Pathogenesis

The development of edema can be explained by considering the various forces that normally control fluid exchange across vessel walls (see Fig. 4-2 and Chapter 4). Local factors include the hydrostatic pressure within the microcirculation and the permeability of vessel walls. Increases in hydrostatic pressure tend to force fluid into the interstitial spaces of the body. For this simple reason, congestion and edema tend to develop together. As explained in the discussion of inflammation, a local increase in the permeability of vessel walls to protein allows these large molecules to escape the vessels, and fluid follows osmotically. Therefore edema is a prominent part of the acute inflammatory reaction. Another local cause of edema formation is obstruction of lymphatic channels, which normally drain the interstitial fluid. When these channels become obstructed for any reason, an important drainage pathway of fluid is lost, leading to accumulation of fluid, which is called *lymphedema*. Lymphedema is present in a variety of inflammatory conditions affecting the lymphatics but is perhaps most frequently encountered after either excision or irradiation of local lymphatics as part of cancer therapy. A specific example of this type of edema is the swelling of the upper extremity, frequently observed after radical mastectomy with dissection of axillary lymph nodes.

Systemic factors may also favor edema formation. Because fluid balance depends on osmotic properties of serum protein, conditions accompanied by a lower concentration of this protein may lead to edema. In nephrotic syndrome, massive amounts of protein are lost in the urine, and the patient becomes hypoproteinemic and edematous. The hypoproteinemia of advanced liver disease may also favor the formation of edema. In famine situations, massive edema may similarly accompany the nutritional hypoproteinemia.

Transudates versus Exudates

Fluid that accumulates in a tissue or space because of increased vascular permeability to protein is called an *exudate*. Thus inflammatory edema is an exudate. Fluid that accumulates in the tissues or spaces for reasons other than changes in vascular permeability is called a *transudate*. Cardiac failure is a leading cause of transudate formation. Sometimes, determining whether a particular fluid accumulation represents a transudate or an exudate becomes clinically important. For example, the presence of an exudate in the pleural cavity (e.g., as a complication of a lung abcess or lung cancer) can result in fibrothrax (i.e., welding together of the parietal and visceral pleura by fibrous adhesions; therefore removal of the exudate with chest tube drainage is necessary). This complication does not occur when the excess pleural fluid is a transudate (e.g., as in congestive heart failure) and does not usually require chest drainage. Exudates, by their very nature, tend to contain more protein that transudates and therefore tend to have higher specific gravities. Additionally, the protein of exudates often includes fibrinogen, which precipitates as fibrin, causing clotting of the exudate fluid. Transudates generally do not clot. Finally, exudates usually contain leukocytes as part of the inflammatory process, whereas transudates tend to be cell-poor.

Morphology

The morphology of edema involves simply a swelling of the affected part because of excess fluid contained within the interstices. The swelling is generally soft, and unless it is largely intracellular, the fluid can be moved about. This latter feature is used clinically in diagnosing subtle degrees of edema. Although a massively swollen ankle is easily diagnosed on sight, a slight degree of edema may be present without being particularly visible. In this instance, gentle pressure of a thumb against the side of the ankle tends to displace some of the edema fluid temporarily, and when the thumb is removed after a few moments, a depression is left in the tissues. This condition is referred to as *pitting edema*. This same mobility of edema fluid within the interstices of tissues accounts for certain postural effects. At times, when first admitted to the hospital, a patient has demonstrably edematous ankles, because in the ambulatory situation the edema moves with gravity toward the lower extremities. However, when the patient has been in bed for a time with the lower extremities not in a dependent position, the ankles may become slimmer and edema may become demonstrable over the sacrum instead.

Effects

Edema is an important indicator of something being amiss. In other words, the swollen ankles per se do not harm the patient other than perhaps in a cosmetic sense, but they do serve as an indicator of protein loss or congestive heart failure. In certain locations, edema itself is extremely important. Edema of the lungs, as in left-sided heart failure, is an acute medical emergency when extensive. When a sufficient number of air spaces in the lungs fill with edema fluid, the patient may literally drown. Massive pulmonary edema can be lethal within minutes.

Lesser degrees of pulmonary edema that can be tolerated in a ventilatory sense may be dangerous to bedridden patients. In such instances, the fluid may collect posteriorly at the lung bases and serve as a focus for the development of bacterial pneumonia, called *hypostatic pneumonia*. Edema is also life threatening when it affects the brain, because the skull is a closed space with no room to spare. As the brain becomes edematous, it swells and is compressed against the bony confines of the skull. At some point, in severe cases, increased intracranial pressure will compromise blood flow within the brain, leading to death.

HEMORRHAGE

Hemorrhage is the escape of blood from the cardiovascular system, with accumulation in tissues or spaces of the body or with actual escape from the body. Special terms are used to designate various types of hemorrhage. An accumulation of blood within tissues is called a *hematoma*. When the blood escapes into various spaces in the body, it is named according to the space, for example, hemopericardium, hemothorax (hemorrhage into the pleural space), hemoperitoneum, and hematosalpinx (hemorrhage into the fallopian tube). Pinpoint hemorrhages visible on cutaneous or mucosal surfaces or on cut surfaces of organs are called *petechiae*. Larger, blotchy areas of hemorrhage are referred to as *ecchymoses*, and a condition characterized by widespread blotchy hemorrhages is referred to as *purpura*.

Etiology

The most common cause of hemorrhage is the loss of integrity of vascular walls, which permits the escape of blood. This action is usually the result of external trauma, such as the injuries everyone occasionally experiences accompanied by bruising. The blood that accumulates in the interstices of the traumatized tissue causes the discoloration of a bruise. Vascular walls may be disrupted as a result of disease as well as of trauma.

Numerous mechanisms exist within the body to counteract hemorrhage (see Part Three). One mechanism of hemostasis involves the blood platelets, which are made in the bone marrow and circulate in the blood in large numbers. Platelets act directly to plug small leaks in vessels by aggregating in the area and blocking the flow. Platelets also lead to hemostasis by triggering the clotting mechanism of the blood. The "backbone" of a blood clot is fibrin, which is precipitated from its circulating precursor, fibrinogen. The precipitation of fibrin is controlled by a number of clotting factors that are activated under certain circumstances (see Chapter 19).

Hemorrhage may be caused by an abnormality of these hemostatic mechanisms. For instance, hemorrhage accompanies a state of *thrombocytopenia*, a deficiency in the number of circulating platelets. Thrombocytopenia may arise because of destruction or suppression of the bone marrow (e.g., by malignancy or some drug), with consequent failure of platelet production. Thrombocytopenia may also occur if circulating platelets are rapidly destroyed, as occurs in certain diseases. When the platelet count in the peripheral blood drops below a certain point, the patient begins to bleed "spontaneously," meaning that the trauma of normal motion leads to widespread hemorrhages. A deficiency of any of the various clotting factors may similarly lead to hemorrhage. This deficiency may be hereditary (e.g., hemophilia) but may also be acquired. Some of the blood-clotting factors are synthesized in the liver, and with advanced hepatic disease, the level of such factors available in the blood may drop precipitously. Paradoxically, in certain situations, excessive clotting of the blood may lead to an acquired deficiency of platelets or clotting factors or both. This usually involves the formation of myriads of tiny clots around the body, *disseminated intravascular coagulation (DIC)*, and the acquired deficiency state is often referred to under the general heading of *consumptive coagulopathy* (see Chapter 19).

Effects

The *local* effects of hemorrhage are related to the presence of extravasated blood in the tissues and can range from trivial to lethal. Perhaps the most trivial local effect is a bruise, which may be of only cosmetic importance. The initial bluish discoloration of the bruise is related directly to the presence of spilled RBCs accumulated in the tissue. These extravasated erythrocytes break down fairly rapidly and are phagocytized by macrophages arriving as part of the associated inflammatory response. These macrophages process the hemoglobin in the same manner as used in the normal recycling of old RBCs but in a much more accelerated, concentrated fashion. As the hemoglobin is metabolized within these cells, an iron-containing complex called *hemosiderin* is formed, along with a non-iron-containing moiety, which in tissues is termed *hematoidin* (although it is chemically identical with bilirubin). Hemosiderin has a rusty-brown color, and hematoidin is light yellow. The interaction of these pigments in a resolving bruise produces the familiar range of colors as the "black-and-blue mark" fades through varying shades of brown and yellow, ultimately to disappear as the macrophages wander off, and restitution of the tissue is complete. Occasionally, when a hematoma is of considerable volume, it may actually organize rather than resolve completely, leaving some degree of local scarring.

At the other extreme, a strictly local hemorrhage may be fatal, even when of small volume, if it is in the wrong place. Thus a relatively small volume of hemorrhage in a vital area of the brain can produce death (Fig. 7-3). Similarly, when a few hundred milliliters of blood are aspirated into the tracheobronchial tree, the patient may suffocate. Another area wherein a relatively small volume of hemorrhage may produce death is the pericardial sac. When hemopericardium develops quickly and the tough, fibrous pericardial sac does not have the opportunity to stretch, pressure within the sac builds up rapidly as blood accumulates. At times, with accumulation of only a few hundred milliliters, the pressure is sufficient to impair diastolic filling of the heart, leading to death by *cardiac tamponade*.

The *systemic* effects of blood loss are related directly to the volume of blood extravasated. When a major portion

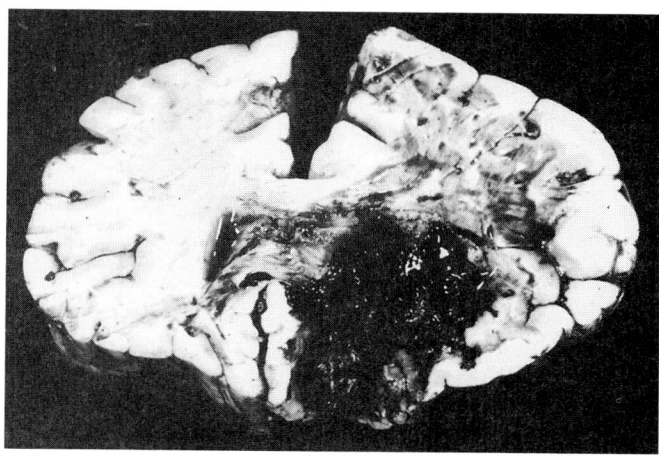

FIG. 7-3   Cerebral hemorrhage. In an instance such as this, a relatively small volume of hemorrhage may lead to death because of local destructive effects.

of the circulatory volume is lost, as with massive trauma, the patient may quickly die of exsanguination. A patient may exsanguinate with absolutely no external evidence of hemorrhage, which occurs when the extravasated blood accumulates within a large body cavity such as the pleural cavity or peritoneal cavity. This type of lethal internal hemorrhage occurs all too often in crushing injuries associated with motor vehicle accidents, when broken ribs lacerate a lung or abdominal trauma results in rupture of the spleen or liver. (In emergency room practice, such internal hemorrhage is identified by needle aspiration of the cavity in question.) The effects of a given volume of hemorrhage are also related to the rate at which the loss occurs, a larger volume loss being better tolerated when it occurs gradually rather than instantaneously.

Short of death, the rapid loss of a sufficient volume of blood may lead to a condition of *shock*. A detailed consideration of the various shock syndromes is beyond the scope of this discussion; however, shock can be produced not only by the loss of blood volume but also by neurogenic causes, cardiac causes, or even accompanying systemic sepsis. Although the various shock syndromes differ in detail, they are all basically accompanied by a decrease in blood pressure and by an element of loss of control over the regulation of blood flow, leading ultimately to inadequate perfusion and oxygenation of the vital tissues of the body.

If a patient survives the acute loss of a given volume of blood, the circulatory volume is then quickly regained by an influx of fluid into the cardiovascular system. This action leads to a relative dilution of the RBC mass remaining, and the patient at that point would be somewhat anemic. Under these conditions, the marrow is stimulated to produce RBCs at an accelerated rate, and the anemia is gradually corrected. Under conditions of chronic loss of even relatively small volumes of blood, the compensatory abilities of the marrow may be exceeded, and the patient may become progressively more anemic. Patients with chronic loss of blood may have signs and symptoms of the anemia rather than of the blood loss itself. Thus many patients with cancer of the colon,

which oozes blood for many months unnoticed into the feces, may ultimately seek medical attention because of fatigue, pallor, or lack of energy. Therefore occult blood loss is a consideration in the investigation of many anemias.

THROMBOSIS

The process of formation of a blood clot or coagulum within the vascular system (e.g., blood vessels or heart) during life is referred to as *thrombosis*. The coagulum of blood is called a *thrombus*. The accumulation of blood that clots outside of the vascular system (e.g., a hematoma) is not referred to as a thrombus. Furthermore, the clots that form after death within the cardiovascular system are not called thrombi, but rather postmortem clots.

Thrombosis is of great adaptive value in case of hemorrhage; a thrombus acts as an effective hemostatic plug. However, thrombosis may also occur inappropriately when the normal control mechanisms are defective and, under these circumstances, prove to be harmful.

Etiology and Pathogenesis

Three sets of factors ordinarily guard against inappropriate thrombus formation. First, the normal vascular system has a smooth, slick lining of endothelial cells to which platelets and fibrin do not readily adhere. Second, the normal flow of blood within the vascular system is fairly streamlined, thus platelets are not hurled against lining surfaces. Finally, the clotting mechanism (see Chapter 19) has built into it a number of chemical checks and balances to control clot formation. Correspondingly, clots form inappropriately in three basic situations: (1) an abnormality exists in the vessel wall and lining; (2) the blood flow is abnormal; and (3) the coagulability of the blood itself is increased.

The flow of blood on the arterial side of the circulation is a high-pressure flow of rapid velocity, and the arteries themselves are rather thick-walled and not easily deformed. For these reasons, the usual cause of arterial thrombosis is disease in the lining and wall of the artery, particularly atherosclerosis (see later discussion). On the venous side of the circulation, the blood flow has a low pressure and relatively low velocity, and the veins are sufficiently thin-walled that they can be deformed readily by external pressures. For these reasons, the usual causes of thrombosis on the venous side of the circulation relate to diminished flow of blood. Finally, chemical changes occur in the blood of patients with a variety of diseases, leading to a hypercoagulable state that may further complicate any of the situations just mentioned.

Morphology and Fate of Thrombi

Thrombi consist of varying combinations of aggregated platelets, precipitated fibrin, and enmeshed RBCs and white blood cells (WBCs, leukocytes). The precise configuration of a thrombus depends on the conditions under which it was formed. When the thrombus begins to form in flowing blood, the first element is often a clump of

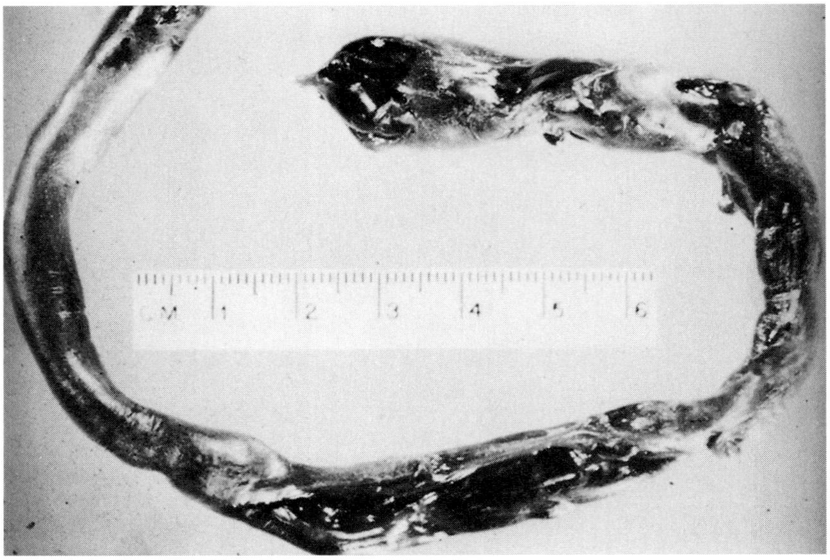

FIG. 7-4 Venous thrombus. This thrombus was extracted from a leg vein at autopsy. Such a finding is unfortunately quite common and is associated with many dire consequences. Reference to the scale emphasizes the magnitude of the clot.

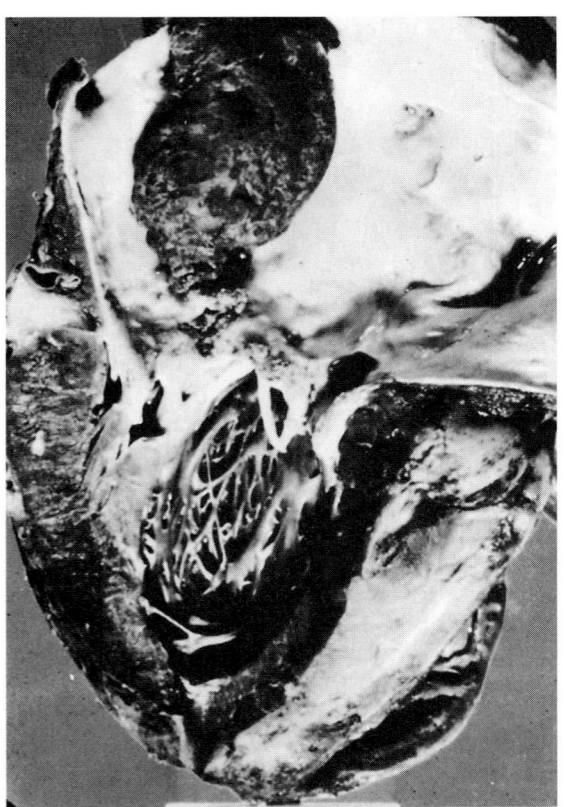

FIG. 7-5 Atrial thrombus. A huge thrombus formed in the left atrium because of malfunction of the scarred mitral valve. The position of this clot renders it a great potential danger.

platelet aggregates soon become surrounded by fibrin and trapped blood cells. Successive waves of events of this type can lead to a complex, ribbed structure of a thrombus. On the other hand, when a thrombus forms in a vessel in which the flow has virtually stopped, the clot may simply consist of a diffuse meshwork of fibrin trapping the formed elements in the blood more or less homogeneously. However, in contrast to the processes just described, postmortem clotting occurs quite slowly, thus the formed elements of the blood layer out before the clot solidifies, giving rise to a stratified structure in which RBCs, WBCs, and fibrin may be quite separate. These postmortem clots tend to be more elastic compared with true thrombi and are much less likely to adhere to vascular walls. These distinctions may become important at autopsy.

Thrombi may occur in any part of the cardiovascular system and for a variety of causes. Fig. 7-4 illustrates a thrombus from a large, deep vein of the leg. Such thrombi are common in patients who are bedridden. Their occurrence is generally related to the decreased rate of flow through these veins, in turn secondary to the loss of pumping action of muscular activity. The situation is aggravated in many instances by sluggish peripheral circulation related to chronic cardiac failure. *Phlebothrombosis*, the formation of thrombi in veins, is an ever-present danger for bedridden or immobilized patients. Such thrombi may develop relatively silently or may be accompanied by signs and symptoms of inflammation of the vein wall, which are presumably secondary to the presence of the thrombus. When inflammatory signs dominate, the condition is called *thrombophlebitis*. The most feared consequence of such venous thrombi is the breaking off of a portion, which is then transported in the bloodstream to lodge at a distant site.

Fig. 7-5 illustrates a thrombus within the left atrium of the heart. In this case, the thrombus formed because of an abnormal flow and a pattern of circulation through the atrium related to stenosis of the mitral valve. Occasionally, this type of atrial thrombus may behave as a

platelets adhering to the endothelium. This action may occur because of abnormal flow allowing platelets to settle against or to be hurled against the endothelium; it also may occur because of a roughening of the endothelial lining, which would produce a nidus for platelet aggregation. As platelets aggregate, they release substances that encourage the precipitation of fibrin thus the

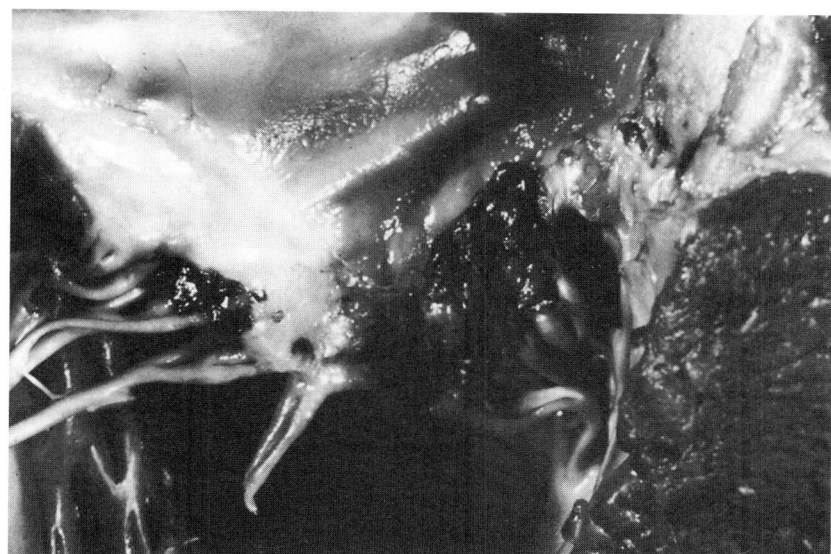

FIG. 7-6 Infective endocarditis. The dark vegetations on this mitral valve are actually thrombotic masses formed around foci of bacterial infection of the valve. The valve was previously scarred (note thickening of leaflets and chordae) and therefore was susceptible to infection during a burst of bacteremia.

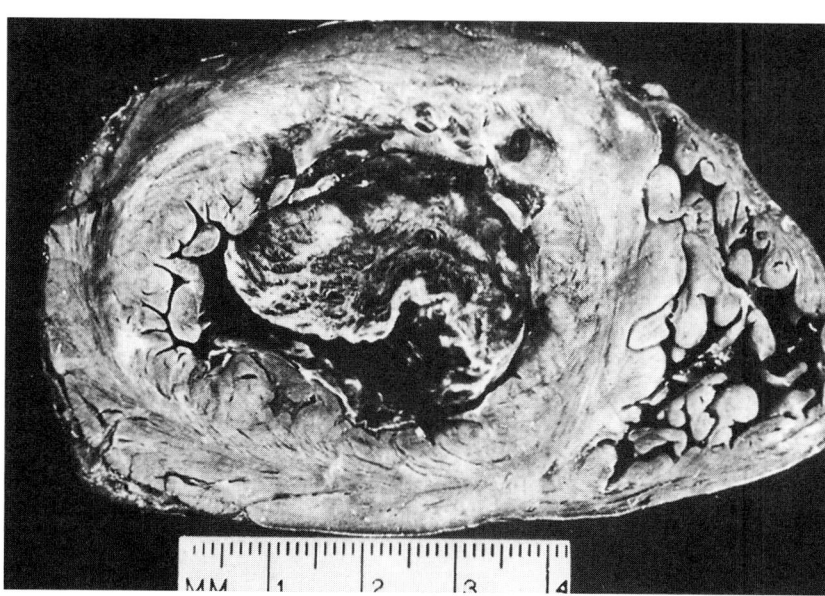

FIG. 7-7 Mural thrombus in heart. In this transverse section a large mural thrombus overlies an area of previous myocardial necrosis in the wall of the left ventricle.

"ball valve," suddenly occluding the atrioventricular orifice and producing instant death. More often, the thrombi act as the source of fragments that are propelled distally in the bloodstream.

Fig. 7-6 illustrates a thrombus on a cardiac valve. In this instance, the cause is bacterial infection of the valve and the thrombus is called a *vegetation*. Vegetations of infective endocarditis are exceedingly dangerous because of local damage to the valve and because fragments may be propelled to other sites in the body, wherein additional vessels may become occluded and infected.

Fig. 7-7 illustrates a thrombus within the left ventricle of the heart. A thrombus such as this that adheres to the wall of the cardiovascular system but does not totally occlude the area is referred to as a *mural thrombus*. The usual reason for the formation of a ventricular mural thrombus is hypokinesis of the heart wall caused by disease or death of the underlying myocardium.

Fig. 7-8 illustrates a thrombus within an artery. Clearly evident are the thickening and roughening of the artery wall that have given rise to the thrombus. The roughening in this instance is caused by a disease (atherosclerosis) and is a precipitating cause of thrombosis.

Frequently, when the subject survives the formation of a thrombus, the thrombus may undergo resolution. The body possesses fibrinolytic mechanisms that, along with the action of leukocytes, may lead to the dissolution of clots. Every individual probably forms tiny thrombi now and then, and these are resolved without reaching the clinical horizon. On the other hand, some large thrombi undergo organization, with granulation tissue growing from an adjacent vascular lining. In these instances, the involved vessel may become permanently plugged by scar tissue. Sometimes the vascular channels within the young granulation tissue organizing a thrombus may anastomose and provide new channels through the area

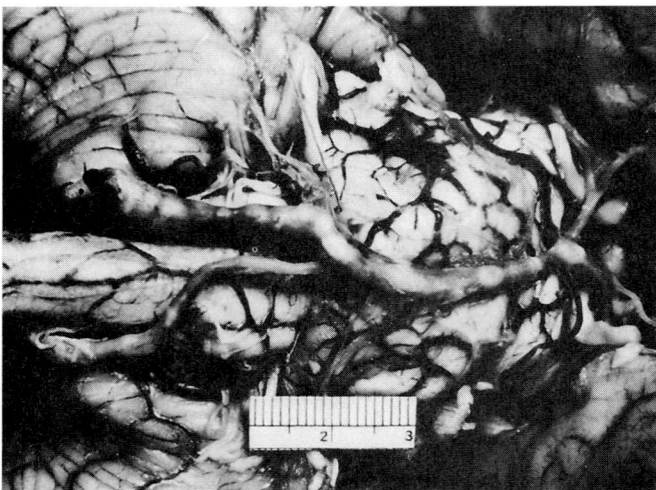

FIG. 7-8 Thrombus in a sclerotic artery. The artery above the brainstem *(left of center)* is atherosclerotic and gnarled. The lumen is occluded by a thrombus that protrudes from the cut end at the left.

occupied by a thrombus. This phenomenon is referred to as *recanalization*. Unfortunately, before the thrombus either organizes or resolves, portions of it often break off and are propelled in the bloodstream, ultimately lodging elsewhere and occluding additional vessels.

Effects

The consequences of thrombosis are perhaps most obvious with arterial thrombi. When an artery is occluded by a thrombus, the tissues served by that artery lose their blood supply. The results of this event may range from functional abnormality of tissue to death of the tissue or death of the subject. The consequences of venous thrombi are somewhat different. When one vein is plugged, the blood is likely to find its way back to the heart via some anastomosing channel. Only when a large vein is occluded by a thrombus do local problems with passive congestion become evident. The most ominous problem associated with venous thrombi is their fragmentation and transport to distant points in the body. Similarly, the effects of cardiac thrombi are largely related to their moving elsewhere within the cardiovascular system.

EMBOLISM

Definition and Types

The transportation of a physical mass in the bloodstream from one place to another with lodgment in the new location is called *embolism*. The physical mass itself is called an *embolus*. The most common emboli in humans are derived from thrombi and are called *thromboemboli*. Many other substances or materials, however, can become embolic. Bits of tissue can embolize when they enter the vascular system, usually with trauma. Cancer cells may embolize, constituting a devastating means of spread of the disease (see Chapter 8). Foreign materials injected into the car-

diovascular system may also embolize. Droplets of liquid that form in the circulation under a variety of circumstances or are injected into the circulation may embolize; even gas bubbles may become embolic.

Pathogenesis, Routes, and Effects

The most common sources of emboli within the body are venous thrombi, most often in the deep veins of the legs or the pelvis. When fragments of such venous thrombi break off and float with the flow of blood, they enter the vena cava and then the right side of the heart. These fragments do not lodge along this path because of the large size of the vessels and cardiac chambers involved. The blood leaving the right ventricle, however, flows into the main pulmonary artery, which branches into right and left pulmonary arteries, which, in turn, branch to smaller vessels. For these anatomic reasons, emboli originating in venous thrombi usually terminate as pulmonary arterial emboli. When a large fragment of a thrombus becomes an embolus, a major portion of the pulmonary arterial supply may suddenly be occluded (Fig. 7-9), which can cause virtually instantaneous death of the subject. On the other hand, smaller pulmonary arterial emboli may be silent, may lead to pulmonary hemorrhage secondary to the vascular damage, or may actually result in necrosis of a portion of lung. Pulmonary emboli of various sizes can be found in a significant number of patients dying after being bedridden; sometimes the pulmonary emboli contribute to the death of the subject, and at other times they are only of incidental importance. Showers of tiny pulmonary emboli over a long period may produce sufficient occlusion of the pulmonary vascular bed to cause the right side of the heart to become overloaded and to fail.

Emboli that lodge on the arterial side of the circulation originate from the "left side" of the circulatory system, either in the left cardiac chambers or in the large arteries. The only way that an embolus originating on the venous side of the circulation might lodge on the arterial side is to bypass the lungs via a defect in the interatrial or interventricular septum of the heart. This situation, called *paradoxical embolism*, is exceedingly rare. Most often, an arterial embolus originates from an intracardiac thrombus or, more rarely, from a mural thrombus in the aorta or one of its large branches.

Gas bubbles may become embolic in a variety of circumstances. One circumstance, called *caisson disease*, is popularly known as "the bends." This situation arises when a subject has been living under markedly increased atmospheric pressure, such as that within a pressurized caisson or in underwater diving gear. In these circumstances, increased amounts of atmospheric gases are dissolved within the bloodstream. When decompression is sufficiently abrupt, the result is analogous to what is seen when a warm bottle of a carbonated beverage is suddenly opened. The myriads of tiny gas bubbles appearing within the circulation are carried to a variety of places in the body, where they lodge in the microcirculation and occlude the blood flow to those tissues. An analogous circumstance may arise when atmospheric air enters venous channels as a result of faulty handling of an intra-

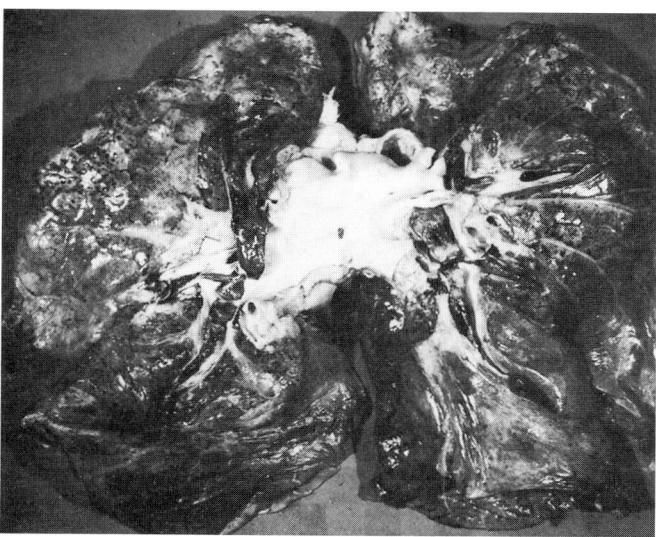

FIG. 7-9 Massive pulmonary emboli. The opened pulmonary arteries supplying these lungs are seen in the center of the photograph. The several dark cylindric masses are emboli that originated from venous thrombus in a leg, similar to that shown in Fig. 7-4. The patient died within moments of lodgment of the emboli.

venous infusion or indwelling vascular catheter, or in the course of a surgical procedure when large vascular channels must be traversed. With massive air embolism, a large *bolus* of air may enter the right side of the heart, and at autopsy, a large, foamy mass of air and blood is observed distending the heart and pulmonary vessels.

An example of embolism of liquid droplets is *traumatic fat embolism*. As the name suggests, these emboli, composed of fat globules, tend to form within the circulation after trauma. The usual point of lodgment is the microcirculation of the lung. Minor degrees of fat embolism likely follow most surgical procedures when fatty tissue is incised and lipidic material is allowed to enter vascular channels. In these circumstances, the few scattered emboli that lodge in the lung are completely silent and trivial. A similar circumstance arises when bones are fractured, apparently with liberation of lipid into the sinusoids of the bone marrow. Again, these scattered pulmonary fat emboli are trivial and clinically inapparent. Occasionally, however, after traumatic injury, fat embolism may be massive. Unclear is whether all the fat droplets in this type of circumstance originate from trauma to adipose cells. Some evidence suggests that in this type of circumstance the lipid normally carried within the bloodstream coalesces. In any event, with sufficiently massive fat embolism, symptoms of respiratory distress may appear, usually in the first day or two after trauma. In severe instances, the emboli lodge in a variety of places in the body beyond the lungs, including the skin and, more importantly, the central nervous system. In both these latter areas, each microscopic fat embolus is associated with a petechial hemorrhage. In the brain, a tiny focus of necrosis surrounds each occluded vessel. In these rare instances, fat embolism can be fatal, usually because of cerebral damage.

ARTERIOSCLEROSIS

Arteriosclerosis, or "hardening of the arteries," is an exceedingly important disease phenomenon in most developed countries. The term *arteriosclerosis* actually encompasses any condition of arterial vessels that results in a thickening or hardening of the walls. Three conditions are generally included under the heading arteriosclerosis: Mönckeberg's sclerosis, arteriolosclerosis, and atherosclerosis.

Mönckeberg's sclerosis involves the deposition of calcium salts in the muscular wall of medium-sized arteries. Although Mönckeberg's sclerosis can be detected grossly and even observed on radiographic films, this form of arteriosclerosis is not clinically significant, because the lining of the involved vessel is not roughened and the lumen is not narrowed.

Arteriolosclerosis refers to a thickening of arterioles and is typically present in patients with elevated blood pressure and, to some extent, is associated with aging. The most important type of arteriosclerosis is atherosclerosis, and when the term arteriosclerosis is used, it is generally used synonymously with atherosclerosis.

Atherosclerosis

Atherosclerosis involves the aorta, its large branches, and medium-sized arteries, such as those supplying portions of the extremities, brain, heart, and major internal viscera. Atherosclerosis does not involve arterioles or the venous side of the circulation. The disease is multifocal, and the unit lesion or *atheroma* (also termed *atherosclerotic plaque*) consists of an elevated mass of fatty material associated with fibrous connective tissue, often with secondary deposits of calcium salts and blood products. The plaques of atherosclerosis begin in the intima or inner layer of the vessel wall and project into the lumen but with growth they may extend to encroach on the media or musculoelastic portion of the vessel wall.

Morphology

The typical gross appearance of moderately severe atherosclerosis is shown in Fig. 7-10. A smooth endothelial lining of vessels is an important protection against thrombus formation, thus realizing why atherosclerosis should involve considerable liability to arterial thrombosis is not difficult. The microscopic appearance of an atheroma is illustrated in Fig. 7-11. The dominance of both fibrous and fatty material in the lesion is evident (*athero* refers to the mushy and *sclerosis* to the hard character of the lesions). In large vessels, such as the aorta, even numerous and severe atheromas generally do not lead to occlusion of the lumen but only to roughening of the lining surface. In smaller vessels, the atheromas may actually become circumferential, leading to marked narrowing of the lumen (Fig. 7-12).

Etiology and Incidence

Many factors contribute to the development of atherosclerosis, and citing a single or dominant cause is therefore

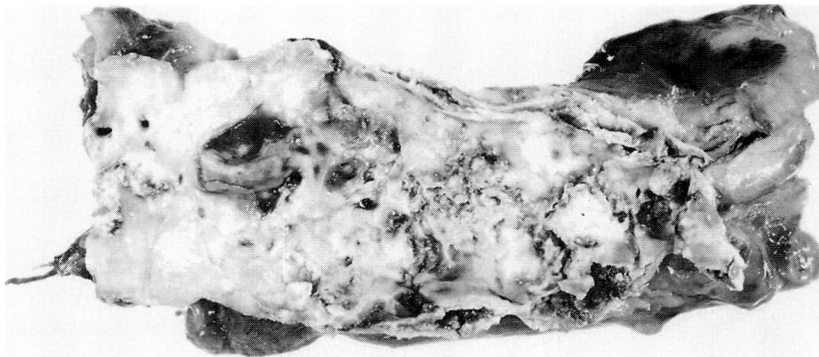

FIG. 7-10 Atherosclerosis of aorta. This photograph depicts the intimal (lining) surface of the opened abdominal aorta. Instead of being pearly and smooth, the surface is a roughened mass of atherosclerotic plaques.

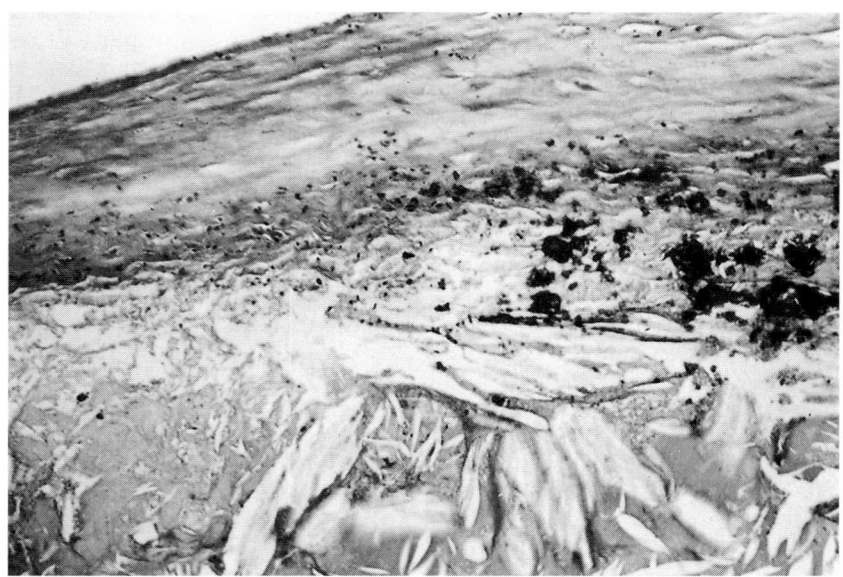

FIG. 7-11 Atherosclerotic plaque. The cleft in the depths of the plaque represents large deposits of cholesterol. The dark material at the right is a dystrophic calcific deposit, and the horizontal band across the top is a fibrous "cap" of the lesion. The elevated rough lesions in Fig. 7-10 have this microscopic appearance.

impossible. The various factors are so widespread in the populations of the more affluent countries that only the youngest individuals are spared by the disease. In fact, autopsies performed on otherwise healthy young adults who died as a result of trauma often reveal lesions of atherosclerosis, occasionally surprisingly severe. The earliest fatty deposits may be seen in young children, and these generally tend to increase with age. A variety of factors influence the rate at which atheromas increase in size and number. Genetic factors are important, and atherosclerosis and its complications often tend to run in families. Subjects with elevated levels of serum cholesterol are often susceptible to accelerated atherosclerosis, as are individuals with diabetes mellitus. Blood pressure is an important factor in the incidence and severity of atherosclerosis. Patients with hypertension are much more likely to have earlier and more severe atherosclerosis; the severity of the disease is correlated with the blood pressure, even in the normal range. Atherosclerosis is not present within the pulmonary arteries (usually a low-

pressure circuit) unless the pressure is abnormally elevated, a state called *pulmonary hypertension*. Another risk factor in the development of atherosclerosis is cigarette smoking, which is a major environmental factor leading to increased severity of atherosclerosis. The precise way in which these various factors contribute to the pathogenesis of the lesions of atherosclerosis has not been completely elucidated.

Consequences

The consequences of atherosclerosis depend in part on the size of the artery involved. When the artery is medium-sized, such as a major branch of the coronary artery, with a lumen perhaps a few millimeters in diameter, atherosclerosis may gradually lead to narrowing or even total obstruction of the lumen.

In contrast to this slowly developing occlusion, complications of atherosclerosis may lead to an abruptly developing occlusion. One such circumstance is throm-

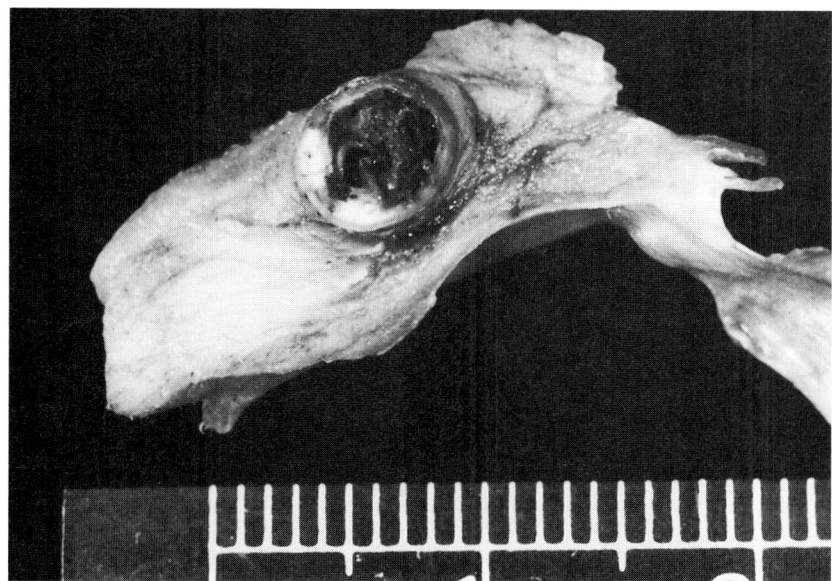

FIG. 7-12   Atherosclerotic coronary artery. The circumferential atheroma has left only a tiny lumen (at 8 o'clock) in this cross section of coronary artery. Consequences in terms of blood flow are obvious.

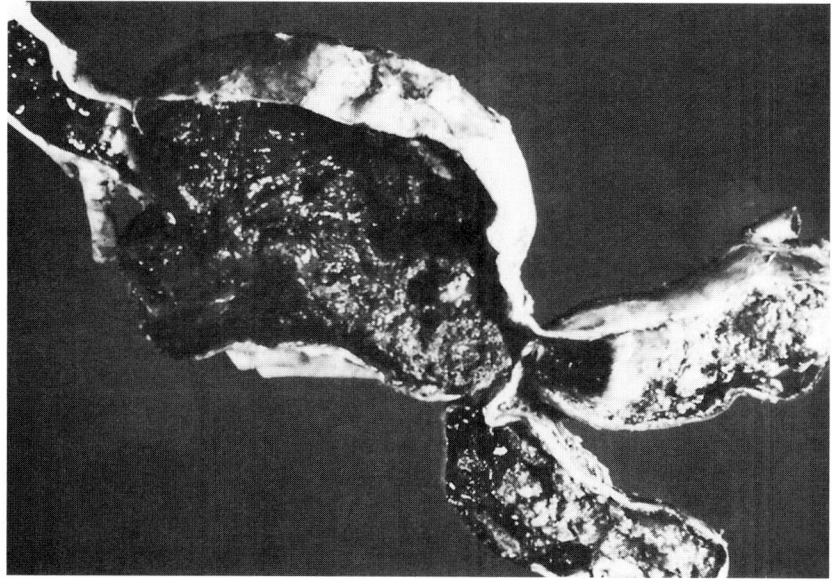

FIG. 7-13   Atherosclerotic aneurysms. A large aneurysm distorts the distal aorta and each iliac artery. The walls of such aneurysms are prone to rupture.

bus formation superimposed on the intimal roughening produced by atherosclerotic plaques. Thrombosis tends to be occlusive in a small or medium-sized artery, but it may be in the form of a relatively thin mural deposit in a large vessel such as the aorta. Another complication of atherosclerosis is hemorrhage in the soft center of the plaque. In a vessel the size of the coronary artery, this may result in swelling of the plaque with sudden occlusion of the lumen. Another complication that may lead to acute arterial occlusion is a rupture of the plaque with welling up of the soft lipidic contents into the lumen and lodgment in a narrower "downstream" segment of

the vessel. Finally, if extensive and severe enough, lesions of atherosclerosis may then encroach on the muscular and elastic wall (the media) of an artery thus weakening it. In the abdominal aorta, a common site of severe atherosclerosis, the result of such medial damage may be the formation of an atherosclerotic *aneurysm,* which is a ballooning of the weakened arterial wall (Fig. 7-13). Although a thrombus may form within this type of aneurysm because of the abnormal swirling of the blood and because of the roughened intima, the most dangerous complication of an aneurysm is rupture with exsanguination.

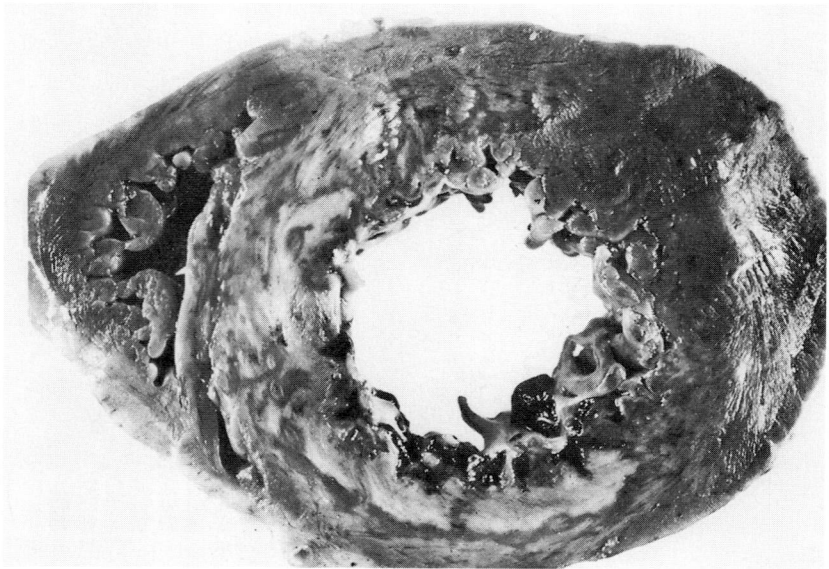

FIG. 7-14 Myocardial infarct. Myocardial ischemia has resulted in coagulative necrosis *(light area)* of much of the septum and ventricular wall.

ISCHEMIA AND INFARCTION

Ischemia is simply an inadequate blood supply in an area. When tissues are rendered ischemic, they are deprived of both the necessary oxygen and nutrients. (In contrast to ischemia, hypoxia is a deprivation of oxygen alone, thus glycolytic energy production can continue by anaerobic metabolism.) The accumulation of metabolic wastes within the poorly perfused tissue may also contribute to tissue damage. Anything that affects the flow of blood may produce tissue ischemia. The most obvious cause is local arterial obstruction related to atherosclerosis, thrombosis, or embolism. Less frequently, venous obstruction may lead to ischemia when the flow of blood through the tissue virtually reaches a standstill. Even systemic causes of tissue ischemia exist. For instance, when heart failure is sufficiently severe, a tissue may become ischemic simply because of the low level of perfusion. Similarly, prolonged shock may lead to significant tissue ischemia.

The effects of ischemia vary, depending on the intensity of the ischemia, the rate of onset, and the metabolic demands of the particular tissue. In some instances of ischemia, usually involving muscular tissues, pain may be a symptom of diminished blood supply. For example, an older person with atherosclerosis of the leg arteries and consequent decrease in blood flow may have sufficient blood supply when at rest but not during activity. When the individual walks briskly, increasing the metabolic demand of the leg muscles, the onset of relative ischemia may cause pain and limping. The same event occurs in the heart muscle with narrowing of the coronary arterial circulation. In this case, with activity, a patient may develop a feeling of oppression or squeezing pain within the chest, a phenomenon referred to as *angina pectoris*. By definition, anginal pain recedes with rest, when the metabolic demand of the heart muscle diminishes to the point at which the narrowed coronary arterial circulation is adequate.

When ischemia is of gradual onset and prolonged duration, another effect is that the involved tissue may atrophy or shrink. A common example of this phenomenon is observed in a patient who has atherosclerosis that diminishes the circulation to the lower extremities. Frequently, the legs exhibit loss of muscle mass, and the skin becomes smooth, thin, and hairless, all the results of chronic ischemia.

The most extreme effect of ischemia is the death of the ischemic tissue. An area of ischemic necrosis is termed an *infarct*, and the process of forming an infarct is termed *infarction*. Whether an ischemic area actually undergoes infarction depends on a variety of local and systemic factors. For example, a degree of arterial occlusion is better tolerated when it occurs slowly, when the metabolic demand of the tissue is low, and when development of collateral circulation occurs (i.e., auxiliary supply of the involved area by branches of neighboring arteries). Additionally, the effects of a given degree of ischemia are worsened when the oxygen transport within the blood is diminished for any reason.

The morphologic features of infarcts vary from organ to organ, but the tissue necrosis produced by ischemia is generally accompanied by an element of hemorrhage from damaged vessels at the edges of the infarcted area. In loose tissues, such as the lung, this hemorrhage is extensive and the infarcted area literally becomes stuffed with blood, producing a hemorrhagic or red infarct. In other organs (e.g., kidney, heart) the hemorrhage accompanying infarction is minimal, and the infarct tends to be pale. In hemorrhagic and in pale infarcts, the basic cause of the damage is ischemia of the tissues. In most infarcts, the necrosis produced by ischemia is coagulative, and the outlines of the tissue are maintained (Fig. 7-14). In the lung, hemorrhage dominates the picture, whereas in the brain, an area of infarction gradually softens and undergoes liquefactive change, resulting in a hole in the tissue (see Fig. 3-6).

The presence of infarcted tissue excites an inflammatory reaction at the margins interfacing with viable tissue.

Neutrophils and macrophages rapidly invade the dead area to begin the job of demolition. Subsequently, the area is gradually organized as demolition proceeds, and the usual outcome is scarring of the infarcted area. In many organs, an infarct itself is not particularly important, given the amount of reserve of that organ. Thus even a moderately large renal infarct will not endanger the person's life because of the ability of one kidney or even part of one kidney to maintain homeostasis. The presence of a pulmonary infarct likewise is not particularly threatening in terms of ventilatory function. In this latter instance, however, the occurrence of pulmonary infarction is somewhat ominous, because it is usually the result of pulmonary embolism. Therefore the ever-present concern is that larger and more threatening emboli may originate from the source of the first embolus. In the brain and myocardium, the results of infarction are more significant because these organs have decreased reserves with each area being important, and because, in particular, no possibility exists of regeneration of infarcted elements in these two areas. Finally, in some areas exposed to bacterial populations, the infarcted tissue will serve as a focus of growth of saprophytic microorganisms. Thus infarcts of the bowel quickly become gangrenous, and infarcts of portions of an extremity are initially recognized as areas of gangrene.

KEY CONCEPTS

- *Congestion (hyperemia)* is an overabundance of blood within a tissue and may be active or passive.
- *Active congestion* is an increase in the amount of blood flowing into an area caused by dilation of the arterioles. Examples are the hyperemia accompanying acute inflammation or increased blood flow to a contracting muscle (functional hyperemia).
- *Passive congestion* occurs when impairment of the drainage of blood from a tissue occurs. Examples include congestion of the lungs in left ventricular failure and liver and systemic congestion in the presence of right ventricular failure. *Chronic passive congestion* may lead to changes in the tissue involved, such as atrophy, fibrosis, and the deposition of certain pigments (e.g., hemosiderin).
- *Edema* is the excess accumulation of fluid between the cells (interstitial fluid compartment) or within the various body cavities.
- *Four basic mechanisms causing edema* may be derived from considering the forces normally controlling fluid exchange across vessel walls: (1) increased hydrostatic pressure (e.g., congestive heart failure); (2) increased permeability of the blood vessels (e.g., acute inflammation); (3) decreased colloid osmotic pressure (e.g., hypoalbuminemia); and (4) lymphatic obstruction (e.g., mastectomy with removal of axillary lymph nodes).
- Exudates accumulate because of increased vascular permeability. *Exudates* contain more leukocytes and protein and have a higher specific gravity than transudates. Exudates may also contain fibrinogen, causing clotting. In contrast, *transudates* accumulate in tissue or spaces for reasons other than increased vascular permeability and contain little protein, have a lower specific gravity, are cell poor, and do not clot.
- Accumulation of significant fluid edema within the lungs or within the brain may cause the death of the individual.
- *Hemorrhage* is the escape of blood from the cardiovascular system with accumulation in the soft tissues, body spaces, or escape from the body and is caused by rupture of the vascular wall or abnormalities of the hemostatic mechanism.
- Local and systemic effects of hemorrhage depend on the location, amount, and rate of blood loss. The loss of a small amount of blood locally may have a trivial effect as in a bruise or may be lethal when in the brain (cerebral hemorrhage), pericardial sac (causing cardiac tamponade), or lungs (causing suffocation). The rapid loss of a large amount of blood from the body may lead to circulatory shock and death; the slow loss of smaller amounts of blood results in anemia.
- *Thrombosis* is the process of the inappropriate formation of a blood clot within the vascular system in a living person and the blood clot is called a *thrombus*. When inflammation dominates, the condition is called *thrombophlebitis*. A thrombus may form in the arterial or the venous system. Thrombus formation occurs when increased coagulability of the blood occurs or when abnormalities of blood flow or of the blood vessel wall or lining are present.
- A piece of the thrombus *(embolus)* may break off and lodge downstream in a smaller branch of the blood vessel, in which case it is called an *embolism*. (Other materials such as fat, cancer cells, foreign materials, or air bubbles may also act as emboli.) *Arterial emboli* originate in the left side of the circulation, either the left cardiac chambers or large arteries. *Venous thrombi* originate in the right side of the circulation, either the right cardiac chambers or more commonly in the deep veins of the pelvis or legs.
- The consequences of an arterial embolus lodging in a cerebral vessel may be a stroke or the loss of a leg when lodging in a branch of the femoral artery. A large embolus from the deep pelvic or leg veins occluding the main pulmonary artery may be lethal.
- *Arteriosclerosis* is a general term meaning "hardening of the arteries" and includes *Mönckeberg's sclerosis* (deposition of calcium salts in the arterial wall), *arteriolosclerosis* (thickening of arteriole walls associated with hypertension), and *atherosclerosis* (formation of fatty plaques in the arterial wall).
- An atherosclerotic plaque narrows the lumen of the artery and favors the formation of a thrombus on its roughened surface. A thrombus that occludes a

medium-sized artery, such as an atherosclerotic coronary artery, will result in *coronary thrombosis* ("heart attack"). Atherosclerosis of a large artery, such as the aorta, may weaken the elastic and muscle layers, causing an *aneurysm* (ballooning of the arterial wall).

■ *Ischemia* is an inadequate blood supply to a tissue, depriving it of *both* oxygen and nutrients and is the most common cause of cell injury. Ischemia tends to injure tissues faster than does *hypoxia* (deprivation of oxygen alone), because the tissue is deprived of substrates for glycolysis thus stopping anaerobic metabolism.

■ The consequences of ischemia vary according to its extent. In a coronary artery narrowed by atherosclerosis, when the individual starts to exercise increasing metabolic demand, the ischemic heart muscle may cause chest pain *(angina pectoris)*. The most extreme effect of ischemia is the death of the ischemic tissue, termed *ischemic necrosis* or *infarct*.

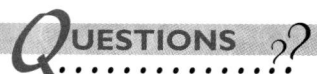

QUESTIONS ??

A sampling of review questions for this chapter appears here. Visit http://www.mosby.com/MERLIN/PriceWilson/ for additional questions.

Answer the following on a separate sheet of paper.

1. Describe how the mechanisms involved in active congestion differ from those in passive congestion.
2. Explain the way in which congestion might be produced by a cardiac problem.
3. What effects do acute passive congestion and chronic passive congestion have on the involved tissue?
4. Define edema.
5. What is the most common cause of a hemorrhage?
6. What are two basic mechanisms for stopping hemorrhage?
7. Describe the local and systemic effects of hemorrhage.
8. Describe two clinical implications of thrombosis.
9. List some local causes of ischemia.
10. Describe possible effects of ischemia.

Disturbances in Growth, Cellular Proliferation, and Differentiation

LORRAINE M. WILSON

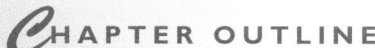
*T*his chapter focuses on a number of extremely diverse conditions that have different causes and consequences. The unifying concept is that each of the conditions discussed is characterized by an abnormality in (1) the size or number of cells in a tissue, (2) the mode of cellular proliferation, or (3) the character of cellular differentiation. These abnormalities may lead to tissues that are smaller or larger than normal and to tissues that have abnormal functional specialization. At the extreme, the abnormal cells may form masses, the behavior of which is generally beyond the influence of normal homeostatic controls.

ORGANS AND TISSUES SMALLER THAN NORMAL

Occasionally, a tissue, organ, or part of the body that is smaller than normal is encountered. This situation can arise in two ways: the organ or tissue may never have grown to normal size, or it may have reached normal size and then shrunk.

Agenesis and Aplasia

In the course of development, the embryonic rudiment of an organ may never form. This phenomenon is called *agenesis*, and the result is the absence of the particular organ; for example, some individuals are born with only a single kidney. A related situation is *aplasia*, in which the embryonic rudiment of an organ fails to grow at all once it has formed. (Some use the terms agenesis and aplasia interchangeably, and little practical difference exists.)

Hypoplasia

Occasionally, the embryonic rudiment forms and grows but never quite reaches definitive or adult size, yielding a dwarfed organ. This phenomenon is called *hypoplasia*. Hypoplasia, as with agenesis and aplasia, may involve any portion of the body, one of a pair of organs, or even both organs of a pair. Minor degrees of hypoplasia of some organ might be well tolerated for long periods, the net effect being some encroachment on the usual degree of reserve of that organ.

Atrophy

Organs that reach definitive size in the course of development and then shrink are referred to as *atrophic*. Atrophy has a variety of causes and, in some instances, can be actually normal, such as when certain parts of the embryo or fetus atrophy in the course of development. Some forms of atrophy are inevitable with advancing age, such as the endocrine atrophy that occurs when hormonal support is withdrawn from a tissue such as the mammary gland. An extremely common cause of atrophy is chronic ischemia. Another common type of atrophy, primarily involving skeletal muscle, is *disuse atrophy*. When a broken leg is placed in an immobilizing cast for weeks or months, the mass of the extremity is significantly reduced because of atrophy of the unused muscle. In this situation, the individual muscle cells are of reduced size, but the state is a reversible one. In other instances of atrophy, actual loss of cellular elements occurs.

ORGANS AND TISSUES LARGER THAN NORMAL

Hypertrophy

Hypertrophy is defined as an enlargement of a tissue or organ because of enlargement of individual cells. Hypertrophy can be present in a variety of tissues but is prominent in various types of muscle. An increased workload on a muscle is a strong stimulus to hypertrophy. The bulging muscles of the weight lifter are an obvious example of muscular hypertrophy. The same type of event occurs as an important adaptive response in the myocardium. When a subject has an abnormal cardiac valve that imposes an unusual mechanical load on the left ventricle or when the ventricle is pumping against an elevated systemic blood pressure, the result is hypertrophy of the myocardium with thickening of the ventricular wall. A similar phenomenon can occur in smooth muscle that is forced to work against an increased load. Thus the wall of the urinary bladder may become hypertrophic when the free outflow of urine is obstructed. In each of these instances, hypertrophic enlargement of cells is actually accompanied by an increase in the contractile elements of the tissue, and thus the response is adaptive. Hypertrophy is stimulus related, thus it tends to regress, at least to some extent, when the abnormal workload is withdrawn.

Hyperplasia

Hyperplasia is an increase in the absolute number of cells within a tissue, leading to an increase in the size of that tissue or organ. This action obviously occurs only in a tissue capable of cell division; in such tissues, hyperplasia may also be accompanied by hypertrophy of individual cells. Hyperplasia occurs in a variety of tissues under many different circumstances, some of them completely physiologic. For example, with the hormonal stimulus of pregnancy and lactation, extensive proliferation of epithelial elements occurs within the breast, with an increase in the size of breast tissue caused by this hyperplasia. An example of nonphysiologic hyperplasia is the enlargement of the prostate gland, often present in aging men. Another example of hyperplasia that is nonphysiologic but still adaptive is a callus, or thickening of skin, developing in response to a mechanical stimulus. Microscopic examination of a callus reveals a marked increase in the number of epidermal cells and layers of cells in the epidermis, clearly an adaptive response.

Many examples of hyperplasia represent "rational" responses of the body to some imposed demand. As with hypertrophy, when the abnormal circumstance is reversed, the signal to cellular proliferation is withdrawn, and the hyperplasia regresses and more normal conditions return. In the previous examples, the enlarged breast shrinks to a more normal size after lactation, and the callus gradually disappears when the mechanical stimulus to the skin is no longer applied. Unfortunately, the stimulus leading to prostatic hyperplasia is not understood, and the excess tissue must often be resected surgically.

ABNORMAL DIFFERENTIATION: DEFINITIONS

Metaplasia

The character of cellular differentiation in a given tissue may also change under abnormal circumstances. *Differentiation* is the process by which the progeny of dividing stem cells become specialized to perform a particular task. For instance, dividing cells in the deepest layer of the epidermis gradually migrate upward, and as they do, they acquire the specialized protective characteristics of outer epidermal cells and produce a proteinaceous substance known as *keratin*. Similarly, within the lining of the respiratory tract, some of the dividing cells in the epithelium develop into tall, columnar cells with cilia on their luminal surfaces.

When differentiating cell systems of this type are placed under adverse circumstances, the pattern of differentiation may change; thus the dividing cells begin to differentiate into types of cells not usually found in the area but that would be normal elsewhere in the body. This phenomenon is referred to as *metaplasia*. For example, when the lining of the uterine cervix is chronically irritated, an epidermis-like squamous epithelium replaces portions of the columnar epithelium (Fig. 8-1). Presumably, this "squamous metaplasia" is adaptive; that is, the squamous epithelium is more resistant to irritation than is the original epithelium. The process of metaplasia appears to be under tight control; that is, the "new" type of differentiation is regular as well as adaptive. Metaplasia is potentially reversible, thus when the cause of the original change can be eliminated, the stem cells once again will differentiate to form the specialized types of cells usually found in that locale.

Dysplasia

Dysplasia is an abnormality in the differentiation of proliferating cells, resulting in an abnormal degree of variation in the size, shape, and appearance of the cells and a disturbance in the usual arrangement of the cells (Fig. 8-2). In dysplasia, a loss of control over the affected cell population occurs. Minor degrees of dysplasia are potentially reversible if the irritant stimulus can be reversed. However, in most instances the stimulus leading to dysplasia cannot be identified and the changes may become progressively more severe, terminating eventually in the development of malignant disease. In the uterine cervix, dysplasia is common and its natural history has been extensively studied. In this location, dysplasia is termed *cervical intraepithelial neoplasia (CIN)*. Dysplasia may progress from mild-to-moderate to moderate-to-severe grades (CIN I to CIN II or III), with severe dysplasia actually representing preinvasive cancer. Destruction of foci of CIN can prevent the development of frankly invasive cancer.

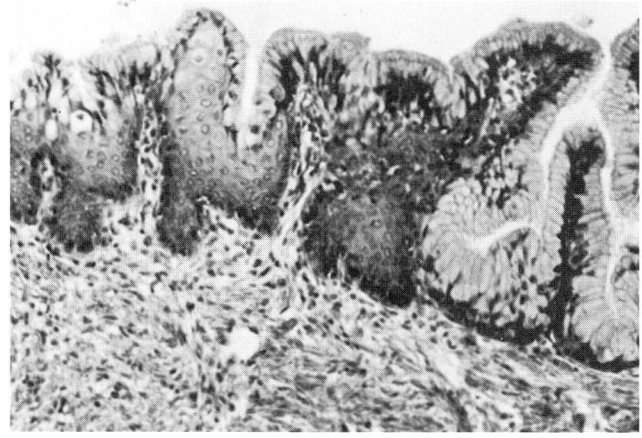

FIG. 8-1   Squamous metaplasia. In this lining epithelium of uterine cervix, the usual cell type is columnar, as at the right. Most of the epithelium has altered its differentiation to form an epidermis-like squamous epithelium. (Photomicrograph, ×200.)

NEOPLASIA

A *neoplasm*, literally a "new growth," is an abnormal mass of proliferating cells. The cells of a neoplasm are derived from previously normal cells; however, in undergoing neoplastic change they acquire a certain degree of autonomy. Neoplastic cells grow at a rate that is uncoordinated with the needs of the host and function quite independently of the usual homeostatic controls. The growth of neoplastic cells is usually progressive; that is, it does not reach equilibrium but results in an ever-increasing mass of cells having the same properties. A neoplasm serves no beneficial adaptive purpose and is often harmful. Finally, because of the autonomous character of neoplastic cells, even when the stimulus that caused the neoplasm is withdrawn, the neoplasm will continue to grow progressively.

The term *tumor* is more or less synonymous with the term *neoplasm*. Originally, tumor meant simply swelling or lump, and occasionally the phrase "true tumor" is used to differentiate a neoplasm from some other sort of lump. Neoplasms are distinguished by their behavior; some are benign, whereas others are malignant. *Cancer* is a general term referring to any malignant neoplasm, and many tumors or neoplasms are noncancerous.

CHARACTERISTICS OF NEOPLASMS

Benign Neoplasms

A *benign* (i.e., noncancerous) neoplasm is strictly a local affair. The proliferating cells that constitute the neoplasm tend to be quite cohesive, thus as the mass of neoplastic cells grows, centrifugal expansion of the mass takes place within a fairly well-defined border. Because the proliferating cells do not fall away from each other, the edges of the neoplasm tend to move outward more or less smoothly, pushing adjacent tissue away in the process. In so doing, benign neoplasms may acquire a capsule of compressed connective tissue that separates them from their surroundings. Above all, as indicated in Fig. 8-3, *A*,

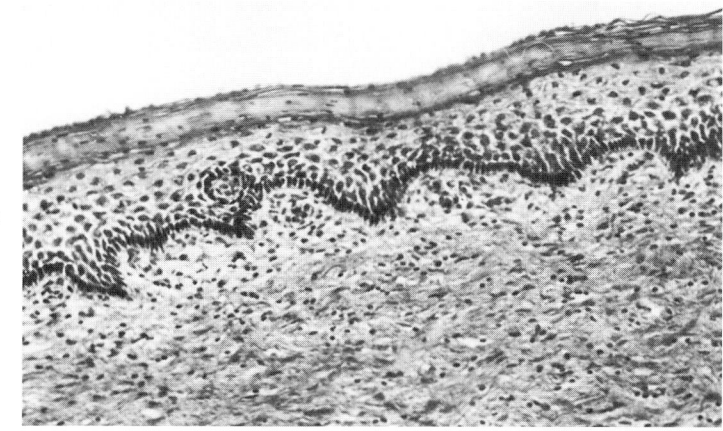
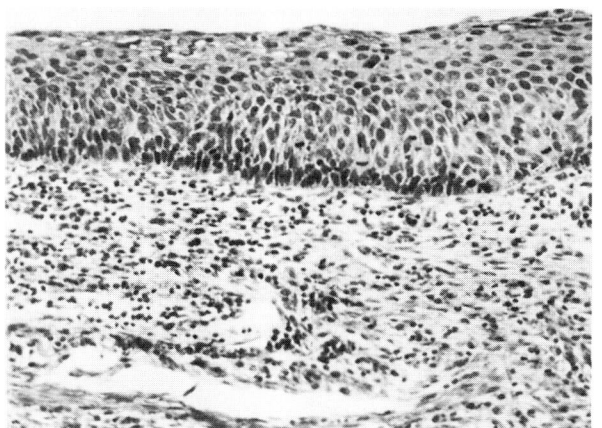

A   B

FIG. 8-2   Dysplasia versus normal cells. **A,** In the normal epithelium the cells are very regular in a given zone and layering is orderly. **B,** In dysplasia there is marked morphologic variation in the cells and layering is disordered. (Photomicrograph, ×200.)

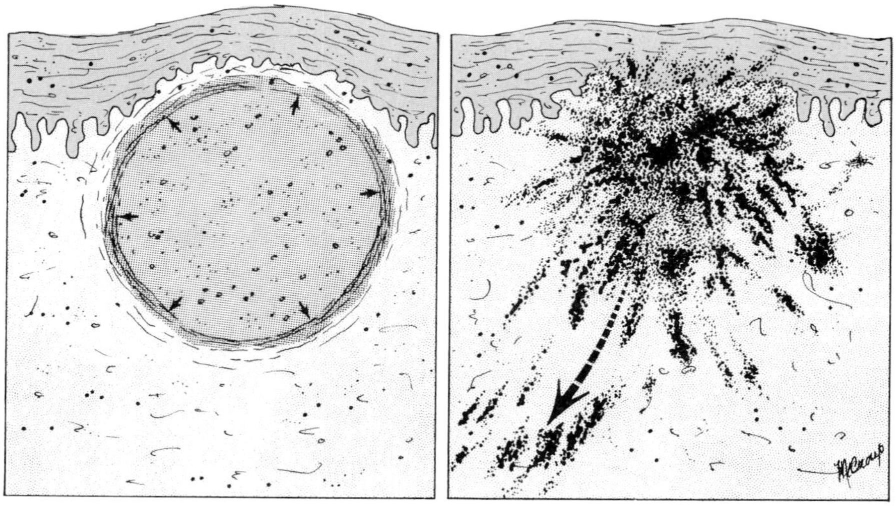

FIG. 8-3 Diagrams of benign versus malignant growth. **A,** "Typical" benign neoplasm is cohesive, centrifugally expanding, smooth bordered, and often encapsulated. Adjacent tissue is compressed. **B,** Malignant neoplasm is less cohesive, has an irregular border, and invades adjacent tissue. Malignant cells are also capable of metastasis *(dotted arrow).*

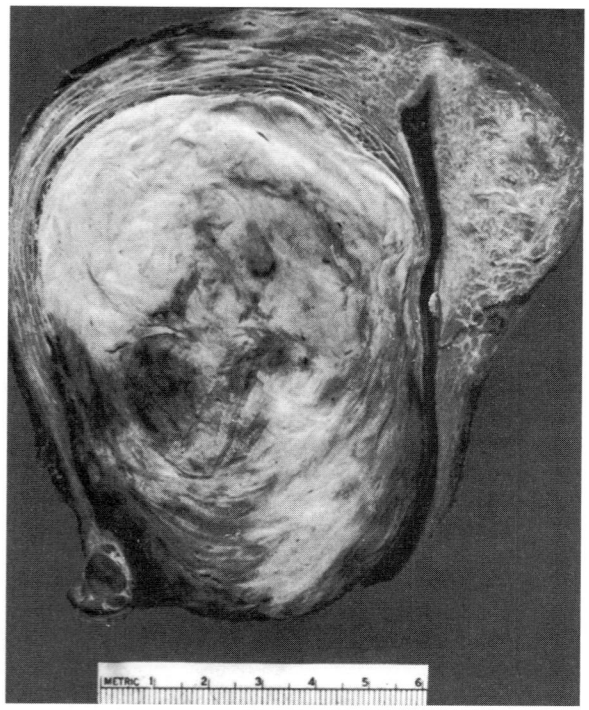

FIG. 8-4 Benign neoplasm. In this section of uterus the right half is normal. On the left is a large, benign neoplasm (leiomyoma).

the benign neoplasm does not spread to a distant site. The rate of growth of benign neoplasms is often rather leisurely, and some seem to plateau and remain at a more or less stable size for many months or years.

Malignant Neoplasms

Many characteristics of malignant neoplasms contrast sharply with those of their benign counterparts. *Malignant* neoplasms generally grow more rapidly than do benign ones and almost always grow in a relentlessly

progressive manner when not removed. The cells of a malignant neoplasm are not cohesive, consequently the pattern of expansion of a malignant neoplasm is often quite irregular (Fig. 8-3, *B*). Malignant neoplasms tend to be unencapsulated, and dissimilar to benign neoplasms, they usually are not easily separable from their surroundings. Malignant neoplasms characteristically invade their surroundings rather than simply push them aside. Malignant cells, whether in clusters, cords, or singly, appear to cut their way through adjacent tissue in a destructive fashion. The gross features of benign and malignant neoplasms are contrasted in Figs. 8-4 and 8-5.

The proliferating cells of malignant neoplasms have the ability to break away from the parent *(primary)* tumor and enter the circulation to float elsewhere. When such embolic cancer cells lodge, they are able to extravasate, continue their proliferation, and form a *secondary* tumor. A single primary focus of cancer can give rise to numerous embolic fragments that, in turn, may form dozens or even hundreds of secondary nodules at considerable distance from the primary. This process of discontinuous spread of malignant neoplasms is referred to as *metastasis,* and the daughter foci or areas of secondary growth are called *metastases* (singular, *metastasis*). Thus cancers or malignant neoplasms are distinguished from noncancerous or benign neoplasms by their ability to invade normal tissue and form metastases. A benign neoplasm has neither of these abilities.

Metastasis can occur by a variety of routes. Invasion of vascular channels gives rise to hematogenous metastasis in a pattern that at first may be quite predictable. When cancer cells originating from a primary location in the wall of the gastrointestinal tract enter the venous drainage of the tract, they are likely to lodge in the liver, because portal venous blood must flow through that organ before returning to the heart. On the other hand, hematogenously borne cells originating from a malignant neoplasm in the leg will flow via the vena cava to the right side of the heart and then to the lungs, where the secondary foci may grow. In an analogous manner,

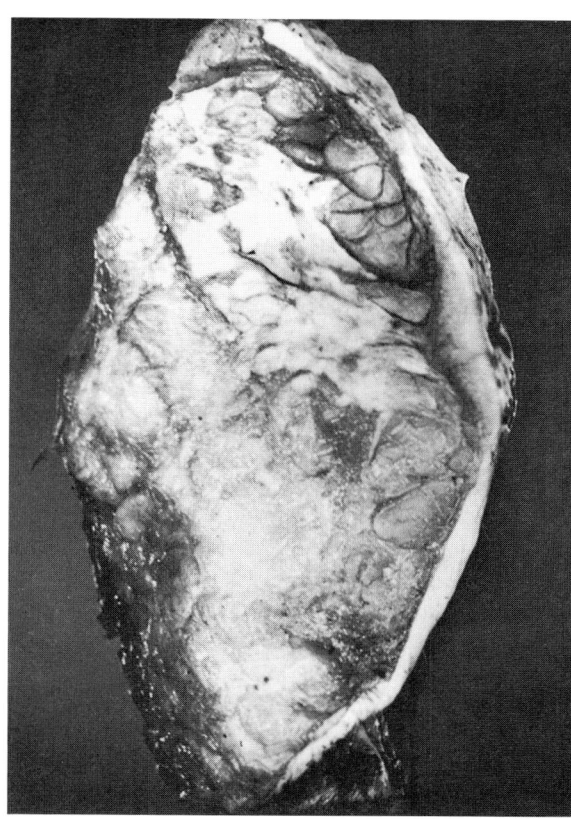

FIG. 8-5 Malignant neoplasm. In this section of breast a whitish tissue infiltrates the breast to the left of center. This is a malignant neoplasm, specifically, a carcinoma. Contrast the gross features of this with the benign neoplasm in Fig. 8-4.

malignant cells may invade lymphatic channels and float with the streaming of lymph. In these instances, metastases would be expected to appear in the regional lymph node group filtering the lymph emanating from a particular organ. Thus lymphogenous metastases from a primary cancer of the breast may be anticipated in the axillary lymph nodes, and lymphogenous metastases from a primary cancer in the oral cavity would be sought in cervical lymph node groups. As cancers progress, floating malignant cells may pass through capillary beds and regional lymph nodes and circulate widely. Then the precise location of metastases depends on the "fit" between the metabolic needs of the embolic cancer cells and the environment provided by a particular tissue. Metastases can become established in virtually any organ of the body. In addition to metastasizing via blood vessels and lymphatics, cancer cells may metastasize directly by being transported across a body cavity (e.g., peritoneal cavity) and implanting on a distant surface of that cavity. In this way, a malignant neoplasm that invades through the entire thickness of the wall of an abdominal organ may "seed" the entire peritoneal cavity, producing literally hundreds of metastases by the direct route. Similarly, when malignant cells are picked up on surgical instruments in the course of a procedure, they may be implanted elsewhere in the incision, ultimately to grow into metastatic foci. Figures 8-6 to 8-8 illustrate metastases encountered at autopsy.

In all likelihood, most cancer cells that enter the blood or lymphatic circulation or various body cavities fail to form progressively growing metastases. This failure is partly because various body defenses (i.e., immunologic defenses) inhibit the growth of such cells; this failure is

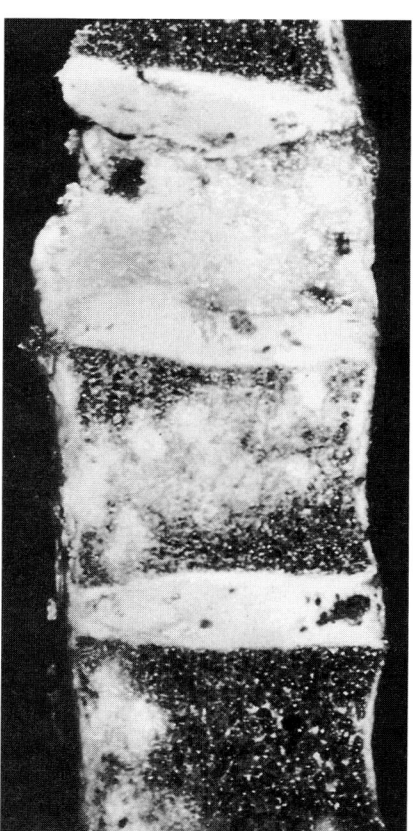

FIG. 8-6 Vertebral metastases. The whitish nodules of metastatic carcinoma within the bone grew from cells originating in the lung and spreading hematogenously.

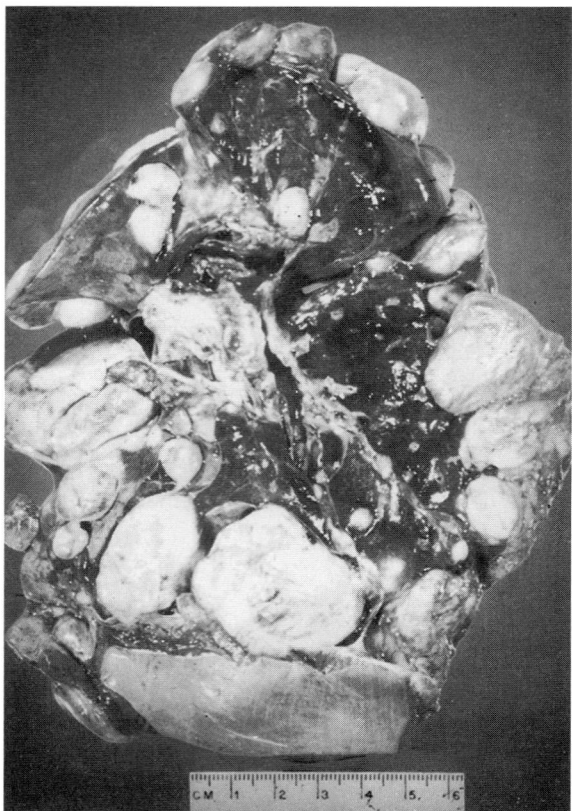

FIG. 8-7 Pulmonary metastases. This lung is extensively replaced (as was the contralateral lung) by a malignant neoplasm that originated in the kidney.

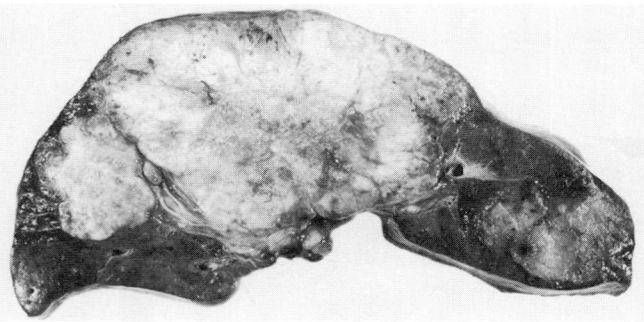

FIG. 8-8 Hepatic metastases. Many neoplasms spread to the liver, particularly, as in this case, those arising in the gastrointestinal tract. The whitish tissue is metastatic carcinoma.

also because growth conditions in an organ of secondary lodgment may be inadequate for the particular cells. On this basis, presumably, many cancers have characteristic patterns of metastases that become important in diagnosis and treatment.

NEOPLASM-HOST INTERACTION

Effects of Neoplasms on the Host

Neoplasms affect the host in a variety of ways. Because benign neoplasms do not invade or metastasize, the problems they cause are generally local, ranging from

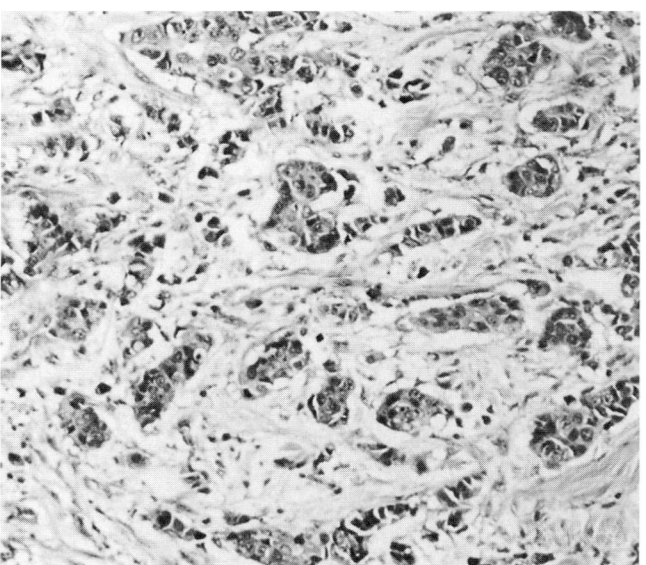

FIG. 8-9 Microscopic structure of a neoplasm. The dark clumps of cells are the actual carcinoma cells (i.e., cells of the malignant clone), while the remaining tissue is a fibrovascular stroma supplied by the host tissue.

trivial to lethal. For example, a small, strictly benign tumor in the loose subcutaneous tissue of the arm might constitute a cosmetic problem but little else. At the opposite end of the spectrum, a perfectly benign tumor growing in a vital area, such as the cranial cavity, might actually kill the patient by exerting pressure on some vital part of the brain as the neoplasm expands locally. For such reasons, "benign" does not necessarily mean inconsequential.

Local problems caused by benign neoplasms might involve plugging of various body passages. A vein or a part of the gastrointestinal (GI) tract might become obstructed by a perfectly benign neoplasm impinging on it. Benign neoplasms can become ulcerated and infected, and they may give rise to significant hemorrhage. Finally, benign tumors can produce striking effects that are not mechanical but are related to the metabolic properties of the tumor cells. For example, the cells of the islets of Langerhans of the pancreas may give rise to a benign neoplasm only a few millimeters in diameter that may never produce mechanical problems. At times, however, such neoplastic cells retain the function of the parent cells and produce insulin. Because neoplasms do not respond appropriately to homeostatic signals, such a neoplasm of islet cells might produce insulin inappropriately and in great excess, causing abnormally low blood sugar levels. Patients with such neoplasms might have a variety of systemic signs and symptoms of hypoglycemia.

Malignant neoplasms do everything that benign tumors do, but they usually do so in a much more aggressive, destructive manner because of the generally faster growth rate of malignant neoplasms and their ability to invade, destroy local tissues, and spread to form distant metastases. Patients with advanced cancers often have the appearance of severe malnutrition, a state referred to as *tumor cachexia*. This condition has a complex origin, probably related to the effects of cytokines generated within the tumor or as part of the response to the tumor.

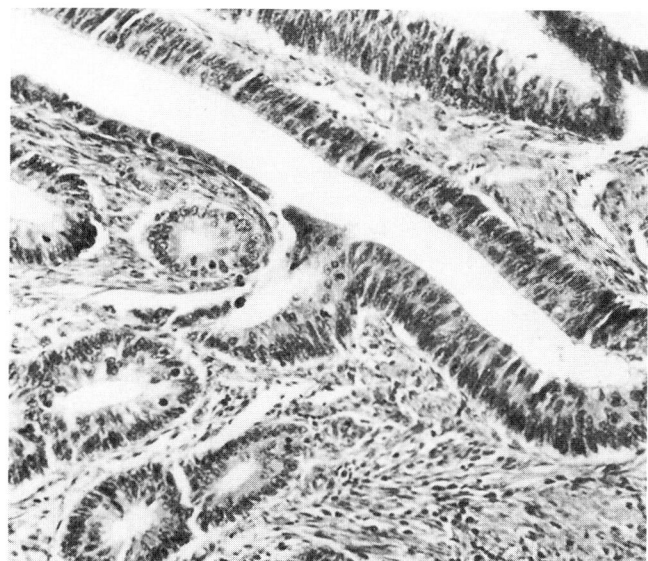

FIG. 8-10 Well-differentiated adenocarcinoma. This carcinoma of the colon resembles the parent tissue to the extent of forming glands that are easily recognizable (see Fig. 6-3); thus it is "well-differentiated." (Photomicrograph, ×200.)

Such debilitated patients with advanced cancer usually succumb to an episode of pneumonia or systemic sepsis.

Host Impact on Neoplasms

Although a key event in the life history of any neoplasm is the development of a "runaway" clone of proliferating cells that are unresponsive to homeostatic signals within the body, even highly malignant neoplasms are not completely autonomous. Neoplasms need a supply of oxygen and nutrients for the proliferating neoplastic cells, and the body must supply these. Neoplastic cells are able to evoke from the neighboring nonneoplastic tissues the formation of a vascular supply to nourish the tumor cells. Thus the supporting framework or *stroma* of neoplasms includes not only a fibrous connective tissue but also numerous finely branching, thin-walled blood vessels (Fig. 8-9). The connective tissue cells and blood vessels are not actually part of the neoplastic clone of cells, but they represent nonneoplastic host cells whose proliferation has been stimulated by substances released from the tumor cells.

Various body processes may modulate the growth of neoplastic cells and, in effect, constitute antineoplastic defenses. Many neoplastic cells are sufficiently different antigenically from the corresponding normal cells that the body may mount an immunologic reaction against the neoplasm. Although such immunologic defenses exist, the current state of knowledge about them does not yet permit the routine widespread use of immunotherapeutic measures. Beneficial immunologic treatments of certain neoplasms have been promising, and the immunologic status of the host is considered in planning and conducting various modes of antineoplastic therapy and even in manipulating the immune system to suppress neoplastic growth.

STRUCTURE OF NEOPLASMS

Neoplasms are made up of proliferating neoplastic cells associated with a support system called a *stroma*. The organization of tumor cells and stroma varies widely among neoplasms, and the relative balance of stromal elements may lend the neoplasm distinctive characteristics. A tumor that contains an extremely dense fibrous stroma is hard grossly and is sometimes referred to as *scirrhous*. A tumor that consists predominantly of neoplastic cells with little stroma is much softer and is sometimes referred to as *medullary*.

Because neoplastic cells are derived from previously normal cell populations, they may have many characteristics of normal cell populations metabolically and microscopically. However, tumors vary in their degree of resemblance to normal tissues. When the microscopic resemblance of tumor cells to their normal ancestors is close, the neoplasm is said to be *well differentiated* (Fig. 8-10). When the resemblance of neoplastic cells to their forebears is slight such that the tumor consists largely of unspecialized proliferating elements, the neoplasm is often termed *poorly differentiated, undifferentiated,* or *anaplastic*. The neoplasm in Fig. 8-9 is rather poorly differentiated. The level of differentiation may be expressed in terms of the structure of individual cells, in terms of the production of some cell products, such as mucin or keratin, or in the arrangement of neoplastic cells in relation to one another. Thus a well-differentiated neoplasm arising from a mucin-producing glandular epithelium may be composed of tumor cells that individually resemble the nonneoplastic glandular tissue, are arranged in a pattern of tubules or glands resembling the parent tissue, and may manifest mucin secretion. An anaplastic tumor arising from such a tissue may lack individual cellular resemblance or glandular arrangement and might manifest no evidence of mucin secretion. Generally, benign neoplasms are well differentiated; they closely resemble parent tissues. Malignant neoplasms occupy a rather broad spectrum with regard to differentiation. Many highly aggressive destructive cancers are poorly differentiated or anaplastic microscopically, but in some instances, even well-differentiated neoplasms may behave in a malignant fashion.

In many malignant neoplasms, individual cells manifest morphologic abnormalities that appear to mirror the malignant behavioral potential of the cells. Many cancer cells have an altered ratio of nuclear volume to cytoplasmic volume, irregular contour of nuclei, and irregular chromatin patterns. These individual cytologic manifestations of malignancy form the basis of cytopathologic examination, that is, the examination of individual cells that have exfoliated or dropped from the surface of tissues into the secretion bathing those tissues or that have been brushed from the surface of a tumor or aspirated from a mass through a fine needle. The familiar Pap smear, named after George Papanicolaou, is a smear made from a sample of cervicovaginal mucus. Specimens for cytologic examination can often be obtained with minimal inconvenience to the patient and provide valuable diagnostic information should morphologically malignant cells be found on the smear. Fig. 8-11 illustrates benign

FIG. 8-11 Benign and malignant cells in vaginal cytologic smears. In **A**, the cells are benign. The ratio of nucleus to cytoplasm is small, and nuclei are regular. In **B**, taken from a patient with carcinoma of the uterine cervix, the ratio of the nucleus to cytoplasm is increased, and the nuclei are irregular. These features allow the diagnosis of malignancy. (Photomicrograph, ×800.)

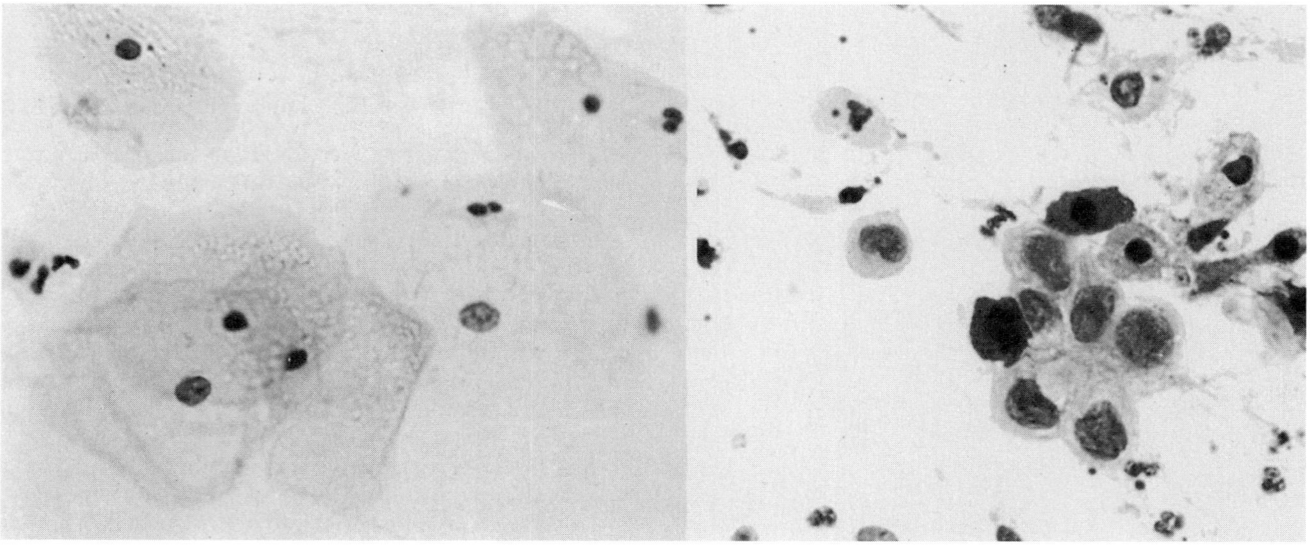

and malignant cells present in a cytologic smear. Even dysplastic cells (CIN) can be identified in Pap smears.

CLASSIFICATION AND NOMENCLATURE OF NEOPLASMS

A classification of neoplasms helps predict the possible or probable course of disease in a particular patient and aids in planning rational modes of therapy. The usual contemporary scheme of classification of neoplasms uses several sets of criteria, the most important of which is the distinction between benign and malignant biologic behavior. A particular neoplasm that has already invaded neighboring nonneoplastic tissue or has produced metastases is obviously malignant. However, even in the absence of such established invasion or metastasis, the pathologist can classify a neoplasm as malignant when its potential for malignant behavior can be predicted; that is, a particular neoplasm will be designated as malignant on the basis of its microscopic appearance alone when experience has shown that neoplasms of that type will invade and metastasize if not treated. Other parts of the classification scheme take into account the cell type of origin of the neoplasm and the organ of origin of the neoplasm. Years of accumulated experience have shown that a tumor with a particular appearance of cells, of a certain level of differentiation, arranged in a certain way, and originating in a certain organ will behave with a degree of predictability. This predictability allows the health care team to plan therapy based on the knowledge of what has happened to many patients with similar neoplasms in the past.

This kind of classification of neoplasms uses a system of naming that serves as a sort of shorthand, condensing abundant information into a relatively few terms. The entire system of tumor nomenclature will not be covered at this point, but a few generalizations are provided here as a basis for further discussion. Abundant specific information is given in subsequent chapters.

Many neoplasms arise from epithelium, which includes cells covering surfaces, lining organs, and forming glands of various kinds. The root *adeno-* denotes a glandular origin. The suffix *-oma* refers to a neoplasm (with some exceptions). Thus, in the usual system of nomenclature, an adenoma is a benign neoplasm of glandular epithelial origin. Examples of such neoplasms would include adenomas of the thyroid gland, the adrenal gland, or the lining glandular epithelium within the GI tract. In the instance of neoplasms arising and projecting from lining epithelia, less specific topographic terms are occasionally used. Thus an adenoma of the colonic lining of the epithelium, which projects into the lumen either as a broad-based mass or hangs into the lumen on a "stem," is often called a *polyp*. Such a growth projecting into the lumen of an organ in fingerlike projections is often referred to as a *papilloma*. These topographic terms are not restricted in their use, however, thus the usual nasal polyp, for instance, is not a neoplasm at all but a polypoid fold of swollen nasal mucosa. A malignant neoplasm arising from epithelium is referred to as *carcinoma*. Various qualifying prefixes and adjectives can then be added to the name. A malignancy of glandular epithelium would be referred to as an *adenocarcinoma*, whereas a malignant neoplasm arising from a squamous epithelium would be called a *squamous cell carcinoma*. The designation of a neoplasm might also include some comment about the level of differentiation, for example, "well-differentiated, mucin-forming adenocarcinoma" or "well-differentiated, keratinizing squamous cell carcinoma." Additionally, topographic descriptors may be used, such as "papillary adenocarcinoma" or "fungating (literally, mushrooming) carcinoma" for a projecting lesion.

Neoplasms derived from the supporting tissues of the body are named according to the specific tissue of origin.

TABLE 8-1

Classification of Neoplasms

Cell or Tissue of Origin	Benign	Malignant
Epithelium—stratified, squamous	Squamous papilloma	Squamous cell carcinoma (epidermoid carcinoma)
Glandular (lining fluid-filled spaces)	Adenoma (cystadenoma)	Adenocarcinoma (cystadenocarcinoma)
Melanocytes	Nevus	Melanoma
Connective tissue		
Fibrous	Fibroma	Fibrosarcoma
Adipose	Lipoma	Liposarcoma
Cartilage	Chondroma	Chondrosarcoma
Bone	Osteoma	Osteosarcoma
Muscle		
Smooth	Leiomyoma	Leiomyosarcoma
Striated	Rhabdomyoma	Rhabdomyosarcoma
Endothelium		
Blood vessel	Hemangioma	Hemangiosarcoma
Lymphatic	Lymphangioma	Lymphangiosarcoma
Nervous tissue		
Nerve sheath	Neurofibroma	Neurofibrosarcoma
Glial cells	—	Glioma, glioblastoma
Meninges	Meningioma	
Lymphoid tissue/bone marrow	—	
Hematopoietic lymphoid tissue	—	
Lymphoid tissue	—	Lymphoma, Hodgkin's disease
	Lymphocytic leukemia	
		Plasmacytoma (multiple myeloma)
Bone marrow	—	Granulocytic (myelogenous, monocytic, erythroleukemia, polycythemia rubra vera)
Germinal tissue	Teratoma	Malignant teratoma, teratocarcinoma, seminoma, embryonal carcinoma

Thus a benign neoplasm of fibrous tissue is termed a *fibroma*, a benign neoplasm of bone is called an *osteoma*, and a benign neoplasm of cartilage is referred to as a *chondroma*. A malignant neoplasm derived from supporting tissue is referred to as a *sarcoma*. The specific tissue of origin is prefixed to this term. Thus a malignant neoplasm arising from fibrous tissue is a *fibrosarcoma*, one arising from bone is an *osteosarcoma*, and one arising from cartilage is a *chondrosarcoma*.

Neoplasms arising from lymphoid tissue are called *lymphomas*. These neoplasms generally behave in a malignant manner, thus the term lymphoma generally is synonymous with malignant lymphoma. Lymphomas may arise from lymphoid tissue anywhere in the body, that is, not only from lymph nodes and spleen but also from lymphoid cells in virtually any organ. Lymphomas may involve the bone marrow extensively, and in many patients the lymphoma cells circulate in the blood in large numbers, giving rise to leukemia. *Leukemia* literally means "white blood" and pertains not only to lymphoid malignancy but also to malignancy of bone marrow cells with circulating malignant elements. The nomenclature of leukemias and lymphomas is discussed more fully in Part Three.

Many special names are used for neoplasms arising in specific sites and from particular specialized tissues. Thus gliomas arise from glial supportive cells in the central nervous system (CNS), mesotheliomas arise from the lining cells of body cavities, retinoblastomas arise within the eye, and so forth. Table 8-1 provides a simplified summary of the classification of neoplasms.

CARCINOGENESIS

Under normal conditions, cell division, proliferation, and differentiation are tightly controlled. A balance exists between cell proliferation and cell death, and cellular division is activated only when cell death or a physiologic need for more cells of a particular type occurs (e.g., in acute infection, a need for more white blood cells develops). Special intercellular signaling systems function to regulate the replication of individual cells in the body. Cell proliferation is largely controlled by chemical factors in the environment, which can increase growth of a particular tissue while simultaneously inhibiting unwanted growth of other cells. A class of proteins, the growth factors, first introduced as examples of signal transduction pathways, is important in promoting or arresting cell division. Growth factors do what their name implies; they stimulate cellular mitosis and hence tissue growth. Cells of different types secrete various growth factors. For example, skin cells secrete what is called epidermal growth factor (EGF). Fibroblast growth factor (FGF) promotes mitosis of connective tissue cells called fibrocytes (cells that make collagen and other connective tissue proteins) and endothelial cells. Platelet-derived growth factor (PDGF) activates fibroblasts in the area of a wound, where platelets will be found as a result of blood vessel trauma.

Cell Replication Regulation

Under normal physiologic conditions, the cell signaling mechanism that initiates cell proliferation can be divided

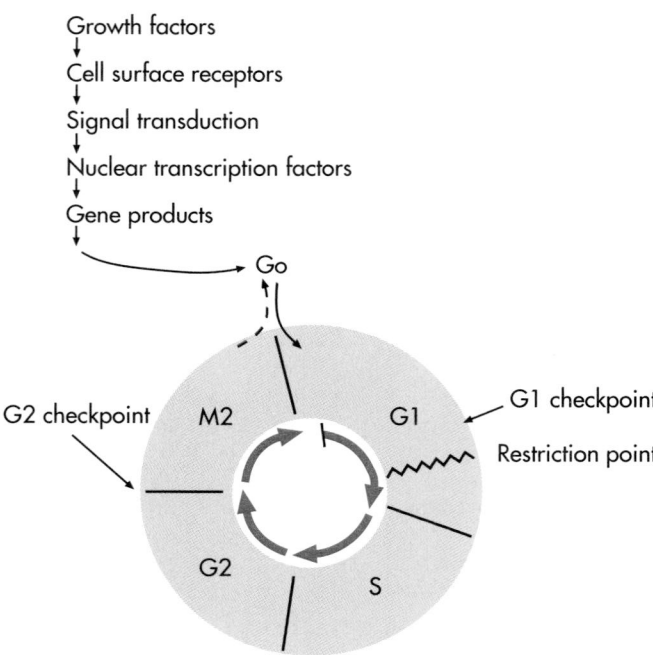

FIG. 8-12 The cell replication cycle begins in the G1 (gap 1) phase after a quiescent cell (Go) responds to an appropriate stimulus and progresses through the S (synthesis), G2, (gap 2) and M (mitosis) phases. Checkpoints control the order and timing of cell cycle transitions and can arrest the cell cycle in response to detection of DNA damage.

into the following steps: (1) a molecule, commonly a *growth factor*, binds to its specific receptor on the cell surface; (2) the *growth factor receptor* is activated, which, in turn, activates several transducing proteins; (3) the signal is transmitted across the cytosol via a *second messenger* to the cell nucleus; and (4) *nuclear transcription factors* that initiate deoxyribonucleic acid (DNA) transcription are activated.

When the conditions are favorable for cell growth, the cell proceeds through the phases of the cell replication cycle (Figure 8-12). The cell cycle can be defined as the orderly duplication of intracellular components, including the cell genome (DNA), followed by division of the cell into two cells. The cell cycle is divided into four phases: G1 (gap 1), S (synthesis), G2 (gap 2), and M (mitosis). Quiescent cells are in a nondividing state called Go. Some cells divide frequently (labile cells, such as epidermal cells of the skin and gut); others occasionally divide (stable cells, such as the parenchymal cells of the glandular organs), although permanent cells never divide once they are formed (e.g., neurons of the CNS or cardiac muscle). During G1 of the cell cycle, enzymes and substrates for DNA replication are synthesized. During the S phase of the cell cycle, DNA synthesis takes place, producing the replicated chromosomes. This event is triggered by the individual cell, which appears to evaluate itself sometime in the G1 phase (G1 restriction point) and determines whether it has the resources to divide. Once started, this process cannot be reversed; the cell is committed to divide. The synthesis of ribonucleic acid (RNA) and proteins needed for mitosis takes place during the G2

phase in preparation for mitosis. Important checkpoint control mechanisms occur late in G1 near the restriction point and at the G2/M border which can arrest the cell cycle if DNA damage is detected. After completing these checkpoints, if all is well, the mitosis or cell division phase begins and ends with the production of two daughter cells.

The cell-replication cycle and its regulation has been the subject of intense study in recent years because of its importance in understanding *carcinogenesis* (the process of cancer development). Increasingly evident is that cancer is a genetic disorder, although most cancer is not inherited. The basic process common to all neoplasms is an alteration of the genes caused by a mutation in a somatic cell. The earliest evidence for the genetic basis of cancer came from the observation that a number of agents such as radiation, certain chemicals, and viruses (carcinogens) were capable of initiating cancer in experimental animals when given the proper exposure. What these carcinogens had in common was that they were mutagenic (i.e., capable of causing genetic mutations). Clearly, in the vast majority of cancers, probably all cancers, mutations (e.g., changes in the sequence of the DNA nucleotides) exist and are critical in causation. The transformed (mutated) cell gives rise to a malignant clone that no longer responds to the normal regulatory control mechanisms and proceeds to proliferate without regard to the needs of the body.

Four classes of genes have been identified that play an important role in regulating the growth factor signaling mechanisms and the cell cycle itself, including protooncogenes, tumor suppressor genes, genes that regulate apoptosis, and DNA repair genes. That mutations in these regulatory genes are responsible for the pathogenesis of cancer is now a well-established fact, although all the details have not been worked out. Fig. 8-13 provides an overview of the interaction of these genes in the pathogenesis of cancer.

Protooncogenes and Oncogenes

Protooncogenes are cellular genes whose functions are to encourage and promote the normal growth and division of cells. The genes are denoted by three letter names such as c-*myc* or *erb*-B1. Cells expressing mutated forms of these genes are called oncogenes and have a high probability of progressing to malignancy after a limited number of cell divisions. Approximately 100 known oncogenes have been identified. When normal protooncogenes mutate to become carcinogenic oncogenes, they are referred to as "activated," and the result is excessive cell multiplication. The term *oncogene* is derived from the Greek word *oncos*, meaning tumor.

Protooncogenes code for proteins involved in the receptor-activated proliferation and differentiation pathways as previously described, which include growth factors, growth factor receptors, proteins involved in signal transduction, nuclear regulatory proteins, and cell cycle regulators. Protooncogenes that code for these various components in the cascade may mutate, becoming oncogenes (producing abnormal oncoproteins) that keep these pathways continuously active when they would

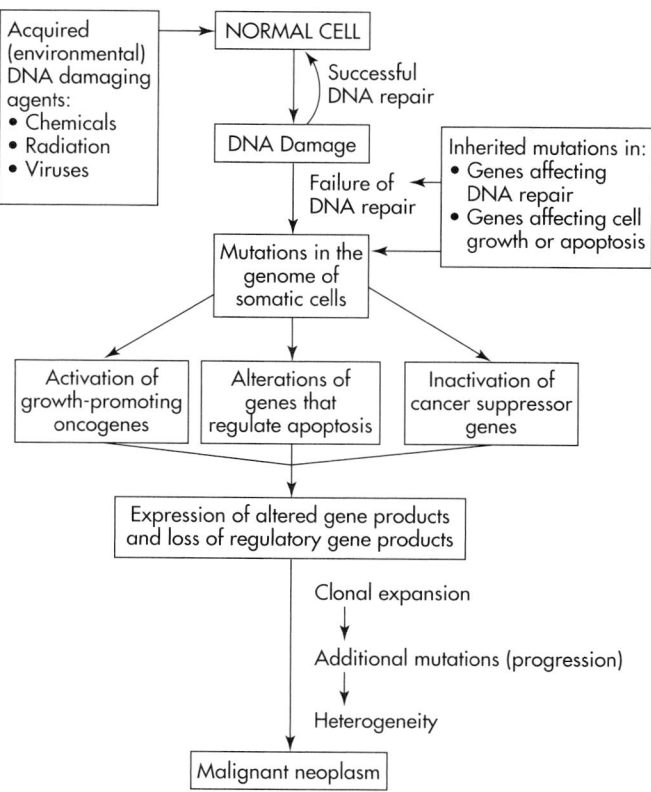

FIG. 8-13   Flow chart depicting a simplified scheme of the molecular basis of cancer. (Redrawn from Cotran RS, Kumar V, Collins T: *Robbin's pathologic basis of disease*, ed 6, Philadelphia, 1999, WB Saunders.)

otherwise be quiescent. The abnormal oncoproteins, which resemble the normal products of protooncogenes, are devoid of important regulatory elements and their production does not depend on growth factors or other external signals. The result may be overproduction of growth factors, flooding of the cell with replication signals, uncontrolled stimulation of the intermediary pathway, or unrestrained cell growth driven by elevated levels of transcription factors. Additionally, mutation of cyclins and cyclin-dependent kinases (CDKs), which normally control progression through the cell replication cycle, may cause dysregulation.

In addition to the functional characteristics of oncogenes already described, oncogenes exhibit a dominant phenotype at the cellular level, with only one copy of the activated oncogene being sufficient to produce its carcinogenic effect. Oncogenes may be transmitted from generation to generation when a protooncogene mutates in the germ line. This action results in a dominantly inherited cancer *predisposition*. Usually more than one mutation in this class of gene is required to change a normal cell line into a tumor or neoplasm.

Protooncogenes can be transformed into oncogenes by four basic mechanisms: point mutation, gene amplification, chromosome rearrangement, and insertion of a viral genome. These mutations result in either a change in gene structure, causing the synthesis of an abnormal gene product (oncoprotein) with aberrant function, or a change in regulation of gene expression, causing inappropriate secretion or enhancement of structurally normal growth promoting protein.

1. *Point mutation.* This mechanism involves a single base substitution in the DNA chain resulting in a miscoded protein that has one amino acid substituted for another. Point mutations have been observed in a large proportion of tumors carrying the *ras* gene, including carcinomas of the colon, pancreas, and thyroid. Normal ras proteins are involved in the regulation of the cytosol signal transduction pathway and in regulation of the cell cycle.

2. *Gene amplification.* This mechanism causes the cell to acquire an increased number of copies of the protooncogene causing overexpression of its protein products. Two interesting examples include neuroblastoma in which the tumor cells contain multiple copies of the N-*myc* gene and in some breast cancers multiple copies of the c-*erb*-B2 gene. The more copies of the gene the cell contains, the more malignant the tumor and the poorer the prognosis.

3. *Chromosomal rearrangements.* Translocation of one chromosome fragment onto another, or deletion of a fragment of a chromosome, leads to a juxtapositioning of genes that are normally distant from each other. Cell growth and differentiation are normal when the protooncogene and its neighbors function together in an orderly manner but may be deranged when this relationship is disturbed. The translocation may bring the protooncogene to a location on another chromosome that stimulates its functions. Alternately, the translocation may bring the gene to a new location where it is freed from the inhibitory genes that formerly controlled its functions. The Philadelphia chromosome, characteristic of chronic myelogenous leukemia, is a prototype example of an oncogene formed by the fusion of two separate genes. In these cases, chromosome 9 is broken in the region of a gene called *abl*, then transposed to a break point on chromosome 22 containing the *bcr* gene so that the *abl* and *bcr* genes are fused. Another example is the translocation of the c-*myc* gene, normally on chromosome 8, to chromosome 14 next to the immunoglobulin (Ig) gene. The Ig gene promotes the activity of the c-*myc* gene, which ultimately results in Burkitt's lymphoma.

4. *Insertion of a viral genome.* Insertion of a viral genome into the host cell genome results in the disruption of normal chromosomal structure and genetic dysregulation. Numerous viruses have been shown to be oncogenic in animals. Several types of viruses, mostly in the form of DNA viruses, have been implicated in the causation of human cancer. Human papillomaviruses (HPV), primarily types 16 and 18, which are sexually transmitted, have been linked to uterine cervical cancer. Hepatitis B and C (HBV and HCV) have been linked to hepatocellular carcinoma. The Epstein-Barr virus (EBV) has been implicated in the pathogenesis of four types of cancers: Burkitt's lymphoma, B-cell lymphomas, nasopharyngeal carcinoma, and some cases of Hodgkin's lymphoma. Only one type of RNA virus, human T-cell leukemia virus type 1 (HTLV-1), is

firmly implicated in the causation of a form of T-cell leukemia/lymphoma common in Japan.

Tumor Suppressor Genes

Whereas protooncogenes encode proteins that promote cell growth, tumor suppressor genes inhibit or "put the brakes on" the cell growth and division cycle. The name of these genes is somewhat misleading because their normal function is to regulate cell growth not prevent tumor formation. One such manifestation of inhibition in a culture of normal cells in the laboratory is *contact inhibition*. Normal cells cease to replicate when they contact other cells, generally forming a monolayer when grown in a culture dish. In contrast, cancer cells continue to grow and pile up on top of one another after they have formed a confluent monolayer. In other words, the cancer cells become autonomous, failing to respond to the normal growth and inhibitory signals in the community of cells.

Mutations in tumor suppressor genes cause the cell to ignore one or more of the components of the network of inhibitory signals, removing the brakes from the cell cycle and resulting in a higher rate of uncontrolled growth—cancer. In a manner similar to that of oncogenes, the protein products of tumor suppressor genes function in all parts of the cell, at the cell surface, in the cytoplasm, and in the nucleus.

Tumor suppressor genes are defined by the impact of their absence and thus tend to be recessive. Both normal alleles must mutate before giving rise to malignant growth. Thus neoplasia is a result of the loss of function of both tumor suppressor genes. The loss or inactivation of a normal suppressor gene may be acquired somatically in a single clone of cells or be constitutionally present in the germ line. Hypotheses suggest that the development of a neoplasm requires two separate mutational events. One of these events may occur in the germline and may be inherited; the second one occurs somatically. Alternately, the two mutational events may occur only in the somatic cell of an individual. This "two-hit hypothesis" has helped to explain the natural history of retinoblastoma and has been extended to other neoplasms.

The Rb gene was the first tumor suppressor gene discovered. Retinoblastoma is a malignant eye tumor in children that occurs in a hereditary and sporadic form. The hereditary form shows a deletion of a segment of the long arm of chromosome 13 where the Rb gene is located. When one copy is deleted, cell growth is still normal, relying on the surviving gene copy. If the remaining copy is mutated or lost, then a tumor occurs in the retina, causing blindness in both eyes. In sporadic retinoblastoma, the child is born with two normal alleles. However, if both these alleles are mutated owing to some exogenous factor and both Rb genes are lost, retinoblastoma will then develop. These tumors are usually unilateral.

The Rb gene codes for the pRb protein, important in the control of the cell cycle at the G1-S checkpoint (see Fig. 8-12) and has been called the master brake. At this checkpoint, the cell commits to either DNA replication or to quiescence or differentiation (or both), depending on the balance between growth promoting and inhibitory signals. Progression through the cell cycle is mediated by the various cyclins, which combine with cyclin-dependent kinases (CDKs). The pRb protein can block cell division by binding transcription factors, preventing them from transcribing growth factors. An inactivating mutation of the Rb gene removes one of the major restraints on cell division. Mutation of the Rb gene is found in bone, bladder, small cell lung cancer, and breast cancers, as well as retinoblastoma. The genes that regulate cell cycle control are frequently disrupted in cancer cells.

If the Rb gene is the master brake of the cell cycle, then the TP53 gene (which codes for the p53 protein) is the emergency brake. The p53 protein is known as the guardian of the G1-S checkpoint but is not usually called upon in the course of normal cell replication. However, when DNA damage occurs, p53 influences transcription to halt the cell cycle (through p21 expression, a CDK inhibitor) and signals the DNA repair genes to correct the damage. If the damage is too great, then p53 induces apoptosis (programmed cell death or suicide). If the TP53 tumor suppressor gene is inactivated by a mutation, a major protection against the propagation of cells with damaged DNA (giving rise to a malignant clone) is lost. Approximately 50% of human cancers are associated with a TP53 mutation, including cancers of the breast, colon, lung, bladder, and skin. The function of TP53 is also critical to the way in which many cancer treatments kill cells. Radiation and chemotherapy act in part by triggering apoptosis in response to DNA damage. This successful response to therapy is greatly reduced in malignancies in which TP53 is mutant, making them difficult to treat.

Other examples of tumor suppressor genes include BRCA1 and BRCA2, associated with breast and ovarian cancer. The APC gene is associated with familial adenomatous polyposis of the colon and the NF1 gene is associated with neurofibromatosis.

Genes that Regulate Apoptosis

Apoptosis (see Chapter 3), or programmed cell death, is an active process by which cells are eliminated from the organism. Similar to cell growth and differentiation, apoptosis requires active and coordinated regulation by specific genes. A large family of genes has been discovered that regulate apoptosis. Some of these genes inhibit apoptosis, similar to the *bcl-2* gene, while others promote apoptosis (such as *bad* or *bax*). The belief is that the proapoptosis and antiapoptosis members of this family of genes act as a rheostat in controlling apoptosis. Overexpression of the bcl-2 gene, caused by a chromosomal translocation, is associated with the majority of B-cell lymphomas of the follicular type. In other words, failure of the cells to die as they should (because apoptosis is suppressed by the mutant bcl-2) leads to the accumulation of B lymphocytes within the lymph nodes and lymphoma.

In addition to the role of the bcl-2 family of genes in regulating apoptosis, at least two other cancer-associated genes can trigger apoptosis: the tumor suppressor gene TP53, described previously, and the protooncogene, *c-myc*. These genes interact with apoptosis-regulating genes in determining whether a cell will respond to an apoptotic stimulus.

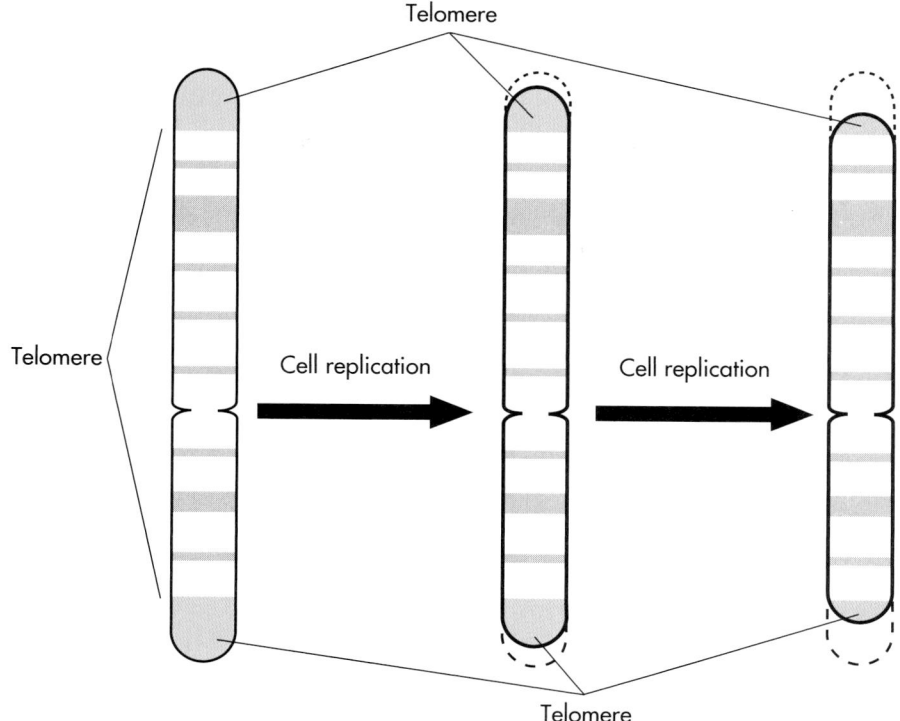

FIG. 8-14   The end caps of chromosomes are called telomeres (analogous to the plastic tips on shoe laces). In most somatic cells, the telomeres become progressively shorter with each cell replication until they reach a critical length that induces replicative senescence. Most cancer cells secrete telomerase, which can restore telomere length and allow them to replicate indefinitely.

DNA Repair Genes

The causes of DNA damage include radiation, chemicals, ultraviolet light, and random errors in DNA replication. DNA repair genes code for proteins, the normal function of which is to correct errors that arise when cells duplicate their DNA before cell division. Mutations in DNA repair genes can lead to failure in DNA repair, which, in turn, allows subsequent mutations in tumor suppressor genes and protooncogenes to accumulate. DNA repair genes, similar to tumor suppressor genes, exist in pairs in homologous chromosomes, and both must be nonfunctional before the repair functions regulated by the genes are compromised (i.e., autosomal recessive pattern of expression).

Individuals born with an inherited mutation of DNA repair genes are at an increased risk of developing cancer because if a spontaneous mutation of the other normal allele occurs, the affected cell is unable to correct DNA replication errors. For example, hereditary nonpolyposis colon cancer (HNPCC) results from mutated DNA mismatch repair genes and accounts for 10% of all colon cancers. These genes normally act as "spell checkers" to ensure that the sequence of DNA is correct as genes are duplicated during the cell cycle. The family history is positive for colon cancer for individuals with HNPCC and the average age at diagnosis is 45 years (compared with 65 years for colon cancer in the general population).

Telomeres, Telomerase, Aging, and Cancer

Telomeres are repeating DNA strings (TTAGGG) that form end caps on chromosomes (Fig. 8-14). Telomeres are essential for chromosomal stability because they protect against end-to-end fusion and degradation during cell replication. Telomeres have been the focus of intense investigation in recent years because of their possible significance to cancer and to aging. During the 1960s Hayflick discovered that normal human cells undergo a finite number of cell divisions (called the Hayflick limit) and ultimately enter a nondividing state called replicative senescence. The mechanism responsible for the Hayflick limit is telomere shortening. Each time a mortal cell divides, its telomeres become shorter. When they reach a preset length, the cell ceases to divide, ages, and dies. Theories suggest that telomere shortening is the molecular clock that counts the number of cell divisions and triggers senescence. This finding led to the telomeric theory of aging (Bodner, 1998). Telomere shortening is prevented in germ cells, including embryonic stem cells, by the sustained action of an enzyme, telomerase, thus explaining their extensive ability to replicate. Telomerase is absent from most somatic cells, thus explaining why they suffer progressive loss of telomeres and senescence. Most cancers arise from somatic cells, but one of the crucial features that distinguishes a cancer cell from a normal cell is its ability to divide indefinitely. Most cancer cells have regained the ability to synthesize telomerase and are thus able to prevent shortening of their telomeres. Telomerase is currently the best and most common marker of cancer cells. Activity has been detected in every major category of human malignant neoplasia tested, exhibiting an overall prevalence of 85% (Meeker and Coffey, 1997).

Multistep Nature of Carcinogenesis

A neoplasm develops from the clonal proliferation of a single transformed (mutated) cell. As has been seen, the initiating event that transforms a normal cell into an abnormal mutated cell may be the introduction of an oncogene, inactivation of a tumor suppressor gene, or failure to repair the DNA or induce apoptosis of the damaged cell. This initiating transformation, however, is insufficient to cause a full-blown malignant tumor. The mutated cell must replicate itself and undergo multiple mutations to achieve full malignancy with the ability to infiltrate local tissues, penetrate vessels, and metastasize.

The classic model of carcinogenesis divides the process into three stages: initiation, promotion, and progression. *Initiation* is the process involving a genetic mutation that becomes permanent in the DNA of the cell. *Promotion* is the stage during which the mutant cell proliferates. Hormones often act as promoters that stimulate growth. For example, estrogen may stimulate growth of breast or ovarian cancer, and testosterone is a growth factor for prostate cancer. Some cancer cells may make their own growth factors and not need external signals. Forced to proliferate, the unstable initiated clone of cells undergoes additional mutations and eventually develops into a malignant tumor. *Progression* is the stage during which the clone of mutant cells acquires one or more characteristics of a malignant neoplasm. As the tumor grows the cells become more heterogenous from additional mutations. Some of these subclones may exhibit more aggressive malignant behavior or are better able to evade attack by the patient's immune system. During the progressive stage, the expanding tumor mass acquires further changes that allow it to invade adjacent tissues, develop its own blood supply (angiogenesis), penetrate blood vessels, and migrate to a distant site (metastasize) to establish secondary tumors.

CLINICAL ASPECTS OF NEOPLASIA

The variety of signs and symptoms that can be produced by neoplasms is virtually endless. Therefore the possibility of neoplasm can be considered with many different modes of patient presentation. Fig. 8-15 provides information about the incidence of various kinds of cancers in different organs in the two sexes. A clue of particular value is the *persistence* (if not progression) of a given manifestation, for example, a *sore that does not heal* or *chronic hoarseness.* The age of the patient must also be considered. For example, hoarseness in a young child suggests a different list of possibilities (and approaches) than the same sign would in a 60-year-old smoker. An iron deficiency anemia in an elderly patient might be associated with a chronically bleeding colonic cancer, whereas the same finding in a teenage girl may be explained by a nutritionally inadequate diet combined with the onset of menstrual blood loss.

Whether the index of suspicion is based on circumstances or on physical findings, the presence of the neoplasm must be definitively confirmed, because nonneoplastic conditions can also produce identical manifestations. In a few instances, certain blood tests may provide additional circumstantial evidence of a particular neoplasm. Ultimately, a space-occupying mass must be identified and delineated, whether by simple palpation during physical examination or by radiography, ultrasonography, radionuclide scanning, or any of several endoscopic procedures for direct visualization of internal structures. A final diagnostic step involves morphologic confirmation by the pathologist based on microscopic examination of the tissue in question. The diagnostic biopsy may be curative, such as when the questionable lump is totally excised and found to be benign. In other cases, a wedge biopsy might be performed, a tiny core

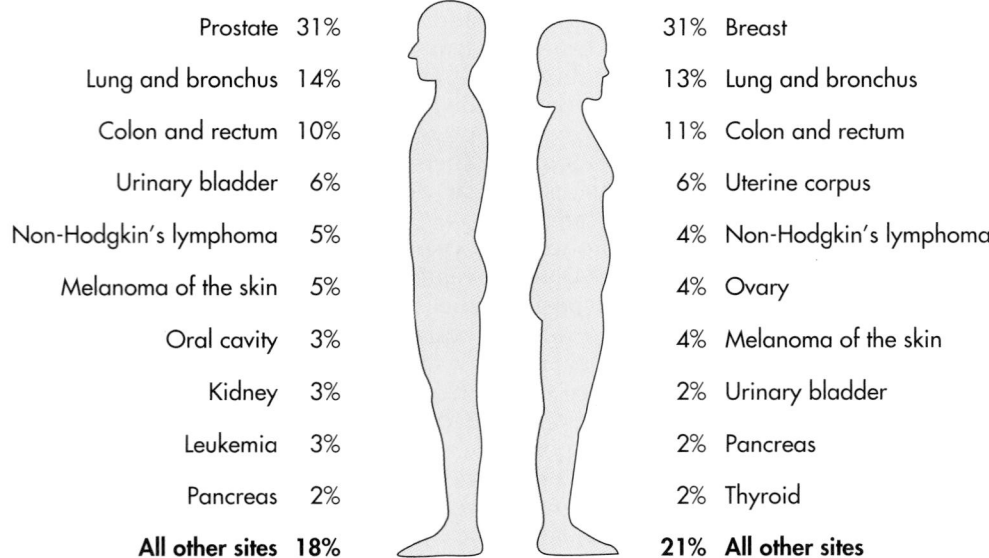

Male			Female
Prostate	31%	31%	Breast
Lung and bronchus	14%	13%	Lung and bronchus
Colon and rectum	10%	11%	Colon and rectum
Urinary bladder	6%	6%	Uterine corpus
Non-Hodgkin's lymphoma	5%	4%	Non-Hodgkin's lymphoma
Melanoma of the skin	5%	4%	Ovary
Oral cavity	3%	4%	Melanoma of the skin
Kidney	3%	2%	Urinary bladder
Leukemia	3%	2%	Pancreas
Pancreas	2%	2%	Thyroid
All other sites	**18%**	**21%**	**All other sites**

FIG. 8-15   Estimated new cancer cases, United States, ten leading sites by gender for 2001. Statistics do not include basal and squamous cell skin cancers and in situ carcinomas except urinary bladder. (From Greenlee RT, Hill-Harmon B, Murray T, Thun M: *Ca J Clin* 51[1]:18, 2001. Redrawn with permission from the American Cancer Society, Michigan Division.)

of tissue might be removed from the mass with a special biopsy needle, or a small amount of fluid containing neoplastic cells might be aspirated by needle from the mass.

A cytologic smear made from some fluid or secretion bathing the area in question may also yield valuable diagnostic information. A cytologic examination indicating the presence of cancer cells is usually confirmed by biopsy before treatment is undertaken. The Papanicolaou smear may contain cancer cells from an area not visible by ordinary examinations (e.g., the upper endocervical canal) and thereby may direct attention to that precise area. Pap smears also provide samples from large numbers of individuals on a routine basis even when signs and symptoms of abnormality may not have been noted. Obviously, routine biopsy of asymptomatic people is not feasible; however, sampling cervicovaginal mucus is an innocuous procedure that may yield some "positives," leading to the diagnosis of dysplasia or possibly of cancer in an early stage.

Microscopic examination of the tissue is essential in distinguishing neoplastic from nonneoplastic and malignant from benign conditions and is of additional value in planning therapy. Precise identification of a cancer allows some important general predictions of its likely behavior, for instance, whether a particular neoplasm might have an extremely high probability of metastases in regional lymph nodes, lungs, or other sites, even in the absence of clinical evidence. In this situation, simple excision of the primary lesion with no additional therapy would generally be unsuccessful. Predictions about certain malignant neoplasms may be more accurate if they take into account the *histologic grade* of the neoplasm, which is based on the microscopic appearance, arrangement, and degree of differentiation of the cancer cells (i.e., the extent to which they resemble normal cells), features that may correlate with the behavioral aggressiveness of the tumor.

These predictions are general and provide correspondingly broad guidelines for therapy. However, determining the clinical stage of the cancer in the patient can refine the decisions regarding treatment. *Staging* is based on an estimate of the progression of the neoplasm within the patient's body. A patient with a small, limited primary tumor would be at an earlier clinical stage and less likely to have metastases in local lymph nodes compared with a patient with a larger, more deeply invasive tumor of the same type. A patient with established lymph nodal metastases would be at a more advanced stage than one without and would be more likely to have occult distant metastases. A patient with overtly evident distant metastases would, of course, be in an extremely advanced stage of the disease. These considerations have led to extensive use of the *TNM system* of staging. In this system, *T* refers to the primary tumor, and a T1 lesion would be smaller than a T4 lesion. *N* is the status of regional lymph nodes, with N0 designating absence of nodal metastases and N1, N2, or N3 indicating increasing metastatic involvement. *M* refers to distant metastasis, with appropriate adscripts. The precise definition of T, N, and M varies for different cancers, but the system provides widely applicable shorthand for tumor staging.

Clinical staging not only helps determine the prognosis but also helps to plan rational therapy, preferably a step ahead of the neoplasm. The patient in a late stage of disease requires an entirely different treatment regimen than does a patient in an early stage, and the regimen may have risks and morbidity that render it undesirable unless the regimen is clearly indicated. Because different types of neoplasms have strikingly different natural histories, the staging schemes and methods vary accordingly. For example, a patient with cervical carcinoma will be staged differently than will a patient with lymphoma in the neck. Staging may involve physical examination, various radiologic techniques, or even surgical biopsy of certain tissues distant from the primary.

Several different modalities of cancer treatment may be employed simultaneously or serially. Each modality attempts to eradicate the cancerous tissue with an acceptable degree of loss or damage to normal tissues.

The oldest and best-known treatment is *surgical removal* of the cancerous tissue. This procedure is extremely effective if excision of the primary tumor, along with a margin of normal tissues and perhaps the regional lymph nodes, eliminates all cancer cells from the body (or, some would claim, reduces the total body load of cancer cells to the point at which host defenses can eliminate the remainder). However, many tumors are "inoperable." In some cases, this is because the primary cannot be totally excised without sacrificing essential local structures. In other cases, distant metastases may be evident; therefore removal of the primary tumor would not eradicate all the neoplasm. Additionally, the natural history of some diseases (e.g., leukemia) renders surgery inappropriate at any stage.

Another mode of treatment is *radiotherapy*, which is the application of ionizing radiation to the neoplasm. Because the lethal effect of radiation is greater on proliferating, poorly differentiated cancer cells than on adjacent normal cells, the normal tissues may be injured to a tolerable, reparable degree, whereas the cancer cells are eliminated. In a favorable situation, a cure can be effected without sacrificing some vital structure. This mode of therapy also has limitations. Some tumors are radioresistant, being no more sensitive to the effects of irradiation than are the surrounding normal cells. Widespread tumors cannot be treated by radiotherapy, because irradiation of broad areas of the body would risk unacceptable morbidity or could be lethal.

A rapidly evolving treatment modality is *chemotherapy*, which exposes proliferating cancer cells and normal cells to a variety of cytotoxic agents. A systemically administered drug of which the toxic effects on normal cells are low enough to be acceptable may eliminate widely disseminated cancer cells beyond the confines of surgical or radiation therapy. However, various cancers are sensitive to different drugs or combinations of drugs, and no one regimen is applicable to all tumors. Unfortunately, chemotherapy is often limited by the toxicity of the agents for rapidly proliferating normal cells, such as the hematopoietic cells or the lining epithelial cells of the bone marrow or the GI tract. However, reports are continually emerging of previously uncontrollable neoplasms proving to be sensitive to new chemotherapeutic approaches.

Immunotherapy is also being tried in the treatment of cancers. Cancer cells often differ antigenically from normal cells to a degree that immunologic reactions may be mounted against them. These reactions are demonstrable in laboratory situations but are not yet controllable at a practical clinical level. However, therapeutic measures aimed at immunologic stimulation of the patient with cancer have shown promise in some instances.

The approach to the patient with cancer is not limited to the use of a single treatment modality, but rather involves a team approach tailored to the unique needs of the individual with a particular neoplasm at a given clinical stage. Even when a neoplasm is deemed "incurable," several modes of therapy may provide dramatic palliation, significantly prolonging the span of comfortable, useful life for the patient.

KEY CONCEPTS

- *Agenesis* is the congenital failure of an organ to develop after organogenesis, and *hypogenesis* is the failure of an organ to develop to adult size.
- *Atrophy* is the shrinkage of an organ or tissue that had previously been of adult size; the cause may physiologic or pathologic. Common causes are decreased workload (disuse atrophy), loss of innervation (denervation atrophy), aging (senile atrophy), loss of endocrine stimulation, ischemia, and inadequate nutrition.
- *Hypertrophy* refers to an increase in the size of an organ or tissue resulting from an *increase in the size of the cells*. The number of cells does not increase. Hypertrophy may be physiologic or pathologic and is caused by increased functional demand or hormonal stimulation, for example, increased size of biceps muscle in a weight lifter (normal physiologic response) or myocardial hypertrophy in a person with chronic hypertension (adaptive but eventually becomes pathologic).
- *Hyperplasia* refers to an increase in the size of an organ or tissue resulting from an *increase in the number of the cells*. Hyperplasia may be physiologic or pathologic. Examples of physiologic hyperplasia include breast and uterine enlargement during pregnancy (hormonal hyperplasia) or compensatory callous formation (e.g., on the hand from repetitive work-related pressure). The cause of pathologic hyperplasia is usually excessive hormonal stimulation as in endometrial hyperplasia in a postmenopausal woman who is taking estrogens; the cause of prostatic hyperplasia, common in older men, is unknown. Pathologic hyperplasia constitutes a fertile soil in which cancerous proliferation may eventually arise.
- *Metaplasia* is the replacement of one mature cell type for another that is not normally present at that site as an adaptation to an adverse environmental stress. For example, the normal ciliated columnar epithelium of the bronchial mucosa is replaced by the more rugged stratified squamous epithelium because of chronic irritation in a habitual smoker. Metaplasia is potentially reversible if the causative factors are removed; without removal, metaplasia may progress to dysplasia.
- *Dysplasia* (disordered growth) is an abnormal change in the size, shape, and organization of mature cells. Minor degrees of dysplasia are potentially reversible if the irritant stimulus can be identified and removed. Epithelial dysplasia almost invariably precedes the appearance of cancer, and when severe, the dysplasia is considered to be a preinvasive neoplasm and is referred to as *carcinoma in situ*.
- A *neoplasm* (new growth or tumor) is an abnormal mass of proliferating cells that serves no beneficial adaptive purpose. Neoplasms are classified as benign or malignant (cancer).
- *Differences between benign and malignant neoplasms* can be compared on the basis of differentiation and anaplasia, rate of growth, local invasion, and metastasis. Differentiation and anaplasia apply to the parenchymal cells of the neoplasm. *Differentiation* refers to the extent to which the parenchymal cells resemble comparable normal cells. Benign neoplasms are generally well differentiated, whereas malignant neoplasms range from well differentiated to undifferentiated (*anaplasia*—resembling embryonic cells). Most benign tumors grow slowly over a period of years and do not usually kill the host, whereas most malignant tumors grow rapidly, at an erratic pace, and eventually kill their host. Nearly all benign tumors grow as cohesive encapsulated masses, whereas the growth of cancers is characterized by progressive infiltration, invasion, and destruction of the surrounding normal tissues (local spread). Finally, malignant neoplasms have the ability to metastasize (distal spread) and cause secondary growths at a distant site, whereas benign neoplasms do not metastasize.
- Dissemination of cancers may occur through three routes: *lymphatic spread* (most common), *hematogenous spread*, and *seeding of body cavities and surfaces*. A fourth possible route is by *direct implantation* of cancer cells on surgical gloves or instruments during biopsy or surgical manipulation of the tumor.
- *Local effects of neoplasms* depend on the location and impingement on adjacent structures and include the following: ischemic necrosis from compression of tissues; secondary infection; obstruction of the airways, intestine, biliary or urinary tract; hemorrhage resulting from an erosion into a blood vessel; pain from compression of sensitive structures; and pathologic fractures resulting from bone metastasis in the case of malignant neoplasms.
- *Systemic effects of malignant neoplasms* include cachexia (wasting syndrome), anemia (from bone marrow suppression or bleeding), and symptoms related to abnormal secretion of hormones.
- Generally, benign neoplasms are designated by attaching the suffix *-oma* to the cell of origin. The

naming of malignant neoplasms follows the same schema with some modifications. A malignant neoplasm of epithelial origin is designated as a *carcinoma*, which may be qualified as an *adenocarcinoma* (when it shows a glandular pattern of growth) or as a squamous cell carcinoma (producing squamous cells). Malignant neoplasms arising in mesenchymal tissue are called *sarcomas*. Specifying the organ of origin (e.g., adenocarcinoma of the lung) is also common practice. Many exceptions to these rules exist.

■ *Carcinogenesis* is initiated by nonlethal genetic damage (mutations) acquired by the action of environmental agents (e.g., radiation, chemicals, viruses) in a somatic cell or may be inherited in the germ line. *A neoplasm develops from the clonal expansion of a single progenitor cell that has incurred the genetic damage.*

■ Four classes of genes that play an important role in regulating the growth factor signaling mechanisms and the cell cycle—*protooncogenes, tumor suppressor genes, genes that regulate apoptosis,* and *DNA repair genes*—are the main targets of genetic damage in carcinogenesis. Cancer cells exhibit antisocial behavior that allow them to ignore growth factor signals from the community of cells thus they proliferate abnormally or fail to respond to repair DNA damage or apoptosis signals.

■ *Telomeres* are the end caps on chromosomes that are essential for chromosomal stability during cell replication. Telomeres shorten with each somatic cell replication until a critical length is reached and the cell is no longer able to replicate. Telomere shortening is believed to be the genetic basis of aging. Cancer cells secrete *telomerase* that repairs telomeres and may be the key to attaining immortality.

■ *Carcinogenesis is a multistep process* involving *initiation* (the original genetic mutation), *promotion* (proliferation of the malignant clone and additional mutations), and *progression* (proliferating clone acquires the behavior of a malignant tumor including infiltration and metastasis).

■ Histologic grading and clinical staging are performed to help establish the prognosis and guide the therapy of malignancies. *Histologic grading* is based on the degree of differentiation of the tumor cells and the number of mitoses is presumed to correlate with the aggressiveness of the malignant neoplasm. The *TNM clinical staging system* is based on the size of the primary lesion, its extent of spread to the regional lymph nodes, and the presence or absence of distant metastases.

■ Common modes of cancer treatment include surgical excision, irradiation, and chemotherapy.

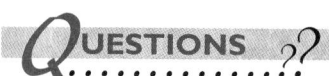

QUESTIONS ??

A sampling of review questions for this chapter appears here. Visit http://www.mosby.com/MERLIN/PriceWilson/ for additional questions.

Match the term in column A with its proper description in column B.

Column A
1. _____ Aplasia
2. _____ Hyperplasia
3. _____ Hypertrophy
4. _____ Metaplasia
5. _____ Dysplasia
6. _____ Neoplasia
7. _____ Anaplasia

Column B
a. Abnormal degree of variation in size, shape, and appearance of the cells with an abnormal arrangement of cells
b. Lack of differentiation or specialization in a group of neoplastic cells; representation as a mass of pleomorphic primitive cells
c. Failure of structure to grow in the course of organogenesis
d. Increase in the absolute number of cells, leading to an increase in the size of that tissue or organ

e. Differentiation of dividing cells into types of cells not ordinarily found in the area but types of cells that would be perfectly reasonable elsewhere
f. Increase in size of existing cells without an increase in their number
g. Formation of an abnormal mass of proliferating cells, possessing a significant degree of autonomy

Fill in the blanks with the correct words.

8. Some causes of atrophy are _____, _____, and _____.

9. Two dangerous properties of malignant neoplasms that distinguish them from benign neoplasms are _____ and _____.

Answer the following on a separate sheet of paper.

10. List at least three pathways by which malignant neoplasms disseminate through the body.
11. How do neoplasms (benign and malignant) affect the host?
12. What are the criteria used in the classification of neoplasms?
13. Explain the importance of cervical intraepithelial neoplasia (CIN) with regard to severe grades of dysplasia (CIN II or III).

14. What is the significance of the condition referred to as tumor cachexia?
15. What is happening at a cellular level during the "transformation" or carcinogenesis?
16. List at least four types of agents that can produce genetic changes that are necessary for malignant transformation.
17. In terms of cellular control mechanism, explain the "phenotypic" expression of malignancy in cells.
18. What is the TNM system for tumor staging?

19. Why is it important to identify the genetic abnormalities that may be inherited in relation to the development of neoplasia in families?
20. What are the means and criteria used to establish the diagnosis and to determine the therapeutic modalities for treatment of neoplasia?

BIBLIOGRAPHY ■ PART ONE

Alberts B, Bray D, Lewis J et al: *Molecular biology of the cell*, ed 4, New York, 1999, Garland Publishing.

Buys CHCM: Telomeres, telomerase, and cancer, *N Eng J Med* 342:1282-1283, 2000.

Cotran RS, Kumar V, Collins T: *Robbin's pathologic basis of disease*, ed 6, Philadelphia, 1999, WB Saunders.

Evan G, Littlewood T: A matter of life and cell death, *Science* 281:1317, 1998.

Fenton RG, Longo DL: Cell biology of cancer. In Fauci AS et al, editors: *Harrison's principles of internal medicine*, ed 14, New York, 1998, McGraw-Hill.

Greenlee RT, Hill-Harmon B, Murray T et al: Estimated new cancer cases, United States, ten leading sites by gender for 2001, *CA J Clin* 51(1):18, 2001.

Goldsby RA, Kindt TJ, Osborne BA: *Kuby immunology*, ed 4, New York, 2000, WH Freeman.

Janeway CJ, Travers P, Walport M et al: *Immunobiology: immune system in health and disease*, ed 4, New York, 1999, Garland Publishing.

Jorde L, Carey J, Barnshard M et al: *Medical genetics*, ed 2, St Louis, 2000, Mosby.

Keane MP, Streiter RM: Chemokine signaling in inflammation, *Crit Care Med* 28(S4):N13-N26, 2000.

Lashley FR: *Clinical genetics in nursing practice*, ed 2, New York, 1998, Springer.

Levinson WE, Jawetz E: *Medical microbiology and immunology*, ed 6, New York, 2000, Lange Medical Books/McGraw-Hill.

McKenna G: Apoptosis, radiosensitivity and the cell cycle. *http://oncolink.upenn.edu*

Meeker AK, Coffey DS: Telomerase: a promising marker of biological immortality of germ, stem, and cancer cells, a review, *Biochemistry (Moscow)* 62(11):1323, 1997.

Moore K, Persaud TVN: *The developing human, clinically oriented embryology*, ed 6, Philadelphia, 1998, WB Saunders.

Nausbaum R, McInnes R, Willard H: *Genetics in medicine*, ed 6, Philadelphia, 2001, WB Saunders.

Oberholzer A, Oberholzer C, Moldawer LL: Cytokine signaling—regulation of the immune response in normal and critically ill states, *Crit Care Med* 28(S4):N3-N12, 2000.

PRR Inc: Oncogene and proto-oncogenes, May 18, 2001. *http://intouchlive.com/cancergenetics/onco.htm*

Samuelson J: Infectious diseases. In Cotran RS, Kumar V, Collins T, editors: *Robbin's pathologic basis of disease*, ed 6, Philadelphia, 1999, WB Saunders.

Skulachev VP: Telomere, telomerase, cancer, and aging, *Biochemistry (Moscow)* 62(11):entire issue, 1997.

Sommers MS: Immunological patient assessment. In Kinney MR, Dunbar SB, Brooks-Bunn N et al, editors: *AACN clinical reference for critical care nursing*, ed 4, St Louis, 1998, Mosby.

Stites DP, Teer AI, Parslow TG: *Medical immunology*, ed 9, Norwalk, Conn, 1997, Appleton & Lange.

Terr AI: Anaphylaxis and urticaria. In Stites DP, Teer AI, Parslow TG, editors: *Medical immunology*, ed 9, Norwalk, Conn, 1997, Appleton & Lange.

PART TWO

IMMUNE SYSTEM DISORDERS

*U*nfavorable effects of immune processes underlie much human disease and may impair the function of any major organ system. In addition, characteristic changes in immune reactants that provide essential diagnostic clues *accompany* many conditions as effects or parallel events. Normal antibody and cell-mediated responses involve a series of steps, each modulated by groups of specific cells. Defects in these control processes may cause excessive or inappropriate immune reactions. Less often, disease results when normally protective immediate and delayed hypersensitivity mechanisms become impaired or fail to develop properly. Various immunologic states may be viewed as a *balance* between the pathogenic effects of potentially harmful foreign agents of disease (e.g., microorganisms) and of the body's defensive responses, which may cause incidental damage or disordered function in "bystander" tissues.

Protective immunity and allergic diseases share common processes of tissue response to substances recognized as "foreign." Immune mechanisms provide essential defense against invasion by injurious organisms and the emergence of malignant tumors, functions that have ensured their retention throughout vertebrate evolution. However, these same processes may be activated by relatively innocuous extrinsic agents and occasionally may focus the reaction on host tissue components. In these circumstances the *net* effects of exposure and host response are unfavorable; patterns of overt illness that result are recognized as immunologic diseases. These conditions are diverse and range from trivial, chronic disorders of the skin or mucous membranes to catastrophic events that may be fatal within seconds. The tissue processes responsible and their relationship to a practical classification of human immunologic disorders are described in Chapter 5. Because these diseases are determined by host reactivity as well as by the type and strength of antigenic exposure, regional differences in their prevalence are prominent. Overall, however, these disorders are remarkably common and their impact on human comfort and productivity is evident universally.

Familiar (IgE-Mediated) Allergic Disorders

Anaphylaxis and the Atopic Diseases

WILLIAM R. SOLOMON

𝒞linical reactions of immediate (antibody-mediated) or delayed (activated lymphocyte-mediated) hypersensitivity can result when prior contact with a specific, chemically characterizable entity ("antigen") has sensitized the individual to that particular agent. Reexposure to the antigen may cause sensitized cells, as well as one or more types of immunoglobulin (antibody), to react in a specific "defensive" response. Clinical hypersensitivity reactions in humans often show more than one immunologic process, each with its specific amplification systems. This complexity is understandable when an antigenically complex "invader" (e.g., microorganism) is involved, but also can be elicited by single, defined proteins (see Chapter 5).

After exposure to a *single* antigen, humoral (antibody-dependent) and cell-mediated immune responses may develop together or separately. The size and form of the antigen and the route of exposure, as well as the respondent's age, health, and prior experience with that sensitizer, will affect the responding immunoglobulin (Ig) class(es). For example, first exposure to an injected agent (e.g., vaccine) usually elicits an IgM response that, within days, changes to IgG synthesis. Reexposure typically elicits only high-level IgG production. Very low antigen often favors IgE synthesis, whereas mucosal exposure promotes an IgA response, often localized to the challenged organ. A single antigen-antibody interaction can also provoke different effects, depending on the indicator system in which it is observed. Human IgG molecules specific for an antigen may separate dissolved antigen from solution, agglutinate insoluble particles coated with

the antigen, or may activate complement proteins after interacting with antigen in either form. Observed effects depend largely on antigen-antibody concentrations, the relative proportions of these reactants, and the presence of additional components, which serve as "indicators" in laboratory tests. When these interactions occur in vivo, their effects reflect similar factors, as well as local tissue responses to the primary antigen-antibody reaction and to activation of secondary amplification mechanisms leading to inflammation (see Chapter 5).

Antigen-binding specificity is determined by paired combining sites on the Fab (antibody) fragment portions of immunoglobulin molecules. Events that follow binding are directed by the "crystallizable" fragment (Fc fragment) portion of antibodies, which is shared by immunoglobulins of a defined class (isotype), that is, IgG molecules. Receptors on phagocytic cells may recognize this region, facilitating adhesion and removal of antigen-antibody complexes and other particles bearing surface-bound immunoglobulins. Activation of the "classic" complement pathway (see Fig. 5-13) also involves the Fc region. As a result, target cell lysis, leukocyte attraction, and release of permeability-enhancing factors may be generated. Additionally, the class-specific properties of immunoglobulins that determine their tissue localization and specificity as antigens (to "antiimmunoglobulin" antibodies) are expressed on the Fc region.

Although levels of IgE are normally the lowest of the five antibody classes, these molecules play a disproportionately major role in human allergic* responses. IgE molecules readily bind to surface receptors of tissue mast cells and blood basophils. As a result, bound IgE is concentrated in the respiratory and gastrointestinal (GI) tracts, as well as in circulating blood and skin. When adjacent,

---

*The term *allergy* was proposed by von Pirquet in 1906 to denote all instances of acquired altered reactivity that promote "supersensitivity." Current usage equates allergy with common, clinically evident responses of immediate or delayed hypersensitivity.

receptor-bound IgE molecules combine with groupings of a multiply reactive antigen, a series of events (Fig. 9-1) can occur with the cell liberating tissue-reactive "mediator" substances, including histamine, leukotrienes, chemoattractants for eosinophils and neutrophils, kinin precursors, and interleukins. Additional products may include an anticoagulant (heparin), proteolytic enzymes (tryptase and chymase), and a highly reactive oxygen radical (superoxide), as well as prostaglandins and related arachidonic acid products. Individual characteristics of some of these agents are summarized in Table 9-1; their combined effects promote dilation and hyperpermeability of small blood vessels (principally venules), spasm of the walls of hollow viscera, and increased secretion by mucous membranes. Heightened venule permeability should lower the circulating blood volume and arterial pressure and promote collection of fluid outside of vessels. In fact, these effects are all observed in clinically significant human responses involving IgE.

The release of mediator substances from mast cell granules is modulated by cellular components, particularly cyclic nucleotides, with cyclic adenosine monophosphate (AMP) depressing and guanosine monophosphate (GMP) facilitating secretion (see Fig. 9-1). Both cholinergic and alpha-adrenergic stimuli increase GMP, whereas beta-adrenergic agents promote adenylate cyclase activity and augment AMP. IgE-dependent cell activation begins

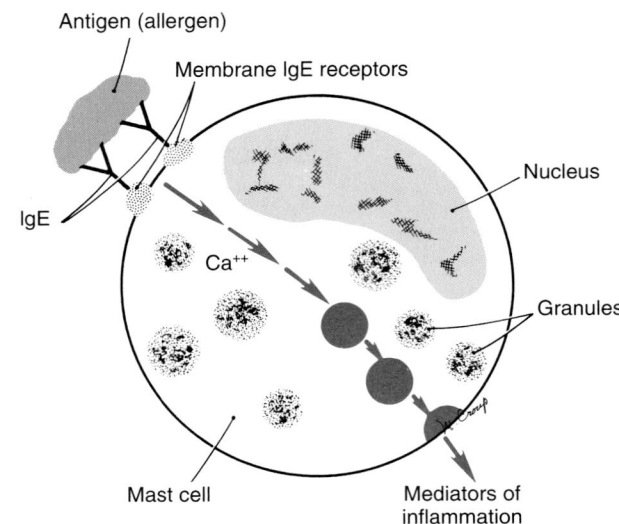

FIG. 9-1 Mast cell secretion provoked by bridging of adjacent IgE molecules by multivalent antigen or allergen. The process is calcium dependent and proceeds after membrane IgE receptors are brought together. The secretion process is affected by levels of cyclic nucleotides (cyclic AMP and GMP) within the mast cell (see Fig. 10-7). Many drugs can affect mast cell activity by effects on cyclic nucleotides, although separate membrane receptors also occur for these and other substances.

TABLE 9-1

Some Mediators of Inflammation Released by Human Mast Cells and Basophils

Mediator*	Chemical Characteristics	Biologic Activity
Histamine	Simple amine; mol wt 111	Contacts visceral smooth muscle; increases permeability of capillaries; increases respiratory mucous gland activity; produces sensation of itching
Prostaglandin D	mol wt 352	Contracts smooth muscle; increases mediator release by basophils
PAF	Phospholipid(s?), mol wt 500-550	Aggregates and degranulates platelets; contracts some smooth muscle; produces wheal and flare skin responses; variably attracts neutrophils
Leukotrienes (C, D, and E)†	Acid lipids	Causes prolonged visceral smooth muscle spasm; dilates and increases permeability of venules
Prostaglandin-generating factor of anaphylaxis	Simple peptide; mol wt 1450	Stimulates production of prostaglandins, leukotrienes, and related products of arachidonic acid
Neutral proteases (including tryptase, chymase, and carboxypeptidase)	Small protein enzymes; mol wt <50,000	Cleaves tissue components, such as collagen and complement factors; may generate kinins
Acid hydrolases (including beta-glucuronidase and arylsulfatase)	Fairly large proteins	Cleaves sugars from complex carbohydrates and glycoproteins
Superoxide dismutase	Enzymatic protein	Converts superoxide (O_2^-) to H_2O_2
Heparin	Peptide chain bearing long-chain sulfated amino sugars	Anticoagulant; modulates activities of other mediators
ECF-A	Pair of acidic tetrapeptides	Attracts eosinophils selectively
NCF-A	Large protein; mol wt >500,000	Causes directed migration of neutrophils
Basophil kallikrein‡	Not defined	Causes formation of bradykinin

ECF-A, Eosinophil chemotactic factor of anaphylaxis; *NCF-A*, neutrophil chemotactic factor of anaphylaxis; *PAF*, platelet-activating factor.
*Serotonin is present in human platelets and in the mast cells of other species.
†Formerly called slow reacting substance of anaphylaxis (SRS-A), many additional arachidonic acid products of activated mast cells (including thromboxanes and prostacyclins) may contribute to tissue inflammation.
‡Released from basophils, but not as yet described from mast cells.

within seconds, releasing mediators such as histamine that are preformed and stored. Minutes later, newly synthesized agents such as leukotrienes appear. Clinically, the resulting "immediate" reactions reach peak intensity in 10 to 20 minutes and then subside. Additionally, "late" IgE-dependent reactions may follow, 4 to 8 hours after the eliciting antigen was introduced. Reappearance of several mediators characterizes late responses, which likely reflect secretion by cells that are newly attracted to the reaction site.

TYPE I DISORDERS

Anaphylaxis

Acute systemic reactions, often fatal, were first recognized in several species during immunization experiments with foreign toxins. In many animals, sensitization did not confer protection; rather, when the toxin was readministered, shock, airway obstruction, and visceral congestion quickly developed in species-specific patterns. The term *anaphylaxis* (*ana-*, against; *-phylaxis*, protection) reflected this paradoxical outcome. Similar human reactions were noted early in the twentieth century and remain the most rapidly developing and dangerous form of allergic response. Acute systemic reactions generally follow the *injection* of a potent antigen (allergen) into a highly sensitive subject, although rarely, reaction may follow the ingestion of an offending agent. In the past, antiserums derived from other species (especially horses) were most often responsible for these reactions. More recently, injected antibiotics have become principal offenders, with serums, insulin, and other drugs less often implicated. Murine (mouse) monoclonal antibodies, used increasingly in organ transplantation, provoke similar problems. Comparable reactions may also follow insect stings and bites in previously sensitized subjects.

Acute systemic reactions generally begin within minutes after exposure to an allergen; a delay longer than 1 hour is distinctly rare. In extreme sensitivity, injection of an allergen may cause death or a sublethal reaction almost instantly, and, generally, the most severe reactions begin most rapidly. Affected individuals report a sense of uneasiness, followed rapidly by light-headedness, which may lead to syncope (loss of consciousness). Itching of the palms and scalp may herald hives (urticaria) that are often extensive. Localized tissue swellings (angioedema) may appear within minutes and distort particularly the eyelids, lips, tongue, hands, feet, and genitalia. These abnormalities involving deeper tissues of skin or mucous membranes are produced by a localized increase in vascular permeability without injury to the small veins and capillaries involved. Angioedema is often reversible within a short period and differs from other forms of swelling (edema) in which abnormal pressure or blood vessel damage promotes passage of fluid into tissues. Edema of the uvula and larynx are less evident to casual inspection but are especially prominent in human anaphylaxis and may cause death by respiratory obstruction. Laryngeal edema induces prominent air hunger, impaired vocal strength, noisy breathing, and a "barking" cough. Respiratory difficulty also may arise because of

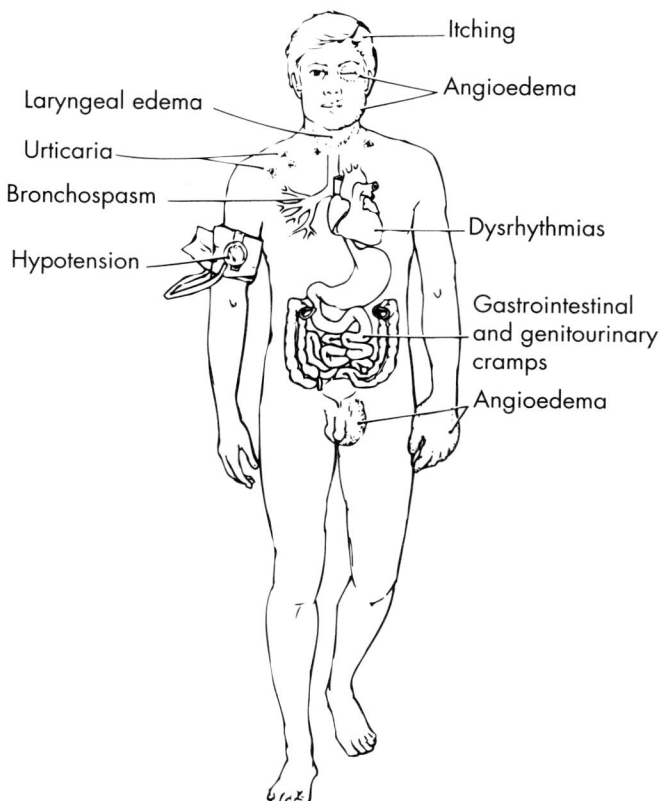

FIG. 9-2 Prominent manifestations of anaphylaxis. Laryngeal edema and profound hypotension usually pose the greatest dangers; cardiac effects may be primary or secondary to profound lowering of blood pressure.

bronchial narrowing, with audible wheezes mimicking spontaneous asthma (see Chapter 10). Less frequently, spasm of the gut, bladder, or uterus is prominent, with cramping pain, loss of visceral contents, or vaginal spotting. Fig. 9-2 summarizes the principal manifestations of human anaphylaxis.

Clinical anaphylaxis involves a sudden multifocal reaction of allergen with mast cell–bound, specific IgE, followed by widespread tissue response to released mediator substances such as histamine and leukotrienes. Many features of these responses, including urticaria, can be induced by injection of agents that *directly* release mediators from mast cells in vivo, although not by injection of histamine alone. Systemic reactions to certain injected agents (e.g., radiologic contrast media) may reflect such nonimmunologic mast cell secretion, because plasma levels of mediators and activated complement components have been shown to rise. Additionally, narcotic analgesics, dextrans, certain antibiotics, and other drugs directly stimulate mediator secretion by mast cells. The resulting nonimmunologic responses, which may closely resemble anaphylaxis, are termed *anaphylactoid*.

The first and most important step in managing an anaphylactic reaction is to ensure a patent airway and to maintain arterial oxygen levels. Careful and continuous observation is essential, because it may become necessary to perform oropharyngeal intubation or tracheostomy to prevent asphyxia from laryngeal edema. Hypotension principally reflects vessels leaking intravascular fluid.

When hypotension is severe or prolonged, it may lead to brain, kidney, or heart damage. Hypotension may be corrected most directly by restoring plasma volume with normal saline solution, one half normal saline solution, or plasma. Several liters of fluid are often required to normalize blood pressure. Vasoconstrictor drugs such as norepinephrine may help, but without adequate volume replacement, they have limited benefit. Epinephrine is the preferred drug to limit and reverse the anaphylactic process. A dose of 0.3 ml of 1:1000 epinephrine may be injected subcutaneously (see Chapter 10) and repeated several times, if needed, at intervals of 15 minutes; small children may receive 0.022 ml/kg to a maximum of 0.3 ml per dose. The absorption of epinephrine from subcutaneous depots is slow with severe hypotension. When shock is present, the drug may be diluted to 1:10,000 and slowly infused intravenously to provide comparable total doses. Injected antihistaminics, such as diphenhydramine, may speed the resolution of urticaria and relieve cramps originating in hollow viscera but do little to mitigate shock. Adrenocortical steroids are often given for their favorable effects on inflammation and abnormal vascular permeability; however, they are not immediately beneficial. Although steroids may be lifesaving in prolonged shock, they should be given after the airway is secure, volume repletion has been initiated, and epinephrine has been administered.

Avoiding known offenders (allergens) for specific individuals is critical in reducing the risk of anaphylaxis (see Chapter 13 for drug considerations). Typical systemic reactions may follow specific foods (e.g., nuts, shellfish) and stings of insects such as bee, wasp, hornet, and yellow jacket and, rarely, insect bites (e.g., deerflies). These IgE-mediated apparent reactions can be fatal without treatment. Besides avoiding situations favored by stinging insects, susceptible individuals are encouraged to carry commercially prepared, preloaded syringes of epinephrine whenever feasible. At-risk individuals must be prepared to self-administer the drug in 0.3 ml subcutaneous doses and to apply a proximal tourniquet when an extremity has been attacked. Immunotherapy (hyposensitization) with incremental injected doses of purified, diluted venoms is extremely effective in reducing risks of sting anaphylaxis when adequate doses are administered over many months. However, scrupulous avoidance is the only proven approach for food-sensitive subjects. *Exercise-induced anaphylaxis* presents the typical syndrome, evoked *inconstantly* by exertion. No premedication has been useful, and affected individuals *must* rest when symptoms appear and carry self-injectable epinephrine; exercising with a "buddy" is advisable. An even rarer problem, *idiopathic anaphylaxis*, lacks obvious precipitants, occurring capriciously. When tolerated, extended corticosteroid treatment is usually beneficial, despite failure of other remedies. As in other anaphylactic events, elevated levels of serum tryptase, a constitutive mast cell component, provides a diagnostic marker in the hours after onset of symptoms.

Atopic Diseases

Anaphylactic sensitization generally requires the injection of potent allergens; certain GI and respiratory parasites also can elicit prominent IgE responses. Additionally, a substantial minority of individuals demonstrate specific IgE responses to mucosal contact (by inhalation or ingestion) with quite innocuous materials, including foods, pollens, and animal emanations (dander). Allergen-specific IgE, fixed to tissue, may be demonstrated by performing skin tests and observing the development (5 to 15 minutes) of redness (erythema), often with a central hive (wheal). Some people, presenting such type I (IgE-mediated) responses also manifest one or more related illnesses, such as allergic rhinitis, allergic (extrinsic) asthma, and *atopic* dermatitis. In these instances, GI allergy, allergic conjunctivitis, and instances of acute urticaria and angioedema may coexist. Individuals with GI allergy may show (in response to specific foods) perioral pruritus (itching), tongue and mucous membrane swelling, difficulty in swallowing (dysphagia), nausea, vomiting, abdominal cramps, diarrhea, and perianal itching, singly or in combination. Food allergy may affect distant organs, including the skin and bronchi, and may rarely underlie generalized reactions. These common conditions are often grouped as *atopic* diseases, and the predisposition that favors their occurrence is termed *atopy.**

The pathophysiologic basis of atopy remains unclear; however, prominent IgE production from mucosal exposure to (benign) allergens is a principal marker and one fundamental characteristic. Additionally, health histories of affected subjects typically include *more than one* of the atopic conditions (e.g., eczema in infancy, then allergic rhinitis or asthma or both). Furthermore, familial clustering of these conditions is prominent, although the atopic tendency or allergen reactivity, rather than any specific form of illness, appears to be heritable. In most North American reports, over 50% of overtly affected subjects have close relatives with atopic conditions, whereas in subjects free of atopic disease, a positive family history is definable in only approximately 10%.

Allergic Rhinitis

Nasal allergy is the most frequently encountered atopic condition, affecting as many as 20% of children and young adults in North America and Western Europe. Elsewhere, rates of this and other atopic illnesses appear to be lower, particularly in less developed countries. Individuals with allergic rhinitis experience prominent nasal stuffiness and may report excessive nasal secretion *(rhinorrhea)* and sneezing occurring in rapid succession. *Pruritus* (Fig. 9-3) of the nasal mucosa, throat, and ears is often distressing and is accompanied by conjunctival redness, ocular pruritus, and lacrimation. The involved mucous membranes show dilation of blood vessels (particularly venules) and extensive edema with prominent eosinophils in both tissue and secretions. Some of these features, including the pruritus, can be duplicated by applying histamine alone to the normal mucosa, and allergic rhinitis may reflect the straightforward tissue effects of recognized mast cell–derived mediator substances (see earlier discussion). A release of histamine, leukotrienes, prostaglandin D, and so on from the

*Atopy is derived from the Greek atopia, which means strange or out of place. The term probably was chosen to express the inappropriateness of an immune response to entirely innocuous environment agents.

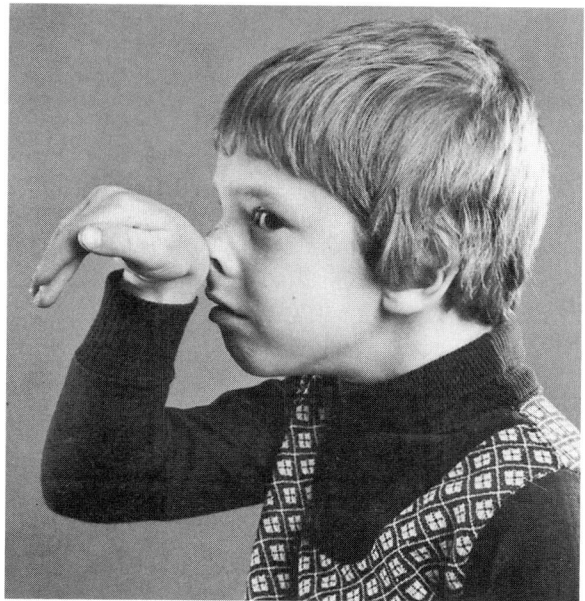

FIG. 9-3 Upward deflection of the nasal tip is a common mannerism among children with allergic rhinitis. This "allergic salute" briefly reduces pruritus and opens the nasal airway.

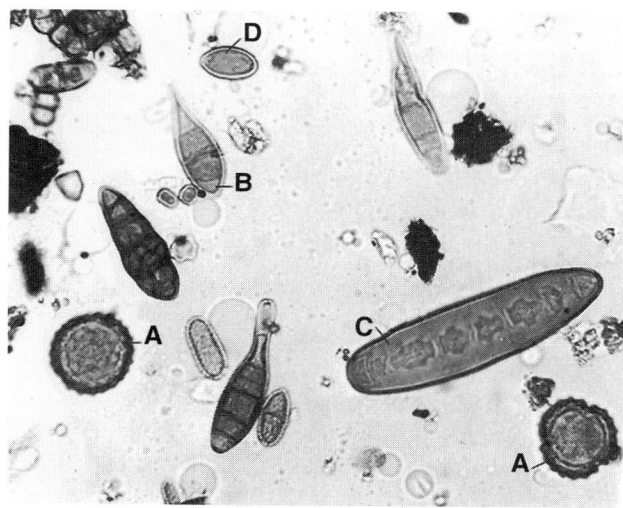

FIG. 9-4 Particles recovered during atmospheric sampling in late summer. Prominent sources of hay fever including ragweed pollen grain **(A)** and fungus spores of *Alternaria* **(B)** and *Helminthosporium* **(C)** species are evident. Many spores, such as those of mushrooms **(D)**, remain to be evaluated as allergens.

mucosa has been shown after direct nasal challenge of sensitive subjects with pollen allergens.

Although no absolute distinction is implied, allergic rhinitis is often divided into "seasonal" and "perennial" forms. Seasonal allergic rhinitis, or "hay fever," connotes a specific period of symptoms in successive years, reflecting sensitivity principally to airborne pollens and fungus spores (Fig. 9-4) with defined schedules of prevalence. Seasonal rhinitis is mild in many individuals who do not seek medical care, but it can be an exhausting illness for some because of continual sneezing, copious rhinorrhea, and unremitting pruritus. Intense pallor and swelling of

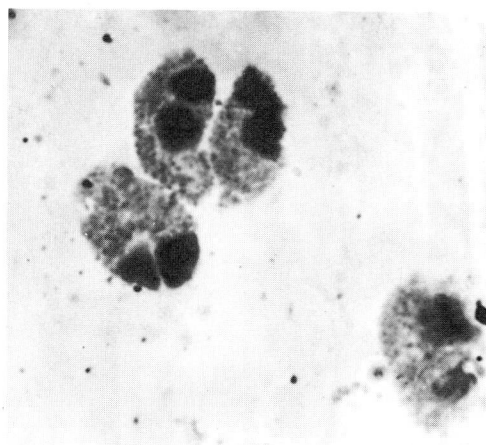

FIG. 9-5 Eosinophils from nasal secretions of a child with florid ragweed hay fever. Bilobed nuclei and discrete, round granules are familiar features of these cells, when suitably stained.

mucous membranes usually accompany these symptoms, and eosinophils abound in nasal secretions (Fig. 9-5). In contrast, perennial rhinitis seldom shows major annual variations in severity, and symptoms are often dominated by chronic nasal obstruction; prominent offenders include house dust mites and animal emanations to which daily exposure is commonplace. Not surprisingly, those with multiple clinical sensitivities often experience perennial rhinitis, as well as one or more predictable seasonal flares.

Perennial allergic rhinitis is rarely a direct source of dramatic symptoms. However, persistent partial nasal obstruction can promote distressing complications, such as mouth breathing, with resulting complaints of snoring and oropharyngeal dryness. Dark circles and redundant tissue often develop under the eyes. Although popularly termed "allergic shiners," these changes occur with longstanding nasal obstruction of any cause. The swollen mucosa readily sustains bacterial infection, and obstruction of paranasal sinuses is common, leading to recurrent or chronic sinusitis. Drainage from foci of nasal infection promotes sore throat and leads to bronchial soiling and bronchitis. Especially with recurrent infection, the swollen nasal mucosa may form local projections, or *polyps*, that further obstruct the airway. Additionally, especially in children, the pharyngeal openings of the eustachian tubes are readily blocked by swollen mucosa, enlarged lymphoid tissue, or exudate. Without normal access to air, the middle ears develop negative pressure and fill with fluid, creating a *chronic serous otitis* with at least transient hearing loss, impaired speech development, and in many cases, recurrent middle ear infection.

Although allergic rhinitis sufferers tend to develop bronchial asthma with above-normal frequency, the extent of this increased risk remains unclear. In one population of subjects with rhinitis, unselected for symptom severity, less than 10% were observed to develop asthma

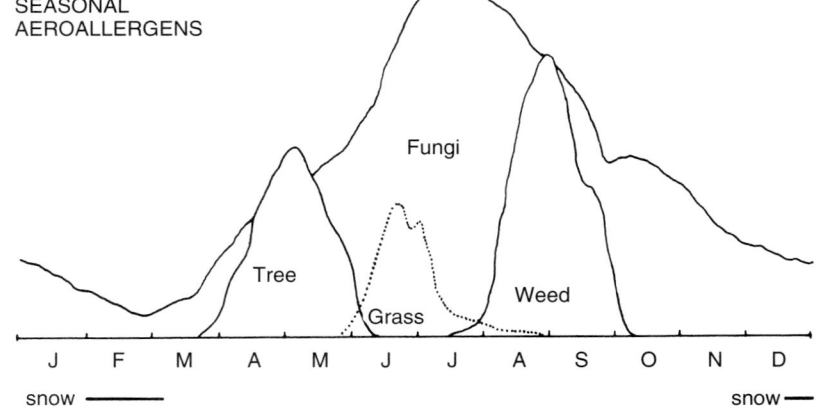

SEASONAL
AEROALLERGENS

FIG. 9-6 Patterns of airborne allergen prevalence typical of central North America. The relationship of the patient's symptoms to tree, grass, fungi, and weed pollen sensitivity can often be deduced from their periods of occurrence.

as a *new* manifestation. However, this sequence has been recorded more often in individuals who were eventually evaluated by an allergist. Generally, the risk of subsequent asthma appears to rise with increasing severity of rhinitis, with prominent sinobronchial infection, and when asthma was present in the past.

Although pruritus, repetitive sneezing, and watery, profuse rhinorrhea of hay fever are characteristic, they are not unique to this disorder, and the symptoms of perennial rhinitis readily mimic those of other conditions. The distinctive feature of allergic rhinitis is that compatible symptoms appear or worsen predictably in response to specific allergen exposures. Therefore, in diagnosis, careful analysis of factors precipitating rhinitis is of overriding importance. Many subjects with nonallergic "vasomotor" rhinitis have similar nasal stuffiness and marked rhinorrhea; some also showing intense nasal eosinophilia. However, this group is without response to identifiable allergens. Rather, their complaints relate largely to airborne irritants, extremes of temperature and humidity, pregnancy, stages of the menstrual cycle, and emotional factors. Long-standing nasal complaints caused by recurrent or chronic infection, nasal polyps, marked deviation of the nasal septum, hypothyroidism, and antihypertensive or ovulatory suppressant drugs also must be distinguished from perennial allergic and nonallergic forms of rhinitis.

A clinical history of symptoms on specific exposures provides a direct indication of offenders in respiratory allergy. Symptom variations during and after travel deserve special attention and the effects of overt exposure to house dust mites, animals and fur products, feathers, seed derivatives, silk, and so forth may be sought directly. When casual observations are insufficient, a history may be "created" by markedly increasing or reducing (or both) specific exposures, such as to foods or house pets, for brief periods to observe the results. The time or place of symptom occurrence may also furnish etiologic clues not readily evident to the individual. Specific pollen sensitivities, for example, may be deduced if the resulting symptoms can be dated precisely and "seasons" of prevalence for local airborne pollens are known (Fig. 9-6). Similarly, recognition of the heavy fungus exposures associated with leaf collection, lawn care, and gardening,

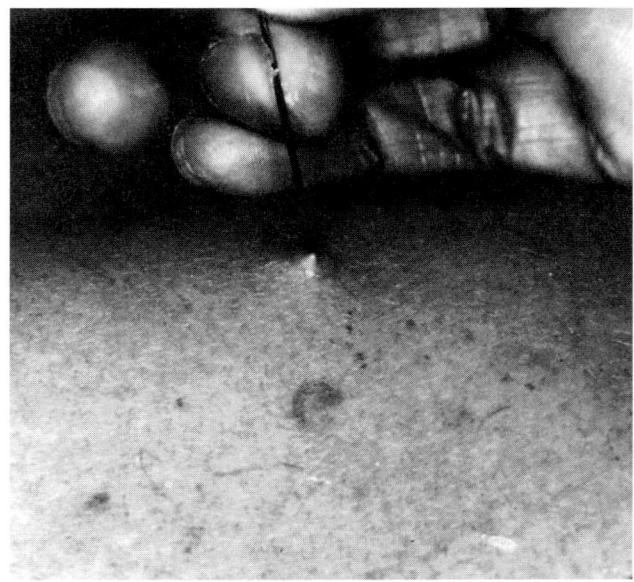

FIG. 9-7 Technique of epidermal (prick) testing using a sterile, straight needle. Because only the epidermis is penetrated, bleeding should not occur.

as well as with hiking in tall vegetation, helps to explain associated symptoms.

Skin tests that elicit a wheal-and-flare reaction provide useful correlates for a detailed clinical evaluation and are widely performed. However, even strongly positive reactions indicate only the immunologic "apparatus" for response and provide no *assurance* that symptoms arise from exposure to the reactive allergens. The ultimate value of skin tests is to support or oppose impressions formed during clinical fact finding. For tests of immediate reactivity, testing is performed by pricking the skin through applied drops of aqueous allergen extracts to produce epidermal or "prick" tests or by injecting small quantities (usually 0.02 ml) intracutaneously (Figs. 9-7 and 9-8, respectively). Because even this volume of highly diluted extract may be hazardous in exquisitely sensitive subjects, prick tests are best performed first, and subjects with negative reactions are considered for intracutaneous (IC) testing. Because occasional persons man-

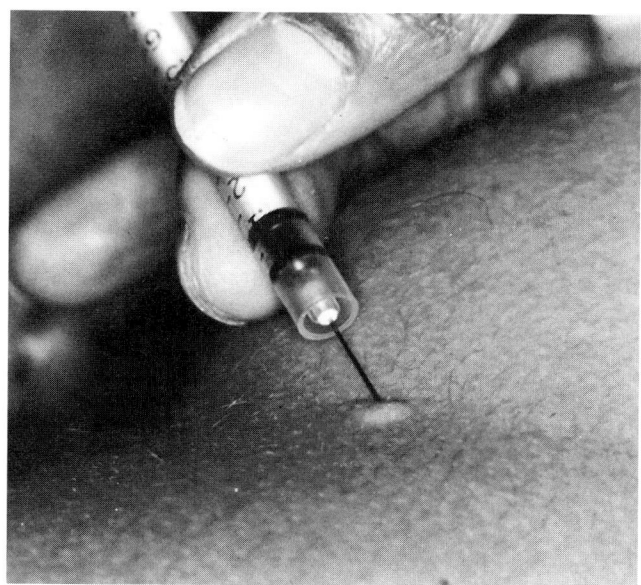

FIG. 9-8   Technique of intradermal (intracutaneous) skin testing. Because the wheal formed may not dissipate in 15 minutes, reactions are read relative to a negative (saline) control.

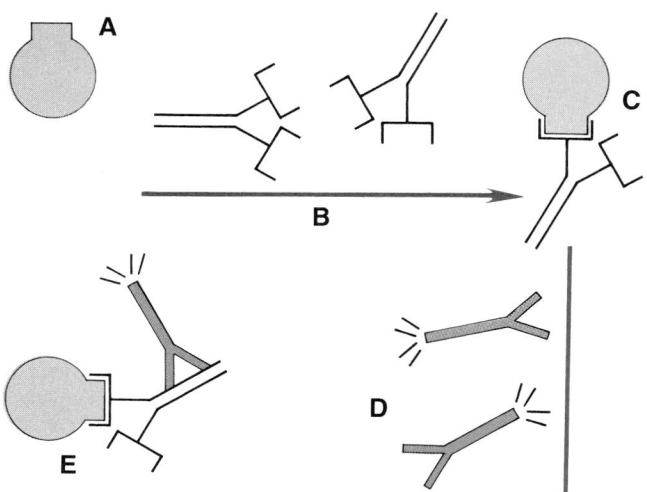

FIG. 9-9   The radioallergosorbent test (RAST), a technique for quantitating *allergen-specific* immunoglobulin E. In this procedure, allergens are linked chemically to carrier particles **(A)**, and the resulting conjugate is reacted with serum presumably containing specific IgE **(B)**. If IgE is bound **(C)**, it will react with and bind radiolabeled antihuman IgE **(D)** to form a radioactive complex **(E)**. By counting radioactivity, the amount of specific IgE originally present may be estimated.

ifest whealing with any skin trauma *(dermographism)*, all reactions must be compared with those at negative control sites tested with sterile diluent alone. Similarly, whealing responses at sites tested with histamine (directly vasoactive) and codeine phosphate (a mast cell activator) confirms normal skin responsiveness. Wheal and erythema reactions may be factitiously reduced by antihistamine drugs (see later in this section). Cortisone-like drugs, by contrast, have little effect on immediate skin reactivity, whereas suppression by theophylline and sympathomimetic amines is trivial, at best.

Few additional test procedures help evaluate respiratory allergy. Initial hopes that levels of *total* serum IgE can distinguish symptomatic atopic patients from others have not been sustained. In vitro measurement of allergen-specific IgE is possible using venous blood. One approach, the radioallergosorbent test (RAST), is diagrammed in Fig. 9-9. Alternative in vitro procedures, such as enzyme-linked immunosorbent assay (ELISA) and fluorescent antibody staining technique (FAST), also are available. However, neither the sensitivity nor the specificity of these approaches now exceeds that of conventional skin tests.

The demonstration of eosinophils as prominent cells in nasal or lacrimal secretions suggests an associated type I allergic inflammatory process but may also occur in nonallergic conditions. In suitably stained material, the bilobed nuclei and abundant, discrete, red, refractile granules of eosinophils are evident by oil-immersion microscopy (see Fig. 9-5).

Three principal considerations dominate the management of allergic rhinitis: (1) efforts to reduce allergen (and irritant) exposure; (2) suppressive medications to mitigate symptom severity nonspecifically; and (3) specific hyposensitization* to reduce responsiveness to

*Generally termed *immunotherapy*.

unavoidable allergens. Avoidance measures are most feasible for allergens associated with home and work situations, such as house dust mites, animal emanations, and agricultural products. However, even pollen exposure can be significantly reduced by the subject remaining indoors with windows closed, a strategy that usually requires air conditioning for success. Avoidance of dust mites is fostered by smooth, simple surfaces that facilitate cleaning (e.g., bare floors, uncluttered table and dresser tops) and by elimination or plastic encasing of bedding and upholstered furnishings (Fig. 9-10). High-efficiency filters are helpful when central forced-air heating is used, but they do not replace a careful antidust program at room level. Avoidance of indoor dampness also effectively limits dust mite populations.

Where symptoms result from sensitivity to animal emanations (dander), total avoidance of the source is usually justified. Although dander is popularly equated with hair, far more potent allergen sources include epidermal scales, saliva, lacrimal secretions, and even urine. House pets are the most persistently troublesome animal allergen sources. However, occupational exposures also may plague laboratory workers, veterinarians, and livestock handlers. Products from animal sources may also retain sensitizing properties for long periods; these include feather- and down-filled materials, fur-trimmed clothing and toys, furniture and rug pads (cattle and horse hair), and raw silk. Mohair (goat) and camel hair fabrics are occasionally implicated as allergen sources, although commercially processed sheep's wool rarely appears to be an offender.

Tobacco smoke is an acknowledged respiratory irritant containing numerous toxic agents but none confirmed as

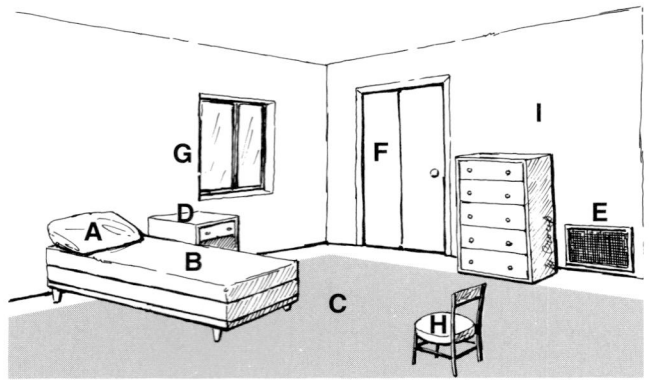

FIG. 9-10 Measures designed to minimize exposure to house dust mites (and other inhalant allergens) as applied to a bedroom. Objectives include covering pillows **(A)** plus mattresses and box springs **(B)** with plastic or microfiber encasings; maintaining a bare floor **(C)** and uncluttered surfaces **(D)**; applying final filters to warm-air ducts **(E)**; keeping closet doors closed **(F)**; and minimizing window coverings **(G)**, upholstered furnishings **(H)**, and wall decorations **(I)**. These empirically derived measures greatly decrease exposure to mite-derived allergens.

allergens. In contrast, plant products such as cottonseed, flaxseed, and castor bean meals are among the most potent industrial sensitizers.

For many decades, antihistaminic drugs (i.e., histamine H_1 receptor blockers) have been the most useful agents in the symptomatic (i.e., nonspecific) treatment of allergic nasal disease. Although many antihistaminics also share anticholinergic, antiserotonin, or tranquilizing properties, their capacity to compete with histamine for tissue receptors appears to underlie their usefulness in hay fever and so on. These drugs are generally effective when given orally and may be administered safely for long periods when necessary. Side effects of older agents are common though seldom severe in normal persons and may include drowsiness, lethargy, mucous membrane dryness, and occasionally, nausea, cramps, or light-headedness. However, because of these symptoms and potential impairment of depth perception, activities involving moving vehicles, dangerous machinery, or fine hand-eye coordination in general must be undertaken cautiously by individuals taking these drugs. Recently, several effective newer agents that do not cross the blood-brain barrier have been shown to produce little or no sedation and are generally preferred. In practice, several antihistaminic agents must often be tried before an optimal (or even satisfactory) one is identified, and the results of such trials defy prediction at the outset. In choosing drugs for comparison by individuals, it must be remembered that many older preparations are merely different forms of a few generic agents (e.g., chlorpheniramine); efficacy trials should compare different chemical species. Patients often report a waning of previous antihistaminic effectiveness, prompting substitution (or addition) of different agents; at times, this reflects suboptimal compliance in drug dosing but is often unexplainable.

Sympathomimetic amines offer additional benefit in relieving nasal stuffiness and are often marketed in combinations with antihistaminic agents. Drugs, principally including ephedrine, isoephedrine, and phenylpropanol-amine act as mucosal decongestants and, by causing more or less psychomotor stimulation, can offset the sedative effects of older antihistaminic agents. Whether oral sympathomimetic drugs significantly affect the release of mediator substances from tissue mast cells is unclear, although (opposing) beta- and alpha-adrenergic effects are possible. These agents also readily produce side effects that may impair ocular, cardiac, GI, and genitourinary function (see Chapter 10). The topical use of sympathomimetic agents as drops, sprays, and vapors is widespread and provides prompt mucosal shrinkage, which is helpful in acute illness such as bacterial sinusitis. Unfortunately, these preparations are easily obtained and often abused. Prolonged overuse results in an irritant effect, thus each dose gives transient decongestion followed by a prolonged obstructive response, prompting further self-medication. In habituated individuals, the resulting mucosal inflammation, or *rhinitis medicamentosa*, causes persistent nasal stuffiness and a congested, or edematous, appearance. Complete withdrawal of topical nasal medication is mandatory, and when possible, oral agents are substituted. In some cases, a topical nasal corticosteroid spray must be given for several weeks to make this change tolerable. Recently introduced agents, including beclomethasone, fluticasone, mometasone, and flunisolide, are locally effective and rapidly metabolized by the liver, making them safe and well tolerated.

Intranasal steroids are useful also in suppressing the primary symptoms of allergic rhinitis and are preferred, particularly for seasonal periods of exquisite severity. Currently, five agents are available for prescription as Freon-propelled or hand-pumped preparations. Additionally, systemic corticosteroids suppress hay fever manifestations when other remedies have failed. However, the widespread side effects of these systemically active agents make their chronic administration for nasal allergy unacceptable.

Except for antibiotics, when indicated, few other drugs offer benefit to rhinitis sufferers. The appropriate topical application of cromolyn sodium (see Chapter 10) can also reduce the symptoms of allergic rhinitis and conjunctivitis. Additional ocular agents (e.g., levocabastine and olopatadine drops) may provide benefit when eye symptoms are prominent.

Immunotherapy (hyposensitization) continues to provide an important allergen-specific treatment approach for respiratory allergy. In this procedure, incremental doses of extracts of a recognized allergen are injected subcutaneously over prolonged periods and serve to modify clinical reactivity. After reaching an empirically indicated "maximal" level, this dosage is maintained, pending evaluation of symptoms, and adjustments in the program are carried out accordingly. Indications for immunotherapy include allergic asthma, as well as allergic rhinitis or conjunctivitis that is inadequately controlled despite optimal avoidance measures and acceptable medication treatment. In each instance, sensitivity to specific, *inhalant* allergens must be confirmed, because any nonspecific benefits of injection treatment are unpredictable; food factors are approached by diet modification exclusively. A typical treatment schedule is illustrated in Fig. 9-11. Properly controlled clinical trials have confirmed the value of immunotherapy for grass and ragweed pollen and strongly suggest that tree pollen, animal dander, *Alternaria* (an important fungus), and dust mite immunotherapy *is* beneficial. Injection treatment for other materials either has been shown to be valueless (e.g., for respiratory bacterial vaccines) or remains incompletely studied (e.g., for most fungi). Trials of pollen extracts also indicate that (1) optimal benefit is reached when the largest well-tolerated doses are given, (2) symptom suppression caused by treatment may carry over to one or more subsequent years in which injections are withheld, and (3) a placebo, or inert material, given by injection may decrease reported symptoms in one third to one half of subjects, which reemphasizes the need for proper controls in evaluating treatment results.

The basis of the efficacy of immunotherapy remains unclear, although several tissue effects that might promote benefit are known. That the procedure induced active immunization against a pollen "toxin" was initially assumed, but this rationale was soon discredited. Although immunotherapy may "turn off" specific IgE production, RAST values and skin test positivity often change little during extended successful treatment, and specific IgE values usually rise early in the injection sequence before any later decline. The appearance in serum of IgG antibodies specific for the injected allergen is well documented, and these factors can compete with IgE for allergen, thus showing "blocking" capabilities. Although a general correlation between blocking antibody titer and clinical improvement is apparent, exceptions (e.g., persons with high titers and unabated rhinitis) imply that other factors must also contribute. Recently described elevations, with immunotherapy, of IgG and IgA (blocking) antibodies in respiratory tract secretions suggest an alternative tissue mechanism. Additionally, blood basophils from subjects receiving high-dose immunotherapy release progressively less histamine on allergen challenge in vitro, in some cases becoming wholly unresponsive. Current interest also surrounds possible treatment-induced changes in the function of allergen-specific T helper lymphocytes (e.g., decreased lymphokine production). Presently therefore, although the clinical value of hyposensitization for selected allergens is clearly established, the responsible mechanisms are not; several effects, varying among patients, are possible.

Although there is no evidence of serious, long-term adverse effects of immunotherapy, significant transient local or systemic reactions can occur. Redness, whealing, and tender swelling lasting up to 36 hours may develop at treatment sites when the dosage is excessive. These reactions usually mandate a reduction in the amount of allergen next injected. However, wiping the needle with a sterile swab before injection to remove adhering extract and applying firm pressure to the injected site to reduce retrograde oozing of fluid along the needle track may decrease their severity. Acute systemic reactions are often preceded by increasingly prominent local swellings but may occur *at any time* during treatment without warning. A generalized reaction may be anaphylactic or may be accompanied by or confined to rhinitis or asthma symptoms; management has been described previously. Additionally, 0.1 to 0.2 ml of epinephrine is usually introduced at the site of the responsible injection to slow allergen absorption. Extract should be given into a site

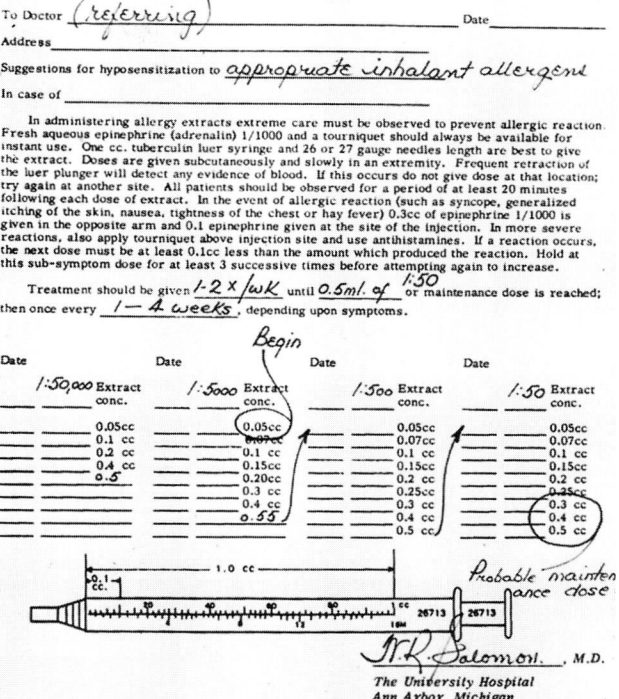

FIG. 9-11   Typical dosage schedule form used at the allergy clinic of the University Hospital, Ann Arbor, Michigan, for patients whose injection treatment will be administered by their personal physicians. Additional dilutions or dosage volumes may be desirable for specific persons.

distal enough to allow for placement of a proximal tourniquet. Although adverse reactions may occur capriciously, their risk increases with conditions that elevate cutaneous blood flow, including high environmental temperature, fever, physical exertion, hyperthyroidism, and pregnancy. Human error is also a factor. Mishaps may occur as a result of misreading previously recorded doses or vial labels; confusion of persons with similar names is a common error. Usually, reactions that will require treatment have onset within 20 to 30 minutes after injection; therefore most clinics require their patients to remain quietly seated in a well-ventilated room for this period after treatment. The low but inescapable risk of systemic reactions and a corresponding need for rapid, complex treatment measures leave *no* justification for self-injection of extract by any patient. Facilities that administer treatment extracts should be prepared to provide epinephrine, oxygen, and intravenous fluids quickly and have personnel competent in cardiopulmonary support available.

Presently, skin testing and on-site injection treatments are carried out with sterile, aqueous extracts containing an antimicrobial agent (e.g., phenol, thimerosal) and a protein stabilizer (e.g., human serum albumin). Attempts to establish standards of biologic activity for these materials have developed slowly, although assays of defined allergens in ragweed and grass pollen extracts are now used as indicators of potency. Other materials are typically rated on a "weight-by-volume" basis. In this system, a 1:500 ragweed pollen extract is the solution resulting when 1 g of defatted ragweed pollen is extracted under defined conditions in 500 ml of fluid. Alternative approaches based on assays of total protein or total nitrogen are no more instructive. Comparisons of extract potency based on ability to inhibit standardized RAST assays or skin test potency in panels of sensitive subjects (e.g., "allergy units") also appear feasible. Currently, alum-precipitated aqueous extracts are available with modestly long-acting properties, although local and systemic adverse reactions can occur. Allergens absorbed to carriers such as formalin or glutaraldehyde continue to hold interest, as do allergen active groups reactive exclusively with T lymphocytes.

KEY CONCEPTS

- Adverse immune processes underlie much human disease and may impair the function of any major organ system. Additionally, changes in immune reactants that provide important diagnostic clues *accompany* many conditions as effects or parallel events.
- Normal antibody- and cell-mediated responses involve a series of steps, each modulated by groups of specific cells. Defects in these control processes may cause excessive or inappropriate immune reactions.
- Immediate (antibody-mediated) or delayed (activated lymphocyte-mediated) hypersensitivity can result when prior contact with a specific, chemically characterizable antigen has sensitized the individual to that particular agent.
- Acute systemic reactions generally follow the *injection* of a potent antigen (allergen) into a highly sensitive subject.
- Clinical anaphylaxis involves a sudden multifocal reaction of allergen with mast cell–bound, specific IgE, followed by widespread tissue response to released mediator substances such as histamine and leukotrienes.
- Individuals presenting type I (IgE-mediated) reactivity (e.g., on skin testing) *may* manifest one or more related illnesses, such as allergic rhinitis, allergic (extrinsic) asthma, and *atopic* dermatitis.
- Prominent IgE production from mucosal exposure to (benign) allergens is a principal marker and one fundamental characteristic of atopy.

- Nasal allergy is the most frequently encountered atopic condition.
- Seasonal rhinitis can be an exhausting illness for some people because of continual sneezing, copious rhinorrhea, and unremitting pruritus.
- Skin tests eliciting a wheal-and-flare reaction provide useful correlates for a clinical evaluation, and support or oppose impressions formed during clinical fact finding.
- Currently, neither the sensitivity nor the specificity of alternative in vitro measurement of allergen-specific IgE using venous blood exceeds that of the conventional skin test.
- Antihistaminic drugs (i.e., histamine H1 receptor blockers) have been the most widely useful agents in the symptomatic (i.e., nonspecific) treatment of allergic nasal disease; poorly absorbed topically active corticosteroids provide complementary benefit.
- Several effective, newer antihistaminics that do not cross the blood-brain barrier have been shown to produce little or no sedation and are generally preferred.
- Immunotherapy (hyposensitization) provides an important allergen-specific treatment approach for respiratory allergy.
- Feasible allergen avoidance should always be a consideration first in treatment programs for allergic disease.

QUESTIONS ??

A sampling of review questions for this chapter appears here. Visit http://www.mosby.com/MERLIN/PriceWilson/ for additional questions.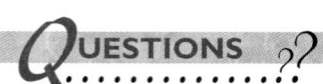

Answer the following on a separate sheet of paper.

1. Differentiate between hypersensitivity and sensitization in the context of immunologic events.
2. Contrast angioedema and lymphedema.

3. Describe the pathogenesis of an acute systemic (anaphylactic) reaction.
4. What are the necessary conditions for anaphylactic sensitization in humans?
5. Describe exercise-induced anaphylaxis as to the typical presentation and treatment.

6. List three principal considerations that dominate the management of respiratory allergy, as exemplified by allergic rhinitis.
7. What measures should be taken to reduce the risk of an anaphylactic reaction?

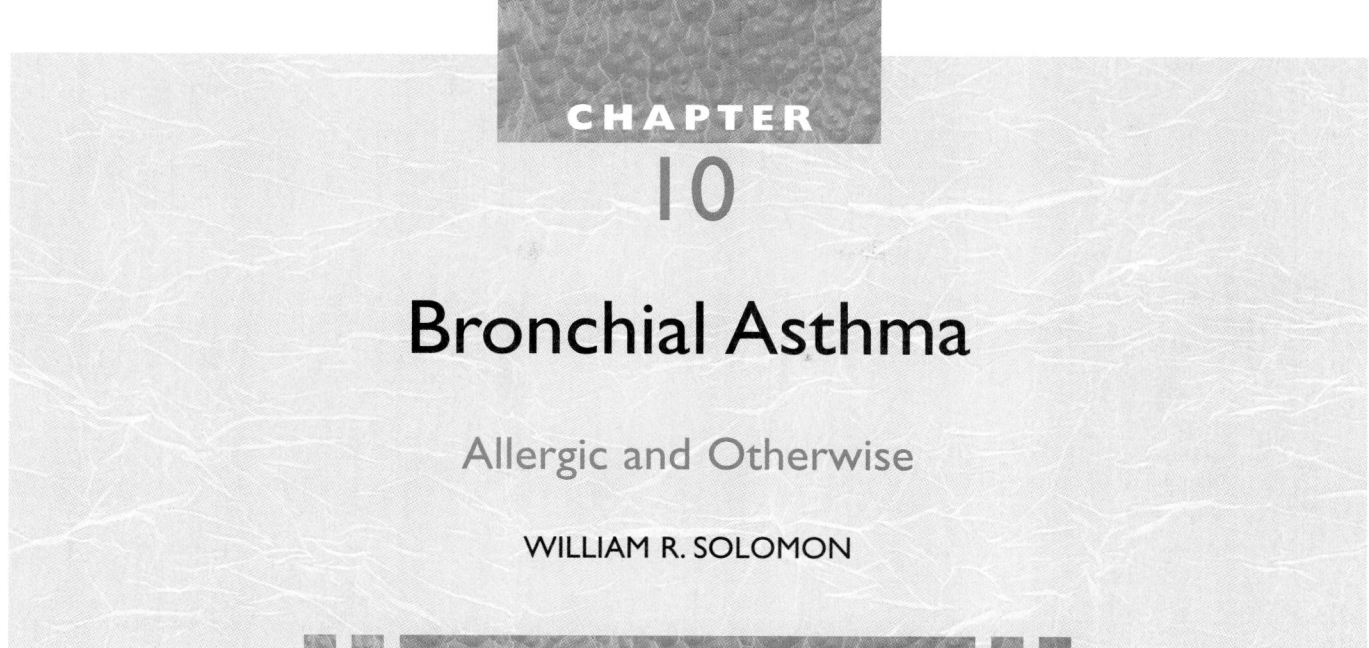

CHAPTER
10

Bronchial Asthma

Allergic and Otherwise

WILLIAM R. SOLOMON

*C*HAPTER OUTLINE

*A*sthma is a clinically defined condition marked by recurrent episodes of reversible bronchial narrowing, often separated by periods of more normal ventilation. These events are readily provoked in asthma-prone subjects by a variety of stimuli, denoting a characteristic state of bronchial hyperreactivity. Allergic factors are evident detriments in some individuals with asthma but absent in others, despite exhaustive study.

Tissue changes in uncomplicated asthma (Fig. 10-1) are confined to bronchial airways and consist of spasm of smooth muscle, mucosal edema and persistent infiltration by inflammatory cells, and hypersecretion of viscid mucus. Airway narrowing and chronic shedding of ciliated bronchial epithelial cells that normally aid in the clearance of mucus compromises mobilization of luminal secretions.

FIG. 10-1   Bronchial changes in chronic asthma. This small bronchus shows increased width of the epithelial basement membrane *(arrow)* and partial loss of mucosal cells. The lumen **(A)** is filled with mucus and cellular debris, and the submucosa **(B)** is densely infiltrated with inflammatory cells, including many eosinophils. (From Sheldon JM, Lovell RG, Mathews KP: *A manual of clinical allergy,* ed 2, Philadelphia, 1967, WB Saunders.)

VENTILATORY DYSFUNCTION

The person experiencing asthma has a fundamental inability to achieve normal rates of airflow during respiration (particularly expiration). This inability is reflected in a lowering of the volume of air produced during the first second of forced expiratory effort (FEV_1) and by other flow-related parameters. Figure 10-2 illustrates these components in relation to the curve (flattened in asthma), which relates total expiratory volume and time. Because many narrowed airways cannot fill and empty quickly enough, uneven lung aeration and a loss of the normal spatial matching of ventilation and pulmonary blood flow occurs (Fig. 10-3). Depending on their severity,

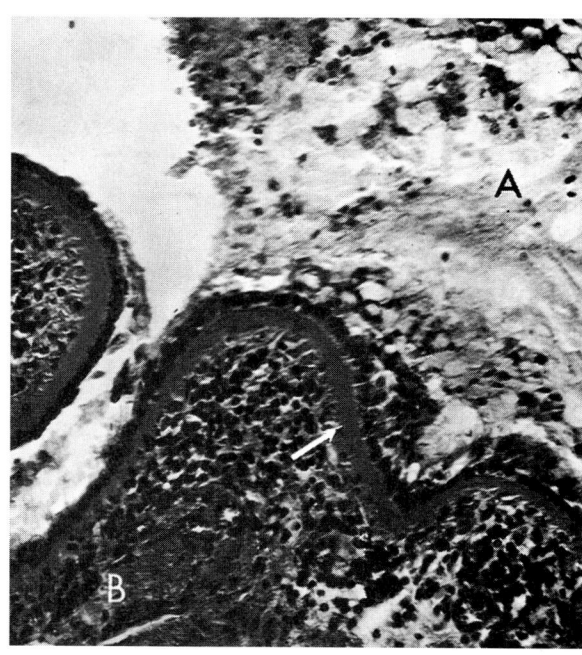

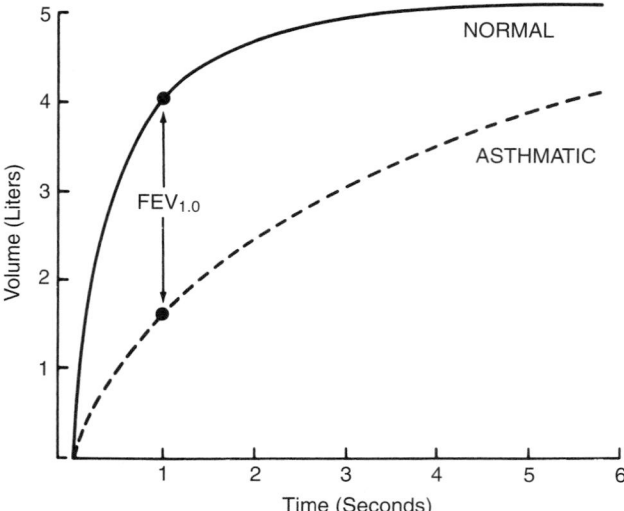

FIG. 10-2 Forced expiratory curves produced by two 20-year-old men—one normal and one with moderately severe asthma. The slope of these curves at any point is equivalent to flow rate. An inability to move air quickly is the major ventilatory defect in asthma, and this is evident most clearly as a prolongation of the forced expiratory time when airways are narrowed.

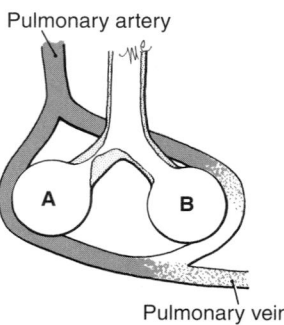

FIG. 10-3 Mismatching of ventilation and perfusion in asthma. Because of narrowing of its bronchus, alveolus *A* does not properly oxygenate its share of pulmonary artery blood; alveolus *B* functions normally. As a result of these contributions, average oxygen saturation of pulmonary venous blood is abnormally low. In asthma a shift of blood flow from *A*-type to *B*-type alveoli occurs secondarily but is usually incomplete. Furthermore, hyperventilation of *B* with room air cannot compensate for the venous-to-arterial "shunting" at *A*.

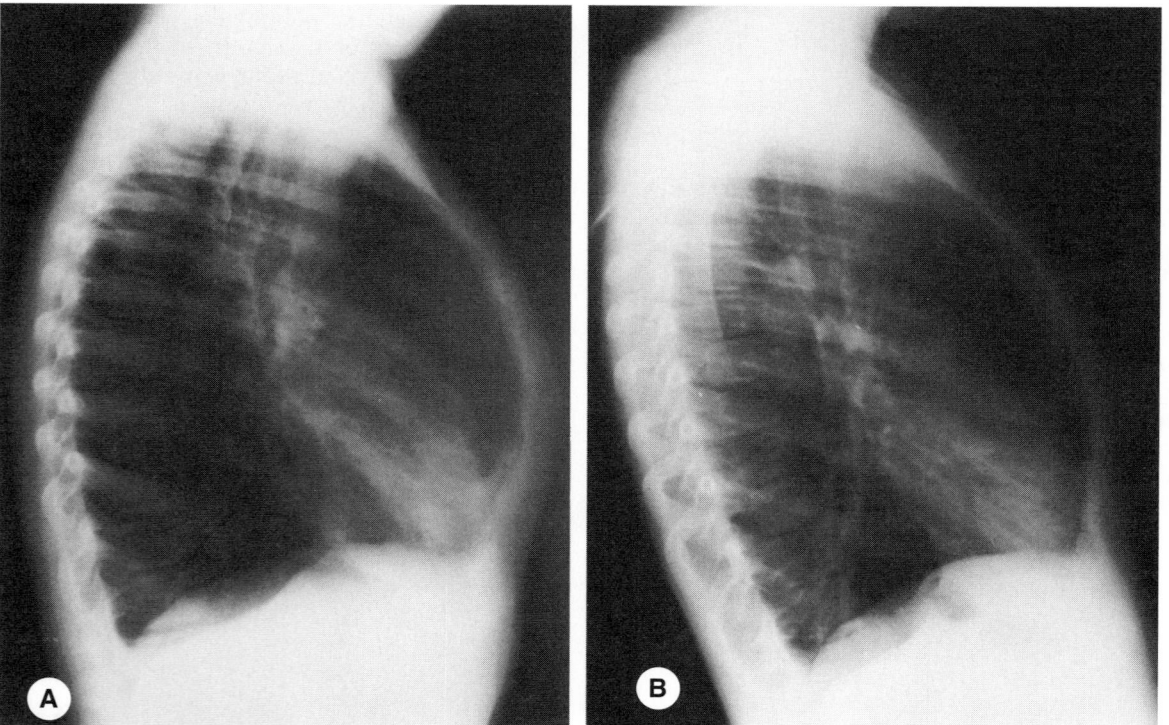

FIG. 10-4 Hyperinflation of the chest of an 8-year-old boy with asthma. **A**, Radiograph taken during a severe status asthmaticus attack that later required mechanical ventilation. (Note especially the broad space between the heart and sternum.) **B**, Radiograph taken during a symptom-free interlude 4 months later, which shows much less severe changes.

these defects may produce no symptoms or merely a sense of tracheal irritation; in other cases, respiratory distress may be intolerable. Air stream turbulence and the vibrations of bronchial mucus lead to audible wheezing during asthmatic attacks; however, this physical sign is also prominent in other obstructive airway problems. With symptomatic asthma, breathing is more rapid than is normal (even though this tends to increase resistance to airflow). Additionally, the chest assumes a position of maximal inspiration that is achieved by effort at first and dilates the airways. This appearance is later sustained because of incomplete emptying of alveoli, which results in progressive hyperinflation of the thorax (Fig. 10-4). In uncomplicated asthma, cough is typically prominent, mainly as attacks resolve, when it serves to clear accumulated secretions. Rarely, "dry" cough may be the only evident manifestation of asthma.* Between bouts of asthma, the patient may be free of wheezing and asymptomatic, although heightened bronchial reactivity and defects in ventilation remain. However, in chronic asthma, interludes with no symptoms decline, leading to a state of continuous distress, often with secondary bacterial infection.

Individuals with asthma, both with and without allergic mechanisms, share an abnormal bronchial lability that promotes airway narrowing by many factors that have no effect on normal persons. The basis of this tendency remains unclear, but it appears to parallel bronchial inflammatory changes. Functionally, asthmatic airways behave as though their beta-adrenergic innervation (which helps preserve airway patency) is incompetent, and evidence suggests that, at least functionally, partial blockage of beta-adrenergic receptors exists in typical asthma. Bronchoconstrictor influences, which are normally mediated by parasympathetic (cholinergic) and alpha-adrenergic pathways, therefore tend to predominate. In clinical practice, the bronchial lability of asthmatic patients may be confirmed by demonstrating their ready airway obstructive responses to extremely low concentrations of inhaled histamine and methacholine (a substance with activity resembling that of acetylcholine). Related mechanisms probably contribute to the bouts of asthma that often follow inhalation of cold air, as well as exposure to diverse mists, dusts, and volatile irritants. Poorly understood nervous pathways also mediate airway closure in response to psychic stimuli. (Asthma that is solely caused by emotional factors is exceptionally rare, however.) In asthma, reflex pathways promoting bronchospasm with forced chest deflation are activated by maneuvers such as laughing, blowing up a balloon, or providing a full expiration for ventilatory testing.

SUBSETS OF ASTHMA

Asthma must be distinguished from two conditions described in detail in Chapter 38. These are *chronic bronchitis*, marked by continuous bronchial hypersecretion, and *emphysema*, in which loss of supporting lung tissues

*This is termed *cough-equivalent asthma.*

allows severe airway narrowing to occur with expiration. Both entities can also produce wheezing and air hunger and worsen symptomatically with infection, exercise, and irritant inhalation. Although atopy is readily implicated in many instances of bronchial asthma, a substantial number of asthmatic subjects lack demonstrable allergic factors. These individuals, including many infants and middle-aged and older adults, experience prominent bronchial hyperactivity (BHR) with essentially *idiopathic* (i.e., unexplained) asthma.

Some adults with idiopathic asthma also manifest nasal polyps, recurrent sinusitis, and severe airway obstructive responses to aspirin in various combinations. Typically, other nonsteroidal antiinflammatory drugs (NSAIDs) such as ibuprofen and indomethacin also precipitate severe attacks in these patients. However, moderate asthma usually persists even when recognized offenders are avoided, and prominent (nonallergic) vasomotor rhinitis frequently ushers in the disease. Accepting the patient's report of respiratory distress after ingesting these drugs is essential, because no simple and safe confirmatory test is available. Additionally, because severe intolerance to aspirin and NSAIDs may begin suddenly, asthmatic adults with polyps or sinusitis or both should recognize the potential risks associated with these agents.

Flares of asthma frequently accompany viral or bacterial respiratory infections and may progress to necessitate inpatient care. When responsible pathogens have been sought in pediatric asthma patients, rhinovirus and parainfluenza virus infections have been especially implicated. Respiratory syncytial virus (RSV) infection often provokes a severe asthmatic event followed by lengthy periods of BHR. The presence of significant secondary infection may be manifested by fever, purulent expectoration, elevated white blood cell count, or recovery of pathogens from sputum. However, persistent asthma often provides the only signal. Many children with infection-triggered asthma in preschool years develop classic nasal allergy or allergic (atopic) asthma in later life, although few indications exist that "bacterial allergy" was responsible. Rather, because invading organisms destroy already compromised ciliated epithelium and localize agents of inflammation in labile bronchi, their adverse effect on asthma is predictable. Animal studies have also suggested that microbial substances may further reduce already inadequate beta-adrenergic activity.

Many asthmatic patients experience increased wheezing and *dyspnea* (abnormal shortness of breath) with exertion. Additionally, a specific form of *exercise-induced asthma* (EIA) is often noted in which significant bronchospasm occurs after several minutes of brisk activity and often well after its termination. EIA is most often evident in children and characteristically appears before exertion in subjects who have no symptoms. Although minimal total energy expenditure is necessary, above this critical level, the risk of symptoms varies with the type of activity. Generally, at comparable work levels, sprint running is most and swimming is least conducive to EIA. Current evidence suggests airway cooling and mucosal water shifts as an important determinant of EIA.

DIFFERENTIAL DIAGNOSIS

Because bronchial asthma is an abnormal pattern of response rather than a discrete disease, differential diagnosis requires attention to the clinical form and major determinants of this syndrome,* as well as to its distinction from other obstructive airway problems. Rarely is asthma suggested in individuals who over-breathe with psychic stress or in children with noisy respiration because of large adenoids, a short neck, or a "floppy" epiglottis. Laryngeal muscle dysfunction producing periods of involuntary vocal cord adduction can also narrow the airway episodically, mimicking (or accompanying) more distal obstruction. The upper airway obstruction produced suggests asthma that is unresponsive to medication. Once the asthma is identified, bouts may be aborted by physical (speech therapy) maneuvers. In adults, airway hyperactivity, at least, may often be excluded by demonstrating a normal test response to inhalation of methacholine, whereas the childhood problems are usually clarified by careful examination, and they may resolve in time with developmental changes. At any age, however, the impaction of a foreign body or growth of a localized tumor in the bronchi (or larynx) may lead to diffuse wheezing, simulating asthma. More typical recurrent symptoms occur in certain forms of diffuse vascular inflammation (vasculitis) and with secreting carcinoid tumors when these are metastatic to the liver (see Chapter 42).

Severe airway obstruction, capable of producing respiratory failure and associated with fever, is characteristic of the bronchiolitis of small children. This illness is often recurrent and frequently results from infection with RSV. Intense local inflammation promotes closure of small, distal airways, although humoral immune mechanisms also may contribute to this process.

A striking picture occasionally occurs in individuals with allergic asthma who acquire a growth of the fungus *Aspergillus fumigatus* in their bronchial lumina. Although little or no tissue invasion occurs, this organism excites an intense, apparently immunologically directed, inflammatory response with fever, pulmonary infiltrates (shadows) on chest x-ray films, and prominent tissue and peripheral blood eosinophilia. Affected subjects experience fatigue, weight loss, severe asthma, and expectoration of bronchial mucus plugs that may show the fungus as minute, dark growth points. Immediate wheal-and-flare skin reactivity to the fungus is striking, and total serum immunoglobulin E (IgE) levels are extremely high. IgG-precipitating antibodies with specificity for this organism also are demonstrable in this group. Suppression of the disease with adequate doses of adrenocortical steroids (see later in this chapter) is feasible and also essential if irreversible bronchial damage (bronchiectasis) is to be averted (Fig. 10-5).

Chronic bronchitis and pulmonary emphysema often require distinction from bronchial asthma when the latter has no evident allergic factors, particularly in older adults. Chronic bronchitis is often a slow progressive condition of bronchial inflammation and hypersecretion that is manifested by cough and sputum production extending

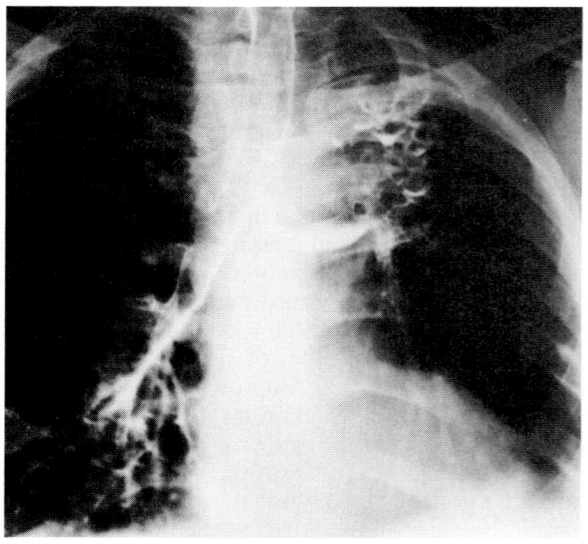

FIG. 10-5   Saccular (saclike) bronchiectasis of the left upper lobe demonstrated by contrast bronchography in an adult with long-standing allergic bronchopulmonary aspergillosis. Bronchi in lower lung fields are essentially uninvolved. A high-resolution CT scan is currently the preferred imaging method because it is noninvasive. (Radiograph courtesy Terry Silver, MD.)

over months and years. A proportion of those with chronic bronchitis also experience episodic bouts of airway obstruction—in effect, idiopathic asthma—late in the disease. Pulmonary emphysema, by contrast, produces prominent, irreversible anatomic changes with diffuse loss of the alveolar walls that normally exert outward traction on bronchi that they surround. Deprived of this elastic support, the airways tend to close in expiration wherever pressure outside their walls exceeds that within. Affected individuals develop predictable periods of dyspnea and wheezing with any increase (usually exertional) in respiratory effort rather than experiencing spontaneous attacks, typical of asthma, which may begin at rest or even during sleep. The prognosis of emphysema is quite unfavorable, with variably increasing disability the rule, and this diagnosis cannot be proposed lightly. However, because asthmatic individuals with recurrent infection also may acquire chronic bronchitis and severely bronchitic patients may ultimately show emphysema as well, a sharp distinction between these disorders is impossible at times. On the other hand, when chest hyperinflation, evident on radiographic or physical evaluation, is casually (and erroneously) designated "emphysema," a grave stigma may be implied without basis. In fact, the hyperinflation and resulting thoracic deformity of young asthmatic persons may be totally reversed with successful treatment, leaving them anatomically and functionally normal.

LONG-TERM TREATMENT CONSIDERATIONS IN BRONCHIAL ASTHMA

The protracted course, typical of asthma and its associated state of bronchial hyperreactivity, defines an extended need for treatment measures. For subjects in whom IgE-

---

*A syndrome is a set of signs and symptoms that characteristically occur together in an illness or related group of illnesses.

mediated factors are evident, efforts to reduce exposure to (and when needed, institution of immunotherapy for) selected inhalant allergens have established value (see Chapter 9). Avoidance of irritants, particularly tobacco smoke, and prompt treatment of unresolved bacterial respiratory infections are beneficial but frequently overlooked imperatives.

Perfumes, aerosol cleaners, cosmetics, strong cooking odors, solvents, and paint fumes also pose potentially avoidable risks that must be considered. Cold air is an additional bronchoconstrictor influence that may be mitigated by wearing a scarf or gauze mask over the nose and mouth as a heat exchanger. Adding moisture to dry indoor air (to maintain a relative humidity of approximately 30%) is desirable, although poorly maintained humidifiers can become sources of microbial aerosols. Programs of regular medication can also effectively reduce bronchial lability and thereby raise the threshold for obstructive airway responses.

Recent evidence that asthma prevalence and mortality are increasing globally and the promise implicit in newer treatment options have prompted an extensive reexamination of asthma care. The resulting guidelines reflect several increasingly accepted principles:

1. The overall severity of impairment caused by asthma differs widely among individuals and typically varies with time in any affected person.
2. Treatment programs of increasing potency (and complexity) are appropriate to control asthma of mounting severity (i.e., a "stepped" approach).
3. Antiinflammatory drugs are fundamental treatment for all but the most minimal forms of asthma.
4. Increasing symptom intensity should prompt a *preplanned* set of remedial behaviors designed to improve the individual's functional status.* Patient education and informed compliance are essential for favorable outcomes.

Beta-adrenergic agents (e.g., metaproterenol, pirbuterol, albuterol) remain the most widely used antiasthmatic drugs. These remedies show predominant beta$_2$-adrenergic effects, primarily airway smooth muscle relaxation with lesser (beta$_1$-adrenergic) increase in cardiac rate and contractile force. However, the latter effects are not absent from current preparations, and muscle tremor, sleeplessness, and psychomotor stimulation are additional, *intrinsic* beta$_2$-induced events. Direct comparisons readily confirm that inhaled preparations produce more rapid and effective asthma relief, with fewer systemic side effects, than do the same agents given orally. This principle, which especially favors beta-adrenergic aerosols, also can be generalized to other drug classes (e.g., corticosteroids, anticholinergics). However, reliance on bronchodilator aerosols leading to *overuse* is potentially harmful and variably linked to excess asthma fatalities. Furthermore, because patients readily control and may become habituated to aerosol use, a substantial abuse potential exists. Current guidelines recognize that beta-agonist aerosols alone suffice for minimal asthma, which occurs, at most, once or twice a week and is rapidly reversed by these agents. More frequent or severe

symptoms require the addition (or substitution) of antiinflammatory medications (see following discussion) on a regular schedule. Combined-drug programs have increasingly used inhaled salmeterol, twice daily, for its extended beta-adrenergic effects, although this agent cannot quickly reverse acute asthma. Leukotriene antagonists (see following discussion) may provide additive benefit. *Oral* beta$_2$-adrenergic drug treatment enjoys less popularity when symptoms are resistant. However, beta$_2$-adrenergic syrups and salmeterol are useful for small children when given for sporadic asthma or specific, short-term circumstances (e.g., respiratory infection, predictable allergen exposure) that provoke symptoms.

Recognition of bronchial inflammation as characteristic of and fundamental to asthma has focused attention increasingly on means to reduce the accumulation and activation of cells in the airway. When these changes follow IgE-mediated mast cell secretion, inhaled cromolyn sodium and nedocromil have demonstrated prophylactic value. The ability of these relatively safe drugs to block airway responses to specific allergens in laboratory-provocative challenges may realistically model their observed clinical benefit. However, whether IgE-based processes alone are affected is unclear, because these agents can often suppress EIA, and additional effects, apparently independent of mast cells, have been suggested.

Whatever the place of cromolyn sodium and nedocromil in drug treatment may be, inhaled corticosteroids are now broadly accepted as medications indicated for most individuals with symptomatic asthma. Several agents, marketed in *metered-dose inhalers (MDIs)*,* offer topical effectiveness and rapid (hepatic) metabolism of any absorbed drug; some of these permit twice-daily (bid) dosing to promote enhanced compliance. The addition of inhaled corticoids to treatment programs has significantly lessened asthma morbidity, measurable bronchial hyperreactivity, and both the numbers and the activation levels of airway inflammatory cells. These effects are almost certainly interrelated and are routinely achieved without the systemic side effects associated with oral or parenteral corticosteroid use. Despite these safety factors, in rare cases extrabronchial effects *can* occur when dosing guidelines are exceeded; hypercorticism may manifest at conservative doses in select patients. Additionally, local side effects can occur at recommended doses and can increase as medication use rises. These side effects include throat irritation, oropharyngeal *Candida* infection, and laryngeal myopathy (muscle dysfunction), producing hoarseness. Patients using corticosteroid inhalers can reduce unfavorable events by briefly washing out their mouths with tap water after drug inhalation.

Atropine and related anticholinergic agents have also demonstrated activity as bronchial muscle relaxants. The inhalation of an aerosolized congener, ipratropium bromide, achieves moderate bronchodilation without the side effects expected of a systemic muscarinic antagonist. Ipratropium is especially used when asthma has complicated chronic bronchitis but can benefit other patients with reactive airway problems. Adverse effects occur

---

*Objective determinations such as patient-determined peak flow values are useful.

*A change from chlorofluorocarbons to more environmentally acceptable propellants is slowly occurring in these aerosol products.

infrequently, and efforts to better define indications for this agent continue.

The benefits of administering antiasthmatic drugs by aerosol are now established beyond reasonable doubt with delivery of agents as micronized, dry powders offering especially favorable airway penetration. Although increasingly potent MDI preparations have been marketed that require fewer inhalations, many patients still underuse these devices. Even more often, faulty inhalation technique limits drug delivery to the tracheobronchial airways and increases deposition on oropharyngeal mucous surfaces from which systemic absorption readily occurs. The principal errors recognized involve the following:

1. Failure to synchronize inhalation and nebulizer discharge
2. Inadequate time before passive exhalation occurs to permit aerosol mixing and deposition in the airways

---

BOX 10-1

Considerations for Users of Metered-Dose Inhalers (MDIs)

1. Shake the inhaler briefly to mix its contents and invert (thus pressurized canister is above mouthpiece) to fill the metering chamber.
2. After complete exhalation, position the mouthpiece two fingerbreadths from the open lips. (Note: When a spacer is used, the lips are closed on its exit port instead.)
3. Activate the MDI synchronously, with slow, full inspiration.
4. Hold the breath for a count of 5 or 10; allow passive exhalation; repeat steps 2 to 4 as indicated.
5. When appropriate (i.e., with corticosteroids), rinse out mouth and throat and discard the washings.
6. Record the number of puffs used. Discard the inhaler when the rated total has been reached; drug-free discharge of propellants may still occur after this point.

---

3. Interception and effective loss of rapidly moving particles by oropharyngeal "baffles" (e.g., teeth, tongue, uvula)

Box 10-1 lists points of technique for optimizing lower airway delivery of aerosols in the seconds after discharge. Many of these deficiencies are reduced when MDIs are used with spacers, which are basically reservoirs for aerosol. These types of devices are essential for children and many adult users and substantially increase lung deposition (Fig. 10-6).

Although not currently asthma remedies of first choice for ambulatory patients, systemically administered drugs still offer useful options when other measures fail to control symptoms. For example, the addition of oral beta-agonists to a program of inhaled agents may restore comfort during brief or extended periods of need (e.g., respiratory infection). For many patients, however, side effects (noted earlier) preclude effective use of these drugs by mouth.

Although used less often, theophylline remains a functional antiasthmatic drug for selected patients. This methylxanthine agent appears to promote bronchodilation by inhibiting airway muscle phosphodiesterase, thereby increasing cyclic adenosine monophosphate (cAMP) levels (Fig. 10-7); however, other effects may contribute (or predominate). Several marketed preparations are well absorbed and active for 8 to 12 hours or as long as 24 hours. Drug effects are closely related to concurrent blood levels, with maximal benefit expected in the range from 8 to 18 μg/ml; below this lesser responses occur. Similarly, the risk of toxicity rises with serum levels; values greater than 20 μg/ml are best avoided. Individual responses vary widely. However, with some patients, toxicity usually causes nausea and vomiting, and potentially fatal seizures and cardiovascular collapse may be the first signs of an excessive dose. Additionally,

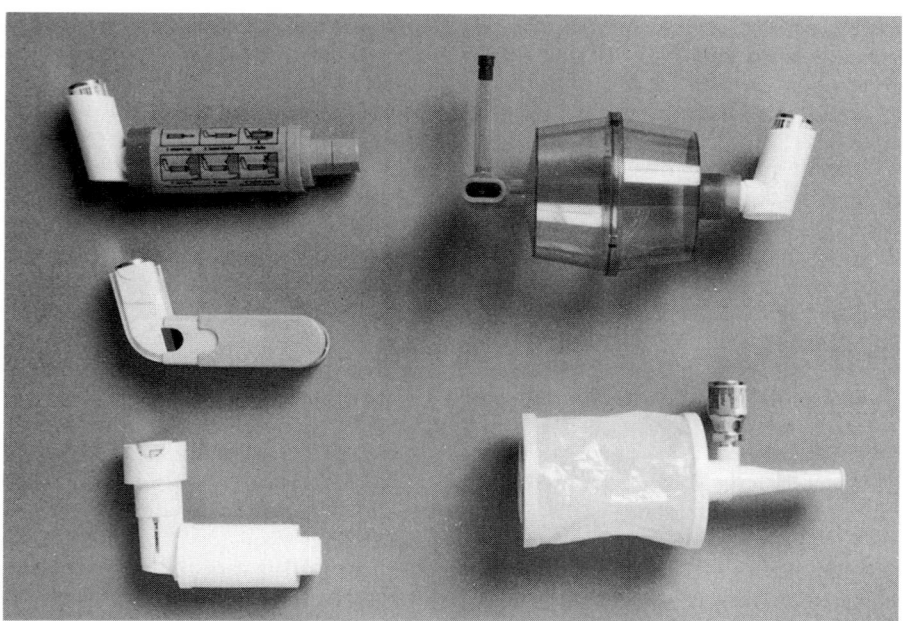

FIG. 10-6 Commercially available "spacing" devices for use with pressurized nebulizers, also called metered-dose inhalers (MDIs). Spacers provide a mixing chamber in which rapidly ejected particles can decelerate, allowing them to be captured more efficiently at the next inspiration.

several drugs (e.g., macrolide antibiotics, cimetidine) predictably elevate serum levels of theophylline by impeding its metabolism. With astute use of serum values, theophylline has remained useful, particularly as a bedtime medication to prevent asthma during sleep.

Corticosteroids provide a host of antiinflammatory activities that ameliorate asthma but also impose serious adverse effects with prolonged administration. This paradox can be resolved for most patients by regular use of inhaled agents (e.g., budesonide, beclomethasone, flunisolide, triamcinolone, fluticasone); however, asthmatic patients, who are dependent on regular oral corticosteroid treatment to maintain acceptable function, are not rare. For these individuals, adequate control of symptoms with the lowest feasible daily dose of a rapidly metabolized agent such as prednisone or methylprednisolone is an appropriate goal. Alternatively, administration of moderate corticosteroid doses *every other day* may be effective while reducing both systemic side effects and suppression of hypothalamic-pituitary-adrenocortical function. The latter benefits must reflect brief periods (beginning more than 36 hours after dosing) when no drug effect remains, because required alternate-day doses are often more than twice those necessary in daily administration.

Persons requiring systemic corticosteroids have special needs for optimization of other drug therapy and of antiallergic management when relevant. Additionally, possible contributions to symptom severity by factors such as chronic paranasal sinusitis, gastroesophageal reflux, and vocal cord dysfunction merit concern.

Because control of asthma may require doses of corticosteroids and other agents imposing unacceptable side effects, an active search for new approaches continues. Fragmentary evidence suggests gold compounds and twice-weekly, low-dose methotrexate as "steroid-sparing" antiasthmatic drugs, although this approach has not gained clinical acceptance.

Many cells in asthmatic airways produce leukotrienes, a group of lipid oxidation products, which promote smooth muscle spasm, vascular fluid leaks, and ingress of neutrophils and eosinophils. Considering these effects, benefit for asthma from drugs that block leukotriene synthesis or tissue effects is not surprising. Zileuton is a drug antagonist of synthesis acting on 5-lipoxygenase, a critical oxidative enzyme. A second group of agents (zafirlukast, montelukast) block receptors for leukotrienes (LTs), particularly LTD_4. These oral drugs are useful for many patients and appear safe, despite extended daily dosage. However, predictive criteria for success in specific individuals do not exist. Liver dysfunction occurs rarely and suggests monitoring of laboratory indicators, at least early in treatment. Currently, montelukast is most widely accepted (as Singulair) but additional antileukotrienes will certainly be introduced.

Antihistamines offer uncertain benefits, even in allergic asthma, and may compound the problem of sputum mobilization because of drying secretions. The expectorant properties of iodides and glyceryl guaiacolate (guaifenesin) remain controversial at doses that do not uniformly produce uniform gastrointestinal irritation. Benefits of simple systemic hydration should not be over-

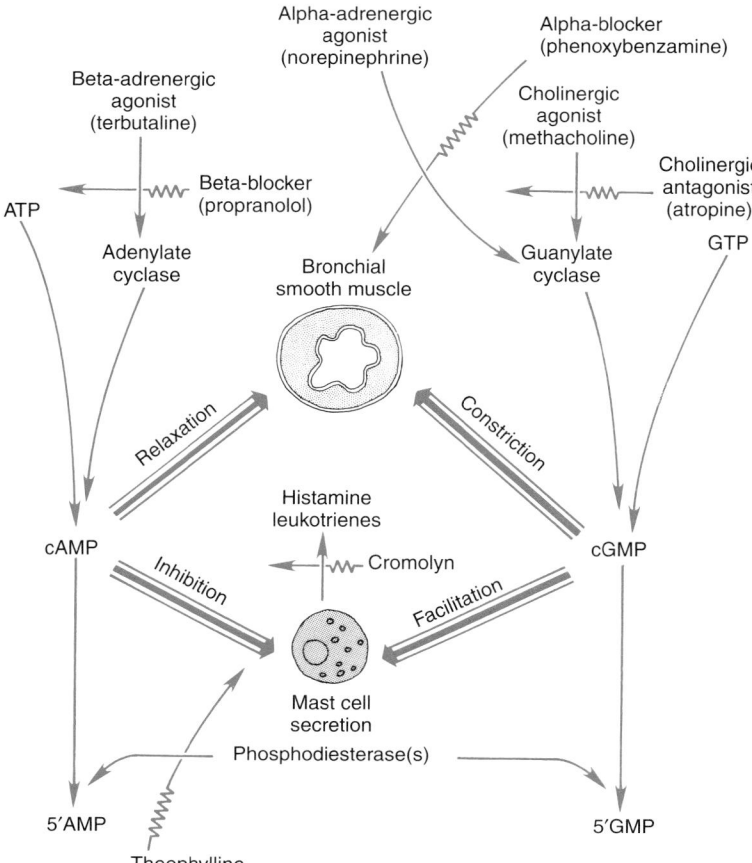

FIG. 10-7 Actions of drugs that affect bronchial patency either directly *(upper portion)* or by modifying mediator substance release from mast cells *(lower portion)*. Smooth lines indicate potentiation of an effect; wavy lines signify inhibitory influences. The central importance and opposing effects of cyclic adenosine monophosphate *(cAMP)* and cyclic guanosine monophosphate *(cGMP)* deserve special attention. cAMP levels are increased by beta-agonists acting on adenylate cyclase and by inhibition of phosphodiesterase effect (e.g., theophylline). cGMP levels are increased by cholinergic agents (e.g., methacholine) and possibly by alpha-adrenergic agents. Effects of theophylline and other drugs on cGMP–active phosphodiesterases are not clear. Bronchoconstrictive effects of alpha-adrenergic agents may reflect inhibition of cAMP or promotion of cGMP synthesis. The scope of corticosteroid effects is uncertain, but they are associated with increased responsiveness to beta-adrenergic agents and reduced inflammatory cell movement into airway tissues.

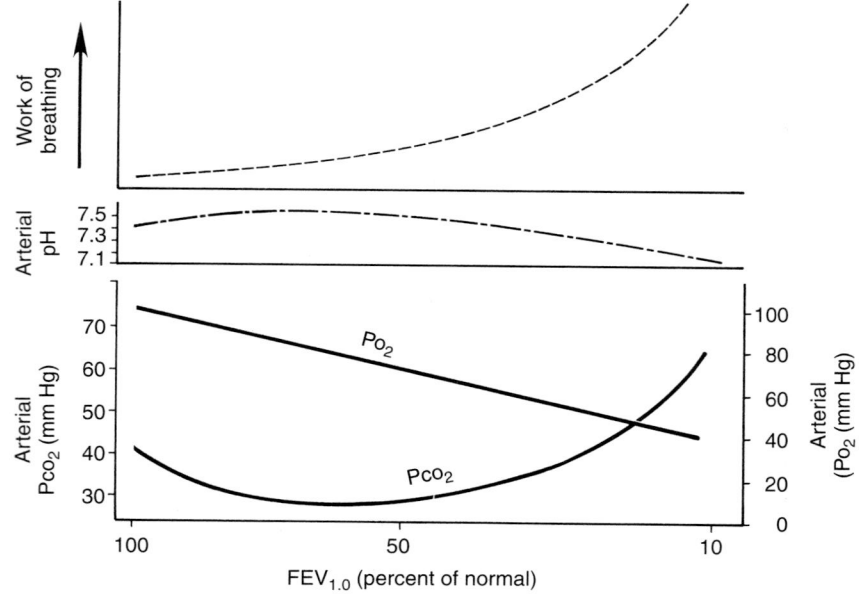

FIG. 10-8   Changes in the work of breathing and in arterial pH, Po_2, and Pco_2 observed in asthmatic patients with increasingly severe airway obstruction *(left to right)*. Hyperventilation is adequate to decrease Pco_2 and raise pH until airway narrowing and plugging are severe.

looked when sputum mobilization is a problem, and many mild asthma attacks may be curtailed if the patient sits calmly, breathes slowly, and sips a warm liquid.

Treatment Approach to Severe Asthma

Although proper management can promote a favorable prognosis for most asthmatic subjects, flares of the disease occur, requiring more intensive treatment or hospitalization and, rarely, resulting in fatalities. A sustained increase in symptoms often follows respiratory infection or the sudden withdrawal of a necessary suppressive medication. However, allergen exposure alone rarely precipitates hospitalization.

Medical aid is often sought only after many days of increasing symptoms. During this period, poor fluid and calorie intake coupled with increased respiratory work and fluid loss may produce significant dehydration and metabolic acidosis, as well as progressive bronchial mucus plugging. As previously emphasized, the extent of airway obstruction is not uniform, and despite vascular compensation, imperfect matching of ventilation and blood flow in local areas of lung is common. Because of these disparities, portions of the pulmonary blood flow escape aeration, which produces hypoxia and tends to impede carbon dioxide (CO_2) clearance. The deficit for CO_2 is overcome easily by respiratory effort, which can clear this readily diffusible gas by hyperventilating a minority of adequately perfused alveoli. Because hyperventilation is typically an early response to increased airway closure, the partial pressure of CO_2 ($Paco_2$) in arterial blood is often below the normal value (40 mm Hg) with asthma of mild or moderate severity. A rise to normal or elevated $Paco_2$ levels therefore signifies that an advanced and perilous stage of obstruction (and of ventilation-perfusion mismatching)

has been reached. Similar compensation is not possible even transiently for deficient oxygen (O_2) uptake. As a result, arterial Pao_2 values fall progressively as asthma worsens. Substantial increases in respiratory work compound these defects by greatly raising the O_2 cost of breathing and its penalty in CO_2 production. Ultimately, ventilation may not suffice even for the metabolic needs of the respiratory system. Figure 10-8 summarizes changes observed in several parameters during increasingly severe asthma.

Epinephrine administration remains an appropriate first step in the urgent treatment of asthma, although inhaled beta-adrenergic agents (e.g., metaproterenol, albuterol) are often equally effective, particularly when nebulized slowly with a compressor. If substantial improvement is not evident in 1 hour or less, other measures must then be substituted. Epinephrine-fast asthma may yield to intravenous (IV) aminophylline, although increasing IV corticosteroids are deployed. Because many hours of self-medication with ephedrine-like drugs or with theophylline may have occurred, an estimate of residual drug activity is mandatory. When possible, rapid determination of theophylline serum levels can be used to predict dosage requirements initially. Individuals without theophylline "on board" may receive 5 to 6 mg/kg of the drug IV by manual injection over at least 10 minutes, or by "drip" infusion. Although care will minimize instances of vomiting, hypotension, and seizures, a treatment facility must be prepared to handle these side effects promptly. Severe asthma that has persisted for at least 24 hours and is not substantially managed by optimal doses of epinephrine and theophylline is often termed *status asthmaticus*. This condition presents a serious threat to life and should prompt intensive inpatient care with high-dose corticosteroid therapy.

Most hospitalized asthmatic patients require supplementary hydration to replace water deficits, which may amount to several liters. The oral route is rarely adequate to achieve proper hydration, and a significant risk of aspiration must be faced unless fluids and medication are given parenterally to patients with air hunger. Without supplementary O_2, hypoxemia is present almost uniformly in status asthmaticus and should be corrected to a level of at least 70 mm Hg after initial arterial blood gas determinations. Supplementary humidified oxygen is best provided by 24% or 28% Venturi mask (Fig. 10-9) or, lacking these units, by nasal prongs.

When bronchial unresponsiveness to epinephrine has been confirmed, this agent is withheld initially, although some patients may benefit from regular doses of inhaled adrenergic agents. The need for antibiotic drugs must also be decided after appropriate cultures are obtained.

Systemic corticosteroids are often lifesavers for patients with status asthmaticus and are usually begun at or before admission. High doses are also given promptly to individuals who have required steroids either to terminate previous bouts of severe asthma or for other indications within the previous 6 to 12 months, as a regular outpatient medication. Preparations of hydrocortisone or methylprednisolone for IV infusion are preferred, although even with these, at least several hours are required for initial therapeutic effects. Frequently, several days of intensive corticosteroid and other treatment elapse before benefit is evident.

A favorable outcome in status asthmaticus necessitates that competent personnel closely monitor the patient's condition, promptly recognize deterioration, and anticipate problems. Prominent complications include pneumothorax, pneumomediastinum, aspiration, drug toxicity or idiosyncrasy, and cardiac failure or rhythm disturbance. Widespread plugging of airways may develop rapidly, which is manifested by a decrease in wheezing and by distant breath sounds over affected areas (an ominous combination). Obvious deterioration is often heralded by drowsiness, confusion, and decreased muscle tone, as well as by a flagging of respiratory effort, signaling general physical exhaustion. This situation readily leads to inadequate alveolar ventilation with mounting hypoxia and rising arterial levels of CO_2. The clinical state and arterial $PaCO_2$ correlate closely, and an upward trend is disquieting, although the absolute value may be normal (i.e., 40 mm Hg) or only minimally elevated. When $PaCO_2$ levels exceed 55 mm Hg despite optimal treatment, mechanical ventilation must be considered to reestablish adequate gas transfer. A volume-cycled ventilator is usually chosen for this purpose after placement of a soft, cuffed endotracheal tube; a tracheostomy is rarely required. Details of respirator care are beyond the scope of this discussion. Ventilatory assistance in status asthmaticus is usually needed for only 24 to 60 hours, when improvement produced by bronchodilators, steroids, antibiotics, and other agents usually has become evident.

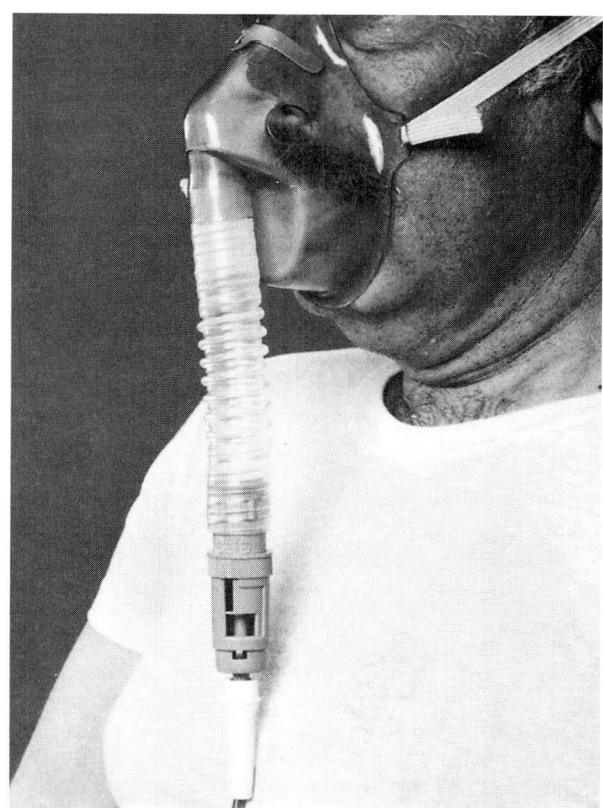

FIG. 10-9   Variable-concentration oxygen mask, using a Venturi effect, helps control O_2 administration. With this particular device, inspired O_2 concentrations between 30% and 55% may be chosen.

For many inpatients with severe asthma, attaining an audibly clear chest is a realistic predischarge goal, even though ventilatory test results (forced expiratory time, FEV_1, maximal midexpiratory flow rate) may remain somewhat abnormal; for others, irreversible bronchopulmonary changes may preclude a wheeze-free state. In either case, intensive treatment is continued until the anticipated maximal benefit is manifest, and then preparations are made for an outpatient program. During recovery, bronchial responsiveness to epinephrine and beta-adrenergic aerosols generally reappears. Sputum production often increases during recovery; however, clearance of secretions may remain difficult despite optimal hydration and use of glyceryl guaiacolate (which have equivocal expectorant properties). Chest physiotherapy (i.e., repetitive manual percussion of the chest with postural drainage) is generally available. This approach appears to promote sputum mobilization and can, at times, dislodge obstinate bronchial plugs, permitting reexpansion of atelectatic areas.

KEY CONCEPTS

■ Asthma is a clinical condition manifested by recurrent episodes of reversible bronchial narrowing, usually separated by periods of more normal ventilation. These events, provoked in asthma-prone subjects by a variety of stimuli, reflect and augment a characteristic state of bronchial hyperreactivity.

■ Asthmatic individuals, experiencing symptomatic periods, are unable to achieve normal rates of airflow during respiration (particularly expiration).

■ Asthmatic subjects, both with and without allergic mechanisms, share an abnormal bronchial lability that promotes airway narrowing by many factors that have no effect on normal persons.

■ Functionally, asthmatic airways behave as though their beta-adrenergic innervation patency is incompetent, and, at least functionally, partial blockage of beta-adrenergic receptors exists in typical asthma.

■ Flares of asthma frequently accompany viral or bacterial respiratory infections and may progress in severity, ultimately requiring inpatient care.

■ Many children with infection-triggered asthma in preschool years go on to develop classic nasal allergy or allergic (atopic) asthma in later life.

■ Many asthmatic patients experience increased wheezing and dyspnea with exertion of any intensity and obstructive airway problems from infection, particularly with respiratory syncytial virus.

■ Chronic bronchitis is often a slowly progressive condition of bronchial inflammation and hypersecretion manifested by cough and sputum production extending over long periods. An asthma component often develops as bronchial changes progress.

■ Pulmonary emphysema produces prominent, *irreversible* anatomic changes with diffuse *loss* of the alveolar walls that normally exert outward traction on bronchi they surround.

■ Antiinflammatory drugs are fundamental treatment for all but the most minimal forms of asthma. Inhaled beta-adrenergic agents (e.g., metaproterenol, pirbuterol, albuterol) remain the most widely used antiasthmatic drugs for "rescue" from acute distress.

■ Several corticosteroid agents, also marketed in MDIs, offer topical effectiveness and rapid (hepatic) metabolism of any absorbed drug.

■ Although proper management can promote a favorable prognosis for most people with asthma, flares of the disease occur, requiring more intensive treatment. A sustained increase in symptoms often follows respiratory infection or the sudden withdrawal of a necessary suppressive medication. Compliance is a critical determinant of treatment success.

■ Epinephrine administration remains an appropriate first step in the urgent treatment of asthma, although inhaled beta-adrenergic agents (e.g., metaproterenol, albuterol) are often equally effective.

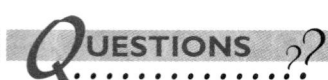

QUESTIONS

A sampling of review questions for this chapter appears here. Visit http://www.mosby.com/MERLIN/PriceWilson/ for additional questions.

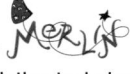

Answer the following on a separate sheet of paper.

1. Define bronchial asthma.
2. What is the pattern of ventilatory dysfunction in asthma?
3. What is the relationship of atopy to bronchial asthma?
4. Describe a postulated basis for the abnormal bronchial lability that is characteristic of asthmatic individuals. In clinical practice, how is this bronchial lability confirmed?
5. Why do flares of asthma typically accompany viral or bacterial respiratory infection?
6. List the principles that reflect the newer treatment options for asthma.
7. Explain why drugs with intrinsic beta-adrenergic effects continue to be useful for acute and long-term management of asthma.
8. Describe the faulty inhalation techniques associated with administering antiasthmatic drugs by aerosol (MDIs). How might these techniques be improved for optimizing lower airway delivery of these aerosols?
9. Explain the role of corticosteroids in the treatment of asthmatic patients who need to maintain an acceptable level of functioning.

Match the disease condition in column A with the appropriate description in column B. More than one letter may be used in column A.

Column A
10. _____ Chronic bronchitis
11. _____ Pulmonary emphysema
12. _____ Bronchial asthma

Column B
a. Irreversible anatomic changes with loss of supporting lung tissue associated with severe airway narrowing with exertion
b. A slowly progressive condition of bronchial inflammation and hypersecretion with or without airway obstruction
c. Predictable periods of dyspnea and wheezing with any increase in respiratory effort
d. Daily cough and increased sputum production extending over months and years
e. Spontaneous attacks of wheezing and dyspnea often occurring at rest; between attacks, patient is typically symptom free

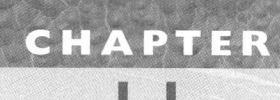

CHAPTER

11

Atopic Dermatitis and Urticaria

WILLIAM R. SOLOMON

CHAPTER OUTLINE

ATOPIC DERMATITIS

Atopic dermatitis is a common, chronic skin disorder (or group of related disorders) observed particularly in individuals with allergic rhinitis and asthma, as well as among their family members. High total serum immunoglobulin E (IgE) levels and multiple positive immediate skin test reactions are typical of this condition. These associations would appear to classify atopic dermatitis as a *de facto* "atopic disease." However, the lesions of atopic dermatitis are not readily explained in terms of the transient wheal-and-flare response associated with IgE-mediated reactions. Rather, established skin lesions of atopic dermatitis show edema and variable infiltration with mononuclear cells and eosinophils, as well as fluid collections within the skin (forming clinically evident vesicles). Rupture of numerous tiny blisters can lead to crusting and scaling. These changes and severe pruritus, which precedes and accompanies the eruption, are associated with excessively dry skin. Sweating is impaired in this condition, and sweat retention often leads to prominent heat-induced itching. Additionally, sebaceous secretions are deficient, and the skin shows both a low threshold for pruritus-inducing stimuli and an abnormal tendency to *lichenification* (thickening of the skin with accentuation of normal creases).

Atopic dermatitis most often appears in response to scratching in the first year of life (as "infantile eczema") with red, raised, pruritic, scaling areas involving the cheeks, scalp, and diaper area. In most children, the condition remits by age 5 but often only after the neck, antecubital and popliteal fossae, wrists, ankles, and waist also have become affected. The latter areas are prominently involved when rash still is present in late childhood or when, following onset in infancy or adolescence, it persists into adult life (Fig. 11-1).

Intractable itching and painful cracks in the skin are major sources of discomfort for eczematous individuals. Additionally, bacteria, particularly staphylococci, and viruses that localize in skin readily infect the abraded, fissured epidermis. As a result, contact with herpes simplex virus, the "cold sore" agent, may produce a generalized eruption (Fig. 11-2), fever, and toxicity. An even more severe illness, eczema vaccinatum, had followed exposure to vaccinia virus.*

As many as one half of children with eczema develop overt respiratory allergies before puberty. Despite this strong association, identifying allergens that substantially determine the activity of any case of atopic dermatitis is rare.† In individuals with strong skin reactivity, factors such as house dust mites and pets may worsen the rash, perhaps acting by direct contact with an abraded epidermis. Foods, particularly egg white, cause skin lesions to flare in a minority of children and deserve careful attention. Although the importance of ingestant allergens appears to decline with increasing age, prolonged avoidance of food offenders identified by well-controlled test challenge is clearly justified.

Because no basis for allergen-specific measures is found in most cases, the approach to treatment of atopic dermatitis remains largely symptomatic (i.e., by nonspecific symptom suppression). Care to avoid potential irritants and topical sensitizers, including those in medications, is essential. Prolonged use of bland, inexpensive lubricants is the foundation of most treatment programs and often keeps the disorder quiescent. Oil-in-water

---

*In the era of compulsory vaccination, the high mortality rate associated with eczema vaccinatum had been substantially reduced by administration of vaccinia immune globulin and by improved supportive care.
†Although sensitivity to staphylococci does not appear to contribute, IgE responses to resident skin yeasts (*Pityrosporum* species) have been demonstrated and may contribute to this chronic inflammatory condition.

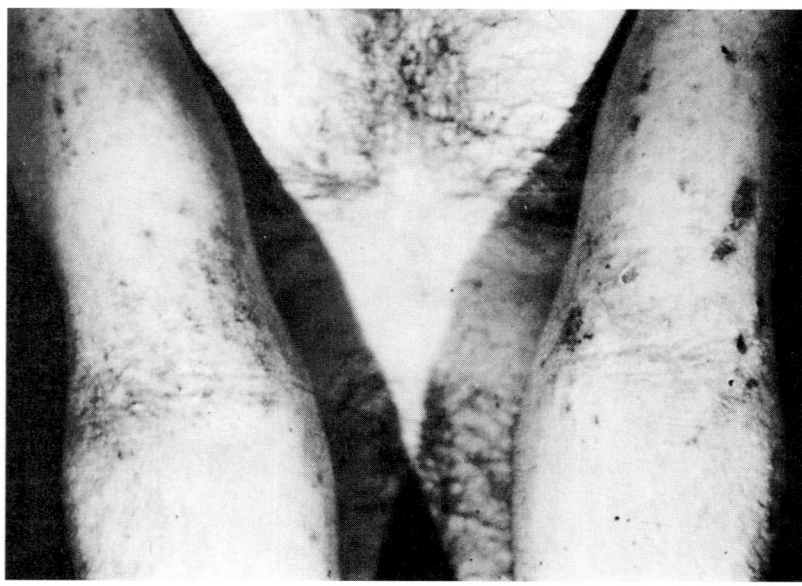

FIG. 11-1   Chronic lesions of atopic dermatitis (atopic eczema) on the flexor surfaces of the arms of a young man; erosions, pigmentary changes and a deepening of skin creases (lichenification) are evident. Additional typical lesions in a child and an adult are shown in Figs. 78-1 and 78-2, respectively. (From Sheldon JM, Lovell RG, Mathews KP: *A manual of clinical allergy*, ed 2, Philadelphia, 1967, WB Saunders.)

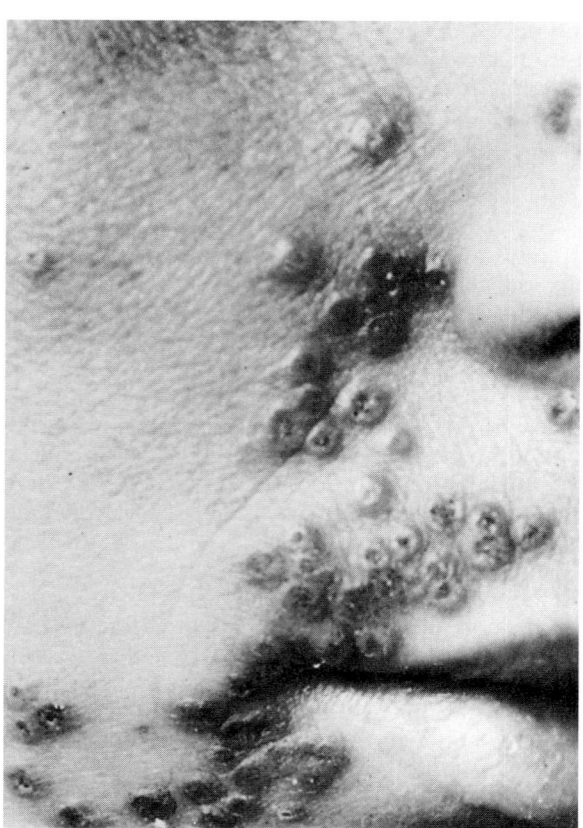

FIG. 11-2   Facial lesions of eczema herpeticum in a young adult with lifelong atopic dermatitis.

emulsions (e.g., water-washable base USP) may be adequate and act as minimally greasy vanishing creams. More effective lubrication can be obtained with water-in-oil emulsions (ointments), including hydrophilic ointment USP, Eucerine, and Aquaphor. Inert oils such as petrolatum provide maximal greasiness and protection from drying, but their occlusive properties often promote retention of debris, causing troublesome pruritus.

Topical corticosteroids are widely useful in atopic dermatitis, but these preparations should be employed for their antiinflammatory properties alone rather than for general lubrication. When indicated, topically applied steroids may be covered with an occluding layer of polyethylene to promote penetration of the drug, a strategy especially feasible at night. Steroids have largely replaced the once-popular coal tar preparations as antiinflammatory agents. Tars are still rarely used to reduce lichenification and cracking, although urea-containing ointments are more cosmetically acceptable agents to promote healing, hydration, and restoration of skin texture.

In managing atopic dermatitis, reduction of pruritus is both an end in itself and a means of interrupting the harmful "scratch-itch" cycle. Oral antipruritic agents such as diphenhydramine (Benadryl) and hydroxyzine (Atarax, Vistaril, or the less sedating Zyrtec) are especially useful at night when subconscious scratch responses can do serious damage. Fingernails and toenails should be kept as short as possible (consistent with comfort) to minimize trauma, and, for young children, soft, padded mittens or restraint of the extremities may be essential to sustain improvement. Well-washed cotton clothing is generally preferred, and as a rule, fibers such as wool and synthetics that "snag" the skin are best avoided. Chapping because of cold dry air is irritating to eczematous individuals, and well-maintained sources of humidification can offset the tendency of the rash to worsen in winter; organic solvents that defat even normal skin must be scrupulously excluded. A more subtle drying effect is inflicted by the regular use of soap and water or by contact with water alone. This problem may be approached in part by using skin cleaners with low emulsifying activity. Additionally, application of topical lubricants after washing or use of emulsified oils in bath water is often helpful. However, frequent bathing by eczematous individuals is rarely desirable, and water temperature should be maintained in a tepid range because body heating usually will increase pruritus.

Acute flares of atopic dermatitis are especially frequent in children, with prominent redness, vesicle formation, and oozing. Brief periods of high-dose systemic corticosteroids will usually speed resolution, and antimicrobial agents may be required because colonization of the affected skin is constant. Cool soaks will also reduce itching and remove cutaneous debris. As acute lesions begin to resolve, topical creams are used, followed by the progressively greasier applications emphasized in chronic care programs.

Several drugs that target T lymphocyte function have shown benefit in atopic dermatitis. Of these, only RU 4885 has been approved (as a topical agent) for prescription; a search for less costly options is in progress.

URTICARIA

Hives (urticaria) are familiar skin lesions that, at some time, may affect at least 25% of the population. Many clinical forms of urticaria exist, which suggests that a variety of determinants will ultimately be recognized. Clearly at present, *some* urticaria reflects immunologic processes, particularly those involving IgE, whereas others remain totally unexplained. This practical reality must be faced, because the resemblance of urticarial wheals to IgE-mediated skin reactions has often prompted the false inference that hives *per se* indicate allergy. Microscopically, most urticarial lesions demonstrate only edema, variable dilation of vessels, and occasional neutrophils and eosinophils. In some patients, however, grossly identical lesions show a definite vasculitis with disruption of blood vessel walls and infiltrating phagocytes. The discrete, raised, pruritic, nontender lesions of urticaria appear most often on the trunk and proximal extremities, and individual wheals rarely last more than 36 hours. Angioedema (see Chapter 9) marked by painless and minimally pruritic swelling of subcutaneous and submucosal tissues may be associated.

Most episodes of urticaria are brief and self-limited, particularly in childhood, when hives are often related to viral infections. However, in a minority of adults (and rarely in children), unexplained hives may persist for many months or years. These individuals should be evaluated for a serious underlying disease promoting urticaria; lymphomas, systemic lupus erythematosus, hyperthyroidism, and non-lymphoid neoplasms are occasionally found. Although chronic foci of bacterial infection and intestinal parasites are often sought in these patients, they are rarely shown to cause the chronic hives.

As with anaphylactic reactions, urticaria alone can result from IgE-mediated responses to protein allergens. In both situations, the implicated agents are usually ingestants, particularly fish, diverse shellfish, and nuts, including the peanut. Drugs and drug metabolites that are complete antigens or are capable of stable bonding to proteins (e.g., penicillin derivatives) are also prominent factors in systemic or urticarial type I reactions (see Chapter 9). However, many drugs also appear to cause urticaria by mechanisms exclusive of IgE. Aspirin is probably the most frequent offender in this group and may worsen nonspecifically in at least 30% of patients with chronic urticaria.

In some patients with chronic urticaria, environmental influences may play a role; cold is probably most frequently implicated. *Cold urticaria* affects particularly young adults and may appear with the most minor chilling. Hives develop in some as skin temperature falls but generally require rewarming for their appearance. Cold urticaria has been associated with elevated plasma histamine levels (e.g., in venous blood from a chilled extremity), and both headache and hypotension may result. This effect has occasionally led to disaster when affected individuals fainted while swimming and subsequently drowned. Urticaria also may be elicited specifically by local heating; lesions may be immediate in some subjects and delayed as long as several hours in others. Total body heating (e.g., in a warm bath) can also worsen pruritus and whealing of diverse additional causes. Furthermore, *cholinergic urticaria* is a clinically distinct condition in which physical exertion, emotional stress, and environmental warmth promptly elicits crops of tiny wheals, each surrounded by a broad border of redness. Affected persons typically show abnormally large whealing or erythematous responses to intradermal methacholine, although the pathogenetic significance of this response remains unclear. A period of sustained running usually elicits typical wheals, which confirm the diagnosis. Local urtication (hive formation) or angioedema may also follow exposure to sustained pressure, various wavelengths of light, or vibratory stimuli. Some of these rare conditions appear to be familial defects. Furthermore, in certain examples of heat-, light-, or cold-induced urticaria, *local* specific reactivity can be conferred on normal subjects by the transfer of IgE in the serum of affected persons. Currently, whether these "passive transfer" phenomena involve classic antigen-antibody reactions or alternative mechanisms is unclear.

Urticaria caused by pressure usually occurs in individuals with *dermographism* (Fig. 11-3), in whom firm stroking will produce definite whealing responses. Dermographism is longstanding in a small proportion of normal people but also may be acquired after adverse drug reactions or in disease states prompting infiltration of the skin by mast cells. Those with dermographism typically develop wheals at pressure points, including the buttocks and soles of the feet, as well as beneath watchbands, belts, and tight underclothing.

Instances of angioedema accompanying acute urticaria are occasionally confused with *hereditary angioedema* (HANE), a familial defect in the control of inflammation. HANE manifests as recurrent bouts of edema involving peripheral structures, as well as the larynx and bowel, the last producing intense abdominal pain and often leading to exploratory laparotomies. These episodes rarely appear before age 10 and may recur indefinitely, although their frequency often decreases after the sixth decade of life. Emotional stress or physical trauma (often quite subtle) may precede the edema, but many bouts are unexplained. Laryngeal edema poses a serious threat to life in these patients, and pedigree analysis usually reveals one or more members in each family who succumbed to asphyxiation. Swelling in this condition develops over

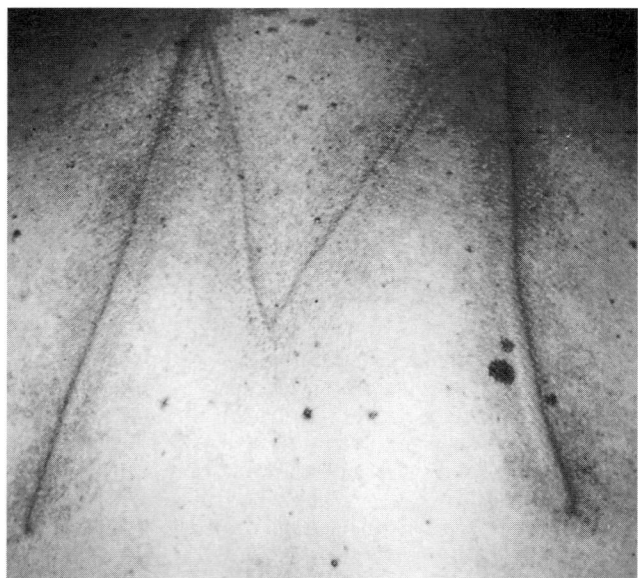

FIG. 11-3 Dermographism evident 2 minutes after the patient's back is lightly stroked with a fingernail. The subject had occasional urticarial wheals at the belt line and on the buttocks after prolonged sitting.

many hours, regresses slowly, and is *not* accompanied by urticaria. Patients with HANE are known to share low activity levels of the factor that normally inhibits the activated first component of the complement system (C1), as well as additional activities concerned with clotting, inflammation, and fibrinolysis. As a result of this deficiency, C1 effects are unopposed, and C1 proceeds to activate and consume the early components of the sequence, C4 and C2, which, on assay, are demonstrably low in this condition. However, as to which of the factors, normally checked by the C1 inhibitor, may be responsible for the swellings in this condition is unknown. Treatment measures are properly focused on preservation of the airway, avoidance of needless laparotomy when bowel edema occurs, and general support. Currently, available drugs contribute little to acute care;

however, regular use of anabolic agents of limited androgenic potency (e.g., danazol, stanozolol) stimulates synthesis of the deficient factor and can greatly reduce frequency of attacks.

A few additional conditions lend confusion to the evaluation of ordinary urticaria and angioedema. IgE-mediated urticaria to rubber latex is problematic, particularly in health care personnel. Exposure may also induce respiratory symptoms or overt anaphylaxis. Occasionally, penetrants such as stinging plant hairs or insects produce troublesome whealing reactions. Chronic, pruritic, raised papules, termed *papular urticaria*, often follow insect bites, particularly on the legs in children, but the persistence and induration (i.e., firm consistency) of these lesions usually sets them apart. Drugs or chemical additives in foods and beverages may be identified as sources of urticaria and should be evaluated carefully, although confirmatory skin or in vitro tests are rarely available. Similarly, a painstaking review of historical details may provide evidence implicating foods, physical agents, or psychogenic factors, but frequently no cause is evident.

Because bouts of hives are generally self-limited and vary in duration and severity, the value of treatment measures is often difficult to evaluate. However, epinephrine speeds the resolution of acute urticaria and angioedema. Agents such as diphenhydramine and hydroxyzine also have treatment value in this condition, although nonsedating alternatives such as loratadine (Claritin), fexofenadine (Allegra), and cetirizine (Zyrtec) are generally preferred. These drugs are considered to inhibit a type of histamine receptor termed H_1. Agents that include cimetidine and ranitidine block a second histamine receptor type (H_2); these may provide additional relief from pruritus. Adrenocortical steroids often benefit patients with severe acute hives but may fail to interrupt longer established disease at tolerable doses. In chronic urticaria, optimal antihistaminic medications are of paramount importance with or without sympathomimetic agents. Although repeated study of such patients is rarely fruitful, all concerned should remain receptive to clues that may ultimately implicate a responsible factor.

KEY CONCEPTS

- Atopic dermatitis is a common, chronic skin disorder observed particularly in individuals with allergic rhinitis and asthma, as well as among their family members.
- High total serum IgE levels and multiple positive immediate skin test reactions are typical of this condition.
- Skin lesions of atopic dermatitis show edema and variable infiltration with mononuclear cells and eosinophils and fluid collections within the skin. Rupture of numerous tiny blisters may lead to crusting and scaling.
- Atopic dermatitis often appears in response to scratching in the first year of life (as "infantile eczema") with red, raised, pruritic, scaling areas. However, in most children, the condition remits by age 5.
- Intractable itching and painful cracks in the skin are major sources of discomfort for eczematous subjects, and the abraded, fissured epidermis is readily infected by bacteria, particularly staphylococci, and by viruses that localize in skin.
- The approach to treatment of atopic dermatitis remains largely symptomatic (i.e., by nonspecific symptom suppression).
- In managing atopic dermatitis, a primary goal in reduction of pruritus, is both an end in itself and a means of interrupting the harmful "scratch-itch" cycle; oral antipruritic agents such as diphenhydramine (Benadryl) and hydroxyzine (Atarax, Vistaril) or cetirizine (Zyrtec) are especially useful.
- Topical (or systemic) corticosteroids are also a mainstay of atopic dermatitis treatment. Tacrolimus (Protopic) ointment is a highly effective (but quite expensive) nonsteroidal antiinflammatory agent recently introduced.

- Hives (urticaria) are familiar skin lesions sometimes reflecting immunologic processes involving IgE or other mechanisms exclusive of IgE.
- Most episodes of urticaria are brief and self-limited, particularly in childhood, when hives often are related to viral infections. However, in a minority of adults, unexplained hives may persist for many months or years.
- As with anaphylactic reactions, urticaria can result from IgE-mediated responses to protein allergens.
- Environmental influences may play a role in chronic urticaria in which cold exposure is probably most frequently implicated. However extensive skin or dietary testing (or both) is rarely instructive.
- Hereditary angiodema (HANE) is a familial defect in the control of inflammation and manifests as recurrent bouts of edema involving peripheral structures, as well as the larynx and gut wall.
- Additional conditions that lend confusion to the evaluation of ordinary urticaria and angioedema include IgE-mediated urticaria to rubber latex. Occasionally, penetrants such as stinging plant hairs or insects produce troublesome whealing reactions.
- Chronic, pruritic, raised papules, termed *papular urticaria*, often follow insect bites, particularly on the legs of children.
- Treatment measures are often difficult to evaluate; however, epinephrine speeds the resolution of acute urticaria and angioedema. Agents such as diphenhydramine and hydroxyzine also have value in this condition, although loratadine (Claritin), fexofenadine (Allegra), and cetirizine (Zyrtec) are generally preferred.

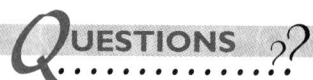

QUESTIONS

A sampling of review questions for this chapter appears here. Visit http://www.mosby.com/MERLIN/PriceWilson/ for additional questions.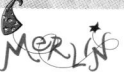

Answer the following on a separate sheet of paper.

1. Describe the similarities between anaphylactic reactions and urticaria.
2. Discuss the treatment measures used for acute urticaria and angioedema.
3. What is the prevalence of urticaria (hives)?
4. Why are treatment modalities for urticaria difficult to evaluate?
5. Name two common characteristics of individuals with atopic (allergic) disease.
6. Differentiate atopic dermatitis (eczema) from allergic eczematous contact dermatitis (AECD).
7. Describe the basic skin characteristics of individuals with atopic dermatitis.
8. Describe the treatment of atopic dermatitis.

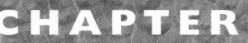

CHAPTER
12

Autoimmune and Immune Complex–Induced Diseases

WILLIAM R. SOLOMON

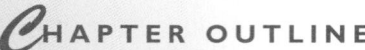
AUTOIMMUNITY AS FAILURE OF NORMAL IMMUNE MECHANISMS

Although illness often results from immune processes, the body's own antibody or specifically sensitive cells rarely attack host tissues. However, antibodies that bind to autologous tissue components can arise and may provide valuable diagnostic markers.

The lack of reaction to "self" components is normal and contrasts with the brisk response induced by (transplanted) tissues of other individuals and species. Selective unresponsiveness to potential antigens characterizes "immunologic tolerance," which may reflect several mechanisms operating singly or in combination. The tissue components that produce tolerance are the same ones responsible for normal immune reactivity and include the following:

1. Antigen-presenting cells (usually macrophages and "dendritic" cells in skin and lymph nodes)
2. T_H (helper T) cells, which assist the antibody production by B cells and promote activities of other T cell subgroups
3. T_S (suppressor T) cells, which inhibit the maturation of B cells, from which antibody-forming cells are derived, and the activity of other T cell subgroups

Most antibody responses require that the antigen be processed by an antigen-presenting cell, be presented to a specific T_H cell, and be transferred with "help-promoting" soluble factors to one or more specifically reactive B cells. The latter multiply and mature into antibody-forming cells, which, as plasma cells, secrete immunoglobulins with the properties of an antibody.

Antigen exposure may also result in T_C (cytotoxic T) lymphocytes, which kill other cells that display a sensitizing antigen, such as a virus or a tumor marker. To be effective in host protection, all the component cell types must be present and functionally mature and must participate in the proper sequence. A failure to respond will occur if a cell subset, cell receptor, or normally secreted factor is missing. The resulting immunologic unresponsiveness can block immune events induced by all or most antigens. However, "tolerance" is antigen specific and implies a *selective* functional inactivity or loss of cells with highly defined reactivity.

Animal studies have shown that tolerance can be established in B cells, in the subsets of T cells, or in both, and is accomplished most easily in fetal life or shortly after birth. Presentation of antigen at these times may promote specific tolerance. When immature lymphocytes (particularly T_H cells) encounter large antigen loads, their function may be suppressed and they may die. With such "clonal deletion," the ability to respond to a specific antigen may be permanently lost.

B cells generally require larger amounts of antigen to produce tolerance. However, B cell clones may be deleted, or intense antigenic stimulation may exhaust their ability to secrete antibody for long periods. Tolerance induced in this way may be sustained if antigen continuously binds all antigen-reactive (immunoglobulin) receptors on clones of specifically responsive B cells. Depending on the amount of antigen present, T_S cells may also develop and restrict reactive T and B cells with the same specificity. Although their roles have not been confirmed, each of these mechanisms appears to contribute to tolerance. Clonal deletion is most easily accomplished in fetal life and is an important function of the thymus. Embryonic T_H and B cells that become constitutively reactive with "self" host antigens are lost or their function is eliminated under extended exposure to these antigens. Regardless, the human infant is born tolerant to normal body components, and the developing individual normally remains so.

The appearance of autoantibodies or autoreactive T_C cells implies either an acquired mutation among immunocompetent cells or activation of cells that had been suppressed but not eliminated. Several mechanisms may result in autoimmunity. With some agents, such as ocular pigment and endocrine gland cell components, the inciting antigens are normally sequestered in closed tissue compartments throughout development; therefore they may remain "foreign" even to mature lymphoid tissues. If injury releases these once locally confined materials, an immune response may then occur, with secondary damage to the injured organ and antigenically related structures. This mechanism appears to operate in certain eye conditions (e.g., sympathetic ophthalmia) and in several endocrine deficiency states. Immune responses to host tissue components can also arise after more subtle injury incident to microbial invasion. The possibility that infecting bacteria and viruses may produce limited changes in host tissue components that render them "foreign" (i.e., "altered self") to immune surveillance has also been proposed. Antibodies (or sensitized lymphocytes) resulting from this process might have specificities broad enough to permit reaction with native and altered tissue determinants. Additionally, autoimmune phenomena might result if an invading organism (or other introduced agent) and normal host tissues shared an antigen or closely similar antigenic group as a result of parallel evolution. Although invoked particularly to explain the pathogenesis of poststreptococcal glomerulonephritis and rheumatic fever, the role of this mechanism remains uncertain. Finally, autoaggressive immune reactions may originate with mutant ("forbidden") clones of lymphoid cells programmed to recognize normal host components as "foreign." Alternatively, disease, including viral invasion, may damage T_S cells that normally prevent such T and B cell responsiveness with "self" components.

Organ-Specific Autoimmune Disease

Human antibody-dependent, autoimmune disorders most often affect formed elements of the blood, with platelets and red blood cells (RBCs) attacked most often. Increasing evidence has linked the disease, *idiopathic thrombocytopenic purpura* (ITP), with circulating immunoglobulin G (IgG) molecules reactive with host platelets. Even when fixed to platelet surfaces, these antibodies do not cause localization of complement proteins or lysis of platelets in the free circulation. However, platelets bearing IgG molecules are more readily removed and destroyed by macrophages bearing membrane receptors for IgG in the spleen and liver. Evidence supporting this mechanism for thrombocytopenia has come from studies of ITP patients and subjects who have shown severe but brief platelet deficits after receiving ITP patients' serum. *Transient thrombocytopenia*, noted in infants delivered by mothers with ITP, is also consistent with IgG-dependent damage caused by placentally transmitted antibody. ITP may follow infections, particularly in childhood, but it often appears without prior event and typically resolves after days or weeks. Persistent ITP can usually be suppressed by corticosteroids, which are thought to reduce platelet removal by the spleen and liver. However, when the disease has lasted 6 or more months, the prospect of prolonged high-dose steroid treatment with its inherent side effects generally prompts a splenectomy. Platelet counts usually rise and may become normal after this procedure, despite continued sequestration by the liver; in either case, lower steroid requirements result in most patients (see Chapter 19). Recently, patients with ITP have been treated with daily high-dose infusions of commercially prepared gamma globulin (human serum immune globulin). This approach usually raises platelet levels and may avert splenectomy for some patients.

RBC membranes carry a host of described antigens, and immunoglobulins reacting with one or more of these appear in ill and in otherwise normal persons. Depending on the type, specificity, and number of antibody molecules involved, fixation to membrane sites may have no effect or may shorten cell life by allowing extravascular removal (e.g., in the spleen) or intravascular lysis. When shortened RBC survival results, signs of increased turnover of heme pigments (see Part Three) can usually be demonstrated, and frank anemia will develop if RBC replacement cannot fully compensate for the losses. Generically, these conditions are often described as *immunohemolytic (IH) processes.* Hemolytic transfusion reactions are a distinctive form of IH process usually occurring when a recipient, already sensitized to "foreign" human RBC antigens by pregnancy or prior transfusion, receives blood containing these antigens. Much less often, transfused blood contains antibodies reactive with the recipient's erythrocytes. However, most IH processes arise through production of antibodies reactive with the body's own RBCs.

The *Coombs' test* provides information central to the description of IH disorders. In this procedure, antibodies derived from another species (e.g., goat) and directed toward human immunoglobulins or complement components or both are mixed with washed human erythrocytes. If these cells have human immunoglobulin or complement factors on their surfaces, the foreign antiserum, by reacting with molecules on adjacent cells, will tend to link the cells and cause them to clump visibly (Fig. 12-1). In practice, the foreign (Coombs') serum is usually mixed directly with cells from drawn blood. A positive (clumping) reaction in this *direct Coombs' test* indicates that circulating cells with significant bound immunoreactive molecules are present. At times, the direct test is negative, despite the presence in a patient's serum of antibodies reactive with human erythrocyte antigens other than those of the host. Incubating the test serum with human RBCs of compatible ABO and Rh types and then adding Coombs' serum may detect these unbound antibodies. RBC agglutination in this *indirect Coombs' test* indicates unsuspected serum antibody. Coombs' reactions are largely performed with antiserums specific for human IgG or the third component of serum complement (C3).

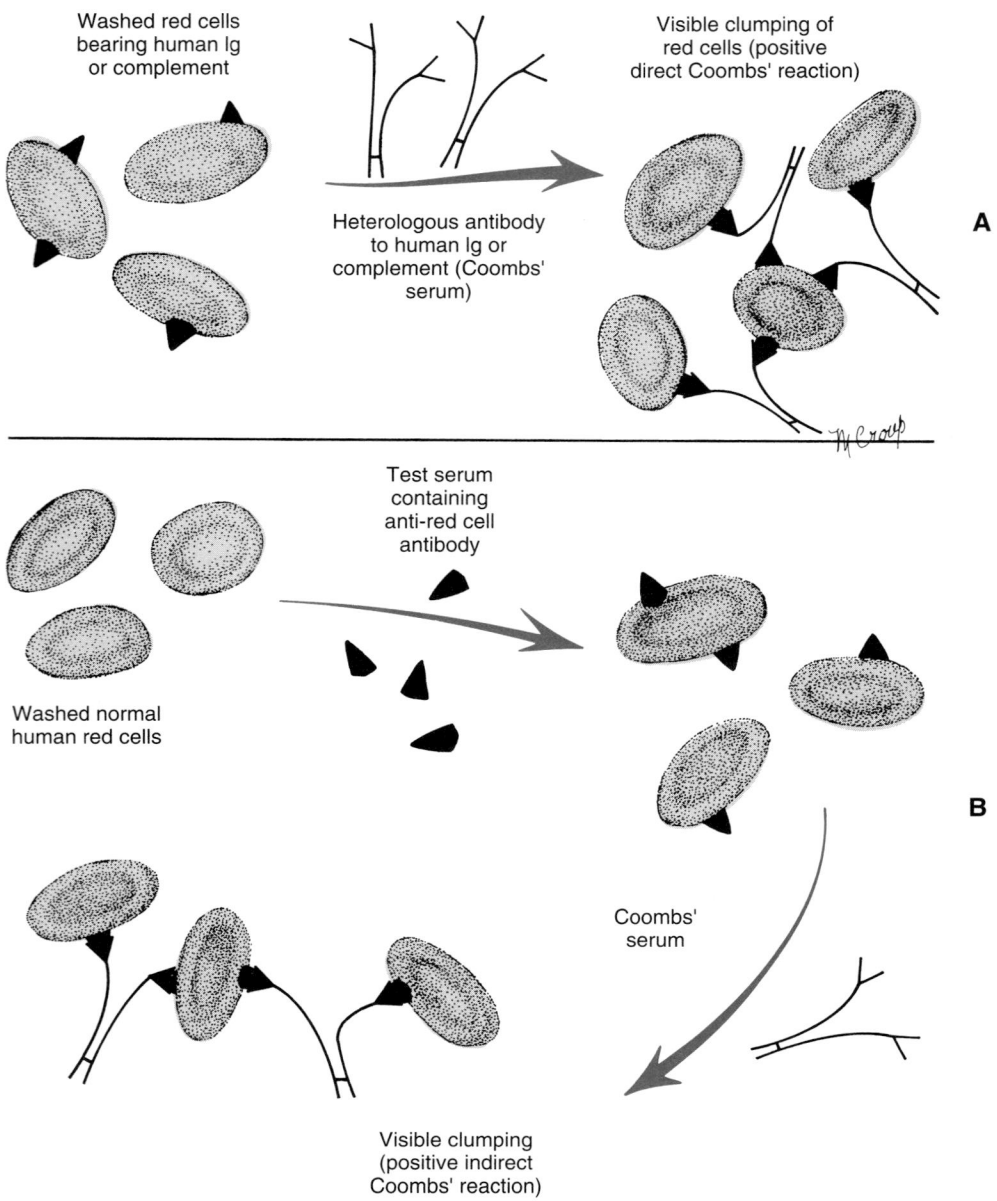

FIG. 12-1 Reaction sequences in the direct **(A)** and the indirect **(B)** Coombs' test.

Hemolytic reactions to transfused blood provide the most dramatic and dangerous IH phenomena observed clinically. These responses almost always appear during infusion of the offending blood and are marked by rapid intravascular lysis of RBCs induced by circulating host antibodies. Individuals at risk include those who are sensitized to RBC antigens by prior pregnancy, transfusion, or unknown factors that may include bacterial or viral infection. Victims of transfusion reactions have chills, fever, and low back pain, occasionally preceded by urticaria or flushing and often by uneasiness and air hunger. When cell lysis is massive, the resulting debris may also trigger widespread clotting within small vessels.* This process reduces blood flow to tissues and con-

sumes clotting factors faster than they can be replaced. Bleeding from wounds and venipuncture sites typically follows. Survivors of severe acute reactions also share a high risk of acute kidney failure promoted by shock and by massive hemoglobinuria (i.e., passage of free hemoglobin into the urine).

Considering these dire consequences, every reasonable measure to prevent or mitigate hemolytic transfusion reactions is justified. Identifying the source and proper recipient of blood products is crucial, and individuals receiving blood, particularly those whose mobility or awareness is impaired, must be under continual observation. If any suggestion of an incipient reaction should occur, the suspect infusion should then be immediately discontinued, intravenous (IV) access should be maintained, and the patient should be closely monitored. A carefully drawn venous sample from the recipient should

---

*This is one example of disseminated intravascular coagulation (DIC) (see Chapter 19).

be checked for serum hemoglobin, a sign of intravascular RBC breakdown, and the compatibility of donor and recipient should be reconfirmed. Without exception, all materials used for transfusion must be saved to facilitate serologic and microbiologic testing. Special precautions to monitor urine output are essential, and examination of serial centrifuged urine specimens for hemoglobin is desirable, because clearance of serum hemoglobin is rapid. Maintenance of adequate hydration and urine flow is important in treatment, and osmotic diuresis with cautiously administered IV mannitol may help in achieving this goal. Safe fluid therapy demands precise and regular evaluation of cardiopulmonary and renal function. Measures to combat shock, pulmonary edema, acute renal failure, and defibrination with bleeding may be required.

In addition to hemolysis, several adverse reactions may accompany transfusion of blood or blood products. Urticaria alone occurs rarely in recipients and, particularly in atopic subjects, may reflect trace amounts of food or other allergens in transfused serum. In patients who are repeatedly requiring blood or after multiple pregnancies, antibodies to human leukocyte membrane antigens often develop. With subsequent transfusion of "foreign" whole blood, these factors agglutinate leukocytes and, at times, platelets. These reactions are the most common source of transfusion-associated *fever*, although vital organs are minimally affected. Suitable blood for patients with leukoagglutinins may be obtained by filtration through nylon fibers or reconstitution from the frozen state; both preparations are essentially free of leukocytes. Recipients of serum containing potent leukoagglutinins have developed fever, cough, shortness of breath, and lung shadows on chest radiographs; several days have been required for full resolution. In addition to these problems, personnel who supervise transfusion therapy must be alert for possible air embolism, volume overload, septicemia from microbial contamination, chilling from excessively cold blood, and calcium or platelet deficiency after massive blood replacement.

Three categories of spontaneously developing IH phenomena have been identified: (1) types associated with medications (see Chapter 13); (2) types with "warm" RBC autoantibodies reacting at 37° C; and (3) a group of conditions with "cold" antibodies that bind at lower temperatures and often only in a range of 4° to 15° C. Warm autoantibodies are usually of the IgG class and are recognized primarily in middle-age adults. In more than one half of these cases, a serious primary disease, such as chronic lymphocytic leukemia, lymphoid (and rarely nonlymphoid) tumors, or systemic lupus erythematosus (SLE), will become evident, and these conditions substantially determine the prognosis for those affected. The IH disorder may be evident only as a positive Coombs' test (using antibody to human IgG), rarely leading to symptoms or even fulminant, fatal hemolysis. Usually, however, shortened RBC life promotes chronic pallor, fatigue, and weakness, as well as recurrent fever and jaundice; dyspnea arising from heart failure, angina pectoris, and vascular thrombosis are also common. Splenic enlargement is frequent, because this organ is the main site of RBC destruction. Splenic trapping of erythrocytes is at a maximal level when both IgG autoantibodies and C3 are present on their surfaces. When treatment is nec-

essary, adrenocortical steroids are a proper first consideration; these induce remissions in more than two thirds of patients, although relapses are common when these drugs are withdrawn. Splenectomy is undertaken when steroids, in acceptable doses, have proved inadequate. Additionally, immunosuppressive (cytotoxic) agents (e.g., cyclophosphamide, azathioprine) may be helpful in highly selected patients. Because warm hemolysins usually react with cells of essentially all potential normal donors, transfusions pose extreme difficulties and are avoided when possible. When no other choice remains, addition of Coombs' serum after incubation of the patient's serum with panels of cells permits the *least* incompatible ones to be chosen.

Cold autoantibodies to RBCs generally bind at temperatures well below 32° C; however, these molecules become dissociated at the warmer levels required for the "fixation" (i.e., cell-surface localization) of complement. Because of this action, hemolysis may be absent and RBC agglutination minimal despite extremely high levels of autoantibody. Immunoglobulin M (IgM) cold agglutinins are frequently found in infectious mononucleosis and *Mycoplasma pneumoniae* infections, although decreased RBC survival rarely results. Chronic cold-dependent hemolysis is observed, however, in some older individuals, many of whom have lymphoid neoplasms and IgM autoantibodies. Besides stigmata of chronic hemolysis, these patients display signs of RBC agglutination (e.g., pain, cyanosis) in the peripheral circulation when they are exposed to cold. Treatment considerations usually focus on the associated malignancy, when present, although corticosteroids or immunosuppressive drugs appear to offer benefit in individual cases.

General (Non–Organ-Specific) Autoimmune Disease

Goodpasture's syndrome is a rare disorder that exemplifies antibody-mediated human autoimmunity that causes major damage to internal organs. The typical clinical picture of recurrent pulmonary hemorrhage (Fig. 12-2) and anemia coupled with progressive kidney failure is described in Part Eight. The relative severity of these features, however, varies among patients. Most instances of Goodpasture's syndrome have no *obvious* cause, although the disease has followed viral and chemical insults to the lungs. Circulating antibodies that are reactive with glomerular (kidney) and alveolar (lung) basement membrane glycoproteins, particularly type 4 collagen, are usually present and, along with complement components, form linear deposits at these sites. The associated tissue damage reflects, in part, complement-mediated cytotoxicity and local effects of recruited neutrophils.*

Antibodies, apparently reactive with normal tissue, are found in many additional human diseases, particularly those involving connective tissue (e.g., dermatomyositis,

---

*Many mononuclear cells have membrane receptors that lead them to sites of IgG deposition. Direct contact with these activated cells causes cytotoxic effects and other tissue damage without complement activation. This process, termed *antibody-dependent cell-mediated cytotoxicity* (ADCC), may play a part in Goodpasture's syndrome and many other hypersensitivity disorders.

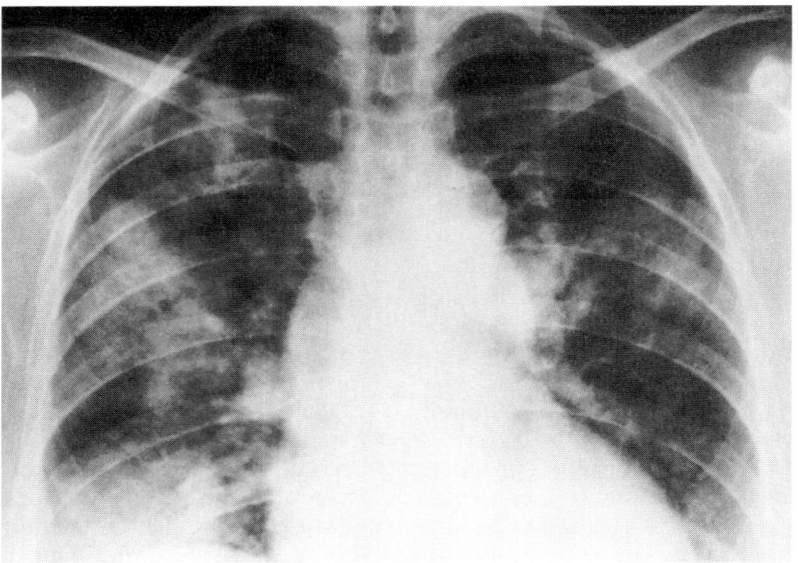

FIG. 12-2 Frontal chest radiograph during active pulmonary involvement in Goodpasture's syndrome. (Radiograph courtesy Terry Silver, MD.)

scleroderma) and thyroid gland inflammations. However, in most of these conditions, antibody-induced damage as such has not been easily demonstrated, although in some instances (e.g., SLE), pathogenic immune complexes are recognized. Complexes that contain antibody to double-stranded deoxyribonucleic acid (DNA) combined with that antigen are important factors in the nephritis of SLE (see later discussion). Additionally, antibodies to organ-specific components and to nuclear and cytoplasmic antigens occur in SLE. Because these various serum factors are currently associated more with diagnostic than pathogenetic considerations, they are discussed briefly in chapters that discuss treating diseases of major organ systems.

SERUM SICKNESS AND OTHER CONDITIONS INDUCED BY CIRCULATING IMMUNE COMPLEXES (TYPE III DISORDERS)

Serum sickness is considered the prototypic immune complex–induced illness. Originally described after administration of large volumes of unfractionated equine antiserums for prophylaxis of diphtheria or tetanus, this condition is most prevalent today after exposure to drugs, such as penicillin and sulfonamides. The development of serum sickness requires exposure (often by injection) to an antigenic material that will remain in the circulation until a specific antibody response occurs, as shown in Figure 12-3. At that time, the slowly diminishing blood levels of antigen drop sharply, signaling the formation of immune (antigen-antibody) complexes that are rapidly cleared from circulation by macrophage-monocyte scavenging and other mechanisms (i.e., "immune elimination"). Complexes form initially in considerable antigen excess, with small aggregates comprising one antibody molecule and two antigen molecules (or determinant groups) predominating. As antibody synthesis and

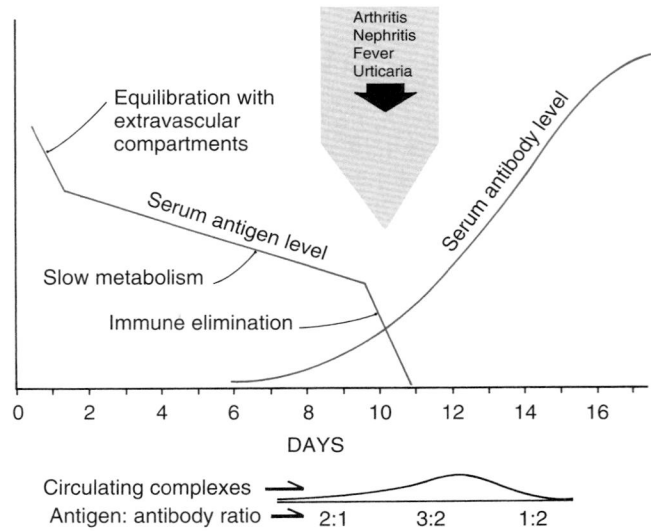

FIG. 12-3 Trends in immune reactants during the course of serum sickness.

immune elimination of antigen proceed, a state of antibody excess progressively develops. Between these extremes is a usually brief period during which modest antigen excess occurs and somewhat larger complexes, with molecular proportions approaching three antigen molecules to two antibody molecules, predominate. These complexes activate complement components and probably other amplification systems that can mediate inflammation. Furthermore, because of their physical properties, these complexes are readily deposited in the walls of small vessels in many organs, including the kidneys; inflammatory changes follow at these sites.

After initial exposure to an appropriate sensitizer, manifestations of serum sickness classically appear in 7 to 14 days; shorter latency periods precede second or subsequent attacks if exposure is repeated. Typically, the

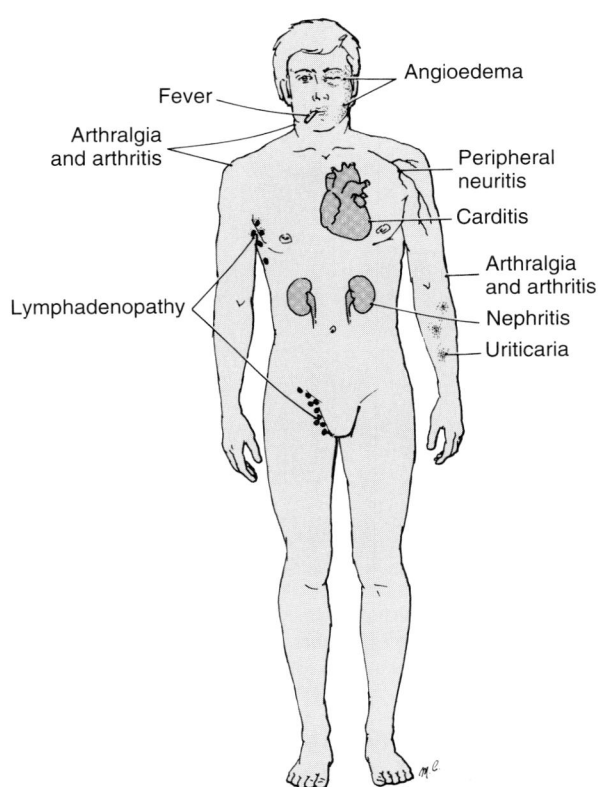

FIG. 12-4   Possible manifestations of serum sickness. Most patients, however, experience only fever with skin or joint problems.

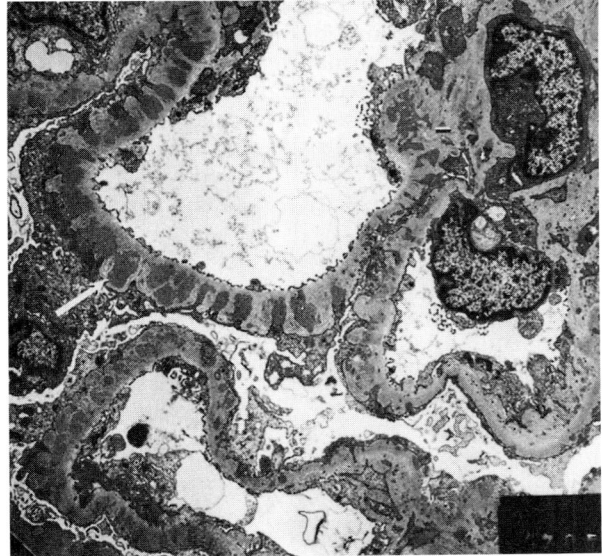

FIG. 12-5   Antigen-antibody complex deposition *(arrow)* in the glomerular basement membrane of a nephritic subject. The irregular "lumps" of material are typical of blood-borne immune complexes in which the antigen is not a kidney component.

most prominent manifestation is urticaria (Fig. 12-4), which is often severe and confluent, and angioedema; however, skin lesions may resemble bruises or the rash of measles. In addition, many persons develop fever, muscle soreness, and fatigue. Lymphadenopathy, with enlarged tender nodes, is often generalized and may be especially striking in node groups draining the site of introduction of the causative agent. Joint pain (arthralgia) may occur alone, or frank arthritis may affect several large joints together or sequentially. Although genitourinary symptoms are rare, urinalysis may reveal excessive excretion of albumin, erythrocytes, and leukocytes. Gastrointestinal complaints of nausea, vomiting, and abdominal pain infrequently dominate the picture, and cardiac and peripheral nerve dysfunction is rare. These diverse manifestations often make the task of distinguishing serum sickness from certain infectious processes (particularly viral) and from such conditions as rheumatic fever, sickle cell crisis, glomerulonephritis, and bacterial endocarditis difficult. Laboratory findings offer limited guidance in this differential process, although modest leukocytosis, elevated RBC sedimentation rate, and transient depression of serum complement activity are typical of serum sickness.

As indicated, complement-fixing immune complexes are strongly implicated in causing serum sickness. Among the complement system products formed (see Chapter 5) are *anaphylatoxins* (C5a and C3a), which can release histamine and other proinflammatory agents from mast cells. Additionally, most affected patients have tissue-fixing antibodies that mediate wheal-and-flare

skin reactivity to the implicated antigen and may contribute additionally to clinical urticaria and angioedema.* Furthermore, growing evidence indicates that mast cell–derived mediator substances that increase the permeability of small vessel walls favor the deposition of complement-fixing complexes. In support of this mechanism are data suggesting that prophylactic use of antihistaminic agents may reduce clinical serum sickness in high-risk populations—an effect also shown in animal models.

Serum sickness is typically a brief illness and may require no medication. However, discomfort may be relieved with regular doses of aspirin for fever and joint pain, as well as antihistaminic drugs and, when needed, epinephrine to suppress urticaria and angioedema. When these measures do not suffice, particularly when urinary tract or neurologic changes are suggested, a brief course of corticosteroid treatment is justified. Careful prospective avoidance of the implicated antigen is essential, because acute systemic reactions and a more prompt reappearance of serum sickness may develop if exposure recurs.

Prolonged antigen exposure in individuals with only modest antibody responses can promote a chronic condition in which complexes formed in relative antigen excess circulate continuously. This situation may be readily produced in laboratory animals and, in humans, occurs with SLE, bacterial endocarditis, and prolonged infections, including malaria, syphilis, and leprosy. Deposition of immune complexes affects the kidney in particular, where antigen, as well as the host antibody and complement (singly or in combination), may be demonstrated along the glomerular basement membrane or between adjacent capillaries (Fig. 12-5). As an apparent result of these

---

*Most of these factors are likely IgE; however, in a few cases studied, this activity may have resided in other immunoglobulin classes.

KEY CONCEPTS

■ Most antibody responses require that the antigen first be processed by an antigen-presenting cell, be presented to a specific T_H cell, and be transferred with "help-promoting" soluble factors to one or more specifically reactive B cells. The latter cells multiply and mature into antibody-forming cells, which, as plasma cells, secrete immunoglobulins (i.e., proteins with the properties of antibody).

■ Antigen exposure may also result in T_c (cytotoxic T) lymphocytes, which kill other cells that display a sensitizing antigen, such as a virus or a tumor marker.

■ A failure to respond will occur when a cell subset, cell receptor, or normally secreted factor is missing; the resulting immunologic unresponsiveness can block immune events induced by all or most antigens.

■ The appearance of autoantibodies or autoreactive T_c cells implies either an acquired mutation among immunocompetent cells or activation of "forbidden" cells that had been suppressed but not eliminated.

■ Human antibody-dependent, autoimmune disorders mainly affect formed elements of the blood, with platelets and RBCs attacked most often.

■ Increasing evidence has linked the disease, *idiopathic thrombocytopenic purpura (ITP)*, with circulating IgG molecules reactive with host platelets.

■ Hemolytic transfusion, reactions are a distinctive form of *immunohemolytic (IH) processes* usually occurring when a recipient, already sensitized to

"foreign" human RBC antigens by pregnancy or prior transfusion receives blood containing these antigens.

■ The *Coombs' test* provides information central to the description of IH disorders.

■ Hemolytic reactions to transfused blood provide the most dramatic and dangerous IH phenomena observed clinically. Considering these dire consequences, every reasonable measure to prevent or mitigate hemolytic transfusion reactions is justified.

■ *Goodpasture's syndrome* is a rare disorder that exemplifies antibody-mediated human autoimmunity causing major damage to internal organs (predominantly lung and kidney).

■ *Serum sickness* is considered the prototypic immune complex–induced illness and requires exposure to an antigenic material that will remain in the circulation until a specific antibody response occurs; deposition in tissue of resulting complexes promotes inflammation.

■ *Delayed-type hypersensitivity (DTH)*, mediated by specifically sensitized lymphocytes, provides a major defense against fungi, viruses, and bacteria adapted to intracellular growth and also deters growth of malignant cells.

■ DTH also underlies responses that seems to lack any current protective function; the most familiar of these is *allergic eczematous contact dermatitis (AECD)*.

QUESTIONS

A sampling of review questions for this chapter appears here. Visit http://www.mosby.com/MERLIN/PriceWilson/ for additional questions.

Answer the following on a separate sheet of paper.

1. What is the significance of the appearance of autoantibodies?
2. Describe the way in which immune responses to tissue components might arise.
3. Describe Goodpasture's syndrome as an apparent example of antibody-mediated human autoimmunity.
4. What are the usual manifestations (signs and symptoms) of transfusion reactions?
5. Evaluate the measures that must be employed to prevent or mitigate hemolytic transfusion reactions.
6. What reactions can occur when serums containing potent leukoagglutinins have been infused?

Match the immunologic mechanisms in column B with the conditions to which they correspond in column A.

Column A	Column B
7. _____ Goodpasture's syndrome	a. Immune complex–induced systemic reaction
8. _____ Serum sickness	b. Non–organ-specific autoimmunity disorder
9. _____ Allergic eczematous contact dermatitis (AECD)	c. Organ specific autoimmune disorder
10. _____ Idiopathic thrombocytopenic purpura (ITP)	d. Delayed-type hypersensitivity reaction

Adverse Reactions to Drugs and Related Substances

WILLIAM R. SOLOMON

𝓜ore than 10% of patients who receive indicated drugs experience unforeseen adverse effects from their medication, which constitutes a substantial public health problem and causes a serious waste of human and material resources.

NONIMMUNOLOGIC REACTIONS

Many adverse responses are unwanted (but recognized) associated effects of drugs, or they represent frank toxicity arising from the dose used or its rate of administration. However, the reactions of some individuals are unique and inappropriate; these are called *idiosyncratic reactions*. Personal response patterns and instances of readily induced toxicity may arise from inborn deficiencies in drug-metabolizing capability or related pharmacogenetic defects. Reactions that mimic immunologic events are observed with drugs that cause direct histamine release from human mast cells (Fig. 13-1). Agents such as morphine alkaloids, thiamine, polymyxin, and *d*-tubocurarine share this property and produce whealing at injection sites or, rarely, generalized hives and flushing after injection. A similar mechanism may be responsible for common adverse events (e.g., flushing, hypotension, urticaria) after intravenous (IV) injection of radiographic contrast media. Local anesthetics often precipitate distressing reactions marked by syncope, hypotension, cardiac rhythm disturbances, and, at times,

convulsions. Although reminiscent of anaphylaxis, these reactions are generally more likely a direct toxic effect of the large drug doses required for local infiltration. High blood levels may result, particularly when these agents are injected with some force into restricted tissue compartments, as often occurs for dental procedures. Many reactions involving skin or internal organs (or both) are otherwise unexplained and are often termed *allergic*;

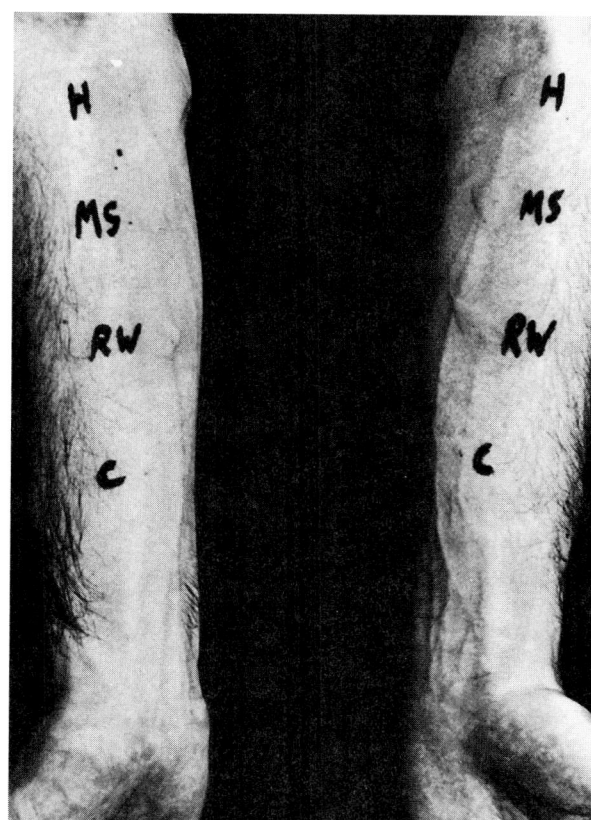

FIG. 13-1   Skin test sites injected intracutaneously with histamine, morphine sulfate (a histamine releaser), ragweed pollen extract, and a saline solution control. Several mechanisms have produced similar wheals in this ragweed-sensitive subject.

however, a causative immunologic process has been established in only a small fraction of these.

IMMUNOLOGIC REACTIONS

Type I reactions, apparently mediated by immunoglobulin E (IgE) antibodies, occur with systemically administered agents, such as foreign sera (e.g., antilymphocyte globulin). These agents act as complete antigens along with those of small molecular size that are capable of stable binding to host proteins. Adverse reactions to penicillins exemplify the latter mechanism, in which a drug or its metabolites (or both) serve as *haptens*. The sensitizing agent may produce anaphylaxis, as well as "late" urticaria, with onset after 24 or 48 to 72 hours; penicillins may also produce immunohemolytic (IH) reactions, serum sickness, and allergic eczematous contact dermatitis (AECD). IgE responses to *injected* antigens are possible in most people; therefore the risk of immediate systemic and urticarial reactions is not confined to, or even concentrated among, the atopic population. In human subjects, penicillin metabolism can proceed along several potential pathways, involving many final and intermediate products, some of which are allergenic. Of the resulting substances, the penicilloyl radical appears to be the predominant sensitizer, and antibodies with this specificity are frequently associated with late urticarial and, at times, acute systemic reactions. By contrast, systemic (anaphylactic) responses with potentially fatal consequences make up a major proportion of the adverse reactions referable to native penicillin G or derivatives that include penicilloic and penilloic acids. Based on the frequency of associated reactions rather than on their relative severity, the penicilloyl radical is often designated as the "major determinant" of penicillin allergy and the others as "minor determinants."

In clarifying the antigens responsible for penicillin sensitivity, efforts were directed to identify reactive subjects. This goal was attained, however, only after development of a skin-reactive but nonsensitizing "major determinant" reagent, through conjugation of numerous penicilloyl groups to the synthetic peptide poly-L-lysine. Skin testing with the product, *benzylpenicilloyl-polylysine* (PPL),* is now widely performed, although minor determinant materials are less readily available. These regents can clarify reported previous reactions and of the future risk of untoward events. In practice, skin tests are performed initially with PPL, a mixture of minor determinants, and saline solution as a control. Penicillin G is applied in a strength of 10,000 units/ml, unless extreme sensitivity is suggested, in which case testing is begun at 10 units/ml. Because higher levels may produce skin irritation, 10,000 units/ml is the highest penicillin G concentration employed for testing. If epidermal sites are negative, intracutaneous tests are then performed (see Chapter 9) with 0.02 ml portions of PPL, penicillin G, other minor determinants, and the control. Persons who react negatively to all these materials have been shown empirically to tolerate therapeutic doses of penicillin G

with essentially no danger of *acute systemic* reactions. A fraction of nonreactors to PPL may show late urticarial responses or ultimately a picture of serum sickness. Additionally, indications suggest that not all persons with positive PPL reactions would have adverse responses to administered penicillin. However, the predictive value of these test procedures is strong, and the high risk associated with positive skin reactivity (particularly to minor determinants) is daunting. Unfortunately, patterns of skin and systemic reactivity to semisynthetic penicillins (e.g., methicillin, ampicillin, carbenicillin) do not always parallel those to penicillin G and its derivatives.

Furthermore, those with previous adverse reactions to penicillins are at increased risk of harm with cephalosporin agents. These issues are especially distressing because only the unmodified, parenteral forms of newer penicillins and cephalosporins are available for testing (usually performed at 6 mg/ml). Additionally, a single set of negative skin tests cannot predict freedom from adverse reactivity months and years later when that drug is repeated.

An immunologic basis can usually be shown by skin testing for acute systemic and urticarial reactions to various immunizing biologicals, penicillins, and cephalosporins but rarely for additional drugs, including aspirin.

In rare instances, autoimmune phenomena are also clearly related to the administration of specific medications. Several drugs, for example, including hydralazine, procainamide, phenytoin, and certain ovulatory suppressants, may promote formation of antinuclear antibodies. Furthermore, some affected persons manifest symptoms that mimic systemic lupus erythematosus and recede slowly only after the offending drug has been withdrawn. Additional agents (e.g. alpha-methyldopa) in some way induce red blood cell (RBC) autoantibodies that lead to positive direct Coombs' tests and, in a few instances, bring on spherocytosis and frank hemolysis. Drug-associated hemolysis has also occurred in patients receiving large IV doses of penicillin because of acquired sensitivity to a penicillin-conjugated RBC substance. Responsible immunoglobulin G (IgG) molecules participate in the direct and indirect Coombs' reactions using, respectively, patients' cells and "penicillinized" normal cells. Hemolysis characteristically begins 1 to 2 weeks after initiation of high-dose penicillin treatment but ceases shortly after drug cessation.

Although hemolysis is not a feature of classic serum sickness, drug-associated circulating complexes are known to facilitate RBC, leukocyte, and platelet destruction in certain situations. These occurrences have been associated prominently with quinidine, antituberculous drugs (p-aminosalicylic acid and isoniazid), and sulfonamides, although other medications have been implicated. Initially, complexes of host IgG or IgM and the drug (or drug-protein conjugate) become attached to one or more blood cell types. Complement components are then localized to these surface sites, and their interaction (see Fig. 5-13) results in discrete membrane lesions or enhanced removal of affected cells from the circulation. In this process, blood elements are injured as "innocent bystanders" rather than as direct participants. After fixation of complement factors, the immune complexes ini-

---

*Available under the trade name Pre-Pen.

tially responsible often dissociate from affected membranes. These cells may show Coombs' reactivity with antisera specific only for human complement (i.e., positive "nongamma" Coombs' tests).*

Many additional forms of adverse drug reactivity are encountered with some frequency; of these, however, only allergic eczematous contact dermatitis (AECD) also has a well-defined immunologic basis, that is, in type IV (cell-mediated) hypersensitivity (see Chapter 12). A remarkably high proportion of topically applied agents are known to elicit contact sensitivity; among the foremost offenders are penicillin, aminoglycoside antibiotics, antihistaminic drugs, and local anesthetics.

ADDITIONAL IMMUNOLOGIC REACTIONS OF UNCERTAIN MECHANISM

Fever is a feature of many drug reactions and is occasionally the sole manifestation of adverse response. Because granulocytes, monocytes, and other cells release substances that indirectly elevate body temperature, not surprisingly, fever accompanies a variety of health problems. Drug-related fever has been noted particularly with penicillin, sulfonamides, iodide, streptomycin, and phenytoin (Dilantin), as well as additional agents.

Nitrofurantoin, a drug often used to treat urinary tract infections, has been associated with distinctive adverse effects centered in the respiratory tract. Affected individuals develop fever, cough, and variable chest discomfort, often with a striking increase in peripheral blood eosinophil numbers. Chest radiographic films obtained during these reactions are often abnormal, showing diffuse lung infiltrates and, at times, fluid in the pleural spaces. These rapidly developing changes tend to resolve completely when nitrofurantoin is promptly discontinued; however, a chronic increase in lung fibrous connective tissue may occur without acute manifestations in patients who are receiving the drug over long periods.

Many drugs are directly *nephrotoxic* (i.e., they cause kidney dysfunction or damage or both). Additionally, several of the penicillins, particularly methicillin, have been implicated in diffuse renal inflammatory reactions, or "interstitial nephritis." Drug-specific antibody responses are often demonstrable, but their significance remains controversial. Kidney damage has been associated frequently with fever and skin rash and may result from immune complex deposition.

The *liver* is a principal site of drug metabolism and often bears the brunt of adverse reactions to therapy. A spectrum of tissue effects is recognized, with certain agents characteristically leading to cholestasis (a failure of bile transport) with little or no inflammation and other agents mimicking florid viral hepatitis in causing necrosis of liver cells and collapse of supporting tissues. Cholestasis is an infrequent complication of treatment with certain anabolic steroids, as well as some oral contraceptives, erythromycin estolate,† chlorpropamide, and

so on. Bile stasis and jaundice also occur in reaction to chlorpromazine; however, pathologically, dense infiltration of portal areas with neutrophils, eosinophils, and macrophages is an additional feature, and progression to permanent liver damage is a possibility. Hepatitis has resulted during treatment with isoniazid, alpha-methyldopa, phenytoin, thiazide diuretics, and additional drugs, including the anesthetic agents halothane and methoxyflurane. These drugs may be associated with acute fatal reactions or may lead to a picture of chronic liver inflammation and scarring (i.e., a form of cirrhosis). In some instances, fever, joint pains, peripheral blood eosinophilia, and skin rashes may precede evidence of liver involvement. Although these manifestations have increased speculation concerning an "allergic" basis for these reactions, the case for immune causation is preliminary, at best.

By far the largest proportion of familiar adverse drug reactions affect the *skin*. The resulting lesions are generally transient and not at all distinctive. Most "drug rashes" consist of macules (flat red spots) or papules (raised red spots), which are pruritic and tend to coalesce into a morbilliform (rubeola-like) eruption. In the case of penicillin, maculopapular rash may be associated with reactions in tissue of drug-specific IgM antibodies; however, this has not been suggested for other agents. Failure to withdraw the responsible medication may lead to an exfoliative dermatitis, in which the skin is effectively shed, leading to serious infection, as well as heat and fluid losses. Additional common manifestations of adverse response to systemic medication include eruptions that are erythematous (diffuse flush), eczematous, vesicular (small blisters), bullous (large blisters), petechial (tiny hemorrhagic spots), purpuric (large hemorrhagic patches), and urticarial. Firm hemorrhagic spots ("palpable purpura") suggest inflammatory lesions of small blood vessels (vasculitis), which can involve diverse organs. Reactions to iodides and bromides may consist of pustules or merely worsening acne vulgaris on the face and upper back. Skin reactions are occasionally confined to discrete patches of rash (i.e., "fixed drug eruptions"), which become inflamed with each administration of the responsible systemic agent.

PREVENTIVE MEASURES

The prevention of adverse drug responses is a serious responsibility that all health care personnel share. An effective approach to this problem requires knowledge of the potential complications of medication and a willingness to consider adverse drug reactivity as a possible cause of *any* unexpected clinical event. Because untoward responses usually recur with reexposure, no drug should be given without first reviewing the individual's prior experience with that agent. Similarly, the clinical database requires no less than a comprehensive assessment of prior drug reactivity. Health care personnel must also be prepared to accept, at face value, reports of previous problems arising from medication until these have been disproved conclusively.

Close surveillance can reveal the earliest stigmata of drug reactions, facilitating prompt withdrawal of the

---

*"Nongamma" Coombs' test reactions are obtained using antiserums to human serum components other than the gamma globulin fraction or specific immunoglobulin classes that it comprises.

†Less often, however, than other salts of erythromycin.

offender and, often, limiting morbidity. Once recognized, adverse reactivity must be clearly indicated in the clinical record (Fig. 13-2), when possible, and made clear to the patient or responsible family members. Documentation (and recall) is aided, for practical purposes, if the patient can carry a card, bracelet, or medallion indicating medications to be avoided. Careful instruction is also necessary when a risk of reaction from related agents exists or when, as with aspirin, the offender has many readily available and poorly identified sources.

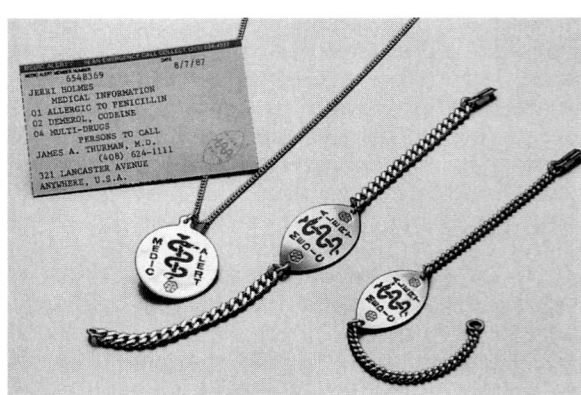

FIG. 13-2 Adverse drug reactivity may be minimized by clearly identifying those at risk. Well-marked health records and personal identification, as shown, complement patient education. (From Judd RL, Ponsell PP: *Mosby's first responder*, ed 2, St Louis, 1988, Mosby.)

KEY CONCEPTS

- More than 10% of patients who receive indicated drugs experience unforeseen adverse effects from their medication, which constitutes a substantial public health problem and causes a serious waste of human and material resources.
- Many adverse responses are unwanted (but recognized) associated effects of drugs, or they represent toxicity arising from the dose used or its rate of administration.
- Idiosyncratic reactions in some individuals are unpredictable "personal" responses that may reflect unique patterns of drug metabolism.
- Reactions that mimic immunologic events are observed with drugs that cause direct histamine release from human mast cells and basophils.
- Many reactions involving skin and internal organs are not otherwise explained and are often termed allergic. However, a causative immunologic process has been established in only a small fraction of these cases.
- Type I reactions, apparently mediated by IgE antibodies, occur with systemically administered agents, such as foreign sera (e.g., antilymphocyte globulin).

- Adverse reactions to penicillins exemplify the latter mechanism, in which a drug or its metabolites (or both) serve as haptens, coupling to body proteins for active antigens (allergens).
- IgE responses to *injected* antigens (e.g., penicillins) are possible in most individuals; the risk of immediate systemic and urticarial reactions is not confined to the atopic population.
- Skin testing with the product, penicilloyl polylysine (PPL), is now widely performed to assist testing for hypersensitivity to penicillin.
- The liver is a principal site of drug metabolism and often bears the brunt of adverse reactions to therapy.
- By far the largest proportion of familiar adverse drug reactions affect the skin in which most drug rashes consist of macules (flat red spots) or papules (raised red spots), which are pruritic and tend to coalesce into a morbilliform (rubeola-like) eruption.
- Close surveillance can reveal the earliest signs of adverse drug reactions, facilitating prompt withdrawal of the offender and, often, limiting morbidity. Eliciting history that provides clues to increased risk and acting accordingly is, however, the most effective safety measure.

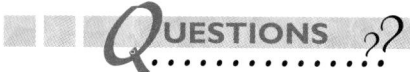

QUESTIONS ⁇

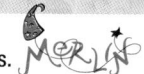

A sampling of review questions for this chapter appears here. Visit http://www.mosby.com/MERLIN/PriceWilson/ for additional questions.

Match the medication in column A with its characteristic reaction in column B. More than one item from column B may be used in column A.

Column A
1. _____ Morphine alkaloids
2. _____ Chlorpropamide
3. _____ Isoniazid
4. _____ Iodides
5. _____ Halothane
6. _____ Penicillin

Column B
a. Bile stasis and jaundice
b. Hepatitis
c. Maculopapular rashes
d. Chronic liver inflammation and scarring
e. Whealing at injection sites
f. Pustules or worsening facial and upper dorsal lesions of acne vulgaris

Answer the following on a separate sheet of paper.

7. Explain the basis of the adverse reactions observed with drug-associated circulating complexes that affect blood elements.

8. List the reactions typically associated with the administration of local anesthetics. What is the probable mechanism of these reactions?

9. Discuss the considerations that are helpful in reducing the prevalence of adverse drug responses.

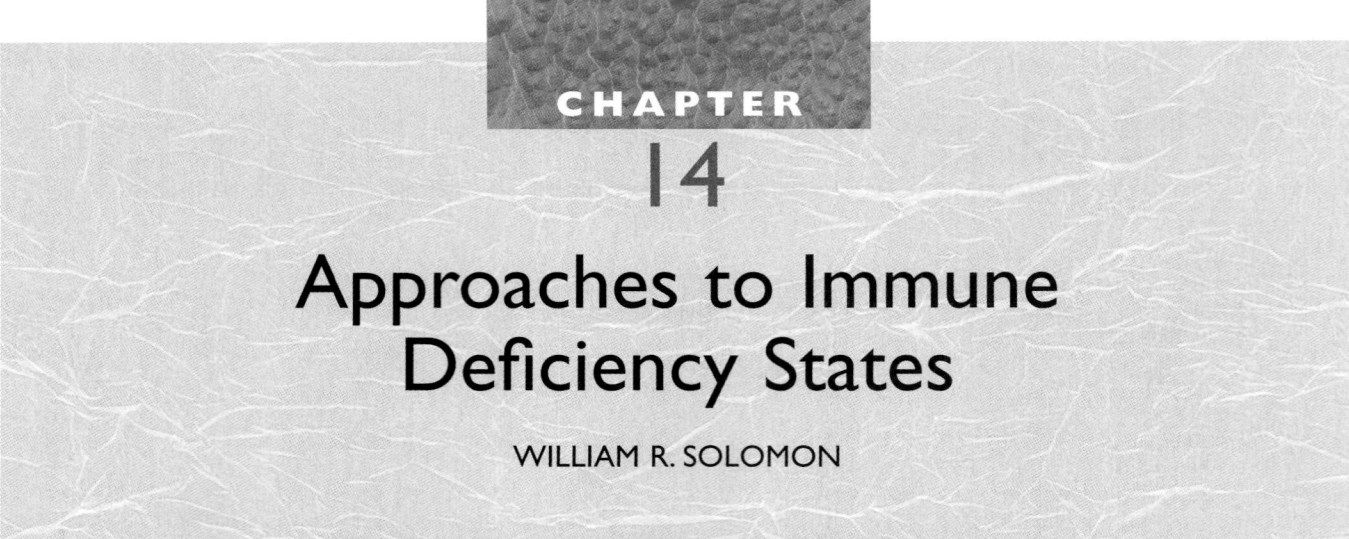

Approaches to Immune Deficiency States

WILLIAM R. SOLOMON

*C*urrent views of immune function emphasize the complex integration of antigen-specific components and effector systems required for normal humoral and cellular hypersensitivity. Both inborn and acquired defects have been recognized; the resulting flaws in immune competence may have no clinical consequences or may open the way for catastrophic infection and neoplastic disease. No attempt is made here to describe or catalog various immunodeficiency disease states; rather, this chapter focuses briefly on methods of evaluating immune function as they relate to these conditions. The related but separate topic of acquired immunodeficiency syndrome (AIDS) is discussed in Chapter 15.

Deficits in humoral (i.e., antibody-mediated) immunity frequently undermine defenses against virulent bacteria, many of which are encapsulated and stimulate pus formation. Hosts with impaired antibody function are likely to have recurrent infections of the skin, middle ear, and meninges, as well as of paranasal sinuses and bronchopulmonary structures. Repeated attacks by bacteria of a single type of antigen are often demonstrable, and, in those with the greatest impairment, naturally acquired viral infections and live viral vaccines may also cause serious disseminated illness.

Assaying serum immunoglobulins by nephelometry now is widely used to measure levels of immunoglobin (Ig)—IgG, IgA, IgM, and IgD—in human serum. By mixing antihuman Ig isotope (e.g., goat antihuman IgA) with serum, immune aggregates are formed and the degree of turbidity produced is measured by their ability to scatter light. Radial immunodiffusion (Fig. 14-1) is an older but more graphic method using the same reagents. In this procedure, test serums and samples of known Ig content are placed in separate wells cut into agar that contains antiserum to human IgA, IgG, IgM, or IgD. As the human serum diffuses outward, a line of precipitation forms at the forward edge, where a favorable ratio of antiserum and specific human Ig is achieved; within this perimeter, an excess of the Ig (here, serving as the antigen) suppresses precipitation.* The ring

diameter around each well is proportional to the Ig content of the test serum added, and absolute levels are derived by referring to assayed "known" samples. (Determination of IgE content requires alternative techniques using radioactive or other amplification markers because of the lower range in which levels of this Ig fall.) Normal total values for specific Ig classes are indicated in Table 14-1. More discrete deficiencies of one or more of the IgG subclasses (i.e., IgG_1 to IgG_4) are also recognized to promote bacterial infection.

Several methods are available to evaluate antigen-specific antibody activity associated with one or more Ig classes, including the following:

1. Determination of naturally occurring (IgM) antibodies to ABO blood group substances that are absent from subjects' red blood cells (RBCs). Normal individuals consistently demonstrate such isohemagglutinins by age 1 year.
2. Schick testing of patients previously immunized with diphtheria toxoid. If adequate levels of specific (IgG) antibody have been produced, then tissue breakdown at the site of toxin injection is prevented.
3. Determination of antibody titers before and after administering nonviable immunizing materials using proteins (tetanus toxoid and influenza vaccines) or pneumococcal polysaccharides (Pneumovax). A pronounced rise in neutralizing antibody should occur. These determinations are generally available from state or large municipal health departments.

Additionally, *immunofluorescent staining* of the Ig molecules that are typically prominent on their cell surfaces is used to estimate the number of circulating B lymphocytes. In the blood of normal individuals, approximately 15% to 20% of lymphocytes bear these markers, identifying them as B lymphocytes. Additional markers, such as CD19* also are useful with quantification using fluorescence-activated cell sorters (FACS).

---

* Outside the ring, the assayed Ig content is too low to allow precipitate to form.

---

* The cluster designation (CD) system is used to define groups (clusters) of cells that bear a particular membrane component as defined by the binding to them of a specific monoclonal antibody. Certain CD-defined specificities may be found on several different types of cells; some are associated with molecules having well-recognized functions.

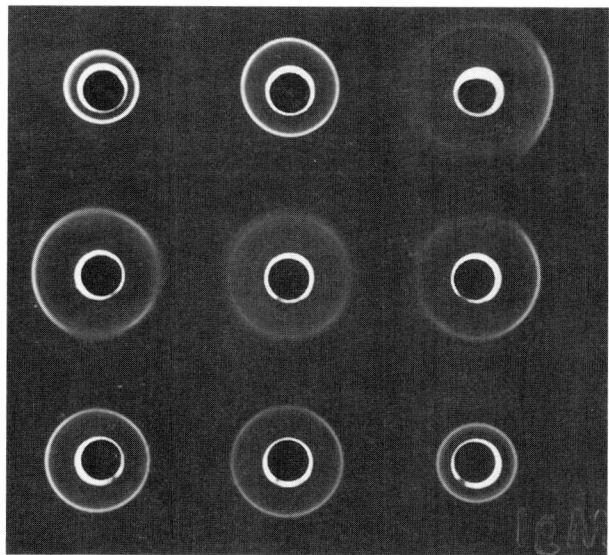

FIG. 14-1 Determination of immunoglobulin (Ig) levels by radial immunodiffusion. The agar plate shown contains goat antihuman IgM. The IgM content of samples added to the wells is evidenced by the diameters of the resulting circles of precipitation. The uppermost row of wells contains known serums of increasing IgM content *(left to right)*, allowing the system to be calibrated. The lower six wells are loaded with sera from individual patients.

TABLE 14-1 ■ ■ ■

Normal Serum Immunoglobulin (Ig) Levels at Various Ages (in years)*

Age	IgG (mg/dl)	IgA (mg/dl)	IgM (mg/dl)	IgE (IU/ml†)
At birth	650-1250	1-6	5-35	1-3
1-3	250-1320	15-160	15-115	10-500
5-10	550-1450	20-220	30-135	15-600
10-15	620-1450	30-230	35-150	20-750
Adult	720-1800	60-300	45-160	25-900

*Values are approximations of expected ranges derived from several sources.
†IU (international unit) = 2.3 nanograms (ng) IgE.

In certain immunodeficiency states, early B cell forms showing either *no* surface Ig or IgM and IgD *alone* may be found. The numbers and functional state of T lymphocytes also affect antibody secretion, because antigen recognition by T cells must precede most antibody (humoral) responses. T helper cells that bear the CD4 membrane marker also drive B cell proliferation and development into Ig-secreting plasma cells. Conversely, T suppressor cells (bearing CD8) may act to down-regulate B cell responses. Determining the numbers of these T cell subsets can provide a clue to factors responsible for defective antibody responses, as well as impaired cell-mediated immunity (CMI). Currently, FACS analysis, using appropriately specific monoclonal antibodies, rapidly accomplishes these assays. In acquired immunodeficiency syndrome (AIDS) (see Chapter 15), the human immunodeficiency virus type 1 (HIV-1) directly attacks the CD4 molecule and progressively destroys the helper

T cells that bear it; as a result, specific antibody responses and CMI are impaired.

The most frequently encountered form of continuing antibody-dependent immunodeficiency is a selective *deficit of IgA*, which is observed in 1 in every 500 to 1000 patients. Serum levels of IgA are less than 5 mg/dl in this condition, and at mucosal surfaces, IgG and IgM typically replace the normal preponderance of IgA. Some affected individuals remain free of evident illness, but many manifest recurrent paranasal sinus and pulmonary infections. Additionally, increased risks of atopic allergic problems and certain rheumatic and gastrointestinal diseases appear to exist in this condition. Replacement of deficient serum IgA is not feasible, and systemic reactions caused by anti-IgA antibodies may follow transfusion of human blood products containing IgA (see Chapter 12).

Male patients with (Bruton's) *X-linked hypogammaglobulinemia* exhibit the most severe selective deficiency of humoral immune function, with virtual absence of circulating immunoglobulins and B cells. These individuals also have marked reduction in the size and structural organization of lymph nodes and lymphoid tissues of the pharynx and gut (see Chapter 5). Recurrent purulent infections usually begin after 4 to 6 months of age, when transplacentally acquired levels of maternal IgG have been cleared and are no longer protective. Otitis media, bronchitis, pneumonitis, meningitis, and skin infections are prominent and often lead to permanent organ damage, such as bronchiectasis. Additionally, viruses, including hepatitis B and attenuated strains present in certain vaccines, may produce severe illnesses, at times with central nervous system damage. Rapidly progressive tooth decay and chronic conjunctivitis often add to patients' discomfort, and an eczematous dermatitis, arthritis resembling rheumatoid disease, and intestinal malabsorption are frequently associated. The administration of commercial gamma globulin by injection controls many of these problems and complements appropriate antibiotic treatment; adequate doses usually approximate 0.2 to 0.4 ml/kg every 2 to 4 weeks. These preparations contain no IgA or IgM and, possibly as a result, fail to control infection in some patients despite maximal doses. Although intramuscular (IM) administration was previously the norm, preparations largely free of molecular aggregates now permit safe, high-dose intravenous (IV) replacement.

Individuals of either sex with low Ig levels and infections beginning after infancy are observed with some frequency. This group with acquired, "common, variable immunodeficiency (hypogammaglobulinemia)" often have prominent lymph nodes and intestinal lymphoid aggregates, as well as normal numbers of circulating B cells. However, Ig synthesis or secretion (or both) tends to be deficient. As a result, these patients experience recurrent and sustained sinopulmonary infections, as well as intestinal malabsorption, often augmented by infection with the protozoan *Giardia lamblia*. Affected patients and their relatives have an increased risk of autoantibodies and related diseases, including idiopathic thrombocytopenic purpura (ITP), immunohemolytic (IH) anemia, pernicious anemia, systemic lupus erythematosus (SLE), and rheumatoid arthritis, as well as lymphatic malignancy. Laboratory evidence of impaired

T cell function has also been obtained in some patients. Appropriate antibiotic therapy and Ig replacement provide substantial benefit in most cases, however.

Humoral immunodeficiency is especially prominent in certain malignant states (e.g., multiple myeloma, chronic lymphocytic leukemia) and becomes a concern whenever tumor cells infiltrate lymphoreticular structures. Similar infectious problems (with pyogenic bacteria) may develop in individuals who are deficient in one or more serum complement factors and those with inadequate leukocyte numbers or function. Serum levels of C3 may be assayed by radial immunodiffusion. Additionally, overall complement activity is usually estimated from the ability of test serums to facilitate hemolysis of optimally sensitized RBCs; this capacity is expressed as "CH_{50} activity." Granulocyte deficiencies may be inborn or may accompany conditions such as alcoholism or corticosteroid excess. Defects in leukocyte function may affect random movement, directed movement (chemotaxis), phagocytosis, formation of enzymatically active vacuoles, and intracellular killing. These modalities can be examined individually with acceptable precision in only a few laboratories. More generally available studies include the white blood cell (WBC) count, leukocyte morphology in peripheral blood smears, and peroxidase stain to confirm the content of myeloperoxidase, a leukocyte enzyme required for intracellular killing of certain ingested organisms.

Additionally, quantitative assay of *nitroblue tetrazolium* (NBT) dye reduction provides a valuable clue to the diagnosis of *chronic granulomatous disease* (CGD) (of childhood). Recurrent infection by the fungus *Aspergillus fumigatus*, as well as *Staphylococcus aureus (Micrococcus pyogenes)*, *Pseudomonas* species, *Escherichia coli*, and organisms normally of low virulence (e.g., *Serratia, Staphylococcus epidermidis, Candida*) are typical of this X-linked disorder.* Offending organisms are ingested normally but escape death and can multiply intracellularly, ultimately destroying the inept phagocytes; a clinical picture of recurrent abscesses, indolent drainage of lymph nodes, osteomyelitis, pneumonia, and persistent diarrhea results. Defective killing appears to reflect impaired leukocyte metabolism with decreased generation of hydrogen peroxide and related substances that inactivate living microorganisms.† The metabolic defect also precludes the normal reduction of NBT to a readily visible blue-black form, a deficit easily quantitated by colorimetric assay, useful as a disease marker, and increasingly subject to confirmation by deoxyribonucleic acid (DNA) analysis; several possible gene defects are described.

Cell-mediated immune function is inadequate in many disease states either as a "primary defect" or secondary to disorders, including sarcoidosis, Hodgkin's disease, certain non-Hodgkin's neoplasms, and uremia; therapy with corticosteroids or cytotoxic drugs (e.g., cyclophosphamide) is also a frequent factor. CMI may also be impaired transiently by viral infections such as rubeola (measles). Of the steadily growing list of conditions associated with abnormalities of T cell function, many also

display some aberrant humoral (i.e., B cell–dependent) function.* Overall, individuals with these disorders are prone to infection by characteristic organisms that include viruses, protozoa (particularly *Pneumocystis carinii*), fungi, and bacteria (particularly intracellular forms). Lymphoreticular malignancies are common terminal complications of many of these disorders.

Relatively complete absence of T cell function occurs when the thymus fails to develop (as in *DiGeorge syndrome*), and affected infants have been restored immunologically to adequate function with grafts of early fetal thymus tissue. The most compromised individuals have *severe combined immunodeficiency (SCID)*, totally lack B cell and T cell function, and often succumb within the first year of life. Transplantation of bone marrow from optimally matched donors has permitted survival, and partial reconstitution has been achieved with early fetal liver or thymus grafts. A variety of other conditions with combined defects are recognized; most often observed are the *Wiskott-Aldrich syndrome* (eczema, platelet deficiency, low IgM level) and *ataxia telangiectasia* (ataxia, spontaneous movements, vascular malformations of skin and conjunctiva, mental retardation), both of which are familial conditions. AIDS also demonstrates severe defects in cellular and humoral immunity because of the assault of the HIV-1 retrovirus on CD4-bearing T lymphocytes and other cells (see Chapter 15).

A serious concern in any individual with profound T cell deficiency is his or her inability to clear foreign cells, including the WBC fraction of transfused blood. If this risk is overlooked, transfused WBCs may then "reject" the recipient, causing skin, gastrointestinal, and liver lesions, which can be fatal. This type of "graft-versus-host" disease is preventable by irradiating all blood before administration to high-risk recipients.

Although numerous correlates and functional components of CMI are recognized, few are widely tested at present. T cell defects may be reflected in decreased numbers of peripheral blood lymphocytes (the majority of which are T cells), and counts consistently less than $1200/\mu l$ ($2000/\mu l$ in infancy) suggest cellular immunodeficiency. Reactivity to *delayed-type hypersensitivity (DTH)* skin tests provides a readily available indicator of cellular immune competence measuring both antigen processing and cellular response. For this purpose, intradermal injections are performed with 0.1 ml portions of substances that elicit DTH and to which a previous sensitizing exposure may be assumed. Frequently used materials include purified protein derivative of the tubercle bacillus (PPD), tetanus toxoid, and antigens from *Candida albicans*, mumps virus, *Histoplasma capsulatum*, and fungi of superficial skin infections. Test sites are observed and palpated after 48 hours, and an indurated area with a diameter of 10 mm or larger generally is regarded as a positive reaction. Using a "battery" of such materials, at least one positive test should be evident in the vast majority of normal individuals (excluding infants). For nonreactors, the next step has become determination of B and T cell categories using monoclonal antibodies to tag their cell

---

*A variant form in females is known to occur rarely.
†Recently, partial correction of this defect has followed treatment with a lymphokine, gamma interferon.

---

*Because T cell competence is essential for much normal B cell function, this should not be surprising.

TABLE 14-2   ■ ■ ■

Some Commonly Determined CD Markers

Marker	Principal Cell Expression	Function
CD3	T cells	Signal transduction
CD4	Helper T cells	Receptor for MHC*II
CD8	Supressor cytotoxic T cells	Receptor for MHC*I
CD10	Immature (some mature) granulocytes, lymphocytes	?– (an endopeptidase)
CD16	Natural killer (NK) cells, macrophages, some granulocytes	Receptor for IgG Activates NK cells
CD18	Leukocytes	Promotes adhesion to blood vessel walls
CD19	Most B cells	Regulates B cell Activation
CD40	B cells	Receptor for T cell Helper factor
CD64	Monocytes, macrophages	Receptor for IgG Facilitates phagocytosis

*MHC, Major histocompatibility class.

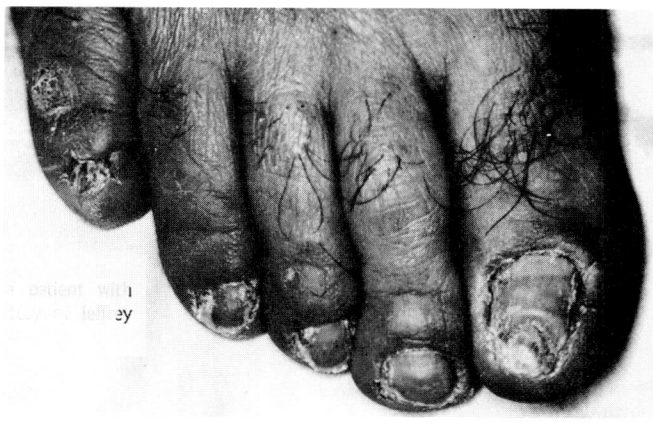

FIG. 14-2   Skin and nail lesions on the foot of a patient with chronic mucocutaneous candidiasis. (Photograph courtesy Jeffrey Callen, MD.)

membrane components. Automated approaches to such assays (i.e., by flow cytometry) can estimate levels of helper-inducer, suppressor-cytotoxic, and null cells, as well as functional subcomponents within these groups (Table 14-2). Additional tests reflecting T cell function may include the following:

1. Response of lymphocytes in short-term tissue culture to antigens and nonspecific agents (e.g., phytohemagglutinin) that stimulate cell division and associated nucleic acid synthesis. An increase in the incorporation of added thymidine tagged with tritium normally is observed in response to these agents.
2. Assays of lymphokines produced in response to appropriate antigens added to lymphocyte preparations (see Chapter 5). Currently available monoclonal antibodies provide an expanding variety of specific reagents.

Antigen-specific defects in CMI also are recognized; perhaps the best-studied example is *chronic mucocutaneous candidiasis* (Fig. 14-2). In this condition, indolent *Candida albicans* infection with granuloma formation occurs. Although systemic dissemination is almost unknown, oral candidiasis (thrush), esophageal involvement with dysphagia (difficulty in swallowing), and *Candida* vaginitis may cause severe distress. Additionally, affected individuals often show autoantibodies reactive with endocrine tissues and defects in endocrine function (particularly adrenal and parathyroid deficiencies) as a possible result. Although CMI to *Candida* is ineffective in this condition, other T cell functions usually are intact. Defective responses to *Candida* antigens vary among patients, being total in some, whereas others show intact lymphocyte mitogenic responses despite negative skin tests at 48 hours; in a few, circulating inhibitors of *Candida*-directed CMI occur. Treatment with azole antifungals and other, newer anti-*Candida* agents has greatly improved the outlook for these patients. Repeated injection of transfer factor (see Chapter 5) prepared from lymphocytes of persons with strong DTH to *Candida* has led to prolonged remissions in some patients but remains an experimental approach.

KEY CONCEPTS

- Deficits in humoral (i.e., antibody-mediated) immunity frequently undermine defenses against virulent bacteria, many of which are encapsulated and stimulate pus formation.
- Hosts with impaired antibody function are likely to have recurrent infections of the gums, middle ear, and meninges, as well as of the paranasal sinuses and bronchopulmonary structures.
- Assay of serum immunoglobulins by nephelometry now is widely used to assess levels of IgG, IgA, IgM and IgD in human serum.
- Methods used to evaluate antigen-specific antibody activity focus on: (1) determination of antibody titers before and after nonviable immunizing materials using proteins (tetanus toxoid and influenza vaccine) pneumococcal polysaccharides (Pneumovax) and Schick testing of persons previously immunized with diphtheria toxoid, and (2) determination of naturally occurring (IgM) antibodies to ABO blood group substances that are absent from subjects' own RBCs.
- The most frequently encountered form of continuing antibody-dependent immunodeficiency is a selective *deficit of IgA*, which is observed in 1 in every 500 to 1000 individuals.
- Male patients with (Bruton's) *X-linked hypogammaglobulinemia* exhibit the most severe selective deficiency of humoral immune function; some T cell defects may occur also.
- Humoral immunodeficiency is especially prominent in certain malignant states, such as multiple myeloma and chronic lymphocytic leukemia and becomes a concern whenever tumor cells infiltrate lymphoreticular structures.
- Cell-mediated immune function is inadequate in many disease states either as a "primary defect" or secondary to disorders, including AIDS, sarcoidosis, Hodgkin's disease, certain non-Hodgkin's neoplasms, and uremia.
- Relatively complete absence of T cell function occurs when the thymus fails to develop (as in *DiGeorge syndrome*), and affected infants have been restored immunologically to adequate function with grafts of early fetal thymus tissue.
- A serious concern in anyone with profound T cell deficiency is their inability to clear foreign cells including the viable WBC of transfused whole blood.

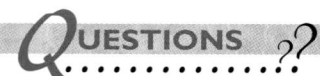

QUESTIONS ??

A sampling of review questions for this chapter appears here. Visit http://www.mosby.com/MERLIN/PriceWilson/ for additional questions.

Answer the following on a separate sheet of paper.

1. List three methods used to evaluate antigen-specific antibody activity associated with one or more Ig classes.
2. Explain the significance of DTH skin tests as an indicator of cellular immune competence.
3. Describe two additional laboratory tests reflecting lymphocyte function.
4. Why is determining the numbers of T cells important in subsets that are involved in antibody (humoral) responses?
5. What are some of the signs of immunodeficiency?
6. Name several types of primary and secondary immunodeficiencies and give an example of each.
7. What is the most common cause of primary selective antibody-dependent immunodeficiency? How is this type of immunodeficiency manifested and what precautions must be taken in administering blood transfusions to an individual with such a condition?

Human Immunodeficiency Virus (HIV) and Acquired Immunodeficiency Syndrome (AIDS)

VIRGINIA MACEDA LAN

Acquired immunodeficiency syndrome (AIDS) first came to the attention of the health community in 1981 after the unusual occurrence of *Pneumocystis carinii* pneumonia (PCP) and Kaposi's sarcoma (KS) in young homosexual men in California (Gottlieb, 1981; Centers for Disease Control, 1981). Epidemiologic evidence suggested that an infectious agent was involved, and in 1983 the human immunodeficiency virus type 1 (HIV-1) was identified as the cause of the disease (Barre-Sinoussi et al, 1983; Gallo, 1984). AIDS comprises a set of defined clinical conditions that are the end result of infection with HIV. The actual cases of AIDS reflect mature, long-standing infection with HIV. Currently, AIDS is found in nearly every country and is a worldwide pandemic.

ETIOLOGY

Formerly called human T cell lymphotrophic virus type III (HTLV-III) or lymphadenopathy virus (LAV), HIV is a cytopathic human retrovirus of the lentivirus family. *Retroviruses* convert their ribonucleic acid (RNA) to deoxyribonucleic acid (DNA) after they enter the host cell. HIV-1 and HIV-2 are cytopathic lentiviruses, with HIV-1 being the most significant cause of AIDS throughout the world.

The HIV genome codes nine proteins essential for every aspect of the life cycle of the virus (Fig. 15-1). In terms of genomic structure, the viruses differ in that the HIV-1 protein, Vpu, which helps in virus release, appears to be replaced by the protein Vpx in HIV-2. Vpx facilitates infectivity and may be a duplication of another protein, Vpr. Vpr is thought to enhance viral transcription. HIV-2, first recognized in serum from West African (Senegalese) women in 1985, causes clinical disease but appears to be less pathogenic compared with HIV-1 (Marlink, 1994).

EPIDEMIOLOGY

HIV-2 is more prevalent in many countries in western Africa, but HIV-1 predominates in central and eastern Africa and the rest of the world. According to the Joint United Nations Program on HIV/AIDS (2000), an estimated 36.1 million people were infected with HIV and AIDS by the end of 2000. Of the 36.1 million cases, 16.4 million were women, and 600,000 were children under 15 years of age. HIV infection has caused approximately 21.8 million deaths since the beginning of the epidemic in the late 1970s to early 1980s. The region of the world most severely affected by HIV and AIDS was Sub-Saharan Africa, where an estimated 25.3 million adults and children were living with the infection and disease at the end of the year 2000 (Fig. 15-2). Another region of concern is South and Southeast Asia, where an estimated 5.8 million people were living with HIV and AIDS during the same period.

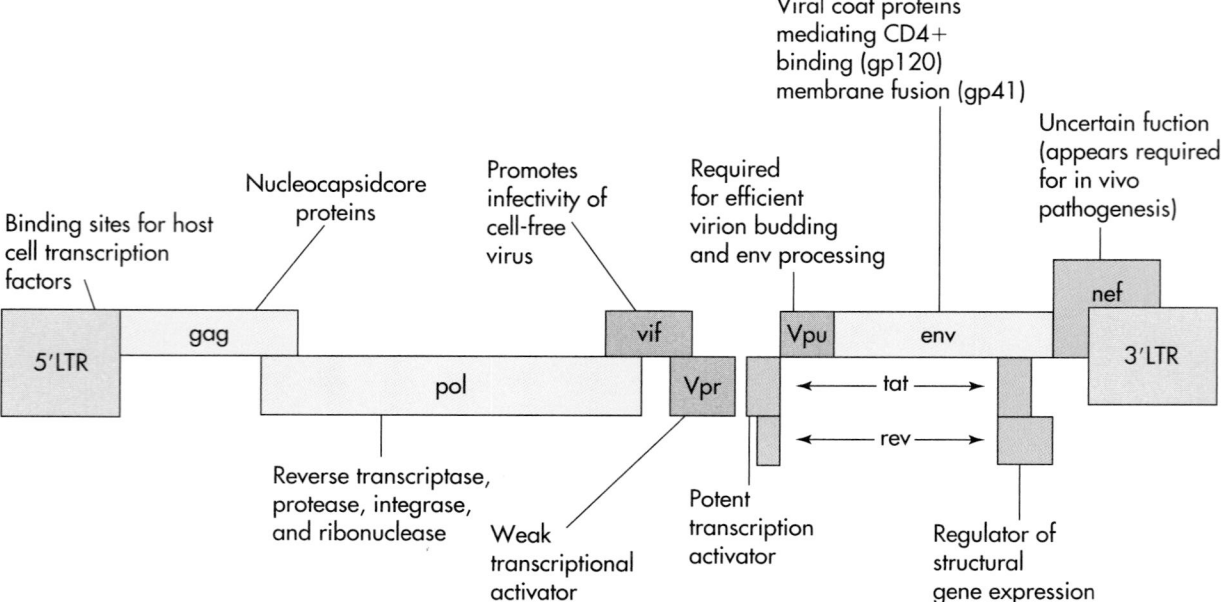

FIG. 15-1 Genomic structure of HIV-1. These genes code for the nine proteins essential for HIV replication. (Modified from Levy J: *HIV and the pathogenesis of AIDS*, Washington, DC, 1994, ASM Press.)

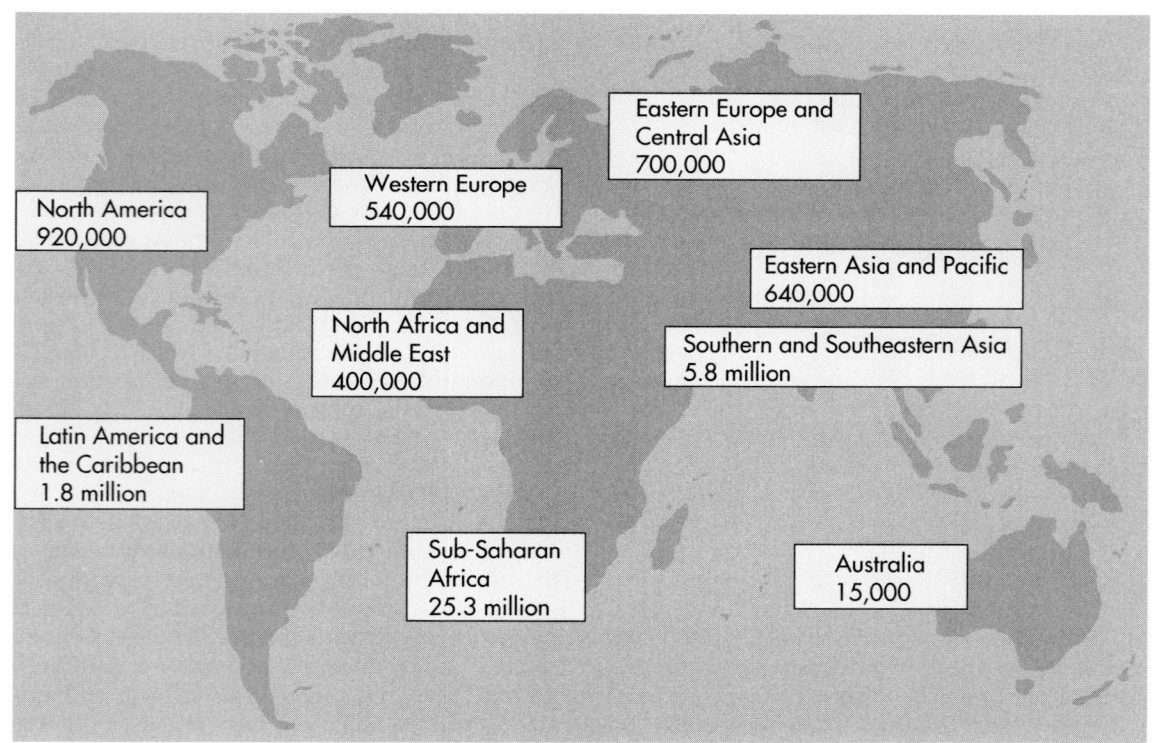

FIG. 15-2 Estimated distribution of adults and children infected with HIV and AIDS at the end of 2000; global total: 36.1 million. (Data from the Joint United Nations Program on AIDS, December 2000.)

Worldwide surveillance is a challenge because no current case definition of AIDS exists that can be used globally (Stanley, Fauci, 1995). Since 1995 the U.S. Centers for Disease Control and Prevention (CDC) case surveillance definition of AIDS was revised three times to reflect new understanding of HIV disease and changes in medical practice. In 1987 wasting syndrome and other conditions were added to the list of indicator diseases diagnosed definitively with laboratory evidence of HIV infection. In 1993 the clinical importance of the CD4+ T lymphocyte count in the categorization of HIV-related clinical conditions was emphasized. This finding led to a revised classification system for HIV infection outlined in Table 15-1. The 1993 expansion of the surveillance

TABLE 15-1 ▪ ▪ ▪

1993 Revised Classification System for HIV Infection and Expanded Surveillance Case Definition Among Adolescents and Adults[*]

CD4+ T Cell Categories	Clinical Categories		
	(A) Asymptomatic, Acute (Primary) HIV, or PGL	**(B)** Symptomatic, Not (A) or (C) Conditions	**(C)** AIDS-Indicator Condition
1. ≥ 500/μl	A1	B1	C1
2. 200-499/μl	A2	B2	C2
3. < 200/μl AIDS indicator T-cell count	A3	B3	C3

Modified from Centers for Disease Control and Prevention: 1993 Revised classification system for HIV infection and expanded surveillance case definition for AIDS among adolescents and adults, *MMWR* 41(RR-17):1-19, December 1992.

[*]The nine-cell matrix combines the three clinical categories associated with HIV infection and three levels of CD4+ lymphocyte counts (see Boxes 15-1 and 15-2). This system replaces the classification system published in 1987. Individuals with AIDS-indicator conditions (C1, C2, C3) and those with CD4+ T-cell counts less than 200/μl (A3, B3) have been counted as AIDS cases since January 1, 1993. Before 1993, individuals in cells A3 and B3 would not have been reportable as AIDS cases.

AIDS, Acquired immunodeficiency syndrome; *HIV,* human immunodeficiency virus; *PGL,* persistent generalized lymphadenopathy.

case definition for AIDS initially resulted in a large increase in the reported AIDS cases for 1993. This increase was a result of the inclusion of individuals diagnosed with severe immunosuppression, which typically occurs before the onset of opportunistic diseases associated with AIDS. By 1997 the CDC reported the first decrease in the number of newly diagnosed AIDS cases attributed to the use of highly active antiretroviral therapy (HAART) in 1996.

Effective January 2000, the CDC's (1999) updated surveillance case definition for HIV infection integrates the reporting criteria for HIV infection and AIDS into a single case definition and incorporates new laboratory tests into the laboratory criteria for HIV case reporting. These new tests are the HIV nucleic acid (DNA or RNA) detection tests that were not commercially available when the AIDS case definition was revised in 1993 (Box 15-1). The 2000 revision takes into consideration the impact of advances in antiretroviral therapy, the implementation of new HIV treatment guidelines, and the increased need for epidemiologic data regarding individuals at all stages of the HIV disease to forecast needed resources and services more accurately.

From 1981 through 2000, 774,467 cumulative AIDS cases have been reported in the United States (CDC, 2000b). Approximately 58% of these cases are known to have died. In December 2000, the CDC reported 127,286 adults and children (under 13 years of age) living with HIV infection and 322,865 with the AIDS disease. This figure includes only individuals diagnosed with HIV infection in states with integrated HIV and AIDS surveillance systems and those diagnosed with AIDS in all states and territories. Of the 322,865 AIDS cases, 79% were men, 61% were African American or Hispanic, and 41% were infected through male-to-male sexual activity. In the early 1980s more AIDS cases occurred among Caucasians. By 1996 more cases occurred among African Americans than any other racial-ethnic groups. Throughout the epidemic, approximately 85% of patients diagnosed with AIDS were aged 20 to 49 years (CDC, 2001a).

The cumulative number of pediatric AIDS cases (children younger than age 13 years) reported to the CDC, as

of December 2000, was 8908. Because pediatric AIDS is predominantly a reflection of prenatal or perinatal infection (vertical transmission), as the rate of HIV in women rises, more infants acquire HIV. The number of perinatally acquired AIDS cases peaked in 1992 and then declined through 1999. The decline was associated with the implementation of Public Health Service guidelines for universal counseling and voluntary HIV testing of pregnant women and the use of zidovudine as a therapy by HIV-infected women and their newborn infants. AIDS among women is transmitted predominantly by the heterosexual mode, followed by injected drug use (CDC, 1999).

PATHOPHYSIOLOGY

Pathogenesis

Transmission and Entry

HIV has been isolated from blood, cerebrospinal fluid, semen, tears, vaginal or cervical secretions, urine, breast milk, and saliva. Transmission occurs most efficiently by means of blood and semen. HIV has also been transmitted via breast milk and vaginal or cervical secretions. The three major means of transmission are blood and sexual and maternal-infant contact. After the virus is transmitted, an elaborate series of steps involved in the infection begins.

Viral Attachment

A mature HIV virion is approximately spherical in shape (Fig. 15-3). Its outer coat, or viral envelope, consists of a lipid bilayer that contains many protein spikes. These spikes include two glycoproteins: gp120 and gp41. Gp refers to the glycoprotein, and the number refers to the mass of the protein in thousands of daltons. Gp120 is the external surface envelope of the spike, and gp41 is the stem or transmembrane portion.

A matrix protein called p17 surrounds the inner segment of the viral membrane. A capsid protein called p24 circumscribes the core. Inside the capsid, p24, are two identical strands of RNA and preformed molecules of

BOX 15-1

CDC Surveillance Case Definition for HIV Infection

The 2000 revised criteria for national reporting combines HIV infection and AIDS in a single case definition. In adults, adolescents, or children aged 18 months* or older, HIV infection surveillance case definition is met if one of the laboratory criteria is positive or clinical evidence exists that is specifically indicative of HIV infection and severe HIV disease (AIDS).

Laboratory evidence of HIV infection consists of repeated positive reactions to antibody screening tests confirmed with supplementary tests (e.g., ELISA, confirmed by the Western blot test) or a positive result or report of a detectable quantity of any of the following HIV virologic or nonantibody tests: (a) HIV p24 antigen test with neutralization assay; (b) HIV viral culture; (c) HIV nucleic acid (DNA or RNA) detection (e.g., polymerase chain reaction or plasma HIV-1 RNA, which is used for infants infected by perinatal exposure).

Clinical criteria include a diagnosis of HIV infection based on the listed laboratory criteria that are documented in a medical record by a physician or conditions that meet criteria included in the case definition for AIDS.

CRITERIA FOR A CASE DEFINITION OF AIDS
A. All HIV-infected individuals with:
  1. CD4+ T cell counts <200/μl or
  2. CD4+ T cell counts <14% of total T cells, regardless of clinical category, symptomatic or asymptomatic
B. Presence of AIDS-related opportunistic infections such as:
  1. Candidiasis of bronchi, trachea, or lungs
  2. Candidiasis, esophageal
  3. Cervical cancer, invasive[†]
  4. Coccidioidomycosis, disseminated or extrapulmonary
  5. Cryptococcus, extrapulmonary
  6. Cryptosporidiosis, chronic intestinal (for more than 1 month duration)
  7. Cytomegalovirus disease (other than liver, spleen, or nodes)
  8. Cytomegalovirus retinitis (with loss of vision)
  9. Encephalopathy, HIV-related
  10. Herpes simplex; chronic ulcer(s) for more than 1 month duration; or bronchitis, pneumonitis, esophagitis
  11. Histoplasmosis, disseminated or extrapulmonary
  12. Isosporiasis, chronic intestinal (for more than 1 month duration)
  13. Kaposi's sarcoma (KS)
  14. Lymphoma, Burkitt's (or equivalent term)
  15. Lymphoma, immunoblastic (or equivalent term)
  16. Lymphoma, primary, of brain
  17. Mycobacterium avium complex or *Mycobacterium kansasii,* disseminated or extrapulmonary
  18. Mycobacterium tuberculosis, any site, pulmonary[†] or extrapulmonary
  19. Mycobacterium, other species or unidentified species, disseminated or extrapulmonary
  20. *Pneumocystis carinii* pneumonia (PCP)
  21. Pneumonia, recurrent
  22. Progressive multifocal leukoencephalopathy
  23. Salmonella septicemia, recurrent
  24. Toxoplasmosis of brain
  25. Wasting syndrome caused by HIV

* Children aged 18 months or older but younger than 13 years are categorized as "not infected with HIV" if they meet other criteria (see CDC [1999], pp. 30-31, for criteria for a child <18 months).
† Added to the 1993 CDC expanded AIDS surveillance case definition.
Modified from Centers for Disease Control and Prevention: 1993 Revised classification system for HIV infection and expanded surveillance case definition for AIDS among adolescents and adults, *MMWR* 41(RR-17):1-17, December, 1992; Centers for Disease Control and Prevention: Guidelines for national human immunodeficiency virus case surveillance, including monitoring for human immunodeficiency virus and acquired immunodeficiency syndrome, *MMWR* 48(RR-13):1-31, December, 1999.

reverse transcriptase, integrase, and protease. HIV is a retrovirus, thus the genetic material is in the form of RNA rather than DNA. *Reverse transcriptase* is the enzyme that transcribes viral RNA into DNA after the virus enters the target cell. Other enzymes accompanying the RNA are integrase and protease.

HIV infects cells by binding to the surface of a target cell that has a CD4 membrane receptor molecule (Fig. 15-4). By far, HIV's preferred target is the CD4-positive T helper lymphocyte, or T4 cell (CD4+ lymphocyte). HIV's gp120 binds tightly to the CD4+ lymphocyte, allowing the gp41 to mediate in the virus-to-cell membrane fusion. Recently, it has been found that two cell surface coreceptors, CCR5 or CXCR4, are necessary for the binding of the gp120 and gp41 glycoproteins to the CD4+ receptor (Doms, Peiper, 1997). These coreceptors cause conformational changes that allow insertion of gp41 into the target cell membrane. Individuals who inherit two defective copies of the CCR5 receptor gene (homozygotes) are resistant to the development of AIDS, despite repeated exposure to HIV (approximately 1% of Caucasian Americans). Individuals who are heterozygotes for the defective gene (18% to 20%) are not protected from AIDS, but the onset of the disease is somewhat delayed. No homozygotes have been found in Asians or African populations, which may help explain their increased susceptibility to HIV infection (O'Brien, Dean, 1997).

Other cells that may be susceptible to HIV infection include monocytes and macrophages. Infected monocytes and macrophages can serve as reservoirs for HIV but are not destroyed by the virus. HIV is polytrophic and may infect a wide variety of human cells (Levy, 1994), such as natural killer (NK) cells, B lymphocytes, endothelial cells, epithelial cells, Langerhans' cells, dendritic cells (which are present on the body's mucosal surfaces), microglial cells, and various body tissues.

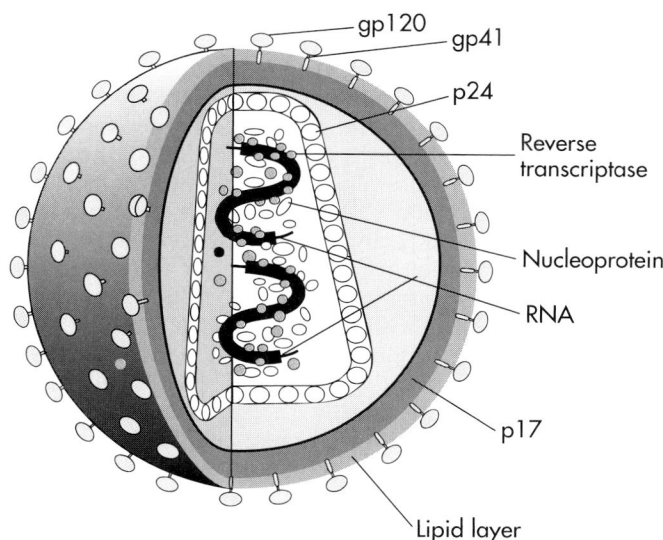

FIG. 15-3   Mature HIV virion structure. Two molecules of viral RNA are shown in the center associated with three important enzymes: reverse transcriptase, integrase, and protease. Surrounding the core is a nucleocapsid composed of p24 proteins. Two glycoproteins, gp120 and gp41, are embedded in the lipid bilayer derived from the cell membrane. (Redrawn from Greene WC: *Sci Am* 269[3]:100, 1993.)

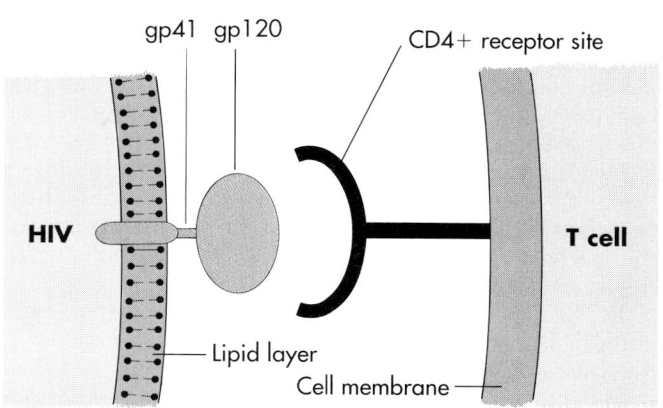

FIG. 15-4   Attachment/binding of gp120 to receptor protein on CD4+ T lymphocyte.

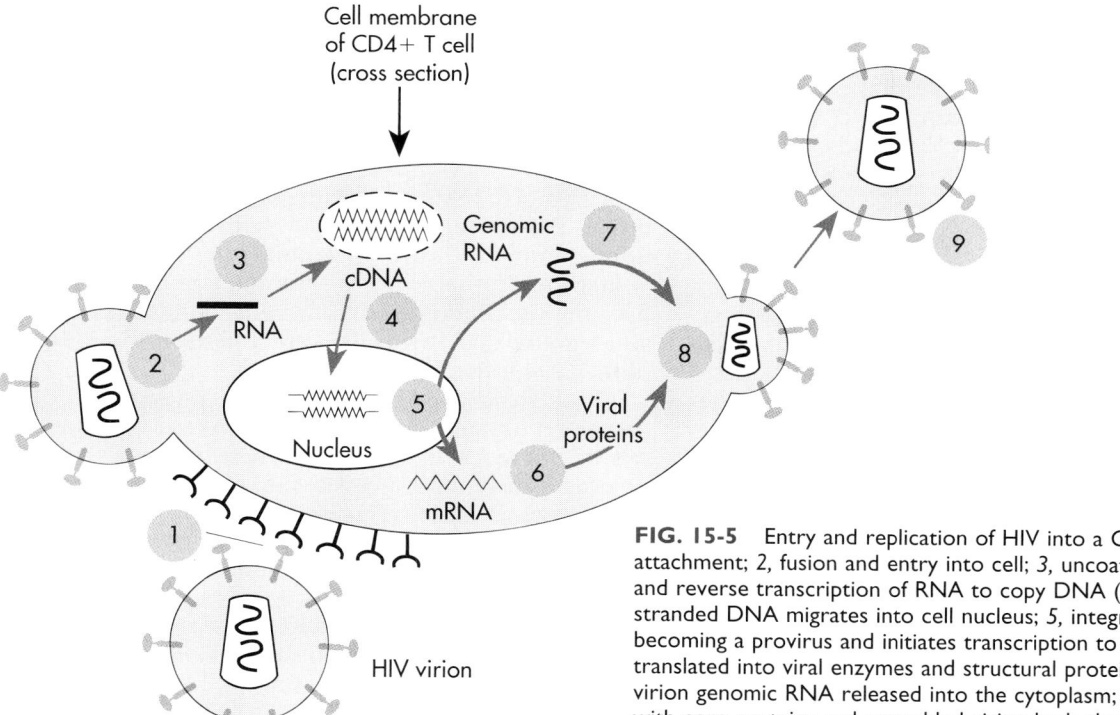

FIG. 15-5   Entry and replication of HIV into a CD4+ T lymphocyte: *1*, attachment; *2*, fusion and entry into cell; *3*, uncoating of the nucleocapsid and reverse transcription of RNA to copy DNA (cDNA); *4*, double-stranded DNA migrates into cell nucleus; *5*, integrates into host DNA becoming a provirus and initiates transcription to mRNA; *6*, viral mRNA translated into viral enzymes and structural proteins in the cytoplasm; *7*, virion genomic RNA released into the cytoplasm; *8*, viral RNA combines with core proteins and assembled virion buds through membrane; *9*, new HIV virion released from infected CD4+ T lymphocyte.

After fusion of the virus to a CD4+ lymphocyte, a complex series of events occurs that, if not interrupted, leads to the production of new virus particles from the infected cell. The infected CD4+ lymphocyte may remain latent in a proviral state or may undergo replication cycles producing multiple viruses. Infection of the CD4+ lymphocyte may also lead to cytopathogenicity through a variety of mechanisms, including *apoptosis* (programmed cell death), *anergy* (prevention of further cell division), or formation of *syncytium* (cell fusion).

Viral Replication

After the virus-cell fusion occurs (Fig. 15-5), viral RNA enters the core of the CD4+ lymphocyte's cytoplasm. After uncoating of the nucleocapsid, *reverse transcription* occurs from a single strand of RNA to double-stranded copy DNA (cDNA) of the virus. The HIV *integrase* aids in the insertion of the viral cDNA into the host nucleus. When the two strands of DNA are integrated into the host cell's chromosomes, they become a *provirus* (Greene, 1993). The provirus produces viral messenger RNA (mRNA), which leaves the nucleus and enters the cytoplasm. Viral proteins are produced from full-length and spliced mRNA as genomic RNA is released into the cytoplasm. The final stage of virus production requires a viral enzyme called *HIV protease*, which cuts and assembles the virus protein into small segments that surround the viral RNA, forming the infectious virus particles that bud from the infected cell. As the virus particles bud from the host cell, they become coated by part of the cell membranes of the infected cell. The newly formed HIV can now attack other susceptible cells throughout the body.

Replication of HIV continues throughout the period of clinical latency, even when minimal viral activity is demonstrated in blood (Embretson et al, 1993; Pantaleo et al, 1993). HIV is found in massive amounts in CD4+ lymphocytes and macrophages throughout the lymphoid system at all stages of infection. Virus particles have also been associated with follicular dendritic cells, which may transmit infection to cells during migration through lymphoid follicles.

Although low levels of viremia and viral replication may be found in peripheral blood mononuclear cells during clinical latency, a true latency does not exist. HIV is continually accumulating and replicating in the lymphoid organs. Some data suggest that an extraordinarily large number of replications and rapid cell turnovers occur, with the composite half-life of plasma virus and virus-producing cells being approximately 2 days (Wei et al, 1995; Ho et al, 1995). This activity indicates that a persistent battle occurs between the virus and the individual's immune system.

Immune Responses to HIV Infection

For a review of the response of the body to immunologic challenge, see Chapter 5. Both humoral and cell-mediated immune responses are involved in HIV infection.

Soon after a person is exposed to HIV, he or she mounts an intense immune defense. B cells produce specific antibodies against the viral proteins. Neutralizing antibodies to regions of the envelope gp120 and to the external portion of gp41 are found. The detection of antibodies is the basis for various HIV tests (e.g., enzyme-linked immunosorbent assay [ELISA]). Both the immunoglobulin G (IgG) and the immunoglobulin M (IgM) classes of antibodies appear in the circulation, but as the IgM titer decreases, in most cases the IgG titer remains high throughout infection. IgG antibodies are the principal antibodies used in HIV testing. Antibodies to HIV can appear within 1 month after initial infection and in most HIV-infected individuals within 6 months of exposure. However, HIV antibodies neither neutralize HIV nor confer immunity against further infection.

Immunoglobulin production is regulated by the CD4+ lymphocyte. As discussed in Chapter 5, the CD4+ lymphocyte is activated by an antigen-presenting cell (APC) to produce cytokines such as interleukin-2 (IL-2), which help stimulate B cells to divide and differentiate into plasma cells. These plasma cells then produce immunoglobulins specific to the stimulating antigen. The cytokine IL-2 is only one of many cytokines that influence both humoral and cell-mediated immune responses. Although the extent of cytokine control, expression, and potential function in HIV infection is still being explored, cytokines are certainly critical in intracellular activities. For example, the addition of the cytokine IL-12 (NK cell stimulatory factor) appears to counter the reduction in NK cell activity and function seen in HIV infection. NK cells are important because they normally recognize and destroy virus-infected cells by secreting perforins similar to those produced by CD8 cells.

Recent research supports the cytotoxic and suppressor roles of CD8 cells in HIV infection. The CD8 cell's cytotoxic role involves binding with the virus-infected cell and releasing perforins, which cause cell death. The cytotoxic activities of CD8 cells are vigorous at the beginning of HIV infection. The CD8 cell can also suppress HIV replication in CD4+ lymphocytes. This suppression has been found to be variable not only among individuals but also within the same person as the disease develops. The antiviral activity of the CD8 cell decreases with disease advancement. As the disease progresses, the number of CD4+ lymphocytes is also depleted. Various hypotheses as to the cause of this gradual loss are discussed later.

The essential regulator function of CD4+ lymphocytes in cell-mediated immunity is irrefutable. As discussed earlier and in Chapter 5, CD4+ lymphocytes release cytokines that expedite processes such as production of immunoglobulins and activation of additional T cells and macrophages. Two specific cytokines produced by CD4+ lymphocytes—IL-2 and gamma interferon—are pivotal in cell-mediated immunity. Under normal conditions, CD4+ lymphocyte release of gamma interferon attracts macrophages and intensifies the immune reaction to the antigen. If the CD4+ lymphocyte is not functioning properly, however, gamma interferon production is then diminished. IL-2 is important in facilitating not only the production of plasma cells but also the growth and antiviral activity of CD8 cells and the self-replication of the CD4+ lymphocyte population.

Although the precise mechanism of the CD4+ lymphocyte cytopathogenicity is as yet unknown, arguments can be made for hypotheses such as apoptosis, anergy, syncytia formation, and lysis of the cell. *Antibody-dependent, complement-mediated cytotoxicity* (ADCC) may be one humoral immune effect that helps remove HIV-infected CD4+ lymphocytes. ADCC is induced by antibodies to the two glycoproteins, gp120 and gp41. Cells such as NK cells then act to kill the infected cells.

Apoptosis is one of several theories offered to explain the marked loss of circulating CD4+ lymphocytes through the course of HIV disease. Many CD4+ lymphocytes appear to commit cellular suicide when stimulated by an activating agent or by a defect in activation signaling (Gougeon, Montagnier, 1993). CD4+ lymphocytes also may fail to divide, resulting in a phenomenon called anergy. Another theory involves the formation of syncytia. In syncytium formation, uninfected CD4+ lymphocytes are fused with infected cells—the "bystander effect" (Weiss, 1993)—thereby eliminating many uninfected cells. Finally, the decrease in the number of CD4+ lymphocytes may result from the budding of new viruses;

they may rupture through the CD4+ lymphocyte membrane, effectively killing it in the process.

No matter which theory supports the loss of CD4+ lymphocytes, depletion of these cells remains a principal feature of HIV infection. The depletion varies among individuals with HIV infection. Some of the factors influencing this variation include function of the host immune system, presence of other host factors (e.g., congenital or metabolic disorders, nutritional deficiencies, additional pathogens), or differences in viral strains (Schattner, Laurence, 1994).

MEASUREMENT OF CD4+ CELLS AND MONITORING LOSS

In an intact immune system, the number of CD4+ lymphocytes ranges from 600 to $1200/\mu l$ (or mm³) of blood. Because CD4+ lymphocyte counts can vary even within a single individual, a baseline count is established as soon as possible after exposure to HIV. Immediately after primary virus infection, the CD4+ lymphocyte count drops below the normal level for the individual. The cell number then increases but to a level somewhat below normal for the individual. A slow decrease in CD4+ lymphocyte count occurs over time and correlates with the clinical course of the disease. External factors such as stress, smoking, drugs, and alcohol can affect hormone and immune functions and may serve as intervening variables. Their effects on CD4+ lymphocyte counts need further evaluation.

Since 1993 the CDC AIDS surveillance case definition includes individuals with "AIDS-indicator conditions" and those with a CD4+ lymphocyte count less than 200/μl (whether asymptomatic or symptomatic) (see Table 15-1). Patients with CD4+ lymphocyte counts less than 200 are severely immunosuppressed and are at high risk for malignancies and opportunistic infections. The body becomes nearly defenseless to invaders such as bacteria, viruses, fungi, protozoa, and parasites.

CLINICAL PROGRESSION

Phases of Infection

AIDS is the final stage in a continuum of immunologic and clinical abnormalities known as the "spectrum of HIV infection" (Fig. 15-6, Table 15-2, Box 15-2). The course of disease is initiated when transmission occurs and the person becomes infected. Not every person who is exposed becomes infected (e.g., homozygotes with a mutant CCR5 gene). Other cofactors to acquisition may exist and are yet to be identified. After initial infection with HIV, an individual may remain seronegative for several months. However, the individual is infectious during this period and can transmit the virus to others. This phase is called the "window" period. Clinical manifestations in the infected individual can be present as early as 1 to 4 weeks after exposure.

Acute infection occurs at the point of seroconversion from negative antibody status to positive. Some people have a virus- or mononucleosis-like ailment that lasts for a few days. Symptoms might include malaise, fever, diarrhea, lymphadenopathy, and a maculopapular rash. A few individuals experience more acute symptoms, such as meningitis and pneumonitis. During this period, high levels of HIV can be detected in the peripheral blood

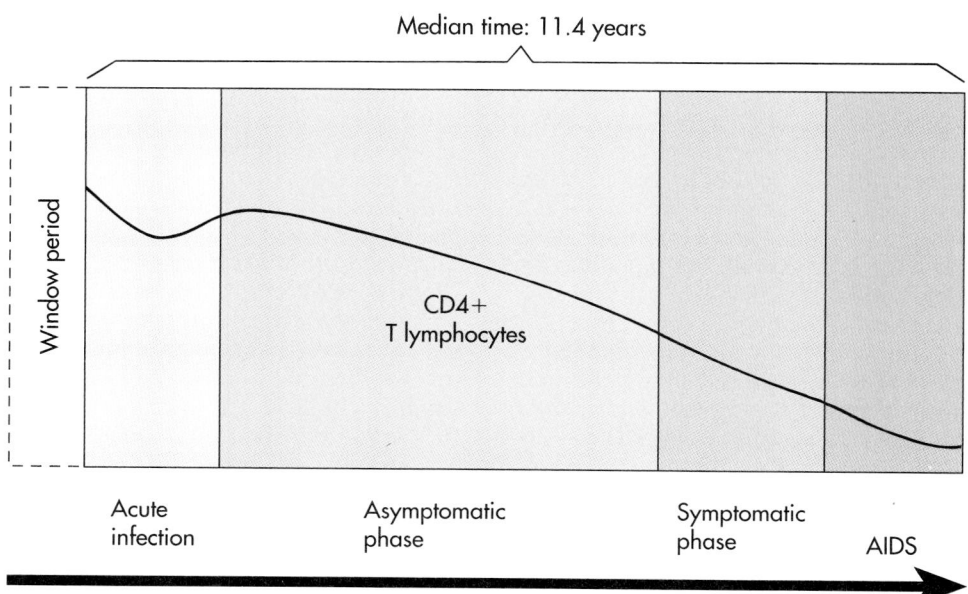

FIG. 15-6   Phases of HIV infection. The period of time between HIV seroconversion and the appearance of symptoms may be about 10 years or less. The median time between seroconversion and death is 11.4 years. (Modified from Grimes D, Grimes R: *AIDS and HIV infection*, St Louis, 1994, Mosby.)

TABLE 15-2 ∎∎∎

CDC Classification of HIV Infection Based on Pathophysiology of the Disease as Immune Function Progressively Worsens

Class	Criteria
Group I	1. Acute infection with HIV 2. Influenza-like symptoms; resolve completely 3. HIV antibody negative
HIV ASYMPTOMATIC	
Group II	1. HIV antibody positive 2. No laboratory or clinical indicators of immunodeficiency
HIV SYMPTOMATIC	
Group III	1. HIV antibody positive 2. Persistent generalized lymphadenopathy

Group IV-A	1. HIV antibody positive
	2. Constitutional disease
	  a. Persistent fever or diarrhea
	  b. Weight loss of greater than 10% of normal body weight

Group IV-B	1. Same as group IV-A and
	2. Neurologic disease
	  a. Dementia
	  b. Neuropathy
	  c. Myelopathy

Group IV-C	1. Same as group IV-B and 2. CD4 + T lymphocyte count of less than 200/μl 3. Opportunistic infection
Group IV-D	1. Same as group IV-C and 2. Pulmonary tuberculosis, invasive cervical cancer, or other malignancy

Data from Centers for Disease Control and Prevention, March 1993.

(Levy, 1994). CD4+ lymphocyte levels drop and then return to a level slightly below the original level for that individual.

Within weeks after the acute infection phase, the person enters an *asymptomatic phase.* At the beginning of this phase, CD4+ lymphocyte levels have generally returned to near normal. However, CD4+ lymphocyte levels decrease gradually over time. During this phase of infection, both the virus and the viral antibodies can be found in the blood. As discussed, replication of the virus is taking place in the lymphoid tissue. The virus itself never enters a period of latency even though the phase of clinical infection may be latent.

In the *symptomatic phase* of the disease course, the individual's CD4+ cell counts have usually dropped below 300 cells/μl (Levy, 1994). Symptoms indicating immunosuppression are present and continue until the person develops an AIDS-related condition. The CDC has defined the symptomatic conditions for this clinical category (see Table 15-2 and Box 15-2).

The CDC has added a CD4+ lymphocyte count of less than 200/μl as a sole criterion for AIDS diagnosis, regardless of clinical category, asymptomatic or symptomatic. The presence of any of the AIDS-indicator conditions, as defined by the CDC, denotes a reportable AIDS case. When the CDC expanded its definition in 1993, three clinical conditions were added: pulmonary tuberculosis, recurrent pneumonia, and invasive cervical cancer. These conditions joined the 23 others contained in the previous case definition published in 1987.

Clinical Manifestations

AIDS comprises a variety of clinical manifestations in the form of characteristic opportunistic malignancies and infections.

Malignancies

Kaposi's sarcoma (KS) is the most common type of malignancy present among homosexual or bisexual HIV-infected men (26%), but it is rare among other adults (less than 2%) and extremely rare in children. KS is a manifestation of excessive proliferation of spindle cells believed to be of vascular origin and has features in common with endothelial and smooth muscle cells. KS generally develops in a multicentric fashion in asymptomatic nodules (i.e., an angiosarcoma). Strong evidence suggests that a sexually transmitted agent, *human herpes virus Type 8 (HHV8)* or *Kaposi's sarcoma-associated herpesvirus,* rather than HIV, causes KS. HHV8 predisposes the infected person to develop KS (similar to the human papilloma virus that predisposes the infected person to develop cervical cancer). Reddish-purple patches occur on the skin, but the color may vary to include violet, dark purple, pink, red, and red-brown (see color plates 1 to 3). In addition to the skin changes observed in KS, common extraneous sites are the gastrointestinal (GI) tract, lymph nodes, and lungs. KS can cause structural and functional damage, such as lymphedema and malabsorption. When KS is localized primarily to the skin, cryosurgery, laser surgery, and surgical excision have been somewhat successful, but radiotherapy is the treatment of choice for local disease. Chemotherapeutic agents such as vinblastine, vincristine, bleomycin, and doxorubicin have been useful to varying degrees. Of the various immune stimulation agents available, interferon has been the most effective because of its antiviral, antiproliferative, and immunostimulating effects.

Most malignant lymphomas are high-grade pathologic B cell tumors, including small, noncleaved lymphoma and Burkitt's or Burkitt-like lymphoma (see color plate 4). A common finding is the occurrence of symptoms that include fever, weight loss, and night sweats, which are probably caused by the malignancy. Patients who have *persistent generalized lymphadenopathy (PGL)* are at significant risk to develop malignant lymphoma.

Initial signs and symptoms of primary central nervous system (CNS) lymphoma include headache, short-term memory loss, cranial nerve palsies, hemiparesis, and personality changes. These impairments may be caused by the location of the tumor, edema, or coexisting diseases. The space-occupying lesion must be differentiated from other lesions, particularly toxoplasmosis.

Invasive cervical cancer is a gynecologic malignancy associated with long-standing HIV disease included in the case definition since 1993. Cervical dysplasia affects 40% of HIV-infected women (Fauci, Lane, 1998). Cervical dysplasia is caused by a human papilloma virus that correlates with the eventual development of invasive cancer. Thus a Papanicolaou smear or colposcopic examination should be performed every 6 months in HIV-infected women to

---

BOX 15-2

1993 Revised HIV Classification System for Adolescents and Adults

The revised CDC classification for HIV-infected adolescents and adults emphasizes the importance of CD4+ T lymphocyte counts in the clinical management of patients who are infected with HIV. This classification is divided into laboratory and clinical categories. By contrast, the usefulness of the classification in Box 15-1 is limited to epidemiologic and surveillance purposes.

LABORATORY CATEGORIES
Category 1: >500 μl CD4+ T lymphocytes/μl
Category 2: 200-499 μl CD4+ T lymphocytes/μl
Category 3: <200 μl CD4+ T lymphocytes/μl

CLINICAL CATEGORIES
Category A
Category A consists of one or more of the following conditions in an adolescent or adult ($\geq$13 years) with documented HIV infection. Conditions listed under categories B and C must not have occurred.
- Asymptomatic HIV infection
- Persistent generalized lymphadenopathy (PGL)
- Acute (primary) HIV infection with accompanying illness or history of acute HIV infection

Category B
Category B consists of symptomatic conditions occurring in an HIV-infected adolescent or adult that are not listed in category C and meet at least one of the following criteria:
1. The conditions are attributed to HIV infection or are indicative of a defect in cell-mediated immunity or both.
2. The conditions are considered by physicians to have a clinical course or management that is complicated by HIV infection.
Selected examples of conditions include the following:
- Bacterial endocarditis, meningitis, pneumonia, or sepsis
- Candidiasis, oropharyngeal (thrush)
- Candidiasis, vulvovaginal, persistent for more than 1 month
- Cervical dysplasia, severe or carcinoma
- Constitutional symptoms such as fever or diarrhea for more than 1 month
- Hairy leukoplakia (oral)
- Herpes zoster (shingles), at least two distinct episodes or more than one dermatome
- Idiopathic thrombocytopenic purpura
- Listeriosis
- Mycobacterium tuberculosis infection, pulmonary
- Pelvic inflammatory disease
- Peripheral neuropathy

Category C
Category C consists of any condition listed in the 1987 surveillance case definition (including the 1993 expansion) affecting an adolescent or adult.
   The conditions in category C are strongly associated with severe immunodeficiency, occur frequently in HIV-infected patients, and cause serious morbidity and mortality.
- According to the proposed classification system, HIV-infected patients would be classified on the basis of both the following:
   1. The lowest accurate (not necessarily the latest) CD4+ T lymphocyte count
   2. The most severe clinical condition diagnosed regardless of the patient's present clinical condition

Modified from Centers for Disease Control and Prevention: 1993 Revised classification system for HIV infection and expanded surveillance case definition for AIDS among adolescents and adults, *MMWR* 41(RR-17):1, December 1992.

---

detect cervical cancer in the early stages. Cervical cancer is especially aggressive in women with AIDS.

Other malignancies have occurred in HIV-infected patients, including multiple myeloma, B cell acute lymphocytic leukemia, T lymphoblastic lymphoma, Hodgkin's disease, carcinoma of the anus, squamous cell carcinoma of the tongue, adenosquamous carcinoma of the lung, adenocarcinoma of the colon and pancreas, and testicular cancer. More research must be completed to generalize impact of an underlying HIV infection on the course of concurrent malignancies or other chronic illnesses that are unrelated to the HIV infection.

Infections

AIDS causes a progressive destruction of immune functioning. The morbidity and mortality, however, result primarily from the major opportunistic infections that develop because of unsuccessful immune surveillance and action.

Patients with AIDS are susceptible to a broad range of protozoal, bacterial, fungal, and viral infections, and some of these are quite rare, such as *Cryptosporidium* and *Mycobacterium avium-intracellulare* (MAI). These infections are persistent, severe, and frequently relapsing. Patients typically have more than one infection at the same time.

Pneumocystis carinii pneumonia (PCP) is the most frequently diagnosed serious infection in patients with AIDS. The presentation is frequently atypical when compared with that of PCP in patients with cancer. In AIDS, the only symptom may be a fever; other symptoms include exercise intolerance, a dry, nonproductive cough, weakness, and shortness of breath at a gradual, indolent rate. A high degree of suspicion of PCP must accompany the clinical evaluation of every HIV-seropositive or suspected positive patient. Prophylactic or suppressive treatment is of the utmost importance because of the severity and frequency of PCP in patients with AIDS.

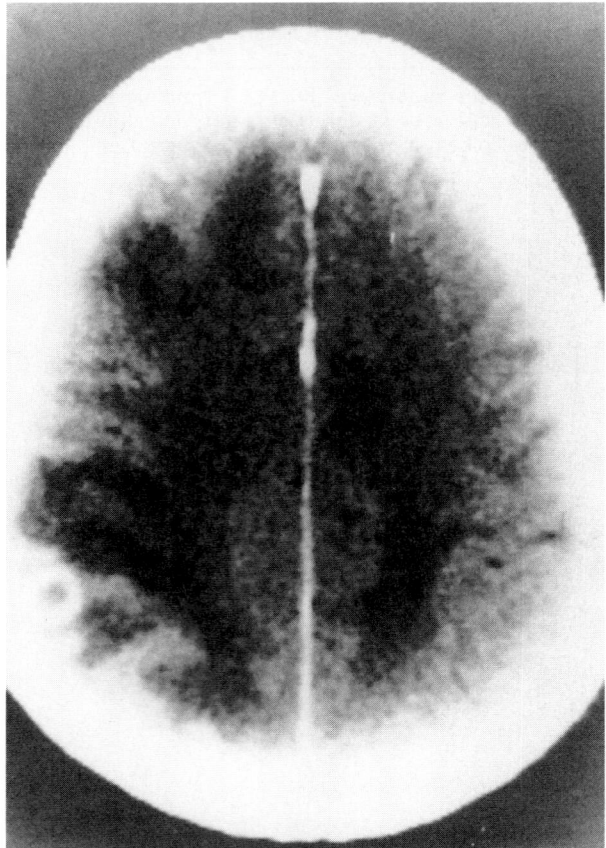

FIG. 15-7 Toxoplasmosis in AIDS patient. Note ring lesion at left. (Courtesy of Bruce Polsky, MD, Memorial Sloan-Kettering Cancer Center.)

Trimethoprim-sulfamethoxazole (Bactrim, Septra) is the drug of choice. Pentamidine is an alternative drug that may be given parenterally or as an aerosol for mild cases.

Infection with *Toxoplasma gondii* is mostly silent in healthy individuals, although some develop lymphadenopathy. No prophylaxis exists. Patients with AIDS have a 30% risk of developing toxoplasmosis over a 2-year period, usually as a reactivation of an earlier infection. Specific agents that determine reactivation are unknown. In patients with AIDS, CNS disease develops, marked by multiple or solitary lesions that can be observed on computed tomographic (CT) scans (Fig. 15-7).

Cryptosporidia, microsporidia, and *Isospora belli* are the most common protozoa that infect the gastrointestinal tract and cause diarrhea in HIV-infected patients. Infection is spread by the fecal-oral route; sexual, food, water, or animal contact. Infection may present in a variety of ways, ranging from a self-limited or intermittent diarrheal illness in the early stages of HIV infection to a severe, life-threatening diarrhea in patients who are severely immunocompromised. In contrast to cryptosporidiosis or microsporidiosis, isosporiasis responds well to trimethoprim-sulfamethoxazole (Bactrim) therapy.

Infection with MAI occurs evenly in all risk groups and is a late complication of AIDS. Although the infection clearly contributes to morbidity, its relationship to mortality is unclear. Symptoms include fever, rigor, diarrhea, and abdominal cramping. Recommended prophylaxis

against MAI is controversial, but the drug most often suggested is rifabutin.

Mycobacterium tuberculosis, the cause of tuberculosis (TB), is endemic in certain geographic locations, and most cases of AIDS-TB are reactivations of prior infection. AIDS-TB is usually an early indication of AIDS, occurring when T cells are fairly high (greater than $200/\mu l$). The manifestation of AIDS-TB is similar to that of normal TB, with 60% to 80% of patients having pulmonary disease. However, extrapulmonary disease develops in 40% to 75% of patients with HIV infections, with lymphatic TB and miliary disease being particularly common. Patients respond well to the traditional drug regimen of isoniazid (INH), rifampin, pyrazinamide, and ethambutol. Patients who are at high risk for TB may benefit from INH prophylaxis. As patients progress to AIDS with decreasing immunocompetence, many HIV-infected individuals become anergic; therefore PPD skin testing poses a particular problem. A positive PPD test in an HIV-infected person is defined as an area of induration greater than or equal to 5 mm in diameter, and a negative test does not rule out TB infection. Additionally, HIV-infected patients with sputum culture-positive and AFB-positive TB may have a normal chest radiograph.

Fungal infections include *candidiasis, cryptococcosis,* and *histoplasmosis.* Oral candidiasis is common in patients with AIDS and causes dry mouth and oral irritation (see color plates 5 to 7). Candidiasis of the bronchi, lungs, trachea, or esophagus is pathognomonic for an AIDS diagnosis. Rarely do patients develop systemic disease. *Cryptococcus neoformans* infections occur in 7% of patients with AIDS, with meningitis being the most common presentation. Treatment with fluconazole provides limited prophylaxis against both oral candidiasis and *Cryptococcus neoformans.* In patients with AIDS, symptoms of infection with *Histoplasma capsulatum* are varied and nonspecific, including fevers, chills, sweats, weight loss, nausea, vomiting, diarrhea, skin lesions, pneumonitis, and bone marrow depressions. Amphotericin B is used for induction therapy, with lower dosages used for maintenance.

Opportunistic infections caused by invasion by viruses are numerous and responsible for further pathologic conditions. Infection with *herpes simplex virus (HSV)* in patients with AIDS usually results in genital or perianal ulcerations that are easily diagnosed by viral cultures. HSV can be spread by direct skin contact. HSV may also result in esophagitis and can cause pneumonia and encephalitis. Acyclovir is the drug of choice for both HSV and herpes zoster.

The development of *herpes zoster (shingles)* may signal progression of illness in an HIV-infected patient. Infections in the skin and eyes may precede opportunistic infections. *Cytomegalovirus (CMV)* is a common finding in patients with AIDS; it causes disseminated disease with four clearly defined illnesses: chorioretinitis (Figs. 15-8 and 15-9), enterocolitis, pneumonia, and adrenalitis. Asymptomatic individuals can shed CMV. CMV pneumonia is difficult to distinguish from other pneumonias and may occur simultaneously with another pathogen such as *Pneumocystis carinii.* Symptoms of adrenal insufficiency may be detected. Treatment with ganciclovir or foscarnet is indicated for CMV-related illnesses (Goldschmidt, Dong, 1995).

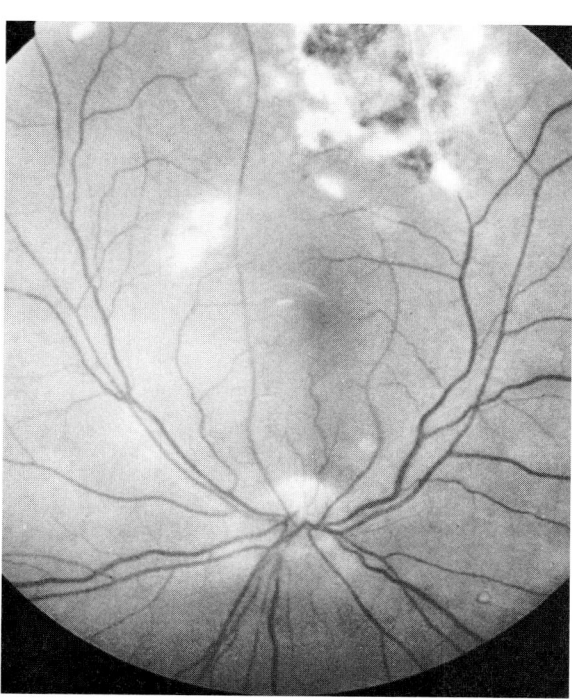

FIG. 15-8 Cytomegalovirus (CMV) retinitis. (Courtesy Bruce Polsky, MD, Memorial Sloan-Kettering Cancer Center.)

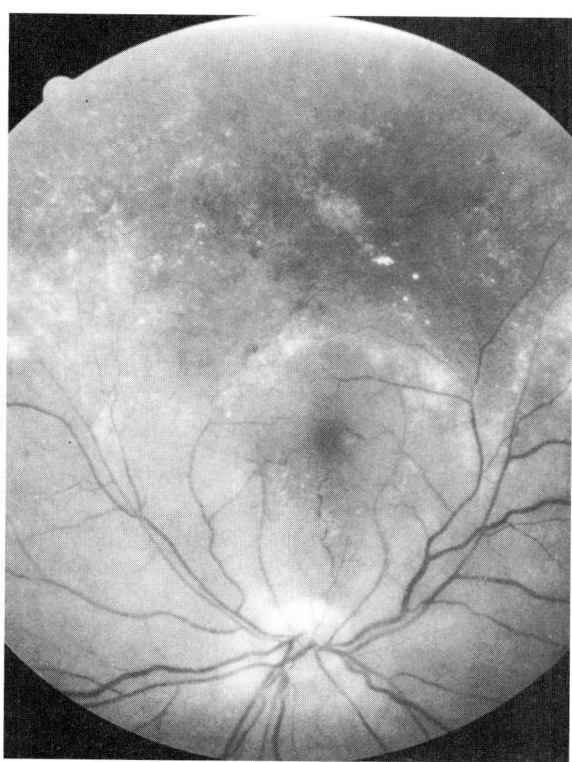

FIG. 15-9 Cytomegalovirus (CMV) retinitis after treatment with ganciclovir (DHPG). (Courtesy of Bruce Polsky, MD, Memorial Sloan-Kettering Cancer Center.)

Progressive multifocal leukoencephalopathy is a rapidly progressive illness caused by a papovavirus. Clinically, the patient has personality changes and motor and sensory deficits. Symptoms may include headache, tremors, coordination and balance difficulties, weakness, and other signs of cerebellar dysfunction. *Epstein-Barr virus (EBV)* is implicated in the development of oral hairy leukoplakia (see color plate 8), pneumonitis in children, and lymphomas and is frequently isolated from the throat washings of patients with AIDS.

Testing

Two tests are typically used for detecting antibodies to HIV. The first, enzyme-linked immunosorbent assay (ELISA), reacts to the presence of antibodies in serum by demonstrating a more intense color as large quantities of viral antibodies are detected. Because false-positive results can be psychologically devastating, positive ELISA studies are repeated, and when both results are positive, a more specific test, *Western blot*, is performed. The Western blot test is also confirmed twice. This test is less likely to give a false-positive or false-negative reading. Inconclusive tests also can occur, such as when ELISA or Western blot is weakly reactive and somewhat suspicious. This may occur in early HIV infection, in developing infection (until all necessary bands on the Western blot studies are completely present), or in the cross-reactivity to another high retrovirus titer, such as HIV-2 or HTLV-I. After confirmation, the person is said to be *HIV seropositive*. At this point, additional clinical and immunologic studies are per-

formed to evaluate the extent of the illness and efforts to control infection are initiated.

HIV can also be detected by other tests, which discern the presence of the virus or viral components before ELISA or Western blot can detect antibodies. These procedures include viral culture, measurement of p24 antigen, and measurement of HIV DNA and RNA by means of the *polymerase chain reaction (PCR)* and plasma HIV-1 RNA. Tests such as these are useful in studies of immunopathogenesis, as disease markers, in early detection of infection, and in neonatal transmission. Infants born to HIV-infected mothers can demonstrate maternal anti-HIV antibodies in their blood for up to 18 months after birth, regardless of whether they are actually infected.

PEDIATRIC AIDS

In the early 1980s children with hemophilia or those receiving blood or blood products were at high risk for HIV infection. With the testing of the blood supply, however, begun in 1985, this mode of transmission is now nearly nonexistent. Currently, HIV in children is predominantly a result of *vertical transmission*—acquired before birth, during delivery, or through breast-feeding.

Infants of HIV-infected women demonstrate antibodies to the virus up to 10 to 18 months after birth because of the transfer of maternal anti-HIV IgG across the placenta. Therefore testing an infant's serum for IgG antibodies is futile, because the test does not discriminate between the infant's and the mother's antibodies. Most of these babies, over time, will stop demonstrating maternal antibodies and will also fail to develop their own antibodies to the virus, indicating a seronegative status. True HIV infection can be measured in many infants through tests such as viral culture, p24 antigen, or PCR analysis for viral RNA or DNA. HIV DNA PCR is the preferred virologic test because of its sensitivity for diagnosing HIV infection during the neonatal period (Working Group on Antiretroviral Therapy, 2001).

Until recently, the mechanism for HIV transfer from mother to fetus remained elusive. Transfer rates vary from approximately 25% in untreated nonbreast-feeding populations in industrialized countries to approximately 40% of untreated nonbreast-feeding populations in developing countries. In the absence of breast-feeding, approximately 20% of infant HIV infections occur in utero and 80% occur during labor and delivery (Stringer, Vermund, 2000). Postpartum transmission may occur through colostrum or breast milk and is believed to confer an additional 15% risk of perinatal transmission.

Maternal factors associated with increased risk of transmission include advanced maternal HIV disease, high serum viral load, and a low CD4+ T cell count. In 1994 the Pediatric AIDS Clinical Trials Group (PACTG) 076 study demonstrated that treating HIV-infected pregnant women with zidovudine reduced the mother-to-infant transmission rate by two-thirds—from 25% to 8% (Conner et al, 1994). The incidence of perinatally acquired AIDS in the United States declined 67% from 1992 through 1997 as a result of prenatal maternal HIV testing and prenatal prophylaxis with zidovudine therapy. Women comprise approximately 20% of the HIV-AIDS cases in the United States. Minority women (African Americans and Hispanics) are disproportionately affected, accounting for 85% of the total AIDS cases. In addition to the administration of oral zidovudine to HIV-positive mothers during pregnancy, other recommended measures to reduce the risk of maternal-child HIV transmission include: (1) a cesarean delivery before the onset of labor and rupture of membranes (reduces transmission rate by 50%); (2) the administration of intravenous zidovudine during labor and delivery; (3) the administration of zidovudine syrup to the infant after birth; and (4) refraining from breast-feeding (Perinatal HIV Guidelines Working Group, 2001; Stringer, Vermund, 2000).

Data indicate that the progression of the disease is accelerated in children. The asymptomatic phase is shorter in children who have contracted the virus through vertical transmission. The median time to onset of symptoms is less in children, and after symptoms appear, progression to death is expedited. In 1994 the CDC revised the classification system for HIV infection in children younger than age 13 years. In this system, infected children are classified into categories according to three parameters: infection status, clinical status, and immunologic status. These categories are mutually exclusive.

Similarities and differences exist in the clinical course of HIV disease in children and in adults. B-cell dysfunction often occurs in children before changes are present in the CD4+ lymphocyte number. As a result of these immune system dysfunctions, children are subjected to recurrent bacterial infections (Krasinski, 1994; Rubinstein, Calvelli,

1995). Invasion by these bacterial pathogens results in the clinical syndrome present in children, such as otitis media, sinusitis, urinary tract infection, meningitis, respiratory infection, GI diseases, and other diseases.

Additional infections observed in children include toxoplasmosis, cryptococcal infection, chronic herpes (simplex and zoster) infection, disseminated cytomegaloviral infection, histoplasmosis, and candidiasis (oral, esophageal, and disseminated). Approximately one half of infants and children with AIDS develop PCP. PCP is the most common opportunistic infection present in HIV-infected children, and their prognosis is typically poor, particularly when additional pathogens are present (Rubinstein, Calvelli, 1994).

Infection with the EBV appears related to the *lymphoid interstitial pneumonitis–pulmonary lymphoid hyperplasia* (LIP-PLH) and the generalized lymphadenopathy present in children. HIV-infected children demonstrate a high incidence of LIP-PLH. In the clinic, lymphadenopathy and parotid swelling, as well as developmental delays, unexplained fever, diarrhea, or failure to thrive, are part of the clinical picture, particularly in older children.

Thrombocytopenia is a common hematologic complication. Progressive encephalopathy is observed in many infants and children and is considered the most severe of the CNS problems associated with HIV infection (Brouwers et al, 1994). KS is rare in children. Malignancies (e.g., lymphomas) in children probably result from the dysfunction in both B and T cells.

ANTIRETROVIRAL THERAPEUTIC INTERVENTION

New and more sensitive tests have shown that HIV virus replication is active throughout the course of the infection and proceeds at levels far higher than previously understood (CDC, 1998d). Many researchers believe that therapeutic intervention and antiretroviral treatment (ART) should be started as early as possible. However, the optimal time to initiate ART is unknown. Current therapies confront the issues of targeting the multiple stages of viral entry and replication, manipulating viral genes to control for production of viral proteins, rebuilding the immune system, combining treatments, and preventing drug resistance. Two laboratory measurements, CD4+ T cell counts and HIV RNA serum levels, are used as tools for monitoring risk for disease progression and the appropriate time to initiate or modify drug regimens (Fig. 15-10). The CD4+ T cell count provides information on the patient's current immunologic status, while the HIV RNA serum level (viral load) predicts the clinical prognosis (status of the CD4+ T cell count in the near future). A HIV RNA count of 20,000 copies/ml (2×10^4) is felt by many experts to be an indication for antiretroviral therapy regardless of CD4+ T cell count. Serial measurements of HIV RNA and CD4+ T cell serum levels are of great value in delineating rates of disease progression, rates of viral turnover, the relationship between immune system activation and viral replication, and the time to development of antiviral drug resistance. All effective forms of antiretroviral treatment are associated with a drop in levels of HIV RNA (Fauci, Lane, 1998).

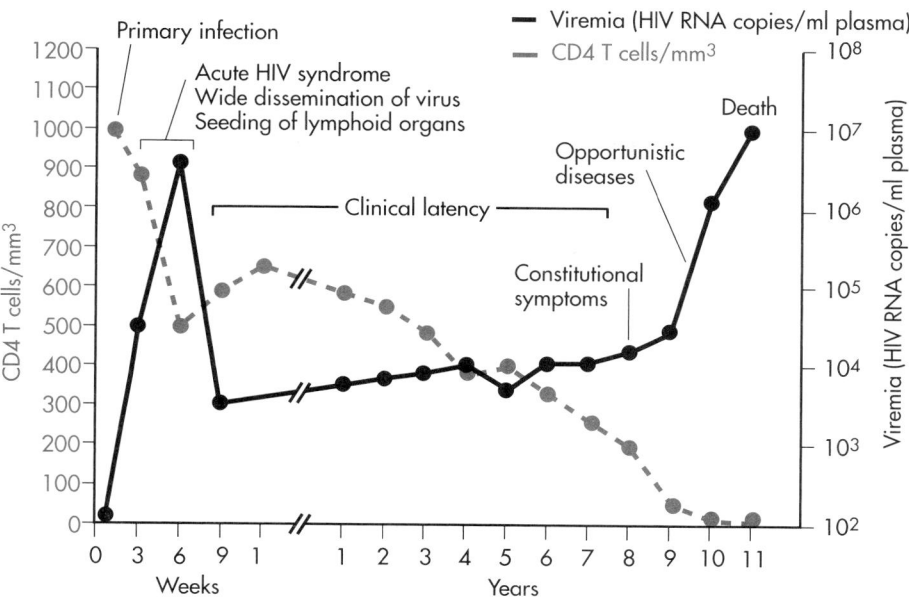

FIG. 15-10   Typical serum CD4+ T cell counts and HIV RNA levels correlated with the phases of HIV infection. Serial measurements are used to predict clinical prognosis and guide drug therapy. (Redrawn from Fauci AS, Lane HC: Human immunodeficiency virus (HIV) disease: AIDS and related disorders. In Fauci AS, et al (eds): *Harrison's principles of internal medicine*, ed 14, New York, 1998, McGraw-Hill).

TABLE 15-3   ■ ■ ■

Highly Active Antiretroviral Therapy (HAART)

Drug Class	Examples
NUCLEOSIDE REVERSE TRANSCRIPTASE INHIBITORS (NRTIs)*	
Zidovudine	ZDV, Retrovir
Didanosine	ddI, Videx
Zalcitabine	ddC, HIVID
Stavudine	d4T, Zerit
Lamivudine	Epivir
Abacavir	Ziagen
NONNUCLEASE REVERSE TRANSCRIPTASE INHIBITORS (NNRTIs)†	
Nevirapine	Viramune
Delavirdine	Rescriptor
Efavirenz	Sustiva
PROTEASE INHIBITORS (PIs)‡	
Indinavir	Crixivan
Ritonavir	Norvir
Nelfinavir	Viracept
Saquinavir	Invirase, Fortovase
Amprenavir	Agenerase
Lopinavir	Kaletra

MECHANISM OF ACTION

*Inhibits HIV reverse transcriptase, thereby terminating the DNA chain growth and HIV replication

†Inhibits the transcription of HIV RNA to DNA, a critical step in the viral replication process

‡Inhibits HIV protease, which prevents maturation of the infectious HIV virus

In the United States (2001), three classes of drugs have been approved by the U.S. Food and Drug Administration (FDA) for HIV infection: (1) *nucleoside reverse transcriptase inhibitors (NRTIs)*; (2) *nonnucleoside reverse transcriptase inhibitors (NNRTIs)*; and (3) *protease inhibitors* (PIs) (Table 15-3). NRTI inhibits the enzymes HIV-RNA–dependent DNA polymerase (reverse transcriptase) and terminates DNA chain growth. Examples of NRTIs are zidovudine, didanosine, zalcitabine, stavudine, lamivudine, and abacavir. NNRTIs inhibit the transcription of HIV-1 RNA to DNA, a critical step in the viral replication process. This type of drug lowers the amount of HIV in the blood (viral load) and increases CD4 lymphocytes. Nevirapine, delavirdine, and efavirenz are examples of NNRTI. PIs inhibit the activity of HIV protease and prevent the cleavage of HIV polyproteins, which are essential for HIV maturation. Instead of mature HIV, immature, noninfectious viral particles are formed. Indinavir, ritonavir, nelfinavir, saquinavir, amprenavir, and lopinavir are examples of PIs. These 15 antiretroviral agents are administered in two to three different combinations according to research findings and specific guidelines developed by the Panel on Clinical Practice and Treatment of HIV Infection convened by the U.S. Department of Health and Human Services (DHHS) and Kaiser Family Foundation (CDC, 1998b). The administration of two to three antiretroviral agents is also called *highly active antiretroviral therapy (HAART)*. Data on the efficacy and durability of HAART reveal that sustained effectiveness is limited in many HIV-infected patients because of drug resistance and poor adherence to complex medication regimens. Drug resistant viral variants emerge when ART does not maximally suppress replication because of the rapidity and magnitude of HIV replication dur-ing all stages of infection (Perelson et al, 1996). Poor adherence to HAART is a common cause of treatment failure because of the sheer volume of drugs that must be taken (8 to 9/day) with special timing and food restrictions and conditions such as homelessness and drug addiction.

BOX 15-3

Summary of Principles of Therapy for HIV Infection

1. Ongoing HIV replication leads to immune system damage and progression to AIDS. HIV infection is always harmful, and true long-term survival free of clinically significant immune dysfunction is unusual.
2. Plasma HIV RNA levels indicate the magnitude of HIV replication and its associated rate of CD4+ T cell destruction, whereas CD4+ T cell counts indicate the extent of HIV-induced immune damage already experienced. Regular periodic measurement of plasma HIV RNA levels and CD4+ T cell counts are necessary to determine the risk for disease progression in an HIV-infected individual and to determine the appropriate time to initiate or modify antiretroviral treatment regimens (see Fig. 15-10).
3. Because rates of disease progression differ among HIV-infected persons, treatment decisions should be individualized by level of risk indicated by plasma HIV RNA levels and CD4+ T cell counts.
4. The use of potent combination antiretroviral therapy to suppress HIV replication to below the levels of detection of sensitive plasma HIV RNA assays limits the potential for the selection of antiretroviral-resistant HIV variants, the major factor limiting the ability of antiretroviral drugs to inhibit virus replication and delay disease progression. Therefore maximum achievable suppression of HIV replication should be the goal of therapy.
5. The most effective means to accomplish durable suppression of HIV replication is the simultaneous initiation of combinations of effective anti-HIV drugs with which the patient has not been previously treated and that are not cross-resistant with antiretroviral agents with which the patient has been previously treated.
6. Each of the antiretroviral drugs used in combination therapy regimens should always be used according to optimal schedules and dosages.
7. The available effective antiretroviral drugs are limited in number and mechanism of action, because cross-resistance between specific drugs has been documented. Therefore any change in antiretroviral therapy increases future therapeutic constraints.
8. Women should receive optimal antiretroviral therapy, regardless of pregnancy status.
9. The same principles of antiretroviral therapy apply to HIV-infected children, adolescents, and adults, although the treatment of HIV-infected children involves unique pharmacologic, virologic, and immunologic considerations.
10. Individuals identified during acute primary HIV infection should be treated with combination antiretroviral therapy to suppress virus replication to levels between the limit of detection of sensitive plasma HIV RNA assays.
11. HIV-infected individuals, even those whose viral loads are below detectable limits, should be considered infectious. Therefore these patients should be counseled to avoid sexual and drug-use behaviors that are associated with either transmission or acquisition of HIV and other infectious pathogens.

From Centers for Disease Control and Prevention: Report of the NIH Panel to define principles of therapy of HIV infection and guidelines for the use of antiretroviral agents in HIV-infected adults and adolescents, *MMWR* 47(RR-5):1, 1998.

The main goals of antiretroviral therapy are maximal and durable suppression of viral load, restoration or preservation (or both) of immunologic function, improvement of quality of life, and reduction of HIV-related morbidity and mortality. A summary of the principles of therapy of HIV infection developed by the NIH (National Institutes of Health) Panel (CDC, 1998b) is available in Box 15-3. The same principles of HAART apply to infected children, adolescents, and adults; however, special considerations are taken with regard to treatment of HIV-infected children because of their growth and development and changes in pharmacokinetic parameters. Other considerations are: (1) acquisition of infection through perinatal exposure and differences in diagnostic evaluation, (2) exposure to zidovudine and other antiretroviral medications in utero, and (3) differences in immunologic markers (i.e. CD4+ T cell count) in young children.

The development of an effective HIV vaccine is a great challenge because of genetic mutations and complex characteristics of HIV. The ideal vaccine would induce both humoral and cellular immunity. Efficacy trials are being initiated (Bolognesi, 1994) and are continuing (CDC, 2001e) as more information about HIV is being discovered. A comprehensive HIV prevention program, however, includes not only vaccine development but also research and education geared toward preventing transmission of the virus.

KEY CONCEPTS

- *Acquired immunodeficiency syndrome (AIDS)* is a retroviral disease characterized by profound immunosuppression that leads to opportunistic infections, secondary neoplasms, and neurologic manifestations.
- AIDS is caused mainly by the *RNA retrovirus HIV-1*, but HIV-2 also causes AIDS and is most common in West Africa.
- By the end of 2000, 36.1 million individuals were infected with HIV-AIDS worldwide, and 70% live in Sub-Saharan Africa.
- HIV-1 is spherical in shape and contains a cone-shaped core surrounded by a lipid bilayer derived from the host cell. The core contains two strands of RNA, with three important enzymes: reverse transcriptase, integrase, and protease. Surrounding the core is a nucleocapsid containing the p24 protein. Two glycoprotein molecules, gp120 and gp41, which project from the viral envelope, are critical for HIV infection of target cells.
- The major target of the HIV virus is the CD4+ receptor present on the cell membrane of T helper cells, as well as on macrophages and follicular dendritic cells contained in the nervous system and lymphoid tissues.
- The HIV virus gains entry to T helper cells by attachment of gp120 to the CD4+ T cell receptor in concert with one of the chemokine coreceptors (CCR5 or CXCR4), taking over cellular metabolism to syn-

thesize new virus. Before entry into the target cell, HIV fusion with the cell membrane occurs with the help of gp41. Once inside the cell, the virus makes a DNA copy of its own RNA by means of *HIV reverse transcriptase*, and the DNA copy is inserted into the genetic material of the target cell, a process assisted by another enzyme, *HIV integrase*. The final stages of virus production requires the help of *HIV protease*, which cuts and assembles the virus into small segments that surround the viral RNA, forming the new HIV viruses that bud from the infected target cell.

- *Transmission of HIV* occurs through sexual intercourse (homosexual or heterosexual), transfusion of infected blood, IV drug abuse, and vertically from mother to infant via the placenta or breast milk.
- The standard screening test for HIV infection is the *enzyme-linked immunosorbent assay (ELISA)*, and the most common confirmatory test is the *Western blot*. Other tests include viral culture, as well as measurement of p24 antigen and of HIV RNA or DNA by means of the polymerase chain reaction (PCR).
- The hallmark of HIV infection is the progressive depletion of CD4+ cells, including T helper cells and macrophages.
- In an intact immune system, the normal number of CD4+ T cells ranges from 600 to 1200/μl or mm^3.
- Both cellular and humoral immune responses are involved in HIV infection.
- Four *clinical phases of HIV infection* include: (1) primary acute infection (seroconversion), (2) asymptomatic phase, (3) early symptomatic phase, and (4) late symptomatic phase.
- After *initial infection* with HIV, an individual may remain seronegative for several months (the *window period*) during which he or she may transmit the virus to others.
- *Acute infection* occurs at the point of seroconversion from negative antibody status to positive. Many patients develop an influenza-like illness, rashes, or lymphadenopathy at this time associated with a transient fall in CD4+ T lymphocytes.
- The *asymptomatic phase* of HIV infection (CDC group II) represents a period of clinical latency, which may last for several years in a relatively intact immune system; however, continuous HIV replication occurs, predominantly in the lymphoid tissues.
- The *early symptomatic phase* of HIV infection is characterized by *persistent generalized lymphadenopathy (PGL)* with significant *constitutional symptoms* (e.g., persistent fever, night sweats, diarrhea, weight loss) and reflects the onset of immune system decompensation, escalation of viral replication, and the onset of the full-blown AIDS disease.
- In the *late symptomatic phase* of HIV infection, there is fully developed immunodeficiency with complications of opportunistic infection, development of

HIV infection of the central nervous system and the development of neoplastic disease.
- A person with a CD4+ T cell count of less than 200/μl, whether symptomatic or asymptomatic, is classified as having the AIDS disease.
- Patients with AIDS are susceptible to a broad range of protozoal, bacterial, fungal, and viral infections because of depressed immune surveillance and function.
- *Pneumocystis carinii pneumonia (PCP)* is the most frequently diagnosed serious opportunistic infection in patients with AIDS, the terminal phase of HIV infection.
- The development of *malignancy* is a common feature of the AIDS disease including *Kaposi's sarcoma (KS)*, high-grade lymphomas of the B-cell type, and invasive carcinomas of the cervix.
- KS produces purple-colored tumors in any organ but most typically in the skin.
- Infection of the CNS by HIV produces an encephalitis that leads to a syndrome of dementia (*AIDS dementia complex*), peripheral neuropathy, and myelopathy in the majority of patients in the late phases of the disease. Opportunistic infections, such as toxoplasmosis or cryptococcosis, and neoplasms may also affect the CNS.
- The median time from seroconversion to death from the AIDS disease is approximately 11 years.
- Infants born to HIV-infected mothers demonstrate antibodies to the virus for 10 to 18 months; consequently, the children's HIV status cannot be diagnosed by the ELISA and Western blot tests; tests for the p24 antigen or HIV RNA are used. HIV antibodies present in the infant do indicate that the mother is HIV-positive.
- The vertical transmission rate to an infant from a HIV-infected mother may be reduced considerably by antiretroviral therapy (oral zidovudine) during pregnancy, IV zidovudine during labor and delivery, cesarean section before labor and rupture of membranes, and, after delivery, zidovudine syrup therapy for the infant and formula feeding rather than breast-feeding.
- Children with AIDS show clinical differences from adults: disease progression is accelerated, and severe bacterial infections are more common with both routine pathogens and a range of opportunistic infections similar to those present in adults.
- Combinations of three classes of drugs are used for highly active antiretroviral therapy (HAART): (1) nucleoside reverse transcriptase inhibitors (NRTIs); (2) nonnucleoside reverse transcriptase inhibitors (NNRTIs); and (3) protease inhibitors (PIs).
- Serial measurements of serum CD4+ T cell counts and HIV RNA viral counts are used to predict clinical prognosis and guide drug therapy.

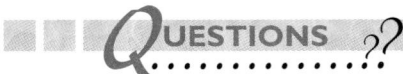

QUESTIONS ??

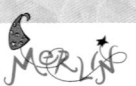

A sampling of review questions for this chapter appears here. Visit http://www.mosby.com/MERLIN/PriceWilson/ for additional questions.

Match the clinical manifestations in column A with the phase of HIV infection in column B with which they are most likely to be associated.

Column A

1. _____ Generally asymptomatic, but CD4+ T cell count gradually decreased below normal value
2. _____ CD4+ T cell count less than 500/mm³, persistent generalized lymphadenopathy, minor opportunistic infections (e.g., thrush from *Candida,* shingles, oral hairy leukoplakia from Epstein-Barr virus [EBV])
3. _____ Mononucleosis-like illness lasting 3 to 6 weeks (e.g., fever, malaise, lymphadenopathy, erythematous maculopapular rash), CD4+ T cell count slightly decreased below normal value
4. _____ Individual infected with HIV but virus cannot be detected using the standard antibody tests; no detectable physiologic response to virus screenings
5. _____ CD4+ T cell count less than 200/mm³, recurrent opportunistic infections such as *Pneumocystis carinii* pneumonia (PCP) and neoplasms

Column B

a. Incubation phase (window period)
b. Acute HIV syndrome soon after initial infection
c. Clinical latency phase
d. Early symptomatic disease
e. Advanced symptomatic disease

Match the AIDS-related illnesses in column A with the most appropriate treatment in column B.

Column A

6. _____ *Pneumocystis carinii* pneumonia (PCP)
7. _____ HIV-positive children and adults (asymptomatic and symptomatic)
8. _____ Kaposi's sarcoma (KS)
9. _____ Cytomegalovirus retinitis
10. _____ Herpes simplex abscesses
11. _____ *Mycobacterium* pulmonary tuberculosis

Column B

a. Zidovudine (ZDV)
b. Ganciclovir
c. Bactrim or Septra
d. Acyclovir
e. Local radiation therapy or chemotherapy or both
f. Isoniazid, rifampin, ethambutol, and pyrazinamide

BIBLIOGRAPHY ■ PART TWO

Barre-Sinoussi F et al: Isolation of a T-lymphocyte retrovirus from a patient at risk for acquired immunodeficiency syndrome (AIDS), *Science* 220:868-871, 1983.

Bierman CW et al: *Allergy, asthma and immunology from infancy to adulthood,* ed 3, Philadelphia, 1996, WB Saunders.

Bernstein IL et al: *Asthma in the workplace,* ed 2, New York, 1999, Marcel Dekker.

Bolognesi D: Prospects for an HIV vaccine, *Sci Am Sci Med* 1:44-53, 1994.

Borkowsky E et al: Correlation of perinatal transmission of human immunodeficiency virus type 1 with maternal viremia and lymphocyte phenotypes, *J Pediatr* 125:345-351, 1994.

Brouwers P et al: Central nervous system involvement: manifestations, evaluation, and pathogenesis. In Pizzo P, Wilfert C, editors: *Pediatric AIDS,* Baltimore, 1994, Williams & Wilkins.

Centers for Disease Control: Pneumocystis pneumonia—Los Angeles, *MMWR* 30:250-252, 1981.

Centers for Disease Control: Revision of the CDC surveillance case definition for acquired immunodeficiency syndrome, *MMWR* 36(No. 1S):3S-15S, 1987.

Centers for Disease Control and Prevention: 1993 Revised classification system for HIV infection and expanded surveillance case definition for AIDS among adolescents and adults, *MMWR* 41(RR-17):1-19, 1993.

Centers for Disease Control and Prevention: 1994 Revised classification system for human immunodeficiency virus infection in children less than 13 years of age, *MMWR* 43(RR-12):1-19, 1994.

Centers for Disease Control and Prevention: Public Health Service Task Force recommendations for the use of antiretroviral drugs in pregnant women infected with HIV-1 for maternal health and for reducing perinatal HIV-1 transmission in the United States, *MMWR* 47(RR-2):1-30, 1998a.

Centers for Disease Control and Prevention: Report of the NIH Panel to define principles of therapy of HIV infection and guidelines for the use of antiretroviral agents in HIV-infected adults and adolescents, *MMWR* 47(RR-5):1-82, 1998b.

Centers for Disease Control and Prevention: Guidelines for national human immunodeficiency virus case surveillance, including monitoring for human immunodeficiency virus infection and acquired immunodeficiency syndrome, *MMWR* 48(RR-13):1-31, 1999.

Centers for Disease Control and Prevention: HIV/AIDS surveillance report, 2000, 12 (No. 1):1-41, 2000a. *http://www.cdc.gov/hiv/stats/hasr1201.pdf*

Centers for Disease Control and Prevention: HIV/AIDS surveillance report, 2000, 12 (No. 2):1-44, 2000b. *http://www.cdc.gov/hiv/stats/hasr1202.pdf*

Centers for Disease Control and Prevention: HIV/AIDS–United States, 1981-2000, *MMWR* 50(21):430-434, 2001a.

Centers for Disease Control and Prevention: The global HIV and AIDS epidemic, 2001, *MMWR* 50(21):434-439, 2001b.

Centers for Disease Control and Prevention: HIV incidence among young men who have sex with men–seven U.S. cities, 1994-2000, *MMWR* 50(21):440-454, 2001c.

Centers for Disease Control and Prevention: Successful implementation of perinatal HIV prevention guidelines, *MMWR* 50(RR06):15-28, 2001d.

Centers for Disease Control and Prevention: *CDC-funded study to examine critical questions in HIV vaccine research*, 2001e. *http://www.cdc.gov/hiv/vaccine/VisLaunchupd-3-30-2.pdf*

Centers for Disease Control and Prevention: *Vaccine development*, April 1999. *http://www.cdc.gov/hiv/vaccine/vudev.htm*

Church JA: The mode of delivery and the risk of vertical transmission of human immunodeficiency virus type 1, *Pediatr* 106:470-471, 2000.

Conner EM et al: Reduction of maternal-infant transmission of human immunodeficiency virus type 1 with zidovudine treatment, *M Eng J Med* 331:1173-1180, 1994.

Darslow TG et al: *Medical immunology*, ed 10, New York, 1996, Lange/McGraw-Hill.

Doms RW, Peiper SC: Unwelcomed guests with master keys: how HIV uses chemokine receptors for cellular entry, *Virology* 235:179, 1997.

Embretson J et al: Massive covert infection of helper T lymphocytes and macrophages by HIV during the incubation period of AIDS, *Nature* 362:359-362, 1993.

Fauci AS, Lane HC: Human immunodeficiency virus (HIV) disease: AIDS and related disorders. In Fauci AS et al, editors: *Harrison's principles of internal medicine*, ed 14, New York, 1998, McGraw-Hill.

Gallo RC et al: Frequent detection and isolation of cytopathic retroviruses (HTLV-III) from patients with AIDS and at risk for AIDS, *Science* 224:500-503, 1984.

Goldschmidt R, Dong B: Current report–HIV: treatment of AIDS and HIV-related conditions, 1995, *J Am Board Fam Pract* 8:139-162, 1995.

Gottlieb MS et al: *Pneumocystis carinii* pneumonia and mucosal candidiasis in previously healthy homosexual men, *N Engl J Med* 305:1425, 1981.

Gougeon M, Montagnier L: Apoptosis in AIDS, *Science* 260:1269-1270, 1993.

Greene W: AIDS and the immune system, *Sci Am* 269(3):99-105, 1993.

Grimes D, Grimes R: *AIDS and HIV infection*, St Louis, 1994, Mosby.

Ho D et al: Rapid turnover of plasma virions and CD4 lymphocytes in HIV-1 infection, *Nature* 373:123-126, 1995.

Hoffman GS, Fauci AS: Emerging concepts in the management of vasculitic diseases, *Adv Int Med* 39:277-304, 1994.

Joint United Nations Programme on HIV/AIDS: AIDS epidemic update, December 2000. *http://www.unaids.org/wac/2000/wad 00/files/WAD_epidemic_report.htm*

Kaplan AP, editor: *Allergy*, ed 2, New York, 1997, Churchill-Livingstone.

Krasinski K: Bacterial infections. In Pizzo P, Wilfert C, editors: *Pediatric AIDS*, Baltimore, 1994, Williams & Wilkins.

Leung DYM, Greaves MW: *Allergic skin disease: a multidisciplinary approach*, New York, 2000, Marcel Dekker.

Levy J: *HIV and the pathogenesis of AIDS*, Washington, DC, 1994, ASM Press.

Lockey RF, Bulcantz SC: *Allergens and allergen immunotherapy*, ed 2, New York, 1999, Marcel Dekker.

Marlink R et al: Reduced rate of disease development after HIV-2 infection as compared to HIV-1, *Science* 265:1587-1590, 1994.

NOVA: *Search for a vaccine*, October 2000. *http://www.pbs.org/wgbh/nova/aids/vaccine.html*

Metcalfe DD, Sampson HA, Simon RA: *Food allergy: adverse reactions to foods and food additives*, ed 2, Cambridge, Mass, 1997, Blackwell Science.

Middleton E Jr, Reed CE, Ellis EF: *Allergy principles and practice*, ed 5, St Louis, 1998, Mosby.

O'Brein SJ, Dean M: In search of AIDS resistance genes, *Scientific Am* 277:46, 1997.

Ochs HD, Smith CIE, Puck JM: *Primary immunodeficiency diseases*, New York, 1999, Marcel Dekker.

Panel on Clinical Practices for Treatment of HIV Infection, convened by US Department of Health and Human Services (DHHS) and the Henry J. Kaiser Family Foundation: *Guidelines for the use of antiretroviral agents in HIV-infected adults and adolescents*. *http://www.hivatis.org/trtgdlns.html*

Pantaleo G et al: HIV infection is active and progressive in lymphoid tissue during the clinically latent stage of disease, *Nature* 362:355-358, 1993.

Perelson AS et al: HIV-1 dynamics in vivo: virion clearance rate, infected cell life span, and viral generation time, *Science* 271:1582-1586, 1996.

Perinatal HIV Guidelines Working Group, Public Health Service Task Force: *Recommendations for the use of antiretroviral drugs in pregnant HIV-1-infected women for maternal health and for reducing perinatal HIV-1 transmission in the US*, January 24, 2001. *http://www.hivatis.org/trtgdlns.html*

Rietschel R, Fowler JF Jr: *Fisher's contact dermatitis*, ed 5, Philadelphia, 2001, Lippincott–Williams & Wilkins.

Rubinstein A, Calvelli T: Pediatric acquired immunodeficiency syndrome. In Frank M et al, editors: *Samter's immunologic diseases*, ed 5, Boston, 1995, Little, Brown.

Sampson HA, Mendelson I, Rosen JP: Fatal and near-fatal anaphylactic reactions to food in children and adolescents, *N Eng J Med* 39:380-384, 1992.

Schattner E, Laurence J: HIV-induced T-lymphocyte depletion, *Clin Lab Med* 14:221-238, 1994.

Stanley SG, Faucie A: Acquired immunodeficiency syndrome. In Frank M et al, editors: *Samter's immunologic diseases*, ed 5, Boston, 1995, Little, Brown.

Stringer JSA, Vermund SH: Prevention of mother-to-child transmission of HIV-1, *Curr Opinion Obstet Gynecol* 11:427-434, 2000.

Wei X et al: Viral dynamics in human immunodeficiency virus type 1 infection, *Nature* 373:117-122, 1995.

Weiss R: How does HIV cause AIDS? *Science* 260:1273-1278, 1993.

Working Group on Antiretroviral Therapy and Medical Management of HIV-Infected Children, convened by the National Pediatric and Family HIV Resource Center (NPHRC), the Health Resources and Services Administration (HRSA), and the National Institutes of Health: *Guidelines for the use of antiretroviral agents in pediatric HIV infection*. *http://www.hivatis.org/guidelines/Pediatric/Aug08_01/pedaug08_01.pdf*

HEMATOLOGIC SYSTEM DISORDERS

*H*ematology deals with blood and the blood-forming tissues. The hematologic system also includes the monocyte-macrophage (mononuclear phagocyte) system, originally described as the reticuloendothelial system (RES), which is located throughout the body, particularly in the spleen, liver, lymph nodes, and bone marrow. The monocyte-macrophage system phagocytizes materials ranging from foreign microorganisms to dying red blood cells from the blood and body tissues. Disorders arising from these systems, called *blood dyscrasias,* range from mild and curable to rapidly progressing and lethal diseases. Diagnosis and treatment focus on the accurate interpretation of historical data, careful physical assessment, and laboratory examination.

This section examines the blood-forming tissues, the blood, and its components, with emphasis on alterations relating to red blood cells, white blood cells, platelets, and the clotting factors.

CHAPTER

16

The Composition of Blood and the Monocyte-Macrophage System

CATHERINE M. BALDY

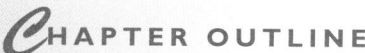HAPTER OUTLINE

COMPONENTS OF NORMAL BLOOD

Blood is a suspension of particulate material in an aqueous colloid solution that contains electrolytes. Blood serves as a medium of exchange between the fixed cells of the body and the external environment, and it possesses properties protective to the organism as a whole and to itself in particular.

The aqueous component of blood, called *plasma*, consists of 91% to 92% water as a transport medium and 8% to 9% solids. The solids include proteins such as albumin, globulins, clotting factors, and enzymes; other organic constituents such as nonprotein nitrogenous substances (urea, uric acid, xanthine, creatinine, amino acids), neutral fats, phospholipids, cholesterol, and glucose; and inorganic constituents, including sodium, chloride, bicarbonate, calcium, potassium, magnesium, phosphorus, iron, and iodine. Even though all the elements play a vital role in homeostasis, the plasma proteins are often involved in blood dyscrasias. Of the three major types, albumin formed in the liver accounts for approximately 53% of the serum protein. The major roles of albumin are in the maintenance of blood volume by providing colloid osmotic pressure, in pH and electrolyte balance, and in the transport of metal ions, fatty acids, hormones, and drugs. Globulins, accounting for 43% of the protein, are formed in the liver and lymphoid tissues.

Antibodies (immunoglobulins) are among the most important globulins. Fibrinogen, accounting for 4% of the protein, is one of the clotting factors.

The cellular component of whole blood consists of red blood cells (RBCs) (erythrocytes, red corpuscles, or RBCs), several different types of white blood cells (WBCs) (leukocytes, white corpuscles, or WBCs), and fragments of cells called platelets (or thrombocytes). RBCs transport or exchange oxygen (O_2) and carbon dioxide (CO_2), WBCs are responsible for infection control, and platelets maintain hemostasis. Because these cells have a finite life span, constant production is necessary to maintain levels required to meet tissue needs. This production, called *hematopoiesis* (formation and maturation of blood cells), takes place in the bone marrow of the skull, vertebrae, pelvis, sternum, ribs, and the proximal epiphyses of the long bones. During periods of increased demand, as in hemorrhage or cell destruction (hemolysis), production may resume in all the long bones, as it does in childhood.

On the basis of sophisticated karyotype (chromosomal) studies, all normal blood cells are thought to derive from a single pluripotent stem cell with mitotic capability. Daughters of stem cells can differentiate into either lymphoid or myeloid stem cells, which become progenitor cells. Differentiation occurs in the presence of colony-stimulating factors such as erythropoietin for red cell production and G-CSF for white cell production. Progenitor cells differentiate along a single pathway. Through a series of divisions and maturational changes, these cells become specific mature cells in the circulating blood (Fig. 16-1). The marrow stem cells continuously replace senescent (aging) blood cells and respond to acute changes, such as hemorrhage or infection, by preferentially differentiating into the specific cell lines needed.

The monocyte-macrophage system is a part of the hematologic system and includes circulating monocytes and their precursor cells in the bone marrow. The more mature tissue monocyte is called a *macrophage* (a specific WBC responsible for phagocytosis in the inflammatory reaction). This system is described in Chapter 4.

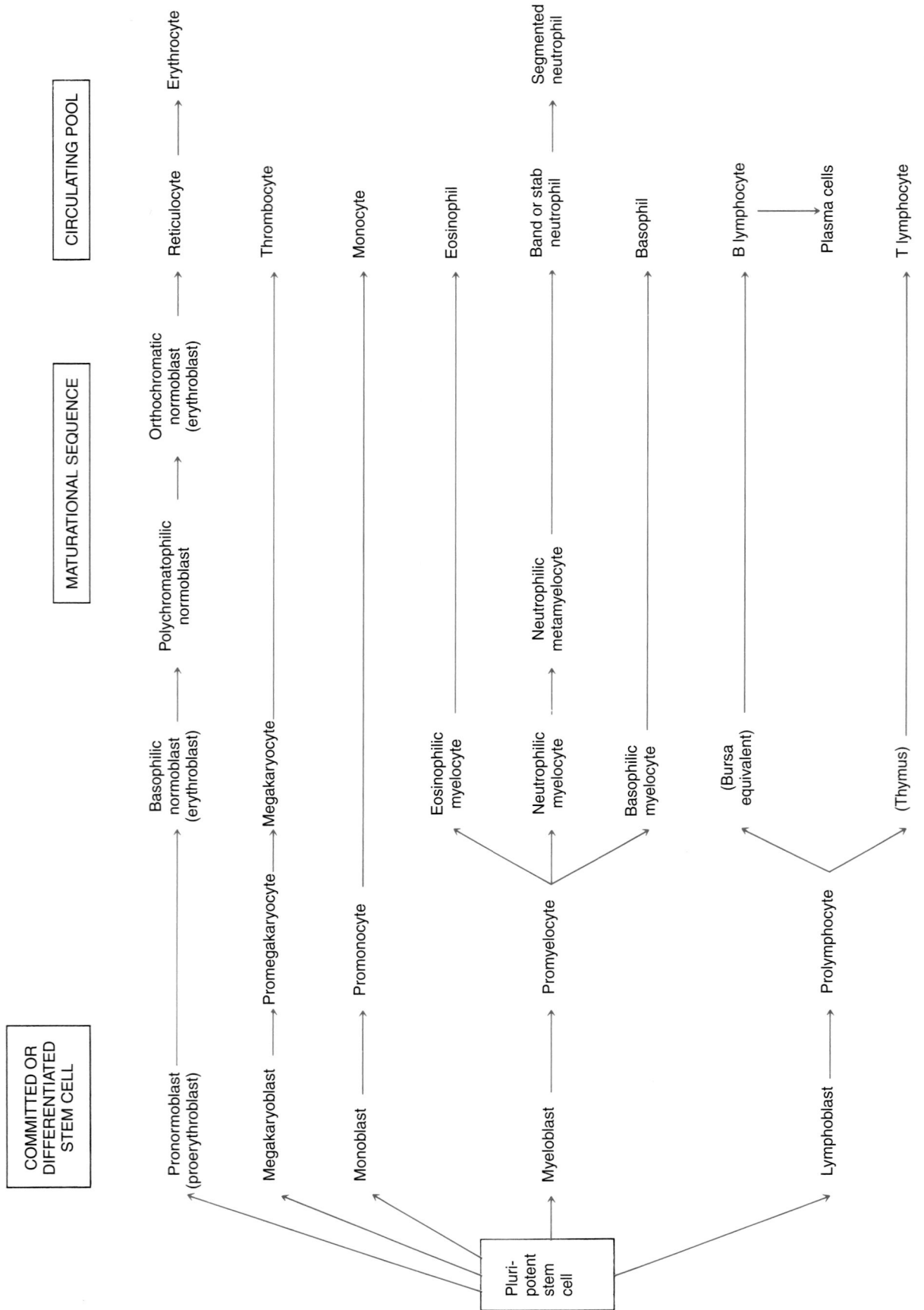

FIG. 16-1 Theory of formation and maturation of blood cells (hematopoiesis).

METHODS FOR STUDYING BLOOD

Inherent in an accurate diagnosis of hematologic disorders (blood dyscrasias) is an in-depth assessment of the individual. This assessment includes a thorough history (i.e., past and current illnesses, drug exposure, bleeding tendencies, nutritional habits, family history), physical examination, and selective diagnostic studies. Specific studies attempt to quantitate the various constituents of blood and bone marrow. This goal may be accomplished by examining a specified volume of blood. For the most accurate results, a blood sample obtained by a venipuncture is preferred. However, capillary blood specimens may be obtained by pricking the free margin of the earlobe or the palmar surface of the fingertips.

Descriptive Terms and Methods of Measurement

Blood cell count refers to an actual count of the number of formed elements (i.e., RBCs, WBCs, and platelets) in a specific volume of blood. RBCs must be lysed (destroyed) before the WBCs can be counted. These counts are usually expressed as a number of cells per cubic millimeter (mm^3) of blood. Abnormal cell counts are a reflection of the body's response or lack of response to certain processes.

Differential blood cell count determines the morphologic characteristics, as well as the numbers of the various blood cells. This information is obtained by extracting a drop of capillary blood from the fingertip or the earlobe and carefully spreading a thin film on a glass slide. The slide is stained with Wright's stain, which imparts different colors to the various cell structures according to their pH. Colors range from blue to pink or red. The various types of WBCs, RBCs, and platelets can be differentiated according to (1) the color they stain, (2) their size and configuration, (3) the structure of the nuclear chromatin, and (4) the presence or absence of nucleoli within the nucleus. An experienced hematologist, hematopathologist, or laboratory technologist can identify the various cells, their maturities, and other characteristics.

The RBCs visible on smears may be characterized according to variations in size and shape (see color plates 9, 10, and 11). The term *anisocytosis* refers to an abnormal variation in the size of the cells. Abnormal variation in shape is *poikilocytosis* and may denote cells shaped as teardrops, pears, helmets, and ovals. Both poikilocytosis and anisocytosis may reflect defective erythropoiesis (formation and development of RBCs).

Spherocytes have a decreased diameter-thickness ratio and are spherical rather than having the normal biconcave disk shape. Spherocytes have increased osmotic fragility and are present in a congenital hemolytic anemia called *congenital spherocytosis*. Sickle cells are characteristic of hemoglobin S and other sickling forms of hemoglobin. The cells assume a sickle shape on deoxygenation.

Polychromasia is a term used when cells vary in their color distribution. *Normochromia* (normal coloration) reflects a normal hemoglobin concentration in cells. The hemoglobin content of the cell determines the coloration. *Hypochromia* denotes a cell that is pale, reflecting a decreased hemoglobin concentration as observed in iron deficiency anemia.

Other variations in RBC structure that can be identified on a stained smear are *siderocytes*, which are cells containing granules of inorganic iron, and *nucleated red blood cells* or *normoblasts* (erythroblasts), which are normally observed in the bone marrow but present in the peripheral blood in response to high erythrocyte demand.

The major component of the RBC is the protein hemoglobin (Hb). Synthesis of hemoglobin in RBCs extends from the normoblast to the reticulocyte stage of development. Hemoglobin's major function is to transport O_2 and CO_2. The hemoglobin concentration of blood is measured by its color intensity, using a photometer, and is expressed as grams of hemoglobin per hundred milliliters of blood (g/100 ml) or grams per deciliter (g/dl).

The type of hemoglobin can also be identified. Approximately 300 variants of hemoglobin, differing in the genetic code and thus the sequence of amino acids, have been identified. Although most types are without clinical significance and are functionally normal, some produce marked morbidity and mortality. Hemoglobin electrophoresis identifies the abnormal hemoglobin. The various types move at different characteristic velocities across paper or starch gel, based on their electrical charge. Hemoglobins are identified by letters or by their place of occurrence and discovery:

Hb A: normal adult hemoglobin
Hb F: fetal hemoglobin
Hb S: hemoglobin found in sickle cell disease
Hb: Memphis

Another measure, the *hematocrit (Hct)* or packed cell volume, indicates the volume of the whole blood that is composed of RBCs. This measurement is the percentage of RBCs in the whole blood after centrifugation of the specimen and is expressed as cubic millimeters of packed cells per dl of blood or in volumes per dl.

The results of the RBC count, its hemoglobin concentration, and the hematocrit are used to calculate the red cell indices, which reflect the size of the RBC, its hemoglobin content, and its concentration. Dividing the hematocrit by the RBC count gives the *mean corpuscular volume (MCV)*. MCV is a size measurement, expressed as cubic micrometers, with the normal range being 81 to 96 μm^3. RBCs in that range are termed *normocytic*, being of normal cell size. An MCV less than 81 μm^3 indicates cells that are microcytic, because they appear smaller than 7 μm on smears, whereas an MCV greater than 96 μm^3 indicates macrocytic cells that are larger than 8 μm on smears.

The *mean corpuscular hemoglobin concentration (MCHC)* measures the amount of hemoglobin in 100 ml (1 dl) of packed RBCs. Determined by dividing the hemoglobin measurement by the hematocrit, MCHC is expressed in grams per 100 ml (g/dl). The normal range is 30 to 36 g/dl of blood, which is termed normochromic; a finding of less than 30 g/dl is hypochromic because these cells appear pale on the smear. The *mean corpuscular hemoglobin (MCH)* measures the amount of hemoglobin present in a single RBC and is determined by dividing the amount of hemoglobin in 1000 ml of blood by the number of red cells per cubic millimeter of blood. The MCH is expressed in picograms of hemoglobin per RBC. The normal value is about 27 to 31 pg per RBC.

The *reticulocyte count*, another important determination, reflects bone marrow activity. A reticulocyte is an

TABLE 16-1 ■■■

Methods for Examining Blood

Measurement	Description
Red blood cell (RBC) count	Number of RBCs in 1 mm³ of blood (millions per cubic millimeter)
Hemoglobin concentration	Amount of hemoglobin in a given volume of blood (expressed as g/dl)
Hematocrit	Percent of blood made up of RBCs (volume %)
Mean corpuscular volume (MCV)	Volume of each individual RBC (μm³): $$MCV = \frac{Hematocrit\ (vol\ \%\ \times\ 10)}{RBC\ count\ (millions/mm^3)}$$
Mean corpuscular hemoglobin concentration (MCHC)	Proportion of each RBC occupied by hemoglobin (concentration measurement): $$MCHC = \frac{Hemoglobin\ (g/dl\ \times\ 100)}{Hematocrit\ (vol\ \%)}$$
Mean corpuscular hemoglobin (MCH)	Amount of hemoglobin present in each RBC (weight measurement): $$MCH = \frac{Hemoglobin\ (g/dl\ \times\ 10)}{RBC\ count\ (millions/mm^3)}$$
White blood cell (WBC) count	Number of WBCs in 1 mm³ of blood
Differential count	Percent of the various types of WBCs seen on examination of a peripheral film (granulocytes including PMNs,* Segs,* eosinophils, and basophils; monocytes; and lymphocytes)
Platelet count	Number of platelets in 1 mm³ of blood
Reticulocyte count	Percent of immature nonnucleated RBCs containing residual RNA

*PMN, Polymorphonuclear neutrohil; Segs, segmented neutrophils.

immature nonnucleated RBC that contains residual ribonucleic acid (RNA) in its cytoplasm. Normally, only 1% to 2% is present in the peripheral blood. A peripheral blood smear, taken as described, is treated with a supravital stain, which imparts a blue color to any RNA within immature RBCs; these cells appear to have a net or "reticulum" inside hence the name reticulocyte (Table 16-1). The residual RNA disappears within the first day or two that the cell is outside the bone marrow, and the cell becomes a mature RBC. An increased number of circulating reticulocytes indicates increased bone marrow activity, whereas a decrease or absence indicates bone marrow failure. Normal values for these measurements are given in Table 16-2.

Study of Bone Marrow

A bone marrow aspiration and biopsy are performed when the preceding studies yield insufficient data or when diseases are suspected that may affect the hematologic system. Aspiration studies are also used to guide the dosages of chemotherapy and radiation therapy in patients with hematologic malignancies.

An accurate bone marrow specimen in an adult can be obtained from the sternum, the spinous processes of the vertebrae, or the anterior or posterior iliac crest. When a biopsy is also required, the latter is the preferred site.

Bone marrow biopsy, as well as aspiration, must be considered a minor surgical procedure and carried out under aseptic conditions. The patient is placed comfortably on his or her side with the back slightly flexed and the knees drawn toward the chest. The posterior iliac crest is cleansed and covered with antiseptic solution. The skin, subcutaneous tissue, and periosteum are anesthetized using 1% to 2% lidocaine (Xylocaine). A 2 to 3 mm incision is made to facilitate penetration with a 14-gauge, 2- to 4-cm bone marrow needle and to avoid introducing

TABLE 16-2 ■■■

Normal Blood Cell Values

Measurement	Men	Women
Red blood cell count (million cells/mm³)	4.7-6.1	4.2-5.2
Hemoglobin (g/dl)	13.4-17.6	12.0-15.4
Hematocrit (vol %)	42-53	38-46
MCV (μm³/RBC)	81-96	
MCHC (g/dl of RBC)	30-36	
MCH (pg/RBC)	27-31	
Total WBC count (cells/mm³)	4000-10,000	
Granulocytes*		
PMNs (%)	38-70	
Eosinophils (%)	1-5	
Basophils (%)	0-2	
Monocytes (%)*	1-8	
Lymphocytes (%)*	15-45	
Platelets (cells/mm³)	150,000-400,000	
Reticulocyte count (%)†	1-2	

PMN, Polymorphonuclear neutrophil; RBC, red blood cell; WBC, white blood cell.
*Percentage of total WBCs.
†Percentage of total RBCs.

a skin plug into the marrow cavity. On entry, the stylet is removed from the needle, a 10-ml syringe is attached, and with a swift, short aspiration, approximately 25 μl of bone marrow is withdrawn. Even though the patient experiences tremendous pressure throughout the procedure, he or she must be warned that a sudden sharp but brief pain may be felt because of the negative pressure that occurs with aspiration. Smears are quickly made with the aspirate, and grayish white particulate matter can usually be observed along with fat vacuoles. A portion of the specimen is allowed to clot and is sectioned for further study. Cell counts and differentials are also obtained from the aspirate.

A biopsy is usually indicated in hematologic malignancies. In this procedure, a special biopsy needle (a Jamshidi needle, 11-cm long with a 3-mm diameter tapering to a 2-mm cutting edge) is used to obtain a bone spicule. This bone spicule is extruded onto a glass slide using a probe inserted through the cutting edge. Several imprints are made by gently touching the slide with the spicule, which can be stained with Wright's stain, as discussed with the peripheral smear. One or two slides may be stained, with Prussian blue reaction depicting stored iron. The biopsy spicule is placed in Bouin's or Zenker's solution, both of which are fixatives. The specimen is then placed in paraffin blocks, sectioned, stained, and studied microscopically.

The bone marrow biopsy is used to study the marrow cellularity without destroying the architecture. Bone marrow of increased activity is termed *hypercellular* or *hyperplastic* (increased number of cells with ↓ fat); marrow with decreased activity is *hypocellular* or *hypoplastic* (decreased number of cells ↑ fat). The ratio of myeloid (bone marrow leukocytes) to erythroid (red blood cell) elements (M/E ratio) is calculated, and the presence of a normal, increased, or decreased number of megakaryocytes (platelet precursors) is noted. Cell distribution, maturation abnormalities, and neoplastic cells can be observed. Status of the bone, such as fibrosis, can also be identified.

Cytogenics

In diagnosing hematologic malignancies, cytogenetic analysis has emerged as one of the most important studies for diagnosing and treating, and is paramount in prognosticating the responsiveness to therapy and the potential for remission or cure, as well as documenting relapse. Cytogenetics is the study of the chromosomal makeup of cells, their normal functions, and any deviation from that norm. The cells are studied during the metaphase stage of mitosis (cell division to depict translocations, inversions, and deletions of genetic material from one chromosome to another). Cytogenetic analysis can be done on tissue obtained during bone marrow aspiration and biopsy, on peripheral blood if the counts are elevated, and on lymph nodes, liver, and spleen. Cytogenetic testing is also performed on amniotic fluid and products of conception to diagnose fetal abnormalities.

Another major test is immunophenotyping, which is used to accurately diagnose hematologic disorders, particularly in differentiating acute lymphocytic leukemia from acute myelogenous leukemia and other lymphatic malignancies. Immunophenotyping is performed by flow cytometry to identify antigen groups known as clusters of differentiation (CDs) on the surface of hematopoietic cells. In this study, specific monoclonal antibodies labeled with a fluorescent marker will associate with its corresponding surface antigen on the cell (Sacher, McPherson, 2000). As the cells flow past an optical detector, they are counted to determine cell volume and cell granularity, identifying the cellular phenotype, size, and cytoplasmic constitution. Normal cells display a variety of cell types and differentiation status. A malignant process disturbs this programmed expression and the aberrant expression of cell surface antigens that distinguishes normal from abnormal cells. Similar to cytogenetics, flow cytometry can be performed on bone marrow, peripheral blood, lymph nodes, liver, and spleen (Radich, Sievers, 2000).

Biochemical Studies

Various studies can be used to measure levels of the elements necessary for cell development, particularly that of red blood cells. These studies include measurements of serum iron (Fe), total iron-binding capacity (TIBC), vitamin B_{12}, and folic acid levels. The iron-binding capacity measures the ability of plasma transferrin to carry iron from the gastrointestinal tract or iron stores to the bone marrow and is elevated in iron deficiency anemia. Erythropoietin radioimmunoassay measures the level of erythropoietin. The glycoprotein hormone preferentially increases the erythrocyte-committed (red cell) unit and decreases the maturation time of the red cells in the marrow (Sacher, McPherson, 2000). Other studies related to hematology include the coagulation studies (see Chapter 19).

KEY CONCEPTS

- Blood is a suspension of particulate material in an aqueous colloid solution containing electrolytes, which is a medium of exchange between the fixed cells of the body and the external environment.
- Plasma is the aqueous component of blood and is a transport medium.
- Solids include proteins such as albumin, globulins, clotting factors, and enzymes; other organic constituents, neutral fats, phospholipids, cholesterol, and glucose; and inorganic constituents.
- The cellular component of whole blood consists of red blood cells (erythrocytes, red corpuscles, or RBCs), several different types of white blood cells (leukocytes, white corpuscles, or WBCs), and fragments of cells called platelets (or thrombocytes).

- RBCs transport or exchange O_2 and CO_2, WBCs are responsible for infection control, and platelets maintain hemostasis.
- Hematopoiesis is the formation and maturation of blood cells.
- All normal blood cells are thought to derive from a single pluripotential stem cell with mitotic capability.
- The monocyte-macrophage system is a part of the hematologic system and includes circulating monocytes and their precursor cells in the bone marrow.
- A macrophage is a specific WBC responsible for phagocytosis in the inflammatory reaction.
- Blood cell count refers to an actual count of the number of formed elements (i.e., RBCs, WBCs, and platelets) in a specific volume of blood.

- Abnormal cell counts are a reflection of the body's response or lack of response to certain processes.
- Anisocytosis is an abnormal variation in the size of the cells.
- Abnormal variation in shape is poikilocytosis.
- Polychromasia reflects RBCs that vary in their color distribution.
- Normochromia reflects a normal hemoglobin concentration in RBCs.
- Hypochromia denotes an RBC that is pale, reflecting a decreased hemoglobin concentration as observed in iron deficiency anemia.
- The major component of the RBC is the protein Hb and its major function is to transport O_2 and CO_2.
- Hemoglobins are identified by the following letters or by their place of occurrence and discovery: (Hb A: normal adult hemoglobin; Hb F: fetal hemoglobin; Hb S: hemoglobin found in sickle cell disease; Hb: Memphis).
- Hematocrit (Hct) or packed cell volume, indicates the volume of the whole blood that is composed of RBCs.
- MCV is a size measurement; normocytic being of normal cell size; microcytic, appear smaller; macrocytic cells are larger.

- The MCH measures the amount of hemoglobin present in a single RBC.
- The reticulocyte count reflects bone marrow activity. A reticulocyte is an immature nonnucleated RBC that contains residual RNA in its cytoplasm.
- Bone marrow aspiration studies are also used to guide the dosages of chemotherapy and radiation therapy in patients with hematologic malignancies.
- In diagnosing hematologic malignancies, cytogenetic analysis is one of the most important studies used in diagnosing and treating, prognosticating the responsiveness to therapy, the potential for remission or cure, and documenting relapse.
- Cytogenetics is the study of the chromosomal make-up of cells, their normal functions, and any deviation from that norm.
- Another major test is immunophenotyping, which is used to diagnose hematologic disorders accurately, particularly in differentiating acute lymphocytic leukemia from acute myelogenous leukemia and other lymphatic malignancies.

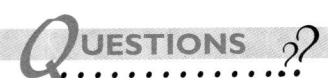

QUESTIONS ??

A sampling of review questions for this chapter appears here. Visit http://www.mosby.com/MERLIN/PriceWilson/ for additional questions.

Answer the following on a separate sheet of paper.
1. Define hematology.
2. Describe the hematologic system.
3. Describe the three major types of cells found in the cellular component of whole blood.
4. Explain the theory of hematopoiesis.
5. Explain how normal cells are thought to derive from a single pluripotential stem cell with mitotic capability.
6. Describe the assessment process applied when diagnosing blood dyscrasias.

Match each descriptive statement in column A with its appropriate measurement in column B.

Column A
7. _____ Red cell count
8. _____ Hematocrit
9. _____ Mean corpuscular volume (MCV)
10. _____ Hemoglobin concentration
11. _____ Mean corpuscular hemoglobin concentration (MCHC)
12. _____ Reticulocyte count
13. _____ White cell count
14. _____ Mean corpuscular hemoglobin (MCH)
15. _____ Differential count
16. _____ Platelet count

Column B
a. Percentage of packed RBCs in a sample of blood (volume percentage)
b. Amount of hemoglobin in a given volume of blood (g/dl)
c. Number of WBCs in 1 mm^3 of blood
d. Number of RBCs in 1 mm^3 of blood (millions/mm^3)
e. The proportion of each RBC occupied by hemoglobin (concentration measurement)
f. Number of platelets in 1 mm^3 of blood
g. Volume of each individual RBC (μm^3)
h. Percentage of the different types of WBCs seen on examination of a peripheral film
i. Percentage of immature nonnucleated RBCs containing residual RNA
j. Amount of hemoglobin present in each RBC (weight measurement)

Red Blood Cell Disorders

CATHERINE M. BALDY

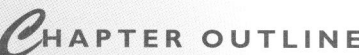
NORMAL STRUCTURE AND FUNCTION

Red blood cells (RBCs), or erythrocytes, are nonnucleated biconcave disks approximately 8 μm in diameter, 2 μm thick at the outer perimeter and decreasing to 1 μm or less at the center (Fig. 17-1). Because these cells are soft and pliable, they change in configuration during passage through the microcirculation. The outer leaflet of the cell membrane contains the blood group antigens A and B and the Rh factor identifying the individual's blood type. The RBC's major component is the protein hemoglobin (Hb), which transports most of the oxygen (O_2) and a small fraction of carbon dioxide (CO_2) and maintains normal pH through a series of intracellular buffers. The Hb molecule consists of two pairs of polypeptide chains (globin) and four heme groups, each one containing an atom of ferrous iron. This configuration allows the most expedient exchange of gases.

The average adult has approximately 5 million RBCs per cubic millimeter of blood , each RBC having an average life span of 120 days. A steady balance is maintained between normal daily losses and replacement. RBC production is stimulated by a glycoprotein hormone, *erythropoietin*, known to originate primarily in the kidney, with 10% coming from liver hepatocytes (Dessypries, 1999). Erythropoietin production is stimulated by renal tissue hypoxia caused by changes in atmospheric O_2 pressure, decreased O_2 content of arterial blood, and decreased hemoglobin concentration. Erythropoietin stimulates the stem cells to initiate the proliferation and maturation of RBCs. Maturation depends on adequate amounts and proper use of nutrients, such as vitamin B_{12}, folic acid, protein, iron, and copper. In the presence of renal disease or absent kidneys, anemia becomes profound because the liver cannot supply enough erythropoietin (Guyton, 2001).

All the steps of hemoglobin synthesis take place in the bone marrow. The late steps continue after the immature RBC is released into the circulation as a reticulocyte.

As the RBC ages, it becomes rigid and fragile, finally rupturing. The hemoglobin is phagocytosed primarily in the spleen, liver, and bone marrow and is reduced to globin and heme. Globin reenters the amino acid pool. Iron is liberated from heme, and the greater part is transported by the plasma protein transferrin to the bone marrow for RBC production. The remaining iron is stored in the form of ferritin and hemosiderin in the liver and other body tissues for future use (Guyton, 2001). The remaining heme portion is reduced to carbon monoxide (CO) and biliverdin. The CO, carried in the form of carboxyhemoglobin, is excreted via the lungs. The biliverdin is reduced to free bilirubin, which, in turn, is slowly released into plasma, where it combines with plasma

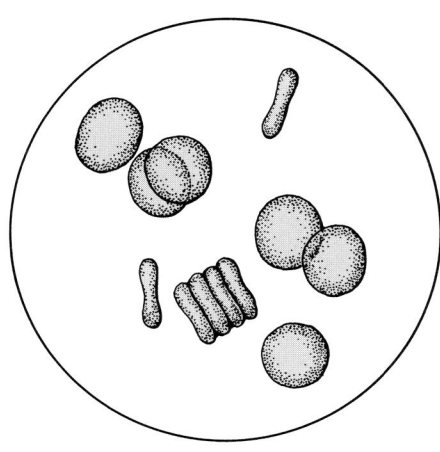

FIG. 17-1   Erythrocytes.

albumin and is transported to the hepatic cells for excretion into the bile canaliculi (Ganong, 1999). In the presence of active RBC destruction, as in hemolysis, the rapid release of large amounts of bilirubin into the extracellular fluids causes the yellowish hue to the skin and conjunctivae called *jaundice* (Guyton, 2001).

ABNORMALITIES OF RBC PRODUCTION

Alterations of the RBC mass produce two distinct entities. When the number of RBCs is insufficient, anemia develops. The opposite condition, too many RBCs, is called polycythemia.

Anemia

By definition, *anemia* is a reduction below the normal level in the number of RBCs, the quantity of hemoglobin, and the volume of packed RBCs (hematocrit) per 100 ml of blood. Anemia thus is not a diagnosis but a reflection of an underlying pathophysiologic alteration revealed by a careful history, physical examination, and laboratory confirmation.

Because all organ systems may be involved, a wide range of clinical manifestations may be present in anemia, depending on (1) the rate at which the anemia develops, (2) the age of the individual, (3) his or her compensatory mechanism, (4) his or her activity level, (5) the underlying disease state, and (6) the severity of the anemia.

As the effective number of RBCs decreases, O_2 delivery to the tissues decreases. Sudden blood loss (30% or more), as in hemorrhage, results in symptoms of hypovolemia and hypoxemia, including restlessness, diaphoresis (cold perspiration), tachycardia, shortness of breath, and rapid progression to circulatory collapse or shock. However, a drop in RBC mass over a period of several months (even as much as a 50% decrease) allows the body's compensatory mechanism to adapt, and the patient is usually asymptomatic, except on exertion. The body adapts by (1) increasing the cardiac output and respirations, thereby increasing the delivery of O_2 to the tissues by the RBCs, (2) increasing the release of O_2 by hemoglobin, (3) expanding plasma volume by pulling fluid from the tissue spaces, and (4) redistributing blood flow to vital organs (Guyton, 2001).

One of the most common signs attributed to anemia is pallor. This condition generally results from decreased blood volume, decreased hemoglobin, and vasoconstriction to maximize O_2 delivery to major vital organs. Skin color is not a reliable index for pallor because of influences such as skin pigmentation, temperature, and depth and distribution of the capillary bed. Nail beds, palms, and mucous membranes of the mouth and conjunctivae are better indicators for assessing pallor. When the creases of the palm are no longer pink, the hemoglobin is generally less than 8 grams.

Tachycardia and cardiac murmurs (sounds caused by increased velocity of blood flow) reflect the increased cardiac workload and output. Angina (chest pain), particularly in older individuals with coronary stenosis, may result from myocardial ischemia. In severe anemia, congestive heart failure may result because the anoxic heart muscle cannot adapt to its increased workload. Dyspnea (difficulty in breathing), shortness of breath, and increased fatigue on exertion are manifestations of decreased O_2 delivery. Headache, dizziness, faintness, and tinnitus (ringing in the ears) may reflect the decreased oxygenation of the central nervous system. Gastrointestinal symptoms such as anorexia, nausea, constipation or diarrhea, and stomatitis (a sore tongue and oral mucous membranes) may also occur in severe anemia; these symptoms are generally associated with deficiency states, such as iron deficiency.

Classification of Anemias

Anemias may be classified according to (1) the morphologic factors of the red blood cell and the indices or (2) the etiology.

In the morphologic classification of anemias, *micro-* or *macro-* refers to the size of the RBCs and *chromic* to their color. Three major categories are recognized. In the first, *normocytic, normochromic* anemia, the RBCs are normal in size and shape and contain the normal amount of hemoglobin (mean corpuscular volume [MCV] and mean corpuscular hemoglobin concentration [MCHC] are normal or low normal). Causes of this type of anemia are acute blood loss, hemolysis, chronic diseases that include infections, endocrine disorders, renal disorders, marrow failure, and metastatic infiltrative diseases of the bone marrow.

The second major category is *macrocytic, normochromic* anemia, in which the RBCs are larger than is normal but are normochromic because the hemoglobin concentration is normal (increased MCV; normal MCHC) (Fig. 17-2). This condition results from disordered or interrupted synthesis of deoxyribonucleic acid (DNA) as observed in deficiency states of vitamin B_{12} or folic acid or both. Normochromic anemia may also occur in cancer chemotherapy because the agents interfere with DNA synthesis.

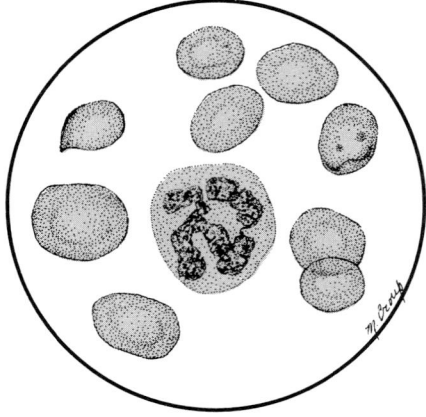

FIG. 17-2 Peripheral blood characteristic of macrocytic anemia. In the upper right, the red blood cells are not as uniformly round (poikilocytosis) as they are in Fig. 17-1, and they are of different sizes (anisocytosis). Most of the cells are either of normal size or too large. The large oval red cells seen in the lower left are called ovalomacrocytes. These cells are characteristic of vitamin B_{12} and folate deficiencies.

The third category is *microcytic, hypochromic* anemia (Fig. 17-3). Microcytic means small cell, and hypochromic means decreased coloration. Because the hue comes from hemoglobin, these cells contain less than the normal amount of hemoglobin (decreased MCV; decreased MCHC). This condition generally reflects either insufficient heme synthesis or lack of iron, as in iron deficiency anemia, sideroblastic states, and chronic blood loss, or impaired globin synthesis, as in thalassemia. Thalassemia involves a mismatch in the amounts of alpha- and beta-chains synthesized, thus the normal tetrameric hemoglobin molecule cannot form.

Anemias may also be classified by etiology. The major causes considered are (1) increased RBC loss and (2) decreased or defective cell production.

Increased RBC loss may be caused by bleeding or by cell destruction. Bleeding may result from trauma or ulcers or from chronic bleeding from polyps in the colon, malignancy, hemorrhoids, or menstruation. Destruction of circulating RBCs, known as *hemolysis*, occurs when a defect in the RBC itself shortens its life (intrinsic defect) or an altered environment leads to its destruction (extrinsic defect) (Sacher, McPherson, 2000). Conditions in which the RBC itself is defective include the following:

1. Hemoglobinopathy or inherited abnormal hemoglobin, such as sickle cell disease
2. Impaired globin synthesis, such as thalassemia
3. RBC membrane defects, such as hereditary spherocytosis and elliptocytosis
4. Enzyme deficiencies, such as glucose 6-phosphate dehydrogenase (G6PD) deficiency and pyruvate kinase deficiency

The foregoing disorders are hereditary. However, hemolysis can also be caused by problems of the RBC environment, which often entail an immune response. An *isoimmune* response involves different individuals within the same species and results from an incompatible blood transfusion. An *autoimmune* response consists of production of antibodies against the body's own RBCs. Autoimmune hemolytic anemia can occur without known cause after the administration of certain drugs, such as alpha-methyldopa, quinine, sulfonamides, or L-dopa, or in other disease states, such as lymphoma, chronic lymphocytic leukemia, lupus erythematosus, rheumatoid arthritis, and viral infections. Autoimmune hemolytic anemias are classified according to the temperature at which the antibody reacts with the RBCs—they may be warm antibody type or cold antibody type.

Malaria is a parasitic disease transmitted to humans by the bite of an infected female *Anopheles* mosquito. Malaria results in severe hemolytic anemia when RBCs become infested by a *Plasmodium* parasite, which causes an irregular surface defect in the RBC. The defective RBCs are then rapidly removed from the circulation by the spleen (Goldsmith, 2001; Beutler, 2001).

Hypersplenism (enlarged spleen) can also cause hemolysis by markedly increased trapping and destroying of RBCs. Because the enlarged spleen sequesters all types of blood cells, a hypersplenic patient will demonstrate pancytopenia and a normal or hypercellular bone marrow. Severe burns, particularly when the capillary bed is disrupted, can also lead to hemolysis. Artificial heart valves also cause hemolysis by mechanical destruction (Linker, 2001).

The second major etiologic classification includes decreased or defective RBC production (dyserythropoiesis). Any condition affecting the bone marrow function falls into this category. Included are (1) metastatic solid tissue malignancies, the leukemias, lymphomas and multiple myeloma; exposure to toxic drugs and chemicals; and irradiation can reduce effective red cell production; and (2) chronic diseases involving the kidneys and liver, as well as infections and endocrine deficiencies. Lack of essential vitamins, such as B_{12}, folic acid, and C, and lack of iron can result in ineffective RBC formation, leading to anemia. To determine the type of anemia, both the morphologic and etiologic considerations must be incorporated.

Aplastic Anemia

Aplastic anemia is a life-threatening disorder of the stem cell in the bone marrow, in which an insufficient number of blood cells are produced. Aplastic anemia may be congenital, idiopathic (unknown cause), or secondary to industrial or viral causes (Hoffbrand, Pettit, 1993). Individuals with aplastic anemia are pancytopenic (deficient in all types of blood cells). Morphologically, the RBCs are normocytic and normochromic, the reticulocyte count is low or absent, and bone marrow biopsy indicates a "dry tap" with marked hypoplasia and replacement with fatty tissue. No abnormal marrow cells exist in the marrow. The idiopathic aplastic anemias are thought to be immunologically mediated, with the patient's T lymphocytes suppressing hematopoietic stem cells.

Secondary causes of aplastic anemia (temporary or permanent) include the following:

1. Systemic lupus erythematosus-autoimmune basis
2. Antineoplastic or cytotoxic agents
3. Radiation therapy
4. Certain antibiotics
5. Miscellaneous drugs, such as anticonvulsants, thyroid medication, gold compounds, and phenylbutazone
6. Chemicals such as benzene, organic solvents, and insecticides (agents thought to damage the marrow directly)
7. Viral diseases such as infectious mononucleosis and human immunodeficiency virus (HIV); aplastic anemia following viral hepatitis is particularly severe and likely to be fatal.

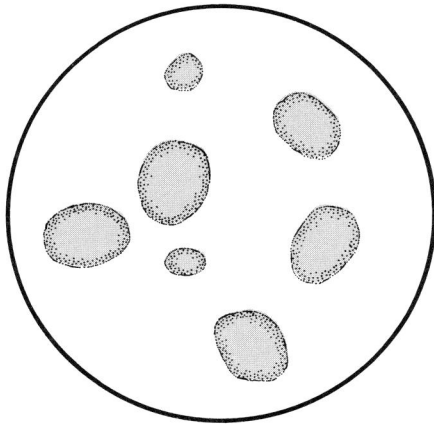

FIG. 17-3   Erythrocytes characteristic of hypochromic anemia.

TABLE 17-1

Hematologic Effects Secondary to Drugs

Generic Name	Trade Name*	Hemolysis	Megalo-blastosis	Aplasia	Leukopenia or Agranulocytosis	Thrombo-cytopenia†	Thrombo-cytopathy†
ANTIBIOTICS							
Chloramphenicol	Chloromycetin	X		XX	X	X	
Erythromycin	Ilosone			X	X	X	
Penicillin	Pen-Vee K	XX		X	X	X	X
Sulfisoxazole	Gantrisin	XX		X	X	XX	
Tetracycline	Sumycin	X		X	X	X	
Cotrimazole	Bactrin	XX		X	X	X	
ANTICONVULSANTS							
Phenytoin	Dilantin	X	X	X	X	X	
Phenobarbital	Luminal	X	X	X		X	
Mephenytoin	Mesantoin	X	X	X	X	X	
Carbamazepine	Tegretol	X		X	X	X	
ORAL HYPOGLYCEMICS							
Tolbutamide	Orinase	X		XX	X	X	
Chlorpropamide	Diabinese			X	X		
ANTIINFLAMMATORY DRUGS							
Acetylsalicylic acid, aspirin	Colsalide	X		X	X	XX	XX
Colchicine	Colqout			X	X	X	X
Gold compounds				X	XX	X	
Indomethacin	Indocin	X		X	X	X	XX
Phenylbutazone	Butazolidin			XX	XX	XX	XX
ANTIHYPERTENSIVES AND DIURETICS							
Chlorothiazide	Diuril	X		X	X	X	
Methyldopa	Aldomet	XX		X	X	X	
Captopril	Capoten			X	X	X	
ANTINEOPLASTICS							
Mechlorethamine hydrochloride	Mustargen			XX	XX	XX	
Cyclophosphamide	Cytoxan			XX	XX	XX	
Cytarabine	Cytosar-U		XX	XX	XX	XX	
Methotrexate	Folex	X	XX	XX	XX	XX	
Mercaptopurine	Purinethol		XX	XX	XX	XX	
Hydroxyurea	Hydrea		XX	XX	XX	XX	
TRANQUILIZERS							
Chlordiazepoxide	Librium			X	X		X
Imipramine	Tofranil			X	XX		X
Chlorpromazine	Thorazine	X	X	X	X	X	X

X, Infrequently occurring; XX, frequently occurring.
*This list is not all inclusive; other equally effective brands may exist.
†Thrombocytopenia is a decrease in platelet numbers; thrombocytopathy is an alteration in platelet function.

Table 17-1 identifies various drugs and their hematologic effects.

The symptom complex in aplastic anemia is caused by the degree of pancytopenia. The signs and symptoms include those of anemia, with fatigue, weakness, and shortness of breath with exertion. Other signs and symptoms are attributable to deficiencies of platelets and white blood cells (WBCs). Platelet deficiency may lead to (1) ecchymoses and petechiae (bleeding into the skin), (2) epistaxis (nosebleed), (3) gastrointestinal bleeding, (4) genitourinary bleeding, and (5) central nervous system bleeding. Deficiency of WBCs increases both the susceptibility and severity of infections, including bacterial, viral, and fungal infection.

Severe aplasia with a decreased (less than 1%) or absent reticulocyte count, a granulocyte count of less than 500/mm^3 and a platelet count of less than 20,000 cause death from infection and or bleeding within weeks or months. Sepsis is the most frequent cause of death (Young, 2000). However, a person who is less severely affected may live for years. Treatment of aplastic anemia dictates the removal, when known, of the causative agent. The major focus of treatment is supportive care until the bone marrow recovers. Because infection and bleeding are the major causes of death, prevention becomes essential. Growth factors such as G-CSF can be used to raise the neutrophil count and prevent or minimize infections. Prevention measures should include a protected environment and good overall hygiene. In the event of bleeding or infection, judicious use of blood component therapy (red cells and platelets) and antibiotics becomes essential. Bone marrow stimulating agents such as androgens may induce erythropoiesis, although their efficacy is uncertain. Patients with chronic aplastic anemia adapt well and can be maintained at hemoglobin levels between 8 and 9 g/dl with periodic blood transfusions.

In young individuals with severe aplastic anemia secondary to stem cell damage, allogeneic stem cell transplantation with compatible donors (siblings with matching human histocompatible leukocyte antigens [HLA] is indicated.) The overall success rate exceeds 80% in patients who were not previously transfused. In older patients with aplastic anemia or those cases considered to be immunologically mediated, antithymocyte globulin (ATG)–containing antibodies against human T cells has been used together with corticosteroids and cyclosporine to benefit 50% to 60% of the patients. Response can be expected within 4 to 12 weeks. Generally, this response is partial but sufficient to raise the counts high enough to protect the patients and allow a comfortable life (Linker, 2001).

Iron Deficiency Anemia

Morphologically, this condition is classified as microcytic, hypochromic anemia with a decrease in the quantity of hemoglobin synthesis. Iron deficiency is the major cause of anemia in the world and is particularly prevalent in women of childbearing age, secondary to menstrual losses and to increased iron demand during pregnancy. Other causes of iron deficiency include (1) inadequate iron intake, for example, infants maintained on milk-only diets for 12 to 24 months and individuals who follow strict vegetarian habits; (2) impaired absorption after gastrectomy; and (3) persistent blood loss, as with slow gastrointestinal bleeding from polyps, neoplasms, gastritis, esophageal varices, aspirin ingestion, and hemorrhoids.

Normally the average adult body contains 4 to 5 g of iron, depending on sex and size. Greater than two thirds of the iron is found in hemoglobin. Iron is released with cell senescence and death and transported via plasma transferrin to the bone marrow for erythropoiesis. With the exception of minute amounts in myoglobin (muscle) and in heme enzymes, the remaining iron is stored for further needs in the liver, spleen, and bone marrow as ferritin and hemosiderin.

Although the average diet contains 10 to 20 mg of iron, only approximately 5% to 10% (1 to 2 mg) is actually absorbed. As iron stores become depleted, more is absorbed from the diet. Ingested iron is converted to ferrous iron in the stomach and duodenum and is absorbed from the duodenum and proximal jejunum. The iron is then transported by plasma transferrin to the bone marrow for hemoglobin synthesis or to the tissue stores.

Each milliliter of blood contains 0.5 mg of iron. Iron losses generally are minute, from 0.5 to 1 mg/day. However, menstruating women lose an additional 15 to 28 mg/month. Although loss to menses ceases during pregnancy, the daily iron requirement increases to meet the demands of the mother's increased blood volume and the formation of the placenta, umbilical cord, and fetus, as well as to compensate for blood lost during delivery.

In addition to the signs and symptoms presented for anemia, individuals with severe iron deficiency (plasma iron less than 40 mg/dl; hemoglobin 6 to 7 g/dl) have brittle, fine hair and nails that are thin, flat, easily broken, and possibly spoon shaped (koilonychia). Additionally, the papillae of the tongue atrophy, resulting in a pale, smooth, shiny, beefy-red appearance, and the tongue becomes inflamed and sore. Angular stomatitis (cheilosis), cracking with redness and pain at the corners of the mouth, may also occur.

Examination of the blood reveals a normal or near-normal RBC count and a reduced hemoglobin level. On peripheral smear, the RBCs are microcytic and hypochromic (decreased MCV, decreased MCHC, and decreased MCH) with poikilocytosis and anisocytosis (see color plate 12). The reticulocyte count may be normal or decreased. The iron level is reduced, whereas the total serum iron-binding capacity is increased.

To treat iron deficiency, the underlying cause of the anemia must be identified and resolved. Surgical intervention may be necessary to inhibit active bleeding from polyps, ulcers, malignancies, and hemorrhoids; dietary alterations may be needed for babies who were fed milk only or for individuals with food idiosyncrasies or those who are taking large doses of aspirin. Although dietary modifications may increase the available iron (e.g., by adding liver), supplemental iron is needed to increase the hemoglobin and restore iron stores. Iron is available in parenteral and oral forms. Most people respond well to oral compounds, such as ferrous sulfate, 325 mg three times a day for at least 6 months to replace iron stores. Parenteral iron preparations are used in patients who cannot tolerate oral preparations or those who are noncompliant. Parenteral iron does have a relatively high incidence of adverse reactions. The patient is administered a test dose and is monitored for an hour. If they do not experience any adverse effects, the remaining dose is then given over 2 hours.

Megaloblastic Anemias

Megaloblastic anemias (large RBCs) are classified morphologically as macrocytic normochromic anemias. Megaloblastic anemias are often caused by vitamin B_{12} and folic acid (folate) deficiencies, which result in disordered DNA synthesis, with failure of nuclear maturation and division (Guyton, 2001). These deficiencies may be secondary to malnutrition, folic acid deficiency, malabsorption, lack of intrinsic factor (as in pernicious anemia and postgastrectomy), parasitic infestations, intestinal disease, and malignancies, as well as being a result of chemotherapeutic agents. In individuals with tapeworm infections (Diphyllobothrium latum) secondary to ingestion of infected freshwater fish, the tapeworm competes with its host for the vitamin B_{12} in ingested food, which leads to megaloblastic anemia (Goldsmith, 2001).

Although pernicious anemia typifies megaloblastic anemias, folate deficiency is more commonly encountered in clinical practice. Megaloblastic anemia is often noted as malnutrition in older adults, alcoholics, or adolescents, and in women during pregnancy, when the demand to meet the needs of the fetus and lactation is increased. This demand is also increased in hemolytic anemias, malignancies, and hyperthyroidism. Celiac

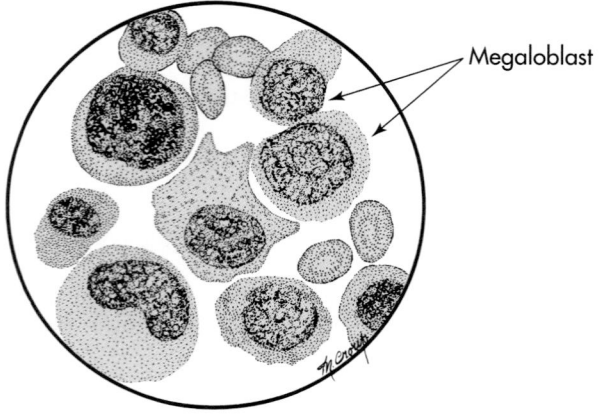

Megaloblast

FIG. 17-4 Bone marrow characteristic of megaloblastic anemia. In the upper left there is one red blood cell precursor that is nearly normal, with a condensed nuclear chromatin pattern. The remaining cells are large and have an open nuclear chromatin pattern. These large cells (two to three times normal size) are also red blood cell precursors. In the lower left is a large white blood cell precursor (metamyelocyte) that is two to three times normal size. This finding indicates that all cell lines develop abnormally in this condition.

disease and tropical sprue also cause malabsorption, and drugs that act as folic acid antagonists interfere with use.

The minimal daily requirement of folate, approximately 50 mg, is easily provided in an average diet. The most abundant sources are red meats, such as liver and kidney, and fresh, leafy green vegetables. However, proper preparation of the food is necessary to ensure adequate nutrition. For example, 50% to 90% of the folate can be lost with cooking in large volumes of water. Folate is absorbed from the duodenum and upper jejunum, weakly bound to plasma proteins, and stored in the liver. In the absence of folate intake, folate stores are usually depleted in approximately 4 months. In addition to the symptoms described for anemias, individuals with megaloblastic anemia secondary to folate deficiency may appear malnourished and experience severe glossitis (inflamed, painful tongue), diarrhea, and loss of appetite. Serum folate levels are also decreased (less than 4 ng/ml). The bone marrow of a patient with megaloblastic anemia is depicted in Fig. 17-4. Color plate 13 illustrates the peripheral blood findings seen in megaloblastic anemia. The reticulocyte count is usually decreased along with the hematocrit and hemoglobin.

As mentioned, treatment depends on identifying and removing the underlying cause. Treatment includes correcting the dietary deficiencies and replacement therapy with folic acid or vitamin B_{12}. Alcoholic patients who are hospitalized often have a "spontaneous" response when given a nutritionally balanced diet.

Sickle Cell Disease

Causes

Sickle cell disease is a hemoglobinopathy resulting from abnormalities in hemoglobin structure. The defect in structure occurs in the globin fraction of the hemoglobin molecule. Globin is constructed of two pairs of polypeptide chains. For example, Hb S differs from normal Hb A

in the substitution of valine for glutamic acid in one pair of chains. In Hb C, lysine is in that position. As noted, many abnormal hemoglobins exist with varying degrees of symptoms, ranging from none to severe.

Sickle cell disease is an autosomal recessive genetic disorder in which an individual inherits the sickle hemoglobin (hemoglobin S) from both parents. The patient is therefore homozygous (Gelehertr, 1999). Heterozygous individuals (abnormal gene inherited from only one parent) are said to have the sickle cell trait. These subjects are generally asymptomatic and have a normal life span. In patients with sickle cell trait, morbidity related to impaired oxygenation, such as that during anesthesia, at high altitudes, and with chronic obstructive pulmonary disease (COPD), has been reported but is extremely rare and not well documented (Beutler, 2001).

The amino acid substitution in sickle cell disease results in major rearrangement of the hemoglobin molecule when deoxygenation (decreased O_2 tension) occurs. The RBCs then elongate and become rigid and crescent- or sickle-shaped (Fig. 17-5).

Deoxygenation can occur for many reasons. Erythrocytes that contain Hb S traverse the microcirculation more slowly than do normal erythrocytes, giving more time for deoxygenation. The Hb S erythrocytes adhere to the endothelium, further retarding blood flow. The increased deoxygenation may take the abnormal red blood cells below a critical point and bring on sickling within the microvasculature. Because of their rigidity and irregular membrane, sickle cells clump together, leading to vascular occlusion, pain crisis, and organ infarctions (Linker, 2001). Repeated episodes of sickling and unsickling cause the cell membranes to become fragile and fragment. The cells are then hemolyzed and removed by the monocyte-macrophage system. The RBC life span is markedly reduced, and an increased demand is put on the bone marrow for replacement. Fig. 17-6 depicts the cycle of sickle cell infarctive crisis.

Sickle cell anemia is the most prevalent form of congenital hemolytic anemia. Affecting approximately 1 in 600 African Americans, sickle cell anemia is the most common form of sickle cell disease. Hb S accounts for 75% to 95% of the hemoglobin; the remainder is Hb F, which accounts for 1% to 20%. The diagnosis is based on the patient's history, physical findings, and a laboratory evaluation. A sickle solubility test is performed to confirm the presence of Hb S in the red blood cell. In this test, RBCs are mixed with a reducing agent and the solution becomes turbid. Hemoglobin electrophoresis further delineates the abnormal hemoglobin. The anemia is generally normocytic and normochromic, with hemoglobin levels ranging between 5 and 10 g/dl. Peripheral smear shows anisocytosis and poikilocytosis (irreversibly sickled cells), leukocytosis (increased WBCs), thrombocytosis, and nucleated RBCs (see Fig. 17-5). The reticulocyte count is markedly increased during periods of hemolysis. Individuals of Mediterranean heritage, Greeks, and Italians are also susceptible to sickle cell disease.

Signs and Symptoms

Signs and symptoms occur as a result of the vascular occlusions that cause infarcts in various organs, such as

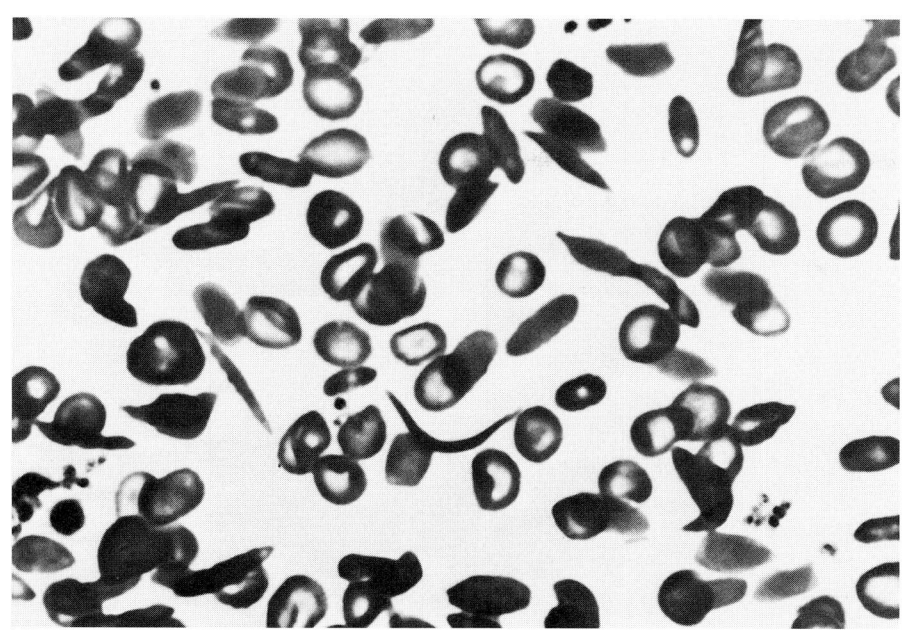

FIG. 17-5   The characteristic sickle- or crescent-shaped red blood cells are shown in a peripheral smear. (Courtesy Kolchi Maeda, MD, Henry Ford Hospital, Detroit, Mich.)

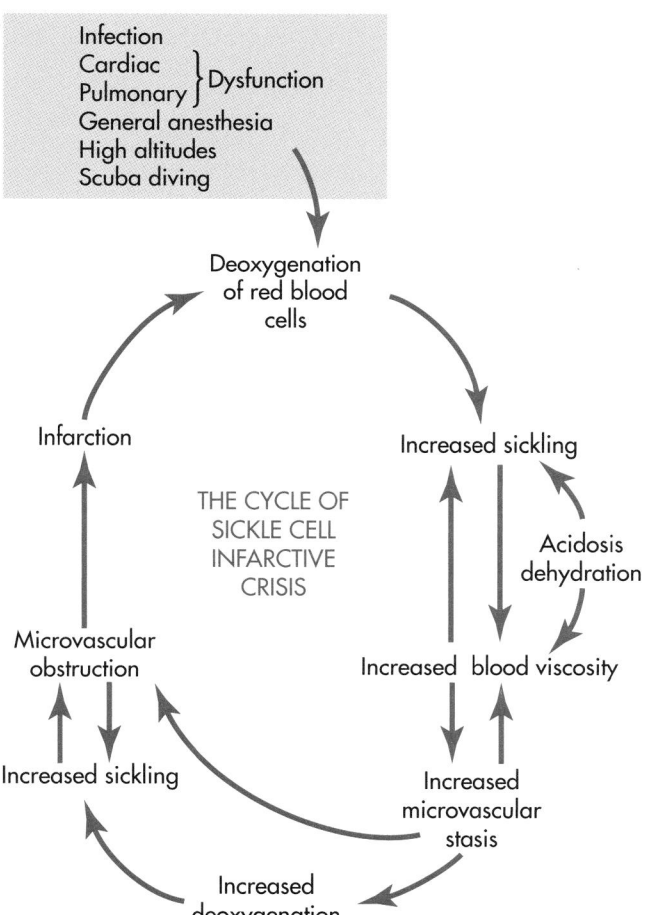

FIG. 17-6   The cycle of a sickle cell infarctive crisis.

kidneys, lungs, and the central nervous system. Infants are usually asymptomatic for 5 to 6 months because of the persistence of fetal hemoglobin (Hb F), which tends to inhibit sickling. Clinical manifestations include failure-to-thrive syndrome, impaired growth and devel-

opment, and frequent episodes of bacterial infections, particularly pneumococcal infections. Initially, the spleen is enlarged; however, owing to repeated infarcts, the spleen becomes atrophied and nonfunctional before the child is 8 years of age. This process is referred to as *autosplenectomy*. Susceptibility to infection persists throughout life. Life expectancy is shortened secondary to infarctions leading to organ failures.

Swollen, painful, inflamed hands and feet (hand-foot syndrome known as *dactylitis*) are present in approximately 20% to 30% of children under 2 years of age. Dactylitis results from ischemia and infarction of the metacarpal and metatarsal bones; the condition is accompanied by fever. Debilitating, recurrent, painful "crises" are the major cause of the morbidity from sickle cell disease. The most frequent sites affected are the abdomen, back, chest, and joints. Crises are exacerbated by infection or dehydration, may mimic other acute illnesses, and last from a few hours to several days. The incidence of the crises decreases with increasing age. Aplastic crisis may also occur, particularly in children, with intermittent cessation of bone marrow function and marked decrease in erythropoiesis and reticulocyte count (see Fig. 17-6). Visceral sequestration crisis with sickling and pooling of blood, particularly in the chest, is a leading cause of death.

Cardiac signs of anemia, such as tachycardia or murmurs, are usually present. Increased heart size and congestive heart failure may also occur. Renal involvement is evidenced by an impaired ability to concentrate urine, and repeated infarctions can lead to papillary necrosis and hematuria. Repeated pulmonary infections or infarctions (or both) impair pulmonary function. Central nervous system infarctions ("strokes"), although rare, can lead to varying degrees of hemiplegia. Chronic leg ulcers above the ankle and along the medial aspect of the tibia are encountered. Because of the increased RBC breakdown, the patients are often icteric (jaundiced) and develop cholelithiasis (gallstones) secondary to increased bilirubin. Physical appearance ranges from the thin

TABLE 17-2

Clinical Manifestations of Sickle Cell Anemia

System	Complications	Signs and Symptoms	Related To
Cardiac	Congestive heart failure	Cardiomegaly, systolic ejection murmur, tachycardia, shortness of breath, dyspnea on exertion, restlessness	Anemia, chronic hemolysis
Pulmonary	Pulmonary infarction, pneumonia (especially *Haemophilus influenzae* and *Streptococcus pneumoniae*), pneumococcal pneumonia	Chest pain, cough, shortness of breath, fever, hemoptysis, restlessness	Infarctive crisis, increased susceptibility to infection, intrapulmonary arteriovenous shunting, functional asplenia
Central nervous	Cerebral thromboses	Hemiplegia, aphasia, drowsiness, convulsions, headache, bowel and bladder dysfunction	Infarctive crisis
Genitourinary	Renal dysfunction	Flank pain, hematuria, isothenuria	Renal papillary necrosis secondary to microinfarcts
	Priapism	Penile engorgement and pain	Infarctive crisis and intravascular sickling
Gastrointestinal	Cholecystitis, hepatic fibrosis, hepatic abscess	Abdominal pain, hepatomegaly, jaundice, fever	Chronic hemolysis, infarctive crisis
Ocular	Retinal detachment, peripheral vessel disease, hemorrhage	Pain, altered vision, blindness	Microinfarcts
Skeletal	Aseptic necrosis of femoral or humeral heads, dactylitis (usually in young children)	Pain, decreased mobility, painful and swollen hands and feet	Infarctions, infection, intramedullary infarction with or without periostitis
Skin	Chronic leg ulcers	Pain, open and draining ulcers	Infarctions, impaired circulation in capillaries, venules caused by intravascular sickling

asthenic to that of normal development. Table 17-2 depicts the clinical manifestations of sickle cell anemia.

Treatment

Currently no known therapy is available that will reverse sickling; therefore treatment is primarily preventive and supportive. Because infections appear to trigger sickle cell crises, emphasis is placed on the prevention, early detection, and prompt treatment of infections. In 1987 the National Heart, Lung, and Blood Institute (NHLBI) recommended prophylactic use of penicillin for young children to reduce the incidence of pneumonia (Mayfield, 1999). Pneumococcal vaccine (Pneumovax) should be offered prophylactically because it decreases the incidence of pneumococcal infections. Treatment includes prompt and vigorous administration of antibiotics and hydration. Oxygen should be administered only when the patient is hypoxic. Daily folic acid supplements are required to replenish the folate stores depleted as a result of chronic hemolysis. The painful crisis that occurs independently or secondary to infection may affect any part of the body. Prompt intervention with hydration and opioid analgesics may abort or decrease the duration and severity of the crisis. Transfusions are necessary during aplastic or hemolytic crises, during pregnancy, for surgery, or to interrupt severe painful crisis. Exchange transfusions are used for patients with repeated crises or neurologic damage. Iron overload becomes a problem, and these patients need deferoxamine to reduce their iron stores.

In February 1998 the U.S. Food and Drug Administration (FDA) approved the use of hydroxyurea (Droxia) for the treatment of patients with sickle cell disease, particularly for patients who are over 18 years of age with frequent crisis. The goal is to increase the hemoglobin F level in the RBC. Hemoglobin F does not sickle. Studies are underway to examine the safety of hydroxyurea in younger patients. Bone marrow or stem cell transplantation in young patients has been successful. However, lack of donors and the potential morbidity of the preparatory phase limit this as a treatment option for most patients (Gelehert, 1998).

Frequent crises have an impact on the entire quality of life for the patient and the family. Patients are often disabled by chronic recurrent pain and vasoocclusive events. A high incidence of drug dependency is present in this population, as well as school and job difficulties. Ongoing teaching and counseling, including genetic counseling, are essential to the prevention and treatment of sickle cell disease.

Polycythemia

The previous discussion has focused on conditions resulting from an insufficient number of RBCs. The condition known as polycythemia results from too many RBCs. Polycythemia means an excess (poly-) of all cell lines (-cythemia), but the name is generally used for conditions in which the volume of RBCs exceeds normal. This condition results in increased whole blood viscosity and increased blood volume. Primary, or polycythemia vera, is a myeloproliferative disorder. The pluripotent stem cell is abnormal. Marked erythrocytosis, with normal or low erythropoietin levels, as well as leukocytosis and thrombocytosis are also observed. Polycythemia vera is a progressive disease of middle age, affecting men slightly more than women. The signs and symptoms are secondary to the increased total blood volume and increased blood viscosity. The plasma volume is usually normal, and vasodilation occurs to accommodate the increased RBC volume. The patient presents with a plethoric (brick red) complexion and blood-shot eyes. The symptoms are nonspecific, ranging from a sensation of "fullness in the head" to headache, dizziness, difficulty in concentrating, visual blurring, fatigue, and pruritus (itching) after bathing. The increased blood volume and viscosity (slow blood flow) along with the elevated platelet numbers and abnormal platelet function predispose the individual to thrombosis and hemorrhage. Thrombosis is the major cause of morbidity and mortality. The disease progresses over a period of 10 to 15 years. During this time, the spleen and liver enlarge, secondary to RBC congestion. The marrow becomes fibrosed and eventually becomes "spent"-nonproductive, or converts to acute myelogenous leukemia, either as a consequence of treatment or the natural course of the disease (Shelton, 2000).

Laboratory studies reveal a persistently elevated hemoglobin greater than 18 g, hematocrit over 60, and an increased total blood volume. The RBC morphology is normal. WBC and platelet counts are also elevated. The reticulocyte count is normal or slightly increased. Vitamin B_{12} levels are generally increased. Leukocyte alkaline phosphatase is elevated, as is the uric acid. Iron stores are often depleted secondary to phlebotomies (removal of a pint of blood by venesection).

Treatment modalities for polycythemia vera include weekly phlebotomies to achieve a hematocrit of less than 45, and then on an "as-needed" basis. The use of radioactive phosphorus and alkylating agents are limited, largely because they are known to be carcinogenic and may play a role in the development of acute leukemia. Short-term use of busulfan (i.e., 4 to 6 weeks) may achieve a potential remission. Hydroxyurea is often used for its ease of administration and tolerance. These drugs, however, cause a generalized myelosuppression. Anagrelide hydrochloride (Agrylin) is used to lower platelet counts.

Secondary polycythemia occurs when the volume of circulating plasma is decreased (hemoconcentrated) but the total volume of circulating RBCs is normal. Therefore the hematocrit rises in men to approximately 57% and to 54% in women. The most likely cause is dehydration. Another form is called pseudo or stress polycythemia. Although the exact cause is unknown, the incidence is highest in middle-aged, obese, highly anxious men with hypertension. Cigarette smoking appears to exacerbate this state because chronic carbon monoxide exposure enhances erythrocytosis (Linker, 2001).

Underlying medical conditions that stimulate erythropoietin production include cardiopulmonary diseases that decrease arterial O_2 saturation or renal tumors that decrease renal blood flow. This condition is also present in people who live at high altitudes in which atmospheric O_2 is decreased. For secondary polycythemia, treatment of the underlying cause is indicated.

KEY CONCEPTS

- RBCs, or erythrocytes, are nonnucleated biconcave disks.
- The RBC's major component is the protein hemoglobin (Hb), which transports most of the O_2 and a small fraction of CO_2 and maintains normal pH through a series of intracellular buffers.
- The average adult has approximately 5 million RBCs per cubic millimeter of blood, and these RBCs have an average life span of 120 days.
- RBC production is stimulated by a glycoprotein hormone, erythropoietin, known to originate primarily in the kidney.
- Alterations of the RBC mass produce two distinct entities: an insufficient number of RBCs (anemia) and too many RBCs (polycythemia).
- Anemia is a reduction below the normal level in the number of RBCs, the quantity of hemoglobin, and the volume of packed RBCs (hematocrit) per 100 ml of blood.
- Anemia is not a diagnosis but a reflection of an underlying pathophysiologic alteration revealed by a careful history, physical examination, and laboratory confirmation.
- Signs and symptoms attributed to anemia include pallor, tachycardia, cardiac murmurs, angina, myocardial ischemia, dyspnea, shortness of breath, and increased fatigue on exertion.

- Anemias may be classified according to (1) the morphology of the RBC and the indices and (2) the etiology.
- Normocytic, normochromic anemia, is a state in which the RBCs are normal in size and shape and contain the normal amount of hemoglobin; macrocytic, normochromic anemia, is a condition in which the RBCs are larger than is normal but are normochromic.
- In microcytic (small), hypochromic (containing less than the normal amount of hemoglobin) anemia, both the MCV and MCHC are decreased.
- The major causes of anemia are increased RBC loss and decreased or defective cell production.
- The second major etiologic classification includes decreased or defective RBC production (dyserythropoiesis) and includes any condition affecting the bone marrow function.
- Aplastic anemia is a life-threatening disorder of the stem cell in the bone marrow, in which insufficient numbers of blood cells are produced.
- Iron deficiency anemia is classified as microcytic, hypochromic anemia with a decrease in the quantity of hemoglobin synthesis. Iron deficiency anemia is the major cause of anemia in the world.
- Megaloblastic anemias (large RBCs) are classified morphologically as macrocytic, normochromic

anemias and are often caused by vitamin B_{12} or folic acid (folate) deficiencies, which result in disordered DNA synthesis.

■ Sickle cell disease is an autosomal recessive genetic disorder whereby an individual inherits the sickle hemoglobin (hemoglobin S from both parents). The patient is therefore homozygous.

■ Heterozygous individuals (abnormal gene inherited from only one parent) are said to have the sickle cell trait.

■ Sickle cell anemia is the most prevalent form of congenital hemolytic anemia. Hb S accounts for 75% to 95% of the hemoglobin; the remainder is Hb F, which accounts for 1% to 20%.

■ Currently, no known therapy is available to reverse sickling; therefore treatment is primarily preventive and supportive.

■ Polycythemia means an excess (poly-) of all cell lines (-cythemia) but is generally used for conditions in which the volume of RBCs exceeds normal.

■ Primary or polycythemia vera is a myeloproliferative disorder in which the pluripotent stem cell is abnormal.

■ Secondary polycythemia occurs when the volume of circulating plasma is decreased (hemoconcentrated) but the total volume of circulating RBCs is normal.

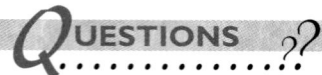

QUESTIONS ??

A sampling of review questions for this chapter appears here. Visit http://www.mosby.com/MERLIN/PriceWilson/ for additional questions. MERLIN

Answer the following on a separate sheet of paper.

1. What are the major components and functions of the normal RBC?
2. Explain the relationship of erythropoietin to RBC production.
3. Define anemia.
4. List the classic signs and symptoms of anemia.
5. State two etiologic factors related to anemia, and give at least two examples of each type.
6. Describe the three morphologic classifications for anemia, and give at least two examples of each type.
7. What are the three major principles to consider when treating anemia?
8. What is polycythemia?
9. Describe the two classifications of polycythemia, and include an example of each type.
10. Draw a normal RBC.
11. Explain why deoxygenation can occur in sickle cell disease.
12. Describe aplastic anemia.
13. What are the secondary causes of aplastic anemia?
14. Describe the treatment modality and survival success rate for young individuals with severe aplastic anemia secondary to stem cell damage.

Complete the following statements by filling in the blanks.

15. An anemia in which the MCV is normal and the MCHC is normal is referred to as _____.

16. The leading cause of death in sickle cell disease is _____.

White Blood Cell and Plasma Cell Disorders

CATHERINE M. BALDY

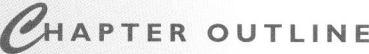
NORMAL STRUCTURE AND FUNCTION

Defense against infection is the major role of leukocytes or white blood cells (WBCs). The normal range for the WBC count is from 4000 to 10,000/mm³. The five types of WBCs identified in the peripheral blood are (1) neutrophils (50% to 75% of the total WBCs), (2) eosinophils (1% to 2%), (3) basophils (0.5% to 1.0%), (4) monocytes (6%), and (5) lymphocytes (25% to 33%).

Neutrophils, eosinophils, and basophils are also called *granulocytes*, which means cells with granules in the cytoplasm (see color plates 14 through 16). Granulocytes range in size from 10 to 14 μm in diameter; their identification depends on the affinity of the granules for certain dyes. Cells whose granules have an eosin affinity, staining red to red-orange, are called *eosinophils*, whereas cells with a blue or basic dye affinity are called *basophils*. The granules of the neutrophils, which are also called *segmented neutrophils* and *polymorphonuclear leukocytes (PMNs)*, have little affinity for either eosin or basic dyes and stain a faint pink or blue surrounded by a light pink cytoplasm. All three types of granulocytes (Fig. 18-1) originate from the pluripotent stem cell in the bone marrow.

Although all the regulatory mechanisms for the differentiation and maturation of the WBCs and all the cell lines are not yet fully understood, the identification of several colony-stimulating factors (CSFs) or hematopoietic growth factors has clarified that process. CSFs are a group of cell-derived glycoproteins that belong to a broader group of WBC regulators called *cytokines*. CSFs are continuously synthesized by a variety of cells, the most important of which are the lymphocyte-macrophage system, fibroblasts, and endothelial cells found in the bone marrow. CSFs have been detected (Bondurant, Kourey, 1999) in various body tissues and in human serum and urine. Detectable levels of CSFs have been found in the serum during periods of inflammation, viral infections, and stress. Further rapid production appears to occur after stimulation by various antigens and microorganisms and their products, such as endotoxins (Bondurant, Kourey, 1999).

CSFs are believed either to act where they are produced or to circulate and attach themselves to specific receptors on the cell surface of the hematopoietic precursors, committing them to differentiation, which, in the case of the WBCs, is to the granulocyte, monocyte, and lymphatic cell lines.

The cells undergo a mitotic (dividing) proliferating phase, followed by a maturation phase. The time required varies for the different leukocytes and ranges from 9 days for the eosinophil to 12 days for the neutrophil. All these phases are accelerated during periods of infection. In the bone marrow, as the cell matures, it becomes smaller, and the round or oval nucleus acquires two to five lobes, surrounded by cytoplasm containing small, evenly distributed granules (see Fig. 18-1). These granules contain enzymes (e.g., myeloperoxidase, muramidase, and cationic antibacterial proteins) that, after degranulation of the WBCs, kill and digest bacteria.

The bone marrow contains a constant reserve of approximately 10 times the quantity of neutrophils produced daily. This reserve is referred to as the storage pool. In the presence of infection, the reserve neutrophils are mobilized and released into the circulation where they remain for approximately 6 to 8 hours and then go into

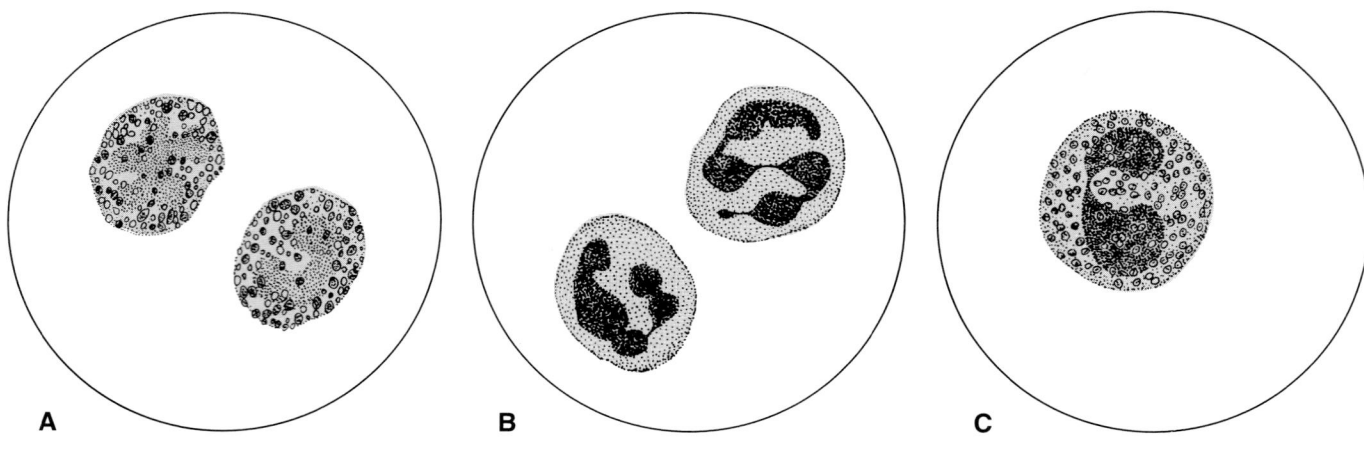

FIG. 18-1   Granulocytes. **A**, Basophils. **B**, Neutrophils. **C**, Eosinophil.

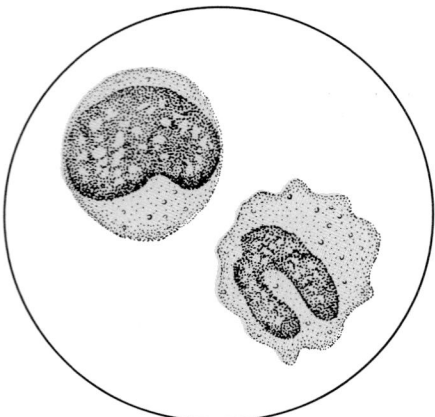

FIG. 18-2   Monocytes.

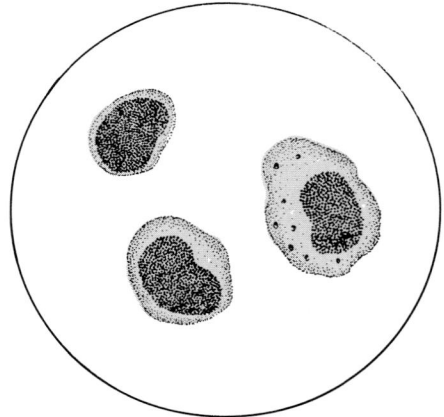

FIG. 18-3   Mature lymphocytes.

the tissues. Neutrophils in the circulation are divided between the circulating pool and the marginating pool (WBCs positioned along the capillary wall). With ameboid movements, the neutrophils move by diapedesis from the marginal pool into the tissues and mucous membranes. Neutrophils are the body's primary defense system against bacterial infection; their method of defense is phagocytosis, which is discussed in detail in Chapter 4. A constant granulocyte pool is maintained, influenced by cell-to-cell interactions, and growth hormones as cytokines are released from inflammatory cells (Sacher, McPherson, 2000).

Eosinophils have a weak phagocytic function that is not clearly understood. Apparently, eosinophils function in antigen-antibody reactions; levels are elevated during asthmatic attacks, drug reactions, and certain parasitic infestations (see Chapter 9). *Basophils* carry heparin and histamine- and platelet-activating factors in their granules to inflamed tissues; their actual function is poorly defined. Elevated levels of basophils (basophilia) are found in myeloproliferative disorders, that is, proliferative disorders of blood-forming cells.

The *monocyte* (Fig. 18-2; see color plate 17) is larger than the neutrophil and has a relatively simple monomorphic nucleus. The nucleus is folded or indented and looks lobulated with brainlike convolutions. The cytoplasm appears more abundant in relation to its nucleus

and stains dull blue-gray with faint, evenly distributed granules. The differentiation, maturation, and release of monocytes occur over 24 days—a much longer period than that for granulocytes.

Monocytes leave the circulation and become tissue macrophages and are a part of the monocyte-macrophage system. The life span of the monocyte is weeks to months. Monocytes have phagocytic functions, removing injured and dead cells, cell fragments, and microorganisms (as in bacterial endocarditis).

The other mononuclear (monomorphonuclear) leukocytes in the blood are the lymphocytes, which have a round or oval nucleus surrounded by a narrow rim of blue-staining cytoplasm containing a few granules. The nuclear chromatin pattern is heavily clumped with a network of inner connections. Lymphocytes (Fig. 18-3; see color plate 18) vary in size from small (7 to 10 μm) to large cells the size of granulocytes and appear to originate from a pluripotent stem cell in the bone marrow and migrate to other lymphoid tissues, including the lymph nodes, spleen, thymus, and the mucosal surfaces of the gastrointestinal tract and the respiratory tract. Two types of lymphocytes include the long-lived, thymus-conditioned, thymus-dependent T lymphocytes and the non–thymus-dependent B lymphocytes. T lymphocytes migrate from the thymus gland to other lymphoid tissue and are typically located in the paracortex of lymph nodes and the periarteriolar lymphoid sheets of the white pulp of the spleen. B lymphocytes are distributed in the follicles of lymph nodes, the spleen, and the medullary cords of the lymph nodes. The T lymphocytes are responsible for cellular immune responses through the production of antigen-reactive cells, whereas B lymphocytes, when properly stimulated, differentiate into immunoglobulin-producing plasma cells responsible for the humoral immune response. Chapter 5 contains a complete discussion of the functions and interrelationships of the T and B lymphocytes.

WBC DISORDERS

Disorders of WBCs can affect any or all of the cell lines and are generally related to production defects or early destruction.

Leukocytosis refers to an increase in the leukocytes, generally exceeding 10,000/mm³. *Granulocytosis* refers to an increase in granulocytes but, in common usage, refers only to an increase in the neutrophils; thus *neutrophilia* is the more accurate term. Leukocytes increase as a physiologic response to protect the body from invading microorganisms. In response to an acute infection or inflammation, neutrophils leave the marginating pool and enter the area of infection; the bone marrow releases its reserves and initiates accelerated granulopoiesis. Because of this increased demand, an increased number of immature forms called *band* (or *stab*) neutrophils enter the circulation, a process referred to as a "shift to the left" (see color plate 19). As the infection subsides, the number of neutrophils decreases and the number of monocytes increases (monocytosis). With progressive resolution, the number of monocytes decreases and mild lymphocytosis (increased lymphocytes) and eosinophilia (increased number of eosinophils) occur. Leukemoid reaction refers to a state of elevated leukocytes, with an increase in immature forms, reaching levels of 100,000/mm³. This condition is in response to infectious, toxic, and inflammatory states and also occurs in malignancy, particularly in breast, kidney, lung, and metastatic carcinomas (Beck, 1991). Disorders in which a general increase in blood-forming cells occurs are called *myeloproliferative disorders*.

Neutrophilia

Neutrophilia also occurs following stresses, such as severe violent exercise or injection with epinephrine. This is a "pseudoleukocytosis" because granulopoiesis in the bone marrow is not accelerated and the number of granulocytes in the body is not actually increased. Rather, granulocytes are mobilized from the marginated pool thus the number of granulocytes that can be drawn into the sampling device is increased. Treatment with corticosteroids also results in a pseudoleukocytosis. Corticosteroids are thought to increase the release of granulocytes from the marrow reserves and to inhibit the margination of granulocytes, which results in a greater amount of circulating leukocytes. Eosinophilia occurs with skin disorders such as mycosis fungoides and eczema, allergy states such as asthma and hay fever, drug reactions, and para-

sitic infestations. Eosinophilia is also present in malignancies and myeloproliferative disorders, as is basophilia.

Monocytosis is observed during the recuperating phase of infection and in chronic granulomatous diseases such as tuberculosis and sarcoidosis. *Lymphocytosis* refers to an elevated lymphocyte count. Lymphocytes activated by viral or antigenic stimuli are transformed into larger atypical lymphocytes. These cells are present in larger numbers in infectious mononucleosis, infectious hepatitis, toxoplasmosis, measles, mumps, some allergic reactions (e.g., serum sickness, drug sensitivities), and the malignant lymphomas (Schrier, 1979). In addition to lymphocytosis, these patients often have an enlarged liver, spleen, and lymph nodes, all of which are areas of lymphocyte maturation.

Leukopenia refers to a decreased number of leukocytes, and *neutropenia* refers to a decrease in the absolute neutrophil count. Because of the role of neutrophils in host defense, an absolute neutrophil count of less than 1000/mm³ predisposes the individual to infection; counts under 500/mm³ predispose the person to serious, life-threatening infections. Neutropenia may result from ineffective and defective neutrophil production, which is found in hypoplastic or aplastic anemias secondary to cytotoxic drugs, toxic substances, and viral infection; starvation; and replacement of normal bone marrow by malignant cells, such as in leukemia.

Agranulocytosis is a serious condition characterized by an extremely low leukocyte count and absence of neutrophils. The causative agent is generally a drug that interferes with cell formation or enhances cell destruction. Drugs commonly implicated are the myelosuppressive (suppress bone marrow) chemotherapeutic agents used to treat hematologic and other malignancies. Increasingly, more commonly used drugs, such as analgesics, antibiotics, and antihistamines, have been identified as capable of causing severe neutropenia or agranulocytosis. This response is either dose-related or an idiosyncratic reaction.

Recurrent chromosomal changes occur in over one half of all cases of leukemia, and they occur only in the malignant hematopoietic cell (Bloomfield, Caligiuri, 2001).

Common symptoms of agranulocytosis are infection and feelings of general malaise (discomfort, lassitude, headache, and muscle aches) followed by ulceration of the mucous membranes, fever, and tachycardia. When agranulocytosis is untreated, sepsis and death ensue. Removal of the offending agent will often inhibit and reverse the process with an increased production of the neutrophils and other normal marrow elements.

Leukemia
Classification

Leukemia, originally described by Virchow in 1847 as "white blood," is a neoplastic disease characterized by differentiation and proliferation of malignantly transformed hematopoietic stem cells, leading to suppression and replacing normal marrow elements (Greer et al, 1999). The most widely used classification of leukemia is the French-American-British (FAB) classification (Box 18-1). This classification is morphologic and is based on the

BOX 18-1

FAB Cooperative Group Classification of Acute Leukemias

ACUTE LYMPHOBLASTIC LEUKEMIA

L-1 Acute lymphocytic leukemia of childhood: homogeneous cell population
L-2 Acute lymphocytic leukemia in adults: heterogeneous cell population
L-3 Burkitt's lymphoma–type leukemia: large cells, homogeneous cell population

ACUTE MYELOBLASTIC LEUKEMIA

M-0 Minimally differentiated
M-1 Granulocytic differentiation without maturation
M-2 Granulocytic differentiation with maturation to promyelocytic stage
M-3 Granulocytic differentiation with hypergranular promyelocytes, associated with disseminated intravascular coagulation
M-4 Acute myelomonocytic leukemia: both granulocytic and monocytic cell lines
M-5a Acute monocytic leukemia: poorly differentiated
M-5b Acute monocytic leukemia: well differentiated
M-6 Predominance of erythroblasts with severe dyserythropoiesis
M-7 Megakaryocytic leukemia

From Gralnick HR et al: Classification of acute leukemia, *Ann Intern Med* 87(6):740-753, 1977; Bennett JM et al: Criteria for the diagnosis of acute leukemia, *Ann Intern Med* 103(3):460-462, 1985; Sacher RA, McPherson R: *Widman's clinical interpretation of laboratory tests*, ed 11, Philadelphia, 2000, FA Davis.

differentiation and maturation of the predominant leukemic cells in the bone marrow, as well as on cytochemical studies (Dabich, 1980; Gralnick et al, 1977). Since its early report by Gralnick, further subclassifications have been added (Bennett et al, 1985).

Advances in cytogenetics, molecular biology and immunology have had a marked impact on distinguishing normal hematopoietic cells from the malignant clone. Immunologic technology has enhanced the classification by identifying the malignant clone as myeloid, B lymphoid, T lymphoid, or biphenotypic (having characteristics of both myeloid and lymphoid cells) (Devine, Larson, 1994; Wujcik, 2000). Cytogenetic analysis has yielded vast knowledge of the chromosomal aberrations present in patients with leukemia. Chromosomal changes can include numeric changes, in which whole chromosomes may be added or deleted, or structural changes, including translocations, deletions, inversions, and insertions. Chromosomal changes can include numeric changes, in which whole chromosomes may be added or deleted, or structural changes, including translocations, deletions, inversions, and insertions. In these situations, two or more chromosomes exchange genetic material, with the development of altered genes thought to be responsible for the start of abnormal cellular proliferation (Sandberg, 1994). The Philadelphia chromosome (Ph) is an example of a cytogenetic change found in 85% of patients with chronic myeloid leukemia and in some patients with acute myeloid or lymphoid leukemia. This action is a translocation of chromosomes 9 and 22, identified as t(9;22). Molecular studies detecting changes at the deoxyribonucleic acid (DNA) level have further delin-

eated the Ph chromosome as varying in the different types of leukemia. More than 90% of children with acute lymphocytic leukemia have been shown to have one or more chromosomal aberrations. Numerous chromosomal aberrations have been identified and are diagnostic for specific types of leukemia. Identification of these changes is predictive of the clinical course, prognosis, and attainment of a remission or relapse (Sandberg, 1994; Wujcik, 2000). These findings have a tremendous impact on treatment modalities and overall prognosis.

Incidence

Although both genders are affected, a slight male to female predominance exists. Acute granulocytic or myelocytic leukemia is observed in adults of all ages, with increases noted after 40 years of age. The mean age is 60 years. Acute lymphocytic leukemia is more prevalent in children under 15 years of age, with a peak between the ages of 2 and 4 years; it may also be present in adults of all ages, with a gradual increase at 60 years of age. Chronic granulocytic or myelocytic leukemia is most frequently found in middle-age patients with a mean age of 60 years, but it can occur in any age-group. Chronic lymphocytic leukemia is usually observed in older individuals.

Etiology

Although the basic cause of leukemia is unknown, both genetic predisposition and environmental factors appear to play a role. Familial leukemias are rare, but a higher incidence of leukemia appears to occur in siblings of affected children, with the incidence increasing to 20% in monozygotic (identical) twins. Individuals with chromosomal abnormalities such as Down syndrome appear to have a twentyfold increased incidence of acute leukemia.

Environmental factors include exposure to high doses of ionizing radiation with manifestations of leukemia occurring years later. Chemicals (e.g., benzene, arsenic, pesticides, chloramphenicol, phenylbutazone, antineoplastic agents) are being implicated with increased frequency, particularly the alkylating agents. The likelihood of leukemia increases in patients treated with both radiation and chemotherapy. Any hypoplastic bone marrow state appears to predispose the individual to leukemia. Patients with myelodysplastic syndrome (stem cell disorder manifested by presence of blasts and pancytopenia found in older adults) often progress to acute nonlymphocytic leukemia.

Therapy is directed toward elimination of the abnormal cell line; 65% of patients, with resumption of normal hematopoiesis, achieve remission of disease. Attaining a complete molecular remission with reversal of all cytogenetic abnormalities is imperative for long-term remission or cure. Table 18-1 lists the chemotherapeutic agents commonly used to treat the hematologic malignancies. The chemotherapeutic agents selected destroy the cells by various mechanisms, such as interfering with cell metabolism and maturation. The same clinical manifestations of pancytopenia accompanying active disease are present after chemotherapy. Infection remains the leading cause of death in patients with acute leukemia. Supportive care is the key to increasing the survival rate

TABLE 18-1

Commonly Used Chemotherapeutic Agents in Hematologic Malignancies

Drug				Toxicity	
Generic Name	Trade Name*	Disease	Administration	Acute	Long-term
ALKYLATING AGENTS					
Mechlorethamine hydrochloride, nitrogen mustard	Mustargen	Hodgkin's lymphoma	IV push	Anorexia; nausea and vomiting: nausea, 30 minutes to 4 hours after injection	Myelosuppression, amenorrhea, male sterility
Cyclophosphamide	Cytoxan, Endoxan	Lymphomas Chronic lymphocytic leukemia Acute leukemia Multiple myeloma Waldenström's macroglobulinemia	PO, IV	Delayed nausea, 6-18 hours	Alopecia, hemorrhagic cystitis, myelosuppression, amenorrhea, male sterility, immunosuppression
Busulfan	Myleran	CGL Polycythemia vera Thrombocythemia	PO	Minimal nausea	Myelosuppression, skin pigmentation, pulmonary fibrosis, addisonian syndrome
Chlorambucil	Leukeran	CLL Hodgkin's lymphoma Lymphomas	PO	Mild anorexia; nausea and vomiting	Myelosuppression
Melphalan	Alkeran	BMT MM	PO	Mild anorexia; nausea and vomiting	Myelosuppression
ANTIMETABOLITES					
Methotrexate	Amethopterin	ALL AGL	PO, IV, IM, IT, IP	Nausea, vomiting	Myelosuppression, stomatitis, diarrhea, alopecia, mucosal ulceration, hepatic-renal dysfunction, immunosuppression
Cytarabine (cytosine arabinoside)	Cytosar-U, Ara-C	AGL Acute myelomonocytic leukemia	IV, SC	Nausea, vomiting	Myelosuppression, GI mucositis, immunosuppression
6-Mercaptopurine	6-MP, Purinethol	ALL	PO, IV	Nausea, vomiting	Myelosuppression, hepatocellular dysfunction, GI mucositis
6-Thioguanine, 6-TG		AGL AGL	PO	Nausea, vomiting	Myelosuppression, photosensitivity, hepatocellular dysfunction
Cladrabine 2-Chlorodeoxyadenosine	Leustatin	Hairy cell leukemia CLL Lymphomas	IV	Mild nausea	Myelosuppression with delayed recovery, especially platelets, rash, fever, malaise, anorexia
Fludarabine hydrochloride	Fludara	B cell CLL	IV	Tumor lysis syndrome, mild nausea	Myelosuppression, mild hair loss, cardiotoxicity and neurotoxicity with high doses, mucositis, malaise
Hydroxyurea	Hydrea	CGL Sickle cell anemia	PO	None	Myelosuppression, anorexia, stomatitis, nausea and vomiting, diarrhea, hallucinations
	Droxia				Hyperpigmentation
NATURAL PRODUCTS, PLANT ALKALOIDS					
Vincristine	Oncovin	ALL AGL Hodgkin's lymphoma	IV	Nausea, local phlebitis	Peripheral neuropathy, myopathy, alopecia
Vinblastine	Velban	Hodgkin's lymphoma Lymphomas	IV	Local phlebitis, mild nausea, stomatitis, glossitis	Leukopenia, rare peripheral neuropathy
Etoposide VP-16	Vepesid	AGL Lymphoma	IV	Orthostatic hypotension, mild nausea, vomiting, anorexia	Myelosuppression, alopecia

CGL, Chronic granulocytic leukemia; *CLL,* chronic lymphocytic leukemia; *ALL,* acute lymphocytic leukemia; *AGL,* acute granulocytic leukemia; *BMT,* bone marrow transplant; *IV,* intravenous; *PO,* by mouth; *IM,* intramuscular; *IT,* intrathecal; *IP,* intraperitoneal; *MM,* multiple myeloma; *SC,* subcutaneous.
*This list is not all-inclusive. Other equally effective brands may exist.

Continued

TABLE 18-1

Commonly Used Chemotherapeutic Agents in Hematologic Malignancies—cont'd

Drug				Toxicity	
Generic Name	Trade Name*	Disease	Administration	Acute	Long-term
ANTIBIOTICS					
Doxorubicin	Adriamycin	Acute leukemia Lymphomas	IV	Severe vesicant with tissue necrosis, nausea	Myelosuppression, alopecia Cardiac toxicity with cumulative doses
Daunorubicin (daunomycin)	Cerubidine	Acute leukemia Lymphomas Hodgkin's lymphoma Multiple myeloma	IV	Severe vesicant with tissue necrosis, nausea	Myelosuppression, alopecia Cardiac toxicity with cumulative doses
Bleomycin	Blenoxane	Lymphomas	IV, IM, SC	Fever, possible anaphylaxis, acute pulmonary edema	Pulmonary fibrosis with cumulative doses Minimal myelosuppression, skin and nail discoloration
Idarubicin hydrochloride	Idamycin	ALL AGL Lymphoma	IV	Nausea, vomiting, vesicant with tissue necrosis	Myelosuppression, cardiotoxicity with cumulative doses, alopecia, mucositis
Mitoxantrone hydrochloride	Novantrone	AGL ALL CLL CGL in blast crisis Lymphoma	IV	Nausea, vomiting, vesicant	Myelosuppression, stomatitis, mild congestive heart failure, alopecia
ENZYMES					
L-asparaginase	Elspar	ALL	IV, IM	Hypersensitivity with potential for anaphylaxis Nausea, vomiting, and anorexia	Hyperglycemia, pancreatitis, hepatotoxicity, general malaise, somnolence, depression
ADRENOCORTICOIDS					
Prednisone	Orasone, Deltasone	ALL AGL Lymphomas Multiple myeloma Waldenström's macroglobulinemia	PO	GI distress, water retention	GI distress, chemical diabetes, water retention, osteoporosis, psychosis
MONOCLONAL ANTIBODIES					
Rituximab	Rituxan	Lymphoma CLL	IV IV	Hypersensitivity Fever, chills, shortness of breath, nausea, leukopenia	Unknown
Gemtuzumab ozogamicin	Mylotarg	AGL	IV	Nausea/vomiting Hypotension, chills, fever, headache, pancytopenia, nausea	Unknown
Campath-1-H		CLL	IV	Hypersensitivity, fever, chills, shortness of breath, mylosupperssion infection	Unknown

of these patients. Care should include assiduous precautions against infection and bleeding. Aggressive antimicrobial therapy must be initiated at the first sign of infection, along with an antifungal prophylaxis. Judicious use of blood component therapy (e.g., platelets, RBCs) will protect the patient against bleeding.

Acute Leukemia

The acute leukemia affecting the myeloid series is termed acute nonlymphocytic leukemia (ANLL), acute myelocytic leukemia (AML), or acute granulocytic leukemia (see color plate 20). The neoplasm is uniclonal and originates with the transformation of a hematopoietic progenitor cell. The exact nature of the transformed cell's neoplastic properties are being delineated through molecular studies, but the critical defect is intrinsic and inheritable by the cell's progeny (Hoffbrand, Petit, l993). Both quantitative and qualitative defects are in all the myeloid cell lines, which proliferate in an uncontrolled fashion and replace normal cells (Linker, 2001).

ANLL accounts for 80% of the acute leukemias in adults. The onset may be abrupt or progressive over a 1- to 3-month period, with short duration of symptoms. Without treatment, ANLL is fatal in approximately 3 to 6 months.

The diagnosis of ANLL can be made based on peripheral blood findings but is verified by a bone marrow aspiration and biopsy. The peripheral blood may be markedly elevated, normal, or decreased with circulating myeloblasts and a decreased absolute granulocyte count. The platelet count is also decreased, with levels often below 50,000. Moderate anemia may be present. The bone marrow is generally hypercellular, with 30% to 90% of the myeloblasts containing Auer rods. *Auer rods* are rodlike structures in the cytoplasm of myeloblasts and are diagnostic for acute myeloid leukemia. The remaining bone marrow elements may be suppressed. Cytogenetic studies most often reveal chromosomal abnormalities. Metabolic alterations are present, with elevations in the uric acid levels and lactic dehydrogenase related to the high levels of WBC turnover.

Clinical manifestations relate to the decrease of normal hematopoietic cells, particularly the granulocytes and thrombocytes. Patients often present with infection or bleeding or both at the time of diagnosis. Chills, fever, tachycardia, and tachypnea are frequently presenting symptoms. Infections can involve all organ systems. Cellulitis, pneumonia, oral infections, perirectal abscesses, and septicemias are a few examples of infections encountered in this patient population. The most common organisms are the gram-negative bacteria such as *E. coli* and pseudomonas, as well as fungal infections. Without prompt treatment, patients with septicemia can die within hours.

Patients who present with markedly elevated WBCs and circulating blasts (counts in excess of 200,000/mm³) may present with symptoms of hyperviscosity. These symptoms include headaches, visual changes, confusion, and dyspnea, requiring emergent leukopheresis (removal of white cells via a cell separator) and prompt chemotherapy (Linker, 2001).

Patients with promyelocytic leukemia (M-3) may present with a bleeding diathesis (disseminated intravascular coagulation [DIC]) and those with monocytic leukemia (M-4 or M-5) often present with gum infiltration.

Thrombocytopenia results in bleeding evidenced by petechiae and ecchymosis, epistaxis, and hematomas in the mucous membranes, as well as gastrointestinal and urinary tract bleeding. Bone pain and tenderness may result from bone infarcts or subperiosteal infiltrates. Anemia is not an early manifestation because of the long life span of the erythrocytes (120 days). When anemia is present, headaches and symptoms of fatigue and dyspnea on exertion are evident, along with marked pallor.

Combination chemotherapy, including the antimetabolite Cytosine arabinoside and an anthracycline antibiotic such as daunorubicin hydrochloride, idaru-

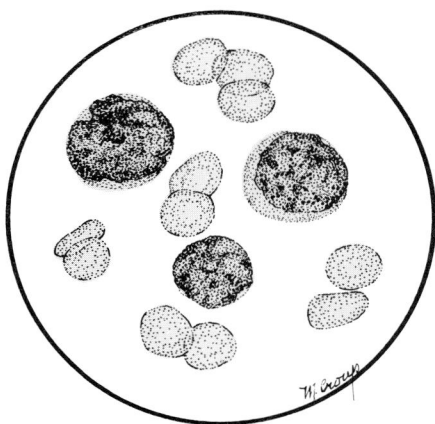

FIG. 18-4   Lymphoblasts.

bicin, or mitoxantrone is the standard of care. Another combination includes etoposide and mitoxantrone or topotecan and mitoxantrone. With the identification of specific antigenic markers (clusters of differentiation [CDs]) such as CD33 on the myeloblasts, a new and promising category of "biologicals," are being developed and in clinical trials. These drugs are monoclonal antibodies that target cells with specific markers. One such drug, Mylotarg is being used in patients with relapsed acute leukemia and targets the cells that are CD33 positive. It is also in clinical trials for newly diagnosed, elderly patients. Patients with acute promyelocytic leukemia (APL) M-3, with the favorable cytogenetic marker t(15;17) have also benefited from advances in therapeutics. These patients present with a bleeding diathesis. With standard chemotherapy, their course was complicated by bleeding from different orifices and including catheter insertions sites, gums, and intercranially, which was, at times, the cause of sudden death. All-trans-retinoic acid (vitamin A) used as a topical antiacne product has proven to be most successful as an oral agent in patients with APL, allowing maturation of the hematopoietic cells with attainment of a remission. This regimen is followed by standard chemotherapy, with long-term remissions and survivals. In the event of relapse, another oral agent is already in clinical trials, arsenic trioxide (approved by the U.S. Food and Drug Administration [FDA]), for patients with APL. Time alone will prove the efficacy and benefits of these treatment modalities. This certainly is an exciting time for medical researchers and health care providers in the fields of hematology-oncology.

Acute Lymphocytic Leukemia

Acute lymphocytic leukemia (ALL) is the most common cancer affecting children under the age of 15 years, with a peak incidence between 3 and 4 years of age. However, a 20% incidence occurs in adults with acute leukemia. ALL is manifested by an abnormal proliferation of lymphoblasts in the bone marrow and extramedullary sites (those outside of the bone marrow, such as lymph nodes and spleen) (Fig. 18-4; see color plate 21). Diagnosis is established through a complete blood cell count (CBC), differential, platelet count, and bone marrow examination. The WBC count is generally markedly elevated, but it may be normal or low, with a lymphocytosis. The platelet, neutrophil, and red blood cell (RBC) counts are generally low. The bone marrow is hypercellular, with infiltrating lymphoblasts. Cytogenetics and immunotyping are also performed to elucidate the malignant clone. Because of the recognized incidence of central nervous system (CNS) involvement, an analysis of the spinal fluid is also included.

Diagnosis and classification of ALL are similarly based on morphologic characteristics using the FAB classification (see Box 18-1). ALL is further subclassified by immunologic criteria. The CDs previously discussed identify T cells with CD5 and CD7 markers; the common ALL antigen (cALLa), now known as CD10, also has CD19 and TdT features; the B cells carry CD19, CD20, CD21, and CD22. The "null" cell represents an immature B cell and thus has no identifying CD marker (Wujcik, 2000).

Clinical manifestations of lymphocytic leukemia resemble those of acute granulocytic leukemia, with signs and symptoms related to suppression of the normal bone marrow elements (Wujcik, 2000). Therefore infection, bleeding, and anemia are major clinical manifestations. One third of the patients present with infection and bleeding at the time of diagnosis. Malaise, fever, lethargy, weight loss, and night sweats may all be presenting symptoms. Because extramedullary sites are also involved, these patients have lymphadenopathy (enlarged lymph nodes) and hepatosplenomegaly (enlarged liver and spleen). Bone pain and arthralgia, although present in adults, are more common in children. CNS involvement may be present in 5% to 10% at diagnosis (Linker, 2001). Signs and symptoms of CNS involvement (most often found during relapse) include headaches, vomiting, seizures, and visual disturbances.

The onset of ALL is usually abrupt and rapidly progresses to death when untreated. Improved survival with treatment has been dramatic. Not only do 90% to 95% of children achieve a full remission but also 60% are cured.

About 80% of adults achieve a complete remission (Devine, Larson, 1994; Linker, 2001), with one third experiencing long-term survival, which is achieved through aggressive chemotherapy directed at the bone marrow, as well as the CNS. Treatment programs use combinations of vincristine, prednisone, L-asparaginase, cyclophosphamide, and an anthracycline such as daunorubicin (see Table 18-1). Because the meninges may harbor leukemia cells, prophylactic intrathecal (into the subarachnoid space) chemotherapy is also included to prevent CNS relapse. Bone marrow transplantation should be considered for adults with aggressive, poor prognosis disease to prolong a disease-free survival. Children with less than 18-month remissions should be considered for bone marrow transplantation (Wujcik, 2000).

Chronic Leukemias
Chronic Granulocytic Leukemia

Chronic granulocytic leukemia (CGL) or chronic myelocytic leukemia (CML), accounting for 15% of the

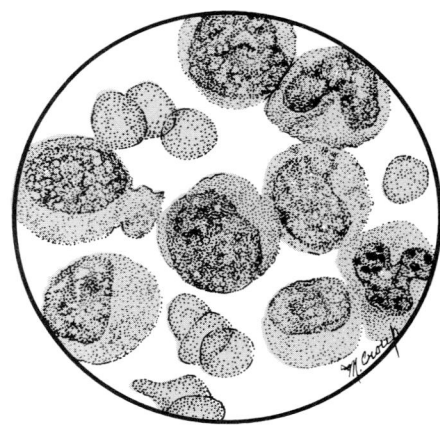

FIG. 18-5 Bone marrow characteristic of chronic granulocytic leukemia.

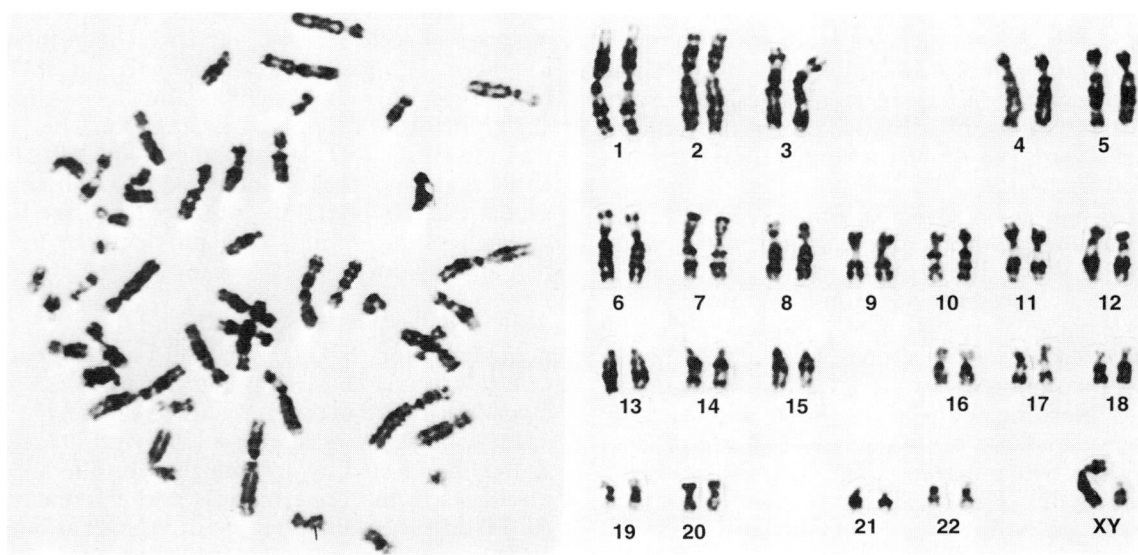

FIG. 18-6 Karyotype of a marrow cell from a male patient with chronic granulocytic leukemia. A fragment has been lost from chromosome 22 and translocated to chromosome 9. The preparation at left is stained with the acetic-saline-Giemsa method 1 to show banding patterns. (Reproduced with permission from Raymond Teplitz, MD.)

leukemias, is most frequently present in middle-age adults but may occur in any age group. Unlike AGL, CGL is insidious in its onset, often discovered during routine examinations and blood screening. CGL is considered a myeloproliferative disorder because the bone marrow is hypercellular with proliferation of all the cell lines (Fig. 18-5; see color plate 22). Granulocyte counts generally are greater than 30,000/mm³. Although maturation is disordered, most of the cells are mature and functional. A left shift occurs with less than 5% blasts in the peripheral blood. Basophils and eosinophils are often present. In 85% of the cases, a chromosomal abnormality referred to as the *Philadelphia chromosome* is present. The Philadelphia chromosome is a translocation of the long arm of chromosome 22 to that of 9 (Fig. 18-6). This chromosomal abnormality affects the hematopoietic stem cell and is therefore present in the myeloid cell lines, as well as some of the lymphoid lines.

Signs and symptoms are related to a hypermetabolic state: fatigue, weight loss, increased diaphoresis, and heat intolerance. The spleen is enlarged in 90% of the cases, which leads to a sensation of abdominal fullness and early satiety. Anemia is not usually observed on presentation, but when anemia is present, the patient may be tachycardic, pale, and short of breath. Bruising may occur secondary to abnormal platelet function. The goal of treatment is to eradicate the Philadelphia chromosome and the oncogene BCR-ABL that forms as a consequence of the 9-to-22 translocation t(9;22). This gene is thought to trigger the uncontrolled growth of the leukemic cells (Wujcik, 2000).

Treatment to date has been with intermittent chemotherapy, using Hydroxyurea and alpha-Interferon. Clinical trials using homoherringtonine, a plant alkaloid, and cytosine arabinoside, an antimetabolite, have proven to be effective in over 65% of patients (O'Brien et al, 1999). Most treatments result in the suppression of hematopoiesis and a reduction in the size of the spleen. Interferon reduces the number of Philadelphia chromosome positive cells, increasing the survival benefits and is now recommended as first line therapy in the chronic phase. Although some long-term survivals have been reported, the median survival rate with or without treatment is approximately 5 to 6 years. Patients invariably progress to a more aggressive, resistant phase with an overwhelming production of myeloblasts (called blast transformation or blast crisis). Death occurs within weeks to months after transformation. Allogenic stem cell transplantation, (peripheral blood stem cells from another individual) performed while the patient is in the stable chronic phase of CGL, offers hope for a cure in an otherwise fatal disease. Although the morbidity and mortality remain high during transplantation, allogenic stem cell transplantation should be considered for all young patients with an HLA-identical sibling or unrelated donor.

The new oral drug STI 571, a tyrosine kinase inhibitor, has been in clinical trials with patients in an aggressive phase of their disease. Although a chronic phase was reestablished, these results were transient. By inhibiting tyrosine kinase, STI 571 inhibited the proliferation of the gene BCR/ABL (DeVita et al, 2001). Currently, the FDA has approved its use in patients with newly diagnosed CGL. The brand name is Gleevec, and thus far it has been well tolerated, with minimal side effects. The goal is to completely eradicate the Philadelphia chromosome t(9;22), as well as the BCR-ABL gene and attain a cure. As with all new treatments, the test of time will verify the anticipated achievement of long-term survival and cure.

Chronic Lymphocytic Leukemia

Chronic lymphocytic leukemia (CLL) is a lymphoproliferative disorder in older individuals (median age 60 years) with a 2:1 male predominance (see color plate 23). CLL is manifested by a proliferation and accumulation of 30% small abnormal mature lymphocytes in the bone marrow, peripheral blood, and extramedullary sites, with levels reaching 100,000+/mm³. In more than 90% of the cases, the abnormal lymphocyte is a B lymphocyte with CD19, CD20, CD23, and CD5 markers. Because the B lymphocyte is responsible for immunoglobulin synthesis, the patients with CLL have insufficient immunoglobulin synthesis and a depressed antibody response. Cytogenetic studies reveal greater than 80% of patients have various cytogenetic changes, which probably indicate a poor prognosis (Kalil, Cheson, 2000). The onset is insidious and is often discovered during routine blood work, showing an elevated absolute lymphocyte count or because of painless lymphadenopathy and splenomegaly. As the disease progresses, the liver also enlarges. Patients with only lymphocytosis and lymphadenopathy may survive 10 years or longer. As organs become involved, particularly the spleen, the prognosis worsens. Early anemia and thrombocytopenia (low platelet count) along with a doubling time of the WBCs in less than a year reflect a very poor prognosis with a median survival of less than 2 years. Approximately 10% of patients experience an aggressive transformation similar to Richter's syndrome (aggressive lymphoma).

Approximately 5% to 10% of the patients develop an autoimmune hemolytic anemia or thrombocytopenia or both, requiring intervention with steroids or chemotherapeutic agents or both.

Signs and symptoms, which are similar to those of CGL, reflect a hypermetabolic state. Massive organ enlargement causes mechanical pressure on the stomach with symptoms of early satiety, abdominal discomfort, and bowel irregularities. Because of insufficient immunoglobulin synthesis and depressed antibody response, their course is complicated by recurrent episodes of infections, involving mainly the lungs and skin. Pneumonia is common, particularly *Pneumocystis carinii* and pneumococcal pneumonia. Viral skin infections such as herpes zoster are frequently present, which affect the patient both physically and emotionally. Treatment of these complications requires prompt intravenous antibiotics and antiviral agents, occasionally requiring the latter prophylactically for the duration of their lives. Intravenous immune globulin prophylaxis monthly is also indicated in patients with frequent episodes of infection requiring hospitalization.

Patients with low-grade disease are observed over time with no active interventions often needed for several years. Treatment is indicated when the patient has increasing pancytopenia with infections, increasing bulky lymphadenopathy and organomegaly, anemia and thrombocytopenia secondary to bone marrow replacement, and changes in his or her quality of life. The treatment is directed toward reducing the lymphocytic mass thus reversing the pancy-

TABLE 18-2 ■ ■ ■

Differential Features of the Leukemias

	Acute Myelogenous (Granulocytic) Leukemia	Acute Lymphoblastic (Lymphocytic) Leukemia	Chronic Myelogenous (Granulocytic) Leukemia	Chronic Lymphocytic Leukemia
Incidence (age)	Adult; 10% in children, peak 60 years	Usually in children <15 years; peak 3-4 years; may occur in adults	Ages 20-60 years Peak 40 years May occur in children	Median 60 years
Gender distribution	Slight M/F predominance 3:2	M/F predominance 5:4	Slight M/F predominance	Male/female predominance 2:1
Implicated causal factors	High ionizing radiation, chemical exposure, genetic aberrations (e.g., Down syndrome) Alkylating agents	Genetic aberrations (e.g., Down syndrome), irradiation, virus	Ionizing radiation, chemical exposure	Unknown
Survival	3-6 months without treatment 1-3 years with treatment Some long-term survivors	3-6 months without treatment Low-risk features (>50% 5+ years survival): null cell*; ages 2-10 years High-risk features (±2 years' survival): T and B cell; children <2 years, teens, young adults	1-10 years; mean 3 years	2-25 years
Signs and symptoms	Variable: ecchymoses, gum and nose bleeding, malaise, fatigue, fever, sternal tenderness, occasional hepatosplenomegaly	Variable: hepatosplenomegaly, lymphadenopathy, 10% mediastinal mass, ecchymoses, low-grade fever, weight loss, sternal tenderness, bone and joint pain, malaise, fatigue	Splenomegaly, bone tenderness, pallor, hypermetabolic symptoms, diaphoresis, weight loss, anorexia	Painless lymphadenopathy, hepatosplenomegaly, acquired hypersensitivity to insect bites
Peripheral blood	Elevated, normal, or decreased WBCs with myeloblasts Thrombocytopenia Anemia	Markedly elevated WBCs with lymphocytosis WBC count may be normal or decreased Thrombocytopenia Anemia	Markedly elevated WBCs, mainly mature granulocytes All developmental stages present, including blasts Basophilia Eosinophilia Early thrombocytosis Thrombocytopenia and anemia (end stage)	Moderately elevated small mature lymphocytes; neutrophils Thrombocytopenia Anemia with progressive disease
Bone marrow	Hypercellular (>50% myeloblasts) Auer rods†	Hypercellular with infiltrating lymphoblasts No Auer rods	Hypercellular (<50% blasts, megakaryocytes)	>30% lymphocytes
Cytogenetics	Nonrandom chromosomal aberrations t(8;21) (q22; q22) +8 t(15;17) (q22; q11)	Variable chromosomal aberrations; 5% Philadelphia chromosome aberrations + 21 t (4;11) (q21; q23) t (9;22) (q34; q11)	85% Philadelphia chromosome aberrations Other chromosomal aberrations t (9;22)	Random unconfirmed chromosomal aberrations t (12;14) del (13q14) t (11;14) del (11q23) t (17;14) del (6q21) Trisomy 12
Immunologic identification	Not identified Lack cALLa‡ antigen Lack T and B cell determinants	85% CD10‡ antigen (lack B or T cell characteristics) CD19, CD20, CD21, CD22, CD24, T cell, ALL CD1, 3, 5, 8	None identified	Majority have B cell markers: CD19, CD20, CD23, CD24 1%-3% have T cell markers

t, Translocation.
*Null cell: lymphocyte that lacks B cell (membrane immunoglobulin) or T cell (E-rosette formation) markers.
†Auer rods: red-staining rods seen in cytoplasm of myeloblasts characteristic of acute myelogenous leukemia.
‡CD$_{10}$: formerly cALLa (common ALL antigen)—a distinct surface membrane glycoprotein complex carried on 70% of non–T cell leukemia lymphoblasts.

topenia and relieving the discomfort caused by the organ enlargement (Hayes, Cartney, 1998). Some patients with medically unresponsive autoimmune hemolytic anemia or thrombocytopenia may require a splenectomy. Alkylating agents, such as chlorambucil and cyclophosphamide, are active in the treatment of CLL. Fludarabine, a purine antimetabolite, given over 3 to 5 days as a single agent, is also effective and can be combined with other active agents

such as cyclophosphamide if the patient becomes refractory. A new approach to the treatment of B cell malignancies such as CLL is the application of biologic therapy, using monoclonal antibodies to specifically attack cells bearing a specific antigenic marker. These monoclonal antibodies include rituximab (anti-CD20) and Campath 1H (anti-CD52), both recently obtaining FDA approval. Table 18-2 presents the differential features of the major leukemias.

TABLE 18-2

Differential Features of the Leukemias—cont'd

	Acute Myelogenous (Granulocytic) Leukemia	Acute Lymphoblastic (Lymphocytic) Leukemia	Chronic Myelogenous (Granulocytic) Leukemia	Chronic Lymphocytic Leukemia
Treatment (see Table 18-1)	Combination chemotherapy including cytosine arabinoside; daunorubicin, idarubicin or mitoxantrone; and topotecan, Mylotarg Blood products and antibiotic support Bone marrow transplant Stem cell transplant	Combination chemotherapy including vincristine and prednisone; methotrexate; L-asparaginase Blood products and antibiotic support Bone marrow transplant	Generally single alkylating agent; melphalan (Alkeran) or hydroxyurea; Gleevec Bone marrow transplant; stem cell transplant Alpha-interferon	When symptomatic alkylating agents, corticosteroids, radiation therapy, fludarabine Rituximab, Campath-1H
Complications	Hemorrhage, sepsis, disseminated intravascular coagulation (DIC)	Hemorrhage, sepsis, CNS involvement	Myelofibrosis, pancytopenia, blast transformation, splenic infarction	Pancytopenia, hemolytic anemia, idiopathic thrombocytopenic purpura (ITP) viral infection

Hairy Cell Leukemia

Hairy cell leukemia is a relatively rare, indolent B cell lymphocytic leukemia. The name identifies the spindle-like microscopic projections on the lymphocytes on stained smears of blood and bone marrow.

Presenting signs and symptoms are fatigue, pancytopenia, and splenomegaly. Although both sexes can be affected, hairy cell leukemia generally occurs in middle-aged men with a 5:1 male to female predominance. CD11 and CD22 antigens are expressed on the lymphocytes. The treatment of choice consists of 7 days of continuous infusion with cladribine (2CdA) resulting in over 80% remissions, often lasting more than 10 years. (Wujcik, 2000; Linker, 2001).

Lymphoma

The lymphomas are malignancies of the lymphatic system. The etiology is unknown, but identified risk factors include immunodeficiency states (congenital or acquired), as well as exposure to herbicides, pesticides, and organic solvents such as benzene. The increased incidence of acquired immunodeficiency syndrome (AIDS) associated with high-grade lymphomas during recent years implicates immunosuppression as a causative factor (Williams et al, 2001). Viruses have also been implicated, particularly the Epstein-Barr virus found in Burkitt's lymphoma and more recently implicated in the possible pathogenesis of Hodgkin's disease (Weinshel, Peterson, 1994).

The initial tumor formation in lymphoma is in the secondary lymphatic tissues (e.g., the lymph nodes or spleen) where abnormal lymphocytes replace the normal structure.

Two broad categories of lymphomas are identified on the basis of the microscopic histopathology of the involved lymph nodes. The categories are Hodgkin's disease and the non-Hodgkin's lymphomas. Although the signs and symptoms of the lymphomas overlap, the treatment and prognosis for cure are different for each kind. Thus establishing an accurate diagnosis is imperative. To achieve this goal, one or more lymph nodes are surgically removed and studied microscopically.

Non-Hodgkin's lymphomas and Hodgkin's disease are differentiated according to the predominant types of cells found in the lymph node, as well as their distribution. The cells may be distributed in a nodular or diffuse manner. These cells destroy the normal architecture of the lymph nodes. Current progress in genetic and molecular biology to identify phenotypic (genetic) markers and chromosomal translocations, along with the clinical features of the disease, differentiates aggressive from indolent lymphomas and guides treatment and progress. B cell lymphomas are noted to be more indolent with long relapse-free survivals, whereas T cell lymphomas of the same histologic type have higher relapse rates with shorter relapse-free survivals (Williams et al, 2001).

The benefits in cytogenetics analysis are found in Burkitt's lymphoma. Burkitt's lymphoma is an example of a high-grade lymphoma, in which a characteristic translocation between the long arms of chromosome 8 and 14, t(8;14), are identified, along with a "protooncogene" c-myc. C-myc is translocated from its normal position on chromosome 8 to 14 and is responsible for its malignant transformation (Linker, 2001). Burkitt's lymphoma is a highly aggressive, high-grade tumor, requiring prompt treatment.

One of the major determinants of treatment, as well as the prognosis, is the clinical stage (extent of disease) of the patient at diagnosis. The staging system developed in Ann Arbor, Michigan, for Hodgkin's disease in the 1970s, was modified in Cotswell, England, in 1989 and is the current internationally used staging system for Hodgkin's and non-Hodgkin's lymphoma. The Cotswell modifications include the subscript X for bulky disease greater than 10 cm; the subscript E for localized extranodal involvement such as lung, pleura, bone, and chest wall. The subscript S designates the spleen (Box 18-2).

After the tissue diagnosis is established, staging procedures must be carried out. These procedures commonly include the following:

1. Complete history including exposures, infections, fevers, night sweats, weight loss in excess of 10% body weight in less than 6 months.
2. Physical examination with particular attention to the lymphatic system (lymph nodes, liver, and

Modified Ann Arbor Cotswell Staging Classification of Hodgkin's Disease and Lymphomas

Stage I	Disease involves a single lymph node region located above or below the diaphragm, or one extralymphatic organ or site (I_E).
Stage II	Disease involves more than two adjacent or two nonadjacent regions on one side of the diaphragm or an extralymphatic organ or site along with one or more lymph node regions on the same side of the diaphragm (II_E).
Stage III	Disease extends above and below the diaphragm but is limited to lymph nodes or involves, additionally, an extralymphatic organ or site (III_E) or the spleen (III_{ES}).
Stage IV	Diffuse or disseminated involvement of one or more extralymphatic organs or tissues, such as bone marrow or liver. Further subclassification indicates absence (A) or presence (B) of systemic symptoms: weight loss exceeding 10% of body weight, fever, and night sweats.

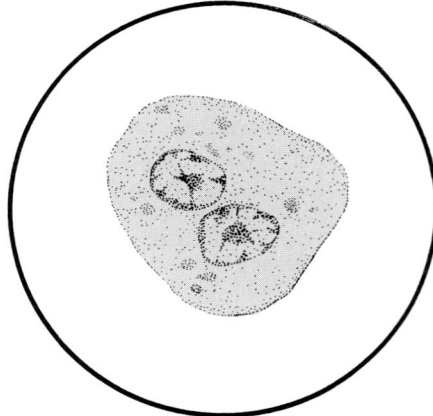

FIG. 18-7 Reed-Sternberg cell.

spleen with size documentation), skin infiltrates, or infections.

3. Routine CBC, differential, and platelet count.
4. Chemistries (liver, kidney function, uric acid, lactic dehydrogenase (LDH), alkaline phosphatase).
5. Chest radiographs looking for hilar adenopathy (enlarged bronchial lymph nodes), pleural effusions, and chest wall thickening.
6. Computed tomography (CT scans) or magnetic resonance imaging (MRI) or both of the chest, abdomen, and pelvis.
7. Bone scan in the presence of bone tenderness.
8. Gallium scans are not routinely performed but may be helpful in identifying residual disease.
9. Bone marrow aspiration and biopsy in stage III and IV disease.
10. Flow cytometry and cytogenetics evaluation.

A gallium scan performed before and after therapy identifies the sites of disease or residual disease in the mediastinum. Bilateral bone marrow biopsies are indicated for patients with systemic symptoms or stage III disease. Bilateral pedal lymphangiography and staging laparotomy, including splenectomy, lymph node biopsy, and open liver biopsy, once routine for staging Hodgkin's disease, is rarely performed because of improved imaging techniques.

Hodgkin's Disease

Hodgkin's disease is a lymphoma that is predominant in young adults between the ages of 18 and 35 years and in those older than 50 years. The cause to date is unknown but may be the culmination to diverse pathologic processes, such as viral infections, environmental exposures, and a genetically determined host response (Weinshel, Peterson, 1994). A 3:2 male-to-female predominance occurs. The Reed-Sternberg cell, which is a malignant, large, binucleated or multinucleated cell that contains two or more large nucleoli, is the characteristic finding in Hodgkin's disease (Fig. 18-7; see color plate 24).

The current classification of Hodgkin's disease is part of the Revised European-American Lymphoma (REAL) classification (Yarbro, 2000). Based on histology and immunophenotyping, the former Rye classification of lymphocyte predominant is now subclassified as a separate entity. The classifications are as follows:

- Nodular lymphocyte-predominant Hodgkin's lymphoma: carries a risk of transformation to non-Hodgkin's lymphoma.
- Classical Hodgkin's lymphoma
  1. Nodular sclerosis Hodgkin's lymphoma
  2. Lymphocyte-rich classical Hodgkin's lymphoma
  3. Mixed cellularity Hodgkin's lymphoma
  4. Lymphocyte-depleted Hodgkin's lymphoma (Lynch et al, 2000)

The most common histologic type is the nodular sclerosis, observed in 60% to 80% of patients with Hodgkin's disease, followed by mixed cellularity, found in 15% to 30% of patients (Yarbro, 2000).

Although histology has been used to predict prognosis, it correlates with the distribution of the disease. Lymphocyte predominant and nodular sclerosis subtypes are generally stage I or II at presentation, whereas lymphocyte depleted is generally stage III or IV. Hilar and mediastinal involvement are more common in the nodular sclerosing subtype.

Clinical manifestations vary. The younger patient generally presents with a nontender, rubbery-feeling enlarged lymph node low in the cervical or supraclavicular area or with a dry cough and shortness of breath secondary to hilar lymphadenopathy.

The general mode of dissemination is an orderly involvement of contiguous sites. Approximately 25% of patients have unexplained persistent fever or night sweats. Constitutional symptoms such as anorexia, cachexia, weight loss, and fatigue are present in disseminated disease and have prognostic significance. In certain cases, the Pel-Ebstein fever (a cyclic pattern of elevated evening temperatures lasting a few days to weeks) is present. Splenomegaly occurs during the course of the disease in 50% of the patients (Hoffbrand, Pettit, 1993). Defects in immunity are present in all phases of Hodgkin's, both during and after therapy, and the incidence of infections, particularly viral and fungal infections, increases. Tuberculosis is also present. Hematologic manifestations depend on the stage of disease and presence of organ involvement (Weinshel, Peterson, 1994).

Accurate clinical and pathologic staging, with appropriate treatment, has improved the prognosis of Hodgkin's disease. For example, 90% cures of patients with asymptomatic stages I and II disease are evident, particularly of the lymphocyte predominant or nodular sclerosis types (see Box 18-2). The ideal treatment of Hodgkin's disease remains controversial but depends on the clinical and pathologic staging. Patients with localized disease, stage IA and IIA, are generally treated with radiation therapy alone to involved or extended fields. Patients with more advanced disease are treated with combined modality of radiation therapy and combination chemotherapy. This approach appears to provide an extended duration of relapse-free survival (Lynch et al, 2000). Although a variety of chemotherapy combinations were studied, the standard of care for many years was MOPP therapy, consisting of nitrogen mustard, Oncovin, prednisone, and procarbazine given over six monthly courses. Long-term complications included secondary malignancies and infertility. ABVD (Adriamycin, Oncovin, bleomycin, and dacarbazine) was found to give superior results with less toxicity over treatments given in combination with MOPP. At this writing, the "gold standard" for treating advanced stage Hodgkin's disease is ABVD.

Although all patients require a great deal of supportive care, the patients in the younger age group are especially needy in this area and require a lot of counseling before, during, and after therapy regarding the potential side effects and complications, particularly that of changes in body image with predictable hair loss, fatigue, fertility issues, and potential secondary malignancies. The latter two are more commonly observed with MOPP therapy. Compliance with the medical regimen is imperative and often depends on patient calls to remind them and encourage them to seek treatments. Delays in treatment and decreases in the dosing of the chemotherapy adversely affect the potential response and cure rates. Studies are continuing in an effort to develop the best mode of therapy without the carcinogenic and sterilizing effects (Lynch et al, 2000). Low-grade lymphomas are indolent but often disseminated at the time of diagnosis. Bone marrow involvement is not unusual.

Non-Hodgkin's Lymphomas

The median age of individuals with non-Hodgkin's lymphomas is 50 years. Classification of the non-Hodgkin's lymphomas is in a state of transition. The widely used Rappaport classification (introduced in 1956) is based on the cytology and the architectural arrangement of the malignant lymphocytes in the lymph nodes. This method divides lymphomas according to (1) the nodular type (N), in which neoplastic cells group in cohesive aggregates that stimulate lymphoid follicles, and (2) the diffuse type (D), in which no aggregation occurs.

The advancement of knowledge in the field of immunology and lymphocyte physiology, such as identifying lymphocytes as B cells or T cells, has led to more definitive classification of the non-Hodgkin's lymphomas, as reflected in the classification by Lukes and Collins. Lukes and Collins demonstrated that 70% of the lymphomas are of B cell origin. The most current classification,

known as the *Working Formulation,* is the result of an international multiinstitutional effort and is based on immunology, lymphocyte physiology, and morphology, as well as the biologic behavior of lymphomas. Three prognostic categories are identified: low-grade, intermediate-grade, and high-grade malignant lymphoma. Table 18-3 presents the Working Formulation, the Rappaport equivalent, the incidence, and median survival rates (Johnson, 1994).

Patients may not require treatment unless they are symptomatic. Treatment and outcome is dependent on the age of the individual, their performance status, the presence or absence of symptoms, staging, and the histology. One of the low-grade lymphomas, mucosa-associated lymphoid tissue (MALT), which is confined to the stomach, is thought to be related to *Helicobacter pylori* infection and responds to antibiotics completely (Linker, 2001). When treatment is indicated for low-grade lymphoma, alkylating agents such as chlorambucil as a single agent, or combination chemotherapy with cyclophosphamide, vincristine, and prednisone, are used. The anti-CD20 monoclonal antibody, Rituxan, has similarly been tested for efficacy in this disease, with promising results in relapsed patients (Patterson, 2000). To date, no known cure for low-grade lymphoma is available. The median life span is 8 to 10 years, but death invariably ensues (Hagemeister, 2001).

Patients with intermediate-grade lymphoma, nodular-lymphocytic type, tend to present at more advanced stages initially, with approximately 60% to 80% incidence of bone marrow involvement. The tonsillar lymphatic tissue in the oropharynx and nasopharynx (referred to as Waldeyer's ring) is also the site of involvement in 15% to 30% of patients (Johnson, 1994). Tissue biopsy, cytochemistry, surface marker studies, gene rearrangement, and cytogenetics are needed to diagnose these lymphomas accurately and give a prognosis. According to the National Comprehensive Cancer Network (NCCN) practice guidelines, CHOP (cyclophosphamide, Adriamycin, Oncovin, and prednisone) should be given for six cycles along with localized radiation therapy (NCCN, 1998).

The Burkitt's and immunoblastic lymphomas are high-grade lymphomas and have a propensity to CNS involvement. The CNS is also a frequent site for relapse in patients with stage IV disease along with sites of previous involvement. These patients require aggressive multidrug chemotherapy, including intrathecal chemotherapy (NCCN, 1998).

Although intermediate- and high-grade lymphomas are highly aggressive and fatal without treatment, they are responsive to chemotherapy and have the potential for cure. Intravenous cytosine arabinoside and methotrexate, which cross the blood-brain barrier or can be given intrathecally, have been incorporated into aggressive combination chemotherapeutic regimens, including alkylating agents and anthracyclines, with good results. The standard treatment to which all combinations are compared is CHOP (cyclophosphamide, Adriamycin, vincristine, and prednisone) (Yarbro, 2000). Monoclonal antibodies are also studied for their potential use in lymphoma. The common chemotherapeutic agents used in hematologic malignancies are listed in Table 18-1.

TABLE 18-3 ∎∎∎

Working Formulation with Rappaport Classification of Malignant Lymphomas

Working Formulation	Non-Hodgkin's Lymphomas (%)	Median Survival (Years)	Rappaport Equivalent
LOW GRADE			
Malignant lymphoma			
Small lymphocytic (SL)	3.6	5.8	Diffuse, well-differentiated lymphocytic (DWDL)
Consistent with CLL			
Plasmacytoid			
Malignant lymphoma, follicular			
Predominantly small cleaved cell (FSC)	22.5	7.2	Nodular, poorly differentiated lymphocytic (NPDL)
Diffuse areas			
Sclerosis			
Malignant lymphoma, follicular			
Mixed, small cleaved and large cell (FM)	7.7	5.1	Nodular, mixed lymphocytic-histiocytic (NM)
Diffuse areas			
Sclerosis			
INTERMEDIATE GRADE			
Malignant lymphoma, follicular			
Predominantly large cell (FL)	3.8	3.0	Nodular histiocytic (NH)
Diffuse areas			
Sclerosis			
Malignant lymphoma, diffuse			
Small cleaved cell (DSC)	6.9	3.4	Diffuse, poorly differentiated lymphocytic (DPDL)
Sclerosis			
Malignant lymphoma, diffuse			
Mixed, small and large cell (DM)	6.7	2.7	Diffuse, mixed lymphocytic-histiocytic (DM)
Sclerosis			
Epithelioid cell component			
Malignant lymphoma, diffuse			
Large cell (DL)	19.7	1.5	Diffuse, histiocytic (DH)
Cleaved cell			
Noncleaved cell			
Sclerosis			
HIGH GRADE			
Malignant lymphoma			
Large cell, immunoblastic (IBL)	7.9	1.3	Diffuse, histiocytic (DH)
Plasmacytoid			
Clear cell			
Polymorphous			
Epithelioid cell component			
Malignant lymphoma			
Lymphoblastic (LBL)	4.2	2.0	Lymphoblastic (LBL)
Convoluted cell			
Nonconvoluted cell			
Malignant lymphoma			
Small noncleaved cell (SNC)	5.0	0.7	Diffuse, undifferentiated (DU)
Burkitt's			Burkitt's
Follicular areas			Non-Burkitt's
MISCELLANEOUS	12.0		
Composite			
Mycosis fungoides			
Histiocytic			
Extramedullary plasmacytoma			
Unclassifiable			
Other			

From Johnson G: Malignant lymphomas. In Mazza J, editor: *Manual of clinical hematology*, Boston, 1994, Little, Brown.

Although constitutional symptoms (fever, weight loss, and night sweats) occur, the incidence is lower than it is in Hodgkin's disease and does not necessarily influence prognosis. Painless diffuse lymphadenopathy is observed and may affect any or all of the peripheral lymph nodes. Hilar adenopathy is not usually present; however, pleural effusions are common. Approximately 20% or more of the patients have symptoms related to retroperitoneal or mesenteric lymph node enlargement and present with abdominal pain or irregularities of bowel movements. Involvement of the stomach and small intestine is common, with symptoms of pain similar to that of peptic ulcer: anorexia, weight loss, nausea, hematemesis (bloody vomiting), and melena. Low-grade lymphomas are indolent but are often disseminated at the time of diagnosis. Bone marrow involvement is not unusual.

PLASMA CELL DYSCRASIAS

Plasma cell dyscrasias are a group of disorders manifested by a proliferation of plasma cells in the bone marrow or peripheral blood or both. Plasma cells are lymphoid in origin (B lymphocyte) and are normally responsible for immunoglobulin synthesis. The five main classes of immunoglobulins are IgA, IgD, IgE, IgG, and IgM (see Chapter 5). In plasma cell dyscrasias, the plasma cells synthesize and secrete an abnormal, structurally homogeneous immunoglobulin called the *M component*. These proteins are found in serum or urine (or both) of affected patients (Foerster, 1999).

Multiple Myeloma

Multiple myeloma is a neoplastic plasma cell dyscrasia arising from a single clone (monoclonal) of plasma cells, manifested by the uncontrolled proliferation of immature and mature plasma cells in the bone marrow. The clinical consequences of the abnormal plasma cells include bone destruction and replacement of normal bone marrow elements, leading to anemia, thrombocytopenia, and leukopenia; altered immune function, with an increased risk for infections; hemostatic abnormalities with bleeding manifestations; and cryoglobulinemia and hyperviscosity related to the abnormal protein *M component*. Bence Jones protein is a light-chain monoclonal protein excreted by the kidneys that plays a role in renal failure (Foerster, 1999).

The exact cause of multiple myeloma is unknown. Genetic susceptibility has been considered as has radiation exposure. The incidence increases with age. The incidence is much higher in people of color than it is in the Caucasian population. The median age at diagnosis is 60 years and is rare in individuals younger than 20 years of age. Diagnosis before the age of 50 years carries a poorer prognosis. At this time, multiple myeloma is an incurable disease.

The diagnostic workup of a patient with suspected multiple myeloma includes (1) a history; (2) a physical examination; (3) skeletal radiographic films and metastatic bone survey; an MRI when spinal cord compression is suspected; (4) hematologic studies including a bone marrow examination, CBC, and differential and platelet count; (5) a monoclonal protein evaluation that includes the serum immunoglobulins and a 24-hour urine collection for Bence Jones proteins; and (6) biochemical studies that assess renal function, albumin, calcium, uric acid, and LDH levels; (7) serum viscosity, which measures the rate of blood flow, denotes "thickness"; slow flow of the blood; and (8) a beta-2 microglobulin, which measures tumor cell mass (Anderson, 1998; NCCN, l998). Positive findings to confirm the diagnosis include the following (Foerster, 1993):

1. Greater than 10% plasma cells in the bone marrow
2. Plasma cells in bone or soft tissue biopsies

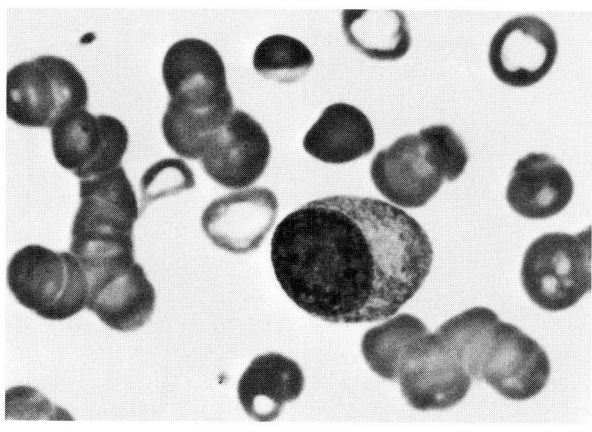

FIG. 18-8 Peripheral blood characteristic of multiple myeloma. Peripheral blood depicting rouleaux formation typically seen in multiple myeloma. The large cell in the center is an immature plasma cell. (Courtesy Rita C. Pohlod, MT [ASCP], SH, Special Hematology Department, Henry Ford Hospital, Detroit, Mich.)

3. Presence of the myeloma protein (M component) on plasma or urine immunoelectrophoresis
4. Presence of "punched-out" lytic bone lesions on skeletal radiographic films
5. Peripheral smear containing myeloma cells

Clinical manifestations vary. Patients with tumor burden (smoldering or indolent myeloma) may be completely asymptomatic. Patients with a high tumor burden, including anemia, hypercalcemia, and high monoclonal proteins, are highly symptomatic. Infection is a common complication of multiple myeloma and is often the cause of death. *Streptococcus*, *Haemophilus influenzae*, *Staphylococcus aureus*, bacteremias, and gram-negative urinary tract infections are common because of the decrease or lack of normal immunoglobulins, as well as the leukopenia secondary to marrow replacement or chemotherapy. Increased levels of abnormal globulins cause increased serum viscosity with visual disturbances, headaches, somnolence, irritability, and confusion. Expanded plasma volume and amyloid infiltration may result in congestive heart failure. The RBCs become coated with proteins, which causes them to stick together similar to stacks of coins (rouleaux) (Fig. 18-8). Bleeding manifestations occur because the protein interacts with the plasma coagulation factors and interferes with platelet function. One of the globulins (cryoglobulin) precipitates in cold temperatures, causing blanching, pain, and ulceration in fingertips and toes (Raynaud's phenomenon). A normochromic normocytic anemia is also present. Fig. 18-9 depicts a peripheral blood smear in multiple myeloma, which illustrates malignant plasma cells (see color plate 25).

Severe disabling bone pain, particularly in weight-bearing areas, is common secondary to bone destruction and pathologic fractures. Simple maneuvers such as turning in bed, coughing, or sneezing can result in fractures of the arms and ribs. Compression fractures of thoracic and lumbar vertebrae cause loss of height. Because of the bone destruction, calcium is mobilized, causing hypercalcemia (increased calcium levels). Symptoms include mental confusion, nausea, vomiting, constipation, polydipsia, and polyuria. Neurologic symptoms range from

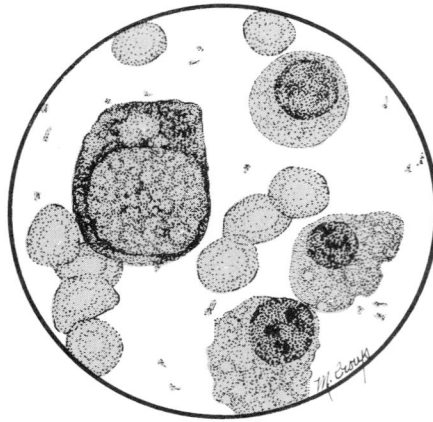

FIG. 18-9 In the upper right field is a normal plasma cell and a plasma cell typical of multiple myeloma; the other cells are malignant plasma cells.

peripheral neuropathy to cord compression. The latter is a medical emergency and, unless treatment is promptly instituted with radiotherapy, chemotherapy, or surgery, the patient will be paralyzed. These patients may have symptoms of renal failure, anorexia, confusion, and coma. When the renal failure is untreated, death occurs. In addition to hypercalcemia, renal impairment may result from the myeloma proteins (referred to as *Bence Jones proteins*), damaging the renal tubules. High uric acid levels secondary to the increased plasma cell turnover may also lead to renal failure. This condition may result from the primary disease or may be secondary to chemotherapy. Dehydration may precipitate actual renal failure.

Newly diagnosed patients with multiple myeloma who present with a high tumor mass, hemoglobin values below 8.5 g, hypercalcemia, serum IgG above 7 g or IgA above 5 g, and renal failure carry a poor prognosis, whereas those with a low tumor mass have a median survival of 5 to 6 years. Response to therapy is also a good prognostic indicator.

Treatment is aimed at reducing the tumor burden (malignant plasma cells and immunoglobulins), preventing and controlling complications (e.g., infections, anemia, hypercalcemia, pathologic fractures), and managing pain. The goal is to maintain as much mobility as possible. Patients with indolent disease are monitored on a regular basis and treatment is initiated when evidence of progression exists and includes monitoring for increases in plasma cells, an increase in immunoglobulins, hypercalcemia, anemia, and increased symptoms, such as pain, fractures, or neurologic changes. First-line therapy consists of prednisone and melphalan (Alkeran). This regimen is administered intermittently every 4 to 6 weeks for 12 months. If the patient attains a remission, he or she is then monitored without ongoing therapy, other than a monthly infusion of one of the biphosphonates. If the patient is no longer responsive or shows progression, multiple drug combinations using 3 to 5 agents are then employed, which includes varying combinations such as carmustine (BCNU), vincristine, melphalan, cyclophosphamide, prednisone or Adriamycin, vincristine, and dexamethasone (Anderson et al, 1998). Thalidomide is the newest agent being tested in refractory multiple myeloma (Nirenberg, 2001). Thalidomide, a new anti-angiogenic drug, is thought to prevent new vascularization needed for survival of tumor cells (Goldman, Bennett, 2001). Approximately 50% of the patients will show a significant tumor reduction. Autologous stem cell transplantation is used in some cases for long-term remissions.

Localized painful bone lesions or other tumor masses are treated with radiation therapy. Because immobility exacerbates bone demineralization and osteoporosis, the patient must maintain a high level of mobility. Supportive garments, walking aids, and judicious use of analgesics may be beneficial. Other preventative measures such as hydration and control of infections and bleeding will limit many of the complications. Biphosphonates (Aredia) are used monthly as an intravenous infusion to minimize bone loss, treat hypercalcemia, and control pain. Intravenous immunoglobulin therapy can be given to avoid recurrent infections. Erythropoietin injections are used in patients with anemia, particularly when they have renal insufficiency (Anderson et al, 1998). Drugs that can adversely affect renal function, such as the nonsteroidal pain medications and imaging contrast, should be avoided.

Waldenström's Macroglobulinemia

Waldenström's macroglobulinemia is a less common plasma cell dyscrasia that affects predominately men older than 50 years of age. Morphologically, Waldenström's macroglobulinemia resembles a malignant lymphoma with B lymphocytes, plasma cells, and plasmacytoid lymphocytes (resembling plasmacytes) infiltrating the bone marrow. As the disease progresses, the clinical pattern is that of a lymphoma or chronic lymphocytic leukemia. Hepatic, splenic, and other lymphoid tissue involvements are common, resulting in enlargement of these organs. The malignant cells rarely produce bone destruction but synthesize and release large quantities of IgM into the intravascular space. This action causes increased plasma volume and severe hyperviscosity. The immunoglobulin is relatively nonfunctional but may suppress production of normal immunoglobulins.

Diagnostic workup is similar to that of multiple myeloma but includes a serum viscosity, and a CT scan of the chest, abdomen, and pelvis. Laboratory findings include an increased sedimentation rate and rouleaux formation (RBCs resemble a stack of coins on a blood smear). Pancytopenia occurs with disease progression. Blood volume and serum viscosity are increased. The bone marrow is often a "dry tap" because of the hypercellularity. The predominant cells are plasmacytoid lymphocytes. These cells are also found in the lymph nodes and spleen. Serum protein electrophoresis depicts an IgM spike (McDermott, Bell, 1999).

Patients may experience general malaise, fatigue, weight loss, and bleeding tendencies for years before diagnosis as the disease progresses (Foerster, 1999). The major clinical manifestations relate to the hyperviscosity syndrome, the abnormal plasma immunoglobulin, and bone marrow infiltration. The symptoms of hyperviscosity are similar to those of multiple myeloma, including a marked increase in plasma volume, vision disturbances, and segmental dilation of retinal veins and hemorrhages. Cold agglutinin disease (agglutination of RBCs at cold temperature) with hemolytic anemia has been described, as has Raynaud's phenomenon and anemia secondary to bone marrow replacement. Bleeding tendency, which is attributed to coating of the platelets with the macroglobulins and interference with the coagulation factors, also occurs and is further aggravated by thrombocytopenia caused by marrow replacement. Lymphadenopathy and splenomegaly may be present. Patients may present with bruising, oral mucous membrane bleeding, and retinal hemorrhages. Polyneuropathies may also occur.

Treatment of Waldenström's macroglobulinemia is aimed at decreasing the IgM plasma load and infiltration of the bone marrow and lymphoid tissues. Because IgM is mainly a circulating intravascular protein, plasmapheresis can be used effectively to decrease the globulin and temporarily reduce the hyperviscosity symptoms. Plasmapheresis is a process whereby plasma is removed by means of a cell separator and replaced with volume expanders. In the anemic patient, this procedure should be performed before RBC infusion, because the RBCs add to the hyperviscosity syndrome. Combination chemotherapy with alkylating agents such as cytoxan, along with steroids, is used monthly. The purine analogues (antimetabolites), Cladribine (Leustatin, 2CdA) and fludarabine are also active in this disorder (NCCN, 1998; McDermott, Bell, 1999). Radiation is used to reduce large lymphoid aggregates. Prevention, early detection, and prompt treatment of infections are imperative because of their high incidence and increased mortality from infection. Asymptomatic patients with stable M component and no hyperviscosity or hematologic changes may live for years without treatment. After the disease progresses, even with appropriate treatment measures, the median survival is only 4 years.

TREATMENT OF HEMATOLOGIC MALIGNANCIES

The major treatment modalities for malignancies over the last several decades have been surgery, chemotherapy, and radiation therapy. In the hematologic malignancies, chemotherapy and radiation therapy have been and continue to be the hallmarks. At this time, a fourth major treatment modality is available in limited but ever-increasing use, with many clinical trials in progress. This group of medications is known as the Biologicals. These are natural substances extracted from natural sources or synthesized in the laboratory to attack specific biologic targets (Finley, 2000). Examples include the monoclonal antibody, Rituxan, which targets B lymphocytes with CD20 cell surface antigen, and Campath-1H, which targets B lymphocytes with CD52 cell surface antigen. Some drugs, such as Thalidomide, interfere with angiogenesis, interfering with the formation of new blood vessels and thereby inhibiting essential nutrients needed for tumor growth, with resultant apoptosis (programmed cell death) (Goldman, Bennett, 2001; Finley, 2000). Vaccines

and gene therapy directed at inhibiting cell division are also in clinical trials (Myers, 1999). These modalities are being used independently or in combination with chemotherapeutic agents. As natural, targeted substances, Biologicals are thought to preserve the hematopoietic stem cells and thus are less toxic and are hailed to be potentially curative.

Current chemotherapeutic regimens consist of single agents or multiple drugs used in combination, which result in more sustained remission rates. In select cases of Hodgkin's disease, lymphoma, and acute leukemia, cures are being achieved. In other diseases such as multiple myeloma, quality of life and length of survival have improved.

All cells go through a series of divisions (mitosis) and maturational stages called a *cell cycle* (see Fig. 8-12). During the mitotic phase, chromosome replication takes place, followed by the first gap or G1 phase with ribonucleic acid (RNA) and protein synthesis. This phase is followed by the S or DNA synthesis phase and then the second gap or G2 phase with resumed RNA synthesis. Mitosis follows, producing two daughter cells (Fischer, Knobf, 1997).

Generally, therapeutic regimens are developed to include drugs acting at different stages of the cell cycle. *Phase-specific agents* arrest or kill dividing cells during a specific phase of this cycle. For example, vincristine arrests cell division, and cytarabine (Cytosar) interferes with DNA synthesis during the S phase. *Cycle-specific drugs* such as cyclophosphamide (Cytoxan) kill proliferating cells more effectively than resting cells, and non–cycle-specific agents such as nitrogen mustard and carmustine (BCNU) kill both proliferating and resting cells.

The drugs are further classified according to their mode of action. *Alkylating agents* are substances in which an alkyl radical (hydrocarbon molecule with an absent hydrogen atom) is substituted for a hydrogen atom, causing cross-linking of DNA strands and abnormal base-pairing, thereby interfering with DNA replication. This category includes nitrogen mustard, cyclophosphamide, phenylalanine mustard, and chlorambucil (Fischer, Knobf, 1997). The *antimetabolites*, such as methotrexate, cytosine arabinoside, and 6-mercaptopurine, interfere with the biologic synthesis of DNA and RNA, and thus the cell metabolism, by either blocking the needed developmental enzymes or actually being incorporated into the DNA or the RNA or both.

The *antibiotic agents*, isolated from microorganisms, appear to inhibit DNA and RNA synthesis. Doxorubicin hydrochloride (Adriamycin) and bleomycin are only two of many antibiotic antitumor agents. Natural products—the vinca alkaloids, vincristine, and vinblastine, derived from the periwinkle plant—interfere with the mitotic spindle formation and arrest cell division at the metaphase stage (Fischer, Knobf, 1997).

The *nitrosourates* are lipid-soluble alkylating agents that inhibit nucleic acid synthesis (DNA or RNA or both). Drugs in this category include lomustine (CCNU) and carmustine (BCNU).

Adrenocorticosteroids are hormone preparations. Although their exact action is unclear, they may influence synthetic processes related to RNA and protein synthesis.

Prednisone is the one most commonly used in the hematologic malignancies and may be part of many combinations.

The commonly used chemotherapeutic agents as presented in Table 18-1 are listed according to their classification. Their adverse reactions are divided according to acute or chronic toxicity. Acute toxicity occurs within minutes to hours after administration; chronic toxicity occurs over a longer period and is generally a cumulative, or dose-related, effect.

KEY CONCEPTS

- Defense against infection is the major role of leukocyte of WBCs.
- Five types of WBCs identified in the peripheral blood are (1) neutrophils, (2) eosinophils, (3) basophils, (4) monocytes, and (5) lymphocytes.
- Several CSFs or hematopoietic growth factors have been identified. CSFs are a group of cell-derived glycoproteins that belong to a broader group of WBC regulators called cytokines.
- Leukocytosis refers to an increase in the leukocyte count generally exceeding 10,000/mm³.
- *Granulocytosis* is an increase in granulocytes but, in common usage, refers only to an increase in the neutrophils; thus *neutrophilia* is the more accurate term.
- Disorders in which a general increase in blood-forming cells occurs are called *myeloproliferative disorders*.
- *Leukopenia* refers to a decreased number of leukocytes, and *neutropenia* refers to a decrease in the absolute neutrophil count.
- *Agranulocytosis* is a serious condition characterized by an extremely low leukocyte count and absence of neutrophils.
- Leukemia is a neoplastic disease characterized by differentiation and proliferation of malignantly transformed hematopoietic stem cells, leading to suppression and replacement of normal marrow elements.
- FAB is a morphologic classification based on the differentiation and maturation of the predominant leukemic cells in the bone marrow, as well as on cytochemical studies.
- Advances in immunology, cytogenetics, and molecular biology have had a marked impact on distinguishing normal hematopoietic cells from the malignant clone.
- Immunologic technology has enhanced the classification of the leukemias by identifying the malignant clone as myeloid, B lymphoid, T lymphoid, or biphenotypic (having characteristics of both myeloid and lymphoid cells).
- The Philadelphia chromosome (Ph) is an example of a cytogenetic change in 85% of patients with chronic myeloid leukemia and in some patients with acute myelocytic or lymphoid leukemia.

- Acute leukemia affecting the myeloid series is termed ANLL, AML, or acute granulocytic leukemia.
- ANLL accounts for 80% of the acute leukemias in adults, and the diagnosis is made on the basis of peripheral blood findings but is verified by a bone marrow aspiration and biopsy.
- Clinical manifestations of acute lymphocytic (ALL) leukemia resemble those of acute granulocytic leukemia, with signs and symptoms related to suppression of the normal bone marrow elements.
- The onset of ALL is usually abrupt and rapidly progresses to death without treatment, but improved survival with treatment has been dramatic, with 90% to 95% of children achieving a full remission and 69% eventually being cured; 80% of adults achieve a complete remission.
- Chronic granulocytic or myelocytic leukemia (CGL or CML), accounting for 15% of the leukemias, is found most frequently in middle-aged adults but may occur in any age group.
- Chronic lymphocytic leukemia (CLL) is a lymphoproliferative disorder in older individuals (median age 60 years) with a 2:1 male-to-female predominance.
- Lymphomas are classified as malignancies of the lymphatic system.
- The initial tumor formation in lymphoma is in the secondary lymphatic tissues (e.g., the lymph nodes or spleen) where abnormal lymphocytes replace the normal structure.
- Two broad categories of lymphomas are Hodgkin's disease and the non-Hodgkin's lymphomas.
- Although the signs and symptoms of the lymphoma overlap, the treatment and prognosis for cure are different for each kind.
- Multiple myeloma is a neoplastic plasma cell dyscrasia arising from a single clone (monoclonal) of plasma cells, manifested by the uncontrolled proliferation of immature and mature plasma cells in the bone marrow.
- Waldenström's macroglobulinemia is a less-common plasma cell dyscrasia that predominately affects men older than 50 years of age.

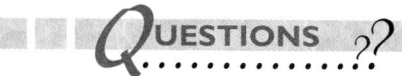

QUESTIONS ??

A sampling of review questions for this chapter appears here. Visit http://www.mosby.com/MERLIN/PriceWilson/ for additional questions. MERLIN

Answer the following on a separate sheet of paper.

1. Explain the role of CSF or hematopoietic growth factors in the differentiation and maturation of WBCs.
2. Describe the FAB classification of leukemia.
3. Cite the importance of the genetic and environmental factors associated with leukemia.
4. What is the goal of therapy in the treatment of leukemia?
5. Formulate a definition of multiple myeloma.
6. Describe the symptoms associated with Hodgkin's disease.
7. What are the aims of the treatment for multiple myeloma and Waldenström's macroglobulinemia?

Complete the following statements by filling in the blanks.

8. _____ refers to a neoplastic disease characterized by an abnormal proliferation and impaired functional capability of the hematopoietic cells.
9. The cells characteristic of Hodgkin's disease are called _____.
10. _____ is a decrease below normal in the leukocyte count.
11. Certain abnormal chromosome patterns, such as the Philadelphia chromosome, are encountered in approximately 85% of the cases of _____.
12. ANLL accounts for _____ % of the acute leukemias in adults.

Fill in the blanks.

13. List the type of WBC count that is elevated in the following conditions:

Condition	Type of Cell
Acute bacterial infection	a. _____
Allergic rhinitis	b. _____
Myeloproliferative disorders	c. _____

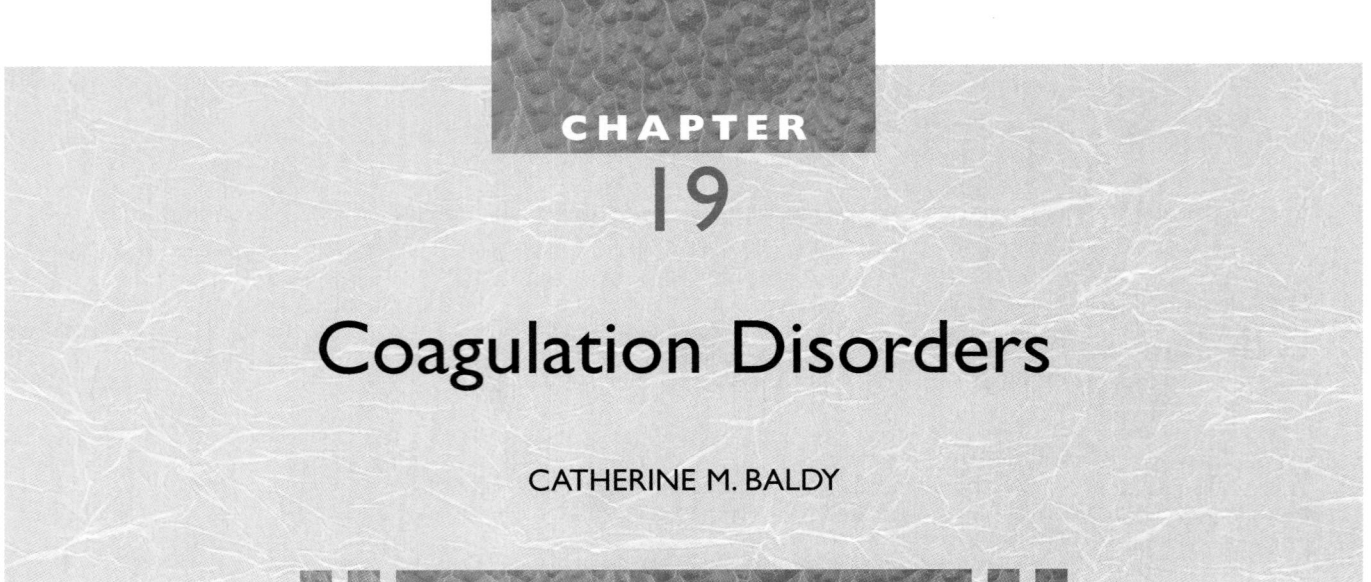

Coagulation Disorders

CATHERINE M. BALDY

NORMAL COAGULATION PROCESS AND PLASMA CLOTTING FACTORS

Hemostasis and coagulation refer to a complex series of reactions that lead to the control of bleeding through the formation of a platelet and fibrin clot at the injury site. Clotting is followed by resolution or lysis of the clot and regeneration of the endothelium. In homeostatic states, hemostasis and coagulation protect the individual from massive bleeding secondary to trauma. In abnormal states, life-threatening hemorrhage or thrombosis occluding the vascular tree can occur.

At the time of injury, three major processes are responsible for hemostasis and coagulation: (1) transient vasoconstriction; (2) platelet reaction consisting of adhesion, release reaction, and aggregation of platelets; and (3) activation of the clotting factors (Box 19-1). The ini-

tial steps occur at the exposed surfaces of the injured tissue, and subsequent reactions occur on surface phospholipids of the aggregated platelets.

Platelets

Platelets, or thrombocytes, are not cells but granular, disk-shaped nonnucleated cell fragments; they are the smallest of the bone marrow cellular elements and are vital to hemostasis and coagulation. Platelets are derived from a noncommitted pluripotent stem cell, which, on demand and in the presence of a platelet-stimulating factor (Mk-CSF [megakaryocyte colony-stimulating factor]), interleukin and TPO (megakaryocyte growth and development factor) (Bagley, Heinrich, 2000), differentiates into the committed stem cell pool to form the megakaryoblast. This cell, through a maturation sequence, becomes a giant megakaryocyte (see Fig. 16-1). Unlike the other cellular elements, megakaryocytes undergo endomitosis, whereby nuclear division occurs within the cell but the cell itself does not duplicate. The cell expands as increased DNA is synthesized. The cell cytoplasm eventually breaks up into individual platelets.

Platelets measure 1 to 4 μm in diameter and have a life span of approximately 10 days. Approximately one third are in the spleen as a reserve pool, and the remainder are in the circulation, numbering between 150,000 and 400,000/mm^3. When Wright's stain is used on a peripheral smear, these cells appear light blue with red-purple granules (see color plate 26). Adsorbed on the platelet membrane are factors V, VIII, and IX, the contractile protein actomyosin, or thrombosthenin, and various other proteins and enzymes. The granules contain the potent vasoconstrictor serotonin, the aggregating factor adenosine diphosphate (ADP), fibrinogen, von Willebrand's factor, platelet factors 3 and 4 (heparin-neutralizing factor), and calcium, as well as enzymes. All these factors are released and activated in response to injury.

Clotting Factors

The clotting factors, with the exception of factors III (tissue thromboplastin) and IV (calcium ion), are plasma

Plasma Clotting Factors

I	Fibrinogen: precursor of fibrin (polymerized protein)
II	Prothrombin: precursor of the proteolytic enzyme thrombin and perhaps other accelerators of prothrombin conversion
III	Thromboplastin: a tissue lipoprotein activator of prothrombin
IV	Calcium: necessary for prothrombin activation and fibrin formation
V	Plasma accelerator globulin: a plasma factor that accelerates the conversion of prothrombin to thrombin
VII	Serum prothrombin conversion accelerator: a serum factor that accelerates prothrombin conversion
VIII	Antihemophilic globulin (AHG): a plasma factor associated with platelet factor III and Christmas factor (IX); activates prothrombin
IX	Christmas factor: serum factor associated with platelet factors III and VIII$_{AHG}$; activates prothrombin
X	Stuart-Prower factor: a plasma and serum factor; accelerator of prothrombin conversion
XI	Plasma thromboplastin antecedent (PTA): a plasma factor that is activated by Hageman factor (XII); accelerator of thrombin formation
XII	Hageman factor: a plasma factor; activates PTA (XI)
XIII	Fibrin stabilizing factor: plasma factor; produces stronger fibrin clot that is insoluble in urea
—	Fletcher factor (prekallikrein): contact-activating factor
—	Fitzgerald factor (high–molecular-weight kininogen): contact-activating factor

proteins that circulate in the blood as inactive molecules. Box 19-1 identifies the coagulation factors, using the internationally accepted and standardized Roman numerals, provides their synonyms, and summarizes their functions. Prekallikrein and high–molecular-weight kininogen (HMWK), along with factors XII and XI, are called *contact factors* and are activated at the time of injury by contact with tissue surfaces; they also play a role in the dissolution of clots once they are formed.

Activation of the coagulation factors is believed to occur as an enzyme splits off a fragment of an inactive predecessor form, for this reason called a *procoagulant.* Each activated factor, except for V, VIII, XIII, and I (fibrinogen), is a protein-cleaving enzyme (serine protease), which thus activates the succeeding procoagulant.

The liver is the site of synthesis of all the coagulation factors except factor VIII and possibly XI and XIII. Vitamin K is essential for the synthesis of the prothrombin factors II, VII, IX, and X. The available evidence suggests that factor VIII is really a complex molecule of three distinct subunits: (1) the procoagulant part, which contains the antihemophilic factor, VIII$_{AHG}$, absent in patients with classic hemophilia; (2) another subunit containing an antigenic site; and (3) von Willebrand's factor, VIII$_{VWF}$, necessary for platelet adhesion to vascular walls (Erslev, Gabuzda, 1985).

Phases of Coagulation

Coagulation is initiated in homeostatic states by vascular injury. Vasoconstriction is an immediate response to the injury, followed by adhesion of platelets to collagen in the vessel wall exposed by the injury. ADP is released by the platelets, causing them to aggregate. Minute amounts of thrombin (created as described later) also stimulate platelet aggregation, serving to amplify the reaction. Platelet factor III, from platelet membranes, also accelerates plasma clotting. In this way, a platelet plug forms, soon to be strengthened by the filamentous protein known as *fibrin.*

Fibrin production begins with conversion of factor X to Xa, as the activated form of a factor is designated. Factor X can be activated by means of two reaction sequences (Fig. 19-1). One requires tissue factor, or tissue thromboplastin, which is released by the vascular endothelium at the time of injury. Because tissue factor is not in the blood, it is an extrinsic element in coagulation hence the name *extrinsic pathway* for this sequence.

The other sequence leading to activated factor X is the *intrinsic pathway,* given the name because it employs factors found within the vascular system of plasma. In this sequence, a "cascade" of reactions occurs, one procoagulant's activation leading to activation of a successor form. The intrinsic pathway is initiated by plasma exposed to skin or collagen within a damaged vessel. Tissue factor is not required, but platelets adhering to the collagen again play a part. As Fig. 19-1 shows, factors XII, XI, and IX must be activated in succession, and factor VIII must be involved before factor X can be activated. The substances prekallikrein and HMWK are participants as well, and calcium ion is needed.

From this point, coagulation proceeds along what has been called the *common pathway.* As the illustration shows, activation of factor X takes place as a result of either extrinsic or intrinsic pathway reactions. Clinical experience suggests that both pathways participate in hemostasis (Handin, 2001).

The next step toward fibrin production is taken when factor Xa, helped by phospholipids from activated platelets, splits prothrombin, creating thrombin. Thrombin, in turn, cleaves fibrinogen to form fibrin. (Small amounts of thrombin are apparently reserved to amplify platelet aggregation.) This fibrin, at first a soluble gel, is stabilized by factor XIIIa and polymerizes into a tight meshwork of fibrin, platelets, and entrapped blood cells. The fibrin strands then shorten (clot retraction), bringing together the edges of the wounded vessel wall and sealing the site.

Termination of Clot Generation

After the formation of a clot, terminating further blood clotting to avoid unwanted thrombotic events that result from excessive systemic clot formation is imperative. Naturally occurring anticoagulants include antithrombin III (heparin co-factor), protein C and protein S. Antithrombin III circulates freely in plasma and inhibits the procoagulant system, by binding thrombin, as well as activated factor Xa, IXa, and XIa, neutralizing their activity and inhibiting clotting (Sacher, McPherson, 2001; Jenny, Mann, 1998). Protein C, a polypeptide, is also a physiologic anticoagulant, produced by the liver, and circulates freely in an inactive form and is activated to become protein Ca. Activated protein C inactivates prothrombin and the intrinsic pathway by cleaving and inactivating factor Va and VIIIa. Protein S accelerates the inactivation of those factors by Protein C. Thrombomodulin, a substance produced by the vessel wall, is necessary for the previously noted neutralizing affect (Jenny, Mann, 1998; Sacher, McPherson, 2001), Deficiencies in Protein C and S lead to thrombotic episodes. Individuals with an abnormal factor V (factor V Leiden) are prone to venous thrombosis, because Factor V Leiden is resistant to degradation by activated Protein C (Linker, 2001).

Clot Resolution

The fibrinolytic system refers to the sequence whereby fibrin is split by plasmin (also called *fibrinolysin*) into fibrin degradation products, leading to the dissolution of the clot. As diagrammatically demonstrated in Fig. 19-2, several interactions are required to convert the specific inactive circulating plasma proteins into the active fibrinolytic enzyme plasmin. Circulating proteins known as *plasminogen proactivators*, in the presence of kinases (enzymes) such as streptokinase, staphylokinase, and tissue kinase, as well as factor XIIa, are catalyzed to plasminogen activators. In the presence of additional

enzymes such as urokinase, the activators convert plasminogen, a plasma protein that has been incorporated within the fibrin clot, into plasmin. Plasmin then splits fibrin and fibrinogen into fragments (fibrin-fibrinogen degradation products), which interfere with thrombin activity, platelet function, and fibrin polymerization, leading to the dissolution of the clot. Macrophages and neutrophils also play a role in fibrinolysis through their phagocytic activities. Fig. 19-3 is a graphic presentation of the sequence of events of the clotting process, as previously discussed.

Diagnostic Approach

The preceding discussion makes evident that abnormalities can occur at any stage of the hemostatic process. Evaluation then includes an in-depth history and physical and laboratory assessments. A carefully elicited history will often lead to the accurate diagnosis and required laboratory studies. This assessment includes family history, coexisting medical problems, medication exposure, prior bleeding episodes (e.g., "spontaneous" or related to surgery or tooth extractions), and the need for blood component therapy.

Careful scrutinizing of the skin and mucous membranes with attention to the type of lesions may suggest the abnormality present.

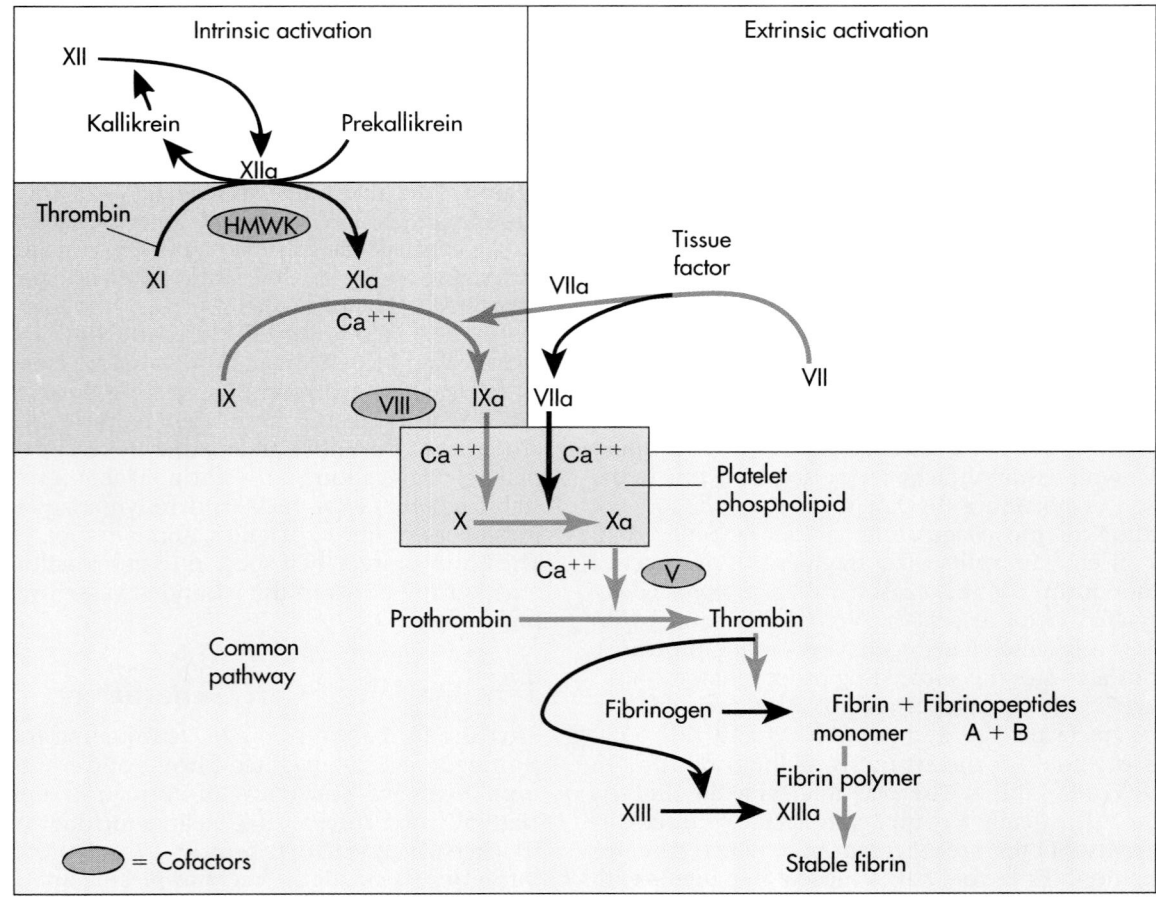

FIG. 19-1 Activation of factor X by the steps in the extrinsic and intrinsic coagulation pathways. (Redrawn from Hoffbrand AV, Pettit JE, Moss P: *Essential haematology*, ed 4, London, 2001, Blackwell Science.)

Telangiectasias are dilated capillaries and venules that are 2 to 3 mm, purple to red-purple macular spots that blanch with pressure and bleed with the slightest trauma. These spots are most commonly observed on the face, lips, mucous membranes, fingertips, and toes. Telangiectasias are viewed as birthmarks, or in a hereditary hemorrhagic disorder, Osler-Weber-Rendu disease. *Arterial spiders*, bright-red lesions with a pulsatile center and threadlike extensions radiating 5 to 10 mm in length, are commonly found in the face and trunk, above the waist-

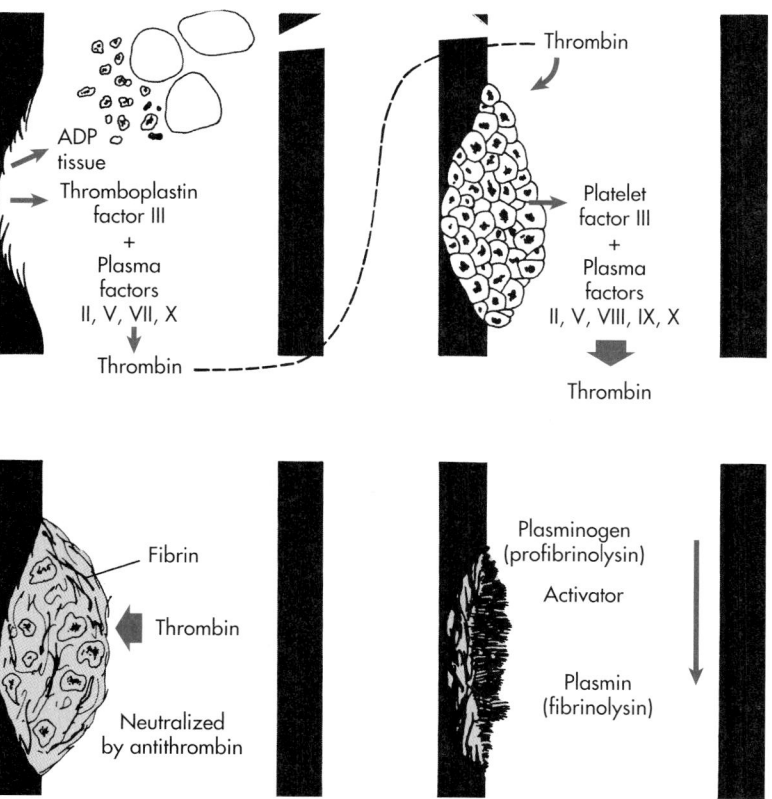

Plasminogen proactivator
(profibrinolysin)

Kinases (including streptokinase, staphylokinase,
←tissue kinase)
←Factor XIIa
←Thrombin

Plasminogen activator

Urokinase
Tissue kinase

Plasminogen → Plasmin (fibrinolysin)

Fibrinogen and fibrin → Fibrin/fibrinogen
degradation
products

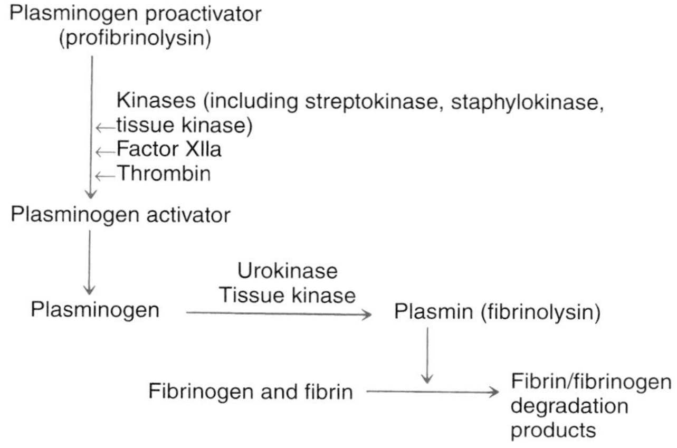

FIG. 19-2 Fibrinolytic system. Antithrombin is a circulating protein that inactivates fibrin and helps maintain blood fluidity.

line. These similarly blanch when pressed at their center and represent vascular anomalies, often present in liver disease.

Petechiae are 1 to 4 mm flat, round, nonblanching, purplish hemorrhagic lesions, which may coalesce to form larger lesions called *purpura*. These lesions are found in the mucous membranes and skin, particularly in the dependent or pressure areas. *Hematomas* (blood blisters) can also be found in mucous membranes.

All of these lesions reflect a platelet abnormality, either in the number of platelets or their function.

Ecchymoses, bruises or black-and-blue marks, are large areas of extravasated blood in the subcutaneous tissues and skin. Fresh bleeding is blue-black and fades to green-brown and yellow on resolution. Although ecchymoses commonly occur with trauma, extensive ecchymoses may reflect a platelet abnormality or a coagulation defect or both.

Laboratory Evaluation

Laboratory evaluation will further delineate and confirm the hemostatic defect. This assessment should always include a peripheral blood smear and a platelet count as previously described. These studies provide morphologic platelet characteristics, as well as numbers.

The *bleeding time* tests both vascular status and platelet number and function; it does not, however, differentiate between the two. A controlled puncture incision is made in the free-hanging earlobe (Duke method) or on the volar surface of the forearm (Ivy method). The length of

ADP
tissue

Thromboplastin
factor III
+
Plasma
factors
II, V, VII, X

Thrombin

Thrombin

Platelet
factor III
+
Plasma
factors
II, V, VIII, IX, X

Thrombin

Fibrin

Thrombin

Neutralized
by antithrombin

Plasminogen
(profibrinolysin)

Activator

Plasmin
(fibrinolysin)

FIG. 19-3 Sequence of events in the clotting process. (Modified from Hiss RG, Penner J: The before and after of blood clotting, *Med Clin North Am* 53[6]:1309-1320, 1969.)

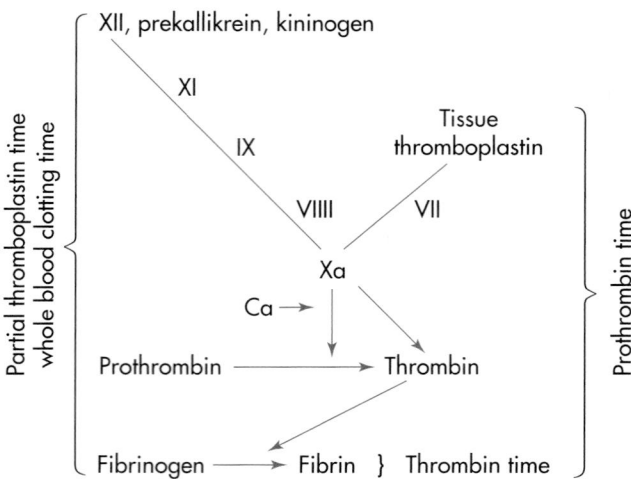

FIG. 19-4 Coagulation tests. (From Nossel HL: Bleeding. In Isselbacher K et al, editors: *Harrison's principles of internal medicine*, ed 9, New York, 1980, McGraw-Hill.)

time for bleeding to cease is recorded. Normal bleeding time is 3 to 7 minutes. Prolongation, such as 10 minutes, may indicate thrombocytopenia (platelet count of less than $100,000/mm^3$) or thrombocytopathy (abnormal platelet function) or both. Aspirin ingestion can interfere with platelet function for 7 to 10 days and should thus be withheld before testing the bleeding time. Although a battery of tests is available to evaluate the coagulation status, screening tests should include the *prothrombin time (PT)*, measuring the extrinsic and common pathway, and the partial *thromboplastin time (PTT)*, measuring the intrinsic and common pathway.

In tests of the PT, an aliquot of the patient's citrated plasma is mixed with phospholipid and tissue thromboplastin. Because calcium has been removed, coagulation does not occur. Next, calcium is added and the time required for clot formation is recorded. Normal plasma requires 11 to 13 seconds to clot under these conditions. Deficiencies of factors VII, X, and V, prothrombin, and fibrinogen will prolong the PT.

In tests of the PTT, phospholipid is added to the patient's citrated plasma, resulting in clot formation in 60 to 90 seconds. Adding a contact-activating agent such as kaolin reduces the variability of the study, as well as the time required for clot formation. This modification gives an *activated partial thromboplastin time (APTT)*. The results are compared with the APTT of normal plasma. The normal range is 26 to 42 seconds. Because the PTT measures the intrinsic and common pathways, it is prolonged by deficiencies of prekallikrein, HMWK, factors V, VIII, IX, X, XI, and XII, prothrombin, and fibrinogen. If only the PT is prolonged, a deficiency or an inhibitor of factor VII can then be assumed. If only the PTT is prolonged, a deficiency or an inhibitor of any intrinsic pathway factor can then be assumed. With prolongation of both, a deficiency or inhibitor of the common pathway factors V and X, prothrombin, and fibrinogen can be assumed. Similarly, liver disease can cause prolongation of both PT and PTT.

In tests of the *thrombin time (TT)* or thrombin clotting time (normally 10 to 13 seconds), exogenous thrombin

is added to citrated plasma, and clotting time is measured. Because this measures the time for transformation of fibrinogen to fibrin and detects abnormalities in fibrin polymerization or low fibrinogen level, this test is used to further delineate the missing clotting factors when both PT and PTT are abnormal. Coagulation tests are depicted in Fig. 19-4, and coagulation studies are presented in Table 19-1. Heparin, a potent anticoagulant, enhances the neutralizing effects of antithrombin III on factors IXa, Xa, XIa, thrombin, and plasmin and thus prolongs the PT, PTT, and TT.

Because of the wide range of interlaboratory variations in PT values, based on the reagents used, the International Normalized Ratio (INR) was developed comparing local reagents against an international reagent and assigning a relative value (International Sensitivity Index). This process results in a normalized value across all laboratories and has become standard for monitoring patients on oral anticoagulant therapy. Oral anticoagulant doses are adjusted to maintain a specific INR, depending on the individual's condition requiring oral anticoagulant therapy. For example, for the prevention or treatment of high-risk venous thrombosis or treatment of pulmonary embolism, prevention of stroke following a myocardial infarction, the recommended INR is between 2.0 and 3.0. Individuals with mechanical prosthetic valves are maintained at an INR of 2.5 to 3.5 (Sacher, McPherson, 2000).

ABNORMALITIES OF HEMOSTASIS AND COAGULATION

Vascular Defects

A wide variety of abnormalities can occur at any level of the hemostatic mechanism. A patient with defects in the vascular system usually presents with cutaneous hemorrhages, often involving the mucous membranes. The hemorrhages can be classified as either nonallergic or allergic purpuras. In both instances, platelet function and the coagulation factors are normal.

Many forms of nonallergic purpura exist, that is, diseases in which no true allergy is present but various forms of vasculitis develop. The most common of these is found in systemic lupus erythematosus. This is a collagen-vascular disease in which the patient develops autoantibodies (see Chapter 72). Vasculitis, or inflammation of vessels, occurs and destroys the integrity of the vessels, resulting in purpura.

Ineffective, deteriorating vascular supportive tissue, which occurs with aging, results in *senile purpura*. Cutaneous hemorrhages generally occur on the dorsum of the hands and forearms and are aggravated by trauma. Except for the cosmetic annoyance, this condition is nonthreatening. A similar cutaneous manifestation is found with long-term corticosteroid therapy, believed to result from the protein catabolism in the vascular supportive tissue. Scurvy, related to malnutrition, and alcoholism similarly affect the integrity of the connective tissue of the vascular wall.

An autosomal dominant form of vascular purpura, *hereditary hemorrhagic telangiectasia* (Osler-Weber-Rendu dis-

TABLE 19-1

Coagulation Studies

Study	Purpose	Normal Values	Clinical Significance
Bleeding time	Measures platelet and vascular function	2-9½ minutes	Prolonged in thrombocytopenia, thrombocytopathy, von Willebrand's disease, aspirin ingestion, anticoagulant therapy, and uremia
Platelet count	Assesses platelet concentration	150,000-400,000/mm³	Decreased in idiopathic thrombocytopenic purpura (ITP) and bone marrow malignancies Drugs, especially chemotherapeutic agents, may cause prolonged bleeding Elevated in early myeloproliferative disorders After splenectomy, may predispose to later thrombotic episodes
Clot reaction	Assesses platelet adequacy to form fibrin clot	Clot retracts to one-half size in 1 hour, firm clot in 24 hours if undisturbed	Poor clot retraction in thrombocytopenia and polycythemia; lysis of clot in fibrinolysis
Lee-White clotting time (coagulation)	Assesses coagulation mechanism—time required for blood to form a solid clot after exposure to glass	6-12 minutes	Relatively insensitive test Prolonged with severe deficiencies of coagulation factors, in excessive anticoagulant therapy, and with selected antibiotics Decreased with corticosteroid therapy
International normalized ratio (INR)	Standardization of prothrombin times	Prevention and treatment of venous thrombus 2.0-3.0	Used as a guide for prescribing oral anticoagulant therapy
Prothrombin time (PT)	Measures extrinsic and common coagulation pathway	11-16 seconds	Prolonged in deficiencies of factors VII and X and fibrinogen, excess dicumarol therapy, severe liver disease and vitamin K deficiency
Activated partial thromboplastin time (APTT)	Measures intrinsic and common coagulation pathway	26-42 seconds	Prolonged in deficiencies of factors VIII to XII and fibrinogen, with circulating anticoagulant therapy, in liver disease and DIC, and in vitamin K deficiency Shortened in malignancies (except liver)
Thrombin time (TT) or thrombin clotting time	Measures fibrinogen to fibrin formation	10-13 seconds	Prolonged with low fibrinogen levels, inhibitors, DIC, and liver disease, anticoagulant therapy, and in dysproteinemias
Thromboplastin generation test (TGT)	Measures ability to form thromboplastin	12 seconds or less	Prolonged in thrombocytopenia, with deficiencies of factors VIII to XII, and with circulating anticoagulants
D-Dimer test	Measures breakdown products of plasma fibrin clots	<500	Elevated in DIC, pulmonary emboli, infarcts, thrombolytic therapy, surgery, trauma
Platelet aggregation test	Tests platelet function	Platelets aggregate within a specified time when exposed to substances such as adenine diphosphate (ADP), collagen, epinephrine	Decreased or absent aggregation in thrombasthenia, aspirin ingestion, myeloproliferative disorders, severe liver disease, dysproteinemias, von Willebrand's disease

ease), presents with profuse intermittent epistaxis and gastrointestinal (GI) bleeding. Diffuse telangiectasia, generally developing in adulthood, is found in the buccal mucosa, tongue, nose, and lips and likely extends throughout the GI tract. Treatment is mainly supportive.

The Ehlers-Danlos syndrome, another hereditary disease, involves decreased compliance of the perivascular tissues, leading to severe hemorrhage.

The *allergic* or *anaphylactoid purpuras*, thought to result from immunologic damage to the vessels, are characterized by petechial hemorrhages on dependent portions of the body and also involve the buttocks. Henoch-Schönlein purpura, a triad of purpura and mucosal bleeding, GI symptoms, and arthritis, is a form of allergic purpura that primarily affects children. The mechanism of this disease is not well understood; its symptoms are often preceded by an infectious state. Patients develop an inflammation of the vascular tree, at the capillary and venous levels, leading to vascular disruption, loss of red blood cells, and bleeding. Glomerulonephritis is a frequent complication. Treatment is supportive, with avoidance of aspirin and its compounds.

Thrombocytosis and Thrombocytopenia

The platelets adhering to the exposed collagen of injured blood vessels, contracting and releasing ADP and platelet factor 3, are important in the initiation of the clotting system. Abnormalities in the numbers or functions (or both) of the platelets can interfere with blood coagulation. Too many or too few platelets can interfere with blood coagulation. The condition, which is characterized by too many, is known as thrombocytosis or thrombocythemia. These terms are used interchangeably (Barui, Finazzi, 1998). *Thrombocytosis* is generally defined as an increase in the platelet counts above 400,000/mm³ and may be primary or secondary. Primary thrombocytosis is present in primary thrombocythemia, in which an abnormal proliferation of megakaryocytes occurs, with platelet counts exceeding 1 million. Primary thrombocytosis is also found with other myeloproliferative disorders, such as polycythemia vera or chronic granulocytic leukemia, in which an abnormal proliferation of the megakaryocytes occurs, along with other cell lines, in the bone marrow. Cytogenic studies are needed to exclude these disorders. Both hemorrhage and thrombosis can occur. The pathophysiology is obscure but thought to be related to intrinsic qualitative abnormality in platelet function, as well as the consequences of the increased platelet mass. The bleeding time is usually prolonged (Rogers, Greenberg, 1999).

When the platelet count exceeds 1 million or the patient is symptomatic, treatment is initiated and aimed at reducing the bone marrow activity through the use of cytotoxic agents such as hydroxyurea, which dramatically lowers the count, in all cell lines. Anogrelide hydrochloride (Agrylin) is added for its specificity in reducing platelet production. In the presence of acute bleeding or thrombosis, platelet pheresis offers temporary relief. Antiplatelet agents such as aspirin and anticoagulants have also been used.

Secondary thrombocytosis occurs as a consequence of other underlying causes, either temporarily after stress or exercise with storage pool release (from the spleen) or it may accompany increased bone marrow demand states as with hemorrhage, hemolytic anemia, or iron deficiency anemia. An increased number of platelets is briefly observed in patients whose spleens have been surgically removed. Because the spleen is the primary site of platelet storage and destruction, removal (splenectomy) without a concomitant decrease in bone marrow production will lead to thrombocytosis, often exceeding 1 million/mm³. Treatment of secondary or reactive thrombocytosis is generally not indicated.

Thrombocytopenia is defined as a platelet count below 100,000/mm³. This low count is a result of either decreased production or increased destruction of platelets. Clinical manifestations, however, are generally absent until the count falls below 100,000/mm³ and are further influenced by other underlying or coexisting conditions such as leukemia or liver disease. Increased ecchy-

mosis and prolonged bleeding with minor trauma occur with levels under 50,000/mm³· Petechiae are the major manifestations, with platelet counts below 30,000/mm³. Mucosal, deep tissue, and intracranial bleeding occur with counts under 20,000 and require immediate intervention to prevent exsanguination and death.

Decreased platelet production, verified by bone marrow aspiration and biopsy, is present in any condition interfering with or inhibiting bone marrow function. This includes aplastic anemia (Chapter 17), myelofibrosis (replacement of bone marrow elements by fibrous tissue), acute leukemia (Chapter 18), and other metastatic carcinomas that replace the normal marrow elements. Deficiency states, as of vitamin B_{12} and folic acid, affect megakaryopoiesis with production of large hyperlobulated megakaryocytes. Chemotherapeutic agents (Chapter 18) are particularly toxic to the bone marrow, suppressing platelet production.

In the event of thrombocytopenia with normal platelet production, excessive destruction or sequestration is usually the cause. Any condition causing splenomegaly (markedly enlarged spleen) may be accompanied by thrombocytopenia, including states such as hepatic cirrhosis, lymphomas, and myeloproliferative diseases. The spleen normally holds one third of the produced platelets, but with splenomegaly, this pool may increase to 80%, decreasing the available circulating pool.

Platelets can also be destroyed by drug-induced antibody production, such as with quinidine and gold (see Table 17-1) or by autoantibodies (antibodies acting against the body's own tissues). These antibodies are present in such disease states as lupus erythematosus, chronic lymphocytic leukemia, certain lymphomas, and idiopathic thrombocytopenic purpura. The last, primarily in young women, is manifested by severe life-threatening thrombocytopenia with platelet counts often below 10,000/mm³. As described in Chapter 12, an Immunoglobulin G antibody is demonstrated on the platelet membrane, resulting in defective platelet aggregation and increased platelet removal and destruction by the macrophage system.

Platelet function can be altered (thrombocytopathy) in various ways, the result being prolonged bleeding. Drugs such as aspirin, indomethacin, and phenylbutazone inhibit platelet aggregation and release reaction thus causing prolonged bleeding in spite of normal platelet numbers. The effects of a single dose of aspirin may last 7 to 10 days.

Plasma proteins, such as those in macroglobulinemia and multiple myeloma coat platelets, interfere with platelet adhesion, clot retraction, and fibrin polymerization. In all these situations, correcting the underlying problem will reverse the abnormal platelet function.

INHERITED PLASMA FACTOR DISORDERS

Hemophilia

Hemophilia is among the most common hereditary or acquired coagulation disorders, manifested by intermittent bleeding episodes. Hemophilia is caused by mutations in either the factor VIII (FVIII) or factor IX (FIX) genes, classified as hemophilia A and hemophilia B. Both genes are located on the X chromosome, making it an X-linked recessive disease (Ginsberg, 2000). Therefore all the daughters of hemophiliac males are carriers of the disease, and the sons are not afflicted. Sons of a carrier female have a 50% chance of being hemophiliacs. Homozygous females with hemophilia (father a hemophiliac, mother a carrier) can occur but are extremely rare. Approximately 33% of the patients have no family history and are presumably from spontaneous mutations (Hoffbrand, Pettit, 1993).

Two clinically identical major types of hemophilia are (1) classic hemophilia, or hemophilia A, in which antihemophilic factor VIII activity is deficient or absent, and (2) Christmas disease, or hemophilia B, in which factor IX activity is deficient or absent. Hemophiliacs are classified as (1) severe, with factor activity levels less than 1%, (2) moderate, with activity levels between 1% and 5%, and (3) mild, when 5% or greater. Spontaneous bleeding occurs with factor activity levels less than 1%. However, with levels of 5% or more, bleeding is generally related to trauma or surgical procedures. Clinical manifestations include bleeding into soft tissues, muscles, and joints, particularly the weight-bearing joints, called hemarthrosis (joint bleeding). Repeated bleeding into the joints leads to articular cartilage degeneration with symptoms of arthritis. Retroperitoneal bleeding and intracranial bleeding are life threatening. The degree of bleeding is related to the amount of factor activity and the severity of injury. Bleeding may occur immediately or hours after the injury. Surgical bleeding is common in all hemophiliacs, and any anticipated surgical procedure requires aggressive preoperative and postoperative factor replacement to greater than 50% activity level.

Laboratory diagnosis includes measuring the appropriate factor level: factor VIII for hemophilia A or factor IX for hemophilia B. Because factors VIII and IX are part of the intrinsic pathway of coagulation, the PTT is prolonged, whereas the PT, which bypasses the intrinsic pathway, is normal. Bleeding time, measuring platelet function, is usually normal, but delayed bleeding may occur because of inadequate fibrin stabilization. The platelet count is normal.

Treatment of hemophilia dictates prophylactic infusions beginning at 1 to 2 years of age in severely deficient children to prevent chronic joint disease (Lusher, 2000). Intervention at the earliest signs or symptoms of bleeding, as well as preoperative factor replacement in preparation for surgical procedures, is essential in the care of these patients. The treatment is aimed at increasing the deficient factor or activity to a normal level and thereby preventing complications. Severity of the bleeding, anticipated surgical complexity, the patient's weight, and the patient's specific factor level will determine the dose of the factor replacement. For minor bleeding events, such as early muscle or joint bleeding, a 20% to 50% activity level maintained for a few days may suffice, whereas for major events such as intracranial bleeding or surgery, 100% activity level should be attained and maintained for a minimum of 2 weeks. Currently available, highly purified, recombinant factor VIII products are *Recombinate* and *Kogenate*. *Monoclate-P* is a pasteurized monoclonal factor VIII product, and *Mononine* is a highly puri-

fied factor IX preparation. Doses for all the factors are calculated in units per kilogram of body weight and infused on a daily basis. A loading dose of factor is administered, followed by twice daily dosing. A continuous infusion may be used in patients with hemophilia who are undergoing major surgical procedures. The patient is monitored with serum factor level determinations and responsiveness to the prescribed therapy.

A marked incidence of human immunodeficiency virus (HIV) infection occurred in the hemophiliac population starting in the 1980s. Additionally, most of the adult population has serologic evidence of hepatitis. Improved donor screening, HIV testing of blood, and the development of virucidal methods and recombinant (genetically engineered) factor preparations, as noted with the previously mentioned factors, have greatly reduced the risk of transmission of blood-borne infections, including acquired immune deficiency syndrome (AIDS) (Andreoli et al, 1993; Bauer et al, 1994). Since 1985 the prophylactic use of the hepatitis vaccination series at the time of diagnosis has further reduced the incidence or eliminated hepatitis B for these patients.

The majority of the patients are now monitored through hemophilia treatment centers in which the global needs of patients are addressed, and they have the benefit of consultation from a comprehensive health care team. Improved preventive care, physical therapy, and teaching good health habits and self-administration of factor concentrates in the home setting have vastly improved the quality of life for this patient population. Life expectancy has increased to greater than 70 years. With the identification of the respective genes for both hemophilia A and B, the condition should be anticipated in the severely afflicted individuals. This information has great implications for genetic and prenatal counseling.

Antibody inhibitors directed against the specific coagulation factor occur in 5% to 10% of patients with factor VIII deficiency and less often in factor IX. Subsequent infusions of the factor stimulate more antibody formation. Immunosuppressive agents, plasmapheresis to remove the inhibitor, and prothrombin complexes that bypass factors VIII and IX inhibitors found in fresh frozen plasma are used to treat these patients. With the use of recombinant products, inhibitors still occur, but most patients spontaneously resolve. A genetic influence may exist in developing inhibitors because a higher incidence in African Americans and Hispanics exists (Lusher, 2000). A synthetic product, DDAVP (1-deamino 8-D-arginine vasopressin) is available for the treatment of mild to moderate hemophilia. Administered by intravenous (IV) infusion, DDAVP can induce a threefold to sixfold increase in the factor VIII activity level. Because DDAVP is a synthetic product, the risk of transmitting harmful viruses such as hepatitis or AIDS is alleviated.

von Willebrand's Disease

von Willebrand's disease is the most common inherited coagulation disorder. Various subtypes are identified, but the most common is type I. Except for types II and III, which are autosomal recessive, all types are inherited as an autosomal dominant trait, occurring in men and women alike. As in hemophilia, cases occur without a family history, and the disorder is thought to occur as a genetic mutation. Depending on the subtype and severity of the disease, the spectrum of bleeding may be infrequent, mild-to-moderate mucocutaneous (skin and mucous membranes) bleeding; bleeding secondary to trauma or surgery; or a life-threatening hemorrhage. GI bleeding, epistaxis, and menorrhagia are common. Most patients are asymptomatic. In von Willebrand's disease, decreased activity of both factor VIII$_{VWF}$ and factor VIII$_{AHG}$ exists (Handin, 2001). von Willebrand's factor is synthesized in endothelial cells and megakaryocytes and is stored in storage organelles. von Willebrand's factor facilitates platelet adhesion to components in the vascular subendothelium under conditions of high flow and shear stress, and it is the intravascular carrier for factor VIII to sites of active hemorrhage (Bauer et al, 1994; Handin, 2001). In von Willebrand's disease, the platelets do not adhere to collagen secondary to deficient or defective von Willebrand's factor.

Diagnostic studies for von Willebrand's disease include an assay of the von Willebrand's factor, showing subnormal levels. A prolonged bleeding time in the presence of factor VIII deficiency and defective platelet aggregation with ristocetin (an antibiotic that causes platelet aggregation) are diagnostic for von Willebrand's disease.

The treatment of von Willebrand's disease varies depending on the type and degree of bleeding. Treatment options include cryoprecipitate, factor VIII concentrates, desmopressin (DDAVP), fresh frozen plasma, and estrogens. The goal is to increase the availability of von Willebrand's factor (Bauer et al, 1994). When cryoprecipitate is used, it should be obtained from carefully selected and repeatedly tested donors according to the Medical and Scientific Council of America.

DDAVP is used in the treatment of types I and IIA of von Willebrand's disease. In most instances, DDAVP can be used to control minor bleeding, and it is used prophylactically before surgical procedures. Now available as a nasal spray the role of DDAVP is the release of von Willebrand's factor from the storage pools. For the replacement of von Willebrand's factor, the newer generation, virus-inactivated factor VIIIs, known to contain the von Willebrand's factor, are used. Patients scheduled for surgical procedures must be evaluated and prepared in advance of and during their procedure by a qualified hematologist.

ACQUIRED PLASMA FACTOR DEFICIENCIES

Acquired plasma factor deficiencies may be related to decreased production of the coagulation factors, as observed in liver disease or vitamin K deficiency, or increased consumption accompanying disseminated intravascular coagulation or fibrinolysis.

Because the liver is the major site of synthesis of factors II, V, VII, IX, and X, severe liver impairment (i.e., cirrhosis) will alter the hemostatic response. Additionally, a decreased hepatic clearing of the activated coagulation factors occurs. Vitamin K assimilation is also impaired, which further impairs the synthesis of the K-dependent coagulation factors. Portal hypertension in liver disease results in congestive splenomegaly with thrombocytopenia, as well as esophageal varices. These conditions, together with coagulation defects, can lead to massive hemorrhage. The PT, PTT, and bleeding time are all prolonged.

Vitamin K, which is obtained from diet and bacterial synthesis, is required for the synthesis of factors II, VII, IX, and X. In cases of malnutrition, malabsorption, or GI sterilization by antibiotics, vitamin K is markedly reduced with a resultant decrease in the biologic activity of the coagulation factors (Beck, 1991). Therapy for severe bleeding requires replacement of the coagulation factors with fresh frozen plasma (which supplies factors II, VII, IX, and X), parenteral vitamin K, and resolution of the underlying disease process.

Disseminated Intravascular Coagulation

Disseminated intravascular coagulation (DIC) is a multifaceted, complex syndrome in which a normally homeostatic and physiologic system of maintaining the fluidity of blood becomes a pathologic system leading to diffuse fibrin thrombi occluding the microvasculature of the body. The fibrinolytic system is activated by circulating thrombin, which cleaves fibrinogen to the fibrin monomer. Thrombin also stimulates platelet aggregation, activates factors V and VIII, and releases plasminogen activator, which generates plasmin. Plasmin cleaves fibrin, generating fibrin-degradation products, and further inactivates factors V and VIII. The excess thrombin activity results in decreased fibrinogen, thrombocytopenia, depletion of the coagulation factors, and fibrinolysis (Linker, 2001), which results in diffuse hemorrhage. DIC is not a disease but the consequence of an underlying disease process. Alteration of any of the components of the vascular system, namely, the vessel wall, plasma proteins, and platelets, can result in a consumptive disorder (Coleman et al, 1993). The introduction of a procoagulant material or activity into the circulating blood initiates the syndrome and can occur in any condition in which tissue thromboplastin is liberated secondary to tissue destruction, with an initiation of the extrinsic clotting pathway. Because the placenta is a rich source of tissue thromboplastin, one of the most common causes of DIC is placental abruption (abruptio placentae, premature separation of the placenta). This condition causes retention of the conceptual products (placenta, fetus), leading to necrosis and further tissue damage. Tumor products, burns, and crushing trauma cause thromboplastin release. In promyelocytic leukemia, the granular promyelocytes exhibit thromboplastin-like activity often when chemotherapy is initiated and the granules are released. Initiation of the intrinsic pathway also occurs with the exposure of intrinsic procoagulants to damaged vascular endothelium as in vasculitis, sepsis, and shock. During the process of coagulation, platelets aggregate and, together with the coagulation factors, are used and depleted. The resultant fibrin thrombi may or may not occlude the microvasculature. Concomitantly, the fibrinolytic system is activated for the dissolution of the fibrin thrombi, producing large numbers of fibrin and fibrinogen degradation products that interfere with fibrin polymerization and platelet function (Guyton, 2001). This action results in the diffuse hemorrhage that is characteristic of DIC.

The clinical manifestations depend on the extent and duration of the fibrin thrombi formation, the organs involved, and the resultant necrosis and hemorrhage. The organs most frequently involved include the kidney, skin, brain, pituitary, lungs, and the adrenals and the mucosa of the GI tract. Mucous membrane and deep-tissue bleeding, as well as bleeding around sites of injury, venipuncture, injection, and every orifice, are noted. Petechiae and ecchymoses are common. Other manifestations include hypotension (shock), oliguria or anuria, convulsions and coma, nausea and vomiting, diarrhea, abdominal pain, back pain, dyspnea, and cyanosis (Guyton, 2001).

Diagnostic tests reveal prolonged PT, PTT, and TT and increased fibrin split products. The fibrinogen level and platelet count are depressed. The peripheral blood smear may show erythrocyte fragmentation with a variety of bizarre shapes secondary to damage by fibrin strands.

Management is aimed at correcting the underlying mechanism, which may require the use of antibiotics and chemotherapeutic agents, cardiovascular support, and, in the event of retained placenta, emptying the uterine contents. Replacement of plasma factors with plasma and cryoprecipitate, as well as platelet and red blood cell transfusions, may be necessary. In the presence of intense bleeding, the role of heparin, a potent antithrombin anticoagulant, is highly controversial. Heparin neutralizes thrombin activity, thereby inhibiting the consumption of the coagulation factors and fibrin deposition. Increasing the concentration of the clotting factors and platelets with infusions of plasma and platelets should then inhibit the bleeding diathesis. Heparin is indicated whenever replacement therapy fails to enhance the coagulation factors and bleeding persists. Heparin is also indicated in the presence of fibrin deposition resulting in dermal necrosis (Logan, 1994). Low-dose heparin has been successfully used concomitantly with chemotherapeutic agents in the treatment of promyelocytic leukemia, preventing DIC secondary to thromboplastin release by the leukocytic granules.

Hypercoagulable states with an increased incidence of thrombosis also occur. These conditions were discussed in Chapter 7 and will not be addressed here.

KEY CONCEPTS

- Hemostasis and coagulation are a complex series of reactions that lead to the control of bleeding through the formation of a platelet and fibrin clot at the injury site.
- Clotting is followed by resolution or lysis of the clot and regeneration of the endothelium.
- In homeostatic states, hemostasis and coagulation protect the individual from massive bleeding secondary to trauma, and in abnormal states, life-threatening hemorrhage or thrombosis occluding the vascular tree can occur.
- At the time of injury, three major processes are responsible for hemostasis and coagulation: (1) transient vasoconstriction; (2) platelet reaction consisting of adhesion, release reaction, and aggregation of platelets; and (3) activation of the clotting factors.
- Platelets, or thrombocytes, are granular, disk-shaped nonnucleated cell fragments.
- Coagulation is initiated in homeostatic states by vascular injury. Vasoconstriction is an immediate response to the injury, followed by adhesion of platelets to collagen in the vessel wall exposed by the injury.
- ADP is released by the platelets, causing them to aggregate. Thrombin stimulates platelet aggregation; platelet factor III also accelerates plasma clotting.
- After the formation of a clot, terminating further blood clotting is imperative to avoid unwanted thrombotic events that result from excessive systemic clot formation.
- Naturally occurring anticoagulants include antithrombin III (heparin co-factor), protein C, and protein S.

- The fibrinolytic system is activated by circulating thrombin, which cleaves fibrinogen to the fibrin monomer.
- Excess thrombin activity results in decreased fibrinogen, thrombocytopenia, depletion of the coagulation factors, and fibrinolysis.
- Thrombocytopenia is defined as a platelet count below $100,000/mm^3$, which is caused by either decreased production or increased destruction of platelets.
- Hemophilia is among the most common hereditary or acquired coagulation disorders, manifested by intermittent bleeding episodes.
- Hemophilia is caused by mutations in either factor VIII (FVIII) or factor IX (FIX) genes, classified as hemophilia A or B. Both genes are located on the X chromosome, making it an X-linked recessive disorder.
- Treatment of hemophilia is aimed at increasing the deficient factor or activity to a normal level and preventing complications.
- von Willebrand's disease is the most common inherited coagulation disorder. The most common is type I.
- Treatment of von Willebrand's disease varies depending on the type and degree of bleeding. The goal is to increase the availability of von Willebrand's factor.
- DIC is a multifaceted, complex syndrome in which a normally homeostatic and physiologic system of maintaining the fluidity of blood becomes a pathologic system leading to diffuse fibrin thrombi occluding the microvasculature of the body.

QUESTIONS ??

A sampling of review questions for this chapter appears here. Visit http://www.mosby.com/MERLIN/PriceWilson/ for additional questions. MERLIN

Answer the following on a separate sheet of paper.

1. Explain the maturation sequence of platelet cells when vascular injury occurs.
2. In proper sequence, list the three ways that platelets contribute to blood coagulation.
3. Which two plasma coagulation factors are shared by both the extrinsic and intrinsic systems?
4. State the mechanism that causes bleeding in primary and secondary thrombocytosis. Cite an example of each.
5. What is von Willebrand's factor? Why is it important in coagulation?
6. What are the treatment options and goals for von Willebrand's disease?
7. Describe the treatment goals for hemophiliacs.
8. Define DIC.
9. Describe the role of heparin in the presence of intense bleeding.
10. What preventive measures are currently being used to reduce the risk of transmission of blood-borne infection, including AIDS?
11. Explain the rationale for using the International Normalized Ratio (INR) for monitoring patients on oral anticoagulant therapy.

BIBLIOGRAPHY ■ PART THREE

Anderson KC et al: NCCN practice guidelines for multiple myeloma: in national comprehensive cancer network proceedings, *Oncology* 12(11A):317-350, 1998.

Bagley GC, Heinrich MC: Growth factors, cytokines and the control of hematopoiesis. In Hoffman R et al, editors: *Hematology basic principles and practice*, ed 3, London, 2000, Churchill Livingston.

Barbui T, Finazzi G: Thrombocytosis. In Loscalzo J, Schafter I, editors: *Thrombosis and hemorrhage*, ed 2, Baltimore, 1998, Williams & Wilkins.

Bauer KA et al: Coagulation/hemostatisis. In Beng EJ, McArthur JR, editors: *Hematology education program*, Nashville, 1994, American Society of Hematology, University of Washington, Smith, Bueklin & Associates.

Beck WS: *Hematology*, ed 5, Cambridge, Mass, 1991, MIT Press.

Bennett JM et al: Criteria for the diagnosis of acute leukemia of M7, *Ann Intern Med* 103(3):460, 1985.

Beutler E: Genetic principles. In Beutler E et al, editors: *Williams hematology*, ed 6, New York, 2001a, McGraw-Hill.

Beutler E: Hemolytic anemia due to infections and microorganisms. In Beutler E et al, editors: *Williams hematology*, ed 6, New York, 2001b, McGraw-Hill.

Bloomfield CD: Acute and chronic myeloid leukemia. In Braunwald E et al, editors: *Harrison's principles of internal medicine*, ed 15, New York, 2001, McGraw-Hill.

Bondurant MC, Koury MJ: Origin and development of blood cells. In Lee RG et al, editors: *Wintrobe's clinical hematology*, ed 10, Baltimore, 1999, Williams & Wilkins.

Dabich L: Adult acute non-lymphocytic leukemias, *Med Clin North Am* 64(4):683, 1980.

Dessypries EN: Erythropoiesis. In Lee RG et al, editors: *Wintrobe's clinical hematology*, ed 10, Baltimore, 1999, Williams & Wilkins.

Devine SM, Larson RA: Acute leukemia in adults: recent developments in diagnosis and treatment, *CA* 44(6):326, 1994.

Diehl V et al: Hodgkin's disease. In DeVita VT et al, editors: *Cancer principles and practice of oncology*, vol 2, ed 6, Philadelphia, 2001, Lippincott, Williams & Wilkins.

Finley RS, Overview of promising agents in oncology, *Oncology Nursing Updates* 7(4):2-14, 2000.

Fischer DS, Knobf M: *The cancer chemotherapy handbook*, ed 5, St Louis, 1997, Mosby.

Foerster J: Waldenström's macroglobulinemia and multiple myeloma. In Lee RG et al, editors: *Wintrobe's clinical hematology*, ed 10, Baltimore, 1999, Williams & Wilkins.

Ganong WF: *Review of medical physiology*, ed 19, Stanford, 1999, Appleton & Lange.

Gelehertr JD et al, editors: *Principles of medical genetics*, Baltimore, 1998, Williams & Wilkins.

Ginsburg W: von Willebrand's disease. In Beutler E et al, editors: *Williams hematology*, ed 6, New York, 2001, McGraw-Hill.

Goldman L et al, editors: *Cecil's textbook of medicine*, ed 21, Philadelphia, 2000, WB Saunders.

Goldsmith RS: Infectious diseases. In Tierney LM et al, editors: *Current medical diagnosis and treatment*, ed 40, New York, 2001, Lange Medical Books, McGraw-Hill.

Gralnick HR et al: Classification of acute leukemia, *Ann Intern Med* 87(6):740, 1997.

Greer JP et al: Acute myelogenous leukemia. In Lee RG et al, editors: *Wintrobe's clinical hematology*, ed 10, Baltimore, 1999, Williams & Wilkins.

Guyton AC, Hall JE: *Textbook of medical physiology*, ed 10, Philadelphia, 2001, WB Saunders.

Hagemeister FB: Newer therapy options for indolent lymphomas: is anyone cured? Paper presented at the Providence Cancer Institute, Southfield, Mich, April 2001.

Handin RJ: Bleeding. In Braunwald E et al, editors: *Harrison's principles of internal medicine*, ed 15, New York, 2001, McGraw-Hill.

Hayes K, McCartney S: Nursing care of the patient with chronic lymphocytic leukemia, *Seminars in Oncology* 25(1):992, 1980.

Hoffbrand AV, Pettit JE: *Essential hematology*, ed 3, London, 1993, Blackwell Scientific Publications.

Jenny NS, Mann KG: Coagulation cascade. In Loscalzo J, Schafer AI, editors, *Thrombosis and hemorrhage*, ed 2, Baltimore, 1998, Williams & Wilkins.

Johnson G: Malignant lymphomas. In Mazza J, editor: *Manual of clinical hematology*, Boston, 1995, Little, Brown.

Kalil N, Cheson BD: Management of chronic lymphocyte leukemia, *Drugs and Aging* 16(1):9, 2000.

Larson RA et al: Acute leukemia; biology and treatment. In Beng EJ, McArthur JR, editors: *Hematology education program*, Nashville, 1994, American Society of Hematology, University of Washington, Smith, Bueklin & Associates.

Linker CA: Blood. In Tierney LM et al, editors: *Current medical diagnosis and treatment*, ed 40, New York, 2001, Lange Medical Books, McGraw-Hill.

Logan L: Hemostasis and bleeding disorders. In Mazza J, editor: *Manual of clinical hematology*, ed 2, Boston, 1994, Little, Brown.

Lusher JM: Advances in the treatment of hemophilia. In Schecter GP, Berliner N, Telen MJ, editors: *Hematology, 2000*, San Francisco, 2000, American Society of Hematology, education program book.

Lynch DC et al: Hodgkin's choice of therapy and late complications. In Schacter GP, Berliner N, Telen MJ, editors: *Hematology, 2000*, San Francisco, 2000, American Society of Hematology, education program book.

Mayfield E: *FDA Consumer Report,* Publication No 99:125, 1999 (February 1,1999).

McArthur JR, editor: *Hematology education program,* Nashville, 1994, American Society of Hematology, Smith, Bueklin & Associates.

McDermott MK, Bell EM: A review of Waldenström's macroglobulinemia, *Clin J Onc Nsg* 3(3):107, 1999.

Meyers JS: *Integrating today's and anticipating tomorrow's therapeutic advances, moving theory into practice.* Symposium, April 27, 1999, 24th Annual Oncology Nursing Society Congress.

Nirenberg A: Thalidomide: when everything old is new again, *Clin J Onc Nsg* 3(3):15, 2000.

O'Brien S et al: Sequential homoherringtonine in the treatment of early chronic phase of chronic myelogenous leukemia, *Blood* 93(12):41, 1999.

Patterson B: *Lymphoma update and standards of care,* Paper presented at the meeting of the Oncology Nursing Congress, San Antonio, May 2000.

Radich J, Sievers E: New developments in the treatment of acute myeloid leukemia, NCCN proceedings, *Oncology* 14(11):125, 2000.

Rogers G, Greenberg CS: Inherited coagulation disorders. In Lee RG et al, editors: *Wintrobe's clinical hematology,* ed 10, Baltimore, 1999, Williams & Wilkins.

Sacher RA, McPherson R: *Widmann's clinical interpretation of laboratory tests,* ed 11, Philadelphia, 2000, FA Davis.

Sandberg AA: Cytogenetics for clinicians, *CA* 44(3):136, 1994.

Schrier SL: Hematology. In Rubestein E, Federman DD, editors: *Scientific American medicine,* New York, 1979, Scientific American Books.

Shelton BK, Solomon AB: Normal and altered leukocyte function. In Bullock B, Henzerg RL, editors: *Focus on pathophysiology,* Philadelphia, 2000, Lippincott, Williams & Wilkins.

Ship, MA et al: NCCN, preliminary non-Hodgkin's lymphoma practice guidelines, NCCN proceedings, *Oncology* 11(11A): 281, November 1997.

Weinshel EL, Peterson BA: Hodgkin's disease, *CA* 44(6):327, 1994.

Williams E: Disseminated intravascular coagulation. In Loscalzo J, Schafer AI, editors: *Thrombosis and hemorrhage,* ed 2, Baltimore, 1998, Williams & Wilkins.

Williams ME et al: Hodgkin's disease and non-Hodgkin's lymphoma. In Beng EJ, McArthur JR, editors: *Hematology education program,* Nashville, 1994, American Society of Hematology and Smith, Bueklin, & Associates.

Wujcik D: Leukemia. In Yarbro CH et al, editors: *Cancer nursing principles and practice,* ed 5, Sudbury, Mass, 2000, Jones & Bartlett.

Yarbro C: Malignant lymphomas. In Yarbro CH et al, editors: *Cancer nursing principles and practice,* ed 5, Sudbury, Mass, 2000, Jones & Bartlett.

Young NS et al: New insights into the pathophysiology of acquired cytopenias. In Schecter GP, Berliner N, Telen MJ, editors: *Hematology, 2000,* San Francisco, 2000, American Society of Hematology, education program book.

FLUID AND ELECTROLYTE DISORDERS

*A*ll the cells and tissues of the human body are bathed in a fluid similar in chemical composition to seawater, reflecting our evolutionary beginnings. The normal functioning of the cell demands that the composition of this fluid be relatively constant. The dynamic equilibrium or homeostasis of water, electrolyte, and acid-base balance in the body is maintained through complex physiologic mechanisms involving the cooperation of multiple body systems.

Fluid and electrolyte and acid-base disorders are common manifestations of underlying illness and, in turn, produce systemic derangements. Recognition and treatment of these disorders are best enhanced through an understanding of normal fluid and electrolyte physiology and pathophysiologic mechanisms involved in their genesis.

Chapter 20 summarizes fluid and electrolyte balance in health and an approach to the assessment of fluid and electrolyte status. Chapter 21 deals with abnormalities of fluid volume, osmolality, and selected electrolytes. Acid-base disorders are discussed in Chapter 22. Fluid and electrolyte and acid-base disorders are discussed throughout the book in subsequent chapters, because they are associated with various diseases and disorders.

Total Body Water in Percentage of Body Weight*

Age	Percentage of Body Weight
Infant (newborn)	75%
Adult Male (20-40 yrs)	60%
Adult Female (20-40 yrs)	50%
Elderly Adult (60+ yrs)	45%-50%

*Data from Maxwell M, Kleeman CR, Narins RG: *Maxwell and Kleeman's clinical disorders of fluid and electrolyte metabolism,* ed 5, New York, 1994, McGraw Hill.

proportionately more fat and a smaller muscle mass than do men, which accounts for their smaller amount of TBW in relation to weight. Older adults also have a higher percentage of body fat than do younger adults. Finally, TBW is highest in a newborn infant, at 75% of total weight. This percentage decreases rapidly to approximately 60% at the end of 1 year and then more gradually until male and female adult proportions are reached during adolescence (Table 20-1).

Major Compartments of Body Fluid

Various membranes (capillary, cell) separate total body fluids into two major compartments. In the adult approximately 40% of body weight or two thirds of TBW is within cells or *intracellular fluid (ICF)*. The remaining one third of TBW or 20% of body weight is found outside of cells or *extracellular fluid (ECF)*. The ECF compartment is further divided into the *interstitial-lymph fluid (ISF)* compartment between the cells (15%) and the *intravascular fluid (IVF)* or plasma compartment (5%). In addition to the ISF and IVF, special secretions, such as the cerebrospinal fluid, intraocular fluid, and gastrointestinal secretions, form a small proportion (1% to 2% of body weight) of the ECF called transcellular fluid. Fig. 20-1 illustrates the volume and distribution of body fluids in a healthy young man.

Major Electrolytes and Their Distribution

The solutes found in body fluids include electrolytes and nonelectrolytes. *Nonelectrolytes* are solutes that do not dissociate in solution and do not carry an electrical charge. Nonelectrolytes include proteins, urea, glucose, oxygen, carbon dioxide, and organic acids. Salts that dissociate in water into one or more charged particles are called *ions* or *electrolytes*. Body electrolytes include sodium (Na^+), potassium (K^+), calcium (Ca^{++}), magnesium (Mg^{++}), chloride (Cl^-), bicarbonate (HCO_3^-), phosphate (HPO_4^-), and sulfate (SO_4^-). Electrolyte solutions conduct an electric current. Ions that carry a positive charge are called *cations*, and those carrying a negative charge are called *anions*. For example, sodium chloride (NaCl) dissociates in solution into Na^+ (cations) and Cl^- (anions). On the other hand, when dissolved in water, glucose does not break down into anything smaller.

The electrolyte concentration of body fluid varies from one compartment to another, and in health it must be in the right compartment in the right amount (Fig. 20-2). The chief cation of the ECF is Na^+, and the chief anions are Cl^- and HCO_3^-; their concentrations are low in the

ICF. In the ICF, K^+ is the chief cation and HPO_4^- is the chief anion, whereas their concentrations are low in ECF. As the most abundant particle in the ECF, Na^+ plays a major role in controlling total body fluid volume, whereas K^+ is important in controlling the volume of the cell. An electrical gradient across the cell membrane is necessary for the generation of nerve and muscle action potentials, and differential K^+ and Na^+ concentrations across the cell membrane are important in its maintenance. Despite the differences in ionic concentration between compartments, the *law of electrical neutrality* states that the sum of negative charges must be equal to the sum of positive charges (measured in milliequivalents) in any particular compartment. The need to maintain electroneutrality is an important determinant of ion transport between the ECF and ICF and in the kidney. Finally, the ionic composition of the ISF and IVF is similar. The main difference is that the ISF contains little protein as compared with the IVF. The higher amount of protein in plasma plays a significant role in maintaining the volume of the IVF.

Units of Solute Measurement

Terminology plays an important role in the interpretation and management of fluid and electrolyte disorders. Thus understanding the units of measurement commonly used is essential. The concentration of a given solute can be expressed in milligrams/deciliter (mg/dl or mg%), millimoles/liter (mmol/L or mM/L), milliequivalents/liter (mEq/L), milliosmoles/kilogram (mOsm/kg), or milliosmoles/liter (mOsm/L). Box 20-1 summarizes the definition of types of measurements and their equivalencies.

The molecular weight of a substance is the sum of the atomic weights of all the elements specified in the formula of that substance. A *mole* (mol) is the molecular (or atomic) weight of a substance expressed in grams, and a *millimole* (mmol) is 1/1000 of a mole, or its weight in milligrams. The terms mole and millimole may be applied to all substances, regardless of whether they are organic or nonorganic or ionized or nonionized, because the terms are independent of valence. Thus 1 mmol of glucose ($C_6H_{12}O_6$) = 180 mg [6(12)+12(1)+6(16)=180]; 1 mmol of NaCl = 58 mg (23+35), whereas 1 mmol of Na^+ ions = 23 mg.

The term *milliequivalent* is 1/1000 of an equivalent or the atomic (or molecular) weight in milligrams divided by its *valence* or *electrochemical combining power* in the reaction. The weight of an element in grams that combines with or replaces 1 g of hydrogen ion (as a standard) would be its equivalent weight. The concept of a milliequivalent is important in discussing the composition of body fluids, because ions combine milliequivalent for milliequivalent and not milligram for milligram or millimole for millimole. The equivalent weight differs from the gram molecular weight because the valence (combining power) of the electrolyte is considered. Clinical laboratory reports are sometimes in milligrams per deciliter or 100 ml (mg/dl or mg%). This value may be converted to mEq/L using the conversion formula in Box 20-1. A final advantage of expressing ion concentrations in mEq/L is that the total number of cations in mEq/L is always equal to the number of anions in mEq/L thus preserving electroneutrality (Table 20-2).

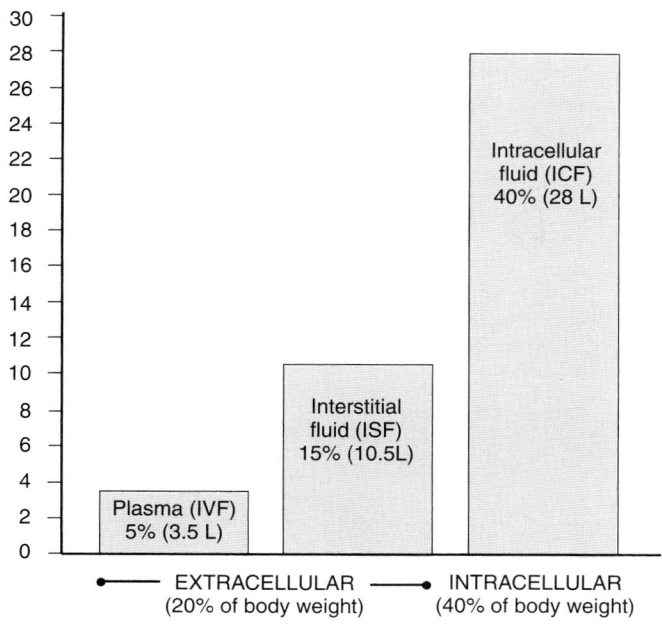

FIG. 20-1   Volume and distribution of body fluids in a healthy young man. Water is 60% of body weight and is distributed in two main compartments: the extracellular and intracellular. The extracellular fluid is subdivided into the interstitial and intravascular (plasma) fluid compartments.

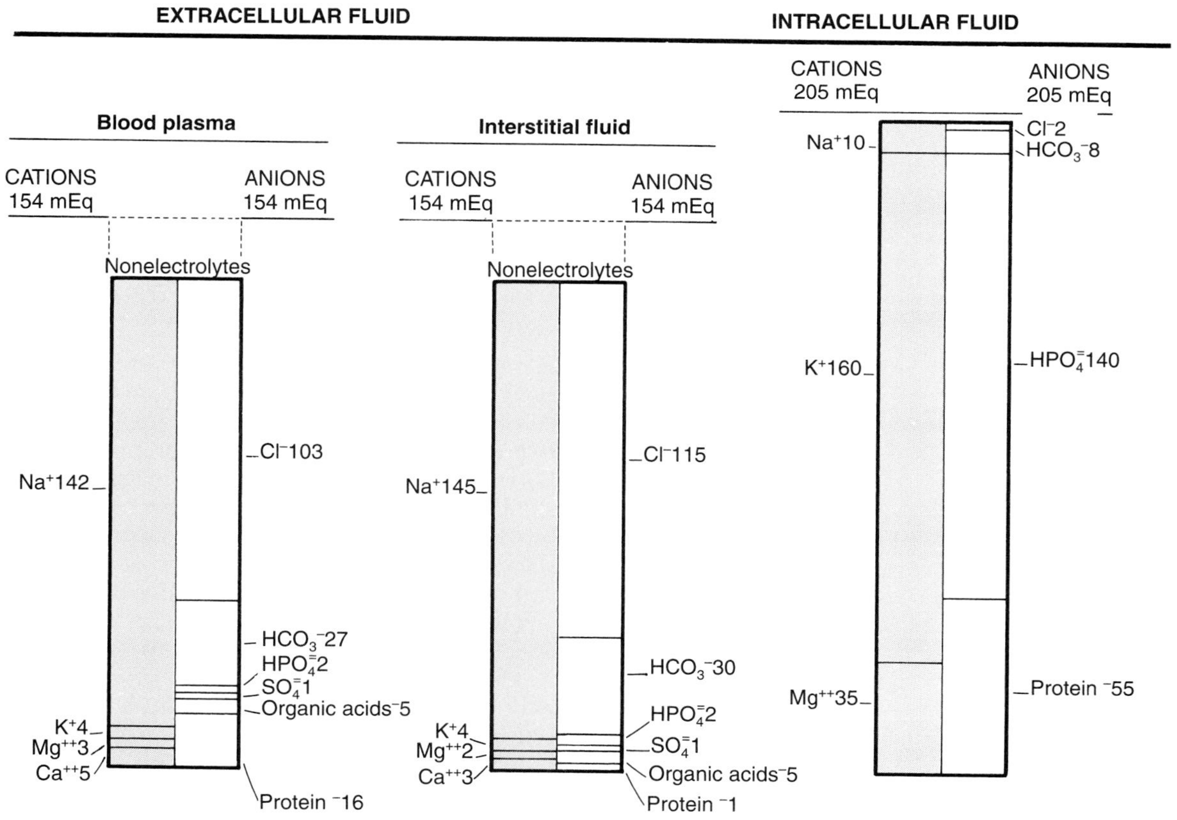

EXTRACELLULAR FLUID

Blood plasma

CATIONS
154 mEq   ANIONS
                 154 mEq

Nonelectrolytes

Na^+142_

_Cl^-103

_HCO_3^-27
$HPO_4^=2$
_$SO_4^=1$
_Organic acids$^-5$

K^+4_
$Mg^{++}3$_
$Ca^{++}5$_

_Protein $^-16$

Interstitial fluid

CATIONS
154 mEq   ANIONS
                 154 mEq

Nonelectrolytes

Na^+145_

_Cl^-115

_HCO_3^-30

$HPO_4^=2$
_$SO_4^=1$
_Organic acids$^-5$

K^+4_
$Mg^{++}2$_
$Ca^{++}3$_

_Protein $^-1$

INTRACELLULAR FLUID

CATIONS
205 mEq   ANIONS
                 205 mEq

Na^+10_

_Cl^-2
_HCO_3^-8

K^+160_

_$HPO_4^=140$

$Mg^{++}35$_

_Protein $^-55$

FIG. 20-2   Electrolyte content of fluid compartments. (Modified from *Fluids and electrolytes*, Abbott Laboratories, 1970, Abbott Park, Ill, pp. 10-11.)

Units of Measure for Body Fluids and Their Conversions

MG/DL = MG OF SOLUTE/100 ML SOLVENT
  Example:
  Serum Ca^{++} = 10 mg/dl

MMOL = MOLECULAR (OR ATOMIC) WEIGHT IN MG
  Examples:
  1 mmol Ca^{++} = 40 mg
  1 mmol Cl^- = 35.5 mg
  1 mmol Na^+ = 23 mg
  1 mmol $NaCl$ = 58.5 mg (23 + 35.5 = 58.5)

$$mEq = \frac{MOL\ (OR\ ATOMIC)\ WEIGHT\ IN\ MG}{VALENCE}$$

  Valence: $Na^+ = 1$; $Ca^{++} = 2$
  Examples:
  Na^+ = 23 mg/L; 23 mg Na^+ = 1 mEq
  Ca^{++} = 40 mg/2; 20 mg Ca^{++} = 1 mEq
  1 mmol Ca^{++} = 2 mEq (2 x 20 mg)

$$mOsm = \frac{MOL\ (OR\ ATOMIC)\ WEIGHT\ IN\ MG}{n\ (PARTICLES\ EXERTING\ OSMOTIC\ PRESSURE)}$$

  Na^+ = 1 particle in solution
  $NaCl$ = 2 particles in solution (Na^+ and Cl^-)
  Examples:
  mOsm Na^+ = 23 mg/1; 23 mg Na^+ = 1 mOsm
  mOsm $NaCl$ = 58.5 mg/2; 29.3 mg $NaCl$ = 1 mOsm
  1 mmol $NaCl$ = 2 mOsm

$$MMOL/L = \frac{MG/DL \times 10}{MOL\ WEIGHT}$$

$$mEq/L = \frac{MG/DL \times 10 \times VALENCE}{MOL\ WEIGHT}$$

  Example:
$$Ca^{++}\ in\ mEq/L = \frac{(10\ mg/dl \times 10 \times 2)}{40\ mg} = 5\ mEq/L$$

  mEq/L = MMOL/L × VALENCE

$$mOsm/KG = MMOL/L \times N = \frac{(MG/DL \times 10)}{MOL\ WEIGHT} = \frac{(mEq/L \times n)}{VALENCE}$$

  Examples:
    For monovalent ions:
    1 mmol Na^+ = 1 mEq = 1 mOsm (1 valence; 1 particle)
    1 mmol $NaCl$ = 2 mEq = 2 mOsm (2 valences; 2 particles)
    For multivalent ions:
    1 mmol $MgSO_4$ = 4 mEq = 2 mOsm (4 valences; 2 particles)
    1 mmol Na_2SO_4 = 4 mEq = 3 mOsm (4 valences; 3 particles)

A *milliosmole* equals 1/1000 of an osmole and is a measure of the number of discrete particles in a solution independent of their valence, electrical charge, or mass. The osmolality of body fluid has a great deal to do with water movement and balance as will be discussed later.

MOVEMENT OF BODY FLUIDS AND ELECTROLYTES

Body fluids and their dissolved substances are in a constant state of mobility. A continual intake and output of fluids occurs within the body as a whole and between the various compartments as the fluids transport nutrients

Plasma and Intracellular Electrolytes

	Plasma	Intracellular
CATIONS		
Sodium (Na^+)	142 mEq	10 mEq
Potassium (K^+)	4 mEq	160 mEq
Calcium (Ca^{++})	5 mEq	
Magnesium (Mg^{++})	3 mEq	35 mEq
TOTAL	154 mEq/L	205 mEq/L
ANIONS		
Chloride (Cl^-)	103 mEq	2 mEq
Bicarbonate (HCO_3^-)	27 mEq	8 mEq
Phosphate (HPO_4^-)	2 mEq	140 mEq
Sulfate (SO_4^-)	1 mEq	
Organic acids	5 mEq	
Proteins	16 mEq	55 mEq
TOTAL	154 mEq/L	205 mEq/L

and oxygen to the cells and remove wastes and manufactured substances from the cells. First, oxygen, nutrients, fluids, and electrolytes are picked up by the lungs and gastrointestinal tract, where they become part of the IVF and are transported to various parts of the body via the circulatory system. Second, IVF and its dissolved substances are rapidly exchanged with the ISF through the semipermeable capillary membrane. Third, ISF and its constituents are exchanged with the ICF through the selectively permeable cell membrane. Even though the situation as a whole is one of incessant replacement and exchange, the composition and volume of the fluid are relatively stable, a state called *dynamic equilibrium* or *homeostasis*. The movement of water and solutes between body compartments involves active and passive transport mechanisms. An *active transport* mechanism involves the expenditure of energy, but a *passive transport* mechanism does not. Diffusion and osmosis are passive transport mechanisms.

Movement of Solutes between Body Fluid Compartments

The primary barrier to the movement of solutes in the body is the cell membrane. The lipid and protein molecules that make up these membranes are arranged such that only certain substances can pass through them. Pores in these membranes allow the passage of water and small water-soluble substances such as ions and glucose, but larger protein molecules do not readily pass. Substances that are lipid-soluble, such as urea, oxygen, and carbon dioxide, can pass directly through the membrane.

Most solutes move by passive transport mechanisms. *Simple diffusion* is the random movement of particles in all directions through a solution or gas. Several factors affect how readily a solute diffuses across capillary and cell membranes, including membrane permeability, concentration, electrical potential, and pressure gradients. *Permeability* refers to the size of the diffusing particles relative to the size of the membrane pores. Small particles, such as water and ions, diffuse through the membrane pores most easily. Large particles, such as glucose and amino acids, must pass through the membrane by a process called *facilitated diffusion*. In facilitated diffusion, a membrane-bound carrier protein combines with the transported molecule, acting as a shuttle in the process. In diffusion, solutes move from an area of higher concentration to one of lower concentration until the concentration is equal on both sides of the membrane. In addition to concentration gradients, the diffusion of charged particles (electrolytes) is affected by the *electrical gradient* or *potential* across the cell membrane. Positively charged particles tend to move to the negative side of the cell membrane (usually the inside of the cell), whereas negatively charged particles tend to move to the positive side (usually the outside of the cell) because like charges repel and opposite charges attract. Concentration and electrical gradients together compose the *electrochemical potential*, which is the force that drives the (passive) movements of electrolytes. The electric potential component, although quite small, is important in excitable tissues. Finally, a *hydrostatic pressure* gradient increases the rate of diffusion of solutes through the capillary membrane (see the discussion of movement of water between the plasma and interstitial fluid).

The movement of solutes across a cell membrane against a concentration or electrical gradient (or both) is called *active transport*. Active transport differs from passive transport in that it requires the expenditure of energy in the form of adenosine triphosphate (ATP). One of the most widely distributed active transport systems is the *Na-K-activated–ATPase system* (also called the *sodium-potassium pump*) located in cell membranes. This single enzyme molecule pumps three Na^+ ions out of the cell in exchange for two K^+, at the expense of one ATP molecule. The Na-K–ATPase system plays an important role in maintaining the proper concentrations of Na^+ and K^+ inside and outside the cell, thus maintaining the membrane electropotential. Important to recall is that ECF Na^+ concentration is high (142 mEq/L), whereas ICF Na^+ concentration is low (10 mEq/L), and the reverse is true for K^+ (4 mEq/L in the ECF and 155 mEq/L in the ICF). Additionally, the resting cell membrane is selectively permeable to K^+ and quite impermeable to Na^+. The membrane potential is created because K^+ diffuses out of the cell, leaving behind most of the negative ions (primarily proteins and phosphate) that are too large to follow. Na^+ also diffuses into the cell down its concentration gradient but at a much slower rate than K^+ exit. The net diffusion of Na^+ and K^+ is balanced by the active transport of these ions in the opposite direction across the cell membrane. K^+ balance is important clinically because of the life-threatening dysrhythmias that develop when either an excess or deficit of this ion occurs.

Movement of Water between Body Fluid Compartments

Unlike electrolytes and other solutes, water freely crosses all body membranes. Two forces control the movement of water between the various fluid compartments: osmotic and hydrostatic pressures.

Osmotic and Hydrostatic Pressures

Osmotic pressure refers to the drawing force for water exerted by solute particles. The concept of osmotic pres-

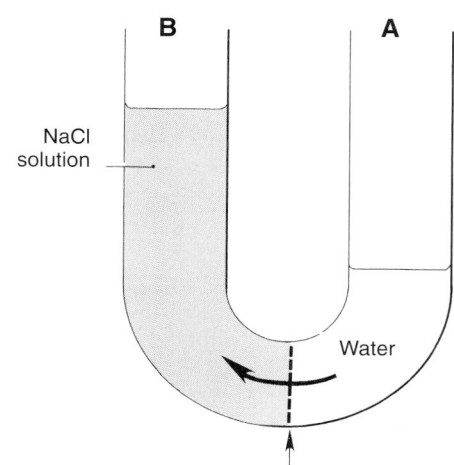

FIG. 20-3   Osmosis. The effect of adding an *impermeable solute* on one side of a semipermeable membrane. Water moves freely from the high solvent on side A to the low solvent on side B, causing the levels of the fluid columns to become farther apart. A hydrostatic pressure is created on side B (measured by the height of this column), which will be equal to the osmotic pressure of this solution at equilibrium. The amount of pressure required to stop osmosis completely is called the *osmotic pressure* of the solution.

sure is most easily grasped by an illustration. Fig. 20-3 shows a U tube, with each arm separated by a semipermeable membrane. A certain volume of a NaCl solution is placed in one arm (side *B*), with an equal volume of pure water in the other arm (side *A*). Water diffuses freely through the membrane, but both Na^+ and Cl^- ions are nondiffusible. Net water movement is from side *A* (pure water) to side *B* (salt solution), the final result being that the total volume is greater in side *B*. The hydrostatic pressure (compression force of a liquid) that would have to be applied over the solution in side *B* to prevent the net diffusion of water to that side is equal to the osmotic pressure of that solution. *Osmosis* is the process of the net diffusion of water caused by a concentration gradient. Net diffusion of water occurs from an area of low solute concentration (dilute solution) to one of high solute concentration (concentrated solution). To put it another way, water diffuses from an area of higher water activity to one of lower water activity. The osmotic pressure of body fluids may be measured by freezing point depression (see Chapter 45) and expressed as either osmolality or osmolarity. The terms osmolality and osmolarity are almost but not quite synonymous. *Osmolality* refers to the number of osmols (the standard unit of osmotic pressure) per kilogram of *solvent* (water) (mOsm/kg). *Osmolarity* refers to the number of osmols per liter of *solution* (mOsm/L). In the first case (osmolality), the total volume will be 1 L of water plus the small volume taken up by the solutes; in the second case (osmolarity), the volume of water will be less than 1 L by an amount equal to the volume of the solute. Osmolality is therefore more exact. However, the terms osmolality and osmolarity are used interchangeably in clinical practice because the difference is negligible with dilute body fluids.

The osmotic concentration of a solution depends only on the *number of particles* without regard to their size, charge, or mass. The solute particles may be crystalloids (substances that form a true solution, such as sodium salts) or colloids (substances that do not readily dissolve into true solutions, such as large protein molecules). For a particle to serve as an *effective osmole*, it must be largely confined to one particular compartment. Na^+ (and its anions) contributes most to the osmolality of the ECF, because it is the most numerous of particles in the ECF and the cell membrane is relatively impermeable to it. K^+ plays this role in the ICF. Although urea and glucose are solutes in the plasma, they freely diffuse across cell membranes and are not important contributors to the plasma osmolality, except under abnormal circumstances.

Movement of Water between the Plasma and Interstitial Fluid

Sodium does not play an important role in the movement of water between the plasma and interstitial fluid compartments because the concentration of sodium is nearly the same in both compartments. The distribution of water between these two compartments is determined by the hydrostatic pressure of the capillary blood, produced mainly by the pumping action of the heart, and the counterbalancing *colloid osmotic pressure (COP)* or *oncotic pressure*, produced primarily by serum albumin. Colloids, such as albumin and other high–molecular-weight serum proteins, act as effective osmoles because they are confined to the intravascular space and do not readily cross the capillary membrane. The process of fluid movement from the capillary to the interstitial space is called *ultrafiltration* because water, electrolytes, and other solutes (except plasma proteins and blood cells) readily cross the capillary membrane. Another example of ultrafiltration in the body is the renal corpuscle (glomerulus).

Fig. 20-4 illustrates Starling's law of the capillaries, which states that the rate and direction of fluid exchange between the capillaries and ISF are determined by the hydrostatic and colloid osmotic pressures of the two fluids. At the arterial end of the capillary, the hydrostatic pressure of the blood (pushing fluid out) exceeds the colloid osmotic pressure (holding the fluid in) thus net movement is from the intravascular to the interstitial

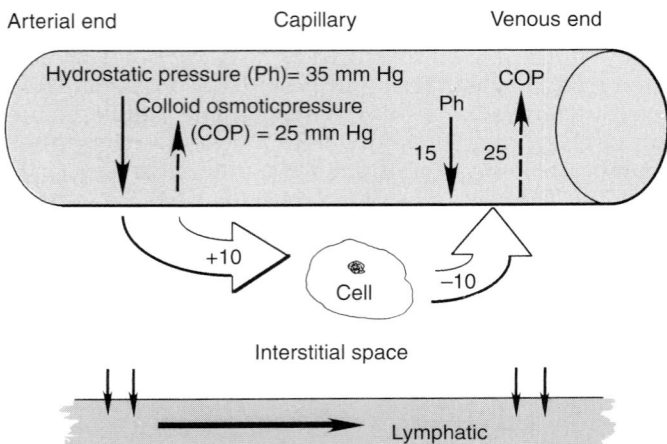

FIG. 20-4 Starling's law of the capillaries. Fluid outflow is favored at the arterial end and fluid resorption at the venous end of the capillary.

compartments. At the venous end of the capillary, fluid moves from the interstitial space to the intravascular space because colloid osmotic pressure exceeds the hydrostatic pressure. This process delivers oxygen and nutrients to the cells and removes carbon dioxide and waste products. The interstitial compartment also has hydrostatic and colloid osmotic pressures, but they are generally quite small and are thus ignored in this illustration. In cases of inflammation or injury causing plasma proteins to leak into the interstitial space, however, the tissue colloid osmotic pressure increases considerably. The lymphatic system normally returns excess ISF and protein to the general circulation. In cases of lymphatic blockage or removal (e.g., surgical removal of axillary lymph nodes for treatment of breast cancer), excess ISF may accumulate.

The accumulation of excess fluid in the interstitial spaces is called *edema*. A review of the capillary dynamics discussed indicates that the following four factors favor edema formation:

1. Increased capillary hydrostatic pressure (as in congestive heart failure with sodium and water retention or venous obstruction)
2. Decreased plasma oncotic pressure (as in nephrotic syndrome or liver cirrhosis, which results in decreased albumin concentration in the plasma)
3. Increased capillary permeability resulting in an increase in ISF colloid osmotic pressure (as in inflammation or injury)
4. Lymphatic obstruction or increased interstitial oncotic pressure

Movement of Water between the ECF and the ICF

Osmotic forces determine movement of water between the ECF and the ICF. Osmosis is the net transfer of water across a semipermeable membrane to the side with the larger concentration of nondiffusible particles. Sodium chloride in the ECF and potassium and organic solutes in the ICF are the major effective nonpenetrating solutes that determine the water concentration on the two sides of the membrane. (Some Na^+ ions do leak into the cell, and some K^+ ions leak out of the cell, but the Na-K pump transfers them to their proper compartments thus they have the effect of nonpenetrating particles.) Because sodium comprises over 90% of the particles in the ECF, it has a major effect on total body water and its distribution, thus the axiom, "water goes where the salt is." Water moves easily and rapidly across most cell membranes until osmotic equilibrium between the two compartments is attained.

The principle of osmosis can be applied in the administration of IV solutions, which are designated as isotonic, hypotonic, or hypertonic, depending on whether their particle concentrations are respectively the same as, less than, or more than the body cell fluids. Basically, an isotonic solution is physiologically isoosmotic with the plasma and cell fluids. The plasma osmolality is normally approximately 287 mOsm/kg.

When red blood cells (RBCs) are placed in an isotonic saline (0.9%) solution, they undergo no change in volume (Fig. 20-5). The osmolal concentration of the saline solution is exactly equal to that of the cell contents (isoosmotic), thus net water diffusion in and out of the cell is zero. Placing RBCs in a hypotonic solution, such as 0.45% saline, causes cell swelling. The solution is hypoosmotic to the RBC, thus net diffusion of water is from the solution into the cell. Conversely, placing RBCs in a hypertonic solution, such as 3% saline, would cause the cells to shrink because the solution is hyperosmotic to the cells. Net diffusion of water is from the RBC to the hypertonic solution. These principles dictate that the safe administration of an IV solution requires that it be nearly isoosmotic with body fluids. For example, IV administration of distilled water (osmolality = 0) would cause RBC swelling and hemolysis. To provide free water to the cells, 5% glucose in water (D_5W) may be given. D_5W is isotonic with body fluids when first infused. As glucose enters cells and is metabolized, the glucose molecule is removed from the ECF. Ultimately, the glucose contributes only carbon dioxide and water as final metabolites. Thus D_5W, isotonic with body fluids at the time of infusion becomes hypotonic as carbon dioxide is removed and water retained. A final point must be made about the terms isotonic and isoosmotic when applied to IV solutions. Even though an isotonic IV solution is isoosmotic, the converse may not be true (Rose, 2001). For example, an isoosmotic solution of urea would cause hemolysis of RBCs if given IV. Both urea (a penetrating molecule) and water equilibrate across the cell membrane (in contrast to saline and glucose, which do not).

The same principles identified in the experiment with RBCs apply to water distribution between the ECF and ICF compartments. When ECF osmolality increases (becomes hyperosmotic), water shifts from the ICF to the ECF, decreasing cell volume. When the ECF osmolality decreases (becomes hypoosmotic), water shifts from the ECF to the ICF, increasing cell volume.

IV administration of isotonic saline results in no change in the ICF volume or osmolality, and the entire volume remains in the ECF (Fig. 20-6). Consequently, isotonic IV fluids may be the first choice for the treatment of hypovolemic shock for the purpose of ECF volume expansion and restoration of perfusion. IV administration of D_5W (isotonic in the bottle but hypotonic when metabolized) provides free water. The volume of the ECF increases by one third of the volume of D_5W infused, the volume of the ICF increases by two thirds of the infused volume, and the osmolality of both ECF and ICF decreases. Hypotonic IV solutions are commonly used to provide for maintaining fluid needs and for replacing fluid losses. Finally, when a hypertonic solution of 3% saline is given IV, the volume of the ECF compartment increases but the volume of the ICF compartment decreases. NaCl remains in the ECF compartment, increasing osmolality. Water leaves the cells by osmosis until the osmolal concentrations of the ECF and ICF are equal. Thus one indication for administering hypertonic saline is for the treatment of cerebral edema.

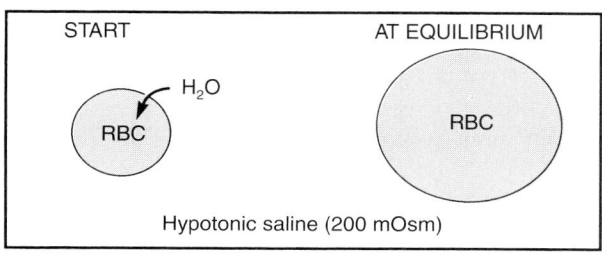
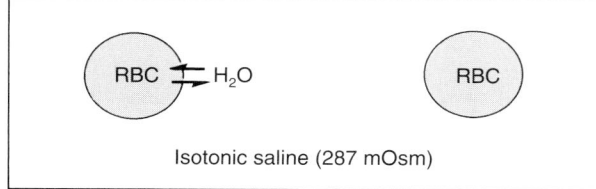
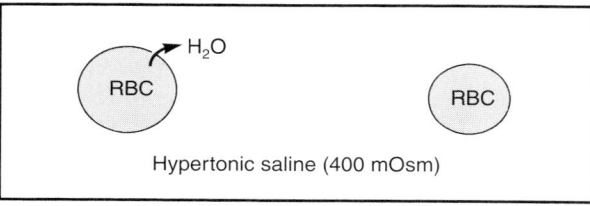

FIG. 20-5   Change of the volume of red blood cells as a result of placing them in hypotonic, isotonic, and hypertonic solutions of sodium chloride (NaCl).

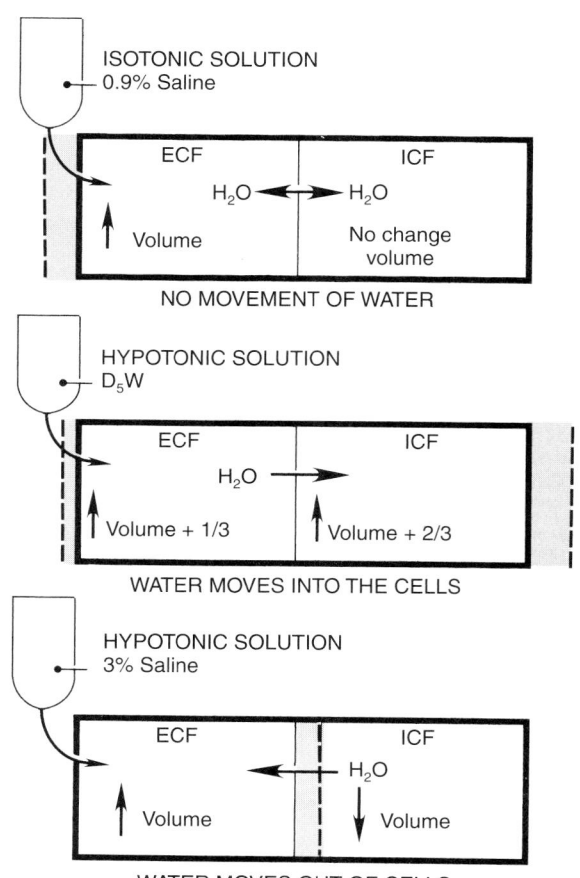

FIG. 20-6   The effect of the intravenous administration of isotonic, hypotonic, and hypertonic solutions on the distribution of water between the body fluid compartments.

Exchange of Water with the External Environment

A balance between intake and output determines TBW (and electrolyte) balance. The normal daily water requirement for healthy adults or infants is approximately 1500 ml/m² of body surface area. Water and electrolytes enter the body via the digestive tract, both in liquids and in food. Water is also formed from the oxidation of food. The oxidation of each 100 calories of food provides approximately 14 ml water. Thus a diet of 2100 calories/day would produce approximately 300 ml of water.

Water is normally lost from the body to the external environment by four routes: kidneys (urine), intestines (feces), lungs (water vapor in the expired air), and skin (through evaporation and sweat). The loss of water through vaporization in the airways and from nonsweating skin is known as *insensible water loss*. This type of water loss should not be confused with the loss of water from sweat, which is low in the basal state but can increase markedly during exercise or exposure to a hot environment. Loss of heat by vaporization of sweat helps to regulate body temperature.

According to the cardinal principle of fluid balance, fluid intake equals fluid output. The normal daily fluid requirements for an adult are approximately 2500 ml (Box 20-2), although this figure can vary considerably and still be considered normal. The minimal water intake is the amount required to replace loss from all body sources, and the maximal intake is the amount that can be excreted by the kidneys. Insensible water loss from the lungs and skin and in the feces (approximately 1 L) is obligatory. *Obligatory losses* are those fluid losses essential for the excretion of body wastes. An obligatory volume of urine output also exists, which is directly related to solute excretion (mostly urea, Na^+, and K^+). The formula for determining minimal urine output is:

$$\frac{\text{Minimum urine output}}{\text{(L/day)}} = \frac{\text{Osmolar load (mOsm/day)}}{\text{Renal concentrating ability (mOsm/L)}}$$

If 600 mOsm of solute is excreted per day and the maximal renal concentrating ability is 1200 mOsm/L, then the minimal obligatory urine output per day is 0.5 L. Fluid intake (from all sources) must equal the total obligatory fluid losses to maintain fluid balance.

BOX 20-2

Typical Daily Fluid Gains and Losses in Healthy Adults

INTAKE		OUTPUT	
Ingested		Kidneys	
liquids	1200 ml	(urine)	1500 ml
Solid foods		Intestines	
(water)	1000 ml	(feces)	200 ml
Food oxidation		Lungs (in	
(water)	300 ml	expired air)	400 ml
Total intake =	2500 ml	Skin (sweat,	
		diffusion)	400 ml
		Total output =	2500 ml

PHYSIOLOGIC REGULATION OF FLUIDS AND ELECTROLYTES

A number of homeostatic mechanisms operate to maintain not only the electrolyte and osmotic concentration of body fluids but also total body fluid volume. Normal body fluid and electrolyte balances are the consequences of dynamic equilibrium among oral fluids and dietary intake and equilibria involving a large number of organ systems. The kidneys, cardiovascular system, pituitary gland, parathyroid glands, adrenal glands, and the lungs are particularly involved.

The kidney mediates the majority of control over fluid and electrolyte levels. TBW and electrolyte concentration are primarily determined by "what the kidney keeps." The kidney, in turn, responds to a number of hormones in its regulatory function.

Sodium and Water

Body water and salt (NaCl) balances are closely related, affecting both the osmolality and volume of the ECF. However, the regulation of sodium and water balances involves different but overlapping mechanisms. Body water balance is primarily regulated by the thirst and antidiuretic hormone (ADH) mechanisms for the purpose of maintaining isoosmotic plasma (near 287 mOsm/kg). Sodium balance, on the other hand, is regulated primarily by aldosterone for the purpose of maintaining the ECF volume and tissue perfusion.

Water Balance and Osmotic Regulation

Osmotic regulation is mediated via the hypothalamus, pituitary, and renal tubules. ADH is a peptide hormone synthesized in the hypothalamus and stored in the pituitary. The hypothalamus also contains the thirst center and osmoreceptors sensitive to the osmolality of the blood. Fig. 44-18 shows that an increase in plasma osmolality stimulates both thirst and ADH release. Thirst stimulates ingestion of water, and ADH alters the permeability of the renal collecting ducts, increasing water reabsorption. The result is an increase in the volume of body water, which restores plasma osmolality to normal and a smaller volume of hyperosmotic (concentrated) urine. A decrease in plasma osmolality results in the opposite response with suppression of thirst and ADH release. The ADH mechanism is so sensitive that the plasma osmolality does not normally vary more than 1% to 2% from the normal 287 mOsm/kg. A relatively large decline in ECF volume (5% to 10%) is required to stimulate thirst or the release of ADH (Rose, 2001). Thus the ADH mechanism is largely concerned with osmoregulation through controlling water balance and is much less sensitive to volume regulation. Because sodium salts (mainly NaCl) comprise 90% of the effective osmoles, hypoosmolality is synonymous with hyponatremia, and hyperosmolality is synonymous with hypernatremia. The plasma osmolality may be estimated by multiplying the measured serum sodium by two. Hypernatremia and hyponatremia indicate intracellular water depletion and excess, respectively, because the ICF and ECF are in osmotic equilibrium.

Sodium Balance and Volume Regulation

Maintaining plasma volume, which is essential for tissue perfusion, is closely related to the regulation of sodium balance. The mechanisms that regulate volume balance respond primarily to changes in the effective circulating volume. *Effective circulating volume* is that part of the ECF volume in the vascular space that effectively perfuses the tissues. In healthy people, the ECF volume generally varies directly with the effective circulating volume and is proportional to the total body sodium stores because sodium is the principal solute that holds water within the ECF. Thus renal mechanisms controlling sodium excretion are primarily responsible for volume regulation in the body.

The renin-angiotensin-aldosterone system is a mechanism of primary importance in the regulation of the ECF volume and renal sodium excretion (Fig. 44-19). Aldosterone is a hormone secreted by the zona glomerulosa of the adrenal cortex. The major stimulus for aldosterone production is a reflex initiated by baroreceptors located in the afferent arteriole of the kidney. A decrease in the effective circulating volume is detected by the baroreceptors, which, in turn, cause the renal juxtaglomerular cells to secrete a protein, *renin*. Renin acts as an enzyme that splits off angiotensin I from the plasma protein angiotensinogen. Angiotensin I is then converted into angiotensin II in the lungs. Angiotensin II stimulates the adrenal cortex to secrete aldosterone. Aldosterone acts on the renal collecting ducts, causing sodium (and water) retention. Additionally, angiotensin II causes vasoconstriction of arteriolar smooth muscles. Both mechanisms help to restore the effective circulating volume. A fall in plasma sodium concentration (Na^+) of only 4 to 5 mEq/L is another stimulus for aldosterone release, but it does not play an important role in normal subjects because Na^+ is held relatively constant by the effects of ADH (Rose, 2001). In fact, even when hyponatremia is present, its effect on aldosterone is often overridden by concomitant changes in the ECF volume. Thus aldosterone secretion is increased in the patient with hyponatremia who is volume-depleted but may be reduced in a patient who is volume-expanded because of the retention of water.

Osmoregulation versus Volume Regulation

The mechanisms regulating plasma osmolality and plasma volume are different. The plasma osmolality (P_{osm}) is determined by the ratio of solutes to water, whereas the ECF volume is determined by the absolute amounts of sodium and water present.

Changes in P_{osm} (primarily determined by the ratio of sodium salts to water or P[Na]) are sensed by osmoreceptors in the hypothalamus, which then affect water intake and water excretion by influencing thirst and the release of ADH. ADH causes water retention and increases urine osmolality by enhancing the permeability of the renal collecting ducts. Thus osmoregulation is achieved by altering water balance, and sodium handling is not affected unless concomitant changes in volume occur.

Volume regulation, on the other hand, maintains tissue perfusion. Different sensors and effectors are involved because renal sodium excretion, but not osmolality, is primarily regulated. The only major overlap between these two mechanisms is the hypovolemic stimulus to ADH secretion.

Regulation of ECF Potassium

Aldosterone is a primary control mechanism for potassium secretion by the distal nephron of the kidney. An increase in secretion of aldosterone causes sodium (and water) reabsorption and potassium excretion. Conversely, a decrease in the secretion of aldosterone causes sodium and water excretion and potassium conservation. The primary stimulus for aldosterone secretion is a decrease in the effective circulating volume, a decrease in serum sodium, or an increase in the serum potassium. Hypervolemia, a decrease in serum potassium, or an increase in serum sodium causes a decrease in aldosterone. Potassium excretion is also influenced by acid-base status and flow rate in the distal tubule. In the presence of an alkalosis, K^+ excretion is increased and in acidosis it is decreased. Within the distal tubule, hydrogen (H^+) ions and K^+ ions compete for excretion in exchange for Na^+ reabsorption to maintain body electroneutrality. When a metabolic alkalosis exists with a deficit of H^+ ions, the tubule exchanges Na^+ for K^+ to conserve H^+ ions. Metabolic acidosis results in an increase in H^+ excretion and a decrease in K^+ excretion. This mechanism explains the reasons for which hypokalemia is often associated with alkalosis and hyperkalemia is associated with acidosis. High rates of urine flow in the distal tubule result in an increase in total K^+ excretion and a low flow rate in a reduced K^+ excretion.

Regulation of ECF Calcium and Phosphate

Normal serum concentrations of Ca^{++} and $HPO_4^=$ ions are maintained by three mechanisms: intestinal absorption, exchange between the ECF and bone, and renal excretion. The homeostasis of these ions is interrelated and under hormonal control. Parathyroid hormone (PTH) and 1,25-dihydroxycholecalciferol (active form of vitamin D_3) act on the intestine, bone, and kidney to maintain normal serum levels. PTH is secreted by the parathyroid glands, four (or sometimes more) structures resembling wheat grains located on the posterior poles of the thyroid gland. The kidneys activate vitamin D_3. Serum levels of calcium and phosphate are reciprocal; thus as levels of one rise, the levels of the other decline. PTH release occurs in response to a decrease in the serum Ca^{++} and then acts to increase serum Ca^{++} in the following three ways:

1. It stimulates bone reabsorption in the presence of permissive amounts of vitamin D_3, resulting in the release of calcium phosphate.
2. It promotes the activation of vitamin D_3 by the kidney, which, in turn, promotes calcium phosphate absorption through the intestinal mucosa.
3. It augments calcium reabsorption in the renal tubule and phosphate excretion in the urine; a rise in the serum Ca^{++} suppresses PTH secretion.

Calcitonin is a hormone produced by the parafollicular cells of the thyroid gland and is released in response to a large increase in serum Ca^{++}. Calcitonin lowers serum Ca^{++} by inhibiting bone reabsorption. However, Ca^{++} fluctuations in the normal range do not influence the secretion of calcitonin, although they clearly affect PTH secretion.

Regulation of ECF Hydrogen Ion Concentration

The blood buffers, lungs, and kidneys play a major role in maintaining acid-base balance by regulating the hydrogen ion concentration ($[H^+]$) of the ECF. Blood buffers are able to accept or donate H^+, thus acting rapidly as sponges to prevent large fluctuations in acid-base balance. The lungs are also vital in maintaining homeostasis. The lungs regulate $[H^+]$ by controlling the level of carbon dioxide (CO_2) in the ECF. Metabolic acidosis causes compensatory hyperventilation, resulting in CO_2 excretion by the lungs, thus reducing the acidity of the ECF; metabolic alkalosis causes compensatory hypoventilation, resulting in CO_2 retention and thus increased acidity of the ECF. Finally, the kidneys play a vital role in acid-base homeostasis by excreting excess H^+ and are able to compensate for respiratory acidosis and alkalosis by increasing or decreasing the reabsorption of bicarbonate.

In summary, it is evident from this brief discussion of the systems that regulate fluids and electrolytes that precise mechanisms exist in the body to maintain homeostasis. The kidneys, more than any other organ, play a critical role in these regulatory processes. Thus renal failure results in multiple fluid and electrolyte disorders (see Part Eight).

ASSESSMENT OF FLUID AND ELECTROLYTE STATUS

History: Clues to Likely Imbalances

The assessment and diagnosis of fluid and electrolyte disturbances require a thorough understanding of normal physiologic mechanisms and conditions likely to cause disturbances. Many illnesses, diseases, and therapeutic modalities may cause fluid and electrolyte disturbances. Additionally, many fluid and electrolyte disturbances produce symptoms that are nonspecific or subtle. Therefore a high degree of suspicion is required to recognize them, particularly when the imbalance is mild or in the early stages.

Metheny (2000) has developed an excellent approach to the assessment of fluid and electrolyte status based on correlation and analysis of history, clinical assessment data, and laboratory tests. Box 20-3 lists six important questions to consider during history taking. The first question requires knowledge about the most likely fluid and electrolyte disturbances associated with particular diseases thus the clinician may anticipate them. For example, respiratory acidosis would be an anticipated electrolyte disturbance in a patient with chronic bronchitis and emphysema because of CO_2 retention. In a patient with end-stage renal failure, one would anticipate fluid volume excess, metabolic acidosis, hyperkalemia, and calcium disturbances because of the inability of the

---

BOX 20-3

Six Critical Questions to Ask When Assessing Fluid and Electrolyte Status

1. Is there a disease process or injury state present that could disrupt fluid and electrolyte balance?
2. Is the patient receiving any medication, parenteral fluid, or other treatment that could disrupt fluid and electrolyte balance? If so, how might this therapy upset fluid balance?
3. Is there an abnormal loss of body fluids and, if so, from what source? What type of imbalance is usually associated with the loss of these fluids?
4. Have any dietary restrictions (e.g., low-sodium diet) been imposed? If so, how might fluid balance be affected?
5. Has the patient taken adequate amounts of water and other nutrients orally or by some other route? If not, how long has the intake been inadequate?
6. How does the total intake of fluids compare with the total fluid output?

From Metheny NM: *Fluid and electrolyte balance: nursing considerations,* ed 4, Philadelphia, 2000, Lippincott, Williams & Wilkins.

---

kidneys to excrete acid metabolites, potassium, and fluids adequately. Calcium disturbance results from phosphate retention and secondary hyperparathyroidism.

Answers to the second question require knowledge about fluid and electrolyte imbalances likely to result from medications and other treatment. For example, one should expect the use of thiazide diuretics to result in hypokalemia and should therefore monitor for its presence and prevent its development.

Answering the third question requires knowledge of the composition of specific body fluids to anticipate the type of imbalance that is likely to occur with their excessive loss. The gastrointestinal (GI) tract is a common site of abnormal fluid loss. Normally, approximately 8 L of GI secretions are produced each day, most of which is reabsorbed (approximately 100 to 200 ml is excreted in the stool). Thus a fluid volume deficit may easily develop in cases of vomiting, gastric suction, diarrhea, or drainage from fistulas or an ostomy. The various GI secretions vary in electrolyte composition, thus their loss produces different imbalances in addition to fluid volume deficit. Gastric secretions are highly acidic (pH = 1 to 3) and contain considerable amounts of sodium and potassium chlorides. Thus vomiting and prolonged gastric suction are often associated with sodium and potassium deficit and metabolic alkalosis. On the other hand, bile and intestinal and pancreatic secretions are quite alkaline (pH = 8) and are high in Na^+, K^+, and HCO_3^-. Thus diarrhea, intestinal suction, fistulas, or T-tube drainage of bile after gallbladder surgery is often associated with fluid volume deficits, Na^+ and K^+ deficits, and metabolic acidosis from the loss of HCO_3^-. Finally, perspiration, a hypotonic fluid, may cause the loss of water in excess of Na^+, resulting in hypernatremia. Losses from perspiration can increase dramatically during heavy exercise and hot environments (up to 1 L/hr). Similarly, water losses in febrile, hyperventilating patients may be higher. Answering all of the six questions should suggest potential fluid and electrolyte disturbances. A detailed list and discussion of the causes of the various imbalances are presented in Chapters 21 and 22.

Clinical Assessment

After a hypothesis is formed about a particular potential fluid and electrolyte imbalance, systematic clinical observations are critical to follow up cues suggested by the history and to arrive at a diagnosis. Systematic clinical observations are also critical for monitoring an actual problem and response to treatment. However, to be valuable, these observations must be planned and based on an understanding of the physiologic aspects of fluid and electrolyte balance. Table 20-3 presents a brief and general guide for making clinical observations related to fluid and electrolyte disturbances. Signs and symptoms commonly associated with specific disorders are presented in Chapters 21 and 22.

Laboratory Values

Finally, because many fluid and electrolyte disturbances produce nonspecific signs and symptoms, only through laboratory data can these disturbances be confirmed. Importantly, however, laboratory values are rarely sufficient by themselves to interpret fluid and electrolyte disturbances; they must always be correlated with history and clinical observations. Also important is to observe trends in measurements and compare them with the patient's baseline values rather than to ascribe undue importance to a single measurement. The intelligent use of laboratory values in identifying and managing fluid and electrolyte imbalances requires a thorough knowledge of pathophysiologic aspects and the limitations of individual tests. Table 20-4 presents normal values for frequently used laboratory measurements used in the evaluation of fluid and electrolyte disturbances. Laboratory tests used to evaluate acid-base status are listed in Chapter 22.

TABLE 20-3

Fluid and Electrolyte Clinical Assessment Guide

Observation	Comments
Monitor weight daily	Rapid losses (or gains) indicate changes in TBW
	1 kg = 2.2 lb = 1 L
	1 lb = 1 pint ≈ 500 ml
	Body weight unchanged when fluid sequestered in a "third space"
	Most accurate method assessing fluid balance
Loss (or gain)	2%: mild fluid volume deficit or excess (2.4 lb in a 120 lb person)
	5%: moderate fluid volume deficit or excess (6.0 lb in a 120 lb person)
	8%: severe fluid volume deficit or excess (9.6 lb in a 120 lb person)
Monitor I/O	Keep accurate records and include all sources of I/O; compare I/O pattern over several days
Observe eyes	
Dry conjunctiva	Fluid volume deficit
Decreased tearing	
Soft eyeballs	
Periorbital edema	Fluid volume excess
Observe lips and oral cavity	
Dry, cracked lips	Fluid volume deficit (or mouth breathing); tongue normally has one longitudinal
Small, multifurrowed tongue	furrow
Observe skin turgor	Pinch skin over sternal area; normally springs back immediately
Decreased skin turgor	Fluid volume deficit
Assess cardiovascular status	
Temperature	Elevated temperature (101°-103° F) increases fluid requirements by 500 ml/day
Tachycardia	Fluid volume deficit
Orthostatic BP drop	Lying/standing systolic BP drop >10 mm Hg sensitive index of fluid volume deficit
Narrow pulse pressure	
Hand veins	Normal filling time 3-5 sec in dependent position; emptying time 3-5 sec when elevated (prolonged filling time in fluid volume deficit; prolonged emptying time in fluid volume excess)
Jugular vein distention (JVD)	Built-in CVP manometer reflecting changes in fluid volume
	Normal: JVD 2 cm above sternal angle in 45-degree position
	Fluid volume deficit: flat neck veins in supine position
	Fluid volume excess: JVD may extend to jaw angle in 45-degree position
Central venous pressure (CVP)	Normally 4-11 cm water in vena cava or 0-4 cm water in right atrium
	Low CVP may indicate hypovolemia
	High CVP may indicate hypervolemia
Cardiac dysrhythmias	May indicate excess or deficits of K^+, Mg^{++}, Ca^{++}
Assess respiratory system	
Moist rales, rhonchi	Pulmonary edema; fluid volume excess
Increased respiratory rate	
Dyspnea	

BP, Blood pressure; *CNS,* central nervous system; *CVP,* central venous pressure; *GI,* gastrointestinal; *ICP,* increased intracranial pressure; *I/O,* intake and output; *JVD,* jugular vein distention; *TBW,* total body weight

Continued

TABLE 20-3 ■■■

Fluid and Electrolyte Clinical Assessment Guide—cont'd

Observation	Comments
Assess GI system	
Absent bowel sounds	Potassium deficit
Nausea, diarrhea	Potassium excess
Assess renal system	
Oliguria (<30 ml/hr)	Renal failure; severe fluid volume deficit
	Normal urinary volume = 40-80 ml/hr
Observe extremities/sacrum for edema	Fluid volume excess
	Grade: 1+, barely perceptible, to 4+, pitting edema
Assess neurologic system	
Depressed CNS	Fluid volume deficit
	Acidosis
Increased intracranial pressure (ICP)	Hyponatremia
Seizures	Hypocalcemia, hypomagnesemia
Assess for neuromuscular irritability/hypoactivity	
Hyperactive reflexes	Hypocalcemia, hypomagnesemia, alkalosis
Carpopedal spasm	
Positive Chvostek's sign	
Hypoactive reflexes	Hypercalcemia, hypermagnesemia, hypokalemia, hyponatremia

TABLE 20-4 ■■■

Selected Laboratory Tests Used to Evaluate Fluid and Electrolyte Status

	Normal Value	Comments
BLOOD TESTS		
Serum potassium	3.5-5.0 mEq/L	Serum K^+ higher in acidosis (because of K^+ shift out of cells) and lower in alkalosis (because of K^+ shift into cells); get repeat measurement if laboratory error suspected; correlate with ECG observations
Serum sodium	135-145 mEq/L	Serum Na^+ usually reflects plasma osmolality because sodium salts provide 90% of ECF solute particles Hyponatremia indicates that body fluids are diluted by an excess of water relative to total solute; it is not equivalent to Na^+ depletion Hypernatremia always indicates that body fluids are hyperosmotic, that there is a deficit of water relative to total solute; rarely due to an absolute sodium excess.
Serum chloride	98-106 mEq/L	Hypochloremia commonly associated with metabolic alkalosis and hypokalemia Hyperchloremia may be associated with some types of metabolic acidosis
Serum calcium	9-10.5 mg/dl (4-5.5 mEq/L)	Interpret in relation to serum albumin and pH, which both affect the ionized (physiologically active) fraction of serum Ca^{++}. Normally about 50% of the total serum calcium is in the ionized form, while the rest is bound to protein, mostly albumin. Total serum calcium drops when the albumin level is decreased, but the ionized fraction does not. Thus symptoms of hypocalcemia rarely develop in the hypoalbuminemic (<4-5 g/dl) patient. Alkalosis can produce symptoms of hypocalcemia even when the total serum calcium is normal, since less calcium is in the ionized form with a high pH.
Serum phosphate	2.5-4.5 mg/dl (1.8-2.6 mEq/L)	Rises during early stage of chronic renal failure, causing hyperparathyroidism and renal osteodystrophy; soft tissue precipitation of calcium phosphate salts occurs when $Ca \times PO_4$ cross-product exceeds 60 in mg/dl (see Part Eight)
Serum magnesium	1.5-2.5 mEq/L (1.8-3.0 mg/dl)	
Serum glucose	70-100 mg/dl	High values cause osmotic diuresis and fluid volume deficit
Hematocrit	Men: 44%-52% Women: 39%-47%	May be elevated in hypovolemia and depressed in hypervolemia
Blood urea nitrogen	10-20 mg/dl	Elevated in renal failure, conditions of increased catabolism, and with hypovolemia; depressed in hypervolemia

TABLE 20-4

Selected Laboratory Tests Used to Evaluate Fluid and Electrolyte Status—cont'd

	Normal Value	Comments
BLOOD TESTS—CONT'D		
Serum creatinine	0.7-1.5 mg/dl	Elevated in renal failure
Serum osmolality $P_{OSM} = 2 \times [Na] + \dfrac{Glucose}{18}$ $\quad\;\; = 2 \times [Na]$	280-295 mOsm/kg	Increased in water deficit (hypernatremia) and decreased in water excess (hyponatremia) Effective plasma osmolality may be estimated by either formula on the left or measured by laboratory tests
Serum proteins Total Albumin Globulin	 6.0-8.0 g/dl 3.5-5.5 g/dl 2.0-3.5 g/dl	
URINE TESTS		
Urinary sodium	100-260 mEq/24 hr (>40 mEq/L in random specimen)	Varies with intake <10 mEq/24 hr in hyponatremia associated with edema or with volume depletion because of extrarenal causes >20 mEq/24 hr if hyponatremia is caused by syndrome of inappropriate antidiuretic hormone (SIADH), salt wasting renal disease, or adrenal insufficiency
Urinary potassium Na/K = 2:1	25-100 mEq/24 hr	Varies with intake Increased in hyperaldosteronism (Na/K ratio may be reversed) Decreased in adrenal insufficiency (Na/K ratio may be 10:1)
Urinary chloride	110-250 mEq/24 hr	<10 mEq/L in metabolic alkalosis caused by diuretics, vomiting, or gastric suction >20 mEq/L in metabolic alkalosis caused by hyperaldosteronism or severe K^+ depletion
Urine osmolality Rough equivalencies: *Sp. gravity Osmolality* 1.000 0 1.003 100 1.010 300 1.025 800 1.035 1200	50-1400 mOsm	Reflects renal concentrating/diluting ability Fixed near 287 mOsm (or 1.010 specific gravity) in renal failure Osmolality measurement more accurate than specific gravity
Urinary pH	4.5-8	

KEY CONCEPTS

- Body fluids are isotonic solutions composed of water and solutes (dissolved substances). Electrolytes are electrically charged particles (ions) when they are in solution.
- Fluid and electrolyte balance means that total body water (TBW) and electrolyte concentrations are normal, as well as their distribution throughout body compartments.
- Fluid and electrolyte imbalances are associated with all major illnesses and even some minor ones.
- TBW, which is the percentage of total body weight composed of water, varies according to sex, age, and body fat. At the beginning of life (infancy) the percentage of body weight that is water is approximately 75%. TBW is approximately 60% in the male adult, 50% in the female adult, and less than 50% in elderly adults. Because fat is essentially water-free, the more fat present, the smaller the percentage of body weight that is water.

- TBW is separated into two major body compartments, the ICF containing 40% (2/3) and the ECF containing 20% (1/3). The ECF is further subdivided into the ISF containing 15% and the IVF containing 5%.
- The chemical composition of body fluids include nonelectrolytes and electrolytes. Nonelectrolytes, such as proteins or glucose, do not carry an electrical charge. Electrolytes are salts that dissociate in water into one or more charged particles and can conduct an electrical current. Cations are electrolytes carrying a positive charge, such as Na^+, K^+, or Ca^{++}, while anions, such as Cl^- and HCO_3^-, carry a negative charge.
- The electrolyte concentration of body fluids varies from one body fluid compartment to another. Na^+ is the major cation of the ECF, and K^+ is the major cation of the ICF. An electrical gradient across the cell membrane is necessary for the generation of

nerve and muscle action potentials and the differential concentrations of Na^+ and K^+ concentrations across the cell membrane are important in its maintenance.

- The concentrations of electrolytes are preferably expressed in milliequivalents (mEq) or combining power.
- The law of electrical neutrality states that the sum of the positive charges must be equal to the sum of the negative charges in any particular body fluid compartment (measured in mEq).
- Movement of water and solutes between the body fluid compartments and the external environment is constant to maintain homeostasis and to deliver nutrients and oxygen to the cells and remove waste products and secreted substances from the cells.
- Movement of solutes across the cell membrane (between the ECF and ICF) is highly selective and occurs by diffusion. Passive transport is affected by concentration and electrical gradients and the permeability of the cell membrane (solute size relative to cell membrane pore size and solubility). In diffusion, solutes move from an area of higher concentration to one of lower concentration until the concentration is equal on both sides of the membrane. Positively charged particles tend to move to the negative side of the cell membrane (usually the inside), and negatively charged particles tend to move to the positive side of the cell membrane (usually the outside). Together the concentration and electrical gradients across the cell membrane provide the driving force for passive transport. A hydrostatic pressure gradient can increase the rate of diffusion.
- Active transport of solutes across the cell membrane against a concentration or electrical gradient requires the expenditure of energy in the form of ATP. The sodium-potassium pump is an example of an active transport mechanism that moves Na^+ from the ICF to the ECF in exchange for K^+.
- Water moves freely across all body membranes, and two forces control its movement: osmotic and hydrostatic pressures.
- Hydrostatic pressure is the compression force of a fluid. Osmotic pressure refers to the drawing force for water exerted by solute particles. These two forces generally oppose each other.
- Osmolality refers to the osmotic concentration of a solution *and depends only on the number of solute particles* and not on their size, mass, or charge. Osmolality, expressed as mOsm/Kg or mOsm/L of water, is actually a measure of water concentration relative to the number of solute particles.
- A solute particle must be confined to a compartment (unable to cross a semipermeable membrane) to influence the movement of water (serve as an effective osmole). In osmosis, the net movement of water across the semipermeable membrane will be from the compartment with the least number of particles (lowest osmotic concentration) to the compartment with the most number of particles (highest osmotic concentration) in solution. To put it another way,

net water movement is from the compartment with the dilute solution (higher water concentration) across the semipermeable membrane to the compartment with the concentrated solution (lower water concentration). Thus osmosis is simply a special case of diffusion.

- Movement of fluid between the IVF compartment and the ISF compartment is called ultrafiltration because water, electrolytes, and other solutes (except plasma proteins and blood cells) readily cross the capillary membrane. Albumin is the effective osmole controlling the movement of fluid between the IVF and ISF because it is confined to the IVF. Albumin generates the COP holding fluid within the blood vessel while opposed by the hydrostatic pressure of the blood tending to push the fluid out. Fluid outflow is favored at the arterial end of the capillary (in which hydrostatic pressure is higher than the COP) and fluid resorption at the venous end of the capillary (in which hydrostatic pressure is lower than the COP); this action is known as Starling's Law.
- Edema is a condition of excess fluid in the interstitial fluid compartment and may be caused by four mechanisms: (1) increased capillary hydrostatic pressure (e.g., congestive heart failure), (2) decreased COP (hypoalbuminemia as in liver cirrhosis), (3) increased capillary permeability as in inflammation, and (4) lymphatic obstruction (e.g., arm edema following mastectomy with excision of the axillary lymph nodes).
- Movement of water between the ECF and the ICF is determined by osmotic forces. Because Na^+ (and Cl^-) comprise over 90% of the particles in the ECF and is largely confined to that compartment, it has a major effect on total body water and its distribution. Water readily crosses the cell membrane between the ECF and the ICF until osmotic equilibrium is achieved. Thus ICF osmolality always equals ECF osmolality, although the volume of the cell may change.
- The principle of osmosis can be applied to the administration of IV solution designated as isotonic, hypotonic, or hypertonic, depending on whether their particle concentrations are the same as, less than, or more than body cell fluids. The plasma osmolality is normally 287 mOsm/kg (isoosmotic or isotonic). When red blood cells (RBCs) are placed in hypotonic saline (<287 mOsm), the RBC swells; when placed in isotonic saline (near 287 mOsm) no change in RBC volume occurs, and when placed in hypertonic saline (>287 mOsm), the RBC shrinks.
- The same principle of osmosis can be applied to the administration of IV fluids and its distribution between the ECF and ICF. When an isotonic IV solution, such as normal saline, is infused, it remains in the ECF compartment thus increasing the intravascular volume (in cases of hypovolemic shock).
- When a hypotonic IV solution such as D_5W is administered, one third of the water remains in the ECF and two thirds is distributed to the ICF. D_5W is the most common type of IV solution chosen for the purpose of providing free water to the cells.
- The administration of a hypertonic IV solution, such

as 3% saline, causes water to shift from the ICF to the ECF. One indication for administering hypertonic saline would be to reduce cerebral edema.

■ TBW (and electrolyte) balance is determined by intake and output. The total intake for an average adult is approximately 2500 ml from ingested liquids, water in foods, and the oxidation of foods. Approximately 2500 ml of water is lost from the body via the urine, feces, lungs, and skin. In health, intake must always be equal to output.

■ Water balance and Na^+ balance are closely related and regulated by different but overlapping mechanisms.

■ Body water balance is regulated primarily by the thirst and antidiuretic hormone (ADH) mechanism for the purpose of maintaining isoosmotic plasma (near 287 mOsm/kg). An increase in the plasma osmolality above 287 mOsm is sensed by the osmoreceptors in the hypothalamus, which then cause the release of ADH from the pituitary. ADH stimulates the thirst center (causing the person to drink) and stimulates the distal tubules of the kidney causing more water to be reabsorbed and a smaller amount of concentrated urine to be excreted. This effect tends to restore the normal plasma osmolality. A decrease in the plasma osmolality below 287 mOsm has the opposite effect.

■ Na^+ balance is primarily regulated by the renin-angiotensin-aldosterone mechanism for the purpose of maintaining ECF volume and tissue perfusion. A decrease in the effective circulating volume (ECV) is sensed by pressure receptors in the afferent arteriole of the kidney causing the release of renin. Renin ultimately causes the production of angiotensin II (which causes vasoconstriction) and aldosterone (which causes the kidney to reabsorb Na^+ along with water). These two effects tend to restore ECF volume and thus blood pressure and tissue perfusion.

■ Aldosterone is the primary regulator of K^+ homeostasis. An increase in aldosterone causes decreased renal reabsorption of K^+ (and greater excretion). A decrease in aldosterone causes increased renal reabsorption of K^+ (and decreased excretion). Aldosterone has the opposite effect on Na^+ reabsorption and excretion.

■ Parathyroid hormone is the primary regulator of ECF Ca^{++} and $HPO_4^=$ homeostasis.

■ The blood buffers, lungs, and kidneys play a major role in maintaining acid-base balance by regulating the hydrogen ion concentration $[H^+]$ of the ECF.

■ The assessment and diagnosis of fluid and electrolyte disturbances requires a thorough understanding of normal physiologic and pathophysiologic mechanisms and conditions likely to cause disturbances. The assessment should always be based on the correlation and analysis of history, clinical assessment data, and laboratory tests.

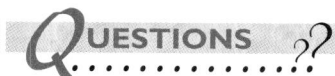

QUESTIONS

A sampling of review questions for this chapter appears here. Visit http://www.mosby.com/MERLIN/PriceWilson/ for additional questions.

Answer the following on a separate sheet of paper.

1. Name the three main fluid compartments of the body.
2. List six critical questions to consider in assessing fluid and electrolyte status.
3. Name the three systems that play a large role in maintaining acid-base homeostasis.

Circle T if the statement is true and F if it is false. Correct any false statements.

4. T F The movement of solutes across a cell membrane against a concentration or electrical gradient is called simple diffusion.

5. T F A subnormal level of the serum albumin in a patient with liver cirrhosis would favor edema formation.

6. T F The serum Ca^{++} level is primarily under the hormonal control of parathyroid hormone.

7. T F The osmolality (or specific gravity) is an indication of the kidney's ability to concentrate or dilute urine (conserve water when a deficit exists or excrete water when an excess exists).

8. T F Increased aldosterone production caused by stress may produce an increased loss of Na^+ in the urine.

9. T F Changes in blood pressure may indicate alterations in the effective circulating fluid volume.

10. T F Accurate daily weights are vital in evaluating TBW changes.

11. T F A loss of 4 lb of body weight after the administration of a diuretic means that approximately 4 L of fluid was lost from the body.

12. T F ECF excess or deficit can be diagnosed from the electrolyte report alone.

13. T F The milliequivalent and millimole measurements are equivalent measures for any given ion, thus they can be used interchangeably.

14. T F Osmotic concentration is determined by the total number of particles confined to a body fluid compartment.

Disorders of Fluid Volume, Osmolality, and Electrolytes

LORRAINE M. WILSON

𝒯hree general categories of changes describe abnormalities of body fluids: (1) volume, (2) osmolality, and (3) composition. Although these disturbances are interrelated, each is a separate entity.

Volume imbalances affect primarily the extracellular fluid (ECF) and involve relatively equal losses or gains of sodium and water leading to an ECF volume deficit or excess. For example, the acute loss of an isotonic ECF fluid, as occurs with diarrhea, is followed by a significant decrease in the ECF volume and little, if any, change in the intracellular fluid (ICF) volume. Fluid will not be transferred from the ICF to the ECF as long as the osmolality in the two compartments remains the same. Clinical signs and symptoms generally identify the ECF volume disturbances.

Osmotic imbalances affect primarily the ICF and involve relatively unequal losses or gains of sodium and water. When water alone is lost or added from the ECF, the concentration of the osmotically active particles will change. Sodium ions and the chloride and bicarbonate ions that electrically balance them together account for 90% of the osmotically active particles in the ECF, and changes in the sodium concentration generally reflect changes in the osmolality of body fluid compartments. If the concentration of sodium in the ECF is decreased, water moves from the ECF to the ICF (causing cell swelling) until osmolality is again equal in the two compartments. Conversely, if the concentration of sodium in the ECF should increase, water moves from the ICF to the ECF (causing cell shrinkage) until osmolality is again equal in the two compartments. Osmotic disturbances are generally associated with hyponatremia and hypernatremia, thus serum sodium values are important in their identification.

The concentration of most other ions within the ECF compartment can be altered without significant changes in the total number of osmotically active particles, thus producing a *compositional change*. For example, a rise in the serum potassium concentration from the normal 4 to 8 mEq/L would have a significant effect on myocardial function, but it would not significantly change the osmolality of the ECF. If the kidneys are functioning normally, fluid and electrolyte disturbances are minimized, particularly when the loss or addition of solute or water is gradual.

A change in the distribution of body fluids may occur, such as the internal loss of ECF into a nonfunctional space. Examples include the sequestration of isotonic fluid in a burn, ascites, or muscle trauma. The functional loss of ECF is sometimes referred to as *third spacing* (non-ECF, non-ICF). Essentially, changes in the distribution of fluids result in ECF volume deficits or excesses, thus they will be considered as subcategories of ECF volume imbalances.

The following discussion focuses on single imbalances of fluids and electrolytes. It is important to realize, however, that in practice a combination of fluid and electrolyte imbalances is far more common than are single disturbances.

VOLUME IMBALANCES

Extracellular Fluid Volume Deficit

ECF volume deficit or *hypovolemia* is defined as the isotonic loss of body fluids, with relatively equal losses of sodium and water. Isotonic fluid volume deficits are often mistakenly referred to as *dehydration,* a term that should be used only to describe relatively pure water depletion leading to hypernatremia.

Pathogenesis

Fluid volume deficit is a common condition that occurs in a wide variety of clinical circumstances and is almost always related to the renal or extrarenal loss of body fluids. Fluid volume depletion occurs more rapidly when the abnormal loss of body fluids is coupled with decreased intake for any reason (Box 21-1).

The most common cause of isotonic fluid volume deficit is the loss of a significant fraction of the 8 L of gastrointestinal (GI) fluids secreted daily. Significant losses may occur through prolonged vomiting, nasogastric suction, massive diarrhea, fistulas, or bleeding. Because the sodium concentration of these fluids is high, their loss causes combined sodium and water deficits. Because gastric secretions also contain large amounts of potassium and hydrogen ions, volume depletion caused by such

---

BOX 21-1

Causes of ECF Volume Deficit

EXTRARENAL LOSSES
Gastrointestinal (GI) losses
  Gastric: vomiting; GI suction
  Intestinal: diarrhea; ileostomies, pancreatic or biliary fistulas
  Bleeding
Skin losses
  Diaphoresis
  Extensive burns (loss by evaporation)
Third-space losses
  Intestinal obstruction
  Peritonitis
  Severe burns
  Ascites
  Pancreatitis
  Pleural effusion
  Crush injury or fractured hip
  Hypoalbuminemia

RENAL LOSSES (POLYURIA)
Causes intrinsic to the kidney
  Renal disease
    Salt-wasting nephritis
    Diuretic phase of acute renal failure
Causes extrinsic to the kidney
  Diuretic excess
  Osmotic diuresis
    Diabetic glycosuria
    Enteral or parenteral hyperalimentation
    Mannitol therapy
Aldosterone deficiency
  Addison's disease
  Hypoaldosteronism

---

losses is often combined with metabolic alkalosis and hypokalemia. The loss of lower GI tract secretions, which contain large amounts of bicarbonate in addition to sodium and potassium, often results in fluid volume deficit combined with metabolic acidosis and hypokalemia.

Other common causes of fluid volume deficit include sequestration of fluid in soft tissue injuries, extensive burns, peritonitis, or within an obstructed GI tract. The accumulation of fluid within these non-ECF and non-ICF spaces is called *third spacing.* Third-space fluid loss refers to a distributional loss of fluids into a space that is not easily exchangeable with the ECF. Fluid is essentially trapped and is unavailable for use by the body. Rapid and extensive fluid volume accumulation in such spaces occurs at the expense of the ECF volume and may reduce the effective circulating blood volume. For example, 5 to 10 L of fluid can accumulate within an obstructed bowel; 4 to 6 L of fluid may accumulate in the peritoneal cavity in acute peritonitis; several liters may accumulate in the interstitial space, primarily during the first 24 hours after extensive burns (Warden, Heinback, 1999).

Sweat is a hypotonic fluid consisting mainly of water, sodium (30 to 70 mEq/L), and chloride. During heavy exercise in hot environments, as much as 1 L of sweat per hour may be lost and contribute to fluid volume deficit if oral intake is inadequate. Large amounts of fluid may be lost during illnesses in which fever, diaphoresis, and inadequate fluid replacement occur. A temperature between 101° and 103° F increases 24-hour fluid requirements by approximately 500 ml, whereas temperatures above 103° F increase this requirement by at least 1000 ml. Finally, large amounts of fluid may be lost from the skin through evaporation when burns are treated by the open method.

Abnormal losses of sodium and water in the urine may occur in several ways. During the recovery (diuretic) phase of acute renal failure or in certain chronic renal diseases primarily involving the tubules (salt-losing nephritis), large amounts of sodium and water may be lost in the urine. However, the usual problem in renal failure is sodium retention (see Part Eight).

Renal loss of sodium and water in the absence of renal disease occurs in three circumstances, the most common being the excessive use of diuretics, particularly the thiazides or potent loop diuretics such as furosemide. An obligatory osmotic diuresis is another common cause of sodium and water loss, which occurs during the marked glycosuria of uncontrolled diabetes mellitus (diabetic ketoacidosis [DKA] or hyperglycemic hyperosmolar nonketotic [HHNK] coma). In the case of high-protein enteral or parenteral alimentation, large amounts of urea are formed and may act as an osmotic agent. An iatrogenic cause of diuresis and fluid volume deficit is the use of mannitol for the treatment of cerebral edema or prerenal azotemia. Finally, excessive loss of sodium and water in the urine may occur in Addison's disease and hypoaldosteronism because of a deficiency of aldosterone.

Hemodynamic Responses to Fluid Volume Deficit

Regardless of the cause of the fluid volume deficit, contraction of the ECF volume (hypovolemia) impairs cardiac output by diminishing venous return to the heart. Clinical manifestations of volume contraction encompass the direct effects of a reduced cardiac output and the secondary effects of homeostatic mechanisms activated to compensate for the falling cardiac output. Because mean arterial pressure (MAP) equals cardiac output (CO) multiplied by the total peripheral resistance (TPR) (MAP = CO × TPR), it follows that the fall in CO lowers blood pressure. The lowered blood pressure is sensed by the cardiac and carotid baroreceptors and communicated to the vasomotor centers in the brain stem, which then induce a sympathetic response. Sympathetic-induced changes include peripheral vasoconstriction, increased heart rate, and increased cardiac contractility, all of which help to restore CO and perfusion of the coronary, cerebral, and pulmonary vascular beds. Diminished renal perfusion results from renal vasoconstriction, mediated, in turn, by activation of the sympathetic nervous system. Diminished renal perfusion activates the renin-angiotensin-aldosterone mechanism. Angiotensin II enhances systemic vasoconstriction, and aldosterone increases renal sodium (and water) reabsorption. These changes increase CO by restoring the effective circulating volume and blood pressure toward normal. When the fluid volume deficit is small (500 ml), activation of the sympathetic response is generally adequate to restore CO and blood pressure to near normal, although the heart rate may still be increased.

When the hypovolemia is more severe (1000 ml or more), sympathetic and angiotensin II–mediated vasoconstriction is increased. Blood is shunted away from the renal, GI, muscular, and cutaneous systems, with the relative preservation of coronary and cerebral blood flow. The intense vasoconstriction may be adequate to maintain systemic blood pressure in a recumbent position, but orthostatic hypotension and dizziness result when assuming a sitting or standing posture.

Clinical Features

The cause of fluid volume deficit can usually be suspected from the history. However, no specific electrolyte test indicates the presence or development of a deficit. Clinical examination of the patient is the best guide to volume abnormalities.

The signs and symptoms of a fluid volume deficit depend on the rapidity and magnitude of its development. The key findings on physical assessment are interstitial and plasma volume depletion (Box 21-2). In the case of a large and rapid loss of volume as in hemorrhage, massive diarrhea, or massive sequestration in a third space, the signs and symptoms are synonymous with circulatory collapse and shock. In most cases, however, the development of a fluid volume deficit occurs more gradually.

General symptoms of moderate-to-severe volume depletion include weakness, lassitude, fatigue, and anorexia. An early sign of plasma volume depletion is orthostatic hypotension, with a decrease in blood pressure of at least 10 mm Hg and an increase in heart rate with postural changes. Tachycardia develops as the heart attempts to maintain tissue perfusion. Arterial pulses are weak and thready. The patient may become dizzy while sitting or standing. The peripheral veins, such as the hand veins, may be collapsed and fill slowly when the hand is held in a dependent position. Other signs of a decrease in

---

BOX 21-2

ECF Volume Deficit: Clinical Features

SIGNS AND SYMPTOMS
Lassitude, weakness, and fatigue (early)
Anorexia
Thirst
Orthostatic hypotension (>10 mm Hg drop in systemic blood pressure)
Tachycardia
Dizziness, syncope
Altered level of consciousness
Decreased body temperature unless infection present
Cold extremities (late)
Prolonged filling time of hand veins (>3-5 seconds)
Flat jugular veins in supine position
Falling central venous pressure (CVP)
Sticky oral mucosa
Dry, furrowed tongue (normally, only one longitudinal furrow in midline)
Poor skin turgor
Oliguria (<30 ml/hr)
Rapid loss of body weight:
    2% loss = mild deficit
    5% loss = moderate deficit
    8% loss = severe deficit

LABORATORY FINDINGS
Increased hematocrit
Increased serum protein level
Normal serum Na^+ (usually)
BUN and serum creatinine ratio >20:1 (normal = 10:1)
Urine specific gravity high
Urine osmolality >450 mOsm/kg
Urine Na^+ <10 mEq/L (extrarenal cause)
Urine Na^+ >20 mEq/L (renal or adrenal causes)

---

the venous volume include flat jugular veins and low central venous pressure, reflecting decreased venous return to the right side of the heart.

Decreased interstitial volume may be recognized by decreased tissue and tongue turgor. Dry mucous membranes, oliguria, and thirst are other signs of fluid volume depletion. The oliguria results from the actions of antidiuretic hormone and of aldosterone, both of which are secreted in response to volume contraction. Weight loss is another cardinal sign of fluid volume deficit, which may be used to estimate the magnitude of the loss, with the exception of third-space sequestration of fluid.

No single diagnostic test confirms fluid volume deficit. Serum laboratory values vary, depending on the underlying cause of the fluid volume deficit. A rise in the blood urea nitrogen (BUN), serum proteins, hemoglobin, or hematocrit may indicate hemoconcentration (unless the condition is caused by hemorrhage, which results in decreased hemoglobin and hematocrit because all blood products are lost). These elevations may be difficult to discern, however, unless baseline values are known. It must be emphasized that in isotonic fluid volume losses, the serum sodium concentration will be normal because equal proportions of sodium and water are lost. Deviations of the serum sodium concentration above or below normal levels indicate disproportionate losses or gains of sodium and water and a disturbance in osmolality. Volume imbalances, however, may be combined with osmolality disturbances (see the discussion of osmolality imbalances).

The response of the kidney to volume depletion is to conserve sodium and water. Consequently, a small volume of concentrated urine (high osmolality or high specific gravity) with a low sodium concentration is excreted when the kidneys are functioning normally. In fact, low urine sodium concentration is virtually pathognomonic of reduced tissue perfusion (Rose, 2001). However, a low urine sodium concentration does not necessarily mean that true fluid volume deficit exists, because some edematous conditions such as congestive heart failure with a decrease in effective circulating volume may result in a low urine sodium concentration. Differentiation between edema states and true volume depletion is easily made from physical assessment. The urinary sodium concentration is helpful in identifying the cause of true fluid volume deficit. With extrarenal losses, urinary sodium is less than 10 mEq/L; the concentration will usually exceed 20 mEq/L when renal or adrenal disorders are at fault.

A final characteristic of moderate-to-severe fluid volume deficit is a rise in the BUN and plasma creatinine, resulting from decreased renal perfusion and glomerular filtration rate (GFR). BUN tends to rise proportionately more than serum creatinine. This finding is termed *prerenal azotemia*. The disproportionate rise in the BUN reflects enhanced renal tubular reabsorption of urea, which accompanies tubular reabsorption of sodium and water. Azotemia in this setting must be regarded as a physiologic trade-off for homeostatic mechanisms otherwise geared to defend the ECF volume by enhancing sodium and water reabsorption. Prolonged renal hypoperfusion and prerenal azotemia may progress to acute renal failure, thus they should be promptly corrected (see Chapter 49).

Treatment

The goal of treatment for an isotonic fluid volume deficit is to restore normovolemia and treat any associated acid-base or electrolyte imbalances. The underlying cause of the fluid volume deficit must also be treated. Bleeding must be controlled. Vomiting may be treated with antiemetics and diarrhea with antidiarrheal drugs.

When a mild volume deficit occurs, increasing dietary sodium and water intake in patients not suffering from GI disorders may be sufficient to correct the imbalance. Severe depletion requires therapy with intravenous (IV) solutions. Isotonic saline (0.9%) is the infusion of choice in patients whose serum sodium concentration is approximately normal, because it will expand the plasma volume. As soon as the patient is normotensive, one-half normal saline (0.45%) may be ordered to provide free water to the cells and help eliminate metabolic waste products.

When the patient with severe fluid volume deficit is oliguric, it is necessary to determine whether the depressed renal function is the result of reduced renal blood flow and secondary to the fluid volume deficit (prerenal azotemia) or, more seriously, secondary to acute tubular necrosis (a form of acute renal failure) from prolonged renal ischemia. In this situation, an initial bolus of IV fluid is given in a fluid challenge test to deter-

---

BOX 21-3

Guidelines for IV Fluid Requirements

GENERAL RULES
1. Provide for maintenance needs and make up for losses
2. Replace concurrent losses volume for volume
3. Administer evenly over 24 hours except in unusual circumstances

24-HOUR VOLUME NEEDED PER SQUARE METER OF BSA
1. Maintenance   1500 ml/m² BSA
2. Moderate fluid volume deficit + maintenance (acute weight loss <5%)   2400 ml/m² BSA
3. Severe fluid volume deficit + maintenance (acute weight loss >5%)   3000 ml/m² BSA

BODY WEIGHT TO BSA CONVERSIONS FOR PERSONS OF AVERAGE BUILD

Weight kg	lb	Approximate BSA in m²
3	6.6	0.20
6	13.2	0.30
10	22.0	0.45
20	44.0	0.80
40	88.0	1.30
50	110.0	1.50
57	125.4	1.60
70	154.0	1.76
85	187.0	2.00

EXAMPLES OF CALCULATIONS
Maintenance needs for a 125-lb woman who is taking nothing by mouth and has no abnormal losses:

24-hour IV fluid needs = 1.60 × 1500 ml = 2400 ml

IV fluid needs for a 70-kg man who has been vomiting for 2 days and has a moderate fluid volume deficit:

24-hour IV fluid needs = 1.76 × 2400 ml = 4224

---

mine whether urine flow will increase, which indicates normal renal function. In the case of prerenal azotemia and normal renal function, the fluid volume deficit is easier to treat, but the treatment becomes more complicated in the case of acute tubular necrosis (see Chapter 49).

The amount of IV solution to be infused cannot be precisely determined. However, the history, intake and output record, and record of daily weights provide an estimate of the magnitude of losses. Box 21-3 provides a general guide for the volume of fluid needed for maintenance and replacement based on body surface area and the severity of the deficit (Metheny, Snively, 1979).

The need to correct other concurrent electrolyte abnormalities may alter the composition of the required infusion. For example, potassium may be added to the IV solution when concurrent potassium depletion occurs. Lactated Ringer's solution may be given to patients with metabolic acidosis and fluid volume depletion. This solution contains sodium lactate, which is slowly metabolized to sodium bicarbonate in the body, and can help correct the acidosis.

Because numerous factors affect the type and rate of IV infusion (e.g., cardiac and renal status) and the required volume cannot be precisely determined, the best approach is to monitor the patient's response to the IV therapy to avoid fluid overload and pulmonary edema.

Metheny (2000) provides detailed guidelines on the care of patients undergoing IV therapy.

Extracellular Fluid Volume Excess

ECF volume excess develops when both sodium and water are retained in roughly the same proportions. As excessive isotonic fluid accumulates in the ECF (hypervolemia), fluid shifts into the interstitial fluid compartment, causing edema. Fluid volume excess is always secondary to an increase in total body sodium content, which, in turn, causes water retention.

Pathogenesis

Edema is defined as an excessive accumulation of interstitial fluid. Edema may be either localized (as occurs with local inflammation or obstruction) or generalized, thus interstitial fluid accumulates in virtually every tissue of the body. In either case, the proximate cause of the edema is always an alteration in one of the critical Starling forces that govern the distribution of fluid between the capillaries and interstitial spaces. Thus edema may result from increased capillary hydrostatic pressure, decreased colloid osmotic pressure, increased capillary permeability, or obstruction to lymphatic flow (see Chapter 20). This discussion focuses on disorders of fluid volume excess associated with generalized edema.

The presence of generalized edema indicates a disturbance in the normal regulation of the ECF. The three most common conditions resulting in generalized edema are congestive heart failure, cirrhosis of the liver, and the nephrotic syndrome (Box 21-4). Each one of these disorders is characterized by a defect in at least one of the Starling capillary forces and by renal retention of sodium and water. The retention of sodium by the kidney in edema-forming states results from one or two basic mechanisms: the response to effective circulating volume depletion or primary renal dysfunction.

Effective circulating volume is an immeasurable entity that refers to the intravascular fluid effectively perfusing the tissues and is generally directly proportional to the CO. Thus, when CO is decreased, the kidney retains sodium and water in an attempt to restore the circulating volume. A decrease in the effective circulating volume is believed to be the mechanism responsible for renal sodium retention in congestive heart failure, liver cirrhosis, and the nephrotic syndrome. In all of these conditions, renal excretory function is intrinsically normal and enhanced renal reabsorption is presumably initiated by the sympathetic nervous system and the renin-angiotensin-aldosterone system. In other words, the kidneys act as if the ECF volume were truly contracted and retain sodium and water despite massive accumulation of fluid in the interstitial space.

In contrast with these mechanisms of edema, edema associated with advanced renal failure results from intrinsic impairment of renal excretory function. Another condition associated with ECF excess includes Cushing's syndrome or corticosteroid therapy because of increased aldosterone activity. Starvation resulting in hypoproteinemia is also associated with edema. Finally, the rapid administration of IV saline may result in hypervolemia.

Clinical Features

Box 21-5 lists the signs and symptoms and laboratory values commonly associated with ECF volume excess. Generally, acute weight gain is the best indicator of ECF volume excess because several liters of fluid can be retained without visible evidence of edema. Gravitational forces that impinge on capillary hydrostatic pressure largely govern the distribution of generalized edema. Thus edema usually develops where capillary hydrostatic pressure is highest (dependent areas, such as the legs or sacral area in a bedridden patient) or where interstitial pressure is lowest (periorbital, facial, scrotal areas). When the finger is pressed over an area of edema, the indentation will remain briefly as the fluid is pushed to another area; this is called *pitting edema*. Fluid then fills the "pit" gradually. The degree of edema may be classified subjectively on a scale of 1+ to 4+ (barely discernible to pitting edema), based on the length of time for fluid to refill the pit.

Pulmonary edema, indicated by moist rales over the lung fields and other signs of respiratory distress, is one manifestation of ECF volume excess that warrants urgent therapy. Pulmonary edema occurs most commonly in patients with left ventricular failure, a condition characterized by elevated hydrostatic pressure within pulmonary capillaries. In edematous disorders mediated by reductions in colloid osmotic pressure (e.g., cirrhosis,

---

BOX 21-4

Causes of ECF Volume Excess

Altered regulatory mechanisms
  CHF
  Cirrhosis of the liver
  Nephrotic syndrome
Renal failure
Cushing's syndrome; corticosteroid therapy
Starvation (hypoalbuminemia)
Rapid infusion of IV saline

BOX 21-5

ECF Volume Excess: Clinical Features

SIGNS AND SYMPTOMS
Jugular venous distention
Elevated central venous pressure (>11 cm water)
Elevated blood pressure
Full, bounding pulse
Slow emptying of hand veins (>3-5 seconds)
Peripheral and periorbital edema
Ascites
Pleural effusion
Acute pulmonary edema (when severe)
  Dyspnea, tachypnea
  Moist rales over lung fields
Rapid weight gain
  2% gain = mild excess
  5% gain = moderate excess
  8% gain = severe excess

LABORATORY FINDINGS
Decreased hematocrit
Low serum proteins
Normal serum Na^+
Low urinary Na^+ (<10 mEq/24 hr)

nephrotic syndrome), frank pulmonary edema is uncommon in the absence of underlying cardiac disease.

Patients with fluid volume excess may accumulate fluid in body cavities. Patients with cirrhosis, in particular, may accumulate fluid in the peritoneal cavity (ascites) because of increased hydrostatic pressure in the portal vasculature. Other signs of fluid volume overload include increased blood pressure, bounding pulse, and slow emptying of hand veins. Jugular venous distention and a rising central venous pressure are other signs of fluid volume excess.

Laboratory findings are not helpful in identifying fluid volume excess. Serum sodium concentration is normal unless an associated osmolality imbalance occurs. Hematocrit is decreased below the patient's baseline level owing to hemodilution. Urine sodium excretion is usually low (<10 mEq/day) because edematous patients are maximally conserving sodium (Schrier, 1997).

Treatment

Treatment of fluid volume excess and edematous states depends on understanding all the factors, both primary and secondary, that caused the problem and treating the underlying causes when possible. Most treatment plans include the restriction of sodium and fluid intake.

Development of acute pulmonary edema with hypoxemia is a life-threatening situation that requires prompt treatment using measures to reduce preload and restore pulmonary gas exchange as rapidly as possible. These measures include positioning the patient in high Fowler's position and administering morphine, a rapidly acting diuretic such as furosemide, and oxygen. In severe cases of acute pulmonary edema, the use of rotating tourniquets to sequester fluid in the limbs may be helpful. To prevent fluid volume excess and acute pulmonary edema, the rate of administration of IV fluids and patient response must be carefully monitored. Patients who are older or those who have compromised cardiac or renal function are particularly vulnerable to acute pulmonary edema. In situations other than acute pulmonary edema, the reduction of edema fluid should be accomplished more slowly.

Congestive heart failure is generally treated with digitalis, diuretics, and dietary sodium restriction. Cirrhosis of the liver is treated with a low-sodium diet and diuretics. Administering corticosteroids to patients with the nephrotic syndrome may diminish proteinuria and thereby correct the hypoalbuminemia, which is the primary mechanism that causes edema. Edema caused by malnutrition responds well to adequate dietary intake, particularly with the addition of protein foods. Conservative measures, such as bed rest and support hose, help mobilize edematous fluid.

OSMOLALITY IMBALANCES

In contrast to the volume disturbances that have been discussed, osmolality imbalances involve the concentration of solutes in the body fluids. Because sodium is the major osmotically active solute in the ECF, in most cases hypoosmolality represents hyponatremia and hyperosmolality represents hypernatremia. One notable exception is the hyperglycemia resulting from uncontrolled diabetes mellitus.

Osmolality imbalances affect the distribution of water between the ECF and ICF compartments because water moves from areas of greater water concentration (i.e., lesser solute concentration, lesser osmolality) to areas of lesser water concentration (i.e., greater solute concentration, greater osmolality). The movement of water between compartments continues until osmotic equilibrium is achieved. Loss or gain of water relative to solute or a loss or gain of solute relative to water causes osmolality imbalances.

Hypoosmolality imbalances are caused by either water excess or sodium depletion. Either a water deficit or ECF sodium excess causes hyperosmolality imbalances. Most osmolality imbalances, however, are caused by a combination of sodium and water excesses and deficits. Hypoosmolality imbalances result in ICF water excess (cell swelling), whereas hyperosmolality imbalances result in ICF water depletion (cell shrinkage).

History, signs and symptoms, and laboratory values, notably the serum sodium concentration are used to identify osmolality imbalances. Treatment of hypoosmolality imbalances involves removal of excess water or sodium replacement; treatment of hyperosmolality imbalances involves replacement of pure water or hypotonic IV solutions or removal of excess sodium or glucose.

Hyponatremia (Hypoosmolality Imbalance)

A serum sodium level less than 135 mEq/L defines hyponatremia (normal serum sodium, 140 ± 5 mEq/L), which may result from two primary mechanisms: water retention or sodium loss. Hyponatremia indicates that an excess of water relative to total solute dilutes the body fluids. Because sodium is the primary ECF ion, hyponatremia is generally associated with plasma hypoosmolality (<287 mOsm/kg). Low plasma osmolality results in water movement into the cells. Swelling of brain cells, which causes increased intracranial pressure, is primarily responsible for associated central nervous system (CNS) symptoms.

Etiology and Pathogenesis

The causes of hyponatremia are presented in Box 21-6. Hyponatremia associated with sodium loss is called *depletional hyponatremia* and is characterized by contraction of the ECF volume. Hyponatremia caused by water excess is called *dilutional hyponatremia* or *water intoxication* and is characterized by expansion of the ECF volume.

Sodium loss that causes depletional hyponatremia can result from renal and nonrenal mechanisms. Common renal causes are diuretics and, less commonly, a salt-losing renal disease. Nonrenal salt loss occurs with fluid volume losses as in vomiting, diarrhea, or adrenal deficiency (low aldosterone). The mechanism of the sodium-loss type of hyponatremia involves two steps. First, the loss of sodium lowers the Na:H_2O ratio. Second, and more indirectly, the loss of sodium results in ECF volume contraction and, as a result, antidiuretic hormone (ADH) release from the posterior pituitary. ADH prevents the excretion of dilute urine and can produce hyponatremia when

Causes of Hyponatremia (Hypoosmolality Imbalance)

LOSS OF SODIUM IN EXCESS OF WATER
Prolonged diuretic therapy with low-salt diet
Excessive GI losses (vomiting, diarrhea, nasogastric [NG] suctioning, irrigation of NG tube with tap water, excessive amounts of ice chips given to patients with NG suction)
Replacement of lost body fluids (as from diaphoresis, hemorrhage, or third-space transudation) with only water or other Na^{++}-free fluids
Renal failure with impaired ability to conserve sodium when necessary
Adrenal deficiency (Addison's disease)

GAIN OF WATER IN EXCESS OF SODIUM
Decreased ability to excrete free water
  Effective circulating volume depletion (CHF, nephrotic syndrome, cirrhosis)
  Renal failure
  Excessive use of diuretics
Excessive IV administration of hypotonic fluids
Excessive administration of tap water enemas
SIADH
Compulsive water drinking (psychogenic polydipsia)
Freshwater drowning

HYPONATREMIA WITHOUT SERUM HYPOOSMOLALITY
Osmotic (hyperglycemia, mannitol)

TYPES OF HYPONATREMIA
Associated with ECF volume depletion (see Box 21-1)
Associated with ECF volume excess and edema (see Box 21-4)
Associated with normal ECF volume

Origin of High ADH in Hyponatremia

INCREASED HYPOTHALAMIC PRODUCTION OF ADH
CNS disorders*
  Head injury, cerebrovascular accidents
  Brain tumors
  Encephalitis
  Guillain-Barré syndrome
Pulmonary disorders
  Pneumonia*
  Tuberculosis
  Mechanical ventilation
Endocrine disorders
  Hypothyroidism
  Addison's disease
Postoperative states* (particularly after heart surgery)
Excessive pain (during postoperative period) and vomiting

ECTOPIC (NONHYPOTHALAMIC) PRODUCTION OF ADH
Malignancies, particularly oat-cell carcinoma of lung*

EXOGENOUS ADMINISTRATION OF ADH
Vasopressin
Oxytocin* (ADH-like agent) for labor induction, particularly when given with sodium-free IV fluids

POTENTIATION OF ENDOGENOUS ADH BY CERTAIN DRUGS
Oral hypoglycemic agents (chlorpropamide* [Diabinese])
Tricyclic antidepressants (amitriptyline [Elavil])
Morphine/barbiturates
Cholinergic (nicotine)
Antineoplastics (vincristine, cyclophosphamide*)
Anticonvulsant (carbamazepine)
Antilipemic (clofibrate)
Isoproterenol (Isuprel)
Prostaglandin inhibitors (aspirin, indomethacin)

*Most common conditions causing SIADH.

water is ingested. Hyponatremia per se is usually of little clinical significance in sodium (volume) depletion. Reduction of serum sodium by more than 10 to 15 mEq/L is rare. The major features are those of ECF volume contraction.

Dilutional hyponatremia (water excess) is commonly observed in conditions characterized by a defect in renal free-water excretion with continued intake, particularly of hypotonic fluids. Effective circulating volume depletion, as in congestive heart failure, nephrotic syndrome, and cirrhosis, provides a central stimulus to ADH release, primarily via low-pressure (venous) receptors, even in the presence of hypoosmolality, thus dilute urine cannot be excreted. ADH also stimulates thirst (water intake must be present to develop hyponatremia). ADH release in this circumstance (low ECF volume) is considered appropriate because ADH release helps maintain tissue perfusion, albeit at the expense of decreasing plasma osmotic concentration and increasing total body water.

ADH release in the absence of hyperosmolality, decreased effective circulating volume, and other physiologic stimuli is said to be "inappropriate." Thus patients with this type of hyponatremia are said to have a syndrome of inappropriate ADH (SIADH) secretion. SIADH is more common than previously recognized and is associated with a large number of neoplastic, pulmonary, and CNS disorders (Box 21-7). The autonomous release of ADH can be caused by abnormal stimulation of the hypothalamus by disease, pain, drugs, or CNS dysfunc-

tion. ADH-like substances may also be produced ectopically in malignancies, particularly oat-cell carcinoma of the lung. In addition, SIADH occurs as a complication of therapy with a large variety of drugs. Some of these drugs augment the hypothalamic release of ADH, whereas others enhance the action of ADH on the renal distal tubule and collecting ducts.

Other causes of dilutional hyponatremia include renal failure, in which impaired ability to dilute the urine occurs, and the excessive use of diuretics (see Box 21-6). Psychogenic polydipsia is a rare neurotic disorder characterized by compulsive water drinking, sometimes as much as 15 to 20 L/day. Although renal function capacity is normal in psychogenic polydipsia, the large intake of water exceeds the normal excretory capacity, resulting in mild hyponatremia. A similar disorder may also occur in excessive beer drinkers with a poor dietary intake. For example, when the maximum urine diluting ability is 50 mOsm/kg in a person who eats a normal diet (solute particles = approximately 750 mOsm/day), the most urine that person can excrete is 15 L/day (750 mOsm/50 mOsm = 15). However, the daily solute load may be only 250 mOsm in an excessive beer drinker who does not eat well, thus maximum daily urine output would be only approximately 5 L (250 mOsm/50 mOsm = 5). Finally, dilutional hyponatremia results when a large volume of water enters the lungs and is rapidly absorbed into the intravascular compartment during freshwater drowning.

Hyponatremia caused by the accumulation of osmotically active solutes in the plasma is the sole exception to the rule that hyponatremia means hypoosmolality. The most common cause of this type of hyponatremia is the hyperglycemia of uncontrolled diabetes and a history of recent administration of mannitol. Plasma sodium is diluted by movement of water from the ICF to the ECF along the osmotic gradient produced by the additional solute particles (glucose or mannitol).

Clinical Features

A high degree of suspicion is mandatory to detect hyponatremia, because the clinical manifestations are mainly nonspecific during the early period when the serum sodium is greater than approximately 120 mEq/L. Hyponatremia is a common electrolyte disorder among hospitalized patients. Patients who present one or more risk factors need to be monitored carefully so that hyponatremia may be identified and treated early in its course before it becomes life threatening.

Signs and symptoms of hyponatremia primarily reflect neurologic dysfunction induced by hypoosmolality. As the serum osmolality falls, water enters brain cells (as well as other cells), causing intracellular overhydration and increased intracranial pressure. The severity of the neurologic symptoms is related to the rapidity and the severity of the reduction of the serum Na^+ concentration. Box 21-8 provides a rough correlation between the signs and symptoms and the degree of reduction in the serum Na^+ concentration. The patient may not have any symptoms with mild hyponatremia (serum Na^+ levels above 125 mEq/L). The earliest symptoms, including lethargy, anorexia, nausea, and muscle cramps, may occur when the serum Na^+ is 120 to 125 mEq/L and progress to convulsions and coma with further reductions. When hyponatremia of this magnitude (<120 mEq/L) develops in less than 24 hours, the mortality rate reaches 50%. By contrast, patients remain relatively asymptomatic when the serum Na^+ is reduced to comparable levels over a period of days to weeks. Slowly developing hyponatremia causes milder symptoms because of the compensatory loss of solutes such as Na^+, K^+, and amino acids from brain cells so that the degree of intracellular swelling is lessened (Rose, 2001).

The diagnosis of hyponatremia, as with other fluid and electrolyte imbalances, involves analysis of findings from the history, clinical signs and symptoms, and laboratory tests. Three simple laboratory tests are helpful in diagnosing the cause of hyponatremia: serum osmolality, urine osmolality, and urine Na^+. Serum osmolality levels will be normal or high when the cause of hyponatremia is renal failure or diabetic hyperglycemia. Urine osmolality level is low (<100 mOsm/kg or specific gravity <1.004) when the cause is primary polydipsia with normal water excretion and high (>100 mOsm/kg or specific >1.004) for other causes of hyponatremia in which water excretion is impaired. Finally, urinary Na^+ is low (<10 mEq/L) when the hyponatremia is associated with edema or volume depletion caused by extrarenal causes; urinary Na^+ is high (>20 mEq/L) when renal salt wasting or SIADH is present.

BOX 21-8
Hyponatremia: Clinical Features

SIGNS AND SYMPTOMS
Serum Na^+ <125 mEq/L:
Anorexia
Impaired taste
Muscle cramps

Serum Na^+ = 115-120 mEq/L:
Headache, personality changes
Weakness and lethargy
Nausea and vomiting
Abdominal cramps

Serum Na^+ <115 mEq/L:
Seizures and coma
Absent or diminished reflexes
Babinski's sign
Papilledema
Fingerprinting edema over sternum

LABORATORY FINDINGS
Serum Na^+ <135 mEq/L (may be very low, <100 mEq/L, in SIADH)
Serum osmolality <287 mOsm/kg
Urine osmolality low (<100 mOsm/kg) with normal water excretion as in psychogenic polydipsia or urine specific gravity <1.004
Urine osmolality or specific gravity inappropriately high (>100 mOsm/kg) with respect to low serum osmolality or specific gravity >1.004 in other causes of hyponatremia
Urinary Na^+ <10 mEq/L when associated with edema or volume depletion from extrarenal causes
Urinary sodium >20 mEq/L when associated with renal salt losses or renal failure with water retention or SIADH

Treatment

The goals of treatment for patients with hypoosmolality and true hyponatremia are to elevate the serum Na^+ toward normal and to treat the underlying cause. The two basic treatments are restricting water or administering Na^+, depending on the severity and underlying cause.

Mild hyponatremia (120 to 135 mEq/L) in patients with true volume depletion from GI or renal losses is treated with oral sodium chloride (NaCl) or normal saline given IV. Correction of the hypovolemia suppresses ADH release, leading to renal excretion of excess water and correction of the hyponatremia. Correction of K^+ depletion is also another important aspect of treatment. In more severe cases of hyponatremia (<120 mEq/L), hypertonic saline may be given at a rate sufficient to raise the serum Na^+ 0.5 mEq/L per hour until a serum Na^+ level of approximately 120 mEq/L is reached and the patient is out of danger. Care must be taken not to raise the serum Na^+ too rapidly, which may cause central pontine myelinosis and irreversible neurologic damage (Rose, 2001).

In addition to correcting the underlying disorder whenever possible, water restriction constitutes the first line of therapy in patients with dilutional hyponatremia and increased ECF because the administration of Na^+ worsens the condition. Restricting water intake to less than urine output is usually sufficient to correct the hyponatremia. In more severe cases, hypertonic saline in combination with a loop diuretic can raise the serum Na^+ more quickly.

Water restriction alone is often an effective treatment for mild cases of SIADH. Removing the cause of the ADH release, such as discontinuing the offending drug or recovering from the offending disease process, may help to resolve the problem. The treatment of severe cases of hyponatremia may require the administration of a small volume of hypertonic saline in addition to restriction of fluid intake and administration of a loop diuretic. In chronic cases caused by the ectopic production of ADH, demeclocycline, a drug that blocks the effect of ADH on the renal tubule, may be given to treat SIADH.

The treatment of the hyponatremia associated with diabetic hyperglycemic states is not directed toward raising the serum Na^+ because this condition does not represent a true hyponatremia. Rather, the treatment involves the administration of insulin and glucose.

Hypernatremia (Hyperosmolality Imbalance)

Hypernatremia is defined by the presence of a serum Na^+ level greater than 145 mEq/L and is always associated with hyperosmolality because Na^+ salts are the main determinants of the plasma osmolality. The rise in serum osmolality causes water to shift from the ICF to the ECF, resulting in cell dehydration and shrinkage. The basic causes are water loss in excess of Na^+ or Na^+ gain in excess of water.

Etiology and Pathogenesis

Box 21-9 lists the major causes of hypernatremia and hyperosmolality. These causes are classified as insufficient water intake with or without loss of water in excess of Na^+ and Na^+ gain. The major protective mechanism against hypernatremia is thirst and renal water conservation stimulated by ADH when the serum solute or Na^+ concentration increases. Hypernatremia rarely occurs except when a disturbance in water intake occurs in combination with hypotonic fluid loss. Inadequate water intake is most common in older adults who have a disturbance in level of consciousness, in the very young who have inadequate access to water, or in a rare instance of a person with a primary disturbance in thirst. Hypotonic water losses may be caused by nonrenal or renal losses that are not replaced. Water loss from the respiratory tract and skin (a hypotonic fluid) is normally slightly under 1 L/day. However, losses may increase dramatically in patients who are febrile and hyperventilating or exposed to a hot environment. Central diabetes insipidus and nephrogenic diabetes insipidus are conditions in which either ADH secretion or its renal effect is impaired, leading to the excretion of large volumes of hypoosmotic urine. Central diabetes insipidus occurs in patients with a CNS lesion, particularly after head injury. Nephrogenic diabetes insipidus is associated with hypokalemia and a number of drugs and disease processes and is not discussed further in this chapter. Osmotic diuresis is another major cause of renal water loss. Glycosuria in uncontrolled diabetes mellitus is the most common cause of osmotic diuresis. Osmotic diuresis may also be caused by the urea produced from high-protein tube feedings or with mannitol administration.

BOX 21-9

Causes of Hypernatremia (Hyperosmolality Imbalance)

INSUFFICIENT WATER INTAKE
Unable to perceive or respond to thirst (e.g., comatose, confused)
Nothing by mouth without sufficient IV maintenance
Unable to swallow (e.g., cerebrovascular accident)

EXCESSIVE WATER LOSS
Nonrenal
    Fever or diaphoresis or both
    Burns
    Hyperventilation
    Prolonged use of mechanical ventilator
    Watery diarrhea
Renal
    Diabetes insipidus (central, nephrogenic)
    Head trauma (particularly basal skull fracture)
    Neurosurgery
    Infection (encephalitis, meningitis)
    Brain neoplasm
    Osmotic diuresis
    Glycosuria in uncontrolled diabetes
    Urea diuresis in high-protein tube feedings
    Mannitol

SODIUM GAIN
Seawater drowning
Excessive use of IV sodium salts
    Hypertonic saline (3% or 5%)
    Excessive IV sodium bicarbonate used to treat cardiac arrest
    Isotonic saline
Accidental replacement of sugar with salt in infant formula
Therapeutic abortion with accidental entry of hypertonic saline into circulation

TYPES OF HYPERNATREMIA
Associated with normal ECF volume
Associated with ECF volume depletion
Associated with ECF volume excess

Hypernatremia caused by an absolute excess of Na^+ is much less common than that caused by water depletion. Some examples that involve intake of Na^+ via the lungs, IV, or orally include seawater drowning (a hypertonic saline solution), IV administration of saline solutions, and accidental ingestion of large amounts of salt orally. Therapeutic abortion has caused a death on rare occasions when the hypertonic saline used to induce the abortion entered the maternal bloodstream.

Hypernatremia may be associated with normovolemia (usually caused by insensible water loss), hypovolemia (loss of water in excess of Na^+), and hypervolemia (relatively greater gain of Na^+ than of water).

Clinical Features

The most prominent manifestations of hypernatremic and hyperosmotic imbalances are neurologic and result from cellular dehydration, particularly of brain cells (Box 21-10). Lethargy, agitation, irritability, hyperreflexia, and spasticity may occur, culminating in coma, seizures, and death. Thirst is the major symptom of hypernatremia, although its absence or the inability to communicate may

Hypernatremia: Clinical Features

SIGNS AND SYMPTOMS
Neurologic
    Early: lethargy, weakness, irritability
    Severe: agitation, mania, delirium, seizures, coma
    Increased deep tendon reflexes
    Nuchal rigidity
Thirst
Elevated body temperature
Flushed skin
Dry, sticky mucous membranes
Tongue rough, red, and dry

LABORATORY FINDINGS
Serum Na^+ >145 mEq/L
Serum osmolality >295 mOsm/kg
Urine osmolality usually >800 mOsm/kg (specific gravity
    >1.030)

be an underlying cause. Other clinical findings include dry, sticky mucous membranes; flushed skin; and a dry, rough, red tongue. Oliguria or anuria may be present, and the patient may be febrile.

The morbidity and mortality of acute hypernatremia in children are high; approximately 45% die, and two thirds of those who survive have serious neurologic sequelae. In adults, acute elevations of the serum Na^+ above 160 mEq/L are associated with a 75% mortality rate, whereas mortality in chronic cases is approximately 60% (Schrier, 1997). The mechanism of brain injury resulting in death is brain hemorrhage from the shrinkage of brain cells, causing tearing of cerebral blood vessels.

The diagnosis of hypernatremia is made from the signs and symptoms and measurement of serum Na^+ and osmolality. The cause can usually be inferred from the history when extrarenal water loss, an osmotic diuresis, or Na^+ excess lead to the condition. In these cases, the urine is hyperosmotic to plasma. The diagnosis of central diabetes insipidus is usually easy to confirm because the patient has a CNS problem plus a history of polyuria (3 to 10 L/day) and polydipsia (excessive thirst, usually preferring cold liquids).

Treatment

The primary goal in the treatment of hypernatremia involves gradually lowering serum Na^+ to the normal range and restoring normal serum osmolality. The therapeutic approach depends on the underlying pathophysiologic mechanism causing the hypernatremia. Free water can be given orally or as IV glucose in water (D_5W) to the patient who is normovolemic and has hypernatremia caused by pure water loss. When the patient is hypovolemic, IV isotonic saline is given to restore normal blood pressure and tissue perfusion, and hypotonic (0.45%) saline may be infused thereafter to provide free water and correct the hypernatremia. When the patient is both hypernatremic and hypervolemic, the goal is to remove the excess Na^+. Removal may be achieved either by the concurrent administration of diuretics and D_5W infusion or by dialysis when renal function is impaired.

Most authors recommend that the plasma Na^+ concentration be lowered to normal at a maximal rate of 2 mEq/hr. Rapid correction of hypernatremia is hazardous because it can induce cerebral edema, convulsions, permanent neurologic damage, and death (Rose, 2001). These complications occur because the administration of a hypotonic infusion renders the ECF temporarily hypoosmotic thus water moves from the ECF to the ICF, causing cerebral edema. Exogenous ADH (usually dDAVP [Desmopressin] in the form of a nasal spray) is administered in the treatment of central diabetes insipidus.

Finally, careful clinical observation of patients at risk for developing hypernatremia must be practiced to detect the condition before serious elevations of the serum Na^+ concentration occur. Serious elevations of serum Na^+ concentration do not usually occur except when the patient is unable to respond to thirst, thus special care must be taken to provide adequate water.

POTASSIUM IMBALANCES

Few of the disturbances in fluid and electrolyte metabolism are as frequently encountered or as immediately life-threatening as are disturbances in K^+ balance. The critical modulating effect of K^+ on neuromuscular conduction, particularly cardiac conduction, accounts for the fatalities and near fatalities that accompany either hypokalemia or hyperkalemia.

Physiologic Considerations

K^+ is the major cation of the intracellular fluid. In fact, 98% of the body's stores (3000 to 4000 mEq) are inside cells, and the remaining 2% (approximately 70 mEq) is located primarily in the ECF compartment. The normal range of serum K^+ is 3.5 to 5.5 mEq/L, in contrast with a concentration of approximately 160 mEq/L inside cells. Because K^+ constitutes a large proportion of the intracellular solute, it plays an important role in keeping fluid inside the cell and maintaining cell volume. The ECF K^+, although a small fraction of the total, greatly influences neuromuscular function. The difference in the concentration of K^+ in the ICF and that of the ECF compartments is maintained by an active Na-K pump in the cell membrane.

The ratio of the ICF to ECF K^+ concentration is the principal determinant of the cell membrane potential in excitable tissues, such as cardiac and skeletal muscle. The resting membrane potential sets the stage for the generation of the action potential that is essential for normal neural and muscular function. Because the concentration of ECF K^+ is so much lower than is the concentration inside the cell, small changes in the ECF K^+ can significantly alter this ratio. Conversely, only large changes in the ICF K^+ influence the ratio significantly. One practical consequence of this relationship is that the toxic effects of a severe hyperkalemia can be mitigated as an emergency treatment by inducing the movement of K^+ from the ECF to the ICF. In addition to playing a primary role in maintaining normal neuromuscular function, K^+ is an important cofactor in a number of metabolic processes.

The homeostasis of K^+ in the body is influenced by the distribution between the ECF and ICF, as well as the balance between intake and output. A number of hormonal and nonhormonal factors play a role in its regulation, including aldosterone, catecholamines, insulin, and acid-base variables.

In the healthy adult, the daily dietary intake of K^+ is approximately 50 to 100 mEq. After a meal, virtually all of the absorbed K^+ is first shifted into cells within minutes; thereafter K^+ excretion occurs primarily by the renal route over a period of hours. A smaller proportion (<20%) may be excreted in the sweat and feces. The shift of K^+ into the cells after a meal until renal excretion can occur is an important mechanism to prevent a dangerous hyperkalemia. Renal K^+ excretion is under the influence of aldosterone, distal tubule Na^+, and the urine flow rate. The secretion of aldosterone is stimulated by the amount of Na^+ reaching the distal tubule and an increase in the serum K^+ level above normal and is suppressed when the level decreases. Most of the K^+ filtered by the glomerulus is reabsorbed in the proximal tubule. Increased aldosterone then causes more K^+ to be secreted into the distal tubule in exchange for Na^+ or H^+ reabsorption. The secreted K^+ is then excreted in the urine. K^+ secretion in the distal tubule is also flow dependent, thus increased distal tubule delivery of fluid (polyuria) favors K^+ excretion.

Acid-base balance and hormones influence the distribution of K^+ between the ICF and ECF. Acidosis tends to shift K^+ out of cells, whereas alkalosis favors movement from the ECF to the ICF. The degree of shift is greater in metabolic acid-base disturbances and greater in alkalosis than it is in acidosis. Several hormones also influence the movement of K^+ between the ICF and ECF. Insulin and epinephrine stimulate K^+ movement into cells. Conversely, alpha-adrenergic agonists impair cellular K^+ uptake. These facts have important clinical implications for the treatment of DKA, which is discussed in Chapter 22.

Hypokalemia

Hypokalemia is defined as a serum K^+ concentration of less than 3.5 mEq/L. Because only 2% of the body K^+ is in the ECF, the serum K^+ value may not always reflect total body K^+. Additionally, the blood pH affects the serum K^+ as previously discussed. For every 0.1 unit fall in pH, the serum K^+ increases 0.5 mEq/L; for every 0.1 unit rise in pH, the serum K^+ decreases by 0.5 mEq/L.

Etiology and Pathogenesis

Box 21-11 lists the principal causes of hypokalemia: GI and urinary losses, inadequate K^+ intake, and K^+ shifts caused by alkalosis or the treatment of DKA with insulin and glucose. Moderate hypokalemia may result from K^+-deficient dietary intake alone or contribute to the hypokalemia caused by GI or renal losses. For example, the older adult who exists on tea and toast has little K^+ intake. The alcoholic who eats infrequently and poorly may likewise have a deficient K^+ intake. All seriously ill patients who are ingesting nothing by mouth should receive K^+ additives in their IV infusions because renal excretion of K^+ continues, even though no intake occurs.

GI disorders characterized by vomiting, nasogastric (NG) suction, diarrhea, or loss of other secretions are perhaps the most frequent causes of hypokalemia. The K^+ depletion that occurs with vomiting or NG suction

---

BOX 21-11

Causes of Hypokalemia

DECREASED DIETARY INTAKE OF K^+
Seriously ill patient with nothing by mouth for several days without K^+ supplement added to IV infusion
Starvation, tea and toast diet
Alcoholism

GASTROINTESTINAL LOSS
Protracted vomiting, NG suction
Diarrhea, chronic laxative abuse
Ileostomy, fistulas
Villous adenoma of colon

RENAL LOSS
Diuretic drugs (thiazides, furosemide)
Some renal diseases
    Diuretic recovery phase of acute renal failure
    Renal tubular acidosis
Diabetic acidosis leading to osmotic diuresis
Healing stage of severe burns
Excessive mineralocorticoid effect
    Primary or secondary hyperaldosteronism
    ECF volume deficit (by far, the most common cause)
    Cushing's syndrome; corticosteroid therapy
    Licorice ingestion (aldosterone-like activity)
    Swallowing chewing tobacco (contains large amounts of licorice)
Antibiotics (carbenicillin, aminoglycosides)
Magnesium (Mg^{++}) depletion

INCREASED LOSS IN SWEAT DURING HEAT STRESS
Heavily perspiring individual not acclimated to heat

SHIFT OF K^+ INTO CELLS
Metabolic alkalosis
Treatment of DKA with insulin and glucose

---

does not occur, primarily because of the K^+ lost in the gastric secretions. The K^+ content of gastric secretions is only 5 to 10 mEq/L. Rather, the hypokalemia associated with vomiting is primarily the result of increased renal excretion of K^+. The increased renal excretion of K^+ appears to involve three mechanisms: (1) loss of gastric acid leads to metabolic alkalosis, which stimulates a shift of K^+ into renal tubular cells; (2) metabolic alkalosis causes more sodium bicarbonate and fluid to be delivered to the distal tubule, and the bicarbonate (HCO_3^-, an anion) augments K^+ excretion; and (3) loss of gastric fluid causes ECF volume contraction, which, in turn, stimulates increased aldosterone secretion via the renin-angiotensin-aldosterone mechanism. Aldosterone stimulates K^+ excretion and helps to maintain the hypokalemia. Large amounts of K^+ can be lost directly from the lower GI tract when diarrhea is present. K^+ content in stool is often in the range of 40 to 70 mEq/L. Additionally, lower GI tract secretions are high in Na^+ and bicarbonate. Loss of large amounts of stool results in ECF volume contraction and metabolic acidosis, as well as K^+ depletion. The K^+ deficit may be difficult to assess because acidosis causes K^+ to shift out of the cells, raising the serum K^+ concentration and obscuring the actual total body deficit. Villous adenomas are potentially malignant tumors of the colon, which are associated with the loss of diarrheal fluid high in K^+ content.

The kidney can be a major site of K⁺ loss. Diuretics are among the most frequent causes of hypokalemia. Thiazides, loop diuretics, and carbonic anhydrase inhibitors all increase K⁺ loss in the urine. Many patients being treated for fluid volume excess have cardiac disease and are also receiving digitalis preparations. Hypokalemia augments the effect of digitalis, often resulting in toxic effects. Thus it is important to encourage eating K⁺-rich foods or to administer K⁺ supplements to these patients or both. Although end-stage renal disease generally results in hyperkalemia, some renal diseases, such as renal tubular acidosis and the diuretic recovery phase of acute renal failure, cause K⁺ loss and hypokalemia. K⁺ excretion is increased during an osmotic diuresis, which leads to K⁺ depletion in DKA. The solutes causing the polyuria are glucose and ketoacid anions. Acidosis and insulin deficiency cause K⁺ to shift from the ICF to the ECF enabling the serum K⁺ to be in the normal range, despite total body K⁺ depletion. When the DKA is corrected by the administration of IV glucose and insulin, a serious hypokalemia may result as the serum K⁺ shifts back into the cells. Patients with severe burns in the healing stage may develop hypokalemia because K⁺ may shift from the cells to the ECF and is then lost in the urine through diuresis.

Patients with primary hyperaldosteronism caused by an adrenal adenoma present with hypokalemia and metabolic alkalosis resulting from renal K⁺ wasting. ECF volume contraction is probably the most frequent cause of secondary hyperaldosteronism and K⁺ wasting, as previously discussed. However, patients with cirrhosis, congestive heart failure, and the nephrotic syndrome are usually not hypokalemic, despite secondary hyperaldosteronism (unless they receive diuretics), probably because decreased effective circulating plasma volume causes less Na⁺ and water to be delivered to the distal tubule. High levels of glucocorticoid hormones can exert a mineralocorticoid (aldosterone) effect, causing hypokalemia. Thus hypokalemia may be associated with Cushing's syndrome or the therapeutic administration of exogenous steroids. Finally, some forms of licorice contain a compound with aldosterone-like activity, which may cause hypokalemia with excessive ingestion. This cause of hypokalemia is not generally a problem in the United States because an artificial licorice flavoring is used. However, chewing tobacco contains large amounts of true licorice, which can cause K⁺ wasting when swallowed.

Certain antibiotics, such as carbenicillin, can cause hypokalemia by acting as an anion and increasing K⁺ excretion. Magnesium depletion can apparently cause K⁺ depletion through urinary and fecal losses, although the exact mechanism is not understood. Hypomagnesemia and hypokalemia frequently occur together in alcoholics.

Normally only a small amount of K⁺ is lost in perspiration. However, the K⁺ content of sweat may increase in persons not acclimated to a hot environment. People who have not acclimated and exercise in a hot environment may lose several liters of fluid per day. Hypokalemia may occur unless K⁺ intake is appropriately increased.

Clinical Features

Box 21-12 lists the signs and symptoms and laboratory findings in hypokalemia. The most prominent features of

---

BOX 21-12

Hypokalemia: Clinical Features

SIGNS AND SYMPTOMS
CNS and neuromuscular
 Early symptoms are vague: fatigue, "not feeling well"
 Paresthesias
 Diminished deep tendon reflexes
 Generalized muscle weakness
Respiratory
 Weak respiratory muscles, shallow respirations (advanced)
Gastrointestinal
 Decreased bowel motility: anorexia, nausea, vomiting, ileus
Cardiovascular
 Postural hypotension
 Dysrhythmias (particularly when digitalis or heart disease present)
 ECG changes
  Broad, progressively flat T waves (sometimes inverted)
  ST segment depression
  Prominent U wave
Renal
 Polyuria, nocturia (concentrating defect)

LABORATORY FINDINGS
Serum K⁺ <3.5 mEq/L
Serum pH >7.45; elevated serum HCO₃⁻ (hypokalemia often associated with metabolic alkalosis)

---

hypokalemia are reflected in the neuromuscular status, and the most serious complication is cardiac arrest, which is more apt to occur when the depletion has been rapid (e.g., treatment of DKA with insulin and glucose without K⁺ additives). Patients with hypokalemia may experience muscle weakness or leg cramps. GI smooth muscle dysfunction results in decreased bowel motility, with progression to paralytic ileus and abdominal distention. The respiratory muscles may be affected with profound hypokalemia. Paresthesias and diminished deep tendon reflexes are other manifestations. Cardiac dysrhythmias and electrocardiogram (ECG) changes are important manifestations of hypokalemia, which become increasingly abnormal and life threatening in rough parallel with the severity of K⁺ depletion. The major effect of hypokalemia on cardiac conduction is prolonged repolarization, resulting in increasingly flattened T waves. The U wave increases in magnitude and ST segment depression occurs with severe hypokalemia (Fig. 21-1). A variety of atrial and ventricular dysrhythmias may occur, particularly in patients receiving digitalis because hypokalemia increases sensitivity to this drug. It is important to remember that patients can be asymptomatic, particularly when hypokalemia develops over a long period.

The cause of hypokalemia is usually evident from the history. A high degree of vigilance in persons at risk is required to detect hypokalemia. The ECG, signs and symptoms of hypokalemia, and serum K⁺ levels should be monitored. Initial and repeat serum K⁺ levels should be obtained to rule out laboratory error.

Treatment

The primary goal with respect to K⁺ should be to prevent an imbalance. *It is important to remember that diuretics, digitalis, and hypokalemia are a potentially lethal combination*

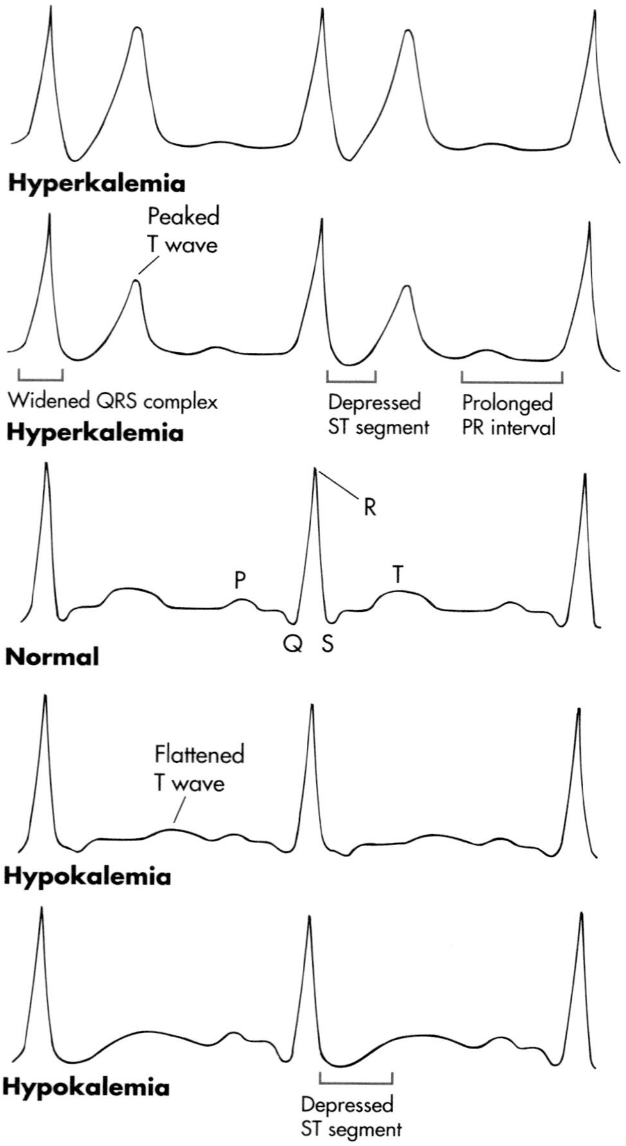

Hyperkalemia

Peaked T wave

Hyperkalemia

Widened QRS complex   Depressed ST segment   Prolonged PR interval

Normal

R

P   T

Q S

Hypokalemia

Flattened T wave

Hypokalemia

Depressed ST segment

FIG. 21-1   ECG changes in potassium imbalances.

because many diuretics cause hypokalemia, and hypokalemia enhances the effect of digitalis. Toxic effects of digitalis and hypokalemia may both cause life-threatening dysrhythmias. Thus serum K^+ and digitalis levels should be monitored in these patients and adequate K^+ intake provided.

When possible, K^+ depletion should be corrected by increased dietary intake of K^+-rich foods or supplementation with K^+ salts. Foods rich in K^+ include fruits (particularly bananas, raisins, and citrus fruits), fruit juices, meats, milk, fresh tomatoes, potatoes, and lentils. Potassium chloride is the supplementary salt of choice, particularly when the patient is alkalotic. IV administration of K^+ is necessary when the patient cannot take K^+ orally or when the K^+ deficiency is severe. K^+ should be given in a nondextrose solution in a severe deficit because dextrose stimulates insulin release, causing K^+ to shift into the cells. The rate of infusion of K^+ should not exceed 20 mEq/hr to avoid a serious hyperkalemia.

BOX 21-13

Causes of Hyperkalemia

RULE OUT PSEUDOHYPERKALEMIA
Poor venipuncture technique; blood cell lysis

INADEQUATE EXCRETION
Renal failure (acute or chronic)
Adrenal insufficiency
  Hypoaldosteronism
  Addison's disease
K^+-sparing diuretics (e.g., spironolactone)

SHIFT OF K^+ OUT OF CELLS INTO ECF
Metabolic acidosis (as in renal failure)
Tissue damage (extensive burns, massive crushing injury, internal hemorrhage)

EXCESSIVE INTAKE
Rapid IV infusion of K^+-containing solutions
Rapid transfusion of aged blood
Ingestion of salt substitutes in patients with renal failure

Hyperkalemia

Hyperkalemia is defined as a serum K^+ concentration of 5.5 mEq/L or greater. Acute hyperkalemia is a medical emergency requiring prompt recognition and treatment to avoid a fatal cardiac dysrhythmia and cardiac arrest.

Etiology and Pathogenesis

The common causes of hyperkalemia are listed in Box 21-13. Although a low serum K^+ concentration can usually be taken at face value, the report from the laboratory of a high serum K^+ concentration does not always represent a true hyperkalemia. A tight tourniquet around an exercising extremity (e.g., opening and closing fist) can elevate the K^+ as much as 2 to 3 mEq/L. Hemolysis of the red blood cells (RBCs) also produces a falsely elevated serum K^+ concentration because blood cells are high in K^+. Therefore ruling out artifacts that produce a falsely elevated serum K^+ or pseudohyperkalemia is important. Serial measurements should be obtained when doubt exists about the veracity of the laboratory measurement. Alternatively, the plasma concentration of K^+ can be measured by obtaining a blood sample in a heparinized tube. The plasma concentration of K^+ will be within normal limits and the serum value elevated in pseudohyperkalemia. K^+ may be falsely elevated with the serum measurement, because the ECF is separated from the red cells *after* clotting has occurred. A small amount of K^+ normally moves out of white cells and platelets during coagulation, and the amount may be much greater when leukocytosis or thrombocytosis is present. Consequently, the measured serum K^+ exceeds the true level in the plasma.

Hyperkalemia can be caused by inadequate excretion, redistribution of K^+ in the body, and increased intake. The most common cause of hyperkalemia is inadequate renal excretion. Because the kidneys excrete 80% to 90% of the K^+, renal failure would be expected to result in hyperkalemia. However, hyperkalemia does not occur until late in the course of chronic renal failure unless the patient is challenged with a K^+ load. This circumstance might occur if a patient with chronic renal failure receives a drug containing K$^+$ or uses a salt substitute (one that contains K$^+$ salts). An endogenous source of K$^+$ overloading might be internal bleeding with the release of K$^+$ during hemolysis of RBCs. People with either Addison's disease or isolated hypoaldosteronism can present with severe hyperkalemia. The latter condition is more common in older adults with renal impairment and diabetes mellitus. K$^+$-sparing diuretics, such as spironolactone, can produce severe hyperkalemia, particularly when they are administered to patients with renal insufficiency who are also taking K$^+$ supplements.

Acidosis and tissue damage that results from burns or a crushing injury cause K$^+$ to shift from the ICF to the ECF and are other causes of hyperkalemia. Finally, K$^+$-containing IV solutions must be given slowly to prevent iatrogenic K$^+$ overload. When possible, fresh blood or packed cells should be used for transfusions because K$^+$ is gradually released from RBCs into the ECF when blood is stored.

A final point must be made about interpreting hyperkalemia. In hypokalemia a rough correlation exists between total body K$^+$ stores and serum K$^+$, but such a correlation does not exist between total body K$^+$ and the serum K$^+$ in hyperkalemia. In most instances of hyperkalemia, total K$^+$ stores are not increased because the body has little capacity for storing K$^+$. In fact, body K$^+$ stores may even be reduced in hyperkalemia. In most types of metabolic acidosis (except lactic acidosis), K$^+$ shifts from the ICF to the ECF, giving rise to moderately severe hyperkalemia when K$^+$ stores are normal and to a normalization of the serum K$^+$ when body K$^+$ stores are depleted.

Clinical Features

Most patients with hyperkalemia are asymptomatic until a marked rise in the serum K$^+$ concentration takes place. The neuromuscular effects of hyperkalemia resemble those of hypokalemia (Box 21-14). Muscle weakness predominates, and symptoms most often begin in the lower extremities and ascend to the trunk and upper extremities. Other signs and symptoms may include listlessness, paresthesias, nausea, intestinal colic, or diarrhea. Cardiac arrest is the most feared complication of hyperkalemia. The progressive disturbance in cardiac conduction can be appreciated from the changes that occur in the ECG. The earliest changes are symmetric peaking, or "tenting" of the T waves (serum K$^+$ >6 mEq/L). Serum levels of 6.5 to 8.0 mEq/L produce more advanced changes, including a prolonged PR interval and widening of the QRS complex. Severe hyperkalemia (serum K$^+$ >8.0 mEq/L) yields a sine wave pattern, an ominous sign of impending cardiac arrest (see Fig. 21-1). It must be emphasized, however, that the progressive ECG changes may not correlate perfectly with the degree of hyperkalemia. Hypocalcemia, hyponatremia, acidemia, and a rapid rise of serum K$^+$ enhance the toxic effects of hyperkalemia (a common combination in renal failure). Hypernatremia and hypercalcemia counteract the effects of hyperkalemia on the membrane potential.

The diagnosis of hyperkalemia cannot be made on the basis of clinical signs and symptoms because they are nonspecific, and many are identical with those of hypokalemia. Rather, the diagnosis is made on the basis

---

BOX 21-14

Hyperkalemia: Clinical Features

SIGNS AND SYMPTOMS
Neuromuscular
  Vague muscle weakness usually first sign
  Ascending muscular weakness progressing to flaccid paralysis in legs, and later in trunk and arms (severe)
  Paresthesias of face, tongue, feet, and hands
Gastrointestinal
  Nausea, intestinal colic, diarrhea
Renal
  Oliguria progressing to anuria
Cardiovascular
  Cardiac dysrhythmias, bradycardia, complete heart block, ventricular fibrillation or cardiac standstill
  ECG changes (invariably present when serum K$^+$ = 7-8 mEq/L)
    High, peaked T waves (early; K$^+$ >6 mEq/L)
    Prolonged PR interval
    Widened QRS

LABORATORY FINDING
Serum K$^+$ level >5.5 mEq/L

---

of the serum K$^+$ and by observing the characteristic ECG changes.

Treatment

Treatment of hyperkalemia varies with the severity of the imbalance. Severe hyperkalemia (>8 mEq/L or advanced ECG changes) requires correction within minutes to bring the serum K$^+$ down to a safe level. Correction is best accomplished by directly counteracting the cardiac effects with calcium, together with redistribution of the K$^+$ from the ECF to the ICF. Three methods are used for the emergency treatment of severe hyperkalemia:

1. 10 ml 10% IV calcium gluconate infused slowly over 2 to 3 minutes with ECG monitoring; onset within 5 minutes but effect lasts only approximately 30 minutes
2. 500 ml 10% glucose with 10 U regular insulin shifts K$^+$ into cells; onset within 30 minutes and lasts several hours
3. 44 to 88 mEq sodium bicarbonate IV corrects acidosis and shifts K$^+$ into cells; onset within 30 minutes and lasts several hours

Emergency treatment of hyperkalemia must be followed with treatment methods to permanently reduce the serum K$^+$. These methods include the use of an exchange resin or dialysis. Sodium polystyrene sulfonate (Kayexalate) is a nonabsorbable ion exchange resin that can be given orally or rectally as an enema. Forty grams given orally in four divided doses will lower the serum K$^+$ by 1 mEq/L over 24 hours. Enemas should be retained for at least 30 minutes to permit exchange. This treatment is often given to patients with renal failure and moderate hyperkalemia. The best method to remove K$^+$ from the body is by peritoneal dialysis or hemodialysis. Intermittent dialysis is used to treat patients with renal failure and chronic hyperkalemia to maintain the serum K$^+$ within an acceptable range (see Part Eight).

The most important aspect of preventing hyperkalemia is to recognize the clinical circumstances that predispose to the condition because hyperkalemia is a predictable consequence of many diseases and the result of the administration of many drugs. Particular care must be taken to avoid rapid infusion of K^+-containing IV solutions.

CALCIUM, PHOSPHATE, AND MAGNESIUM IMBALANCES

Although imbalances of calcium, phosphate, and magnesium are less common than those of K^+ and Na^+, the consequences can be major. Because abnormalities of these three electrolytes are closely linked, excesses and deficits of these ions will be discussed together.

Calcium Homeostasis

Total body calcium in adults is approximately 1 to 2 kg. Approximately 99% of body calcium is found in the bones and teeth in the form of calcium phosphate salts, approximately 1% is found in the ECF, and 0.1% is found within the cytosol. Calcium has two important physiologic roles: maintaining the structural integrity of the skeleton and participating in many vital cellular processes.

Osteoclastic resorption of existing bone and *osteoblastic formation* of new bone are tightly coupled and take place throughout life (Fig. 21-2). Bone resorption always precedes new bone formation, and the length of one replacement sequence is approximately 4 to 5 months in adults. The three major influences on the equilibrium of bone tissue are (1) mechanical stress stimulating osteoblastic activity, (2) calcium and phosphate levels in the ECF, and (3) hormones and local factors influencing resorption and formation.

In the ECF and cytosol, ionized calcium (Ca^{++}) is essential for a variety of cellular processes. Calcium is an important constituent of cell membranes, affecting their permeability and electrical properties. For example, lowering the ECF Ca^{++} causes increased permeability and excitability of the cell membrane. Ionized calcium also affects neuromuscular activity. A decrease in ECF Ca^{++} increases the excitability of nerve tissue and can stimulate muscle contraction. In fact, Ca^{++} acts as a coupling factor between muscle excitation and contraction of actomyosin. Ionized calcium influences cardiac contractility and automaticity via slow calcium channels in the heart muscle (see Chapter 29). Calcium is involved in the release of preformed hormones from endocrine cells and in the release of acetylcholine at neuromuscular junctions. It also participates in the mechanism of action of hormones within the cells. For example, calcium is an important component in the action of cyclic adenosine monophosphate (cyclic AMP or cAMP), the secondary intracellular messenger. Calcium is important in the property of adhesiveness that binds cells together, in enzyme activity, and in blood coagulation. Because of these various and important functions, the level of ionized calcium in the ECF must be carefully maintained within a narrow range.

The concentration of the total serum calcium is normally 9.0 to 10.5 mg/dl (4.5 to 5.5 mEq/L). The calcium in plasma is in three forms: bound to proteins (principal-

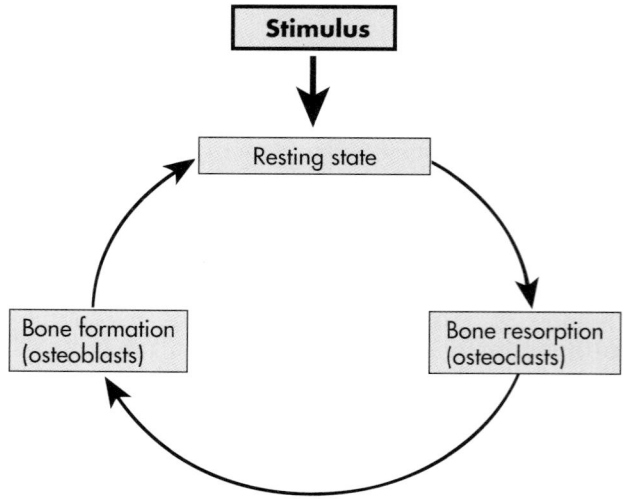

FIG. 21-2 Bone maintenance.

ly albumin), complexed with small ligands (phosphate, citrate, and sulfate), and ionized Ca^{++} (Fig. 21-3). The ionized and complexed forms are diffusible, accounting for 47% and 13% of total calcium, respectively, whereas the protein-bound calcium is not. The ionized calcium in plasma is physiologically active and clinically important in defining hypocalcemia and hypercalcemia. Ionized calcium can be measured directly using a calcium-specific electrode, but the total serum calcium is usually measured. When only the total serum calcium measurement is available, it must be evaluated in relation to the serum albumin. A decrease in the serum albumin of 1 g/dl (assuming 4 g/dl as normal) will decrease the total serum calcium by 0.8 mg/dl. A frequently used formula for estimating the total serum calcium is the following:

$$\text{Total serum Ca (mg/dl)} = \text{measured total Ca (mg/dl)} + 0.8 \times (4 - \text{measured albumin}) \text{ (g/dl)}$$

For example, if the measured total serum Ca^{++} is 8.0 mg/dl (subnormal) and the serum albumin is only 2.0 (subnormal), the corrected total calcium would then be $8.0 + (2 \times 0.8) = 9.6$ mg/dl (normal range). However, this formula is not valid in conditions that alter serum pH. Calcium binding declines with a reduction of pH so that more of the total serum calcium is ionized and less is bound to albumin in conditions of acidosis. Alkalosis (higher pH) produces the converse situation with less ionized Ca^{++} and more bound to albumin. Thus signs and symptoms of hypocalcemia are more likely to occur when associated with alkalosis but are masked when associated with acidosis.

The serum calcium depends on the balance between calcium input and output from the ECF. Calcium input is determined by the amount ingested and the amount mobilized from the skeletal pool. The average intake of calcium for a North American adult is 600 to 1000 mg/day; the major sources are dairy products. Calcium absorption occurs principally in the duodenum and upper jejunum by an active transport process. Generally, less than one half of the ingested calcium is absorbed. Calcium loss from the ECF occurs through secretion into

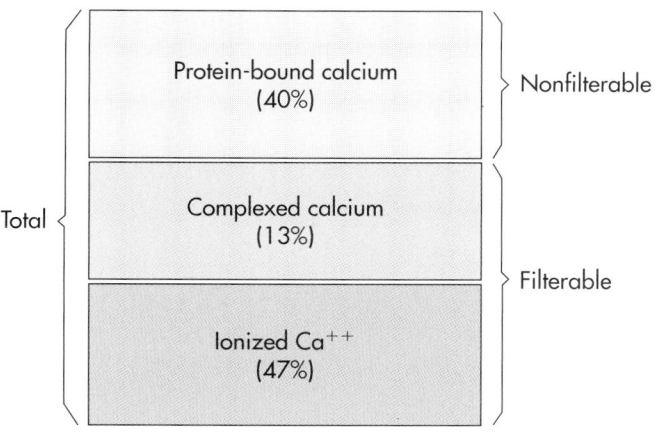

FIG. 21-3   Distribution of calcium in plasma.

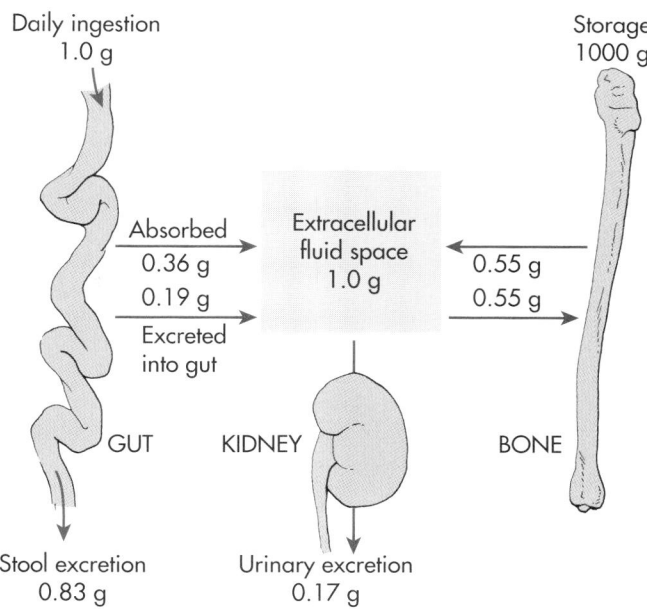

FIG. 21-4   Outline of calcium intake, absorption, excretion, and storage in humans. In conditions of calcium balance, rates of calcium release and uptake into bone are equal and calcium excretion via urine and feces is equal to intake.

the GI tract, urinary excretion, and deposition in bone (Fig. 21-4).

The level of ionized calcium in the ECF is homeostatically maintained within the narrow normal range of 9 to 10.5 mg/dl by an effective balance of bone formation and bone resorption, calcium absorption, and calcium excretion. The principal sites of this regulation are in the bones, kidneys, and GI tract under the control of three hormones: parathyroid hormone, calcitonin, and calcitriol or 1,25-dihydroxycholecalciferol (1,25[OH]$_2$D$_3$).

Parathyroid hormone or *parathormone (PTH)* is a polypeptide secreted by the parathyroid glands, which are located in the neck behind the lobes of the thyroid gland. The four parathyroid glands include one right superior, one left superior, one right inferior, and one left inferior. PTH secretion occurs in response to hypocalcemia and is suppressed by hypercalcemia. PTH acts directly on bone and kidney and indirectly on the GI tract through stimulating dihydroxyvitamin D$_3$ synthesis. PTH stimulates osteoclastic bone resorption, thereby releasing both calcium and phosphate into the ECF. PTH also stimulates increased renal tubular reabsorption of calcium (thus returning it to the blood) and increases the excretion of phosphate. Finally, PTH acts directly on the kidney to modulate the synthesis of 1,25(OH)$_2$D$_3$, the most active metabolite of vitamin D, which, in turn, causes increased calcium and phosphate absorption from the gut. The net effect is that PTH raises the plasma ionized calcium concentration while having little effect on the plasma phosphate concentration, because changes in the phosphate handling in bone, intestine, and kidney tend to balance out. Excessive PTH causes hypercalcemia and hypophosphatemia, and deficiency of PTH causes hypocalcemia and hyperphosphatemia.

Calcitonin is a hormone produced by the C cells, or parafollicular cells, of the thyroid gland. Calcitonin is released in response to hypercalcemia. Its main effect is to lower serum calcium by inhibiting osteoclastic bone resorption. The actual physiologic role of calcitonin in the minute-to-minute regulation of calcium levels has not been clarified. The hypothesis that calcitonin functions to prevent postprandial hypercalcemia and prevents postprandial urinary loss of calcium (particularly in the milk-drinking infant) will require further investigation.

Vitamin D and its metabolites are not vitamins but *steroid hormones.* Vitamin D works in concert with PTH in the regulation of serum calcium levels. *Vitamin D$_3$,* or *cholecalciferol,* is either ingested with the diet* or is synthesized from *7-dehydrocholesterol* in the skin by ultraviolet radiation from the sun. Vitamin D$_3$ is absorbed in the ileum and jejunum and is subsequently metabolized to its active form, first in the liver and ultimately in the kidney. The metabolism of vitamin D$_3$ involves sequential hydroxylations. In the liver, vitamin D$_3$ is converted to *25-hydroxycholecalciferol* and in the kidney to *calcitriol* or 1,25(OH)$_2$D$_3$ (Fig. 21-5). PTH is a potent stimulator of vitamin D$_3$ activation (as well as hypophosphatemia). The major target sites of 1,25(OH)$_2$D$_3$ are intestine and bone. In the intestine, 1,25(OH)$_2$D$_3$ promotes absorption of ingested calcium and phosphate, and in the bone it acts in concert with PTH to enhance bone resorption, releasing calcium and phosphate into the ECF. The net effect is the elevation of both serum calcium and phosphate (in contrast to PTH, which only raises the serum calcium). These actions are consistent with the two major functions of 1,25(OH)$_2$D$_3$, which are to ensure the availability of calcium and phosphate for new bone formation and to prevent hypocalcemia and hypophosphatemia. A deficiency of 1,25(OH)$_2$D$_3$ results in inadequate mineralization of bone matrix, called *rickets* in children and *osteomalacia* in adults. The latter condition is common in chronic renal failure (see Chapter 47). Fig. 21-6 illustrates the regulation of calcium and phosphate metabolism by PTH and 1,25(OH)$_2$D$_3$.

---

*Another source of dietary vitamin D is vitamin D$_2$ (ergocalciferol), found in irradiated milk, vitamin supplements, fish, and liver.

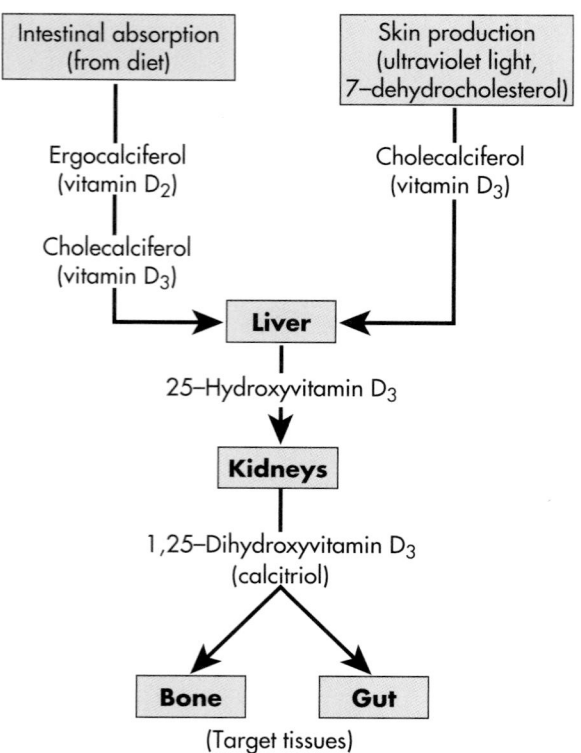

FIG. 21-5 Overview of the metabolism of vitamin D.

Phosphate Homeostasis

Phosphorus is the most abundant constituent of all tissues in the body and is involved in a large number of essential biologic processes. Along with calcium, phosphorus is an essential component of bones and teeth and is an important constituent of phospholipids that are components of cell membranes. Phosphorus is the primary anion in ICF, and it is essential in the metabolism of proteins, fats, and carbohydrates. Virtually all metabolic processes require phosphorus, including the provision of high-energy phosphate bonds in the form of adenosine triphosphate (ATP). Phosphorus plays an essential role in muscle function, neurologic function, and formation of 2,3-diphosphoglycerate in RBCs, which facilitate oxygen delivery to the tissues (see Chapter 35). Phosphorus in the form of inorganic phosphate plays a major role in maintaining acid-base balance through its action as a urinary buffer in excreting a large portion of the daily acid load (see Chapters 22 and 44).

Of the average 700 g of phosphorus in the body, 85% is in the bones and teeth, 15% is in soft tissues, and 0.1% is in the ECF. Plasma phosphorus exists largely as *inorganic phosphate* ions ($HPO_4^=$ and $H_2PO_4^-$) with only 10% bound to proteins and the remainder freely diffusible and in equilibrium with intracellular and bone phosphorus. Normally the serum phosphate levels range from 2.5 to 4.5 mg/dl (1.8 to 2.6 mEq/L) in an adult. Serum phosphate has a wide physiologic range and varies with age. Infants and young children have higher levels than do adults because of the influence of growth hormone and their increased rate of skeletal growth.

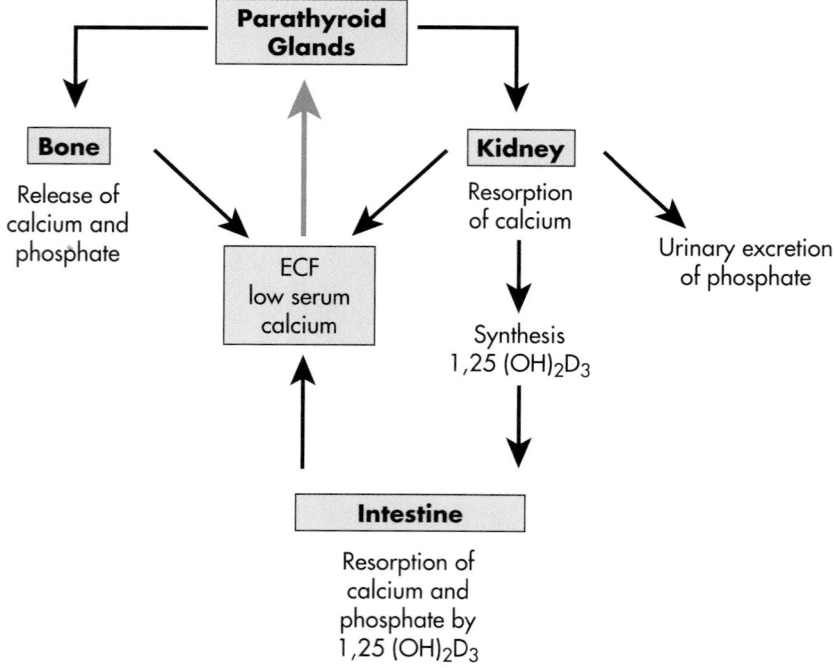

FIG. 21-6 Mechanism of the action of parathyroid hormone (PTH). The principal function of PTH is to defend against hypocalcemia. In response to a low serum calcium, PTH is released, which acts directly on bone and kidneys and indirectly on the gut through stimulating 1,25(OH)$_2$D$_3$ synthesis by the kidneys (most active form of vitamin D hormone). All three effects favor elevation of the serum calcium. PTH secretion is suppressed by elevated levels of serum calcium.

The average diet contains 1000 to 1600 mg of phosphorus, and phosphorus is present in a large variety of foods thus consuming less than is needed is nearly impossible. Phosphate absorption occurs largely in the jejunum by passive diffusion and by active transport under the influence of $1,25(OH)_2D_3$. Intestinal absorption varies with intake but can be impaired by certain drugs such as phosphate-binding antacids and by malabsorption syndromes. The major route for phosphate excretion is the kidneys (90%) under the control of PTH. PTH causes increased renal calcium reabsorption and decreased phosphate reabsorption. Because calcium and phosphate interact in a reciprocal relationship, urinary excretion of phosphates increases or decreases in inverse proportion to serum calcium levels. Normally the serum $Ca^{++} \times HPO_4^=$ cross product (in mg/dl) is maintained at approximately 30 to 40 (e.g., $9.5 \times 3.5 = 33.25$), allowing precipitation of calcium phosphate salts in the bone but not in the soft tissues. If both the serum calcium and the serum phosphate should rise simultaneously such that their cross product exceeds 60 to 70, soft tissue deposition of calcium salts, or *metastatic calcification*, can occur. The latter condition is possible when secondary hyperparathyroidism develops in chronic renal failure (see Chapter 47).

Magnesium Homeostasis

Magnesium (Mg^{++}) is the fourth most abundant cation in the body. Similar to potassium, magnesium is found primarily in the ICF. Magnesium is an important regulator of cellular processes that are essential for life. The best-defined function of magnesium is the activation of a wide variety of enzyme systems. For example, all ATPases require magnesium for activation. Magnesium is required for the synthesis of nucleic acids and proteins, and it affects muscle directly by decreasing acetylcholine release at the neuromuscular junction and at sympathetic ganglia, resulting in a curarelike effect. This effect can be antagonized by an excess of calcium or by the simultaneous administration of potassium. Magnesium plays a role in maintaining normal calcium and potassium homeostasis; it facilitates the transportation of sodium and potassium across the cell membrane (accounting for the secondary hypokalemia that occurs in hypomagnesemia), and it influences intracellular calcium levels through its effect on PTH secretion. Hypomagnesemia interferes with the release of PTH and with its effect on target tissue thus hypocalcemia may develop as a result of hypomagnesemia.

The human body contains approximately 2000 mEq of magnesium. Approximately 67% of this amount is in the bones, 31% is intracellular, and less than 2% is in the ECF. The normal serum level of Mg^{++} is 1.8 to 3.0 mg/dl (1.5 to 2.5 mEq/L). Of the total plasma magnesium, approximately 35% is protein-bound, 55% is free, and 15% is complexed to phosphates, citrates, and other ligands. Only the free ionized Mg^{++} is available for biochemical processes. Normally an exchange occurs between ECF Mg^{++} and bone Mg^{++} in response to an excess or deficit of this ion. Mg^{++} exists in two forms inside cells: bound to organic components and in solution, which is in equilibrium with the free Mg^{++} form in plasma. Because most Mg^{++} inside cells is bound to ATP, MgATP is in equilibrium with free Mg^{++} ions. Thus shifts in free Mg^{++} may help to regulate stores of ATP. Because ATP is critical to all metabolic processes, a normal concentration of serum Mg^{++} is essential to maintain stores of this important nucleotide. Considering that magnesium is predominantly an intracellular cation, its serum levels may not always reflect total body stores of magnesium.

The normal diet supplies approximately 25 mEq of magnesium daily, mostly in meat, green vegetables rich in chlorophyll (a chelator of magnesium), whole grains, and nuts. Approximately 10 mEq of the dietary intake is absorbed in the jejunum and ileum, an equal amount is excreted in the urine, and the remainder is excreted in the feces. Regulation of magnesium metabolism is not well understood. Under conditions of hypomagnesemia, more magnesium is absorbed in the intestine and less is excreted in the urine. Renal conservation of Mg^{++} is so efficient that the total loss of urinary Mg^{++} can be reduced to only 1 mEq.

Hypocalcemia

Hypocalcemia is defined as a total serum calcium level less than 9 mg/dl (4.5 mEq/L) or ionized calcium less than 4.5 mg/dl. Box 21-15 lists some of the causes of hypocalcemia. These causes include deficiency in the production, secretion, or actions of PTH or $1,25(OH)_2D_3$ or both.

Occasionally, hypocalcemia is caused by malabsorption of calcium or hyperphosphatemia. Idiopathic hypoparathyroidism (causing a PTH deficit) is a rare condition that can result from autoimmune destruction of the parathyroid glands. The serum calcium is low, serum phosphate is normal or increased, and $1,25(OH)_2D_3$ is low because of the lack of PTH. Hypoparathyroidism may be secondary to accidental removal of the parathyroid glands with thyroidectomy, but this is less common today because hyperthyroidism is more commonly treated by radioactive iodine ablation rather than by surgery. More commonly, hypoparathyroidism follows a subtotal parathyroidectomy, although the hypocalcemia is generally only transitory until the remaining parathyroid tissue can increase PTH secretion. A deficiency of magnesium (<1 mg/dl) can cause hypocalcemia by interfering with PTH secretion, as well as its peripheral action.

Hypocalcemia is a common feature of vitamin D deficiency that may occur because of inadequate intake, lack of exposure to sunlight, or malabsorptive disease. Some causes of intestinal malabsorption include sprue, chronic pancreatitis, partial gastrectomy, intestinal bypass surgery for obesity, biliary cirrhosis, and prolonged abuse of laxatives. Alcoholic liver disease may interfere with the 25-hydroxylation of vitamin D_3, and a number of factors may interfere with the final hydroxylation to $1,25(OH)_2D_3$ in the kidney. Chronic renal failure is the most common cause of hypocalcemia. The hypocalcemia is the result of several factors, including hyperphosphatemia (causing a reciprocal drop in serum calcium), impaired sensitivity of the skeleton to the bone-resorbing action of PTH, reduced production of $1,25(OH)_2D_3$ by surviving renal tissue, and decreased intestinal absorption. Patients develop secondary hyperparathyroidism and hyperplasia

---

■ **BOX 21-15**
■ **Causes of Hypocalcemia**

PTH DEFICIT
Hypoparathyroidism
  Idiopathic
  Postsurgical*
Hypomagnesemia*

ABNORMAL METABOLISM OF VITAMIN D
Deficiency
  Inadequate intake
  Poor exposure to sunlight
  Malabsorption disease
Impaired 25-hydroxylation in liver
  Alcoholic liver disease
Impaired renal hydroxylation
  Chronic renal failure*
  Hypoparathyroidism
  Hypophosphatemic rickets
  Pseudohypoparathyroidism
  Vitamin D–dependent rickets, type I
Impaired response to $1,25(OH)_2D_3$
  Anticonvulsant drugs
  Vitamin D–dependent rickets, type II

OTHER FACTORS
Alkalosis*
Hypoalbuminemia
Hyperphosphatemia
Neonatal hypocalcemia
Osteoblastic metastases
Medullary thyroid carcinoma
Acute pancreatitis
Drugs
  Chemotherapy
  Phosphates (IV, oral, enema)
  Citrate-buffered blood
  Loop diuretics (e.g., furosemide)
  Mg^{++}-lowering drugs
  Radiographic contrast media

*Most common conditions causing hypocalcemia.

■ **BOX 21-16**
■ **Hypocalcemia: Clinical Features**

SIGNS AND SYMPTOMS
Cardiovascular
  ECG changes
  Dysrhythmias
  Decreased sensitivity to digitalis
Neuromuscular
  Paresthesias (circumoral, hands, feet)
  Hyperactive reflexes
  Tetany
    Trousseau's sign
    Chvostek's sign
    Muscle tics or spasms of face, extremities
    Laryngospasm
Central nervous system
  Altered mood, impaired memory, confusion
  Convulsive seizures
Gastrointestinal
  Diarrhea, loose stools
  Malabsorption and steatorrhea
Skin
  Dry, scaly skin
  Coarse, dry hair
  Brittle nails
Ocular
  Cataracts

LABORATORY FINDINGS
Total serum Ca^{++} <8.5 mg/dl
  Evaluate serum albumin: suspect ionic hypocalcemia
    when decreased calcium in presence of normal albumin
  Evaluate serum pH: suspect ionic hypocalcemia when
    normal calcium in presence of severe alkalosis (pH >7.55)
Ionic serum Ca^{++} <4.5 mg/dl

---

of the parathyroid glands, and with autonomous parathyroid function, they may eventually develop hypercalcemia and metastatic calcification (see Chapter 47). Hypophosphatemic rickets, pseudohypoparathyroidism, and vitamin D–dependent rickets (types I and II) are rare hereditary disorders in which either impaired production of $1,25(OH)_2D_3$ or resistance to its effect occurs. Hypocalcemia, rickets, or osteomalacia may occur in patients with epilepsy who are receiving treatment with anticonvulsant drugs, which interfere with the peripheral actions of $1,25(OH)_2D_3$.

Alkalosis can cause symptoms of hypocalcemia as a result of decreased ionized Ca^{++} in the serum, although the total serum calcium may be normal. Hypoalbuminemia, as occurs in the nephrotic syndrome or cirrhosis of the liver, results in decreased total serum calcium although the ionized fraction may be normal. Some causes of hyperphosphatemia that lead to hypocalcemia include administration of phosphates and hematologic malignancies either because of high cell turnover as part of the malignancy or because of cell destruction when chemotherapy is instituted. Hypocalcemia may develop in neonates who are fed cow's milk. The cause has been attributed to two mechanisms: physiologic hypofunction

of the parathyroids and hyperphosphatemia from the high phosphate content of cow's milk compared with human milk. Hypocalcemia may develop in patients with malignant neoplasms of the prostate, lung, and breast with osteoblastic (bone-forming) metastases. Medullary thyroid carcinoma may cause hypocalcemia if calcitonin is secreted by the carcinoma. Acute pancreatitis may result in severe hypocalcemia, possibly the result of precipitation of calcium soaps in the abdomen caused by enzymatic fat necrosis. Multiple transfusions of banked blood buffered with sodium citrate may cause hypocalcemia. The excess citrate not only can bind calcium ions but also may cause alkalosis when it is metabolized to form bicarbonate. Other drugs that can lower serum calcium include loop diuretics (increase Ca^{++} excretion), drugs that lower magnesium such as cisplatin and gentamycin (decrease Ca^{++} mobilization from bone), and certain radiographic contrast media (form complexes with Ca^{++}).

Clinical Features

Symptoms of hypocalcemia depend on the degree, duration, and rate of its development. Hypocalcemia may be asymptomatic. Box 21-16 outlines the clinical manifestations of hypocalcemia that are primarily caused by an increase in neuromuscular irritability. Tetany is the most characteristic sign of hypocalcemia. *Tetany* is characterized by involuntary muscle spasms and may involve muscles of the upper and lower extremities, causing car-

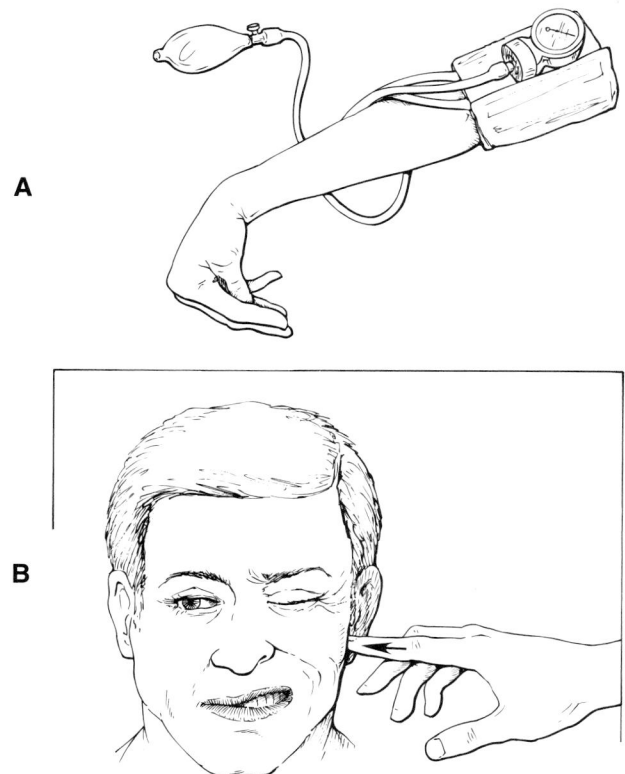

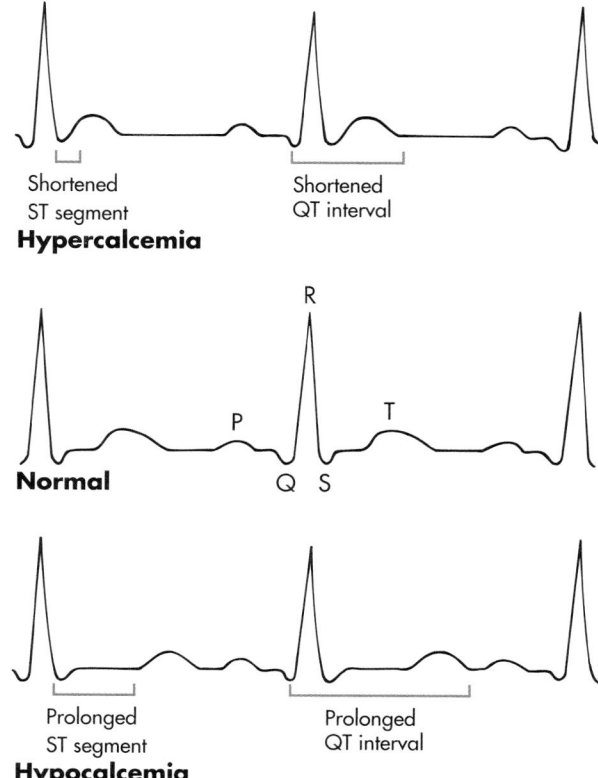

FIG. 21-7 Checking for latent tetany. **A**, Trousseau's sign: carpal spasm induced by inflating a blood pressure cuff above systolic pressure. **B**, Chvostek's sign: contraction of facial muscles induced by a light tap over the facial nerve.

FIG. 21-8 ECG changes in calcium imbalances. In hypocalcemia the QT interval and ST segment may be prolonged. Hypercalcemia causes shortening of the QT interval and ST segment.

popedal spasms, as well as paresthesias of the hands and feet and around the mouth. Latent tetany can be demonstrated by testing for Trousseau's sign. A blood pressure cuff is placed on the upper arm and inflated above systolic pressure for 1 to 4 minutes. *Carpopedal spasm* (adducted thumb, flexed wrist and metacarpophalangeal joints, and extended interphalangeal joints with fingers together) indicates a positive *Trousseau's sign.* Latent tetany may also be demonstrated by tapping over the facial nerve immediately anterior to the ear and observing for ipsilateral contraction of the facial muscles, called *Chvostek's sign* (Fig. 21-7). Hyperactive deep tendon reflexes are additional signs that may be elicited indicating increased neuromuscular irritability. Severe hypocalcemia may result in convulsive seizures or in laryngospasm.

Patients with hypocalcemia usually experience a variety of neuropsychiatric disturbances, including irritability, emotional instability, impairment of memory, and confusion. Patients with hypocalcemia often have diarrhea or loose stools and may even develop intestinal malabsorption and steatorrhea (excess fecal fat). Prolonged hypocalcemia, as observed in idiopathic hypoparathyroidism, may cause changes in the skin, hair, nails, teeth, and lenses. The skin may be coarse, dry, and scaly, and alopecia may develop with patchy or absent eyelashes and eyebrows. The teeth in young children may erupt late and appear hypoplastic. Cataracts may develop within a few years of untreated hypocalcemia.

Hypocalcemia classically produces prolongation of the QT interval and ST segment, which are frequently present when serum calcium is 7 mg/dl and consistently present when serum calcium is 6 mg/dl or less (Chan, Gill, 1990; Fig. 21-8). Heart block and dysrhythmias may develop. The heart may be refractory to digitalis.

Treatment

Treatment of hypocalcemia focuses on correcting the imbalance and the underlying cause. Severe symptomatic hypocalcemia with tetany or seizures is a medical emergency and is treated with 10 ml of 10% calcium gluconate administered IV over a 4-minute period followed by an additional calcium infusion (e.g., 30 to 60 ml of 10% calcium gluconate mixed in 1000 ml of D_5W) given over 6 to 12 hours (Kokko, Tannen, 1996). The serum calcium and ECG should be monitored frequently during the treatment to avoid hypercalcemia. The most common situation associated with severe symptomatic hypocalcemia is following parathyroidectomy.

Chronic mild hypocalcemia is treated by administering calcium salts and vitamin D. Calcium salts are available as calcium gluconate, calcium lactate, or calcium carbonate. Giving 10 to 15 g of calcium gluconate or calcium lactate daily is usually necessary. Vitamin D is given in doses of 50,000 to 150,000 units/day. 1,25-Dihydroxycholecalciferol is given in doses of 0.25 μg/day. When patients are treated with the proper combination of calcium and vitamin D, serum calcium can be maintained within the normal range. The treatment of the calcium and phosphate disturbances associated with chronic renal failure is discussed in Chapter 48.

■ **Causes of Hypercalcemia**

HYPERPARATHYROIDISM
Primary hyperparathyroidism
Secondary hyperparathyroidism
    Chronic renal failure
    Vitamin D malabsorption

MALIGNANCIES
Solid tumors without bone metastasis
    Squamous cell carcinoma of the lung, head, and neck;
        carcinoma of the ovary, kidney
Solid tumors with bone metastasis
    Carcinoma of the breast
Hematologic malignancies
    Multiple myeloma
    Lymphomas
    Acute leukemia

ABNORMAL VITAMIN D METABOLISM
Sarcoidosis
Tuberculosis

ENDOCRINE
Hyperthyroidism
Adrenal insufficiency

PROLONGED IMMOBILIZATION

DRUGS
Thiazide diuretics
Lithium
Vitamin A intoxication
Vitamin D intoxication
$1,25(OH)_2D_3$ intoxication
Milk-alkali syndrome

Hypercalcemia

Hypercalcemia exists when the total serum calcium exceeds 10.5 mg/dl (5.5 mEq/L). In 90% of the cases, hypercalcemia is caused by either primary hyperparathyroidism or cancer. The causes of hypercalcemia are outlined in Box 21-17.

Many conditions may lead to hypercalcemia, but PTH excess is by far the most common cause. Excessive production of PTH may result from primary hyperparathyroidism or secretion of a PTH-like peptide by nonparathyroid malignancies. Additionally, hypercalcemia may be associated with severe secondary hyperparathyroidism observed in chronic renal failure and after dialysis or renal transplantation. Primary hyperparathyroidism is usually caused by a benign adenoma of the parathyroid glands (but may be caused by hyperplasia of all four glands). The incidence has risen dramatically since the introduction of automated analysis and frequent measurement of calcium by laboratories. The condition occurs more frequently in women than it does in men, and the occurrence rises with age. Hypercalcemia results from the PTH-mediated mobilization of calcium from bone and the PTH-enhanced renal reabsorption of calcium. Some patients have elevated $1,25(OH)_2D_3$, which, in turn, causes increased intestinal absorption that may cause *hypercalciuria* (excessive loss of calcium in the urine). PTH causes increased renal phosphate excretion, thus patients with primary hyperparathy-

roidism often have either a low or normal serum phosphate. These patients also have increased renal cAMP, and measurements of this nucleotide are often used to diagnose primary hyperparathyroidism.

A malignant neoplasm is the single most common cause of hypercalcemia, and this complication often occurs during an advanced stage of the disease. Common malignancies associated with hypercalcemia include squamous cell carcinoma of the lung, head, or neck; carcinoma of the kidney, ovary, or pancreas; breast cancer; and hematologic malignancies such as multiple myeloma, lymphomas (particularly T-cell lymphoma), and acute leukemia. These malignancies can be divided into three classes (see Box 21-17): (1) solid tumors without bone metastasis, called *humoral hypercalcemia of malignancy,* (2) solid tumors with bone metastasis, and (3) hematologic malignancies. Two mechanisms causing the hypercalcemia of malignancy are localized bone destruction from osteolytic metastasis and humoral factors that stimulate osteoclastic bone resorption. In the past, the assumption was made that tumor invasion of the bone with localized destruction was the predominant mechanism causing the hypercalcemia of malignancy. Certainly, extensive bone destruction occurs in patients with multiple myeloma, lymphomas, and breast cancer with bone metastasis. However, research has revealed that humoral factors produced by these tumors play a major role in causing the hypercalcemia of malignancy whether bone invasion or bone metastasis occurs or not (Chan, Gill, 1990). Some of these humoral factors include PTH-related peptide (PTHrP), tumor necrosis factor (TNF), transforming growth factors (TGF-alpha and beta), interleukin-1 (IL-1), prostaglandin E, and lymphotoxin. All of these humoral factors cause increased bone resorption and, when PTHrP is present, increased renal calcium reabsorption. Additionally, some lymphoma cells synthesize $1,25(OH)_2D_3$, resulting in both increased osteoclastic bone resorption and increased gut absorption of calcium.

Hypercalcemia occasionally occurs in sarcoidosis and in pulmonary tuberculosis, and the mechanism involves extrarenal synthesis of $1,25(OH)_2D_3$. Hypercalcemia occurs in 8% to 22% of patients with hyperthyroidism, but the serum calcium is only mildly elevated (Chan, Gill, 1990). Increased bone turnover in hyperthyroidism takes place. PTH secretion is suppressed, as well as $1,25(OH)_2D_3$, accounting for the characteristically high urinary and fecal calcium. Hypercalcemia sometimes occurs in adrenal insufficiency (Addison's disease) caused by glucocorticoid deficiency and ECF volume deficit. Glucocorticoid deficiency stimulates prostaglandin synthesis and increased bone resorption. The ECF volume deficit decreases the glomerular filtration rate thus more of the filtered calcium is reabsorbed. Prolonged immobilization, as occurs in individuals with quadriplegia or paraplegia, invariably leads to bone loss and hypercalciuria because of the uncoupling of bone remodeling so that bone resorption exceeds bone formation. Usually the calcium released from bone is excreted in the urine and does not lead to hypercalcemia.

A number of drugs can cause hypercalcemia. Thiazide diuretics act directly to increase calcium release from bone and increase its renal tubular reabsorption. Chronic lithium administration, commonly used to treat manic-

BOX 21-18
Hypercalcemia: Clinical Features

SIGNS AND SYMPTOMS
Cardiovascular
  Hypertension
  ECG changes
    Dysrhythmias
    Bradycardia
    Heart block
  Increased sensitivity to digitalis
Neuromuscular
  Generalized muscular weakness
  Depressed deep tendon reflexes
  Metastatic calcification in soft tissues
Central nervous system
  Impaired concentration, confusion
  Altered state of consciousness: lethargy → stupor → coma
Gastrointestinal
  Polydipsia
  Anorexia
  Nausea and vomiting
  Weight loss
  Constipation
Renal
  Polyuria
  Nephrolithiasis
  Nephrocalcinosis
  Renal failure
Skeletal (secondary to hyperparathyroidism)
  Bone resorption
  Formation of bone cysts
  Subperiosteal erosion of long bone (see Fig. 21-9)
  Osteitis fibrosa cystica
Skin
  Pruritus
Ocular
  Band keratopathy

LABORATORY FINDINGS
Total serum calcium >10.5 mg/dl
  Evaluate serum albumin and calculate true serum calcium

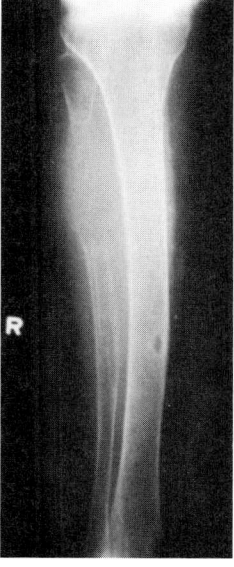

FIG. 21-9   Lesions of osteitis fibrosa cystica in the tibia and fibula of a patient with hyperparathyroidism.

become dehydrated, confused, and lethargic. The clinical features are summarized in Box 21-18.

Hypercalcemia depresses neuromuscular irritability and release of acetylcholine at the myoneural junction, giving rise to symptoms such as muscular weakness, anorexia, nausea, and constipation. Neuropsychiatric signs may be prominent when the serum calcium is greatly elevated (>15 mg/dl), and the patient may show mental confusion, slurred speech, and lethargy progressing to coma. Polyuria and polydipsia, with clinical signs of ECF volume deficit, may accompany excessive urinary loss of calcium, phosphate, and sodium. Renal colic caused by *nephrolithiasis* (kidney stones) is common. Widespread precipitation of calcium salts in the kidney, *nephrocalcinosis*, may lead to obstructive uropathy and renal failure. When bone disease is present, x-ray studies may show a generalized decrease in bone density, fractures, cysts, and subperiosteal bone erosion (Fig. 21-9). Precipitation of calcium salts in the skin may cause *pruritus* (itching) and in the eye, band keratopathy (see Fig. 47-4). Cardiovascular changes in hypercalcemia include systolic hypertension, bradycardia, shortening of the QT interval and the ST segment (see Fig. 21-8), and dysrhythmias. Cardiac arrest may occur when the serum calcium is approximately 18 mg/dl (hypercalcemic crisis). Hypercalcemia can also precipitate digitalis toxicity, because sensitivity to its effects is increased.

The diagnosis of primary hyperparathyroidism is based on the demonstration of a high serum level of calcium and a low level of phosphate together with an elevated level of PTH. Measuring the serum albumin is important, because hypoalbuminemia may mask an increase in ionized calcium. PTH radioimmunoassay directed to the intact molecule or its *N*-terminal portion is the most reliable test. In cases other than primary hyperparathyroidism, serum phosphate levels may be elevated and PTH depressed. The urine may show an increased calcium content (normally <275 mg/day in males and <250 mg/day in females), and urinary excretion of cyclic AMP (cAMP) is increased in primary hyperparathyroidism, as well as in some other causes of hypercalcemia.

depressive illness, is sometimes associated with both mild hypercalcemia and hypermagnesemia. Excess intake of vitamin A results in increased bone resorption. Excess intake of the standard vitamin D_2 (ergocalciferol) or the active $1,25(OH)_2D_3$ (Rocaltrol) can lead to hypercalcemia and hypercalciuria. The milk-alkali syndrome can occur in persons who ingest large amounts of milk and alkali (e.g., sodium bicarbonate or calcium carbonate) to relieve the symptoms of peptic ulcer disease. The syndrome is characterized by alkalosis, hypercalcemia, hyperphosphatemia, soft tissue deposition of calcium salts, and progressive renal failure. Because this form of treatment for peptic ulcers is no longer used, the syndrome is seldom encountered.

Clinical Features

Signs and symptoms of hypercalcemia vary greatly, depending on the rapidity of onset and the degree of elevation of calcium levels. In mild cases, patients may be completely asymptomatic and the hypercalcemia is discovered through routine laboratory investigation. On the other hand, in severe cases with marked elevation of serum calcium levels, patients deteriorate rapidly and

BOX 21-19
Management of Hypercalcemia

GENERAL MEASURES
Hydration
Restriction of calcium intake
Withholding of drugs that potentiate hypercalcemia (vitamin A and D; thiazide diuretics)
Maintenance of weight bearing/avoidance of immobilization
Dialysis

ENHANCE URINARY CALCIUM EXCRETION
IV saline
Diuretics
   Furosemide
   Ethacrynic acid

INHIBIT BONE RESORPTION
Calcitonin
Diphosphonates
Glucocorticoids
Plicamycin (Mithracin)
Gallium nitrate
Phosphates

TREAT UNDERLYING DISEASE

BOX 21-20
Causes of Hypophosphatemia

DECREASED INTAKE-INTESTINAL ABSORPTION
Deficiency of dietary phosphate
Antacid abuse
Various malabsorption states
Vitamin D deficiency

SHIFT FROM ECF INTO CELLS AND BONE
Respiratory alkalosis
Total parental nutrition (TPN)
Diabetic ketoacidosis (DKA)
Glucose-insulin infusion
Nutritional recovery syndrome
Severe burns
Hungry bone syndrome
Alcohol withdrawal

INCREASED URINARY LOSSES
Hyperparathyroidism
Renal tubular disorders

Treatment

When possible, the treatment of hypercalcemia is directed toward reversing the underlying pathogenic disorder. For example, primary hyperparathyroidism is usually treated by surgery, and antineoplastic therapy may improve malignancy-related hypercalcemia. Symptomatic or severe hypercalcemia (>14 mg/dl) requires medical treatment, as outlined in Box 21-19. Treatment goals are directed toward improving hydration, promoting urinary excretion of calcium, and inhibiting bone resorption. The first priority in severe hypercalcemia is hydration with isotonic saline at the rate of 3 to 4 L/day until ECF volume is restored. The saline also promotes urinary calcium excretion by inhibiting its reabsorption. Once the ECF is restored, a diuretic such as furosemide is given to promote further excretion of calcium. In life-threatening hypercalcemia, particularly in persons with renal insufficiency, hemodialysis or peritoneal dialysis with a dialysate containing little or no calcium may rapidly restore serum calcium to normal levels.

A variety of drugs may be used to inhibit bone resorption, the usual source of the excess serum calcium. Calcitonin inhibits bone resorption and increases renal calcium excretion. This drug may be given when a rapid decrease of serum calcium is required. Diphosphonates, such as etidronate or pamidronate, are potent inhibitors of osteoclastic bone resorption and are of great value in the treatment of primary hyperthyroidism and cancer. Gallium nitrate reduces the osteolytic response to PTH and is used to treat cancer-related hypercalcemia. Gallium nitrate is a nephrotoxic drug, so the patient must be well hydrated and have adequate renal function before taking this drug. Plicamycin (Mithracin) is a cytotoxic antibiotic that inhibits bone resorption, but it is rarely given because of its high toxicity. Glucocorticoids block bone resorption, decrease intestinal absorption of calcium, and increase its urinary excretion and are quite effective in the treatment of hypercalcemia from a number of causes. Finally, sodium phosphate can rapidly decrease serum calcium when given IV but is potentially dangerous because a fatal hypocalcemia may result. Another danger is metastatic calcification caused by precipitation of calcium phosphate in the soft tissues. These risks are diminished when it is given orally.

Hypophosphatemia

Hypophosphatemia is defined as a serum phosphate level less than 2.5 mg/dl (normal, 2.5 to 4.5 mg/dl) although symptoms do not usually occur until serum phosphate is less than 1.0 mg/dl. A low serum phosphate level does not necessarily indicate a deficiency of total body phosphate because only 1% is in the ECF. Because phosphate is available in so many foods and is easily absorbed, hypophosphatemia is unusual unless (1) reduced oral intake, (2) a shift of phosphate from the ECF into the cells or bone, or (3) excessive renal loss of phosphate occurs. Some of the most common causes of hypophosphatemia are listed in Box 21-20.

Phosphate absorption is under the influence of $1,25(OH)_2D_3$, and renal phosphate excretion is under the control of PTH. Thus vitamin-D deficiency, intestinal malabsorption, and hyperparathyroidism are causes of hypophosphatemia. Excess ingestion of antacids (e.g., aluminum hydroxide) for the treatment of peptic ulcer disease, for example, can cause hypophosphatemia. The antacids bind phosphate in the gut, after which it is excreted in the feces. Fanconi's syndrome is a descriptive phrase for a group of inherited or acquired renal tubular transport disorders that may result in excess phosphate excretion (as well as bicarbonate, glucose, and amino acids), resulting in hypophosphatemia and metabolic acidosis.

One of the most common causes of severe hypophosphatemia is prolonged, intense hyperventilation causing respiratory alkalosis. Gram-negative bacteremia, alcohol withdrawal, heat stroke, and acute salicylate poisoning are examples of clinical situations leading to respiratory alkalosis. Intracellular alkalosis occurs in respiratory alkalosis, because carbon dioxide (CO_2) is readily diffusible across the cell membrane but bicarbonate is not. Intracellular alkalosis activates phosphofructokinase and increases phosphorylation of glucose, and serum phosphate moves into the cells to be consumed in the process. Total parenteral nutrition without adequate phosphate replacement, treatment of DKA with glucose and insulin, and refeeding persons with severe protein-calorie malnutrition all cause phosphate movement into cells as anabolism occurs and can result in severe hypophosphatemia.

Severe hypophosphatemia is common in patients with extensive burns. Because nearly all severely burned patients hyperventilate, respiratory alkalosis and the resulting accelerated glycolysis are a likely cause.

Increased deposition of calcium phosphate salts in bone following parathyroidectomy, called the *hungry bone syndrome,* is a factor in both the hypophosphatemia and hypocalcemia frequently found after this surgery.

Finally, hypophosphatemia develops in approximately one half of patients hospitalized for withdrawal from alcohol abuse (Schrier, 1997). Several factors are responsible for the phosphate depletion in alcoholics, including poor dietary intake, vomiting, diarrhea, ingestion of antacids, and hypomagnesemia. Chronic alcoholism causes magnesium deficiency, which, in turn, may cause phosphaturia. These patients may also be given glucose infusions, causing phosphate to move from the ECF into cells.

Clinical Features

Most of the clinical features of hypophosphatemia (Box 21-21) can be attributed to the deficiency of ATP or 2,3-diphosphoglycerate (2,3-DPG) or both. A deficiency of ATP impairs active cellular processes that require it as an energy source, and a deficiency of 2,3-DPG impairs oxygen delivery to the tissues.

Hypophosphatemia may be associated with depletion of ATP in RBCs, WBCs, and platelets, reducing their function and survival time. Leukocyte dysfunction results in impaired chemotaxis, phagocytosis, and intracellular killing, with consequent increased susceptibility to bacterial and fungal infections. Platelet dysfunction may result in a bleeding tendency because of impaired aggregation. The RBC is the only tissue in the body that produces 2,3-DPG. Severe phosphate deficiency can reduce RBC content of 2,3-DPG, causing RBCs to become rigid spherocytes that hemolyze easily and whose shape impairs capillary perfusion. Both ATP and 2,3-DPG facilitate dissociation of oxyhemoglobin in the RBC and promote oxygen delivery to the tissues. Reduced 2,3-DPG and ATP in the RBC enhance affinity of oxygen for hemoglobin and reduce tissue oxygenation.

In the muscles, severe phosphate depletion may be associated with muscle weakness manifested as respiratory insufficiency when the respiratory muscles are affected and as congestive cardiomyopathy when the heart muscle is affected. *Rhabdomyolysis,* disintegration of skeletal muscle fibers with excretion of myoglobin in the urine, may occur in people with chronic alcoholism who become acutely hypophosphatemic during the course of alcohol withdrawal.

Phosphate depletion has multiple effects on renal function, including increased excretion of urinary calci-

---

BOX 21-21

Hypophosphatemia: Clinical Features

SIGNS AND SYMPTOMS
Hematologic
  RBC dysfunction and hemolysis
  Leukocyte dysfunction
  Platelet dysfunction
Neuromuscular
  Weakness
  Rhabdomyolysis
Cardiovascular
Cardiomyopathy
  Reduction in cardiac output
  Hypotension
Respiratory insufficiency
  Respiratory acidosis
  Hypoxia
Renal
  Increased calcium, HCO_3^-, Mg^{++} excretion
  Increased $1,25(OH)_2D_3$ synthesis
  Metabolic acidosis
Central nervous system
  Irritability, apprehension
  Paresthesias
  Dysarthria
  Confusion
  Obtundation
  Seizures
  Coma
Skeletal (long-term effects)
  Osteomalacia or rickets

LABORATORY FINDINGS
Mild: serum phosphate 1.5-2.5 mg/dl
Severe: serum phosphate 1.0 mg/dl or less

---

um, bicarbonate, and magnesium and increased synthesis of $1,25(OH)_2D_3$. Severe hypophosphatemia may also result in metabolic acidosis through two mechanisms. The hypophosphatemia results in decreased urinary phosphate excretion, thereby limiting H^+ excretion as NaH_2PO_4. The conversion of ammonia (NH_3) to ammonium (NH_4), another mechanism for acid excretion, is also depressed in phosphate deficiency.

CNS function may be impaired in hypophosphatemia, with symptoms of irritability, paresthesias, weakness, and encephalopathy progressing from confusion to coma. These symptoms usually occur in the setting of refeeding (e.g., victims of famine in a war-torn country) or hyperalimentation-induced hypophosphatemia that develops over the course of 8 to 10 days (Knochel, 1998).

Hypophosphatemia causes calcium and phosphate to be mobilized from bones and muscle and causes hypercalciuria. A consequence of long-term phosphate depletion includes osteomalacia or rickets.

Treatment

Treatment of hypophosphatemia should be primarily preventive. Adequate phosphate supplements must be given when hyperalimentation containing high glucose concentrations is administered. The treatment of hypophosphatemia varies with the cause. Phosphate depletion is rapidly reversible by correcting the underlying disorder and by phosphate therapy. Milk is an excellent source of phosphorus, supplying approximately 240 mg

DECREASED RENAL PHOSPHATE EXCRETION
Renal failure*
Hypoparathyroidism
Endocrine disorders
   Acromegaly
   Adrenal insufficiency
   Hyperthyroidism
Biphosphonate therapy

REDISTRIBUTION FROM ICF TO ECF
Chemotherapy for neoplasms
Respiratory or metabolic acidosis
Rhabdomyolysis
Hemolysis

INCREASED INTAKE-INTESTINAL ABSORPTION
Excess use of phosphate-containing laxatives or enemas
IV phosphate
Vitamin D intoxication
   Vitamin D medication
   Sarcoidosis
   Tuberculosis

*Most common cause.

per cup. Alternately, sodium phosphate and potassium phosphate tablets containing 250 mg of inorganic phosphate can be given in divided doses. In rare circumstances, phosphate may be given IV for severe hypophosphatemia. However, hypocalcemia and metastatic calcification may result as a complication.

Hyperphosphatemia

In adults, hyperphosphatemia is defined as an elevation of serum phosphate above 4.5 mg/dl. Hyperphosphatemia may be caused by decreased renal phosphate excretion, redistribution from the ICF to the ECF, and increased intake and intestinal absorption. The degree of hyperphosphatemia is a function of the rate of entry of phosphate into the ECF and the renal excretion of phosphate. When renal function is normal, clinically significant hyperphosphatemia seldom occurs. Some of the most common conditions causing hyperphosphatemia are listed in Box 21-22.

Acute or chronic renal failure is by far the most important cause of hyperphosphatemia, and it regularly occurs when the glomerular filtration rate (GFR) falls to 25% to 50% of normal (see Chapter 47). Decreased PTH secretion in hypoparathyroidism results in decreased urinary phosphate excretion. Acromegaly or administration of growth hormone causes modest hyperphosphatemia. Finally, biphosphonate therapy for malignancy-related hypercalcemia may result in hyperphosphatemia as a complication because of increased renal tubular reabsorption of phosphate.

Because phosphate is contained largely within cells, conditions causing transcellular shifts from the ICF to the ECF can result in hyperphosphatemia. Chemotherapy, especially for hematologic malignancies, causes cell lysis and the release of phosphate. Muscle contains large phosphate stores, and the breakdown of muscle in rhab-domyolysis, as sometimes occurs in withdrawal from alcohol, can cause hyperphosphatemia. Acidosis reduces phosphorylation and may cause phosphates to diffuse out of the cell. Phosphate is likewise released from RBCs in hemolysis.

Hyperphosphatemia may be produced from excess intake of phosphate-containing laxatives or enemas (e.g., Sal-Hepatica or Fleet enema) or from IV phosphate administration. Overmedication with vitamin D or the abnormal secretion of vitamin D in sarcoidosis or tuberculosis can cause an increased intestinal absorption of phosphate.

Clinical Features
Few signs and symptoms can be attributed to hyperphosphatemia alone. When symptoms do occur they can usually be attributed to the accompanying hypocalcemia. An acute rise in serum phosphate tends to result in an acute fall in serum calcium because of the reciprocal relationship of these two ions. Symptoms of hypocalcemia include paresthesias, muscle spasms, and tetany (see previous discussion of hypocalcemia). However, renal failure patients rarely have symptoms of hypocalcemia, because they generally have a metabolic acidosis that causes more serum calcium to exist in the ionized form. Long-term consequences of hyperphosphatemia may include precipitation of calcium phosphate salts around joints and in the soft tissues of the body.

Treatment
Therapy for hyperphosphatemia is directed at the underlying cause. The hyperphosphatemia of renal failure is treated by restriction of dietary phosphate and by the administration of calcium carbonate, a phosphate binder. Phosphate-binding antacids such as aluminum hydroxide (Amphojel) or aluminum carbonate (Basaljel) are used less frequently than they were in the past because of the danger of aluminum toxicity. Magnesium hydroxide (Maalox) should never be used for the treatment of hyperphosphatemia in patients with renal failure because a fatal hypermagnesemia may result.

Hypomagnesemia

Hypomagnesemia is defined as serum magnesium less than 1.5 mEq/L or 1.8 mg/dl, the lower limits of normal. Like other electrolytes that are largely intracellular, serum values of Mg^{++} may not accurately reflect total body deficits or excesses. When symptomatic hypomagnesemia is present, the serum magnesium is usually less than 1 mEq/L. Magnesium deficiency rarely occurs alone. When any of the three major intracellular ions (potassium, magnesium, or phosphate) is lost, losses of the others usually follow. Hypocalcemia also frequently accompanies hypomagnesemia because a magnesium deficit interferes with the release of PTH. The most common cause of hypomagnesemia is chronic alcoholism and alcoholic withdrawal. Studies have shown that hypomagnesemia is also common in critically ill patients, although it has often been overlooked in this population (Chan, Gill, 1990). Hypomagnesemia results from insufficient dietary intake, excessive loss in GI fluids or urine, or movement from the ECF to the ICF (Box 21-23).

BOX 21-23
Causes of Hypomagnesemia

DECREASED INTAKE
Deficiency of dietary magnesium
Starvation or malnutrition
Chronic alcoholism*
Total parenteral nutrition or IV fluids without magnesium
   replacement

GASTROINTESTINAL LOSSES
Malabsorption syndromes
   Nontropical sprue
   Biliary fistulas
   Chronic pancreatic insufficiency
Prolonged vomiting or nasogastric suction
Prolonged diarrhea

INCREASED URINARY LOSSES
Acute tubular necrosis (diuretic phase)
Diabetic ketoacidosis
Hyperparathyroidism
Hypoparathyroidism
Phosphate depletion
Aldosteronism
Syndrome of inappropriate antidiuretic hormone (SIADH)
Following renal transplantation
Drugs
   Alcohol
   Diuretics
   Aminoglycosides
   Amphotericin B
   Cyclosporine
   Antineoplastics (cisplatin)
   Vitamin D intoxication
   Citrated blood

SHIFT FROM ECF INTO CELLS/BONE
Alcoholic withdrawal*
Hungry bone syndrome following parathyroidectomy
Refeeding syndrome after starvation

*Most common causes.

Producing clinically symptomatic magnesium deficiency by dietary deficiency alone is difficult, unless other factors such as GI or renal losses occur simultaneously; a subclinical deficiency is more likely. However, magnesium deficiency can occur under conditions of prolonged malnutrition (e.g., chronic alcoholics who eat poorly), prolonged starvation, or prolonged administration of magnesium-free parenteral fluids without oral food intake.

Intestinal malabsorption is a common cause of magnesium loss, particularly when steatorrhea is present. Both calcium and magnesium form insoluble fatty acid soaps that are then excreted in the feces, resulting in both hypomagnesemia and hypocalcemia. Prolonged diarrhea in inflammatory bowel disease (e.g., Crohn's disease or ulcerative colitis), as well as prolonged vomiting or nasogastric suction, can cause magnesium depletion.

Excess renal loss of magnesium can occur during the diuretic phase of acute tubular necrosis (a type of acute renal failure) or from the diuresis following renal transplantation. Renal transplant patients are also given cyclosporine to prevent organ rejection; this drug causes increased renal tubular excretion of magnesium. The most common cause of excess urinary loss of magnesium is the prolonged administration of diuretics, particularly loop diuretics, such as furosemide or ethacrynic acid. Excessive urinary loss of magnesium also occurs in DKA, hyperaldosteronism, primary hyperparathyroidism and other hypercalcemic states, and the syndrome of inappropriate antidiuretic hormone (SIADH). Hypomagnesemia is frequently found in patients with hypoparathyroidism who have increased loss of Mg^{++} in their urine and feces. Other drugs causing excess renal magnesium wasting include aminoglycosides (e.g., gentamycin, tobramycin), amphotericin B, cisplatin (an antineoplastic drug), and vitamin-D overdosage. Transfusion with citrated blood may cause both hypomagnesemia and hypocalcemia because of the formation of complexes with the citrate.

Several factors play a role in the hypomagnesemia associated with chronic alcoholism and alcohol withdrawal. Chronic alcoholics are often malnourished from poor dietary intake and have reduced intake of foods that contain magnesium. Diarrhea is common in alcoholism, resulting in loss of intestinal fluids rich in magnesium. Alcohol has a direct effect on the kidney, causing increased urinary excretion of magnesium. The mild hypomagnesemia associated with chronic alcohol abuse may become severe during alcoholic withdrawal because of a shift of magnesium into the cells superimposed on the net deficit. Respiratory alkalosis and insulin release, stimulated by the administration of IV glucose, act in concert to incorporate phosphate into cells. Increased ATP synthesis as a result of phosphate moving into cells may cause increased magnesium binding and worsen the hypomagnesemia. For hypomagnesemia, hypophosphatemia, and hypokalemia to coexist during alcohol withdrawal is common. Hypocalcemia may also be present during alcohol withdrawal because a deficit of magnesium interferes with the secretion and action of PTH.

Other situations besides alcohol withdrawal that cause hypomagnesemia because of transcellular shifts of magnesium include refeeding after starvation and the hungry bone syndrome following parathyroidectomy. The rapid deposition of magnesium in the newly formed bone salts following parathyroidectomy or into muscle tissue during the refeeding syndrome causes a reduction in the serum magnesium.

Clinical Features

The clinical manifestations of magnesium deficiency are difficult to define because of other electrolyte abnormalities, such as hypokalemia and hypocalcemia, which frequently accompany depletion of this ion. Signs and symptoms usually involve the neuromuscular, central nervous, cardiovascular, and GI systems (Box 21-24).

Magnesium plays an important role in neuromuscular transmission. Consequently, in magnesium depletion, signs and symptoms of neuromuscular irritability are prominent and similar to those found in hypocalcemia (which may also be present). These signs and symptoms include paresthesias (numbness and tingling of fingertips or around the mouth), dysphagia, muscle weakness, cramps and tremors, occasional positive Chvostek's or Trousseau's signs, and hyperactive deep tendon reflexes.

CNS manifestations of magnesium deficit include personality changes such as agitation, apathy, or memory

BOX 21-24
Hypomagnesemia: Clinical Features

SIGNS AND SYMPTOMS
Neuromuscular
  Muscle weakness, fatigue
  Dysphagia
  Paresthesias
  Muscle cramps, twitching
  Gross tremors
  Chvostek's sign
  Trousseau's sign
  Hyperactive deep tendon reflexes
Central nervous system
  Apathy, depression, poor memory
  Mild to severe delirium
    Confusion
    Disorientation
    Hallucinations
    Delusions
  Vertigo and ataxia
  Convulsive seizures
  Coma
Gastrointestinal
  Anorexia, nausea and vomiting
  Paralytic ileus
Cardiovascular
  Tachycardia
  Dysrhythmias
  ECG changes
    Prolonged PR and QT intervals
    Widening of QRS complex
    Flat or inverted T wave
    Depressed ST segment
Metabolic
  Hypokalemia (caused by renal loss)
  Hypocalcemia (caused by decreased PTH
    secretion/action)

LABORATORY FINDINGS
Serum magnesium <1.5 mEq/L (1.8 mg/dl) (clinical manifestations occur when serum Mg^{++} <1.0 mEq/L)

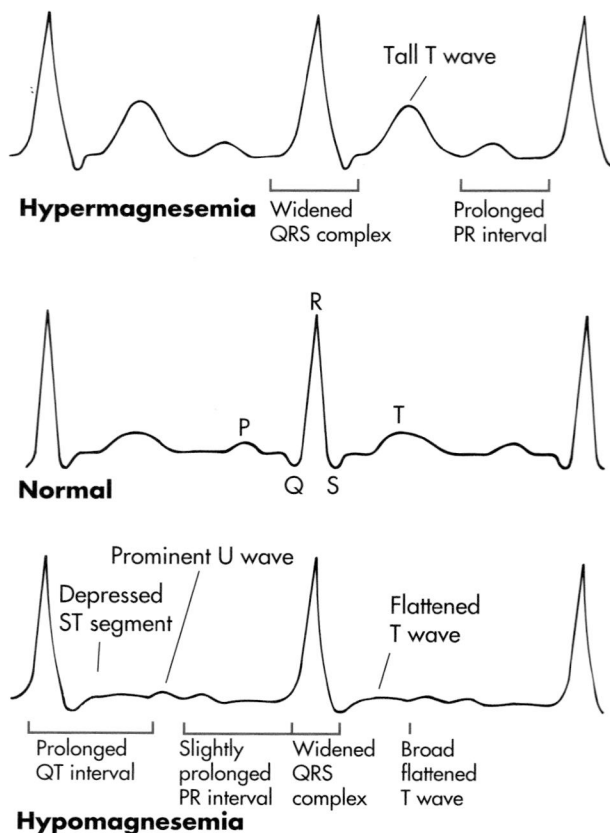

FIG. 21-10 ECG changes in magnesium imbalances. A prolonged PR interval, widened QRS complex, flattened T waves, and ST segment depression are changes that may be seen in hypomagnesemia. A prolonged PR interval, widened QRS complex, and peaked T waves may be seen in mild hypermagnesemia (< 9 mEq/L). Complete heart block and cardiac arrest occur at higher levels.

loss. The patient may have vertigo and ataxia and various degrees of delirium, convulsions, and coma. *Delirium tremens,* a term describing the neuromuscular irritability and CNS signs and symptoms, commonly occurs during acute alcohol withdrawal.

GI changes include decreased contractility of smooth muscle, which may lead to anorexia, nausea and vomiting, and even paralytic ileus. The cardiovascular abnormalities observed as a result of magnesium depletion may result from the malfunction of the many enzyme systems activated by magnesium or from the hypokalemia and hypocalcemia (or both) that are often present. Cardiac dysrhythmias include premature ventricular contractions (PVCs) and atrial or ventricular fibrillation; ECG changes that may be noted include prolonged PR and QT intervals, widened QRS complex, flat or inverted T waves, and ST segment depression (Fig. 21-10). Some of the ECG changes are similar to those present in hypokalemia and hypocalcemia, which may play a role in their creation. An increased sensitivity to digitalis may also occur that may require a decreased dosage to avoid toxicity.

A magnesium deficit affects the sodium-potassium pump, often resulting in hypokalemia, and an associated hypocalcemia may occur because hypomagnesemia suppresses PTH secretion and target organ action.

Treatment
Treatment seeks to correct the magnesium imbalance and identify and treat the underlying disorder. Any associated potassium, calcium, and phosphate deficiencies must be anticipated and corrected. Assessing renal function before administering magnesium is important because dosage should be reduced in the presence of renal insufficiency or failure.

A mild magnesium deficit may be treated by the administration of foods high in magnesium (green vegetables, meat, beans, nuts) and possibly daily oral magnesium salts in liquid or tablet form. Treatment with oral magnesium salts is limited because of the resultant diarrhea. When hypomagnesemia is severe with seizures or cardiac dysrhythmias, magnesium sulfate or chloride can be administered by intramuscular injection or by IV infusion. When magnesium is given IV, it must be given slowly (maximal infusion rate is 150 mg/min) with careful monitoring of serum electrolytes, vital signs, deep tendon reflexes (e.g., knee jerk), and ECG to detect and prevent hypermagnesemia and possible cardiac arrest.

Hypermagnesemia

Hypermagnesemia is defined as a serum magnesium greater than 2.5 mEq/L (3.0 mg/dl), the upper limit of normal. Hypermagnesemia is uncommon and is caused by either decreased renal excretion or increased intake of magnesium. When hypermagnesemia occurs, it is almost always in patients with renal failure who have ingested magnesium-containing drugs (e.g., antacids, such as Maalox or Riopan, or laxatives, such as milk of magnesia). Patients with renal insufficiency have limited ability to excrete magnesium, and a fatal hypermagnesemia may result. Phosphate-binding antacids administered to patients with chronic renal failure to prevent secondary hyperparathyroidism should be limited to magnesium-free antacids (Amphojel, Basojel, or calcium carbonate). The parenteral administration of magnesium to treat hypomagnesemia or *eclampsia* (toxemia of pregnancy) is another situation that could result in hypermagnesemia if not carefully monitored. Magnesium is a standard form of therapy for preeclampsia and eclampsia and may cause intoxication in both the mother and neonate. Other less common causes of hypermagnesemia include untreated DKA, Addison's disease (hypoadrenalism), and hemodialysis using hard water high in magnesium.

Clinical Features

The predominant clinical manifestations of hypermagnesemia involve the neuromuscular and cardiovascular systems. Magnesium excess produces a sedative effect on the neuromuscular system, causing muscular weakness. The eventual result is ventilatory arrest from paralysis of the respiratory muscles. Magnesium excess produces this effect mainly by suppressing the release of acetylcholine at the myoneural junction, thus blocking neuromuscular transmission and reducing muscle cell excitability. Excess magnesium also reduces the responsiveness of the postsynaptic membrane, displacing calcium from binding sites and preventing its action.

Hypermagnesemia impairs cardiac function by interfering with atrioventricular conduction, producing a variety of disturbances in the ECG that may eventually culminate in complete heart block and cardiac arrest. Magnesium excess causes hypotension by relaxing vascular smooth muscle and reducing vascular resistance by displacing calcium from the vascular wall surface (Chan, Gill, 1990). Table 21-1 depicts a rough correlation between the total serum magnesium levels and the clinical findings. No general agreement in the literature exists concerning the precise magnesium levels related to specific signs and symptoms.

When the serum magnesium is between 3 and 5 mEq/L, facial flushing may be present because of cutaneous vasodilation that may be accompanied by a sensation of heat and thirst. The patient may complain of muscular weakness and nausea and vomiting, and the deep tendon reflexes are diminished.

When the serum magnesium level is approximately 5 to 9 mEq/L, the patient becomes increasingly drowsy and

TABLE 21-1 ■ ■ ■

Hypermagnesemia: Clinical Features

Serum Mg^{++} (mEq/L)	Signs and Symptoms
1.5-2.5	Normal
3-5	Facial flushing with sensation of heat and thirst Muscular weakness Diminished deep tendon reflexes (DTRs) Nausea and vomiting
5-9	Lethargy, drowsiness Peripheral vasodilation, hypotension Increasing weakness and paralysis of all muscles Respiratory compromise Absent deep tendon reflexes (DTRs) ECG: bradycardia, prolonged PR interval, peaked T waves, widened QRS complex
10-12	Coma
15-20	ECG: Complete heart block Cardiac arrest Respiratory arrest

lethargic and becomes comatose at higher levels. The patient may be hypotensive because of peripheral vasodilation, and deep tendon reflexes (DTRs) may be completely absent. Increasing weakness and finally a curarelike paralysis of all the muscles occur. Respiratory compromise occurs because of respiratory center depression and involvement of the respiratory muscles. Fig. 21-10 depicts some of the ECG changes that may occur with magnesium excess.

When serum magnesium levels reach 15 to 20 mEq/L, complete heart block and cardiac arrest, as well as respiratory arrest, may occur.

Treatment

Avoiding the administration of magnesium-containing medications to persons with renal insufficiency should prevent hypermagnesemia. Patient education is particularly important with respect to achieving this goal. When magnesium is administered parenterally, the nurse must closely monitor the rate of administration and assess the patient frequently for any signs or symptoms of magnesium excess.

When hypermagnesemia is mild, the only treatment that may be necessary is to discontinue magnesium administration. Instituting peritoneal dialysis or hemodialysis with magnesium-free dialysate may be the treatment of choice for patients with renal failure. In patients with normal renal function, saline and furosemide may be given to provide hydration and promote diuresis with elimination of excess magnesium. When cardiac conduction or respiratory effects occur, emergency care is required. Calcium gluconate (a magnesium antagonist) may be given under ECG monitoring to reverse the effects of magnesium temporarily, and the patient may be placed on a ventilator.

KEY CONCEPTS

- The three basic classes of fluid and electrolyte disturbances include (1) isotonic ECF volume imbalances (hypovolemia and hypervolemia), (2) osmotic imbalances, caused primarily by unequal gains or losses of Na^+ and water and affecting the ICF (hypoosmolality and hyperosmolality), and (3) changes in the composition of the ECF (excesses or deficits of electrolytes, such as K^+, Ca^{++}, Mg^{++}, and H^+ [acid-base disturbances]). A change in the distribution of body fluids may also occur, such as into a non-ECF, non-ICF space, resulting in ECF volume deficits or excesses.

- ECF volume deficit (hypovolemia) is the loss of fluids isotonic to the plasma with relatively equal losses of Na^+ and water. This type of fluid loss is commonly referred to as dehydration although this is erroneous because the fluid loss is isotonic. Because the Na^+ to water ratio remains unchanged, osmolality is not affected.

- ECF volume deficit may be caused by extrarenal or renal losses of fluid. Extrarenal losses include the following: GI tract losses, which can be large because GI secretions are approximately 8 L/day (vomiting, NG suction, diarrhea, ileostomies); losses from the skin because of diaphoresis or extensive burns; and distribution losses (third spacing, as in ascites or bowel obstruction). Renal losses (polyuria) can occur as a result of intrinsic renal disease (e.g., salt wasting nephritis) or as a result of causes extrinsic to the kidney (e.g., use of potent diuretics, osmotic diuresis, aldosterone deficiency).

- The signs and symptoms of an ECF volume deficit depend on the rapidity and magnitude of the deficit. When the fluid loss is rapid and large, such as hemorrhage, severe diarrhea or massive sequestration in a third space, the signs and symptoms are synonymous with circulatory shock. More commonly the fluid loss develops more slowly and is less severe. Generalized symptoms of a moderate ECF deficit include weakness, lassitude, fatigue, and anorexia. Cardiovascular signs include orthostatic hypotension (early sensitive sign), flat jugular veins in the supine position, and prolonged filling time of the hand veins. The tongue and mucous membranes are dry and skin turgor is poor. Analysis of daily weight and intake and output records is essential. Acute weight loss of 1 lb equals a fluid loss of approximately 500 ml. A 2% loss of total body weight equals a mild ECF deficit; a 5% loss is moderate, and a 8% loss is severe.

- Laboratory finding are of little help in diagnosing an ECF volume deficit. The hemoglobin and hematocrit may be elevated, but ECF volume deficit is difficult to interpret unless baseline values are known. Serum Na^+ will be normal unless an osmolality imbalance is also present. The urine will be concentrated (high specific gravity or osmolality) and scanty. Urine Na^+ will be low (<10 mEq/L) if the cause of the deficit is extrarenal and high (>20 mEq/L) if the cause is intrarenal (salt-losing nephritis) or aldosterone deficiency (as in Addison's disease).

- The goal of treatment for an ECF volume deficit is to restore normovolemia and treat any associated acid-base or electrolyte imbalances, as well as the underlying cause. When the patient is hypotensive, the IV fluid of choice is an isotonic solution (such as 0.9% saline) because it will expand the plasma volume and restore tissue perfusion. This application should be followed by a hypotonic IV solution to provide free water to the cells.

- When adequate fluid cannot be taken by mouth, the general rules for IV therapy are to provide for maintenance needs and make up for losses, replace concurrent losses volume for volume, and administer the fluid evenly over 24 hours, except in unusual circumstances.

- IV fluid requirements are based on body surface area (BSA), which can be obtained from a nomogram in most drug handbooks. Multiply the BSA by 1500 ml for 24-hour maintenance needs, by 2400 for a moderate deficit (<5% acute weight loss), and by 3000 for a severe deficit (>5% acute weight loss).

- ECF volume excess (hypervolemia or circulatory overload) develops when both Na^+ and water are retained in roughly the same proportions (isotonic to the plasma). As isotonic fluid accumulates, fluid shifts into the interstitial space causing edema. The proximate cause of edema is always a disruption of one of the Starling forces discussed in Chapter 20. ECF volume excess is always secondary to an increase in total body Na^+ content, which, in turn, causes water retention.

- Common conditions associated with ECF volume excess are congestive heart failure (CHF), cirrhosis of the liver, nephrotic syndrome, and renal failure. The mechanism responsible for the first three conditions is believed to be a decrease in the effective circulating volume with activation of the renin-angiotensin-aldosterone mechanism, resulting in renal retention of Na^+ and water. In the case of renal failure, the cause of the ECF volume excess and edema is impairment of renal excretory function. Cushing's syndrome, starvation (hypoalbuminemia), and rapid infusion of IV saline are additional causes of hypervolemia.

- Signs and symptoms of ECF volume excess include jugular venous distention, rising central venous pressure, elevated blood pressure, slow emptying of hand veins, peripheral and periorbital edema, acute pulmonary edema (if gain is severe or rapid), moist rales, rapid weight gain, and intake and output records showing intake greater than output.

- The treatment of ECF volume excess depends on the cause. Most treatment plans include the restriction of Na^+ and fluid intake. Acute pulmonary edema requires prompt treatment using measures to reduce preload, such as positioning in high Fowler's position and administering a potent diuretic and oxygen.

- Osmolality imbalances involve the concentration of solutes in body fluids (or the solute-to-water ratio).
- Because Na^+ is the major osmotically active solute particle of the ECF, in most cases, hypoosmolality represents hyponatremia, and hyperosmolality represents hypernatremia. One notable exception is the hyperglycemia of uncontrolled diabetes mellitus. Because of insulin deficiency, the glucose is unable to enter the cell, thereby acting as an osmotically active solute particle.
- Hyponatremia (hypoosmolality) is caused by water excess or Na^+ depletion.
- Hypernatremia (hyperosmolality) is caused by either a water deficit or Na^+ excess.
- Because water passes readily between the ECF and ICF until equilibrium is achieved, *the osmolality of the ECF and ICF are always equal.* Water moves from an area of lesser solute concentration (lower mOsm) to an area of higher solute concentration (higher mOsm).
- However, a change in the ECF serum Na^+ has a profound effect on *ICF fluid volume and cell size.*
- Hyponatremia (hypoosmolality) imbalances cause cell swelling (because net water movement is from the ECF to the ICF).
- Hypernatremia (hyperosmolality) imbalances cause cell shrinkage (because net water movement is from the ICF to the ECF).
- The most serious and life-threatening clinical manifestations of hyponatremia or hypernatremia are neurologic and are related to brain cell swelling (cerebral edema) or shrinkage of brain cells, respectively.
- Plasma Na^+ is a measure of concentration (osmolality) and not of ECF volume because it reflects the Na^+-to-water ratio, not the absolute amount of either solute or water. Therefore plasma Na^+ should not be used to assess ECF volume disturbances but should be used to assess osmolality and ICF volume disturbances.
- Assessing the urinary Na^+ concentration is important to determine the cause of hyponatremia. Urinary Na^+ of less than 10 mEq/L/24 hours occurs when hyponatremia is associated with edema or with volume depletion resulting from extrarenal causes. Urinary Na^+ greater than 20 mEq/L/24 hours occurs when hyponatremia is associated with SIADH, salt-wasting renal disease, or renal failure with water retention.
- The general principles of treatment for osmolality imbalances are (1) hypoosmolality—remove excess water or replace Na^+ and (2) hyperosmolality—replace water or remove excess Na^+ (or glucose).
- Osmolality imbalances and ECF volume imbalances may be combined with six possible combinations:
  1. Hyponatremia with ECF volume depletion
  2. Hyponatremia with ECF volume excess
  3. Hyponatremia with normovolemia
  4. Hypernatremia with ECF volume depletion
  5. Hypernatremia with ECF volume excess
  6. Hypernatremia with normovolemia

- Hyponatremia (serum Na^+ <135 mEq/L) caused by a loss of Na^+ in excess of water loss is called *depletional hyponatremia.* A common cause is people on prolonged diuretic therapy with a low-salt diet. Other causes include GI losses, excessive sweating, salt-losing nephritis, and adrenal insufficiency.
- Hyponatremia caused by a gain of water in excess of Na^+ is called *dilutional hyponatremia* or *water intoxication.* Dilutional hyponatremia may occur in conditions in which the ability to excrete free water is impaired because of activation of the renin-angiotensin-aldosterone mechanism resulting from decreased effective circulating volume, such as in CHF, liver cirrhosis, and the nephrotic syndrome. SIADH, excessive hypotonic IVs, psychogenic polydipsia, and freshwater drowning are other causes.
- Hyponatremia without hypoosmolality may occur in DKA and with mannitol administration.
- The clinical signs and symptoms of hyponatremia are primarily neurologic and related to cerebral edema (brain cell swelling) and increased intracranial pressure (ICP). The signs and symptoms depend on the rapidity and magnitude of the decrease in serum Na^+. A serum Na^+ of 125 to 135 mEq/L is usually asymptomatic, and the cause is usually depletional hyponatremia. Symptoms with moderate hyponatremia (115 to 125 mEq/L) may result in complaints of anorexia, impaired taste, and muscle cramps. Severe hyponatremia (<115 mEq/L) is serious and life threatening and may result in headache, lethargy, nausea and vomiting, abdominal cramps, papilledema, hypoactive tendon reflexes, Babinski's sign, seizures and coma (all related to increased ICP), and fingerprinting over the sternum.
- The treatment goals for hyponatremia are to raise the serum Na^+ to normal without causing ECF volume excess and to treat the underlying cause.
- Mild depletional hyponatremia (120 to 135 mEq/L) in patients with true ECF volume depletion from GI or renal losses is treated with oral NaCl or IV normal saline. Correction of the hyponatremia suppresses ADH release allowing the kidney to excrete the excess water.
- Mild dilutional hyponatremia can usually be treated by water restriction alone.
- Syndrome of the inappropriate secretion of ADH (SIADH) is a special type of dilutional hyponatremia that is more apt to be severe and life threatening. The basic cause is the sustained secretion of ADH by the hypothalamus or release of ADH by an ectopic source (commonly oat cell carcinoma of the lung).
- In SIADH, aldosterone secretion is decreased because of the increased ECF volume, thus the kidneys excrete Na^+ inappropriately in the presence of low serum osmolality. Higher priority is given to ECF volume control over osmolality regulation when the two are in conflict. The combination of both water retention and Na^+ loss in the urine lowers the serum Na^+, causing a progressively severe hyponatremia.
- The most common situations associated with SIADH are head injuries (including facial trauma),

- pneumonia, postoperative states, particularly after open-heart surgery, and in oat cell lung cancer. Oxytocin (Pituitrin), when added to Na^+-free IV fluids to induce labor, can cause SIADH. (Normal saline should be used.)
- In more severe cases of hyponatremia (<120 mEq/L) usually associated with SIADH, hypertonic saline (3%) may be given slowly to raise the serum Na^+ at a rate of 0.5 mEq/hour until a level of 120 mEq/L is reached and the patient is out of danger. This treatment is combined with fluid restriction.
- Declomycin is used to treat chronic SIADH from an ADH-secreting tumor as in oat cell lung cancer.
- Hypernatremia (serum Na^+ >145 mEq/L) causes hyperosmolality, resulting in ICF dehydration and cell shrinkage. The basic causes are loss of water in excess of Na^+ or gain of Na^+ in excess of water.
- The most common situation causing loss of water in excess of Na^+, resulting in hypernatremia is inadequate provision of water intake for a patient who is unable to communicate thirst, confused, unable to swallow, or comatose. Other conditions include diabetes insipidus (lack of ADH) in patients with CNS trauma, loss of a hypotonic body fluid (fever and diaphoresis, tracheobronchitis), osmotic diuresis (high-protein tube feedings without adequate water or hyperglycemic osmotic diuresis in DKA).
- Hypernatremia caused by a gain of Na^+ in excess of water is uncommon; seawater drowning is probably the most common situation (seawater Na^+ = 500 mEq/L).
- The most serious clinical manifestations of hypernatremia are neurologic as a result of brain cell shrinkage, which may result in permanent brain damage caused by subarachnoid hemorrhage or brain contraction. Lethargy, weakness, and irritability are early symptoms that may progress to severe agitation, delirium, nuchal rigidity, and coma as the magnitude of hypernatremia increases. The tongue is red and rough, mucous membranes are dry and sticky, and the skin is flushed with a rubbery turgor. The temperature is elevated and oliguria is present. The patient will complain of extreme thirst when able to communicate.
- Laboratory findings include a serum Na^+ >145 mEq/L. A serum Na^+ of 160 mEq/L in adults is associated with a mortality rate of 75%. The serum osmolality is usually high (>295 mOsm/Kg) and the urine is concentrated and scanty as the kidneys try to conserve water.
- The treatment goal for hypernatremia is to reduce the serum Na^+ before a critical level (>160 mEq/L) is reached, gradually lowering the serum Na^+ and hyperosmolality to normal. The treatment depends on the underlying pathophysiologic mechanism causing the hypernatremia. Hypernatremia with normovolemia is treated with water orally or IV D_5W. Hypernatremia with hypervolemia is treated with IV D_5W and diuretics. Central diabetes insipidus is treated with Desmopressin (dDAVP) nasal spray (synthetic ADH).

- K^+ is the major cation of the ICF (160 mEq/L), the normal ECF range of which is 3.5 to 5.5 mEq/L; this concentration differential plays a major role in maintaining the electrical gradient across the cell membrane necessary for the normal function of nerve action potentials and muscle contraction, particularly cardiac impulse conduction and cardiac muscle contraction. Consequently, signs and symptoms of hypokalemia or hyperkalemia are manifested primarily in the neuromuscular and cardiac status.
- Normal dietary intake of K^+ is 50 to 150 mEq/day, and 90% of the output is in the urine. K^+ is poorly conserved, and approximately 5% of the stores are lost when the patient takes nothing by mouth. Polyuria favors K^+ loss. High concentrations of K^+ are present in the gastric mucosa and in intestinal secretions, thus vomiting or diarrhea favors the loss of K^+.
- The renal excretion of K^+ is regulated by aldosterone. Increased aldosterone causes K^+ excretion in the urine, and decreased aldosterone causes K^+ reabsorption.
- The distribution of K^+ between the ICF and ECF is influenced by the acid-base status and hormones.
- Hypokalemia is usually associated with alkalosis because alkalosis causes K^+ to move from the ECF to the ICF in exchange for H^+.
- Hyperkalemia is usually associated with acidosis because acidosis causes K^+ to move from the ICF to the ECF in exchange for H^+. K^+ may be lost in the osmotic diuresis associated with DKA; the acidosis may be masking an actual hypokalemia when the serum K^+ is in the normal range. Administration of insulin for the treatment of DKA will cause K^+ to move from the ECF to the ICF and may unmask a serious hypokalemia when the acidosis is corrected.
- Manifestations of hypokalemia and hyperkalemia are evident on the EKG tracing. Hypokalemia (serum K^+ <3.5 mEq/L) causes flattening of the T wave, ST segment depression, increased height of the U wave, and various dysrhythmias. Hyperkalemia (serum K^+ >5.5 mEq/L) causes peaking of the T wave, ST segment depression, prolonged PR interval, widening of the QRS, ventricular fibrillation, and death from cardiac arrest.
- The most common causes of hypokalemia (serum K^+ <3.5 mEq/L) are from GI losses (e.g., vomiting, NG suction, diarrhea) enhanced by the lack of K^+ intake. Diuretic therapy is the most common cause resulting in renal loss of K^+. Other causes of the renal loss of K^+ are DKA leading to osmotic diuresis, the healing stage of severe burns, and Mg^{++} depletion. Heat stress may cause excessive K^+ loss in sweat. Metabolic alkalosis that accompanies prolonged vomiting or NG suction, causes K^+ to shift into the cells and contributes to the hypokalemia.
- Early signs and symptoms of hypokalemia are vague, such as fatigue and generalized muscular weakness. Manifestations of hypokalemia affect primarily the neuromuscular and cardiovascular systems and may

include paresthesias, weak respiratory muscles, paralytic ileus, and postural hypotension; EKG changes are likely the most sensitive and earliest signs of hypokalemia.

- Laboratory findings in hypokalemia include serum K^+ <3.5 mEq/L, often accompanied by metabolic alkalosis (serum pH >7.45, HCO_3^- >26 mEq/L).

- The treatment goal for hypokalemia is to restore normokalemia. *It is important to remember that diuretics, digitalis, and hypokalemia are a potentially lethal combination.* Many diuretics cause hypokalemia, and hypokalemia enhances the effect of digitalis. The toxic effect of both digitalis and hypokalemia may cause life-threatening cardiac dysrhythmias. When possible, K^+ depletion should be corrected by increased intake of K^+-rich foods or by K^+ supplements. Potassium chloride (KCl) should be added to the IV if the patient cannot take K^+ orally and particularly in cases of metabolic alkalosis or for the treatment of DKA. The rate of infusion should not exceed 20 mEq/hour to avoid serious hyperkalemia. A bolus of KCl should *never* be given directly into an IV line because instant cardiac arrest would result.

- The most common cause of hyperkalemia (serum K^+ >5.5 mEq/L) is renal failure (because 90% is excreted in the urine). Hypoaldosteronism (as in Addison's disease), serious burns, and crushing injuries, and K^+-sparing diuretics are other causes.

- Signs and symptoms of hyperkalemia are primarily manifested in the neuromuscular and cardiac systems and are similar to those of hypokalemia and difficult to differentiate clinically. EKG changes are likely the earliest and most reliable signs of hyperkalemia.

- Laboratory findings in hyperkalemia are an elevated K^+ (serum K^+ >5.5 mEq/L), often accompanied by metabolic acidosis (serum pH <7.35, HCO_3^- <22 mEq/L).

- The treatment of hyperkalemia varies with its severity. When the serum K^+ is dangerously high (7 to 8 mEq/L) or when ECG changes are advanced indicating imminent cardiac arrest, the serum K^+ must be reduced to a safe level within minutes. The serum K^+ can be reduced within 5 minutes by the slow IV administration of 10 mL of 10% calcium gluconate with ECG monitoring or within 30 minutes by the administration of 500 ml of 10% glucose with insulin.

- When hyperkalemia is less severe, a short-term treatment of hyperkalemia is to administer Kayexalate (a nonabsorbable ion exchange resin) orally or by enema. Finally, the long-term treatment of hyperkalemia and renal failure is intermittent peritoneal dialysis or hemodialysis. Serial measurement of K^+ should be obtained for all patients with renal insufficiency or failure for early detection of hyperkalemia and early treatment to prevent cardiac arrest.

- Imbalances of calcium, phosphate, and magnesium are closely linked as well as their regulation.

- Calcium has a structural and functional role. Structurally, 99% of the body's calcium is stored in bone (along with phosphate). Calcium resorption and deposition is important in growth, and the constant bone remodeling is required to adapt to changing mechanical stresses. Functionally, Ca^{++} plays a central role in nerve function and muscle contraction, modulating enzyme function, and serving as an important intracellular signaling system.

- The normal total serum calcium is 4.5 to 5.5 mEq/L or 9.0 to 10.5 mg/dl. Only approximately 50% of the serum Ca^{++} is in the physiologically active ionized form; the remainder is bound to albumin or complexed with small ligands. A decrease in albumin will result in a low total serum calcium, while the ionized Ca^{++} will remain normal. To correct for this discrepancy, the following formula should be used: corrected total serum Ca (mg/dl) = 4 − serum albumin (g/dl) × 0.8 + measured serum Ca (mg/dl). Alkalemia increases the binding of calcium to albumin and may result in a functional hypocalcemia. Acidemia decreases the binding of calcium to albumin and increases the ionized Ca^{++}.

- The normal dietary intake of calcium is approximately 1000 mg/day, and absorption in the gut requires calcitriol (1,25-dihydroxycholecalciferol). Calcium loss occurs through fecal and urinary excretion and deposition in bone.

- The normal serum $HPO_4^=$ is 1.8 to 2.6 mEq/L or 2.0 to 4.5 mg/dl.

- The serum calcium and phosphate have a reciprocal relationship. A rise in the serum Ca^{++} causes a fall in the serum $PO_4^=$; a rise in the serum $PO_4^=$ causes a fall in serum Ca^{++}. The adaptive purpose of this relationship is to allow deposition of calcium in bone and to prevent precipitation of calcium salts in the soft tissues of the body. In the presence of vitamin D and alkaline phosphatase, when the Ca and PO_4 cross product is greater than 30 (in mg/dl) $CaPO_4$ precipitates in the osteoid framework (immature weak bone) to form calcified mature bone. If both Ca^{++} and $PO_4^=$ should rise and their cross product exceeds 60 to 70 (in mg/dl) as in primary or secondary hyperparathyroidism, calcium salts would then precipitate in the soft tissues of the body, around the joints, and in the kidney.

- Serum Ca^{++} (and phosphate) is closely regulated by the coordinated action of parathyroid hormone (PTH) and vitamin D_3 (1,25-dihydroxycholecalciferol, the most potent form of vitamin D). The kidneys, bone, and gut are the target organs. In response to a decrease in the serum Ca^{++}, PTH is released and helps to restore serum Ca^{++} to its normal range. The actions of PTH are to (1) mobilize $CaPO_4$ from bone, (2) stimulate the kidneys to convert 25-OH vitamin D_3 to it most potent form, 1,25-dihydroxycholecalciferol, and (3) increase the renal excretion of $PO_4^=$ which, in turn, raises serum Ca^{++} (because of their reciprocal relationship). The actions of 1,25-dihydroxycholecalciferol are to (1) increase calcium absorption by the gut, (2) augment $CaPO_4$ mobilization from bone, and (3) increase renal absorption of calcium.

- Hypocalcemia is defined as a total serum calcium level less than 9 mg/dl or ionized calcium of less than 4.5 mEq/L. Any disorder that leads to decreased effective PTH or 1,25-dihydroxycholecalciferol can cause hypocalcemia and bone disease. Chronic renal failure is the most common cause of hypocalcemia resulting from several factors: phosphate retention (causing a reciprocal drop in serum Ca^{++}), impaired sensitivity to the bone-resorbing action of PTH, reduced renal hydroxylation of vitamin D to its most potent form (1,25-dihydroxycholecalciferol) leading to decreased intestinal absorption. Hypomagnesemia can interfere with the PTH secretion and cause hypocalcemia. Hypoparathyroidism and hypocalcemia can follow subtotal parathyroidectomy until the remaining parathyroid tissue can increase PTH secretion.

- Alkalosis can also cause symptoms of hypocalcemia as a result of decreased serum ionized Ca^{++}, although the total serum calcium may be normal.

- Symptoms of hypocalcemia depend on the degree, duration, and rate of its development. The most prominent signs and symptoms are caused primarily by increased neuromuscular irritability. Tetany (involuntary muscle spasms) is the most characteristic sign of hypocalcemia demonstrated by a positive Trousseau's sign or Chvostek's sign. The total serum calcium is less than 8.5 mg/dl (<4.5 mEq/L) or ionized Ca^{++} is less than 4.5 mg/dl. Hypocalcemia produces prolongation of the QT interval on the ECG when serum Ca^{++} is 7 mg/dl and is consistently present when serum Ca^{++} is 6 mg/dl or less.

- Treatment of hypocalcemia focuses on correcting the imbalance and the underlying cause. Acute severe hypocalcemic tetany is treated with 10 ml of 10% calcium gluconate IV with continuous ECG monitoring.

- In 90% of the cases, hypercalcemia (total serum calcium >10.5 mg/dl [5.5 mEq/L]) is caused by either primary hyperparathyroidism or cancer. Additionally, hypercalcemia may be associated with severe secondary hyperparathyroidism observed in chronic renal failure.

- Signs and symptoms of hypercalcemia vary greatly, depending on the rapidity of onset and degree of the elevation of calcium levels. In mild cases, patients may be asymptomatic. The predominant effects of hypercalcemia involve the CNS, the kidney, and the neuromuscular system. Confusion, lethargy, and stupor frequently accompany hypercalcemia. Polyuria and volume depletion may accompany excessive urinary loss of calcium. Nephrocalcinosis may occur in chronic hypercalcemia. Generalized muscular weakness may be quite marked. Shortening of the QT interval may be evident on the ECG.

- Treatment of hypercalcemia is directed toward correcting the underlying cause. Severe life-threatening hypercalcemia (>14 mg/dl) is treated with IV saline, diuretics, or dialysis. Etidronate, pamidronate, gallium, and corticosteroids inhibit bone resorption and promote calcium excretion and are useful for cancer-related hypercalcemia.

- Common causes of hypophosphatemia are prolonged hyperventilation, resulting in respiratory alkalosis, total parenteral nutrition without adequate phosphate replacement, and withdrawal from alcohol abuse.

- The most common cause of hyperphosphatemia (>4.5 mg/dl) is chronic renal failure. The hyperphosphatemia of renal failure is treated by restriction of dietary phosphate and by the administration of calcium carbonate, a phosphate binder.

- Hypomagnesemia (<1.5 mEq/L or 1.8 mg/dl) results from decreased intake (total parenteral nutrition or IV therapy without Mg^{++} replacement), excessive GI or renal losses, or movement of Mg^{++} from the ECF to the ICF (as in alcohol withdrawal or refeeding syndrome after starvation). Hypokalemia and hypocalcemia frequently accompany hypomagnesemia, making the clinical manifestations specific to hypomagnesemia difficult to define. Hypomagnesemia causes decreased blood pressure and may result in cardiac dysrhythmias. Hypomagnesemia may be treated with intramuscular (IM) or IV magnesium salts.

- Hypermagnesemia (>2.5 mEq/L or 3.0 mg/dl) is uncommon and is caused by either decreased renal excretion or increased intake of magnesium; hypermagnesemia most commonly occurs in patients with renal failure who have ingested drugs containing magnesium (e.g., antacids, such as Maalox or Riopan, or laxatives, such as milk of magnesia). Patients with renal insufficiency should not be given drugs containing magnesium.

QUESTIONS ??

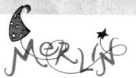

A sampling of review questions for this chapter appears here. Visit http://www.mosby.com/MERLIN/PriceWilson/ for additional questions.

Circle the letter preceding the item below that correctly answers each question or completes the statement. More than one answer may be correct.

1. The most sensitive assessment parameter for the early detection of fluid volume deficit is:
   a. Orthostatic hypotension and tachycardia
   b. Blood pressure of 100/70 mm Hg in the supine position
   c. Lassitude, weakness, and fatigue
   d. Prolonged filling time of the hand veins
   e. Decreased serum Na$^+$ concentration

2. A previously healthy 45-year-old man is admitted to the hospital with a history of nausea, vomiting, and diarrhea over 4 days and a diagnosis of gastroenteritis from eating contaminated food in a restaurant. Physical assessment reveals the following: oral temperature, 97.0° F; pulse, 110 beats/min; respirations, 20 breaths/min; blood pressure, 120/80 mm Hg supine and 90/60 mm Hg sitting; neck veins flat in the supine position; decreased skin and tongue turgor. His weight is 66.0 kg (normal = 70 kg). He is lethargic and weak. Laboratory tests on the blood serum reveal the following: Na$^+$, 143 mEq/L; Cl$^-$, 106 mEq/L; K$^+$, 3.3 mEq/L; BUN, 35 g/dl; creatinine, 1.5 mg/dl; hematocrit, 55%. Urinary findings reveal the following: urine output, 25 ml/hr; specific gravity, 1.038; urinary Na$^+$, 8 mEq/L. These findings indicate:
   a. The patient has an isotonic fluid volume deficit
   b. The patient has combined hyperosmolality disturbance and fluid volume deficit
   c. The patient has a moderate (5%) fluid volume deficit with the loss of approximately 4 L of body fluid
   d. The patient has hyperkalemia
   e. The low urinary Na$^+$ indicates that the fluid loss is extrarenal

3. Which of the following IV solutions would be preferred initially to help correct the patient's problem in Question 2?
   a. Isotonic saline (0.9% NaCl)
   b. Isotonic saline with added 20 mEq KCl/L

   c. Half-normal saline (0.45% NaCl)
   d. D$_5$W

4. Approximately how much fluid should be given to the patient in Question 2 over the next 24 hours?
   a. 1500 ml
   b. 2500 ml
   c. 3000 ml
   d. 4000 ml

Answer the following on a separate piece of paper.

5. What effect would the loss of 3 L of isotonic fluid (e.g., diarrhea fluid or gastric fluid) have on the following parameters?
   a. Effective circulating blood volume
   b. Plasma osmolality
   c. Plasma Na$^+$ concentration
   d. ADH secretion
   e. Urine osmolality and specific gravity
   f. Thirst
   g. Blood pressure

6. What would happen to the plasma osmolality if the patient in Question 5 ingested a large amount of pure water?

7. Compare the effects of the loss of pure water caused by insensible losses (from the lungs because of hyperventilation or renal loss in diabetes insipidus) to the loss of an equal volume of isotonic fluid (as in vomiting or diarrhea) on the following:
   a. ECF volume and blood pressure
   b. Plasma osmolality
   c. ICF volume of brain cells

8. Why is normal saline the IV infusion of choice for the treatment of hypovolemic shock rather than D$_5$W?

Circle the letter preceding the item below that correctly answers each question or completes the statement. More than one answer may be correct.

9. A middle-aged woman is started on a thiazide diuretic for the treatment of hypertension. After taking the drug for 3 weeks, she complains of weakness, muscle cramps, and postural dizziness. She is alert and oriented to time, place, and person. Physical findings include the following: blood pressure, 130/90 mm Hg (previously 170/100 mm Hg); decreased skin turgor; decreased filling time of hand

veins; flat neck veins in the supine position. Laboratory serum tests reveal the following: Na$^+$, 115 mEq/L; Cl$^-$, 66 mEq/L; K$^+$, 2.1 mEq/L; plasma osmolality, 240 mOsm/kg; HCO$^-_3$, 32 mEq/L. Urine tests reveal the following: Na$^+$, 4 mEq/L; K$^+$, 20 mEq/L; urine osmolality, 540 mOsm/kg. Which of the following has contributed to this patient's hyponatremia?
   a. The thiazide diuretic
   b. ECF volume depletion
   c. Increased ADH secretion
   d. Water ingestion and retention
   e. K$^+$ depletion

10. The appropriate treatment for the patient in Question 2 should include which of the following:
    a. Water restriction alone
    b. Rapid administration of D$_5$W
    c. Isotonic (0.9%) saline
    d. KCl
    e. Half-isotonic (0.45%) saline

11. Mr. Rogers, a business executive, was involved in a private airplane accident along an isolated section of the seacoast. While awaiting rescue, he drank large amounts of ocean water. When admitted to a local hospital, his condition was complicated by salt intoxication. Which of the following signs, symptoms, and laboratory values might this patient exhibit?
    a. Hot, flushed skin
    b. Mental confusion and agitation
    c. Hypoactive tendon reflexes
    d. Dry, red tongue and dry, sticky oral mucosa

12. The nurse administers injections of magnesium sulfate for the treatment of a patient with toxemia of pregnancy and preeclampsia. Which of the following signs or symptoms observed during assessment would indicate that the patient is developing Mg^{++} toxicity?
    a. Progressively decreased deep tendon reflexes
    b. Hyperactive deep tendon reflexes
    c. Marked fall in blood pressure
    d. Increase in blood pressure
    e. Prolongation of the PR interval

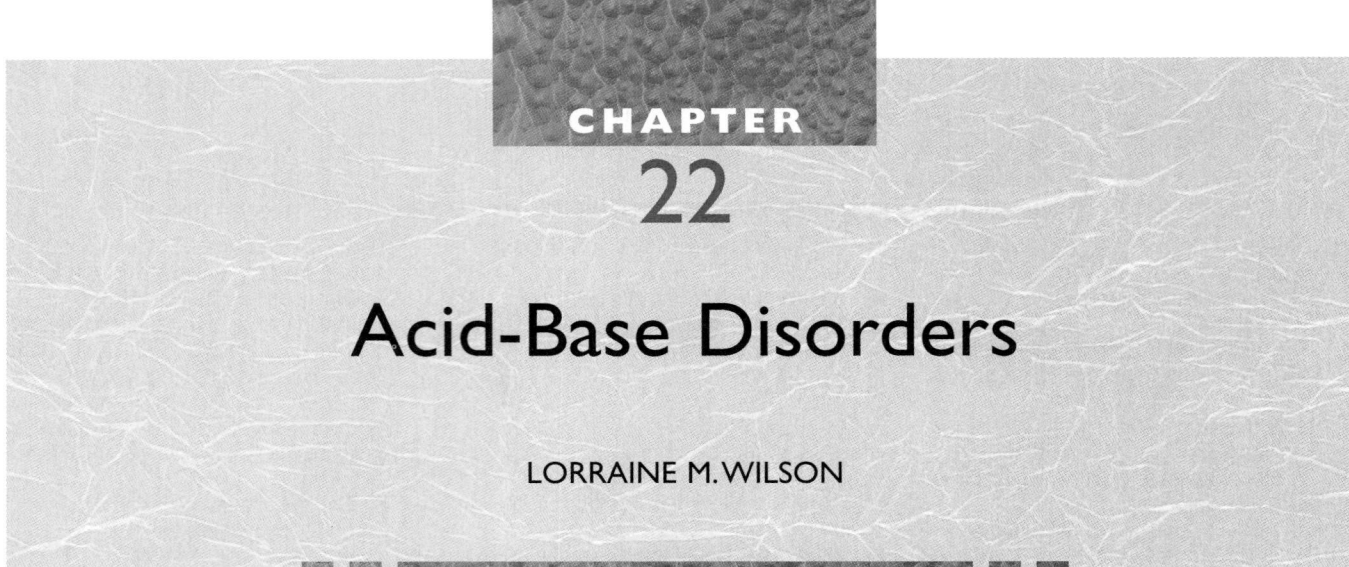

CHAPTER
22

Acid-Base Disorders

LORRAINE M. WILSON

𝒟isturbances in acid-base balance are common clinical problems that range in severity from mild to life threatening. This chapter reviews the basic principles of acid-base physiology, the general mechanisms by which abnormalities can occur, and an approach to the clinical assessment of acid-base disturbances. A more detailed discussion of the four primary acid-base disorders—metabolic acidosis, metabolic alkalosis, respiratory acidosis, and respiratory alkalosis—and mixed acid-base disorders follows this review.

PHYSIOLOGIC CONSIDERATIONS

Acid-base balance refers to the homeostasis of the hydrogen ion concentration ($[H^+]$) in body fluids. Acids are produced continuously from normal metabolism. Despite the large addition of acids from metabolism, the $[H^+]$ of body fluids is low. The normal H^+ concentration of the arterial blood is 0.00000004 (4×10^{-8}) mEq/L or about one millionth of the concentration of Na^+. Despite this low concentration, the maintenance of a stable $[H^+]$ is required for normal cellular function, because small fluctuations have important effects on the activity of cellular enzymes. Because of these effects on cellular enzymes, only a relatively narrow range of $[H^+]$ is compatible with life.

pH Scale

An increase in the $[H^+]$ makes a solution more acid, and a decrease makes a solution more alkaline. Because the $[H^+]$ is a small quantity, the pH scale was devised by chemists as a means to express it. The pH is defined as the negative log of the hydrogen ion concentration (pH = $-\log [H^+]$). Thus a $[H^+]$ of 0.0000001 g/L equals 10^{-7} g/L equals pH 7. Thus the pH and the $[H^+]$ are inversely related. As the $[H^+]$ increases, the pH decreases; as the $[H^+]$ decreases, the pH increases. A low pH means that a solution is more acidic, whereas a high pH means that a solution is more alkaline or basic. Water, a liquid having a pH of 7, is neutral because at that pH, the number of (acid)

TABLE 22-1   ■ ■ ■

Relationship between the pH and the Hydrogen Ion Concentration in the Physiologic Range

pH	[H$^+$] nmol/L
7.80	16
7.70	20
7.60	26
7.50	32
7.45	35
7.40	40
7.35	45
7.30	50
7.20	63
7.10	80
7.00	100
6.90	125
6.80	160

hydrogen ions (H$^+$) is exactly balanced by the number of (basic) hydroxyl ions (OH$^-$). An acid solution has a pH less than 7; an alkaline or basic solution has a pH greater than 7. The pH scale ranges from 1 (most acid) to 14 (most alkaline).

The mean pH of the blood or extracellular fluid (ECF) is slightly alkaline at 7.4. The normal range of the blood pH is from 7.38 to 7.42 (1 standard deviation [SD] from the mean) or 7.35 to 7.45 (2 SD from the mean).

Rather than use the pH scale, some medical centers prefer to express the [H$^+$] in nanomoles per liter (nmol/L). Table 22-1 contains a pH to nanomoles conversion table. This table illustrates that a log scale such as the pH scale may obscure the magnitude of a change in the [H$^+$] when one is not mathematically inclined. For example, it is evident that when the [H$^+$] increases from 40 to 80 nmol/L, a doubling of [H$^+$] has occurred, but this may not be evident when the pH changes from 7.4 to 7.1.

Acids

An acid is a substance containing one or more H$^+$ ions that can be liberated in solution (proton donor). A strong acid, such as hydrochloric acid (HCl), is almost completely dissociated in solution, thus liberating more H$^+$ ions. A weak acid, such as carbonic acid (H$_2$CO$_3$), is only partially dissociated in solution thus fewer H$^+$ ions are liberated.

Metabolic processes in the body result in the formation of two types of acids: volatile and nonvolatile. A *volatile acid* can change between liquid and gaseous states. Carbon dioxide—a major end product in the oxidation of carbohydrates, fats, and amino acids—can be regarded as an acid by virtue of its ability to react with water to form H$_2$CO$_3$, which in turn can dissociate to form H$^+$ and HCO$_3^-$:

$$CO_2 + H_2O \rightleftharpoons H_2CO_3 \rightleftharpoons H^+ + HCO_3^-$$

Because carbon dioxide (CO$_2$) is a gas that can be eliminated by the lungs, it is often called a volatile acid.

All other sources of H$^+$ are considered to be *nonvolatile* or *fixed acids*. Nonvolatile acids cannot be converted to a

gaseous form to be excreted by the lungs but must be excreted by the kidneys. Nonvolatile acids may be inorganic or organic. Sulfuric acid is the end product of the oxidation of sulfur-containing amino acids, whereas phosphoric acid is formed from the metabolism of phospholipids, nucleic acids, and phosphoproteins. Because organic acids, such as lactic acid and ketoacids, are formed during the metabolism of carbohydrates and fats and are further oxidized to CO$_2$ and water, they do not normally affect the body pH. However, these organic acids may accumulate in certain abnormal circumstances. Lactic acid accumulates in the absence of oxygen, as in circulatory shock or cardiac arrest. In uncontrolled diabetes mellitus, ketoacids (acetoacetic and beta-hydroxybutyric acids) may accumulate because of increased lipid metabolism. Approximately 20,000 mmol of H$_2$CO$_3$ and 80 mmol of nonvolatile acids are produced in the body each day and eliminated by the lungs and kidneys, respectively.

Bases

In contrast to an acid, a base is a substance that can capture or combine with H$^+$ from a solution (proton acceptor). A strong base, such as sodium hydroxide (NaOH), is highly dissociated in solution and reacts strongly with an acid. A weak base, such as sodium bicarbonate (NaHCO$_3$), is only partially dissociated in solution and reacts less vigorously with an acid.

Buffers

The term *buffer* describes a chemical substance that minimizes the pH change in a solution caused by the addition of either an acid or a base. A buffer is a mixture of a weak acid and its alkali salt (or a weak base and its acid salt). A buffer is most effective in defending the [H$^+$] against acids or bases when it is 50% dissociated (having an equal amount of undissociated acid and its salt). The pH at which an acid or base is 50% dissociated is known as its pK. The effectiveness of a given buffer is determined by its concentration and its pK relative to the pH of the compartment in which it is active.

Four main buffer pairs or systems in the body help to maintain the constancy of the pH:
1. Bicarbonate–carbonic acid system (NaHCO$_3$ and H$_2$CO$_3$)
2. Disodium–monosodium phosphate buffer system (Na$_2$HPO$_4$ and NaH$_2$PO$_4$)
3. Hemoglobin-oxyhemoglobin buffer system in red blood cells (RBCs) (HbO$_2^-$ and HHb)
4. Protein buffer system (Pr$^-$ and HPr)

The bicarbonate–carbonic acid buffer system is quantitatively the largest in the body and operates in the ECF, contributing more than one half of the buffering capacity of whole blood. The remaining nonbicarbonate buffer systems operate primarily in the intracellular fluid (ICF). The phosphate buffer system is an important buffer in RBCs and in renal tubule cells. The H$^+$ ions excreted in the urine buffered by phosphate is referred to as *titratable acid*. Hemoglobin is an effective buffer of H$^+$ ions produced within the RBC in the course of transporting CO$_2$ from the tissues to the lungs in the form of bicarbonate

(HCO_3^-). Because reduced hemoglobin has a strong affinity for H^+ ions, most of these ions become bound to hemoglobin. In this manner, only a few H^+ ions remain free, thus the acidity of venous blood is only slightly greater than that of arterial blood. As venous blood passes through the lungs, hemoglobin becomes saturated with oxygen and its ability to bind H^+ ions decreases. The H^+ ions are released, whereupon they react with HCO_3^- to give CO_2, which is then expired by the lungs. In effect, the hemoglobin-oxyhemoglobin system actually buffers the bicarbonate–carbonic acid buffer system. The protein buffer system is predominant in tissue cells and also operates in the plasma. More than one half of the 70 mmol of H^+ ions derived from the diet is initially buffered intracellularly.

Regulation of the ECF pH

Because various acids and bases continually enter the blood from absorbed foods and from catabolism of foods, some kind of mechanism is necessary for neutralizing or eliminating these substances. Actually, the constancy of the pH is maintained by the integrated action of the body buffers, lungs, and kidneys. These three regulatory mechanisms vary in the rapidity and effectiveness of defending the constancy of the pH when acids or bases are added or lost from the body.

The immediate response (within seconds) to an increase or decrease in $[H^+]$ is the chemical buffering of H^+ ions by both the ECF and ICF buffer systems. Buffering, however, is only a temporary measure in restoring normal pH.

A second line of defense that stabilizes the H^+ ion concentration consists of the respiratory control of the CO_2 level in the body fluids through changes in alveolar ventilation. This response is fairly rapid, taking only minutes to be fully operative.

Ultimately, the restoration of normal pH during acid-base disturbances depends on the renal regulation of the HCO_3^- level of body fluids. This response is relatively slow, taking several days to complete the correction.

Bicarbonate–Carbonic Acid Buffer System

The bicarbonate–carbonic acid buffer system is of central importance in understanding the physiologic processes involved in normal acid-base equilibrium and its abnormalities; it is the major ECF buffer, and the assessment of its components provides the basis for the clinical evaluation of the patient's acid-base status. The following equation describes the components of the bicarbonate–carbonic acid buffer system and the relationships among them:

$$\overset{CA}{CO_2 + H_2O \rightleftharpoons H_2CO_3 \rightleftharpoons H^+ + HCO^-}$$
$$(40 \text{ mm Hg}) \quad (1.2 \text{ mEq/L}) \quad (pH\ 7.4) \quad (24 \text{ mEq/L})$$

The bidirectional arrows indicate that the reaction can proceed in either direction with equal facility, depending on the concentrations of the components in each section of the equation. This reaction readily occurs in RBCs because of the presence of the catalyzing enzyme carbonic anhydrase (CA). Because this enzyme is absent in blood plasma, the reaction is slowed there. It is evident from this equation that the $[H^+]$ is a function of the ECF

$[HCO_3^-]$ and the carbon dioxide gas dissolved in the blood (Pco_2). *Acidemia* (an increase in $[H^+]$) occurs when there is either a fall in $[HCO_3^-]$ or an increase in Pco_2 (both displace the equation to the *right*, generating additional H^+). Conversely, *alkalemia* (a fall in the $[H^+]$) occurs when either an increase in the $[HCO_3^-]$ or a decrease in Pco_2 occurs (both of which displace the equilibrium to the *left*). The $[H^+]$, $[HCO_3^-]$, and Pco_2 are thus the three parameters controlling the acid-base status of the ECF.

The left side of the buffer equation is the respiratory component: $CO_2 + H_2O \rightleftharpoons H_2CO_3$. The respiratory component is controlled primarily by the lungs through variations in alveolar ventilation. When the Pco_2 is above or below normal, the amount of alveolar ventilation is inadequate (hypoventilation) or excessive (hyperventilation). The Pco_2 is regulated by pulmonary function and reflexes in the brainstem, which control respiratory drive (see Chapter 35).

The right side of the equation is the renal-metabolic component: $H_2CO_3 \rightleftharpoons H^+ + HCO_3^-$. The H_2CO_3 formed by the hydration of CO_2 gas dissociates into H^+ ions and HCO_3^- ions. Primarily the kidneys regulate this half of the equation. The kidneys contribute to acid-base balance by regulating the plasma $[HCO_3^-]$ in two ways: (1) by reabsorbing the filtered HCO_3^- and preventing its loss in the urine and (2) by excreting the daily load of excess H^+ produced by metabolism. Two thirds of the excess H^+ is excreted in the form of ammonium ions (NH_4^+); one third is excreted in the form of phosphoric acid (H_3PO_4) or sulfuric acid (H_2SO_4). The latter process results in the generation of new HCO_3^- to replace that HCO_3^- lost in buffering the daily H^+ load. Thus the kidneys are able to retain or eliminate HCO_3^- as needed, either with Na^+ and K^+, or in exchange for Cl^-.

Although several buffer systems operate simultaneously in the body, only one of them needs to be measured to analyze acid-base disorders. The *isohydric principle* states that all buffer systems in a solution are in equilibrium with the same H^+ ions. For practical purposes, then, changes in one buffer system accurately reflect changes in the others. Clinically, the bicarbonate-carbonic acid system is the one chosen for analysis because it is the largest buffer system of the ECF and is easiest to measure.

Henderson-Hasselbalch Equation

At equilibrium, the relationship between the reactants of the bicarbonate–carbonic acid buffer system may be expressed by the law of mass action:

$$[H^+] = 24 \times \frac{Pco_2}{[HCO_3^-]}$$

or by the Henderson-Hasselbalch equation:

$$pH = pK + \log \frac{[HCO]}{[H_2CO_3]}$$

where pK is the carbonic acid dissociation constant, HCO_3^- is the plasma HCO_3^- concentration, and H_2CO_3 is the plasma carbonic acid concentration. Because the Pco_2 in the plasma is proportional to the concentration of carbonic acid and dissolved carbon dioxide in the plasma, the Henderson-Hasselbalch equation can be rewritten:

$$pH = pK + \log \frac{[HCO_3^-]}{S \times P_{CO_2}}$$

$$= 6.1 + \log \frac{24 \text{ mEq/L}}{0.03 \times 40 \text{ mm Hg}} = \frac{24}{1.2}$$

$$= 6.1 + \log \frac{20}{1}$$

$$7.4 = 6.1 + 1.3$$

where S is the CO_2 solubility constant and has a value of 0.03. The pK for the bicarbonate–carbonic acid buffer system is a constant with a value of 6.1. Substituting in the normal plasma values for the HCO_3^- (24 mEq/L) and P_{CO_2} (40 mm Hg) and solving the equation, the result is the normal pH of 7.4. This equation shows that the ratio of the HCO_3^- to H_2CO_3 determines the pH. At a body pH of 7.4 the ratio of HCO_3^- to H_2CO_3 must be 20:1 as shown. As long as the 20:1 ratio is maintained, regardless of the absolute values, the pH will be 7.4.

Overview of the Primary Acid-Base Imbalances

Figure 22-1 illustrates the normal range of blood pH near 7.4 and the widest range compatible with life from 6.8 to 7.8 or an interval of one pH unit. The normal range of pH is from 7.38 to 7.42 when one uses the more sensitive value of one standard deviation (SD) from the mean of 7.4. Most clinicians, however, use the less sensitive value of 7.35 to 7.45, which is two SD from the mean. A blood pH of less than 7.35 is called *acidemia,* and the process causing it is called *acidosis.* A pH of 7.25 or less is life threatening, and a pH of 6.8 is incompatible with life. Similarly, a blood pH greater than 7.45 is called *alkalemia,* and the process causing it is called *alkalosis.* A pH

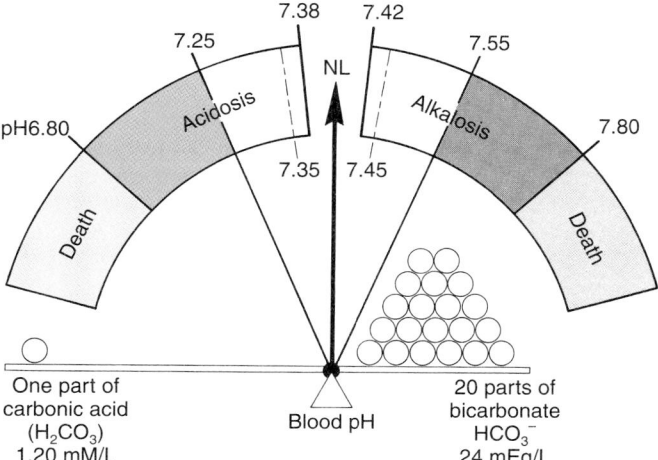

FIG. 22-1 Normal blood pH is 7.40 ± 0.02 (one standard deviation [SD]) or ± 0.05 (two SD). Acid-base balance occurs when the ratio of bicarbonate to carbonic acid is 20:1. Any change in this ratio tips the balance and swings the pointer to the acidosis or alkalosis side. A pH below 7.25 or above 7.55 is life-threatening, and the extremes of 6.8 or 7.8 cause death.

greater than 7.55 is life threatening, and a pH greater than 7.8 is incompatible with life.

The four primary acid-base disturbances and their compensations may be visualized using a simplified version of the Henderson-Hasselbalch equation:

$$pH \propto \frac{[HCO_3^-]}{P_{aCO_2}} = \frac{20 \text{ (metabolic component controlled by kidneys)}}{1 \text{ (respiratory component controlled by lungs)}}$$

This equation emphasizes the fact that the ratio of base to acid must be 20:1 to maintain the pH in the normal range. The equation also emphasizes the ability of the kidneys to alter the base bicarbonate through metabolic processes and the ability of the lungs to alter the P_{aCO_2} (partial pressure of CO_2 in the arterial blood) through respiration.

Metabolic imbalances are those in which the primary disturbance is in the concentration of bicarbonate. Because HCO_3^- appears in the numerator of the Henderson-Hasselbalch equation, an increased HCO_3^- concentration causes increased pH, which is called *metabolic alkalosis.* A decrease in the HCO_3^- concentration causes a decrease in the pH, which is called *metabolic acidosis.* Respiratory imbalances are those in which the primary disturbance is in the concentration of CO_2 (carbonic acid). The CO_2 concentration appears in the denominator of the Henderson-Hasselbalch buffer equation. An increase in the P_{aCO_2} lowers the pH and is called *respiratory acidosis* (also referred to as alveolar hypoventilation, or hypercapnia). A decrease in the P_{aCO_2} raises the pH and is called *respiratory alkalosis* (also referred to as alveolar hyperventilation or hypocapnia). Notably, the 20:1 bicarbonate–carbonic acid ratio is altered in each of the four primary acid-base imbalances, which causes a deviation in the pH from the normal 7.4. Metabolic or respiratory acidosis lowers the 20:1 bicarbonate–carbonic acid ratio, whereas metabolic or respiratory alkalosis raises it. Thus all four of the primary acid-base disturbances may be identified by examining the relationship be-tween bicarbonate and carbonic acid in the Henderson-Hasselbalch equation. Various combinations of the primary acid-base disturbances are called *mixed acid-base disturbances.* An example would be respiratory acidosis and metabolic acidosis.

Compensatory Responses to Alterations in pH

After the pH is altered by a primary acid-base disorder, the body immediately uses compensatory responses to bring the pH back to normal. Three compensatory responses as discussed previously include (1) ECF and ICF buffering, (2) respiratory alteration of the P_{aCO_2} by hypoventilation or hyperventilation, and (3) renal alteration of the $[HCO_3^-]$ or $[H^+]$. ECF and ICF buffering may involve the shift of H^+ into or out of the cells in exchange for K^+ and is discussed later. The respiratory and renal compensatory responses are easily analyzed in terms of the Henderson-Hasselbalch equation.

A primary metabolic acidosis (decreased $[HCO_3^-]$) is compensated by respiratory hyperventilation, thus reducing the P_{aCO_2} and restoring the pH toward normal. Primary metabolic alkalosis (increased $[HCO_3^-]$) is compensated by respiratory hypoventilation, thus increasing the P_{aCO_2} and restoring the pH toward normal. The

TABLE 22-2 ▪▪▪

Simple Acid-Base Disorders

Acid-Base Disorder	Cause	Bicarbonate–Carbonic Acid Ratio 20:1	Compensation
Respiratory acidosis	Hypoventilation (retained CO_2)	Ratio <20:1	Renal: retention of HCO_3^-; excretion of acid salts; increased ammonia formation
Respiratory alkalosis	Hyperventilation (excessive loss of CO_2)	Ratio >20:1	Renal: excretion of HCO_3^-; retention of acid salts; decreased ammonia formation
Metabolic acidosis	Retention of fixed acids Loss of base bicarbonate	Ratio <20:1	Lungs: hyperventilation Renal: as in respiratory acidosis
Metabolic alkalosis	Loss of fixed acids Gain of base bicarbonate K^+ depletion	Ratio >20:1	Lungs: hypoventilation Renal: as in respiratory alkalosis

respiratory compensatory response occurs within minutes. In contrast, the kidneys compensate for primary respiratory acidosis (increased $Paco_2$) or alkalosis (decreased $Paco_2$) by retention or excretion of HCO_3^- or H^+ ion. However, renal compensation is slower so no effects are noticeable for about 24 hours. Full compensation takes approximately 2 to 3 days. Thus respiratory acidosis is classified as *acute* when renal compensation has not yet occurred and the HCO_3^- is still normal; when renal compensation has occurred and the HCO_3^- is increased, it is classified as *chronic*. Primary respiratory alkalosis may also be classified as acute or chronic, depending on whether renal compensation is partial or complete. In terms of the Henderson-Hasselbalch equation, when the numerator increases, the denominator must increase to maintain the 20:1 ratio and minimize deviations of the pH from the normal. Compensation always involves a compensatory change in the numerator (or denominator) that is in the same direction as the primary disturbance. Table 22-2 presents a simplified overview of the four primary acid-base disorders.

ASSESSMENT OF ACID-BASE IMBALANCE

Diagnosis and treatment of acid-base disorders require a thorough understanding of the pathogenesis and pathophysiologic aspects of these disturbances. Many authors have developed various methods to simplify the interpretation of the respiratory and metabolic components of the arterial blood gas values to identify the primary major imbalance (whether acute or compensated) or a mixed disorder. These methods include the use of acid-base nomograms and the use of standard bicarbonate, with the base excess and base deficit as a method of identifying metabolic disorders. Importantly, however, none of these methods are foolproof, and all are subject to misinterpretation. The acid-base nomogram uses confidence bands to identify the acute and compensated primary acid-base disorders, with mixed disorders falling between the confidence bands. It is possible for the pH to be normal in the presence of an acid-base disturbance such as a mixture of respiratory acidosis and metabolic alkalosis. This mixture, in turn, would be hard to differ-

entiate from a well-compensated chronic respiratory acidosis without the appropriate clinical information.

The standard HCO_3^- and base deficit or excess is another popular method devised to assist interpretation of acid-base disturbances. The standard HCO_3^- is supposed to represent a measure of the true plasma HCO_3^- in place of the classic carbon dioxide content measure. The latter contains the respiratory or H_2CO_3 component (although small).

The base excess or deficit may be calculated from the standard HCO_3^- and is supposedly a sure way of evaluating the metabolic component of an acid-base disorder. Many authors, however, have severely criticized the use of the standard HCO_3^- and base excess or deficit values (Rose, Post, 2001; Schwartz, Relman, 1963). These authors point out that the standard HCO_3^- is also an estimate of the true plasma HCO_3^- and offers no advantage over the CO_2 content measure. Using the base deficit or excess is not recommended because these values may be misleading.

A final warning about the interpretation of laboratory values in the diagnosis of acid-base disturbances needs to be emphasized. The $Paco_2$ cannot be regarded solely as an indicator of a respiratory disturbance nor can the $[HCO_3^-]$ be viewed exclusively as an index of metabolic disorders. A low $Paco_2$ may indicate a primary respiratory alkalosis or may result from the expected respiratory compensation for a metabolic acidosis. Similarly, an increased $[HCO_3^-]$ may reflect the presence of a primary metabolic alkalosis or may be a compensatory response to chronic respiratory acidosis. To further complicate the picture, most acid-base disturbances are partially compensated when first detected and mixed disorders occur frequently. In summary, no easy shortcuts exist as to the accurate assessment of acid-base disorders. The acid-base laboratory variables cannot stand alone but must be interpreted in the context of a thorough knowledge of the clinical situation, experience, good judgment, and a sound understanding of acid-base physiology.

With these caveats in mind, Box 22-1 presents a systematic guide for the assessment of acid-base disorders. Assessment begins with a high degree of clinical suspicion because acid-base disorders may be difficult to detect unless severe, and signs and symptoms tend to be vague and nonspecific. The clinical history, signs and symptoms, and other laboratory data that suggest a disease process associated with an acid-base disorder are

BOX 22-1

A Systematic Approach to the Assessment of Acid-Base Disturbances

BEGIN WITH A HIGH DEGREE OF CLINICAL SUSPICION
1. Examine the *clinical history* for disease processes that may lead to simple acid-base disorders.
    a. This requires knowledge of the pathogenesis of the various acid-base disorders.
    b. For example, one might expect a person with advanced chronic obstructive pulmonary disorder (COPD) to develop respiratory acidosis.
2. Note *clinical signs and symptoms* that suggest an acid-base disorder.
    a. Unfortunately, many of the signs and symptoms of an acid-base disorder are subtle or nonspecific.
    b. For example, Kussmaul respirations in a diabetic patient may represent respiratory compensation for metabolic acidosis.
3. *Examine laboratory reports of the electrolytes and other data* that suggest disease processes associated with acid-base disorders.
    a. For example, hypokalemia is often associated with metabolic alkalosis.
    b. For example, an elevated serum creatinine level indicates renal insufficiency, and renal insufficiency and failure are usually associated with metabolic acidosis.

EVALUATE ACID-BASE VARIABLES TO IDENTIFY THE TYPE OF DISORDER
1. First, *examine the arterial blood pH* to determine the direction and magnitude of the acid-base disturbance.
    a. If decreased, the patient has acidemia with two potential causes: metabolic acidosis or respiratory acidosis.
    b. If increased, the patient has alkalemia with two potential causes: metabolic alkalosis or respiratory alkalosis.
    c. Helpful to note is that the renal and respiratory compensations rarely return the pH to normal, thus a normal pH in the presence of changes in the $Paco_2$ and HCO_3^- suggests a mixed disorder; for example, a person with a combined respiratory acidosis and metabolic alkalosis might have a normal pH.
2. *Examine the respiratory ($Paco_2$) and metabolic (HCO_3^-) variables in relation to the pH* to tentatively characterize the primary disturbance as a respiratory, metabolic, or mixed disorder.
    a. Is the $Paco_2$ normal (40 mm Hg), increased, or decreased?
    b. Is the HCO_3^- normal (24 mEq/L), increased, or decreased?
       Optional: Is there a base excess or deficit?
    c. In a simple acid-base disorder, the $Paco_2$ and HCO_3^- are always altered in the same direction.
    d. Deviation of the $Paco_2$ and HCO_3^- in opposite directions indicates the presence of a mixed acid-base disorder.
    e. Make a tentative decision about the primary disturbance by correlating the findings with the clinical situation.
3. *Estimate the expected compensatory response to the primary acid-base disorder.*
    a. Use Table 22-4 to determine the expected respiratory or metabolic compensatory response to the primary disorder.
    b. If the compensatory response is greater or less than expected, a mixed acid-base disorder is suggested (an acid-base nomogram may also be used to help identify a mixed acid-base disorder).
    c. Calculate the plasma anion gap.
       If increased (>16 mEq/L), metabolic acidosis is most likely.
    d. Compare the magnitude of fall in plasma $[HCO_3^-]$ with the increase in the anion gap; these should be similar in magnitude.
       (1) The anion gap that has risen less than the fall in $[HCO_3^-]$ suggests that a component of the metabolic acidosis is a result of HCO_3^- loss.
       (2) The increase in anion gap that is much greater than the fall in $[HCO_3^-]$ suggests a coexistent metabolic alkalosis.
4. *Make the final interpretation.*
    a. Simple acid-base disorder
       (1) Acute (uncompensated) or
       (2) Chronic (partially or fully compensated)
    b. Mixed acid-base disorder
    c. Normal or wide anion gap: metabolic acidosis

---

noted. The common causes and symptoms of the specific acid-base disorders are discussed later.

Next, clinical suspicions are confirmed with a systematic examination of the acid-base variables. Table 22-3 presents the normal values of the arterial blood parameters used in analyzing acid-base disorders, as well as some useful formulas. The first step is to examine the pH to determine whether acidemia or alkalemia is present and, if so, its magnitude. The second step is to examine the $Paco_2$ and $[HCO_3^-]$ in relationship to the pH in an attempt to characterize the disturbance as a primary respiratory or metabolic or mixed acid-base imbalance. The Henderson-Hasselbalch equation or an acid-base nomogram (Fig. 22-2) may be helpful in making a tentative decision. Knowledge of the clinical situation is essential in making a decision. The third step is to estimate the expected compensatory response to the primary acid-base disorder. Table 22-4 may be helpful in this regard, as well as suggesting possible mixed acid-base disorders when the compensatory response is less than or greater than expected.

The acid-base nomogram may also be helpful. The anion gap should also be calculated to determine whether a metabolic acidosis is the result of the retention of fixed acids associated with an increased anion gap:

$$[Na^+] - ([HCO_3^-] + [Cl^-])$$

Actually, an anion gap does not exist in reality because an equal number of positive and negative ions are required for body electroneutrality. Rather, the anion gap represents unmeasured anions because the sum of the plasma chloride plus HCO_3^- concentrations is less than the serum Na^+ concentration:

$$140 \text{ mEq/L} - (104 \text{ mEq/L} + 24 \text{ mEq/L}) = 12 \text{ mEq/L} =$$
$$\text{Normal anion gap}$$

The increase in the anion gap should also be compared with the decrease in the $[HCO_3^-]$ to detect a mixed disorder such as a metabolic alkalosis combined with the metabolic acidosis. A reduced anion gap provides an index to cer-

TABLE 22-3 ∎∎∎

Arterial Blood Parameters Used for the Analysis of Acid-Base Status

Parameter	Normal Value	Definition and Implications

Pa_{O_2}	80-100 mm Hg	Partial pressure of oxygen in arterial blood (decreases with age)
		In adults <60 yr:
		  60-80 mm Hg = mild hypoxemia
		  40-60 mm Hg = moderate hypoxemia
		  <40 mm Hg = severe hypoxemia

pH	7.40 (±0.05 [2 SD]) 7.40 (±0.02 [1 SD])	Identifies whether there is acidemia or alkalemia; the value using 2 standard deviations (SD) from the mean is the common clinical value. pH <7.35 = acidosis; pH >7.45 = alkalosis
$[H^+]$	40 (±2) nmol/L or nEq/L	The hydrogen ion concentration may be used instead of the pH
Pa_{CO_2}	40 (±5.0) mm Hg	Partial pressure of CO_2 in the arterial blood Pa_{CO_2} <35 mm Hg = respiratory alkalosis Pa_{CO_2} >45 mm Hg = respiratory acidosis
CO_2 content	25.5 (±4.5) mEq/L	Classic method of estimating $[HCO_3]$; measures HCO_3^- + dissolved CO_2 (latter is generally quite small except in respiratory acidosis)
Standard HCO_3^-	24 (±2) mEq/L	Estimated HCO_3^- concentration after fully oxygenated arterial blood has been equilibrated with CO_2 at a P_{CO_2} of 40 mm Hg at 38° C; eliminates the influence of respiration on the plasma HCO_3^- concentration.
Base excess	0 (±2) mEq/L	Reflects pure metabolic component Base excess = 1.2 × deviation from 0 Negative in metabolic acidosis Positive in metabolic alkalosis Misleading in respiratory and mixed acid-base disturbances Not essential for interpretation of acid-base disturbances
Anion gap	12 (±4) mEq/L	Anion gap (or delta) reflects the difference between the unmeasured cations (K^+, Mg^{++}, Ca^{++}) and unmeasured anions (albumin, organic anions, HPO_4^-, $SO_4^=$); useful in identifying types of metabolic acidosis; value >16-20 indicates acidosis is caused by retention of organic acids (e.g., diabetic ketoacidosis)

USEFUL FORMULAS

Plasma anion gap = $[Na^+] - ([HCO_3^-] + [Cl^-])$

Calculation of third acid-base parameter when two are known:

$$[H^+] = 24 \times \frac{Pa_{CO_2}}{[HCO_3^-]}$$

Conversion of pH into $[H^+]$ (use conversion in Table 22-1 or formulas below):
pH of 7.4 = $[H^+]$ of 40 mEq/L
For every 0.1 increase in pH above 7.4, multiply 40 × 0.8
For every 0.1 decrease in pH below 7.4, multiply 40 × 1.25
For example, pH of 7.60 = 40 × 0.8 × 0.8 = [H+] of 26 mEq/L

TABLE 22-4 ∎∎∎

Expected Compensatory Responses in Primary Acid-Base Disorders

Disorder	Expected Response	Possible Mixed Disorder
Metabolic acidosis	For every 1 mEq decrease in HCO_3^-, 1.2 mm Hg decrease in Pa_{CO_2}	Fall in Pa_{CO_2} > expected Superimposed respiratory alkalosis + metabolic acidosis Fall in Pa_{CO_2} < expected Superimposed respiratory acidosis + metabolic acidosis
Metabolic alkalosis	For every 1 mEq increase in HCO_3^-, 0.7 mm Hg increase in Pa_{CO_2}	Rise in Pa_{CO_2} > expected Superimposed respiratory acidosis + metabolic alkalosis Rise in Pa_{CO_2} < expected Superimposed respiratory alkalosis + metabolic alkalosis
Respiratory acidosis		
Acute	For every 10 mm Hg increase in Pa_{CO_2}, 1 mEq/L increase in HCO_3^-	Rise in HCO_3^- > expected Secondary metabolic alkalosis + respiratory acidosis
Chronic	For every 10 mm Hg increase in Pa_{CO_2}, 3.5 mEq/L increase in HCO_3^-	Rise in HCO_3^- < expected Superimposed metabolic acidosis + respiratory acidosis
Respiratory alkalosis		
Acute	For every 10 mm Hg decrease in Pa_{CO_2}, 2 mEq/L decrease in HCO_3^-	Fall in HCO_3^- > expected Secondary metabolic acidosis + respiratory alkalosis
Chronic	For every 10 mm Hg decrease in Pa_{CO_2}, 5 mEq/L decrease in HCO_3^-	Fall in HCO_3^- < expected Secondary metabolic alkalosis 1 respiratory alkalosis

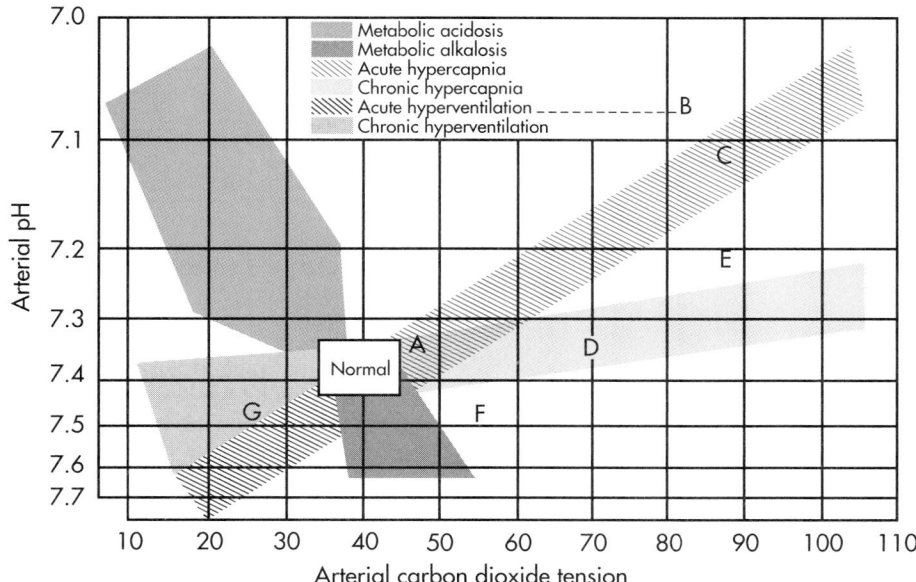

FIG. 22-2 Nomogram for acid-base disturbances. This graph displays the quantity and direction of changes in pH and $PaCO_2$ in various types of acid-base disturbances. The shaded areas represent the range of variability in persons with pure acid-base disorders. See Chapter 41 for explanation of lettered points (Modified from Burrows B, Knudson RJ, Kettel LJ: *Respiratory insufficiency*, Chicago, 1975, Mosby.)

tain other disorders. For example, the serum Na^+ may remain normal while the serum HCO_3^- and Cl^- increase, which occurs most commonly in hypoalbuminemia.

The final step in the assessment of an acid-base disorder is identifying the primary imbalance and characterizing it as acute or chronic (compensated) or as a mixture of two or more disturbances. Metabolic acidosis should be classified as a normal or an increased anion gap.

METABOLIC ACIDOSIS

Metabolic acidosis (HCO_3^- deficit) is a systemic disorder characterized by a primary decrease in the plasma HCO_3^- concentration that results in a decrease of the pH (increase in the [H^+]). The ECF [HCO_3^-] is less than 22 mEq/L, and the pH is less than 7.35. Respiratory compensation begins immediately to lower the $PaCO_2$ by hyperventilation so that metabolic acidosis seldom develops acutely.

Causes and Pathogenesis

The basic causes of metabolic acidosis are either gains of fixed (noncarbonic) acid, failure of the kidneys to excrete the daily acid load, or a loss of base bicarbonate. The causes of metabolic acidosis are commonly divided into two groups according to whether the anion gap is normal or increased. As stated previously, the anion gap is calculated by subtracting the sum of the plasma concentrations of Cl^- and HCO_3^- from the Na^+ concentration. The normal value is 12. The cause of high anion gap metabolic acidosis is an increase in unmeasured anions such as sulfate, phosphate, lactate, and other organic acids. When the acidosis is caused by the loss of HCO_3^- (e.g., diarrhea) or gain of a chloride acid (e.g., administration

of ammonium chloride), the anion gap will be normal. Conversely, when the acidosis is caused by increased production of an organic acid (e.g., lactic acid in circulatory shock) or the retention of sulfuric or phosphoric acid (e.g., in renal failure), the concentration of unmeasured anions (anion gap) increases (Fig. 22-3).

Box 22-2 lists some of the common causes of metabolic acidosis. In normal anion gap metabolic acidosis, HCO_3^- loss may occur via the gastrointestinal (GI) tract or kidneys. Diarrhea, small bowel fistula, and ureterosigmoidostomy cause significant losses of HCO_3^-, whereas renal reabsorption of HCO_3^- is decreased in proximal renal tubular acidosis or in persons taking carbonic anhydrase inhibitors such as acetazolamide. Because Cl^- combines with Na^+ in competition with HCO_3^-, it is related to the acid-base balance of the body. When HCO_3^- is lost from the body, reducing the serum [HCO_3^-], the plasma [Cl^-] rises in compensation because the total number of anions and cations in the ECF must be equal to maintain electroneutrality. The result is *hyperchloremic metabolic acidosis.* Administration of excess chloride salts (e.g., NH_4Cl) also causes hyperchloremic metabolic acidosis. The acidosis caused by the rapid administration of IV saline is usually mild and temporary and is called *dilutional acidosis.*

Conditions associated with high anion gap metabolic acidosis are listed in Box 22-2. The most common condition is shock or inadequate tissue perfusion from any number of causes, resulting in the accumulation of large amounts of lactic acid. Diabetic ketoacidosis (DKA), starvation, and ethanol intoxication cause elevation of the anion gap because of the formation of ketoacids; renal failure causes such elevation by the retention of sulfuric and phosphoric acids. Poisoning by salicylate overdose, methanol, or ethylene glycol produces increased anion gaps by elevation of their organic acid counterparts (salicylate, formate, oxylate).

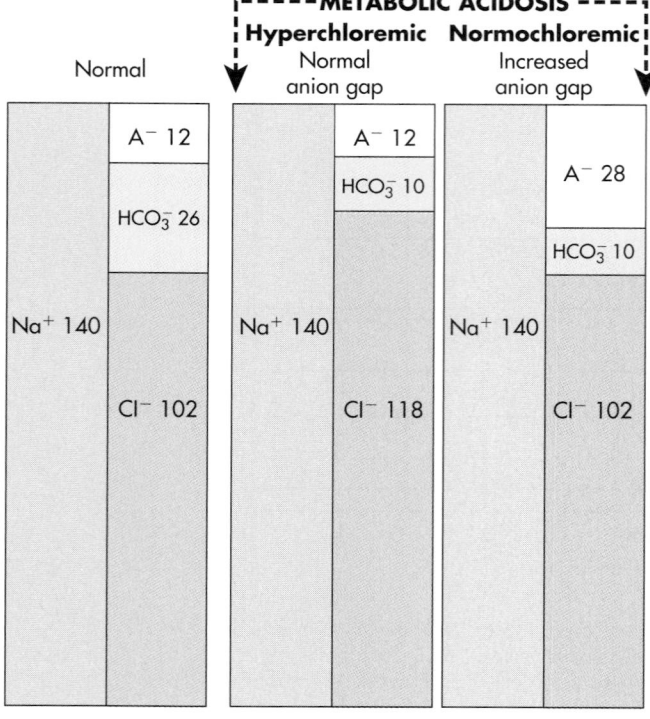

FIG. 22-3 Classification of metabolic acidosis arrived at by using the anion gap. Values are given in milliequivalents per liter. The bar on the left shows the normal relationship of the unmeasured anions (A-) to the plasma electrolytes. To maintain electroneutrality, the number of cations and anions must be equal. Normally, the number of sodium (Na+) ions exceeds the number of chloride (Cl−) and bicarbonate (HCO₃⁻) ions, called the anion gap (normally 12). The anion gap is made up of anions such as sulfate and organic acids such as ketones not normally measured in routine laboratory tests. The anion gap is significant because it gives the level of unmeasured anions. The bar in the middle depicts hyperchloremic (or normal anion gap) acidosis usually caused by renal or GI loss of bicarbonate, with a compensatory increase in chloride ions to preserve electroneutrality. The bar on the right depicts normochloremic (or high anion) acidosis caused by an increase in unmeasured anions as, for example, in diabetic ketoacidosis or lactic acidosis.

Compensatory Response to Acid Load in Metabolic Acidosis

The immediate response to the H^+ load in metabolic acidosis is ECF buffering by HCO_3^-, thus reducing the plasma $[HCO_3^-]$. Excess H^+ also enters the cells and is buffered by proteins and phosphates (which provide 60% of the buffering). To maintain electroneutrality, the entry of H^+ into cells is accompanied by movement of K^+ out of the cells into the ECF. Thus the serum K^+ rises in conditions of acidosis. When a patient with acidosis has normokalemia or hypokalemia, K^+ depletion is present and must be corrected along with the acidosis.

The second mechanism activated within minutes in metabolic acidosis is respiratory compensation. The increased arterial $[H^+]$ stimulates chemoreceptors in the carotid bodies, which, in turn, stimulate increased alveolar ventilation (hyperventilation). Consequently, the $Paco_2$ is lowered and the pH restored toward 7.4.

BOX 22-2
Causes of Metabolic Acidosis

NORMAL ANION GAP (HYPERCHLOREMIC)
Bicarbonate loss
  GI loss
    Diarrhea*
    Ileostomy; pancreatic, biliary, or intestinal fistulas
    Ureterosigmoidostomy
  Renal loss
    Proximal renal tubular acidosis (RTA)
    Carbonic anhydrase (CA) inhibitors (acetazolamide)
    Hypoaldosteronism
Increased acid load
    Ammonium chloride ($NH_4Cl \rightarrow NH_3 + HCl$)
    Hyperalimentation fluids
Other
    Rapid administration of IV saline

INCREASED ANION GAP
Increased acid production
    Lactic acidosis*: lactate (inadequate tissue perfusion or oxygenation as in shock or cardiopulmonary arrest)
    Diabetic ketoacidosis*: Beta-hydroxybutyrate
    Starvation: increased ketoacids
    Alcohol intoxication: increased ketoacids
Ingestion of toxic substances
    Salicylate overdose: salicylate, lactate, ketones
    Methanol or formaldehyde: formate
    Ethylene glycol (antifreeze): oxylate, glycolate
Failure of acid excretion: diminished NH_4^- excretion; retention of sulfuric and phosphoric acids
    Acute or chronic renal failure*

*Most common causes.

The renal compensatory response provides the final means of correcting the metabolic acidosis, although the response is slow and may require several days. This process takes place by several mechanisms. Excess H^+ is secreted into the tubule and excreted as NH_4^+ or as titratable acid (H_3PO_4). Increased NH_4^+ excretion is accompanied by increased HCO_3^- resorption, but H_3PO_4 excretion results in the formation of new HCO_3^-. Renal insufficiency or failure decreases the effectiveness of H^+ elimination.

Clinical Features and Diagnosis

Signs and symptoms of metabolic acidosis tend to be vague, and the patient may be asymptomatic unless the serum $[HCO_3^-]$ falls below 15 mEq/L. Kussmaul breathing (deep, rapid respirations indicating compensatory hyperventilation) may be more prominent in the acidosis of diabetic ketoacidosis than in that of renal failure. The major signs and symptoms of metabolic acidosis are manifested as abnormalities in cardiovascular, neurologic, and bone function. When the pH is less than 7.1, cardiac contractility and the inotropic response to catecholamines are reduced. Peripheral vasodilation may be present. These effects may lead to hypotension and cardiac dysrhythmias.

Neurologic symptoms range from lethargy to coma related to the fall in pH of the cerebrospinal fluid. Nausea and vomiting may be present. Neurologic symptoms are less severe in metabolic acidosis than in respiratory acidosis because the lipid-soluble CO_2 crosses the blood-brain barrier more rapidly than does the water-soluble HCO_3^-.

The buffering of H^+ by bone bicarbonates in the metabolic acidosis of chronic renal failure retards growth in children and may lead to a variety of bone disorders (renal osteodystrophy).

The diagnosis of metabolic acidosis is made on the basis of clinical features and confirmed by laboratory measurement of the pH, Pa_{CO_2}, and HCO_3^- using a systematic approach as outlined previously. The pH is less than 7.35, HCO_3^- is less than 22 mEq/L, and the Pa_{CO_2} is less than 40 mm Hg but rarely falls to less than 12 mm Hg. The expected degree of compensation should be calculated to determine whether a mixed acid-base disorder exists.

Treatment

The treatment goal for metabolic acidosis is to raise the systemic pH to a safe level and treat the underlying cause of the acidosis. Only a small increase in the plasma pH to 7.20 or 7.25 is necessary to restore the patient to a safe range. The HCO_3^- must be less than 15 mEq/L and the pH less than 7.20 to cause serious disruption of physiologic processes. The metabolic acidosis should be corrected slowly to avoid the following complications of intravenous (IV) $NaHCO_3$ administration:

1. Increased pH of cerebrospinal fluid (CSF) and suppressed respiratory drive, resulting in less respiratory compensation.
2. Respiratory alkalosis because patients tend to hyperventilate for several hours after the ECF acidosis is corrected.
3. Shift of the oxyhemoglobin dissociation curve to the left in the event of a complicating respiratory alkalosis, which increases the affinity of oxygen for hemoglobin and possibly reduces oxygen delivery to the tissues (see Fig. 35-13).
4. Metabolic alkalosis (because no loss of potential HCO_3^- occurs, and the ketoacids can be metabolized back to lactate) in a patient with diabetic ketoacidosis (DKA). Insulin alone will usually restore acid-base balance; however, monitoring the serum K^+ while the acidosis is being corrected is important because the acidosis may be masking K^+ deficit.
5. Serious metabolic alkalosis as a result of overcorrection of lactic acidosis resulting from cardiac arrest. Some investigators found that the serum pH reached 7.9 and the serum HCO_3^- 60 to 70 mEq/L with the indiscriminate infusion of $NaHCO_3$ during CPR (Mattar et al, 1974).
6. Functional hypocalcemia from administering IV $NaHCO_3$ to a renal failure patient with severe metabolic acidosis (the acidosis may be masking a hypocalcemia because calcium (Ca^{++}) is more soluble in an acid medium; Ca^{++} is less soluble in an alkaline medium), resulting in tetany, convulsions, and death. Hemodialysis is the usual treatment for renal metabolic acidosis.
7. Serious circulatory overload (hypervolemia) in patients who already have an ECF fluid volume excess, such as those with congestive heart failure or renal failure.

IV lactated Ringer's solution is generally the fluid of choice to effect the correction of normal anion gap metabolic acidosis and the ECF fluid volume deficit that often accompany this condition. The sodium lactate is slowly metabolized to $NaHCO_3$ in the body and corrects the acidosis slowly.

Treatment of high anion gap metabolic acidosis is generally directed toward correcting or ameliorating the causative factor. Treatment of the acidosis itself is required only when it causes serious organ dysfunction ($HCO_3^- < 10$ mEq/L). In these cases, sufficient $NaHCO_3$ is given to raise the HCO_3^- to 15 mEq/L and a pH of about 7.20 over a period of 12 hours (Schrier, 1997).

METABOLIC ALKALOSIS

Metabolic alkalosis (HCO_3^- excess) is a systemic disorder characterized by a primary increase in the plasma HCO_3^- concentration, resulting in an increase in the pH (decrease in the $[H^+]$). The ECF $[HCO_3^-]$ is greater than 26 mEq/L, and the pH is greater than 7.45. Metabolic alkalosis is frequently accompanied by ECF volume contraction and hypokalemia. Respiratory compensation consists of raising the Pa_{CO_2} by hypoventilation; however, the degree of hypoventilation is limited because respiration continues to be driven by hypoxia.

Causes and Pathogenesis

Box 22-3 lists common causes of metabolic alkalosis, which are net loss of H^+ (and Cl^- ions) or excess retention of HCO_3^-. HCl may be lost from the GI tract, as in prolonged vomiting or nasogastric suction, or in the urine because of the administration of loop or thiazide diuretics. Sustained metabolic alkalosis caused by the oral or parenteral ingestion of HCO_3^- is rare because the HCO_3^- load is excreted in the urine unless a Cl^- deficit also exists.

The pathogenesis of metabolic alkalosis is best understood as occurring in three stages: generation, maintenance, and recovery. Metabolic alkalosis is generated by the net loss of H^+ from the body with the consequent elevation of the ECF HCO_3^- (or by the addition of exogenous HCO_3^-). The maintenance of a sustained metabolic alkalosis occurs because the base excess cannot be excreted. A variety of factors (Cl^- and K^+ deficit, ECF volume [Na^+ and water] depletion, and aldosterone excess) may cause this condition. Cessation of the event that caused the metabolic alkalosis (e.g., vomiting) is not necessarily accompanied by resolution and recovery from the alkalosis. The specific therapy required is evident by understanding the factors that maintain alkalosis.

The depletion of Cl^- is crucial, both in the generation and the maintenance of *hypochloremic metabolic alkalosis*. Na^+ is the primary cation in the ECF, balanced by an equal number of anions, mainly Cl^- and HCO_3^-. Additionally, Cl^- and HCO_3^- have a reciprocal relationship: a decrease in Cl^- results in an increase in HCO_3^-, and an increase in Cl^- causes a decrease in HCO_3^-. The purpose of this relationship is to balance the total negative and positive charges to maintain ECF electroneutrality. Thus, when HCL is secreted into the stomach, an equimolar

NET LOSS OF H⁺ FROM THE ECF
GI loss (ECF volume depletion)
  Vomiting or nasogastric suction*
  Chloride-losing diarrhea
Renal loss
  Loop or thiazide-type diuretics* (NaCl restriction + ECF depletion)
  Mineralocorticoid excess*
  Hyperaldosteronism
  Cushing's syndrome; exogenous corticosteroid therapy
  Excess licorice ingestion
  High-dose carbenicillin or penicillin
H⁺ movement into cells
  Hypokalemia*

RETENTION OF HCO₃⁻
Excess administration of sodium bicarbonate
Milk-alkali syndrome (antacids, milk, NaHCO₃)
Massive (>8 units) bank blood (citrate)
Posthypercapnia metabolic alkalosis (after correction of chronic respiratory acidosis)
  Mechanical ventilation: rapid decrease in $PaCO_2$ but HCO_3^- remains high until kidneys can excrete excess

CHLORIDE-RESPONSIVE METABOLIC ALKALOSIS (URINARY CL⁻ <10 MEQ/L)
Usually associated with ECF volume contraction
  Vomiting or nasogastric suction
  Diuretics
  Posthypercapnia

CHLORIDE-RESISTANT METABOLIC ALKALOSIS (URINARY CL⁻ >20 MEQ/L)
Usually not ECF volume contracted
  Mineralocorticoid excess
  Edematous states (congestive heart failure; cirrhosis; nephrotic syndrome)

*Most common causes.

amount of HCO_3^- is secreted into the ECF. Metabolic alkalosis is commonly initiated by vomiting or nasogastric suction, with the consequent loss of fluids rich in chlorides (HCl) and deficient in HCO_3^-. KCl and NaCl and water are lost as well. The result is an increase in the serum HCO_3^-, K⁺ depletion, and fluid volume depletion.

The immediate compensatory response to metabolic alkalosis is intracellular buffering. H⁺ exits the cells to buffer the excess ECF HCO_3^-. K⁺ moves into cells in exchange for the H⁺. Additionally, lactic acid production is slightly increased within cells to produce more H⁺. Consequently, a paradoxic ICF acidosis and an ECF alkalosis occur.

The increased pH is sensed by the chemoreceptors in the carotid bodies, which, in turn, cause a reflex decrease in alveolar ventilation. However, the magnitude of the respiratory compensation is generally quite small. The degree of hypoventilation and rise in the $PaCO_2$ is limited by the need for oxygen and rarely exceeds 50 to 55 mm Hg.

The final renal correction of metabolic alkalosis requires the excretion of the excess HCO_3^-. Producing a sustained metabolic alkalosis from the ingestion of HCO_3^- is difficult because the kidneys normally have a great capacity to excrete HCO_3^-.

Research findings by Galla and Luke (1987) suggest that Cl⁻ depletion plays the major role in preventing the renal excretion of HCO_3^-. In contrast to previous theories positing a major role for ECF volume depletion and secondary hyperaldosteronism, these authors claim that intrarenal mechanisms responsible for Cl⁻ depletion can account for the maintenance of metabolic alkalosis, regardless of the status of the ECF volume. According to the findings of Galla and Luke, Cl⁻ depletion stimulates the renin-angiotensin-aldosterone mechanism, increased renal K⁺ and H⁺ excretion, and increased reabsorption of HCO_3^- independent of the Na⁺. In addition to Cl⁻ depletion as a cause of the perpetuation of metabolic alkalosis, fluid volume depletion stimulates the renin-angiotensin-aldosterone mechanism. Aldosterone causes increased Na⁺ and water reabsorption in an effort to restore the ECF volume. Protection of the ECF volume takes precedence over correction of the alkalosis, because the excretion of Na⁺ along with HCO_3^- is required. When Cl⁻ depletion occurs, insufficient Cl⁻ is available to absorb with Na⁺, thus more Na⁺ is reabsorbed in exchange for H⁺, both in the proximal and the distal tubule (via aldosterone). In fact, H⁺ secretion can increase to the point at which all of the filtered HCO_3^- is reabsorbed and additional HCO_3^- is generated. The result of the increased H⁺ secretion is paradoxically acid urine in the presence of an alkalosis. Aldosterone also stimulates K⁺ excretion. K⁺ depletion, in turn, promotes H⁺ excretion and accelerated HCO_3^- reabsorption. In summary, Cl⁻ depletion, fluid volume depletion, hyperaldosteronism, and K⁺ depletion all contribute to the maintenance of metabolic alkalosis.

Clinical Features and Diagnosis

No specific signs and symptoms in metabolic alkalosis are evident. The disorder should be suspected in patients with a history of vomiting, nasogastric suction, or diuretic therapy or patients recovering from hypercapnic respiratory failure. Signs and symptoms of hypokalemia and fluid volume deficit, such as muscle cramps and weakness, may be present. Severe alkalemia (pH >7.6) can cause cardiac dysrhythmias in normal persons and particularly in those with cardiac disease. When the patient is hypokalemic, particularly when digitalized, electrocardiogram (ECG) abnormalities or a cardiac dysrhythmia may develop. Occasionally, tetany may occur in a patient when the serum Ca^{++} is borderline low and the alkalosis has developed rapidly. Ca^{++} is more closely bound to albumin in an alkaline pH, and the drop in ionized Ca^{++} may be sufficient to produce tetany or a seizure.

Diagnosis of metabolic alkalosis is made on the basis of the history and appropriate laboratory studies. Plasma pH is elevated above 7.45, and the HCO_3^- is greater than 26 mEq/L. The $PaCO_2$ may be normal or slightly elevated; the expected compensatory rise is 0.7 mm Hg for every 1 mEq increase in the HCO_3^-. The serum K⁺ will usually be less than 3.5 mEq/L, and the serum Cl⁻ may be less than 98 mEq/L (hypokalemic hypochloremic metabolic alkalosis). Measurement of the urinary Cl⁻ helps determine the cause and appropriate treatment. Patients with *chloride-responsive metabolic alkalosis* and ECF volume depletion have a urinary Cl⁻ of less than 10 mEq/L. Those with urinary Cl^- greater than 20 mEq/L are not usually fluid volume depleted and have *chloride-resistant metabolic alkalosis* (see Box 22-3). The latter type of alkalosis is much less common and is associated with aldosterone excess.

Treatment

Mild *chloride-responsive metabolic alkalosis* may be corrected by replacing the ECF deficit with parenteral isotonic saline with added KCl. The provision of Cl^- allows increased Na^+ reabsorption in the proximal tubule, with less Na^+ presented to the distal tubule. As the amount of Na^+ reabsorbed in the distal tubule decreases, the alkalosis begins to resolve because less H^+ is secreted and less HCO_3^- is generated. Additionally, H^+ secretion is decreased further as hypokalemia is corrected because more K^+ is now available to exchange with Na^+. A dilute HCl IV solution (100 to 200 mEq/L) may be given when the alkalosis is severe and life threatening (pH >7.55) and an immediate need for correction exists. Other acidifying agents that are occasionally administered for severe alkalosis include IV ammonium chloride (NH_4Cl) or arginine HCl.

Chloride-resistant metabolic alkalosis caused by excess adrenal steroids in hyperaldosteronism or Cushing's syndrome is corrected by treating the underlying disorder. Acetazolamide, a carbonic anhydrase inhibitor that enhances HCO_3^- excretion, may be given to patients who have fluid volume excess (e.g., a patient with congestive heart failure who is taking diuretics). KCl is also helpful for treating and preventing alkalosis and hypokalemia.

RESPIRATORY ACIDOSIS

Respiratory acidosis (H_2CO_3 excess) is characterized by a primary rise in the Pa_{CO_2} (hypercapnia), resulting in a decrease of the pH. The Pa_{CO_2} is greater than 45 mm Hg and the pH is less than 7.35. Renal compensation results in a variable increase in the serum HCO_3^-. Respiratory acidosis may be acute or chronic. Hypoxemia (low Pa_{O_2}) invariably accompanies respiratory acidosis when the patient is breathing room air.

Causes and Pathogenesis

The fundamental cause of respiratory acidosis is alveolar hypoventilation, a term virtually synonymous with CO_2 accumulation. Normally, 15,000 to 20,000 mmol of CO_2 are produced each day by tissue metabolism and eliminated by the lungs. Most of the CO_2 is transferred to the lungs in the form of blood HCO_3^- (see the bicarbonate-buffer equation). When tissue CO_2 enters the blood, it causes an increase in the $[H^+]$, which, in turn, stimulates the respiratory center, resulting in increased ventilation. Normally, this process is efficient to the extent that the Pa_{CO_2} and pH are kept within a normal range. CO_2 accumulation is nearly always caused by impairment of the rate of alveolar ventilation rather than overproduction of CO_2 from hypermetabolism.

Box 22-4 lists some common causes of respiratory acidosis. Acute respiratory acidosis usually stems from acute airway obstruction as in laryngospasm, foreign body

---

BOX 22-4

Causes of Respiratory Acidosis (Basic Cause = Hypoventilation)

INHIBITION OF THE MEDULLARY RESPIRATORY CENTER
Drugs: opiate, sedative, anesthetic overdose (acute)
Oxygen therapy in chronic hypercapnia
Cardiac arrest (acute)
Sleep apnea

DISORDERS OF THE RESPIRATORY MUSCLES AND CHEST WALL
Neuromuscular disease: myasthenia gravis, Guillain-Barré syndrome, poliomyelitis, amyotrophic lateral sclerosis
Chest cage deformity: kyphoscoliosis
Extreme obesity: pickwickian syndrome
Chest wall injury such as fractured ribs

DISORDERS OF GAS EXCHANGE
COPD (emphysema and bronchitis)*
End-stage diffuse intrinsic pulmonary disease
Severe pneumonia or asthma
Acute pulmonary edema
Pneumothorax

ACUTE UPPER AIRWAY OBSTRUCTION
Aspiration of foreign body or vomitus
Laryngospasm or laryngeal edema, severe bronchospasm

*Most common cause of chronic respiratory acidosis.

---

aspiration, or central nervous system (CNS) depression of the medullary respiratory center, such as that from barbiturate or opiate overdose. In severe acute respiratory acidosis, as in asphyxia or cardiopulmonary arrest, the resulting respiratory acidosis is worsened by an accompanying metabolic acidosis from the rapid accumulation of lactic acid produced during cellular anaerobic glycolysis. High-concentration oxygen therapy may depress the respiratory drive, particularly in patients with chronic hypercapnia. Other causes of acute respiratory acidosis include disorders of the respiratory muscles or chest wall injury. The terminal stage of respiratory failure because of any number of causes always involves hypercapnia in addition to hypoxemia.

The most common cause of chronic respiratory acidosis by far is chronic obstructive pulmonary disease (COPD). In these patients, acute respiratory failure is often superimposed on chronic CO_2 retention when they develop an acute bronchitis secondary to a viral or bacterial lung infection. Kyphoscoliosis, the pickwickian syndrome, and sleep apnea are other causes of chronic respiratory acidosis. All of these conditions are discussed in detail in Part Seven.

The arterial pH and plasma HCO_3^- are different in acute and chronic respiratory acidosis. In response to acute respiratory acidosis, only the cellular buffering defense has time to be used because the renal compensatory mechanism will not be significant for 12 to 24 hours. Plasma proteins provide ECF buffering, but this process is minor. (Because the increased H_2CO_3 is a member of the major ECF buffer pair HCO_3^- and H_2CO_3, the pair does not directly participate in the buffer defense in respiratory acidosis.) Hemoglobin provides the major ICF buffering. As CO_2 enters the RBCs (producing H^+), HCO_3^- moves out in exchange for Cl^-. The expected rise of the serum HCO_3^- is approximately 1 mEq/L for every 10 mm Hg rise in the CO_2. Cellular buffering alone is ineffective in restoring a normal pH. Thus acute respiratory acidosis is poorly compensated and the pH is seriously reduced.

Chronic respiratory acidosis, in contrast to acute respiratory acidosis, is well compensated because the renal compensatory mechanism has had time to become operational. The kidneys increase secretion and excretion of H^+, accompanied by the resorption and generation of new HCO_3^-. The compensatory increase in plasma HCO_3^- requires 2 to 3 days for complete expression. Conversely, a 2- to 3-day lag time in renal HCO_3^- excretion occurs, resulting in posthypercapnia metabolic alkalosis, as discussed previously. Thus patients with respiratory acidosis, which is relatively well compensated, as evidenced by a nearly normal pH, should not be treated overzealously. Lowering their $Paco_2$ too rapidly leaves them with a sizable HCO_3^- excess and shifts their acid-base balance into acute alkalosis. The expected compensatory rise of the plasma HCO_3^- in chronic respiratory acidosis is 3.5 mEq/L for every 10 mm Hg rise in the $Paco_2$ above 40 mm Hg.

Clinical Features and Diagnosis

The signs and symptoms of CO_2 retention are nonspecific and, generally, have an unpredictable relationship to the level of the $Paco_2$. Additionally, because both acute respiratory acidosis and chronic respiratory acidosis are always accompanied by hypoxemia, the hypoxemia itself is responsible for many of the clinical characteristics of CO_2 retention. Generally, the greater the magnitude and the faster the rate of rise in $Paco_2$, the more severe the symptoms will be. An acute rise in the $Paco_2$ to 60 mm Hg or above results in somnolence, mental confusion, stupor, and eventually coma. Because a high $Paco_2$ produces a kind of metabolic brain syndrome, asterixis (flapping tremor) and myoclonus (muscle jerking) may be present. Because CO_2 retention causes cerebral vasodilation, the consequent cerebral vascular congestion leads to increased intracranial pressure (ICP). Increased ICP may be manifested as papilledema (swelling of the optic disc visible on examination with the ophthalmoscope). The laboratory findings in acute respiratory acidosis reveal a low Pao_2, pH below 7.35, and $Paco_2$ above 45 mm Hg, with a small compensatory rise of the HCO_3^- (less than 30 mEq/L). Of course, in acute airway obstruction, respiratory distress symptoms related to hypoxemia may completely dominate the clinical picture.

Chronic respiratory acidosis appears to be tolerated much better than does acute respiratory acidosis. Few signs and symptoms related to the CO_2 retention and acidosis may be present unless the $Paco_2$ is greater than 60 mm Hg. The $Paco2$ is greater than 45 mm Hg and the HCO_3^- is greater than 30 mEq/L, indicating renal compensation. The serum pH may be normal or slightly decreased in a well-compensated chronic respiratory acidosis. A compensatory polycythemia commonly occurs in states of chronic hypercapnia. Hemoglobin levels may reach 16 to 22 g/L. The signs and symptoms of COPD, with or without cor pulmonale, generally predominate (see Part Seven). Acute respiratory acidosis and chronic respiratory acidosis are differentiated on the basis of the history and analysis of the arterial blood gases.

Treatment of Acute and Chronic Respiratory Acidosis

Treatment of acute respiratory acidosis is restoration of effective ventilation as soon as possible by administering oxygen therapy and treating the underlying cause. The Pao_2 must be raised to a minimal level of 60 mm Hg and the pH above 7.2 to avoid the development of cardiac dysrhythmias. High concentration oxygen (>50%) may be given safely to patients for 1 to 2 days when no history of chronic hypercapnia is present. When patients with chronic hypercapnia develop an acute rise in the $Paco_2$, attention should be directed toward identifying factors, such as pneumonia or pulmonary embolism, which may have aggravated the underlying disorder and precipitated the crisis. Mechanical ventilation may be necessary to deal with the crisis. Great caution must be exercised in administering oxygen to patients with chronic hypercapnia. In these patients, hypoxia replaces hypercapnia as the major stimulus for respiration. Thus, when the oxygen therapy raises the Pao_2 above the patient's normal level, it will remove the hypoxic drive to respiration and result in even further reduction in alveolar ventilation. Consequently, the correct approach in treating these patients is to start with the lowest possible concentration of oxygen (24% to 28%) to raise the Pao_2 to 60 to 70 mm Hg. Arterial blood gases must be monitored carefully during the treatment to detect signs of increasing $Paco_2$ and deterioration of alveolar ventilation. The $Paco_2$ is lowered, but achievement of a normal value is not the goal.

▒ RESPIRATORY ALKALOSIS

Respiratory alkalosis (H_2CO_3 deficit) is characterized by a primary decrease in the $Paco_2$ (hypocapnia), resulting in an increase in the pH. The $Paco_2$ is less than 35 mm Hg, and the pH is greater than 7.45. Renal compensation consists of decreased excretion of H^+ and consequently less absorption of HCO_3^-. The serum HCO_3^- is reduced in varying amounts, depending on whether the condition is acute or chronic.

Causes and Pathogenesis

The fundamental cause of respiratory alkalosis is alveolar hyperventilation or excess excretion of CO_2 in expired air. Hyperventilation should not be confused with an increased respiratory rate (tachypnea), which may or may not be associated with hyperventilation. Hyperventilation can occur with a normal respiratory rate when tidal volume is increased. Hyperventilation can be positively identified only by a decreased $Paco_2$. Respiratory alkalosis may well be the most common acid-base imbalance, although it is often not recognized. Hyperventilation may be difficult to recognize clinically, and the diagnosis is often made only by blood gas determination.

Box 22-5 lists some of the common causes of respiratory alkalosis. Respiratory alkalosis may occur as a result of stimulation of the medullary respiratory center. The most common cause by far is functional hyperventilation caused by anxiety and emotional stress (hyperventilation syndrome or psychogenic hyperventilation). When all the stressful life situations that humans encounter are considered, both within a hospital environment (e.g., pain, awaiting a potential diagnosis of a malignancy) and in the community, not surprisingly, hyperventilation syndrome is common. Nearly everyone has experienced hyperventilation syndrome at some time during his or her life. Other conditions causing stimulation of the respiratory center include hypermetabolic conditions caused by fever or thyrotoxicosis and CNS lesions, such as cerebral vascular accidents, meningitis, head trauma, or brain tumors. Salicylates are the most important drugs that cause respiratory alkalosis, presumably by direct stimulation of the medullary respiratory center. Hypoxia is a common cause of primary hyperventilation in association with pneumonia, pulmonary edema or fibrosis, or congestive heart failure. Generally, a reduction of the PaO_2 below 60 mm Hg is necessary to stimulate ventilation. Correction of the tissue hypoxia results in rapid resolution of the respiratory alkalosis. Chronic hyperventilation occurs in the acclimation response to high altitudes (low ambient oxygen tension). Respiratory alkalosis is commonly produced iatrogenically by mechanical ventilation with a volume-cycled or pressure-cycled ventilator. Respiratory alkalosis is commonly associated with gram-negative sepsis and hepatic cirrhosis. Finally, although hyperpnea is an adaptive response to increased oxygen demand during physical exercise, transitory respiratory alkalosis may be produced occasionally.

The immediate response to an acute reduction in the $PaCO_2$ is intracellular buffering. H^+ is released from the intracellular tissue buffers, which minimizes the alkalosis by lowering the plasma HCO_3^-. Acute alkalosis also stimulates lactic acid and pyruvate production within the cells and helps to provide more H^+ for release into the ECF. Extracellular buffering by plasma proteins is minor. The effect of ECF and ICF buffering is a small decrement in the plasma HCO_3^-. When hypocapnia is sustained, renal adjustments yield a much larger decrement in plasma HCO_3^-. Renal tubular reabsorption and generation of new HCO_3^- are inhibited. As in respiratory acidosis, compensation for chronic respiratory alkalosis is much more complete than it is for the acute condition. In the acute condition, the expected fall in plasma HCO_3^- is 2 mEq/L for every 10 mm Hg fall in the $PaCO_2$; the expected decrease of HCO_3^- is 5 mEq/L for every 10 mm Hg fall in the $PaCO_2$ in the chronic condition.

Clinical Features and Diagnosis

The breathing pattern in anxiety-induced hyperventilation syndrome varies from an apparently normal respiratory pattern to obviously frequent, deep, sighing respirations. Frequent yawning may often be observed. Patients are surprisingly unaware of their hyperventilation. When symptoms are referable to respirations, the complaint is usually "unable to get enough air" or "unable to catch my breath," despite the fact that unimpaired overbreathing is taking place. Other prominent symptoms include "light-headedness," circumoral paresthesias, numbness and tin-

---

BOX 22-5

Causes of Respiratory Alkalosis (Basic Cause = Hyperventilation)

CENTRAL STIMULATION OF RESPIRATION
Psychogenic hyperventilation caused by emotional stress*
Hypermetabolic states: fever, thyrotoxicosis
CNS disorders
Head trauma or vascular accidents
Brain tumors
Salicylate intoxication (early)

HYPOXIA
Pneumonia, asthma, pulmonary edema
Congestive heart failure
Pulmonary fibrosis
High-altitude residence

EXCESSIVE MECHANICAL VENTILATION

UNCERTAIN MECHANISM
Gram-negative sepsis
Hepatic cirrhosis

EXERCISE

*Most common cause.

---

gling of the fingers and toes, and when the alkalosis is sufficiently severe, manifestations of tetany such as carpopedal spasm. The patient may complain of chronic exhaustion, palpitations, anxiety, dry mouth, and sleeplessness. The palms of the hands and soles of the feet may feel cold and clammy to the examiner's touch and may indicate emotional tension. Severe respiratory alkalosis may be associated with inability to concentrate, mental confusion, and syncope.

The basis of the neuromuscular signs and symptoms may be attributed to the alkalosis because it directly enhances neuromuscular irritability. Additionally, less calcium is ionized in an alkaline medium thus a functional hypocalcemia may contribute to manifestations of tetany. CNS symptoms may be related to cerebral hypoxia. Alkalosis not only shifts the oxyhemoglobin dissociation curve to the left (causing hemoglobin to have a greater affinity for oxygen), but also reduces cerebral blood flow. Both of these mechanisms may induce cerebral hypoxia. Cerebral blood flow is reduced approximately 40% at a $PaCO_2$ of 20 mm Hg. In fact, hyperventilation and acute hypocapnia are such potent producers of cerebral vasoconstriction that they are deliberately induced on a mechanical ventilator as a treatment for cerebral vascular congestion and increased ICP. Although some cerebral hypoxia may be induced, the benefits of reducing the cerebral edema outweigh this adverse effect.

As stated, laboratory findings in acute respiratory alkalosis consist of a pH above 7.45 and a $PaCO_2$ below 35 mm Hg. If the $PaCO_2$ should rapidly drop to 20 mm Hg, for example, the drop in plasma HCO_3^- should then be no greater than approximately 4 mEq/L because of cellular buffering. In chronic metabolic alkalosis, the plasma HCO_3^- would be expected to drop approximately 10 mEq/L with the same degree of hypocapnia. A greater than expected fall in the plasma HCO_3^- suggests coexistent metabolic acidosis; when the fall is less than expected, a coexistent metabolic alkalosis may be present.

Other laboratory findings may include a reciprocal hyperchloremia and a hypokalemia. The diagnosis of respiratory alkalosis is made based on the history, signs, and symptoms and confirmed by evidence of the laboratory findings.

Treatment

The only successful treatment for respiratory alkalosis is elimination of the underlying cause. Hyperventilation with mechanical ventilators may be corrected by reducing minute ventilation when excessive or by adding dead space. If this goal cannot be achieved without compromising oxygenation, a gas mixture containing 3% CO_2 may then be used for a short time (Schrier, 1997).

When severe anxiety produces the hyperventilation syndrome, air rebreathing with a paper bag held tightly around the nose and mouth generally terminates the acute attack. These patients may need stress management counseling.

MIXED ACID-BASE DISORDERS

Mixed acid-base disorders are conditions in which at least two of the more simple acid-base disturbances coexist. Given the large number of pathophysiologic processes that can alter the $PaCO_2$ or HCO_3^-, not surprisingly, one acid-base disorder does not preclude the existence of another that has independent effects on acid-base balance. In fact, the existence of some acid-base disturbances increases the likelihood that another will develop. Mixed acid-base disturbances frequently occur in the presence of complex medical problems, thus the clinical features are difficult to distinguish from the underlying illness.

Table 22-5 lists four combinations of the primary acid-base disorders and examples of diseases and clinical situations implicated in their pathogenesis. These mixed disturbances include (1) metabolic acidosis and respiratory acidosis, (2) metabolic alkalosis and respiratory alkalosis, (3) metabolic acidosis and respiratory alkalosis, and (4) metabolic alkalosis and respiratory acidosis. Any of the simple acid-base disturbances may be superimposed on another or may follow another in sequence. The individual components may have either additive or offsetting effects on the plasma acidity, as evidenced by the combinations of mixed acid-base imbalances, thus the resulting change in pH may be profoundly severe or deceptively mild.

Metabolic Acidosis and Respiratory Acidosis

The most common situation leading to metabolic acidosis and respiratory acidosis is untreated cardiopulmonary arrest. Respiratory arrest with absent alveolar ventilation results in the rapid accumulation of CO_2, and the tissue hypoxia from lack of oxygenation results in activation of anaerobic metabolism with the consequent accumulation of lactic acid. Another example is a person with COPD (chronic respiratory acidosis) who goes into shock (metabolic acidosis). A third example is a patient with chronic renal failure (metabolic acidosis) complicated by respiratory insufficiency secondary to fluid overload and pulmonary edema. Patients with chronic renal failure often

TABLE 22-5

Common Mixed Acid-Base Disorders

Dual Mixed Disorder	Common Causes
ADDITIVE EFFECT ON pH CHANGE	
Metabolic acidosis + Respiratory acidosis $PaCO_2$ too high HCO_3^- too low pH very low	Cardiopulmonary arrest Patient with COPD goes into shock Chronic renal failure with fluid volume excess and pulmonary edema Patient with DKA receives potent opiate or barbiturate
Metabolic alkalosis + Respiratory alkalosis $PaCO_2$ too low HCO_3^- too high pH very high	Patient with previously compensated respiratory acidosis caused by COPD overventilated on mechanical respirator Hyperventilating patient with CHF or hepatic cirrhosis who is vomiting or is treated with potent diuretics or nasogastric suction Head trauma patient with hyperventilation treated with diuretics
OFFSETTING EFFECT ON pH CHANGE	
Metabolic acidosis + Respiratory alkalosis $PaCO_2$ too low HCO_3^- too low pH near normal	Lactic acidosis complicating septic shock Hepatorenal syndrome Salicylate intoxication
Metabolic alkalosis + Respiratory acidosis $PaCO_2$ too high HCO_3^- too high pH near normal	Patient with COPD who is vomiting or who is treated with NG suction or potent diuretics Adult respiratory distress syndrome

CHF, Congestive heart failure; *COPD,* chronic obstructive pulmonary disease; *DKA,* diabetic ketoacidosis; *NG,* nasogastric.

find that compliance with their sodium-restricted diet is difficult and may indulge in a pizza binge, with resulting fluid overload and pulmonary edema. A less obvious situation that produces this mixed disorder is a patient with diabetic ketoacidosis who receives an opiate or a potent sedative, which causes depression of the respiratory center.

In each of these examples, the respiratory disorder prevents a compensatory fall in the $PaCO_2$ for the metabolic acidosis and the metabolic disorder prevents buffering and renal mechanisms from raising the HCO_3^- in response to the respiratory acidosis. Consequently, the laboratory data show an increased $PaCO_2$ and a decreased HCO_3^-, with a profound drop in the plasma pH. The clue to recognizing this mixed disorder is that the respiratory and metabolic components of the buffer equation change in opposite directions. The clinical history provides obvious clues to the diagnosis in the case of cardiopulmonary arrest, but recognition of this mixed disorder may not be as obvious in the case of a person with COPD (chronic respiratory acidosis) who develops diabetic ketoacidosis.

Therapy for mixed respiratory and metabolic acidosis is directed toward treatment of each of the underlying disorders. In the case of cardiopulmonary arrest, the goal is to restore tissue perfusion and oxygenation by restoring heart and lung function. Administering a small amount of $NaHCO_3$ may be necessary to raise the pH to a more optimal level (7.2) such that cardiac function will respond to resuscitation efforts.

Metabolic Alkalosis and Respiratory Alkalosis

The combination of metabolic and respiratory alkalosis is one of the most common mixed acid-base disorders according to Schrier (1997). A common clinical example is a person with COPD (compensated respiratory acidosis with increased HCO_3^-) who is hyperventilated on a respirator. The respiratory acidosis is thus rapidly converted to a respiratory alkalosis, which combines with the metabolic alkalosis produced by the original compensatory rise in HCO_3^-. Another example is a person with congestive heart failure who is hyperventilating (respiratory alkalosis) and treated with potent diuretics (metabolic alkalosis and hypokalemia) or has prolonged vomiting or nasogastric suction. The same aggravating factors in a person with hepatic cirrhosis who is hyperventilating might produce similar consequences. Another example is a person with central neurogenic hyperventilation from brainstem trauma who receives diuretics.

Each acid-base disorder blocks the appropriate compensatory response of the other when alkalotic acid-base disturbances are combined. Consequently, the pH is significantly increased. The $Paco_2$ and the HCO_3^- deviate from the normal range in opposite directions. In addition to the history, other laboratory findings that provide clues to recognition of this mixed disorder include hypokalemia.

In the case of the person placed on a ventilator, great care must be taken in adjusting the ventilation and oxygen concentration to keep the Pao_2 at a minimally safe level of approximately 60 to 70 mm Hg, and at the same time the $Paco_2$ is reduced very slowly, giving the kidneys time to reduce the elevated HCO_3^-. Patients with chronic hypercapnia depend on a hypoxic stimulus for breathing and are relatively insensitive to CO_2 as a stimulus. Thus raising oxygen tension and lowering CO_2 tension to normal values in patients with COPD may depress the respiratory drive, resulting in a deterioration of their condition. The other mixed disorders mentioned are treated with NaCl and KCl to reduce the HCO_3^- and restore a safe pH level because it would be difficult, if not impossible, to direct attention toward elevating the $Paco_2$.

Metabolic Acidosis and Respiratory Alkalosis

A mixed metabolic acidosis and respiratory alkalosis can be identified when plasma HCO_3^- and $Paco_2$ are both low and the pH is normal or nearly normal, because these two disorders tend to offset each other.

Primary respiratory alkalosis can coexist with various types of metabolic acidosis, commonly occurring with lactic acidosis complicating septic shock. The latter condition is associated with hyperventilation. Primary respiratory alkalosis also occurs with renal acidosis in the hepatorenal syndrome and with organic acidosis in salicylate intoxication.

In a mixed metabolic acidosis and respiratory alkalosis, the drop in the $Paco_2$ is greater than would be expected as a compensation for a primary metabolic acidosis, and the drop in HCO_3^- is greater than would be expected as a compensation for primary respiratory alkalosis. The treatment must be directed at the specific entities causing the mixed acid-base imbalance because the pH is normal or nearly normal.

Metabolic Alkalosis and Respiratory Acidosis

A diagnosis of mixed respiratory acidosis and metabolic alkalosis can be made when the plasma HCO_3^- and the $Paco_2$ are both elevated and the pH is normal or nearly normal. This mixed disorder is quite common and occurs most often when patients with COPD (chronic respiratory acidosis) are treated with potent diuretics or have other conditions causing metabolic alkalosis, such as vomiting, nasogastric suction, or steroid therapy. This dual acid-base disturbance also occurs in adult respiratory distress syndrome (ARDS).

The detection of even small degrees of metabolic alkalosis is important in patients with COPD and chronic hypercapnia because their respiratory drive depends in part on the accompanying acidosis. Thus any reduction in H^+ (increase in pH) from an accompanying elevated HCO_3^- will depress ventilation and cause a further rise in the $Paco_2$ and a fall in the Pao_2. In such cases, treatment of the alkalosis can significantly improve ventilation. Increasing dietary Cl^- or KCl therapy will help lower the plasma HCO_3^-.

OTHER MIXED ACID-BASE DISTURBANCES

Although the four possible dual mixed acid-base disturbances have been reviewed, another common imbalance, *acute-on-chronic respiratory acidosis*, is important to keep in mind. Common precipitating factors are intercurrent pulmonary infection or administration of sedative in a patient with COPD and chronic hypercapnia. This situation causes a marked acute rise in the $Paco_2$ and a seriously low pH. $Paco_2$ levels above 70 mm Hg may depress respirations and cause stupor, coma (CO_2 narcosis), and hypoxemia. Treatment is directed at the factors causing the respiratory failure. Mechanical ventilation may be necessary to correct the hypercapnia, acidosis, and more importantly, the hypoxemia. On the other hand, care must be taken to gradually lower the $Paco_2$ so that a posthypercapnic metabolic alkalosis is not precipitated.

In summary, acid-base disturbances can be complex. A thorough understanding of acid-base physiology and pathophysiology, coupled with a systematic approach as outlined at the beginning of this chapter, is a necessary prerequisite for recognizing these conditions. Particularly, recognizing offsetting mixed acid-base disorders requires an accurate history and ancillary laboratory data.

KEY CONCEPTS

- Acid-base balance refers to the homeostasis of the hydrogen ion concentration [H$^+$]. The normal [H$^+$] in arterial blood is 4×10^{-8}. This number is expressed as the pH (negative log of the [H$^+$]). Body fluids are classified as acids or bases according to their H$^+$ ion concentration.

- Human metabolism produces 50 to 100 mEq of H$^+$ ions per day, yet the mean blood pH is 7.4 and is kept within a narrow range. A stable pH is necessary for normal enzyme and cardiac function.

- Acid-base balance is maintained in the normal 7.35 to 7.45 range when the ratio of carbonic acid (H_2CO_3) to bicarbonate (HCO_3^-) is 1:20. A blood pH under 7.35 is called acidemia or acidosis; blood pH above 7.45 is called alkalemia or alkalosis. A blood pH under 6.8 or above 7.8 is incompatible with life.

- An acid is a proton [H$^+$] donor and a base is a proton acceptor. Strong acids or bases are completely dissociated in solution; weak acids or bases are only partially dissociated.

- Volatile acids, such as H_2CO_3, can change into a gaseous form ($CO_2 + H_2O$) and be excreted by the lungs. Nonvolatile (fixed) acids, such as sulfuric and phosphoric acids, cannot change into a gaseous form so must be excreted by the kidneys.

- A buffer is similar to a chemical sponge and reacts with either an acid or base to minimize the change in pH of the solution. A buffer may be a weak acid and its basic salt or a weak base and its acid salt.

- The pK of a buffer system is the pH at which the buffer is 50% dissociated and the most effective in defending pH changes when acids or bases are added to the system.

- Four main buffer pairs within the body help maintain the pH within normal limits:
  1. Bicarbonate–carbonic acid buffer system ($NaHCO_3$ and H_2CO_3), which operates mainly in the ECF
  2. Disodium–monosodium phosphate buffer system (Na_2HPO_4 and NaH_2PO_4), which is an ICF buffer
  3. Hemoglobin-oxyhemoglobin buffer system (HbO_2^- and HHb), which is an ICF buffer within the RBCs
  4. Protein buffer system: Pr$^-$ and HPr, which is mainly an ICF buffer but is also an ECF buffer

- Defense of the normal blood pH is achieved by the integrated action of the blood buffers, lungs, and kidneys. Chemical buffers in the ECF and ICF can act within seconds by combining with acids or bases added to the system to prevent deviation of the pH from normal. Buffering is only a temporary measure in restoring normal pH. The lungs are the second line of defense (acting within minutes) protecting the normal pH by controlling the excretion of CO_2 by increasing or decreasing alveolar ventilation. The kidneys are the third line of defense restoring normal pH by regulation of the ECF HCO_3^- level but may take 1 to 3 days to make the correction.

- As the major ECF buffer, the bicarbonate–carbonic acid buffer system is of central importance in understanding and assessing acid-base balance and imbalances. This buffer system is a reversible chemical reaction and can proceed to the left or to the right:

$$\underset{(40 \text{ mm Hg})}{\text{(lungs) } CO_2 + H_2O} \overset{1}{\rightleftharpoons} \underset{(1.2 \text{ mEq/L})}{H_2CO_3} \overset{20}{\rightleftharpoons} \underset{(\text{pH } 7.4)}{H^+} + \underset{(24 \text{ mEq/L})}{HCO_3^- \text{ (kidneys)}}$$

As long as the ratio of H_2CO_3 to HCO_3^- is 1:20, a pH of 7.4 can be maintained. The left side of the equation is the respiratory component controlled through variations in alveolar ventilation. The lungs represent a spigot at one end that can increase or decrease CO_2 by hyperventilation ("blowing off" CO_2) or hypoventilation (retaining CO_2) thus shifting the equation to the left or right respectively and influencing the [H$^+$]. The right side of the equation is the renal-metabolic component. The kidneys represent a spigot at the other end that can regulate the HCO_3^- by conserving or excreting HCO_3^- (this is accomplished by controlling H$^+$ secretion into the renal tubule).

- The Henderson-Hasselbalch equation expresses the pH of a buffer equation at equilibrium. This equation states that the pH equals the pK of a buffer system plus the log of the base over the acid. When applied to the bicarbonate–carbonic acid buffer system the equation becomes:

$$pH \propto 6.1 + \log \frac{20}{1} \frac{[HCO_3^-] \text{ controlled by the kidneys}}{Pa_{CO_2} \text{ controlled by the lungs}} =$$
$$6.1 + 1.3 = 7.4$$

The pK of the bicarbonate–carbonic acid buffer system is a constant at 6.1. The numerator in the equation is HCO_3^-, the base concentration, normally 24 mEq/L. The partial pressure of CO_2 in the arterial blood (Pa_{CO_2}) is used in the denominator (multiplied by a constant) as the acid (rather than H_2CO_3, which is not usually measured) and is controlled by the lungs. This equation emphasizes that as long as the ratio of HCO_3^- to Pa_{CO_2} is 20 to 1, the pH will be maintained at 7.4.

- The four primary acid-base disturbances and their compensations can be easily visualized using the Henderson-Hasselbalch equation:
  - Metabolic acidosis: ↓ [HCO_3^-] in numerator, compensated by lungs by ↓ Pa_{CO_2} in denominator
  - Metabolic alkalosis: ↑ [HCO_3^-] in numerator, compensated by lungs by ↑ Pa_{CO_2} in denominator
  - Respiratory acidosis: ↑ Pa_{CO_2} in denominator, compensated by kidneys by ↑ HCO_3^- in numerator
  - Respiratory alkalosis: ↓ Pa_{CO_2} in denominator, compensated by kidneys by ↓ HCO_3^- in numerator

The compensation for the primary disturbance is always in the same direction so as to maintain the 20:1 base-to-acid ratio to minimize deviation from the normal pH of 7.4. The compensatory response in the opposite direction to the primary distur-bance indicates that a mixed acid-base disorder may be present.

■ The diagnosis and treatment of acid-base disorders requires the clinician to develop a systematic assessment approach. No easy shortcuts to accurate assessment are available. The acid-base variables cannot stand alone but must be interpreted in the context of a thorough knowledge of the clinical situation, experience, good judgment, and a thorough knowledge of acid-base physiology.

■ Metabolic acidosis is characterized by $[HCO_3^-]$ under 22 mEq/L and a pH under 7.35. Respiratory compensation begins immediately to lower the $Paco_2$ by hyperventilation.

■ The basic causes of metabolic acidosis are (1) gains of fixed acids (e.g., diabetic ketoacidosis, lactic acidosis as in cardiac arrest or shock, aspirin overdose), (2) failure of the kidney to excrete the daily acid load (e.g., acute or chronic renal failure), or (3) loss of base HCO_3^- (e.g., diarrhea).

■ Metabolic acidosis is classified as wide anion gap metabolic acidosis (normochloremic, caused by retention of fixed acids) or normal anion gap metabolic acidosis (hyperchloremic, caused by loss of HCO_3^- or gain of Cl^-). Anion gap = $[Na^+] - ([HCO_3^-] + [Cl^-]$. The normal anion gap is 8 to 16 mEq/L. The primary significance of determining the type of metabolic acidosis is the treatment implications.

■ The immediate response to the excess [H+] in metabolic acidosis is ECF buffering by HCO_3^-, thus lowering ECF $[HCO_3^-]$. ICF buffering occurs as H^+ enters cells in exchange for K^+, which moves from the ICF to the ECF. Thus serum K^+ rises in conditions of acidosis. When a patient with acidosis has normokalemia, the acidosis may be masking an actual hypokalemia, which must be corrected when the acidosis is treated. The respiratory compensation for metabolic acidosis is hyperventilation ("blowing off" CO_2). The final correction of metabolic acidosis is the renal excretion of the excess H^+ as NH_4^+ or H_3PO_4 and takes several days.

■ The signs and symptoms of metabolic acidosis tend to be vague and the patient may be asymptomatic unless the serum $[HCO_3^-]$ falls below 15 mEq/L. The major clinical features are manifested as abnormalities of the following body systems: (1) cardiovascular: dysrhythmias, decreased cardiac contractility, peripheral and cerebral vasodilation when the pH is 7.1 or less; (2) neurologic: lethargy progressing to stupor and coma as the acidosis becomes more severe; (3) respiratory: hyperventilation manifested by Kussmaul respirations (most commonly present in DKA); and (4) alteration in bone function: in chronic metabolic acidosis, as in renal failure, bone bicarbonates may be used to buffer the acidosis, thus contributing to renal osteodystrophy in adults and growth retardation in children.

■ The treatment goal for metabolic acidosis is to raise the blood pH to a safe level (7.20 to 7.25) and treat the underlying cause of the acidosis. IV $NaHCO_3$

may be used when the pH is less than 7.2 or $[HCO_3^-]$ is less than 15 mEq/L. The IV fluid of choice to treat normal anion gap metabolic acidosis is lactated Ringer's solution (the lactate is slowly metabolized to $NaHCO_3$ in the body). Treatment of wide anion gap metabolic acidosis involves correcting the underlying disorder.

■ Hazards of excessive IV $NaHCO_3$ administration include (1) suppression of the respiratory drive, (2) respiratory alkalosis, (3) shift of oxyhemoglobin dissociation curve to the left, possibly causing tissue hypoxia, (4) metabolic alkalosis in a patient with DKA, (5) overcorrection of the acidosis causing a life-threatening metabolic alkalosis during resuscitation for cardiac arrest, (6) hypocalcemia, tetany, and seizure in patients with renal failure, and (7) serious circulatory overload in patients with congestive heart failure.

■ Metabolic alkalosis is characterized by $[HCO_3^-]$ above 26 mEq/L and a pH above 7.45 and is frequently accompanied by ECF volume deficit and hypokalemia. Respiratory compensation consists of raising the $Paco_2$ by hypoventilation. The final renal correction consists of excretion of the excess HCO_3^-.

■ The causes of metabolic acidosis include (1) net loss of H^+ (and Cl^- ions) from the GI tract (vomiting or nasogastric suction), renal (diuretics; aldosterone excess), or shift of H^+ from ECF to the ICF in hypokalemia; (2) retention of HCO_3^- (e.g., posthypercapnic metabolic alkalosis following the correction of chronic metabolic acidosis with mechanical ventilation).

■ The immediate response to metabolic alkalosis is intracellular buffering. H^+ moves from the ICF to the ECF in exchange for K^+, which moves from the ECF to the ICF. Respiratory compensation consists of hypoventilation to raise the $Paco_2$ but is a limited response because of the need for oxygen. The final renal correction requires the excretion of HCO_3^-, but this cannot occur until the ECF volume deficit and hypokalemia are corrected.

■ Cl^- depletion, fluid volume deficit, and K^+ depletion all contribute to the pathogenesis and maintenance of metabolic acidosis. Cl^- depletion is crucial in the generation metabolic alkalosis usually caused by the loss of chloride-rich (HCO_3^--poor) fluids, as in vomiting or nasogastric suction; K^+ and ECF volume depletion result as well. The loss of Cl^- causes a compensatory increase in HCO_3^- (these two anions have a reciprocal relationship) resulting in primary HCO_3^- excess. Cl^- depletion again plays a major role in the maintenance of the metabolic alkalosis by stimulating the renin-angiotensin-aldosterone mechanism, causing increased K^+ and H^+ excretion, and increased HCO_3^-, Na^+, and water reabsorption. The ECF volume deficit also stimulates aldosterone secretion with the same results previously described. Hypokalemia (from loss in urine and movement from the ECF to the ICF) also stimulates aldosterone secretion.

■ Metabolic alkalosis presents no specific signs and symptoms. Signs and symptoms of fluid volume deficit and hypokalemia, such as muscle cramps and weakness, may be present. Severe alkalemia (pH >7.6) may cause cardiac dysrhythmias. ECG abnormalities may result from the hypokalemia, particularly when the patient is taking digitalis. Paresthesias, tics, and muscle cramps may be present from functional hypocalcemia (more Ca^{++} is bound to albumin in an alkaline medium).

■ Measurement of urinary Cl^- helps to determine the cause and appropriate treatment for metabolic alkalosis. When the urinary Cl^- is less than 10 mEq/L, the cause of the metabolic alkalosis is ECF volume and Cl^- depletion. When the urinary Cl^- is greater than 20 mEq/L, the cause is usually primary aldosterone excess (as in adrenal adenoma) or secondary aldosterone excess (as in congestive heart failure [CHF], nephrotic syndrome, or liver cirrhosis).

■ The treatment goals for metabolic alkalosis are to eliminate the process that generated the condition or to treat the processes that maintain it. Cl^--responsive metabolic alkalosis (urinary Cl^- <10 mEq/L) is treated with IV normal saline (0.9% NaCl) with added KCl; this treatment removes the aldosterone stimulus and allows excretion of $NaHCO_3$ because K^+ is now available to exchange for Na^+ in the renal tubule. Cl^--resistant metabolic alkalosis (urinary Cl^- >20 mEq/L) is caused by aldosterone excess (but not an ECF volume deficit) thus patients are not given IV saline; the underlying disorder is treated and the physician may order acetazolamide (Diamox, a diuretic).

■ Respiratory acidosis is characterized by an elevated $Paco_2$ (>45 mm Hg) and a pH under 7.35. Renal compensation consists of retention and elevation of the HCO_3^-. Respiratory acidosis may be acute (poorly compensated) or chronic and is invariably accompanied by hypoxemia (decreased Pao_2).

■ The basic cause of respiratory acidosis is always hypoventilation (CO_2 retention). Specific causes of respiratory acidosis include (1) inhibition of the medullary respiratory center (e.g., sedative overdose, cardiac arrest), (2) disorders of the chest wall or respiratory muscles (e.g., fractured ribs, myasthenia gravis), (3) disorders of gas exchange (e.g., COPD), and (4) acute upper airway obstruction (e.g., aspiration of foreign body or vomitus, laryngoedema, tongue falling back and occluding airway in a comatose patient).

■ Little ICF or ECF buffering occurs in respiratory acidosis. Renal compensation by HCO_3^- elevation is not significant for 12 to 24 hours thus acute respiratory acidosis is poorly compensated, although chronic respiratory acidosis is generally well compensated.

■ The signs and symptoms of respiratory acidosis are nonspecific, and those attributed to the accompanying hypoxemia may dominate the clinical picture, particularly in acute respiratory acidosis resulting from obstruction of the airways. In chronic respiratory acidosis, rising $Paco_2$ levels (>60 mm Hg) may cause progressive somnolence progressing to coma. Increased $Paco_2$ levels also cause cerebral vasodila-

tion leading to increased ICP, resulting in headache and papilledema.

■ Treatment of acute respiratory acidosis is restoration of effective ventilation as soon as possible by administering oxygen therapy and treating the underlying cause. The Pao_2 must be raised to a minimum of 60 mm Hg and the pH above 7.2 to avoid the development of cardiac dysrhythmias. High concentrations of oxygen (50%) may be given to patients for 1 to 2 days when no history of chronic hypercapnia is present. When patients with COPD and chronic hypercapnia develop an acute rise in $Paco_2$, attention is directed to identifying the factors causing the deterioration, such as pneumonia. Oxygen therapy consists of using the lowest possible concentration (beginning with 24% to 28%) sufficient to raise the Pao_2 to a safe level (60 mm Hg) and gradually reducing the $Paco_2$.

■ Respiratory alkalosis is characterized by a decrease in the $Paco_2$ (<35 mm Hg) and an increase in the serum pH (>7.45) and it may be acute or chronic. Renal compensation consists of increased retention of H^+ and increased excretion of HCO_3^-.

■ The basic cause of respiratory alkalosis is always hyperventilation ("blowing off" CO_2 excessively). The most common specific cause by far is psychogenic hyperventilation resulting from stress and anxiety. An iatrogenic cause is mechanical ventilation. Other conditions that stimulate the respiratory center include hypoxemic states such as pneumonia or CHF, hypermetabolic states (fever), strokes, early stage of aspirin poisoning, and gram-negative septicemia. The compensatory hyperventilation of metabolic acidosis may continue for some time after correction of metabolic acidosis causing respiratory alkalosis.

■ Patients with hyperventilation and respiratory alkalosis are not usually aware that they are overbreathing. Hyperventilation can only be diagnosed by measuring the arterial blood gases (ABGs) and not by observing the respiratory rate. Frequent yawning and sighing may be observed, and the patient may complain of breathlessness. The presenting signs and symptoms are often those of anxiety (e.g., dry mouth, palpitation, exhaustion, cold and clammy hands and soles of feet). The patient often complains of paresthesias, muscle twitches, and tetany (presumably caused by the functional hypocalcemia caused by the alkalosis). Alkalosis also causes cerebral vasoconstriction and shifts the oxyhemoglobin curve to the left resulting in cerebral hypoxia and complaints of light-headedness and inability to concentrate.

■ The only successful treatment of respiratory alkalosis is elimination of the underlying cause. When acute anxiety produces the hyperventilation syndrome, air rebreathing with a paper bag held tightly around the nose and mouth may relieve an acute attack. Hyperventilation with mechanical ventilators can be corrected by reducing minute ventilation, adding dead space, or breathing 3% CO_2 for a short period.

- Four possible combinations of mixed acid-base imbalances have been identified, two of which have additive effects on pH change and two of which have offsetting effects on the pH. Discerning more than two coexisting acid-base imbalances is difficult.
- Mixed acid-base disorders are suspected from the history and clinical situation. The key to diagnosing a mixed acid-base disorder is a deviation from the expected compensatory response for the primary disorder. The expected compensatory change can be calculated, or an acid-base nomogram may be used to interpret the acid-base laboratory measures.
- Mixed acid-base imbalances that have an additive effect and cause a profound change in the pH include:

1. Metabolic acidosis and respiratory acidosis (e.g., cardiopulmonary arrest)
2. Metabolic alkalosis and respiratory alkalosis (e.g., COPD patient with chronic respiratory acidosis overventilated on a mechanical ventilator)
- Mixed acid-base imbalances that have an offsetting effect such that the pH may be in the normal range.
1. Metabolic acidosis and respiratory alkalosis (e.g., aspirin poisoning)
2. Metabolic alkalosis and respiratory acidosis (e.g., ARDS; COPD patient who is vomiting or treated with nasogastric suction or diuretics)

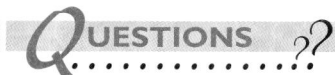 UESTIONS ??

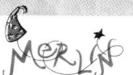

A sampling of review questions for this chapter appears here. Visit http://www.mosby.com/MERLIN/PriceWilson/ for additional questions.

Answer the following on a separate sheet of paper.

1. Why does the body maintain a critical pH range?
2. Define the following terms: pH, acid, base, pK, and buffer.
3. Differentiate between a volatile and a nonvolatile acid. Name some volatile and nonvolatile acids. How are they excreted?
4. Name the four major blood buffer systems. Which are intracellular, and which are extracellular?

5. List the two main functions of the kidneys in maintaining acid-base balance.
6. What is the role of the lungs in maintaining acid-base balance? Define hypoventilation and hyperventilation.
7. What is the anion gap? How is it calculated? What is its significance in describing an acid-base imbalance?
8. What is the isohydric principle, and what is its significance?
9. How do the CO_2 content, $Paco_2$, and standard HCO_3^- differ? What are their normal values? What is base excess?

10. Outline the steps in the systematic assessment of acid-base status.
11. How is calculation of the expected compensatory response of a primary acid-base disturbance helpful in assessment?
12. Describe several hazards of rapidly correcting metabolic acidosis or chronic respiratory acidosis by $NaHCO_3$ administration.

Renal mechanisms compensate for respiratory insufficiency, and, conversely, respiratory mechanisms partially compensate for metabolic acid-base disturbances. Tell how this mechanism works in each of the following cases by filling in the blanks with the correct word(s).

13. When respiratory acidosis occurs, the kidneys compensate by increasing excretion of _____ and conserving _____.
14. When respiratory alkalosis occurs, the kidneys compensate by decreasing excretion of _____ and increasing excretion of _____.
15. When metabolic acidosis occurs, the lungs are able to compensate by _____.
16. When metabolic alkalosis occurs, the lungs are able to partially compensate by _____.

Analyze data from the following cases by answering the following questions used in the systematic assessment presented at the beginning of the chapter. You may use the acid-base nomogram to assist when desired.

a. What acid-base disturbance is suggested by the history?
b. What do the signs and symptoms suggest?
c. Analyze $Paco_2$ and HCO_3 in relation to the pH. What primary acid-base disorder is suggested?
d. What is the expected compensation for this disorder?
e. Calculate the anion gap.
f. What is your final conclusion?

17. A 36-year-old woman is seen after several days of severe diarrhea. She complains of weakness and postural dizziness. Her blood pressure is 100/60 mm Hg when recumbent and 80/50 mm Hg when standing. Her resting pulse is 100 beats/min and regular. Her neck veins are flat in the recumbent position. Skin turgor is poor, and mucous membranes are dry. Laboratory data included: plasma Na^+, 142 mEq/L; K^+, 3.9 mEq/L; Cl^-, 118; pH, 7.27; HCO_3^-, 12 mEq/L; $Paco_2$, 28 mm Hg; urine Na^+, 4 mEq/L.
18. A 40-year-old woman has chronic renal failure. The following laboratory data were obtained: plasma Na^+, 137 mEq/L;

K^+, 6.0 mEq/L; Cl^-, 102; pH, 7.14; HCO_3^-, 8 mEq/L; $Paco_2$, 24 mm Hg; creatinine, 9.6 mEq/L; blood, urea, nitrogen (BUN), 110 mg/dl.

19. A previously stable patient with chronic renal failure was admitted to the hospital renal unit in a moribund state. The chest radiograph and lung auscultation were suggestive of pulmonary edema. The patient had skipped the last two hemodialysis sessions while on a vacation trip. Weight gain was 10 lb since the last dialysis. The following laboratory data were obtained: plasma pH, 7.02; HCO_3^-, 15 mEq/L; $Paco_2$, 60 mm Hg; Pao_2, 40 mm Hg.

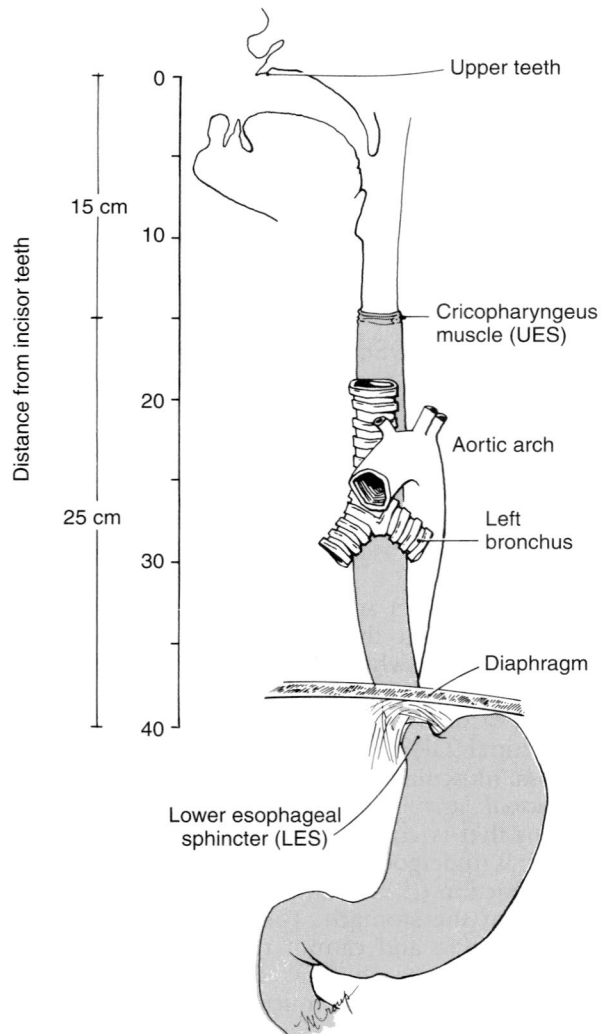

FIG. 23-1   Gross structure and anatomic relationships of the esophagus.

The function of the enteric nervous system is independent of the extrinsic nerves. Stimulation of the parasympathetic and sympathetic systems can activate or inhibit GI function. Perivascular and free nerve endings are also found within the esophageal submucosa and the myenteric ganglia. These nerve endings are thought to serve as mechanoreceptors, thermo-osmo, and chemoreceptors in the esophagus. Mechanoreceptors receive mechanical stimuli such as touch, and chemoreceptors receive chemical stimuli within the esophagus. Thermo-osmo receptors can be affected by body temperature, smell, and changes in osmotic pressure.

Blood distribution to the esophagus follows a segmental plan. Branches from the inferior thyroid and subclavian arteries supply the upper portion. Segmental branches from the aorta and from bronchial arteries supply the middle portion, and the left gastric and inferior phrenic arteries supply the subdiaphragmatic portion.

Venous drainage also follows a segmental pattern. The cervical esophageal veins drain into the azygos and hemiazygos veins; and below the diaphragm, the esophageal veins enter the left gastric vein. Communication between the portal and systemic veins allows for bypass of the liver in cases of portal hypertension. Collateral flow through the esophageal veins causes the formation of *esophageal varices* (varicose veins of the esophagus). These enlarged veins may rupture, causing hemorrhage that may be fatal. This complication is common in patients with cirrhosis of the liver and is discussed in detail in Chapter 27.

Swallowing

Swallowing is a complex physiologic act whereby food or liquid passes from the mouth to the stomach; it is a highly coordinated muscular sequence initiated by a voluntary movement of the tongue and completed by a series of involuntary reflexes in the pharynx and esophagus. The afferent side of this reflex arc involves fibers in the fifth, ninth, and tenth cranial nerves. A swallowing, or *deglutition,* center is present in the medulla. Under the coordination of this center, impulses pass outward in a flawlessly timed sequence via the fifth, tenth, and twelfth cranial nerves to the muscles of the tongue, pharynx, larynx, and esophagus.

Although swallowing is a continuous process, it occurs in three phases: oral, pharyngeal, and esophageal. During the *oral phase* of swallowing, a mouthful of chewed food, called a *bolus,* is thrown backward against the posterior wall of the pharynx by a voluntary movement of the tongue. The impact of the bolus against the pharynx is the stimulus that triggers the reflex movements of swallowing.

During the *pharyngeal phase,* the soft palate and uvula reflexively close off the nasal cavity. Simultaneously, the larynx is elevated and the *glottis* is closed, keeping food from entering the trachea. Contractions of the pharyngeal constrictor muscles move the bolus past the *epiglottis* to the lower pharynx and into the esophagus. Retroversion of the epiglottis over the laryngeal orifice further protects the respiratory pathway, but primarily, the closure of the glottis prevents food from entering the trachea. Respirations are simultaneously inhibited to decrease the possibility of aspiration. In fact, voluntarily inhaling and swallowing at the same time is nearly impossible.

The *esophageal phase* begins as the cricopharyngeus muscle relaxes briefly and allows the bolus to enter the esophagus. After this brief relaxation, a *primary peristaltic wave,* beginning in the pharynx, is transmitted to the cricopharyngeus, causing it to contract. The peristaltic wave continues throughout the body of the esophagus, propelling the bolus to the LES, which relaxes briefly to allow entry into the stomach. The primary peristaltic wave moves at the rate of 2 to 4 cm/second, thus swallowed food reaches the stomach within 5 to 15 seconds. Beginning at the level of the aortic arch, a *secondary peristaltic wave* occurs when the primary wave fails to empty the esophagus and is triggered by distention of the esophagus from remaining food particles. The primary peristaltic wave is essential for conveying food and liquids through the upper esophagus but is less important in the lower esophagus. The upright posture and the force of gravity facilitate lower esophageal transport, but peristalsis makes it possible to drink water while standing on one's head or while in outer space with zero gravity.

During swallowing, pressure changes occur within the esophagus, which reflect its motor function. In the resting state, pressure in the body of the esophagus is slightly below atmospheric pressure, reflecting intrathoracic pressure. In the regions of the UES and LES, areas of high pressure exist. These high-pressure zones prevent aspiration and reflux of the gastric contents. The pressure decreases when each sphincter area relaxes during swallowing and then increases when the peristaltic wave passes through.

It is evident that the complex series of movements that make up the act of swallowing may be upset by a number of pathologic processes. These processes involve interference either with transport or with the prevention of gastric reflux.

SYMPTOMS OF ESOPHAGEAL DISORDERS

Dysphagia, difficulty swallowing ingested material from the pharynx, is a major symptom of disease of the pharynx or esophagus. Dysphagia should not be confused with *globus hystericus* (the feeling of a "lump in the throat"), which may be emotional in origin and occurs without swallowing.

Dysphagia occurs in nonesophageal disorders that result from muscular or neurologic disease. These diseases include cerebrovascular accidents (CVAs, strokes), myasthenia gravis, muscular dystrophy, and bulbar poliomyelitis. These conditions predispose individuals to an increased risk of choking on fluids or food that become lodged in the trachea or bronchia.

Esophageal dysphagia may be of obstructive or motor origin. Obstructive causes include esophageal stricture and tumors extrinsic or intrinsic to the esophagus, resulting in narrowing of the lumen. Motor causes of dysphagia may result from diminished, absent, or disordered peristalsis or dysfunction of the UES or LES. Common motor disorders that produce dysphagia are achalasia, scleroderma, and diffuse esophageal spasm.

Pyrosis (heartburn) is another common symptom of esophageal disease characterized by a hot, burning sensation, usually felt high in the epigastrium or behind the xiphoid process and radiating upward. Heartburn may be caused by reflux of gastric acid or bile secretions into the lower esophagus; both of these are irritating to the mucosa. Persistent reflux is caused by incompetence of the LES and may occur with or without hiatus hernia or esophagitis. Heartburn is a common complaint during pregnancy.

Odynophagia is defined as pain induced by swallowing and may occur with dysphagia and may be experienced as a sensation of tightness or as a burning pain, indistinguishable from heartburn, in the midchest. Odynophagia may result from esophageal spasm induced by acute distention, or it may be secondary to inflammation of the esophageal mucosa.

Regurgitation refers to the backflow or welling up of gastric or esophageal contents into the oral cavity. Differing from vomiting in that it is effortless and not accompanied by nausea, regurgitation is felt in the throat as a sour or bitter-tasting hot liquid. This effortless regurgitation is quite common in infants as a result of incomplete development of the LES. In adults, regurgitation reflects both LES incompetence and failure of the UES to serve as a regurgitation barrier. *Water brash* is reflex salivary hypersecretion in response to peptic esophagitis or dysphagia and should not be confused with regurgitation. Water brash occurs approximately 15% of the time in individuals with dysphagia (Lundquist, 1998).

DIAGNOSTIC PROCEDURES

In addition to taking a careful history and performing a physical examination, special diagnostic measures that are helpful in detecting esophageal disease include barium radiologic studies, esophagoscopy with biopsy and possibly cytologic studies, manometric or motility studies, and acid reflux tests.

Barium Radiologic Studies

Radiologic examination of the esophagus as a routine is usually combined with that of the stomach and duodenum (upper GI tract radiologic series) using barium sulfate in a liquid or creamy suspension that is swallowed. The swallowing mechanism may be directly visualized by fluoroscopy, or the radiographic image may be recorded using motion picture techniques (cineradiography). When esophageal disease is suspected, the radiologist may place the patient in various positions to bring out in greater detail alterations in form and function. Tumors, polyps, diverticulitis, strictures, hiatus hernia, large esophageal varices, uncoordinated swallowing, and weak peristalsis may all be detected using this method.

Other Radiology and Imaging Studies

Radiologic imaging of the esophagus also includes computed tomography (CT) and endoscopic ultrasonography (US). Endoscopic US is preferred to CT to evaluate abnormal thickening of esophageal lesions and for visualization of vascular anatomy. Endoscopic US is used for esophageal carcinoma imaging and for assessment of the degree of infiltration of the tumor before surgery. Magnetic resonance imaging (MRI) provides thin tomographic slices of the esophagus and does not involve radiation. MRIs are useful for the staging of esophageal malignancies; and Doppler echocardiography along with the MRI can be used to assess submucosal blood flow. Endoscopy with cytology screening (biopsy) is the primary means of diagnosing esophageal tumors.

Esophagoscopy

Direct inspection of the esophageal mucosa is important in diagnosing esophageal disorders. Flexible fiberoptic instruments have made this procedure much simpler and safer for the patient. Inflammation, ulcers, tumors, and esophageal varices may be visualized, photographed, and biopsied. Cell washings may be

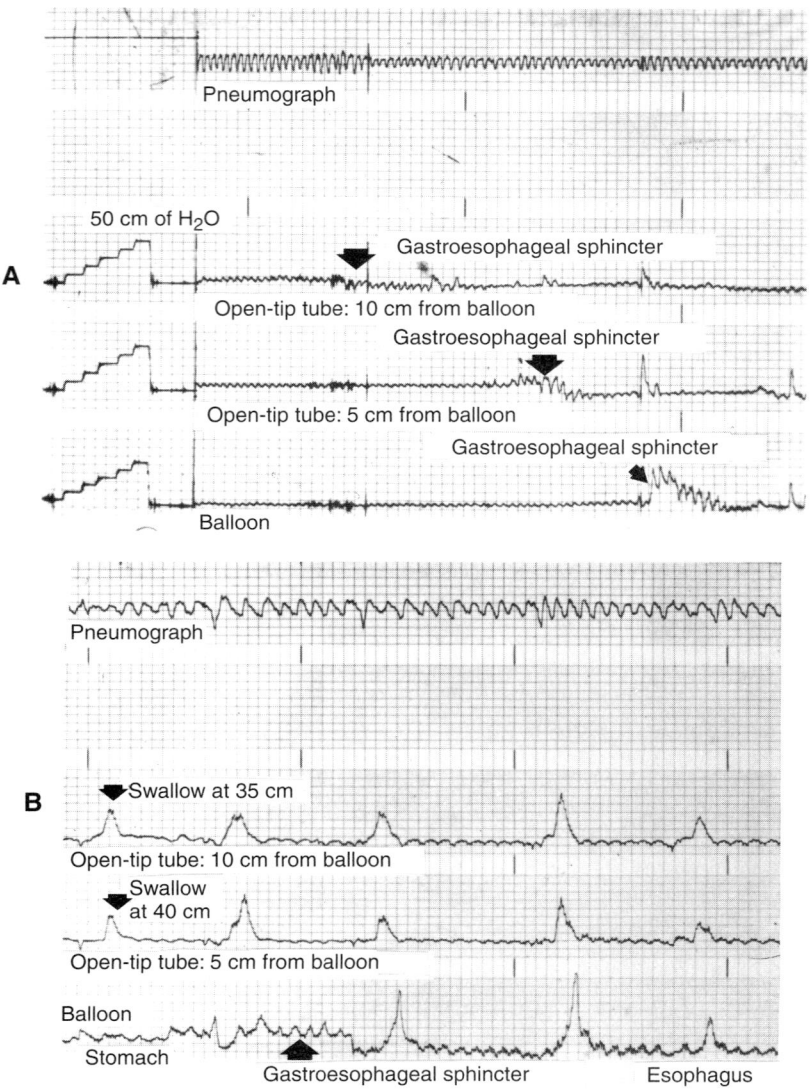

FIG. 23-2 **A,** Esophageal manometric recordings. The pressure is recorded by three catheters spaced 5 cm apart. The catheters are pulled from the stomach into the esophagus. Note the zone of high resting pressure at the junction between the stomach and the esophagus (LES). **B,** Normal swallowing. Swallowing produces a single contraction; at the same time, the sphincter zone relaxes.

obtained for cytologic studies, which can be highly accurate in diagnosing esophageal carcinoma. Infections, such as *Helicobacter pylori* (*H. pylori*) can be diagnosed by noninvasive serologic tests and urea breath tests (Kandel, 2000).

Preparation for esophagoscopy includes 6 hours of fasting and various forms of premedication, often spraying the throat with a local anesthetic. Endoscopic examinations of the esophagus, stomach, and duodenum are often combined in one examination.

Motility Studies

Motor function of the esophagus may be studied by placing three pressure-sensitive catheters or miniature balloons in the stomach and then drawing them back incre-

mentally. Pressures are then transmitted to a transducer located outside the patient. Measurements of pressure changes in the esophagus and stomach at rest and during swallowing have greatly increased understanding of esophageal activity both in health and in disease. Esophageal motility studies are helpful in the diagnosis of achalasia, diffuse esophageal spasm, scleroderma, and other motor disorders of the esophagus.

Fig. 23-2, *A* and *B*, show normal motility in a recording of the esophagus in the resting state and during swallowing. The function of the LES is of particular interest to the gastroenterologist. Normally a zone of high pressure (15 to 30 cm of water above that of the intragastric pressure) exists in this region; this prevents reflux of gastric contents into the esophagus. Reflux may occur if the sphincter fails to maintain a pressure above the intraabdominal pressure.

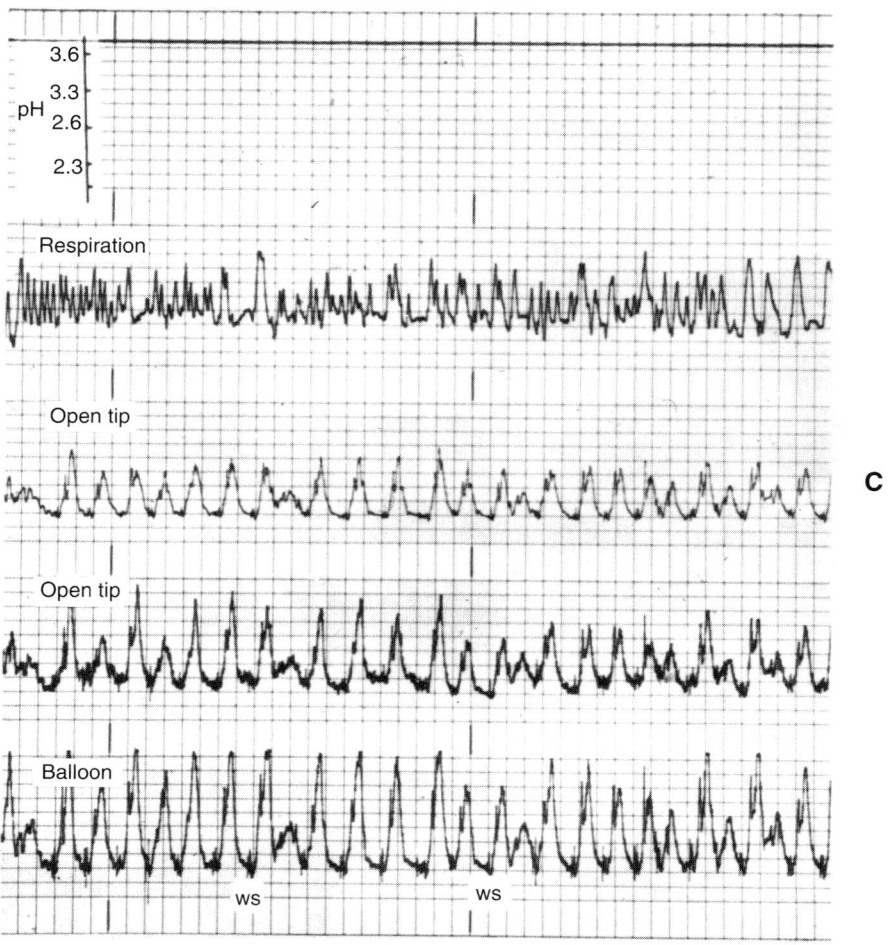

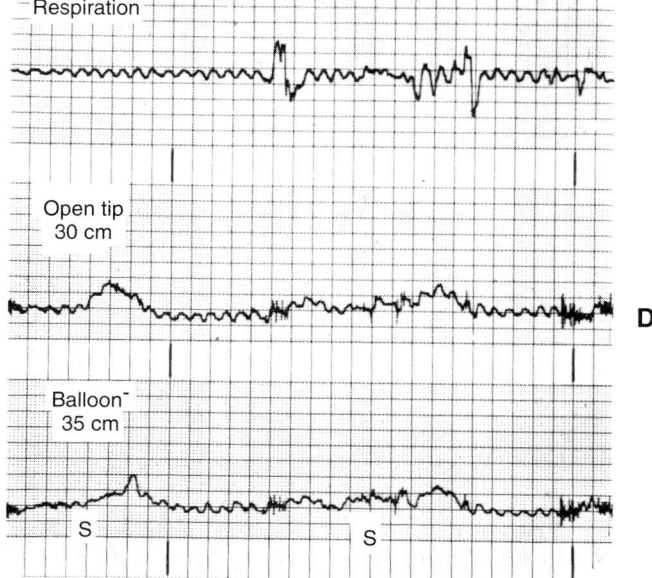

FIG. 23-2—cont'd   C, Diffuse esophageal spasm. Repetitive nonprogressive contractions independent of water swallowing *(ws)* occur. **D,** Scleroderma. The contractions produced by swallowings *(S)* are low in amplitude.

Acid Reflux Tests

The *acid perfusion test (Bernstein test)* is used to differentiate between chest pain that is cardiac in origin and pain resulting from acid-induced esophageal spasm, because the symptoms may be identical.

In the acid perfusion test, 0.1 N hydrochloric acid (HCl) is permitted to drip through a catheter at 6 to 15 ml/minute into the distal esophagus (the HCl is of the same concentration as that of normal gastric acid). When the patient has esophageal pain or heartburn, the test result is positive. Rapid cessation of the pain after instillation of a neutral or alkaline solution confirms that the esophageal mucosa is the site of acid-induced pain. The most common finding in a positive result is reflux esophagitis, but any disease that causes a break in mucosal continuity may cause a positive result. The person with chest pain of cardiac origin is unable to distinguish between saline and acid perfusion.

Other reflux tests include monitoring of the pH within the esophagus to detect the reflux of acid contents from the stomach, fluoroscopic observation of the esophagus to detect the reflux of barium from the stomach into the esophagus, and fluoroscopic observation of the esophagus during the ingestion of a mixture of HCl and barium to detect momentary disorders in peristaltic activity. All the currently available tests for acid reflux have possible false-positive and false-negative results; therefore a combination of two or more of these studies is used to make a diagnosis in difficult cases.

DISORDERS OF ESOPHAGEAL MOTILITY

Achalasia

Achalasia, formerly called cardiospasm, is an uncommon hypomotility disorder characterized by weak and uncoordinated peristalsis or aperistalsis within the body of the esophagus, elevated LES pressure, and failure of the LES to relax completely during swallowing. Consequently, food and fluids accumulate in the lower esophagus and then slowly drain as the hydrostatic pressure increases. The body of the esophagus loses its tone and may become greatly dilated (Fig. 23-3).

The exact etiology of achalasia is unknown, but evidence suggests that degeneration of Auerbach's plexus causes the loss of neurologic control. As a result, primary peristaltic waves do not reach the LES to stimulate relaxation. *Primary* idiopathic achalasia accounts for most of

the cases in the United States. *Secondary* achalasia may be caused by gastric carcinoma invading the esophagus, by irradiation, and by certain toxins and drugs.

Achalasia is more common in adults than it is in children. The onset is usually insidious, and the most prominent symptom is dysphagia for liquid and solid foods. Meals may be interrupted by the necessity to regurgitate. Nocturnal regurgitation may result in aspiration, resulting in chronic pulmonary infections or sudden death. The stasis of food in the esophagus may lead to inflammatory changes, erosions, and in some cases, cancer of the esophagus, although this is usually a late complication.

The diagnosis is made based on the history and the characteristic radiographic appearance. When barium is swallowed, the peristaltic wave is weak, and the collection of barium in the lower esophagus gives the structure a funnel-like appearance. The administration of small doses of a cholinergic or parasympathomimetic drug causes marked contraction and emptying of the esophagus and confirms the diagnosis. Esophageal motility studies may be helpful in the early diagnosis of achalasia. Manometric measurements in these studies reveal that the LES fails to relax with swallowing. The resting pressure of the LES is usually elevated (35 mm Hg versus the normal pressure of 15 to 30 mm Hg).

Treatment of achalasia is palliative and consists of measures to relieve the obstruction of the lower esophagus. No known method of restoring normal peristalsis to the body of the esophagus is available. Two forms of therapy that effectively relieve the symptoms are dilation of the LES and esophagomyotomy. Dilation may be achieved by passing a mercury-filled tube called a *bougie*

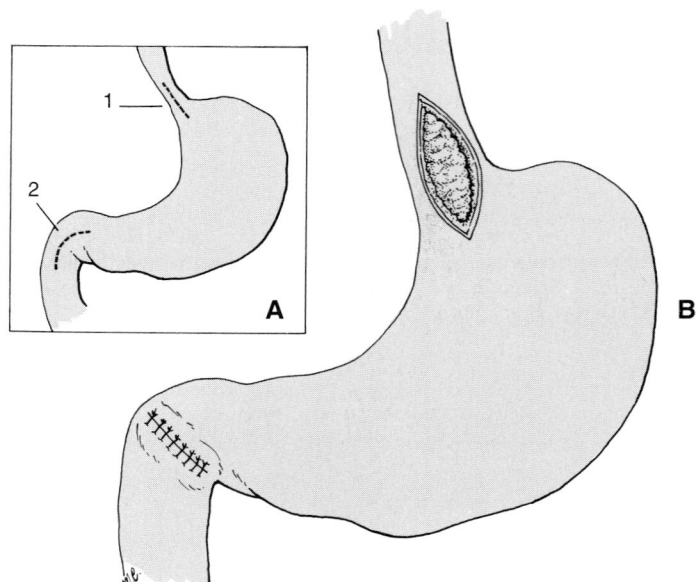

FIG. 23-4 Surgical treatment of esophageal achalasia. **A**, Longitudinal incision for Heller esophagomyotomy, *1*, and pyloroplasty, *2*. **B**, The esophageal incision is made through the muscle layers to allow pouching of the mucosa, thus relieving the esophageal obstruction. A gastric drainage procedure (pyloroplasty) often accompanies the esophagomyotomy to prevent esophageal reflux. The pyloric incision is sutured in the opposite direction to enlarge the gastric outlet.

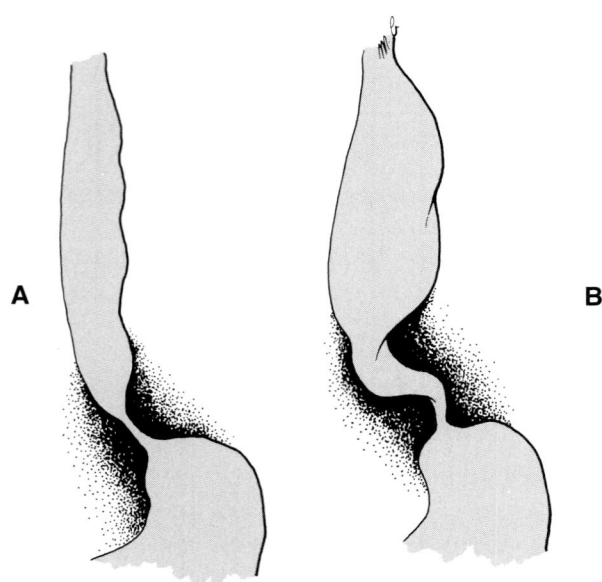

FIG. 23-3 Esophageal achalasia. **A**, Early stage, showing tapering of lower esophagus. **B**, Advanced stage, showing dilated, tortuous esophagus.

(the procedure is *bougienage*) or, more often, by placing a pneumatic bag in the area of the LES and forcefully dilating it. When dilation fails to relieve the symptoms, surgical intervention may be indicated.

The surgery most frequently performed for achalasia or esophageal stricture is the *Heller esophagomyotomy*, which consists of dividing the muscle fibers of the gastroesophageal junction. A *pyloroplasty* (enlargement of gastric outlet) frequently accompanies this procedure to allow rapid emptying of stomach contents and prevent reflux into the esophagus (Fig. 23-4).

Drug therapy is currently reserved for patients who are not considered suitable for either pneumatic dilation or surgery. Isosorbide (long-acting nitrate) and nifedipine (calcium channel antagonist) lower LES pressure and have been used with some success to treat achalasia. Other helpful measures to minimize symptoms include slow eating and avoidance of alcohol and hot, cold, or spicy foods. Patients should be instructed to sleep with the head elevated to avoid aspiration.

Diffuse Esophageal Spasm

Diffuse esophageal spasm is a fairly common condition characterized by uncoordinated, nonpropulsive contractions (tertiary peristalsis) of the esophagus in response to swallowing. Although most prominent in the lower two thirds of the organ, diffuse esophageal spasm may involve the entire esophagus. The two sphincters operate normally. This disease is of unknown cause and is present more frequently in older patients. Similar motility disturbances may be secondary to reflux esophagitis or obstruction of the lower esophagus, as in carcinoma (results of manometric studies in early carcinoma are usually normal).

Primary diffuse spasm of the esophagus usually occurs in patients over 50 years of age. Nonperistaltic responses to swallowing are common findings on barium radiologic studies and increase with aging. These radiologic findings are referred to as "corkscrew esophagus," "rosary bead esophagus," "curling," and a variety of other descriptive names that are usually of little clinical significance. The pathogenic basis for the diffuse spasm is poorly understood and may represent a degeneration of local neurons, because some patients have a positive response to cholinergics, as occurs in achalasia.

Diffuse esophageal spasm is usually asymptomatic, but in a few cases, the contractions may give rise to symptoms. The most common symptoms include intermittent dysphagia and odynophagia, which are aggravated by ingestion of cold foods and large boluses and by nervous tension. When the patient has intermittent chest pain, diffuse esophageal spasm may be confused with angina pectoris, particularly when the symptoms are not associated with eating. To add to this confusion, the pain caused by diffuse spasm is often relieved by nitroglycerin. Consequently, some patients with diffuse esophageal spasm have been misdiagnosed as having cardiac disease. Motility studies reveal a hypermotile pattern of nonperistaltic contractions and aid in the diagnosis (see Fig. 23-2, *C*).

Treatment consists of dietary manipulations (small meals, avoidance of cold foods), antacids, sedatives, and nitroglycerin to relieve the spasm. If symptoms are persistent and distressing, esophageal dilation may then be recommended. As a last resort, a longitudinal myotomy of the distal esophagus may be performed.

Scleroderma

Esophageal motor dysfunction occurs in more than two thirds of patients with *progressive systemic sclerosis (scleroderma)*. The basic abnormality in the GI tract is atrophy of the smooth muscle of the lower portion of the esophagus. The diagnosis is suspected on barium swallow radiographic examination but is confirmed by manometric findings. Aperistalsis or weak peristalsis of the distal one half to two thirds of the esophagus and diminished pressure of the LES characterize scleroderma (see Fig. 23-2, *D*).

Incompetence of the LES often leads to reflux esophagitis with subsequent stricture formation in the lower esophagus. Although gastroesophageal reflux and esophagitis occur often with scleroderma, heartburn is not a common symptom. Dysphagia becomes a prominent symptom when esophagitis has led to stricture formation (see following discussion).

ESOPHAGITIS

Inflammation of the esophageal mucosa may be acute or chronic and is found in a variety of circumstances, including the motility disorders previously discussed. An innocuous type of esophagitis follows the ingestion of hot liquids. The substernal burning sensation is usually of short duration and may be associated with superficial edema and esophagospasm. The most common significant form of esophagitis is caused by acid reflux from the stomach, often in association with hiatus hernia. Infectious forms of esophagitis may also occur, including those caused by *Candida albicans* (thrush), herpes simplex virus, varicella-zoster virus, cytomegalovirus (occurring only in immunocompromised patients), human immunodeficiency virus (HIV), and *Helicobacter pylori*. Infectious esophagitis is common in people with severe immunodeficiency, such as in acquired immunodeficiency syndrome (AIDS).

An acute, severe form of esophagitis follows the ingestion of strong alkalis or acids. Strong alkalis are typically found in most households in the form of drain cleaners, which will produce a severe liquefying necrosis of the mucosa if ingested. Accidental ingestion of these substances occurs most often in small children, but these substances are occasionally used in suicide attempts. Immediate symptoms include severe odynophagia, fever, toxicity, and possible esophageal perforation with consequent infection of the mediastinum and death. Long-term effects include scarring and esophageal stricture that requires periodic dilation with bougies for the remainder of the patient's life. Treatment must be prompt and vigorous and includes the use of antibiotics, steroids, intravenous fluids, and possibly surgery. Vomiting should not be induced for the emergency treatment of individuals with a caustic injury because this will reinjure the esophagus and oropharynx.

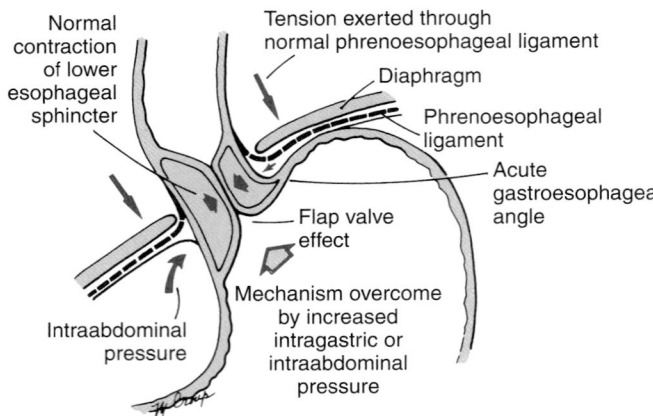

FIG. 23-5 Mechanisms preventing esophageal reflux: high-pressure zone at the LES; acute gastroesophageal angle causing a flap valve effect; and phrenoesophageal (PE) ligament causing a pinchcock valve effect.

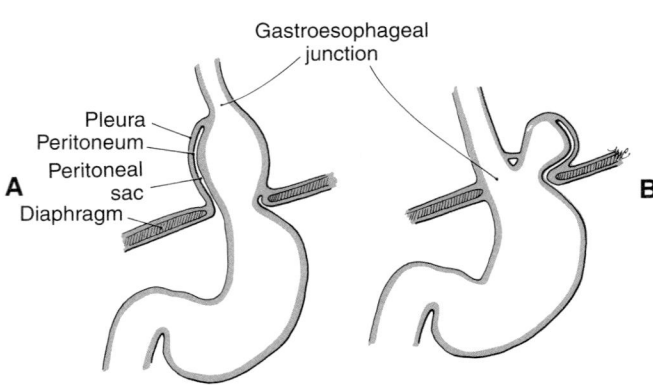

FIG. 23-6 **A**, Sliding or direct hiatus hernia. **B**, Rolling or paraesophageal hiatus hernia.

Chronic Reflux Esophagitis and Hiatus Hernia

Chronic reflux esophagitis is the most common form of esophagitis encountered clinically and is caused by incompetence of the LES and reflux of acid gastric or alkaline intestinal juice into the esophagus over a long period. The sequelae of reflux are inflammation, ulcer formation, bleeding, and scarring with stricture formation. Chronic reflux esophagitis is often associated with hiatus hernia. Little correlation exists between the severity of symptoms and the degree of esophagitis. Some patients with heartburn have minimal evidence of esophagitis, whereas others with chronic reflux may be asymptomatic until stricture formation develops.

Patients over the age of 40 years with significant complaints of heartburn for over 10 years should be considered for esophagoscopy to detect Barrett's esophagus. *Barrett's esophagus* is the progressive replacement of distal eroded squamous mucosa with metaplastic epithelium, which is more resistant to peptic digestion. Metaplastic epithelium is more prone to malignant transformation and esophageal carcinoma.

Mechanisms Preventing Reflux

Fig. 23-5 illustrates the mechanisms that normally prevent reflux of gastric contents into the esophagus. The high-pressure zone at the gastroesophageal junction (or LES) is probably the most important mechanism for preventing reflux. The tone of this sphincter is affected not only by a variety of drugs but also by influences of hormones such as gastrin and secretin, which may play an important role in maintaining the integrity of the sphincter. The importance of the anatomic configuration of the esophagogastric junction is unknown at present. The acute angle between the esophagus and stomach may be an important mechanism for preventing reflux, because this creates an arrangement similar to a flap valve, which would prevent material from regurgitating.

Also suggested is that the short segment of the esophagus below the diaphragm is kept closed by intraabdominal pressure. Displacement of this lower esophageal segment into the chest, as occurs in hiatus hernia, would eliminate this barrier to reflux and may explain the reason for which an association appears to exist with reflux esophagitis. However, the role of a sliding hiatus hernia is thought to be not as important as once thought.

Hiatus Hernia

Hiatus hernia is defined as a herniation of a portion of the stomach into the chest through the esophageal hiatus of the diaphragm. Two distinct types of hiatus hernia have been identified (Fig. 23-6). The most common form is the *direct* or *sliding hiatus hernia,* in which the gastroesophageal junction slides into the thoracic cavity, particularly when the patient assumes a supine position. The competency of the LES may be destroyed, resulting in reflux esophagitis. Sliding hiatus hernia is often asymptomatic and is discovered only accidentally during a search for the cause of a variety of epigastric symptoms or on routine GI tract radiographs.

In *paraesophageal* or *rolling hiatus hernia,* part of the gastric fundus rolls through the hiatus, and the gastroesophageal junction remains below the diaphragm. No insufficiency of the LES mechanism occurs, and consequently, reflux esophagitis does not occur. The major complication of paraesophageal hernia is strangulation.

Sliding and rolling hiatus hernias are diagnosed through radiography or endoscopy. The important clinical question is whether esophageal reflux exists, because this has serious consequences, including esophagitis with ulceration and stricture, asthma, and aspiration pneumonia. Continuous monitoring of esophageal pH with a miniaturized pH meter has been helpful in demonstrating reflux and correlating reflux with symptoms.

Treatment of sliding hiatus hernia is directed toward prevention of reflux, neutralizing refluxate, and protecting the esophageal mucosa. The patient is instructed to eat small, frequent meals and to take antacids. H_2 blockers such as ranitidine and a protective agent such as sucralfate may be helpful. The overweight patient is instructed to lose weight. Calcium channel blockers and anticholinergic drugs should not be given because they delay gastric emptying and relax the LES. Metoclopramide, a derivative of procainamide, increases the tone of the LES and is useful in the treatment of selected cases of reflux. Omeprazole, a drug that suppresses gastric acid secretion, may be given to patients with resistant conditions. Nicotine, which decreases LES tone, should be avoided. The patient should avoid activities that involve stooping forward, particularly after meals. The head of the bed generally should be elevated during sleep to prevent reflux. Surgical repair may be indicated if medical treatment fails and if evidence exists of persistent reflux esophagitis or stricture formation.

TUMORS

Benign tumors of the esophagus are rare. The most common type, however, is a *leiomyoma* (smooth muscle tumor). Leiomyomas may occasionally bleed but are usually of little clinical significance and are discovered incidentally.

Cancer of the esophagus, however, is not rare and has caused approximately 4% of all cancer deaths in the United States from 1990 to 1996. Cancer of the esophagus is estimated to cause 23% of cancers involving the digestive system (American Cancer Society, 1999). Men between ages 50 and 70 years are affected most frequently. Predisposing factors include heavy smoking, alcohol abuse, and chronic gastric reflux (Barrett's esophagus). *Squamous cell carcinoma* is the most common type of tumor and is highly malignant. Tumors can occur in any part of the esophagus, but most develop in the lower two thirds.

Barium radiologic and cytologic studies and esophagoscopy with biopsy are important in the diagnosis. The 5-year survival rate is less than 10%. The reason for the poor prognosis is the early lymphatic spread and the late development of symptoms. The first symptom is generally dysphagia, but this does not generally occur until the tumor involves the entire circumference of the esophagus.

Irradiation and surgical resection are the major forms of treatment. Lesions in the upper portion of the esophagus may be impossible to resect and are treated by irradiation. Bougies may be passed to dilate the lumen, or a plastic prosthesis may be inserted to enable the patient to continue eating. A newer form of palliation is the use of a laser beam to vaporize the core of the obstructing tumor and thus reestablish the lumen and allow passage of food.

KEY CONCEPTS

- The esophagus is a cylindrical tube that extends from the hypopharynx to the cardiac portion of the stomach; its function is to transport ingested material. A sphincter regulates each end of the esophagus. The *upper esophageal sphincter (UES)*, formed by the *cricopharyngeus muscle*, is normally in a contracted state except during swallowing. The *lower esophageal sphincter (LES)* serves as barrier to reflux of stomach contents. The wall of the esophagus consists of a mucosa, submucosa, muscularis, and an adventitia layer. The pH of the esophagus is slightly alkaline, and it poorly tolerates the acid gastric contents.
- Deglutination, or swallowing, is a complex physiologic act involving the passage of materials from the mouth to the stomach and occurs continuously in three phases. The first, known as the *oral phase*, consists of a bolus of food being forced backward by a voluntary movement of the tongue. During the *pharyngeal phase*, the bolus moves past the epiglottis to the lower pharynx and on to the esophagus. In the final *esophageal phase*, a *primary peristaltic wave* beginning in the pharynx, continues through the esophagus moving the bolus to the LES, which briefly relaxes, allowing the bolus to enter the stomach.
- Symptoms of esophageal disorders include *dysphagia*, the subjective awareness of an impairment in the transport of ingested material; *pyrosis*, or heartburn;

odynophagia, pain induced by swallowing; and *regurgitation*, which is the effortless backflow of gastric contents into the oral cavity.
- Some diagnostic measures that are helpful in detecting esophageal diseases include barium radiologic and imaging studies, esophagoscopy with biopsy and cytologic studies, motility studies, and acid reflux tests.
- *Achalasia*, also known as cardiospasm, is an uncommon hypomotility disorder characterized by weak, uncoordinated peristalsis within the body of the esophagus. Signs and symptoms include elevated LES pressure and failure of the LES to relax during swallowing. *Primary achalasia* is believed to be a result of degeneration of Auerbach's plexus (intrinsic nerve plexus, which coordinates esophageal peristalsis). *Secondary achalasia* is associated with a number of disorders, including diabetic neuropathy and cancer of the esophagus. Treatment may involve pneumatic dilation of the LES or (Heller) esophagomyotomy.
- *Diffuse esophageal spasm* is characterized by uncoordinated, nonpropulsive contractions of the esophagus in response to swallowing (tertiary peristalsis). The cause is unknown, and it is found more frequently in older patients. This disease is usually asymptomatic; however, some symptoms may

include intermittent dysphagia and odynophagia (pain from swallowing). Diffuse esophageal spasm may be confused with angina pectoris because nitroglycerin often relieves the pain.

- *Scleroderma* involves an atrophy of the smooth muscle of the lower portion of the esophagus. The diagnosis can be suspected following a barium swallow radiographic examination but must be confirmed by manometric findings. Characteristics include weak peristalsis of the distal half of the esophagus and diminished pressure of the LES. Gastroesophageal reflux and esophagitis often occur with scleroderma because of LES incompetence.

- Inflammation of the esophageal mucosa, *esophagitis*, may be acute (ingestion of hot liquids, infections) or chronic (acid reflux from the stomach). Infectious forms are common in patients with severe immunodeficiency, such as AIDS.

- An acute, severe form of esophagitis occurs following the ingestion of strong alkalis or acids found in drain cleaners. Symptoms include severe odynophagia, fever, toxicity, and possible esophageal perforation. Perforation can result in mediastinal infection and possible death. Vomiting should not be induced for the emergency treatment of persons with a caustic injury because this will reinjure the esophagus and oropharynx.

- Chronic reflux esophagitis is the most common form of esophageal inflammation encountered clinically. Incompetence of the LES and reflux of gastric acid or alkaline intestinal juice cause it over a long period. Common causes are esophageal motility disorders and sliding or direct hiatal hernia. Sequelae from chronic gastroesophageal reflux include Barrett's esophagus (predisposing to carcinoma), ulceration, bleeding, scarring, and stricture (leading to obstruction).

- *Mechanisms normally preventing gastroesophageal reflux* are (1) the normal contraction of the LES creating a high pressure zone (most important); (2) the acute gastroesophageal angle creating a flap-valve effect; and (3) tension created through the phrenicoesophageal ligament creating a pinchcock valve effect.

- *Hiatus hernia* is a herniation of a portion of the stomach into the chest through the esophageal hiatus of the diaphragm. The most common type is *direct* or *sliding hiatus hernia* in which the gastroesophageal junction slides into the thoracic cavity destroying the competence of the LES. Reflux esophagitis is the most common complication of sliding hiatus hernia. The other form is *periesophageal* or *rolling hiatus hernia* in which part of the gastric fundus rolls through the hiatus and the gastroesophageal junction remains below the diaphragm; the most common complication is strangulation.

- Benign tumors of the esophagus are rare; however, cancer in this area is not. Men are affected most. Heavy smoking, alcohol abuse, and Barrett's esophagus (metaplasia and dysplasia of mucosa from chronic gastroesophageal reflux) are predisposing factors. Barium, cytology, and endoscopy with biopsy studies are the primary diagnostic tools.

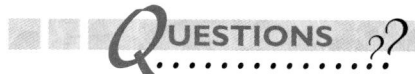

QUESTIONS ??

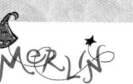

A sampling of review questions for this chapter appears here. Visit http://www.mosby.com/MERLIN/PriceWilson/ for additional questions.

Answer the following on a separate sheet of paper.

1. Describe the function of the esophagus.
2. How does regurgitation differ from vomiting?
3. What is usually the first symptom of malignant esophageal tumor?
4. What is an esophagomyotomy? What is a pyloroplasty? Why are these two procedures often combined? What condition is often treated by esophagomyotomy and pyloroplasty?
5. What kind of instructions would you give to patients with the following conditions to minimize symptoms and prevent complications: diffuse esophageal spasm, scleroderma, and sliding hiatus hernia?
6. Sketch the anatomic relations of the gastroesophageal junction, and briefly describe the three mechanisms preventing reflux.
7. Describe the consequences of chronic esophageal reflux.
8. Why do patients with achalasia and sliding hiatus hernia often have chronic pulmonary infections?
9. Why is chronic reflux esophagitis occasionally difficult to identify? What test is used to assist in the diagnosis?

Match each of the following symptoms in column A with its proper definition or description in column B.

Column A
10. _____ Dysphagia
11. _____ Regurgitation
12. _____ Odynophagia
13. _____ Pyrosis
14. _____ Globus hystericus
15. _____ Swallowing

Column B
a. Hot, burning sensation usually felt high in the epigastrium
b. "Lump in the throat" present during the absence of swallowing
c. Subjective awareness of difficulty in swallowing
d. Pain in middle chest induced by swallowing
e. Effortless welling up of esophageal or gastric contents into the mouth
f. A complex physiologic act whereby ingested food or liquid passes from the mouth to the stomach

Match each of the following esophageal motor disorders in column A with its common findings in motility studies in column B.

Column A
16. _____ Diffuse esophageal spasm
17. _____ Achalasia
18. _____ Scleroderma

Column B
a. Loss of contractile power in lower distal portion of esophagus
b. Characterized by a hypermotile pattern of ineffective contractions
c. Absence of peristalsis in body of esophagus and incomplete relaxation of the LES
d. Characterized by resting pressure lower than normal at the LES
e. Characterized by resting pressure higher than normal at the LES

Disorders of the Stomach and Duodenum

GLENDA N. LINDSETH

ANATOMY

The stomach lies obliquely from left to right across the upper abdomen directly beneath the diaphragm. When empty, the stomach resembles a J-shaped tube and, when full, a giant pear. The normal capacity of the stomach is 1 to 2 L. Anatomically, the stomach is divided into the *fundus*, the *body*, and the *pyloric antrum*, or *pylorus* (Fig. 24-1). The concave *lesser curvature* forms the upper right border of the stomach, and the convex *greater curvature* forms the left and lower borders. Sphincters at each end of the stomach regulate inflow and outflow. The *cardiac sphincter*, or lower esophageal sphincter (LES), allows food to flow into the stomach and prevents the reflux of gastric contents into the esophagus. The area of the stomach into which the cardiac sphincter opens is known as the *cardiac*

region. The terminal *pyloric sphincter* relaxes to permit food to enter the duodenum, and when contracted, it prevents backflow of intestinal contents into the stomach.

The pyloric sphincter is of particular clinical interest because obstructive narrowing (stenosis) may occur as a complication of peptic ulcer disease. Abnormalities of the pyloric sphincter may also occur in infants. *Pyloric stenosis* or pylorospasm results when hypertrophied or spastic muscle fibers surrounding the opening fail to relax sufficiently to permit food to pass easily from the stomach to the duodenum. The infant vomits the food instead of digesting and absorbing it. These conditions may be corrected by surgery or by adrenergic drugs that relax the muscle fibers.

The stomach is composed of four layers. The *serosa*, or outer layer, is a part of the visceral peritoneum. The two layers of the visceral peritoneum come together at the lesser curvature of the stomach and duodenum and extend upward to the liver, forming the *lesser omentum*. Peritoneal folds reflected from one organ to another are distinguished as ligaments. Thus the lesser omentum (also known as the hepatogastric and hepatoduodenal ligaments) suspends the stomach along its lesser curvature to the liver. At the greater curvature, the peritoneum continues downward as the *greater omentum*, draping over the intestines as a large apron. The lesser omental sac is a common site for the accumulation of fluid (pancreatic pseudocyst) as a complication of acute pancreatitis.

Unlike other areas of the digestive tract, the stomach's *muscularis* is composed of three rather than two layers of smooth muscle: an outer longitudinal layer, a middle circular layer, and an inner oblique layer. This unique arrangement of fibers provides the variety of contractions necessary to break food into small particles, churn and mix it with gastric juices, and propel it into the duodenum.

The *submucosa* is composed of loose areolar tissue that connects the muscularis and mucosal layers, permitting the mucosa to move with peristaltic motion. This layer also contains the nerve plexuses, blood vessels, and lymph channels.

The *mucosa*, the inner layer of the stomach, is arranged in longitudinal folds called *rugae*, which allow for dis-

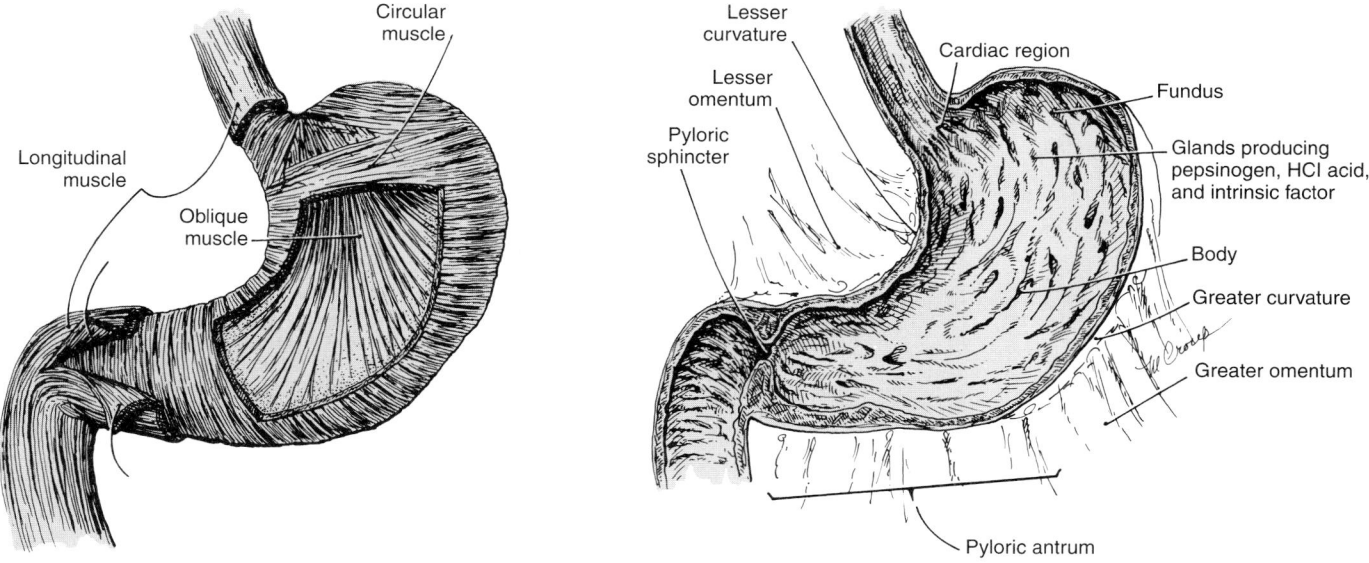

FIG. 24-1   Anatomy of the stomach.

tention as the stomach becomes filled with food. Several types of glands are located in this layer and are categorized according to the anatomic portion of the stomach in which they are located. *Cardiac glands* lie near the cardiac orifice and secrete mucus. The *fundic* or *gastric glands* are located in the fundus and over the greater part of the body of the stomach. Gastric glands have three main types of cells. *Zymogenic* or *chief cells* secrete *pepsinogen*. Pepsinogen is converted into *pepsin* in an acid environment. *Parietal cells* secrete hydrochloric acid (HCl) and intrinsic factor. *Intrinsic factor* is necessary for the absorption of vitamin B_{12} in the small intestine. A lack of intrinsic factor results in pernicious anemia. *Mucous (neck) cells* are found in the neck of the fundic glands and secrete mucus. G cells located in the pyloric region of the stomach produce the hormone *gastrin*. Gastrin stimulates the gastric glands to produce HCl and pepsinogen. Other substances secreted in the stomach include enzymes and various electrolytes, particularly sodium, potassium, and chloride ions.

The stomach receives its extrinsic nerve supply entirely from the autonomic nervous system. The parasympathetic nerve supply for the stomach and duodenum is conveyed to and from the abdomen through the vagus nerves (Fig. 24-2). Gastric, pyloric, and celiac branches emerge from the vagal trunks. Understanding this anatomy is especially important, because selective vagotomy is of primary importance in the surgical treatment of duodenal ulcers and is discussed in greater detail later in this chapter.

Sympathetic innervation is supplied via the greater splanchnic nerves and the celiac ganglia. The afferent fibers conduct pain impulses stimulated by distention, muscle contraction, and inflammation and are felt in the epigastric region of the abdomen. Efferent sympathetic fibers inhibit gastric motility and secretion. The *myenteric* (Auerbach's) and the *submucosal* (Meissner's) *nerve plexuses* form the intrinsic innervation within the wall of the stomach and coordinate its motor and secretory activity.

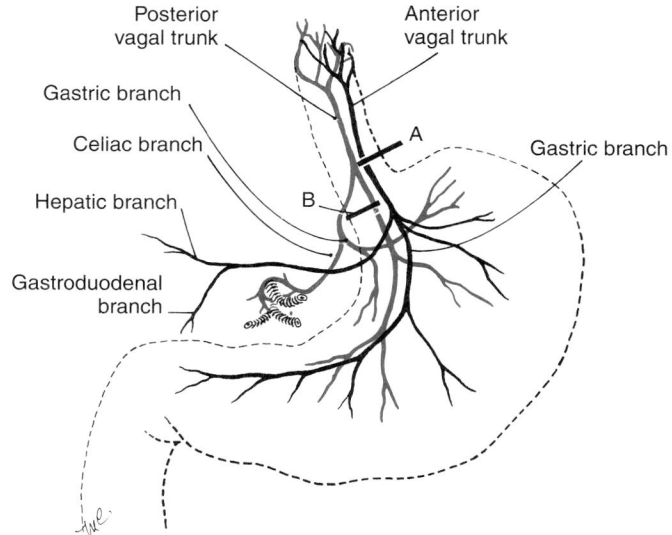

FIG. 24-2   Parasympathetic (vagal) innervation of the stomach. It is possible to sever the vagal nerve branches supplying the stomach at points *A* and *B*, leaving intact those branches supplying other abdominal structures (selective vagotomy). Selective vagotomy is an important aspect of the surgical treatment of duodenal ulcers.

The entire blood supply of the stomach and pancreas (as well as the liver, gallbladder, and spleen) is derived mainly from the celiac artery or trunk, which gives off branches supplying the lesser and greater curvatures. Two arterial branches of particular clinical significance are the *gastroduodenal* and the *pancreaticoduodenal* (retroduodenal) *arteries*, which course along the posterior duodenal bulb (Fig. 24-3). Ulcers of the posterior duodenal wall may erode into these arteries and cause hemorrhaging. The venous blood from the stomach and duodenum, as well as that from the pancreas, spleen, and the remainder

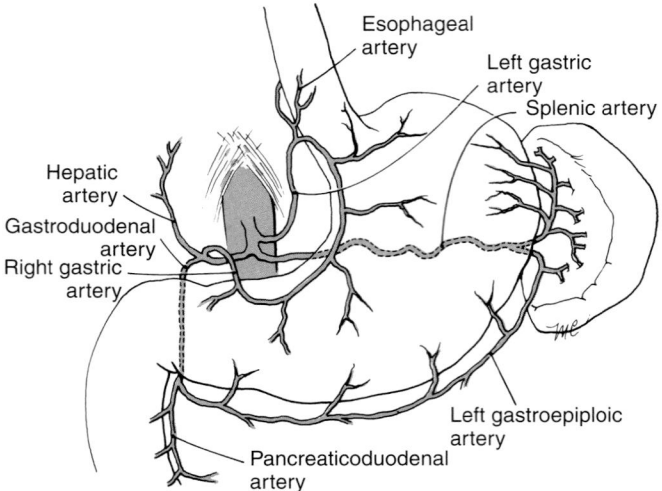

FIG. 24-3 Blood supply of the stomach and duodenum.

of the gastrointestinal (GI) tract, is conveyed to the liver by the portal vein.

PHYSIOLOGY

The digestive and motor functions of the stomach are summarized in Box 24-1. The types of secretions have been discussed. Motor functions include storing, mixing, and emptying *chyme* (a semifluid mass of partly digested food mixed with gastric secretions) into the duodenum. Understanding the regulation and control of gastric secretions is essential for a rational understanding of the pathogenesis and treatment of peptic ulcer disease.

Control of Gastric Secretion

Gastric secretion may be divided into three phases: cephalic, gastric, and intestinal. The *cephalic phase* occurs even before food enters the stomach, resulting from the site, smell, thought, or taste of food. This initial phase is mediated entirely by the vagus nerve and is eliminated by vagotomy. Neurogenic signals causing the cephalic phase may originate in the cerebral cortex or in the appetite center. Efferent impulses are then transmitted via the vagus nerves to the stomach. As a result, the gastric (oxyntic) glands are stimulated to secrete HCl, pepsinogen, and increased amounts of mucus. The cephalic phase of secretion accounts for approximately 10% of the gastric secretions normally associated with a meal.

The *gastric phase* is initiated by the presence of food in the pyloric antrum. Distention of the antrum can also result in the mechanical stimulation of receptors in the wall of the stomach. Impulses travel to the medulla over vagal afferents and return to the stomach over vagal efferents; these impulses stimulate the release of the hormone gastrin and also directly stimulate the gastric glands. Gastrin is released from the antrum and is then carried by the bloodstream to the gastric glands, causing secretion. Gastrin release is also stimulated by an alkaline pH, by bile

salts in the antrum, and especially by protein foods and alcohol. Parietal cell membranes in the fundus and body of the stomach contain receptors for gastrin, histamine, and acetylcholine, which stimulate the acid secretion. After meal consumption, gastrin can act on the parietal cells directly for acid secretion and can also stimulate release of histamine from the enterochromaffin cells of the mucosa for acid secretion. Table 24-1 lists the effects of gastrin.

The gastric phase of secretion accounts for more than two thirds of the total gastric secretion after a meal is eaten and thus accounts for most of the total daily gastric secretion of about 2000 ml. The gastric phase can be affected by surgical resection of the pyloric antrum, because this is the site of gastrin production.

The movement of chyme from the stomach to the duodenum initiates the *intestinal phase*. This phase of gastric secretion is believed to be largely hormonal. The presence of partially digested proteins in the duodenum apparently stimulates the release of enteric gastrin, a hormone that causes the stomach to continue to secrete small amounts of gastric juice. However, the role of the small intestine as an inhibitor of gastric secretion is of much greater importance.

Distention of the small intestine initiates the *enterogastric reflex*, which inhibits gastric secretion and emptying and is mediated through the myenteric plexus, sympathetic nerves, and vagus nerve. The presence of acid (pH less than 2.5), fat, and protein breakdown products causes the release of several intestinal hormones. *Secretin,*

TABLE 24-1   ▪▪▪

Actions of Gastrin

Actions	Physiologic Significance
Stimulates acid and pepsin secretion	Promotes digestion
Stimulates secretion of intrinsic factor	Promotes vitamin B_{12} absorption in small intestine
Stimulates pancreatic enzyme secretion	Promotes digestion
Stimulates increase in flow of hepatic bile	Promotes digestion
Stimulates release of insulin	Promotes glucose metabolism
Stimulates gastric and intestinal motility	Promotes mixing and propulsion of ingested food
Promotes receptive relaxation of stomach	Stomach can greatly increase volume without increasing pressure
Increases resting tone of LES	Prevents gastric reflux during active mixing and churning
Inhibits gastric emptying	Allows time for thorough mixing of gastric contents before delivery to intestine

LES, Lower esophageal sphincter.

cholecystokinin (CCK), and *gastric-inhibiting peptide (GIP)* all have inhibitory effects on gastric secretions.

During the *interdigestive period*, when digestion is not occurring in the gut, HCl secretion continues at the low rate of 1 to 5 mEq/hour. This process is called the *basal acid output (BAO)* and may be measured by analysis of gastric secretions after a 12-hour fast. The normal gastric secretions during the interdigestive period are composed mainly of mucus and contain little pepsin and acid. Strong emotional stimuli, however, can increase the BAO via the parasympathetic (vagus) nerves and are believed to be one of the factors in the development of peptic ulcers.

DIAGNOSTIC PROCEDURES

Diagnostic procedures that help identify gastric and duodenal disease include barium radiologic studies, breath tests, serology testing, gastric analysis, and endoscopy using a flexible fiberoptic gastroscope. Photography, biopsy, and exfoliative cytology may be performed through the gastroscope. *Exfoliative cytology*, or collection of cells by lavage with normal saline solution, is a valuable technique for identifying malignancies that may not be directly visible through the gastroscope. Malignant cells exfoliate (slough off) more readily than do normal cells. The collected solution should be placed on ice and taken to the laboratory immediately for analysis. Delay will result in destruction of the exfoliated cells by the digestive enzymes. Cytologic washings are approximately 90% accurate in the diagnosis of stomach cancer.

Diagnosis of gastric pathogens, such as *Helicobacter pylori* (*H. pylori*), can be made by use of endoscopic, serologic, and urea breath testing. The urea breath test is a diagnostic method based on the principle that urea is converted by *H. pylori* urease in the stomach into ammonia and carbon dioxide (CO_2). The CO_2 is rapidly absorbed through the gastric wall and can be detected in expired air. Serologic testing is also reliable for diagnosing the presence of *H. pylori* infection; however, the test may remain positive for several months after the *H. pylori* infection is eradicated. By comparison, the urea breath test is the most efficient noninvasive test.

Upper GI endoscopy permits stomach evaluation with side-viewing scopes that makes this a method of choice. Lesions of the stomach can be evaluated by endoscopic ultrasound, a technique that combines diagnostic ultrasound (US) with endoscopy. In secondary tumors that are not diagnosable through mucosal evaluation, visualization may be completed by US or computed tomography (CT). Magnetic resonance imaging (MRI) can be useful for imaging some abdominal masses.

Gastric analysis of acid secretion is another important technique in the diagnosis of gastric disease. A nasogastric tube is inserted into the stomach, and the fasting contents are aspirated for analysis. The *basal analysis* measures BAO in the absence of stimulation. This test is valuable in the diagnosis of *Zollinger-Ellison syndrome*, in which a tumor of the pancreas secretes large amounts of gastrin, which, in turn, causes marked hyperacidity and multiple recurrent peptic ulcers. Duodenal ulcers are usually associated with a high BAO, whereas the BAO is normal to low in gastric ulcer and carcinoma.

Stimulation analysis may be performed by measuring *maximum acid output (MAO)* after administration of a drug that stimulates acid secretion, such as histamine; betazole hydrochloride (Histalog), a histamine analogue; or pentagastrin, a synthetic, gastrinlike peptide. *Achlorhydria* is defined as a lack of acid secretions after administering a maximal dose of one of the stimulating drugs, provided the analysis is accurate and no reflux of duodenal contents has occurred into the stomach, which would neutralize the acid. If a patient is achlorhydric and has a gastric ulcer, then the ulcer likely represents cancer and is not related to acid secretions. Patients with pernicious anemia are also achlorhydric as a result of atrophy of the secretory cells in the stomach. Without intrinsic factor, vitamin B_{12} absorption is impaired and the serum levels of vitamin B_{12} will be low.

NAUSEA AND VOMITING

Nausea and vomiting are common signs and symptoms accompanying GI disorders, as well as many other illnesses. Several theories concerning the cause of nausea and vomiting have evolved, but no agreement exists on a definitive cause or treatment. Nausea and vomiting can be considered a phenomenon that occurs in three stages: (1) nausea, (2) retching, and (3) vomiting. The first stage, *nausea*, may be described as a highly disagreeable feeling experienced in the back of the throat and the epigastrium, often resulting in vomiting. Various changes in digestive tract activity have been associated with nausea, such as increased salivation, decreased gastric tone, and peristalsis. An increase in duodenal and jejunal tone results in a reflux of duodenal contents into the stomach. However, no evidence suggests that these events cause nausea. Signs and symptoms of nausea often include pallor, increased salivation, queasiness, faintness, sweating, and tachycardia.

Retching, an involuntary attempt to vomit, often follows nausea and precedes vomiting, consisting of spasmodic respiratory movements against the glottis and inspiratory movements of the chest wall and diaphragm. Expiratory abdominal muscle contractions control the inspiratory movements. The distal antrum and pylorus contract while the fundus relaxes.

The last stage, *vomiting,* is defined as a reflex causing the forceful expulsion of the contents of the stomach or intestine or both through the mouth. The vomiting center receives input from the cerebral cortex, vestibular organs, *chemoreceptor trigger zone (CTZ),* and afferent fibers, including those of the GI system. Vomiting is the result of stimulation of the *emetic center,* which is located in the area postrema of the medulla in the floor of the fourth ventricle. Vomiting can be stimulated through the afferent neural pathways by vagal and sympathetic nerve stimulation or by an emetic stimulus that leads to vomiting by activating the CTZ. The efferent pathways relay the signals that lead to the coordinated respiratory, GI, and abdominal muscle expulsive movements and accompanying emetic epiphenomena called vomiting. Because the vomiting center is anatomically near the salivation and respiratory centers, hypersalivation and respiratory movements often occur with vomiting.

Vomiting is considered important because it can be an indicator of various conditions, such as intestinal obstruction, infections, pain, metabolic diseases, pregnancy, labyrinthine and vestibular disorders, exogenous emetic substances such as poisons, uremia or kidney failure, radiation sickness, psychologic conditions, migraines, myocardial infarction, and circulatory syncope. Because nausea and vomiting can result from many different illnesses, distinguishing among characteristics of the symptoms is important. Symptoms that have been present for a few hours or days may indicate an acute infection, inflammatory conditions, or pregnancy. Nausea and vomiting that have been present for weeks may indicate obstructive, carcinogenic, or psychogenic origins. Factors that should be considered include timing of the nausea and vomiting, relationship to meals, content and odor of the vomitus, and associated symptoms such as pain, weight loss, fever, menstruation, abdominal mass, jaundice, headache, and other factors that may influence the patient's diagnosis and care. Vomiting can also lead to life-threatening complications because of its relationship with the autonomic and sympathetic nervous systems, as well as the impact of nausea and vomiting on the body's fluid and electrolytes.

GASTRITIS

Gastritis is an inflammation or hemorrhagic condition of the gastric mucosa that may be acute, chronic, diffuse, or localized. The two most common types of gastritis are acute superficial and chronic atrophic.

Acute Superficial Gastritis

Acute gastritis is a common, usually benign, and self-limiting disease that represents the response of the gastric mucosa to a variety of local irritants. Bacterial endotoxins (after the ingestion of contaminated food), caffeine, alcohol, and aspirin are common offending agents. *H. pylori* infection is more frequently being considered as a cause of acute gastritis. The organism attaches to gastric epithelium and destroys the protective mucosal layer, leaving areas of denuded epithelium. Other drugs, such as nonsteroidal antiinflammatory drugs (NSAIDs; e.g., indomethacin, ibuprofen, naproxen), sulfonamides, steroids, and digitalis, have also been implicated. Bile acids, pancreatic enzymes, and ethanol are also known to disrupt the gastric mucosal barrier.

When alcohol is ingested in combination with aspirin, the effect is more deleterious than is the effect of either taken alone. *Diffuse hemorrhagic erosive gastritis* is known to occur with heavy alcohol and aspirin use and may lead to the necessity of gastric resection. This serious condition is considered with stress ulcers, because many similarities exist between the two. Destruction of the gastric mucosal barrier is believed to be the pathogenic mechanism responsible for the injury and is considered later.

In superficial gastritis, the mucosa is reddened and edematous and covered with adherent mucus; small erosions and hemorrhages are common. The degree of inflammation is highly variable.

Clinical manifestations of acute gastritis may range from vague abdominal complaints, such as anorexia, eructation (belching), or nausea, to more severe symptoms, such as epigastric pain, vomiting, bleeding, and hematemesis. In some patients, when symptoms are prolonged and resistant to treatment, additional diagnostic measures, such as endoscopy, mucosal biopsy, and gastric analysis, may be needed to clarify the diagnosis.

Acute superficial gastritis usually resolves when the offending agent is removed. Antiemetic drugs may help relieve the nausea and vomiting. If vomiting persists, it may then be necessary to correct fluid and electrolyte imbalances with intravenous (IV) infusions. The use of H_2 blockers (e.g., ranitidine) to decrease acid secretion, antacids to neutralize secreted acid, and sucralfate to coat inflamed or ulcerated areas may facilitate healing.

Chronic Atrophic Gastritis

Chronic atrophic gastritis is characterized by progressive atrophy of the glandular epithelium with loss of parietal and chief cells. The gastric wall becomes thin, and the mucosa has an unusually smooth surface. Chronic gastritis is classified into two categories: Type A (atrophic or fundal) and Type B (antral) gastritis.

Type A chronic gastritis may be referred to as *atrophic* or *fundal gastritis* (because it involves the stomach's fundus). Type A chronic gastritis is an autoimmune disease resulting from the presence of autoantibodies to the gastric gland parietal cells and intrinsic factor and is associated with the loss of chief cells and parietal cells, which decreases acid secretion and results in high gastrin levels. In the most severe cases, production of intrinsic factor is lost. Pernicious anemia is often present in these individuals because intrinsic factor is unavailable to facilitate vitamin B_{12} absorption in the ileum.

Type B chronic gastritis is referred to as *antral gastritis* because it generally involves the antrum region of the stomach and is much more common than is Type A chronic gastritis. Type B chronic gastritis occurs more often in the elderly. This form of gastritis has near normal acid secretion and is not associated with pernicious anemia. Low serum gastrin levels are often present. A major cause of Type B chronic gastritis is chronic infection by *H. pylori*. Other etiologic factors in chronic gastritis are heavy alcohol intake, smoking, and chronic bile reflux along with the *H. pylori* cofactor.

Chronic atrophic gastritis may predispose the patient to the development of gastric ulcers and carcinoma. The incidence of gastric cancer is particularly high in patients with pernicious anemia (10% to 15%). Symptoms of chronic gastritis are generally varied and vague; they may include a feeling of fullness, anorexia, and vague epigastric distress. The diagnosis is suspected when the patient has achlorhydria or a low BAO or MAO, and the diagnosis is confirmed by the typical histologic changes on biopsy.

The treatment of chronic atrophic gastritis varies, depending on the suspected cause of the disorder. When duodenal ulcer lesions are present, antibiotics may be given to eliminate *H. pylori*. However, lesions are not typically present with chronic gastritis. Alcohol and drugs known to irritate the gastric mucosa are avoided. Iron deficiency anemia (caused by chronic bleeding), when present, is corrected. Vitamin B_{12} and other appropriate therapy are given in the case of pernicious anemia.

PEPTIC ULCER DISEASE

Peptic ulcers are circumscribed breaks in the continuity of mucosa, extending below the epithelium. Strictly speaking, breaks in the mucosa not extending below the epithelium are called *erosions*, although they are often referred to as "ulcers" (e.g., stress ulcers). *Chronic ulcers*, as opposed to acute ulcers, have scar tissue at the base (Fig. 24-4).

By definition, peptic ulcers can be located in any part of the GI tract exposed to the acid-pepsin gastric juice, including the esophagus, stomach, duodenum, and after gastroenterostomy, the jejunum. Although the peptic digestive activity of gastric juice is an important etiologic factor, evidence indicates that many factors are important in the pathogenesis of peptic ulcer disease. For example, the *H. pylori* bacterium is present in approximately 90% of individuals with duodenal ulcers. Mucosal bicarbonate secretions, genetic characteristics, and stress are also causes of peptic ulcer. Because many similarities and differences exist between gastric and duodenal ulcers, some aspects of these two entities are considered together for convenience, and special problems relating to each are discussed separately. Gastric erosions or stress ulcers are considered last. Table 24-2 lists some of the differences between the various types of peptic ulcers.

Pathogenesis

Because pure acid gastric juice is capable of digesting all living tissues, one of the major questions is, "Why doesn't the stomach digest itself?" Two factors appear to protect the stomach from autodigestion: the gastric mucus and the epithelial barrier.

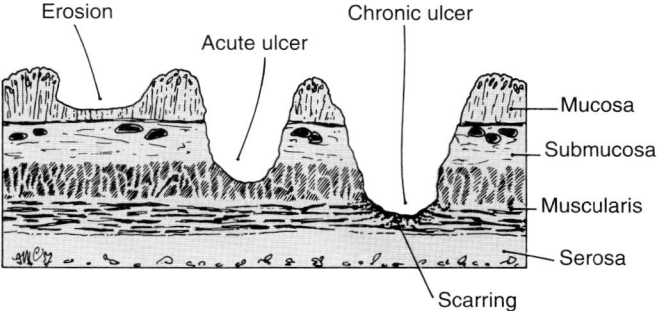

FIG. 24-4   Peptic ulcers, illustrating an erosion, an acute ulcer, and a chronic ulcer. Acute and chronic ulcers may penetrate the entire wall of the stomach.

Gastric Mucosal Barrier

According to Hollander's *two-component mucous barrier* theory, the thick, tenacious layer of gastric mucus constitutes the first line of defense against autodigestion. This layer provides protection against mechanical trauma and chemical agents. NSAIDs, including aspirin, produce qualitative changes in the gastric mucus that may facilitate its degradation by pepsin. Prostaglandins are present in abundant quantities in the gastric mucus and appear to play an important role in gastric mucosal defense.

The *gastric mucosal barrier* is important to the protection of the stomach and duodenum. Although the exact nature of this barrier is not understood, it probably involves the mucous lining, the lumen of the columnar epithelial cells, and the tight junctions at the apices of these cells. Normally this mucosal barrier allows little back diffusion of hydrogen ions (H^+) from the lumen to the blood, even though a large concentration gradient exists (gastric acid with a pH of 1.0 versus blood with a pH of 7.4).

Destruction of Gastric Mucosal Barrier

Aspirin, alcohol, bile salts, and other substances injurious to the gastric mucosa alter the permeability of the epithelial barrier, which allows back diffusion of HCl with resultant injury to underlying tissues, particularly blood vessels (Fig. 24-5). Histamine is liberated, which stimulates further acid and pepsin secretion and increased capillary permeability to proteins. The mucosa becomes edematous, and large amounts of plasma proteins may be lost. The mucosal capillaries may be damaged, resulting in interstitial hemorrhage and bleeding. The mucosal barrier is unaffected by vagal inhibition or atropine, but back diffusion is inhibited by gastrin.

Destruction of the gastric mucosal barrier is believed to be an important factor in the pathogenesis of gastric ulcers. Evidence suggests that the antral mucosa is more susceptible to back diffusion than that of the fundus, which explains why gastric ulcers are often located in the antrum. Also suggested is that the low level of acid recovered in gastric analysis of patients with gastric ulcer is caused by increased back diffusion, not lower production. This pathogenic mechanism may also be important in patients with acute hemorrhagic gastritis caused by alcohol, aspirin, and severe stress.

TABLE 24-2 ■ ■ ■

Differentiating Features of Duodenal, Gastric, and Stress Ulcers

	Duodenal Ulcer	Gastric Ulcer	Stress Ulcer
Incidence	Peak age: 40 years Duodenal/gastric ulcer: 4:1 Prevalence: 10% of population Men/women: 1:1	Peak age: 50-60 years Men/women: 2:1 Lifetime prevalence: 10%	Related to severe stress, trauma, sepsis, burns, head injuries No gender difference
Pathogenesis	Hyperacidity important factor Gastric colonization with *Helicobacter pylori* reported in 90%-95% of patients Associated diseases: hyperparathyroidism, chronic pulmonary disease, chronic pancreatitis, alcoholic cirrhosis Ulcerogenic drugs, alcohol, tobacco Blood group O: higher frequency Psychosocial stress and chronic anxiety possible factors in exacerbations	Disruption of mucosal barrier seems important factor Normal to low HCl production Presence of *H. pylori* gastritis Ulcerogenic drugs, alcohol, tobacco Chronic bile reflux Not related to blood group More common in laboring groups Familial predisposition may be due to intrafamilial *H. pylori* infection	Head injuries: hypersecretion of HCl All others: ischemia of gastric mucosa, disruption of mucosal barrier, back diffusion of HCl, acute gastritis Hemorrhagic gastric erosions possibly drug induced; alcohol and aspirin most common offenders
Pathology	90% in duodenal bulb	90% in antrum and lesser curvature	Usually multiple, diffuse erosions; more often located in stomach, especially fundus
Complications	About 10% of patients; most respond to medical therapy	More common than with duodenal ulcer	
Hemorrhage	Common in posterior wall of duodenal bulb	25% occurrence	Most frequent complication; high mortality
Perforation	More common when located in anterior wall of duodenum	More common in anterior wall of stomach	Common
Obstruction	Common	Rare	
Malignancy	Almost never	Incidence about 4%	
Clinical features	Pain-food-relief pattern of pain Patient usually well nourished Seasonal exacerbations Night pain possible	Food-pain pattern of pain Anorexia, weight loss common Night pain possible	May be asymptomatic until serious complication such as hemorrhage or perforation

The resistance of the duodenum to peptic ulceration is believed to be a function of *Brunner's glands* (submucosal duodenal glands in the intestinal wall), which produce a highly alkaline, viscid, mucoid secretion that neutralizes the acid chyme. Patients with duodenal ulcers often have excessive acid secretion, which appears to be the most important pathogenic factor. The normal mucosal defense mechanisms may be overwhelmed. The factor of decreased tissue resistance is implicated in both gastric and duodenal ulcers, although it appears to be more important in gastric ulcers.

In addition to the mucosal and epithelial barriers, tissue resistance also depends on an abundant vascular supply and continued, rapid regeneration of epithelial cells (normally replaced every 3 days). Failure of this mechanism may also play a role in the pathogenesis of peptic ulcer.

Other Factors

Although the incidence of duodenal ulcers is decreasing, currently about 500,000 new cases occur each year, with 10% to 15% of the population affected. Duodenal ulcers generally occur in a much younger age group than do gastric ulcers. The lower incidence of peptic ulcers in women appears to indicate a gender-linked influence.

Certain drugs such as aspirin, alcohol, indomethacin, phenylbutazone, and corticosteroids may have a direct irritating effect on the gastric mucosa and produce ulceration. If these drugs do have an effect, it may be caused by a disruption of one of the protective barriers in the stomach. Caffeine-containing drinks and smoking should be avoided because they stimulate acid production.

Most peptic ulcers occur "downstream" from the source of acid secretion. More than 90% of duodenal ulcers are located on the anterior or posterior wall of the first part of the duodenum, within 3 cm of the pyloric ring. Although gastric ulcers may occur anywhere in the stomach, 90% are situated along the lesser curvature and in the pyloric gland region.

Approximately 40% to 60% of patients with ulcers have a family history of ulcer disease. Genetic factors or the intrafamilial transmission of *H. pylori* infections are possible explanations. Individuals with blood type group O appear to be more susceptible to duodenal ulcers. A possible explanation is that *H. pylori* binding is enhanced with epithelial cells that bear the group O antigen (Cotran et al, 1999).

A number of diseases appear to be associated with peptic ulcer formation, including alcoholic liver cirrhosis, chronic pancreatitis, chronic lung disease, hyperparathyroidism, and Zollinger-Ellison syndrome.

Abnormal pyloric sphincter function resulting in bile reflux has been proposed as a pathogenic mechanism in

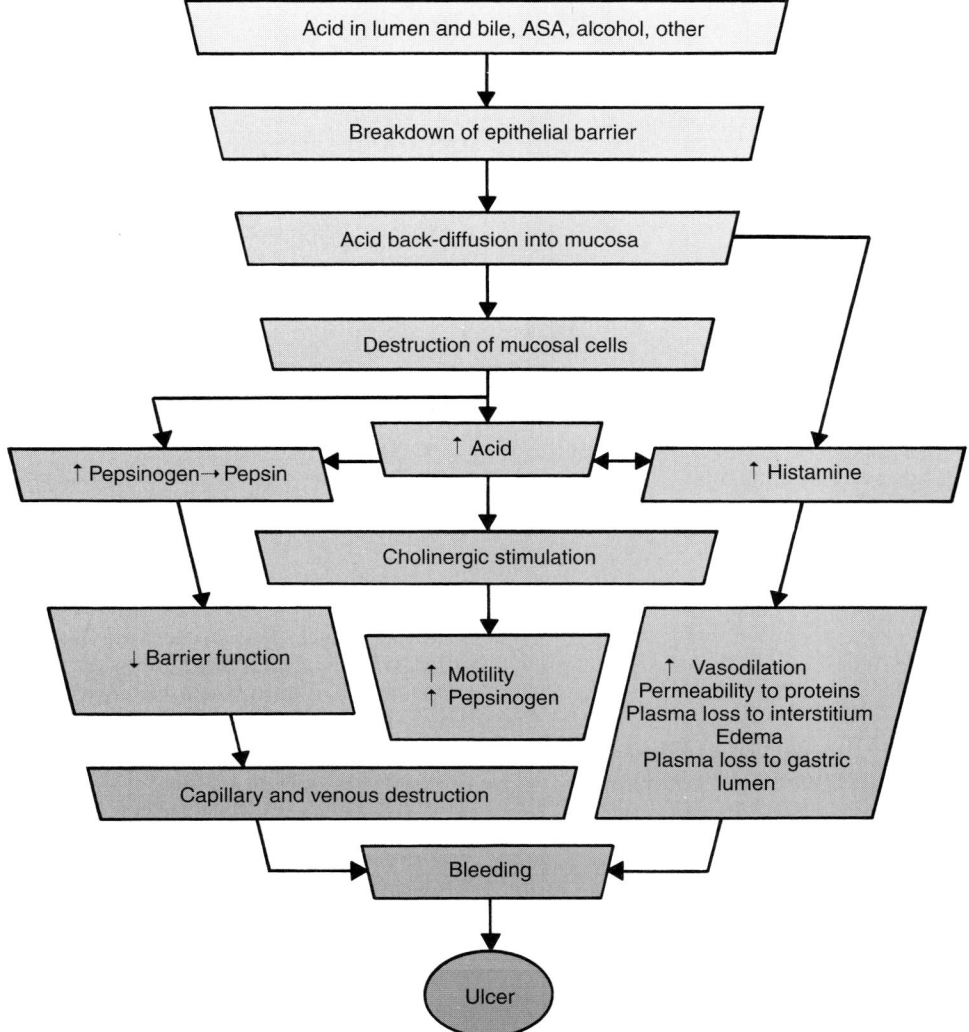

FIG. 24-5   Pathophysiologic consequences of back diffusion of acid through the damaged mucosal barrier.

the development of gastric ulcer. The bile disrupts the gastric mucosal barrier, causing gastritis and increased susceptibility to ulcer formation. The damaged mucosa is ultimately eroded and digested by the action of acid and pepsin.

Zollinger-Ellison Syndrome

Zollinger-Ellison syndrome is a condition caused by a noninsulin secreting pancreatic tumor that secretes excess amounts of gastrin. The excess gastrin stimulates the stomach to secrete large amounts of HCl and pepsin, which promotes an ulcer located in the duodenal bulb and that responds poorly to ulcer therapies. The diagnosis is usually made by serum gastrin and acid secretory studies. Symptoms typically include diarrhea (present in almost one third of the cases), hypercalcemia (a result of hyperparathyroidism), and pituitary dysfunction (a complication resulting from the tumor mass). The disorder appears to be genetic with a family history predisposing the patient. Some individuals present with enlarged gastric folds when visualized by radiographic or endoscopic examination. Zollinger-Ellison syndrome is commonly

associated with extremely high serum gastrin levels and very high HCl secretion. Zollinger-Ellison syndrome tumors are usually malignant (60%). Treatment might include total gastrectomy or excision of the pancreatic tumor if metastasis is not too extensive. Approximately 50% of these patients die within 10 years, usually as a result of metastases.

Clinical Features

The principal clinical feature of peptic ulcer is chronic, intermittent epigastric pain typically relieved by food or antacids. Pain usually occurs 2 or 3 hours after a meal or at night when the stomach is empty. Peptic ulcer pain is often described as gnawing, burning, or nagging in nature. Approximately one fourth of patients with ulcers experience bleeding, although it is more common with duodenal ulcer. Signs and symptoms may also include vomiting, red or "coffee-ground" emesis, nausea, anorexia, and weight loss. Persistent upper abdominal pain is rarely a symptom of peptic ulcers; exacerbation and remissions are more characteristic of peptic ulcers. The

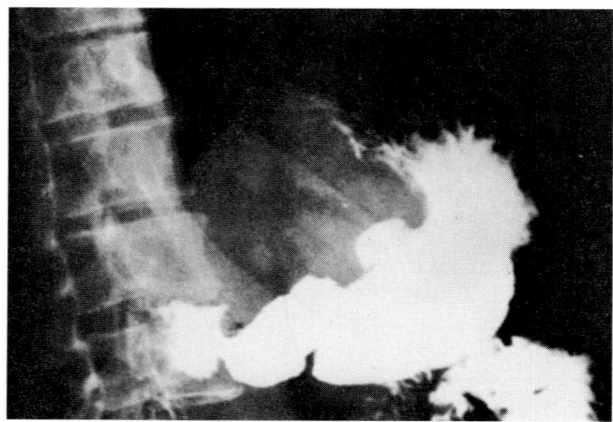

FIG. 24-6 Barium radiographic appearance of gastric ulcer. Note the large, nodular-shaped protrusion on the lesser curvature of the stomach.

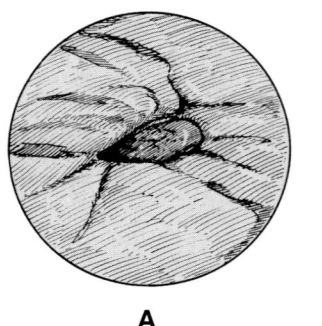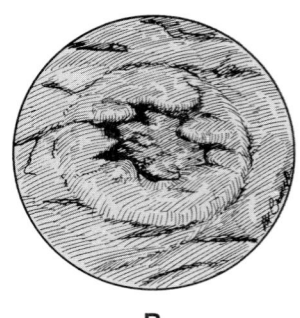

A   B

FIG. 24-7 Gastroscopic appearance of, **A**, a benign gastric ulcer and, **B**, a malignant gastric ulcer (carcinoma). The benign ulcer has a sharp, well-defined margin. The malignant ulcer has an irregular margin that fades into the surrounding tumor mass.

pain-food-relief pattern may not be typical with gastric ulcers. In fact, with gastric ulcers, food occasionally aggravates the pain.

Diagnosis

An important criterion in the diagnosis of duodenal ulcer is a positive serology or urea breath test for *H. pylori* infection, because it is a factor or cofactor in up to 90% of duodenal ulcers. A history of the typical *pain-food-relief pattern* is also a strong indicator. The history is not as informative in patients with gastric ulcer, because vague symptoms of epigastric distress occur more often. Distinguishing between gastric and duodenal ulcers on the basis of history alone is usually impossible.

The diagnosis of peptic ulcer is usually confirmed by barium meal radiography (Fig. 24-6). When barium radiography fails to reveal an ulcer in the stomach or duodenum but characteristic symptoms persist, endoscopic examination is indicated. Serum gastrin levels may be assayed if Zollinger-Ellison syndrome is suspected.

Benign versus Malignant Ulcers

Although duodenal ulcers are almost never malignant, approximately 4% of gastric ulcers turn out to be carcinoma of the stomach. The gastroenterologist must therefore differentiate between a benign and a malignant gastric ulcer. Generally, malignant ulcers have a shaggy, necrotic base, whereas benign ulcers have a smooth, clean base with a distinct margin (Fig. 24-7). Biopsy and cytologic studies are also helpful in distinguishing a benign from a malignant ulcer.

Medical Treatment

The primary objective in the medical treatment of peptic ulcer is to inhibit or buffer acid secretions to relieve symptoms and promote healing. Measures that achieve these ends are antacids, dietary management, anticholinergics, H_2 blockers (cimetidine, ranitidine, famotidine), antimicrobial therapy, and physical and emotional rest. Antibacterials are considered a primary treatment for eliminating documented *H. pylori* infection.

Antacids are given to neutralize the acid gastric contents by keeping the pH high enough such that pepsin is not activated, thus protecting the mucosa and relieving the pain. The most widely used antacid preparations are mixtures of aluminum hydroxide and magnesium hydroxide. Dietary management of peptic ulcers should include eating small, frequent meals to neutralize gastric contents; high fiber intakes may also be of some benefit. Milk, cream, and bland diets that were used in the past are no longer recommended. Milk products can stimulate acid secretion. Stimulants of acid secretion, such as alcohol and caffeine, are avoided. Anticholinergic drugs, such as propantheline bromide (Pro-Banthine) and atropine (from *Atropa belladonna*), inhibit the direct effect of the vagus nerve on the acid-secreting parietal cells. Anticholinergics also inhibit gastric motility and emptying time, and many physicians therefore do not prescribe this type of drug for patients with gastric ulcers. H_2 blockers have rapidly become the most common drugs used to treat duodenal ulcers because of their ability to reduce acid secretion by 70%. Another drug, sucralfate, not only forms an acid-impermeable membrane that adheres to injured mucosa but also accelerates mucosal cell production (a cytoprotective effect).

Providing a quiet environment, listening to the patient's problems, and offering emotional support help promote physical and emotional rest. Small doses of sedatives may be prescribed.

The response of gastric ulcers to the classic therapy of Pepto-Bismol, metronidazole, and tetracycline for 14 days has resulted in eradication rates of *H. pylori* of near 90%. The use of omeprazole may further increase *H. pylori* eradication (Walsh, Fass, 1997). Close monitoring of progress is required because drugs may relieve the symptoms of malignant gastric ulcers, thus masking the symptoms that lead to a diagnosis.

Complications

Complications of peptic ulcer disease include hemorrhage, perforation, pyloric obstruction, and intractability. Any of these complications is an indication for surgical treatment.

Hemorrhage

Bleeding is the most frequent complication of peptic ulcer and occurs in 15% to 25% of patients at some time during the course of the disease. Although ulcers in any site may bleed, the most common site of hemorrhage is in the posterior wall of the duodenal bulb, because erosion into the pancreaticoduodenal or gastroduodenal artery may occur in that location.

The symptoms associated with bleeding ulcer depend on the rapidity of blood loss. Mild, chronic blood loss may lead to iron deficiency anemia. The stools may be positive for occult blood (positive guaiac test) or may be black and tarry (melena). Massive bleeding may lead to *hematemesis* (vomiting blood) and the development of shock and may require blood transfusions and emergency surgery. Relief of pain often follows bleeding as a result of the buffering effect of blood. The mortality in these patients ranges up to 10%, with patients over age 50 years having a higher mortality rate. This group represents about 20% to 25% of the total deaths attributable to ulcer disease.

Perforation

Approximately 2% to 3% of all ulcers perforate, and this complication accounts for about 65% of deaths from peptic ulcer disease (see Fig. 4-11). The ulcers are usually on the anterior wall of the duodenum or stomach. The primary cause of perforation is thought to be excess acid secretion and often is a result of ingestion of NSAIDS, which deplete the cells of adenosine triphosphate (ATP), rendering them vulnerable to oxidant stress. This delayed cellular repair leads to perforation.

Most patients with perforation present in a characteristically dramatic fashion. A sudden onset of excruciating pain in the upper abdomen occurs. Within minutes, a chemical peritonitis develops because of the escaping gastric acid, pepsin, and food, causing intense pain. The patient fears to move or breathe. The abdomen becomes silent to auscultation and assumes a boardlike rigidity to palpation. Acute perforation can usually be diagnosed on the basis of the symptoms alone. The diagnosis is confirmed by the presence of free gas within the peritoneal cavity, presenting as a translucent crescent between the liver and diaphragm shadows; the air has entered the peritoneal cavity through the perforated ulcer. The treatment is immediate surgery with gastric resection or simple suture of the perforation, depending on the patient's condition.

Occasionally a gastric or duodenal ulcer breaks through the wall but remains sealed off by a contiguous structure and is called a *penetrating ulcer*. A classic example of a penetrating ulcer is a duodenal ulcer of the posterior wall that penetrates into the pancreas and is walled off (Fig. 24-8). Clinically, the pain becomes intractable and may radiate to the back. The patient may present with pancreatitis.

Obstruction

Obstruction of the gastric outlet as a result of inflammation and edema, pylorospasm, or scarring occurs in approximately 5% of patients with peptic ulcer. Obstruction occurs more often in patients with duodenal ulcer but occasionally occurs when a gastric ulcer is located close to the pyloric sphincter.

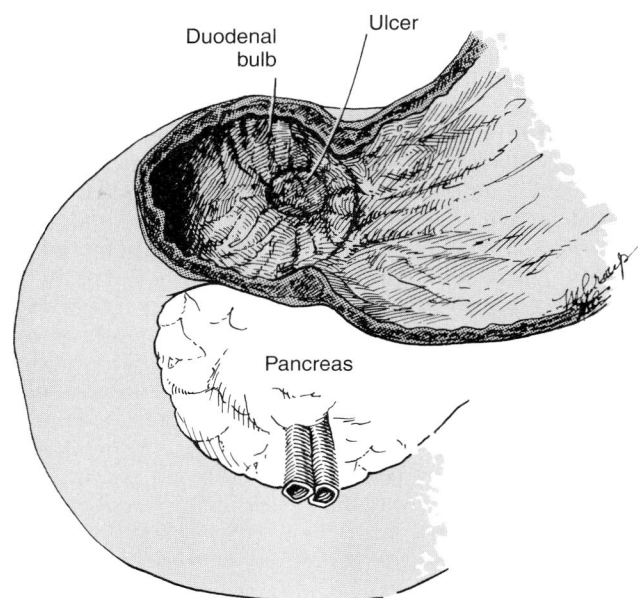

FIG. 24-8   Duodenal ulcer of the posterior wall, penetrating into the head of the pancreas and resulting in a walled-off perforation.

Anorexia, nausea, and bloating after eating are common symptoms; weight loss often results. When the obstruction becomes severe, pain and vomiting may occur.

Treatment is directed toward restoring fluids and electrolytes, decompressing the stomach by insertion of a nasogastric tube, and surgically correcting the obstruction (pyloroplasty).

Intractability

Another complication of peptic ulcer is intractability, which simply means that medical therapy fails to control the symptoms adequately, resulting in frequent, rapid recurrences. Patients may have their sleep interrupted by pain, lose time from work, require frequent hospitalization, or simply be unable to follow a medical regimen. Surgery is typically recommended for intractability. Malignant transformation is not an important consideration in either gastric or duodenal ulcer. Approximately 4% of gastric ulcers that start out benign are later diagnosed as malignant.

Surgical Treatment

Patients who do not respond to medical therapy or who develop other complications such as perforation, hemorrhage, or obstruction are treated surgically by one of two procedures, vagotomy or gastrectomy, or sometimes by both. Many variations of these two procedures exist, and the type of surgery elected depends on many factors, including the nature of the pathology and the patient's age and general condition.

The common aim in the surgical treatment of duodenal ulcers is to reduce permanently the stomach's capacity to secrete acid and pepsin. This objective can be achieved in at least four ways:

I. *Vagotomy* is the division of the vagus nerve branches to the stomach, thus eliminating the cephalic phase of gastric secretion. *Conventional truncal vagotomy* not only diminishes gastric secretions but also decreases gastric motility and emptying. Consequently, a "drainage" procedure is required to prevent gastric retention—either a gastrojejunostomy or pyloroplasty. Truncal vagotomy also denervates the hepatobiliary tract, pancreas, small intestine, and proximal colon. Two other types of vagotomy, selective and superselective vagotomy, are being used with increasing frequency. With *selective vagotomy*, only the branches of the vagus nerve that supply the stomach are transected, resulting in more complete vagotomy, less ulcer recurrence, and fewer postvagotomy complications. Because the antrum and pylorus are denervated, a drainage procedure is still required. *Superselective* or *parietal cell vagotomy* denervates only the acid-secreting portion of the stomach, sparing the branches that supply the antrum, which makes a gastric drainage procedure (e.g., pyloroplasty) unnecessary. More recently, the posterior truncal vagotomy and anterior lesser curve *seromyotomy* have come into use as a surgical treatment for chronic duodenal ulcer. The procedure results in denervation of the entire lesser curvature of the stomach while reducing acid secretion rates with no alteration in gastric emptying. This procedure is also gaining popularity because it can be performed using laparoscopic technique, making this surgery a minimally invasive procedure.

2. *Antrectomy* is the removal of the entire antrum of the stomach, thus eliminating the hormonal or gastric phase of gastric secretion.

3. *Vagotomy plus antrectomy* eliminates both the cephalic and the gastric phases of gastric secretion. Thus neural stimulation is interrupted, drainage is enhanced, and the major site of gastrin production is removed. This approach is thought to be superior to some of the more extensive surgical procedures.

4. *Partial gastrectomy* is the removal of the distal 50% to 75% of the stomach, thus removing a substantial portion of the acid-secreting and pepsin-secreting mucosa. After gastric resection, anastomosing the gastric remnant to the duodenum (*gastroduodenostomy*, or *Billroth I procedure*) or to the jejunum (*gastrojejunostomy*, or *Billroth II procedure*) restores GI continuity.

Fig. 24-9 illustrates some of the common surgical procedures for treating peptic ulcers. Most surgeons treat gastric ulcer by partial gastrectomy and a gastroduodenal anastomosis. The line of resection is usually proximal to the gastric ulcer. A vagotomy usually is not performed, because these patients have normal to low gastric acid production.

Postoperative Sequelae

Although modern surgery for peptic ulcer is effective in the treatment of ulcer complications and in the prevention of ulcer recurrence, numerous postoperative sequelae may occur. *Dumping syndrome* is a complication that occurs after eating in approximately 20% of patients after peptic ulcer surgery and is believed to result from the rapid emptying of hyperosmotic chyme into the intes-

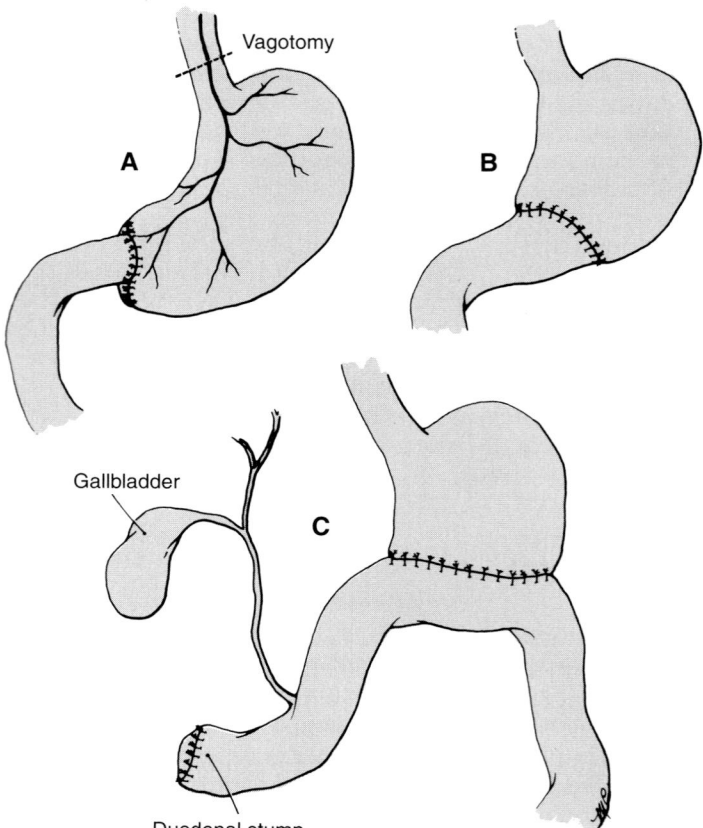

FIG. 24-9 Common surgical procedures for treating peptic ulcers. **A**, Vagotomy plus antrectomy (removal of pyloric antrum). **B**, Billroth I procedure (gastroduodenostomy anastomosis after resection). **C**, Billroth II procedure (gastrojejunostomy anastomosis after resection).

tine. The hypertonic contents of the intestine then cause a rapid fluid shift from the vascular compartment into the intestinal lumen. The decrease in plasma volume results in hypotension, which causes dizziness and weakness. The hypotension initiates reflex tachycardia, diaphoresis, and vasoconstriction of the skin, resulting in pallor. Feelings of fullness, nausea, vomiting, and diarrhea are common. Symptoms of *early dumping syndrome* occur during or within minutes after a meal.

Late dumping syndrome is a complex of similar symptoms occurring approximately 90 minutes to 3 hours after eating as a result of hypoglycemia in response to excessive insulin secretion. The increased insulin secretion is stimulated by an abrupt increase in blood glucose secondary to the rapid emptying of simple carbohydrates into the proximal intestine. The hyperosmolar material in the proximal intestine causes excessive release of enteroglucagon, which sensitizes the beta cells of the pancreatic islets so that large amounts of insulin are released. This action, in turn, overcorrects the hyperglycemia, resulting in hypoglycemia and related symptoms. Treatment consists of eating frequent, small meals that are low in carbohydrate and high in protein and restricting liquids at mealtimes. Restricting fluids at mealtime delays the emptying time of stomach contents into the small intestine. The stomach empties more rapidly after gastric resection because of decreased acid-secreting activity. For patients who have had gastric surgery, gastric emptying and limiting the hyperosmolarity of food intake are ongoing problems that often correct themselves over time. Antimuscarinic medications have been used for patients who fail to benefit from diet therapy.

Other sequelae after peptic ulcer surgery include recurrent ulcer caused by incomplete vagotomy or incomplete antrectomy; bile reflux gastritis; diarrhea, especially after truncal vagotomy; megaloblastic anemia caused by vitamin B_{12} malabsorption; osteomalacia and osteoporosis caused by malabsorption of calcium and vitamin D; general malabsorption and weight loss; and increased incidence of stomach cancer.

Acute Stress-Induced and Drug-Induced Ulcers

The term *stress ulcer* has been used to describe gastric or duodenal erosions that occur as a sequela to prolonged psychologic or physiologic stress. The stress may take many forms, such as hypotensive shock after traumatic injury and major surgery, sepsis, hypoxia, severe burns (Curling's ulcers), or cerebral trauma (Cushing's ulcers). Any seriously ill patient in an intensive care setting is susceptible to the development of a stress ulcer. Acute erosive and hemorrhagic gastritis induced by an alcoholic bout, aspirin or other ulcerogenic drugs, and bile reflux are often grouped with stress ulcers, because the lesions are similar.

Acute stress ulcers are usually shallow, irregular, punched-out lesions that may be large and multiple and are often located in the stomach. The lesions may bleed slowly, causing melena, and are often asymptomatic or are overshadowed by the serious illness in the patient. Because these lesions are superficial, they are not usually evident on radiographic examination.

Stress ulcers are clinically apparent when massive gastric hemorrhage or perforation occurs. In fact, stress ulcers account for 5% of all cases of peptic ulcer bleeding. Massive bleeding resulting from alcohol-induced acute erosive gastritis is also a common problem (see color plate 27).

Pathogenesis

Stress ulcers are generally divided into two different groups, based on probable pathogenic mechanisms. *Cushing's ulcers* associated with serious brain injury are characterized by marked hyperacidity, which is possibly mediated by vagal stimulation (cerebral injury → vagal stimulation → hyperacidity → acute peptic ulcer). On the other hand, stress ulcers associated with *shock, sepsis, burns,* and *drugs* are not characterized by gastric acid hypersecretion.

The mechanisms that provoke stress ulcerations of the gastric mucosa are much debated and still to be fully defined. Most investigators agree that ischemia of the gastric mucosa is the central etiologic factor leading to destruction of the gastric mucosal barrier and ulceration (Fig. 24-10). The mechanism by which ischemia is related to the formation of these lesions, however, is not fully understood. On the most simplistic level, the gastric mucosa is an organ of high metabolic activity requiring a

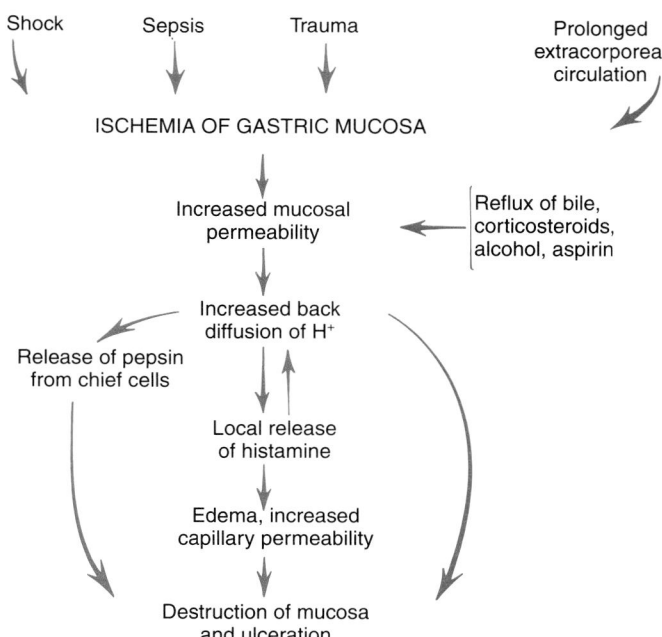

FIG. 24-10 Pathogenesis of "stress" ulcers. (Modified from Silen W, Skillman, JJ: *Advances in internal medicine,* Vol 19, Chicago, 1974, Mosby.)

consistent delivery of oxygen and substrate to maintain cellular integrity and its high renewal rate. Without the maintenance of adequate gastric mucosal blood flow, delivery of these nutrients must diminish. Consequently, mucosal cellular integrity must suffer with resultant cell death and a halt to cell renewal.

Other factors contributing to mucosal erosion include gastric acid in the stomach, reflux of bile, and decreased prostaglandins. Because stress ulcers occur in situations in which both increased gastric hyperacidity (Cushing's ulcers) and normal to decreased gastric acidity (e.g., Curling ulcers) occur, the volume of gastric acid may not be the key. Rather, the concentration of the luminal acid may be a more important factor in determining whether lesions will form; similar to the more common peptic ulcerations, it may serve as a pH facilitator for the action of pepsin in the digestion of the mucosa. Prostaglandins are resident in the gastric mucus and are known to have a protective effect on the mucosa. Aspirin and other NSAIDs cause their major effects mainly by inhibiting an enzyme, cyclooxygenase, which plays a key role in the synthesis of prostaglandins; this antiprostaglandin effect may explain the role of NSAIDs in irritating the gastric mucosa. Gastric ulcers develop in 10% to 30% of patients receiving chronic NSAID treatment (Friedman, Peterson, 1998).

Treatment

Recent studies reveal that the presence of erosive gastritis (stress ulcers) is a common finding in critically ill patients. Approximately 80% of severely burned patients have evidence of occult blood in their stools. Other studies have revealed an even higher incidence of stress ulcers identified by gastroscopy in critically ill patients. Most of these patients have no symptoms until massive bleeding takes place, which occurs in approximately 5% of cases.

This condition has led to the prophylactic treatment of high-risk patients with H_2 blockers, antacids, or sucralfate. The other 95% heal with little or no residual effects.

When bleeding is serious, some patients have been treated successfully by continuous intraarterial perfusion with vasopressin, a powerful vasoconstrictor. Vasopressin infusion is accomplished by inserting a catheter into an artery supplying the bleeding site and thereby controlling arterial bleeding. Vasopressin may also be infused into a peripheral vein to control bleeding from varices. The bleeding site is identified by arteriography, after which a vasopressin infusion is started. Thermal devices have been tested and are being used for hemostasis. Methods using these coagulation devices include electrocoagulation and photocoagulation (laser coagulation).

When these conservative methods of treatment fail, surgery may be the only method of treatment, even though these patients are critically ill and poor surgical risks. The most effective surgical procedure is total gastrectomy, because these erosions are multiple or diffuse and tend to rebleed.

STOMACH CANCER

Carcinoma of the stomach is the fourth most common form of GI neoplasm and accounts for approximately 2.4% of all cancer deaths (American Cancer Society, 1999). Men are more frequently affected than are women, and most cases occur after age 40.

The cause of stomach cancer is unknown, but certain predisposing factors are recognized. Genetic factors appear to be important, because gastric cancer is more common in persons with blood group A compared with other blood groups. Geographic or environmental factors also appear to be important, because gastric cancer is common in Japan, China, Thailand, Finland, Ireland, and Colombia. A carcinogenic factor in foods, such as smoked meats, pickled foods, and high nitrates, is associated with increased incidence of gastric cancer. For unknown reasons, gastric cancer has been declining in the United States during the last 60 years, occurring more often in lower socioeconomic groups. One of the most important predisposing factors is the presence of atrophic gastritis or pernicious anemia, as previously discussed. *H. pylori* infection is becoming more accepted as a factor in chronic atrophic gastritis and is, in turn, being associated with the increased risk of gastric cancer. A history of

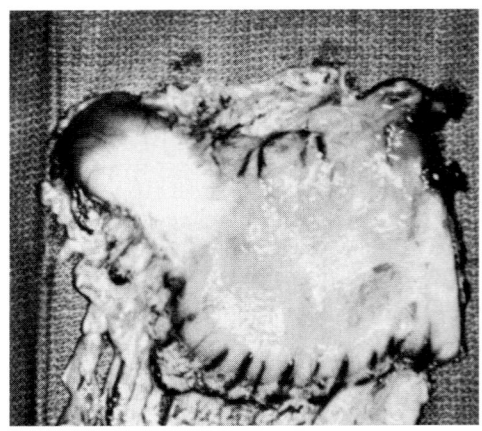

FIG. 24-11 Surgical specimen of gastric infiltrative carcinoma. The entire wall is cartilaginous and stiff.

nonhealing gastric ulcers is also associated with increased risk for stomach cancer.

Approximately 50% of gastric cancers are located in the pyloric antrum. The rest of the lesions are distributed throughout the body of the stomach.

Gastric carcinoma is classified under three general forms. *Ulcerating carcinoma* is the most common type and must be differentiated from a benign gastric ulcer. *Polypoid carcinoma* appears as a cauliflower-like mass protruding into the lumen and may arise from an adenomatous polyp. *Infiltrating carcinoma* may penetrate the entire thickness of the stomach wall and is responsible for the inflexible "leather bottle stomach" *(linitis plastica)* (Fig. 24-11).

Carcinoma of the stomach is seldom diagnosed in an early stage because symptoms develop late or are vague and indefinite. Early symptoms may include a mild feeling of discomfort in the upper abdomen or a feeling of fullness after eating. Eventually, the patient has anorexia and weight loss. When the tumor is located near the cardia, dysphagia may be the first major symptom. Vomiting from pyloric obstruction may occur when the tumor is near the gastric outlet.

Radiologic studies, exfoliative cytology, and endoscopy with biopsy are all important methods in the diagnosis of gastric cancer. Surgical excision is the only effective therapy. Because of the usually late diagnosis, the prognosis is poor, with a 10% 5-year survival rate.

*K*EY CONCEPTS

- The stomach is divided into the fundus, the body, and the pyloric antrum or pylorus. The cardiac sphincter, or lower esophageal sphincter (LES), lets food enter the stomach and prevents gastric reflux into the esophagus. The terminal pyloric sphincter relaxes and contracts to permit food to enter the duodenum and prevents backflow.

- The stomach is composed of four layers. The serosa (outer layer) is part of the visceral peritoneum. The muscularis is composed of three layers: an outer longitudinal layer, a middle circular layer, and an inner oblique layer.
- The submucosa is composed of loose areolar tissue connecting the muscularis and mucosal layers. The

inner layer, the mucosa, is arranged in longitudinal folds called *rugae* that allow for distention as the stomach fills.

- The stomach receives its extrinsic nerve supply from the autonomic nervous system. The parasympathetic nerve supply is conveyed through the vagus nerves, which give way to gastric, pyloric, and celiac branches. Sympathetic innervation is supplied via the greater splanchnic nerves and the celiac ganglia. The intrinsic nerve network of the stomach (which is continuous throughout the entire GI tract) is formed by Auerbach's (myenteric) and Meissner's nerve plexuses, allowing communication and coordination of GI motility and secretion. For example, the gastrocolic reflex (peristaltic wave in colon induced by entry of food or hot liquids into an empty stomach) is based on the intrinsic innervation of the GI tract.
- The motor functions of the stomach include the storing, mixing, and emptying of a semifluid mass of partly digested food mixed with gastric secretions. This substance is known as *chyme*.
- Cardiac glands that lie near the cardiac orifice of the stomach secrete mucus. Gastric glands in the fundus and body of the stomach have three types of cells: *parietal cells* secrete HCl and intrinsic factor (necessary for vitamin B_{12} absorption in the ileum); *chief cells* secrete pepsinogen, which is activated to pepsin in the presence of an acid pH; and *mucous neck cells* secrete mucus. *G cells* in the pyloric region secrete the hormone, gastrin.
- Gastric secretion is divided into three phases. The first is the *cephalic phase*, during which gastric glands are stimulated by the sight, smell, thought, or taste of food and account for 10% of gastric acid secretion. The second, *gastric or hormonal phase*, accounts for 67% of gastric acid secretion. When food enters the stomach, the alkaline pH and stomach wall distention stimulate the vagus nerve both chemically and mechanically. Vagal impulses stimulate the parietal cells and the G cells to release gastrin, causing secretion of HCl and pepsinogen. The final, *intestinal phase*, is initiated by the movement of chyme from the stomach to the duodenum and is largely inhibitory by hormones.
- Nausea and vomiting, common symptoms accompanying GI disorders, occur in three stages. The first is nausea, a highly disagreeable feeling in the back of the throat and the epigastrium. Retching, the next phase, is an involuntary attempt to vomit. The last stage, vomiting, is a reflex causing the forceful expulsion of stomach contents through the mouth.
- Gastritis is an inflammation or hemorrhagic condition of the gastric mucosa. The two most common types are acute superficial and chronic atrophic. *Acute gastritis* is a common benign disease resulting from a variety of factors that include *H. pylori* infection and local irritants, such as caffeine, alcohol, or aspirin. Chronic atrophic gastritis is characterized by progressive atrophy of the glandular epithelium, loss of parietal and chief cells, and hypochlorhydria or

achlorhydria. The gastric wall becomes thin, and the mucosa has an unusually smooth surface. *Type A chronic gastritis* is considered to be an uncommon autoimmune disease associated with the loss of intrinsic factor and pernicious anemia. *Type B chronic gastritis* is not associated with pernicious anemia and is largely caused by *H. pylori* infection.

- Peptic ulcers are circumscribed breaks in the mucosa, extending below the epithelium. Chronic ulcers, as opposed to acute ulcers, have scar tissue at the base.
- Pure acid gastric juice is capable of digesting all living tissues. Both the *gastric mucus* (containing prostaglandins) and the *epithelial barrier* protect the stomach from digesting itself. The gastric mucosal barrier also prevents back diffusion of H^+ from the lumen to the blood.
- When the permeability of the epithelial barrier is altered, a backflow of HCl with resultant injury to underlying tissues results. The mucosa becomes edematous and plasma proteins may be lost. The mucosal capillaries may be damaged, resulting in interstitial hemorrhage and bleeding. The destruction of the *gastric mucosal barrier* is believed to be a prime factor in the pathogenesis of gastric ulcers.
- Gastric or duodenal ulcers may be diagnosed by direct visualization using endoscopy. Cytologic examination of gastric washings is important to differentiate carcinoma of the stomach from a gastric ulcer. *H. pylori* infection is believed to be the cause of a large proportion of peptic ulcers. Methods used to detect *H. pylori* infection include the urea breath test and serologic testing methods.
- Chronic intermittent epigastric pain, usually 2 to 3 hours after a meal or at night, is the principal clinical feature of peptic ulcers. Food or antacids typically relieve the condition, which forms a "pain-food-relief pattern", the most important criterion in the diagnosis of these ulcers.
- The *Zollinger-Ellison syndrome* is an uncommon cause of peptic ulcers caused by a gastrin-secreting neoplasm, which results in extreme gastric hyperacidity. Peptic ulcers associated with this syndrome are often multiple and refractory to treatment. The ideal treatment is surgical excision of the neoplasm if it can be located.
- The medical treatment of peptic ulcers consists of measures to inhibit or buffer acid secretions to allow healing. Antacids, H_2 blockers (e.g., ranitidine) or gastric acid pump inhibitors (e.g., omeprazole), and antimicrobial therapy in the case of documented *H. pylori* infection may all be administered.
- Complications of peptic ulcers include *intractability* (most common), *hemorrhage*, *perforation*, and *obstruction*. Ulcers of the posterior duodenal wall are more apt to hemorrhage (because of erosion into the gastroduodenal or pancreaticoduodenal arteries), and ulcers of the anterior wall are more apt to perforate.
- The surgical treatment of peptic ulcers usually includes some type of vagotomy and partial gastrectomy. Antrectomy is the removal of the entire

antrum of the stomach, thus eliminating the gastric or hormonal phase of gastric secretion. A *Billroth I* or *gastroduodenostomy* procedure involves a partial gastrectomy with anastomosis of the remnant to the duodenum or with anastomosis of the remnant to the jejunum (*Billroth II* or *gastrojejunostomy*). Postoperative sequelae include the *dumping syndrome*, particularly with the Billroth II surgery.

■ Gastric or duodenal erosions that occur as a sequela to prolonged physiologic stress are referred to as *stress ulcers* and are divided into two groups. Cushing's ulcers are associated with serious brain injury and characterized by marked hyperacidity. Those associated with shock, sepsis, burn, and drugs are not characterized by gastric acid hypersecretion. Stress ulcers associated with burn injury are called Curling's ulcers. The central etiologic factor in the development of stress ulcers is believed to be ischemia of the gastric mucosa.

■ Genetic, geographic and environmental factors, and the presence of atrophic gastritis or pernicious anemia are all predisposing factors for carcinoma of the stomach, which can take on three general forms: *ulcerating carcinoma*, *polypoid carcinoma*, and *infiltrating carcinoma*.

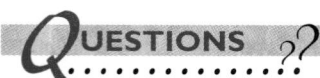

QUESTIONS ??

A sampling of review questions for this chapter appears here. Visit http://www.mosby.com/MERLIN/PriceWilson/ for additional questions.

Answer the following on a separate sheet of paper.

1. Sketch the stomach and indicate the location of the following: fundus, body, pyloric antrum, pyloric sphincter, cardiac region, lesser curvature, greater curvature, and glands secreting HCl and pepsin, intrinsic factor, and gastrin.
2. What are the lesser and greater omenta? Where are they located?
3. What are rugae and what is their purpose in the stomach?
4. How is pepsinogen activated in the stomach? What is the action of pepsin?
5. Describe the extrinsic and intrinsic innervation of the stomach and the function of each.
6. Name the truncal artery and its major branches supplying the stomach.
7. Why is hemorrhaging a more frequent complication in duodenal ulcers of the posterior wall?
8. List three motor functions of the stomach.
9. List three diagnostic procedures that can assist in identifying gastric and duodenal ulcers.
10. Why do patients become anemic when a deficiency or absence of intrinsic factor occurs?
11. What controls the mixing and emptying activities of the stomach?
12. What prevents the stomach from digesting itself? Explain your answer using the theories of gastric mucosal defense formulated by Hollander and Davenport. What drugs or chemicals may alter mucosal defense? What protects the duodenum from the actions of acid and pepsin?
13. List five effects of gastrin and the physiologic significance of each.
14. What is acute superficial gastritis? Do you think you have ever had this condition? What are the symptoms?
15. Explain how gastric secretions are controlled during the three phases of gastric secretion.

Match the following gastric acid analysis tests in column A with their diagnostic value in column B.

Column A
16. _____ Basal acid output (BAO)
17. _____ Maximum acid output (MAO)

Column B
a. Especially useful in the diagnosis of Zollinger-Ellison syndrome
b. May be used to determine if true achlorhydria is present

Match the following differentiating features of gastric and duodenal ulcers in column B with the type of peptic ulcer in column A.

Column A
18. _____ Gastric ulcer
19. _____ Duodenal ulcer

Column B
a. Symptomatic improvement with antacids
b. Nocturnal pain possible
c. Always should be treated surgically
d. Obstruction an infrequent problem
e. More common in people with blood type O
f. Higher frequency in persons subjected to stress

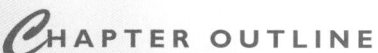

CHAPTER
25

Disorders of the Small Intestine

GLENDA N. LINDSETH

CHAPTER OUTLINE

ANATOMY

The small intestine is a complex, folded tube extending from the pylorus to the ileocecal valve. Approximately 12 feet (3.6 m) in length in a living person and nearly 22 feet (6.6m) in a cadaver (as a result of relaxation), the small intestine is contained in the central and lower part of the abdominal cavity. The proximal end is approximately 1.5 inches (3.8 cm) in diameter, but the diameter gradually diminishes to approximately 1 inch (2.5 cm) at the lower end.

The small intestine is divided into the duodenum, jejunum, and ileum. This division is rather imprecise and is based on slight modifications in structure and relatively more important differences in function. The *duodenum* is approximately 25 cm (10 inches) in length and extends from the pylorus to the jejunum. The division between the duodenum and jejunum is marked by the *ligament of Treitz*, a musculofibrous band that originates from the right crus of the diaphragm near the esophageal hiatus and attaches to the junction of the duodenum and jejunum, acting as a suspensory ligament. Approximately two fifths of the remaining intestine is the jejunum, and the terminal three fifths is the ileum. The *jejunum* lies in the left midabdominal region, and the *ileum* tends to lie in the right lower abdominal region. The *pyloric sphincter* controls entry of chyme into the small intestine, and the *ileocecal valve* controls exit of digested materials into the large intestine. The ileocecal valve also prevents reflux of contents from the large intestine into the small intestine.

The *vermiform appendix* is a blind tube approximately the size of the little finger located in the ileocecal region at the apex of the cecum. Inflammation or rupture of this structure is an important cause of morbidity in young people, although it is a less frequent cause of death now than it was in the preantibiotic era.

The wall of the small intestine is composed of four basic layers. The outer, or serous, coat is formed by the peritoneum. The *peritoneum* has a visceral and a parietal layer, and the potential space between these layers is called the *peritoneal cavity*. The peritoneum is reflected over and almost completely envelops the abdominal viscera.

Special names have been given to the folds of the peritoneum. The *mesentery* is a broad, fanlike fold of peritoneum that suspends the jejunum and ileum from the posterior abdominal wall and allows considerable motion of the bowel. The mesentery supports the blood and lymph vessels supplying the intestine. The *greater omentum* is a double layer of peritoneum that hangs from the greater curvature of the stomach and descends in front of the abdominal viscera similar to an apron. The omentum usually contains fat in considerable amounts and lymph nodes, which aid in protecting the peritoneal cavity against infection. The *lesser omentum* is the fold of peritoneum that extends from the lesser curvature of the stomach and upper duodenum to the liver, forming the hepatogastric and hepatoduodenal suspensory ligaments. One of the important functions of the peritoneum is to prevent friction between contiguous organs by secreting a serous fluid that acts as a lubricant. Inflammation of the peritoneum is called *peritonitis* and may be a serious sequela to inflammation or perforation of the bowel. *Adhesions* (fibrous bands) may develop after peritonitis or abdominal surgery, sometimes causing obstruction of the bowel.

The muscular coat of the small intestine has two layers: an outer, thinner layer of longitudinal fibers and an inner layer of circular fibers. This arrangement aids the peristaltic action of the small intestine. The submucosal layer is composed of connective tissue, and the inner mucosal layer is thick, vascular, and glandular.

Three structural features that greatly increase its surface area and aid in its primary function of absorption characterize the small intestine. The mucosal and submucosal layers are arranged in circular folds called *valvulae conniventes* (Kerckring's folds), which project approximately 3 to 10 mm into the lumen of the tube. These folds are prominent in the duodenum and jejunum and disappear near the midileum. Kerckring's folds are responsible for the feathery appearance of the small intestine on barium radiographs. The *villi* are fingerlike projections of mucosa numbering approximately 4 or 5 million and are present in the entire length of the small intestine (see Fig. 6-2). The villi are 0.5 to 1.5 mm in length (barely visible to the naked eye) and account for the velvetlike appearance of the mucosa. The *microvilli* are fingerlike projections approximately 1.0 μ in length along the outer surface of each individual villus, visible by electron microscopy and appearing as a *brush border* on light microscopy. If the lining of the small intestine were smooth, the surface area would then be approximately 2000 cm². The valvulae conniventes, villi, and microvilli combine to increase the total absorbing surface to 1.6 million cm², which is approximately a 1000-fold increase. Diseases of the small intestine (e.g., sprue) that cause atrophy and flattening of the villi greatly reduce the surface area for absorption, resulting in malabsorption.

Structure of the Villus

Fig. 25-1 illustrates the structure of a villus, which is the functional unit of the small intestine. Each villus consists of a central lymph channel called a *lacteal*, surrounded by a network of blood capillaries held together by connective tissue. This structure, in turn, is surrounded by columnar epithelial cells. After food has been digested, it passes into the lacteals and capillaries of the villi. The villous epithelium consists of two cell types: *goblet cells*, which produce mucus, and *absorptive cells* (with microvilli projecting from the surface), which are responsible for absorption of nutrients. Enzymes are located on the brush border and complete the process of digestion as absorption is taking place.

Surrounding each villus are several small pits called the *crypts of Lieberkühn*. These crypts are intestinal glands that produce secretions containing digestive enzymes. Undifferentiated cells in the crypts of Lieberkühn proliferate rapidly and migrate upward toward the tip of the villus, where they become absorptive cells. At the tip of the villus, these cells are shed into the intestinal lumen. Maturation and migration from the crypts to the tip of the villus require only 5 to 7 days. An estimated 20 to 50 million epithelial cells are extruded into the intestinal lumen each minute. Because of this high cell-turnover rate (fastest in the body), the intestinal epithelium is especially vulnerable to alterations in cell proliferation. Cytotoxic drugs given to treat cancer or leukemia inhibit cell division, resulting in mucosal atrophy and shortening of both crypts and villi. Patients receiving these drugs often develop ulcerations of the gastrointestinal (GI) mucosa. Villi may be flattened or absent in sprue.

Blood Supply and Innervation

The *superior mesenteric artery*, arising from the aorta immediately below the celiac artery, supplies all of the small intestine except the duodenum, which is supplied by the gastroduodenal artery and its branch, the superior pancreaticoduodenal artery. Blood is returned via the superior mesenteric vein, which unites with the splenic vein to form the portal vein.

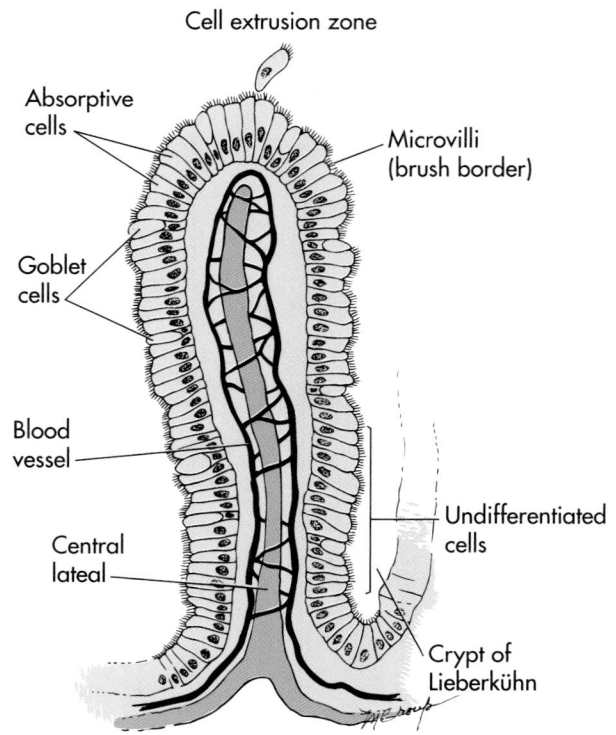

FIG. 25-1 Structure of a villus of the small intestine.

Both branches of the autonomic nervous system innervate the small intestine. Parasympathetic impulses stimulate secretory activity and motility, and those of the sympathetic system relay pain, whereas those of the parasympathetic regulate intestinal reflexes. The intrinsic nerve supply, which initiates motor function, passes through Auerbach's plexus in the muscular layer and Meissner's plexus in the submucosal layer.

PHYSIOLOGY

The small intestine has two primary functions: (1) digestion, the process of breaking down food into an assimilable form through the actions of various enzymes in the GI tract, and (2) absorption of ingested nutrients and water. All other activities either regulate or facilitate this process. The digestive process is initiated in the mouth and stomach by the actions of ptyalin, hydrochloric acid (HCl), pepsin, mucus, renin, and gastric lipase on the ingested food. The process is continued in the duodenum primarily by the action of pancreatic enzymes, which hydrolyze carbohydrates, fats, and proteins into simpler substances. The presence of bicarbonate in the pancreatic secretion helps neutralize the acid and provide an optimal pH for the action of the enzymes. Mucus also provides some protection from the acid. The secretion of bile from the liver aids the digestive process by emulsifying fats thus a greater surface area is presented for the action of pancreatic lipase.

The action of bile results from the detergent properties of conjugated bile acids, which solubilize lipid material by the formulation of micelles. *Micelles* are aggregates of bile acids and fat molecules. Fats form the hydrophobic core, and the bile acids, being polar molecules, form the surface of the micelles, with the hydrophobic end pointing inward and the hydrophilic end pointing outward toward the aqueous medium. The center of the micelle also dissolves fat-soluble vitamins and cholesterol. Thus free fatty acids, glycerides, and fat-soluble vitamins are kept in solution until they can be absorbed by the epithelial cell surface.

The process of digestion is completed by a number of enzymes present in the intestinal juice (succus entericus). Many of these enzymes are located on the brush border of the villi, and they digest food substances as they are being absorbed. Table 25-1 lists the principal digestive enzymes.

TABLE 25-1   ■■■

Principal Digestive Enzymes

Enzyme	Source	Substrate	Products	Optimal pH	Volume of Secretion* (Daily)
Salivary amylase (ptyalin)	Salivary glands	Starch	Maltose (a disaccharide and smaller carbohydrate polymer; minor physiologic role)	6-7	1-1.5 L
Pepsin	Chief cells of stomach	Protein	Proteoses, peptones	1.5-2.5	2-4 L
Gastric lipase	Stomach	Fat	Fatty acids, glycerides (minor physiologic role)	—	
Enterokinase	Duodenal mucosa	Trypsinogen	Trypsin		
Trypsin	Exocrine pancreas	Denatured proteins and polypeptides	Small polypeptides (also activates chymotrypsinogen to chymotrypsin)	8	0.6-0.8 L
Chymotrypsin		Proteins and polypeptides	Small polypeptides	8	
Carboxypeptidases		Polypeptides	Smaller polypeptides (removes C-terminal amino acid)	—	
Nucleases		Nucleic acids	Nucleotides	—	
Pancreatic lipase		Fat	Glycerides, fatty acids, glycerol	8	
Pancreatic amylase		Starch	Disaccharides	6.7-7	
Bile acids (not an enzyme)	Liver	Unemulsified fats	Emulsified fats (formation of micelles; action is physical)	7.5	0.8-1 L
Aminopeptidases	Intestinal glands	Polypeptides	Smaller polypeptides (removes N-terminal amino acid)	8	2-3 L
Dipeptidase		Dipeptides	Amino acids	—	
Maltase		Maltose	Glucose	5-7	
Lactase		Lactose	Glucose + galactose (all monosaccharides)		
Sucrase		Sucrose	Glucose + fructose		
Intestinal lipase		Fat	Glycerides, fatty acids, glycerol	8	
Nucleotidase		Nucleotides	Nucleosides, phosphoric acid	8	

*All secretions are reabsorbed, except about 100 ml water normally excreted in stool per day.

Two hormones are important in the regulation of intestinal digestion. Fat, in contact with the duodenal mucosa, causes the gallbladder to contract, which is mediated by the action of *cholecystokinin*. Products of partially digested proteins and fatty acids in contact with the duodenal mucosa stimulate the secretion of pancreatic juice rich in enzymes, which is mediated by the action of *pancreozymin*. Pancreozymin and cholecystokinin are considered to be the same hormone having two different effects; it is called *CCK* (some textbooks still refer to this hormone as CCK-PZ). This hormone is produced by the duodenal mucosa.

Gastric acid in contact with the intestinal mucosa causes the release of another hormone, *secretin*, and the amount released is proportional to the amount of acid flowing through the duodenum. Secretin stimulates the secretion of the bicarbonate-containing juice from the pancreas and bile from the liver and also potentiates the action of CCK.

Segmental movements of the small intestine mix ingested materials with pancreatic, hepatobiliary, and intestinal secretions, and peristaltic movements propel the contents from one end to the other at a rate suitable for optimal absorption and continuing entry of gastric contents.

Absorption

Absorption is the transfer of the end products of carbohydrate, fat, and protein digestion (simple sugars, fatty acids, and amino acids) across the intestinal wall to the vascular and lymphatic circulation for use by the body cells. Additionally, water, electrolytes, and vitamins are absorbed. Absorption of the various substances takes place by both active and passive transport mechanisms that are, for the most part, poorly understood.

Although many substances are absorbed throughout the entire length of the small bowel, principal sites are responsible for absorption for specific nutrients. Knowledge of these absorption sites is necessary to understand the way in which disease of the intestine may cause specific nutritional deficiencies (Fig. 25-2).

The absorption of sugars, amino acids, and fats is largely complete by the time the chyme reaches the mid-jejunum. Iron and calcium are absorbed primarily in the duodenum and jejunum, and absorption of calcium requires vitamin D. Absorption of the fat-soluble vitamins (A, D, E, and K) is facilitated by bile acids and occurs in the duodenum and upper jejunum. Most water-soluble vitamins are absorbed in the upper small intestine. The absorption of vitamin B_{12} takes place in the terminal ileum by a special transport mechanism requiring gastric intrinsic factor. Most of the bile acids released by the gallbladder into the duodenum to aid in the digestion of fats are reabsorbed in the terminal ileum and recirculated to the liver. This circuit is termed the *enterohepatic recirculation of bile salts* and is important in maintaining the bile pool. The bile acids or salts thus perform their action in relation to fat digestion many times before being excreted in the feces. Disease or resection of the terminal ileum may thus cause deficiency of bile salts and interference with fat digestion. The entry of large amounts of bile salts into the colon causes colonic irritation and diarrhea.

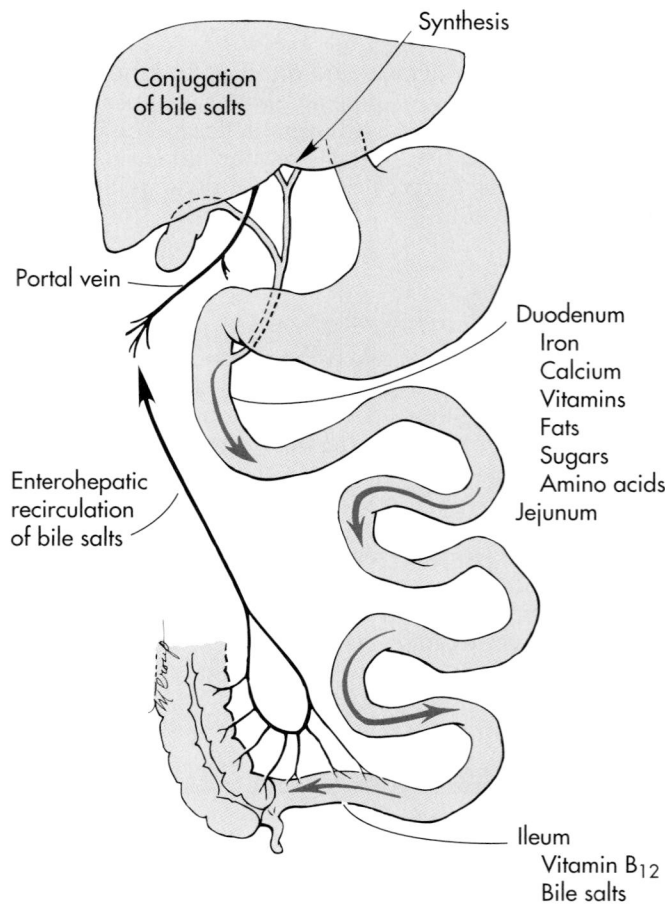

FIG. 25-2 Primary absorption sites of the major nutrients and the enterohepatic recirculation of bile salts for reconjugation by the liver.

MALABSORPTION

Diseases of the small intestine are often accompanied by alterations in function manifested by the malabsorption syndrome. *Malabsorption* is the condition in which intestinal mucosal absorption of single or multiple nutrients is impaired, resulting in inadequate movement of digested food from the small intestine into the blood or lymphatic system.

Distinguishing between malabsorption and maldigestion is important, because increased loss of nutrients in the stool may be a reflection of either process. *Maldigestion* refers to a breakdown of the chemical processes of digestion that take place in the intestinal lumen or at the brush border of the intestinal mucosa, resulting in a failure to absorb nutrients.

Causes

Box 25-1 lists some of the more common causes of the malabsorption syndrome. The basic causes of maldigestion are included in the first three categories. Gastrectomy, particularly the Billroth II procedure, causes poor mixing of chyme with gastric secretions. Hepatobiliary disease may result in insufficiency of intraluminal bile acids. Failure of the pancreas to produce or release sufficient enzymes may result from a number of pancreatic disorders. Failure of the release of CCK, which stimulates pancreatic secretion, may occur in Zollinger-Ellison syndrome as a result of excessive acidification of the duodenum or may result from disease of the intestinal mucosa itself, as in sprue. Disease of the terminal ileum or ileal resection for treatment of regional enteritis may cause a deficiency of bile salts by interfering with ileal resorption. Bacterial overgrowth in the duodenal stump (blind or afferent loop created in the Billroth II procedure) causes vitamin B_{12} malabsorption by using this vitamin and causes fat maldigestion by deconjugating bile salts. Unconjugated bile salts are effective to a lesser extent in forming micelles and are absorbed less in the ileum. Lack of intrinsic factor causes inability to absorb vitamin B_{12}; lack of B_{12} causes pernicious anemia. A hereditary lack of lactase causes selective malabsorption of lactose (a milk disaccharide) and is common in Hispanics, African Americans, and Southeast Asian populations. Mesenteric atherosclerosis (abdominal angina) may cause malabsorption and is a source of discomfort in older adults but is infrequently diagnosed. Chapter 27 deals with pancreatic and hepatobiliary disorders, and this chapter discusses a few of the more common intestinal disorders associated with malabsorption.

Signs and Symptoms

The signs and symptoms of malabsorption may be divided into two groups: those resulting from abnormal content in the intestinal lumen and those resulting from deficiency of dietary nutrients. Weight loss, diarrhea, steatorrhea (fatty stools), flatulence, and nocturia are the most common signs and symptoms and all are caused by abnormal intestinal luminal content. Table 25-2 lists the signs and symptoms of malabsorption and their pathophysiologic basis.

Detection

Most of the tests useful in the diagnosis of malabsorption indicate the presence of either malabsorptive or maldigestive disturbances. Only a few of the tests distinguish between these two entities. A combination of tests is often necessary to make a diagnosis.

Stool Fat

The oldest and most reliable test for documenting the presence of steatorrhea, and thus malabsorption, is the quantitative determination of stool fat. Qualitatively, the stool can be examined for neutral fat, split fats, and undigested muscle fibers. This screen can be reliable for steatorrhea and a means of differentiating between celiac sprue and pancreatic insufficiency. Normal individuals excrete less than 6 g of fat in the stool per day. Fat excretion in excess of 6 g is considered excessive and is termed *steatorrhea.* In severe cases, the stools are abnormal to the naked eye and appear pale, greasy, and frothy and may float; they may stick to the side of the toilet and not flush away easily.

A 72-hour stool collection for quantitative fat determination is routinely used to eliminate errors resulting from daily variations. Testing stools for fat is essential in

BOX 25-1
Some Causes of Malabsorption Syndrome

PRIOR GASTRIC SURGERY
Total gastrectomy
Billroth II gastrectomy
Pyloroplasty
Vagotomy

PANCREATIC DISORDERS
Chronic pancreatitis
Pancreatic cancer
Cystic fibrosis
Pancreatic resection
Zollinger-Ellison syndrome

HEPATOBILIARY DISEASE
Biliary tract obstruction
Cirrhosis and hepatitis
Biliary fistula

DISEASE OF THE SMALL INTESTINE
Primary disease of small bowel
    Nontropical sprue
    Tropical sprue
    Regional enteritis
    Massive bowel resection
    Bacterial overgrowth from stasis in afferent loop after
        Billroth II gastrectomy
Ischemic disease of small bowel
    Mesenteric atherosclerosis
    Chronic congestive heart failure
Infections and infestations of small bowel
    Acute enteritis
    Giardiasis
Systemic disease involving small bowel
    Whipple's disease
    Amyloidosis
    Sarcoidosis
    Scleroderma
    Lymphoma

HEREDITARY DISORDER
Primary lactase deficiency

DRUG-INDUCED MALABSORPTION
Neomycin
Calcium carbonate

the diagnosis of nontropical sprue, after extensive gastrectomy, and in other malabsorptive disorders. This test does not differentiate between maldigestion as in pancreatic disorders and malabsorption caused by an intestinal disease such as nontropical sprue. However, the level of undigested meat fibers in the stool is significantly increased in pancreatic insufficiency that is not usually present in nontropical sprue.

D-xylose Absorption Test

D-xylose is a relatively inert five-carbon monosaccharide (pentose) that is absorbed in the proximal bowel without digestion, passes through the liver, and is then excreted by the kidneys. Measurement of the amount of D-xylose excreted in the urine therefore gives an indication of the absorptive capacity of the small intestinal mucosa. This test is useful to assess for carbohydrate absorption. The test is carried out after the patient has fasted for 12 hours. At least 20% of a 25 g dose of

TABLE 25-2

Signs and Symptoms of Malabsorption Syndrome

Sign or Symptom	Pathophysiology
Weight loss and generalized malnutrition	Impaired absorption of carbohydrate, fat, and protein leading to loss of calories
Diarrhea	Excess load of fluids and electrolytes introduced into colon, which may exceed its absorptive capacity; bile acids and fatty acids in colon cause decreased colonic absorption of sodium and water and laxative effect from colonic irritation
Steatorrhea (bulky, frothy, voluminous stools)	Excess fat content of feces
Flatulence, abdominal distention	Undigested lactose → fermentation → gas formation
	Undigested lactose → osmotic effect → shift of extracellular fluid into gut → diarrhea (may be caused by primary lactase deficiency or secondary damage to brush border from intestinal lesions)
Nocturia	Delayed absorption and excretion of water (may be pooled in gut during day)
Weakness and easy fatigability	Anemia; electrolyte depletion caused by diarrhea (hypokalemia, hypomagnesemia)
Edema	Impaired absorption of amino acids → protein depletion → hypoproteinemia
Amenorrhea	Protein depletion → secondary hypopituitarism
Anemia	Impaired absorption of iron, folic acid, and vitamin B_{12}
Glossitis, cheilosis	Deficiency of iron, folic acid, vitamin B_{12}, and other vitamins
Peripheral neuropathy	Deficiency of vitamin B_{12}, thiamine
Bruising, bleeding tendency	Vitamin K malabsorption, hypoprothrombinemia
Bone pain, skeletal deformities, fractures	Calcium malabsorption → hypocalcemia; protein depletion → osteoporosis; vitamin D malabsorption → impaired calcium absorption
Tetany, paresthesias	Calcium malabsorption → hypocalcemia; magnesium malabsorption → hypomagnesemia and hypokalemia
Eczema	Cause uncertain

D-xylose given orally should be excreted in the urine in 5 hours, providing that renal function is normal. Excretion of less than this amount or blood levels of D-xylose lower than 30 mg/dl indicates malabsorption. Abnormal D-xylose test results are found most frequently in disorders affecting the proximal bowel, such as sprue. The results are normal in maldigestive disorders such as chronic pancreatitis.

Schilling Test for Vitamin B_{12} Absorption

The Schilling test is a valuable measure of vitamin B_{12} absorption and is frequently carried out in stages to determine the specific cause of the malabsorption. When urine collection is adequate, low excretion of ^{60}Co-tagged vitamin B_{12} indicates impaired absorption as a result of a lack of intrinsic factor (pernicious anemia), bacterial overgrowth in the proximal small bowel after Billroth II gastrectomy, diseased ileal mucosa as in regional enteritis, or pancreatic insufficiency. Correction of the malabsorption with intrinsic factor confirms intrinsic factor deficiency, which causes pernicious anemia. If the Schilling test returns to normal after antibiotic therapy, this result helps to confirm the diagnosis of malabsorption as a result of bacterial overgrowth in the proximal bowel after Billroth II gastrectomy (the bacteria take up vitamin B_{12} thus preventing its absorption). Malabsorption of vitamin B_{12} as a result of pancreatic insufficiency may be corrected by the administration of pancreatic enzymes. Vitamin B_{12} malabsorption resulting from regional enteritis involving the terminal ileum is not corrected by any of the measures mentioned.

Culture of Duodenal and Jejunal Contents

The most reliable test for confirming the presence of bacterial overgrowth in the proximal bowel is aspiration and culture of the contents. The proximal small bowel normally contains less than 10^5 organisms/ml, and these are generally of the oropharyngeal variety. The most important mechanisms keeping the proximal bowel bacteriologically sterile are the normal peristalsis that sweeps bacteria distally, the gastric acid, and the secretion of immunoglobulin A (IgA) into the gut. Consequently, any condition that causes stasis of proximal intestinal contents, such as the blind loop after Billroth II surgery, may result in macrocytic anemia (because of use of vitamin B_{12} by organisms), diarrhea, and steatorrhea (because of deconjugation of bile salts by bacteria). Gastric achlorhydria and hypogammaglobulinemia are other conditions that may cause bacterial overgrowth.

GI Barium Radiologic Studies

The radiographic appearance of the small bowel may be nonspecific or diagnostic. Characteristic features in the malabsorption syndrome are the loss of the feathery pattern of the barium and increased flocculation of the barium with segmentation and clumping. This finding is common in sprue but is also found in other malabsorptive disorders. In regional enteritis, the ileal lumen may be narrowed (i.e., the "string sign").

Biopsy of the Small Intestine

The biopsy is a useful test to examine abnormalities in diseases such as sprue because a biopsy of the intestinal mucosa can reveal atrophy of villi. The biopsy may be performed through the use of a sighted endoscope or the less commonly used suction capsule endoscope along with radiography to identify mucosal lesions.

Breath Tests

The human body does not normally produce hydrogen gas (H_2), which is, however, a normal by-product of bacterial carbohydrate metabolism. The fasting patient normally has a low baseline concentration of expired H_2. This principle has been used to design several noninvasive breath tests that assist in the diagnosis of various malabsorption disorders.

The *lactose breath test* is a sensitive test for detecting lactase deficiency (see later discussion). Fifty grams of lactose is given by mouth, and the patient's breath H_2 is monitored. Normally, the lactose is absorbed and, in the absence of bacterial overgrowth of the small intestine, the patient's breath H_2 does not increase significantly. Malabsorption of lactose produces high peaks of H_2 excretion caused by colonic fermentation. The *lactulose breath test* and the *^{14}C-cholylglycine (bile acid) breath test* are used to detect bacterial overgrowth within the small bowel. Ingestion of lactulose (a nonabsorbable disaccharide) normally produces a sharp increase in H_2 when it arrives in the cecum and it is sometimes used in this way to estimate the intestinal transit time. An earlier peak of breath H_2 after lactulose ingestion suggests small bowel bacterial overgrowth. In the bile acid breath test, ^{14}C-labeled bile acid is given by mouth and is normally absorbed intact and undergoes enterohepatic circulation. Consequently, little $^{14}CO_2$ is released in the breath. If degraded by bacteria, the ^{14}C is metabolized and eventually exhaled as $^{14}CO_2$. An early peak of breath $^{14}CO_2$ is typical of a patient with proximal bowel bacterial overgrowth, although raised levels also occur with bile salt malabsorption (as in regional enteritis) as a result of degradation by colonic bacteria.

PRIMARY SMALL INTESTINAL DISORDERS ASSOCIATED WITH MALABSORPTION

Nontropical Sprue (Celiac Disease)

Idiopathic steatorrhea in adults and celiac disease in children are the most important causes of severe malabsorption in nontropical areas. Both of these conditions are considered phases of the same disease. Sprue is characterized by marked atrophy of the villi in the proximal small intestine, induced by ingestion of gluten-containing foods (see color plate 28).

Pathophysiology

Gluten is a high–molecular-weight protein found in rye, oats, barley, and particularly wheat. Found in bread, bread products, beer, and many other processed foods, gluten or gluten breakdown products or both (particularly gliadin) are toxic to patients with this disease. Symptoms disappear when gluten is withdrawn from the diet and reappear when it is reintroduced. The characteristic lesion of the bowel mucosa induced by gluten is blunting or loss of the villi and elongation of the crypts, which cause the mucosa to appear flat. The loss of villi causes a marked reduction of absorptive surface.

Although the mechanism of gluten toxicity is not understood, it has been suggested that these patients lack a specific peptidase that would normally detoxify a noxious peptide of gluten. This hypothesis is supported by the fact that a strong familial and genetic tendency exists in occurrence. Also proposed is that gluten or its metabolites cause a hypersensitivity reaction in the intestinal mucosa. This theory is supported by the fact that circu-

lating antibodies to gliadin have been found in patients with this disease and that partial improvement of symptoms is provided by corticosteroid therapy.

Clinical Features

Presumably, patients with nontropical sprue are born with the disease tendency but may not develop symptoms for many years, even though they include gluten in the diet. Factors that precipitate the clinical onset are unknown. The onset generally occurs in infants between ages 6 months and 2 years and in adults between ages 20 and 50 years. The symptoms seldom begin during childhood or adolescence.

In infants, anorexia, irritability, and diarrhea with pale, bulky stools are soon followed by weight loss. If the infant is not treated, failure to grow is then soon obvious. Diarrhea, lassitude, weakness, and steatorrhea are the most common symptoms in adults, but patients may have any of the signs and symptoms of malabsorption syndrome listed in Table 25-2. Adults frequently have a history suggesting sprue during childhood.

The diagnosis is established by evidence of malabsorption, typical small-bowel biopsy changes, and clinical improvement on a gluten-free diet.

Treatment

The treatment of nontropical sprue by a gluten-free diet is generally successful, provided the patient adheres to the diet. Response to the gluten-free diet is noted by the return of normal color to the stools, disappearance of diarrhea, and increase in weight. The minority of patients who do not respond to a gluten-free diet may respond to corticosteroids; however, those who do not may have a dismal prognosis. Mortality was 20% before discovery of the gluten-free dietary treatment during World War II, but it is now almost nil in gluten-sensitive cases.

Tropical Sprue

Tropical sprue occurs in tropical regions such as Puerto Rico, India, and southwestern Asia. The signs and symptoms are similar to those of nontropical sprue, and the biopsy changes are similar but less severe. The condition is a malabsorptive disorder with the cause not really known. Malabsorption of at least two nutrients is considered essential for the diagnosis. Patients are usually deficient in iron, as well as vitamin B_{12} and folate. Most patients improve after combined treatment with folic acid and a broad-spectrum antibiotic, such as tetracycline.

Lactase Deficiency

As indicated in the previous discussion, hydrolysis of disaccharides to monosaccharides occurs within the brush border of the intestinal mucosa. Deficiency of specific enzymes that hydrolyze disaccharides may be present as a result of a genetic defect or may be secondary to a wide variety of GI diseases that damage the mucosa of the small intestine.

Lactase deficiency is the most common type of the disaccharide deficiency syndromes. Lactase is an enzyme that normally splits lactose (a disaccharide) into glucose and galactose (monosaccharides) at the intestinal brush border so that absorption may take place. Because lactose is the principal carbohydrate in milk, many persons showing milk intolerance prove to be lactase deficient. Significant racial variation exists in primary lactase deficiency. Approximately 5% to 10% of the Caucasian population is lactase deficient, but the incidence is as high as 80% to 90% among African Americans, Hispanics, Asians, and Bantus. Although lactase deficiency appears to be hereditary, milk intolerance may not become clinically apparent until adolescence. Secondary lactase deficiency is associated with a large number of conditions that cause intestinal mucosal injury, such as nontropical and tropical sprue, regional enteritis, viral and bacterial infections of the intestinal tract, giardiasis, cystic fibrosis, and ulcerative colitis.

Typical symptoms of lactase deficiency are abdominal cramps, bloating, and diarrhea after milk ingestion. The pathogenic mechanism explaining the diarrhea is as follows. When unhydrolyzed lactose enters the large intestine, an osmotic effect is produced, causing the entry of water into the colonic lumen. Colonic bacteria also ferment the lactose, producing lactic and fatty acids that are irritating to the colon. The result is increased motility, which is caused by colonic irritation, and an explosive diarrhea.

A history of intolerance to milk or milk products and a decreased fecal pH of 6.0 (normal pH 7.0 to 7.5) are strongly suggestive of lactase deficiency. The diagnosis is confirmed by the lactose breath test, as described earlier, or by the lactose tolerance test. The *lactose tolerance test* consists of giving 50 g of lactose and then measuring the blood glucose level as for a glucose tolerance test; in lactase deficiency, the blood sugar fails to rise more than 20 mg/dl above the fasting level. Treatment consists of eliminating milk and milk products from the diet. However, patients are often able to tolerate yogurt because it contains bacterial-derived lactases.

Postgastrectomy Malabsorption

Malabsorption and weight loss are well-recognized features after a gastrectomy and are the rule after total gastrectomy, common after the Billroth II procedure, and rare after the Billroth I procedure. Increased fat loss in the stools occurs in many patients after the Billroth II procedure, particularly when the duodenal stump (afferent or blind loop) is long. The principal causes of the steatorrhea are the following: (1) poor mixing of food and enzymes because of rapid emptying of the gastric remnant (low concentration of digestive secretion and food particles too large for the enzymes); (2) reduced pancreatic output because the duodenum is bypassed and has less stimulation by the acid chyme to release secretin and CCK; (3) stasis of intestinal contents in the afferent loop, resulting in abnormal bacterial proliferation, which uses up vitamin B$_{12}$ and deconjugates bile salts; and (4) the loss of stomach reservoir function, which may result in a more rapid intestinal transit time with resultant diarrhea.

If malabsorption is severe, the patient may then be at risk to develop symptoms as a result of the nutritive deficiencies listed in Table 25-2. Identification of the mechanism responsible for the malabsorption is essential for optimal treatment of postgastrectomy malabsorption. Broad-spectrum antibiotics such as tetracycline may be given when the cause is bacterial overgrowth. Pancreatic enzyme therapy may be helpful with functional pancreatic deficiency (a condition of insufficient production of pancreatic enzymes that are required for protein digestion). Smaller meals that are low in carbohydrates and taken without fluids may help delay rapid gastric emptying (dumping syndrome).

Regional Enteritis (Crohn's Disease)

Regional enteritis, ileocolitis, or *Crohn's disease* is a chronic, relapsing granulomatous inflammatory disease of the intestinal tract. Classically the terminal ileum is affected, although any portion of the GI tract may be involved. The condition usually develops in young adults in the second or third decade of life and is more prevalent again in the sixth decade. Men and women are equally affected. Crohn's disease tends to be familial and is most common in Caucasian and Jewish populations.

The etiology of regional enteritis is unknown. Although no autoantibodies have been demonstrated, it has been speculated that regional enteritis may represent a hypersensitivity reaction or may be caused by an infectious agent that has yet to be identified. These theories are suggested by the granulomatous lesions, which are similar to those found in fungal and tubercular lesions of the lung.

Some interesting similarities exist between regional enteritis and ulcerative colitis. Both are inflammatory diseases, although the lesions of each are distinct. Both diseases have extragastrointestinal manifestations, including uveitis, arthritis, and skin lesions that are identical. Smoking is a strong risk factor for Crohn's disease but not for ulcerative colitis (Rubin, Hanauer, 2000). Further similarities and differences are discussed in Chapter 26.

Pathology

The terminal ileum is involved in regional enteritis in approximately 75% of the cases. In approximately 35% of the cases, lesions occur in the colon. The esophagus and stomach are less frequently affected. In some instances, "skip" lesions occur; that is, portions of diseased bowel are separated by areas of normal bowel a few inches or several feet long.

Lesions are believed to begin in the bowel wall or in the lymph nodes next to the small bowel, with eventual obstruction of the lymphatic channels of drainage. The submucosal coat of the intestine becomes greatly thickened as a result of the hyperplasia of the lymphoid tissue and lymphedema. With progress of the pathologic process, the affected segment of the bowel becomes thickened to such a degree that it is as stiff as a garden hose (Fig. 25-3). The lumen of the bowel may become greatly narrowed, so that it admits only a thin stream of barium, giving rise to the "string sign" observed radiographically. The entire thickness of the bowel wall is typically involved. The mucosa is usually inflamed and ulcerated with grayish white exudate. These ulcerated patches can contain fissures and cobblestone granulomas.

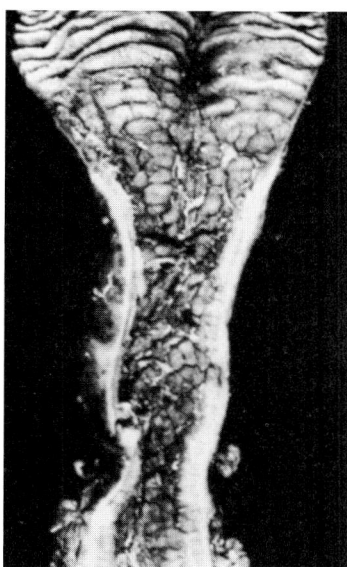

FIG. 25-3 Regional enteritis (Crohn's disease). The gut wall has been thickened by inflammation and scarring, causing marked narrowing of the lumen. The mucosa at the top is more normal looking. Extending downward are longitudinal ulcers that cross the transverse folds, giving the mucosa a cobblestone appearance. (Courtesy Henry D. Appleman, MD, Associate Professor of Pathology, University of Michigan.)

Clinical Features

The signs and symptoms of regional enteritis vary a great deal according to whether the disease is early or late and according to what parts of the GI tract are involved. Mild intermittent diarrhea, flatulence, fever, colicky pain in the lower abdomen, and malaise increasing over a period of years are typical symptoms. Patients with more severe forms of the disease may have frequent liquid stools with blood and pus. Some patients develop steatorrhea, weight loss, anemia, and other manifestations of malabsorption. Low-grade fever is common.

Certain complications are typical of regional enteritis. The development of stenosis may cause symptoms of vomiting and other signs of intestinal obstruction. Similarly, right ureteral obstruction and hydronephrosis may occur as a result of external compression of the ureter by the ileal mass. An ulcerous lesion may perforate through the intestinal wall, causing peritonitis. More frequently, the perforation is closed, and fistulas are formed between loops of bowel, or less frequently, it involves the bladder or vagina. Ulcers, abscesses, and fistulas often occur in the perianal and perirectal regions. External fistulas to the anterior abdominal wall may also occur. High fever is usually associated with extensive inflammation or complications such as fistulas and abscesses.

Up to 30% of patients with ileal disease eventually develop gallstones. The presence of extensive ileal disease, resulting in bile salt malabsorption, is associated with a decreased bile salt pool and increased bile lithogenicity. The patient is also predisposed to urinary oxalate stone formation caused by increased colonic absorption of dietary oxalate. Diarrhea resulting in dehydration is an additional risk factor for renal stone formation.

Extragastrointestinal manifestations of the disease, such as arthritis, uveitis, and skin lesions, occur but are less frequent than they are in ulcerative colitis.

The diagnosis is established based on the clinical presentation, the characteristic radiographic changes, and in the case of colonic or rectal involvement, biopsy changes showing granulomatous lesions. Laboratory examination is not typically used in diagnosis as much as it is for measuring malabsorption and extent of the inflammatory process.

Treatment and Prognosis

No specific or curative treatment exists for regional enteritis. The initial management of most patients is medical, supportive, and palliative, aimed at attaining remission of the disease. Corticosteroid, azathioprine (Imuran), 6-mercaptopurine (6-MP), and sulfasalazine (Azulfidine) are used to promote remission and control suppurative complications. Anticholinergic drugs, such as propantheline bromide (Pro-Banthine), and antidiarrheal drugs, such as diphenoxylate with atropine (Lomotil), may help reduce cramping, abdominal pain, and diarrhea. These drugs are contraindicated if bowel obstruction occurs. Nutrient deficiencies and steatorrhea are treated by the appropriate replacements and a low-fat, low-residue diet. Blood volume and fluid and electrolyte imbalances may be restored by intravenous (IV) fluids, hyperalimentation or blood replacement.

Surgical treatment is generally avoided because recurrence and spread of the lesion is usual after surgical resection. Nevertheless, surgical intervention is usually necessary sometime during the course of the disease to treat complications.

When regional enteritis is characterized by an acute onset, as many as 90% of the patients can achieve remission. However, regional enteritis has an insidious onset in most patients. Approximately 75% of the patients experience relapses. Mortality as a direct result of the disease is low.

APPENDICITIS

Appendicitis is the most common major surgical disease. Although it may occur at any age, appendicitis is most common in adolescents and young adults. Before the era of antibiotics, the mortality from this disease was high.

Pathogenesis

The *vermiform appendix* is the remnant of the apex of the cecum and has no known function in humans. This structure is a long, narrow tube (approximately 6 to 9 cm) and contains the appendicular artery, which is an end artery.

In the usual position, the appendix is located on the abdominal wall under McBurney's point. *McBurney's point* is located by drawing a line from the right anterior superior iliac spine to the umbilicus. The midpoint of this line locates the root of the appendix (Fig. 25-4).

Appendicitis is an inflammation of the appendix involving all layers of the wall of the organ (see color plate 29). The primary pathogenic hallmark is obstruction of the lumen, usually by a *fecalith* (hardened stool typically formed around vegetable fibers). Obstruction of the outflow of mucous secretions then results in swelling, infection, and ulceration. The increased intraluminal pressure may cause occlusion of the appendicular end artery. When the condition is allowed to progress, necrosis, gangrene, and perforation usually result. Current research indicates that appendicitis begins with ulceration of the mucosa in approximately 60% to 70% of the cases, rather than luminal obstruction. The cause of the ulceration is unknown, but a viral origin has been speculated. An infection by the *Yersinia enterocolitica* is the most recently speculated cause.

Clinical Features

In the classic case of acute appendicitis, the initial symptoms are mild periumbilical pain or discomfort. These symptoms generally develop over 1 or 2 days. Within hours the pain shifts to the lower right quadrant, followed by anorexia, nausea, and vomiting. Tenderness to palpation over McBurney's point may also be present. Later, muscle spasm and rebound tenderness may be present. A low-grade fever and moderate leukocytosis are usual findings. When rupture of the appendix occurs, signs of the perforation may include pain, tenderness, and spasm. This event often follows a brief dramatic relief from pain.

Diagnostic Problems

The diagnosis of even the classic case of appendicitis is complicated because many disorders present a similar clinical picture of an acute abdominal condition and must be differentiated from acute appendicitis. Some of these conditions include the following:

1. Acute gastroenteritis (probably the most common)
2. Mesenteric lymphadenitis in children
3. Ruptured ectopic pregnancy

4. Mittelschmerz (pain caused by rupture of ovarian follicle during ovulation)
5. Pelvic inflammatory disease
6. Regional enteritis
7. Inflammation of Meckel's diverticulum (persistence of a duct that, in the fetus, extends from the ileum to the umbilicus; this condition is rare) (see color plate 30)

Further diagnostic difficulties result from the fact that some individuals, particularly infants and older adults, deviate from the classic presentation. When doubt exists, performing surgery is usually safer because the penalty of delay may be a ruptured appendix and peritonitis. Hospitalization is then prolonged, and some patients may die from the peritonitis.

Treatment

After the diagnosis of appendicitis is made, the patient is prepared for surgery and the appendix is promptly removed at any time of the day or night. When surgical removal is carried out before rupture and before the signs of peritonitis occur, the postsurgical course is generally uncomplicated. Antibiotics are usually indicated. The time until the patient is discharged from the hospital depends on how early the appendicitis was diagnosed, the degree of inflammation, and whether a laparoscopic or open surgical method was used.

PERITONITIS

Inflammation of the peritoneum (a serous membrane lining the abdominal cavity and covering the viscera) is a serious complication that may occur in both acute and chronic forms. The condition usually results from spread of infection from abdominal organs (e.g., appendicitis, salpingitis), from perforation of the alimentary tract, or from penetrating abdominal wounds. The most common infecting organisms are the colon group (in the case of a ruptured appendix) that might include *Escherichia coli* or *Bacteroides*. Other organisms such as staphylococci or streptococci are often introduced from outside sources.

The initial reaction of the peritoneum to invasion by bacteria is the outpouring of a fibrinous exudate. Pockets of pus (abscesses) form between the fibrinous adhesions, which glue the surrounding surfaces together and thus localize the infection. The adhesions usually disappear when the infection disappears but may persist as fibrous bands that may later lead to intestinal obstruction.

If the infecting material is distributed widely over the surface of the peritoneum or if the infection spreads, generalized peritonitis may then result. As generalized peritonitis develops, peristaltic activity diminishes until a state of paralytic ileus results; the intestine then becomes atonic and distended. Fluids and electrolytes are lost into the lumen of the bowel, leading to dehydration, circulatory failure, oliguria, and possibly shock. Adhesions may form between the distended loops of intestine and may impede the return of intestinal motility and result in intestinal obstruction.

Signs and symptoms vary with the extent of the peritonitis, its severity, and the type of organisms responsible. Typically, fever, leukocytosis, abdominal pain (usu-

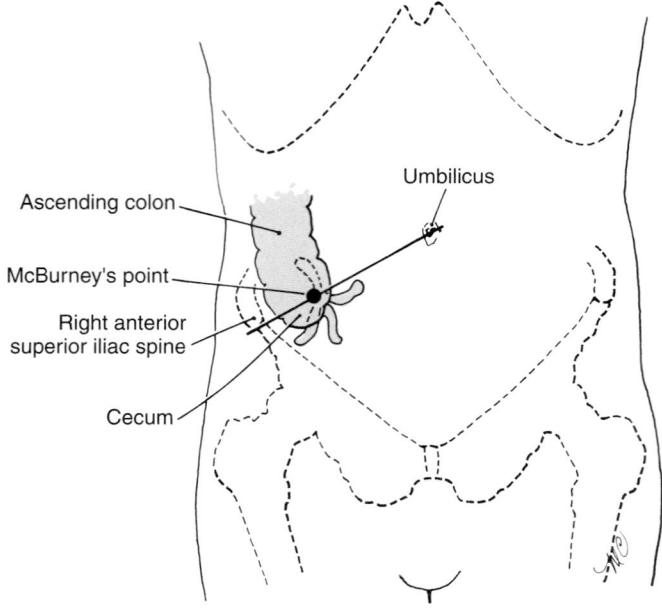

Ascending colon

McBurney's point

Right anterior superior iliac spine

Cecum

Umbilicus

FIG. 25-4 McBurney's point and several common positions of the appendix.

ally continuous), vomiting, and a tense, rigid abdomen with rebound tenderness are present; bowel sounds are often absent. In chronic peritonitis, little or no rebound tenderness is found. Fever and leukocytosis are typical.

The prognosis is good in localized and mild forms of peritonitis and grave in generalized peritonitis caused by virulent organisms.

The general principles of treatment include administration of a suitable antibiotic, decompression of the GI tract by nasogastric or intestinal suction, IV repletion of fluid and electrolyte losses, bedrest in a medium Fowler's position, removal of the septic focus (appendix, etc.) or other cause of inflammation, when possible, and measures to relieve pain.

INTESTINAL OBSTRUCTION

Intestinal obstruction may be defined as an interference (from whatever cause) with the normal flow of intestinal contents through the intestinal tract. Intestinal obstruction may be acute or chronic, partial or complete. Chronic bowel obstruction usually involves the colon as a result of a carcinoma or tumor growth and is slow in development. Most obstructions involve the small bowel. Complete obstruction of the small bowel is a grave condition that requires early diagnosis and emergency surgical intervention if the patient is to survive.

Intestinal obstruction is divided into two types: (1) *nonmechanical* (e.g., *paralytic ileus* or *adynamic ileus*), in which intestinal peristalsis is inhibited as a result of toxic or trau-

matic affectation of autonomic control of motility, and (2) *mechanical*, in which intraluminal obstruction or mural obstruction occurs caused by extrinsic pressure.

Mechanical obstruction is further classified as *simple mechanical obstruction*, in which only one point of obstruction exists, and *closed-loop obstruction*, in which at least two points of obstruction exist. Because a closed-loop obstruction cannot be decompressed, intraluminal pressure is rapidly increased, leading to compression of blood vessels, ischemia, and infarction (strangulation) (see Fig. 3-9). Fig. 25-5 illustrates some of the mechanical causes of bowel obstruction.

Etiology

Nonmechanical obstruction or adynamic ileus typically follows abdominal surgery in which reflex inhibition of peristalsis results from handling of the abdominal viscera. This reflex inhibition of peristalsis is often called *paralytic ileus*, although paralysis of peristalsis is not complete. Another condition that is a common cause of adynamic ileus is peritonitis. Intestinal atony and gaseous distention accompany a wide variety of traumatic conditions; they may especially follow rib fracture, concussion of the spinal cord, or fracture of the spine.

The causes of mechanical obstruction are related to the age group affected and the site of the obstruction. Approximately 50% of all obstructions occur in adults and result from adhesions from previous surgery. Malignant tumors, diverticulitis, and volvulus are the most common causes of obstruction of the large intestine in

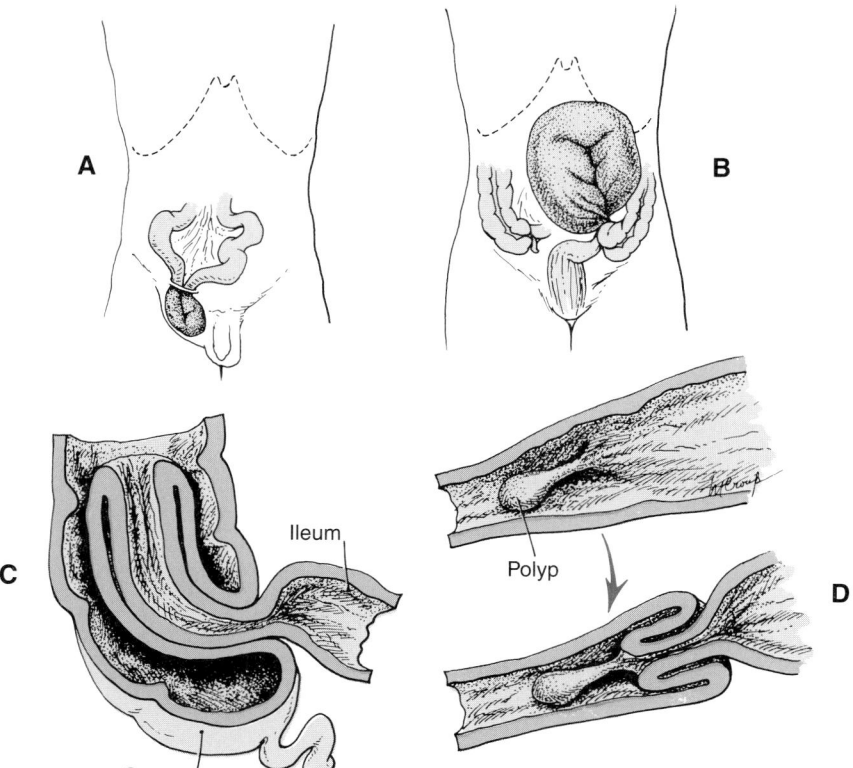

FIG. 25-5   Mechanical causes of bowel obstruction. **A,** Strangulated inguinal hernia. **B,** Volvulus of the sigmoid colon. **C,** Ileocecal intussusception. **D,** Enteroenteric intussusception caused by pedunculated polyp.

middle-age and older people; they account for approximately 90% of the obstructions. *Volvulus* is twisting of the intestine on itself, occurring most frequently in elderly men and usually involving the sigmoid colon. Incarceration of a loop of bowel in an inguinal or femoral hernia is a common cause of small bowel obstruction. *Intussusception* is invagination of one section of the intestine into the next section and is a cause of obstruction encountered almost exclusively in infants and young children. A common site for intussusception is invagination of the terminal ileum into the cecum. Foreign bodies and congenital anomalies are the other common causes of obstruction in infants and children.

Pathophysiology

The pathophysiologic events that occur after intestinal obstruction are similar, whether they result from me-

chanical or functional causes. The main difference is that in paralytic obstruction, peristalsis is inhibited from the start, whereas in mechanical obstruction, peristalsis is accentuated at first, is then intermittent, and is finally absent.

The major pathophysiologic alterations that occur in intestinal obstruction are presented in Fig. 25-6. The wall of the intestine proximal to the obstructed segment is progressively distended by the accumulation of liquid and gas (70% from swallowed air) in the lumen. Severe distention of the wall reduces the flux of water and ions from the intestinal lumen into the blood. Because approximately 8 L of fluid are secreted into the GI tract each day, nonabsorption can lead to rapid intraluminal accumulation. Vomiting and intestinal suction after treatment has begun are major sources of fluid and electrolyte loss. The net effect of these losses is contraction of the extracellular fluid compartment leading to shock, that is,

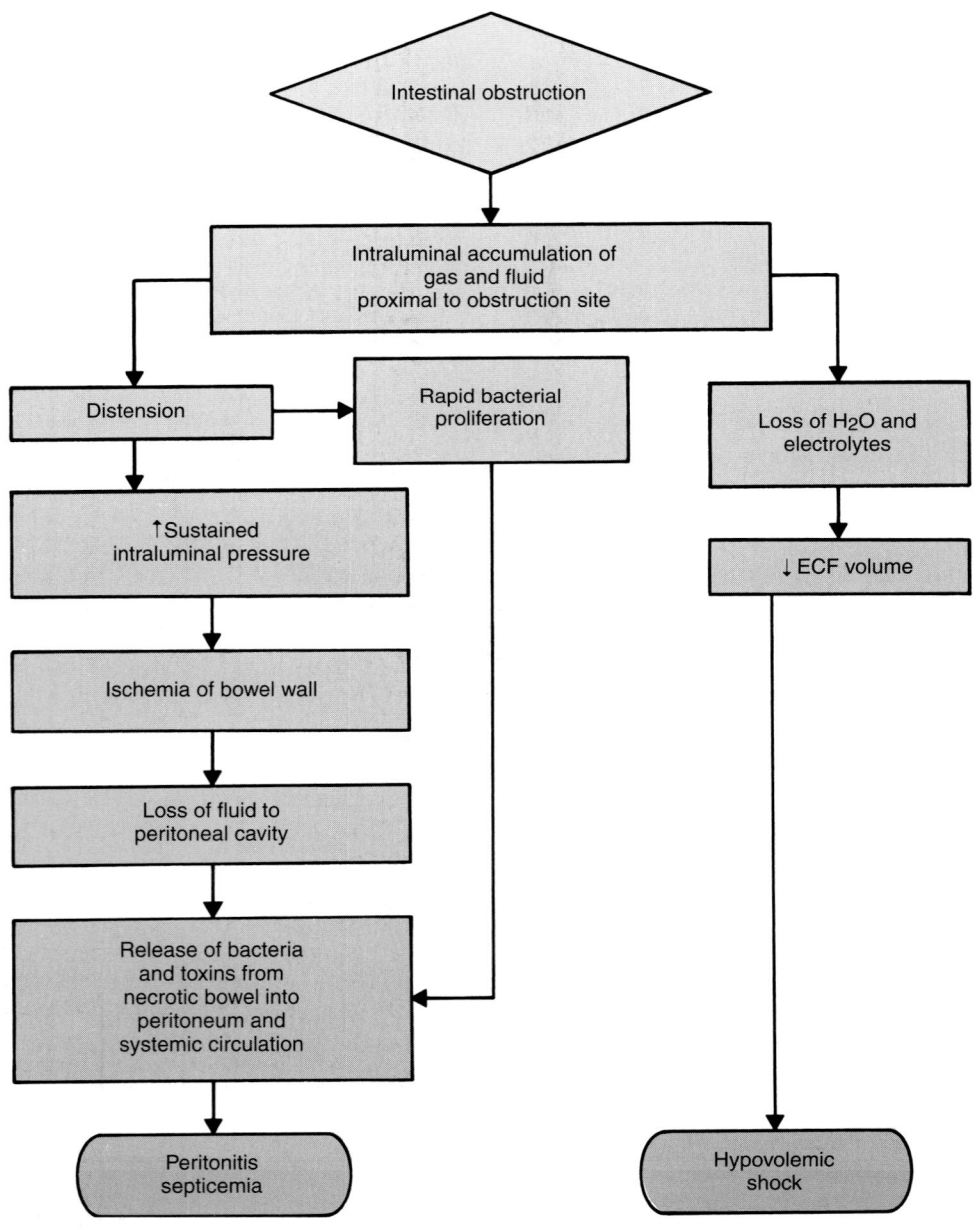

FIG. 25-6 Pathophysiology of intestinal obstruction.

hypotension, reduced cardiac output, decreased tissue perfusion, and metabolic acidosis. Continuing bowel distention results in a vicious cycle of decreased fluid absorption and increased fluid secretion into the bowel. The local effects of bowel distention are ischemia from distention and increased permeability caused by necrosis, with absorption of bacterial toxins into the peritoneal cavity and systemic circulation.

Signs and Symptoms

The cardinal symptoms of small bowel obstruction are abdominal distention, pain, vomiting, and absolute constipation. Pain is usually cramping and midabdominal (typically paraumbilical) and becomes more severe when the obstruction is higher. The abdomen may also be tender. The frequency of vomiting varies with the site of obstruction. When the obstruction is high in the small bowel, vomiting is more prevalent than when the obstruction is in the ileum or large intestine. Absolute constipation is likely to occur early in large bowel obstruction, but flatus and feces may be passed early during the course of small bowel obstruction.

The abdominal radiograph is extremely important in the diagnosis of intestinal obstruction. Mechanical obstruction of the small bowel is characterized by air in the small intestine but not in the colon, whereas colonic obstruction is characterized by gas throughout the colon but with little or no gas in the small intestine. When the plain films are inconclusive, a barium radiograph may be performed to locate the site of obstruction.

Treatment

Treatment principles for bowel obstruction include correction of fluid and electrolyte imbalances, relief of distention and vomiting by intubation and decompression, control of peritonitis and shock when present, and removal of the obstruction to restore normal bowel continuity and function.

Many cases of adynamic ileus are cured by tubal decompression alone. A small bowel obstruction is much more serious and rapid in development than is colonic obstruction. Mortality for nonstrangulating obstruction is 5% to 8%, provided surgical intervention occurs in time. Delay in surgical intervention or the development of strangulation or other complications raises the mortality to approximately 35% to 45%.

KEY CONCEPTS

- The small intestine is a complex, folded tube extending from the pylorus to the ileocecal valve and is divided into the duodenum, jejunum and ileum. The two primary functions are digestion and absorption of ingested nutrients and water.
- *Villi* and *microvilli* are fingerlike projections of mucosa present in the entire length of the small intestine; these structures create a 1000-fold increase in the absorptive surface. Each villus consists of a central lymph channel called a *lacteal* that is surrounded by capillaries. After food has been digested, it passes into the lacteals and capillaries of the villi.
- Enzymes are located on the brush border and complete the process of digestion as absorption is taking place. Surrounding each villus are several small pits called the *crypts of Lieberkühn*. These crypts are intestinal glands that produce secretions containing digestive enzymes.
- Segmental movements of the small intestine mix ingested materials with pancreatic, hepatobiliary, and intestinal secretions. Peristaltic movements propel the contents from one end to the other at a rate suitable for optimal absorption and continuing entry of gastric contents.
- Absorption is the transfer of the end products of carbohydrate, fat, and protein digestion (simple sugars, fatty acids, and amino acids) across the intestinal wall to the vascular and lymphatic circulation for use by the body cells. Additionally, water, electrolytes, and vitamins are absorbed. Absorption of the various substances takes place by both active and passive transport mechanisms.
- Absorption of sugars, amino acids, and fats is largely complete by the time these nutrients reach the midjejunum. Iron and calcium are absorbed primarily in the duodenum and jejunum, and absorption of calcium requires vitamin D. Absorption of the fat-soluble vitamins (A, D, E, and K) is facilitated by bile acids and occurs in the duodenum and upper jejunum. Most water-soluble vitamins are absorbed in the upper small intestine. The absorption of vitamin B_{12} takes place in the terminal ileum by a special transport mechanism requiring gastric intrinsic factor.
- Most of the bile acids released by the gallbladder into the duodenum to aid in digesting fats are reabsorbed in the terminal ileum and recirculated to the liver. This circuit is termed the *enterohepatic circulation of bile salts* and is important in maintaining the bile pool for fat digestion.
- *Malabsorption* occurs when intestinal mucosal absorption of single or multiple nutrients is impaired. Nontropical sprue (celiac disease), tropical sprue, lactase deficiency, postgastrectomy malabsorption, and regional enteritis are disorders associated with malabsorption.
- *Nontropical (celiac) sprue* is a malabsorptive syndrome characterized by flattening of the small intestinal villi caused by sensitivity to gluten found in bread (wheat, rye, oats, barley), beer, and many processed foods. The classic presentation includes diarrhea (pale bulky stools), flatulence, weight loss, and fatigue. Both infants and adults are affected and a familial predisposition is typical. Withdrawal of

gluten from the diet generally reverses or greatly ameliorates the symptoms. *Tropical sprue* is common in the Caribbean and may have an infectious cause because it responds to treatment with antibiotics.

■ *Lactase deficiency* is a malabsorptive disorder involving intolerance to milk and milk products (containing lactose) because of a deficiency of the brush border enzyme, lactase; it is particularly common in African Americans. Typical symptoms of lactase deficiency are abdominal cramps, bloating, and diarrhea after milk ingestion. When unhydrolyzed lactose enters the colon, it produces an osmotic effect, causing water to enter the colon. Colonic bacteria ferment the lactose producing lactic and fatty acid that are irritating to the colon resulting in increased motility and an explosive diarrhea.

■ *Postgastrectomy malabsorption* commonly follows total gastrectomy or the Billroth II procedure. Steatorrhea, weight loss, and macrocytic anemia characterize the condition. The causes are (1) poor mixing of food and enzymes and maldigestion caused by rapid emptying of the stomach remnant, (2) reduced pancreatic exocrine secretion resulting in maldigestion because the duodenum is bypassed, (3) stasis of intestinal contents in the blind loop resulting in bacterial overgrowth, which, in turn, deconjugates bile salts and uses up vitamin B_{12}, and (4) loss of stomach reservoir function resulting in rapid intestinal transit time and diarrhea.

■ *Crohn's disease,* also referred to as *regional enteritis,* is a chronic, relapsing granulomatous inflammatory disease of the intestinal tract that is characterized by "skip" lesions where portions of the diseased bowel are separated by sections of normal bowel. Typical symptoms are colicky abdominal pain and intermittent diarrhea. Complications include intestinal obstruction, perirectal fistulas, abscesses, and fistulas between loops of bowel, to the bladder, or to the external abdominal wall. Extragastrointestinal manifestations include pyoderma gangrenosum, uveitis, and arthritis.

■ Disease or resection of the terminal ileum may cause deficiency of bile salts and interference with fat digestion, as well as macrocytic anemia from interference with vitamin B_{12} absorption.

■ *Appendicitis* is the inflammation of the appendix (remnant of the apex of the cecum, which has no function) involving all layers of the wall of the organ. Appendicitis is the most common surgical disease and occurs more frequently in adolescents and young adults. The earliest symptom is paraumbilical pain, which later localizes to the right lower quadrant of the abdomen.

■ *Peritonitis* is inflammation of the peritoneum, usually resulting from spread of infection from abdominal organs, perforation of the appendix or the alimentary tract, or penetrating abdominal wounds.

■ *Intestinal obstruction* is an interference with the normal flow of intestinal contents through the intestinal tract. There are two types: (1) nonmechanical obstruction (paralytic or adynamic ileus) in which intestinal peristalsis is inhibited and (2) mechanical obstruction caused by intramural obstruction or external pressure on the bowel; mechanical obstruction is further classified as simple (one-point obstruction) or closed loop (two-point obstruction). Bowel obstruction may be acute or chronic, partial or complete, and most commonly involves the small intestine.

■ *Nonmechanical or functional bowel obstruction (paralytic ileus)* results from the handling of the abdominal viscera and some degree of inhibition of peristalsis follows surgery, particularly abdominal surgery. Paralytic ileus is also associated with a wide variety of traumatic injuries (e.g., fractured ribs or vertebrae)

■ The most common cause of mechanical bowel obstruction is *adhesions from prior surgery* (fibrous bands of scar tissue). Other causes are *intussusception* (telescoping of the bowel), *volvulus* (twisting of the intestine on itself usually involving the sigmoid colon), and *incarceration or strangulation* of bowel loop in inguinal or femoral hernia.

■ Pathophysiologic changes in bowel obstruction include the following: (1) intraluminal accumulation of gas and fluid proximal to the obstruction site; (2) abdominal distention; (3) sustained intraluminal pressure causing ischemia of the bowel wall; (4) loss of fluid into the peritoneal cavity; (5) release of bacteria and toxins from the necrotic bowel into the peritoneum and systemic circulation; and (6) peritonitis and septicemia. The loss of water and electrolytes from the ECF compartment into the bowel (third spacing) leads to hypovolemic shock. Treatment of bowel obstruction includes correction of the fluid and electrolyte imbalances, relief of distention and vomiting by nasogastric intubation and decompression, control of peritonitis and shock when present, and removal of the obstruction to restore normal bowel continuity. Many cases of adynamic ileus are cured by tubal decompression alone.

A sampling of review questions for this chapter appears here. Visit http://www.mosby.com/MERLIN/PriceWilson/ for additional questions.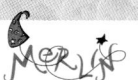

Answer the following on a separate sheet of paper.

1. Why is the gastrointestinal mucosa especially vulnerable to side effects such as ulceration and bleeding from the administration of cytotoxic drugs such as cyclophosphamide (Cytoxan) and mercaptopurine?
2. Describe the function of bile in the digestion and absorption of fats and fat-soluble vitamins.
3. Differentiate between maldigestion and malabsorption.

4. Describe the appearance and characteristics of stool from a patient that would cause you to suspect steatorrhea.
5. What are the characteristics of regional enteritis that have led theorists to suspect that hypersensitivity might be responsible in its pathogenesis?
6. Name the three structures that greatly increase the absorptive surface area of the small bowel.
7. List four causes of steatorrhea in a patient following total gastrectomy or gastrojejunostomy.

8. Describe the pathophysiologic events leading to death from small bowel obstruction. Explain why early diagnosis and surgical intervention are important in mechanical obstruction of the small bowel.

Fill in the blanks with the correct word(s).

9. The major artery supplying the small bowel (except the duodenum) is the _____ artery.
10. The _____ sphincter controls the entry of chyme into the small bowel, and the _____ valve controls the exit of digested material into the large intestine.
11. The fanlike fold of peritoneum that suspends the jejunum and ileum from the posterior abdominal wall is called the _____.
12. The fold of peritoneum that drapes over the small bowel as an apron is called the _____. This structure has sometimes been called the policeman of the abdomen because one of its important functions is to localize _____.
13. The musculofibrous band extending from the diaphragm to the duodenojejunal juncture and acting as a support for this portion of the small bowel is called the _____ of _____.
14. The structures responsible for giving the barium radiograph of the small bowel a feathery appearance are the _____.
15. The structures that account for the velvetlike appearance of the small bowel are the _____.
16. Several small pits surrounding each villus are the _____ of _____.
17. The lymphatic channel of the villus where fat absorption takes place is called the _____.
18. McBurney's point is located at the midpoint on a line between the _____ and the anterior superior _____ spine; it is the point where the _____ is normally located.

Disorders of the Large Intestine

GLENDA N. LINDSETH

ANATOMY AND PHYSIOLOGY

The large intestine or colon is a hollow muscular tube approximately 5 feet (1.5 m) in length, extending from the cecum to the anal canal. The diameter of the large intestine is noticeably larger than that of the small intestine, the average of which is approximately 2.5 inches (6.5 cm), but its diameter decreases toward the lower end of the tube.

The large intestine is divided into the cecum, colon, and rectum, as illustrated in Fig. 26-1. The *cecum*, containing the ileocecal valve and with the appendix attached to its apex, constitutes the first 2 or 3 inches of the large intestine. The ileocecal valve controls the flow of chyme from the ileum into the cecum and prevents backflow of fecal material from the large intestine into the small intestine. The colon is subdivided into the *ascending, transverse, descending,* and *sigmoid* colon. The points

at which the colon makes a sharp turn at the right and left upper abdomen are called the *hepatic* and *splenic flexures*, respectively. The sigmoid colon begins at the level of the iliac crest and describes an S-shaped curve. The lower part of the curve bends toward the left as it joins the rectum and is the anatomic reason for placing a patient on the left side when giving an enema. In this position, gravity aids the flow of water from the rectum into the sigmoid flexure. The last major portion of the large intestine is called the *rectum* and extends from the sigmoid colon to the *anus* (opening to the outside of the body). The terminal inch of the rectum is called the *anal canal* and is guarded by internal and external sphincter muscles. The length of the rectum and anal canal is approximately 5.9 inches (15 cm).

Throughout most of its length, the large intestine exhibits the four morphologic layers found in the remainder of the gut. Several features, however, are peculiar to the large intestine. The longitudinal muscle coat is incomplete, being collected into three bands called the *taenia coli*. The taenia coalesce in the distal sigmoid, thus the rectum has a complete longitudinal muscle coat. The taenia coli are shorter than is the intestine, causing it to pucker and form small sacs called *haustra*. The *epiploic appendages* are small, fat-filled sacs of peritoneum attached along the taenia. The mucosal layer of the large intestine is much thicker than that of the small intestine and contains no villi or rugae. The crypts of Lieberkühn (intestinal glands) are deeper and have more goblet cells than do those of the small intestine.

The large intestine is clinically divided into right and left halves, based on the blood supply. The *superior mesenteric artery* supplies the right half (cecum, ascending colon, and proximal two thirds of the transverse colon), and the *inferior mesenteric artery* supplies the left half (distal one third of the transverse colon, descending and sigmoid colon, and proximal part of the rectum). Additional blood supply to the rectum is provided by the middle and inferior hemorrhoidal arteries, which arise from the abdominal aorta and internal iliac arteries.

Venous return from the colon and superior rectum is via the superior and inferior mesenteric veins and superior hemorrhoidal veins, which become a part of the por-

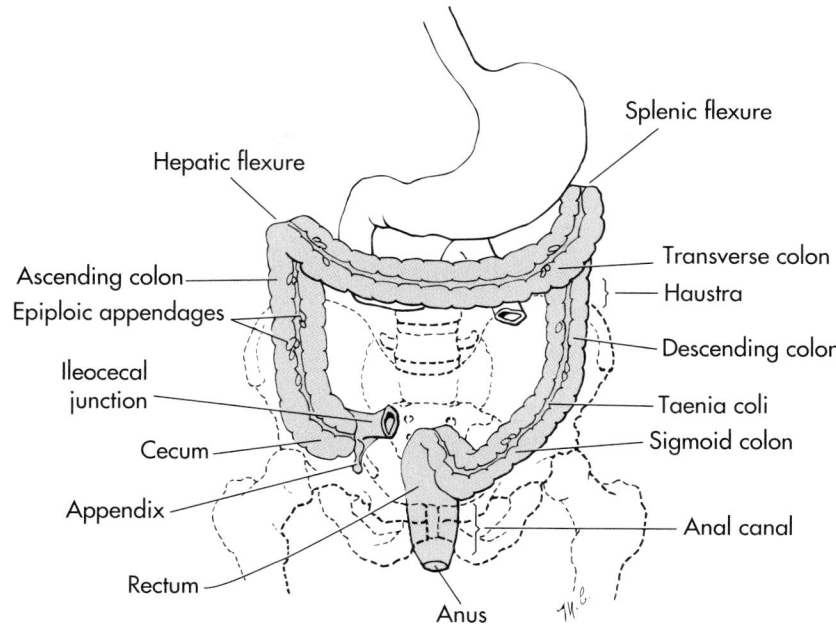

FIG. 26-1   Anatomic relationships of large intestine.

tal system delivering blood to the liver. The middle and inferior hemorrhoidal veins drain into the iliac veins and, consequently, are part of the systemic circulation. Anastomoses exist between the superior and the middle and inferior hemorrhoidal veins, thus increased portal pressure may cause backflow into these veins, resulting in hemorrhoids.

The nerve supply to the large intestine is provided by the autonomic nervous system, with the exception of the external sphincter, which is under voluntary control. Parasympathetic fibers travel via the vagus nerve to the mid-transverse colon, and pelvic nerves of sacral origin supply the distal part. Sympathetic fibers leave the sympathetic trunk via the splanchnic nerves. These fibers synapse in the celiac and aorticorenal ganglia, from which postganglionic fibers reach the colon. Sympathetic stimulation causes inhibition of secretion and contraction and stimulates the rectal sphincter, whereas parasympathetic stimulation has the opposite effect.

The large intestine has a variety of functions, and all are related to the final processing of intestinal contents. The most important function is the absorption of water and electrolytes, which is largely completed in the right side of the colon. The sigmoid colon is a reservoir for the dehydrated fecal mass until defecation takes place.

The colon absorbs approximately 800 ml of water/day compared with approximately 8000 ml absorbed by the small intestine. The absorption capacity of the large intestine, however, is approximately 1500 to 2000 ml/day. When this amount is exceeded by excessive delivery of fluid from the ileum, diarrhea results. The final daily excreted feces weighs approximately 200 g, of which approximately 80% to 90% is water. The remainder is made up of nonabsorbed food residue, bacteria, desquamated epithelial cells, and unabsorbed minerals.

The small amount of digestion that occurs in the large intestine results from bacterial rather than enzymatic action. The large intestine secretes an alkaline mucus that

contains no enzymes. The mucus lubricates and protects the mucosa (see Fig. 6-3).

The bacteria of the large intestine synthesize vitamin K and several vitamins of the B group. Bacterial putrefaction of remaining proteins to amino acids and simpler substances results in the formation of peptides, indole, skatole, phenol, and sulfur compounds. When fatty acids and hydrochloric acid (HCl) are neutralized by bicarbonate, carbon dioxide (CO_2) is produced. The formation of NH_3, CO_2, H_2, H_2S, and CH_4 contributes to flatus (gas) in the colon. Some of these substances are expelled with the feces, and others are absorbed and carried to the liver where they are changed to less toxic compounds and excreted in the urine.

Bacterial fermentation of the remaining carbohydrates with the release of CO_2, H_2, and CH_4 also contributes to flatus in the colon. Approximately 1000 ml of flatus is normally expelled each day. An excess of gas occurs with *aerophagia* (excessive swallowing of air) and with an increase in intraluminal gas frequently related to the diet. "Gassy foods" such as navy beans have a high content of indigestible carbohydrates.

Generally, the movements of the large intestine are slow. A movement characteristic of the large intestine is *haustral churning*. The pouches or haustra become distended, and, from time to time, the circular muscles contract and cause them to empty. The movements are not progressive but cause the contents to move back and forth in a kneading action, thus allowing time for absorption. Propulsive peristalsis is divided into two types: (1) slow, irregular contractions that arise in a proximal segment and move forward, obliterating a few haustra; and (2) *mass peristalsis*, which is a contraction involving a large segment of the colon. Mass peristalsis moves the fecal mass forward, eventually stimulating defecation, which occurs two or three times a day and is stimulated by the gastrocolic reflex after eating, particularly after the first meal of the day.

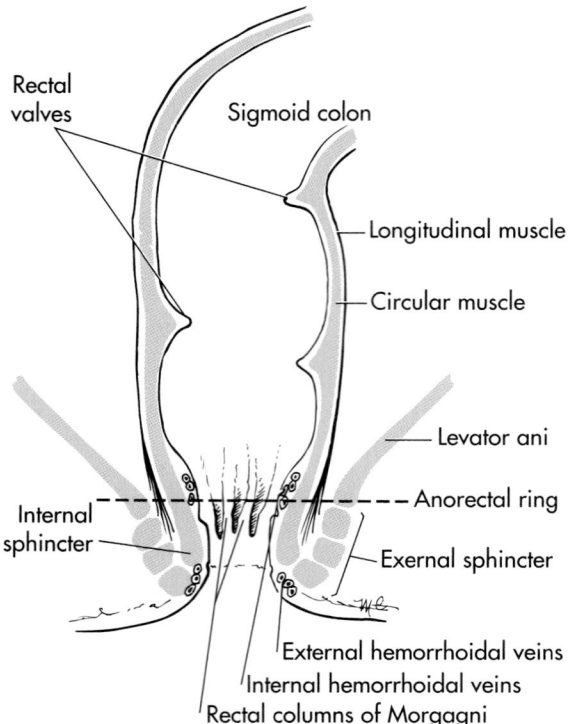

FIG. 26-2 Anatomy of rectum and anus.

Propulsion of feces into the rectum results in distention of the rectal wall and stimulation of the *defecation reflex*. Fig. 26-2 illustrates the basic anatomy of the rectum and anus. The internal and external anal sphincters control defecation. The autonomic nervous system controls the internal sphincter, and the external sphincter is under voluntary control. The defecation reflex is integrated in the second to fourth sacral segments of the spinal cord. Parasympathetic fibers reach the rectum via the pelvic splanchnic nerves and are responsible for contraction of the rectum and relaxation of the internal sphincter. As the distended rectum contracts, the levator ani muscle relaxes, causing the anorectal ring and angle to disappear. The internal and external sphincter muscles relax as the anus is pulled up over the fecal mass. Defecation is facilitated by an increase in intraabdominal pressure brought about by voluntary contraction of the chest muscles on a closed glottis and simultaneous contraction of the abdominal muscles (Valsalva's maneuver or straining). Defecation can be inhibited by voluntary contraction of the levator ani and external sphincter muscles. The rectal wall gradually relaxes, and the urge to defecate passes.

The rectum and anus are the sites of some of the most common disorders known to humans. A common cause of simple constipation is failure to empty the rectum when mass peristalsis occurs. When defecation is not completed, the rectum relaxes and the desire to defecate disappears. Water continues to be absorbed from the fecal mass, causing it to become hard, thus subsequent defecation is increasingly difficult. When a hardened mass of feces is congregated in one area and cannot be expelled, it is known as *fecal impaction*. Excessive straining at the stool causes congestion of the internal and external

hemorrhoidal veins and is one of the important causes of hemorrhoids (varicose veins of the rectum). Incontinence of stool may result from damage to sphincter muscles or from damage to the spinal cord. The anorectal area is a frequent site of abscesses and fistulas. The colon and rectum are the most frequent sites of cancer of the gastrointestinal (GI) tract.

DIAGNOSTIC PROCEDURES

Diagnosis of pathology associated with the large intestine relates mainly to symptoms associated with elimination. Constipation, diarrhea, alteration in size or color of stool, and the presence of blood in the stools are all important symptoms that focus attention on the colon and rectum. Pain of colonic origin is lateralized to the left or right side of the abdomen, as opposed to pain of small intestinal origin, which is usually paraumbilical.

The history and the physical examination are important diagnostic procedures. Abdominal masses may be palpated, and digital examination is important, because approximately 15% of all rectal carcinomas are within reach of the examiner's finger. When incontinence is a problem, integrity of the sphincter should be assessed. Examination of the stools, sigmoidoscopy, colonoscopy, radiologic examination (ultrasound, computed tomography, magnetic resonance imaging) are essential diagnostic tools in the assessment of suspected colonic disease.

The *barium enema radiograph* is a common test carried out on patients for identification of disorders of the colon. Preparation or prior cleansing of the intestine is important for a proper examination, but in the presence of an obstructing lesion or active ulcerative colitis, the use of strong cathartics may be hazardous or life threatening to the patient. Neoplasms, strictures, diverticulosis, and polyps may all be visualized. The cecum and ascending colon may be visualized 3 to 5 hours after a barium swallow. The barium enema radiograph should always precede the barium swallow. The addition of air-contrast with the barium enema radiograph is accurate in up to 90% of examinations. However, endoscopic examination of the colon has been shown to be more accurate in detecting and evaluating lesions than using radiography.

The flexible sigmoidoscope has generally replaced the 25-cm rigid sigmoidoscope. Direct visualization of the terminal 40 to 60 cm of the rectum and sigmoid colon is possible with minimal preparation and less discomfort to the patient. Sixty percent of all the tumors of the large intestine can be visualized directly using this instrument. In addition to visual inspection of the area, bacteriologic, parasitologic, and cytologic studies can be made on the washings through the instrument, and biopsy of suspicious lesions is easy to perform. The *flexible fiberoptic colonoscope* allows visualization and biopsy of lesions of the entire colon. Experienced examiners may be able to insert the instrument as far as the terminal ileum.

Ultrasound (US), computed tomography (CT), and magnetic resonance imaging (MRI) are newer diagnostic tests used for colonic assessment, particularly abdominal masses. The CT, while being more expensive, is effective for lower abdominal evaluations with inflammatory masses. Patients with complications from diverticula can also be accurately imaged using these diagnostic technologies. The MRI can give accurate information on the anatomic extent of invasive rectal cancers and of blood flow in patients with vascular disorders.

DIVERTICULAR DISEASE OF THE COLON

Diverticulosis is a condition of the colon characterized by herniation of the mucosa through the muscularis to form flask-shaped saccules. When one or more of the saccules become inflamed, the condition is called *diverticulitis*.

Pathophysiology

The overall incidence of diverticulosis is high; it affects approximately 10% of the population, according to most necropsy studies. Diverticulosis is rare in people younger than 35 years but increases with age, thus at age 85, two thirds of the population are afflicted. The most common site for diverticula to occur is in the sigmoid colon, which is involved in approximately 90% of the cases.

Although the cause of diverticulosis is unknown, recent motility and pressure studies have done much to support the possibility that diverticular disease may result from a disordered motility pattern of the colon. Fig. 26-3 illustrates the normal motility pattern in the colon and the proposed pathogenic mechanism of diverticulosis. Diverticula-bearing zones of the colon are prone to strong contractions of the circular muscles, which build up high intraluminal pressures. Likely, these high pressures are responsible for herniations of the mucosa through the muscle coat, which become diverticula. The usual position for the diverticula is at the mesenteric attachment of the colon, where the entry of blood vessels weakens the wall. The pressure changes in diverticular disease are similar to those found in spastic or irritable colon syndrome.

A factor of even greater importance in the etiology of diverticular disease relates to the amount of roughage in the diet. Diverticulosis is rare in those who eat a diet high in roughage but is common in Europeans and North Americans (of all races) who eat a low-roughage diet. The tension or strain on the wall of a hollow organ is related to the pressure within and to the diameter of the organ. If a tube such as the colon is habitually of narrow bore (as the result of a low-fiber diet), the strain on the wall from a buildup of pressure is then greater than if it were filled with feces.

Clinical Features and Complications

Most patients with diverticulosis have no symptoms, and the problem remains unidentified unless a barium enema radiographic or colonoscopic study is performed in the investigation of some unrelated condition. When diverticula are discovered, ruling out carcinoma is important. This differentiation is made by the radiographic appearance, colonoscopic examination, and biopsy. A barium enema radiographic study is dangerous during an attack of acute diverticulitis because of the danger of perforation. Flat abdominal radiographs and CT can also be

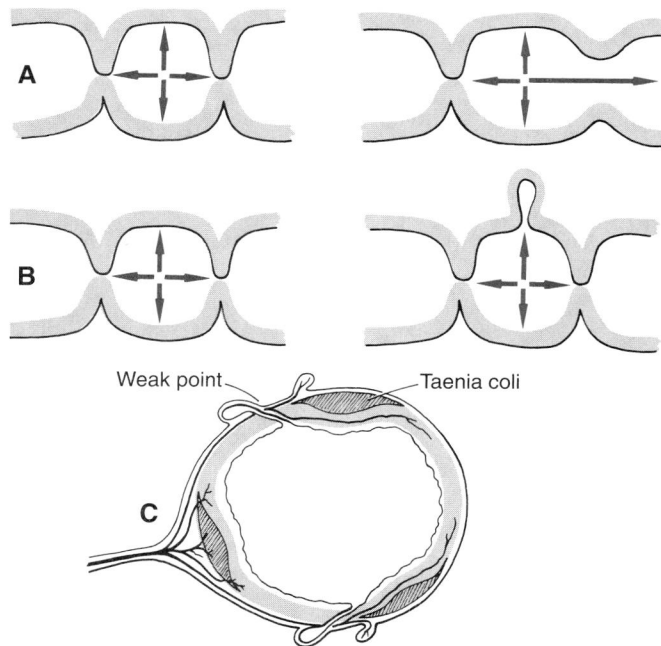

FIG. 26-3 Pathogenesis of diverticular disease. **A,** Normal motility pattern. **B,** Abnormal motility pattern in which there is failure of relaxation and buildup of high intraluminal pressure, resulting in the formation of a diverticulum. **C,** Cross section of colon showing that the weak point in the circular muscle is where a blood vessel pierces the muscle. Herniation of the lining mucosa and the formation of diverticuli develop at these points.

effective in evaluating inflammation and masses in patients with diverticular complications.

In many patients, symptoms are mild and consist of flatulence, intermittent diarrhea or constipation, and discomfort in the lower left quadrant of the abdomen. These symptoms can usually be attributed to the irritable colon syndrome that may precede the development of diverticulosis in some patients.

The complications of diverticular disease are the result of acute or chronic diverticulitis, which may result in bleeding, perforation and peritonitis, abscess and fistula formation, or intestinal obstruction from stricture (Fig. 26-4).

In the case of acute diverticulitis, fever, leukocytosis, and pain and tenderness in the lower left quadrant of the abdomen are present. During a bout of acute inflammation, bleeding may occur from vascular granulation tissue and is usually minor. In rare instances, bleeding may be massive as a result of erosion of the large penetrating blood vessel next to the diverticula. Bleeding is usually treated conservatively, but on rare occasions a bowel resection is necessary.

Sometimes acutely inflamed diverticula rupture. If the perforation is small, the result may be abscess formation next to the perforated diverticulum. If the perforation is large, fecal material may enter the peritoneum and cause a most severe form of peritonitis with a high mortality. Symptoms of perforation are similar to those of a perforated ulcer, except that pain, rigidity, and tenderness are most marked in the lower left quadrant.

The term *chronic diverticulitis* applies to a bowel subjected to repeated attacks of inflammation. The result

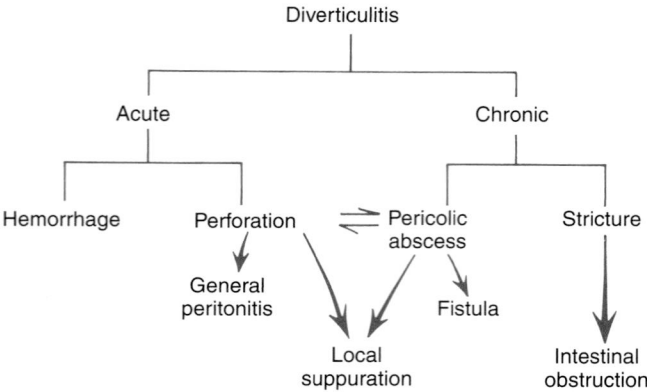

FIG. 26-4 Complications of diverticulitis.

may be fibrosis and adhesions of the surrounding structures. When chronic inflammation has caused significant narrowing of the lumen, chronic incomplete bowel obstruction may result, giving rise to symptoms of constipation, ribbonlike stools, intermittent diarrhea, and abdominal distention. The final obstructive picture may be precipitated by a superimposed acute attack, leading to a pericolic abscess that narrows the already occluded lumen. A fistula may also form as a complication of a pericolic abscess. The most common type is the vesicosigmoid fistula. The flow is usually from the colon to the bladder, and the complaint is *pneumaturia,* or the passage of air bubbles (gas) in the urine. The fistula may also lead to the small bowel or peritoneum.

Treatment

When diverticula are discovered incidentally and the patient is asymptomatic, they are not generally treated. However, 90% of patients with diverticulitis are treated medically. Individuals with mild cases without signs of perforation are treated with a liquid diet or intravenous (IV) fluids, stool softeners, bedrest, and a broad-spectrum antibiotic. Antibiotics effective against gram-negative anaerobic bacteria may be given to patients with suspected perforation or abscess. Incision and drainage of abscesses may be necessary. After the acute phase, a high-residue diet is indicated.

Surgical intervention is needed only for severe and extensive disease or in the event of complications. The essential surgical treatment is resection of the diseased colon with anastomosis to restore continuity. In the absence of complications, the surgery may be carried out in one stage. In other cases, the surgeon may perform a temporary colostomy (diversion of the colon to the abdominal surface). Anastomosis and closure are then carried out at a later date.

INFLAMMATORY DISEASE OF THE LARGE INTESTINE

Chronic inflammatory disease of the large bowel is divided into two major entities: nonspecific ulcerative colitis and Crohn's disease of the large bowel (granulomatous colitis). Although these two conditions have many fea-

tures in common, enough differences exist to separate them into two distinct clinical entities. Table 26-1 lists the differentiating features of these two diseases. Sufficient overlapping features exist to lead some investigators to believe that both diseases may represent variations in response to the same etiologic agent.

Ulcerative Colitis

Ulcerative colitis is a nonspecific inflammatory disease of the colon generally following a prolonged course characterized by alternating periods of remissions and exacerbations. Abdominal pain, diarrhea, and rectal bleeding are the cardinal signs and symptoms. The essential lesion is an inflammatory reaction of the subepithelial zone developing at the base of the crypts of Lieberkühn, which may eventually produce ulceration of the mucosa (see color plate 31). The peak onset of the disease is between ages 15 and 40 years, and the disorder is equally distributed between the genders. The incidence of ulcerative colitis is approximately 1 per 10,000 Caucasian adults per year. Crohn's disease is approximately one fourth as common as is ulcerative colitis. Both diseases are less common in non-Caucasians.

Etiology and Pathogenesis

The cause of ulcerative colitis, as with that of Crohn's disease, is unknown. Genetic factors appear to be involved in the origin, because a definite familial relationship exists among ulcerative colitis, Crohn's disease, and ankylosing spondylitis.

Several theories about the causes of ulcerative colitis have been produced, but none have been proven. The most popular theory is that the body's immune system reacts to a virus or a bacterium resulting in ongoing inflammation in the intestinal wall. Individuals with ulcerative colitis do have abnormalities of the immune system, but whether these are a cause or an effect of the disease is unknown. Ulcerative colitis is not caused by emotional distress or food sensitivities, but these factors may trigger symptoms in some people (NIDDK, 1998).

The initial pathologic lesion is confined to the mucosal layer and consists of abscess formation in the crypts, as opposed to Crohn's disease, which involves the entire thickness of the bowel wall. Early in the disease, edema and congestion of the mucosa occur. The edema may lead to extreme friability, thus bleeding occurs from any minor trauma, such as the surface being lightly rubbed.

In more advanced stages of the disease, the crypt abscess breaks through the wall of the crypt and spreads in the submucosa, undermining the mucosa. The mucosa is then shed into the bowel lumen, leaving areas of denuded mucosa (ulcers). Ulceration is at first scattered and shallow, but at a later stage, the mucosal surface is lost over wide areas, leading to considerable loss of tissue, protein, and blood.

Clinical Features

The three common clinical types of ulcerative colitis are related to frequency of symptoms. The *acute fulminating* ulcerative colitis is characterized by an abrupt onset, with severe, bloody diarrhea (10 to 20 stools/day), nausea, vomiting, and fever, which causes a rapid depletion of

TABLE 26-1   ■■■

Differentiating Features of Ulcerative Colitis and Crohn's Disease

Characteristic Feature	Ulcerative Colitis	Crohn's Disease
Depth of involvement	Mucosa and submucosa	Transmural
Granulomatous inflammatory response	Rare	Common
Rectal involvement	95%	50%
Small bowel involvement	Usually normal	80%
Right colon involvement	Occasional	Frequent
Distribution of lesion	Continuous with rectum	Discontinuous "skip" lesions
Inflammatory mass	Rare	Usually palpable
Diarrhea	Common	Common
Rectal bleeding	Common, continuous	Rare
Internal fistulas	Rare	Common
Anal abscesses	Occasional	Common
Anorectal fissures and fistulas	Rare	Common
Cobblestone appearance of mucosa	Unusual (pseudopolyps, granular, shaggy)	Common
Toxic megacolon	Occasional	Rare
Malignant potential	High after 10 years	Low
Extragastrointestinal manifestation (e.g., arthritis, eye and skin involvement)	Occasional	Less frequent than in ulcerative colitis
Strictures	Occasional, mild	Common
Finger clubbing	Rare	Common
Relative frequency	Three to four times more common than Crohn's disease	
Familial and Jewish association	Yes	Yes
Autoantibodies	Frequent	Not found

fluids and electrolytes. The entire colon may be involved, with undermining and stripping of the mucosa, causing loss of considerable blood and mucus. This type of colitis occurs in approximately 10% of the patients. The prognosis is poor, and toxic megacolon is a frequent complication.

Most patients with ulcerative colitis have the *chronic intermittent (recurrent)* type of colitis. The onset tends to be insidious, occurring over months to years. The mild form of the disease is characterized by short attacks occurring at intervals of months to years and lasting 1 to 3 months. Little or no fever or constitutional symptoms may occur, and usually only the distal colon is affected. Fever and systemic symptoms may accompany the more severe form, and the attack may last 3 or 4 months, occasionally passing into the *chronic continuous* type of disease. In the chronic continuous disease, the patient continues to have diarrhea after the initial attack. As compared with the intermittent type, more of the colon tends to be involved and complications are more frequent.

In mild forms of ulcerative colitis, diarrhea may be mild and bleeding is intermittent and slight. In severe disease, more than six stools occur per day with considerable blood and mucus. The chronic loss of blood and mucus may lead to anemia and hypoproteinemia. Severe, colicky pain may be present in the lower abdomen and is relieved somewhat by defecation. Few deaths occur directly from this disease, but it may be mildly or severely disabling.

The diagnosis of ulcerative colitis is usually straightforward. Diarrhea with passage of blood occurs, and sigmoidoscopy reveals a friable and intensely inflamed mucosa with exudate. In 95% of the cases, the rectosigmoid area of the colon is involved. The disease may extend from this area but always in a continuous fashion, in contrast to Crohn's disease, which tends to skip. Barium radiographic studies of the colon aid in determining the extent of more proximal changes but should not be performed during an acute attack, because they may precipitate toxic megacolon and perforation. Colonoscopy and biopsy can often differentiate ulcerative colitis from granulomatous colitis. Endoscopic ultrasound (EUS) can show imaging of the GI tract wall and adjacent structures. EUS is more accurate than MRI in assessing abscesses and can help differentiate ulcerative colitis from Crohn's disease.

Complications

Complications of ulcerative colitis may be local or systemic. Rectal fistulas, fissures, and abscesses are not as common as they are in granulomatous colitis. Occasionally, a rectovaginal fistula forms. A few patients may have narrowing of the bowel lumen as a result of fibrosis, which is generally mild, as compared with Crohn's disease.

One of the more serious complications is *toxic dilation*, or *megacolon*, in which paralysis of the motor function of the transverse colon is involved, with rapid dilation of that segment of the bowel. Toxic megacolon is most frequently associated with pancolitis. The mortality rate is approximately 30%, and perforation of the bowel frequently results. The treatment for this complication is emergency colectomy. Massive hemorrhage is another complication, sometimes requiring emergency colectomy.

Another significant complication is carcinoma of the colon, which occurs with increasing frequency after the patient has had the disease for more than 10 years. After patients have had total colon involvement with ulcerative colitis for 25 years, the probability of cancer is increased to 40%.

The systemic complications are diverse, and relating some of them causally to the colonic disease is difficult.

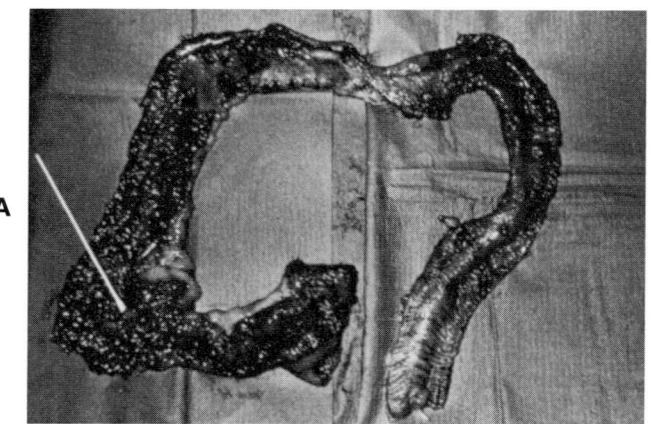

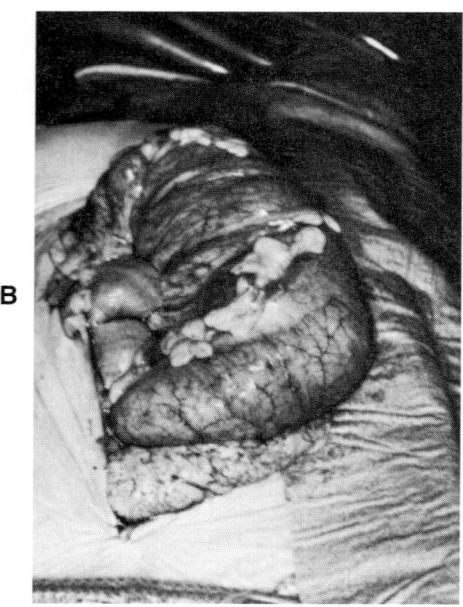

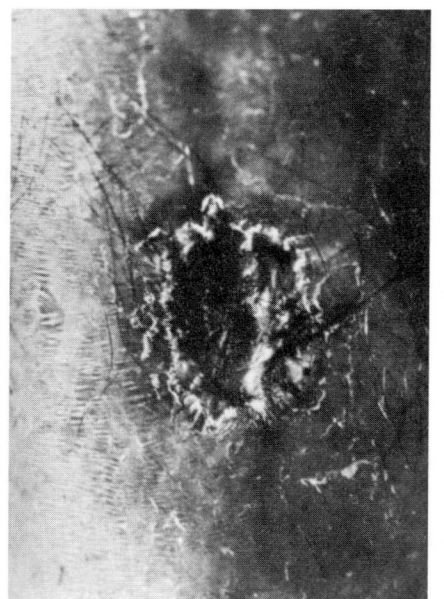

FIG. 26-5 Some complications of ulcerative colitis. **A,** Hemorrhage: surgical specimen of large intestine removed from a patient with ulcerative colitis to control bleeding. The probe is at the site of a small perforation. **B,** Toxic megacolon: the large, dilated colon protruding through a surgical incision. **C,** Pyoderma gangrenosum: a necrotic skin ulcer found in association with inflammatory bowel disease. (Courtesy Daniel J. Fall, MD, St. Joseph Mercy Hospital, Ypsilanti, Mich.)

These complications include pyoderma gangrenosum, episcleritis, uveitis, arthritis, and ankylosing spondylitis. Disordered hepatic function is common in ulcerative colitis. The presence of severe systemic complications may be an indication for surgical treatment of the colitis, even when the colonic symptoms are mild (Fig. 26-5; see color plate 32).

Treatment

No cure or specific medical treatment exists for ulcerative colitis. The aims of therapy are to control the inflammation, maintain the patient's nutritional status, provide symptomatic relief, and prevent infection and other complications.

Corticosteroid drugs are given to reduce inflammation and induce clinical remission. Sulfonamide drugs are given, but their mechanism of action is poorly understood. A low-residue diet causes diminution in the number of stools and thereby makes the patient more comfortable. The diet must also be high in protein to compensate for that lost in the exudative lesions; the diet should be high in vitamins and minerals with lactose restriction to avoid lactose intolerance associated with diarrhea. During exacerbations, tincture of opium and paregoric are occasionally given to control diarrhea. Anticholinergic drugs may also help relieve the abdominal cramps and diarrhea. Agents to control diarrhea should be used with caution to avoid precipitating colonic dilation and toxic megacolon. Malnourished patients may require total parenteral nutrition (TPN). Emotional support and reassurance are important aspects of treatment.

When medical management fails and when the condition becomes intractable, surgical intervention is indicated. The most common procedure performed is total colectomy and the creation of a permanent ileostomy. Some physicians also recommend a colectomy for all patients who have had total colon involvement for several years, because the incidence of carcinoma of the colon in these patients is very high. Colon cancer is difficult to diagnose in these patients, because symptoms such as weight loss or bloody stools may be regarded as another exacerbation of the ulcerative colitis rather than as signs of cancer.

NEOPLASMS OF THE LARGE INTESTINE

Neoplasms of the colon and rectum may be benign or malignant. True benign neoplasms (lipomas, carcinoid tumors, and leiomyomas) are rare in the colon. Colonic polyps, however, are common and occupy an intermediate position between benign and malignant neoplasms.

Colonic Polyps

A *polyp* is a growth that arises from a mucosal surface and extends outward. Colonic polyps are divided into three recognized patterns: pedunculated adenomas, villous adenomas, and familial polyposis.

Pedunculated adenomas (also called adenomatous polyps or polypoid adenomas) are globelike structures attached to the mucous membrane by a thin stalk. This type of polyp occurs in both genders and in all age groups, although they become increasingly common with advancing age. Autopsy and sigmoidoscopy studies indicate that approximately 9% of the population over age 45 years is afflicted. Although pedunculated polyps may occur in any part of the colon, they are more frequently located in the distal 10 to 12 inches (25 to 30 cm). Pedunculated polyps may be singular or multiple; they are usually 0.2 to 0.4 inches (0.5 to 1.0 cm) in diameter but may be as large as 1.6 to 2.0 inches (4 or 5 cm). Histologically, these polyps consist of proliferating glands. The relationship of adenomatous polyps to cancer of the colon is a subject of great controversy, because they have much the same distribution in the colon as does cancer and are often associated with cancer. The prevailing opinion is that they are harmless. However, when the polyps are multiple or when the head is greater than 1 cm in diameter, the chances of malignancy are increased.

Another form of pedunculated polyp occurring most frequently in children younger than 10 years of age is the *juvenile polyp.* Juvenile polyps are often large and vascular and have long pedicles. Believed to be inflammatory in origin, these polyps may present by bleeding or prolapse through the anus. Juvenile polyps occasionally occur in adults.

The *villous adenoma* (villous papilloma, sessile adenoma), in contrast to the pedunculated adenoma, is a sessile (broad-based) tumor. The surface is distinctly papillary to the naked eye and appears as a nodular mass. Histologically, the lesion is composed of fingerlike (villous) projections and is usually solitary and located in the sigmoid colon or rectum. Villous adenomas are generally large (greater than 5 cm) and are approximately one eighth as frequent as are pedunculated adenomas. Malignancy is much more likely to occur in these tumors (with a 25% chance) than it is in the pedunculated adenomas.

Familial polyposis is a rare disorder transmitted genetically as an autosomal dominant trait and characterized by the presence of hundreds of adenomatous polyps, both pedunculated and sessile, throughout the large intestine. Both genders are equally affected. The polyps are not present at birth but usually appear about the time of puberty. The probability of the development of cancer increases with age and is nearly 100% by age 40.

Clinical Features

Most adenomatous polyps are asymptomatic and are found incidentally on examination by sigmoidoscopy, by barium enema, or on autopsy. When polyps do give rise to symptoms, these generally consist of overt or occult bleeding. Occasionally, a large polyp may initiate an intussusception and cause bowel obstruction (see Fig. 25-5, *D*). Diarrhea and mucous discharge may be associated with large villous adenomas and familial polyposis.

Treatment

The treatment of colonic polyps is influenced by the debate concerning their malignant potential. Because the malignant potential in familial polyposis is unquestionable, this condition is treated by total proctocolectomy and permanent ileostomy or subtotal resection with ileorectal anastomosis. When the rectum is preserved, it is examined periodically for cancer.

The guidelines for the treatment of pedunculated or villous adenomas are not as clear. Generally, polyps that are greater than 2 cm in diameter, multiple, or villous are regarded with a high degree of suspicion and should be removed. Polyps that are pedunculated, singular, and less than 1 cm in diameter are rarely malignant and can be observed periodically.

Polyps may be excised from below through the sigmoidoscope or colonoscope. Larger lesions and villous adenomas are treated by laparotomy and segmental resection.

Carcinoma of the Colon and Rectum

The colon (including the rectum) is the most common site for malignancy of the GI tract. Cancer of the colon is the third most common cause of all cancer deaths in both men and women in the United States (American Cancer Society, 2001). Cancer of the large intestine is usually a disease of older people, with peak incidence in 50- and 60-year-old adults. Colon cancer is rare in people younger than age 40, except in those with a history of ulcerative colitis or familial polyposis. The genders are affected about equally. Approximately 60% of all the cancers of the bowel occur in the rectosigmoid portion, thus the lesions may be either palpated during a rectal examination or viewed with a sigmoidoscope. The cecum and ascending colon are the next most common sites. The transverse colon and flexures are least likely to be affected.

The tumor may be a *polypoid,* bulky, fungating mass projecting into the lumen and may quickly become ulcerated; it may extend around the bowel as an *annular* (ringlike) stricture (see color plate 33). Annular lesions are more common in the rectosigmoid portion of the bowel, whereas polypoid flat lesions are more common in the cecum and ascending colon. Histologically, nearly all the large bowel cancers are *adenocarcinomas* (composed of glandular epithelium) and may secrete mucus to a varying degree. The tumor may spread (1) by direct infiltration of adjacent structures, as into the bladder;

(2) by lymphatics to the pericolic and mesocolic lymph nodes; and (3) by the bloodstream, usually to the liver, because the colon is drained by the portal system. The prognosis is relatively favorable when the lesion is confined to the mucosa and submucosa at the time of surgical resection and much less favorable when lymph node metastasis has occurred.

Etiology

Although the causes of cancer of the large bowel, as with other cancers, have not been established, certain predisposing factors have been identified. The relationship between ulcerative colitis, certain types of colonic polyps, and cancer of the bowel has been discussed.

Another important predisposing factor may relate to dietary habits, because cancer of the bowel (as with diverticulosis) is approximately 10 times more common in Western populations, who eat foods high in refined carbohydrates and low in roughage, than it is in emerging populations (e.g., in Africa) who eat foods high in roughage. Burkitt (1971) proposed that a low-fiber, highly refined carbohydrate diet leads to alterations in fecal flora and changes in the degradation of bile salts or of the breakdown products of protein and fat, some of which may be carcinogenic. A low-fiber diet allows concentration of these potential carcinogens into a smaller volume of stool. Additionally, the transit time is increased. The net result is prolonged contact time of potential carcinogens with the bowel mucosa. Initial research indicates that a diet high in phytochemically rich foods containing nutrients such as fiber, vitamins C, E, and carotene can improve colon function, and may be protective from cancer-producing mutagens.

Screening

Because colorectal cancer causes approximately 57,000 deaths per year in the United States, some organizations (e.g., National Cancer Institute, American Cancer Society, American College of Physicians) have endorsed guidelines for screening to detect colorectal cancer at a curable stage so as to help reduce morbidity and mortality of this disease. Strategies for screening of asymptomatic persons are recommended as follows: (1) men and women over 40 years of age should receive annual digital rectal examinations, and (2) people over 50 years of age should have a fecal occult blood test annually and a sigmoidoscopy examination every 3 to 5 years after two initial examinations a year apart. People at high risk because of family history should also have the total colon examined by either an air-contrast barium enema or colonoscopy every 3 to 5 years. An individual with family history of colorectal cancer should be especially vigilant with frequent screenings. Analysis for specific *ras* protooncogene mutations from deoxyribonucleic acid (DNA) recovered from the stool of patients with a history of colorectal cancer is also looking effective as a screening mechanism (Mayer, 1998).

Clinical Features

The most common symptoms of cancer of the bowel are changes in bowel habits, bleeding, pain, anemia, anorexia, and weight loss. The signs and symptoms vary according to the location and are usually divided into those affecting the right and left halves of the large bowel.

Carcinoma of the left colon and rectum tends to cause a change in bowel habits as a result of irritation and reflex responses. Diarrhea, cramplike pain, and distention are common. Because lesions of the left colon tend to encircle, obstruction is a common problem. Stool may be narrow and ribbonlike in shape. Both mucus and gross blood are often visible on the feces. Anemia may result from chronic blood loss. A sigmoid or rectal growth may involve nerve roots, lymphatics, or veins, producing symptoms in the legs or perineum. Hemorrhoids, low back pain, rectal urgency, or urinary frequency may develop as a result of pressure on these structures.

Carcinoma of the right colon, where the bowel contents are liquid, tends to remain occult until far advanced. The tendency to obstruct is small because the bowel lumen is larger and the feces are liquid. Anemia caused by bleeding is common, but the blood is occult and can be detected only by a guaiac test (a simple test that may be performed on the clinical unit). Because bleeding may be intermittent, an endoscopic or full-bowel radiographic examination may be indicated when anemia persists. Mucus is similarly not visible because it is well mixed in the stool. In the thin person, a tumor of the right colon may sometimes be palpated, but this is atypical at an early stage. The patient may have vague abdominal discomfort that is sometimes epigastric.

Treatment

The treatment of carcinoma of the colon and rectum is surgical removal of the tumor and its lymphatic drainage. The most common procedures performed are right hemicolectomy, transverse colectomy, left hemicolectomy or anterior resection, and abdominoperineal resection. Surgical resection of patients without metastasis is highly curable. Radiation and chemotherapy in selected cases can improve survival. Follow-up measurement of carcinoembryonic antigen (CEA) is a sensitive marker for otherwise undetectable tumor recurrence. The overall 5-year survival rate is approximately 50%.

ANORECTAL DISORDERS

Hemorrhoids

Hemorrhoids, or "piles," are varicose veins of the anal canal and are divided into two classes, internal and external. *Internal hemorrhoids* are varices of the superior and middle hemorrhoidal veins, and *external hemorrhoids* are varices of the inferior hemorrhoidal veins. As the terms imply, external hemorrhoids appear external to the sphincter ani muscles, and the internal hemorrhoids appear above (or alternately, proximal to) the sphincter.

Both types of hemorrhoids are common and are present in approximately 35% of the population over age 25 years. Although the condition is not life threatening, it may cause considerable discomfort.

Hemorrhoids result from venous congestion caused by interference with venous return from the hemorrhoidal veins. Several etiologic factors have been implicated, including constipation or diarrhea, straining, pelvic congestion associated with pregnancy, enlargement of the prostate, uterine fibroids, and tumors of the rectum. Chronic liver disease associated with portal hypertension frequently results in hemorrhoids, because the superior hemorrhoidal veins drain into the portal system (see Fig. 27-2). Additionally, the portal system is valveless, thus backflow readily occurs.

External hemorrhoids are classified as acute or chronic. The *acute* form appears as a bluish, rounded swelling at the anal verge and is actually a hematoma, although it is referred to as an acute external thrombosed hemorrhoid. These areas are often quite painful and pruritic because the nerve endings in the skin are pain receptors. Occasionally, evacuating the clot under local anesthesia is necessary, or it may be treated by hot sitz baths and analgesics. A *chronic* external hemorrhoid or *skin tag* is usually the sequela to an acute hematoma. Anal skin tags consist of one or more folds of anal skin composed of connective tissue and a few blood vessels.

Internal hemorrhoids are classified as first, second, and third degree. *First-degree (early)* internal hemorrhoids do not protrude through the anal canal and can be detected only by proctoscopy. These hemorrhoids are usually located in the right and left posterior and right anterior positions, following the distribution of the tributaries of the superior hemorrhoidal vein and appear as globular reddish swellings. *Second-degree* hemorrhoids may prolapse through the anal canal after defecation; they may recede spontaneously or can be reduced manually. *Third-degree* hemorrhoids are permanently prolapsed. The most common symptom of internal hemorrhoids is painless bleeding, because no pain fibers exist in this area. Most cases of hemorrhoids are of the mixed variety rather than being strictly internal or external.

The most common complications of hemorrhoids are bleeding, thrombosis, and strangulation. A strangulated hemorrhoid is a prolapsed one in which the blood supply is cut off by the anal sphincter.

Diagnosis of hemorrhoids is made by inspection, digital examination, and viewing through a proctoscope or anoscope. Ruling out carcinoma when hemorrhoids occur in the middle and later years is important.

Most patients with hemorrhoids need not undergo surgery. Medical treatment includes sitz baths, or other forms of moist heat, bed rest, stool softeners to prevent constipation, high-roughage diet, and the use of soothing suppositories. Surgical excision may be indicated when persistent bleeding, prolapse, or intractable pruritus and anal pain occur.

Anal Fissure (Fissure in Ano)

An *anal fissure (fissure in ano)* is a crack in the lining of the anus caused by stretching from the passage of hard fecal matter; therefore constipation is a common cause. Diarrhea or trauma from childbirth also causes an anal fissure. The most prominent symptom is severe burning pain after defecation, and the bowel movement is usually accompanied by a small amount of bright-red blood. These patients are nearly always constipated; because the bowel movement is so painful, the constipation becomes progressively worse because patients fear to have a bowel movement. Anal fissures are often found in association with the skin tags of external hemorrhoids. Treatment is

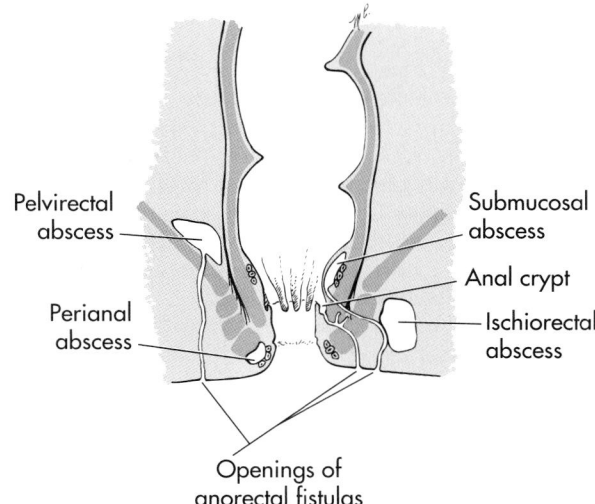

FIG. 26-6   Common sites of anorectal abscesses and fistulas. Inflammation often begins in the anal crypts.

surgical excision of the tract if local dilations, ointments, and cleansing do not help.

Anorectal Abscess and Fistula in Ano

An *anorectal abscess* is a localized infection with the collection of pus in the anorectal area. The infecting organisms are usually *Escherichia coli*, staphylococci, or streptococci. A *fistula in ano* is a chronic granulomatous tract that proceeds in a linear path from the anal canal to the skin outside the anus or from an abscess to the anal canal or the perirectal area. An anorectal fistula is often preceded by abscess formation. Fig. 26-6 illustrates the sites of abscess and fistula formation. The perianal abscess is the most common type of anorectal abscess, followed by the ischiorectal, submucous, and pelvirectal locations. The perianal abscess is usually obvious as a red, painful swelling close to the anal verge. Sitting or coughing aggravates the pain. A submucous or ischiorectal abscess may be palpated as a swelling on rectal examination. A pelvirectal abscess may be more difficult to identify. Discharge of pus from an anorectal fistula may be the first sign. Occasionally, a fistula may be palpated or its course determined by the gentle passage of a probe from the external opening, with a finger of the other hand in the anal canal.

Anorectal abscesses typically begin as an inflammation of the anal crypts, which are located at the lower end of the columns of Morgagni (see Fig. 26-2). The anal glands open into these crypts. Obstruction or trauma to their ducts gives rise to stasis and predisposes to infection. Mucosal tears from hard, constipated stools may be a predisposing factor. In a few cases, a predisposing local lesion such as an ulcerated hemorrhoid or anal fissure may be present.

When symptoms of diarrhea are associated with recurrent anorectal fistulas, Crohn's disease must be suspected, because as many as 50% of patients with Crohn's disease develop a fistula in ano.

The treatment of anorectal abscesses and fistulas is incision and drainage of the abscess and excision of any associated fistulas.

KEY CONCEPTS

- The large intestine or colon is a hollow muscular tube extending from the cecum to the anal canal and is divided into the cecum, colon (ascending, transverse, descending, and sigmoid) and rectum. The ileocecal valves control entry of chyme into the colon, and the internal and external sphincter muscles control exit of feces from the anal canal.

- The large intestine is clinically divided into right and left halves based on blood supply. The superior mesenteric artery supplies the cecum, ascending colon, and proximal two thirds of the transverse colon (right half). The inferior mesenteric artery supplies the distal one third of the transverse colon descending and sigmoid colon and proximal part of the rectum (left half).

- The large intestine has a variety of functions; the most important of which is the absorption of water and electrolytes. This absorption is largely completed in the right side of the colon. The sigmoid colon is a reservoir for the dehydrated fecal mass until defecation takes place. The absorptive capacity of the colon is approximately 1500 to 2000 ml. When this amount is exceeded by excessive delivery of fluid from the ileum, diarrhea results.

- The small amount of digestion that occurs in the large intestine results from bacterial rather than enzymatic action. Bacteria of the large intestine synthesize vitamin K and several vitamins of the B group. Bacterial fermentation of some carbohydrates in the colon also takes place. Approximately 1000 ml of flatus (mostly from swallowed air) is expelled each day.

- A movement characteristic of the large intestine is haustral churning. These nonprogressive kneading movements cause contents to move back and forth, allowing time for absorption. Propulsive peristalsis of feces into the rectum results in distention of the rectal wall and activation of the defecation reflex.

- Pathologic concerns of the large intestine tend to be associated with elimination symptoms. Constipation, diarrhea, alteration in size or color of stool and the presence of blood in the stools are all important signs and symptoms related to the colon and rectum.

- Diverticulosis is a condition of the colon characterized by herniation of the mucosa through the muscularis to form disk-shaped saccules. Herniation commonly occurs at the weakest point, where entry of the blood vessel weakens the colon wall. The sigmoid colon is the most common site for diverticula to develop. When one or more of the saccules become inflamed, the condition is called *diverticulitis*. The pathogenesis of diverticulosis is believed to be related to eating a low-fiber diet, disordered motility, and the build-up of high intraluminal pressures that cause herniation of the mucosa. Greater pressures can build up in a person eating a low-fiber diet because the colon has a narrower lumen compared with one filled with feces when the diet is high in fiber. Complications of diverticulitis include inflammation, abscess formation, bleeding, intestinal obstruction, perforation, and peritonitis.

- Ulcerative colitis is a nonspecific inflammatory disease of the colon generally following a prolonged course of exacerbations and remissions. Inflammatory lesions involve the mucosa and submucosa, eventually causing ulceration and bleeding. The disease process usually begins in the rectosigmoid area and may then spread proximally to involve the entire colon (no skip lesions as in Crohn's disease). Cardinal signs and symptoms are colicky abdominal pain and bloody, mucus-filled diarrhea. Potentially fatal complications include toxic megacolon, hemorrhage, and carcinoma of the colon. Extragastrointestinal manifestations (arthritis, eye and skin involvement) are similar to those of Crohn's disease.

- The lesions of Crohn's disease involve the colon in approximately 35% of the cases.

- Colonic polyps are common and occupy an intermediate position between benign and malignant neoplasms. Polyps occur most frequently in the sigmoid colon and increase with aging. A polyp is a growth that arises from a mucosal surface and extends outward. *Pedunculated adenomas* (adenomatous polyps or polypoid adenomas) are globelike structures attached to the mucous membrane by a thin stalk. Adenomatous polyps that are multiple or greater than 1 cm in diameter are considered to pose an increased cancer risk. A *juvenile polyp* occurs most commonly in children, have extremely long stalks, and are believed to be inflammatory in origin. *Villous adenomas* are sessile (broad-based with no stalk) neoplasms (cauliflower-shaped mass), usually solitary and large (>5 cm) and have a greater than 25% chance of being malignant. *Familial polyposis* is an autosomal dominant genetic disease characterized by the presence of hundreds of pedunculated and sessile polyps throughout the colon; the probability of colon cancer is 100% by the age of 40 years.

- Cancer of the colon and rectum is the third leading cause of cancer death in both men and women; approximately 60% occur in the rectosigmoid area of the colon, thus they may be either palpated during a rectal examination or detected by a sigmoidoscope. Approximately 25% of colon cancers are located in the cecum and ascending colon and can be detected by colonoscopy. Histologically, nearly all colon cancers are adenocarcinomas. Structurally, colon cancers are polypoid in shape (more common in cecum) or annular (ringlike) in shape (more common in the rectosigmoid area).

- Signs and symptoms of cancer of the colon and rectum vary according to location and are generally divided into cancer of the left colon (descending, sigmoid and rectum) and right colon (cecum, ascending, right transverse). Signs and symptoms of cancer of the left colon include: (1) distinct change in bowel habits (constipation or diarrhea, pencil or ribbon-shaped stools, tenesmus); (2) gross blood in the stool; (3) pain (rectal, back, lower left quadrant);

(4) anemia and weight loss; and (5) palpable mass detected by digital or endoscopic examination. Signs and symptoms of cancer of the right colon include: (1) occult blood in stool; (2) pain referred to the umbilicus or back; (3) anemia and weight loss; and (4) palpable abdominal mass in the right lower quadrant. Change in bowel habits is unlikely because the stool is liquid. Cancer of the right colon is generally diagnosed later than is cancer of the left colon and consequently has a poorer prognosis.

- Hemorrhoids or "piles" are varicose veins of the anal canal ands are divided into two classes, internal and external. Internal hemorrhoids are varices of the superior and middle hemorrhoidal veins, located above the internal rectal sphincter. External hemorrhoids are varices of the inferior hemorrhoidal veins, located outside the anal sphincter. The direct cause of hemorrhoids is interference with venous return from the hemorrhoidal veins commonly associated with pregnancy, constipation or diarrhea or both, rectal cancer, and cirrhosis of the liver. Complications of hemorrhoids include bleeding, thrombosis, and strangulation.

- The *acute external hemorrhoid* appears as a bluish, rounded swelling at the anal verge and is actually a hematoma. A chronic external hemorrhoid or *anal skin tag* is usually the sequela to an acute hematoma. External hemorrhoids often cause pruritus.
- *Internal hemorrhoids* are classified as first degree (globular swelling felt inside the anal canal), second degree (prolapse through the anal canal during defecation but recede or can be manually pushed back into the anal canal), and third degree (permanently prolapsed through the anal canal). When hemorrhoids appear in a middle-aged or older patient, cancer of the rectum must be ruled out.
- An *anal fissure* (fissure in ano) is a crack in the lining of the anus caused by stretching from the passage of hard fecal matter.
- An *anorectal abscess* is a localized infection with the collection of pus in the anorectal area. A *fistula in ano* is a chronic granulomatous tract that proceeds directly from the anal canal to the skin outside of the anus or from an abscess to the anal canal or the perirectal area. Anorectal fistulas are present in 50% of patients with Crohn's disease.

QUESTIONS

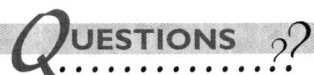

A sampling of review questions for this chapter appears here. Visit http://www.mosby.com/MERLIN/PriceWilson/ for additional questions.

Answer the following on a separate sheet of paper.

1. Draw a picture of the large intestine in the abdominal and pelvic cavities, and label the parts with the following terms: appendix; cecum; ascending, transverse, descending, and sigmoid colon; rectum; anal canal; anus; hepatic and splenic flexures; haustra; and taenia coli.
2. What are the most important functions of the large bowel?
3. Discuss the differences in structure between the small and large bowel. How do these differences in structure lead to differences in function?
4. Briefly summarize the mechanical operation of the large bowel (haustral churning, mass peristalsis).
5. List five common anorectal disorders.
6. List the most common diagnostic procedures used for the detection of disease of the large bowel. What can be detected with each disease?
7. Do all cases of acute diverticulitis require surgical intervention? If not, what is the medical treatment for acute diverticulitis?
8. Identify three predisposing factors in the pathogenesis of cancer of the colon or rectum.
9. What is Burkitt's hypothesis concerning the relationship of diet to the development of cancer of the bowel?
10. Why are hemorrhoids a frequent manifestation of hepatic cirrhosis and portal hypertension?
11. Define fissure in ano and fistula in ano. Is there any relationship between these two disorders and hemorrhoids? What disease of the GI tract is often associated with anorectal fistulas?

Fill in the blanks with the correct word(s) or circle the correct option.

12. _____ is a condition in which herniation of the mucosa occurs through the muscularis of the large bowel to form flask-shaped saccules. The condition is called _____ when the saccules become inflamed.
13. _____ adenoma or adenomatous polyp is a globelike structure on a pedicle arising from a mucosal surface. _____ polyps have very long pedicles and often occur in children. A _____ adenoma is a broad-based tumor composed of villous projections. _____ _____ is a hereditary disease characterized by the presence of hundreds of polyps throughout the colon.
14. An encircling or _____ form of cancer growth is more common in the left colon, whereas the shape is more likely to be _____ in the cecum.
15. Three routes of spread of cancer of the bowel are _____, _____, and _____.
16. Internal hemorrhoids are varicosities of the _____ and _____ hemorrhoidal veins and are located (inside) (outside) the anal sphincters. The _____ hemorrhoidal veins are involved in external hemorrhoids.
17. Three common complications of hemorrhoids are _____, _____, and _____.

ANATOMY AND PHYSIOLOGY

The liver, biliary tract, and pancreas develop as offshoots of the fetal foregut in a region that later becomes the duodenum; all are intimately associated with the physiology of digestion. Considering these structures together is reasonable because of their anatomic proximity, their closely related functions, and the similarity of the symptom complexes induced by many of their disorders.

Liver

The liver is the largest gland in the body, averaging approximately 1500 g (3 lbs) or 2% of the body weight in a normal adult (Fig. 27-1). The liver is a soft, pliable organ that is molded by the surrounding structures. The superior surface is convex and lies beneath the right dome and part of the left dome of the diaphragm. The lower portion of the liver is concave and provides a roof over the right kidney, stomach, pancreas, gallbladder, and intestines. The two principal lobes are the right and the left lobes. The *right lobe* is divided into anterior and posterior segments by the right segmental fissure, not observed from the exterior. The *left lobe* is divided into medial and lateral segments by the externally visible falciform ligament. The *falciform ligament* passes from the liver to the diaphragm and the anterior abdominal wall. The surface of the liver is covered by visceral peritoneum, except for a small area on the posterior surface that is attached directly to the diaphragm. Several ligaments that are reflections of the peritoneum help support the liver. Beneath the peritoneum is a dense, connective tissue layer called the *capsule of Glisson*, which covers the surface of the entire organ, with the thickest parts around the porta hepatis, forming a framework for the branches of the portal vein, hepatic artery, and bile ducts. The *porta hepatis* is the fissure of the liver whereby the portal vein and hepatic artery enter and the hepatic duct leaves.

Microscopic Structure

Each lobe of the liver is divided into structures called *lobules*, which are the microscopic and functional units of the organ (Fig. 27-1, *B*). Each lobule is a hexagonal body

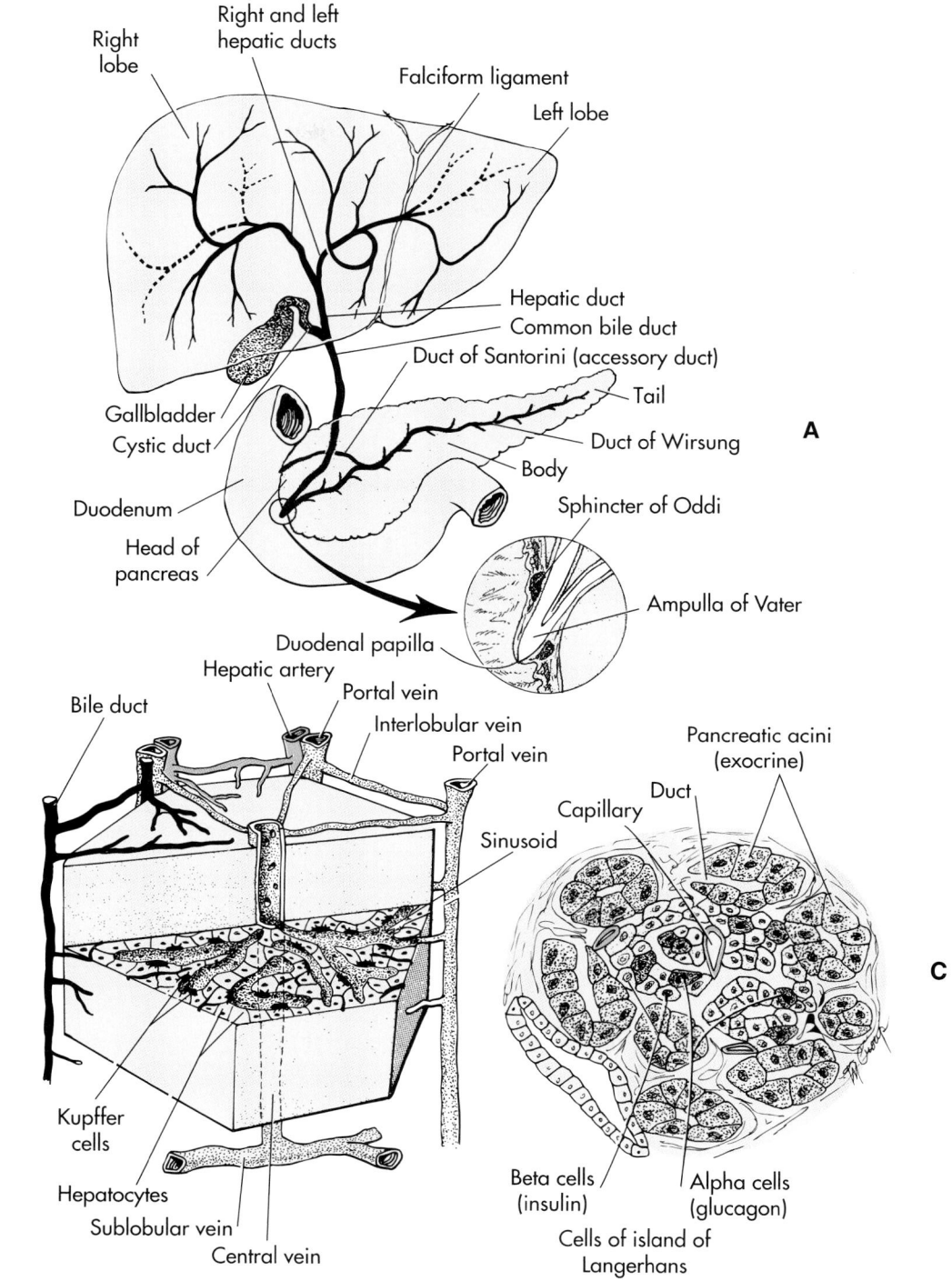

FIG. 27-1   A, Liver, gallbladder, and pancreas. **B**, Microscopic structure of hepatic functional unit (liver lobule). **C**, Pancreatic acinar units.

composed of plates of cuboidal hepatic cells arranged in a radial fashion around a central vein that drains the lobule. Human livers may have up to 100,000 lobules. Between the plates of hepatic cells are capillaries called *sinusoids*, which are branches of the portal vein and hepatic artery. The sinusoids, unlike other capillaries, are lined with phagocytic, or Kupffer, cells. *Kupffer cells* belong to the monocyte-macrophage system, and their main function is to engulf bacteria and other foreign par-

ticles in the blood. As many as 50% of all macrophages are found in the liver as Kupffer cells; thus the liver is one of the principal organs of defense against bacterial invasions and toxic agents. In addition to branches of the portal vein and hepatic artery encircling the periphery of the liver lobule, bile ducts are also present. The interlobular bile ducts form small bile capillaries called *canaliculi* (not shown), which course within the center of the liver cell plates. Bile formed in the hepatocytes is excreted into

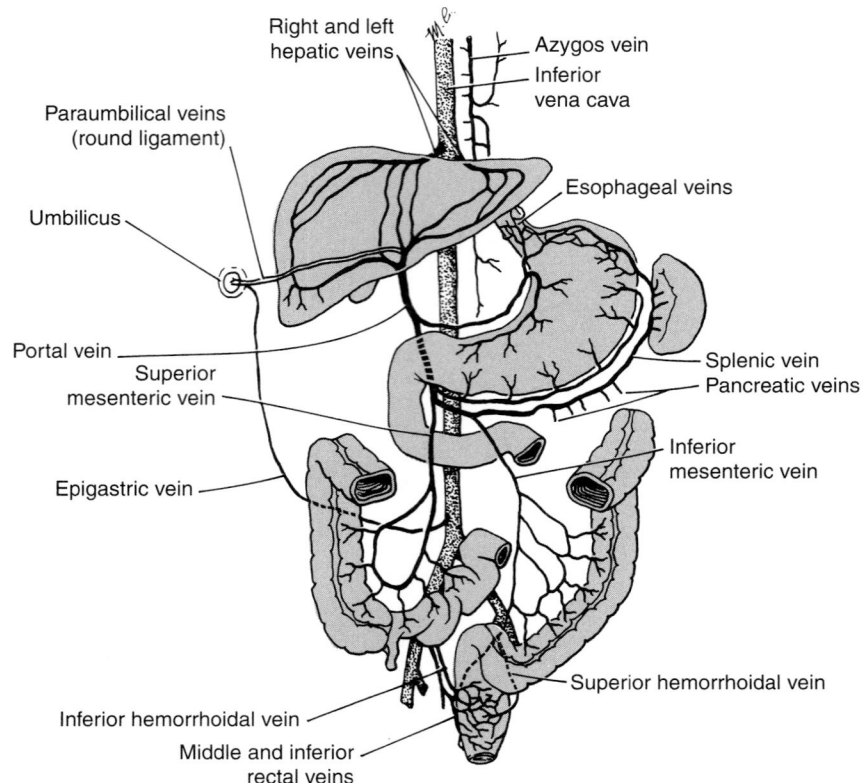

FIG. 27-2 Hepatic portal system. Blood is carried from the stomach, intestines, spleen, and pancreas into the liver sinusoids. Hepatic veins convey blood to the inferior vena cava. Clinically significant sites of anastomosis between the hepatic and systemic circulations are (1) the esophageal veins (portal tributary), which anastomose with the azygos veins (systemic tributary); (2) the paraumbilical veins in the round ligament, which originate in the left branch of the portal vein and connect with the superficial veins of the anterior abdominal wall (systemic tributaries) in the area of the umbilicus; (3) the superior rectal or hemorrhoidal veins (portal tributaries), which anastomose with the middle and inferior rectal veins (systemic tributaries); and (4) the portal tributaries to the intestines, pancreas, and liver, which anastomose with the phrenic, renal, and lumbar veins (systemic tributaries not shown). In portal hypertension and chronic liver disease, blood may be backed up in these veins and shunted around the liver through the points of anastomosis.

the canaliculi, which join to form larger and larger bile ducts until the common bile duct is reached.

Circulation

The liver has a dual blood supply: from the digestive tract and the spleen via the *hepatic portal vein* and from the aorta via the *hepatic artery*. Approximately one third of the incoming blood is arterial, and two thirds is venous from the portal vein. A total volume of 1500 ml passes through the liver each minute and is drained via the right and left *hepatic veins*, which empty into the inferior vena cava (Fig. 27-2).

The portal vein is unique in that it is interposed between two capillary beds, one in the liver and the other in the digestive area that it drains. On entering the liver, the portal vein divides into branches that come into contact with the circumference of the liver lobules. These branches then give off interlobular veins, which run between the lobules. These veins give rise to the sinusoids, which run between the plates of hepatocytes to enter the central veins. Central veins from several lobules join to form the sublobular veins, which, in turn, join to form the hepatic veins (see Fig. 27-1, *B*). The smallest

branches of the hepatic artery also empty into the sinusoids, making the blood composition unique in that it is a mixture of arterial blood from the hepatic artery and venous blood from the portal vein. Fig. 27-2 illustrates the origin of blood flowing into the portal system; increased pressure in this system is a common manifestation in liver disorders, with serious consequences involving the vessels in which the portal blood originates. Several points of portacaval anastomosis are of clinical significance. In cases of obstruction to flow in the liver, portal blood may be shunted around the liver to the systemic venous system. The consequences of portal hypertension and shunting are discussed in greater detail later in this chapter.

Liver Function

In addition to ranking first in size as a parenchymal organ, the liver also ranks first in the number, complexity, and variety of its functions. The liver is essential for the maintenance of life, is involved in nearly every metabolic function of the body, and is specifically responsible for more than 500 separate activities. Fortunately, the liver has a large reserve capacity and needs only 10% to 20% of its

TABLE 27-1

Major Functions of the Liver

Function	Comments
Formation and excretion of bile	
Bile salts metabolism	Bile salts are essential for the digestion and absorption of fats and fat-soluble vitamins in the intestine.
Bile pigment metabolism	Bilirubin, the main bile pigment, is a metabolic end product from the processing of old red blood cells; it is conjugated in the liver and excreted in bile.
Carbohydrate metabolism	The liver plays an important part in maintaining the normal blood glucose level and providing energy for the body; carbohydrates are stored in the liver as glycogen.
Glycogenesis	
Glycogenolysis	
Gluconeogenesis	
Protein metabolism	Serum proteins synthesized by the liver include albumin and the alpha and beta globulins (not gamma globulin).
Protein synthesis	Blood-clotting factors synthesized by the liver include fibrinogen (I), prothrombin (II), and factors V, VII, IX, and X; vitamin K is a necessary cofactor in the synthesis of all these factors except V.
Urea formation	Urea is formed exclusively in the liver from ammonia (NH_3), which is then excreted in the urine and feces; NH_3 is formed from deamination of amino acids and action of intestinal bacteria on amino acids.
Protein (amino acid) storage	
Fat metabolism	Triglycerides, cholesterol, phospholipids, and lipoproteins (absorbed from intestine) are hydrolyzed to fatty acids and glycerol.
Ketogenesis	
Cholesterol synthesis	The liver plays a major role in cholesterol synthesis, most of which is excreted in the bile as cholesterol or cholic acid.
Fat storage	
Vitamin and mineral storage	Fat-soluble vitamins (A, D, E, K) are stored in the liver, as are vitamin B_{12}, copper, and iron.
Steroid metabolism	The liver inactivates and excretes aldosterone, glucocorticoids, estrogen, progesterone, and testosterone.
Detoxification	The liver is responsible for biotransformation of substances that are potentially harmful (e.g., drugs) into harmless substances that are then excreted by the kidneys.
Flood chamber and filter action	Liver sinusoids provide a depot for blood backed up from venae cavae (right-sided heart failure); the phagocytic action of Kupffer cells removes bacteria and debris from blood.

functioning tissue to sustain life. Complete destruction or removal of the liver results in death in less than 10 hours. The liver has an impressive regenerative ability. In most patients, partial surgical removal will stimulate hepatocyte growth to replace the dead or diseased cells. The regeneration process is essentially complete in 4 to 5 weeks. In some individuals, normal liver mass has been restored within 6 months. This phenomenon is important in the transplantation of a liver segment.

Table 27-1 lists the major functions of the liver. Understanding these functions is a prerequisite to understanding liver pathophysiology.

The formation and excretion of *bile* represent a major function of the liver; the bile ducts transport and the gallbladder stores and releases bile into the small intestine as needed. The liver secretes approximately 500 to 1000 ml of yellow bile each day. The basic components of bile are water (97%), electrolytes, bile salts, phospholipids (mainly lecithin), cholesterol, inorganic salts, and bile pigments (mainly conjugated bilirubin). *Bile salts* are essential for fat digestion and absorption in the small intestine. After being acted on by bacteria in the small intestine, most of the bile salts are reabsorbed in the ileum, recirculated to the liver, and reconjugated and re-secreted (see Chapter 25). Although *bilirubin* (bile pigment) is a metabolic end product and has no physiologically active role, it is nonetheless important as an indicator of liver and biliary tract disease, because it tends to color the tissues and fluid with which it comes in contact. Most bilirubin conjugates are waste products and are excreted through feces. Normal bilirubin metab-

olism and jaundice as a sign of disease are discussed later in this chapter.

The liver plays an essential role in the metabolism of three macronutrients delivered by the portal vein after absorption from the intestines: carbohydrates, proteins, and fats. Monosaccharides from the small intestine are converted into glycogen and stored as such in the liver *(glycogenesis)*. The release of glucose from this storage depot of glycogen *(glycogenolysis)* is varied in a controlled manner so as to meet the body's changing requirements for glucose. Some of the glucose is metabolized in the tissues to produce heat and energy, and the remainder is converted either into glycogen and stored in the muscles or into fat and stored in the subcutaneous tissues. The liver is also capable of synthesizing glucose from proteins and fat *(gluconeogenesis)*. The role of the liver in protein metabolism is essential to survival. The plasma proteins, except gamma globulin, are synthesized by the liver. These proteins include albumin, which is necessary for the maintenance of the colloid osmotic pressure, and prothrombin, fibrinogen, and other clotting factors. Additionally, most degradation of amino acids begins in the liver with *deamination*, or the removal of an amino group (NH_2). The ammonia (NH_3) released is then synthesized into urea and excreted by the kidneys and intestines. NH_3 formed in the gut by the action of bacteria on protein is also converted to urea in the liver.

Other metabolic functions of the liver include the metabolism of fat; the storage of vitamins, iron, and copper; the conjugation and excretion of adrenal and gonadal steroids; and the detoxification of numerous endogenous and exogenous substances. Liver enzymes that oxidize, reduce, hydrolyze, or conjugate the potentially harmful substance, rendering it physiologically inactive, accomplish this detoxification function. Endogenous substances, such as indol, skatole, and phenol, which are produced by the action of bacteria on amino acids in the large intestine, and exogenous substances, such as morphine, phenobarbital, and other drugs, are detoxified in this manner. When substances such as ethyl alcohol are ingested, approximately 80% is metabolized in the liver. The remaining alcohol is absorbed in the stomach or excreted through the kidneys, lungs, and skin. Alcohol is transported to the liver and metabolized in a two-step process involving alcohol dehydrogenase. Acetaldehyde and acetate are formed. Some of the resulting acetate combines with coenzymes to form acetyl CoA, which can be biosynthesized into fatty acids and can potentially result in fatty liver disease, hepatic stenosis, or other toxic effects on liver cells and their function. Alcohol abuse can further increase levels of acetaldehyde and perpetuate alcoholic liver injury. Women appear to be more predisposed to alcohol-induced liver damage than are men.

Finally, the liver functions as a "flood chamber" and "filter" because of its strategic position between the intestinal and general circulation. In cases of right-sided heart failure, the liver may become passively congested with a large amount of blood. The Kupffer cells in the sinusoids filter bacteria and other injurious materials from the portal blood by phagocytosis.

Gallbladder

The gallbladder is a pear-shaped hollow sac resting directly beneath the right lobe of the liver (see Fig. 27-1). Bile, which is secreted continuously by the liver, enters the small bile ducts within the liver. The small bile ducts join to form two larger ducts, which emerge from the undersurface of the liver as the *right* and *left hepatic ducts*, but which immediately join to form the *common hepatic duct*. The hepatic duct merges with the *cystic duct* from the gallbladder, forming the *common bile duct*. In many individuals, the common bile duct merges with the pancreatic duct to form the *ampulla of Vater* (dilated portion in common channel) before opening into the small intestine. The terminal parts of both ducts and the ampulla are surrounded by circular muscle fibers known as the *sphincter of Oddi* (see Fig. 27-1, *A*, inset).

The principal function of the gallbladder is the storage and concentration of bile, and it is capable of holding approximately 40 to 60 ml of bile. Hepatic bile may not immediately enter the duodenum; rather, after passing down the hepatic duct, it may be diverted into the cystic duct and gallbladder. In the gallbladder, the lymphatics and blood vessels absorb water and inorganic salts, thus gallbladder bile is up to five times as concentrated as is hepatic bile. At intervals the gallbladder contents are emptied into the duodenum by simultaneous contraction of the muscular coat and relaxation of the sphincter of Oddi. The hormone cholecystokinin (CCK), released from duodenal cells in response to the presence of digestive products from dietary lipids and proteins, stimulates gallbladder contraction.

Pancreas

The pancreas is a long, slender organ approximately 6 to 8 inches (15 to 20 cm) in length and $1\frac{1}{2}$ inches (3.8 cm) in width. The pancreas lies retroperitoneal and is divided into three major segments: the head, body, and tail (see Fig. 27-1). The head lies in the concavity formed by the duodenum, and the tail touches the spleen.

The pancreas is made up of two basic types of cells having entirely different functions (see Fig. 27-1, *C*). The *exocrine cells*, clustered into groups called *acini*, produce the components of the pancreatic juice (see Table 25-1). The *endocrine cells*, or *islets of Langerhans*, produce the endocrine secretions insulin and glucagon, which are important for carbohydrate metabolism.

The pancreas is a compound tubuloalveolar gland. As a whole, the pancreas resembles a bunch of grapes, the branches of which are the ducts terminating into the main pancreatic duct *(duct of Wirsung)*. Small ducts from each acinus empty into the main ducts. The main duct, extending throughout the length of the gland, often joins the common bile duct at the ampulla of Vater before entering the duodenum. An accessory duct, the *duct of Santorini*, is frequently found extending from the head of the pancreas into the duodenum, approximately 1 inch (2.5 cm) above the duodenal papilla.

OVERVIEW

Pathologic changes in diseases of the liver, gallbladder, and pancreas may be broadly categorized into three types: *inflammatory, fibrotic,* and *neoplastic changes*. Hepatitis, cholecystitis, and pancreatitis show evidence of acute or chronic inflammation of the involved tissues. Gallstones and biliary tract obstruction are frequently associated with cholecystitis and pancreatitis. Fibrotic changes occur with cirrhosis of the liver and in chronic inflammatory conditions. Although primary benign or malignant tumors of the liver or gallbladder are rare, pancreatic cancer is not. Widespread destruction of parenchymal cells resulting from inflammation, fibrosis, neoplasms, or obstruction interferes with secretory and excretory functions. *Jaundice* (yellow coloration of the body tissues) is a common symptom and results from interference with the excretion of bilirubin. Portal hypertension, ascites, esophageal varices, and hepatic encephalopathy are common complications in advanced cirrhosis and hepatic failure.

DIAGNOSTIC TESTS

Table 27-2 lists some of the most common diagnostic tests used to detect disordered function of the liver, biliary system, and pancreas. No single test or procedure is capable of measuring the total function of the liver, because it is involved in nearly every metabolic process in the body and has a large functional reserve. A battery of diagnostic tests is typically used.

Table 27-3 summarizes radiologic methods useful in diagnosing disorders of the liver, biliary system, and pancreas. Other diagnostic methods include *esophagoscopy*, which allows direct visualization of esophageal varices;

TABLE 27-2 ∎∎∎

Liver, Biliary, and Pancreatic Function Tests

Test	Normal	Clinical Significance
BILIARY EXCRETION		Measures ability of liver to conjugate and excrete bile pigment.
Direct serum bilirubin (conjugated)	0.1-0.3 mg/dl	Elevated when excretion of conjugated bilirubin is impaired.
Indirect serum bilirubin (unconjugated)	0.2-0.7 mg/dl	Elevated in hemolytic conditions and Gilbert's syndrome.
Total serum bilirubin	0.3-1.0 mg/dl	Both direct and total serum bilirubin elevated in hepatocellular disease.
Urine bilirubin	0	Conjugated bilirubin excreted in urine when elevated in serum, suggesting liver cell or biliary tract obstruction; urine appears brown; foam appears yellow when shaken (simple bedside test).
Urine urobilinogen	1.0-3.5 mg/24 hr	Decreased when bile excretion is impaired, as in liver damage, biliary obstruction, or inflammation; increased when amount produced exceeds ability of liver to reexcrete it, as in hemolytic jaundice.
DYE EXCRETION		
Sulfobromophthalein sodium (Bromsulphalein, BSP) clearance test	<5% retention in 45 minutes	Rate of intravenously administered sulfobromophthalein clearance from plasma is used in evaluating liver function; excretion depends on functional liver cells, patent biliary ducts, and hepatic blood flow; BSP test is a sensitive index of liver function, useful in detecting early liver cell damage and recovery from infectious hepatitis, but because of occasional toxic reactions, it is not widely used.
PROTEIN METABOLISM		
Total serum protein	6-8 g/dl	Most of serum proteins and coagulation proteins are synthesized by liver and are therefore decreased in a variety of liver impairments.
Serum albumin	3.2-5.5 g/dl	
Serum globulin	2.0-3.5 g/dl	
Prothrombin time	11-15 seconds	Increased with decreased prothrombin synthesis resulting from liver cell damage or decreased vitamin K absorption in biliary obstruction; vitamin K is essential for prothrombin synthesis.
Blood ammonia (NH_3)	80-100 μg/dl	Liver converts NH_3 to urea; level increases in hepatic failure or large portal-systemic shunts.
CARBOHYDRATE METABOLISM		
Serum amylase	60-180 Somogyi units/dl	Obstruction and inflammatory disease of pancreas interfere with normal flow of amylase into intestinal tract and result in increased serum levels; value increases greatly in acute pancreatitis; also increases in parotid gland disease and other conditions.
Urine amylase	35-260 Somogyi units/hr	Urine amylase remains high longer than serum amylase (1 week); values >300 indicate pancreatitis.
FAT METABOLISM		
Serum lipase	<1.5 units/ml (Cherry-Crandall method)	Pancreatic digestive enzymes are released into blood with breakdown of acinar cells in obstructive or inflammatory conditions of pancreas.
Serum cholesterol	<200 mg/dl	Increased in bile duct obstruction, decreased in liver cell damage; values >200 increase risk for coronary heart disease.
Fecal fat test	5 gm/24 hours Fat retention ≥95%	Performed to confirm diagnosis of steatorrhea. Obstruction of pancreatic ducts interferes with secretion of pancreatic enzymes resulting in lack of fat digestion and absorbtion and steatorrhea.
SERUM ENZYMES		
AST (SGOT)	5-35 units/ml (Frankel)	Aspartate aminotransferase (AST), formerly serum glutamic-oxaloacetic transaminase (SGOT); alanine aminotransferase (ALT), formerly serum glutamic-pyruvic transaminase (SGPT); and lactic dehydrogenase (LDH) are intracellular enzymes concentrated in the heart, liver, and skeletal tissue; released from damaged tissue (necrosis or altered cell permeability); increased in liver cell damage and in other conditions, especially myocardial infarction.
ALT (SGPT)	5-35 units/ml (Frankel)	
LDH	200-450 units/ml (Wrobleski)	
Alkaline phosphatase	30-120 IU/L *or* 2-4 units/dl (Bodansky)	Manufactured in bone, liver, kidneys, and intestine and excreted into bile; level increases in biliary obstruction, as well as bone disease and liver metastasis.

Continued

TABLE 27-2   ■ ■ ■

Liver, Biliary, and Pancreatic Function Tests—cont'd

Test	Normal	Clinical Significance
SERUM ENZYMES		
Secretin-CKK test	Volume: 2-4 ml/kg in 80 min HCO3: 90-130mEq/L Amylase: 6.5-35.2 U/kg	Direct stimulation of pancreas by IV infusion of secretin and CCK followed by collection of duodenal contents allows assesment of pancreatic enzyme and bicarbonate output. Abnormal test suggests chronic pancreatic damage.
IMMUNOLOGIC TESTS		Key diagnostic tests are for viral hepatitis (see Table 27-5).

TABLE 27-3   ■ ■ ■

Radiologic Methods in Diagnosis of the Liver, Biliary, and Pancreatic Disorders

Test	Comments
Plain radiograph of abdomen	May reveal calcific densities in gallbladder, biliary tree (gallstones), pancreas, and liver; may also reveal splenomegaly or gross ascites.
Ultrasonography	Preferred method for detecting gallstones; reliable in detecting dilated bile ducts and cystic and solid masses of liver and pancreas; noninvasive and inexpensive.
Computed tomography (CT)	Provides high-resolution images of liver, gallbladder, pancreas, and spleen; reveals stones, solid masses, cysts, abscesses, and structural abnormalities; often used with contrast media.
Magnetic resonance imaging (MRI)	Same applications as CT scan but greater sensitivity; can also detect blood flow and blood vessel patency; noninvasive but expensive.
Barium swallow/meal (see Fig. 27-3, A)	Reveals esophageal varices in more than 70% of cases; tumors often produce displacement of duodenum (reverse-3 sign common).
Oral cholecystography	Conjugation and excretion of dye by liver allow visualization of gallbladder and bile ducts, thus revealing gallstones; poor or no visualization of contrast medium may be caused by liver cell disease or biliary obstruction; often used with extracorporeal shock wave lithotripsy and dissolution therapy for cholelithiasis treatment.
Percutaneous transhepatic cholangiogram (THC) (see Fig. 27-3, B)	Dye given by percutaneous puncture and blind probing for a bile duct into which dye is injected; may help to distinguish intrahepatic ducts and causes of biliary obstruction or cholestasis; hazards involve bile leakage, hemorrhage, and sepsis.
Endoscopic retrograde cholangiopancreatography (ERCP) (see Fig. 27-3, B)	Endoscopic insertion of a catheter into duodenal papilla and injection of contrast medium through catheter into pancreatic or biliary ductules allow visualization of these structures.
Technetium-99m (^{99m}Tc) biliary radioisotope scan	Reveals cholestasis, acute or chronic obstruction, bile leaks, fistulas, and cysts.
Radioisotope liver scan with radio-tagged blood cells, ^{99m}Tc-labeled sulfur colloid, or gallium scanning (see Fig. 27-3, C)	Reveals anatomic changes in liver tissue; lesions appear as filling defects (tumors, cysts, abscesses).
Selective celiac axis angiography (see Fig. 27-3, D)	Visualization of pancreatic, hepatic, and portal circulation possible; reveals tumor masses, disruption as in cirrhosis, and portal collateral circulation including hepatic lesions.
Portal pressure measurement (see Fig. 27-3, E)	Principal procedures are by direct measurement through portal vein catheterization or indirectly by intrasplenic pressure or wedge hepatic pressure determinations; portal pressure elevated in cirrhosis; procedures often combined with injection of contrast medium.
Splenoportogram (see Fig. 27-3, E)	Demonstrates size and patency of portal and splenic collaterals.

duodenoscopy, which allows visualization of the papilla of Vater and involves insertion of a catheter to inject contrast medium directly into the biliary or pancreatic system; *peritoneoscopy,* which involves insertion of a peritoneoscope through an abdominal stab wound and allows direct visualization of the anterior surface of the liver and gallbladder; and *electroencephalography,* which may reveal abnormal patterns in hepatic encephalopathy. Finally, percutaneous liver biopsy is a common procedure performed at the bedside.

Percutaneous liver biopsy is a valuable method of diagnosing diffuse parenchymal diseases, such as cirrhosis, hepatitis, and lymphoma. Before performing the procedure, the patient's capacity to clot blood is evaluated, and cross-matched blood is provided in case of need. The procedure itself is brief. The skin is cleansed and anes-

thetized. As a patient holds his or her breath in expiration to bring the liver and diaphragm to the highest position, the needle is inserted into the liver in the eighth or ninth intercostal space or subcostally and withdrawn (Fig. 27-3, F). The specimen is then expelled into formalin for later histologic examination. Patients must understand that they are to hold their breath and not move during the procedure to prevent laceration of the liver. The procedure is contraindicated in patients who cannot meet this requirement. For patients at high risk or those who cannot hold their breath, a transvenous liver biopsy may be performed. This procedure involves placement of an intravenous (IV) catheter transjugularly into the hepatic vein.

To prevent hemorrhage after the procedure, the patient lies on the right side for several hours to splint the

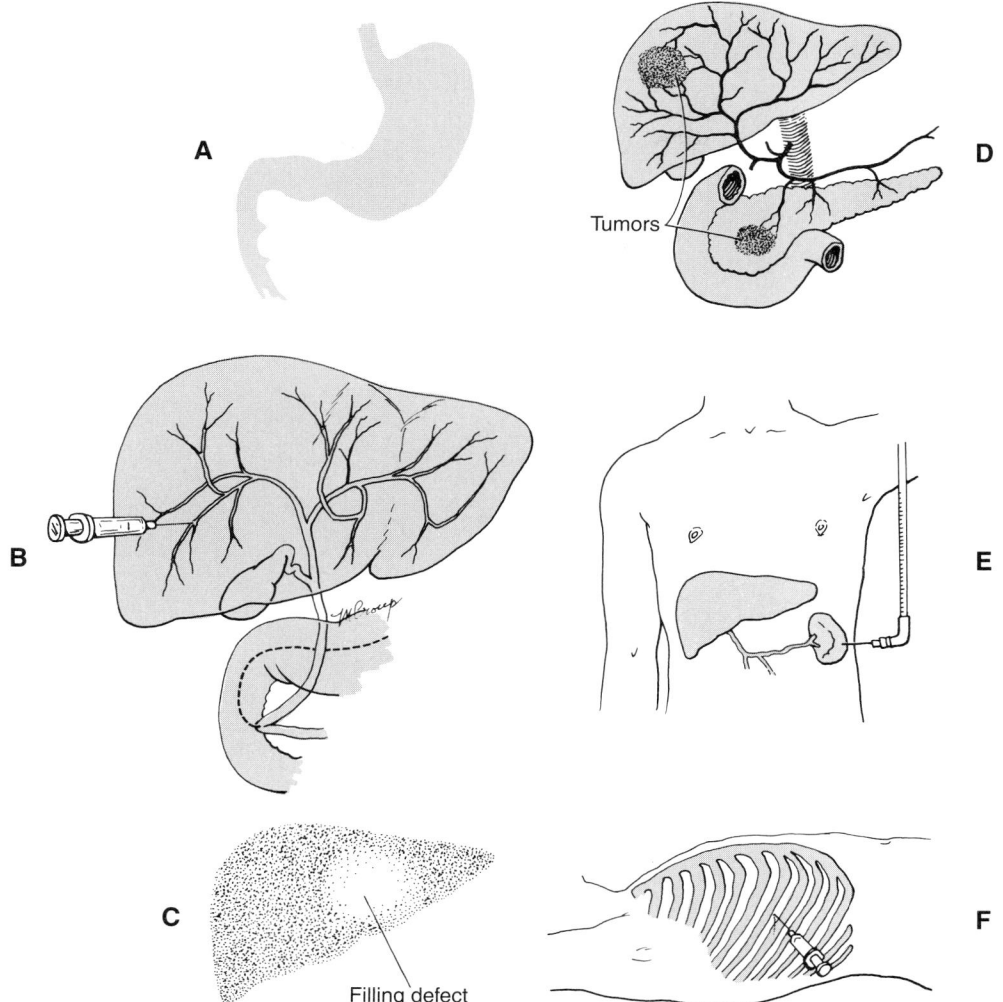

FIG. 27-3   Tests useful in the diagnosis of liver, biliary, and pancreatic disorders. **A,** Barium radiograph of the gastrointestinal tract. **B,** Transhepatic cholangiogram in which contrast material is injected percutaneously. The hepatic or pancreatic ductal systems may also be approached from below by inserting a catheter into the papilla of Vater and injecting contrast material (endoscopic retrograde cholangiopancreatography, ERCP). **C,** Liver scan. **D,** Selective celiac axis angiography. **E,** Splenoportogram and measurement of portal pressure. **F,** Liver biopsy. (See Table 27-3 and text for explanation of tests.)

chest. Although rare, complications of liver biopsy can be dangerous. The chief danger is intraperitoneal hemorrhage (0.4% of cases), which results from penetration of a large blood vessel. Bile peritonitis is a rare but serious complication that requires immediate surgical intervention. Vital signs are checked every 15 minutes until stable and then every 1 or 2 hours for the first 24 hours after the procedure. The dressing is checked frequently for local bleeding, and a pressure dressing is applied when necessary. Severe abdominal pain may indicate bile peritonitis and should be carefully evaluated. A "directed" rather than a "blind" liver biopsy may be performed with the use of computed tomography (CT) scan, magnetic resonance scan, or ultrasonography. The use of new and improved noninvasive diagnostic methods such as ultrasound and CT scan has obviated the need for biopsy in many circumstances. Fig. 27-3 illustrates some of the diagnostic procedures useful in liver, biliary, and pancreatic disorders.

BILIRUBIN METABOLISM AND JAUNDICE

The accumulation of bile pigments in the body causes yellow discoloration of the tissues called *jaundice.* Jaundice can usually be detected in the sclerae (whites of eyes) or skin or by a darkening of the urine when the serum bilirubin reaches 2 to 3 mg/dl. The normal serum bilirubin is 0.3 to 1.0 mg/dl. Surface tissues richest in elastin, such as the sclerae and the undersurface of the tongue, usually become stained first.

A consideration of the mechanisms of jaundice involves an understanding of the formation, transportation, metabolism, and excretion of bilirubin.

Normal Bilirubin Metabolism

In the normal individual, bilirubin formation and excretion proceed smoothly through the steps outlined in

RETICULOENDOTHELIAL SYSTEM

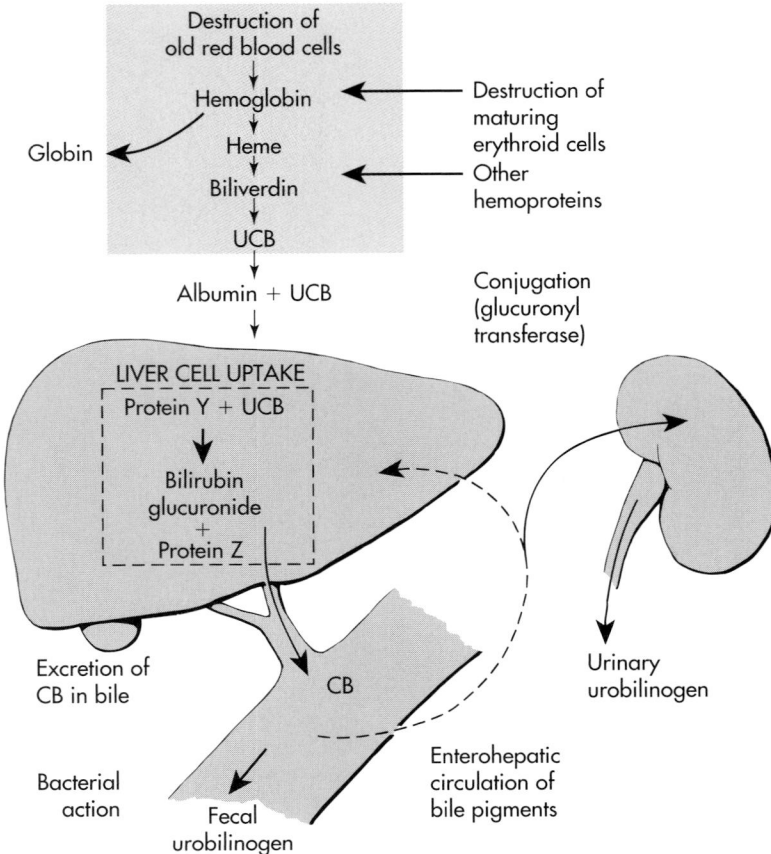

FIG. 27-4 Normal bilirubin metabolism. *CB,* Conjugated bilirubin; *UCB,* unconjugated bilirubin.

Fig. 27-4. Approximately 80% to 85% of the bilirubin is produced by the breakdown of senescent red blood cells (RBCs) in the monocyte-macrophage system. The average life span of an RBC is 120 days. Each day, approximately 50 ml of blood is destroyed, and 250 to 350 mg of bilirubin is produced. Approximately 15% to 20% of total bile pigment does not depend on this mechanism but is derived from destruction of maturing erythroid cells in the bone marrow (ineffective hematopoiesis) and from other hemoproteins, notably those in the liver.

In the catabolism of hemoglobin (largely occurring in the spleen), globin is first dissociated from heme, after which the heme is converted to biliverdin. Unconjugated bilirubin is then formed from biliverdin. *Biliverdin* is a greenish pigment formed by oxidation of bilirubin. Unconjugated bilirubin is lipid soluble, water insoluble, and incapable of being excreted in the bile or the urine. Unconjugated bilirubin, bound to albumin in a water-soluble complex, is transported in the blood to the liver cells. Hepatic metabolism of bilirubin involves three steps: uptake, conjugation, and excretion. Uptake by the liver cell involves two hepatic proteins, designated Y and Z (see Fig. 27-4). Conjugation of bilirubin with glucuronic acid is catalyzed by the enzyme *glucuronyl transferase* in the endoplasmic reticulum. Conjugated bilirubin is lipid insoluble, water soluble, and capable of being excreted in both the bile and the urine. Transport of con-

jugated bilirubin across the cell membrane into the bile by an active process is the final step in hepatic bilirubin metabolism. Unconjugated bilirubin is not excreted into the bile, except after photooxidation or photoisomerization (see the following discussion).

Intestinal bacteria reduce conjugated bilirubin to a series of compounds called *stercobilin* or *urobilinogen*. These substances account for the brown color of stool. Approximately 10% to 20% of the urobilinogen undergoes enterohepatic circulation, and a small fraction is excreted in the urine.

Pathophysiologic Mechanisms in Jaundice States

The four general mechanisms by which hyperbilirubinemia and jaundice can occur include:

1. Excess production of bilirubin
2. Impaired hepatic uptake of unconjugated bilirubin
3. Impaired conjugation of bilirubin
4. Decreased excretion of conjugated bilirubin into bile because of either intrahepatic or extrahepatic factors that may be functional or caused by mechanical obstruction

The first three mechanisms result in predominantly unconjugated hyperbilirubinemia, whereas the fourth results in predominantly conjugated hyperbilirubinemia.

Excess Bilirubin Production

Hemolytic disease, or an increased rate of RBC destruction, is the most common cause of excess bilirubin production. The resultant jaundice is customarily called *hemolytic jaundice.* Conjugation and transfer of bile pigment proceed normally, but the supply of unconjugated bilirubin is greater than the liver can handle. Consequently, the level of unconjugated bilirubin in the blood rises. The serum bilirubin level, however, rarely exceeds 5 mg/dl in patients with severe hemolysis, and the jaundice is a mild pale yellow. Because unconjugated bilirubin is water insoluble, it cannot be excreted in the urine and bilirubinuria does not occur. However, increased production of urobilinogen (caused by the increased bilirubin load presented to the liver and increased conjugation and excretion) occurs, which, in turn, results in increased fecal and urinary excretion. The urine and stool may thus be darker.

Some common causes of hemolytic jaundice are abnormal hemoglobins (hemoglobin S in sickle cell anemia), abnormal RBCs (hereditary spherocytosis), antibodies in the serum (Rh or transfusion incompatibility or as a result of autoimmune hemolytic disease), administration of some drugs, and increased hemolysis. Hemolytic jaundice can occasionally result from a process referred to as *ineffective erythropoiesis.* Essentially, this process increases destruction of RBCs or their precursors in the bone marrow (thalassemia, pernicious anemia, and porphyria).

In the adult, chronic overproduction of bilirubin may lead to the formation of gallstones predominantly composed of bilirubin; otherwise, the mild hyperbilirubinemia is not generally harmful. Treatment is directed toward correction of the hemolytic disease. In infancy, however, unconjugated bilirubin levels greater than 20 mg/dl may lead to kernicterus (see the following discussion).

Impaired Uptake of Bilirubin

The uptake of albumin-bound unconjugated bilirubin by liver cells involves the dissociation and binding of bilirubin to acceptor proteins. Only a few drugs have been shown to influence the uptake of bilirubin by the liver: flavaspidic acid (used to treat tapeworms), novobiocin, and some cholecystographic dyes. The unconjugated hyperbilirubinemia and jaundice usually disappear when the offending drug is withdrawn. Previously, neonatal jaundice and some cases of Gilbert syndrome were believed to involve a deficiency of acceptor protein and a defect in hepatic uptake. In most of these cases, however, a deficiency of glucuronyl transferase has been demonstrated; these conditions are best considered as a defect in bilirubin conjugation.

Impaired Conjugation of Bilirubin

The mild unconjugated hyperbilirubinemia (less than 12.9 mg/dl) that develops between the second and fifth days of life is called *physiologic jaundice of the newborn.* This normal neonatal jaundice results from immaturity of the enzyme glucuronyl transferase. The activity of glucuronyl transferase normally increases within several days to 2 weeks after birth, and the jaundice disappears.

When unconjugated bilirubin levels exceed 20 mg/dl in the newborn, a condition called kernicterus develops.

This condition might occur when a hemolytic process (e.g., erythroblastosis fetalis) is superimposed on the normal glucuronyl transferase deficiency in the newborn. *Kernicterus,* or bilirubin encephalopathy, results from the deposition of unconjugated bilirubin in the lipid-rich basal ganglia. If untreated, death or serious neurologic damage occurs. The current treatment approach to unconjugated hyperbilirubinemia in the newborn is phototherapy. *Phototherapy* involves the application of intense fluorescent or blue light (wavelength of 430 to 470 nm) on the infant's exposed skin. Exposure to the light leads to a structural change in the bilirubin (photoisomerization) to water-soluble polarized isomers that are rapidly excreted in the bile without the prior need for conjugation.

Three hereditary conditions represent progressive deficiency of glucuronyl transferase: Gilbert syndrome and type I and type II Crigler-Najjar syndrome. *Gilbert syndrome* is considered as a benign familial condition characterized by mild (2 to 5 mg/ml) and chronic unconjugated hyperbilirubinemia and jaundice. Current research has identified two forms of Gilbert syndrome. One group includes patients with evidence of hemolysis and increased bilirubin turnover; the other has decreased bilirubin clearance and no hemolysis. Both forms can occur at the same time in the same patient (Isselbacher, 1998). In Gilbert's syndrome, the degree of jaundice fluctuates and is often aggravated by prolonged fasting, infection, stress, surgery, and excessive alcohol intake. The onset is most common during adolescence. Gilbert syndrome is common and may affect up to 5% of the male population. Liver function tests and fecal and urinary urobilinogen levels are normal. Bilirubinuria is absent. Studies reveal that these patients have a partial deficiency of glucuronyl transferase. The condition may be treated by the administration of phenobarbital, which stimulates glucuronyl transferase enzyme activity.

Type I *Crigler-Najjar syndrome* is a rare hereditary disorder caused by a recessive gene in which a complete absence of glucuronyl transferase from birth occurs. Because conjugation of bilirubin cannot take place, the bile is colorless and unconjugated bilirubin levels exceed 20 mg/dl, resulting in kernicterus. Phototherapy may temporarily reduce the unconjugated hyperbilirubinemia, but infants generally die within the first year of life. Type II Crigler-Najjar syndrome represents a milder form of the disease transmitted as a dominant genetic trait in which only a partial deficiency of glucuronyl transferase occurs. Serum unconjugated bilirubin levels are lower (6 to 20 mg/dl) and jaundice may not be manifested until adolescence. Phenobarbital, which induces increased glucuronyl transferase activity, often causes jaundice to disappear in these patients.

Decreased Excretion of Conjugated Bilirubin

Impaired excretion of bilirubin, whether caused by functional or obstructive factors, results in predominantly conjugated hyperbilirubinemia. Because conjugated bilirubin is water soluble, it is excreted in the urine and gives rise to bilirubinuria and dark urine. Fecal and urinary urobilinogen are commonly decreased, thus the stools are pale. Elevated conjugated bilirubin levels may be accompanied by other evidence of hepatic excretory

TABLE 27-4

Differentiating Features of Hemolytic, Hepatocellular, and Obstructive Jaundice

Feature	Hemolytic	Hepatocellular	Obstructive
Skin color	Pale yellow	Mild or deep orange-yellow	Mild to deep yellow-green
Urine color	Normal (may darken with urobilin)	Dark (conjugated bilirubin)	Dark (conjugated bilirubin)
Stool color	Normal or dark (more stercobilin)	Pale (less stercobilin)	Clay colored (no stercobilin)
Pruritus	None	Not persistent	Usually persistent
Serum bilirubin, indirect or unconjugated	Increased	Increased	Increased
Serum bilirubin, direct or conjugated	Normal	Increased	Increased
Urine bilirubin	Absent	Increased	Increased
Urine urobilinogen	Increased	Slight increase	Decreased

failure, such as elevated serum levels of alkaline phosphatase, aspartate aminotransferase, cholesterol, and bile salts. The presence of elevated bile salts in the blood adds the new dimension of itching to the jaundice. Jaundice resulting from conjugated hyperbilirubinemia is usually deeper than that resulting from unconjugated hyperbilirubinemia. The color change ranges from a mild or deep orange-yellow to a yellow-green in cases of complete obstruction of biliary outflow. These changes are evidence of *cholestatic jaundice*, which is another name for *obstructive jaundice*. Cholestasis may be either *intrahepatic* (involving the liver cell, canaliculi, or cholangioles) or *extrahepatic* (involving bile ducts outside the liver). Similar biochemical disturbances are present in both.

The most common causes of intrahepatic cholestasis are *hepatocellular diseases* in which the hepatic parenchymal cells are damaged by viral hepatitis or the various types of cirrhosis. In these diseases, swelling and disorganization of the liver cells can compress and block the canaliculi or cholangioles. Hepatocellular disease usually interferes with all phases of bilirubin metabolism—uptake, conjugation, and excretion—but because excretion is usually impaired to the greatest extent, conjugated hyperbilirubinemia predominates. Other less common causes of intrahepatic cholestasis include certain drugs and the rare hereditary disorders of the Dubin-Johnson and Rotor's syndromes. In these conditions, interference with transfer of bilirubin across the hepatocyte membrane appears to occur, causing retention of bilirubin within the cell. Common offending drugs include halothane (anesthetic), oral contraceptives, estrogens, anabolic steroids, isoniazid, and chlorpromazine.

The most common causes of extrahepatic cholestasis are impaction of a gallstone, usually at the lower end of the common bile duct; carcinoma of the head of the pancreas, producing extrinsic pressure on the bile duct; and carcinoma of the ampulla of Vater. Less common causes are strictures from previous inflammation or surgery and enlarged lymph nodes in the porta hepatis. Intrahepatic lesions such as a hepatoma may occasionally obstruct the right or left hepatic duct.

Intrahepatic versus Extrahepatic Cholestasis

The most important diagnostic decision for the physician and surgeon in conjugated hyperbilirubinemia is to determine whether the obstruction to bile flow is intra-

hepatic or extrahepatic. Patients with extrahepatic cholestasis may benefit from surgery, whereas surgery on those with hepatocellular disease (intrahepatic cholestasis) may exacerbate the illness and even lead to death. The differentiation is not easy, because all forms of cholestasis produce the same clinical syndrome of jaundice, itching, increased transaminases, increased alkaline phosphatase, defective excretion of cholecystographic dyes, and nonvisualization of the gallbladder. Although the ultimate judgment is a clinical one, evaluating the degree of obstruction will facilitate making the differentiation. Intrahepatic obstruction is seldom as complete as extrahepatic obstruction. Consequently, intrahepatic cholestasis generally results in only moderate elevations of alkaline phosphatase, and small amounts of pigment appear in the stools or urobilinogen in the urine compared with these values in extrahepatic cholestasis. Liver biopsy or duodenal or transhepatic cholangiography may be used to clarify difficult cases. Table 27-4 lists some of the differentiating features of the common types of jaundice.

VIRAL HEPATITIS

Viral hepatitis is an important public health problem not only in the United States but also throughout the world. The Centers for Disease Control and Prevention (CDC) estimates that approximately 300,000 hepatitis B virus infections occur each year in the United States. Although mortality from hepatitis is low, extensive morbidity and economic loss are associated with the disease. Acute viral hepatitis is an infectious disease that is generalized in its distribution, although the predominant effect is on the liver.

Six or seven categories of viral agents have been identified as causal agents, as follows:
1. Hepatitis A virus (HAV)
2. Hepatitis B virus (HBV)
3. Hepatitis C virus (HCV)
4. Hepatitis D virus (HDV)
5. Hepatitis E virus (HEV)
6. Hepatitis F (HFV)
7. Hepatitis G (HGV)

Although these viruses are discernible through their antigenic markers, they produce clinically similar illnesses, ranging from subclinical asymptomatic infections to fatal acute infections. Hepatitis F and hepatitis G viruses are listed in the nomenclature; however, further research is being conducted because many details associated with both viruses are unknown.

The best-known forms of the disease are HAV and HBV. These terms are preferred to the former terminology of "infectious" and "serum" hepatitis because both may be transmitted through parenteral and nonparenteral routes. Differential features of HAV through HEV are listed in Table 27-5 and are discussed later.

Viral hepatitis that could not be designated as A or B by serology was formerly called non-A, non-B hepatitis (NANBH) and more recently, hepatitis C. With the discovery of two non-A, non-B agents, one parenterally transmitted and the other enterically transmitted, these were further designated as PT-NANBH and ET-NANBH, respectively. More recently, proposed nomenclature would designate PT-NANBH as hepatitis C and ET-NANBH as hepatitis E.

Delta virus, or hepatitis D (HDV), is a defective ribonucleic acid (RNA) virus that causes infection only in the presence of HBV. HDV may occur as a coexistent infection with HBV or as a superinfection in an HBV carrier.

Etiology and Epidemiology

Hepatitis A (HAV)

HAV is a small RNA virus 27 nm in diameter that can be detected in the liver, bile, feces, and blood during the late incubation and preicteric phase of the illness. With the onset of jaundice, antibody to HAV (anti-HAV) becomes measurable in the serum. Initially, the level of anti-HAV antibody of the immunoglobulin M (IgM) class rises sharply, making it an accurate and simple diagnostic measure of HAV infection. After acute illness, anti-HAV antibody of the immunoglobulin G (IgG) class predominates and persists indefinitely, indicating past HAV infection and immunity. A carrier state has not been demonstrated.

HAV is the most common type of viral hepatitis in the United States. However, cases of HAV in this country have declined since the 1970s. HAV is common among children and young adults. A seasonal increase in the incidence of the disease occurs in autumn and winter.

HAV is transmitted primarily through oral ingestion of material that has been contaminated with feces. Transmission by blood transfusion has been reported but occurs infrequently (CDC, 2000). The disease is typically spread among children or from contact with an infected individual through the fecal contamination of food or water or by ingestion of inadequately cooked shellfish that may harbor the virus. Sporadic cases occur, and epidemics may arise from the spread of the disease in overcrowded areas such as day-care centers and mental institutions. Travelers to highly endemic areas such as Southeast Asia, North Africa, and the Middle East are at greater risk if they bypass the usual tourist routes. Transmission is facilitated by poor sanitation, poor personal hygiene, and intimate (intrahousehold or sexual) contact. The average incubation period is 30 days. Greatest infectivity is during the 2-week period immediately before the onset of jaundice.

An approved HAV vaccine can be given for use by international travelers and provides long-term protection compared with immune globulin, which provides protection for approximately 5 months, depending on the dosage (Marwick, 1995).

Hepatitis B (HBV)

HBV is a 42 nm, double-shelled deoxyribonucleic acid (DNA) virus that possesses a surface coat and an inner core (Fig. 27-5). The typical serologic markers associated with HBV are listed in Table 27-5. The first serologic marker used to identify HBV is the surface antigen (HBsAg, formerly called the "Australia antigen" [HAA]), which is positive for approximately 2 weeks before the onset of clinical symptoms and generally disappears during early convalescence but may persist for 4 to 6 months. In approximately 1% to 5% of patients with chronic hepatitis, HBsAg persists for more than 6 months, and these patients are said to be "carriers" for HBV (Dienstag, 1998). The presence of HBsAg means that the patient can transmit HBV to others and infect them.

The next marker to appear is usually the antibody to "core" antigen (anti-HBc). The core antigen itself (HBcAg) is not detectable routinely in the serum of patients with HBV infection because it is sequestered within the HBsAg coat. Anti-HBc becomes detectable soon after the appearance of clinical hepatitis and persists indefinitely; it is the clearest marker of immune status acquired from HBV infection (not vaccination). Anti-HBc may be further fractionated into IgM and IgG portions. IgM anti-HBc appears early during infection and persists longer than 6 months; it is a reliable marker of current or recent infection. Predominance of IgG anti-HBc indicates either recovery from HBV in the remote past (6 months) or chronic HBV infection.

The next antibody to appear is that to surface antigen (anti-HBs). Anti-HBs develops after a resolved infection and is responsible for long-term immunity. After vaccination (which immunizes only to surface antigen), the anti-HBs level is measured to assess immunity. Measurement of anti-HBc levels best ascertains immunity from a spontaneous infection.

The "e" antigen (HBeAg) represents a soluble portion of HBV and appears concurrently or shortly after HBsAg and disappears a few weeks before HBsAg disappears. HBeAg is present in all acute infections and indicates viral replication and that the patient is highly infectious to others. The persistence of HBeAg may indicate chronic replicative infection. Antibody to HBeAg (anti-HBe) develops in most HBV infections and correlates with the loss of replicating virus and with lower infectiousness.

Finally, an HBV carrier is defined as a person who either tests positive for HBsAg on at least two occasions at least 6 months apart or tests positive for HBsAg and negative for IgM anti-HBc when a single specimen is tested. The degree of infectiousness is best correlated with testing positive for HBeAg. The consensus holds that carrier status is directly related to the person's age when HBV is acquired. For example, in endemic areas, HBV is often acquired early in childhood by vertical transmission from the carrier mother or by horizontal transmission through contact with open wounds. In low endemic

TABLE 27-5

Differential Features of Hepatitis A through E

Virus	Synonym	Agent	Transmission Mode	Incubation Period	Age
HAV	Infectious hepatitis	Single-stranded RNA virus	Fecal-oral, food, water-borne, parenteral (rare), sexual (possible), blood-borne (rare)	15-45 days (shorter) Average: 30 days	Children, young adults
HBV	Serum hepatitis	Double-shelled DNA virus	Parenteral, sexual, perinatal, blood-borne	50-180 days Average: 60-90 days	Any age
HCV RNA virus	Formerly NANBH	Single-stranded RNA virus	Primarily blood-borne, also sexual and perinatal	15-160 days Average: 50 days	Any age
HDV RNA virus (requires HBV to replicate)*	Delta agent or HDV (delta)	Single-stranded RNA virus	Primarily blood-borne but some sexual and parenteral	30-60 days, 21-140 days Average: 35 days	Any age
HEV RNA virus	Major causal agent for NANBH worldwide	Unenveloped single-stranded RNA virus	Fecal-oral; water-borne	15-60 days Average: 40 days	Young to middle aged adults

EIA, Enzyme immunoassay; *HAV*, hepatitis A virus; *HBIG*, hepatitis B immune globulin; *HBV*, hepatitis B virus; *HCV*, hepatitis C virus; *HDV*, hepatitis D virus; *HEV*, hepatitis E virus; *IG*, immune globulin; *IV*, intravenous; *NANBH*, non-A, non-B hepatitis; *PCR*, polymerase chain reaction; *RIBA*, recombinant assay.
*HDV (delta virus) causes infection only in the presence of HBV and is diagnosed by HDV antigen during early infection and by infection and by antibody to HDV during or after viruses were formerly NANBH or HCV. Currently, two viruses are identified: blood-borne NANBH (HCV) and enterically transmitted NANB.

areas, however, only a small percentage of those acquiring HBV after 6 years of age become chronic carriers.

HBV infection is a major cause of acute and chronic hepatitis, cirrhosis, and liver cancer throughout the world; it is endemic in the Far East, most Pacific islands, most of Africa, parts of the Middle East, and in the Amazon basin. HBV infection is not overly endemic in the United States, with infection occurring primarily during adulthood. The CDC estimates that 200,000 to 300,000 individuals, primarily young adults, are infected with HBV each year. Only approximately 25% of these become jaundiced, 10,000 require hospitalization, and approximately 1% to 2% die with fulminant disease. The estimated number of carriers in the United States is 800,000 to 1 million. Approximately 25% of these carriers develop chronic active hepatitis, which often pro-

Transmission Risks	Carrier State Chronicity	Chronic Disease	Laboratory Test	Prophylaxis
Poor sanitation, overcrowded areas such as day-care centers and mental institutions, infected food handlers, health care workers, international travelers, drug users, sexual contact of infected persons, endemic areas such as American Indian reservations or Alaska native villages are at increased risk	No	No	Anti-HAV IgM: acute infection Anti-HAV IgG: past infection, immune to HAV HAV-RNA: detects infectivity	HAV vaccine Hepatitis IG vaccine administered before or after exposure
Homosexual activity, multiple sexual partners, injection drug use, chronic hemodialysis, health care workers, blood transfusion (currently rare because of routine testing), infants born to infected mothers	Yes	Yes	HBsAg: in onset and acute infection; carriers of the HBV HBeAg: correlates with high infectiousness Anti-HBs: confers immunity to HBV HBcAg: in hepatocytes, not easily detected in serum Anti-HBc IgM: appears in recent infection up to 6 mo Anti-HBc IgG: appears in screening of infection beyond 6 mo Anti-HBe: appears shortly after resolution of acute infection HBV DNA: detects infectivity	HBIG vaccine Vaccines use noninfectious HBsAg
Injecting drug users, hemodialysis patients, health care workers, sexual contact of infected persons, persons with multiple sexual partners, recipients of transfusions before July 1992, recipient of clotting factors made before 1987, infants born to infected women	Yes	Yes	HCV RNA: detected in serum from 1-3 wk of elevated transaminases Anti-HCV and HCV RNA: detects infectivity EIA and RIBA detects positivity of anti-HCV Screening of blood, organ, or tissue donors is critical	No vaccine in known
IV drug users Persons with hemophilia Those receiving clotting factor concentrates	No	Yes	IgM anti-HDV: recent HDV exposure IgG anti-HDV antibody: (IgG antibody) detected by competitive radioimmunoassays Reverse transcription PCR: detection of viral genome in serum HDAg: HDV detected in liver biopsy specimens (method of choice) Detection of IgM against both HDAg and HBcAg: denotes acute co-infection of HDV and HBV IgM anti-HDV: persists in longer, chronic infections HBsAg: chronic hepatitis arising from HDV superinfection	HDV-HBV co-infection can be prevented with exposure before or after prophylaxis for HBV (none for HBV carriers)
Contaminated drinking water, travelers (especially to high HEV-endemic areas) High mortality rate (up to 20%) among pregnant women	No	No	Reverse transcription PCR: detection of HEV RNA and HEV in stool and liver specimens with recent HEV exposure IgM anti-HEV: elevated titers are simultaneous with rising serum transaminaces IgG anti-HEV titers: elevated after resolution of symptoms	Research is being done, but presently no effective vaccine is known

gresses to cirrhosis. Additionally, the risk of developing primary cancer of the liver increases significantly in carriers. An estimated 25% to 40% of people who have had acute HBV are at substantial risk for cirrhosis and hepatocellular carcinoma.

The main route for the transmission of HBV is parenteral and across mucous membranes, particularly by sexual intercourse. The average length of the incubation period is 60 to 90 days. HBsAg has been found in nearly every body fluid from infected individuals: blood, semen, saliva, tears, ascites, breast milk, urine, and even feces. At least some of these body fluids, particularly blood, semen, breast milk, and saliva, have been shown to be infectious.

Although HBV infection occurs infrequently in the general adult population, certain groups and people

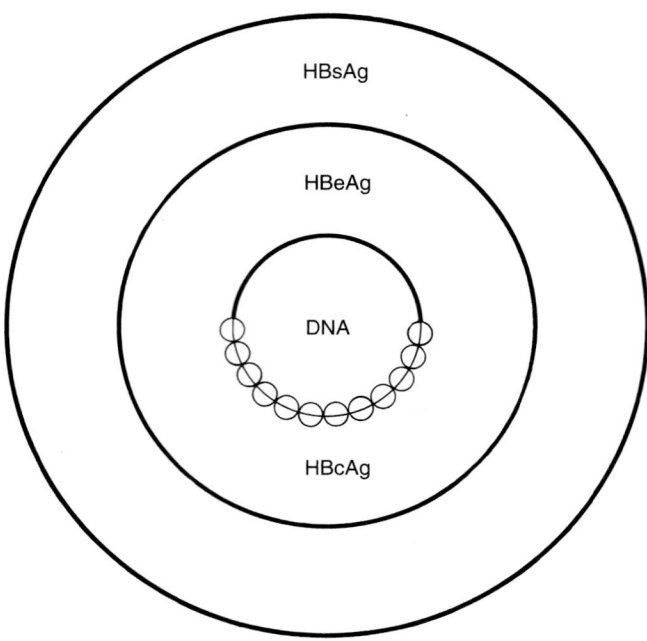

FIG. 27-5 Components of the hepatitis B virus (HBV). Diagram shows that HBV has an incomplete ring of circular DNA within a core particle (HBcAg) surrounded by a surface protein coat (HBsAg). The virus also contains the "e" antigen (HbeAg).

with certain lifestyles carry a high risk, including the following:

1. Immigrants from areas where HBV is endemic
2. IV drug users who share common needles and syringes
3. Persons who engage in heterosexual activity with multiple partners or infected persons
4. Sexually active homosexual men
5. Patients in custodial institutions for developmentally disabled persons
6. Male prisoners
7. Hemodialysis patients and hemophiliac patients receiving certain plasma-derived products
8. Household contacts of HBV carriers
9. Health care workers, especially those in frequent contact with blood
10. Newborn infants of infected mothers, who can acquire infection during or soon after birth.

Hepatitis C (Formerly Non-A, Non-B Hepatitis)

The existence of a non-A, non-B form of infectious hepatitis has been known since 1975. In 1988, after years of intense research, the causal agents were identified. Two forms of non-A, non-B viral hepatitis have been identified, one blood borne and the other enterically transmitted. These two distinct viruses are currently known as hepatitis C virus (HCV) and hepatitis E virus (HEV).

HCV is a linear, single-stranded RNA virus approximately 50 to 60 nm in diameter. A second-generation enzyme immunoassay has been used to detect antibodies to HCV (anti-HCV) but has resulted in many false-negative tests; therefore a supplemental recombinant assay (RIBA) is also being used. Anti-HCV was introduced as a blood donor test in May 1990 and has lowered the rate of trans-

fusion-related HCV significantly. Because HCV has been cloned, work on a vaccine is a goal.

HCV, as with HBV, is believed to be transmitted primarily by the parenteral route and is attributable mainly to IV drug use and blood transfusions. Risk of sexual transmission is controversial but appears low. The incubation period ranges from 15 to 160 days, with an average of 50 days. HCV-related (nor HBV) infection via blood transfusion is no longer a major problem because all blood is tested before transfusion. However, HCV used to account for most of the transfusion-related cases of hepatitis. Chronic hepatitis develops in over 80% of HCV infected individuals, and approximately 70% of these eventually develop cirrhosis of the liver. Chronic HCV is also strongly associated with the development of primary liver cancer. Research has confirmed the existence of a carrier state for HCV, which may be present in approximately 1% to 6% of volunteer blood donors.

Hepatitis D

The hepatitis D virus (HDV, delta virus) is a 35- to 37-nm RNA virus that is unusual in that it requires HBsAg to serve as the outer shell of the infectious particle. Thus only patients who are positive for HBsAg can become infected with HDV. Serologic markers for the antigen (HDAg), which indicates acute early infection, and for the antibody (anti-HDV), which indicates present or past infection, are commercially available. Transmission occurs primarily by serum, and in the United States, the disease occurs mainly among IV drug users. One third or two thirds of individuals who are HBV positive also are positive for the anti-HDV. In Mediterranean countries, HDV infection is endemic with HBV. The incubation period is believed to be similar to that of HBV, approximately 1 to 2 months. HDV may present itself as an acute infection, chronic infection, or coinfection or superinfection with HBV.

Hepatitis E

The hepatitis E virus (HEV) is a small, 32- to 34-nm, nonenveloped, single-stranded RNA virus. HEV is a water-borne type of non-A, non-B hepatitis that is enterically transmitted by the fecal-oral route. Currently, serologic testing for HEV can be performed using a specially encoded enzyme immunoassay. This method has been effective in discriminating antibody to HEV (anti-HEV) activity in sera. HEV infection is rarely encountered in the United States and is much more prevalent in India and the Indian subcontinent. To date, cases in Western countries have been related to travel to endemic areas. Young to middle-aged adults are most often affected, with an approximate mortality of 1% to 2% in the general population and an unusually high (20%) mortality among pregnant women. The incubation period is approximately 6 weeks.

Possible Hepatitis F and G

An ongoing debate in hepatitis research is whether a hepatitis F virus exists. The original debate arose when Fagan (1994) reportedly found several viral (non-A, non-B, non-C, and non-E) particles, which he injected into Indian rhesus monkeys. As a result, these monkeys developed a viral infection, which became known as hepatitis F

(HFV). Unfortunately, no other cases have shown these findings. Although the HFV nomenclature remains, it has not been confirmed that a hepatitis F virus really exists.

The hepatitis G virus (HGV) is a RNA flavivirus that possibly causes fulminant hepatitis. HGV is transmitted primarily through blood-borne means, but sexual transmission is also possible. Risk groups include individuals who have undergone blood transfusions, had accidental needle-stick exposures, injecting drug users, or hemodialysis patients. Currently, polymerase chain reaction (PCR) testing is the only available method for detecting HGV. Some researchers believe that HGV does not cause clinically significant hepatitis, thus they no longer regard the virus as a hepatitis virus (Yeo, 2000; Lefrere, 1999).

Pathology

The morphologic changes in the liver are often similar for the various categories of viral hepatitis agents. In the classic case, the liver appears normal in size and color but is sometimes slightly edematous, enlarged, and "tender edged" to palpation. Histologically, hepatocellular disarray, varying degrees of liver cell injury and necrosis, and periportal inflammation are present. These changes are completely reversible when the acute phase of the disease subsides. In a few cases, submassive or massive necrosis may lead to fulminant hepatic failure and death.

Clinical Features

Infection with a hepatitis virus can result in a range of effects, from fulminant hepatic failure to anicteric (without jaundice) subclinical hepatitis. The latter is more common in HAV infections, and the patient often mistakes it for the "flu." HBV infections tend to be more severe than HAV infections are, and the incidence of massive necrosis and fulminant hepatic failure is more common compared with HAV.

The vast majority of HAV and HBV infections are mild with complete recovery, and the clinical features are similar. *Prodromal symptoms* occur in all patients and may be present 1 or 2 weeks before the onset of jaundice (although not all patients develop jaundice). The main features at this time are malaise, lassitude, anorexia, headache, low-grade fever, and, for smokers, the loss of desire to smoke. Many patients experience arthralgias, arthritis, urticaria, and transient skin rashes. These extrahepatic manifestations of viral hepatitis may represent a syndrome similar to that of serum sickness and may be caused by circulating immune complexes. Additionally, the patient may have discomfort in the right upper quadrant, usually attributed to stretching of the liver capsule.

The prodromal phase is followed by the *icteric phase* and the onset of jaundice. This phase usually lasts 4 to 6 weeks but may start to subside within a few days. A few days before the jaundice, the patient generally has an improved feeling of well-being. The patient's appetite returns after a couple of weeks. As the fever subsides, the urine becomes darker, and the stools somewhat paler. The liver is moderately enlarged and tender, and the spleen is palpably enlarged in approximately one fourth of patients. A tender lymphadenopathy is often present.

The earliest biochemical abnormality is an elevation of aspartate aminotransferase (AST) and alanine aminotransferase (ALT) levels, which precedes the onset of jaundice by 1 or 2 weeks. Urine examination at the onset reveals the presence of bilirubin and an excess of urobilinogen. The bilirubinuria persists throughout the illness, but the urine urobilinogen may disappear temporarily when an obstructive phase caused by cholestasis occurs; later in the course of the illness, a secondary rise in urine urobilinogen may occur.

The icteric phase is associated with hyperbilirubinemia (both conjugated and unconjugated fractions), which is usually less than 10 mg/dl. The serum alkaline phosphatase level is usually normal or only moderately elevated. Atypical lymphocytes are common in acute viral hepatitis, and the prothrombin time may be prolonged. HBsAg is found in the serum during the prodromal phase and definitely establishes HBV hepatitis.

In the uncomplicated case, recovery begins 1 or 2 weeks from the onset of jaundice and lasts 2 to 6 weeks. Easy fatigability is a common complaint. The stools rapidly regain their normal color, the jaundice lessens, and urine color lightens. Splenomegaly, when present, subsides rapidly, but hepatomegaly may resolve only after several weeks. Abnormal laboratory findings and liver function tests may persist for 3 to 6 months.

Complications

Not every patient with viral hepatitis has an uneventful course. A few patients (less than 1%) show rapid clinical deterioration after the onset of jaundice as a result of fulminant hepatitis and massive liver necrosis. *Fulminant hepatitis* is characterized by signs and symptoms of acute liver failure: shrinking liver size, rapidly rising serum bilirubin levels, marked prolongation of prothrombin time, and hepatic coma. The outcome is death in 60% to 80% of these patients. Death may occur within days in some patients, and others may survive for weeks when the damage is less extensive. HBV accounts for more than 50% of the cases of fulminant hepatitis and is often associated with HDV infection. The delta agent (HDV) is able to cause hepatitis when it is present in the body along with the HBsAg. Fulminant hepatitis is less frequently a complication of HCV and is rarely associated with HAV.

The most common complication of viral hepatitis is a more prolonged course that can range from 2 to 8 months. This type is called *chronic persistent hepatitis* and occurs in 5% to 10% of patients. Despite the delayed convalescence in chronic persistent hepatitis, patients nearly always recover.

Approximately 5% to 10% of patients with viral hepatitis have a relapse after recovering from the initial episode, which may be associated with individuals who are in high-risk categories (e.g., substance abusers, carriers). Usually, the jaundice of a relapse is not as marked, and the liver function tests do not show the same degree of abnormality as in the initial episode. Further bed rest is usually followed by an uneventful recovery.

After acute viral hepatitis, a few patients may develop *chronic active* or *aggressive hepatitis*, in which piecemeal destruction of the liver occurs and cirrhosis develops. The condition is distinguished from chronic persistent hepatitis by liver biopsy. Corticosteroid therapy may retard the progression of hepatic injury, but the prognosis is poor. Death often occurs within 5 years in more than one half of these patients as a result of hepatic failure or the complications of cirrhosis. Chronic active hepatitis may develop in as many as 50% of patients with HCV; a much smaller proportion (approximately 1% to 3%) of patients with HBV develop these complications after successful therapy. In contrast, chronic hepatitis does not occur as a complication of HAV or HEV. Not all cases of chronic active hepatitis follow acute viral hepatitis. Drugs may be involved in the pathogenesis of this disorder. Specific drugs implicated include alpha-methyldopa (Aldomet), isoniazid, sulfonamides, and aspirin.

Finally, a significant late complication of hepatitis is the development of primary hepatocellular carcinoma. Although uncommon in the United States, primary liver cancer is quite common in many developing countries. Two major causal factors have been implicated in the pathogenesis: chronic HBV infection and related cirrhosis. HCV-related cirrhosis and chronic HCV infection also have been associated with primary liver cancer.

Treatment

No specific treatment exists for acute viral hepatitis. Bed rest during the acute phase is important, and a diet low in fat and high in carbohydrates is generally the most palatable for these patients. IV feeding may be necessary during the acute phase when the patient has persistent vomiting. Some limitation of physical activity is usually necessary until symptoms have subsided and the liver function tests return to normal.

The treatment of choice for chronic hepatitis B or symptomatic chronic hepatitis C is antiviral therapy with interferon-α. Antiviral therapy for chronic hepatitis D remains the subject of experimental trials. These types of chronic hepatitis have the highest risk of progressing to cirrhosis. Response rates are variable and more likely to be successful with shorter duration of the infection. Immunosuppressed patients with chronic hepatitis B and children infected at birth appear to be unresponsive to interferon therapy. Liver transplantation is a possible option for end-stage disease, although the likelihood of reinfection of the new liver is high.

Prevention

Because effective treatment of viral hepatitis is limited, emphasis is placed on prevention through immunization. Currently, passive and active immunization are available for both HAV and HBV. The CDC (2000) has published recommendations for preexposure and postexposure immunization practices.

In February 1995, the first vaccine against HAV was approved for licensure by the U.S. Food and Drug Administration (FDA). The vaccine is being distributed with recommendations for a two-dose administration schedule for adults 18 years of age and older and for the second dose to be given 6 to 12 months after the first. Children over age 2 years and adolescents are given three doses; the second dose is given 1 month after the first dose, and the third dose is given 6 to 12 months later.

Children under age 2 years are not vaccinated. Route of administration is by intramuscular (IM) injection in the deltoid muscle.

Immune globulin (IG), formerly called immune serum globulin, is administered to provide protection before or after exposure to HAV. All preparations of IG contain anti-HAV. Preexposure prophylaxis is recommended for international travelers to countries in which HAV is endemic. When this type of travel lasts less than 3 months, a single IM dose of IG (0.2 ml/kg body weight) is given; if longer travel is anticipated, 0.06 ml/kg should be given every 4 to 6 months.

The postexposure use of IG is effective in preventing or decreasing the severity of HAV infection. A dose of 0.02 ml/kg is given as soon as possible or within 2 weeks after exposure. Inoculation with IG is indicated for household members, day-care center staff, workers at custodial institutions, and travelers to tropical and developing countries.

Both high-titer HBV immune globulin (HBIG) and a vaccine are available to prevent and treat HBV. Preexposure prophylaxis is recommended for people who are at risk for developing HBV, including the following:
1. Health care workers
2. Clients and staff of custodial institutions for developmentally disabled persons
3. Hemodialysis patients
4. Sexually active homosexual men
5. IV drug users
6. Recipients of blood products on a chronic basis
7. Household or sexual contacts of HBsAg carriers
8. Sexually active heterosexuals with multiple partners
9. International travelers to areas in which HBV is endemic
10. Adoptees or refugees from areas in which HBV is endemic

The newer, genetically engineered vaccine made from recombinant DNA has largely replaced the original 1982 HBV vaccine derived from HBV carriers. The vaccine contains noninfectious HBsAg particles. A series of three injections produces antibodies to HBsAg in 95% of individuals who have been vaccinated but has no effect on those who are carriers.

HBIG is the drug of choice for short-term postexposure prophylaxis. Concurrent HBV vaccine may be given to provide long-term immunity, depending on the circumstances of the exposure. The CDC recommends that both HBIG and HBV vaccine be given within 12 hours after birth to infants with HBsAg-positive mothers. The CDC further recommends routine HBsAg prenatal testing of all pregnant women because pregnancy may result in severe disease for the mother and chronic infection for the newborn. Infants born to HBsAg-positive and HBeAg-positive mothers have a 70% to 90% risk for HBV infection; 80% to 90% of infected infants become chronic HBV carriers, and more than 25% of these carriers die from primary hepatocellular carcinoma or cirrhosis of the liver.

HBIG (0.06 ml/kg) is the treatment of choice for preventing HBV infection after percutaneous (needle stick) or mucosal exposure with HBsAg-positive blood. HBV vaccine should also be initiated within 7 to 14 days when the exposed person has not been vaccinated. Exposed individuals who have already been vaccinated should have their anti-HBs antibody level measured. If the anti-HBs antibody level is adequate, then no treatment is necessary; if inadequate, then a booster dose of vaccine should be given.

Personnel engaged in high-risk contact, as in hemodialysis, exchange transfusions, and parenteral therapy, must exercise great care in the handling of equipment and the avoidance of needle puncture.

Community measures that are important in the prevention of hepatitis include the provision of a safe food and water supply, as well as effective sewage disposal. Careful attention to general hygiene, hand washing, and safe disposal of the urine and feces of infected patients are important. The use of disposable catheters, needles, and syringes eliminates an important source of infection. All blood donors should be screened for the presence of HAV, HBV, and HCV before being accepted on the donor panel.

CIRRHOSIS

Cirrhosis is a chronic disease of the liver characterized by distortion of the normal hepatic architecture by bands of connective tissue and by nodules of regenerating liver cells unrelated to the normal vasculature. The regenerating nodules may be small (micronodular) or large (macronodular). Cirrhosis may interfere with intrahepatic blood circulation, and in far-advanced cases, it causes gradual failure of liver function.

The incidence of this disease has increased significantly since World War II, establishing cirrhosis as one of the most prominent causes of death in men. This increase is partly the result of a corresponding increase in the incidence of viral hepatitis but more significantly to an enormous increase in the intake of alcohol. Alcoholism is the single most important cause of cirrhosis. Alcoholic cirrhosis was the ninth leading cause of death in 1998 in the United States, accounting for 28,000 deaths (NIAAA, 1998).

Etiology, Pathology, and Pathogenesis

Although the cause of many forms of cirrhosis is poorly understood, three characteristic patterns account for the majority of cases: Laënnec's, postnecrotic, and biliary cirrhosis.

Laënnec's Cirrhosis

Laënnec's cirrhosis (also called alcoholic, portal, and nutritional cirrhosis) is a peculiar pattern of cirrhosis associated with chronic abuse of alcoholic beverages, accounting for approximately 75% or more of the cases of cirrhosis. Ten to 15% of alcoholics develop cirrhosis.

The exact relationship between alcohol abuse and Laënnec's cirrhosis is unknown, although a clear and unmistakable association exists. The first change in the liver caused by alcohol is the gradual accumulation of fat within the liver cells (fatty infiltration) (see Fig. 3-3; see color plate 34). A similar pattern of fatty infiltration is also present in *kwashiorkor* (a disorder common in developing countries as a result of severe protein deficiency),

hyperthyroidism, and diabetes. Most authorities agree that alcoholic beverages exert a direct toxic effect on the liver. The accumulation of fat reflects a number of metabolic disturbances, including excess formation of triglycerides, the decreased export of triglycerides from the liver, and the decreased oxidation of fatty acids from inhibition of the citric acid cycle. A person who ingests excessive amounts of alcohol also may not eat properly. The primary cause of liver damage appears to be the direct effect of alcohol on the liver cell, which is increased by malnutrition. These patients may have several nutritional deficiencies, including thiamin, folic acid, pyridoxine, niacin, ascorbic acid, and vitamin A. Bone loss often occurs from decreased calcium intake and faulty metabolism. Vitamin K, iron, and zinc intakes also tend to be deficient in these patients. Protein-calorie deficiencies are also common.

Uncomplicated fatty degeneration of the liver, as might be present in early alcoholism, is reversible, provided the person ceases ingestion of alcohol; few cases of this relatively benign condition progress to cirrhosis. Grossly, the liver is enlarged, fragile, and greasy in appearance and may be functionally deficient because of the large accumulation of fat.

When the habit of alcohol abuse persists, particularly when it becomes more severe, an event may occur (although uncertainty remains as to what causes it) to tip the whole process in favor of widespread scar formation. Some authorities believe that the critical lesion in the development of cirrhosis of the liver may be alcoholic hepatitis. Hepatocellular necrosis, ballooned cells, and polymorphonuclear neutrophil leukocyte (PMN) infiltration of the liver together histologically characterize *alcoholic hepatitis*. However, not all patients who develop the lesion of alcoholic hepatitis progress to full-blown cirrhosis of the liver.

In far-advanced cases of Laënnec's cirrhosis, thick fibrous bands form at the periphery of many lobules, partitioning the parenchyma into fine nodules. These nodules may enlarge somewhat as a result of regenerative activity as the liver attempts to replace damaged cells. The liver appears to consist of tightly packed nests of degenerating and regenerating liver cells encased in thick, fibrous capsules. On this basis, the condition is often referred to as *fine nodular cirrhosis*. In the final stages, the liver is shrunken, hard, and nearly devoid of normal parenchyma, which results in portal hypertension and hepatic failure. Patients with Laënnec's cirrhosis have an increased risk of developing primary liver cell (hepatocellular) carcinoma.

Postnecrotic Cirrhosis

Postnecrotic cirrhosis presumably follows patchy necrosis of liver tissue. Hepatocytes are surrounded and partitioned by scar tissue, with excessive loss of liver cells and interspersion with normal liver parenchyma. Approximately 75% of the cases tend to progress and result in death within 1 to 5 years. Postnecrotic cirrhosis accounts for approximately 10% of the cases of cirrhosis. Approximately 25% to 75% of the cases have a prior history of viral hepatitis. Many patients have positive test results for HBsAg, indicating that chronic active hepatitis may be an essential event. HCV accounts for approximately 25% of cirrhosis cases. A small percentage of cases stem from documented intoxication with industrial chemicals, poisons, or drugs, such as yellow phosphorus, oral contraceptives, methyldopa, arsenicals, and carbon tetrachloride.

A peculiar feature of postnecrotic cirrhosis is that it appears to predispose the patient to the occurrence of a primary hepatic neoplasm of the liver (hepatocellular carcinoma). The risk is increased by almost tenfold in HBV carriers compared with noncarriers (Hildt, 1998).

Biliary Cirrhosis

Liver cell destruction that begins around the bile ducts gives rise to a pattern of cirrhosis known as *biliary cirrhosis*, which accounts for approximately 2% of deaths from cirrhosis.

The most common cause of biliary cirrhosis is posthepatic biliary obstruction. Stasis of bile causes its accumulation within the liver substance with destruction of liver cells. Fibrous bands begin forming around the periphery of the lobule, but they rarely transect a lobule as in the pattern of Laënnec's cirrhosis. The liver is enlarged, firm, and finely granular and has a green hue. Jaundice is always an early and primary part of the syndrome, as are pruritus, malabsorption, and steatorrhea.

Primary biliary cirrhosis presents a pattern somewhat similar to that of secondary biliary cirrhosis just described but is much more rare. The cause of this condition, which is associated with lesions of the intrahepatic bile ductules, is unknown. Primary biliary cirrhosis occurs most commonly in women between 30 to 65 years of age and is associated with a variety of autoimmune disorders, such as autoimmune thyroiditis or rheumatoid arthritis. Circulating antimitochondrial antibodies (AMA) are present in 90% of patients. The bile capillaries and ductules contain bile plugs, and the liver cells frequently contain a green pigment. The extrahepatic biliary tract is not involved. Portal hypertension as a complication is rare. Osteomalacia occurs approximately 25% of the time in patients with primary biliary cirrhosis (because of decreased vitamin D absorption).

Clinical Features

The clinical features and complications of cirrhosis are common to all forms of the disease, regardless of the cause, although individual types of cirrhosis may have additional distinctive clinical and biochemical features. The period during which cirrhosis presents as a clinical problem is generally only a small fraction of the total life history of the disease. Cirrhosis is latent for many years, the pathologic changes progressing slowly until major symptoms induce awareness of the disease. During the long latency period, gradual deterioration of liver function occurs.

Early symptoms are vague and nonspecific and include lassitude, anorexia, dyspepsia, flatulence, a change in bowel habits (either constipation or diarrhea), and slight weight loss. Nausea and vomiting, particularly in the morning, are common. A dull ache or heavy feeling in the epigastrium or right upper quadrant is present in approximately one half the patients. In most cases, the liver is hard and palpable, regardless of whether it is enlarged or atrophied.

Liver failure and portal hypertension are two major manifestations of cirrhosis that develop late in the disease process. Hepatocellular failure is evidenced by jaundice, peripheral edema, bleeding tendencies, palmar erythema (red palms), spider angiomas, hepatic fetor (a mousy odor to the breath when liver impairment occurs), and hepatic encephalopathy. Portal hypertension often results in splenomegaly, esophageal and gastric varices, and other evidence of abnormal collateral circulation. Ascites (fluid in the peritoneal cavity) can be considered as a manifestation of both hepatocellular failure and portal hypertension. Fig. 27-6 illustrates the primary clinical manifestations of cirrhosis (see the following discussion).

Manifestations of Hepatocellular Failure

Jaundice occurs in at least 60% of patients at some time during the course of cirrhosis and is usually minimal. Hyperbilirubinemia without jaundice is more common. The patient may become jaundiced during a phase of decompensation with reversible deterioration of liver function. For example, the patient with cirrhosis may become jaundiced after a heavy drinking episode. Intermittent jaundice is a characteristic feature of biliary cirrhosis and occurs with active inflammation of the liver bile ductules *(cholangitis)*. Patients dying from hepatic failure are usually jaundiced.

Endocrine disturbances are common in cirrhosis. Hormones of the adrenal cortex, testes, and ovaries are metabolized and inactivated by the normal liver. Spider angiomas are present on the skin, particularly around the neck, shoulders, and chest. Spider angiomas consist of a central arteriole from which many small vessels radiate. Spider angiomas, testicular atrophy, gynecomastia, pectoral and axillary alopecia, and palmar erythema are a result of an excess of circulating estrogen. Increased pigmentation of the skin is believed to result from excessive activity of melanocyte-stimulating hormone (MSH).

Hematologic disorders common in cirrhosis include bleeding tendencies, anemia, leukopenia, and thrombocytopenia. Nosebleeds, gingival bleeding, heavy menstrual bleeding, and easy bruising may occur, and the prothrombin time may be prolonged. These manifestations are the result of decreased hepatic production of the clotting factors. The anemia, leukopenia, and thrombocytopenia are believed to result from hypersplenism. Not only is the spleen enlarged *(splenomegaly)*, but also it is more active in the removal of blood cells from the circulation. Other mechanisms contributing to the anemia include folate deficiency, vitamin B_{12} deficiency, iron deficiency secondary to blood loss, and increased hemolysis of RBCs. The patient is also more susceptible to infection.

The peripheral edema that generally occurs after the development of ascites may be explained by the hypoalbuminemia and abnormal salt and water retention. The failure of the liver cells to inactivate aldosterone and antidiuretic hormone (ADH) contributes to sodium and water retention.

Hepatic fetor is a musty, sweetish odor that may be detected on the patient's breath, particularly in hepatic coma, and is believed to result from the liver's inability to metabolize methionine.

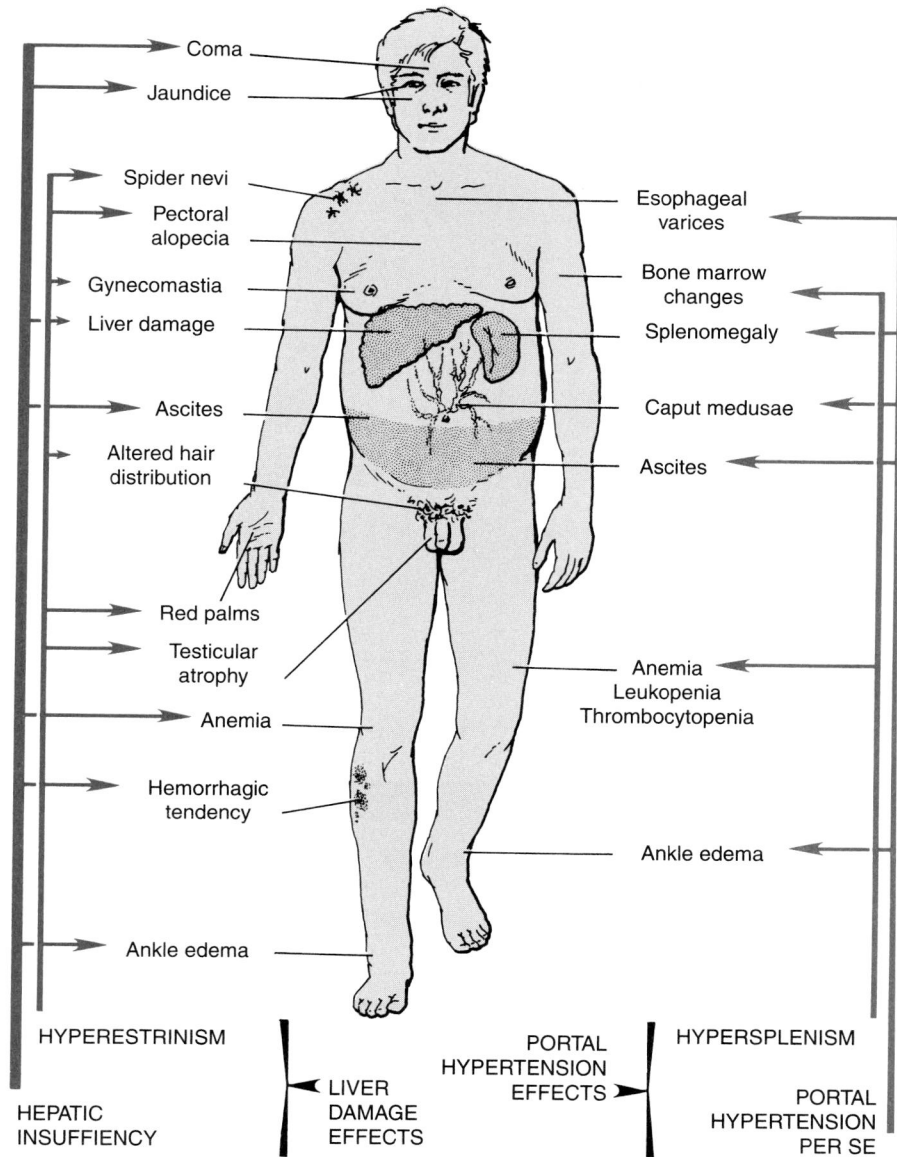

FIG. 27-6   Clinical manifestations of cirrhosis.

The most serious neurologic disorder in advanced cirrhosis is *hepatic encephalopathy* (hepatic coma), which is believed to result from abnormalities in the metabolism of NH_3 and increased cerebral sensitivity to toxins. The development of hepatic encephalopathy is often a terminal event in cirrhosis and is discussed in greater detail later.

Manifestations of Portal Hypertension

Portal hypertension is defined as a sustained elevation of pressure in the portal vein above the normal level of 6 to 12 cm water. The primary mechanism for inducing portal hypertension, regardless of the disease, is increased resistance to blood flow through the liver. Additionally, an increase in splanchnic arterial flow usually occurs. The two factors of decreased outflow through the hepatic vein and increased inflow combine to overload the portal circuit. This overload of the portal circuit stimulates the development of collateral channels (varices), which circumvent the hepatic obstruction. The back pressure in

the portal system causes splenomegaly and is partly responsible for the accumulation of ascites.

Ascites is an intraperitoneal accumulation of watery fluid containing small amounts of protein. Key factors in the pathogenesis of ascites are the increased hydrostatic pressure in the intestinal capillary bed (portal hypertension) and the decreased colloid osmotic pressure from hypoalbuminemia. Other contributing factors include abnormal sodium and water retention and increased synthesis and flow of hepatic lymph (see the later discussion).

The important collateral channels that develop as a result of cirrhosis and portal hypertension are found in the lower esophagus. The shunting of blood through this circuit to the venae cavae causes dilation of these veins *(esophageal varices)*. These varices occur in approximately 70% of patients with advanced cirrhosis. Bleeding from these varices is a common cause of death (Fig. 27-7).

The collateral circulation also involves the superficial veins of the abdominal wall, and its development leads to

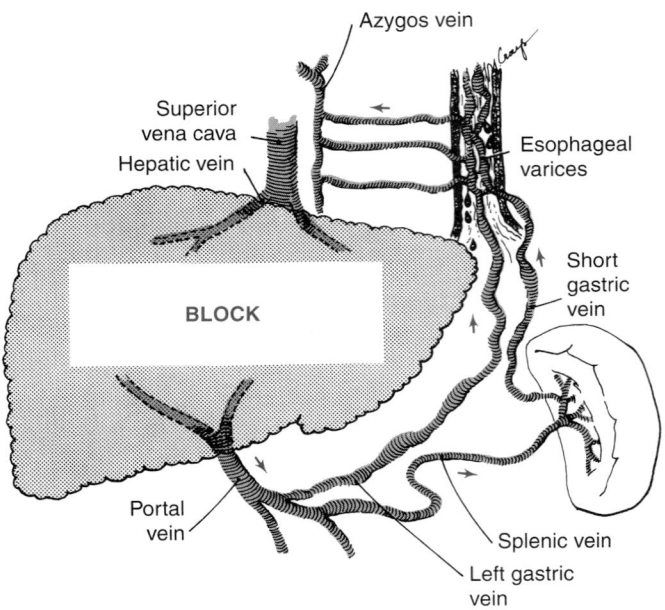

FIG. 27-7 Hemodynamic changes in liver cirrhosis, leading to the development of esophageal varices.

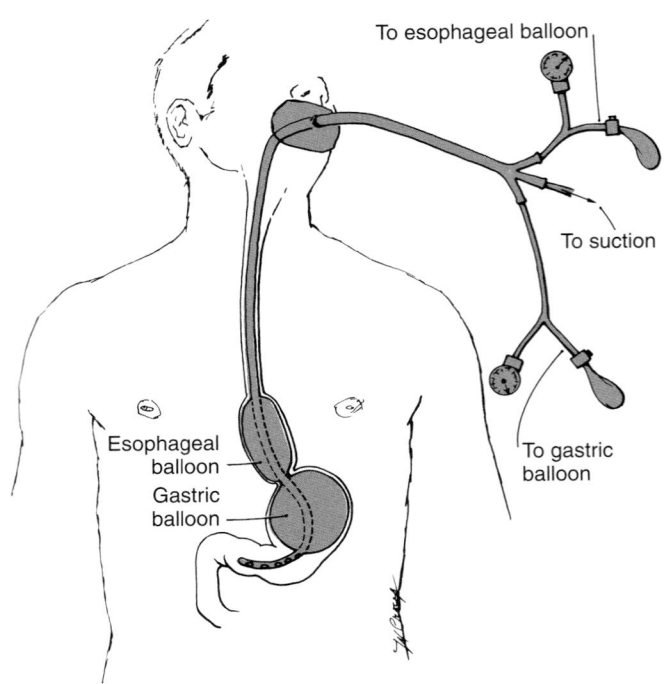

FIG. 27-8 Sengstaken-Blakemore tube in place for the emergency treatment of hemorrhage from esophageal varices. The tube has three openings for (1) gastric aspiration, (2) inflating the esophageal balloon, and (3) inflating the gastric balloon. The esophageal balloon is inflated to a pressure of 20 to 40 mm Hg (monitored by attachment to a gauge or a sphygmomanometer) that compresses the esophageal veins. The gastric balloon, inflated with 250 cc of air, applies pressure to the fundal veins when slight traction is applied.

dilated veins around the umbilicus (caput medusae). Because the rectal venous system helps decompensate portal pressure, the veins dilate and may lead to the development of internal hemorrhoids (see Fig. 27-2 to review points of anastomoses). Serious hemorrhage from the rupture of hemorrhoids does not usually occur because the pressure is not as high in this area as it is in the esophagus because of the greater distance from the portal vein.

Splenomegaly in cirrhosis can be explained on the basis of chronic passive congestion as a result of backup and higher pressure of blood in the splenic vein.

Treatment and Complications

The treatment of cirrhosis is unsatisfactory. No pharmacologic agents arrest or reverse the fibrotic process. Therapy first deals with the underlying cause, such as alcohol abuse or bile duct obstruction, and then treats the various complications, including gastrointestinal (GI) bleeding, ascites, and hepatic encephalopathy.

GI Bleeding

The most common and the most serious cause of GI bleeding in cirrhosis is bleeding from esophageal varices, which accounts for approximately one third of all deaths from cirrhosis. Other causes of bleeding include acute gastric erosions, a generalized bleeding tendency as a result of prolonged prothrombin and thrombocytopenia, and, less often, gastric and duodenal ulcers.

The patient has either melena or hematemesis. Occasionally, a sign of bleeding is hepatic encephalopathy. Depending on the amount and rapidity of the blood loss, the patient may have hypovolemia and hypotension.

A variety of measures have been used for the immediate control of bleeding. Tamponade with apparatuses such as the Sengstaken-Blakemore (triple-lumen) tube (Fig. 27-8) and Minnesota (quadruple-lumen) tube can temporarily stop the hemorrhage. The veins can be visualized with fiberoptic instruments and injected with a solution that will cause a clot to form in the vein, thus stopping the hemorrhage. Most clinicians believe this has a temporary effect and is not effective for long-term management. Vasopressin (Pitressin) has been used to control bleeding. The drug decreases portal pressure by decreasing splanchnic blood flow, although the effect is only temporary. The overall mortality rate of bleeding varices is near 35% because of liver failure and complications.

If the patient recovers from the bleeding, a portacaval shunt procedure may then be performed to reduce the portal pressure by anastomosing the portal vein (high pressure) to the inferior vena cava (low pressure). The shunt procedure represents drastic therapy for this major complication of cirrhosis and lessens the chance of further esophageal bleeding, but at the price of an increased risk of hepatic encephalopathy. The procedure does not increase the patient's life expectancy, which is still determined by the progress of the liver disease.

GI bleeding is one of the important precipitating causes of hepatic encephalopathy. The encephalopathy results when ammonia (NH_3) and other toxins enter the systemic circulation. The source of NH_3 is the bacterial breakdown of protein in the GI tract. Hepatic encephalopathy will follow if the blood is not removed by gastric aspiration, saline cathartics, and cleansing enemas and if the bacterial breakdown of the blood protein is not prevented by the administration of neomycin or a similar antibiotic. These measures are discussed in more detail later.

Ascites

As mentioned, ascites is the accumulation of serous fluid within the peritoneal cavity. Ascites is a cardinal manifestation of cirrhosis and other severe forms of liver disease. Several factors are involved in the pathogenesis of ascites in liver cirrhosis: (1) portal hypertension, (2) hypoalbuminemia, (3) increased production and flow of hepatic lymph, (4) sodium retention, and (5) impaired water excretion. The primary mechanism for inducing portal hypertension, as described, is resistance to blood flow through the liver. This action causes an increase in the hydrostatic pressure in the intestinal vascular bed. Hypoalbuminemia develops because of its reduced synthesis by impaired liver cells. Hypoalbuminemia results in decreased colloid osmotic pressure. The combination of increased hydrostatic pressure and decreased colloid osmotic pressure in the intestinal vascular bed favors transudation of fluid from the intravascular space to the interstitial space according to the law of Starling forces (the peritoneal space in the case of ascites). The portal hypertension further increases the production of hepatic lymph, which "weeps" from the liver into the peritoneal cavity. These mechanisms may contribute to the high-protein content in the ascitic fluid, thus raising the colloid osmotic pressure in the peritoneal cavity fluid and promoting the transudation of fluid from the intravascular space to the peritoneal space. Finally, sodium retention and impaired water excretion are important factors in perpetuating ascites. Sodium and water retention are caused by secondary hyperaldosteronism (decreased effective circulating volume activates the renin-angiotensin-aldosterone mechanism). Decreased hepatic inactivation of circulating aldosterone also may occur because of hepatocellular failure.

A sign of ascites is increased abdominal girth. More pronounced accumulation of fluid may cause shortness of breath because of the elevated diaphragm. As peritoneal fluid accumulates, amounts greater than 500 ml can be demonstrated during a physical assessment by shifting dullness, a fluid wave, and bulging flanks. Smaller quantities may be revealed by ultrasound examination or paracentesis.

Salt restriction is the primary method of treating ascites. Diuretics may also be used in conjunction with a low-sodium diet. Various diuretics and diuretic programs are available, but the essential feature is to introduce the diuretics gradually to avoid too brisk a diuresis. A loss of no more than 1.0 kg/day of fluid is recommended when ascites and peripheral edema are present. Electrolyte imbalance must be avoided, and even then, diuretics may precipitate hepatic encephalopathy.

Paracentesis is the insertion of a cannula into the peritoneal cavity to remove ascitic fluid. In the past, paracentesis was a common form of treatment for ascites but is no longer considered desirable because of its deleterious effects. Danger of inducing hypovolemia, hypokalemia, hyponatremia, hepatic encephalopathy, and renal failure exists. Because ascitic fluid may contain 10 to 30 g of protein/L, serum albumin is further depleted, promoting hypotension and reaccumulation of the ascitic fluid. Therefore IV replacement of albumin may be given during paracentesis to avoid these complications. Paracentesis is usually performed only for diagnostic purposes and when ascites causes prominent respiratory difficulty as a result of a large volume of fluid. Some patients with ascites also develop pleural effusions, particularly in the right hemithorax. The fluid is thought to enter the chest through tears that develop in the tendinous portion of the diaphragm because of the increased abdominal pressure.

Hepatic Encephalopathy

Hepatic encephalopathy (hepatic coma), a neuropsychiatric syndrome in a patient with severe liver disease, is characterized by mental confusion, muscle tremors, and a peculiar flapping tremor called *asterixis*. The mental changes may begin with alterations in personality, memory loss, and irritability and may progress to death in a deep coma. Hepatic encephalopathy ending in coma is the mechanism of death in approximately one third of the fatal cases of cirrhosis.

Pathogenesis

In the simplest terms, hepatic encephalopathy can be described as a form of cerebral intoxication caused by intestinal contents that have not been metabolized by the liver. This condition may occur when either liver cell damage or shunting (pathologic or surgically created) occurs that permits large amounts of portal blood to reach the systemic circulation without traversing the liver.

The metabolites responsible for the encephalopathy have not been identified with certainty. The basic mechanism appears to be intoxication of the brain by breakdown products of protein metabolism produced by bacterial action in the gut. These products are able to bypass the liver because of liver cell disease or shunting. NH_3, normally converted into urea by the liver, is one of the known toxic substances and is believed to interfere with brain metabolism (Fig. 27-9).

Hepatic encephalopathy is usually precipitated by events such as GI bleeding, excessive protein intake, diuretics, paracentesis, hypokalemia, acute infections, surgery, azotemia, and the administration of morphine, sedatives, or NH_3-containing drugs. *Azotemia* is the retention of nitrogenous substances (e.g., urea) in the blood that are normally filtered by the kidneys. The harmful effects of many of these can be traced to mechanisms that cause large amounts of NH_3 to form in the bowel. Encephalopathy that follows potassium depletion or paracentesis is probably related to excessive NH_3 formed by the kidneys and acid-base balance alterations. Table 27-6 summarizes factors that may precipitate hepatic encephalopathy and the possible physiologic mechanisms involved.

Clinical Features

Clinical signs and symptoms of hepatic encephalopathy may arise quickly and progress to coma when hepatic failure occurs in a patient with fulminating hepatitis. In cirrhotic patients, the progress usually is much slower and is reversible in the early stages if detected in time.

Progression of hepatic encephalopathy to coma is usually divided into four stages.

The signs in *stage I* are subtle and may be easily missed. Danger signals include slight personality and behavioral changes, including an unkempt appearance, vacant stare, slurred speech, inappropriate laughter, forgetfulness, and inability to concentrate. Patients may appear to be perfectly rational but uncooperative or disrespectful at times. Careful observation may reveal that patients are more lethargic or sleep more than is usual or that their sleep rhythms are reversed. Because of close association with this type of patient, the nurse is in a strategic position to notice these changes and should enlist the help of the family to detect subtle personality changes.

The signs in *stage II* are more prominent than those of stage I and are easily detected. Behavior may be inappropriate, and sphincter control is not maintained. Generalized muscle twitching and asterixis are characteristic findings. *Asterixis*, or flapping tremor, is elicited by having the patient raise both arms with forearms fixed, wrists hyperextended, and fingers separated. This maneuver causes involuntary rapid flexion and extension movements of the wrists (flapping) and metacarpophalangeal joints. Asterixis is a peripheral manifestation of impaired cerebral metabolism; it may also occur in the uremic syndrome. During this stage, the lethargy and personality and behavioral changes become increasingly marked.

Constructional apraxia is another prominent feature of hepatic encephalopathy. The patient cannot write clearly or draw figures such as stars or houses. A serial record of handwriting or figure construction is a useful method of determining the progress of the encephalopathy.

In *stage III*, the patient may have pronounced confusion and inappropriate behavior. If the patient is given a sedative at this time rather than treatment to reverse the toxic process, then the encephalopathy will probably progress to coma, and the outcome may be fatal. Hyperventilation and hypothermia may be observed before the onset of coma. During this stage, the patient may sleep much of the time. The electroencephalogram (EEG) begins to change in stage II and is definitely abnormal in stages III and IV.

In *stage IV*, the patient fades into a coma from which he or she cannot be aroused. Hyperactive reflexes and a positive Babinski's sign appear. Occasionally, a musty, sweetish odor (hepatic fetor) may be detected on the patient's breath or by simply entering the room. Hepatic fetor is a grave prognostic sign, and the intensity of the odor correlates well with the degree of somnolence and confusion. Elevation of the blood NH_3 level is an additional laboratory finding that may be helpful in the detection of encephalopathy.

Treatment

The steps in treatment of hepatic encephalopathy have been suggested in discussing the mechanisms that cause the condition. Monitoring for any precipitating factors is most important, such as GI bleeding or overenthusiastic diuretic therapy, and providing corrective treatment.

The initial treatment is to exclude all protein from the diet and inhibit the action of bacteria on protein sub-

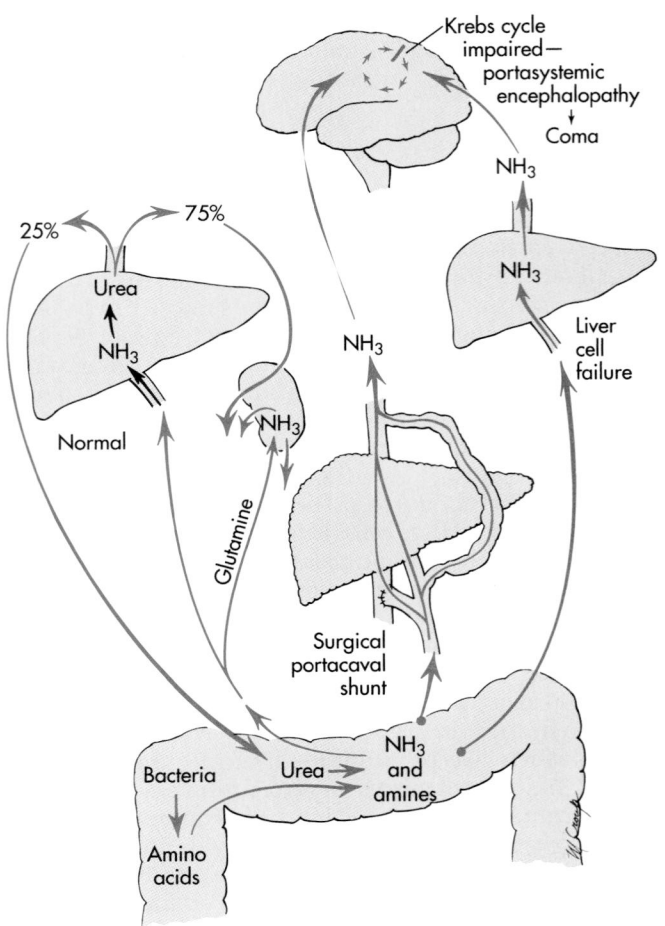

FIG. 27-9 Normal and abnormal circulation of ammonia (NH_3). The left side of the diagram shows the normal metabolism of NH_3. Ingested proteins are transformed into NH_3 and amines by the action of gut bacteria, are absorbed into the portal venous system, and are detoxified by conversion into urea by the hepatocytes. Urea is mostly excreted by the kidney (75%), but 25% is excreted into the intestine. The kidney also produces varying amounts of NH_3, largely by the deamination of glutamine. Normally, very little NH_3 enters the systemic circulation. The right side of the diagram shows the two major mechanisms causing hyperammonemia in liver cirrhosis: (1) failure of the liver to form urea as a result of hepatocellular damage and (2) portosystemic shunting (bypassing the liver) via portosystemic collaterals in the presence of portal hypertension. A portocaval surgical shunt as shown in the diagram can have the same effect. Excess NH_3 in the blood readily crosses the blood-brain barrier, where it causes a toxic effect on the brain called hepatic encephalopathy or hepatic coma.

stances in the bowel, because the breakdown of protein in the bowel is the source of NH_3 and other nitrogenous substances. Neomycin, a minimally absorbed antibiotic, is usually the drug of choice for the inhibition of gut bacteria. The usual dosage is approximately 4 to 12 g/day for adults. Intestinal bacteria may also be lowered through use of lactulose.

Lactulose also lowers stool pH when it is fermented to organic acids by colonic bacteria. The lowered pH traps NH_3 in the colon as nondiffusible ammonium ions (NH_4^+), which are then excreted in the stool. If the patient

TABLE 27-6

Common Factors That May Precipitate Hepatic Encephalopathy (HE)

Precipitating Factor	Possible Mechanisms Leading to HE
INCREASED NITROGENOUS LOAD GI bleeding Excess dietary protein Azotemia (increased BUN) Constipation	Excess blood in GI tract (10 to 20 g protein/dl) or excess dietary protein provides substrate for increased ammonia (NH_3) production. Action of gut bacteria on protein produces NH_3, which is absorbed and normally detoxified in the liver by conversion to urea. Increased NH_3 enters the systemic circulation when there is *hepatocellular failure* or *portosystemic shunting*. NH_3 (and possibly other toxic metabolites) readily crosses the blood-brain barrier, where it has a direct toxic effect on the brain. Impaired renal function and increased BUN causes more urea to diffuse into the gut, where it is converted to NH_3 by gut bacteria. Constipation favors increased production and absorption of NH_3 because of prolonged contact of protein substrates with gut bacteria.
ELECTROLYTE IMBALANCES Alkalosis Hypokalemia Hypovolemia	Alkalosis and hypokalemia, often caused by hyperventilation and vomiting, favor the diffusion of NH_3 from extracellular fluid to intracellular fluid, including brain cells, where it exerts a toxic effect. In alkalosis, more of the NH_3 produced from glutamine in the kidney reenters the systemic circulation rather than being excreted as ammonium ions (NH_4^+). Hypovolemia, caused by GI hemorrhage, excessive use of diuretics, or paracentesis, may precipitate HE by causing renal failure and azotemia, which in turn lead to increased blood NH_3.
MEDICATIONS Diuretics Tranquilizers, narcotics, sedatives, anesthetics	Overzealous use of diuretics can cause electrolyte imbalances, including alkalosis, hypokalemia, and hypovolemia. Thus potassium-depleting diuretics in particular should be avoided. Sedatives and other drugs that cause central nervous system depression act synergistically with NH_3. Impaired metabolism of these drugs also occurs from hepatocellular failure.
MISCELLANEOUS Infection Surgery	Infection or surgery causes increased tissue catabolism, leading to increased BUN and NH_3 production. Hyperthermia, dehydration, and impaired renal function may potentiate NH_3 toxicity.

Modified from Greenberger NJ: *Gastrointestinal disorders: a pathophysiologic approach*, ed 4, St Louis, 1989, Mosby.
BUN, Blood urea nitrogen; *GI*, gastrointestinal; *HE*, hepatic encephalopathy.

has had recent GI bleeding (source of protein), magnesium sulfate or enemas may then be given to purge the bowel. Correcting fluid and electrolyte imbalance is important, particularly hypokalemia, which exacerbates encephalopathy. Sedatives, tranquilizers, and diuretics are avoided, and the use of diuretics is minimized, particularly potassium-depleting diuretics. Nourishment is given in the form of sweetened fruit juices or IV glucose. These measures are usually successful when instituted early in the course of precoma and when the liver damage is not too far advanced.

Several measures are used to prevent encephalopathy in the patient who has a portacaval shunt or who has recovered from encephalopathy. These measures include a diet with modest amounts of protein, maintenance doses of neomycin, avoidance of potassium-depleting diuretics and NH_3-containing medications, avoidance of sedatives and narcotics, avoidance of constipation, and prohibition of all dietary protein if the symptoms should recur.

CHOLELITHIASIS AND CHOLECYSTITIS

The two most prominent diseases of the biliary tree, from the standpoint of frequency, are stone formation (*cholelithiasis*) and an associated chronic inflammation (*cholecystitis*). Although either of these conditions may occur alone, they are usually associated and are discussed together.

Pathology

Gallstones are essentially precipitates of one or more components of bile: cholesterol, bilirubin, bile salts, calcium, protein, fatty acids, and phospholipids (see Fig. 3-10). Of these substances, cholesterol is nearly insoluble in water and bilirubin is poorly soluble. Gallstones are divided by composition primarily into three types: pigment, cholesterol, and mixed stones. *Pigment stones* are composed of calcium salts and one of four of the following anions: bilirubinate, carbonate, phosphate, or long-chain fatty acids. These stones tend to be small, multiple, and black to brown in appearance. Black pigment stones are associated with chronic hemolysis and brown pigment stones with chronic biliary infection. These gallstones are less common. "Pure" *cholesterol stones* usually present a large, solitary, round or oval structure that is pale yellow in color and often contain some calcium and pigment. *Mixed cholesterol stones* constitute a larger category and are the most common. These stones have features of both cholesterol and pigment stones and are multiple and dark brown in color. Gallstones of mixed composition are frequently visible radiographically, whereas those of pure composition may not be.

Etiology and Pathogenesis

Gallstones are unusually common in the United States, with as many as 20% of the population affected. Each year, several hundred thousand of these patients undergo biliary tract surgery. Although gallstones are relatively uncommon during the first two decades of life, women who take oral contraceptives or are pregnant are at increased risk for gallstones, even in the teenage years and 20s. Racial and familial factors appear to be associated with a higher incidence of gallstones. Native Americans have an unusually high incidence, followed by Caucasians and then African Americans. Pathologic conditions associated with a higher incidence of gallstones include diabetes, cirrhosis of the liver, pancreatitis, cancer of the gallbladder, and ileal disease or resection. Other risk factors correlating with gallstone occurrence include obesity, multiparity, increasing age, female gender, and the sudden ingestion of low-fat or low-calorie (fasting) diets.

Gallstones are nearly invariably formed in the gallbladder and rarely in other parts of the biliary tree. The etiology of gallstones is still not completely understood, but the most important predisposing factors appear to be metabolic disturbances that cause changes in the composition of bile, bile stasis, and gallbladder infection.

Changes in the composition of bile are probably the most important factor in gallstone formation. A number of studies have indicated that the liver of patients with cholesterol gallstone disease secretes bile that is supersaturated with cholesterol. This excess cholesterol is precipitated (in a manner that is not yet fully understood) to form gallstones.

Stasis of bile in the gallbladder can lead to progressive supersaturation, changes in the chemical composition, and precipitation of the constituents. Disordered contractility of the gallbladder, spasm of the sphincter of Oddi, or both can cause stasis. Hormonal factors, particularly during pregnancy, may be related to delayed gallbladder emptying and may account for the higher incidence in this group.

Bacterial infection within the biliary tract can play a role in stone formation. Mucus increases the viscosity of bile and the cellular elements or bacteria may serve as a nidus for precipitation. However, infection probably is more often a result of the formation of gallstones than it is a cause of them.

Clinical Features

As many as 75% of people with gallstones are asymptomatic. Most symptoms occur when stones obstruct the flow of bile, frequently because small stones pass into the common bile duct. Patients with gallstones often have symptoms of acute or chronic cholecystitis. The acute form is characterized by the sudden onset of agonizing pain in the epigastrium or right upper quadrant; the pain may radiate to the back and right shoulder. The patient may break out in a profuse sweat or walk the floor or roll from side to side in the bed. Nausea and vomiting are common, and a fever may be present. The pain may last for several hours or may recur after a partial remission. As the pain subsides, tenderness may be noted over the gallbladder region. Acute cholecystitis is often associated with impaction of a stone in the cystic duct and is frequently referred to as *biliary colic.*

The symptoms of chronic cholecystitis are similar to those of acute cholecystitis, but the severity of the pain and the presence of physical signs are less marked. The patient often has a history of vague dyspepsia, fat intolerance, heartburn, or flatulence over a prolonged period.

After gallstones are formed, they may lie quietly in the gallbladder and cause no trouble, or they may cause complications. The most common complications are inflammation of the gallbladder (cholecystitis) and obstruction of the cystic or common bile ducts by a stone. Such obstruction may be temporary, intermittent, or permanent. Rarely, stones may penetrate through the wall of the gallbladder and cause severe inflammation, often leading to peritonitis, or they may cause the gallbladder walls to become thin and rupture.

Diagnosis and Treatment

The diagnosis of both the acute and the chronic forms of cholecystitis and cholelithiasis often relies on ultrasound to reveal the presence of stones or malfunctioning of the gallbladder (Fig. 27-10). Acute cholecystitis can also be successfully diagnosed using cholescintigraphy, a method that uses an IV radioactive agent. The biliary tract is then scanned for images of the gallbladder and biliary tree. When ultrasound equipment is unavailable, oral cholecystography is used. An endoscopic retrograde cholangiopancreatography (ERCP) may be used to detect ductal stones. Gallstones may be visible on plain radiographs if sufficiently calcified.

Palliative treatment for these patients is the avoidance of offending foods, such as those with high fat content. In the acute phase, many patients with cholecystitis initially achieve remission with rest, IV fluids, nasogastric suction, analgesia, and antibiotics. Oral bile acids may be used to dissolve cholesterol of mixed gallstones. According to studies, partial or complete dissolution of these stones has been successful approximately 50% to 60% of the time. Through a method called *lithotripsy,* gallstones may be fragmented by extracorporeal shock waves generated by electromagnetic types of devices in patients with (1) biliary colic, (2) radiolucent stones, (3) functioning gallbladder with normal emptying, (4) up to a maximum of three stones, and (5) absence of complications, such as infection, obstruction, and pancreatitis.

The common treatment of cholecystitis and cholelithiasis is surgical removal of the gallbladder (*cholecystectomy*) or removal of stones from the common bile duct (*choledocholithotomy*), which can be expected to affect a cure in approximately 95% of patients. In patients who have acute cholecystitis with severe symptoms and suspicion of pus formation, some surgeons perform surgery immediately, whereas others do so only when improvement does not occur within a few days. Currently, the traditional open method of abdominal surgery is used approximately 20% of the time, with a laparoscopic method of abdominal surgery used for cholecystectomies approximately 80% of the time. In cases of empyema or when the patient is in poor condition, the gallbladder may not be removed but merely drained (*cholecystotomy*).

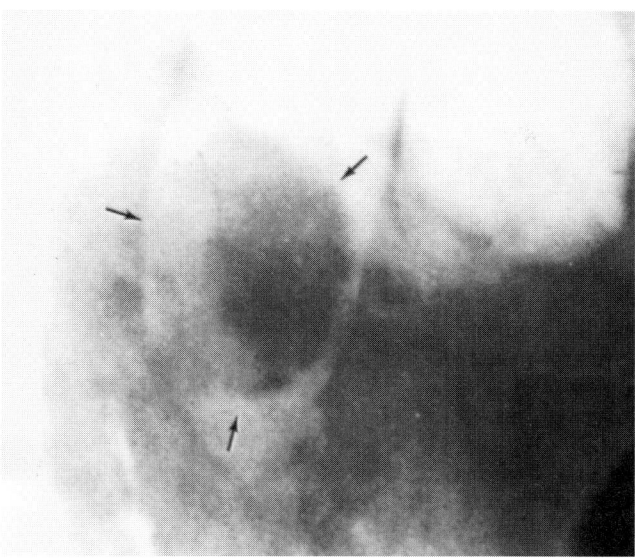

FIG. 27-10 Gallstone.

PANCREATITIS

The pancreas is unusual in that this organ functions as both an endocrine and an exocrine gland. A primary endocrine disorder of the pancreas is diabetes (see Chapter 63). The exocrine products of the pancreas contain powerful enzymes that normally digest proteins, fats, and carbohydrates in ingested food (Table 27-7). However, these potent enzymes that are so effective in digestion in the lumen of the small intestine may also serve as a source of great danger to the organism when they are activated within the substance of the pancreas itself. The autodigestion theory suggests that this event is essentially what happens in pancreatitis. Pancreatitis is typically divided into acute and chronic forms.

Acute Pancreatitis

Acute pancreatitis is an acute inflammatory process involving the pancreas and characterized by varying degrees of edema, hemorrhage, and necrosis of the acinar cells and blood vessels (see color plate 35). The mortality and clinical symptoms vary with the degree of the pathologic process. In 85% to 90% of patients with acute pancreatitis, symptoms usually cease 3 to 7 days after treatment is started. The mortality rate with acute pancreatitis is 10%, whereas the rate with severe necrotizing pancreatitis is approximately 50%. Surgery appears to decrease mortality rates.

Etiology and Pathogenesis
The main etiologic factors in acute pancreatitis are biliary tract disease and alcoholism. Less common causes include trauma (particularly bullet or knife wounds), penetrating duodenal ulcer, hyperparathyroidism, hyperlipidemia, viral infection, and certain drugs, such as sulfonamides and thiazide diuretics. Frequently, a precipitating cause cannot be found.

Pancreatitis is quite common in adults but is rare in children. In men, pancreatitis is more frequently associated with alcoholism, and in women, it is associated more often with gallstones.

Virtually universal agreement exists that the common pathogenetic mechanism in pancreatitis is *autodigestion*, but the process by which the pancreatic enzymes become activated is unclear. In the normal pancreas, a number of protective mechanisms safeguard against inadvertent activation of enzymes and autodigestion. First, the enzymes that digest protein are secreted as inactive precursors (zymogens) that must be activated by trypsin. *Trypsinogen*, the inactive form of trypsin, is normally converted into trypsin by the action of enterokinase in the small intestine. After *trypsin* is formed, it is the key that activates all the other proteolytic enzymes. Trypsin inhibitors are present in the plasma and in the pancreas; they can bind and inactivate any trypsin inadvertently produced, thus proteolytic digestion is unlikely to occur in the normal pancreas.

Reflux of bile and duodenal contents into the pancreatic ducts has been proposed as a possible mechanism for the activation of pancreatic enzymes. Reflux may occur when a common channel is present and a gallstone becomes impacted at the ampulla of Vater. Atony and edema of the sphincter of Oddi might permit duodenal reflux. Obstruction of the pancreatic ducts and pancreatic ischemia may also play a role. Alcohol can stimulate spasm of the sphincter of Oddi causing back pressure and blocking secretion through the pancreatic ducts and ampulla of Vater, which may lead to activation of pancreatic enzymes within the pancreas. Fig. 27-11 summarizes the proposed mechanism of pancreatic autodigestion.

The two activated enzymes believed to play a critical role in pancreatic autodigestion are elastase and phospholipase A. *Phospholipase A* may be activated by trypsin or bile acids and digests the phospholipids of cell membranes. *Elastase* is activated by trypsin and digests the elastic tissue of blood vessel walls, causing hemorrhage. The activation of *kallikrein* by trypsin is believed to play a role in the development of local damage and systemic hypotension. Kallikrein causes vasodilation, increased vascular permeability, invasion of white blood cells, and pain.

Clinical Features
The most prominent symptom of acute pancreatitis is severe abdominal pain that is sudden in onset and continuous. The pain is usually felt in the epigastrium but may be accentuated to the right or left of the midline. Radiation of the pain to the back is common, and the patient may obtain some relief by sitting forward. A supine position or walking appears to worsen the pain. Nausea, vomiting, sweating, and weakness often accompany the pain. The pain is usually severe for approximately 24 hours and then decreases over a period of days.

Physical examination may reveal varying degrees of shock, tachycardia, leukocytosis, and fever. Mild jaundice may be present if biliary obstruction occurs. Tenderness and guarding of the abdominal muscles are present, with distention, rigidity, and other evidence of peritonitis occurring when the inflammation involves the peritoneum. Bowel sounds may be reduced or absent. Severe retroperitoneal bleeding may manifest as bruising in the flanks or around the umbilicus.

The diagnosis of acute pancreatitis is usually established by the finding of an increased serum amylase level. The serum amylase level is elevated during the first 24 to

TABLE 27-7 ∎∎∎

Pancreatic-Secreted Enzymes, Normal and Altered Function

Pancreatic Enzyme	Normal Function	Characteristics of Altered Function
Amylase	Splits or hydrolyzes starch to produce glucose, maltose, and dextrins. Activity is dependent on calcium and other ions.	Increased enzyme levels are a result of pancreatic inflammation. Deficiency of amylase results in intolerance of starch-containing food.
Lipase	Acts preferentially on insoluble micelles or emulsions of tryglycerides, hydrolyzing glycerol-fatty acid ester and yielding free fatty acids and monoglycerides. Concentrated bile salts in the duodenum inhibit lipase activity; however, activity is restored in the presence of the precursor form (colipase), which is activated by removal of pentapeptide by trypsin.	Considered one of the best single enzymes measured for acute pancreatitis. Increased levels are seen in pancreatic inflammation. Deficiency results in steatorrhea and malabsorbtion of fat.
Carboxyl ester hydrolase	A lipolytic that represents about 4% of the protein in pancreatic fluid. Releases free cholesterol and free fatty acid. Requires bile salts for activation.	Interstitial localization of secretory lipolytic enzymes can be found during the necrotizing inflammatory process in pancreatitis.
Phospholipase A	Secreted by the pancreas in an inactive form and activated by trypsin after proteolytic cleavage of an activation peptide. Catalyzes hydrolysis of a phospholipid.	Increased activity is usually seen late in course of disease after clinical course has deteriorated considerably. Is a sensitive test for acute pancreatitis.
Kallikrein	Part of the enzymatic content of the pancreatic fluid; catalytic action results in the release of kinins from kininogens. Serum kinins activated in tissue function as mediators of inflammation. Normally present in body tissue in its inactive state. When activated, one of the most potent vasodilators.	Is implicated in various inflammatory diseases such as pancreatitis. However, research is being conducted on its potential use for therapeutic intervention in diseases such as asthma, pancreatitis, and rheumatoid arthritis.
Trypsin	A hydrolyzing enzyme is released from trypsinogen by cleavage of an "activation peptide" process stimulated by estrokinase. Trypsinogen is synthesized by pancreatic ribosomes.	Increased levels are seen in pancreatic inflammation. Elevated in acute pancreatitis. Decreased amounts are seen in pancreatic deficiency syndromes.
Chymotrypsin	Produced by the pancreas and functions in the small intestine. With trypsin, protein is hydrolysed to peptones.	Increased levels of this enzyme are seen in gross pancreatic hemorrhage. Can serve as an agent in the spread of cancer. Is deficient in children with cystic fibrosis and usually present in most healthy children's stool tests.
Elastase	Produced in the acinar portion of pancreas and is activated by trypsin. Particularly effective in the breakdown of elastin—a structural protein in connective tissue and blood vessels. Can also be a factor in systemic disease process.	Two types: cationic elastase 1 and anionic elastase 2. Elastase 1 is one of the best cationic markers for acute and chronic pancreatitis.
Carboxypeptidase	Metalloprotein that requires zinc for enzymatic activity. A protein-hydrolyzing enzyme that is activated in the duodenum by trypsin.	Dramatic increase of carboxypeptidase in serum follows pancreatitis.
Nucleases (DNase and RNase)	Secreted enzyme that breaks down nucleic acid chains.	RNase is present in patients with pancreatitis. DNase inhibitor input may be an early detector of pancreatic inflammation.

72 hours, and values are often over two times greater than is normal. Urinary amylase levels are elevated as long as 2 weeks after an episode of acute pancreatitis. Serum bilirubin may be mildly elevated. Other biochemical changes include elevation of the serum lipase level, hyperglycemia, hypocalcemia, and hypokalemia. The serum lipase is elevated for several days following the acute phase. Hypocalcemia is a common finding caused by marked fat necrosis with the formation of calcium soaps; it may be severe enough to cause tetany.

Complications of acute pancreatitis include the development of diabetes mellitus, severe tetany, pleural effusion (particularly in the left hemithorax), and a pancreatic abscess or pseudocyst. *Abscesses* are defined as collections of liquid secretory and necrotic products within the pancreas, whereas collections that occur outside the gland are called *pseudocysts*. A *phlegmon*, a solid mass of swollen, inflamed pancreas, often containing patchy areas of necrosis, may be present for 1 to 2 weeks after onset.

Pancreatic abscesses and pseudocysts often occur during the second or third week after the onset of pancreatitis. A common site of a pancreatic pseudocyst is within the lesser omental sac. Secondary infection of these collections of fluid is frequently present.

The most common sequelae of acute pancreatitis are recurrent acute attacks and the development of chronic pancreatitis.

Treatment

The primary early treatment of acute pancreatitis is medical, with surgery limited to treatment of biliary obstruction or specific complications such as a pancreatic pseudocyst. Treatment objectives include relief of pain,

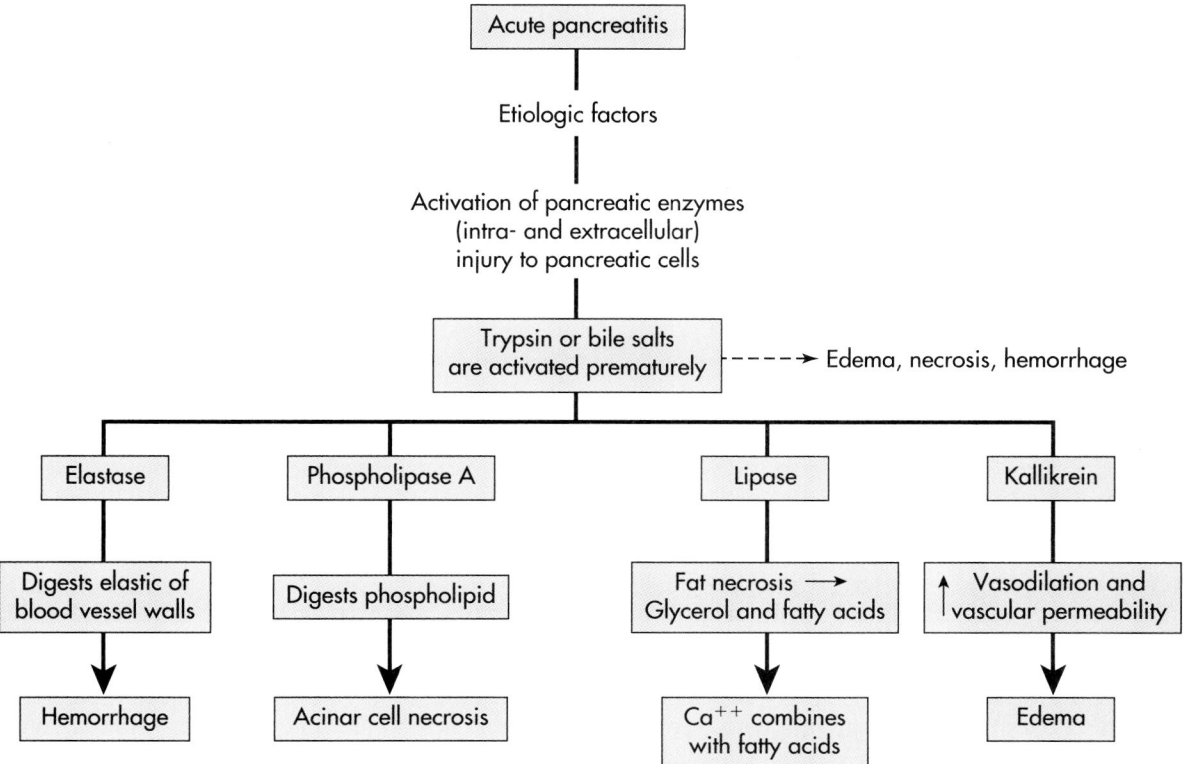

FIG. 27-11   Mechanism of pancreatic autodigestion.

reduction of pancreatic secretions, prevention and treatment of shock, restoration of fluid and electrolyte balance, and treatment of secondary infection. Shock and hypovolemia are treated with plasma and electrolyte infusions using the hematocrit, central venous pressure, and urine output as indexes of adequate volume replacement. Meperidine (Demerol), rather than opiates, is used to relieve the pain because meperidine causes less spasm of the sphincter of Oddi. Elimination of all oral intake and constant gastric suction reduce intestinal distention and prevent acid contents from entering the duodenum and stimulating pancreatic secretion. Antibiotic treatment of established infection is essential to minimize the risks of secondary infections. According to more recent studies, treatment of mild or moderate acute pancreatitis routinely with antibiotics has been ineffective; however, antibiotic therapy for severe pancreatitis with extensive necrosis reduces mortality. Protease inhibitors may also reduce pancreatic damage (Greenberger, Toskes, Isselbacher, 1998).

Pancreatic abscesses are treated by surgical drainage through the anterior abdominal wall or flank. Pseudocysts are managed by internal drainage between the anterior wall of the cyst and the posterior wall of the gastric antrum.

After the acute phase of the illness subsides, oral feedings may begin. As bowel sounds return, clear liquids are given and the patient progresses to a low-fat, high-carbohydrate diet so that pancreatic secretions are minimally stimulated. Attempts are made to determine the cause of the inflammation. The patient is advised against

consuming alcohol for at least 3 months, and when the pancreatitis is believed to be alcohol induced, abstinence should be permanent and total.

Chronic Pancreatitis

Chronic pancreatitis is characterized by progressive destruction of the gland, with fibrotic replacement that may result in stricture and eventual calcification. The etiologic factors are the same as those in acute pancreatitis, although approximately 75% of adult patients with chronic pancreatitis in the United States are alcoholics; cystic fibrosis is the most common cause in children. The clinical course may be one of recurrent episodes of acute pain, each leaving the patient with a lower-functioning pancreatic mass, or it may be a slow advance. Steatorrhea, malabsorption, weight loss, and diabetes are manifestations of advanced destruction. Chronic pancreatitis may follow acute pancreatitis but may begin insidiously in many patients.

The most sensitive test for detecting chronic pancreatitis is the determination of *bicarbonate concentration and output* in the duodenum after stimulation with secretin. Other useful diagnostic measures include fecal fat determination, fasting blood glucose levels to determine islet cell damage, and arteriography and radiographic examinations to detect fibrosis and scattered calcification. Unfortunately, invasive pancreatic carcinoma can produce the same pathophysiologic findings as those produced by chronic pancreatitis and thus presents a major problem for the physician in the differential diagnosis.

The treatment of chronic pancreatitis is directed toward the relief of two major problems: pain and malabsorption. Relief of pain may require large and frequent doses of meperidine (Demerol). Occasionally, local resection of the pancreatic gland may relieve the pain. Pancreatic enzymes have also been effectively used in selected patients to decrease the abdominal pain of chronic pancreatitis. Steatorrhea is managed with a low-fat diet and oral administration of fat-soluble vitamins and pancreatic enzymes. Diabetes requires control with either oral hypoglycemic agents or insulin. Alcohol ingestion is contraindicated.

CANCER OF THE LIVER, GALLBLADDER, AND PANCREAS

Primary cancer of the liver and gallbladder are relatively uncommon tumors in the United States. However, primary cancer of the liver is quite common in Africa and Japan. Both of these malignancies have a poor prognosis.

Malignant tumors primary to the liver arise from either parenchymal cells or bile duct epithelium. The former, known as *hepatocellular carcinoma*, comprises 80% to 90% of primary liver malignancies; the latter is *cholangiocarcinoma*. Approximately 75% of patients who develop hepatocellular carcinoma have underlying cirrhosis of the liver, primarily the alcoholic and postnecrotic types. The most important diagnostic cues are unexplained deterioration in a cirrhotic patient and rapid enlargement of the liver.

The most common neoplasm of the liver is a malignant tumor that has metastasized from some other site. Metastasis to the liver can be detected in more than 50% of all cancer deaths. This is particularly true of GI malignancies, but many others also show this tendency (e.g., cancers of the breast, lung, ovaries, and pancreas) (see Fig. 8-8).

Most cancers of the gallbladder are *adenocarcinomas*, and as many as 90% of these patients have gallstones. Diagnosis is generally late because the early symptoms are insidious and resemble those of chronic cholecystitis and cholelithiasis.

Cancer of the pancreas is a relatively common tumor. Nearly 29,000 persons died of pancreatic cancer in 1999, making it the fourth leading cause of cancer-related mortality (American Cancer Society, 1999). Smoking is the major risk factor; incidence is more than twice as high for smokers versus nonsmokers. Diets high in meats and fats increase the risk. The disease is more common in men than it is in women, and it occurs more often in African Americans than in it does in Caucasian Americans (American Cancer Society, 2001). The peak incidence is in the advanced years. Approximately 60% arise in the head of the pancreas, usually obstructing the biliary tract and causing jaundice and a palpably enlarged gallbladder. Cancers arising in the body and tail often remain silent until far advanced. Other signs and symptoms include abdominal pain, weight loss, anorexia, and nausea. Differential diagnosis from chronic pancreatitis may be difficult. Diagnostic assessment can be made with CT scan, ultrasound, ERCP, and other imaging techniques. Fine needle aspiration biopsy and percutaneous transhepatic cholangiography are some of the procedures used for tumor diagnosis. Some tumor markers that may be useful for diagnosis include CA-19, CA-50, carcinoembryonic enzyme (CEA), and several others (Lott, 1997). Because of the difficulties in diagnosis, the tumor is usually not discovered until it has already spread beyond hope of local resection.

The average life expectancy is less than 1 year after the diagnosis of cancer of the liver, gallbladder, or pancreas is established.

ℋEY CONCEPTS

- The liver is the largest parenchymal organ in the body (approximately 3 lbs) and is divided into right and left lobes; it is held in place by a complex series of ligaments, the most important of which is the *falciform ligament*, which connects its anterior surface to the diaphragm and anterior abdominal wall.
- The liver substance is divided microscopically into functional units called *lobules*—hexagonal rows of liver cells called *hepatocytes* arranged around a central vein that drains the lobule. Between the plates of hepatic cells are capillaries called *sinusoids*, which are branches of the portal vein and hepatic artery. The sinusoids are lined with *Kupffer cells*, phagocytic cells whose function is to remove bacteria and foreign particles from the blood. Bile formed in the hepatocytes is excreted into *canaliculi*, which join to form larger and larger bile ducts until the common bile duct, is reached.

- In addition to being the largest parenchymal organ, the liver ranks number one in the number and complexity of its functions. The liver has the enormous task of maintaining homeostasis of the metabolic functions of the body, which includes the metabolism of carbohydrates, fats, proteins, and vitamins; synthesis of serum proteins, including the clotting factors; formation of urea; formation and excretion of bile; inactivation of steroid hormones; and the detoxification of numerous endogenous and exogenous substances. The liver also acts as a flood chamber for blood backed up when right ventricular heart failure occurs.
- The gallbladder is responsible for the concentration and storage of bile. Bile is released from the gallbladder via the *cystic duct*, which merges with the *hepatic duct* to become the *common bile duct*. The common bile duct often merges with the pancreatic

duct to form the *ampulla of Vater* before opening into the duodenum. The ampulla of Vater is surrounded by circular muscle fibers known as the *sphincter of Oddi.*

- The pancreas is divided into three sections: the head, body, and tail. Two types of cells are present in the pancreas: the exocrine and endocrine cells. The exocrine cells produce the components of pancreatic juice, and the endocrine cells secrete insulin and glucagon, which are important for carbohydrate metabolism.

- The liver has a dual blood supply: from the digestive tract and spleen via the hepatic *portal vein* and from the aorta via the *hepatic artery.* Blood from the portal vein and the hepatic artery mixes as it flows through the liver and is eventually collected into the *right and left hepatic veins,* which drain into the vena cava. Approximately one third of the cardiac output courses through the liver each minute. In cases of obstruction to blood flow through the liver, portal blood must be shunted around the liver to the systemic venous circulation. Several points of portacaval anastomosis to shunt blood around the liver in cirrhosis are of clinical significance: (1) esophageal veins; (2) paraumbilical veins; and (3) the superior hemorrhoidal veins.

- *Portal hypertension* can be defined as a sustained elevation of pressure in the portal vein above the normal level of 6 to 12 cm of water and is often a result of resistance to blood flow through the liver. Splenomegaly and esophageal and gastric varices are the main effects of portal hypertension.

- One of the most important functions of the liver is the formation and excretion of bile—approximately 500 to 1000 ml/day. Bile is transported to the gallbladder and released into the small intestine as needed. Bile is composed of cholesterol, phospholipids, bile salts, bile pigments (mainly conjugated bilirubin), water, and electrolytes. *Bile salts* are essential for fat digestion and absorption in the small intestine. After being acted on by bacteria in the small intestine, most of the bile salts are reabsorbed in the ileum, recirculated to the liver, reconjugated, and resecreted. *Bile pigments* are formed from the breakdown of RBCs by the cells of the monocyte-macrophage system. Although bilirubin (a bile pigment) has no physiologically active role, it is an important indicator of liver and biliary disease because it colors the tissues.

- The accumulation of bile pigments in the skin or sclerae causes a yellow discoloration called *jaundice* or *icterus.* Bilirubin is a bile pigment, which is the end product of the degradation of old RBCs by the monocyte-macrophage system. The normal total serum bilirubin is approximately 1 mg/dl; roughly one half is unconjugated and the other half is conjugated. When the serum bilirubin exceeds a value of approximately 3 mg/dl, jaundice is visible.

- A review of the steps in bilirubin metabolism allows an understanding of the pathophysiologic mecha-

nisms causing jaundice. Normal bilirubin metabolism takes place in the following steps:

1. Heme (from hemoglobin) is converted to unconjugated bilirubin (mainly in the spleen). Hemolytic conditions causing *excess bilirubin production* can cause predominantly unconjugated hyperbilirubinemia and *hemolytic jaundice,* such as sickle cell anemia or *kernicterus* in an infant, as in erythroblastosis fetalis.
2. Unconjugated bilirubin is transported to the liver bound to albumin (because it is fat soluble but water insoluble). Competitive binding by drugs may cause jaundice.
3. Carrier protein (Y and Z) hepatic uptake of unconjugated bilirubin after dissociation from albumin; impaired uptake of unconjugated bilirubin interfered with by some drugs.
4. Conjugation of bilirubin with *glucuronic acid* (catalyzed by *glucuronic transferase*) to produce bilirubin glucuronide, which is now water-soluble and can be excreted; impaired conjugation can occur when deficiency of the enzyme glucuronyl transferase occurs, as in transient neonatal jaundice, Gilbert syndrome, or type I and II Crigler-Najjar syndrome. Phototherapy can convert unconjugated bilirubin to the water-soluble conjugated form, which can be excreted in the treatment of transient neonatal jaundice.
5. Excretion of conjugated bilirubin into the bile canaliculus; hepatocellular diseases such as hepatitis, cirrhosis, or intrahepatic cholestasis can interfere with excretion causing predominantly conjugated hyperbilirubinemia, dark urine, and clay-colored stools.
6. Passage of conjugated bilirubin down the biliary tree; extrahepatic cholestasis (obstructive jaundice); liver metastasis, gallstones, or stricture of extrahepatic bile ducts; and cancer of the head of the pancreas may all cause jaundice.
7. Reduction of conjugated bilirubin to urobilinogens by gut bacteria
8. Enterohepatic circulation of unconjugated bilirubin and urobilinogens
9. Renal excretion of urobilinogen and conjugated bilirubin

- Viral hepatitis has been divided into six categories, ranging from Hepatitis A through G. Hepatitis F, a possible seventh causal agent, exists in the nomenclature; however, its existence as a hepatitis virus is debated. Hepatitis G is not considered pathogenic.

- HAV infection is generally a benign self-limited disease and does not cause chronic hepatitis or a carrier state and only rarely causes a fulminant hepatitis. HAV is transmitted primarily through the fecal-oral route and is most common in institutional settings (e.g., prisons, child-care agencies) and endemic in countries with poor sanitation or substandard hygiene. A reliable serologic marker of acute infection is anti-HAV IgM; anti-HAV IgG indicates immunity. A HAV vaccine is available.

- HBV is a double-shelled DNA virus with a surface coat (HBsAg), a precore region (HBeAg), and an inner core (HBcAg). HBV is a more serious infection with a carrier state and may cause chronic hepatitis ending in cirrhosis or hepatocellular carcinoma. HBV infection is transmitted primarily through the parenteral route and close physical contact (particularly sexual contact). High-risk groups include IV drug users, homosexual males, infants of infected mothers, and health care workers, particularly those in frequent contact with blood. Reliable serologic markers of acute infection include HBsAg, HBeAg, or HBV DNA. The carrier state is indicated by the presence of HBsAg in the serum more than 6 months after the initial infection. Chronic HBV infection is indicated by the persistence of HBsAg, HBeAg, and HBV DNA, usually with anti-HBc. Immunity is indicated by anti-HBs IgG (after recovery from the infection or vaccination). A HBV vaccine is available.
- HCV infection is transmitted in the same manner as is HBV and was once responsible for the majority of blood transfusion infections but is no longer a major problem because all blood is tested before transfusion. Chronic hepatitis develops in 80% of all HCV-infected individuals; 50% of these develop cirrhosis. A strong predisposition also exists for developing hepatocellular carcinoma. HCV RNA is present in acute infection and in chronic infection. Episodic elevations in serum transaminases occur with chronic infection. A carrier state exists and is present in 1% to 6% of volunteer blood donors.
- HDV infection does not exist independently but always occurs with HBV infection as a coinfection or superinfection. Transmission is similar to that of HBV. Simultaneous HBV and HDV infection increases the risk of a fatal fulminant hepatitis or chronic infection. HDV RNA indicates acute infection or anti-HDV IgM (recent exposure).
- HEV infection is uncommon in the United States but occurs primarily in Asia, India, and Sub-Saharan Africa. Transmission occurs primarily by the fecal-oral route and by contaminated water. A characteristic feature of HEV infection is the 20% mortality rate among pregnant women.
- Cirrhosis is a chronic liver disease characterized by distortion of the normal hepatic architecture (fibrosis and liver cell nodules replacing the normal parenchyma) and loss of function. The term *cirrhosis* is a synonym for *end-stage liver disease or failure*; it is irreversible and incurable except by liver transplantation. Cirrhosis is one of the leading causes of death in the Western world.
- The most important causes of cirrhosis are chronic alcoholism (Laënnec's cirrhosis), viral hepatitis (postnecrotic cirrhosis, particularly with chronic HCV or HBV infections), and biliary disease (biliary cirrhosis).
- Regardless of the cause, the clinical manifestations of cirrhosis at the end stage are much the same and can be divided into two categories: (1) hepatocellular failure and (2) portal hypertension.

- *Hepatocellular failure manifestations in cirrhosis* are all related to a failure of remaining liver cells to perform their normal functions including: (1) jaundice (resulting from decreased ability of liver cells to conjugate and excrete bilirubin); (2) endocrine disturbances, such as spider angiomas, palmar erythema, gynecomastia, pectoral alopecia, and testicular atrophy (resulting from failure of liver cells to inactivate estrogen); (3) hematologic disturbances, such as thrombocytopenia, leukopenia, anemia (resulting from hypersplenism), and a bleeding tendency (resulting from decreased production of clotting factors); (4) peripheral edema related to hypoalbuminemia; (5) hepatic fetor (sweetish odor to breath resulting from a failure to metabolize methionine); (6) metabolic disturbances, such as hypokalemia, hyponatremia, hypoalbuminemia, and hyperammonemia; and (7) hepatic encephalopathy (hepatic coma), a neuropsychiatric syndrome associated with high serum NH_3 levels is often a terminal event.
- *Portal hypertension manifestations* in cirrhosis are related to increased resistance to flow through the increasingly fibrotic liver resulting in portal hypertension and return of blood to the vena cava through collateral (portacaval anastomoses) routes. These manifestations include: (1) ascites or the accumulation of fluid in the peritoneal cavity; (2) esophageal varices, which may cause a fatal hemorrhage; (3) splenomegaly resulting from chronic passive congestion; (4) caput medusae (dilated veins around the umbilicus) resulting from collateral flow through the superficial veins of the abdominal wall; and (5) hemorrhoids resulting from collateral flow through the rectal veins that connect with the mesenteric veins and the portal vein.
- GI bleeding is a major precipitating factor resulting in hepatic encephalopathy. NH_3 is produced by the action of gut bacteria on the blood protein, which bypasses the liver because of shunting or fails to be metabolized into urea so it can be excreted in the urine because of liver cell failure. Neomycin or lactulose is given as a treatment to decrease NH_3 absorption to prevent hepatic encephalopathy.
- Ascites is a cardinal manifestation of cirrhosis and other severe forms of liver disease. Several factors are involved in the pathogenesis of ascites in liver cirrhosis: (1) portal hypertension; (2) hypoalbuminemia; (3) increased production and flow of hepatic lymph; (4) sodium retention; and (5) impaired water excretion. The primary mechanism for inducing portal hypertension is resistance to blood flow through the liver.
- The two most frequently occurring diseases of the biliary tree are stone formation (cholelithiasis) and an associated chronic inflammation (cholecystitis). Gallstones are essentially precipitates of one of more components of bile: cholesterol, bilirubin, bile salts, calcium, protein, fatty acids, and phospholipids.
- Acute pancreatitis is characterized by severe continuous epigastric pain radiating to the back resulting from inflammation and enzymatic necrosis of the

pancreas. Varying degrees of shock, tachycardia, leukocytosis, and fever may be present. The diagnosis is usually established by the finding of an elevated serum amylase. The two leading causes of acute pancreatitis are alcoholism and biliary tract disease. Most authorities agree that the common pathogenic mechanism is *autodigestion*, activation of the pancreatic digestive enzymes within the pancreas itself, causing digestion of pancreatic tissue. Complications of acute pancreatitis include pancreatic abscess (collection of liquid secretory and necrotic products within the pancreas) and pancreatic pseudocyst (collection of liquid secretory and necrotic products within the lesser omental sac).

- Progressive destruction and fibrotic replacement of the pancreas characterize chronic pancreatitis. Signs and symptoms include recurrent episodes of acute pain (often precipitated by alcohol ingestion), steatorrhea, malabsorption, weight loss, and diabetes mellitus.
- Cancer of the pancreas is the fifth leading cause of cancer death in the United States. Primary cancer of the liver and gallbladder are rare in the United States, but the liver is a common site of metastasis.

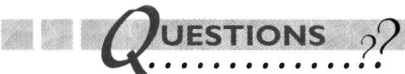

QUESTIONS

A sampling of review questions for this chapter appears here. Visit http://www.mosby.com/MERLIN/PriceWilson/ for additional questions. MERLIN

Answer the following on a separate sheet of paper.

1. Explain the way in which blood circulation through the liver is unusual.
2. Briefly describe the structure and function of the gallbladder and pancreas. What hormones control the release of bile and the exocrine pancreatic secretions?
3. List the eight major functions of the liver. Why is the liver a major organ of defense? Why is the liver called a flood chamber? How does the liver perform its detoxification functions (what are the mechanisms involved)? What is the role of the liver in carbohydrate, fat, and protein metabolism?
4. List the four general pathogenetic mechanisms of jaundice.
5. What is kernicterus? What is its significance?
6. Why do newborns often have a slight transient jaundice during the first few days after birth?
7. Does immune globulin (IG) have any value in the treatment of existing hepatitis? Why or why not?
8. Enumerate measures that might help prevent the spread of viral hepatitis in the community, in the home, and in the clinical unit.
9. What percentage of liver destruction is still compatible with life? How long can a person live after a total hepatectomy?

Fill in the blanks with the correct word(s) or circle the correct word option when indicated.

10. a. The liver is roughly _____ in shape, weighs approximately (150) (1500) g, and is located in the _____ quadrant of the abdomen.
    b. The right lobe forms a roof over the right _____ and _____.
    c. The left lobe forms a roof over two important digestive organs, the _____ and the _____.
    d. The _____ ligament divides the medial and lateral segments of the left lobe of the liver and is attached to the anterior abdominal wall.
    e. The liver is enveloped by dense connective tissue called the _____, and the stretching of this capsule in cases of hepatic enlargement is believed to cause tenderness or dull pain.

11. a. The chief excretory product of the liver is _____, which exits from the liver through the right and left _____ ducts, which immediately merge to form the common _____ duct.
    b. Bile enters the gallbladder through the _____ duct and enters the duodenum through the common _____ duct.
    c. This terminal bile duct joins with the main _____ duct before entering the duodenum through the ampulla of _____.
    d. The sphincter of _____ encircles the common channel and controls the entry of secretions into the duodenum.

12. a. Blood is supplied to the liver by the _____ artery and the _____ vein; it is drained by the right and left _____ veins, which enter the inferior _____.
    b. The paraumbilical veins form a potential pathway from the umbilicus to the _____ vein, allowing passage of a catheter and direct measurement of pressure in this vein.
    c. In cases of right-sided heart failure, blood may back up through the _____ veins, causing passive congestion of the liver but rarely cirrhosis.
    d. When blood flow through the liver is blocked in cirrhosis, blood may back up in the splenic vein, causing enlargement of the _____; blood may be shunted around the liver through the _____ veins, causing varices; blood may be shunted through the _____ veins, causing varices; or blood may be shunted through the _____ veins, causing hemorrhoids.

13. a. The structural and functional unit of the liver is called the _____;
it is hexagonal in shape and composed of plates of liver cells.
   b. Mixed arterial and portal venous blood flows through liver capillaries called
_____, which are lined with phagocytic cells called
_____ cells, and drains into a central vein at the center of the
structural unit.
   c. Bile capillaries course between the hepatocytes and are called
_____.

— ∙ — ∙ — ∙ — ∙ — ∙ — ∙ — ∙ — ∙ —

Answer the following on a separate sheet of paper.
14. What is alcoholic hepatitis and what is its significance in relation to cirrhosis of the liver?
15. Why is cirrhosis of the liver not usually diagnosed until it is advanced?
16. What is portal hypertension? What is the basic mechanism involved in its development?
17. Describe two emergency methods of treatment for bleeding esophageal varices. Why is removing the blood from the GI tract important? Describe the surgical treatment of esophageal varices to prevent recurrent bleeding. Why does the patient often develop hepatic encephalopathy after this type of surgery?
18. What is hepatic encephalopathy? How is it related to portosystemic shunting and liver cell failure? Why is detecting hepatic encephalopathy in its early stages important?
19. What is asterixis? How is it determined?
20. What is constructional apraxia and what is its significance?
21. Make a table that outlines the four progressive stages of hepatic encephalopathy and gives the major clinical features of each stage.
22. Compare the clinical features of acute and chronic cholecystitis.
23. Why is the liver such a common site of metastasis of malignant tumors?
24. Describe the pathogenesis, signs and symptoms, and treatment of ascites.

ℬIBLIOGRAPHY ▪ PART FIVE

Aggarwal R, Krawczynski K: Hepatitis E: an overview and recent advances in clinical and laboratory research, *J Gastroenterol Hepatol*, 15(1):9-20, 2000.

Aldoori WH, Giovannucci EL, Rockett HR, Sampson L, Rimm EB, Willett WC: A prospective study of dietary fiber types and symptomatic diverticular disease in men, *J Nutrition* 128(4):714-9, 1998.

American Cancer Society: Cancer facts and figures—1999: C-1-C-2, 2-3, 2001, The Society.

American Cancer Society: Expected new cancer cases and deaths, by sex, for leading sites, 1999, *Vital Statistics—Cancer; Heart Disease*, 902.

Bond JH: Colorectal cancer update. Prevention, screening, treatment, and surveillance for high-risk groups. *Med Clin North Am* 84(5):1163-82, 2000.

Bruce B, Spiller GA, Klevay LM, Gallaher SK: A diet high in whole and unrefined foods favors altered lipids, antioxidant defenses, and colon function. *J Am Coll Nutr*, 19(1):61-7, 2000.

Burkitt DP: Epidemiology of colon and rectum cancer, *Cancer*, 28:3-13, 1971.

Castell DO, Richter JE: *The esophagus*, ed 3, Philadelphia, 1999, Lippincott, Williams & Wilkins.

Centers for Disease Control and Prevention: Hepatitis C: diagnosis, clinical management, and prevention, *An Interactive Videoconference by Satellite*, 2000.

Centers for Disease Control and Prevention: www.cdc.gov, Viral hepatitis A, B, C, D, E, F, September 2000.

Chan H, Springman EB, Clark JM: Expression and characterization of human tissue kallikrein variants, *Protein Expression Purif* 12(3):361-370, 1998.

Cotran RS, Kumar V, Collins T: *Robbin's pathologic basis of disease*, ed 6, Philadelphia, 1999, Saunders.

Crabb DW: Pathogenesis of alcoholic liver disease: newer mechanisms of injury, *Keio J Med* 48(4):184-188, 1999.

Crabb L: Alcoholic liver diseases. In Kelley WN, editor: *Textbook of internal medicine*, ed 3, Philadelphia, 1997, Lippincott-Raven Publishers.

Crawford JM: The gastrointestinal tract. In Cotran RS, Kumar V, Collins T, editors: *Robbin's pathologic basis of disease*, ed 6, Philadelphia, 1999, Saunders.

de Boer W, Driesen W, Jansz H, Tytgat G: Effect of acid suppression on efficacy of treatment for *Helicobacter pylori* infection, *Lancet* 345(8953):817-820, 1995.

Dienstag J, Isselbacher KJ: Acute viral hepatitis. In Fauci AS et al, editors: *Harrison's principles of internal medicine*, ed 14, New York, 1998, McGraw-Hill.

Diseases: Hepatitis D, E, G fact sheet: www.hopkins-id.edu, 2000.

Ellett ML: Hepatitis A, B, and D, *Gastroenterol Nurs* 22(6):236-244, 1999.

Fagan EA: Acute liver failure of unknown pathogenesis: the hidden agenda, *Hepatology* 19(5):1307-1312, 1994 (editorial).

Fallah MA, Prakash C, Edmundowicz S: Acute gastrointestinal bleeding. *Med Clin North Am* 84(5):1183-1208, 2000.

Friedman LS, Peterson WL: Peptic ulcer and related disorders. In Fauci AS et al, editors: *Harrison's principles of internal medicine*, ed 14, New York, 1998, McGraw-Hill, 1596-1616.

Glickman RA: Inflammatory bowel disease (Ulcerative colitis and Crohn's disease). In Fauci A, et al, editors: *Harrison's principles of internal medicine*, ed 14, New York, 1998, McGraw-Hill.

Goldberg DM: Proteases in the evaluation of pancreatic function and pancreatic disease, *Clinical Chim Acta* 291(2):201-221, 2000.

Goyal RK: Diseases of the esophagus. In Fauci AS et al, editors: *Harrison's principles of internal medicine*, ed 14, New York, 1998, McGraw-Hill.

Goyal RK, Silarao DV: Functional anatomy of swallowing and esophageal motility. In Castell DO and Richter JE editors: *The esophagus*, ed 3, Philadelphia, 1999, Williams & Wilkins.

Greenberger NJ, Isselbacher KJ: Disorders of absorption. In Fauci AS, et al, editors: *Harrison's principles of internal medicine*, ed 14, New York, 1998, McGraw-Hill.

Greenberger NJ, Toskes PP, Isselbacher KJ: Acute and chronic pancreatitis. In Fauci AS et al, editors: *Harrison's principles of internal medicine*, ed 14, New York, 1998, McGraw-Hill.

Hildt E, Hofschneider PH: The PreS2 activators of the hepatitis B virus: activators of tumour promoter pathways, *Recent Results I Cancer Res* 154:315-329, 1998.

Hosking SW et al: Duodenal ulcer healing by eradication of *Helicobactor pylori* without antacid treatment: randomized controlled trial, *Lancet* 343:508-510, 1994.

Isselbacher KJ: Bilirubin metabolism and hyperbilirubinemia. In Fauci AS, et al, editors: *Harrison's principles of internal medicine*, ed 14, New York, 1998, McGraw-Hill.

Isselbacher KJ, Podolsky DK: Disorders of the alimentary tract. In Fauci AS, et al, editors: *Harrison's principles of internal medicine*, ed 14, New York, 1998, McGraw-Hill.

Kandal G: *Helicobacter* and disease: Still more questions than answers. *Can J Surg* 43(5):339-346, 2000.

Katzka DA, Rustgi AK: Gastroesophageal reflux disease and Barrett's esophagus, *Med Clin North Am* 84(5):1137-1161, 2000.

Kelley WN: *Textbook of internal medicine*, ed 3, Philadelphia, 1997, Lippincott-Raven Publishers.

Lefrere JJ, Roudot-Thoraval F, Morand-Joubert L, Petit JC, et al: Carriage of GB virus C/hepatitis G virus RNA is associated with a slower immunologic, virologic, and clinical progression of human immunodeficiency virus disease in coinfected persons, *J Infect Dis* 179(4):783-789, 1999.

Lichtenstein GR: Advances in gastroenterology. Introduction, *Med Clin North Am* 84(5):xiii-xv, 2000.

Lohlun J, Margolis M, Gorecki P, Schein M: Fecal impaction causing megarectum-producing colorectal catastrophes. A report of two cases. *Dig Sur* 17(2):196-8, 2000.

Lott JA, *Clinical pathology of pancreatic disorders*, Totowa, NJ, 1997, Humana Press.

Lundquist A, Olsson R, Ekberg O: Clinical and radiological evaluation reveals high prevalence of abnormalities in young adults with dysphagia, *Dysphagia*, 13(4):202-207, 1998.

Marrone A, Shih JW, Nakatsuji Y, Alter HJ, et. al: Serum hepatitis G virus RNA in patients with chronic viral hepatitis, *Am J Gastroenterol* 92(11):1992-96, 1997.

Marwick C: Hepatitis A vaccine set for 2-year-olds to adults, *JAMA* 273(12):906-907, 1995.

Mayer R: Pancreatic cancer. In Fauci AS et al, editors: *Harrison's principles of internal medicine*, ed 14, New York, 1998, McGraw-Hill.

Mayer R: Colorectal cancer. In Fauci AS, et al, editors: *Harrison's principles of internal medicine*, ed 14, New York, 1998, McGraw-Hill.

Modahl LE, Lai MM: Hepatitis delta virus: the molecular basis of laboratory diagnosis, *Crit Rev Clin Lab Sci* 37(1):45-92, 2000.

National Institute on Alcohol Abuse and Alcoholism: *Facts about alcohol abuse and dependence*, Bethesda, MD, November 1998, The Institute.

National Institute of Diabetes and Digestive and Kidney Diseases: *Ulcerative colitis*, Bethesda, MD, 1998, National Digestive Disease Information Clearinghouse.

Nevalainen TJ, Hietaranta AJ, Gronroos JM: Phospholipase A2 in acute pancreatitis: new biochemical and pathological aspects, *Hepatogastroenterol* 46(29):2731-2735, 1999.

Ott DJ: Radiology of the oropharynx and esophagus. In Castell DO and Richter JE, editors: *The esophagus*, ed 3, Philadelphia, 1999, Williams & Wilkins.

Rizzetto M: Hepatitis D: Virology, clinical and epidemiological aspects, *Acta Gastro-enterologica Belgica* 63(2):221-224, 2000.

Rubin DT, Hanauer SB: Smoking and inflammatory bowel disease. *Eur J Gastroenterol Hepatol* 12(8):855-62, 2000.

Sarkola T, Makisalo H, Fukunaga T, Eriksson CJ: Acute effect of alcohol on estradiol, estrone, progesterone, prolactin, cortisol, and luteinizing hormone in premenopausal women, *Alcohol Clin Exp Res* 23(6):976-982, 1999.

Silen W: Acute appendicitis. In Fauci AS, et al, editors: *Harrison's principles of internal medicine*, ed 14, New York, 1998, McGraw-Hill.

Silen W: Acute intestinal obstruction. In Fauci AS, et al, editors: *Harrison's principles of internal medicine*, ed 14, New York, 1998, McGraw-Hill.

Sleisenger, Fordtran: *Gastrointestinal and liver disease*, ed 6, vol 2, Philadelphia, 1998, Saunders.

Stotland BR, Stein RB, Lichtenstein GR: Advances in inflammatory bowel disease. *Med Clin North Am* 84(5):1107-1124, 2000.

Thulstrup AM, Sorensen HT, Steffensen FH, Vilstrup H, et al: Changes in liver-derived enzymes and self reported alcohol consumption, *Scand J Gastroenterol* 34(2):189-193, 1999.

Wald A: Constipation, *Med Clin North Am* 84(5):1231-1246, 2000.

Wallach MD: *Interpretation of diagnostic tests*, ed 6, Boston, 1996, Little Brown.

Walsh JH, Fass R: Acid peptic disorders of the gastrointestinal tract. In Kelly WN, editor: *Textbook of internal medicine*, ed 3, Philadelphia, 1997, Lippincott-Raven.

Yeo AE, Matsumoto A, Shih JW, Alter HJ, et. al: Prevalence of hepatitis G virus in patients with hemophilia and their steady female sexual partners, *Sex Transm Dis* 27(3):178-182, 2000.

CARDIOVASCULAR SYSTEM DISORDERS

*C*ardiovascular disease in the United States is epidemic. Nearly 6 million Americans are afflicted with some disease of the heart or blood vessels. Cardiovascular disease is the leading cause of death in the United States: each year, nearly 1 million people die from a cardiovascular disorder. According to the American Heart Association, more deaths are attributable to cardiovascular disease than are the next seven leading causes of death combined. This translates to one death from cardiovascular disease every 33 seconds.

A common misconception is that cardiovascular disease occurs primarily in men. The fact of the matter is that in the United States, cardiovascular disease is the number one killer of *both men and women*. Not only is cardiovascular disease the most common killer of both men and women but also in each of the last 15 years, cardiovascular disease has claimed the lives of *more* women than it has men. This female preponderance also holds true in subsets of the population (African Americans, Caucasians, Hispanics, and American Indian/Alaska natives). Health care providers must be cognizant of these statistics because nearly one out of every two Americans will die of cardiovascular disease.

A major disparity between the genders is the age of disease onset. According to the American Heart Association, men have a one in three chance of developing a major cardiovascular disease before the age of 60 years. For women, this risk is one in ten. The presence of estrogen before the onset of menopause is thought to be a major protective factor in keeping cardiovascular disease, and coronary heart disease and stroke in particular, at bay.

Primary prevention—the early identification and modification of risk factors for the development of cardiovascular disease—is crucial in reducing the associated mortality, morbidity, and disability rates. Research as to the pathogenesis of these disease entities is ongoing, as is research concerning the most effective management strategies. The subsequent chapters present a discussion of these advances as they relate to coronary heart disease, valvular heart disease, heart failure, hypertension, and peripheral vascular disease.

Anatomy of the Cardiovascular System

LINDA COUGHLIN DeBEASI

$\mathcal{T}$he apparent simplicity in the design of the cardiovascular system belies the intricate, yet logical, interdependence of circulatory structure and function in health and disease. Each portion of the cardiovascular system is uniquely adapted to contribute to highly integrated cardiovascular responses to disease processes. Therefore an understanding of cardiovascular anatomy is prerequisite to the examination of cardiovascular disease mechanisms and the capabilities and limitations of circulatory compensatory responses.

ANATOMIC RELATIONSHIPS

The heart lies within the mediastinal space of the thoracic cavity between the lungs. The pericardium encloses the heart and is composed of two layers: the inner layer, or *visceral pericardium,* and the outer layer, or *parietal pericardium.* The two pericardial layers are separated by a small amount of lubricating fluid, which reduces the friction created by the pumping action of the heart. The parietal pericardium is attached anteriorly to the sternum, posteriorly to the vertebral column, and inferiorly to the diaphragm. These attachments hold the heart firmly in place. The visceral pericardium is in direct contact with the surface of the heart. The pericardium also provides protection against the spread of infection or neoplasms from surrounding organs to the heart. The heart itself is composed of three layers: the outer layer, or *epicardium;* the middle, muscular layer, or *myocardium;* and the inner, endothelial layer, or *endocardium* (Fig. 28-1).

The upper chambers of the heart, the *atria,* and the great vessels, the aorta and pulmonary artery, form the base of the heart. The atria are anatomically separated from the lower chambers, the *ventricles,* by a fibrous ring in which the four cardiac valves are situated and to which both the valves and the musculature attach. Functionally, the heart is divided into right-sided and left-sided pumps, which propel venous blood into the pulmonary circulation and oxygenated blood into the systemic circulation, respectively. This functional division facilitates conceptualization of the anatomic sequence of blood flow: venae cavae, right atrium, right ventricle, pulmonary artery, lungs, pulmonary veins, left atrium, left ventricle, aorta, arteries, arterioles, capillaries, venules, veins, and back to the venae cavae (Fig. 28-2).

However, the schematic conception of the right and left sides of the heart shown in Fig. 28-2 is anatomically misleading. The heart is actually rotated to the left, with its apex tilted anteriorly. This rotation places the right side of the heart anteriorly beneath the sternum, with the left side of the heart relatively posterior. The apex of the heart can be palpated at the midclavicular line at the fourth or fifth intercostal space (Fig. 28-3).

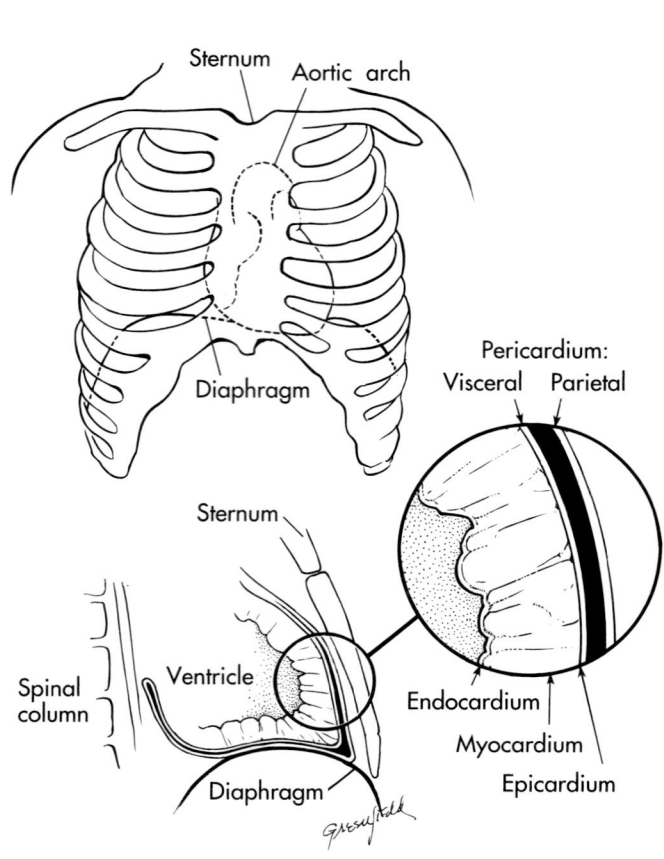

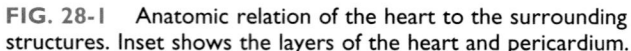

FIG. 28-1 Anatomic relation of the heart to the surrounding structures. Inset shows the layers of the heart and pericardium.

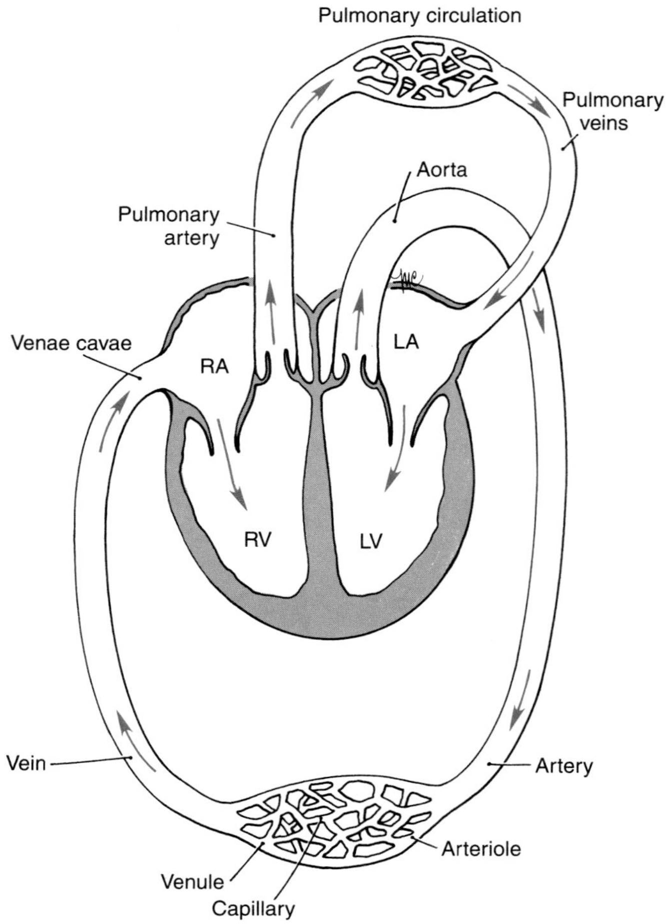

FIG. 28-2 Schematic representation of blood flow through the cardiovascular system. *RA*, Right atrium; *LA*, left atrium; *RV*, right ventricle; *LV*, left ventricle.

Right Atrium

The thin-walled right atrium (RA) functions as a reservoir and a conduit for systemic venous blood flowing to the right ventricle (RV). Venous blood enters the RA via the superior vena cava, the inferior vena cava, and the coronary sinus. No true valves are within the orifices of the venae cavae; only rudimentary valvular folds or muscular bands separate the venae cavae from the atrial chamber. Therefore elevation in right atrial pressure as a result of right-sided congestion is reflected backward into the systemic venous circulation.

Approximately 75% of the venous return to the RA flows passively into the RV through the tricuspid valve. An additional 25% of ventricular filling occurs during atrial contraction; this active contribution to ventricular filling is called the *atrial kick*. Loss of the atrial kick in certain cardiac dysrhythmias can reduce ventricular filling and consequently decrease ventricular output.

Right Ventricle

During ventricular contraction, each ventricle must generate adequate force to propel the blood received from the atrium into either the pulmonary or systemic circula-

tion. The RV has a unique crescent-shaped design and generates a low-pressure, bellowslike contraction that propels blood into the pulmonary artery. The low-pressure pulmonary circulation offers much less resistance to blood flowing into it from the RV than does the high-pressure systemic circulation encountered by the left ventricle (LV). Thus the workload of the RV is much less than that of the LV. Consequently, the wall thickness of the RV is only one third that of the LV (Fig. 28-4).

In the face of gradually increasing pulmonary pressures, as with progressive pulmonary hypertension, the RV undergoes muscular hypertrophy to increase its pumping force to overcome the elevated pulmonary resistance to ventricular emptying. However, in the event of an acute elevation in pulmonary resistance (e.g., in massive pulmonary embolization), the pumping capability of the RV can be overwhelmed, and death may result.

Left Atrium

The left atrium (LA) receives oxygenated blood from the lungs via the four pulmonary veins. No true valves separate the pulmonary veins from the LA. Therefore alterations in left atrial pressure are readily reflected retro-

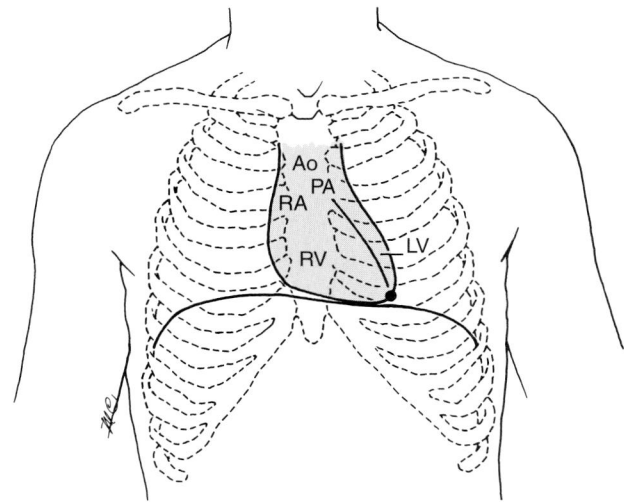

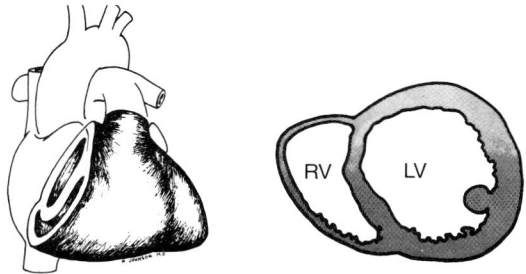

FIG. 28-4   Schematic drawings of the heart to illustrate the differences in shape of the right ventricle *(RV)* and the left ventricle *(LV)*. *Left,* Ventricles in approximate anatomic positions. *Right,* Cross section illustrating the greater wall thickness and nearly circular shape of the left ventricle.

FIG. 28-3   Orientation of the heart within the thorax. *Ao,* Aorta; *RA,* right atrium; *PA,* pulmonary artery; *RV,* right ventricle; *LV,* left ventricle. The black dot marks the normal location of the apical impulse in the fifth left intercostal space near the midclavicular line.

grade into the pulmonary vasculature, and acute elevations in left atrial pressure will cause pulmonary congestion. The LA is a thin-walled, low-pressure chamber. Blood flows from the LA into the LV across the mitral valve.

Left Ventricle

The LV must generate high pressures to overcome the resistance of the systemic circulation and sustain blood flow to peripheral tissues. The thick musculature and circular configuration of the LV facilitate the development of high pressure during ventricular contraction. Even the interventricular septum separating the ventricles contributes to the powerful compression exerted by the entire ventricular chamber during contraction.

Left ventricular pressure exceeds right ventricular pressure approximately fivefold during contraction; if an abnormal communication exists between the ventricles, as with rupture of the interventricular septum after myocardial infarction, blood will then be shunted from left to right through the defect. As a result, normal forward blood flow from the LV through the aortic valve to the aorta will be decreased.

CARDIAC VALVES

The four cardiac valves function to maintain unidirectional blood flow through the chambers of the heart. These valves are of two types: the *atrioventricular (AV) valves,* which separate the atria from the ventricles, and the *semilunar valves,* which separate the pulmonary artery and the aorta from the corresponding ventricles. The valves open and close passively in response to pressure and volume changes within the cardiac chambers and vessels.

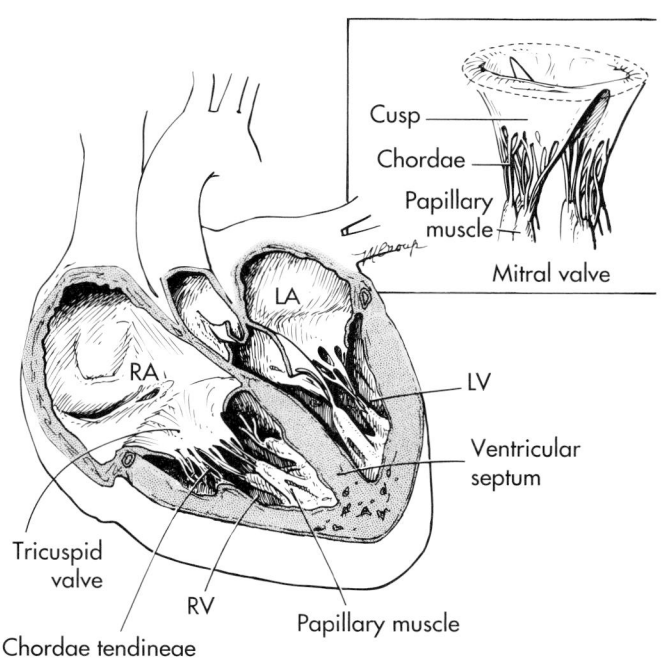

FIG. 28-5   Anatomy of the atrioventricular (AV) valves. *LA,* Left atrium; *LV,* Left ventricle; *RA,* Right atrium; *RV,* right ventricle.

Atrioventricular Valves

The leaflets of the AV valves are delicate but durable. The *tricuspid valve,* located between the RA and RV, contains three cusps, or leaflets. The *mitral valve,* separating the LA and LV, is a bicuspid valve with two valve cusps, or leaflets.

The cusps of both valves are attached to thin strands of fibrous tissue called *chordae tendineae.* The chordae tendineae extend to *papillary muscles,* which are muscular projections arising from the ventricular wall (Fig. 28-5). During ventricular contraction, the papillary muscles contract, "tugging" on the chordae tendineae, preventing eversion of the valve cusps into the atria. Rupture of the chordae tendineae, or ischemia and infarction of the papillary muscles supporting a valve, permits backflow or regurgitation of blood into the atrium during ventricular contraction.

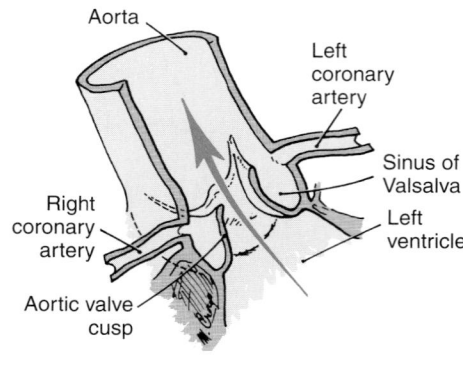

FIG. 28-6 Sinuses of Valsalva.

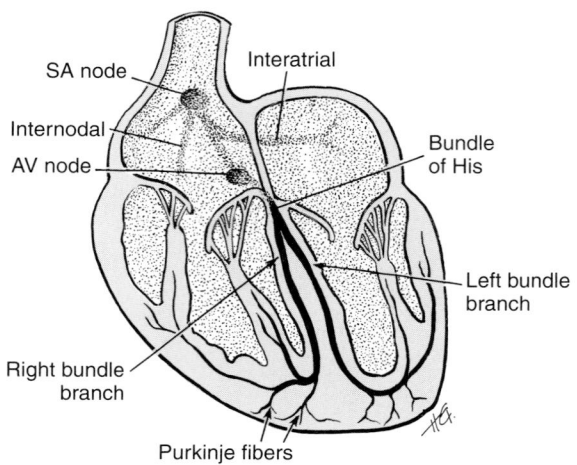

FIG. 28-7 The conduction system of the heart. *SA*, Sinoatrial; *AV*, atrioventricular.

Semilunar Valves

Both semilunar valves are of similar configuration; they consist of three symmetric cuplike cusps secured to a fibrous ring. The *aortic valve* is situated between the LV and the aorta, whereas the *pulmonic valve* is positioned between the RV and the pulmonary artery. The semilunar valves prevent backflow from the aorta or pulmonary artery into the ventricles during ventricular relaxation.

Immediately above the cusps of the valves are outpouchings of the aortic and pulmonary walls called the *sinuses of Valsalva* (Fig. 28-6). The orifices to the coronary arteries are located within the outpouchings of the aortic wall. These sinuses protect the coronary orifices from occlusion by the valve leaflets when the aortic valve opens.

CONDUCTION SYSTEM

The fibrous ring between the atria and ventricles isolates these chambers electrically, as well as anatomically. To ensure rhythmic and synchronized excitation and contraction of the heart muscle, specialized conduction pathways exist within the myocardium. This conduction tissue exhibits the following properties:

1. *Automaticity:* the ability to generate impulses spontaneously
2. *Rhythmicity:* the regularity of impulse generation
3. *Conductivity:* the ability to transmit impulses
4. *Excitability:* the ability to respond to stimulation

Because of these properties, the heart spontaneously and rhythmically initiates impulses that are transmitted throughout the conduction system to excite the myocardium and stimulate muscular contraction.

The cardiac impulse normally originates in the *sinoatrial (SA) node* (Fig. 28-7). The SA node therefore is referred to as the "natural pacemaker" of the heart. The SA node is located in the posterior wall of the RA near the entrance of the superior vena cava.

The cardiac impulse then spreads from the SA node to specialized atrial conduction pathways and to the atrial muscle. An interatrial pathway, Bachmann's bundle, facilitates impulse spread from the RA to the LA. Internodal pathways—anterior, middle, and posterior pathways—connect the SA node with the atrioventricular node.

The electrical impulse then reaches the *atrioventricular (AV) node,* which is positioned to the right of the inter-

atrial septum in the RA near the opening of the coronary sinus (see Fig. 28-7). The AV node is the normal route of impulse transmission between the atria and ventricles.

Impulse transmission is relatively slow across the AV node because of the relative thinness of the fibers in this region and the low concentration of gap junctions. Gap junctions are specialized cell-to-cell communication mechanisms that facilitate impulse conduction. The net result is a 0.9-second delay in impulse conduction through the AV node. The delay in conduction through the AV node allows for synchronization of atrial contraction before ventricular contraction, optimizing ventricular filling. Loss of this synchronization with cardiac arrhythmias, such as atrial fibrillation or heart block, can reduce cardiac output by 25% to 30%. The AV delay also protects the ventricles from bombardment by abnormal atrial impulses. Normally no more than 180 impulses per minute are permitted to reach the ventricles. This is critical during certain abnormal cardiac rhythms such as atrial fibrillation, when the atrial rate can exceed 400 beats per minute. In summary, the AV node performs two critical functions—optimization of ventricular filling time and limitation of the number of impulses that can be conducted to the ventricles.

Extending from the AV node is the *bundle of His,* which pierces the fibrous sheath that isolates the atria from the ventricles (see Fig. 28-7). Normally, the AV node-bundle of His is the only route for the spread of impulses from the atria to the ventricles and typically only in the antegrade direction—that is, from atria to ventricles. The bundle of His travels down the right side of the interventricular septum for about 1 cm and then bifurcates into the *right and left bundle branches.* The left bundle branch travels perpendicularly through the interventricular septum and further branches into a thin *anterior division* and a relatively thick *posterior division.* The right and left bundle branches then divide into the Purkinje fibers.

Impulse transmission through the *Purkinje fibers* is almost immediate. These fibers are relatively large in diameter and provide little resistance to the spread of conduction. Purkinje fibers also have an action potential characterized by a rapid upstroke in phase zero, which, as will be explained in the next chapter, is associated with rapid conduction velocity. Finally, Purkinje fibers contain a large concentration of gap junctions that are maximally aligned, further promoting rapid impulse transmission. Conduction time through the Purkinje system is approximately 150 times faster than conduction through the AV node.

Spread of conduction through the Purkinje fibers begins on the endocardial surface of the heart before plunging one third of the way into the myocardium, at which point the impulse is transmitted to ventricular muscle fibers. The impulse then continues to be spread rapidly to the epicardium. The net result of this structure is an almost immediate activation and near synchronous contraction of the ventricles.

Therefore the normal sequence of excitation through the conduction system is as follows: SA node, atrial pathways, AV node, bundle of His, bundle branches, and Purkinje fibers (see Fig. 28-7).

Anomalous anatomic connections bypassing portions of the conduction system have been identified in some individuals. These "bypass tracts" or connections can produce premature excitation of the ventricles by bypassing the intrinsic delays in conduction within the normal pathways of the conduction system. The Wolff-Parkinson-White (WPW) syndrome is an example of a preexcitation syndrome produced by impulse conduction via a bypass pathway directly connecting the atria and ventricles and bypassing the AV node.

Excitation normally originates in the SA node because the SA node exhibits the fastest intrinsic rate of impulse generation, approximately 60 to 100 bpm. However, in the event of SA node failure or its inability to generate impulses at an adequate rate, other sites can assume the role of pacemaker. The AV node is capable of generating impulses at a rate of approximately 40 to 60 bpm, and ventricular sites in the Purkinje system can generate impulses at rates of approximately 15 to 40 bpm. These lower, or "escape," pacemakers serve a critical function in the prevention of cardiac standstill (asystole) if the natural pacemaker fails in disease states or fails because of adverse effects of medication.

SYSTEMIC CIRCULATION

The systemic circulation supplies blood to all the tissues of the body with the exception of the lungs. Eighty-four percent of the total blood volume is contained in the systemic circulation. The remaining 16% of blood volume is contained in the heart and lungs. The systemic circulation can be divided into five anatomic and functional categories: (1) arteries, (2) arterioles, (3) capillaries, (4) venules, and (5) veins (Fig. 28-8). With the exception of the capillaries and venules, the vessel walls are composed of similar components: a single layer of endothelial cells, elastic tissue, smooth muscle cells, and fibrous tissue. The proportion of each of these components varies according to the function of each particular vessel.

Arteries

The walls of the aorta and large arteries are composed of much elastic tissue and some smooth muscle. The LV

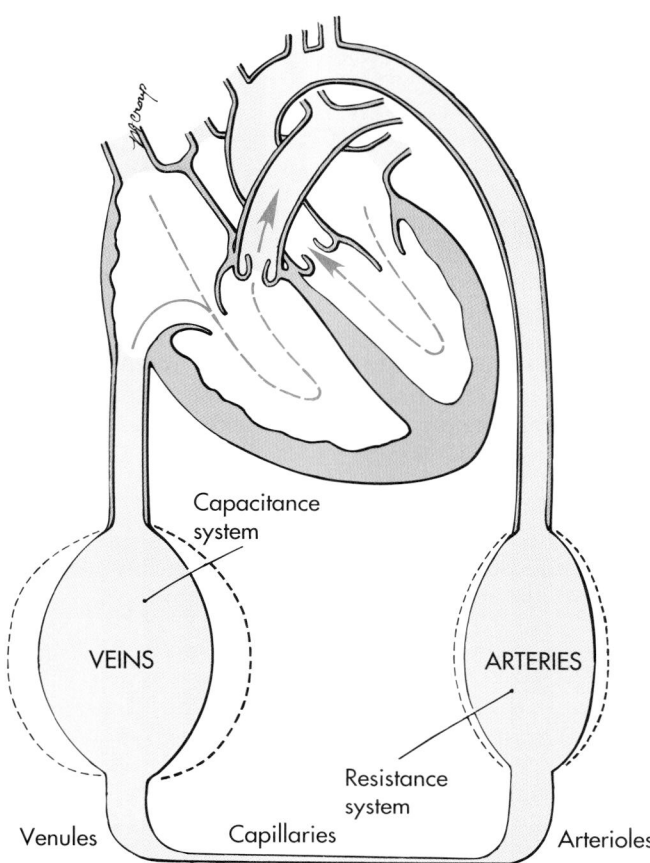

FIG. 28-8   Schematic illustration of the systemic circulation. The arterial system may be considered as a resistance circuit (low volume, high pressure), whereas the venous system may be considered as a capacitance circuit (high volume, low pressure).

ejects blood into the aorta under high pressure. This sudden expulsion of blood distends the elastic arterial walls; during ventricular relaxation, the elastic recoil of the arterial walls propels blood forward throughout the circulatory system. Peripherally, the branches of the arterial system proliferate and subdivide into smaller vessels. As a result of the distensibility of the arterial wall, blood flow changes from pulsatile to smooth and continuous flow by the time the blood reaches the smaller vessels.

The arterial bed contains approximately 15% of the total blood volume at one time. Therefore the arterial system is considered a low-volume, high-pressure circuit. Because of these volume-pressure characteristics, the arterial tree is called a *resistance circuit*.

Arterioles

At the arteriole level, the vascular wall is primarily smooth muscle with some elastic fiber. The muscular wall of the arteriole is highly responsive and can significantly alter the radius of the vessel, resulting in either constriction or dilation. When constricted, the arterioles are the major sites of resistance to flow in the arterial tree. Fully dilated, the arteriole offers almost no resistance to blood flow. At the junction between the arterioles and capillaries of some tissues is a *precapillary sphincter*, which is subject to intricate physiologic control.

Capillaries

The capillary wall is thin, consisting of only a single layer of endothelial cells. Nutrients and metabolites diffuse across this thin, semipermeable membrane and through capillary pores from areas of high concentration to areas of lower concentration. Oxygen and nutrients therefore leave the vessel to enter the interstitial space and the cell; carbon dioxide and metabolites diffuse in the opposite direction. Net fluid movement between the blood vessel and the interstitial space depends on the relative balance between hydrostatic and osmotic pressures at the capillary bed.

Venules

The venules function as collecting tubules and are composed of endothelial cells and fibrous tissue.

Veins

The veins are relatively thin-walled conduits for transport of blood from the capillary bed through the venous system to the RA. Venous flow to the heart is unidirectional as a result of valves strategically located within the venous channels. The veins are the most distensible vessels of the systemic circulation; they can accommodate large volumes of blood under relatively low pressure. Because of these low-pressure, high-volume characteristics, the venous system is referred to as a *capacitance system*.

Approximately 64% of the total blood volume is contained within the venous system. The capacity of the venous bed can be altered. For example, venoconstriction reduces the capacity of the venous bed, forcing blood forward to the heart as needed. The movement of the blood towards the heart is also influenced by venous compres-

sion of skeletal muscles, as well as by thoracic and abdominal pressures. The venous system terminates in the inferior and superior venae cavae. From there, all venous blood flows into the right atrium. Pressure within the right atrium is commonly referred to as the *central venous pressure (CVP)* or *right atrial pressure (RAP)*.

CORONARY CIRCULATION

The efficiency of the heart as a pump depends on adequate oxygenation and nourishment of the heart muscle by the coronary circulation. The coronary circulation courses over the epicardial surface of the heart, carrying oxygen and nutrients to the myocardium via small intramyocardial branches. The distribution of the coronary arteries in relation to specific portions of the myocardium and conduction system must be understood to recognize the consequences of coronary artery disease. Having knowledge of the components of the arterial wall is also important to appreciate the process and treatments of atherosclerosis. Both the distribution of the coronary arteries and the structure of the coronary artery wall are discussed in the following sections.

Distribution of Coronary Arteries

The coronary arteries are the first branches of the systemic circulation. The coronary orifices are located behind the right and left cusps of the aortic valve in the sinuses of Valsalva (see Fig. 28-6). The coronary circulation consists of the *right coronary artery* and the *left coronary artery*. The left coronary artery, or the *left main*, travels several millimeters before bifurcating into two major branches: the *left anterior descending (LAD) artery* and the *left circumflex (LCx) artery* (Fig. 28-9).

The LAD supplies the large anterior wall of the left ventricle, while the LCx supplies the lateral wall of the left ventricle. The right coronary artery (RCA) supplies the RA

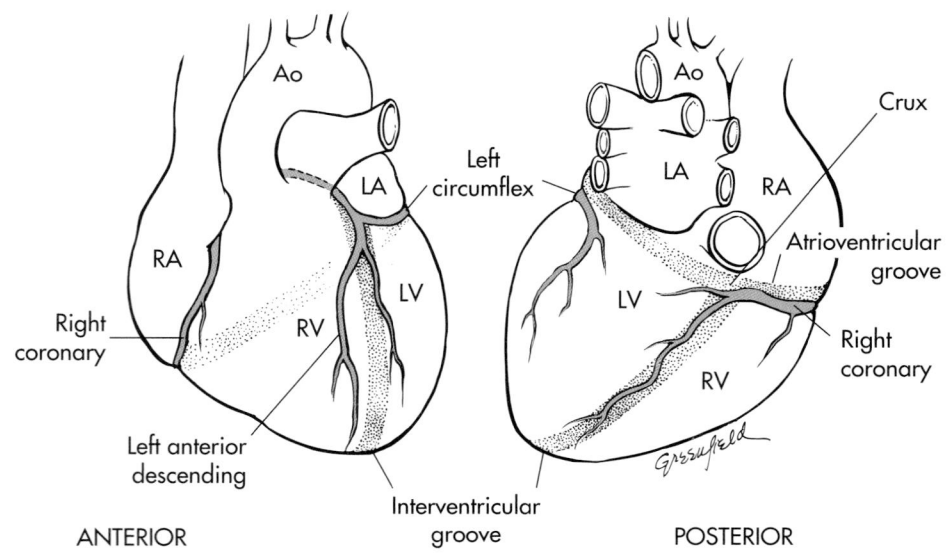

FIG. 28-9 Coronary arteries supplying the anterior and posterior aspects of the heart. *Ao,* Aorta; *RA,* right atrium; *LA,* left atrium; *RV,* right ventricle; *LV,* left ventricle.

and RV. In 85% of the population, the RCA gives rise to the posterior descending artery (PDA) and the posterior left ventricular (PLV) branches. These vessels supply the posterior and inferior walls of the LV, respectively. These individuals are said to have *right-dominant systems*. Of the remaining 15% of the population, one half has either *left-dominant systems* or *mixed dominance*. In people with left dominant systems, the LCx gives rise to both the PDA and PLV. In mixed dominant systems, the RCA gives rise to the PDA, and the LCx gives rise to the PLV.

Each major coronary vessel gives off characteristic epicardial and intramyocardial branches. The LAD gives rise to *septal* branches supplying the anterior two thirds of the septum and *diagonal* branches coursing over the anterolateral surface of the LV. *Obtuse marginal* branches of the LCx supply the lateral surface of the LV.

Portions of the conduction system are also supplied by different coronary arteries. In approximately 60% of the population, the SA node is supplied by the RCA. In slightly under 40% of the population, the LCx supplies the SA node. The AV node is supplied by the RCA in 90% of the population and by the LCx in the other 10% of the population. The right bundle branch and the posterior division of the left bundle branch have a dual blood supply—the LAD and RCA. The anterior division of the left bundle branch receives its nourishment from the septal branches of the LAD.

Knowledge of blood supply to particular areas of the myocardium and conduction system is useful clinically in the anticipation and early identification of clinical complications. For instance, an individual with ischemic changes in the inferior and posterior leads on a 12-lead electrocardiogram (ECG) would be suspected of having an occluded RCA. Conducting both a physical examination and a right-sided ECG would be prudent to assess for RV failure. AV conduction disturbances can also be anticipated. Individuals with occlusion of the LAD are more likely to have problems with the pumping function of the LV, because the LAD supplies the large anterior wall of the LV. Narrowing of the left main coronary artery is always worrisome, but it takes on particular significance for those with a left dominant system because the entire LV is jeopardized.

Collateral Circulation

Anastomoses between very small arterial branches exist within the coronary circulation. Although these intercoronary channels are not functional in the normal circulation, they become critically important as routes for alternative or *collateral circulation* to nourish myocardium deprived of blood flow. Following sudden occlusion, these "collaterals" may take several days or longer to become functional. With gradual narrowing of blood vessels, as with atherosclerosis, large, functional vessels can form over time between occluded and nonoccluded vessels. These collateral vessels are often critical in preserving myocardial function in the region of vessel occlusion.

Components of Coronary Arterial Wall

The arterial wall is composed of three layers: the intima, the media, and the adventitia (Fig. 28-10). All types of arteries have these three layers, with similar components, but the proportion of each component varies according to the function of the particular artery.

Intima

The *intima* is the innermost portion of the arterial wall and is in direct contact with the blood supply. The intima is composed of a single layer of *endothelial cells*. Endothelial cells once were thought to be inert cells, allowing movement of substances in and out of the arterial cell wall. The current understanding is that endothelial cells are quite dynamic, having a variety of functions. As will be discussed in the section on atherosclerosis, endothelial cell function also changes with endothelial injury.

One of the major functions of the endothelium is to provide a barrier between the blood stream and the interior of the vessel wall. Tight junctions and gap junctions, which selectively control the movements of substances in and out of the vessel wall, connect endothelial cells. Substances may also gain access to the subintimal area via the process of endocytosis or, if lipid-soluble, through the lipid membrane.

The endothelium also provides a *nonthrombotic surface*, thus preventing vessel occlusion. The endothelium performs this function by secreting two substances: *prostacyclin (PGI$_2$)* and *nitric oxide (NO)*. PGI$_2$ inhibits platelet aggregation, while NO inhibits both platelet aggregation and adhesion. Additionally, the endothelial cells are negatively charged and therefore naturally repel the like-charged particles. A heparin sulfate coating on the surface of the endothelial cells further assists inhibition of blood clot formation.

Endothelial cells also secrete *vasoactive substances* that affect vasodilation and vasoconstriction. Both PGI$_2$ and NO resist formation of blood clots and are also potent vasodilators, with NO being the most potent vasodilator

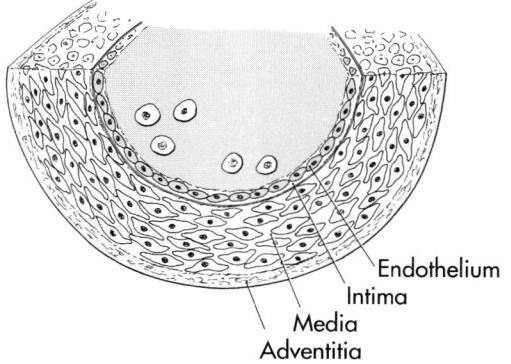

FIG. 28-10   Arterial wall. The normal arterial wall consists of three layers: the intima, the media, and the adventitia. The *intima*, lined by a single layer of endothelial cells, provides a thromboresistant barrier for the vessel and is also a source of vasoactive substances. The *media* is composed of smooth muscle cells that control vasomotor tone by contracting or dilating in response to vasoactive substances. The *adventitia*, composed of connective tissue, provides major strength to the vessel wall and contains nerve fibers and blood vessels.

thus far discovered. Endothelial cells also secrete the most potent known vasoconstrictor: *endothelin I.* Other substances secreted by endothelial cells include the vasoconstrictors, *thromboxane A₂, prostaglandin H₂,* and *angiotensin-2,* as well as the mitogen *platelet-derived growth factor (PDGF).*

Endothelial cells are capable of regeneration following injury. However, only endothelial cells at the margin of the injury are able to participate in the regeneration process. This feature has implications for areas of the arterial tree that suffer repetitive injury and is discussed in the section on atherosclerosis. Endothelial cells line up on a basement membrane interspersed with various proteins and a few smooth muscle cells. This area is known as the internal elastic laminae and forms the outer boundary of the *media.*

Media

The media is the middle portion of the arterial wall and is composed of spiraling layers of *smooth muscle cells.* Each smooth muscle cell is surrounded by a noncontinuous basement membrane, similar in makeup to that supporting the endothelial cells. Smooth muscle cells provide structural integrity to the vessel wall; they are also responsible for the maintenance of arterial wall tone by their slow, continuous contractions. Smooth muscle cells respond to various vasoactive substances either by dilating or contracting, resulting in either vasodilation or vasoconstriction.

Because of the presence of receptor cells for various substances (low-density lipoprotein [LDL], insulin, growth stimulators, and growth inhibitors), current understanding holds that smooth muscle cells may be involved in growth and development. Smooth muscle cells also play a role in the process of atherosclerosis as their function and location within the arterial wall changes.

Adventitia

The adventitia is the outermost portion of the arterial wall, which provides the major strength to the vessel wall and is composed of bundles of collagen fibrils, elastic fibers, fibroblasts, and some smooth muscle cells. The adventitia also contains nerve fibers and blood vessels.

Cardiac Veins

The three subdivisions to the venous system of the heart include the coronary sinus, the anterior coronary veins, and the thebesian veins. The *coronary sinus* and its branches comprise the largest, most significant venous system, draining the bulk of the myocardial venous blood through the ostia of the coronary sinus and into the RA. The *anterior cardiac veins* drain a large portion of right ventricular venous blood directly into the RA. The *thebesian veins* drain a small portion of venous blood from all areas of the myocardium directly into the chambers of the heart.

LYMPHATIC CIRCULATION

The lymphatic capillary network in the interstitial spaces collects excess fluid and protein filtered through the systemic capillaries. This capillary filtrate is then returned to the systemic circulation via collecting vessels located in close proximity to the veins. Lymph is propelled upward through unidirectional valves by a combination of two dynamic influences: (1) external compression by muscles and arterial pulsations and (2) intrinsic peristalsis. Lymphatic fluid is collected in the thoracic duct and the right lymphatic duct and then empties into the venous system via the internal jugular and subclavian veins.

PULMONARY CIRCULATION

The pulmonary circulation is described in depth in Part Seven. However, significant differences between the systemic and the pulmonary circulation warrant mention. The pulmonary vasculature has thinner walls and less smooth muscle compared with the systemic vasculature. The pulmonary circuit therefore is more distensible and offers less resistance to flow. Pressure in the pulmonary circuit is approximately one fifth that in the systemic circuit. The walls of the pulmonary vasculature are much less reactive to autonomic and humoral influences, whereas alterations in oxygen and carbon dioxide content of the blood and alveoli profoundly alter flow through the pulmonary vasculature. These differences make the pulmonary circuit particularly well suited to fulfill its physiologic function of oxygen uptake and carbon dioxide removal.

INNERVATION OF THE CARDIOVASCULAR SYSTEM

The cardiovascular system is richly innervated by fibers of the autonomic nervous system (ANS). The two divisions of the ANS are the *parasympathetic system* and the *sympathetic system,* which exhibit opposite effects and operate reciprocally to effect changes in heart rate. For instance, stimulation of the sympathetic system is usually coupled with inhibition of the parasympathetic system; conversely, parasympathetic stimulation and sympathetic inhibition are typically concurrent events. This reciprocal action increases the precision of neural regulation by the ANS.

ANS regulation of the cardiovascular system requires the following components: (1) sensors, (2) afferent pathways, (3) an integration center, (4) efferent pathways, and (5) receptors.

Sensors are divided into two primary groups: the baroreceptors and the chemoreceptors. The *baroreceptors* (or pressoreceptors), located in the aortic arch and carotid sinus, are sensitive to the stretch or distortion of the vessel wall caused by alterations in arterial pressure. Stimulation of these receptors by elevation of arterial pressure signals the cardiovascular control center to inhibit cardiac activity; conversely, reduction of arterial pressure initiates reflex augmentation of cardiac activity. The *chemoreceptors,* located in the carotid bodies and aortic bodies, are stimulated by reduction in arterial oxygen concentration, elevation of carbon dioxide tension, and elevation in hydrogen ion concentration (reduced blood pH). Activation of the chemoreceptors stimulates the cardiovascular control center to augment cardiac activity. Other receptors, which are sensitive to stretch resulting from alterations in blood volume, are located at the juncture between the great veins and atria. Two reflex responses occur on stimulation of these receptors: an increase in heart rate (Bainbridge reflex) and diuresis, resulting in decreased volume.

Afferent pathways in the vagus and glossopharyngeal nerves carry the neural impulses from the receptors to the brain. The *cardiovascular control center*, or *vasomotor center*, is located in the medulla and lower pons. The center receives impulses from the baroreceptors and chemoreceptors and transmits impulses to the heart and vessels via the parasympathetic and sympathetic nerve fibers. Higher centers of the brain, such as the cerebral cortex and hypothalamus, can also influence ANS activity via the medulla. The efferent pathway from the cardiovascular control center to the heart is mainly through the vagus nerves for the parasympathetic fibers, whereas the sympathetic fibers travel by way of the cardiac nerves. Receptors are located in the conduction system of the heart, the myocardium, and the smooth muscle of the blood vessels. Stimulation of the receptors alters the heart rate, the speed of AV conduction, the strength of myocardial contraction, and the diameter of blood vessels.

The parasympathetic fibers innervate the SA node, the atrial musculature, and the AV node via the vagus nerves. Parasympathetic fibers also extend to the ventricular muscle, but the functional significance of these pathways appears limited. Stimulation of parasympathetic fibers causes the release of acetylcholine. *Acetylcholine* mediates the transmission of the neural impulse to the cardiac receptors. Parasympathetic stimulation restrains cardiac action by reducing the heart rate, the speed of impulse conduction through the AV node, and the force of atrial and perhaps ventricular contraction. This response to parasympathetic stimulation is also referred to as a *cholinergic response* or a *vagal response*. The vagal response is rapid and powerful and capable of achieving beat-to-beat regulation of heart rate. Intense cholinergic or vagal stimulation is capable of reducing the heart rate to zero.

The sympathetic fibers extend to the entire conduction system and myocardium, as well as to the smooth muscle of the vasculature. *Norepinephrine* is the sympathetic neurotransmitter. Sympathetic or *adrenergic* stimulation also causes the release of *epinephrine* and some norepinephrine from the adrenal medullae. Epinephrine and norepinephrine are then carried to all parts of the body via the blood stream. The response of the heart to sympathetic stimulation is mediated by the binding of norepinephrine and epinephrine to specific adrenergic receptors: the *alpha receptors* (α) and the *beta receptors* (β_1 and β_2). Stimulation of the α receptors, located primarily on smooth muscle cells of the vasculature, results in vasoconstriction. Stimulation of the β_1 receptors, which are primarily located on the SA node, AV node, and myocardium, results in increased heart rate, increased speed of conduction across the AV node, and increased force of myocardial contraction. Stimulation of the β_2 receptors results in vasodilation.

Selective stimulation of these receptors, combined with variations in the intensity of sympathetic activity, regulates the degree of vasoconstriction, thereby controlling the capacity of the vascular bed and influencing the vascular resistance to blood flow and thus arterial pressure. For example, arterial constriction increases arterial pressure and the peripheral resistance to blood flow. Venoconstriction reduces the capacity of the venous bed and increases venous return to the heart. As is discussed in the next chapter, an increase in venous return results in a more forceful contraction of the heart, further contributing to an increase in arterial blood pressure.

The interplay of the sympathetic and parasympathetic nervous system operate to stabilize arterial pressure and cardiac output to deliver blood flow relative to body needs. Cardiac output and arterial pressure can be increased by sympathetic stimulation and parasympathetic inhibition, resulting in an elevation of heart rate, increased force of contraction, and vasoconstriction. Conversely, abnormal elevations of blood pressure will result in reflex slowing of heart rate, reduced contractility, and vasodilation.

*K*EY CONCEPTS

- The pericardium holds the heart in place and provides protection from the spread of infection and neoplasms from surrounding organs.
- The heart is composed of three layers: the outer layer (epicardium), the middle layer (myocardium), and the innermost layer (endocardium).
- The heart consists of four chambers: the right and left atria and the right and left ventricles.
- The anatomic sequence of blood flow is venae cavae, right atrium, right ventricle, pulmonary artery, lungs, pulmonary veins, left atrium, left ventricle, aorta, arteries, arterioles, capillaries, venules, veins, and back to the venae cavae.
- The atria function as reservoirs for blood. No valves exist between the right atria and the venae cavae or between the left atria and the pulmonary artery.

- Therefore changes in right or left atrial pressures are reflected into the systemic and pulmonary circulations respectively.
- The right ventricle (RV) ejects its contents into the low pressure, pulmonary circulation. Little resistance exists to right ventricular ejection. In contrast, the left ventricle (LV) ejects its contents into the high pressure, systemic circulation, offering high resistance to ventricular ejection, which explains the reason for which the left ventricular mass is three times that of the right ventricle (RV).
- Atrioventricular (AV) valves consist of the mitral valve (bicuspid) and the tricuspid valve. The mitral valve is located between the left atrium (LA) and LV, while the tricuspid valve is located between the right atrium (RA) and RV. Each cusp is attached to the

chordae tendineae, which are subsequently attached to the papillary muscles. The chordae tendineae and papillary muscles prevent eversion of the cusps into the atria during ventricular contraction.

■ Semilunar valves (aortic valve and pulmonic valve) contain three cusps. The aortic valve is located between the LV and aorta. The pulmonic valve is located between the RV and the pulmonary artery. The semilunar valves function to prevent backflow of blood from the pulmonary artery and aorta into the ventricles.

■ Cardiac impulses originate in the SA node and move through the conduction system as follows: through the interatrial and internodal pathways, to the AV node, through the Bundle of His, through the right and left bundle branches, and on through the Purkinje system.

■ Conduction of cardiac impulses is somewhat delayed through the AV node. This delay allows for synchronization of atrial contraction prior to ventricular contraction, optimizing ventricular filling and for ventricular protection against rapid impulses originating in the atria.

■ Conduction through the Purkinje fibers is near instantaneous and aids in the almost immediate activation and near synchronous contraction of the ventricles.

■ The SA node, AV node, and Purkinje fibers have the ability to generate impulses spontaneously (automaticity). Impulses are generated more quickly in the SA node, and therefore the SA node is the dominant pacemaker of the heart.

■ The systemic circulation, which includes the blood supply to all tissues, with the exception of the lungs, can be subdivided into five anatomic categories: arteries, arterioles, capillaries, venules, and veins.

■ The arterial system is known as the resistance circuit because it contains low volume carried under high pressure. The venous system is known as the capacitance system, because it contains a high volume (64% of blood volume) carried under low pressure.

■ The major coronary arteries are the right coronary artery (RCA) and the left main coronary artery. The left main coronary artery bifurcates to form the left anterior descending (LAD) artery and the left circumflex (LCx) artery. Knowledge of the typical distribution of the coronary arteries is useful to clinicians in anticipating complications following occlusion of a coronary artery.

■ Coronary arteries are composed of three layers: intima, media, and adventitia. The intima is composed of endothelial cells, which protect the integrity of the arterial wall and secrete vasoactive substances. The media is composed of smooth muscle cells that respond to vasoactive substances by either contracting or dilating. The adventitia provides strength to the vessel wall.

■ The cardiovascular system is innervated by the parasympathetic and sympathetic nervous systems. These two systems exhibit opposite effects and operate reciprocally to effect change in cardiovascular functioning.

■ Parasympathetic stimulation via the vagus nerve decreases firing of the SA nose, decreases the speed of conduction across the AV node and decreases the force of atrial contraction. Inhibiting the parasympathetic nervous system results in the opposite effects.

■ Sympathetic fibers extend to the conduction system, the myocardium, and to the smooth muscle cells of the vasculature. Stimulation of the sympathetic nervous system causes release of both norepinephrine and epinephrine from the adrenal medullae. These substances selectively bind to α receptors and β_1 and β_2 receptors to cause vasoconstriction of blood vessels, increased firing of the SA node, increased speed of conduction across the AV node, and increased force of ventricular contraction. Inhibiting the sympathetic nervous system results in the opposite effects.

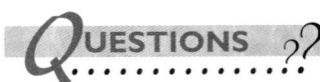

QUESTIONS ??

A sampling of review questions for this chapter appears here. Visit http://www.mosby.com/MERLIN/PriceWilson/ for additional questions. MERLIN

Answer the following on a separate sheet of paper.

1. Trace the anatomic sequence of blood flow through the cardiovascular system, naming the structures traversed.
2. Describe the two critical functions of the atrioventricular (AV) node.
3. Discuss the differences in the wall thickness of the RV and LV in terms of function. Relate the relative wall thickness to differences in the systemic and pulmonary circulations.
4. What is the function of the chordae tendineae and papillary muscles?
5. How many valve cusps are there on the valve between the LV and aorta? Name this valve. Name the outpouchings above the valve cusps. What is the function of these outpouchings?
6. Identify the layers of the pericardium. What does the space between the layers contain, and what is its function?
7. How is lymph propelled in lymphatic vessels?
8. Contrast the vascular effects of sympathetic stimulation of the α receptors and β receptors. Differentiate between β_1 and β_2 receptors.

Fill in the blanks with the correct word or phrase.

9. The conduction tissue of the heart exhibits the following properties:
   _____, the ability to spontaneously generate impulses;
   _____, the ability to respond to stimulation;
   _____, the ability to transmit impulses; and
   _____, the regularity of impulse generation.
10. Elevations of right atrial pressure or left atrial pressure readily result in neck vein distention and pulmonary congestion, respectively, because the venae cavae and pulmonary veins, unlike most systemic veins, have no true _____.
11. In cases of coronary artery occlusion, _____ circulation may protect the involved muscle tissue from ischemia or necrosis.
12. Lesions of the _____ artery are associated with the highest incidence of right ventricular failure. Lesions of the _____ artery are more apt to interfere with the pumping function of the left ventricle.
13. The intrinsic rate of the SA node is _____, the rate of the AV node is _____, and the ventricular rate is _____.
14. The vascular wall of the arterioles is composed primarily of _____, which allow for changes in arteriolar _____.

Physiology of the Cardiovascular System

LINDA COUGHLIN DeBEASI

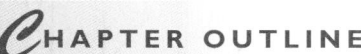
CARDIAC CYCLE

Each cardiac cycle consists of a sequence of interdependent electrical and mechanical events. The wave of electrical excitation spreading from the sinoatrial (SA) node through the conduction system and to the myocardium stimulates muscular contraction. This electrical excitation is referred to as *depolarization;* it is followed by electrical recovery, or *repolarization.* The mechanical responses are *systole*, or muscular contraction, and *diastole*, or muscular relaxation. Fig. 29-1 illustrates the correlation between ventricular depolarization and ventricular contraction. Systole comprises one third of the cardiac cycle.

The electrical activity of the cell, recorded graphically via intracellular electrodes, exhibits a characteristic configuration, the *action potential* (Fig. 29-2, *A*). The summated electrical activity of all myocardial cells can be visualized on an *electrocardiogram (ECG)* (see Fig. 29-2, *B*). The waves on the ECG reflect the spread of electrical excitation and recovery through the atrial and ventricular myocardium. The significance of the waveforms is discussed in subsequent sections.

Electrophysiology

The electrical activity of the heart results from the flow of sodium, potassium, and calcium ions (Na$^+$, K$^+$, and Ca^{++}) across the cardiac cell membrane (Fig. 29-3). As in all cells of the body, Na$^+$ and Ca^{++} are primarily extracellular ions, and K$^+$ is primarily an intracellular ion. Movement of these ions across the cardiac cell membrane is controlled by a variety of forces, including passive diffusion, voltage and time dependent gates, and the Na$^+$, K$^+$-ATPase pump.

Action Potential

The net result of transmembrane ionic movement is an electrical difference across the cell membrane that can be graphically displayed over time as an *action potential* (Fig. 29-4, *A*). The action potential depicts the electrical charge of the interior of the cell in relation to the electrical charge of the exterior of the cell, the *transmembrane potential.* The transmembrane potential changes with ionic movement and is depicted as phase 0 through phase 4 (see Fig. 29-3). The two major types of action potentials are the fast response and the slow response action potentials (see Fig. 29-4, *A* and *B*). These two types are classified according to the primary forces of depolarization, either *fast Na$^+$ channels* or *slow Ca^{++} channels.*

Fast Response Action Potential

Fast response action potentials are observed in the atrial and ventricular muscle cells, as well as the Purkinje fibers. Transmembrane potential in these cells at rest is −90 mV—the *transmembrane resting potential* (designated as RP in Fig. 29-4, *A*). Several factors maintain the negative transmembrane resting potential. The first factor is the selective permeability of the cell membrane to K$^+$ as compared with Na$^+$ ions. Potassium is allowed to move freely down its concentration gradient to the exterior of the cell (see Fig. 29-3, *A*). At the same time, although both the concentration and electrical gradients favor the movement of Na$^+$ to the interior of the cell, cell membrane permeability permits only small quantities of Na$^+$ to leak in.

A second important contributor to the negative transmembrane resting potential is the presence of the Na$^+$,

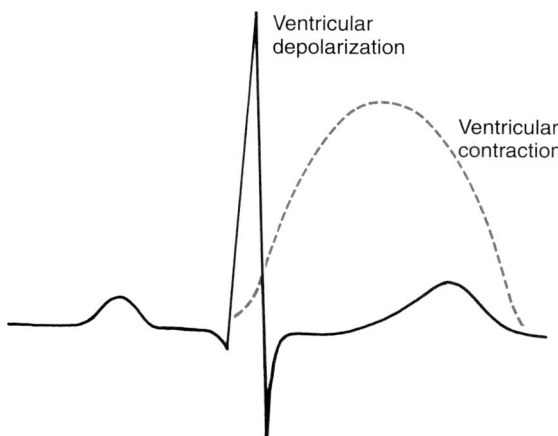

FIG. 29-1   Correlation between ventricular depolarization and ventricular contraction.

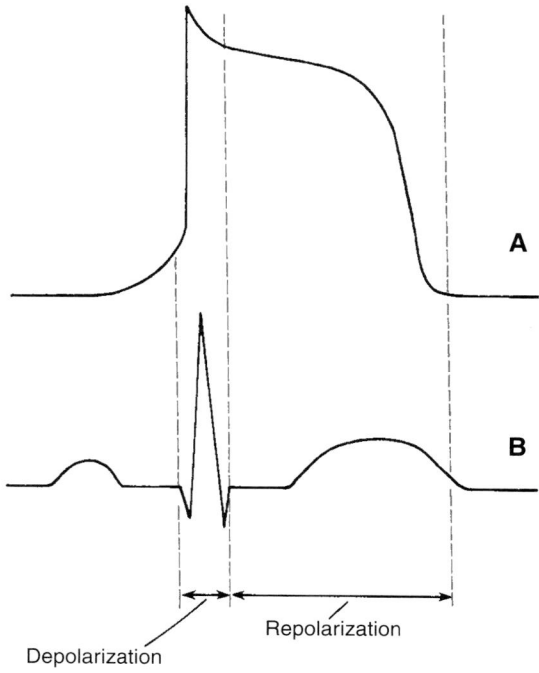

FIG. 29-2   Electrical activity of the heart. **A**, Recording of the intracellular potential of a single cardiac cell during a complete cardiac cycle. **B**, Standard electrocardiographic (ECG) recording from the body surface, representing the summated electrical activity of all the myocardial cells. The time periods within the dashed lines represent depolarization and repolarization of the ventricles.

K^+-ATPase pump. This metabolic pump sits within the cell membrane and continuously pumps both Na^+ and K^+ against their respective concentration gradients. Sodium is moved out of the cell and K^+ into the cell in a 3:2 ratio, further amplifying the electrical difference across the cell membrane.

Phases of Fast Response Action Potential. Stimuli that raise the transmembrane potential to –65 mV, also known as *threshold potential* (designated as TP in Fig. 29-4, *A*), set into play forces that initiate depolarization. A transmembrane potential of –65 mV is required to open the *activation gates* in the fast Na^+ channels. As the activation gates open, Na^+ pours into the cell according to both electrical and concentration gradients. This rapid positive change in transmembrane potential correlates with depolarization, or *Phase 0*, of the action potential. The positive change in transmembrane potential to 0 mV causes the inactivating gates of the Na^+ channel to close but not before a slight "overshoot" in voltage is present. In examining the action potential (see Fig. 29-4, *A*), it is clear to see the sharp upstroke of phase 0, which represents how quickly the gates of the fast Na^+ channels are activated. The amplitude and velocity of phase 0 correlate with the velocity at which the action potential is propagated to other cells.

Following depolarization, an initial repolarization of the cell membrane occurs that is depicted by *Phase 1* of the action potential (see Fig. 29-4, *A*). Phase 1 demonstrates the return of negativity as K^+ moves out of the cell according to both electrical and chemical gradients (see Fig. 29-3, *C*). The electrical movement is unopposed for only a short period until the voltage dependent slow Ca^{++} channels have a chance to open. Slow Ca^{++} channels receive their name because although they are activated during Phase 0, when the transmembrane potential reaches approximately –10 mV, the movement of Ca^{++} into the cell is not apparent until *Phase 2*. During phase 2, a *plateau* in the transmembrane potential occurs as Ca^{++} moves into the cell and electrically neutralizes the effect of K^+ movement out of the cell (see Fig. 29-3, *D*). The plateau lasts for a relatively long period as the slow Ca^{++} channels are both slow to open and to close. Calcium entering the cardiac cell during this period is also

involved in cardiac contraction (excitation-contraction coupling), which is discussed later.

Once Ca^{++} channels have closed, K^+ continue to move out of the cell unopposed (see Fig. 29-3, *E*). This action allows a return in negativity of the transmembrane potential as depicted by *Phase 3*, also known as *final repolarization*. Transmembrane potential continues to fall until resting potential (–90 mV), also known as *Phase 4*, has been reached (see Fig. 29-4).

Refractory Period. From the onset of phase 0 until the middle of phase 3, the cardiac cell cannot be restimulated. This period is known as the *effective or absolute refractory period*. During this period, the fast Na^+ channels are inactivated and cannot be reactivated despite the strength of the stimulus. Toward the middle of phase 3 and immediately before phase 4, a stimulus stronger than is normal will result in the development of an action potential, as the fast Na^+ channels begin to recover from inactivation. This period is known as the *relative refractory period*. After phase 4 is reached, any stimulus that is capable of reaching threshold is able to generate an action potential—the *all or nothing phenomenon*.

Slow Response Action Potential

Both the SA and the atrioventricular (AV) nodes display slow-response action potentials. Cells of these nodes have fewer K^+ channels and are much more leaky to Na^+. As such, the transmembrane resting potential is much less negative (–60 mV), which is noted as RP in Fig. 29-4, *B*. At this transmembrane potential, voltage-dependent fast

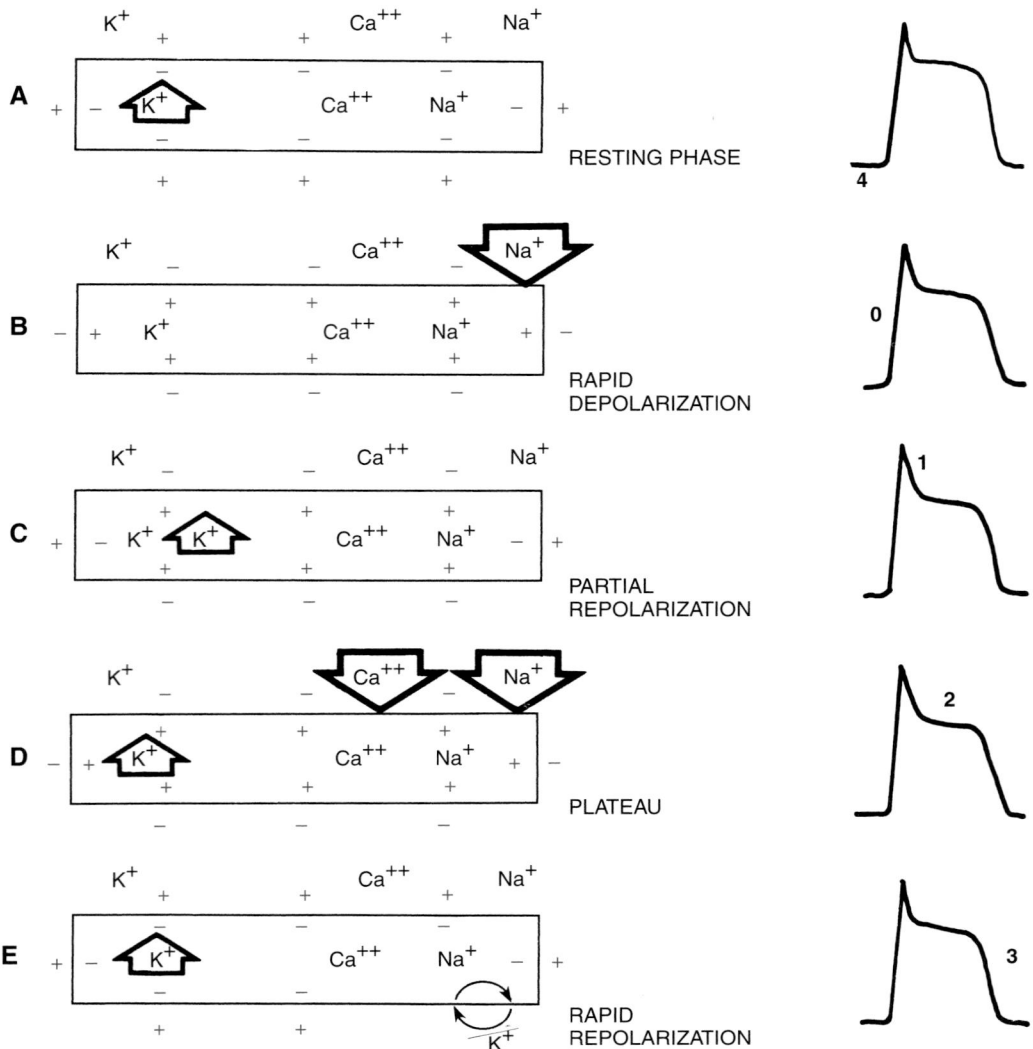

FIG. 29-3   Cellular electrophysiology. **A**, Resting phase. **B**, Rapid depolarization. **C**, Partial repolarization. **D**, Plateau. **E**, Rapid repolarization. K^+, Potassium; Ca^{++}, calcium; Na^+, sodium.

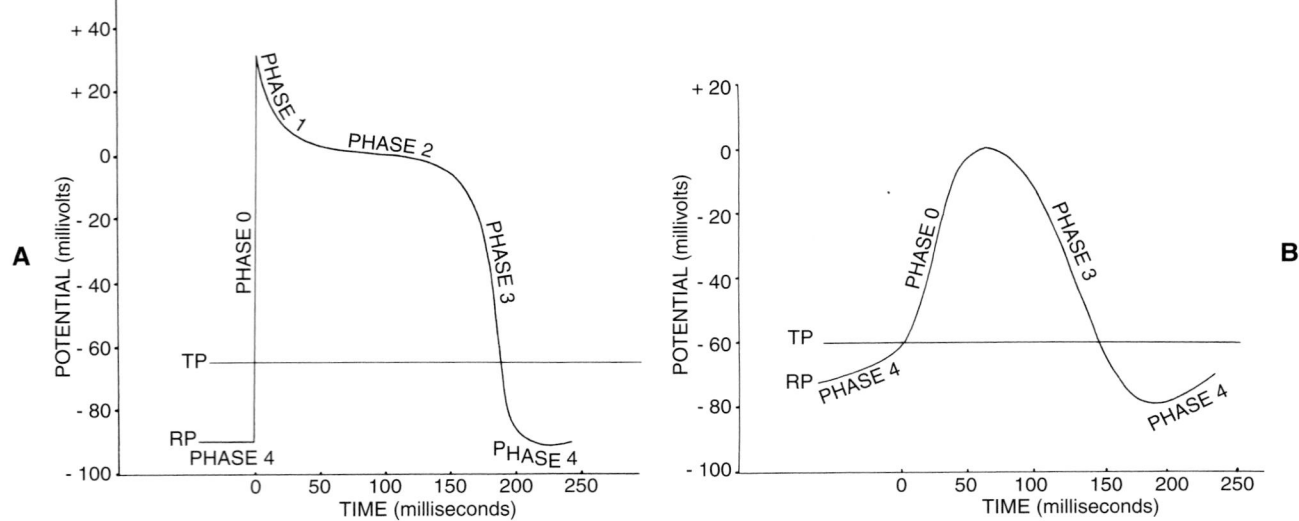

FIG. 29-4   Configuration of action potential. **A**, Fast response. **B**, Slow response. (Modified from Berne RM, Levy MN: *Phsiology*, ed 3, St Louis, 1993, Mosby.)

Na⁺ channels remain inactivated. Despite this state, other channels in the cell membrane are inherently leaky to Na⁺, causing large quantities of Na⁺ to leak into the cell. Transmembrane potential eventually reaches –40 mV, which is threshold potential in slow response cells and is designated as TP in Fig. 29-4. Voltage-dependent slow response Ca⁺⁺ channels become activated, and the influx of Ca⁺⁺ results in cellular depolarization.

Phases of Slow Response Action Potential. The shape of the slow response action potential varies from that of fast response action potential (see Fig. 29-4, *A* and *B*). Depolarization, or phase 0, is much less steep in slow response cells. No phase 1 occurs. Phase 2 is not distinct from phase 3. Phase 3 immediately follows phase 0 as slow Ca⁺⁺ channels become inactivated. At the same time, large quantities of K⁺ moves out of the cell unopposed, causing resting membrane potential to return to –55 to –60 mV (phase 4), at which point the K⁺ channels become less permeable to K⁺. Na⁺ continues to leak into the cell, causing transmembrane potential to rise to –40 mV, and the cycle begins again.

Pacemaker Cells

Fibers of the heart's specialized conduction system (SA node, AV node, and Purkinje fibers) have the characteristic of *automaticity*, which means that they are capable of self-excitation, or the spontaneous generation of an action potential. The SA node is the dominant pacemaker of the heart, because it is capable of self-excitation at a rate quicker than that of the AV node or Purkinje fibers. However, if the SA node becomes injured, the AV node and Purkinje fibers can then take over the role of pacemaker but at a slower rate (40 to 60 bpm and 15 to 40 bpm, respectively).

Ionic movement during phase 4 determines automaticity in both the SA and the AV nodes. Slow depolarization occurs throughout phase 4 as Na⁺ moves into the cell, relatively unopposed by K⁺. This movement raises the transmembrane potential to threshold, with the subsequent development of an action potential. This action occurs repeatedly in a regular, cyclical manner, describing another characteristic of SA and AV node firing—*rhythmicity*.

Muscle Ultrastructure

The *sarcomere*, which is the basic contractile unit of the myocardium (Fig. 29-5), is composed of two sets of overlapping myofilaments: thick *myosin* filaments and thin *actin* filaments. Myosin filaments contain cross-bridges. Actin filaments are composed of three protein components: actin, tropomyosin, and troponin. Muscle contraction occurs when active sites on the actin filaments link with myosin cross-bridges, causing actin filaments to be pulled toward the center of the myosin filaments, shortening the sarcomere.

Calcium is essential for actin-myosin linkage. In the absence of calcium, tropomyosin and troponin cover the active sites on the actin filament, preventing linkage with myosin. The result is cardiac muscle relaxation. In the presence of calcium, the inhibitory effect of tropomyosin and troponin is itself inhibited, allowing active sites on the actin filament to link with myosin cross-bridges. This action results in shortening of the sarcomere and cardiac muscle contraction.

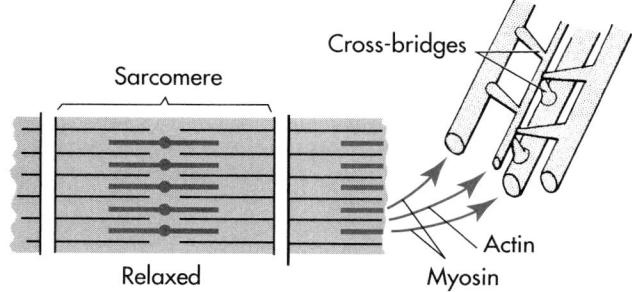

FIG. 29-5   Muscle ultrastructure. The myofibrils are composed of thick myosin filaments and thin actin filaments. Cross-bridges are observed at regular intervals between the actin and myosin filaments, forming linkages during muscle contraction. The amount of overlap between the actin and myosin filaments is decreased during muscle relaxation and increased during contraction. This causes a corresponding increase or decrease in the sarcomere length.

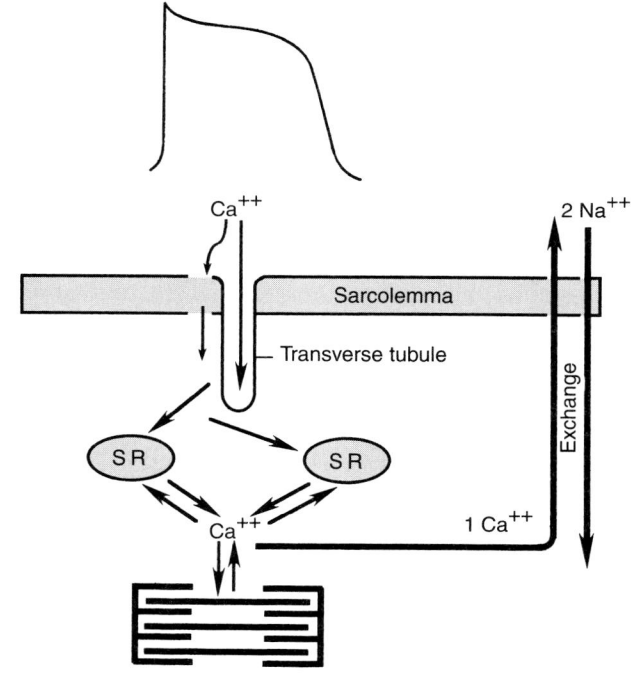

FIG. 29-6   Movement of calcium in excitation-contraction coupling in cardiac muscle. The influx of calcium ions (Ca⁺⁺) from the interstitial fluid during excitation (plateau of action potential) triggers the release of Ca⁺⁺ from the sarcomplasmic reticulum *(SR)*. The free cytoplasmic Ca⁺⁺ activates contraction of the myofilaments (systole). Relaxation (diastole) occurs as a result of Ca⁺⁺ uptake by the SR and the extrusion of intracellular Ca⁺⁺ by sodium-calcium exchange. (From Berne RM, Levy MN: *Cardiovascular physiology*, ed 6, St. Louis, 1991, Mosby.)

The calcium necessary for actin-myosin linkage is provided during the electrical stimulation of the cardiac cell, that is, during the propagation of an action potential. As an action potential is propagated across the cell membrane, slow Ca⁺ channels on the cell membrane become activated. This corresponds with the plateau period of the action potential (see Fig. 29-3, *D*, and Fig. 29-6). Calcium moves across the *sarcolemma* (cell membrane) and *transverse tubules* (extension of the cell membrane). Movement of calcium to the interior of the cell liberates large quantities of stored calcium from the *sarcoplasmic reticulum*. Calcium then inhibits the inhibitory effect of tropomyosin-troponin, allowing actin-myosin linkage to occur, shortening the sarcomere and causing myocardial contraction (see Fig. 29-6). The energy required for this contractile process comes from the degradation of adenosine triphosphate (ATP) to adenosine diphosphate (ADP).

Contraction lasts as long as the plateau period of the action potential (see Fig. 29-6). As slow Ca^+ channels close, calcium is simultaneously pumped out of the cell into the sarcoplasmic reticulum and transverse tubules. In the absence of calcium, the tropomyosin-troponin-system, once again, exerts an inhibitory effect on actin, and myocardial relaxation occurs.

The entire atrial or ventricular myocardium is stimulated simultaneously and then contracts simultaneously resulting from the rapid spread of the action potential across individual cardiac cell membranes and across *intercalated discs*. Intercalated discs are portions of the cardiac cell membranes that connect one cell to the next and offer almost no resistance to flow of the action potential. Therefore stimulation of one cardiac cell results in simultaneous stimulation of all cardiac cells—the *all or none phenomenon*.

The importance of calcium for the concomitant electrical excitation *and* contraction of the cardiac muscle is known as *excitation-contraction coupling*. Clinically, this mechanism is important in understanding the consequences of various medical therapies that alter intracellular calcium concentration. For instance, this action explains the reason for which the administration of a calcium channel blocker for heart rate control may result in the worsening of congestive heart failure. Conversely, the administration of intravenous catecholamines can augment both heart rate and the force of myocardial contraction.

Phases of the Cardiac Cycle

The cardiac cycle describes the sequence of ventricular contraction and emptying *(systole)*, and ventricular relaxation and filling *(diastole)*. Clinically, systole can also be conceptualized as the period between heart sounds S_1 and S_2, and diastole can be conceptualized as the period between S_2 and S_1 (Fig. 29-7). S_1 and S_2 are generated by the closure of the AV and the semilunar valves, respectively. An important factor to keep in mind is that cardiac valves open and close passively in response to pressure gradients. Equally important is that the sequence of mechanical events during the cardiac cycle occurs simultaneously on the right and left sides of the heart. However, for the purpose of clarity, this description will focus on the events occurring on the left side of the heart.

Early in diastole, blood flows rapidly from the atria, across the mitral valve, and into the ventricle. As the pressure between the atria and ventricle begins to equalize, blood flow from the atria to the ventricle slows. This action is called the period of *diastasis* (see Fig. 29-7). Atrial contraction then occurs, contributing an additional 20% to 30% to ventricular filling. Ventricular contraction then begins, and because the pressure in the ventricle is greater than that in the atria, the mitral valve closes (S_1). This action begins systole and, specifically, the period of *isovolumic contraction*. This period is so named because despite an increase in left ventricular pressure, intraventricular volume remains constant because both the mitral and the aortic valves are closed.

As ventricular contraction continues, pressure within the left ventricle rises until it exceeds the pressure within the aorta. The pressure gradient forces the aortic valve open, and blood pours out of the ventricle. This action is known as the period of *ventricular ejection*. Approximately 70% of ventricular emptying occurs during the first one third of the ejection period. Thus the first one third of the ventricular ejection period is known as *rapid ven-*

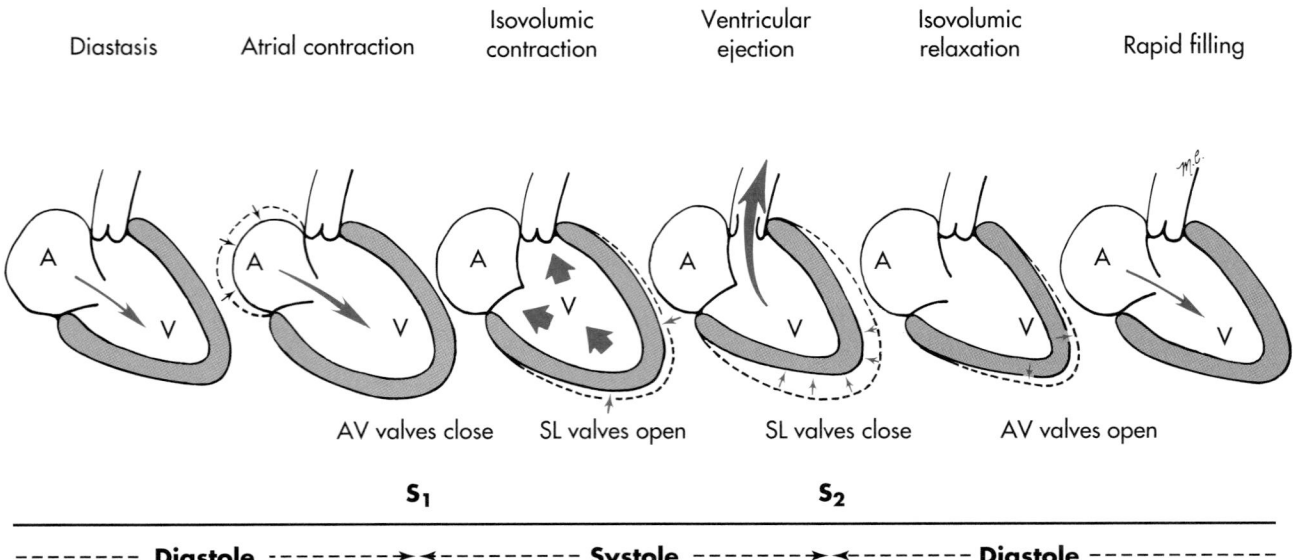

| Diastasis | Atrial contraction | Isovolumic contraction | Ventricular ejection | Isovolumic relaxation | Rapid filling |

AV valves close — SL valves open — SL valves close — AV valves open

S_1 — S_2

- - - - - - - **Diastole** - - - - - - - → ← - - - - - - **Systole** - - - - - - → ← - - - - - **Diastole** - - - - - - - - -

FIG. 29-7 Phases of the cardiac cycle. *A,* Atria; *V,* ventricles; S_1, first heart sound; S_2, second heart sound; *AV,* atrioventricular; *SL,* semilunar.

tricular ejection. The remaining two thirds of the ventricular ejection period is known as *slow ventricular ejection,* because only 30% of ventricular emptying occurs during this period. The ventricle then begins to relax. Ventricular relaxation causes the pressure in the ventricle to fall below that in the aorta, and the aortic valve closes (S_2), heralding the onset of diastole.

With both the aortic and mitral valves closed, the volume of blood in the left ventricle remains constant. Left ventricular pressure declines as the ventricle begins to relax. This decrease in left ventricular pressure, despite a constant left ventricular volume, is known as the period of *isovolumic relaxation.* While ventricular pressure decreases, atrial pressure builds resulting from a venous return against a closed mitral valve. This pressure gradient results in the opening of the mitral valve and subsequent pouring of blood from the atria to the ventricle. Thus the period of *rapid ventricular filling* ensues, and the cardiac cycle begins again.

Correlation of Electrical Events with the Cardiac Cycle

As described in the section on muscle ultrastructure, a linkage exists between cardiac electrical events and cardiac mechanical events (excitation-contraction coupling). Electrical events in the heart precede and, in fact, initiate the mechanical events. The correlation of the electrical events with the subsequent mechanical events—phases of the cardiac cycle—is depicted in Table 29-1. The correlation of electrical events in the heart to specific ECG waveforms is also depicted. The significance of the ECG waveforms is described in subsequent chapters.

An understanding of the cardiac cycle and the linkage between the electrical and mechanical events in the heart is crucial to a full appreciation of the consequences of specific disease states and the benefit of specific medical therapies. For instance, left ventricular contraction in the presence of an incompetent mitral valve results in the ejection of blood both into the aorta and into the left atrium. Atrial fibrillation results in the loss of atrial contraction, with subsequent decrease in left ventricular filling by 20% to 30%. Both of these states have a deleterious effect on cardiac output. After an acute myocardial infarction, a severely failing heart can be supported by the placement of an intraaortic balloon pump, reducing aortic end-diastolic pressure. This therapy decreases the intraventricular pressure required to open the aortic valve during isovolumic contraction, thereby decreasing the work of the heart.

CARDIAC OUTPUT

Definitions

The result of the synchronized, rhythmic myocardial contraction is the ejection of blood into the pulmonary and systemic circulations. The volume of blood ejected by each ventricle per minute is the *cardiac output.* An average cardiac output is 5 L/min. However, cardiac output varies to meet the needs of the peripheral tissues for oxygen and nutrients. Because cardiac output requirements also vary according to body size, a more accurate indicator of cardiac function is the cardiac index. The *cardiac index* is the cardiac output divided by body surface area; it is approximately 3 L/min/m² of body surface.

Stroke volume is the volume of blood ejected by each ventricle per beat. Approximately two thirds of the volume of blood in the ventricle at the end of diastole *(end-diastolic volume)* is ejected during systole. This portion of blood ejected is known as the *ejection fraction;* the residual ventricular volume at the end of systole is referred to as the *end-systolic volume.* Depression of ventricular function impairs the ability of the ventricle to empty, thereby reducing stroke volume and the ejection fraction with a consequent elevation of residual ventricular volumes.

Determinants of Cardiac Output

Cardiac output depends on the relationship between two variables: heart rate and stroke volume.

$$\text{cardiac output} = \text{heart rate} \times \text{stroke volume}$$

Despite alterations in one variable, cardiac output can be held remarkably constant by compensatory adjustments in the other variable. For instance, when the heart rate slows, the period of ventricular relaxation between heartbeats is longer, and ventricular filling time is thereby increased. Consequently, ventricular volumes are greater, and more blood can be ejected per beat. Conversely, when stroke volume drops, increasing the heart rate can stabilize cardiac output. These compensatory adjustments can maintain cardiac output only within limits. The alteration and stabilization of cardiac output depend on control mechanisms regulating heart rate and stroke volume.

Control of Heart Rate

Heart rate is largely under the extrinsic control of the autonomic nervous system; parasympathetic and sympa-

---

TABLE 29-1 ■■■

Correlation of Electrical Events with Mechanical Events in the Heart*

Electrical Events of Conduction System	ECG Waveform	Phases of Cardiac Cycle
Impulse originates in sinus node and is spread through the atria (atrial depolarization)	P wave	Ventricular filling Atrial contraction
Impulse spreads from atria, through the AV node to bundle of His (AV delay)	PR interval	
Impulse spreads through bundle branches and Purkinje fibers (ventricular depolarization)	QRS complex	Isovolumic contraction Ventricular ejection Rapid ejection Slow ejection
Ventricles recover (ventricular repolarization)	T wave	Isovolumic relaxation Ventricular filling Rapid filling Diastasis

*Note that electrical events slightly precede mechanical events, or phases, in the cardiac cycle.

thetic fibers innervate the SA node and the AV node, influencing the rate and speed of impulse conduction. Stimulating the parasympathetic fibers decreases the heart rate, whereas sympathetic stimulation increases the heart rate. In the normal resting heart, the influence of the parasympathetic system appears to dominate in maintaining the heart rate at approximately 60 to 80 bpm. If all neural and hormonal influences on the heart were blocked, the intrinsic rate would then be approximately 100 bpm.

Control of Stroke Volume

Three variables influence stroke volume: the *preload*, *afterload*, and *contractility* of the heart.

Preload

Preload is the degree of myocardial fiber stretch immediately before contraction. Myocardial fiber stretch depends on the volume of blood distending the ventricle at end-diastole. The venous return of blood to the heart determines ventricular end-diastolic volume. An increase in venous return increases end-diastolic ventricular volume, which, in turn, enhances the stretch of myocardial fibers.

The *Frank-Starling mechanism* states that within physiologic limits, the greater the stretch of myocardial fiber at end-diastole is, the stronger the force of contraction during systole will be (Fig. 29-8). Stretch of the myocardial fibers at end-diastole results in optimal overlap between actin and myosin myofilaments, promoting maximal cross-bridge linkage during systole. Cross-bridge linkage and subsequent contractile forces are greatest when the sarcomere is between 2.0 and 2.4 μm in length (Fig. 29-9, A).

The average end-diastolic sarcomere length is between 2.0 and 2.2 μm. Thus a reserve in sarcomere length exists, as well as a reserve in the resultant contractile forces.

When the sarcomere length is less than 2.0 μm, a decrease in the contractile force occurs. Rather than actin overlapping myosin, actin excessively overlaps adjacent actin filaments within the sarcomere. This action reduces the number of sites available for cross-bridge linkages (see Fig. 29-9, B). When the sarcomere length is greater than 2.4 μm, a decrease in the contractile force also occurs. In this situation, however, this state occurs because actin and myosin filaments are stretched further away from each other, again limiting the number of cross-bridge linkages (see Fig. 29-9, C).

Optimal myofilament overlap is only one reason that end-diastolic stretch is important in determining the force of contraction. An additional reason is that end-diastolic stretch increases the sensitivity of the myofilaments to calcium. Although the mechanism is not fully understood, this enhanced sensitivity to calcium results in a more forceful contraction.

The relationship between myocardial fiber length and the force of contraction is represented by a *ventricular function curve* (Fig. 29-10, A). This curve depicts the change in contractility that occurs with any change in preload. The curve demonstrates an initial ascending limb of improved function as the heart fills. Eventually, the curve flattens, or plateaus, indicating that additional increments in ventricular volume will not improve function further; optimal fiber length has been achieved. The normal heart operates on the ascending limb of the ventricular function curve. Considerable cardiac reserve

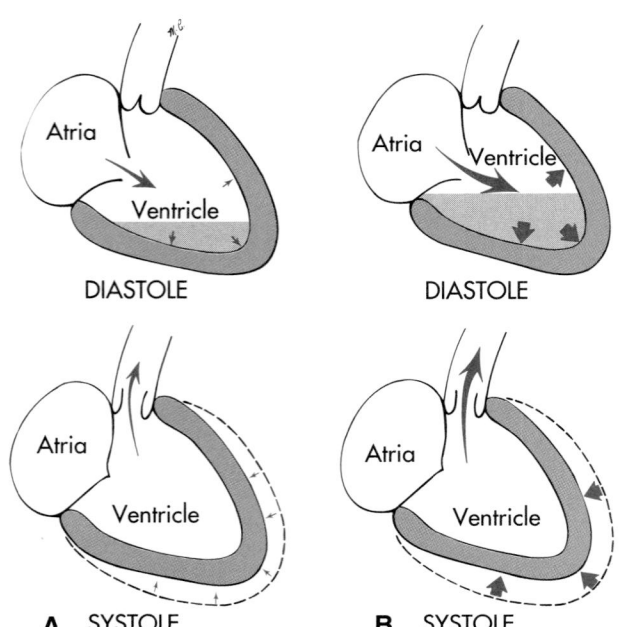

FIG. 29-8 Starling's law of the heart. **A,** Normal filling during diastole causes normal fiber stretch and normal contractile force and stroke volume. **B,** Increased filling during diastole causes increased fiber stretch, increased force of contraction, and increased stroke volume.

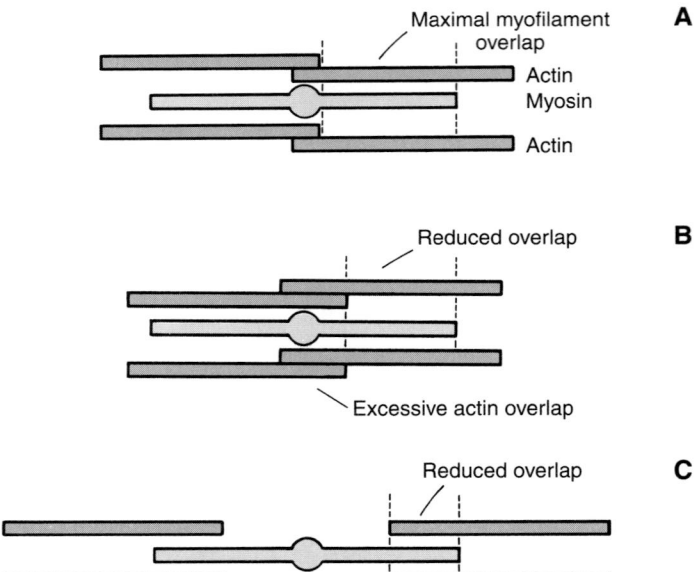

FIG. 29-9 Effect of sarcomere length on myofilament overlap. **A,** Sarcomere length 2.0 – 2.4 micrometers; normal to maximal actin-myosin overlap. **B,** Sarcomere length <2.0 micrometers; excessive overlap between adjacent actin myofilaments. **C,** Sarcomere length >2.4 micrometers; reduced actin-myosin overlap.

exists to move beyond that point with further improvements in cardiac function. In summary, up to a point, increased preload will increase the force of contraction and consequently the volume of blood ejected from the ventricle.

Afterload

Afterload is a second determinant of stroke volume. Afterload is the tension the myocardial fibers have to develop to contract and eject blood. The factors that influence afterload can be explained in a simplified version of the *Laplace equation:*

$$\text{wall tension} = \frac{\text{intraventricular pressure} \times \text{radius}}{\text{ventricular wall thickness}}$$

The Laplace equation indicates that when either intraventricular pressure or ventricular radius increases, a corresponding increase occurs in ventricular wall tension. The equation also demonstrates the inverse relationship between wall tension and ventricular wall thickness: ventricular wall tension decreases as ventricular wall thickness increases.

The Laplace equation is useful in understanding the way in which specific clinical situations can adversely affect afterload and consequently impair stroke volume. For example, an elevation in arterial blood pressure increases the resistance to ventricular ejection. To achieve a stable stroke volume, intraventricular pressure increases to overcome this resistance to ejection. This translates to an increase in wall tension. Wall tension is also increased in dilated cardiomyopathy. In this condition, the radius of the ventricle is increased. To maintain a stable stroke volume, ventricular wall tension must also

increase (Fig. 29-11). The inverse relationship between wall tension and wall thickness is demonstrated when a thickening in the ventricular myocardium occurs, as with hypertrophic cardiomyopathy. In this condition, the ventricle hypertrophies, and, proportionally, less wall tension must therefore be developed by the ventricle to generate pressure and eject blood.

Contractility

Contractility is the third determinant of stroke volume. Contractility refers to changes in the developed force of contraction that occur independent of changes in myocardial fiber length. Increased contractility is the result of intensification of the interaction of the actin-myosin cross-bridge linkages in the sarcomere. The strength of these interactions relates to the intracellular concentration of free Ca^{++} ions. Myocardial contractility is directly proportional to the amount of intracellular calcium present.

An increase in heart rate can enhance the strength of contraction. When the heart is beating more frequently, calcium accumulates within the cardiac cell, resulting in an increased force of contraction. Stimulation of the heart by the sympathetic nervous system, specifically, the binding of norepinephrine to the beta-1 receptors, liberates additional intracellular calcium, increasing the force of contraction. Increased contractility, regardless of the cause, elevates stroke volume enhancing cardiac output. Conversely, decreased contractility, as can occur as with myocardial infarction, beta-blocker therapy, or acidosis, decreases stroke volume and adversely affects cardiac output.

A "family" of ventricular function curves demonstrates the effect of altered contractility on stroke volume, which is independent of myocardial fiber stretch (see Fig. 29-10). Alterations in the position of the ventricular function curve reflect changes in the developed force of contraction. A shift of the curve upward and to the left reflects improvement in ventricular function—improved contractility, as can occur with sympathetic nervous

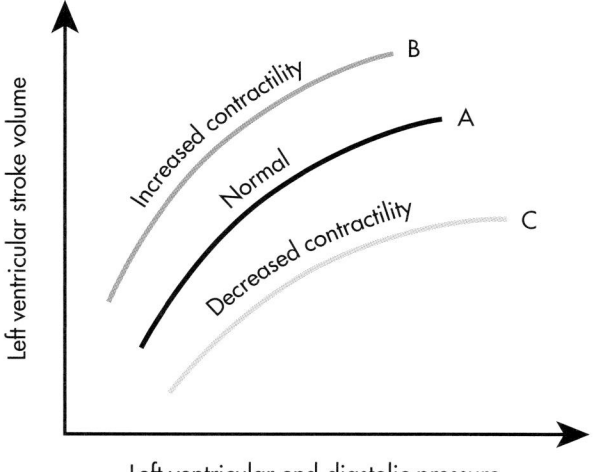

FIG. 29-10   Ventricular function curves. **A,** Normal ventricular function curve. Note that increasing end-diastolic pressure (volume) increases stroke volume up to a point. **B,** Displacement of the curve upward and to the left represents improved ventricular function, as would be seen with sympathetic nervous system stimulation. **C,** Displacement of the curve downward and to the right represents depressed myocardial function, as would be seen with myocardial infarction or beta-blocker therapy.

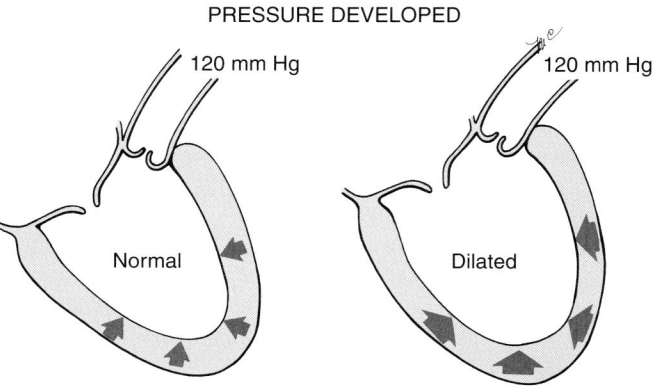

FIG. 29-11   Effect of ventricular size on afterload. The dilated ventricle on the right must generate more tension than the normal ventricle on the left to generate the same stroke volume and arterial blood pressure.

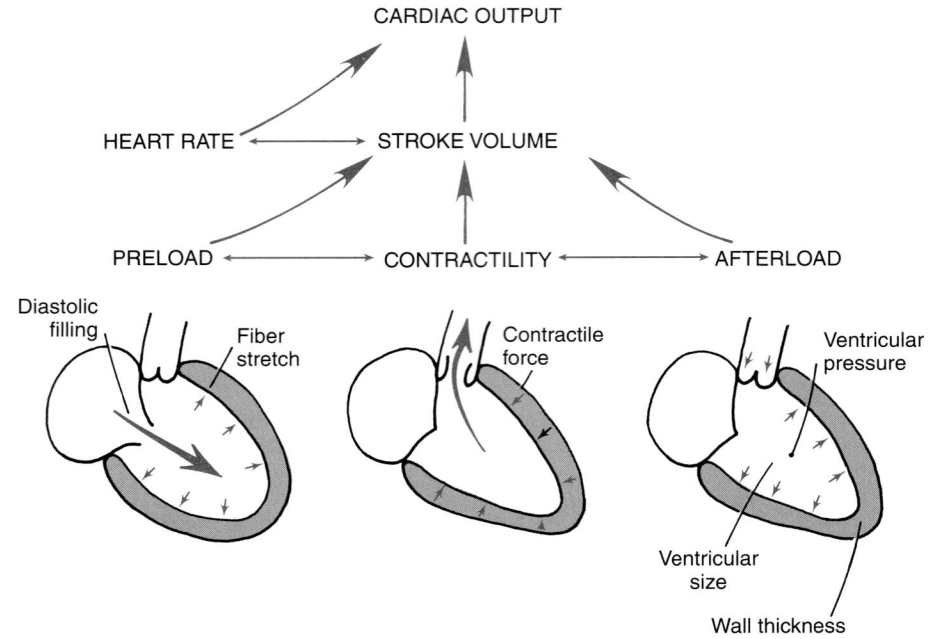

FIG. 29-12 Control of cardiac output.

stimulation (see Fig. 29-10, *B*). A shift downward and to the right represents deterioration in function—depressed contractility, as can occur with myocardial infarction and beta-blocker therapy (see Fig. 29-10, *C*).

In summary, stroke volume is determined by three variables: preload, afterload, and contractility. Although each of these variables has been discussed separately, they are not independent of one another. For instance, an increase in afterload may result in a smaller quantity of blood being ejected from the heart during systole. The volume of blood remaining in the heart after systole contributes to the preload of the next cardiac contraction. In accord with the Frank-Starling mechanism, increased preload stretches the myocardial fiber, delivering a more forceful contraction. The increase in contractile force increases the stroke volume achieved in the subsequent beats. The integration of preload, afterload, and contractility, in conjunction with heart rate, determines cardiac output (Fig. 29-12).

BLOOD FLOW TO THE PERIPHERY

The dynamics of peripheral blood flow are perhaps the most critical element of circulatory physiology for two reasons. First, the distribution of the cardiac output within the periphery depends on properties of the vascular bed. Second, the volume of cardiac output depends on the amount of blood returning to the heart. Essentially, the heart ejects a volume of blood equivalent to its venous return.

Principles of Blood Flow

Blood flow through a vessel depends on two opposing variables: the pressure difference between the two ends of

the vessel and the resistance to flow. *Ohm's law* can best represent the relationship of these two variables with regards to blood flow: $Q = \Delta P \div R$ (where Q = blood flow, ΔP = pressure difference, and R = resistance). Blood flow increases as the pressure difference between the two ends of the vessel increases; inversely, blood flow decreases as resistance increases. Important to note is that the pressure difference, or *pressure gradient*, not the absolute pressure within the vessel, determines blood flow. Overall blood flow within the circulation is called cardiac output.

Blood flows throughout the entire circulation from the arterial to the venous end in response to the pressure gradient. The pressure gradient is established by the *mean arterial blood pressure (MAP)* and the *right atrial pressure (RAP)*, or *central venous pressure (CVP)*. The MAP is defined as the pressure developed in large arteries over time and is a reflection of the average blood volume and compliance in the arterial system. RAP depends on a balance between venous return and right atrial pumping function. MAP is normally 100 mm Hg and can be approximated from the systolic blood pressure (SBP) and the diastolic blood pressure (DBP) using the following formula:

$$MAP = (SBP + ([2 \times DBP]) \div 3$$
$$\text{or } MAP = DBP + [(SBP - DBP) \div 3]$$

RAP is close to 0 mm Hg. The pressure gradient between the arterial and venous ends of the systemic circulation is approximately 100 mm Hg (MAP – RAP). Alterations in either the MAP or the RAP will influence blood flow by changing the pressure gradient between these two points—the larger the pressure gradient is, the greater the blood flow will be.

Resistance is the impediment to blood flow. Resistance is strongly, and inversely, related to the radius of the vessel lumen; that is, small changes in radius result in large changes in resistance. Blood flow is extremely sensitive to alterations in the lumen or radius of the blood vessel as is demonstrated by *Poiseuille's law*:

$$Q = \pi \, \Delta \, Pr^4 \div 8\eta l$$

From this formula, the radius to the fourth power (r^4) influences blood flow; slight changes in radius result in dramatic changes in blood flow: $R \propto 1 \div r^4$.

The arteriole is the major site of vascular resistance. Alterations in the arteriolar smooth muscle tone, under the guidance of the nervous system and local tissue conditions, regulate the radius of the blood vessel. Changes in the radius of the arterioles changes the resistance to blood flow and, ultimately, the amount of blood flow to the capillary bed.

Other factors that may affect resistance and thus blood flow include the length of the vessel and the viscosity of the blood. These factors are denoted in the Poiseuille's law as l and η, respectively. However, because these properties are relatively constant, their influence is normally insignificant. An exception to this characteristic is a change in blood viscosity that occurs with abnormalities in hematocrit. For example, the increase in blood viscosity accompanying polycythemia vera increases resistance and therefore decreases blood flow. In individuals with compromised cardiac function, performing phlebotomy may be critical to decrease the number of red blood cells and therefore improve blood flow.

In summary, according to Ohm's law ($Q = \Delta \, P \div R$), flow is directly proportional to the pressure gradient and inversely proportional to vascular resistance. Differences in pressures at the arterial and venous ends of the circulation determine the pressure gradient. Resistance is a function primarily of the radius of the blood vessels, altered most significantly at the arteriolar level. Of the three variables in the formula, resistance is the only variable that cannot be measured directly. Resistance can, however, be calculated by rearranging the algebraic formula such that: $R = \Delta \, P \div Q$. By measuring MAP, RAP, and cardiac output (CO), systemic vascular resistance (SVR) may be calculated:

$$SVR = \frac{MAP - RAP}{CO}$$

and potentially manipulated by medical therapies as needed.

Velocity of Blood Flow

The velocity of blood flow throughout the vascular system depends on the cross-sectional area of the blood vessels. Velocity *(V)* of blood flow *(Q)* decreases as the cross-sectional area *(A)* increases. This inverse relationship is expressed as follows:

$$V = \frac{Q}{A}$$

As blood flows into the peripheral arterial system, velocity decreases because of the progressive branching and relative increase in cross-sectional area of the vascular tree. At the capillary level, a profound increase in cross-sectional area occurs, significantly reducing flow velocity. This slowing facilitates the eventual exchange of nutrients and metabolites at the capillary level.

Distribution of Blood Flow

Blood flow is distributed among the multiple organ systems according to the metabolic needs and functional demands of the tissues. Because tissue requirements are continually changing, blood flow must be continually readjusted. As tissue metabolism increases, blood flow must increase to supply oxygen and nutrients and to remove the end products of metabolism. For instance, during strenuous exercise, flow to the exercising skeletal muscle must increase. Dual control of the distribution of cardiac output is possible through extrinsic and intrinsic regulatory mechanisms.

Extrinsic Control

Blood flow to a given organ system can be increased either by increasing cardiac output or by shunting blood from a relatively inactive organ system to the more active organ. The activity of the sympathetic nervous system can produce both responses. First, sympathetic stimulation augments cardiac output by increasing heart rate and force of contractility. Second, sympathetic adrenergic fibers also extend to the peripheral vasculature, particularly the arteriole. Selective alterations in sympathetic discharge will stimulate alpha and beta receptors, preferentially constricting some arterioles and dilating others to redistribute blood to capillary beds according to need. Within any capillary bed, considerable reserve exists for increased flow because only a portion of the capillaries is perfused at a given time. Therefore flow can be increased by opening nonperfused capillaries and by further arteriolar dilation of perfused capillaries.

Skeletal muscle vasculature is uniquely capable of vasodilation because sympathetic cholinergic fibers originating in the cerebral cortex innervate these vessels. These fibers release acetylcholine, resulting in relaxation of vascular smooth muscle. Parasympathetic cholinergic fibers innervate only selected, small portions of the peripheral vasculature; therefore parasympathetic activity does not significantly influence the distribution of cardiac output or total peripheral resistance.

In addition to neural control, humoral agents exert an extrinsic influence on peripheral resistance and flow. The adrenal medulla secretes the catecholamines epinephrine and norepinephrine in response to sympathetic activity. These hormones elicit sympathetic responses in the peripheral vasculature. Other blood-borne agents—vasopressin, angiotensin and endothelin—also play a role in vasoconstriction. Additionally, blood-borne agents such as bradykinin and histamine act as vasodilators.

Intrinsic Control

Intrinsic control of blood flow, which is an alteration in blood flow in response to changes in local tissue conditions, plays a particularly important role in tissues that have a limited tolerance for a reduced blood supply, such as the heart and the brain. The level of oxygen and other nutrients is a critical indicator of adequacy of blood flow. Because of intrinsic control mechanisms, a decrease in oxygen or nutrient availability (because of either a decrease in supply or an increase in demand) is met by an increase in blood flow to the tissue.

Currently, two theories explain this change in blood flow related to oxygen or nutrient deprivation. The first is the *vasodilator theory*, which states that when either metabolism is increased or nutrient delivery is decreased, an increase in vasodilator substances produced by the tissues takes place. Some of the proposed vasodilator substances include adenosine and carbon dioxide, as well as K^+ and hydrogen ions. The second theory is the *oxygen or nutrient lack theory*, which states that nutrients are essential in maintaining vascular tone produced by smooth muscle cell contraction. When nutrients are lacking, either because of inadequate delivery or because of increased metabolism, smooth muscle cells are not able to contract. The natural result is vasodilation. Possibly, the vasodilator theory and the oxygen or nutrient lack theory are not mutually exclusive; that is, they act in concert to optimize vasodilation.

Tissues also have the ability to control blood flow in response to a change in perfusion pressure (arterial blood pressure). As perfusion pressure changes, the blood vessels of the affected tissue undergo a change in resistance to maintain a constant blood flow (Ohm's law, $Q = \Delta P \div R$). An increase in perfusion pressure is met by a decrease in resistance, and, conversely, a decrease in perfusion pressure is met by an increase in resistance. The ability to maintain constant blood flow in the face of a changing perfusion pressure is referred to as *autoregulation*.

Although functional in many organs of the body, the exact mechanism for autoregulation is unclear. One explanation put forth is the *myogenic mechanism*. Under this mechanism, an increase in perfusion pressure and concomitant increase in blood flow is followed by contraction of the arteriolar smooth muscle cells, resulting in vasoconstriction. Vasoconstriction returns blood flow to its previous level. Conversely, under the myogenic mechanism, a decrease in perfusion pressure and concomitant decrease in blood flow is followed by relaxation of the arteriolar smooth muscle cells, resulting in vasodilation. Vasodilation returns blood flow to its previous level.

Another factor affecting arteriolar smooth muscle cell relaxation is the release of substances from the endothelium itself. Endothelial cells react to increases in shear stress, as with an increase in velocity of blood flow, by releasing nitric oxide. Nitric oxide is the most potent vasodilator thus far discovered.

Mechanisms related to nutrient delivery and perfusion pressure thus far discussed act to regulate the minute-to-minute flow of blood to the tissues. Other factors act over an extended period—days to months—to regulate blood flow. These factors include collateral blood vessel development (as discussed in Chapter 28) and *angiogenesis*. Angiogenesis is the growth of new blood vessels from existing small vessels following the secretion of vascular growth factors. Some of these vascular growth factors include vascular endothelial growth factor, fibroblast growth factor, and angiogenin. These vascular growth factors are released in response to a change in metabolic demand of the tissue. The development of new blood vessels results in an augmentation of nutrient delivery and waste removal.

In addition to these control mechanisms designed to increase oxygen delivery to the tissues, the tissues can increase oxygen supply by extracting more oxygen from the arterial blood. In most organs, with the notable exception of the heart, the tissue extracts only a small proportion of the oxygen (about 25%) that is available in the arterial blood. When an oxygen deficit develops in the tissues, the concentration gradient of oxygen between the arterial blood and the tissue increases. This action causes more oxygen to diffuse from the intravascular to the extravascular space, thereby increasing oxygen delivery to the cells.

In contrast, the heart is extremely efficient in extracting oxygen from the arterial blood (about 80%) under normal resting conditions. Therefore, during times of enhanced metabolic activity, increased oxygen demand can be met only by increasing arterial blood flow. This characteristic is the reason for which intrinsic control mechanisms are important for maintaining adequate oxygen delivery to the heart.

CARDIAC RESERVE

Normally, the heart possesses the ability to increase its pumping capacity significantly above resting levels. This cardiac reserve enables the normal heart to increase output approximately fivefold. The increase in cardiac output can occur through increments in heart rate or stroke volume (cardiac output = heart rate × stroke volume).

Heart rate can normally increase from resting levels of 60 to 100 bpm to approximately 180 bpm, primarily through sympathetic stimulation. Rates greater than this level can be deleterious for two reasons. First, as heart rate increases, the duration of diastole shortens, and ventricular filling time is reduced; eventually stroke volume falls, negating the advantage of further rate increments. Second, rapid heart rates can adversely affect myocardial oxygenation because cardiac work is increased while the diastolic period, during which most coronary flow occurs, is reduced.

Stroke volume can increase either by increased ventricular emptying resulting from increased contractility or by increased diastolic filling and a subsequent rise in ejection volume. However, both increased force of contraction and increased ventricular volumes will elevate cardiac work and oxygen demand. Additionally, the degree of myocardial fiber stretch limits the effect of increased diastolic filling on contractility and stroke volume.

When the heart is subjected to chronic volume or pressure overload, the ventricular muscle may *dilate* to increase contractile force, according to Starling's law, or *hypertrophy* to increase muscle mass and pumping force. Both responses, although compensatory in nature, eventually contribute to further cardiac decompensation. According to *Laplace's law*, dilation increases cardiac work because a distended heart requires more energy to maintain the same stroke volume. As ventricular diastolic pressure increases, the ability of the sarcomere to adapt may be exceeded and contractile force decreased. Hypertrophy increases the muscle mass requiring a nutrient supply, thereby increasing oxygen demand.

KEY CONCEPTS

- Electrical excitation is referred to as *depolarization,* and electrical recovery is referred to as *repolarization.*
- Electrical excitation in the heart depends on the movement of Na^+, K^+, and Ca^{++} across the cardiac cell membrane. The movement of these ions results in an electrical difference across the cell membrane, which can be graphically displayed as an *action potential.*
- Two major types of action potentials—fast response and slow response—are classified according to the primary forces of depolarization, either fast Na^+ channels or slow Ca^{++} channels. *Fast response action potentials* are observed in the atrial and ventricular muscle cells and the Purkinje fibers. *Slow response action potentials* are observed in both the SA and AV nodes.
- The *effective* or *absolute refractory period* and the *relative refractory period* refer to phases of the action potential during which it is difficult to restimulate cardiac cells.
- The *ECG* depicts the summation of simultaneous electrical activity in cardiac cells.
- The SA node, AV node, and Purkinje fibers are capable of *self-excitation (automaticity).* The SA node is the dominant pacemaker of the heart and has an intrinsic rate of 60 to 100 bpm. The intrinsic rate of the AV node and Purkinje fibers is 40 to 60 bpm and 15 to 40 bpm, respectively.
- Cardiac contraction relies on linkage between actin and myosin myofilaments. Calcium is required for this linkage to occur and is made available to the cell during the plateau phase of the action potential. This relationship between electrical stimulation and mechanical contraction of the heart is known as *excitation-contraction coupling.*
- The *cardiac cycle* describes the sequence of ventricular contraction and emptying (systole) and ventricular relaxation and filling (diastole). The unidirectional flow of blood through the heart depends on the presence of cardiac valves, which open and close in response to the development of pressure gradients.
- *Cardiac output* is the amount of blood ejected by each ventricle per minute. Average cardiac output is 5 L/min. Cardiac output is determined by the relationship of heart rate and stroke volume (CO = heart rate × SV). Stroke volume is determined by the interaction of three variables: preload, afterload, and contractility.
- *Preload* is the degree of myocardial stretch immediately before contraction. Within physiologic limits, the greater the stretch of myocardial fibers at end-diastole is, the stronger the force of contraction during systole will be (Frank-Starling mechanism).
- *Afterload* is the tension that the myocardial fibers have to develop to contract and eject blood. Factors that increase afterload may negatively affect stroke volume.
- *Contractility,* which is the inherent ability of the myocardial fibers to contract, is independent of afterload and preload and dependent on the level of intracellular calcium.
- *Blood flow* through a vessel depends on two opposing variables: the pressure difference between the two ends of the vessel and the resistance to flow. The relationship of these variables can best be represented by Ohm's law: $Q = \Delta P \div R$.
- According to *Ohm's law,* blood flow, or cardiac output, is a function of the pressure differences within the vasculature (MAP minus RAP), and the state of the resistance vessels (arterioles). Dilation of the arterioles provides a decrease in resistance and an increase in blood flow. Conversely, constriction of the arterioles provides an increase in resistance and a decrease in blood flow.
- Blood flow through the periphery is under the influence of extrinsic and intrinsic control mechanisms. The *extrinsic control mechanism* is primarily the sympathetic nervous system. *Intrinsic control of blood flow* is regulated by local tissue conditions and is especially important in optimizing blood flow to the brain and heart.
- The heart has the ability to increase its pumping capacity significantly above resting levels by changing heart rate and the force of contraction, both of which are under control of the sympathetic nervous system.

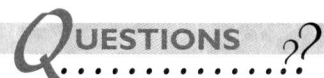

QUESTIONS

A sampling of review questions for this chapter appears here. Visit http://www.mosby.com/MERLIN/PriceWilson/ for additional questions. MERLIN

Answer the following on a separate sheet of paper.

1. What are the two major mechanical phases of the cardiac cycle, and what does each represent? What does an electrocardiogram represent, and how is it different from an action potential? What is the relationship between the electrical and mechanical events of the cardiac cycle?

2. State the Frank-Starling mechanism of the heart. What is the relationship between the mechanism and the ventricular function curve?

3. State Ohm's law as it applies to blood circulation. How would you calculate the systemic blood pressure gradient?

4. Hemodynamic measurements on a 46-year-old woman with a body surface area of 1.5 m² reveal the following data: CO, 4.5 L/min; left ventricular EDV, 100 ml; left ventricular end-systolic volume (ESV), 30 ml. What is her left ventricular stroke volume (SV)? What is her cardiac index and left ventricular ejection fraction (EF)? Are these values normal?

Match each of the hemodynamic parameters in column A with its equivalent in column B.

Column A

5. _____ Cardiac output
6. _____ Mean arterial pressure
7. _____ Stroke volume
8. _____ Ejection fraction
9. _____ Cardiac indexes
10. _____ Blood flow

Column B

a. End-diastolic volume − end-systolic volume

b. $\dfrac{\text{Cardiac output}}{\text{Body surface area}}$

c. $\dfrac{\text{SBP} + 2 \times (\text{DBP})}{3}$

d. Heart rate × stroke volume

e. $\dfrac{\text{Stroke volume}}{\text{End-diastolic volume}}$

f. $\dfrac{\text{Mean arterial pressure} - \text{right atrial pressure}}{\text{Resistance}}$

Fill in the blanks with the correct word or phrase or circle the correct option.

11. The _____ period is the time in the cardiac cycle during which the myocardium will not respond to any stimulus. The myocardium is capable of responding to a strong stimulus during the _____ refractory period.

12. In the resting state, the inside of the cell is _____ charged with respect to the outside. During the repolarization of a cell the Na^+, K^+-ATPase pump moves _____ into the cell and _____ out of the cell.

13. During the ventricular filling phase of the cardiac cycle the AV valves are (open) or (closed), and the semilunar valves are (open) or (closed).

14. During the ventricular ejection phase of the cardiac cycle, the AV valves are (open) or (closed), and the semilunar valves are (open) or (closed).

15. During the phase of ventricular filling, the cardiac impulse is delayed at the _____.

16. Loss of _____ can decrease left ventricular filling by 20% to 30%. Clinically, this action is known as loss of _____.

Match each of the phases of the fast-response action potential in column A with the appropriate descriptive phrase(s) in column B.

Column A

17. _____ Phase 0
18. _____ Phase 1
19. _____ Phase 2
20. _____ Phase 3
21. _____ Phase 4

Column B

a. Slow influx of Ca^{++} is primarily responsible for the plateau during this phase.

b. Rapid decrease in electronegativity of the cell membrane is caused by change of permeability to Na^+ and its rapid influx into cell.

c. Partial repolarization is caused by abrupt inactivation of fast sodium channels and outward movement of potassium.

d. This phase corresponds to the end of the absolute refractory period.

e. The inside of the cell is negative with respect to the outside, and the ionic concentrations of Na^+ and K^+ on either side of the cell membrane are maintained at a steady state by the Na^+, K^+-ATPase pump.

f. Rapid repolarization is caused by cessation of inward currents of Ca^{++} and Na^+ and rapid efflux of K^+ from the cell.

Diagnostic Procedures in Cardiovascular Disease

SUSAN T. DiMATTIA

*I*ncreasingly sophisticated diagnostic techniques are available to detect heart disease and its clinical sequelae. However, the use of these techniques and the interpretation of test results are adjuncts to the systematic clinical assessment of the patient, not substitutes for a thorough history and physical examination. Thus a brief overview of the systematic bedside assessment of the patient with heart disease must precede a description of common diagnostic procedures.

CLINICAL ASSESSMENT

A systematic clinical assessment includes a complete history and physical examination using the techniques of inspection, palpation, percussion, and auscultation. Examination of the cardiovascular system must include the heart and the peripheral vascular system. A detailed discussion of the peripheral vascular examination and related diagnostic tests is presented in Chapter 34.

History

The history must include an assessment of the individual's lifestyle and the impact of heart disease on the activities of daily living if the patient, rather than the disease, is to be treated. The patient's history should also include a history of the family and the incidence of cardiovascular disease in the first-degree relatives (parents and siblings). The following signs and symptoms of heart disease are typically elicited during the history of the patient with heart disease:

1. *Angina*, or chest pain, resulting from a lack of myocardial oxygen, or ischemia. Some patients deny chest "pain" and describe a tightness, squeezing, pressure, or heaviness in their chest without pain per se. Angina may present as *referred pain*, or pain that the body interprets as coming from the jaw, upper arms, or middle of the back. Angina may also be "silent" and without discomfort but associated with a feeling of weakness and fatigue
2. *Dyspnea*, or an awareness of uncomfortable breathing caused by increased respiratory effort associated with pulmonary vascular congestion and alterations in lung distensibility; *orthopnea*, or difficulty in breathing in the recumbent position; *paroxysmal nocturnal dyspnea*, or dyspnea that occurs during sleep because of left ventricular failure and is relieved by sitting up on the side of the bed
3. *Palpitations*, or an awareness of the heartbeat caused by changes in the rate, regularity, or force of cardiac contraction
4. *Peripheral edema*, or swelling caused by fluid accumulation in the interstitial spaces, usually noted in dependent areas as a result of the effect of gravity and preceded by weight gain
5. *Syncope*, or transient loss of consciousness, a result of inadequate cerebral blood flow
6. *Fatigue and weakness*, often a consequence of low cardiac output and reduced peripheral perfusion

Factors that precipitate and relieve symptoms must be determined. Angina is usually precipitated by exertion and relieved by rest. Dyspnea is typically associated with exertion; however, changes in body position and the consequent redistribution of body fluid by gravity may pre-

New York Heart Association Patient Classification Guidelines

Class I:	Asymptomatic with ordinary physical exertion
Class II:	Symptomatic with ordinary physical exertion
Class III:	Symptomatic with less than ordinary physical exertion
Class IV:	Symptomatic at rest

Canadian Cardiovascular Society Angina Classification

Class 0	Patient does not experience angina or angina-equivalent symptoms.
Class I	Ordinary physical activity (e.g., walking, climbing stairs) does not cause angina or angina-equivalent symptoms. Symptoms occur only with strenuous, rapid, or prolonged exertion at work or recreation.
Class II	Patient experiences slight limitation of ordinary activity because of angina. For example, symptoms are provoked with the following:

ACTIVITY	SETTING
Walking	Walking/climbing rapidly
Climbing one flight of stairs	After meals
	In cold weather
Walking more than two blocks on level ground	In wind
	Under emotional stress
	During first few hours after awakening
Walking uphill	
Climbing more than one flight of stairs	At a normal pace

Class III	Patient experiences marked limitation of activity because of angina. For example, symptoms are provoked with walking one to two blocks on level ground or climbing one flight of stairs or less in normal conditions and at a normal pace.
Class IV	Patient develops angina at rest or with any physical activity.

cipitate dyspnea. Orthopnea can be relieved by elevation of the trunk with pillows. Additionally, the degree of disability associated with the elicited symptoms must be determined. The New York Heart Association has developed guidelines for the classification of patients according to the level of physical activity required to produce symptoms (Box 30-1). The categories range from class I patients, asymptomatic with ordinary physical exertion, to class IV patients, symptomatic at rest. The *New York Heart Association classification* is most often used to determine the effects of congestive heart failure on physical exertion. The Canadian Cardiovascular Society Angina Classification is most often used to determine the degree of angina (Box 30-2).

Physical Examination

Simple inspection yields a wealth of information regarding the patient's physical and psychologic status. Obser-

vations such as color, body build, respiratory pattern, work of breathing, and general appearance must be incorporated into the clinical picture. Palpation, coupled with inspection, furthers and substantiates the cumulative database. Skin temperature, turgor, and moistness can be evaluated. Severity of edema can be quantified on a scale of 1+ to 4+ according to persistence of the indentation left by the palpating finger in the edematous area (1+ indicates a slight depression that disappears rapidly; 4+ indicates a deep depression that disappears slowly). Depressing the tip of the nail bed until blanching is observed, releasing the pressure, and noting the length of time required for color to return can evaluate capillary refill. Normally, immediate refill is observed. The following structures are systematically examined: arteries, veins, and anterior chest wall.

Arterial Pulse and Pressure

The arterial pulse is palpated to elicit the following information: (1) rate, (2) regularity, (3) amplitude, and (4) quality. Certain cardiac dysrhythmias can be detected by alterations in the *rate* or *regularity* of the arterial pulse. Irregularities of cardiac rhythm are associated with variability in pulse *amplitude*. When the interval between cardiac impulses is irregular, the ventricular filling time and thus the stroke volume vary with each beat. For instance, shortening the interval between beats reduces filling time and stroke volume; consequently, the amplitude of the peripheral arterial pulsation is reduced for that beat. For this reason, irregular rhythms are occasionally associated with a "radial pulse deficit," or a palpated radial rate slower than the auscultated apical rate. This difference simply indicates that the ventricular filling time was short to the extent that the volume of blood ejected into the periphery for some beats was too small to be palpated in the peripheral bed.

The *quality* of the arterial pulses is an important index of peripheral perfusion. A consistently weak, thready pulse may indicate a low stroke volume or increased peripheral vascular resistance. Conversely, a forceful, bounding pulse correlates with high stroke volumes and reduced peripheral resistance. The contour of the arterial pulse can be appreciated best by light palpation of the carotid artery. Palpation of a small pulse with a slow upstroke would characterize aortic stenosis—a lesion that impedes blood flow through the aortic valve. This pulse is described as an *anacrotic pulse* (Fig. 30-1); the slow upstroke is also referred to as *pulsus tardus*. The valvular lesion of aortic regurgitation produces a bounding, rapidly rising and collapsing pulse referred to as a *water-hammer pulse*.

Pulsus alternans and pulsus bigeminus are both characterized by alternating strong and weak pulsations at regular intervals. *Pulsus alternans* occurs at regular intervals and reflects left ventricular failure, whereas *pulsus bigeminus* is produced by alteration in pulse volume caused by a bigeminal (every second beat) pattern of premature beats in the cardiac rhythm (see Fig. 30-1). *Pulsus paradoxus* is an exaggerated fall in systolic pressure greater than 10 mm Hg during inspiration. Normally, systolic pressure falls slightly on inspiration because the reduction in intrathoracic pressure is transmitted to the pulmonary vasculature and produces a slight increase in pulmonary blood volume and a corresponding decrease in venous return to the left side of the heart. Cardiac tamponade or constrictive pericarditis can compromise cardiac filling further and exaggerate this inspiratory fall, producing the paradoxical pulse.

An impression of the consistency of the arterial wall can be obtained best by rolling a peripheral artery under the examining fingers; hardening or thickening of the

walls can be detected. A full cardiovascular examination includes palpation of arterial pulsations for quality and equality at multiple sites: (1) dorsalis pedis, (2) posterior tibialis, (3) popliteal, (4) femoral, (5) radial, (6) brachial, and (7) carotid. Pulses at each site should be compared with the contralateral pulse. The quality of peripheral pulses is graded on a scale of 0 to 4+ (Box 30-3). Auscultation over arterial sites for bruits may be indicated if localized narrowing is suspected.

Auscultation of blood pressure for systolic and diastolic components concludes the arterial examination. Arterial blood pressure is measured by listening for the onset and disappearance of sounds referred to as *Korotkoff sounds* (sometimes spelled Korotkov) in an artery occluded by a blood pressure cuff (Fig. 30-2). The timing of these sounds is correlated with pressure readings on a mercury manometer. Initially, the pressure in the cuff is increased to exceed systolic pressure in the artery such that no flow through the artery occurs and no sound is heard. To assist in the determination of systolic pressure, the brachial pulse should be palpated as the bladder of the cuff is rapidly inflated. The level at which the pulse disappears and subsequently reappears as the cuff is deflated should be noted to provide a preliminary approximation of the blood pressure. This technique will avoid underinflation of the cuff in the case of auscultatory

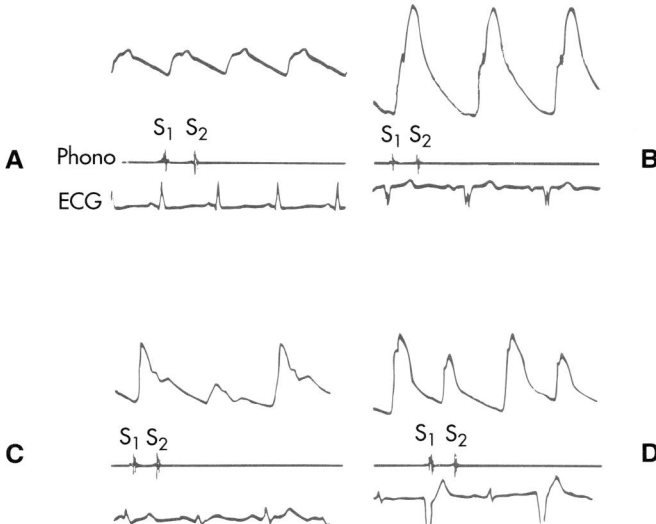

FIG. 30-1 Characteristic arterial pulse wave sphygmograms with simultaneously recorded phonogram and electrocardiogram (ECG). **A**, Anacrotic pulse. **B**, Waterhammer pulse. **C**, Pulsus alternans. **D**, Pulsus bigeminus. S_1, First heart sound; S_2, second heart sound. (From Sana JM, Judge RD: *Physical appraisal for nursing practice,* ed 2, Boston, 1982, Little, Brown.)

BOX 30-3

Grading of Pulses

4+	Normal
3+	Slightly reduced
2+	Greatly reduced
1+	Barely palpable
0	Pulse absent

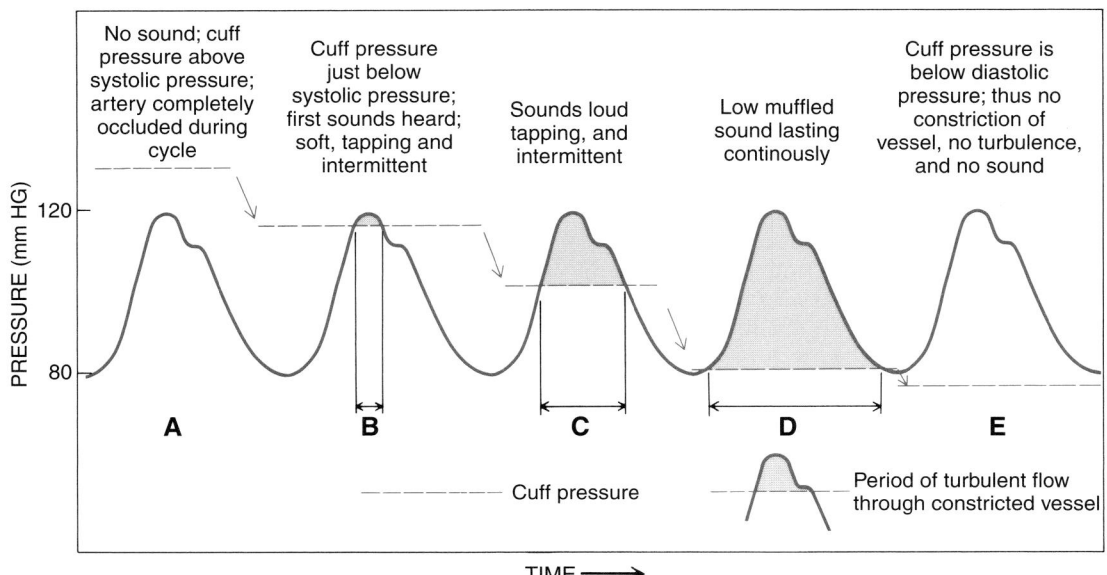

FIG. 30-2 Korotkoff sounds. Systolic blood pressure is recorded at B when the first sounds are heard during a blood pressure measurement. Diastolic pressure is recorded at the point of sound muffling or disappearance, D or E. (From Vander A, Sherman J, Luciano D: *Human physiology: the mechanisms of body function,* ed 8, New York, 2001, McGraw-Hill.)

432

PART SIX CARDIOVASCULAR SYSTEM DISORDERS

gap or overinflation in individuals with low blood pressure. As pressure in the cuff is gradually reduced below systolic pressure, flow begins. However, the flow is turbulent because it occurs through a constricted lumen; turbulent flow produces sound. The onset of turbulent flow is heard as the first Korotkoff sound and correlates with systolic pressure. Further reductions in cuff pressure produce characteristic alterations in the sound as flow increases through the arterial lumen until the sound disappears. Either abrupt muffling or disappearance of sound correlates with diastolic pressure. The American Heart Association (AHA) recommends reporting both diastolic values.

Pressures should be recorded in both arms. If postural hypotension is suspected, measurements should then be compared in the supine, sitting, and standing positions. The normal arterial blood pressure is approximately 120/80 mm Hg. Generally, *hypertension* is designated as a diastolic pressure over 90 mm Hg or a systolic pressure over 140 mm Hg (see Chapter 31). *Hypotension,* for a given individual, is best evaluated in terms of adequacy of peripheral perfusion. In elderly adults or patients with chronic hypertension, hypotension may be manifested as altered brain function resulting from decreased cerebral blood flow (e.g., confusion, dizziness, lethargy). Early signs of inadequate peripheral perfusion may be a decreased urine output and cold, pale skin with reduced peripheral pulses. The kidneys and skin are less metabolically active organs; therefore, as arterial pressure falls, blood is shunted from these organs to the more vital organs, the heart and brain.

The *pulse pressure* is the difference between the systolic and diastolic blood pressure. For example, a blood pressure of 120/80 mm Hg corresponds to a pulse pressure of 40 mm Hg. If arterial pressure falls and sympathetic compensatory vasoconstriction occurs, the pulse pressure is then reduced or narrowed. A fall in pressure to 105/90 mm Hg narrows the pulse pressure to 15 mm Hg. Stroke volume and peripheral resistance influence the pulse pressure most significantly. A narrow pulse pressure indicates a low stroke volume or a high peripheral resistance, or both. A falling blood pressure and narrowing pulse pressure is an ominous sign of left ventricular dysfunction. *Mean arterial pressure (MAP)* is the average peripheral perfusion pressure. This value is not simply the average of the diastolic and systolic pressures because the duration of diastole exceeds the duration of systole at normal heart rates. Consequently, MAP is estimated by doubling the diastolic pressure, adding the systolic pressure, and dividing the total by three.

Venous Pressure and Pulsations

Jugular venous pressure and pulsations reflect the function of the right side of the heart. The internal jugular veins are examined to estimate central venous pressure and to analyze pulsations. To estimate *central venous pressure,* the internal jugular veins are examined with the trunk elevated approximately 15 to 30 degrees. Normally, the highest point of venous pulsation ascends no more than 3 cm above the sternal angle, or angle of Louis (i.e., juncture between manubrium and body of

the sternum). Abnormal elevation of the venous pressure, as in failure of the right side of the heart, can be estimated by measuring the vertical distance between the level of jugular venous pulsation and the sternal angle. With extreme elevations of pressure, usually greater than 25 cm water (H_2O), the jugular veins remain distended to the angle of the jaw with trunk elevations of 90 degrees.

Venous pressure normally fluctuates with respiration; inspiration produces a fall in venous pressure because intrathoracic pressure decreases, favoring venous return to the heart. A paradoxical increase in venous pressure with inspiration, known as *Kussmaul's sign,* indicates an impediment to venous return to the right side of the heart, as in severe right heart failure.

The *hepatojugular reflux test* is an important diagnostic clue to the pressure of right heart failure. Manually sustained pressure is applied for approximately 30 to 60 seconds over the right upper quadrant of the abdomen; the neck veins are observed simultaneously. The abdominal pressure increases venous return to the heart. The normal heart is able to adapt and immediately accept the increased venous return. However, the failing right side of the heart is unable to readily accept this increased load; therefore the distention of the jugular veins increases and the level of venous pulsations rises in the neck. This response of the jugular veins is referred to as a *positive* hepatojugular reflux test.

The anatomic basis for the hepatojugular reflux test may be understood by recalling that the liver functions as a "flood chamber" in its strategic location between the intestinal and general circulation. The liver sinusoids hold a large amount of blood, which is forced into the inferior vena cava through the hepatic veins when pressure is applied over the liver during the reflux test (see Fig. 27-2 and Table 27-1).

The pulsations of the jugular veins are also analyzed to evaluate function of the right side of the heart. At normal venous pressures, maximal venous pulsation can best be observed with trunk elevation of approximately 15 to 30 degrees. The venous waves are gentle and undulating, with three positive components: the *a, c,* and *v* waves (Fig. 30-3, *A*). The *a* wave is produced by atrial contraction; the *c* wave correlates with the onset of ventricular contraction and appears to result from the bulging of the tricuspid valve into the right atrium; and the *v* wave corresponds to the period of atrial filling during ventricular ejection before the tricuspid valve opens. The *c* wave is difficult to distinguish in the jugular veins because of its low amplitude.

Predictable alterations in waveform configuration result from tricuspid valve disease. Tricuspid stenosis impedes the blood flow from the right atrium into the right ventricle, forcing the right atrium to generate more pressure during contraction and creating "giant *a* waves" (see Fig. 30-3, *B*). Tricuspid valvular regurgitation during ventricular systole produces a retrograde flow wave distorting the *c* and *v* waves, referred to as a "significant *v* wave" (see Fig. 30-3, *C*). Certain cardiac dysrhythmias also alter the configuration of the venous waves by disrupting the sequential, synchronized contraction of the atria and ventricles.

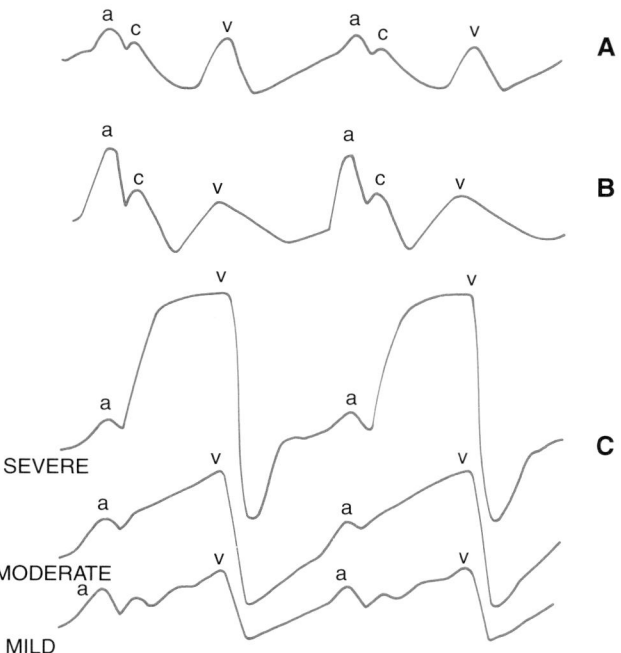

FIG. 30-3   Jugular venous waveforms. **A**, Normal waves, low amplitude and undulating. The *a* wave is produced by atrial contraction; the *c* wave is produced by ventricular contraction and the consequent bulging of the tricuspid valve into the right atrium; and the *v* wave is produced during atrial filling before the opening of the tricuspid valve. **B**, Giant *a* waves seen in tricuspid stenosis. **C**, Mild, moderate, and severe tricuspid regurgitation; the *c* and *v* waves summate into huge *v* waves.

Precordial Movements

Physical examination of the anterior chest involves inspection and palpation of the precordium. Because of the anatomic rotation of the heart in the thorax, the right ventricle lies immediately beneath the sternum (see Fig. 28-3). The thoracic movements are inspected for symmetry and visible pulsations. The chest is then palpated for normal and abnormal pulsations. The apical impulse is produced by the thrust of the left ventricular apex against the chest wall during systole. Normally, this *point of maximal impulse (PMI)* can be palpated as a rhythmic, brief tap approximately 1 cm in diameter, located in the fifth intercostal space at the midclavicular line.

With left ventricular hypertrophy compared with normal heart function, the apical impulse becomes more sustained, more forceful, and larger. The PMI is displaced laterally to the left and downward. Right ventricular hypertrophy characteristically produces a *substernal heave,* or a systolic lift of the sternum, as the contractile force of the anterior right ventricle increases. Abnormal pulsations are also noted with coronary atherosclerotic disease; damaged myocardial fibers with limited or absent contractile force bulge passively outward during systole, creating paradoxical precordial movements. Additionally, the turbulent flow associated with heart murmurs can create palpable precordial vibrations known as "thrills."

Heart Sounds

Auscultation of the chest permits identification of normal heart sounds, abnormal heart sounds, murmurs, and extracardiac sounds. Normal heart sounds result from vibrations of the blood volume and the surrounding chambers with valve closure. The first and second heart sounds are in correlation with the closure of the atrioventricular (AV) valves and the semilunar valves, respectively. Thus the *first heart sound* (S_1) is heard at the onset of ventricular systole as ventricular pressures rise above atrial pressures and close the mitral and tricuspid valves. An abnormal accentuation of S_1 is noted in mitral stenosis as a result of the stiffening of the valve leaflets.

The *second heart sound* (S_2) is audible at the beginning of ventricular relaxation as ventricular pressure falls below the pressure within the pulmonary artery and aorta, closing the pulmonic and aortic valves. Typically, right ventricular ejection lasts slightly longer than does left ventricular ejection, resulting in asynchronous valve closure. Therefore the aortic valve closes before the pulmonic valve, producing a normal physiologic splitting or separation of the valve closure sounds. Inspiration accentuates physiologic splitting because venous return to the right side of the heart increases, thus producing an increment in the volume of right ventricular ejection. During expiration, splitting becomes less pronounced or disappears.

Abnormal *paradoxical splitting* signifies closure of the pulmonic valve before closure of the aortic valve. A paradoxical response to respiration is noted; that is, splitting is most pronounced with expiration and subsides with inspiration. Paradoxical splitting is observed during delayed activation of the left ventricle, as in left bundle branch block, or with prolonged left ventricular ejection, as in aortic stenosis.

Two additional heart sounds can be heard occasionally during ventricular diastole. The *third* and *fourth heart sounds* (S_3, S_4) can be physiologic manifestations but are usually heard in conjunction with heart disease; the pathologic appearance of S_3 or S_4 is referred to as a *gallop rhythm.* This term is applicable because the addition of another heart sound simulates the rhythm of a horse's gallop. S_3 occurs during the period of rapid ventricular filling and is consequently referred to as a *ventricular gallop* when it is abnormal. Although the sound can occur normally in children and young adults, it is usually a pathologic finding produced by cardiac dysfunction, particularly ventricular failure.

S_4 occurs during atrial systole and is referred to as an *atrial gallop.* Normally the sound is faint or inaudible, occurring immediately before S_1. The atrial gallop is audible when ventricular resistance to atrial filling increases as a result of either reduced ventricular wall distensibility or increased ventricular volumes.

Heart murmurs are the result of turbulent flow within the cardiac chambers and vessels. Turbulent flow is produced either by flow through structural abnormalities (narrowed valvular orifices, incompetent valves, dilated arterial segments) or by high-velocity flow through normal structures. Murmurs are described according to (1) timing relative to cardiac cycle, (2) intensity, (3) location or region of maximal audibility, and (4) characteristics.

Diastolic murmurs occur after S_2 during ventricular relaxation. The murmurs of mitral stenosis and aortic regurgitation occur during diastole. *Systolic murmurs* are designated as either ejection murmurs, occurring during midsystole after the early phase of isovolumetric contraction, or regurgitant murmurs, occurring throughout systole. Murmurs that occur throughout systole are referred to as *pansystolic* or *holosystolic*. The murmur of aortic stenosis typifies an ejection murmur, whereas mitral regurgitation produces a pansystolic murmur.

The loudness of a murmur is graded on a scale of I to VI, with grade I representing a faint murmur and grade VI representing a murmur audible with the stethoscope off the chest wall. Five standard areas of the chest wall, illustrated in Fig. 30-4 as aortic, tricuspid, pulmonic, and mitral (or apical) regions and Erb's point, are typically used to localize the region of maximal murmur audibility. The murmur is loudest in regions that lie in the direction of blood flow through the valves rather than in anatomically correct valvular locations. Specification of unique sound characteristics, such as pitch, quality, duration, or radiation, is also included in the description of a heart murmur.

Finally, identification and description of *extracardiac sounds* are essential. Normally, the opening of the heart valves is silent; however, the stiff, thickened valve cusps in mitral stenosis produce an audible "opening snap" in early diastole. A pericardial "friction rub," caused by pericardial inflammation, is audible as a rough sandpaper sound.

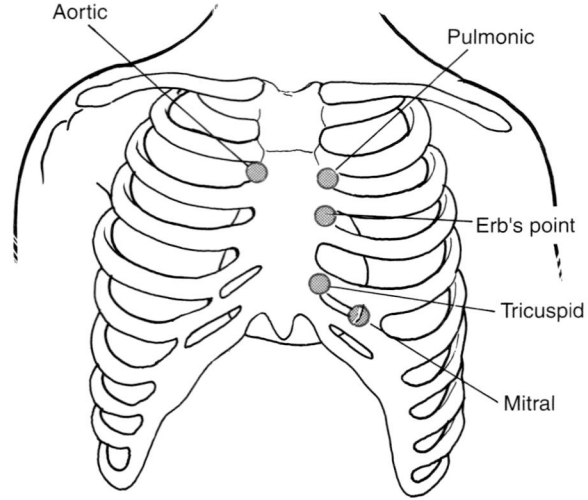

FIG. 30-4 Positions for auscultation of heart sounds: (1) aortic area (second right interspace close to sternum); (2) pulmonic area (second left interspace close to sternum); (3) third left interspace close to sternum, sometimes called Erb's point, where murmurs of both aortic and pulmonic origin may be heard; (4) tricuspid area (fifth left intercostal space close to sternum); and (5) mitral (apical) area (fifth left intercostal space just medial to the midclavicular line).

NONINVASIVE DIAGNOSTIC PROCEDURES

Surface Electrocardiogram

The electrocardiogram (ECG) is the graphic recording of the heart's electrical activity. Characteristic waveforms on the ECG, arbitrarily designated as P wave, QRS complex, and T wave, correlate with the spread of electrical excitation and recovery through the conduction system and myocardium (Fig. 30-5, *A*). These waves are recorded on graph paper with a horizontal time scale and a vertical

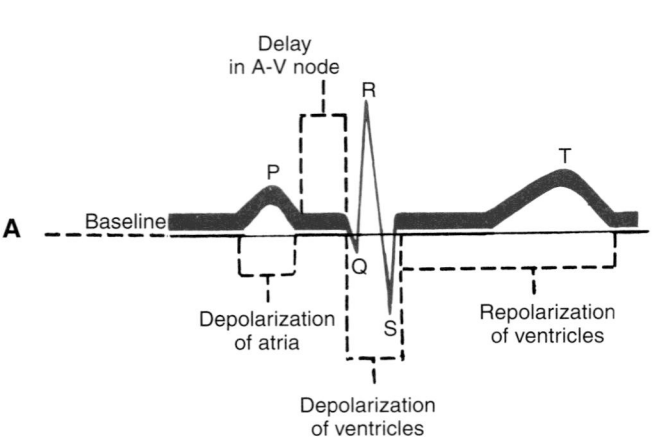

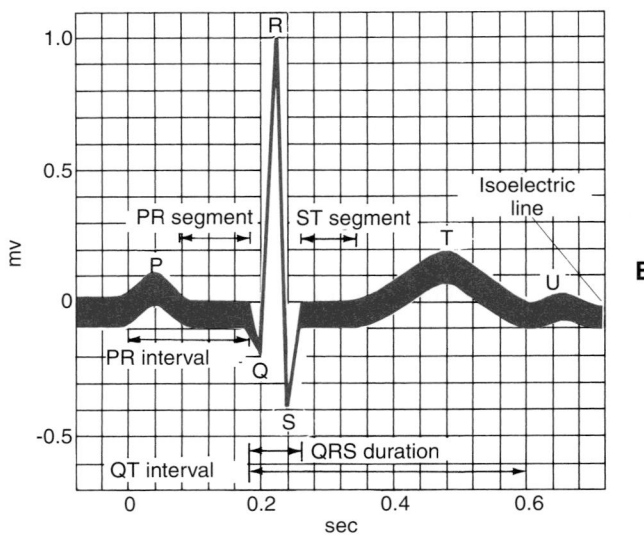

FIG. 30-5 **A,** Correlation between waves of the electrocardiogram (ECG) and impulses that spread through the heart. **B,** Normal recording of ECG on graph paper. Amplitude (in millivolts) is represented on the vertical axis while the horizontal axis represents time (in seconds). Each small square represents 0.04 second, with five small squares equaling 0.2 second. Normal intervals are PR, 0.12 to 0.20 second; QRS, 0.06 to 0.10 second; and QT, 0.36 to 0.44 second. The ventricular rate may be calculated by counting the number of R waves in 6 seconds and multiplying by 10 or counting the number of small squares between two complexes (R to R) and dividing this number into 1500.

voltage scale (see Fig. 30-5, *B*). The significance of the waveforms and intervals on the ECG is as follows:

1. *P wave.* The P wave corresponds to atrial depolarization. The normal stimulus for atrial depolarization originates in the sinus node; however, the magnitude of electrical current associated with excitation of the sinus node is too small to be visualized on the ECG. The P wave is normally gently rounded and upright in most leads. Atrial enlargement may increase the amplitude or width of the P wave and alter its configuration. Cardiac dysrhythmias can also change the P wave configuration. For instance, rhythms originating near the AV junction may cause inversion of the P wave because the direction of atrial depolarization is reversed.

2. *PR interval.* The PR interval is measured from the beginning of the P wave to the onset of the QRS complex. This interval includes impulse transmission time through the atria and the delay of the impulse at the AV node. The normal interval is 0.12 to 0.20 second. Abnormal prolongation of the PR interval is indicative of an impulse conduction disturbance, referred to as *first-degree heart block.*

3. *QRS complex.* The QRS complex represents ventricular depolarization. The amplitude of this wave is great as a result of the large muscle mass traversed by the electric impulse. However, impulse spread is rapid; normally the duration of the QRS complex is 0.06 to 0.10 second. Prolongation of impulse spread through the bundle branches, known as *bundle branch block,* widens the ventricular complex. Abnormal cardiac rhythms that originate in the ventricles, such as ventricular tachycardia, also widen and distort the QRS complex because the specialized pathways that speed impulse spread through the ventricles are bypassed. Ventricular hypertrophy increases the amplitude of the QRS complex as the muscle mass enlarges. Atrial repolarization occurs during the period of ventricular depolarization. However, the magnitude of the QRS complex obscures any ECG evidence of atrial recovery.

4. *ST segment.* This interval is interposed between the wave of ventricular depolarization and repolarization. The initial phases of ventricular repolarization occur during this period; however, the changes are too subtle to be apparent on the ECG. Abnormal depression or elevation of the ST segment is associated with myocardial ischemia and infarction, respectively. Digitalis administration characteristically produces sagging of the segment.

5. *T wave.* Ventricular repolarization generates the T wave. Normally, the T wave is slightly asymmetric, rounded, and upright in most leads. Inversion of the T wave is associated with myocardial ischemia. Hyperkalemia, or serum potassium elevation, causes peaking and elevation of the T wave.

6. *QT interval.* This interval is measured from the beginning of the QRS complex to the end of the T wave, encompassing ventricular depolarization and repolarization. The average QT interval ranges from 0.36 to 0.44 second and varies with heart rate. The QT interval is prolonged with the administration of certain antidysrhythmic drugs, such as quinidine, procainamide, sotalol (Betapace), and amiodarone (Cordarone).

The electrical currents generated within the heart during depolarization and repolarization are conducted to the body surface, where electrodes in contact with the skin can record them. By convention, nine recording electrodes are placed on the extremities and chest wall with a ground electrode, used to reduce electrical interference, attached to the right leg. Varying combinations of these electrodes produce 12 standard leads. Each of the 12 leads records the electrical events of the entire cardiac cycle. However, each lead views the heart from a slightly different perspective; therefore waveforms look slightly different in each lead. Three categories of leads are typically designated (Fig. 30-6) as follows:

1. *Standard limb leads (leads I, II, III).* These leads measure the difference in electrical potential between two points; thus the leads are bipolar, with one negative and one positive pole. Electrodes are placed on the right arm, left arm, and left leg. Lead I views the heart from the axis connecting the right arm and left arm, with the left arm as the positive pole; lead II, from the right arm and left leg, with the left leg positive; and lead III, from the left arm and left leg, with the left leg positive (see Fig. 30-6, *A*).

2. *Augmented limb leads (aVR, aVL, aVF).* These leads are electrically adjusted to measure the absolute electrical potential at one recording site (i.e., electrical potential of a positive electrode placed on the extremities) creating, in essence, a unipolar lead. This event is accomplished by electrically canceling out the effect of the negative pole and establishing an "indifferent" electrode at zero potential. Adjustments are made automatically within the ECG machine to join the other limb electrodes, creating a common indifferent electrode with essentially no effect on the positive record-

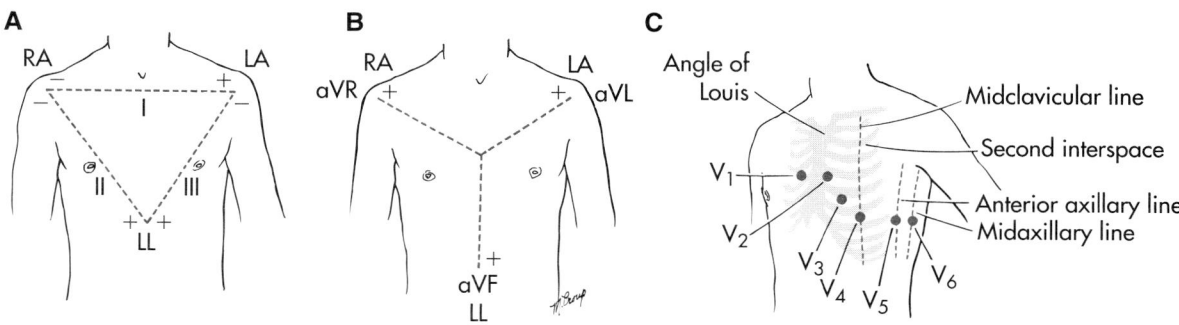

FIG. 30-6   Electrode positions for the standard 12-lead electrocardiogram. **A,** Standard limb leads (I, II, III). **B,** Augmented limb leads (aVR, aVL, aVF). **C,** Precordial leads (V₁ to V₆).

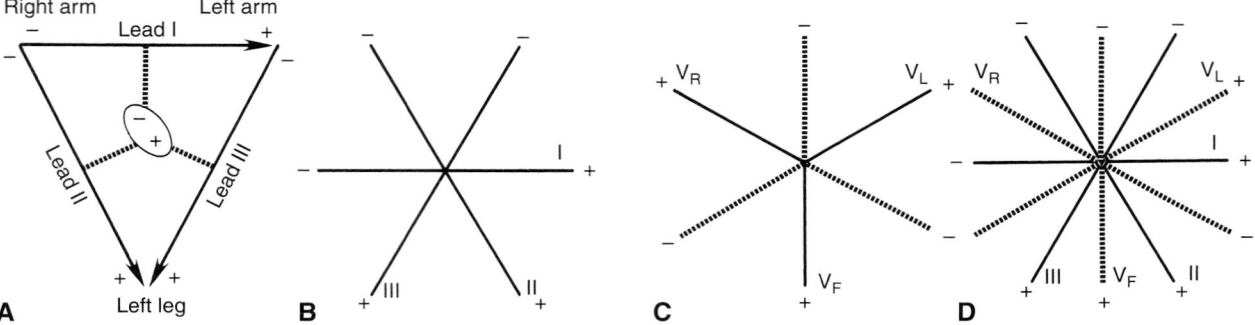

FIG. 30-7 Derivation of the hexaxial reference system. **A**, Einthoven's triangle, showing the axes of the standard limb leads with the heart at the center of the triangle. **B**, The axes of the limb leads are moved to the center of the triangle, forming a triaxial reference system. **C**, The axes of the augmented (unipolar) limb leads. **D**, The axes of the standard and unipolar limb leads are superimposed, forming a hexaxial reference system.

ing electrode. The voltage recorded from the positive electrode is then amplified, or "augmented," to produce a selected, unipolar limb lead tracing. The three augmented limb leads include the following: aVR, recording from the right arm; aVL, from the left arm; and aVF, from the left leg (the aVF location can be easily remembered by associating the "F" with "foot") (see Fig. 30-6, *B*).

3. *Precordial or chest leads (leads V_1 to V_6).* These leads are unipolar leads that record the absolute electrical potential of sites on the anterior chest wall, or precordium. Identification of the following landmarks facilitates accurate placement of the precordial electrodes: (1) angle of Louis, the sternal protuberance at the juncture between the manubrium and body of the sternum; (2) the second intercostal space, adjacent to the angle of Louis; (3) the left midclavicular line; and (4) the anterior and midaxillary lines (see Fig. 30-6, *C*). Electrodes are placed sequentially on the chest wall at six different sites, as follows:

V_1: located in the fourth intercostal space to the right of the sternum
V_2: located in the fourth intercostal space to the left of the sternum
V_3: located midway between V_2 and V_4
V_4: located in the fifth intercostal space in the midclavicular line
V_5: horizontal to V_4 in the anterior axillary line
V_6: horizontal to V_5 in the midaxillary line

The standard limb leads and augmented limb leads view the heart in the frontal plane. The relative perspective of each lead is conceptualized most easily using a schematic diagram, known as the *hexaxial reference system.* This reference system is derived in the following manner (Fig. 30-7):

1. Connecting the lead axes of leads I, II, and III forms an equilateral triangle, referred to as *Einthoven's triangle.* The heart is considered the electrical center of the triangle.
2. Positioning the lead axes such that each radiates from the center of the triangle creates a second diagram, known as the *triaxial reference system.*
3. Combining the triaxial reference system diagram with the schematic representation of the augmented limb

leads radiating from the electrical center of the thorax produces the hexaxial reference system.

The hexaxial reference system is an invaluable aid to ECG interpretation, permitting calculation of the average direction of electrical activity within the heart. The average direction of electrical activation calculated from the ECG is referred to as the *electrical axis* of the heart.

Other modified leads are often used in special situations. A modified lead V_1 (MCL$_1$) is frequently used for bedside monitoring to facilitate dysrhythmia detection and analysis. This lead is a bipolar lead, with the positive electrode positioned in the standard V_1 position (fourth intercostal space to the right of the sternum) and the negative electrode positioned near the left shoulder beneath the clavicle.

The waveform configurations apparent in each lead depend on the orientation of the particular lead relative to the path of cardiac electrical activity. The leads of the hexaxial reference system view the heart in the frontal plane; the six precordial leads offer another perspective from the horizontal plane. Waves will be positive (i.e., deflected upward) when the electrical activity of the heart approaches the positive electrode of a given lead. For example, in Fig. 30-8, the P wave and QRS complex of lead II are positive because the wave of depolarization approaches the positive left leg electrode of lead II. Conversely, the same waves in lead aVR are negative because the path of electrical activity is moving away from the positive right arm electrode. Additionally, the amplitude of waves varies among leads. As a rule, wave amplitude will be greatest in a lead lying parallel to the path of depolarization. Lead II in Fig. 30-8 demonstrates the greatest wave amplitude, indicating that lead II most closely parallels the path of depolarization in this ECG. The ECG permits detection of abnormalities in cardiac rate and rhythm, chamber enlargement, myocardial ischemia or infarction, drug and electrolyte effects, and shifts in the direction of electrical activation.

Conventional bedside monitoring techniques have been extended to ambulatory monitoring *(telemetry)* and continuous 24-hour ECG recording *(Holter monitoring)* and event monitoring. Patients can wear an *event monitor* at home and can record a 30- to 60-second ECG strip when activated by the patient. The event monitor is useful

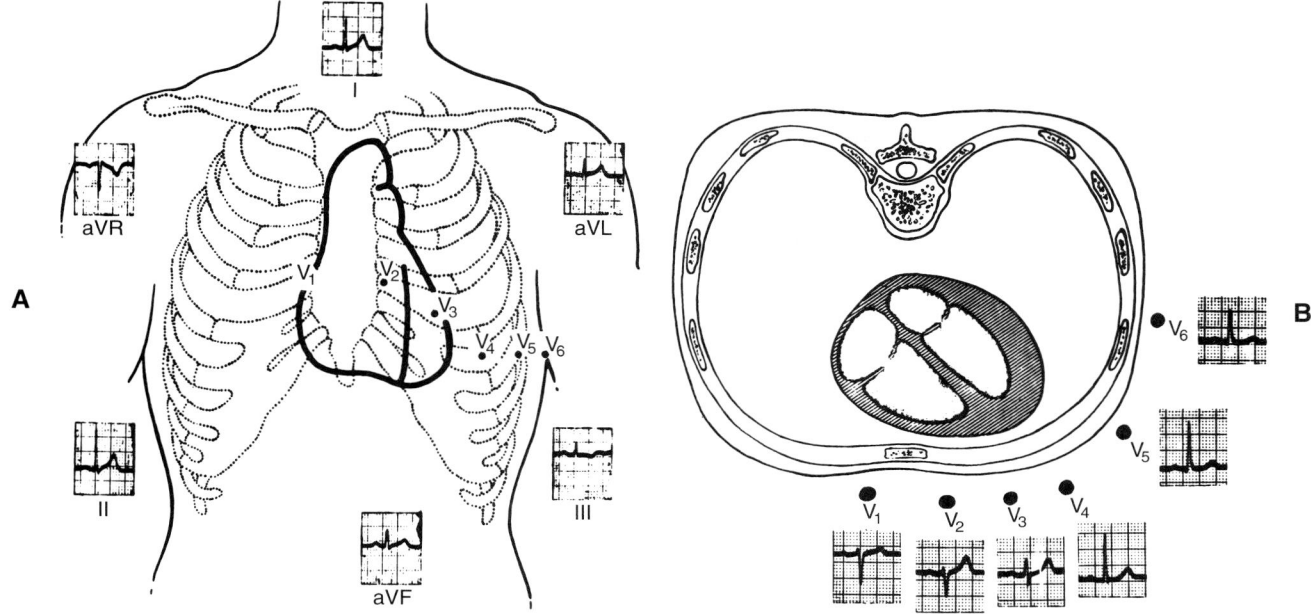

FIG. 30-8   **A**, Normal ECG patterns in the frontal plane (standard leads I, II, and III and augmented unipolar leads aVR, aVL, and aVF). **B**, Normal ECGpatterns in the horizontal plane (precordial leads V₁ to V₆). (From Goldman MJ: *Principles of clinical electrocardiography,* ed 9, Los Altos, Calif, 1976, Lange.)

when monitoring the effects of antidysrhythmic medication or correlating ECG findings with patient symptoms when symptoms are infrequent (Sheffield et al, 1995).

Relative Merits of Imaging Techniques

Multiple noninvasive and invasive imaging techniques are available for diagnosing cardiovascular disease. Each type of study allows varying amounts of information to be obtained for each type of pathologic condition. Additionally, angiography also carries risks to the patient associated with the procedure that the noninvasive studies do not. Table 30-1 presents the strengths and weaknesses of each type of study in diagnosing various types of cardiovascular disease. The amount of information obtained versus the risks involved in the test ultimately determines which test is used. The diagnostic tools are discussed next.

Echocardiography

Echocardiographic procedures use ultrasound as the examination medium. A transducer that emits ultrasonic waves, or high-frequency sound waves beyond the audible range, is applied to the chest wall and directed at the heart (Fig. 30-9). As the ultrasonic beam traverses the heart, ultrasonic waves are reflected back to the transducer whenever the beam crosses a boundary between tissues of different densities or acoustic impedances. The mechanical energy from these reflected sound waves, or cardiac "echoes," is converted to electrical energy by the transducer and displayed in the form of a cardiac image on an oscilloscope or strip chart recorder.

Echocardiography provides significant information about the structure and movement of the heart cham-

TABLE 30-1   ■ ■ ■

Relative Merits of Imaging Techniques

Disorder	CXR	Echo/ Doppler	Angio	Radionuclides	MRI
Ischemic	1	2	4*	3	2
Valvular	2	4*	4*	2	3
Congenital	2	4*	4*	2	3
Traumatic	2	2	3*	2	2
Cardiomyopathy	1	4*	3	2	3
Pericardial	1	3	2	0	4*
Endocarditis	1	4*	2	0	3
Masses	0	4*	3	0	3

From Skorton DJ et al: Relative merits of imaging techniques. In Baunwald E: *Heart disease,* ed 4, Philadelphia, 1992, Saunders.
CXR, Chest x-ray film; *echo,* echocardiography; *angio,* angiography; *MRI,* magnetic resonance imaging.
Range of information provided by test: 0, no information, to 4(*), best test.

bers, valves, and any unusual masses. The test has overcome the previous limitations with the addition of two-dimensional echocardiography, Doppler flow imaging, and the transesophageal approach to the heart. The transesophageal approach virtually eliminates the positioning problems associated with obesity, chest trauma, chronic lung disease, and mechanical or calcified valves. The *M mode* is the most common of the display modes. In the M mode, the echoes are displayed as undulating lines composed of dots of varying intensity (see Fig. 30-9). The movement of the lines corresponds to the motion of each structure. The lines are arranged sequentially in layers on the screen. These layers correspond to the anatomic structures traversed by the ultrasonic beam.

FIG. 30-9 Normal echocardiogram. Path of ultrasound beam *(USB)* is shown schematically on the left. On the right is a diagram of the corresponding echocardiogram for this direction of the transducer. *RV,* Right ventricle; *Se,* septum; *LV,* left ventricle; *ALMV,* anterior leaflet of the mitral valve; *PLMV,* posterior leaflet of the mitral valve; *S,* systole; *D,* diastole; *E,* peak of rapid anterior opening of mitral valve during beginning of diastole; *A,* peak of anterior movement of leaflet into the ventricle produced by atrial systole; *F,* position of leaflet during rapid ventricular filling. (From Gazes PC: *Clinical cardiology,* Chicago, 1975, Mosby.)

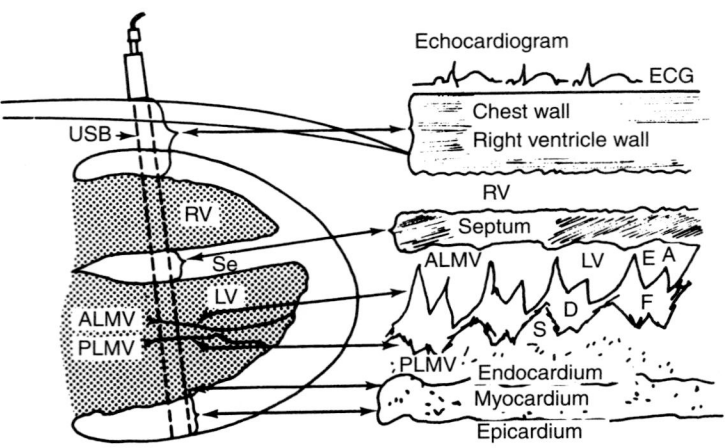

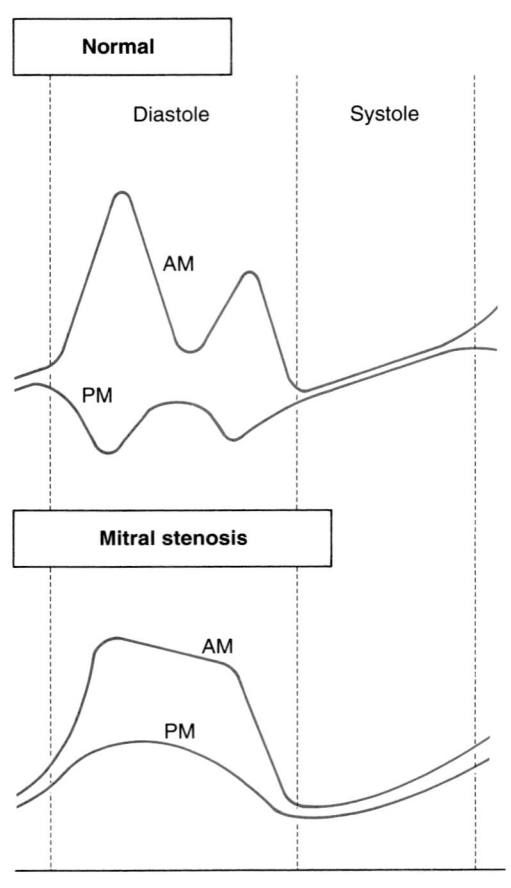

FIG. 30-10 Mitral valve echocardiogram. *Above,* Normal leaflet motion. *Below,* Abnormal leaflet motion with mitral stenosis. *AM,* Anterior mitral valve leaflet; *PM,* posterior mitral valve leaflet. (Modified from Duchak JM, Chang S, Feigenbaum H: The posterior mitral valve echo and echocardiographic diagnosis of mitral stenosis, *Am J Cardiol* 29:631, 1972.)

M-Mode Echocardiography

M-mode echocardiography provides an "icepick" view of the dimensions and motion of the tissues in the path of the ultrasonic beam. The ECG is typically displayed with the echocardiogram on a horizontal time axis, permitting correlation of the electrical and mechanical events of the cardiac cycle. Moving the transducer in several directions can scan the precordium. Fig. 30-9 illustrates one standard M-mode view.

M-mode echocardiography is of particular value for evaluation of chamber volumes and regional abnormalities, such as the abnormal mitral valve leaflet motion characteristic of mitral stenosis. Fig. 30-10 illustrates the normal motion of the anterior and posterior mitral valve cusps relative to the restricted motion of stenotic, diseased mitral leaflets. However, the one-dimensional scanning path limits the application of the M-mode technique in the evaluation of global cardiac function.

Two-Dimensional Echocardiography

Two-dimensional (2-D) echocardiography captures an image of a pie-shaped wedge of the heart (Fig. 30-11). During this procedure, the ultrasonic transducer on the chest rapidly sweeps along a predetermined examination plane. As the beam scans multiple sites (approximately 30 per second), images from the reflected echoes at each site are stored. After the scan is completed, the composite echoes are displayed on a video screen and valve movement, ventricular contraction, and any abnormalities (e.g., thrombus) may be observed in real time. The resultant image is a full transverse section of the heart. A complete 2-D echocardiogram includes images obtained in multiple planes. This 2-D ultrasonic imaging technique can be coupled with Doppler blood flow studies to obtain information about the velocity and direction of blood flow within the cardiovascular system.

Doppler Echocardiography

The technique for Doppler studies is similar to that for echocardiographic studies. Ultrasonic waves of known frequency are directed at the heart through the chest wall. As the beam strikes the tissue interfaces, reflected waves echo back to the transducer. In addition to analyzing the amplitude of the echo as with conventional echocardiography, the frequency of the reflected signal is evaluated and compared with that of the emitted signal. The frequency of the reflected wave is different from that of the emitted wave when the targeted structure is moving. This change in wave frequency is known as a *Doppler shift.* The direction of the shift (i.e., increased or decreased wave frequency) depends on the direction that the target is moving relative to the transducer.

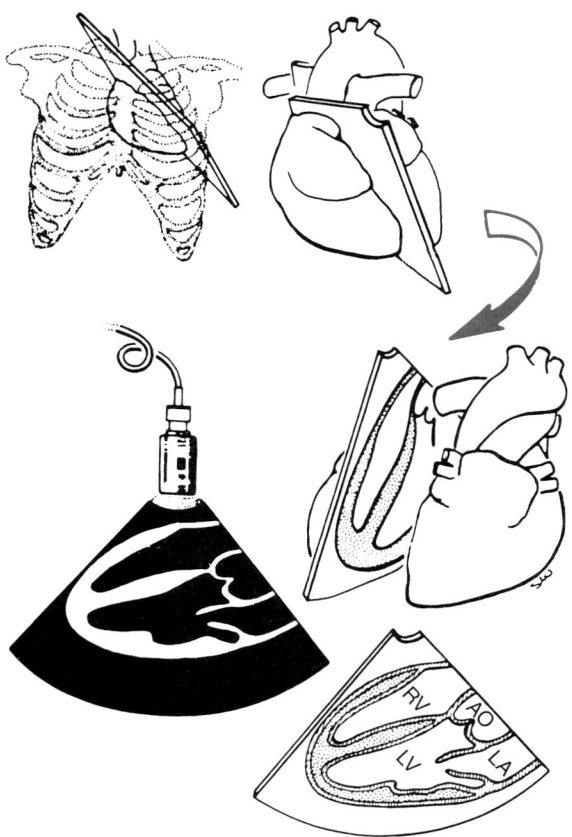

FIG. 30-11   Two-dimensional (2-D) echocardiogram. In contrast to the M-mode, one-dimensional "ice pick" view, 2-D echocardiography simultaneously detects all cardiac structures lying within the plane of examination, displaying the image on a video screen. *AO,* Aorta; *LV,* left ventricle; *RV,* right ventricle; *LA,* left atrium. (From Ream AK, Pogdall RP, editors: *Acute cardiovascular management: anesthesia and intensive care,* Philadelphia, 1982, Lippincott.)

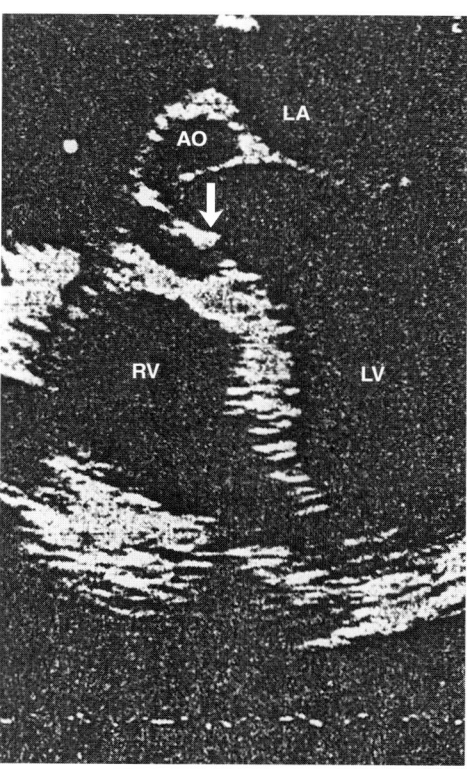

FIG. 30-12   Transesophageal echocardiogram of a patient with a small vegetation *(arrow)* on the aortic valve. *AO,* Aorta; *LA,* left atrium; *RV,* right ventricle, *LV,* left ventricle. (From Braunwald E, Zipes DP, Libby P: *Heart disease: a textbook of cardiovascular medicine,* ed 6, Philadelphia, 2001, Saunders.)

Red blood cells (RBCs) are the primary ultrasound targets for *Doppler blood velocity studies.* The movement of RBCs can be distinguished from the motion of cardiac structures because the signals reflected by blood and tissue differ in frequency and amplitude. The signals reflected by the tissues can be filtered out so that blood flow can be analyzed selectively. Consequently, the velocity and direction of flow can be determined from the Doppler shift. Doppler measures are of particular interest in the evaluation of valvular regurgitation and intracardiac shunts.

The reflected ultrasound generates an audible signal, which varies with changes in the frequency of the reflected signal. The amplitude and frequencies of the signal can also be displayed on a strip chart recording, monitor, or video screen. The video display can be color-coded to distinguish the direction or magnitude of flow.

Doppler flow imaging is the superimposition of Doppler information on a 2-D echocardiographic image. Doppler and 2-D echo information is obtained simultaneously from multiple sites in the plane of examination by rapid computerized scanning. The data are stored, and the Doppler information is superimposed on the pie-shaped 2-D image at the completion of the scan. The addition of color to this technique creates *color flow mapping.*

Transesophageal Echocardiography

In some instances, high-quality echocardiographic images cannot be obtained when the ultrasound transducer is applied to the chest wall. This exclusion most frequently occurs when a patient is obese or has chronic obstructive pulmonary disease, because the ultrasound waves are unable to penetrate the heart. Other circumstances that may limit transthoracic echocardiography include limited access because of chest trauma, inability of patients to lie on their left side, and during interventional cardiac procedures or cardiac surgery. Transesophageal echocardiography (TEE) may be performed by placing the ultrasound transducer into the esophagus in a procedure similar to an endoscopy. TEE has extended the utility of echocardiography by providing high quality studies with increased resolution. Additional structures that can be assessed include the vena cava, coronary sinus, pulmonary veins, pulmonary artery, atrial septum, atrial appendages, and the ascending and descending aorta. TEE is also the method of choice to assess the function of prosthetic mitral valves and to visualize vegetation or abscess (Fig. 30-12).

Computed Tomography

Tomo- is a Greek word element meaning "section or cutting." Consequently, a *tomograph* is an image of a cross-sectional slice of the body. A 2-D echocardiogram is an example of a tomograph. Computed tomography (CT) has extended cardiac imaging from 2-D to three-dimensional (3-D) imaging. To construct this 3-D image, a camera rotates in a 360-degree arc around the chest, recording 2-D images at multiple angles. X-rays are transmitted through the body to detectors on the opposite side. Each x-ray image captures a thin anatomic slice of the body. From these x-ray images, a computer constructs a composite 3-D image. A small amount of contrast material, usually containing iodine, is injected via a peripheral site to increase the contrast between the cardiac structures and the blood.

Computed Emission Tomography

CT can be used with radionuclide imaging (see following discussion) to construct 3-D images. This application of tomography is referred to as computed *emission* tomography (CET), rather than the computed (transmission) tomography described previously. The CET image is based on detection of radiation emitted from decaying radionuclides rather than detection of x-rays transmitted through the body.

Two forms of CET are used: *single-photon emission computed tomography (SPECT)* and *positron emission tomography (PET)*. SPECT is simply CT in combination with thallium or technetium imaging. Both of these radionuclides are *single-photon emission* radionuclides, meaning that a single packet of energy, or photon, is emitted for each atomic decay. *Positrons*, or positively charged electrons, can also be emitted and detected as atoms decay. However, radionuclides that emit positrons must be produced on site in a cyclotron. Consequently, PET of the heart is cost-prohibitive for most centers, particularly given the quality of information available with other noninvasive techniques.

Radionuclide Imaging

Basic Principles

The *nucleus* of an atom is composed of positively charged *protons* and electrically neutral *neutrons*. Negatively charged *electrons* orbit the nucleus. *Radionuclides* are nuclei that are inherently unstable and tend to decay to a more stable form, emitting radiation in the process. The energy emitted during the decay of atoms can be detected and counted by gamma cameras.

Radionuclide imaging of the cardiovascular system involves the intravenous injection of small quantities of radioactive isotopes into a peripheral vein. The isotope either binds to blood elements or is selectively taken up by normal myocardium or infarcted myocardium, thereby acting as a radioactive tracer. The isotope's affinity for either blood or myocardium depends on the properties of the radioactive substance selected.

Two radionuclide techniques are currently used:

1. *Myocardial perfusion imaging* with thallium-201 (^{201}Tl) or technetium-99m–(^{99m}Tc)sestaMIBI or ^{99m}Tc-teboroxime to evaluate myocardial perfusion
2. *Infarct-avid imaging* with ^{99m}Tc–indium-111 (^{111}In) leukocytes, or ^{111}In antimyosin, to detect acute myocardial necrosis

The distribution of radioactive tracers can be detected by gamma cameras from the radiation emitted as the radionuclides decay.

Myocardial Perfusion Imaging

The radioactive isotopes mentioned are currently being used to measure myocardial perfusion and detect ischemia. Each of these radioactive isotopes accumulates within the myocardium in proportion to myocardial blood flow. The most appropriate use of these isotopes is in conjunction with stress testing for evaluation of ischemic heart disease. During stress testing, myocardial blood flow is decreased in areas of the heart supplied by stenosed blood vessels. At peak exercise, the radioactive isotope is injected. The tracer is carried to the myocardium by blood, and areas of decreased perfusion will be supplied with less isotope than are areas with adequate blood flow. These areas are detected as "cold spots" on the images. All three isotopes can detect ischemia. However, ischemia can be differentiated from infarction only by using ^{201}Tl. After ^{201}Tl is injected, the isotope equalizes into viable (live) tissue and does not perfuse into necrotic (dead) tissue. Those areas that do not perfuse are reported as "fixed defects" and may indicate areas of prior myocardial infarction. When the defect "reperfuses" after resting, the area is ischemic.

Infarct Imaging

Infarct imaging can be performed using three isotopes: ^{99m}Tc Sn-pyrophosphate, indium-111 antimyosin, and indium-111 leukocytes. Imaging with ^{99m}Tc Sn-pyrophosphate differs from that with thallium because ^{99m}Tc accumulates selectively in acutely damaged myocardium, permitting identification of the site and evaluation of the extent of necrosis. Areas of concentrated uptake appear as "hot spots" on the scan. The patterns of tracer uptake can be observed within 12 to 72 hours after infarction and persist for 10 to 14 days.

Indium-111 antimyosin is a monoclonal antibody specific for intracellular use. The radioactive antibodies attach themselves to cardiac myosin, which becomes exposed as myocardial cellular membrane integrity is destroyed during progressive myocardial ischemia. This methodology offers advantages over other infarct-imaging agents in that these antibodies are thought to be necrosis-specific and therefore allow more accurate quantification of infarct size. Similarly, indium-111 leukocytes are useful in detecting infarct size 2 to 3 days after a myocardial infarction, during which white blood cell migration occurs.

Magnetic Resonance Imaging

Magnetic resonance imaging (MRI), previously referred to as "nuclear magnetic resonance" (NMR), is a tomographic imaging technique that does not require the administration of radionuclides. This technique is based on analysis of the magnetic behavior of nuclei. Certain types of nuclei possess an inherent *spin*. As the charged nucleus spins, a magnetic field is generated around the atom.

During MRI, an external magnet surrounds the body. The interactions between the external magnetic field and the magnetic fields of the nuclei shift from random positions to alignment with or against the external magnetic field. An average direction for the magnetic field of the nuclei, or a *magnetization vector*, can be determined.

Pulses of energy, in the form of *radiofrequency* waves, are then applied. These pulses disturb the magnetization vector. As the pulses are turned off, signals are emitted as the atoms return to resting positions within the external magnet. MRI has been shown to be effective and useful in diagnosing a wide variety of cardiovascular diseases. Gating the images to the ECG (similar to CT scanning) is essential to minimize artifacts that myocardial contraction produces. MRI is useful in determining ventricular mass, global and regional wall motion, and valvular insufficiency. Additionally, MRI is useful in evaluating extracardiac disease (e.g., aortic aneurysm or dissection) and pericardial thickening. Recently, MRI has been used to evaluate native coronary artery stenosis and quantify coronary blood flow. With further software and hardware improvements, MRI may prove to be a comprehensive noninvasive diagnostic tool.

Exercise Testing

Exercise testing with a treadmill or bicycle ergometer permits evaluation of exercise-induced symptoms or ECG changes. Multiple ECG leads are monitored continuously, and blood pressure is measured frequently during the test. Patients are instructed to report any symptoms immediately. The test is terminated if the patient becomes fatigued, develops anginal symptoms, or abnormalities of the ECG or vital signs. The rationale behind stress testing is that by increasing work performed by the patient through exercise (via treadmill, arm ergometer, or through pharmacologic stress), the work of the cardiovascular system is also increased. This increase in work requires an increase in myocardial oxygen consumption, which requires increased coronary blood flow. Narrowed coronary arteries prevent the increase in coronary blood flow and may result in chest pain or ECG changes, or both. The patient is typically asked to exercise to at least 85% of the maximal age-predicted heart rate. This level allows for sufficient stress on the cardiovascular system and enables changes in myocardial perfusion to become evident (Myer, 1999). Combining radionuclide imaging with exercise testing is significantly more accurate for the diagnosis of coronary disease than is exercise testing alone. Comparisons are made between the nuclear image obtained at rest and that obtained during exercise, thus localizing areas of ischemia or preinfarction.

Pharmacologic Stress Tests

If a patient is unable to exercise or if diagnostic images are required during stress testing, adenosine or dipyridamole may then be administered to produce an ischemic response. Adenosine and dipyridamole produce a vasodilatory effect in normal arteries. Myocardial areas perfused by stenotic vessels are hypoperfused because the vessels cannot dilate. Thus ischemia is produced. Pharmacologic studies are most frequently performed with the addition of radioactive isotopes to quantify blood flow to ischemic areas. Both adenosine and dipyridamole are contraindicated in patients with restrictive or bronchospastic lung disease. Aminophyllin is a direct antagonist to these medications and is used to reverse any adverse effects from their administration.

Stress Echocardiography

A *"stress echo"* may be performed to evaluate the effect of ischemia on left ventricular function. During stress test-

ing, echocardiography is performed, and left ventricular wall abnormalities are detected at peak exercise and after resting. The decrease in contractility is related to significant narrowing of the coronary arteries.

Chest Radiography

A series of chest radiographs in four standard positions is useful in the cardiac diagnostic workup (Fig. 30-13): (1) posterior-anterior or frontal position; (2) left lateral position with left side forward; (3) right anterior oblique position with the body rotated approximately 60 degrees to the left, which places the right shoulder anterior; and (4) left anterior oblique position with the left shoulder anterior. In each position, a different anatomic perspective of the heart is visible. The contour of the heart contrasts with the radiolucent air-filled lungs.

The following findings can be detected on the chest radiograph: (1) generalized cardiac enlargement, or cardiomegaly; (2) localized chamber enlargement; (3) calcification in valves or coronary arteries; (4) pulmonary venous congestion; (5) interstitial or alveolar edema; and (6) enlargement of the pulmonary artery or dilation of the ascending aorta.

An impression of generalized cardiac enlargement can be noted in chest radiographs; however, precise estimation of the degree of enlargement is of questionable accuracy. In contrast, chamber enlargement distinctly alters the contour of the heart, permitting specification of the involved chamber. In the posterior-anterior position, the right border of the heart consists of the superior vena cava with the right atrium below. An angle appears at the juncture between the two areas. The structures comprising the left border, from top to bottom, are the aorta, pulmonary artery, and left ventricle. This projection permits identification of right atrial, left ventricular, and pulmonary arterial enlargement. Right atrial enlargement, for example, displaces the right boundary outward to the right, rounding the curvature of the cardiac contour.

In the left lateral position, the anterior border is primarily the right ventricle, with the posterior border consisting of the left atrium superiorly and the posterior wall of the left ventricle inferiorly. The esophagus lies behind the posterior boundary. Right ventricular and left atrial enlargement are best appreciated in this view. Outlining the esophagus with swallowed barium facilitates the diagnosis of left atrial enlargement, which produces an esophageal indentation with posterior displacement.

Radiologic examination of the lungs demonstrates the effects of cardiac dysfunction on the pulmonary vasculature. Left heart failure or mitral valve disease increases pulmonary venous congestion, dilating the pulmonary veins in characteristic patterns. Excessive elevation of venous pressure results in transudation of fluid into the interstitial space and eventually into the alveoli. Fluid seepage from the intravascular space, or pulmonary edema, produces a clouding, or haziness, of the vascular shadows, progressively whitening the normally dark shadows of the radiolucent lungs.

Characteristic findings typify particular cardiac lesions. For example, in mitral stenosis (a lesion that impedes blood flow from the left atrium to the left ventricle), left atrial enlargement and pulmonary venous congestion would be noted. Valvular calcification might also be observed.

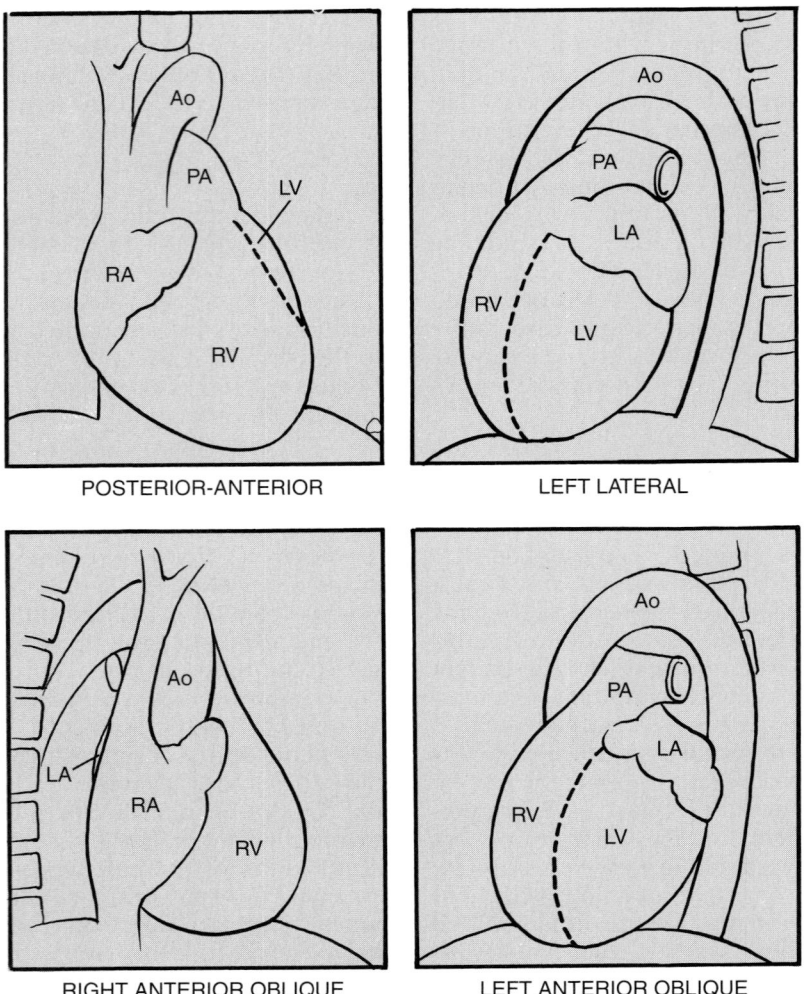

POSTERIOR-ANTERIOR

LEFT LATERAL

RIGHT ANTERIOR OBLIQUE

LEFT ANTERIOR OBLIQUE

FIG. 30-13 Orientation of the heart in four standard positions for cardiac radiography. In the posterior-anterior position the borders of the right atrium *(RA)* and left ventricle are displayed. The right ventricle *(RV)* and left atrium are not visible on the borders of the silhouette. *Ao,* Aorta; *PA,* pulmonary artery. In the left lateral position the silhouette of the RV is seen anteriorly and the left atrium *(LA)* posteriorly. *LV,* Left ventricle. In the right anterior oblique position the RV and the LA are again seen in silhouette. In the left anterior oblique position the RV and LV are seen in silhouette. The LA can be discerned in this projection. (Modified from Rushmer RF: *Cardiovascular dynamics,* ed 3, Philadelphia, 1976, Saunders.)

INVASIVE DIAGNOSTIC PROCEDURES

Electrophysiology Studies

Intracardiac ECG techniques, or *electrophysiology (EP) studies,* permit a more detailed analysis of the mechanisms of cardiac impulse formation and conduction than do standard ECG recordings. As the action potential sweeps through the conduction system and the myocardium, the body surface ECG records the summated signals of atrial and ventricular activation, represented by the P wave and QRS complex, respectively. The amplitude of signals generated by specific sites in the conduction system, such as the sinus node or the bundle of His, is too small to be detected on the body surface. An intracardiac ECG can record deflections from these sites via recording electrodes positioned close to the regions of interest in the conduc-

tion system or myocardium. Fig. 30-14 compares the body surface and intracardiac ECG data.

EP studies are used for the following purposes: (1) to assess sinus node function, (2) to evaluate AV node conduction, (3) to analyze complex atrial and ventricular tachycardias, and (4) to determine the efficacy of pharmacologic or pacemaker therapy for refractory dysrhythmias. (EP testing for refractory ventricular dysrhythmias is discussed in Chapter 31.)

Several catheters, usually two to five, with multiple electrodes are advanced through peripheral veins under fluoroscopic guidance to the desired intracardiac sites. The sites selected depend on the purpose of the study. Fig. 30-15 illustrates a common catheter placement. These electrodes can be used for intracardiac recording or stimulation. Electrical stimulation of the atria or ventri-

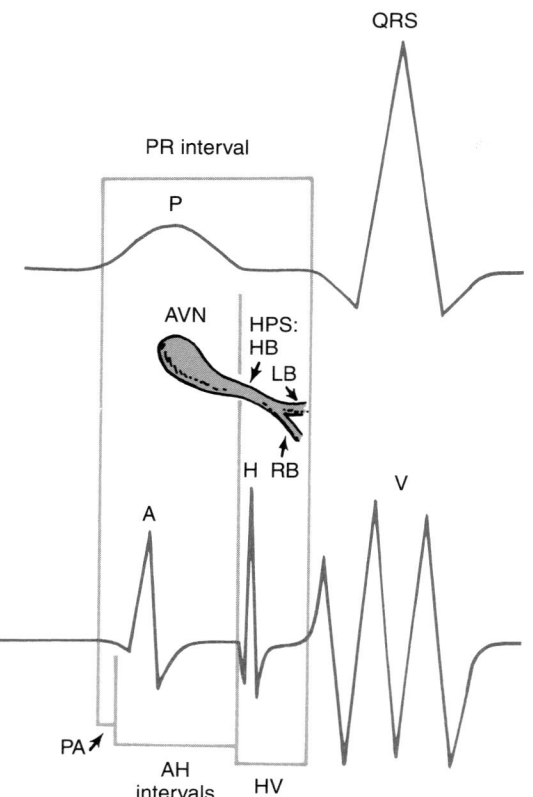

FIG. 30-14   Surface versus intracardiac ECG. Depicted are simultaneously recorded surface *(top)* and intracardiac *(bottom)* ECGs along with the anatomic structures of the atrioventricular (AV) specialized conduction system involved in normal impulse transmission. The surface ECG shows a P wave (atrial muscle depolarization) and a QRS complex (ventricular muscle depolarization). A PR interval can be measured and represents the following conduction times: intraatrial; AV nodal *(AVN)*, His bundle *(HB)*, right bundle *(RB)*, and left bundle *(LB)* branches; and Purkinje fiber. In contrast, the single intracardiac tracing from the AV junction shows three deflections: *A* (low atrial muscle depolarization), *H* (bundle of His activation), and *V* (ventricular muscle depolarization). Three intervals can be measured when the surface and intracardiac ECGs are compared: (1) the PA interval—measure of intraatrial conduction time, as impulse traverses from its exit from the sinus node (near superior vena cava) to the intracardiac recording site low in the right atrium at the AV junction; (2) the AH interval—approximation of AVN conduction time (penetration of the AVN is assumed to occur simultaneously with the arrival of the impulse at the low right atrium, anatomic site of the AVN); and (3) the HV interval—measure of conduction time through the His-Purkinje system (*HPS*, bundle of His, right and left bundles, and Purkinje network) to its exit at the ventricular muscle. From the aforementioned three intervals, conduction delays that exhibit as first-degree AV block (prolonged PR interval) can be differentiated as resulting from delay in the atria, AVN, or HPS. Sites of higher degrees of AV block can also be determined and isolated to one of those areas. (From Gilber CJ, Masgood A: *Heart Lung* 9(1):85-92, 1980.)

cles with an external programmable pulse generator may be indicated to induce or terminate tachydysrhythmias or to evaluate sinus or AV node responses.

Fig. 30-14 illustrates the use of an intracardiac recording to localize the site of AV block. For this study, a

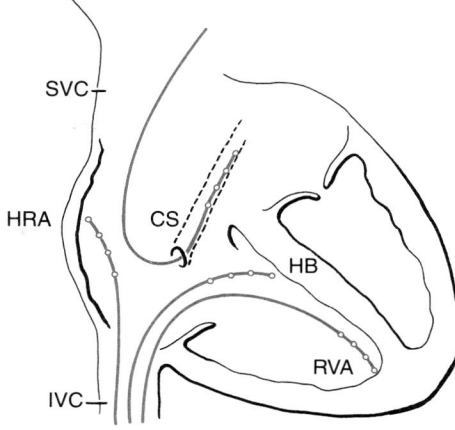

FIG. 30-15   Catheter placement for electrophysiologic (EP) testing. Quadripolar catheters to the high right atrium *(HRA)*, the right ventricular apex *(RVA)*, and the bundle of His *(HB)* are usually inserted via the femoral veins and inferior vena cava *(IVC)*. Left atrial recording and stimulation are usually performed with a catheter in the coronary sinus *(CS)*. *SVC*, Superior vena cava.

recording catheter with multiple electrodes is positioned across the tricuspid valve beside the membranous interventricular septum. The electrodes record deflections as the wave of electrical activation moves from the atria through the AV node to the bundle of His and right ventricle. The site of delays in conduction can be localized by comparing the conduction time as the impulse moves through the AV node to the bundle of His (AH interval) with that from the bundle of His through the ventricular Purkinje fibers (HV interval).

Cardiac Catheterization

Cardiac catheterization is the insertion of catheters into the cardiovascular system to study the anatomy and function of the heart in the presence of suspected or documented heart disease. Depending on the location of a suspected lesion and the degree of myocardial dysfunction, selected studies are performed, including (1) measurement of pressures in the cardiac chambers and vessels, (2) analysis of the waveform configuration of recorded pressures, (3) sampling of the oxygen content in selected regions, (4) opacification of the cardiac chambers or coronary arteries (or both) with contrast material, and (5) determination of cardiac output. Fig. 30-16 illustrates normal pressures, waveform configurations, and oxygen contents.

Two general approaches to the heart are currently used: right-sided heart catheterization and left-sided heart catheterization. *Right-sided heart catheterization* requires insertion of a catheter into the venous system, usually via an antecubital vein in the right arm or the femoral vein. The catheter is progressively advanced through the peripheral venous system to the vena cava and into the right atrium, right ventricle, and pulmonary artery. Advancing the catheter farther into a distal segment of the pulmonary arterial bed eventually produces a "wedging," or lodging, of the catheter tip in the vessel lumen. This wedge position is referred to as the *pulmonary capillary position* and reflects pressures in the cardiovascu-

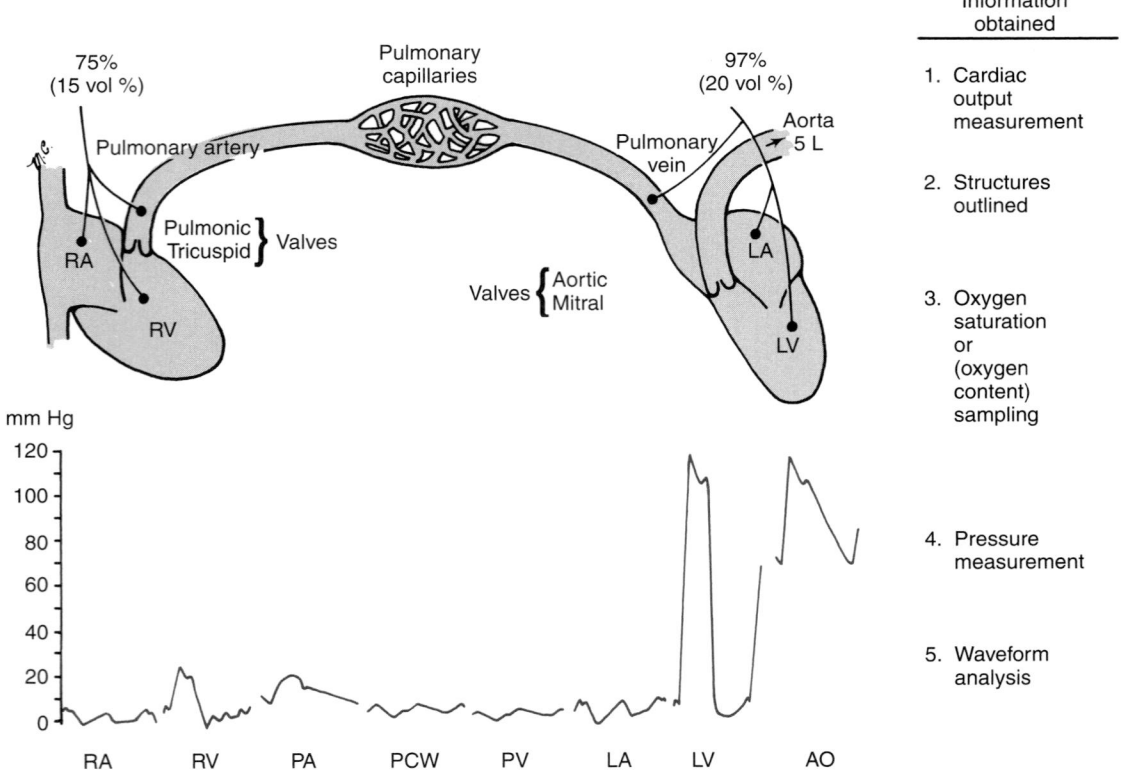

FIG. 30-16 Data obtained during cardiac catheterization. *RA*, Right atrium; *RV*, right ventricle; *PA*, pulmonary artery; *PCW*, pulmonary capillary wedge pressure; *PV*, pulmonary vein; *LA*, left atrium; *LV*, left ventricle, *AO*, aorta.

lar system from the left atrium. Left-sided heart catheterization involves the retrograde passage of the catheter through the arterial system to the aorta, across the aortic valve, and into the left ventricle. The catheter is usually inserted into either the brachial or the femoral artery. Passage of the catheter into the aorta also permits selective cannulation and study of the coronary arteries.

Catheterization in Coronary Atherosclerotic Disease

Coronary angiography, or injection of contrast material into the coronary arteries, is most often used to determine the location, extent, and severity of blockages within the coronary arteries. Additional indications for coronary angiography include evaluation of atypical angina and coronary revascularization results. The catheterization procedure involves the opacification of both coronary arteries, followed by a left ventriculogram, or injection of the contrast medium into the left ventricle, to evaluate left ventricular function (Fig. 30-17).

Coronary angiography provides the following information: (1) location of the lesion or lesions, (2) degree of obstruction, (3) presence of collateral circulation, (4) extent of disease in the distal arterial bed, and (5) type of lesion morphology. After the location and extent of disease are determined, the most appropriate intervention can be planned. Certain lesions identified at the time of catheterization are considered high-risk lesions. One example of a high-risk lesion is significant stenosis of the left main coronary artery, which may require relatively

urgent surgical intervention. Single, discrete lesions within the coronary artery may be best treated with percutaneous transluminal coronary angioplasty (PTCA), stenting, rotational arthrectomy (PTCRA), and directional coronary arthrectomy (DCA). Coronary bypass surgery is reserved for disease in three major vessels or in the left main coronary artery (see Chapter 31).

Two recent developments in interventional cardiology allow a more specific measurement of a given coronary lesion. These assessments are fractional flow reserve (FFR) and intravascular ultrasound.

Fraction flow reserve allows assessment of the clinical significance of a given lesion. Pressure measurements are obtained through a guidewire placed within the lesion. Maximal myocardial blood flow is determined in the presence of coronary stenoses and is compared with the expected normal flow. The value is expressed as a fraction. FFR of less than 0.75 is generally clinically significant and has been shown to correlate with ischemia on noninvasive testing (Pijils, 1995).

Intravascular ultrasound allows direct visualization of vascular anatomy through a transducer placed on a catheter tip. This measurement is useful in delineating plaque morphology distribution; it may also provide a rationale to guide catheter-based intervention and optimal device selection. After stent placement, it can be used to complete stent expansion (Stone et al, 1997).

The evaluation of left ventricular function is an important adjunct to coronary angiography. Injection of contrast material into the left ventricle permits visualization

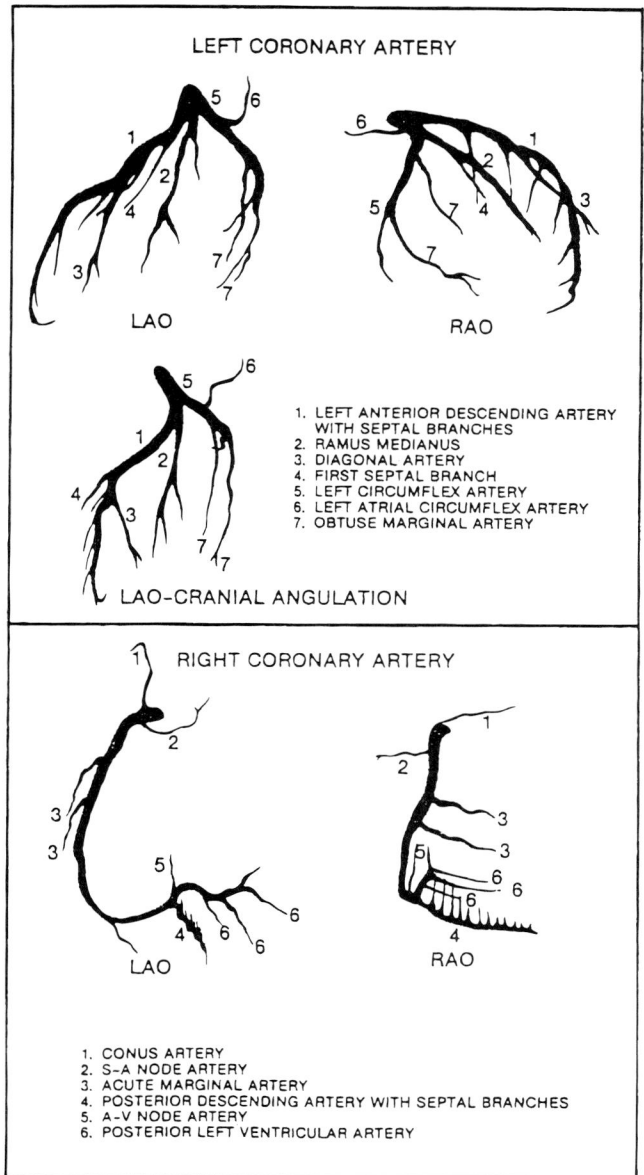

FIG. 30-17   Detailed anatomy of the normal coronary vasculature revealed by angiography. (From Braunwald E, Zipes DP, Libby P: *Heart disease: a textbook of cardiovascular medicine,* ed 6, Philadelphia, 2001, Saunders.)

of ventricular wall movement and chamber size; areas of absent motion *(akinesis),* reduced motion *(hypokinesis),* or asynchronous contraction *(dyskinesis)* or bulging are noted. Rupture of a necrotic interventricular septum after myocardial infarction would also be detected during left ventriculography. Because the pressures are higher on the left side of the heart than they are on the right side, blood would be shunted through the interventricular defect, opacifying the right ventricle. Additionally, oxygen sampling would demonstrate abnormal elevation of oxygen content in the right ventricle as a result of the recirculation of oxygenated blood through the defect. Measurement of left ventricular pressure, arterial pressure, cardiac output, and ejection fraction completes the overall assessment of left ventricular function.

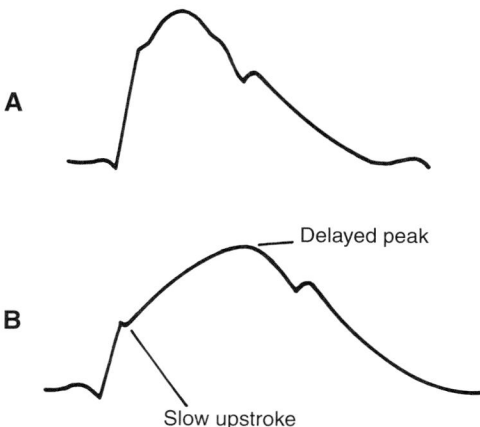

FIG. 30-18   Carotid artery pressure tracing. **A,** Normal. **B,** Aortic stenosis.

Catheterization in Valvular Heart Disease

Catheterization is useful to confirm the presence of valvular stenosis or regurgitation, to estimate the severity of the disease, and to establish or exclude the presence of associated pathology. The approach to diagnosing these two pathologic conditions—*stenosis* (valvular obstruction to blood flow) and *regurgitation* (backward blood flow through the valve)—differs.

Valvular regurgitation is documented by injecting contrast material into the chamber beyond the diseased valve; when regurgitation is present, opacification of the chamber proximal to the valve will occur when the valve fails to close securely. For example, with mitral regurgitation, the contrast medium injected into the left ventricle would appear in the left atrium during the next ventricular contraction as blood and contrast material flow backward through the diseased valve. The severity of the regurgitation is estimated according to the degree of left atrial opacification and the time required for the contrast material to disappear from the left atrium. Aortic regurgitation is detected by injecting contrast material into the ascending aorta, with subsequent opacification of the left ventricle during ventricular relaxation.

Regurgitation is also associated with abnormalities in the pressures within the cardiac chambers and alterations in waveform configuration. Mitral regurgitation creates a volume overload for the left atrium, elevating left atrial and pulmonary pressures. Additionally, the typical low-amplitude undulating left atrial waveform exhibits an abrupt increase in amplitude during ventricular contraction as blood flows backward through the valve.

Valvular stenosis can be visualized by injecting contrast material into the chamber proximal to the diseased valve; as the opacified blood flows through the restricted orifice, the valve boundaries are outlined. Typical alterations in pressures and waveforms are present with valvular stenosis. For instance, the aortic pressure tracing associated with aortic stenosis demonstrates a slow upstroke and delayed peak as a result of the resistance to ventricular ejection into the aorta (Fig. 30-18). Elevations in pressure in the chambers proximal to a stenotic lesion also occur. For example, mitral stenosis elevates left atrial and pulmonary venous pressures. These pressure elevations

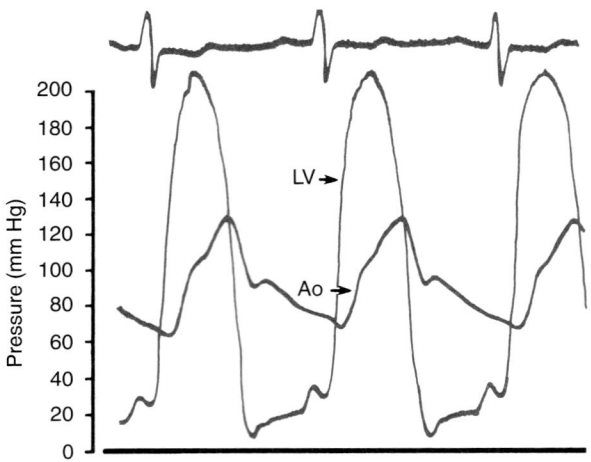

FIG. 30-19 Left ventricular *(LV)* and aortic *(Ao)* pressure tracings in severe aortic stenosis. (Modified from Grossman W: *Cardiac catheterization and angiography,* Philadelphia, 1980, Lea & Febiger.)

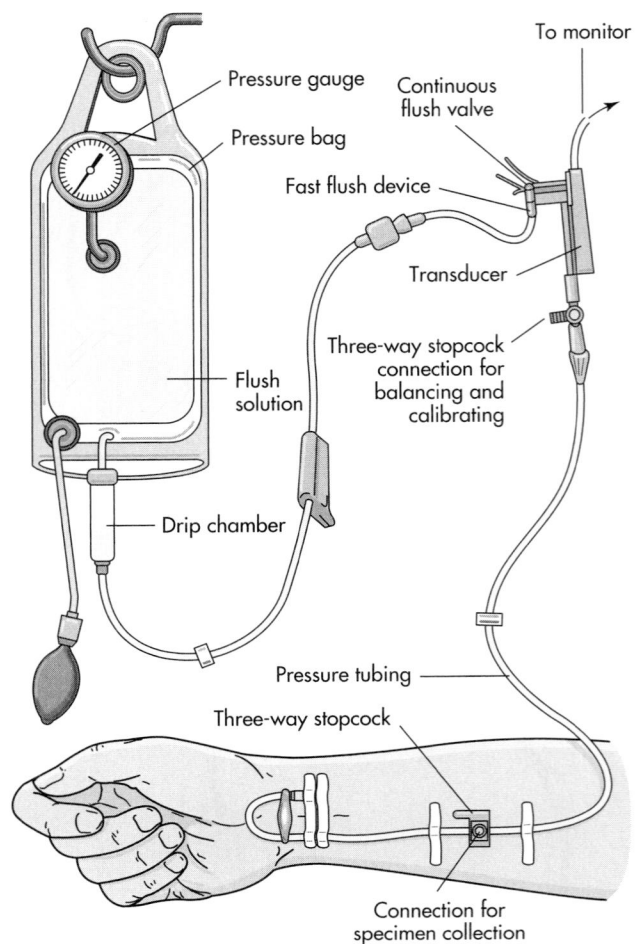

FIG. 30-20 Components of a pressure monitoring system. (From Phipps WJ et al: *Medical-surgical nursing: health and Illness perspectives,* ed 7, St Louis, 2003, Mosby.)

are reflected retrograde through the lungs and detected most easily via a catheter in the wedge position in the pulmonary artery. This pressure measurement is known as the *pulmonary capillary wedge pressure (PCWP)* and reflects left atrial pressure.

Valvular stenosis produces a *pressure gradient,* or difference in pressure, between the chambers on either side of the valve. The pressure gradient results because the chamber proximal to the stenotic valve must generate increased pressure to force blood through the obstructed valve. Fig. 30-19 shows an example of a pressure gradient resulting from severe aortic stenosis. The large pressure discrepancy is important to note, with the left ventricle generating pressures up to 210 mm Hg to force blood through the aortic valve to sustain an aortic systolic pressure of 130 mm Hg. The pressure gradient in this example is 80 mm Hg; normally, the pressure gradient is less than 5 mm Hg.

In addition to the measurement of the pressure gradient, using a formula to calculate the area of the valve orifice is necessary. Determining the pressure gradient across the valve and estimating the valve area are the two most critical indicators of the severity of stenosis.

Hemodynamic Monitoring

Bedside monitoring of selected intracardiac and intravascular pressures permits ongoing evaluation of cardiovascular status. The following hemodynamic parameters can be monitored in critical care units: (1) right atrial or central venous pressure (RAP or CVP) and left atrial pressure (LAP), (2) right ventricular pressure (RVP) and (indirectly) left ventricular end-diastolic pressure (LVEDP), (3) pulmonary artery pressure (PAP) and pulmonary capillary wedge pressure (PCWP), (4) arterial pressure, and (5) cardiac output (CO).

The basic components of the pressure monitoring system (Fig. 30-20) include (1) intravascular catheter, (2) fluid-filled extension tubing and stopcocks, (3) continuous flush device, (4) pressure transducer, and (5) pressurized flush solution. Depending on the pressures to be monitored, the catheter may be either of a single-lumen design, such as a radial arterial catheter, or of a multiple-lumen design, such as the Swan-Ganz balloon-tipped pulmonary arterial catheter.

The most frequently used pulmonary arterial catheter contains four separate lumens (Fig. 30-21). One lumen is for the inflation of the balloon at the tip of the catheter, which is used for positioning the catheter. The distal and proximal lumens are used for the monitoring of PAP or PCWP and the RAP, respectively. The final lumen is for CO measurement.

The catheter is connected to the pressure transducer by stopcocks and noncompliant pressure tubing filled with fluid. The hemodynamic pressures and pulsations are transmitted through this fluid column to the pressure transducer. The pressure transducer converts the mechanical pulsation to an electrical signal, which can be displayed on the bedside monitor.

To maintain the patency of the catheter, a continuous flush device is interposed between the catheter and the

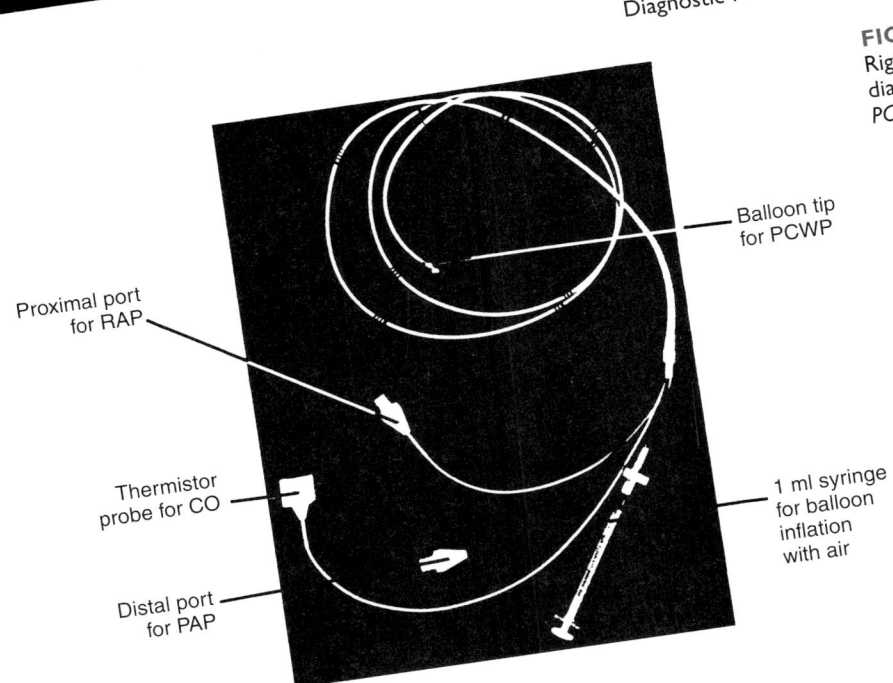

FIG. 30-21 Pulmonary artery catheter. *RAP,* Right atrial (central venous) pressure; *CO,* cardiac output; *PAP,* pulmonary artery pressure; *PCWP,* pulmonary capillary wedge pressure.

transducer. The continuous flush device is designed in a Y configuration to permit simultaneous pressure recording via the transducer and continuous flushing with solution. The device is connected to a bag of heparinized saline solution surrounded by an inflatable bag used to pressurize the solution such that it can flow against the higher intravascular or intracardiac pressures.

To interpret the significance of recorded hemodynamic pressures and waveform configurations, referring to the electrical and mechanical events of the cardiac cycle discussed in depth in Chapter 29 is necessary. Fig. 29-1 illustrates the interdependent relationship between electrical stimulation of the myocardium and the mechanical response. The five mechanical phases of the cardiac cycle are also reviewed. Each of these mechanical phases produces characteristic alterations in the contour of the waveforms recorded within the cardiovascular system. Fig. 30-22 summarizes the relationship between the phases of the cardiac cycle and the characteristic waveforms of the left side of the heart.

Atrial waveforms are normally of low amplitude, given the low pressures generated by these chambers. RAPs average from 0 to 10 mm Hg, with LAPs approximating 3 to 15 mm Hg. Left heart pressures normally exceed right heart pressures because of the higher resistance to ejection posed by the systemic circuit relative to the pulmonary circulation. Direct measurement of left atrial pressure is usually restricted to postoperative cardiac surgical intensive care units.

Atrial pressures reflect changes in the volume status of the heart, as well as alterations in cardiac function and structure. A reduction in atrial pressure is produced by hypovolemia; conversely, hypervolemia elevates atrial pressure. Atrial pressures are also valuable in assessing ventricular function, in the absence of AV valve dysfunction. As the ventricles fill during diastole, the atrial and ventricular chambers are in direct communication. At the end of diastole, the pressures between these two chambers have equilibrated; therefore atrial pressures are equal to ventricular pressures at the end of diastole. Right or left ventricular failure produces increases in right ventricular end-diastolic pressure (RVEDP) or LVEDP as residual ventricular volumes rise because of impaired ventricular function. A change in ventricular end-diastolic pressure is immediately reflected backward to the atrium, where a corresponding rise in atrial pressure is observed.

Atrial waveforms are characterized by three positive components—the *a, c,* and *v* waves—that correspond to three events in the mechanical cycle that increase atrial pressure (see Fig. 30-3). The *a* wave corresponds to atrial contraction, the *c* wave is produced by the backward bulging of the AV valve with the onset of isovolumetric contraction, and the *v* wave results from atrial filling during ventricular ejection (the AV valves normally remain closed at this time).

Predictable alterations in the atrial configuration are observed with changes in cardiac function and structure, as discussed earlier in this chapter. For example, loss of atrial contraction during atrial fibrillation is manifested as loss of *a* waves. Asynchronous contraction of the ventricles and atria, as with complete heart block, intermittently superimposes the *a* wave on the *c* and *v* waves, producing large "cannon" *a* waves (Fig. 30-23). Increased resistance to atrial contraction, as with AV valve stenosis or ventricular failure, increases the size of the *a* wave. Regurgitation of blood through an incompetent AV valve during ventricular systole superimposes an abnormal pulsation on the *c* and *v* waves, referred to as a "significant *v* wave" (see Fig. 30-3). The characteristic changes of AV valve dysfunction will be apparent in either the right atrial or the left atrial trace, depending on whether the tricuspid or mitral valve is affected.

Ventricular pressures and waveforms are not routinely monitored at the bedside. In certain settings, such as right ventricular failure secondary to chronic obstructive lung disease, a multilumen pulmonary artery catheter with a

FIG
um; ι

drugs
dopaɪ
In ι
pressuɪ
This pɪ
fusing
periphe
The ι
been diɪ
duced by
ated wit
caused b
caused by
(5) pulsus
CO can
tion (Fig. .
tutes a knoɪ
the injectat... ɪɪɪɪs technique requires insertion of the

...systemic vascular
...vascular resistance equals the dif-
...ce between MAP and RAP divided by CO, multiplied by a correction factor of 80). Calculation of systemic vascular resistance is valuable for administering vasodilators and vasoconstrictors.

KEY CONCEPTS

- History of a patient with suspected heart disease should include assessment for symptoms of angina, dyspnea, palpitations, peripheral edema, syncope, and fatigue.
- Blood pressure is measured by listening for the onset and disappearance of sounds referred to as Korotkoff sounds.
- Jugular veins are analyzed to evaluate the function of the right side of the heart.
- Left ventricular hypertrophy produces a larger and more forceful PMI that is laterally displaced. Right ventricular hypertrophy produces a substernal heave or systolic lift of the sternum.
- The first heart sound (S_1) is the onset of ventricular systole, and the second heart sound (S_2) is ventricular relaxation.
- The ECG waveform, the P wave, the QRS complex, and the T wave correlate with the spread of electrical excitation and recovery throughout the myocardium. Waveforms can be obtained through the use of a traditional 12-lead ECG, ambulatory telemetry monitoring, Holter monitoring, or through the event recorder.

- Echocardiography provides significant information about the structure and movement of the heart chambers, valves, and any unusual masses.
- Stress testing is a useful noninvasive test to determine possible ischemia or prior infarction in a given patient. The test can be performed through traditional exercise or through the use of pharmacologic stress.
- Electrophysiology testing is an intracardiac ECG that allows for more detailed analysis of conduction. During the procedure, information is obtained that may guide further need for interventions, such as catheter ablation or pacemaker implantation.
- Coronary angiography allows visualization of coronary arteries. The process may identify a discrete stenosis amenable to percutaneous intervention such as PTCA, PTCRA, DCA, or stent.
- Intravascular ultrasound or FFR may assist in determining clinical significance of a given coronary stenosis.
- Atrial pressures reflect change in volume status of the heart, as well as alteration in cardiac function.

QUESTIONS

A sampling of review questions for this chapter appears here. Visit http://www.mosby.com/MERLIN/PriceWilson/ for additional questions.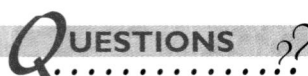

Answer the following on a separate sheet of paper.

1. Mr. H. is a 59-year-old accountant who has been diagnosed as having atherosclerotic heart disease. Recently, he found it necessary to resign from the manufacturing firm because of weakness, fatigue, and inability to climb the stairs to his second-floor office without precipitating an episode of chest pain. At home, Mr. H. is able to perform light housework but experiences shortness of breath or chest pain (or both) when he attempts to mow the lawn with a power mower. How would this patient's heart disease be categorized according to the New York Heart Association guidelines?

2. Palpation of the carotid arteries on a 68-year-old woman with a blood pressure of 178/100 mm Hg reveals that the left carotid pulse has much lower amplitude than the right. Explain the possible significance of this finding. What is this patient's mean arterial pressure (MAP)?

3. How is the hepatojugular reflux test performed? How would you determine whether the test was positive? What is the possible significance of a positive test?

4. What is a hexaxial reference system, and how is it derived?

5. Discuss the type of data and evaluation of the cardiovascular status that may be obtained from cardiac catheterization.

6. List the indications for performing coronary angiography.

Match each of the terms in column A with its definition in column B.

Column A	Column B
7. _____ Angina	a. Awareness of increased breathing effort
8. _____ Palpitations	b. Difficulty in breathing in the recumbent position
9. _____ Orthopnea	c. Chest pain caused by myocardial ischemia
10. _____ Syncope	d. Heartbeats sensed by the patient
11. _____ Dyspnea	e. Accumulation of fluid in the interstitial spaces
12. _____ Edema	f. Transient loss of consciousness
	g. Abnormal chest pulsations noticed by the patient

Match each of the abnormal heart sounds in column A with its probable cause in column B.

Column A	Column B
13. _____ Midsystolic murmur	a. May be produced by aortic stenosis
14. _____ Pansystolic murmur	b. May be produced by pulmonic regurgitation
15. _____ Middiastolic murmur	c. May be produced by mitral stenosis
16. _____ Opening snap in early diastole	d. May be produced by mitral regurgitation

Match the ECG waveform in column A with the electrical events in column B.

Column A	Column B
17. _____ P wave	a. Ventricular repolarization
18. _____ QRS complex	b. Atrial depolarization
19. _____ T wave	c. Ventricular depolarization
	d. Atrial repolarization

Match each ECG abnormality in column A with its possible cause in column B.

Column A	Column B
20. _____ Depression of the ST segment	a. Slow conduction time through the AV node
21. _____ Elevation of the ST segment	b. Myocardial ischemia
22. _____ Inversion of the P wave	c. Hyperkalemia
23. _____ Inversion of the T wave	d. Myocardial infarction
24. _____ Peaking of the T wave	e. AV nodal dysrhythmia
25. _____ Prolonged PR interval	f. Amiodarone effect
26. _____ Prolonged QT interval	

Fill in the blanks with the correct word or phrase.

27. During cardiac catheterization, contrast material is injected into the heart chamber distal to the diseased valve to confirm the diagnosis of valvular _____.

28. The pressure gradient between the left ventricle and the aorta is normally less than _____. A large pressure gradient indicates _____.

29. Heart murmurs are the result of _____ blood flow within the cardiac structures.

TREATMENT ALGORITHM

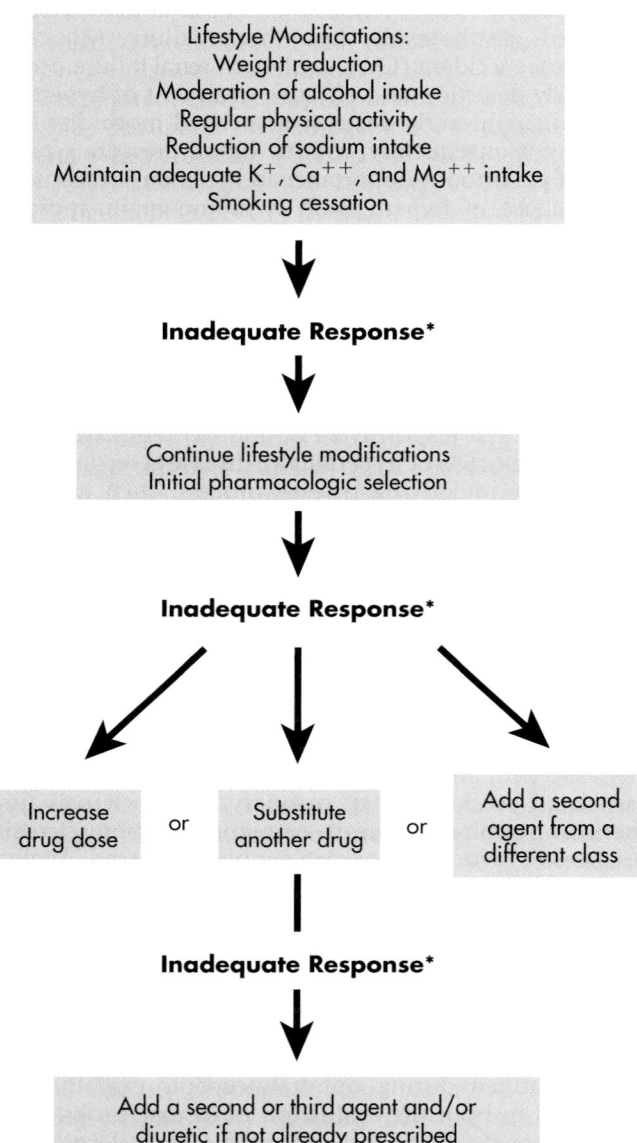

Lifestyle Modifications:
Weight reduction
Moderation of alcohol intake
Regular physical activity
Reduction of sodium intake
Maintain adequate K^+, Ca^{++}, and Mg^{++} intake
Smoking cessation

Inadequate Response*

Continue lifestyle modifications
Initial pharmacologic selection

Inadequate Response*

Increase drug dose   or   Substitute another drug   or   Add a second agent from a different class

Inadequate Response*

Add a second or third agent and/or diuretic if not already prescribed

FIG. 31-4 Treatment algorithm for hypertension. *Adequate response** means patient achieved goal blood pressure or is making considerable progress toward this goal. (Redrawn from *Sixth report of the joint national committee on prevention, detection, evaluation, and treatment of high blood pressure,* NIH Pub No 98-4080, National Heart, Lung, and Blood Institute, Washington, DC, 1997, National Institutes of Health.)

changes are inadequate to attain the blood pressure desired, drug therapy should be initiated. A single drug should be prescribed initially. The primary medication may be a diuretic, beta-adrenergic receptor blocker, calcium channel blocker, angiotensin-converting enzyme (ACE) inhibitor, or alpha-adrenergic receptor blocker, depending on multiple patient considerations, including (1) cost (diuretics are generally the least expensive drug), (2) demographic characteristics (generally, African Americans are more responsive to diuretics and calcium channel

blockers than they are to beta blockers or ACE inhibitors), (3) concurrent diseases (beta blockers may worsen asthma, diabetes mellitus, and peripheral ischemia but may improve angina, certain cardiac dysrhythmias, and migraine headache), and (4) quality of life (some antihypertensive drugs may cause undesirable side effects, such as impairment of sexual function). Secondary hypertension (i.e., hypertension caused by a specific organ defect, such as renal disease, Cushing's syndrome, pheochromocytoma, or primary hyperaldosteronism) is treated by attempting to reverse the underlying disease process.

Other Modifiable Factors

The risk of cigarette smoking is related to the number of cigarettes smoked per day, not to the length of time that the patient has smoked. An individual smoking more than one pack a day is twice as susceptible to coronary atherosclerotic disease as is a nonsmoker. The effect of nicotine on catecholamine release by the autonomic nervous system appears to be the mechanism responsible. The effect, however, is noncumulative; ex-smokers appear to revert to the low risk of nonsmokers.

Patients with diabetes tend to have a greater prevalence, prematurity, and severity of coronary atherosclerosis. Diabetes mellitus induces hypercholesterolemia and significantly increases the development of atherosclerosis. Diabetes mellitus is also associated with proliferation of smooth muscle cells in coronary arteries; the synthesis of cholesterol, triglycerides, and phospholipids; elevated levels of LDL-C; and low levels of HDL-C. The presence of the extensive diffuse atheromatous disease found in these patients is believed to be related to the smooth muscle proliferation (see discussion of pathogenesis). When hyperlipidemia is present, therapy has become aggressive. For example, the new NCEP guidelines (2001) advocate that all patients with diabetes be treated aggressively to get LDL-C levels lower than 100 mg/dl, even in patients without documented CHD. Even in these patients, the absence of autonomic nerve integrity and concomitant altered perception of pain associated with diabetes is believed responsible for the occurrence of "silent myocardial infarctions" or "silent ischemia." Estrogen appears to protect premenopausal women from the same prevalence of heart disease present in men of comparable ages because, in the absence of diabetes, severe hyperlipidemia or severe hypertension, Caucasian men have a five times greater mortality from ischemic heart disease than do Caucasian women. This difference in rates of CHD disappears after menopause.

Homocysteine is a naturally occurring amino acid produced by the body in small amounts; a normal level is 5-15 μmol/L. When present in high levels (>15 μmol/L), hyperhomocystinemia is associated with premature vascular disease and causes endothelial dysfunction and interferes with the vasodilator and antithrombotic functions of the vascular wall (Box 31-3). Deficiencies of folic acid and vitamins B_6 and B_{12} may be factors in the development of mild to moderate hyperhomocystinemia.

The typical American diet—high in calories, total fat, saturated fat, sugar, and salt—contributes to the development of hyperlipidemia and obesity. Obesity increases cardiac work and oxygen demand and contributes to a sedentary lifestyle. Excess body fat (particularly abdominal obesity) and physical inactivity promote the development of insulin resistance.

Finally, physical inactivity increases the risk of CHD comparably with hyperlipidemia or cigarette smoking, and physically inactive individuals have a 30% to 50% greater risk of developing hypertension. In addition to an improved sense of well-being and ability to manage stress, the benefits of regular aerobic exercise include increased levels of HDL-C, lower levels of LDL-C, decreased blood pressure, obesity reduction, decreased resting heart rate and myocardial oxygen (MVO_2) consumption from conditioning, and a decreased insulin resistance.

The list of contributing risk factors expands as additional biologic-environmental correlates with coronary heart disease are identified. At present, psychosocial stress appears contributory. Rosenman and Friedman have popularized an interesting relationship between the so-called type A behavior pattern and accelerated atherogenesis. The type A personality elicits intense competitiveness, ambition, aggressiveness, and a sense of time urgency. Typically acknowledged is that catecholamine release accompanies stress; however, the question arises as to whether stress is atherogenic or simply precipitates the attack. A theory of stress-induced atherogenesis might postulate neuroendocrine influences on circulatory dynamics, serum lipids, or blood clotting.

Atherosclerosis is a multifactorial disease, and substantiated evidence indicates certain risk factors accelerate atherogenesis. The complexity of the process is highlighted by the fact that the susceptibility to atherogenesis in the presence of more than one risk factor is not simply additive; the factors are synergistic. The interaction of multiple factors significantly accelerates the disease process.

PATHOGENESIS OF ATHEROSCLEROSIS

The pathogenesis of atherosclerosis is a complex process set of interactions and, as yet, remains incompletely understood. The interaction and response of components of the vessel wall with the unique impact of various stressors, many known as risk factors, are considered primary. The theory of pathogenesis that encompasses these concepts is the widely held *response-to-injury hypothesis*, in which some form of intimal injury initiates chronic inflammation of the arterial wall and results in the development of atheromas (Ross, 1999).

The vascular wall is exposed to a variety of potential and actual irritants on a daily basis. Among these are hemodynamic factors, hypertension, hyperlipidemia, and cigarette smoke derivatives and toxins (e.g., homo-

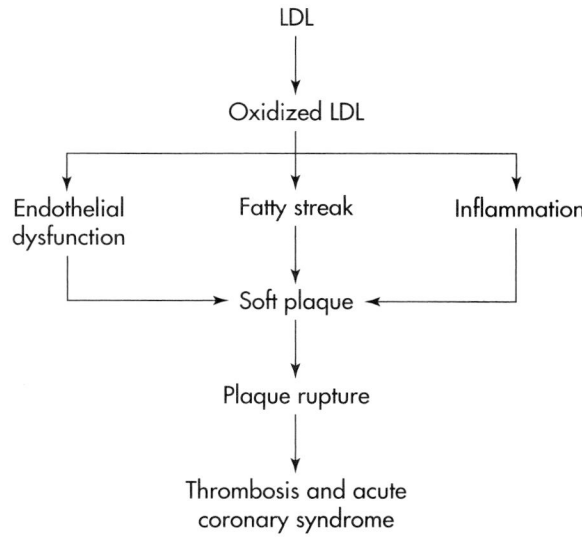

FIG. 31-5 Role of LDL in artherosclerosis. Schematic representation of the effects of LDL and oxidized LDL in the pathogenesis of atherosclerosis. Other coronary risk factors, low HDL levels, smoking, hypertension, diabetes mellitus, and estrogen deficiency also enhance the oxidation of LDL. (From Rackley CE: *UpToDate* 17, 2000.)

cysteine or oxidized LDL-C). Infectious agents (*Chlamydia pneumoniae*) may also cause injury. Of these agents, the synergistic effects of the hemodynamic disturbances that accompany normal circulatory function combined with the adverse effects of hypercholesterolemia are considered most important in the pathogenesis of atherosclerosis. Figure 31-5 highlights the role of LDL-C in the pathogenesis of atherosclerosis.

The essence of the response-to-injury theory of pathogenesis is chronic endothelial injury resulting in a chronic inflammatory response of the arterial wall and development of atherosclerosis. The variable levels of shear stress associated with the turbulence of normal circulation and enhanced in the presence of hypertension are believed to cause focal areas of endothelial dysfunction. For example, the ostia of existing vessels, branch points, and the posterior wall of the descending and abdominal aorta, are well recognized as being primary sites for the development of atherosclerotic plaques.

Figure 31-6 illustrates normal arterial structure and the cellular events in the development of an atheromatous plaque and its complications. The arterial wall consists of three concentric layers in which the endothelial cells, smooth muscle cells, and an extracellular matrix with collagen and elastic fibers can be clearly identified. These three layers are the intima, media, and adventitia (see Fig. 31-6, *A*). The *intima* is composed of *endothelial cells* lining the artery and is the only part of the vessel wall that interacts with the blood components. Important properties of the endothelium are: (1) contains receptors for LDL-C and acts as a highly selective permeability barrier; (2) provides a nonthrombogenic surface by a heparin coating and by secretion of PGI_2 (a potent vasodilator and inhibitor of platelet aggregation), as well as by plasminogen secretion; (3) secretes nitric oxide, a potent vasodilator; and (4) interacts with platelets,

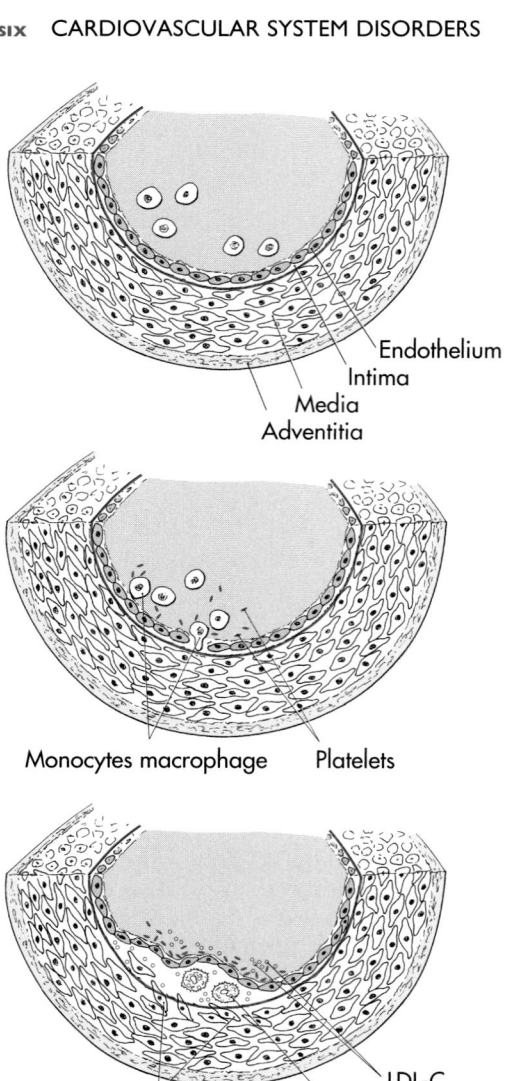

A, Normal arterial structure: (1) *intima,* innermost layer, lined by the endothelium; atherosclerotic lesions form in the intima; (2) *media* or middle layer, composed of smooth muscle cells; (3) *adventitia,* collagen-rich outer-most layer of artery including vasa vasorum.

Endothelium
Intima
Media
Adventitia

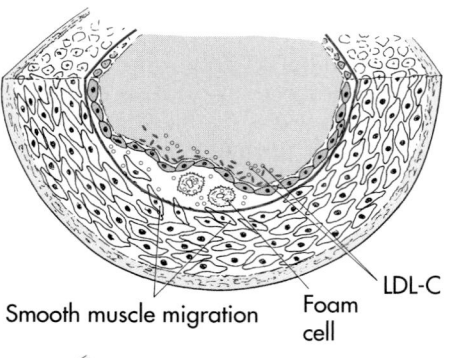

B, Endothelial injury and dysfunction: ↑ leukocyte and platelet adhesiveness, ↑ permeability, ↑ coagulability, inflammation, migration of monocytes into artery wall; oxidized LDL-C can enter intima by a receptor-independent pathway.

Monocytes macrophage   Platelets

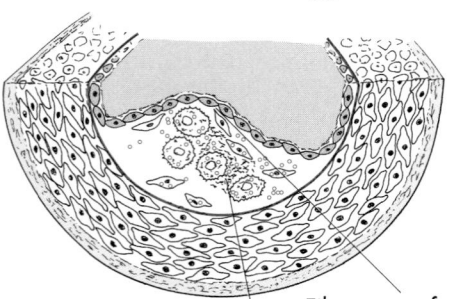

C, Fatty streak formation: Fatty streaks consist of lipid-laden macrophages (foam cells) and T lymphocytes. Later the release of growth factors from activated macrophages and platelets causes the migration of smooth muscle from the media into the intima and the proliferation of matrix; these processes convert the fatty streak into a mature atheroma.

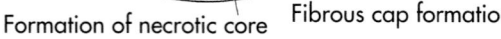

Smooth muscle migration   Foam cell   LDL-C

D, Formation of advanced complicated lesion of atherosclerosis: fatty streaks advance to intermediate and advanced lesion and tend to form a fibrous cap that walls off the lesion from the blood vessel lumen; it is a mixture of leukocytes, debris, foam cells, and free lipid that may form a necrotic core. Deposition of calcium into the fibrous plaque may cause it to harden.

Formation of necrotic core   Fibrous cap formation

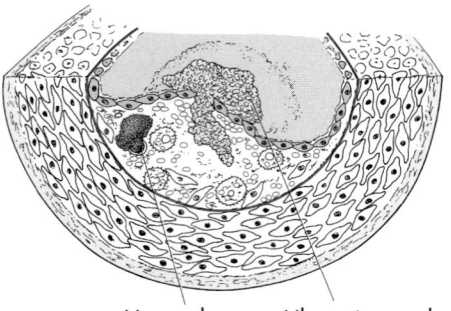

E, Atheromatous plaque complications: Thrombosis may occur from platelet adhesion to the rough edges of the atheroma; ulceration and sudden rupture of the fibrous cap can occur with subsequent occlusion of the artery; alternately hemorrhage within the atheroma from the vasa vasorum or from the endothelium may occlude the artery.

Hemorrhage   Ulceration and plaque rupture

FIG. 31-6 Cellular processes in the response to injury hypothesis of atherosclerosis.

monocytes, macrophages, T lymphocytes, and smooth muscle cells via various cytokines and growth factors. The *media* is the muscular part of the arterial wall and is composed of *smooth muscle cells*, collagen, and elastin. The intima protects the media from the blood components. The media is responsible for the contractility and vasoaction of the vessel. The *adventitia* is the outermost layer of the blood vessel wall and is composed of some smooth muscle cells and fibroblasts; it also contains the *vasa vasorum*, tiny blood vessels that distribute the blood supply to the vessel wall. In atherosclerosis, the integrity of the intima and media are disrupted, leading to the development of an atheroma. The response-to-injury hypothesis postulates that the initial step in atherogenesis is injury and consequent dysfunction of arterial endothelium with increased permeability to blood lipids and monocytes.

Hypercholesteremia by itself is believed to impair endothelial function by increasing production of oxygen free radicals. These radicals deactivate nitric oxide, the primary endothelial-relaxing factor. When hyperlipidemia is chronic, lipoproteins accumulate within the intima at sites of increased endothelial permeability. This exposure to free radicals in the arterial wall endothelial cells results in oxidation of LDL-C, which contributes to and exacerbates the development of atheromatous plaques. LDL-C oxidation is enhanced by low levels of high-density lipoprotein cholesterol (HDL-C), diabetes mellitus, estrogen deficiency, hypertension, and the presence of cigarette smoke derivatives. In contrast, high levels of HDL-C are protective against the development of CAD when it constitutes at least 25% of the total cholesterol. Hypercholesteremia promotes monocyte adhesion, subendothelial migration of smooth muscle cells, and the accumulation of lipids within the macrophages and smooth muscle cells. When exposed to oxidized LDL-C, macrophages become *foam cells*, which aggregate in the intima, where they are macroscopically visible as fatty streaks. Eventually, additional deposition of lipids and connective tissue convert these fatty streaks into mature fibrofatty atheromas, which have the potential to rupture. Rupture exposes the inner core of the plaque to the oxidized LDL-C and the increased adherence of cellular elements, including platelets. Eventually, additional deposition of lipids and connective tissue convert the fibrous plaques to atheromas, which may hemorrhage, ulcerate, calcify or thrombose, and result in an MI.

PATHOPHYSIOLOGY

Ischemia

Oxygen demand in excess of the capacity of the diseased vessels to supply oxygen results in localized *myocardial ischemia*. Transient ischemia causes reversible changes at the cellular and tissue levels, depressing myocardial function.

The lack of oxygen forces the myocardium to shift from aerobic metabolism to anaerobic metabolism. *Anaerobic* metabolism via glycolytic pathways is a much less efficient means of energy production than is *aerobic* metabolism via oxidative phosphorylation and the Krebs cycle; the production of high-energy phosphate is reduced considerably. The end product of anaerobic metabolism—lactic acid—accumulates, reducing cellular pH.

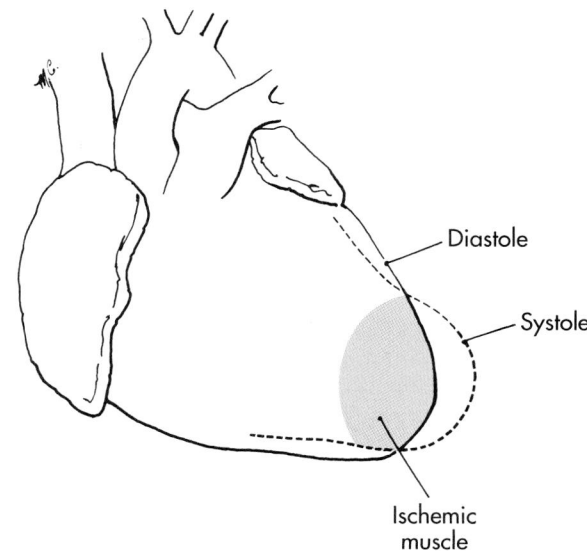

FIG. 31-7 Ischemic wall bulging during systole.

The combination of hypoxia, reduced energy availability, and acidosis rapidly impairs left ventricular function. The strength of contraction in the affected myocardial region is reduced; the fibers shorten inadequately with less force and velocity. Additionally, the wall motion of the ischemic segment is abnormal; the segment passively bulges outward with each ventricular contraction (Fig. 31-7).

The reduced contractility and impaired wall motion alter hemodynamics. The hemodynamic response is variable, depending on the size of the ischemic segment and the degree of reflex compensatory response by the autonomic nervous system. Depression of left ventricular function may lower cardiac output (CO) by reducing stroke volume (SV), the amount of blood ejected per beat). Reduction in systolic emptying increases ventricular volumes. As a result, left-sided pressures—the left ventricular end-diastolic pressure (LVEDP) and pulmonary capillary wedge pressure (PCWP)—rise. This pressure elevation is magnified by changes in wall compliance or distensibility induced by ischemia. A reduction in compliance occurs, accentuating the elevation in pressure for a given ventricular volume (Fig. 31-8).

During ischemia, the manifest hemodynamic pattern is usually that of mild increments in blood pressure and heart rate before the onset of pain. Apparently, this pattern represents a sympathetic compensatory response to the depression of myocardial function. With the onset of pain, further sympathetic activation occurs. A depression of blood pressure suggests ischemic involvement of a large area of myocardium or a vagal response.

Myocardial ischemia is typically associated with two characteristic electrocardiographic (ECG) changes resulting from alterations in cellular electrophysiology: T wave inversion and ST segment depression (Fig. 31-9). A variant form of angina (also known as *Prinzmetal's angina*) resulting from coronary artery spasm is associated with ST segment elevation.

Ischemic attacks usually subside within minutes if the imbalance between oxygen supply and demand is

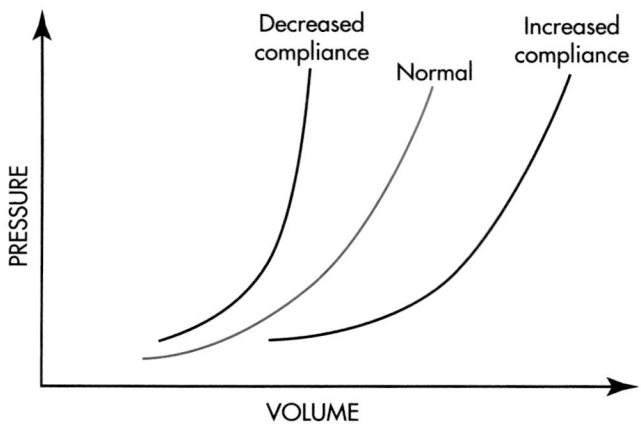

FIG. 31-8 Ventricular compliance, or the pressure-volume rela-tionship of the ventricles. The line in the center indicates the typi-cal relationship between pressure and volume. As volume is increased initially, only a small rise in pressure occurs. As volume increase continues, the rise in pressure is greater. The other lines indicate an alteration in pressure-volume relationships: decreased compliance on the left and increased compliance on the right. This represents a greater or lesser degree of stiffness of the ventricle in relation to the filling volume. Ventricular compliance is a dynamic phenomenon, and this property can change rapidly.

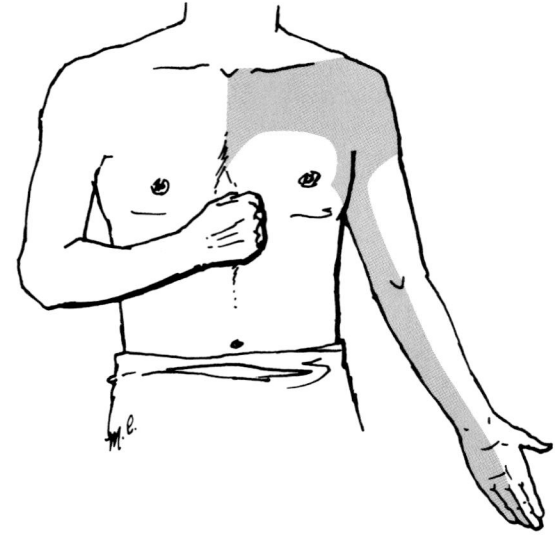

FIG. 31-10 Typical pattern of referred pain in angina pectoris.

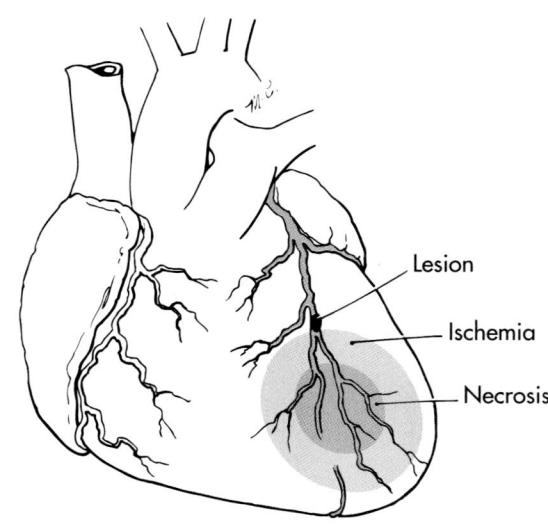

FIG. 31-11 Zones of necrosis and ischemia.

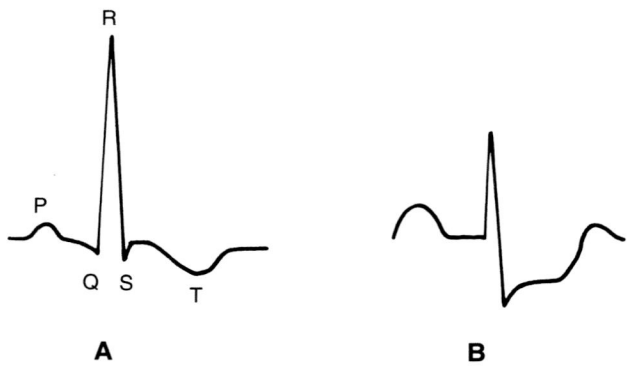
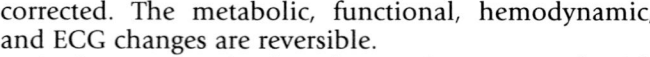

FIG. 31-9 Classic ECG changes with ischemia. **A,** T wave inver-sion. **B,** ST segment depression.

corrected. The metabolic, functional, hemodynamic, and ECG changes are reversible.

Angina pectoris is the chest pain associated with myocardial ischemia. The exact mechanism by which ischemia produces pain is unclear. Apparently, neural pain receptors are stimulated by the accumulated metabolites, by an unidentified chemical intermediary, or by local mechanical stress resulting from abnormal myocardial contraction. Typically, the pain is described as a substernal pressure, occasionally radiating down the medial aspect of the left arm. A clenched fist placed on the sternum graphically illustrates the classic pattern (Fig. 31-10). However, many patients never experience typical angina; anginal pain may mimic indigestion or a toothache. Classically, angina is precipitated by activities increasing myocardial oxygen demand, such as exercise, and is relieved within minutes by rest or nitroglycerin.

The less common Prinzmetal's angina typically occurs at rest rather than during exertion and is caused by a local-ized spasm of an epicardial artery. The etiologic mecha-nism remains unclear. Patients with diabetes often have "silent ischemia" and "silent MIs" resulting from auto-nomic neuropathy.

Infarction

Prolonged ischemia longer than 30 to 45 minutes causes irreversible cellular damage and muscle death or necro-sis. Permanent cessation of contractile function occurs in the necrotic or infarcted area of the myocardium. A zone of ischemic, potentially viable tissue surrounds the infarct (Fig. 31-11). The ultimate size of the infarct depends on the fate of this ischemic zone; necrosis of this marginal area extends the infarct size, whereas reversal of

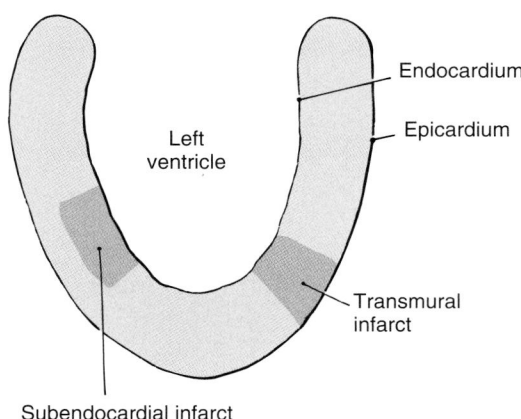

FIG. 31-12   Transmural and subendocardial infarction.

TABLE 31-3   ■■■

Correlation Among Ventricular Surfaces, ECG Leads, and Coronary Arteries

Surface of Left Ventricle	ECG Leads	Coronary Artery Usually Involved
Inferior Wall	II, III, aVF	Right coronary
High Lateral Wall	I, aVL	Left circumflex
Anterior Wall	V_2-V_4	Left anterior descending
Septal	V_1-V_2	Left anterior descending
Anterior/Septal Wall	V_1-V_4	Left anterior descending
Low Lateral Wall (Apical)	V_5-V_6	Left anterior descending
Posterior Wall	V_1-V_2 (reciprocal* changes)	Left circumflex

*Reciprocal changes indicate ST-segment depression and large R waves.

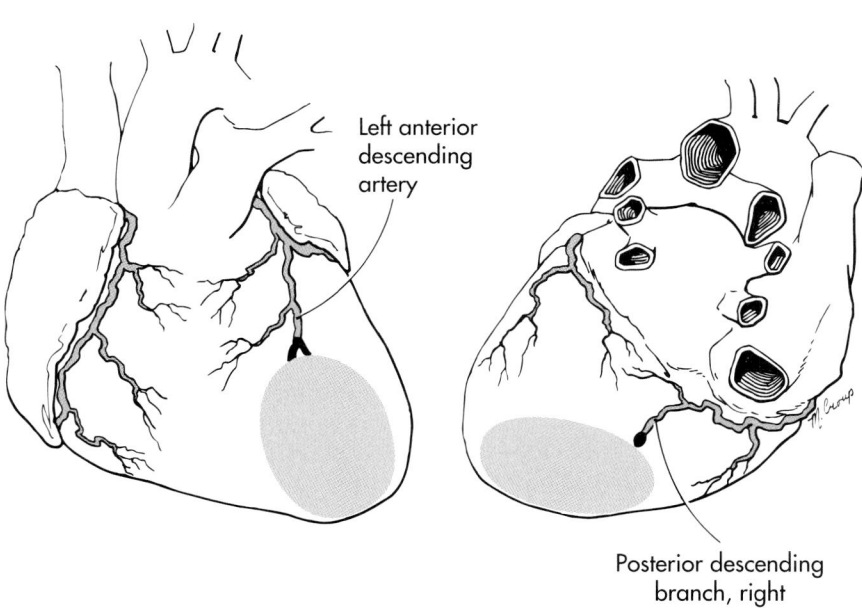

FIG. 31-13   Localization of infarcts on the ventricular wall. *Left,* Infarct of the anterior wall caused by occlusion of the left anterior descending artery. *Right,* Inferior wall infarction caused by occlusion of the posterior descending branch of the right coronary artery.

the ischemia minimizes the residual necrosis. Reversal of ischemia and reestablishment of coronary flow can be achieved either by administering thrombolytic agents or by primary percutaneous transluminal coronary angioplasty (PTCA) (see later section on therapeutic interventions). If the reversal of ischemia is successful, the area of necrosis and the size of the infarction are then minimized. In the absence of these interventions, necrosis of this ischemic zone increases the size of the infarction.

MI usually affects the left ventricle. A *transmural infarction* involves the full thickness of the wall; a *subendocardial infarction* is limited to the inner half of the myocardium (Fig. 31-12). Infarctions are described further according to location on the ventricular wall (Fig. 31-13). For instance, an anterior MI involves the anterior wall of the left ventricle. Other common infarct sites are designated as inferior, lateral, posterior, and septal.

Extensive infarctions involving large portions of the ventricle are described accordingly, that is, as anteroseptal, anterolateral, or inferolateral. MI of the posterior wall of the right ventricle is also observed in approximately one fourth of left ventricular inferior wall infarctions. Biventricular compromise should be anticipated in this situation.

The infarct location correlates with disease in a particular region of the coronary circulation (Table 31-3). For example, anterior wall infarctions result from lesions in the left anterior descending artery. Knowing the coronary anatomy and the location of the infarct is of critical importance in anticipating complications associated with MI. For example, inferior wall infarction, usually the result of right coronary artery lesions, can be associated with variable degrees of heart block. This result is to be expected because the atrioventricular (AV) node receives its nutrient supply from the same vessel that nourishes the inferior wall of the left ventricle.

The infarcted muscle undergoes a sequence of changes during the healing process. Initially, the infarcted muscle appears bruised and cyanotic as a result of regional stagnation of blood. Cellular edema and an inflammatory response with leukocytic infiltration ensue within 24 hours. Cardiac enzymes are released from the cells. Tissue degradation and removal of all necrotic fibers begin by the second or third day. During this phase, the necrotic wall is relatively thin. By approximately the third week, scar formation begins. Gradually, fibrous connective tissue replaces the necrotic muscle and undergoes progressive thickening. By the sixth week, the scar is well established.

MI significantly depresses ventricular function as a result of the loss of contractility in the necrotic muscle and the impaired contractility in the surrounding ischemic muscle. Functionally, MI results in changes similar to those noted with ischemia: (1) reduced contractility, (2) abnormal wall motion, (3) altered ventricular wall compliance, (4) reduced SV, (5) diminished ejection fraction, (6) elevated ventricular end-systolic and end-diastolic volumes, and (7) increased LVEDP.

A wide spectrum of left ventricular dysfunction is apparent after MI. The degree of functional impairment depends on a number of factors, including the following:

1. *Infarct size.* Infarcts of more than 40% of the myocardium are associated with a high incidence of cardiogenic shock.
2. *Infarct location.* Anterior wall infarction is more likely to significantly depress mechanical function compared with inferior wall damage.
3. *Function of uninvolved myocardium.* Old infarcts compromise residual myocardial function.
4. *Collateral circulation.* Collateral circulation, via either preexisting arterial anastomoses or new channels, can develop in response to chronic ischemia and regional hypoperfusion, improving blood flow to the threatened myocardium.
5. *Cardiovascular compensatory mechanisms.* Reflex compensatory mechanisms operate to maintain CO and peripheral perfusion.

Reflex sympathetic augmentation of the heart rate and contractility can improve ventricular function. Generalized arteriolar constriction increases total peripheral resistance (TPR), thereby increasing mean arterial pressure (MAP). Venoconstriction reduces venous capacity, increasing venous return to the heart and ventricular filling. Increased ventricular filling elevates the force of contraction and subsequent ejection volumes up to a point, beyond which the curve flattens. This process is best illustrated by comparing the normal ventricular function curve with that of the compromised myocardium (Fig. 31-14). With depression of ventricular function, higher diastolic filling pressures are necessary to maintain SV. Elevation of diastolic filling pressure and ventricular volume stretches myocardial fibers, increasing the force of contraction according to Starling's law. Circulatory filling pressures can be increased further by renal retention of sodium and water. As a result, MI is often associated with transient left ventricular enlargement caused by compensatory cardiac dilation. When necessary, compensatory cardiac hypertrophy can also occur to increase the force of contraction and ventricular emptying.

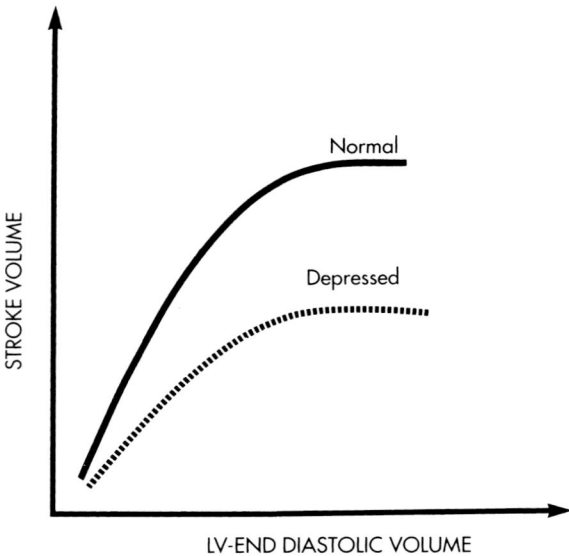

FIG. 31-14 Depression of the ventricular function curve. Normal curve *(solid line)* represents the relationship of stroke volume to left ventricular end-diastolic volume for the normal heart shown in Fig. 29-10. The failing heart *(depressed curve)* must increase the end-diastolic volume to maintain stroke volume. Therefore cardiac dilation occurs.

In summary, a battery of reflex responses are available to forestall deterioration of CO and perfusion pressure: (1) augmentation of heart rate and contractility, (2) generalized vasoconstriction, (3) sodium and water retention, (4) ventricular dilation, and (5) ventricular hypertrophy. However, all compensatory responses can eventually contribute to further myocardial deterioration by increasing myocardial oxygen demand.

The hemodynamic presentation after MI is maintained at normal levels. Heart rate is usually not persistently elevated unless extensive myocardial depression occurs. Blood pressure is a function of the interaction between myocardial depression and autonomic reflexes. The autonomic response to MI is not always the predictable sympathetic support of the compromised circulation. Pain or stimulation of parasympathetic ganglia in the myocardium, particularly in the inferior wall, complicates the hemodynamic response. Parasympathetic stimulation, most often present in inferior MI, reduces the heart rate and blood pressure, adversely affecting CO and peripheral perfusion. This type of response is known as *vasovagal*.

MI is classically associated with a characteristic diagnostic triad: patient presentation, ECG changes, and elevation of chemical biomarkers. First, the typical patient presentation includes complaints of severe, prolonged chest discomfort (often described as pressure, heaviness, or fullness) frequently associated with sweating, nausea, vomiting, and a sense of impending doom. However, between 20% and 60% of nonfatal MIs are "silent" or asymptomatic. Approximately one half of these MIs are truly silent rather than atypical in presentation and are diagnosed only as the result of a routine ECG or postmortem examination.

Second, certain ECG changes that are indicative of acute MI are classified as Q-wave or non–Q-wave infarc-

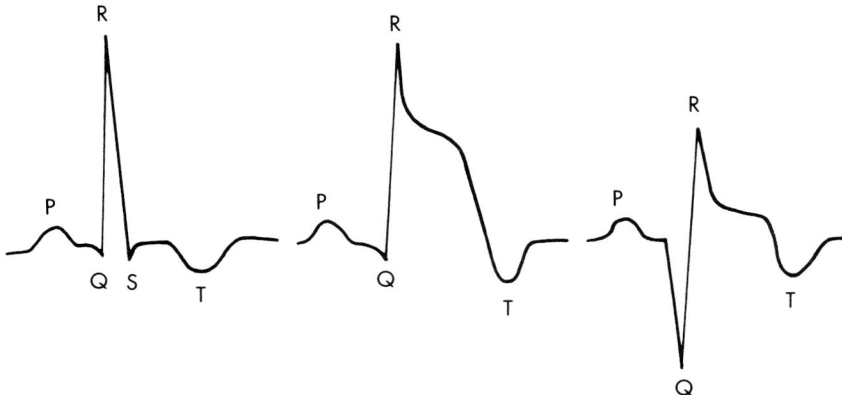

FIG. 31-15 ECG changes overlying an area of MI. T wave inversion *(left)*, ST segment elevation *(middle)*, and pronounced Q waves *(right)*. Q waves may develop early in an infarct, and if they are truly indicative of necrosis, they are irreversible. The ST segment and T wave changes result from the ischemic injury and disappear over time.

tion. The ECG changes associated with a *Q-wave MI* include ST segment elevation, T wave inversion, and the development of pronounced Q waves in the leads overlying the infarcted myocardium. Over time, the ST and T wave changes revert to normal, with only the Q waves persisting as a permanent ECG indication of the previous Q-wave MI (Fig. 31-15). However, only one half to two thirds of patients present this classic evolution of an acute MI. A *non–Q-wave MI (NQWMI)* occurs in approximately 30% of patients diagnosed with an MI. The presence of a Q wave is often related to the duration of ischemia in the infarct-related artery. For instance, patients who receive thrombolytics often have a NQWMI. The ECG manifestations of a NQWMI are transient ST segment depression or T wave inversion (or both) in the leads overlying the infarction. These changes persist up to 72 hours and then revert to normal, leaving no permanent indication of the MI on the ECG.

Transmural infarction is often present when the ECG demonstrates Q waves or loss of R waves; nontransmural infarctions are often present when the ECG shows only transient ST segment and T wave changes. However, because the correlation between the ECG and the infarction characteristics are far from perfect, the terms Q-wave and non–Q-wave infarction are preferred over the terms transmural and nontransmural (or subendocardial), respectively.

The final diagnostic tool in the triad is the release and elevation of serum biochemical markers of cardiac cellular injury. Two biochemical markers (biomarkers) are currently used in the diagnosis of acute myocardial injury. These are *creatinine kinase (CK)* and its isoenzyme *creatinine kinase MB (CK-MB)*, and the troponins: *cardiac-specific troponin T (cTnT)* and *cardiac-specific troponin I (cTnI)*.

Creatinine kinase is an enzyme released in the presence of muscle injury and has three isoenzyme fractions: CK-MM, CK-BB, and CK-MB. CK-BB is most prevalent in brain tissue and is not usually present in serum. CK-MM is found in skeletal muscle and accounts for most of the circulating CK. Muscle injury, such as in a fall, an intramuscular injection, or in certain disease processes (e.g., muscular dystrophy) cause elevations in the CK and CK-MM. CK-MB is present predominantly in the myocardium; however, it is also present in small amounts in skeletal muscle. A rise and fall in the CK and CK-MB is the most specific biomarker of myocardial injury as in MI.

TABLE 31-4 ▪ ▪ ▪

Biomarkers of Cardiac Cellular Injury (Elevation in serum levels)

Biomarker	Rise	Peak	Duration
Creatinine Kinase (CK)	4-6 hours	18-24 hours	2-3 days
Creatinine Kinase-MB (CK-MB)	4-6 hours	18-24 hours	2-3 days
Cardiac-specific Troponin T (cTnT)	4-6 hours	18-24 hours	10 days
Cardiac-specific Troponin I (cTnI)	4-6 hours	18-24 hours	10 days

Following an acute MI, the CK and CK-MB rise within 4 to 6 hours, peak within 18 to 24 hours, and fall back to normal after 2 to 3 days (Table 31-4). Since CK-MB is also present in skeletal muscle, the diagnosis of myocardial injury is based on the rise and fall pattern.

The cardiac-specific troponins, cTnT and cTnI, are also indicative of myocardial injury. These troponins are regulatory proteins that control the calcium-mediated interaction of actin and myosin; elevated serum levels are specific for release from the myocardium. The troponins will rise 4 to 6 hours after myocardial injury and will persist for 10 days after the event and are considered highly specific in situations in which only a small CK elevation occurs (see Table 31-4). In contrast, negative troponins in the presence of an elevated CK tend to exclude an MI. Unlike CK, the healthy general population has no detectable levels of troponins in the blood in the absence of myocardial injury. Of note, serum troponins can be elevated in the presence of congestive heart failure, hypertension, left ventricular hypertrophy, myocarditis, and with chemotherapy that is toxic to the myocardium.

C-reactive protein (CRP) is also currently considered a biomarker of myocardial injury. The current hypothesis holds that the progression of atherosclerotic lesions from plaque destabilization results from inflammatory processes. An acute inflammatory event, such as unstable angina, causes an increase in CRP. The diagnosis of acute MI is therefore dependent on all three variables in the diagnostic triad: the patient presentation, the ECG findings, and the elevation in the serum cardiac markers, CK-MB and the cardiac-specific troponins.

Complications of Ischemia and Infarction

Congestive Heart Failure

Congestive heart failure is a state of circulatory congestion produced by myocardial dysfunction. The location of the congestion depends on the ventricle involved. Left ventricular dysfunction, or left heart failure, produces pulmonary venous congestion, whereas right ventricular dysfunction, or right heart failure, results in systemic venous congestion. Failure of both ventricles is referred to as *biventricular failure*. Failure of the left side of the heart is the most common mechanical complication after MI.

MI compromises myocardial function by reducing contractility, producing abnormal wall motion, and altering chamber compliance. As the ability of the left ventricle to empty effectively lessens, SV falls and residual ventricular volumes rise. Consequently, left ventricular pressures rise. This pressure elevation is transmitted backward into the pulmonary venous circuit. When the hydrostatic pressure in the pulmonary capillary bed exceeds the vascular oncotic pressure, fluid transudation into the interstitium results. Further elevation of pressure eventually causes pulmonary edema because of fluid seepage into the alveoli.

The fall in SV elicits a compensatory sympathetic response. Heart rate and contractile force increase to maintain CO. Peripheral vasoconstriction occurs to stabilize arterial pressure and redistribute blood flow away from the nonvital organs, such as the kidney and skin, to maintain perfusion of the vital organs. Venoconstriction increases venous return to the right side of the heart, further augmenting contractile force according to Starling's law of the heart. Activation of the renin-angiotensin-aldosterone system in response to the fall in renal blood flow and glomerular filtration rate results in renal retention of sodium and water. This action further increases venous return.

The clinical manifestations of heart failure reflect the degree of myocardial compromise and the efficacy and magnitude of compensatory responses. The following findings are frequently noted during left heart failure:

1. *Signs and symptoms:* dyspnea, oliguria, weakness, fatigue, pallor, and weight gain
2. *Auscultation:* rales, third heart sound (resulting from dilation and noncompliance of the ventricle during rapid filling)
3. *ECG:* tachycardia
4. *Chest radiograph:* cardiomegaly, pulmonary venous congestion, and vascular redistribution to the upper lobes

Failure of the left side of the heart can progress to failure of the right side as pulmonary vascular pressures rise, stressing the right ventricle. In addition to this indirect route of compromise via the pulmonary vasculature, left ventricular dysfunction directly affects right ventricular function via shared anatomic and biochemical features. The two ventricles share a common wall—the interventricular septum—and lie within the pericardium. Additionally, biochemical changes, such as depletion of myocardial stores of norepinephrine during failure, can adversely affect both ventricles. Finally, infarction of the right ventricle can occur, particularly in association with inferior wall infarction of the left ventricle. Right ventricular infarction obviously predisposes the right side of the heart to failure. The systemic venous congestion produced by right heart failure is manifested by findings such as engorged neck veins, hepatomegaly, and peripheral edema.

Cardiogenic Shock

Cardiogenic shock results from profound left ventricular dysfunction after a massive infarction, usually involving more than 40% of the left ventricle. Despite the advent and success of early thrombolytic treatment and primary revascularization by PTCA in many hospital settings, cardiogenic shock remains the leading cause of death in hospitalized patients with MI. Cardiogenic shock is a vicious, self-perpetuating cycle of progressively irreversible hemodynamic changes, including (1) reduced peripheral perfusion, (2) reduced coronary perfusion, and (3) increased pulmonary congestion. Hypotension, metabolic acidosis, and hypoxemia further depress myocardial function. The incidence of cardiogenic shock is 10% to 15%, and the mortality can be as high as 68% when untreated. The use of thrombolytics, an intraaortic balloon pump (IABP), and early revascularization by angioplasty or coronary artery bypass graft (CABG) can decrease the mortality (see Chapter 33 for a detailed discussion).

Papillary Muscle Dysfunction

Closure of the mitral valve during ventricular systole depends on the functional integrity of the left ventricular papillary muscles and chordae tendineae. Ischemic dysfunction or necrotic rupture of a papillary muscle impairs mitral valve function and permits varying degrees of leaflet eversion into the atria during systole (Fig. 31-16). Valvular incompetence results in retrograde flow from the left ventricle into the left atrium with two consequences: a reduction in forward aortic flow and an elevation in left atrial and pulmonary venous congestion. The volume of regurgitant flow depends on the extent of papillary muscle disease; ischemia typically causes mild to moderate congestive heart failure. However, papillary

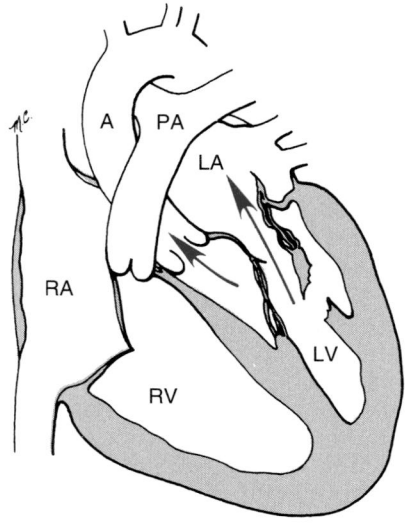

FIG. 31-16 Papillary muscle rupture. *A,* Aorta; *PA,* pulmonary artery; *LA,* left atrium; *RA,* right atrium; *LV,* left ventricle; *RV,* right ventricle.

muscle necrosis and rupture is a catastrophic event with rapid deterioration into pulmonary edema and shock. Although much less common, papillary muscle rupture may also occur in the right ventricle. Severe tricuspid regurgitation and right ventricular failure would result.

Ventricular Septal Defect

Necrosis of the interventricular septum can result in rupture of the septal wall, which creates a ventricular septal defect. Because the septum receives a dual blood supply from arteries descending the anterior and posterior surfaces of the interventricular groove, septal rupture may indicate extensive CAD involving more than one artery.

Essentially, the rupture establishes a second outflow tract from the left ventricle. During each ventricular contraction, competitive outflow occurs through the aorta and the septal defect (Fig. 31-17). Because pressures on the left side of the heart are much greater than pressures on the right side, blood will be shunted through the defect from left to right, from the area of greater pressure to the area of lesser pressure. Great volumes of blood can be shunted over to the right side of the heart, reducing the amount of blood available to be ejected via the aorta. Significant reductions in CO with concurrent elevations in right ventricular work and pulmonary congestion result.

Cardiac Rupture

Although rare, rupture of the ventricular free wall may occur early in the course of transmural infarction during the phase of necrotic tissue removal before scar formation. The thin, necrotic wall ruptures, resulting in massive bleeding into the pericardial sac. The relatively inelastic pericardial sac is unable to distend. Thus the blood-filled pericardial sac compresses the heart, producing *cardiac tamponade* (Fig. 31-18). Cardiac tamponade reduces venous return and CO. Death usually occurs within a few minutes unless the condition is quickly recognized and relieved by a transthoracic pericardiocentesis (needle tap).

Ventricular Aneurysm

Transient paradoxical bulging of the ischemic myocardium is common, and a sustained ventricular aneurysm occurs in approximately 15% of patients. The aneurysm is usually on the anterior or apical surface of the heart. Ventricular aneurysms balloon outward with each systole, passively distended by a portion of what should have been the SV (Fig. 31-19). Ventricular aneurysms can produce three problematic consequences: (1) chronic congestive heart failure, (2) systemic embolization of mural thrombi, and (3) refractory ventricular dysrhythmias.

Thromboembolism

Thromboembolism is a clinically apparent complication of acute MI in approximately 10% of the cases (particularly with large infarcts of the anterior wall). Two-dimensional echocardiography reveals that about one third of patients with anterior infarcts have thrombi in the left ventricle but

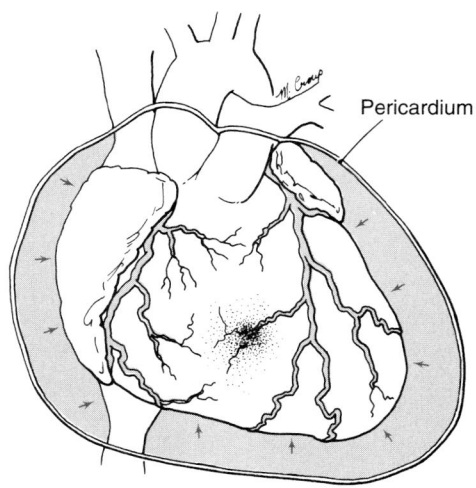

FIG. 31-18 Cardiac tamponade (blood within pericardial space).

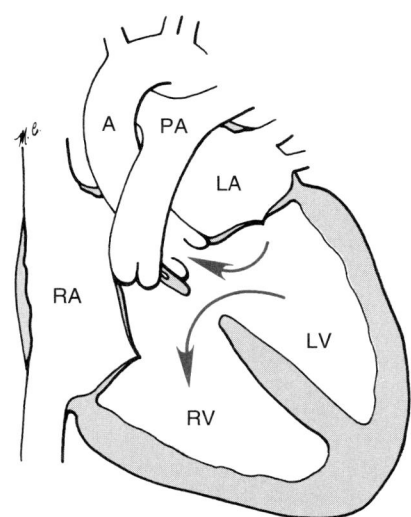

FIG. 31-17 Ventricular setpal defect. (See Fig. 31-16 for abbreviations.)

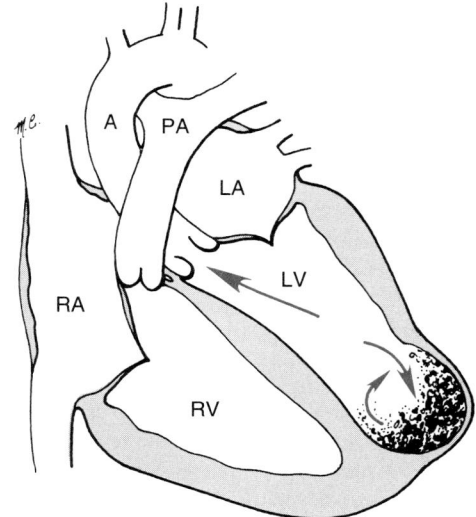

FIG. 31-19 Ventricular aneurysm. (See Fig. 31-16 for abbreviations.)

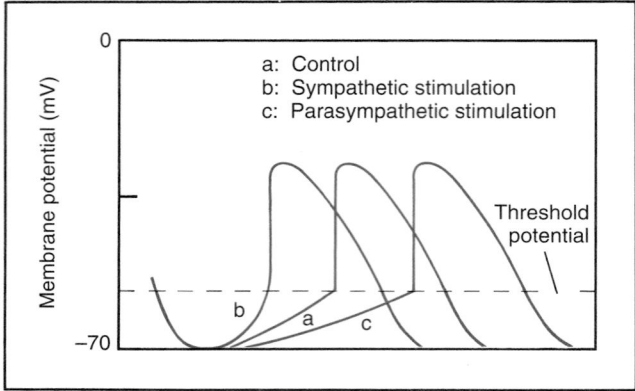

FIG. 31-20   Effects of sympathetic and parasympathetic stimulation on the slope of the action potential of a sinoatrial node cell. (From Vander A, Sherman J, Luciano D: *Human physiology: mechanisms of body function,* ed 8, New York, 2001, McGraw-Hill.)

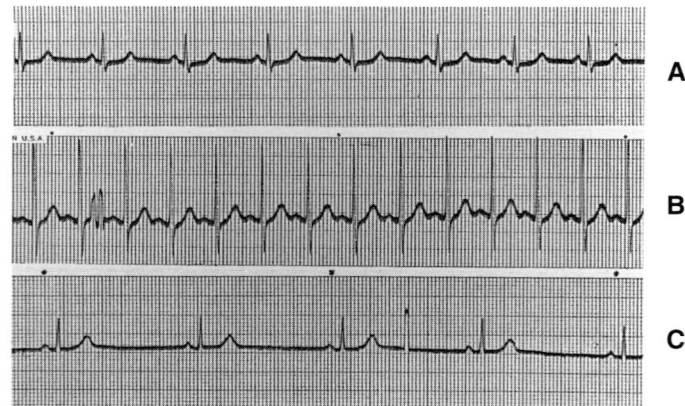

FIG. 31-21   **A,** Normal sinus rhythm (NSR), heart rate of 69. **B,** Sinus tachycardia, heart rate of 125. **C,** Sinus bradycardia, heart rate of 41.

are rare in patients with inferior or posterior infarcts. Thromboembolism is considered to be an important contributing factor in the death of 25% of infarct patients who die after hospitalization. Arterial emboli originate from mural thrombi in the left ventricle and may cause a stroke when they lodge in the cerebral circulation. Most pulmonary emboli arise in the leg veins and confinement to bed increases the risk (see Chapter 40).

Pericarditis

A Q-wave MI (usually a transmural infarction) can involve damage to the epicardial layer of the myocardium in contact with the pericardium, creating the potential for irritation and inflammation of the myocardium. Pericarditis is characterized by severe chest discomfort associated with patient movement.

Diagnosis is by patient presentation and ECG evidence of global ST segment elevation and PR segment depression. Occasionally, a "pericardial rub" (a harsh scratching sound) can be auscultated over the precordium. Rarely, a pericardial effusion, or fluid accumulation, occurs. Fluid accumulation is rarely significant to cause hemodynamic compromise, such as cardiac tamponade.

Dressler's Syndrome

This post-MI syndrome is a benign inflammatory response with pleuropericardial pain. Theories suggest that Dressler's syndrome represents a hypersensitivity reaction to the necrotic myocardium.

Dysrhythmia

A disturbance of cardiac rhythm, or dysrhythmia, is the most common complication during MI, with ventricular premature beats occurring in nearly all patients and complex beats occurring in most patients. Dysrhythmias result from alterations in myocardial cellular electrophysiology. The electrophysiologic alteration is manifested by a change in the configuration of the action potential, which is the graphic recording of cellular electrical activity. For instance, sympathetic stimulation increases the slope of spontaneous depolarization, thereby increasing the heart rate (Fig. 31-20). Clinically, dysrhythmia diagnosis is based on interpretation of the ECG.

Multiple predisposing factors account for the high incidence of dysrhythmias in the setting of coronary atherosclerotic disease: (1) tissue ischemia, (2) hypoxemia, (3) autonomic nervous system influences (e.g., parasympathetic stimulation that decreases heart rate), (4) metabolic derangements (e.g., lactic acidosis caused by compromised tissue perfusion), (5) hemodynamic abnormalities (e.g., reduction in coronary perfusion associated with hypertension), (6) drugs (e.g., digitalis toxicity), (7) electrolyte imbalance (e.g., hypokalemia with excessive diuresis), and (8) sudden reperfusion from the administration of a thrombolytic agent during an acute MI.

Cardiac rhythm abnormalities can be categorized according to the following basic mechanisms: abnormal automaticity, abnormal conduction, or a combination of the two.

The normal heart rate (HR) is between 60 and 100 bpm. A HR less than 60 bpm is referred to as a *bradycardia,* whereas a *tachycardia* indicates a HR greater than 100 bpm (Fig. 31-21). Both rate abnormalities can adversely affect cardiac function. Because HR is a primary determinant of CO (CO = HR × SV), extreme increments or reductions in HR can lower CO. Tachycardias lower CO by reducing ventricular filling time and SV, and bradycardias lower CO by reducing the frequency of ventricular ejection. As CO falls, arterial pressure and peripheral perfusion decrease. Furthermore, tachycardias can aggravate myocardial ischemia by increasing myocardial oxygen demand, while simultaneously reducing the duration of diastole, the period of greatest coronary flow, thereby compromising coronary oxygen supply.

Any cardiac impulse originating outside of the sinus node is considered abnormal and is referred to as an *ectopic beat.* Ectopic beats can originate in the atria, the AV junction, or the ventricles under two conditions: (1) failure or excessive slowing of the sinus node or (2) premature activation of another cardiac site. Ectopic beats resulting from sinus node failure serve a protective function by initiating a cardiac impulse before prolonged cardiac standstill can occur (Fig. 31-22). These beats are called *escape beats.* If the sinus node fails to resume normal function, the ectopic site will then assume the role of pacemaker and sustain the cardiac rhythm, referred to as

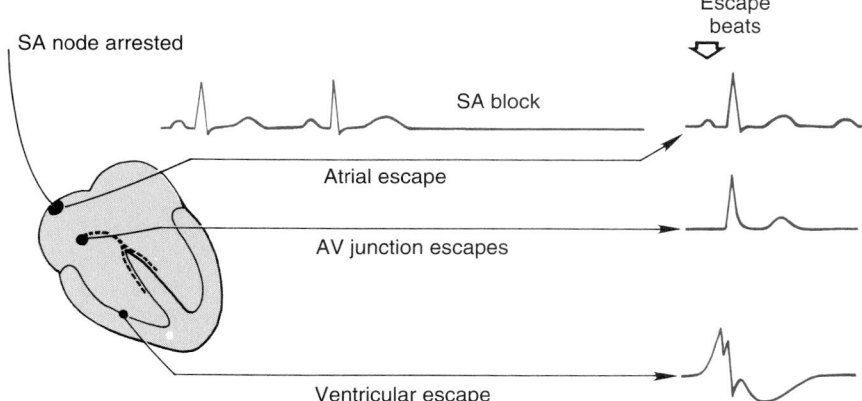

Escape beats

FIG. 31-22   Escape beats. A period of cardiac asystole may result when the sinoatrial *(SA)* node fails to send impulses to the atria unless the lower pacemakers, or escape pacemakers, take over to maintain the cardiac rhythm. If the first beat after the sinus arrest originates in the AV node, it is called a junctional or nodal escape beat. If the impulse after sinus arrest originates in the ventricles, it is called a ventricular escape beat.

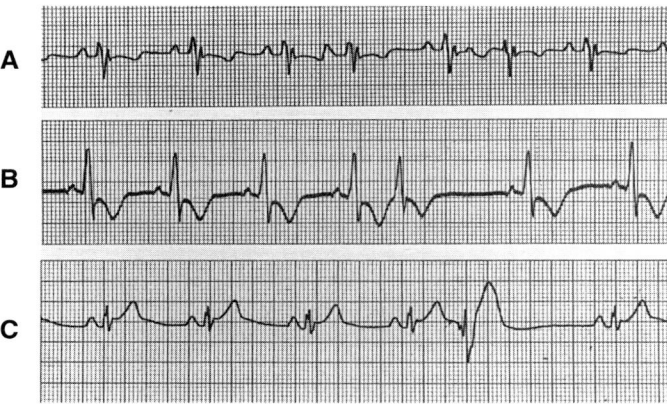

FIG. 31-23   Premature beats. **A**, This is NSR with two premature atrial beats (the fourth and sixth P waves are premature and obviously not sinus-conducted beats). **B**, Junctional premature beat (fifth complex). **C**, This is NSR with one premature ventricular complex (PVC) followed by a full compensatory pause. (From Conover MB: *Understanding electrocardiography*, ed 7, St Louis, 1996, Mosby.)

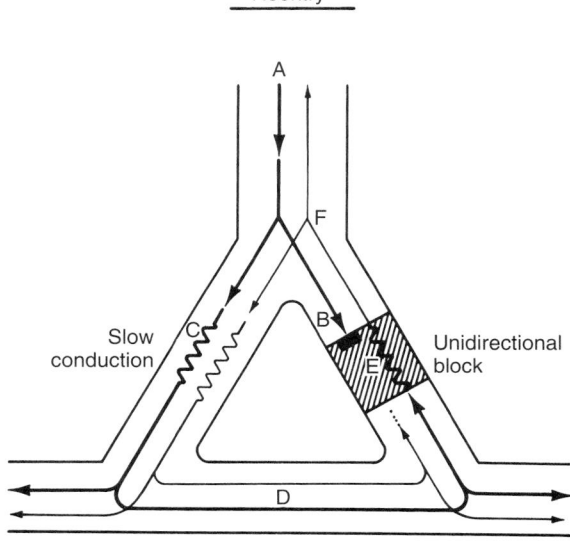

Reentry

FIG. 31-24   Features of reentry. An impulse is shown entering both limbs of an available circuit at point A. The impulse encounters antegrade (unidirectional) block in the shaded area at point B because the effective refractory period of this region exceeds that of the tissue in region C. The impulse is conducted with delay through region C, traverses region D distal to the site of unidirectional block, and retrogradely penetrates in region E, resulting in completion and perpetuation of the reentry circuit. Slow conduction in regions C or E allows sufficient time for recovery of excitability to occur in region F, following its previous depolarization by the initiating (antegrade) impulse. A delicate balance of conduction delay and differential refractoriness must coexist in two limbs of the circuit for reentry to be initiated and sustained. Exit into and excitation of the surrounding myocardium by the reentrant impulse may occur at any point in the circuit. The rate of the resulting dysrhythmia is determined both by the conduction time within the reentry circuit and by the refractory period of the surrounding myocardium. (Modified from Berne RM, Levy MN: *Physiology*, ed 3, St Louis, 1993, Mosby.)

an *escape rhythm*. After the sinus node resumes normal function, the escape focus is suppressed.

Premature activation of cardiac sites other than the sinus node disrupts the normal cardiac cycle; impulses occur prematurely before the sinus node recovers sufficiently from one beat to initiate another (Fig. 31-23). These beats are referred to as *premature beats*. Premature beats are produced by two basic mechanisms: (1) increased automaticity or (2) reentry, a form of abnormal conduction. Reentry is by far the more common mechanism. During *reentry*, illustrated in Figure 31-24, a single cardiac impulse reenters and excites a myocardial region previously activated, producing a premature beat. These sites can produce isolated premature beats or sustained tachycardias; dysrhythmias can develop in the atria, AV junction, or ventricles and are designated accordingly. For instance, an atrial premature beat originates in the atria, whereas ventricular tachycardia is ventricular in origin.

Ventricular premature beats are the most common form of dysrhythmia (Fig. 31-25, *A* and *B*). However, ventricular irritability can degenerate into life-threatening ventricular tachycardia or ventricular fibrillation. *Ventricular*

tachycardia severely reduces CO as a result of the rapid rate, usually greater than 120 bpm, and the loss of mechanical synchrony between atrial and ventricular contraction (see Fig. 31-25, *C*). *Ventricular fibrillation* results in the abrupt cessation of effective ventricular contraction; the ventricles quiver without coordination (see Fig. 31-25, *D*).

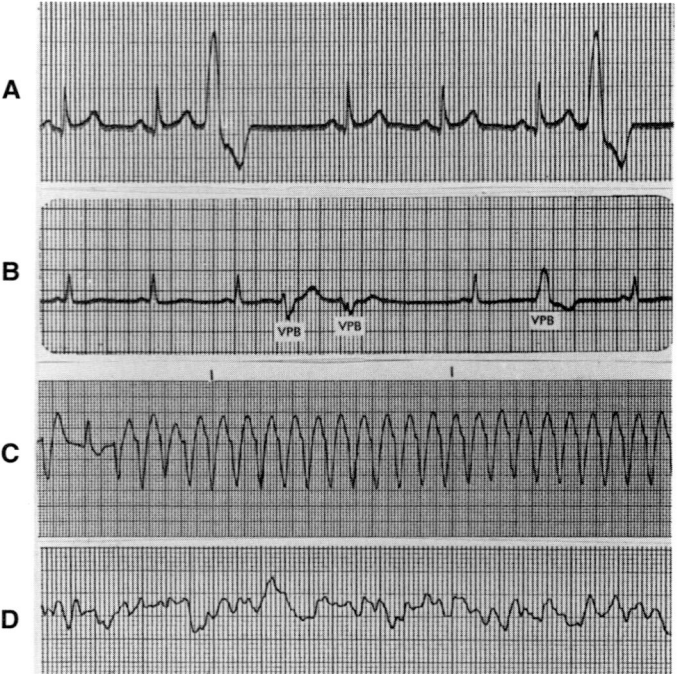

FIG. 31-25 Ventricular dysrhythmias. **A,** Unifocal ventricular premature beats or premature ventricular complexes (*VPBs* or PVCs); since the VPBs are similar in shape, they originated from the same ectopic focus. **B,** Multifocal VPBs have different shapes in the same lead. **C,** Sustained ventricular tachycardia (VT). **D,** Ventricular fibrillation (VF). (From Goldberger AL: *Clinical electrocardiography: a simplified approach,* ed 6, St Louis, 1999, Mosby.)

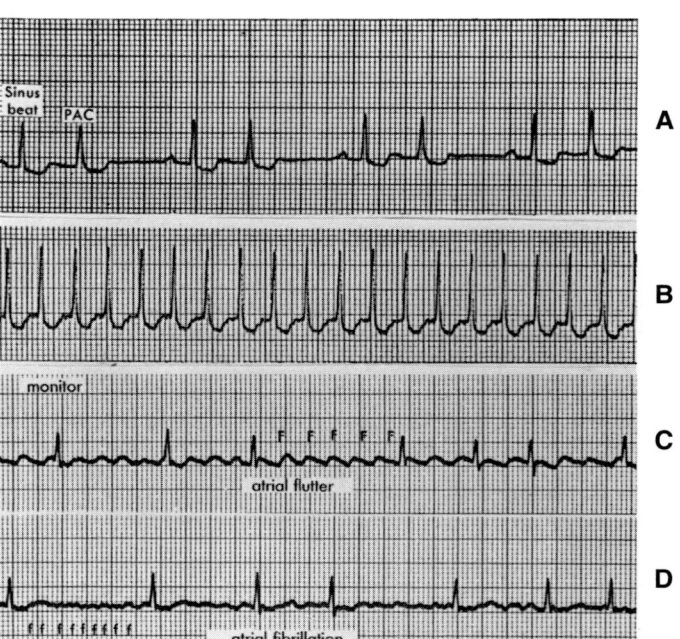

FIG. 31-26 Atrial dysrhythmias. **A,** Atrial bigeminy. Each sinus beat is followed by an atrial premature beat or premature atrial complex (PAC). **B,** Paroxysmal atrial tachycardia (PAT). **C,** Atrial flutter. Note the sawtooth flutter *(F)* waves. **D,** Atrial fibrillation. Note the fine fibrillatory *(f)* waves. (From Goldberger AL: *Clinical electrocardiography: a simplified approach,* ed 6, St Louis, 1999, Mosby.)

Atrial dysrhythmias can be conceptualized along a continuum of rate acceleration associated with progressive reduction in atrial function: (1) *premature atrial beat,* (2) *atrial tachycardia*—atrial rate approximately 150 bpm, (3) *atrial flutter*—atrial rate approximately 300 bpm, and (4) *atrial fibrillation*—quivering, uncoordinated atrial activity (Fig. 31-26). To protect the ventricles from responding to extremely rapid atrial stimulation, the AV node does not normally conduct atrial impulses at rates greater than 180 bpm. For instance, in atrial flutter with an atrial rate of 300 bpm, only every second or third atrial impulse is conducted; consequently, the ventricular rate is 100 to 150 bpm. The hemodynamic response to atrial dysrhythmias depends on the ventricular rate and the efficacy of atrial contraction. For instance, in atrial fibrillation, the atrial musculature is unable to contract effectively and actively contribute to ventricular filling, thus CO may fall.

Heart block is a delay or interruption in impulse conduction between the atria and the ventricles. The cardiac impulse normally spreads from the sinus node along internodal pathways to the AV node and ventricles within 0.20 second (normal PR interval); ventricular depolarization occurs within 0.10 second (normal QRS duration). Heart block occurs in three progressively severe forms. In *first-degree heart block,* all impulses are conducted through the AV junction; however, conduction time is abnormally prolonged. In *second-degree heart block,* some impulses are conducted to the ventricles, but some impulses are blocked. Second-degree heart block consists of two types. Wenckebach (Mobitz I) is characterized by repetitive cycles of progressively lengthening AV conduction time, culminating in the nonconduction of one beat. The second type, Mobitz II, involves conduction of some impulses with a constant AV conduction time and nonconduction of other impulses. In *third-degree heart block,* no impulses are conducted to the ventricles. Cardiac standstill is the result unless *escape pacemakers,* which are either junctional or ventricular in origin, begin to function (Fig. 31-27). *Bundle branch block* is an interruption of conduction in the bundle branches that prolongs ventricular depolarization time beyond 0.10 second.

THERAPEUTIC INTERVENTION

Primary Prevention

The most critical therapeutic intervention in the setting of coronary atherosclerosis is the primary prevention of the disease. Disease prevention is essential for many reasons, including the following:

1. Clinically apparent disease is preceded by a long latent period with silent progression of disease, apparently in early adulthood. Lesions considered as precursors of atherosclerotic disease have been identified in the coronary arterial walls of children and young adults.

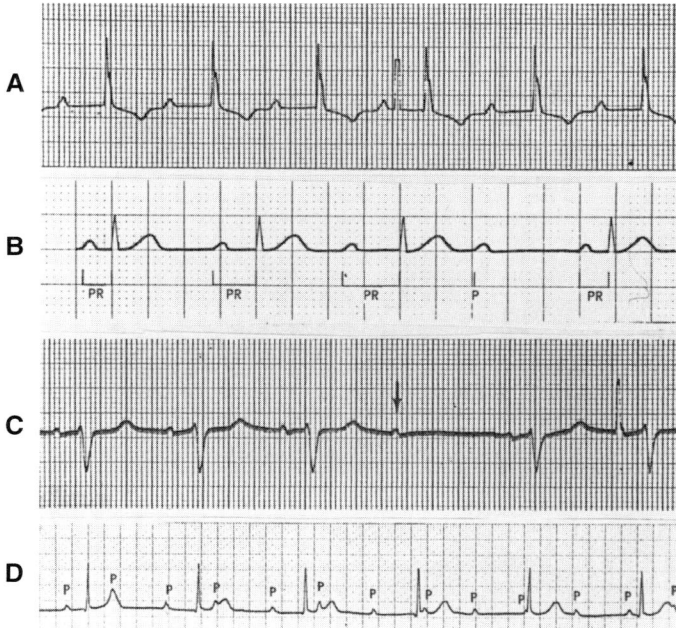

FIG. 31-27   Heart block. **A**, First-degree heart block with uniform prolonged PR intervals of 0.38 second. **B**, Second-degree heart block—Wenckebach or Mobitz I. The PR interval lengthens progressively with successive beats until one P wave is not conducted at all. **C**, Second-degree heart block—Mobitz II. **D**, Third-degree or complete heart block characterized by independent atrial *(P)* and ventricular (QRS) activity. The PR intervals are completely variable. (From Goldberger AL: *Clinical electrocardiography: a simplified approach*, ed 6, St Louis, 1999, Mosby.)

2. No curative therapy exists for coronary atherosclerotic disease. After the disease is recognizable clinically, therapy is essentially palliative, undertaken to minimize the severity of clinical sequelae and potentially to slow disease progression.

3. The consequences of coronary atherosclerosis can be catastrophic. MI often occurs with little or no warning. More than one half of the deaths associated with MI occur during the first few hours of infarction, before hospitalization.

4. Coronary atherosclerosis is the leading cause of death in the United States. According to the American Heart Association, approximately 466,101 deaths were attributable to CHD in the United States in 1997.

Because the precise pathogenesis of atherosclerosis is still undefined, the control of risk factors known to increase susceptibility to atherogenesis is the crux of disease prophylaxis. The risk factors amenable to modification are (1) hyperlipidemia, (2) hypertension, (3) smoking, (4) obesity, (5) sedentary lifestyle, (6) diabetes mellitus, (7) psychosocial stress, and (8) hyperhomocystinemia. Measures should be initiated to eliminate or control these risk factors in every individual, with major emphasis on the first three.

When should risk factor surveillance and control be initiated? Currently, the concept of disease prophylaxis has been applied primarily to "coronary-prone" adults, those with identified risk factors and individuals with evidence of disease. However, control of risk factors earlier in life appears more likely to prevent atherogenesis or retard disease progression so that a substantive reduction in cardiac morbidity and mortality can be achieved. The emphasis must be on health education with early detection and control of risk factors rather than on treatment of the clinical sequelae of established disease.

Treatment

Ischemia and Infarction

The therapeutic aim with acute myocardial ischemia is to prevent myocardial damage by maintaining a balance between myocardial oxygen consumption and oxygen supply (Fig. 31-28). Oxygen supply is maintained by preventing platelet aggregation and thrombosis, which is best achieved by treatment with aspirin, heparin, glycoprotein IIb/IIIa agents, and intravenous (IV) thrombolytics. Aspirin is given as soon as possible after patient presentation and continued on a daily basis indefinitely. The primary goal of aspirin therapy (an antiplatelet agent) is to maintain the patency of the infarct-related artery and reduce the patient's tendency to thrombosis and the likelihood of mural thrombosis formation or deep venous thrombosis, which can result in pulmonary embolism. Sublingual or IV nitroglycerin is the therapeutic mainstay for reversal of ischemia by (1) peripheral vasodilation of the arterial and venous beds, which, in turn, decreases preload and by (2) improving distribution of coronary blood flow to ischemic areas by dilating epicardial arteries and increasing collateral blood flow to ischemic myocardium.

Arterial vasodilation reduces arterial pressure, thereby decreasing the systemic resistance to ventricular ejection and afterload. Dilation of the veins increases the capacity of the venous blood with pooling of blood in the periphery. As a result, venous return to the heart falls, decreasing ventricular volume and size. Consequently, oxygen demand is reduced. IV and long-acting nitrates exhibit similar effects and are useful for reducing ischemia. In the patient with acute MI, sublingual nitroglycerin should be given initially unless the systolic blood pressure is less than 90 mm Hg. If the patient continues to have ischemic pain, the sublingual nitroglycerin may then be repeated until an IV line has been inserted. IV nitroglycerin is then given and titrated to control the patient's pain and blood pressure. Administration of nitrates is not generally recommended in patients with right ventricular infarction because of the resultant decrease in venous return and consequent decrease in right ventricular filling pressure and SV.

Beta-adrenergic blocking agents interrupt ischemia by selectively inhibiting the effects of the sympathetic nervous system on the heart; these effects are mediated by beta receptors. Beta-receptor stimulation increases HR and force of contraction. Beta-blocking agents block these effects, reducing HR and force of contraction, thereby reducing myocardial oxygen requirements. The reduced contractile force produces a mild increment on ventricular size by lowering SV. However, in the absence of heart failure, this slight increment in oxygen demand is greatly outweighed by the reduced demand prompted by blockade of the sympathetic effects on HR and contractility. If sinus tachycardia and hypertension occur in the setting of an acute MI, IV metoprolol tartrate (Lopressor) is then used to decrease myocardial oxygen demand, thereby limiting infarct size and decreasing ischemic pain. Contraindications for the

Acute Ischemia Pathway

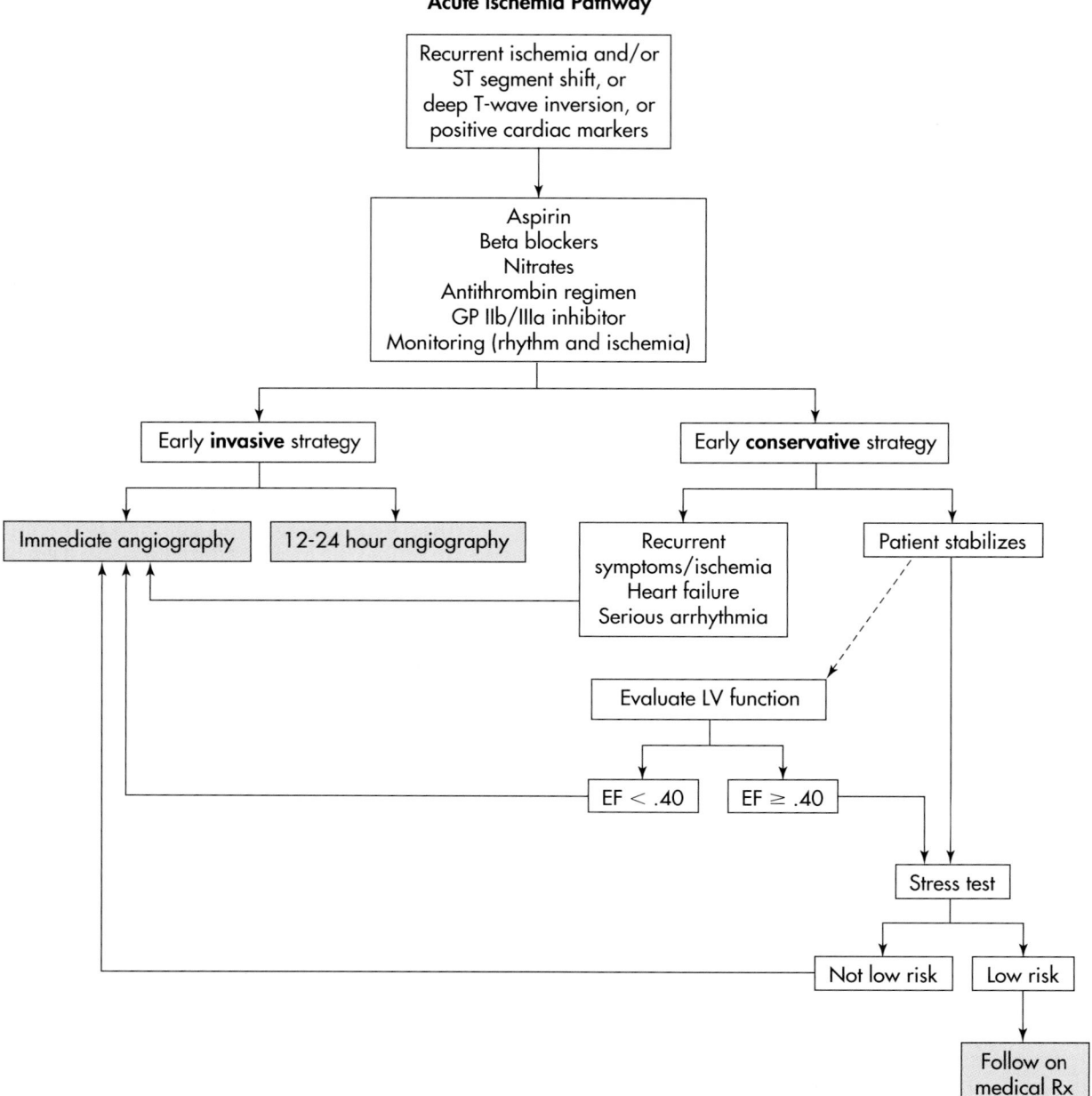

FIG. 31-28 Acute ischemic pathway. *Rx* indicates therapy. (From Braunwald E, Antman EM, Beasley JW, et al: ACC/AHA guidelines for the management of patients with unstable angina: a report of the American College of Cardiology/American Heart Association Task Force on Practice Guidelines (Committee on the Management of Patients with Unstable Angina), *J Am Coll Cardiol* 36:970-1062, 2000.)

use of beta-blocking agents in the treatment of acute MI include the following: HR less than 60 bpm, systolic blood pressure less than 100 mm Hg, moderate to severe left ventricular failure, AV block, and severe chronic obstructive pulmonary disease.

Other pharmacologic interventions similarly act on the determinants of myocardial oxygen demand to correct the oxygenation imbalance. Morphine sulfate is administered in the setting of an acute MI or acute pulmonary congestion. Morphine sulfate decreases myocardial oxygen demand by relieving pain and agitation. Diuretics reduce blood volume and venous return to the heart, thereby reducing ventricular volume and size. Vasodilators, ACE

inhibitors, and calcium channel blockers decrease arterial pressure and resistance to ventricular ejection. Consequently, afterload is reduced. ACE inhibitors act by selectively suppressing renin-angiotensin I to angiotensin II; dilation of arterial and venous vessels occurs. Calcium channel blockers act by inhibiting calcium ion reflux across the cell membrane in cardiac and smooth muscle, thus producing relaxation and vasodilation of coronary and peripheral arteries. Sedatives can also reduce stress-related angina.

Thrombolytic Therapy

Based on the premise that acute MI is caused by coronary thrombosis in most patients, interventions have been aimed at dissolving coronary thrombosis soon after the onset of acute MI to salvage the myocardium, reducing the ultimate size of the infarction. Initiation of treatment within 3 to 6 hours from the onset of symptoms has been widely accepted as a limiting factor for the application of thrombolytic therapy because myocardial necrosis will occur if coronary reperfusion is not carried out before irreversible damage occurs.

The mainstay of acute coronary reperfusion rests with a group of agents called *fibrinolytics*. These agents include drugs such as streptokinase, urokinase, tissue plasminogen activator (TPA), and reteplase recombinant (Retavase). These agents activate the fibrinolytic system, thereby producing clot lysis. By various mechanisms, these agents promote conversion of plasminogen to plasmin, a proteolytic enzyme capable of lysing fibrin clot. By fibrin degradation by plasmin, clot lysis occurs and flow is reestablished to the acutely occluded coronary artery. After fibrinolytic therapy, anticoagulation with heparin and antiplatelet therapy with aspirin are usually carried out to prevent thrombosis.

The current algorithm for the "acute ischemic pathway" (see Fig. 31-28) recommends treatment with *Glycoprotein IIb/IIIa inhibitors* to facilitate thrombolysis and reduce the rate of reocclusion of reperfused vessels. Glycoprotein IIb/IIIa (GP IIb/IIIa) receptors are abundant on a platelet surface. Platelet activation by plaque rupture activates these GP IIb/IIIa receptors, which, in turn, undergo changes in configuration and stimulate a chain of events that leads to fibrinogen binding and platelet aggregation. Currently, three commercial GP IIb/IIIa inhibitors are available: abciximab (ReoPro), tirofiban (Aggrastat), and eptifibatide (Integrilin) (Table 31-5). Abciximab, a monoclonal antibody, binds nonselectively to the GP IIb/IIIa receptors and lasts several days after discontinuing the drug. Studies have shown that abciximab is the most effective of the GP IIb/IIIa inhibitors in decreasing morbidity and mortality; however, it leads all agents in causing thrombocytopenia and bleeding complications. Tirofiban and eptifibatide are small-molecule agents that bind selectively to the GP IIb/IIIa receptors and have a half-life of 2 to 3 hours. The EPIC and EPISTENT trials demonstrated that treatment with abciximab resulted in a 24% to 35% reduction in death of patients with acute MI.

Primary Angioplasty

Angioplasty as a primary treatment for MI is available in some major teaching hospitals. The Primary Angioplasty in Myocardial Infarction (PAMI) Trial found a significant decrease in mortality compared with thrombolytic therapy. Although this therapy is not available for most patients experiencing MI and treated in a community hospital where acute cardiac catheterization is not available, it may be lifesaving in specific cases when thrombolytic therapy is contraindicated (see later discussion).

Two potential consequences of myocardial dysfunction that can further the reduction in myocardial oxygen supply are hypoxemia and hypotension. In the setting of *hypoxemia*, oxygen administration can increase the oxygen content of arterial blood and, consequently, myocardial oxygen delivery. *Hypotension* reduces coronary perfusion pressure. This result is particularly worrisome because diseased coronary vessels, unable to dilate to increase flow, are "pressure dependent" to maintain flow. A reduction in coronary perfusion pressure can perpetuate the ischemic

TABLE 31-5 ■■■

Glycoprotein IIb/IIIa Inhibitors

	Abciximab	Tirofiban	Eptifibatide
Half-life	1-2 days	2-3 hours	2-3 hours
Binding to GP IIb/IIIa receptors	Nonselective	Selective	Selective
Cost	Expensive	Inexpensive	Inexpensive

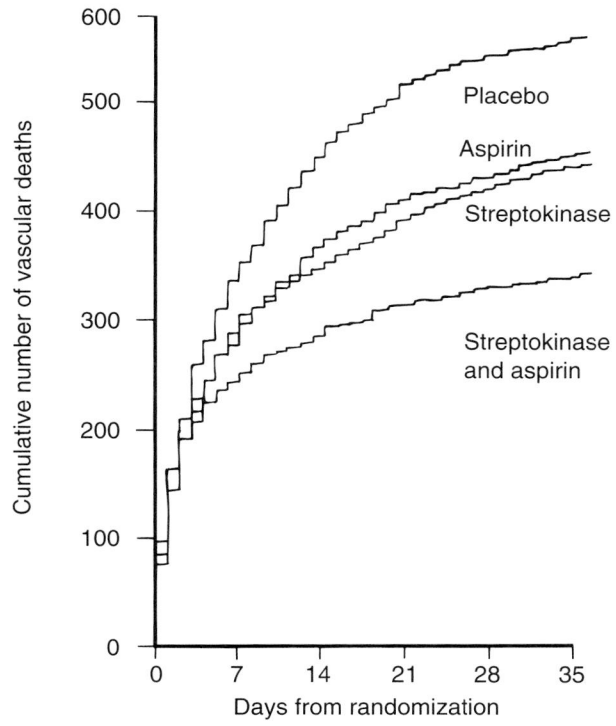

FIG. 31-29 Cumulative vascular mortality of 17,187 patients during the first 5 weeks after MI randomly assigned to four treatment groups: placebo (control) group, aspirin group, streptokinase group; and aspirin plus streptokinase group. Both aspirin alone or streptokinase alone significantly reduced mortality, but the reduction was greatest when these two drugs were given in combination. Deaths in the placebo group were 13.2% (568/4300), 10.7% in the aspirin group (461/4295), 10.4% in the streptokinase group (448/4300), and 8% in the aspirin plus streptokinase group (343/4292). (Redrawn from ISIS-2 [Second International Study of Infarct Survival] Collaborative Group: *Lancet* 8607:354, 1988.)

imbalance. Therefore, in cases complicated by cardiogenic shock, vasopressors to maintain arterial pressure or volume administration to maintain adequate ventricular filling pressures and SV may be indicated. Dysrhythmias can also adversely affect coronary perfusion by reducing cardiac output (CO) and arterial pressure; therefore antidysrhythmics (primarily IV lidocaine) may be helpful.

Aspirin therapy, used as an antiplatelet aggregant, is begun after MI whether patients have been treated with thrombolytics. Data from the Second International Study of Infarct Survival (ISIS-2) trial (Fig. 31-29) show that aspirin alone was able to reduce mortality after MI when compared with a placebo. After MI, rest with monitored return to daily activities through a cardiac rehabilitation program is the primary therapy, allowing the infarcted tissue to heal, thus reducing the incidence of complications and salvaging the ischemic zone surrounding the infarct, thereby reducing the ultimate size of the infarct.

Coronary Revascularization

Either surgically redirecting flow around the obstruction with a bypass graft or increasing flow in the native vessel by a catheter-based treatment can improve blood flow to myocardium beyond an atherosclerotic lesion in the coronary artery. The first *coronary artery bypass graft (CABG)* was performed in 1969 by Favaloro. For nearly a decade, cardiac surgical bypass techniques were unrivaled as the preferred method for myocardial revascularization. In 1977, however, Gruentzig performed the first catheter-based treatment of the coronary arteries with the introduction of *percutaneous transluminal coronary angioplasty (PTCA)*. These techniques for coronary revascularization are discussed in greater detail in the next section. Notable, however, the relative indications for these interventions, either alone or in combination, are constantly evolving as technology changes and as results of outcome studies are known.

Catheter-Based Revascularization

Catheter-based revascularization therapy offers an alternative to CABG surgery for many patients whose atherosclerotic CAD has resulted in unstable angina and acute ischemic syndromes. Additionally, catheter-based therapies offer treatment options to patients who have already undergone CABG surgery. These catheter interventions are performed in the cardiac catheterization laboratory under fluoroscopy. A small catheter is passed through the skin into the femoral artery (percutaneous) and over a guide wire into the narrowed section of the coronary artery (transluminal) via the aorta. Several different types of intervention techniques have been developed to achieve revascularization including *percutaneous transluminal coronary angioplasty (PTCA), percutaneous transluminal coronary rotablator atherectomy (PTCRA), stent* placement, *directional coronary atherectomy (DCA), AngioJet, brachytherapy,* and *laser therapy.*

PTCA involves inflation of a balloon at the site of the lesion, which compresses and splits the atherosclerotic plaque within the intimal layer of the coronary artery. Additionally, stretching and partial disruption of the medial and adventitial layers occur, which increases the overall diameter of the artery (Fig. 31-30). Stents are wire mesh tubes that are often placed at PTCA treatment sites to act as mechanical scaffolding to prevent elastic recoil of the artery (and restenosis) or to treat coronary dissections. Vein graft lesions in patients who have already undergone CABG surgery are often treated with coronary stents. The intima grows over the stent within 1 month, making it a permanent part of the vessel wall.

PTCRA is used to restore patency to vessels when the atherosclerotic lesion is calcified or totally occludes the lumen. The PTCRA has a diamond-tipped burr that rotates quickly and pulverizes the plaque into particles the size of red blood cells. The DCA has a blade that shaves off and mechanically removes plaque. The plaque is then shoved into the nose cone of the catheter and removed from the vessel with the catheter. AngioJet uses an irrigation and aspiration device within the catheter to remove coronary occlusions associated with large

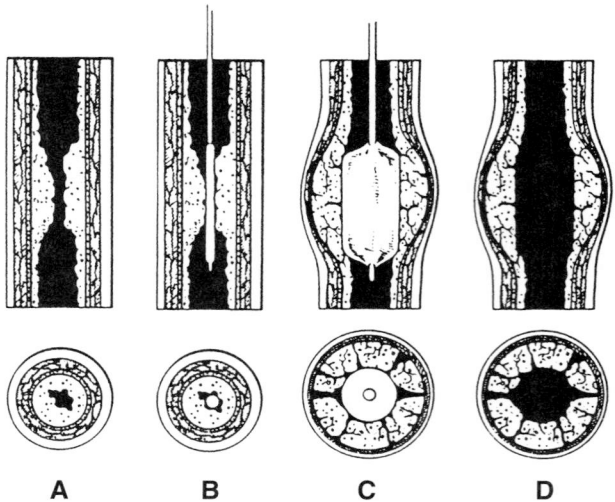

FIG. 31-30 Percutaneous transluminal coronary angioplasty (PTCA). Serial panels show the baseline stenosis (**A**), passage of the deflated balloon catheter (**B**), balloon inflation (**C**), and the postdilation appearance (**D**), as drawn in longitudinal and cross-sectional views. Balloon inflation (**C**) is associated with fracture and outward displacement of the atherosclerotic plaque, as well as stretching of the media and adventitia. The result (**D**) is enlargement of the lumen because of the expansion of the entire vessel wall rather than compaction of the atherosclerotic material. (From Casteneda-Zuniga WR et al: The mechanism of balloon angioplasty, *Radiology* 135:565, 1980.)

amounts of blood clot. This procedure is used primarily to treat vein graft lesions with clot, as well as to remove coronary artery thrombi in the acute MI setting.

Laser angioplasty uses the heat of the laser beam to destroy or vaporize contingent plaque. Brachytherapy involves the use of local radiation to treat vessels that repeatedly renarrow (restenosis) after catheter-based treatments. The procedure involves delivery of local radiation via the temporary insertion of radioactive beads at the treatment site. A radiation oncologist delivers an appropriate radiation dose based on body size. Brachytherapy has shown great success in preventing further restenosis.

Initially, PTCA was recommended only for patients with single-vessel disease. Improved catheter technology and growing experience with the procedure, however, have enabled patients with accessible multivessel disease to also be considered acceptable candidates for PTCA in some centers. An estimated 680,000 angioplasty procedures were performed in the United States in 1997. If the procedure fails because dilations were unsuccessful or complications occurred, emergency surgical vascularization or placement of a metal scaffold (known as a stent) is then necessary to control the dissected coronary artery. Because of this risk, all patients undergoing PTCA must be able to tolerate the rigors of cardiac surgery and should be candidates for CABG surgery (described later). In approximately 20% to 30% of patients undergoing PTCA, clinical *restenosis* or narrowing of the vessel may recur within 6 months; the incidence may be even higher, depending on the location of the stenosis (higher in left anterior descending [LAD] and ostial lesions) or the presence of cardiovascular risk factors, such as elevated

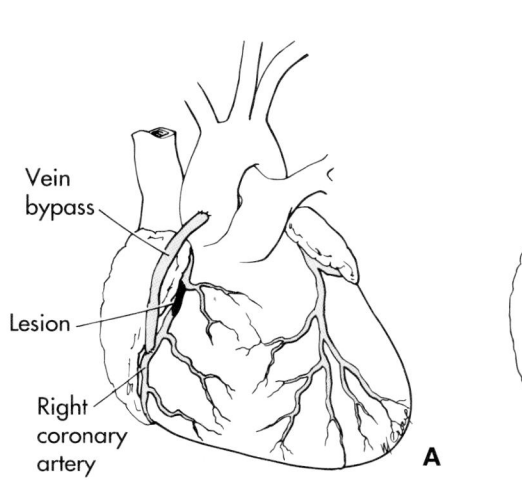
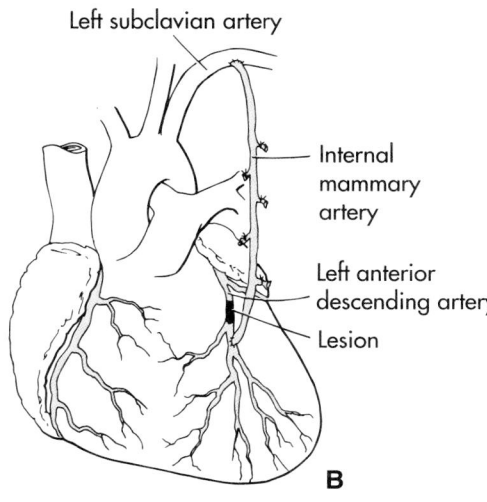

FIG. 31-31   Coronary artery revascularization procedures. **A**, Saphenous vein is sutured to the ascending aorta and to the right coronary artery at a point distal to the blockage so that flow distal to the blockage is again established. **B**, The internal mammary artery is anastomosed to the anterior descending branch of the left coronary artery, bypassing the lesion.

LDL-C or diabetes mellitus. Restenosis can usually be treated with a second intervention.

With angioplasty, patients are treated more quickly, at a lower cost, and without the risks and complications of open-heart surgery. However, patients with left main CAD or complex diffuse narrowing in more than two major epicardial arteries are probably best treated by CABG surgery.

Surgical Revascularization

The standard conduits for CABG procedures are the greater saphenous vein from the leg and the left internal mammary artery (LIMA) from the chest. With saphenous vein bypass grafting, one end of the vein segment is anastomosed to the ascending aorta, and the other end is attached beyond the site of vessel obstruction (Fig. 31-31, *A*). Therefore a vascular conduit is created to shunt blood around the lesion to the myocardium at risk. With LIMA grafting, the origin of the LIMA at the subclavian artery usually remains intact and the distal end of the vessel is sectioned and anastomosed to the coronary artery (see Fig. 31-31, *B*).

Each procedure offers distinct advantages and disadvantages. The saphenous vein bypass graft provides higher flow rates because of the larger vessel caliber. The area is easily accessible from the leg and can be positioned with greater latitude on the surface of the heart. However, a significant incidence of late graft closure is caused by fibrous overgrowth of the intimal wall of the vein. The late patency rate of the internal mammary bypass grafts is superior to that of the saphenous vein making it the vascular conduit of choice. Other advantages of this procedure include the absence of a leg incision and the need for one, rather than two, anastomoses. Given its anterior location, the internal mammary artery is most frequently used to bypass the LAD artery, and saphenous vein segments are used for lesions of the right and circumflex coronary arteries and their branches.

Current indications for elective surgical revascularization include the following: (1) significant triple-vessel coronary artery stenosis and (2) significant left main coronary artery occlusion. Surgery is considered whenever documented evidence exists of large territories of myocardium at risk for infarction. Single- and double-vessel CAD may be an indication if PTCA is not technically possible or has failed to ensure long-term patency of the arteries. Patients with ischemia-induced failure, but not those with chronic ventricular failure, are candidates for surgery.

Urgent surgical revascularization is considered for patients with unstable angina or postinfarction angina who are not PTCA candidates. Surgery is the treatment of choice when CAD has led to significant mitral valve dysfunction, ventricular septal rupture, or ventricular aneurysm. Revascularization is performed in conjunction with repair of the mechanical defect.

Complications
General Principles

Early detection and prevention of complications are essential after treatment of coronary disease. Two categories of complications must be anticipated: electrical instability or dysrhythmias and mechanical dysfunction or pump failure. ECG monitoring is initiated immediately. Dysrhythmia management follows logical principles:

1. Parasympathetic stimulation (e.g., carotid sinus massage), antidysrhythmic drugs (e.g., verapamil), or electrical cardioversion, when necessary, decelerate tachycardias. Drugs that inhibit parasympathetic effects (e.g., atropine) can accelerate bradycardias when they compromise perfusion. Electrical pacing may be indicated when drugs are ineffective.
2. Escape beats, which result from sinus node failure, must be differentiated from premature beats to effectively treat rhythm disturbances originating in sites other than the sinus node. To treat escape rhythms, drugs are administered to speed the normal pacemaker, the sinus node; drugs must not be given to suppress the escape pacemaker, because cardiac standstill can result.

Ventricular dysrhythmias associated with ischemia usually respond best to lidocaine (Xylocaine); otherwise, procainamide is the drug of choice. Ventricular fibrillation requires immediate defibrillation with cardiopulmonary resuscitative maneuvers. Managing refractory ventricular dysrhythmias is reviewed later.

Administering an antidysrhythmic drug best controls atrial dysrhythmias. Amiodarone is currently the drug of choice for treating atrial fibrillation. Electrical cardioversion may be indicated to restore the normal rhythm when the dysrhythmia persists and is poorly tolerated.

3. Therapy of heart block is directed at restoring or simulating normal conduction, by either administering drugs to speed conduction and HR, such as atropine, or external pacing as a bridge to a permanent pacemaker.

Mechanical dysfunction produces a clinical spectrum ranging from mild congestive heart failure to cardiogenic shock. *Congestive heart failure (CHF)* prompts efforts to (1) reduce intravascular volume (preload) and congestion and the associated fluid transudation into the lungs and to (2) improve myocardial function by preventing ventricular remodeling, which is the central feature in the progression of heart failure. IV diuretics, such as furosemide, and IV vasodilators, such as nitroglycerin and nitroprusside, promptly decrease preload by decreasing venous return in acute CHF or pulmonary edema. Long-term treatment for heart failure includes dietary sodium restriction and digoxin.

Angiotensin-converting enzyme (ACE) inhibitors have become mainstays of treatment. ACE inhibitors work by inhibiting the conversion of angiotensin I to angiotensin II. Angiotensin II has a twofold effect: (1) it causes peripheral vascular vasoconstriction and elevation of blood pressure, and (2) it stimulates the production of aldosterone, which, in turn, increases preload by causing renal sodium and water retention.

When the angiotensin II mechanism is stimulated in the setting of hypovolemic trauma, such as severe blood loss from a knife wound, the effects are beneficial. However, when angiotensin II is produced in response to a low CO from CHF (decreased effective circulating volume), a vicious cycle occurs, resulting in refractory heart failure. Recent studies have demonstrated a decrease in mortality when patients with heart failure or MI are treated with ACE inhibitors; thus ACE inhibitors are becoming an integral treatment for both patient populations to prevent ventricular remodeling.

An older drug, spironolactone (Aldactone), is enjoying resurgence as a front-line treatment for CHF. Spironolactone is an angiotensin I receptor antagonist or aldosterone receptor antagonist, which recent studies have shown to decrease mortality in patients with CHF. Although ACE inhibitors decrease the amount of circulating angiotensin II, an "aldosterone escape phenomenon" is observed, indicating that other pathways form angiotensin II. Studies suggest that aldosterone is responsible for the ventricular remodeling, observed in CHF patients, by stimulating cardiac collagen synthesis and tissue proliferation. Spironolactone is believed to decrease mortality by inhibiting this high collagen turnover and subsequent remodeling. The Randomized Aldactone Evaluation Study (RALES) shows an overall 30% decrease in mortality in CHF patients already treated with ACE inhibitors, digitalis, and diuretics when spironolactone was added to the treatment regimen.

Progression of left ventricular failure to *cardiogenic shock*, characterized by inadequate tissue perfusion, is an ominous development. This syndrome, with a mortality rate approaching 68%, remains a therapeutic dilemma. (See Chapter 33 for a detailed discussion of cardiogenic shock.)

Pacing Therapy

The use of pacemakers has become increasingly sophisticated. Both temporary and permanent implantable pulse generators have been developed with a variety of pacing characteristics. Current pulse generators are capable of pacing either the atria or the ventricles or pacing both atria and ventricles sequentially. Pacing stimuli can be delivered in demand or fixed-rate modes. In *demand pacing* the pacer fires on demand as determined by the patient's intrinsic rate. By contrast, *fixed-rate pacing* delivers a stimulus at a predetermined, fixed rate. An international classification system has been developed to standardize pacemaker coding (Table 31-6). Temporary pacing may be performed transcutaneously, when necessary after an acute MI. Skin pads with leads to the pacemaker are placed on the patient's chest in the anterior and posterior positions. The ECG is sensed through these leads and conveyed to the pulse generator of the pacemaker. When the ventricular heart rate falls below a preset limit (40 bpm), the pulse generator will deliver an electrical stimulus through the skin pads, producing a ventricular contraction.

Management of Refractory Ventricular Dysrhythmias

The presence of recurrent, malignant ventricular dysrhythmias that are unresponsive to standard pharmacologic therapy is an indication for *electrophysiologic (EP) evaluation*. These dysrhythmias are usually present in the setting

---

TABLE 31-6 ■ ■ ■

The North American Society of Pacing and Electrophysiology/British Pacing and Electrophysiology Group Generic Pacemaker Code*

Position I: Chamber Paced†	Position II: Chamber Sensed	Position III: Mode of Response	Position IV: Programmable Functions; Rate Modulation	Position V: Antitachyarrhythmia Functions
O = None	O = None	O = None	O = None	O = None
A = Atrium	A = Atrium	T = Triggers pacing	P = Programmable rate and/or output	P = Pacing (antitachyarrhythmia)
V = Ventricle	V = Ventricle	I = Inhibits pacing	M = Multiprogramability of rate, output, sensitivity, etc.	S = Shock
D = Dual (A + V)	D = Dual (A + V)	D = Dual (T + I) Triggers/inhibits pacing	C = Communicating functions (telemetry)	D = Dual (P + S)
			R = Rate modulation	

From Bernstein AD et al: *PACE* 10:794, 1987.
*Positions I to III are used exclusively for antibradyarrhythmia pacing.
†Manufacturers use S for single chamber (atria or ventricles). When designing adaptive rate pacing modes (DDDR, VVIR), four positions will be required.

of chronic ischemic heart disease. Ventricular aneurysms or previous ventricular surgery may predispose the patient to the development of refractory ventricular dysrhythmias. Before the initial EP study, all antidysrhythmic drugs are discontinued when possible. Catheters with multiple electrodes are then positioned within the right atrium, right ventricle, and coronary sinus under fluoroscopic guidance (see Fig. 30-15 for catheter placement). A stimulation protocol is followed to induce ventricular tachycardia; this programmed stimulation can consist of progressively more premature ventricular stimuli, double-ventricular extrastimuli, or bursts of rapid ventricular pacing. Intracardiac recordings of the dysrhythmia are obtained. The dysrhythmia is terminated with another burst of rapid ventricular pacing or countershock when required.

The purposes of EP testing are (1) to diagnose the type of dysrhythmia and its mechanism, (2) to localize and map the site of the dysrhythmia, and (3) to determine the best course of treatment, depending on the previous information. The options for treatment include (1) pharmacologic; (2) device implantation—antitachycardia pacing or implantable cardiac defibrillators (ICDs) or both; and (3) radiofrequency ablation using a transvenous or transarterial approach.

When drug trials are ineffective in treating the dysrhythmia, alternate therapies such as electrical therapy or surgery are considered. Radiofrequency catheter ablation (Fig. 31-32) or ICDs may be used in selected patients. If discrete sites of electrical activation can be found, radiolfrequency catheter ablation is delivered. With the use of high-frequency sound waves, a scar is created in the circuit causing the dysrhythmia. An attempt to reproduce the dysrhythmia is made after the radiofrequency ablation is completed. The ablation is considered successful when the dysrhythmia cannot be reproduced.

Electrical therapy for ventricular tachycardia is now available in the form of a programmable antitachycardia device. EP testing is performed to determine the most effective mode of therapy before device implantation. The currently available devices offer antitachycardia pacing. When the dysrhythmia is responsive to pace termination, the device can be programmed for the following two types of termination methods:

1. *Ramp pacing.* The cycle length of the stimulus is "captured" or "paced" for a predetermined time. Pacing is then terminated with the hope that the mechanism of the tachycardia is interrupted and normal sinus rhythm restored.
2. *Burst pacing.* A rapid sequence of pacing is initiated to interrupt and terminate the dysrhythmia.

The device is capable of being programmed to sense ongoing or recurrent ventricular tachycardia and will cardiovert the heart with the lowest amount of electrical stimulation possible to depolarize a critical mass of myocardium. When the stimulus is ineffective, countershocks are delivered until a successful countershock is given or the programmed number of shocks has been delivered.

Surgical Repair of Mechanical Defects

Aneurysmectomy is the removal of the noncontractile, paradoxically bulging scar. Three indications for aneurysm resection include (1) chronic congestive heart failure, (2) systemic embolization of mural thrombi, and (3) recurrent ventricular dysrhythmias. Aneurysms are

associated with a high incidence of malignant, refractory ventricular dysrhythmias, perhaps resulting from the persistent mechanical strain at the boundary between the normal myocardium and the scarred, outpouching segment. The aneurysm is excised through the left ventricular scar with removal of mural thrombi. Removal of the aneurysm and subsequent reduction of ventricular size improves the mechanical efficiency of the heart. Intraoperatively, the site causing recurrent ventricular dysrhythmias can be localized and excised or sectioned.

A *ventricular septal defect* can be repaired either by simple closure of the hole in the septum or by insertion of a patch graft; access to the septum is gained via the infarct in the ventricle. On closure of the left ventricular incision, a portion of the noncontractile left ventricular scar is frequently excised, a procedure referred to as *infarctectomy.*

Dysfunction of the mitral valve resulting from papillary muscle rupture or malfunction necessitates *mitral valve replacement* with excision of the papillary muscles.

Cardiac transplantation can be lifesaving for patients considered inoperable or unsalvageable with less aggressive surgical intervention. Patients with end-stage heart disease are considered for transplantation. The procedure involves removal of the diseased heart and replacement with a normal donor heart. Technically, the surgery is uncomplicated, requiring reanastomoses of the separated vessels with the donor heart. Cardiac transplantation is discussed in more detail in Chapter 33.

Rehabilitation

The ultimate goal of therapeutic intervention in coronary atherosclerotic disease is to restore the cardiac patient to

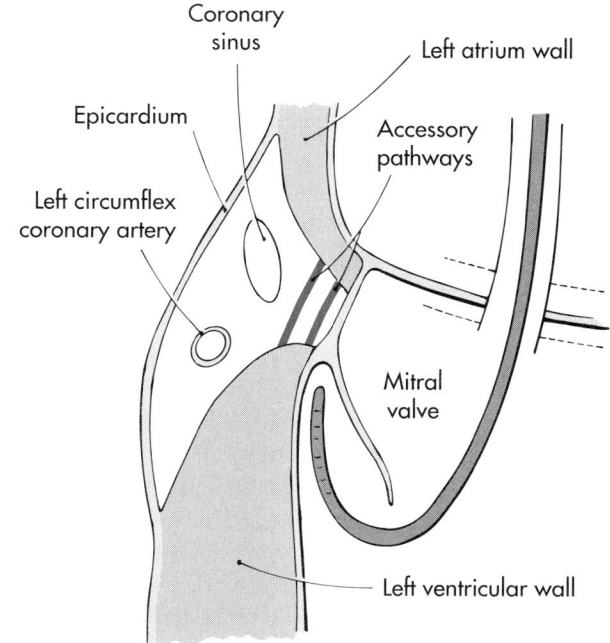

FIG. 31-32 Procedure for radiofrequency catheter ablation of an accessory pathway that is causing a refractory dysrhythmia. A cross section of the left ventricular wall is shown at the level of the atrioventricular groove. (Redrawn from Wagshal AB, Pires LA, Huang SK: Management of cardiac arrhythmias and radiofrequency catheter ablation, *Arch Intern Med* 155(2):137, 1995.)

a productive and satisfying lifestyle. The long-term consequences of MI—physical, psychologic, social, and vocational invalidism—have long been ignored with devastating impact. The complications of myocardial disease are not restricted to the hospital setting, and the responsibility of health professionals for the ultimate well being and coping ability of patients does not terminate on their discharge from the hospital. As early as clinically feasible, patients should be enrolled in an inpatient cardiovascular rehabilitation program that will continue after hospital discharge within an outpatient setting.

Cardiac rehabilitation, as defined by the American Heart Association and the Task Force on Cardiovascular Rehabilitation of the National Heart, Lung, and Blood Institute, is the process of restoring and maintaining the physical, psychologic, social, educational, and vocational potentials of the patient.

Patients must be assisted to progressively resume a level of activity consistent with physical limitations and to be relatively unhampered by psychologic stressors. Many patients can resume all normal activities. Explicit, individualized patient and family education about diet; medications; activity progression, particularly regarding resumption of sexual relations; and risk factor reduction and modification is essential. Every patient and family requires guidance and education during the transition from the dependence of illness to the independence of health.

KEY CONCEPTS

- The determinants of *myocardial oxygen demand* include heart rate, contractile force, muscle mass, and ventricular wall tension.
- Local tissue *hypoxia* is the most potent stimulus to increasing coronary blood flow.
- *Ischemia* is a transient, reversible state of inadequate blood flow.
- Prolonged ischemia will lead to tissue death or *necrosis*.
- *Coronary atherosclerosis*, an inflammatory response to endothelial injury, is the most common cause of coronary artery disease (CAD).
- *CAD* causes myocardial ischemia and dysfunction when the lesion obstructs more than 75% of the vessel lumen.
- *Fatty streaks* are flat, nonobstructive yellowish patches on the endothelial surface of a vessel; they do not necessarily lead to CAD.
- *Fibrous plaques* are palpable elevated areas of intimal thickening that can lead to *complicated lesions* when their fibrous cap is vulnerable and ultimately lead to coronary thrombosis and an MI.
- Plaque rupture can cause vasoconstriction of the coronary artery and thrombosis leading to an *acute ischemic syndrome*.
- *Major modifiable risk factors* for coronary atherosclerotic disease include elevated LDL-C, low HDL-C, hypertension, cigarette smoking, diabetes mellitus, sedentary lifestyle, obesity (particularly the abdominal type), and elevated homocysteine levels.
- The therapeutic National Cholesterol Education Program (NCEP) therapeutic guidelines recommend a treatment goal of *LDL-C* less than 100 mg/dl for patients with CAD.
- A class of drugs called *HMG CoA reductase inhibitors* have demonstrated regression and delayed progression of CAD; they inhibit an enzyme, 3-hydroxy-3-methylglutaryl coenzyme A (HMG CoA), that decreases LDL-C synthesis and enhances its clearance by the liver.
- *Hypertension* is defined as a systolic BP greater than 140 mm Hg or a diastolic BP greater than 90 mm Hg or both; it may be managed by lifestyle changes, such as decreasing dietary sodium, increasing dietary potassium, weight loss, cessation of smoking, stress management, and increasing aerobic activity, as well as with pharmacologic agents, such as diuretics, beta blockers, and ACE inhibitors. ACE inhibitors are particularly helpful in patients with the co-morbidities of diabetes mellitus, renal insufficiency, and heart failure.
- *Diabetes* is the most potent risk factor for atherosclerotic heart disease in women.
- The normal level for *homocysteine* is 5 to 15 μmol/L. Increased levels of homocysteine blocks the production of nitric oxide in the cells of blood vessels, leading to less pliable and reactive coronary vessels and initiation of plaque buildup.
- An MI is termed either a *Q-wave infarction* or a *non-Q-wave infarction (NQWMI)*. The ECG changes in a Q-wave MI consist of pronounced Q waves, ST-segment elevation, and inverted T waves. The ST-segment and T wave changes will revert back to normal, leaving the Q waves as a permanent ECG manifestation of the MI. In an NQWMI, only transient ST depression or T wave inversions return to normal within 72 hours. A NQWMI leaves no permanent ECG manifestation.
- *Myocardial ischemia* leads to impaired wall motion and altered *hemodynamics*. As a result, left-sided heart pressures, such as pulmonary capillary wedge pressure (PCWP), rise. Myocardial ischemia is typically shown as ST-segment depression or T wave inversions (or both) on the ECG.
- The *biomarkers, creatinine kinase (CK)* and *troponins*, are used to diagnose an MI. Both are elevated in the setting of an MI. CK is an enzyme released in the presence of muscle injury and has three enzyme fractions: CK-MM, CK-BB, and CK-MB. The CK-MB enzyme is specific for myocardial damage. The cardiac troponins, cTnT and cTnI, are also indicative of myocardial injury.
- The diagnosis of *MI* depends on the presence of three variables: the patient presentation, the ECG findings, and elevations of the biochemical markers, CK-MB and cardiac troponins.

- *Pericarditis* is an inflammation of the pericardial sac and is diagnosed by patient presentation and the ECG evidence of global ST-segment elevation and PR-segment depression.
- *Cardiogenic shock* may be caused by a profound loss of 40% of the myocardium after a massive MI and can lead to refractory CHF and death.
- Consequences of *MI* can include CHF, pericarditis, papillary muscle dysfunction, ventricular septal defect, and cardiac rupture.
- The last step in an acute ischemic syndrome is the development of a clot. *Thrombolytic agents*, such as tissue plasminogen activator (TPA), streptokinase, and reteplase recombinant, when given within the

first 6 hours of an MI, will limit and even possibly abort the MI.
- The long-term consequence of *CHF* is ventricular remodeling and refractory failure. The pharmacologic agents, ACE inhibitors, and spironolactone can prevent remodeling.
- Catheter-based therapies, such as *angioplasty* and coronary stents, offer an alternative to CABG surgery for many patients with atherosclerotic CAD.
- *ACE inhibitors* are used in the treatment of hypertension and CHF; they prevent the conversion of angiotensin I to angiotensin II, thereby decreasing afterload and preload.

QUESTIONS ??

A sampling of review questions for this chapter appears here. Visit http://www.mosby.com/MERLIN/PriceWilson/ for additional questions. MERLIN

Answer the following on a separate sheet of paper.
1. Explain why the left ventricle is most vulnerable to ischemia and infarction.
2. What are the most common sites of coronary arterial occlusion?
3. Name five factors that affect the degree of functional impairment after an acute MI.
4. What is a vasovagal response, and what might cause this response after an acute

MI? How does it affect the compensatory response?
5. Name three important diagnostic findings associated with MI.
6. Explain why either tachycardias or bradycardias may hemodynamically impair cardiac function.
7. Identify three hemodynamic factors that may be modified to reduce oxygen demand in the treatment of myocardial ischemia.

8. Explain "silent ischemia" and its etiologic factors.
9. What are the two chemical biomarkers used in diagnosing myocardial injury?
10. How do ACE inhibitors work in the treatment of CHF?
11. Why is rehabilitation an important aspect of the treatment of patients with atherosclerotic heart disease?

Fill in the blanks with the correct word or circle the correct word.
12. In MI, an area of _____ surrounds the area of infarction.
13. A reduction in ventricular wall compliance (increases) (decreases) pressure for a constant ventricular volume.
14. Arrange in correct order the following changes that occur after an acute MI.
   a. Removal of necrotic tissue
   b. Bruised and cyanotic tissue
   c. Scar formation
   d. Polymorphonuclear neutrophil infiltration

Match the characteristics in column A with the disorders in column B.

	Column A	Column B
15. _____	ST-segment depression typical	a. Myocardial ischemia
16. _____	ST-segment elevation typical	b. Myocardial infarction (MI)
17. _____	Deep Q waves	
18. _____	Pain relieved by nitroglycerin	
19. _____	Muscle death	
20. _____	Muscle hypoxia	
21. _____	If prolonged, results in necrosis	
22. _____	Reversible	
23. _____	Irreversible	

Match each of the dysrhythmias in column A with its possible therapeutic intervention in column B.

	Column A	Column B
24. _____	Sinus bradycardia	a. Carotid sinus massage
25. _____	Atrial tachycardia	b. Defibrillation
26. _____	Multiple premature ventricular beats	c. Lidocaine
27. _____	Ventricular fibrillation	d. Atropine

Valvular Heart Disease

MADELINE M. O'DONNELL AND PENNY FORD CARLETON

𝒱alvular disease causes abnormalities in blood flow across the cardiac valves. Normal valves demonstrate two critical flow characteristics: unidirectional flow and unimpeded flow. The valves open when the pressure in the chamber proximal to the valve exceeds the pressure in the chamber or vessel beyond the valve. Closure occurs when the pressure beyond the valve exceeds pressure in the proximal chamber. For instance, the atrioventricular valves open when atrial pressures exceed ventricular pressures and close when ventricular pressures exceed atrial pressures. The valve leaflets are so responsive that even a slight pressure difference (less than 1 mm Hg) between chambers will open and close the leaflets.

A diseased valve can produce two types of functional derangements: (1) *valvular regurgitation*—the valve leaflets fail to close securely, permitting backward flow (*valvular insufficiency* and *valvular incompetence* are synonymous terms) and (2) *valvular stenosis*—the valve orifice becomes restricted, impeding forward flow. Regurgitation and stenosis can occur together in the same valve as a "mixed lesion," or either one can occur alone as a "pure lesion."

Valvular dysfunction increases cardiac work. Valvular regurgitation forces the heart to pump the additional regurgitant volume of blood, thus producing an increment

in *volume work.* Valvular stenosis necessitates the generation of increased pressure to overcome the increased resistance to flow, thereby elevating *pressure work.* The characteristic myocardial responses to increased volume work and pressure work are chamber dilation and muscular hypertrophy, respectively. Myocardial dilation and hypertrophy are compensatory mechanisms intended to increase the pumping capability of the heart.

PATHOGENESIS

Valvular heart disease was once considered to be almost entirely rheumatic in origin; however, today, new types of valve disease are becoming increasingly more prevalent. The most common condition is degenerative valve disease, which is related to the increased life span of people living in industrialized countries compared with those in developing countries. Despite the declining incidence of rheumatic fever, rheumatic damage is still a common cause of valvular deformity requiring surgical correction. *Acute rheumatic fever* is a sequela of a group A beta-hemolytic streptococcal pharyngitis. Rheumatic fever develops only when a significant immunologic or antibody response to the antecedent streptococcal infection occurs. Approximately 3% of pharyngeal streptococcal infections are followed within 2 to 4 weeks by attacks of rheumatic fever. Initial attacks of rheumatic fever are typically observed during childhood and the early teenage years. The incidence of streptococcal infection, and therefore of rheumatic fever, is directly related to factors predisposing to the development and transmission of infection; socioeconomic factors, such as living conditions and access to medical care and antibiotic therapy, are foremost in this regard. Both rheumatic fever and mitral stenosis remain common in developing nations, with a higher incidence among the urban poor compared with the rural poor. Currently, a vaccine to protect against streptococcal nasopharyngeal infections is being developed.

The precise pathogenesis of rheumatic fever is unknown. Two possible mechanisms are (1) a hyperimmune response, either autoimmune or allergic in nature, and (2) a direct effect of the streptococcal organisms or its toxins. An immunologic explanation is considered most plausible, although the latter mechanism cannot be entirely ruled out. An autoimmune reaction to a streptococcal infection would hypothetically produce tissue damage, or manifestations of rheumatic disease, as follows:

1. Group A streptococcus would produce pharyngeal infection.
2. Streptococcal antigen would result in antibody production in a hyperimmune host.
3. Antibodies would react with the streptococcal antigen and with host tissues that are antigenically similar to streptococcus (i.e., antibodies are unable to distinguish streptococcal antigen from cardiac tissue antigen).
4. Autoantibodies reacting with host tissues would produce tissue damage.

Whatever the pathogenesis of this disease, the presentation of acute rheumatic fever is that of a diffuse, inflammatory process affecting the connective tissue of many organs, particularly the heart, joints, and skin. Signs and symptoms are nonspecific and include fever, migratory arthritis, arthralgia, skin rash, chorea, and tachycardia. Cardiac involvement is most significant for two reasons: (1) mortality during the acute phase, although extremely low, is attributed exclusively to cardiac failure and (2) residual disability results primarily from valvular deformity.

Acute rheumatic fever can produce inflammation of all cardiac layers, referred to as *pancarditis*. Endocardial inflammation typically involves the valvular endothelium, causing leaflet swelling and erosion of the cusp edges. Beadlike vegetations are deposited along the leaflet borders (Fig. 32-1). These acute changes may interfere with effective valve closure, producing valvular regurgitation; stenosis is not encountered as an acute lesion. The appearance of a murmur is the most common clinical manifestation of acute valvular involvement.

With myocardial involvement, characteristic nodular lesions, referred to as *Aschoff's bodies*, appear in the cardiac walls. Myocarditis may result in cardiac enlargement or congestive heart failure; however, clinical progression to failure is unusual during initial attacks. When present, failure is usually associated with concomitant valvular involvement. Pericarditis, usually observed with myocarditis and valvulitis, occurs infrequently. An exudative pericarditis with thickening of the pericardial layers is characteristic of acute rheumatic fever. Pericarditis typically presents with a friction rub, although pericardial effusions may develop. Progression to cardiac tamponade is rare.

Initial attacks of rheumatic carditis usually subside with little residual damage. However, recurrent attacks produce progressive valvular deformity. The pathologic changes of chronic rheumatic valvular disease are the product of healing with scar formation, recurrent inflammatory insults, and progressive deformity with hemodynamic stress and aging.

Given the gradual progression of chronic rheumatic valvular disease, symptoms generally do not appear for years after the initial attack; this latent period can last into the third, fourth, or fifth decade of life. Cusp thickening and leaflet fusion along the commissures (the junction between the leaflets) characterize the eventual deformity that produces valvular stenosis. These changes narrow the valvular orifice and reduce leaflet motion,

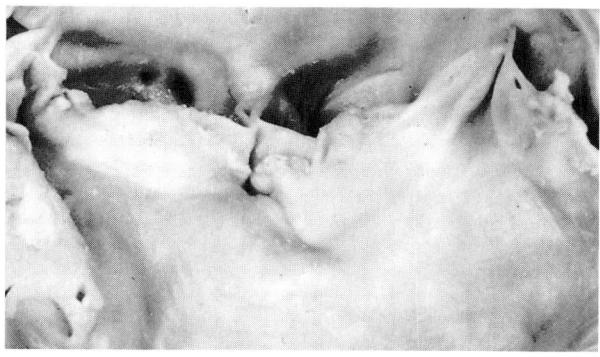

FIG. 32-1 Acute rheumatic endocarditis of the aortic valve. The vegetations form a beadlike row of deposits that tends to conform to the line of closure. (From Hurst JW: *The heart,* ed 3, New York, 1974, McGraw-Hill.)

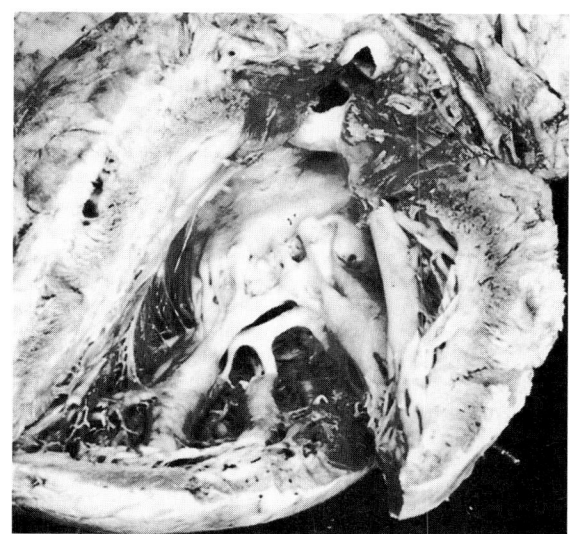

FIG. 32-2 Mitral valve viewed from below in a case of mitral valve stenosis. The valve is converted into a funnel-shaped structure, the apex of which is in the left ventricle. (From Hurst JW: *The heart,* ed 3, New York, 1974, McGraw-Hill.)

thus producing an obstruction to forward blood flow. The chordae tendineae of the atrioventricular (AV) valves may also thicken and fuse (Fig. 32-2), creating a fibrous tunnel below the cusps and further impeding flow.

The lesion associated with valvular regurgitation consists of shrunken, retracted cusps that inhibit cusp contact and shortened, fused chordae tendineae that restrain the AV valve leaflets (Fig. 32-3). These changes impair valve closure, thereby permitting backward flow through the valve.

Calcification and sclerosis of valvular tissue with aging contribute to the ultimate deformity in valves with rheumatic malformation. Chronic disease with ventricular failure and enlargement can also disrupt the function of the AV valves. As the ventricular shape alters, the ability of the papillary muscles to approximate the valvular leaflets during valve closure is reduced. Additionally, the valve orifice can enlarge, further compromising valve clo-

FIG. 32-3 Two examples of rheumatic endocarditis with aortic insufficiency. **A,** The valve leaflets are thickened and shortened to a relatively minor degree. The shortening creates a small triangular-shaped orifice in the center of the aortic valve, which persists during diastole. **B,** The aortic valve leaflets are significantly reduced in size, producing a wide triangular-shaped orifice. (From Hurst JW: *The heart,* ed 3, New York, 1974, McGraw-Hill.)

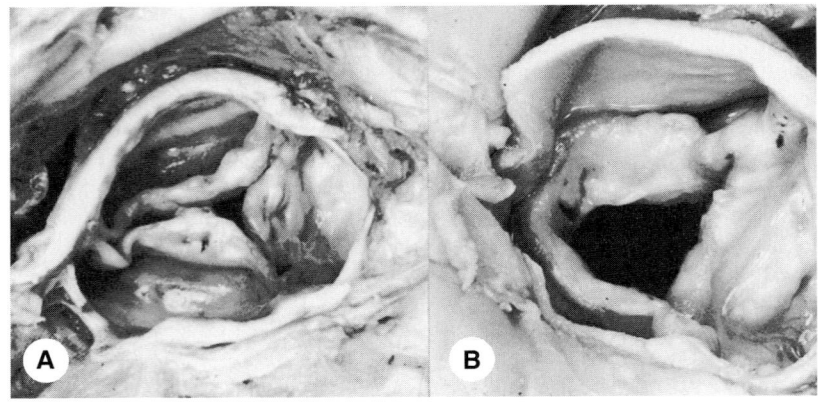

sure. Valvular regurgitation can result. This type of valvular regurgitation occurring secondary to chamber enlargement is known as *functional regurgitation.*

The incidence of valvular disease is highest in the mitral valve, followed by that in the aortic valve. The predominance of left-sided valvular disease is attributed to the relatively greater hemodynamic stress experienced by these valves. Theories suggest that hemodynamic stress increases the degree of acquired valvular deformity. The incidence of tricuspid disease is relatively low. Pulmonic disease is rare. Disease of the tricuspid or pulmonic valves is usually associated with other valvular lesions, whereas aortic or mitral disease is frequently observed as an isolated lesion.

In addition to rheumatic disease, other causes of valvular deformity and malfunction are being recognized with increasing frequency. Other significant causes of valvular heart disease are (1) valve destruction by infective endocarditis, (2) inborn defects of connective tissue, (3) dysfunction or rupture of the papillary muscles as a result of coronary atherosclerosis, and (4) congenital malformations.

Many organisms can cause *infective endocarditis,* including bacteria, fungi, and yeast. Bacterial infections are the most common; consequently, the entity is frequently referred to as *bacterial endocarditis.* Endocarditis may present in an acute or subacute form. *Acute* endocarditis is caused by infection with a highly virulent organism, such as staphylococci, and typically follows a rapidly fulminating course with early valvular destruction. Normal valves may be affected. *Subacute* bacterial endocarditis (abbreviated SBE when bacterial in origin) is caused by organisms of less virulence, such as streptococci, and has a more gradual presentation and course. Nonspecific signs and symptoms, including fever, joint pain, myalgias, and skin manifestations, are frequently reported. Typically, valves with preexisting abnormalities or mechanical prosthetics are involved. Endocarditis produces vegetations along the cusp edges; vegetations may extend to involve the valve and even the myocardium. Subsequently, the cusps may fibrose, erode, or perforate, causing typically regurgitant valvular dysfunction.

Mitral valve prolapse is a congenital syndrome characterized by redundancy of the valve leaflets and elongation of the chordae tendineae. The cusps prolapse or balloon into the atrium to varying degrees during ventricular systole; mitral regurgitation may result. These functional changes are caused by alterations in the collagen structure of the cusp. The exact incidence of mitral valve prolapse is estimated to be 5% to 10%. The course of this syndrome can be benign, although endocarditis prophylaxis is usually indicated.

Papillary muscle dysfunction or *rupture* can lead to a wide spectrum of valvular dysfunction. Papillary muscle abnormalities may be intermittent, may be secondary to ischemia, and may produce only episodic mild regurgitation. However, if rupture of a necrotic papillary muscle occurs after myocardial infarction, acute mitral regurgitation results.

Congenital malformations can occur in any valve. For example, approximately 1% to 2% of aortic valves are bicuspid rather than tricuspid.

Certain valvular lesions strongly suggest the underlying cause of dysfunction. For example, isolated mitral stenosis is usually rheumatic, whereas isolated aortic stenosis usually results from premature calcification and degeneration of a congenitally bicuspid valve. Isolated tricuspid or pulmonic disease is almost invariably a congenital defect. Combined valvular lesions suggest rheumatic causation.

PATHOPHYSIOLOGY

Mitral Stenosis

Mitral stenosis impedes blood flow from the left atrium to the left ventricle during ventricular diastole (Fig. 32-4). To adequately fill the ventricle and maintain cardiac output, the left atrium must generate more pressure to propel blood beyond the valvular obstruction. Therefore the pressure difference, or *pressure gradient*, between the chambers rises; normally the pressure gradient is minimal.

The left atrial musculature hypertrophies to increase its pumping force. The active contribution of atrial contraction to ventricular filling becomes increasingly important. The primary function of the left atrium ceases to be that of a passive reservoir and conduit for blood flowing to the ventricle. Atrial dilation occurs as the left atrial volume rises because of the inability of the chamber to empty normally.

The rise in left atrial pressure and volume is reflected backward into the pulmonary vasculature—pressure in the pulmonary veins and capillaries rises. A spectrum of

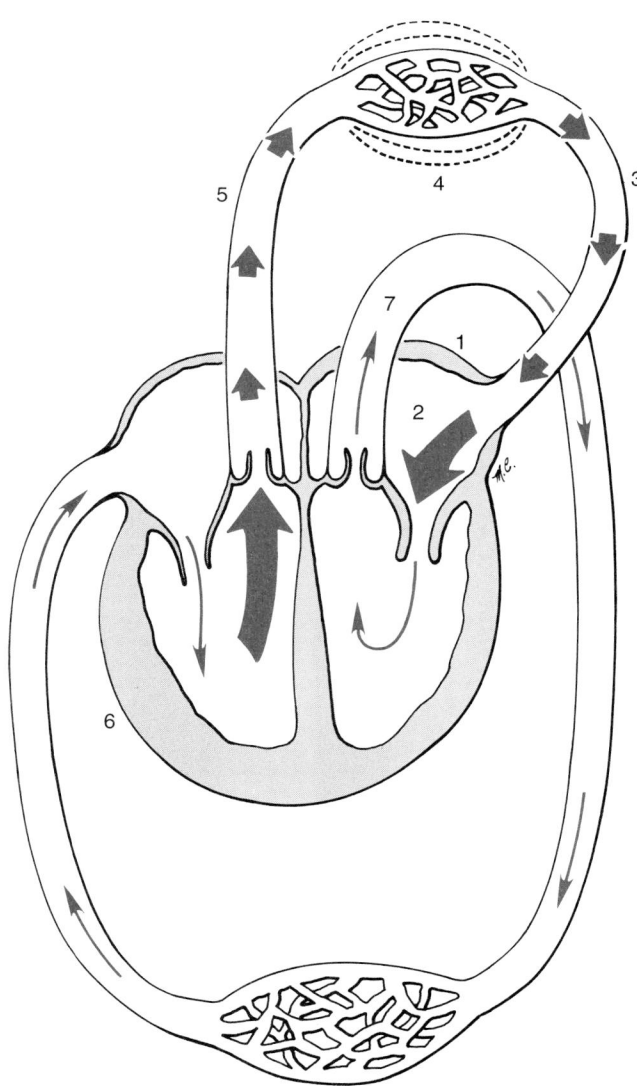

FIG. 32-4 Pathophysiology of mitral stenosis: *1*, left atrial hypertrophy; *2*, left atrial dilation; *3*, pulmonary venous congestion; *4*, pulmonary congestion; *5*, pulmonary hypertension; *6*, right ventricular hypertrophy; *7*, fixed cardiac output.

narrow the vessel lumen, elevating pulmonary vascular resistance. This arteriolar constriction, or *reactive pulmonary hypertension,* significantly elevates pulmonary arterial pressure. Pulmonary pressure can progressively climb to excessive levels approximating systemic pressure.

The right ventricle is poorly suited to perform as a high-pressure pump over long periods. Therefore the right ventricle eventually fails. Right ventricular failure is reflected backward into the systemic circulation, producing systemic venous congestion and peripheral edema. The right-sided failure can be compounded by functional regurgitation of the tricuspid valve as a result of right ventricular enlargement.

Over a period of years, the lesion of mitral stenosis narrows the valve orifice. Symptoms do not characteristically appear until the valve orifice has been reduced by more than 50% from a normal area of 4 to 5 cm^2 to less than 2.5 cm^2. With this degree of valvular restriction, left atrial pressure rises to maintain ventricular filling and cardiac output; consequently, pulmonary venous pressure rises, producing dyspnea. A diastolic heart murmur, indicative of abnormal flow through the restricted orifice, is usually noted much earlier in the course of the disease. The presence of neck vein distension, ascites, and edema on physical examination indicates that pulmonary hypertrophy producing right ventricular overload has developed. Valvular dimensions of less than 1 cm^2 reflect critical mitral stenosis.

The clinical picture can differ depending on the underlying hemodynamics; however, the earliest symptom is usually *dyspnea on exertion.* Two hemodynamic changes associated with exertion are poorly tolerated in mitral stenosis: (1) tachycardia (rapid heart rate) and (2) elevated left atrial pressure. Tachycardia reduces the duration of diastole, the period of ventricular filling from the atria. The duration of diastole is critically important in mitral stenosis because the lesion itself impairs ventricular filling and, consequently, atrial emptying. As ventricular filling time falls with tachycardia, cardiac output is reduced further and pulmonary congestion is increased. The elevation of left atrial pressure with exertion resulting from increased venous return further compounds pulmonary congestion. Because forward flow is restricted, the pressure elevation is transmitted backward to the lungs. Thus dyspnea on exertion is the result of pulmonary congestion. Weakness and fatigue are also prominent early symptoms as a result of the fixed, and eventually reduced, cardiac output.

As the disease progresses, respiratory symptoms become more pronounced. Susceptibility to pulmonary infection is high. Orthopnea and paroxysmal nocturnal dyspnea at rest may be noted. Transmission of the elevated pulmonary vascular pressures to the bronchial capillaries may result in capillary or bronchial vein rupture and mild hemoptysis. Eventually, the lungs become fibrotic and noncompliant. The distribution of blood flow within the lungs shifts. Normally, perfusion of the lower lobes is relatively greater than that of the upper lobes because of the effect of gravity on blood flow. In mitral stenosis, flow predominates in the upper lobes, presumably as a result of greater pulmonary vascular disease and interstitial edema in the lower lobes.

Atrial fibrillation frequently develops as a result of chronic atrial hypertrophy and dilation. With the onset

pulmonary congestion results, ranging from mild venous congestion to interstitial edema with occasional fluid transudation into the alveoli.

Eventually, pulmonary arterial pressure must rise in response to the chronic elevation of pulmonary venous resistance. This response ensures an adequate pressure gradient for blood flow through the pulmonary vasculature. However, pulmonary hypertension increases the resistance to right ventricular ejection into the pulmonary artery. The right ventricle responds to this increased pressure work with muscular hypertrophy.

The pulmonary vasculature may undergo anatomic changes apparently designed to protect the pulmonary capillaries from excessively high right ventricular pressures and pulmonary flow. Structural changes—medial hypertrophy and intimal thickening—occur in the walls of the small arteries and arterioles. The mechanism mediating this anatomic response is unclear. These changes

of atrial fibrillation, severe exacerbation of symptoms can occur. The quivering atrial musculature is incapable of coordinated muscular contraction. This loss of the active atrial kick reduces ventricular filling. Ventricular filling is further reduced by the rapid ventricular response to atrial fibrillation (heart rates approximate 150 bpm unless treated). The abrupt onset of rapid atrial fibrillation can result in low cardiac output and pulmonary edema. Hemodynamic adaptation occurs, usually with pharmacologic assistance (e.g., digoxin). However, the onset of atrial fibrillation exacerbates the risk of thrombus formation and systemic embolization because of stasis of blood in the left atrium proximal to the stenotic valve. Palpitations may also be noted with atrial fibrillation.

End-stage mitral stenosis is associated with right heart failure with consequent systemic venous engorgement, hepatomegaly, peripheral edema, and ascites. Right heart failure and chamber dilation can result in functional tricuspid regurgitation. However, mitral stenosis need not progress to this extreme. With the onset of symptoms, the disease can be managed medically, with eventual surgical correction.

The following findings are typically noted in mitral stenosis:

1. *Auscultation:* low-frequency diastolic murmur (rumble) and accentuated first heart sound (AV valve closure) and opening snap resulting from the loss of leaflet pliability
2. *Echocardiography:* the main noninvasive diagnostic tool for assessing the severity of mitral stenosis. The echocardiogram usually gives an accurate calculation of the valve area.
3. *Electrocardiogram:* left atrial enlargement (widened and notched P wave, most prominent in lead II, known as "P mitrale"), when rhythm is normal sinus; right ventricular hypertrophy; atrial fibrillation common but not specific for mitral stenosis
4. *Chest radiograph:* left atrial and right ventricular enlargement; pulmonary venous congestion; interstitial pulmonary edema; pulmonary vascular redistribution to the upper lobes; mitral valve calcification
5. *Hemodynamic findings:* elevated pressure gradient across the mitral valve; elevated left atrial pressure and pulmonary capillary wedge pressure with prominent *a* waves; elevated pulmonary artery pressure; low cardiac output; elevated right-sided heart pressures and jugular venous pressure with significant *v* waves in right atrial trace or jugular veins if tricuspid regurgitation is present

Mitral Regurgitation

Mitral regurgitation permits retrograde blood flow from the left ventricle to the left atrium as a result of incomplete valve closure (Fig. 32-5). During systole, the ventricle simultaneously ejects blood forward into the aorta and backward into the left atrium. The volume work of both the left ventricle and the left atrium must increase to preserve cardiac output.

The left ventricle must pump a sufficient volume of blood to maintain a normal forward flow into the aorta and the regurgitant flow through the mitral valve. For instance, the normal ventricular output per beat (stroke

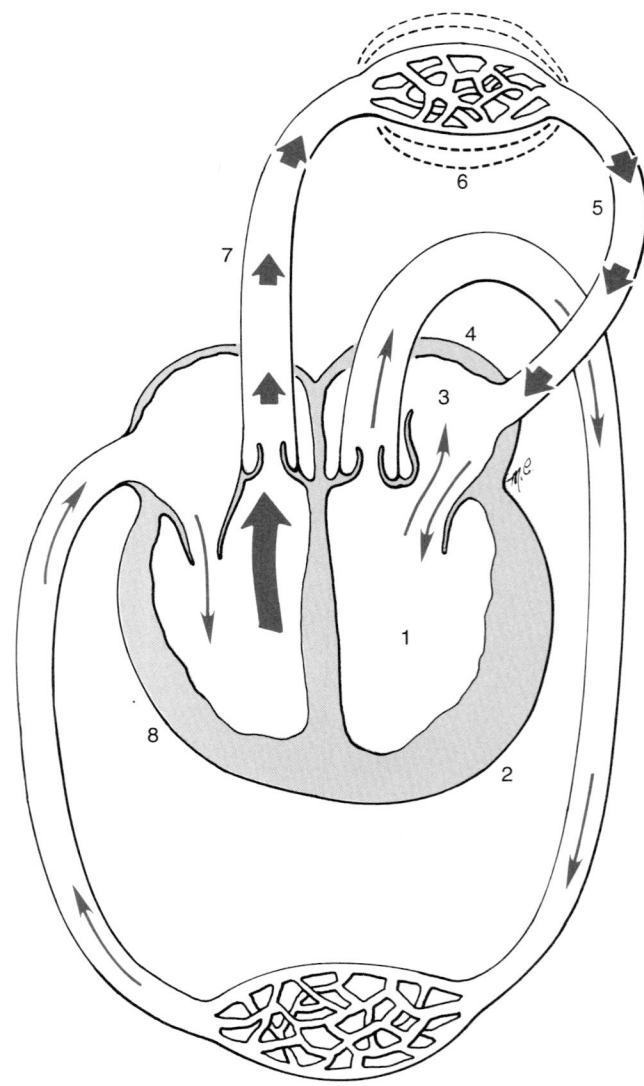

FIG. 32-5 Pathophysiology of mitral regurgitation: *1*, left ventricular dilation; *2*, left ventricular hypertrophy; *3*, left atrial dilation; *4*, left atrial hypertrophy; *5*, pulmonary venous congestion; *6*, pulmonary congestion; *7*, pulmonary artery hypertension; *8*, right ventricular hypertrophy.

volume) is 70 ml. If the regurgitant flow is 30 ml/beat, the ventricle must then pump 100 ml/beat to maintain a normal stroke volume. The additional volume load created by the regurgitant valve prompts ventricular dilation. According to Starling's law of the heart, ventricular dilation increases myocardial contractility. Eventually, the ventricular wall hypertrophies to further increase contractile force.

In the early stages of chronic mitral regurgitation, the left ventricle is able to compensate for the increased volume load. Even though total ventricular output (including both forward and regurgitant flows) increases, the afterload or amount of wall tension the ventricle must develop during systole to eject blood is reduced. Afterload reduction occurs because the ventricle ejects a portion of the stroke volume into the low-pressure left atrium. Paradoxically, this reduction in afterload via re-

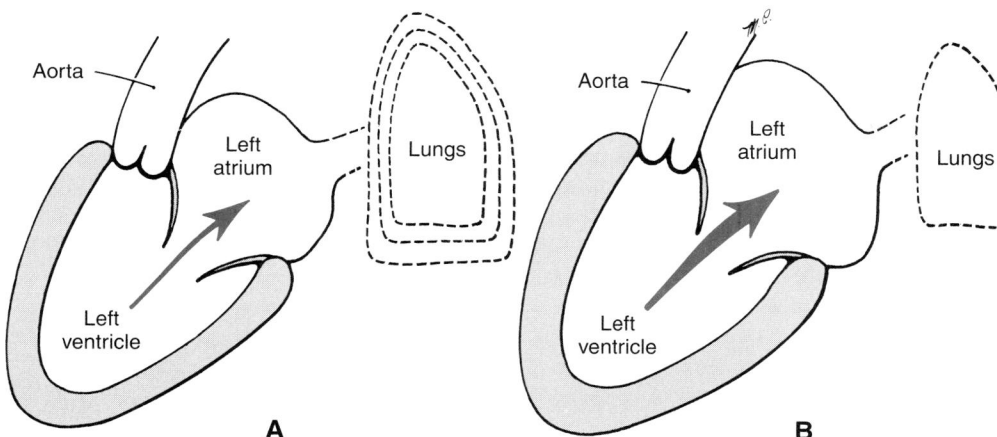

FIG. 32-6 **A**, Acute and **B**, chronic mitral regurgitation. Note that in chronic mitral regurgitation, greater dilation and hypertrophy of the left atrium and ventricle occur. Acute mitral regurgitation causes greater pulmonary congestion because the left atrium is less pliable or distensible.

gurgitant flow improves the ventricular compensatory ability to maintain forward flow. Eventually, however, the ventricle begins to fail, reducing cardiac output and increasing residual ventricular volumes and regurgitant flow.

Regurgitation creates a volume load not only for the left ventricle but also for the left atrium. The left atrium dilates to accommodate the increased volume and to increase the force of atrial contraction. Subsequently, the atrium hypertrophies to further increase atrial contractile force and output. Initially, increased left atrial compliance permits accommodation of increased volume without significant pressure elevation. Thus, for a while, the left atrium buffers the effect of the regurgitant volume, protecting the pulmonary vasculature and limiting pulmonary symptoms.

However, mitral regurgitation is a self-perpetuating lesion. As ventricular volumes and dimensions increase, valve function worsens. Chamber enlargement increases the degree of regurgitation by displacing papillary muscles and dilating the mitral orifice, thus reducing leaflet contact during valve closure.

As the lesion worsens, the ability of the left atrium to distend and protect the lungs is exceeded. Left ventricular failure is usually the prelude to accelerated cardiac decompensation. The left ventricle becomes overburdened, and forward flow through the aorta falls, with a simultaneous rise in backward congestion. Gradually the predictable sequence of pulmonary and right heart involvement ensues: (1) pulmonary venous congestion, (2) interstitial edema, (3) pulmonary arterial hypertension, and (4) right ventricular hypertrophy. These changes are less pronounced than changes with mitral stenosis. Mitral regurgitation can culminate in right heart failure, although less frequently than does mitral stenosis.

The course of the disease is profoundly altered when the onset of mitral regurgitation is acute, as in papillary muscle rupture after myocardial infarction, rather than chronic. Acute mitral regurgitation is poorly tolerated. Normally, the left atrium is relatively noncompliant and therefore unable to abruptly distend and accommodate the regurgitant volume (Fig. 32-6). Thus the sudden increase in volume and pressure is transmitted directly to the pulmonary vasculature. Within hours, fulminating pulmonary edema and shock can develop.

The earliest symptoms of mitral regurgitation are (1) weakness and fatigue caused by the reduction in forward flow, (2) exertional dyspnea, and (3) palpitations. Severe symptoms are precipitated by left ventricular failure with consequent low cardiac output and pulmonary congestion. The following findings are typically associated with chronic, severe mitral regurgitation:

1. *Auscultation:* murmur throughout systole (holosystolic or pansystolic murmur)
2. *Echocardiography:* confirms enlargement of the chamber, the color-flow examination of the mitral valve establishes the pattern of disturbed flow caused by regurgitation across the mitral valve
3. *Electrocardiogram:* left atrial enlargement (P mitrale), when rhythm is normal sinus; atrial fibrillation; left ventricular hypertrophy
4. *Chest radiograph:* left atrial enlargement; left ventricular enlargement; variable pulmonary vascular congestion
5. *Hemodynamic findings:* increased left atrial pressure with significant *v* waves; elevated left ventricular end-diastolic pressure; variable elevations of pulmonary pressures

Aortic Stenosis

Aortic stenosis obstructs blood flow from the left ventricle into the aorta during ventricular systole. As the resistance to ventricular ejection increases, the pressure work of the left ventricle rises. In response, the left ventricle hypertrophies to generate more pressure and maintain peripheral perfusion; a marked pressure gradient develops between the left ventricle and the aorta (Fig. 32-7). Hypertrophy reduces ventricular wall compliance, and the wall becomes relatively stiff. Thus, despite the maintenance of normal cardiac output and ventricular volumes, ventricular end-diastolic pressure is slightly elevated.

The reserve pumping capability of the left ventricle is considerable. For instance, the left ventricle, which normally generates a systolic pressure of 120 mm Hg, can develop pressure up to approximately 300 mm Hg during ventricular contraction. To compensate and maintain cardiac output, the left ventricle not only generates higher pressure but also prolongs the duration of ejection. Therefore, despite the progressive restriction of the aortic orifice

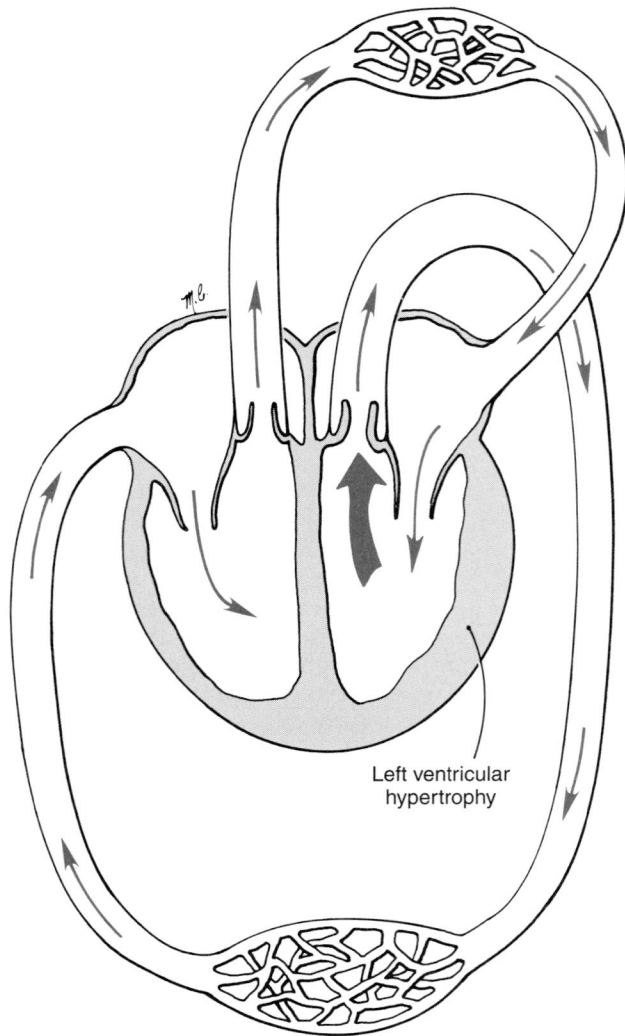

Left ventricular
hypertrophy

FIG. 32-7 Pathophysiology of aortic stenosis.

and a consequent elevation of ventricular work, the mechanical efficiency of the heart is maintained for long periods. Eventually, however, the adaptive ability of the left ventricle is overwhelmed. The onset of progressive symptoms heralds a critical point in the course of aortic stenosis. Critical aortic stenosis corresponds to a reduction in valvular orifice from 3 to 4 cm^2 to less than 0.8 cm^2; generally a pressure gradient does not develop across the valve until this orifice is reduced by approximately 50%.

A characteristic triad of symptoms is associated with aortic stenosis: (1) angina, (2) syncope, and (3) left ventricular failure. When unheeded, these symptoms indicate a poor prognosis, with an average survival of less than 5 years. The onset of *left ventricular failure*, indicating cardiac decompensation, is particularly ominous. *Angina* is produced by an imbalance in myocardial oxygen supply and demand; demand increases with hypertrophy and increased myocardial work, whereas supply is potentially reduced by the powerful systolic compression of the coronary arteries by the hypertrophied muscle. Additionally, with myocardial hypertrophy, the ratio of cap-

illaries to muscle fiber mass may be reduced. The oxygen diffusion distance is therefore increased, potentially limiting myocardial oxygen availability. The subendocardial layer of the left ventricle is the most vulnerable. Death may ensue within 5 years after the onset of angina. *Syncope* occurs primarily with exertion because of the inability to increase the cardiac output sufficiently to maintain cerebral perfusion or the precipitation of a vasodepressor response. Survival after the onset of syncope has been estimated at 3 to 4 years.

Progressive ventricular failure impairs ventricular emptying. Cardiac output falls, and ventricular volumes rise. Ventricular dilation, occasionally associated with functional mitral regurgitation, ensues. Advanced aortic stenosis is associated with severe pulmonary congestion. Right ventricular failure and systemic venous congestion are indicative of end-stage disease. Aortic stenosis infrequently progresses to this extreme. The infrequent occurrence of right heart failure is probably the result of the high mortality rate associated with left heart failure earlier in the course of the disease. Additionally, a significant incidence of sudden death occurs in symptomatic patients with severe aortic stenosis. The pathogenesis of sudden death is controversial but is usually precipitated by strenuous exertion.

The prominent signs of severe aortic stenosis are as follows:

1. *Auscultation:* harsh systolic ejection murmur; paradoxical splitting of second heart sound; ejection click
2. *Echocardiography:* tool of choice for the assessment of leaflet mobility, leaflet thickness, leaflet calcification, subvalvular fusion, calculation of the valve area, and appearance of the commissures
3. *Electrocardiogram:* left ventricular hypertrophy; conduction defects
4. *Chest radiograph:* poststenotic dilation of the ascending aorta (resulting from local trauma from blood ejected under high pressure and striking the aortic wall); valvular calcification (best observed on lateral or oblique views)
5. *Hemodynamic findings:* significant aortic gradient (50 to 100 mm Hg); elevated left ventricular end-diastolic pressure; delayed carotid upstroke

Aortic Regurgitation

Aortic regurgitation produces a reflux of blood from the aorta into the left ventricle during ventricular relaxation (Fig. 32-8). In essence, the peripheral bed competes with the left ventricle for the blood ejected by the ventricle during systole. The magnitude of forward flow, or "runoff," into the periphery relative to retrograde flow into the ventricle depends on the degree of valve closure and the relative resistance to flow between the periphery and the ventricle. Characteristically, peripheral vascular resistance is low in aortic regurgitation, apparently as a compensatory mechanism to maximize forward flow. However, late in the course of the disease, peripheral resistance rises, increasing retrograde flow through the aortic valve and accelerating the disease progression.

The clinical course of chronic aortic regurgitation is the least understood and the most variable of the valvu-

Angina may also be noted with left ventricular hypertrophy and low arterial diastolic pressures, which increase oxygen demand and decrease oxygen supply, respectively. However, substernal pain unrelated to myocardial ischemia may occur. Heart failure precipitates a downhill course of falling cardiac output and rising ventricular volume with retrograde left atrial and pulmonary congestion.

The following signs are associated with chronic aortic regurgitation:

1. *Auscultation:* diastolic murmur; characteristic Austin Flint murmur or diastolic rumble; systolic ejection click caused by increased ejection volume
2. *Electrocardiogram:* left ventricular hypertrophy
3. *Chest radiograph:* left ventricular enlargement; dilation of proximal aorta
4. *Hemodynamic findings:* rapid upstroke and collapse of arterial pulse; widened pulse pressure with elevated systemic and lowered diastolic pressures
5. *Cardiac catheterization:* opacification of the left ventricle during injection of contrast material into the aortic root

Characteristic findings are noted in the peripheral circulation as a result of the hyperdynamic myocardial action and the low peripheral resistance. The forceful, high-volume, left ventricular ejection followed by the rapid forward runoff of blood into the periphery and backward into the left ventricle through the diseased valve creates a rapid distention of the vasculature, leading to a sudden collapse. These cardiovascular dynamics can be manifested by (1) water-hammer pulses (or *Corrigan's pulse*), characterized by a rapid rise and collapse of the arterial pulse; (2) pistol-shot pulses (or *Duroziez's murmur*), audible on auscultation of the femoral artery; (3) *Quincke's capillary pulsation,* visible as alternating flushing and paling of the nail bed capillaries; and (4) systolic head bobbing as the collapsed neck vessels fill rapidly (or *de Musset's sign*).

Tricuspid Valve Disease

Stenosis of the tricuspid valve restricts blood flow from the right atrium into the right ventricle during diastole. This lesion is usually associated with disease of the mitral and aortic valves secondary to severe rheumatic heart disease. Tricuspid stenosis increases the work of the right atrium, forcing the chamber to generate more pressure to maintain flow across the obstructed valve. The right atrium has a limited ability to compensate and thus dilates rapidly. As right atrial volumes and pressures rise, systemic venous engorgement and pressure elevation result (Fig. 32-9).

The classic findings of right heart failure ensue: (1) venous distention with large *a* waves, (2) peripheral edema, (3) ascites, (4) hepatic enlargement, and (5) nausea and anorexia resulting from gastrointestinal engorgement. The following signs are associated with tricuspid stenosis:

1. *Auscultation:* diastolic murmur
2. *Electrocardiogram:* right atrial enlargement (tall, peaked P waves, known as *P pulmonale*)
3. *Chest radiograph:* right atrial enlargement
4. *Hemodynamic findings:* pressure gradient across the tricuspid valve and elevated right atrial and central venous pressures with large *a* waves.

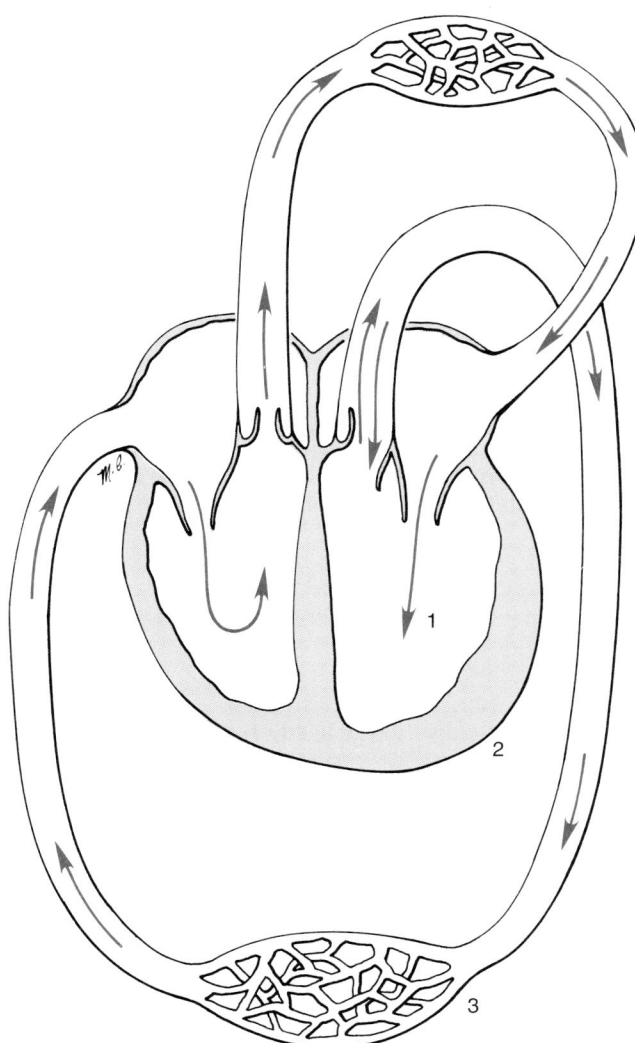

FIG. 32-8 Pathophysiology of aortic regurgitation: *1*, left ventricular dilation; *2*, left ventricular hypertrophy; *3*, hyperdynamic peripheral circulation.

lar lesions. However, the disease obviously imposes a severe volume load on the left ventricle. With each contraction, the ventricle must eject a quantity of blood equal to the normal stroke volume plus the regurgitant volume. The left ventricle dilates greatly and eventually hypertrophies, assuming a distinctive globular shape. An associated increase in wall compliance enables the ventricle to tolerate increased diastolic volumes without abnormal pressure elevations.

The marked left ventricular compensatory ability in combination with a competent mitral valve maintains ventricular function for a long period. Symptoms rarely develop until left ventricular decompensation occurs, which is occasionally compounded by functional mitral regurgitation. Irreversible left ventricular damage, resulting from the prolonged ejection of the volume overload against systemic resistance, can be sustained. The point of significant deterioration is poorly defined. Early symptoms are palpitations, fatigue, and dyspnea on exertion.

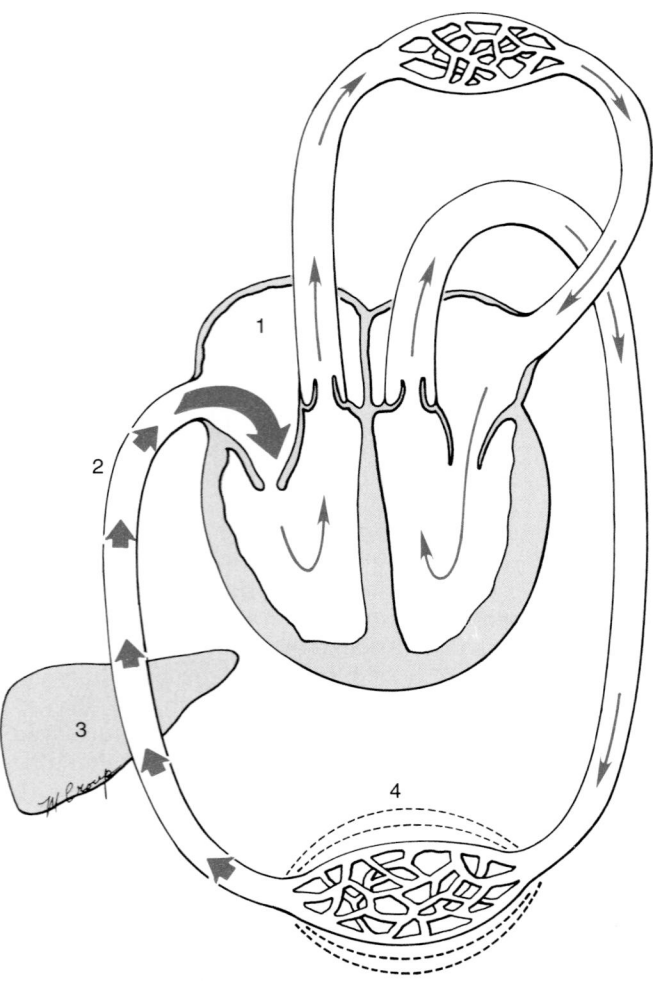

FIG. 32-9 Pathophysiology of tricuspid stenosis: *1*, right atrial dilation; *2*, venous congestion; *3*, hepatomegaly; *4*, systemic congestion.

Pure tricuspid regurgitation is usually the consequence of advanced left heart failure or severe pulmonary hypertension, resulting in right ventricular deterioration. As the right ventricle fails and enlarges, functional regurgitation of the tricuspid valve is produced. Tricuspid regurgitation is associated with right heart failure and the following findings:

1. *Auscultation:* murmur throughout systole
2. *Electrocardiogram:* right atrial enlargement (tall and narrow P wave, or P pulmonale), when rhythm is normal sinus; atrial fibrillation; right ventricular hypertrophy
3. *Chest radiograph:* right atrial and ventricular enlargement
4. *Hemodynamic findings:* elevated right atrial pressure with significant *v* waves

Pulmonic Valve Disease

The incidence of pulmonic valvular lesions is extremely low. Pulmonic stenosis is usually congenital rather than rheumatic. Stenosis of the pulmonic valve increases right ventricular pressure work, producing right ventricular hypertrophy. Symptoms result when right ventricular failure occurs, producing systemic venous engorgement and its clinical sequelae.

Functional pulmonic regurgitation can occur as a sequela to left-sided valvular dysfunction with chronic pulmonic hypertension and dilation of the pulmonic valve orifice. However, this lesion is rarely present.

Compound Valvular Disease

Mixed lesions, consisting of stenosis and regurgitation in the same valve, frequently occur. These lesions are to be expected because a stenotic, immobile valve is often unable to close completely. *Combined lesions,* or multivalvular disease, are often present because rheumatic heart disease typically affects multiple valves.

Mixed lesions and combined lesions compound the valvular dysfunction described for isolated or *pure lesions,* altering to a variable degree the physiologic consequences. Compound lesions can either magnify or buffer a physiologic consequence of a pure lesion. For instance, mixed mitral regurgitation and aortic stenosis increase the volume load and pressure work of the left ventricle and greatly intensify the left ventricular strain. As a result, this combination is associated with a rapidly progressive downhill course.

However, the combination of aortic stenosis and mitral stenosis, in essence, protects the left ventricle from the magnitude of left ventricular strain associated with isolated aortic stenosis. This protective effect results from the reduction in left ventricular filling caused by the restriction to blood flow through the mitral valve. Diminished ventricular filling reduces the volume of the blood that the left ventricle must force through the restricted aortic orifice.

THERAPEUTIC INTERVENTION

Rheumatic fever and subacute bacterial endocarditis are two disease processes that can be prevented, thus reducing the incidence or severity of acquired valvular lesions. Rheumatic fever can be prevented by early detection and treatment of group A beta-hemolytic streptococcal infections with penicillin. Early diagnosis and treatment of acute rheumatic fever are also essential. The diagnosis of acute rheumatic fever can be complicated because no single clinical or laboratory finding is pathognomonic for this disease; many of the findings are nonspecific. The modified Jones criteria are useful in the diagnosis of acute rheumatic fever (Box 32-1). These criteria are designated as major or minor according to their relative importance as diagnostic indicators. The presence of two major criteria or one major and two minor criteria indicates a high probability of acute rheumatic fever. Evidence of an antecedent streptococcal infection is also prerequisite to the diagnosis; elevated antistreptolysin (ASO) levels are frequently used to establish the presence of streptococcal antibodies.

Treatment of acute rheumatic fever is palliative and includes (1) antibiotics, such as penicillin or erythromycin, to eliminate any residual streptococcal organisms; (2) antiinflammatory agents, such as salicylates or corticosteroids; (3) analgesics, when indicated for arthritic pain; and (4) restriction of physical activity according to the degree of carditis. Associated cardiac failure might necessitate salt restriction, digoxin, and diuretics. Beta blockers or calcium channel blockers may be of benefit in patients

Guidelines for Diagnosis of Initial Attack of Rheumatic Fever (Jones Criteria, 1992 Update)*

MAJOR MANIFESTATIONS
1. Carditis
2. Polyarthritis
3. Chorea
4. Erythema marginatum
5. Subcutaneous nodules

MINOR MANIFESTATIONS
Clinical findings
1. Arthralgia
2. Fever

Laboratory findings
1. Elevated levels of acute-phase reactants
   a. Erythrocyte sedimentation rate (ESR)
   b. C-reactive protein (CRP)
2. Prolonged PR interval

SUPPORTING EVIDENCE OF ANTECEDENT GROUP A STREPTOCOCCAL INFECTION
1. Positive throat culture or rapid streptococcal antigen test results
2. Elevated or rising streptococcal antibody titer (ASO titer)

From The Special Writing Group of the Committee on Rheumatic Fever, Endocarditis, and Kawasaki Disease of the Council on Cardiovascular Disease in the Young of the American Heart Association, *JAMA* 268(15):2070, 1992.
*If supported by evidence of preceding group A streptococcal infection, the presence of two major manifestations or of one major and two minor manifestations indicates a high probability of acute rheumatic fever.

with sinus rhythm who have exertional symptoms, when the symptoms occur with rapid heart rates.

After the initial attack of rheumatic fever, susceptibility to recurrent attacks is extremely high. Consequently, antibiotic prophylaxis must begin as soon as the diagnosis is established. Single monthly injections of penicillin are effective and offer a distinct advantage over daily oral therapy in terms of patient compliance. Antibiotic prophylaxis must continue at least into adulthood to avoid potentially crippling deformity of heart valves produced by recurrent attacks of rheumatic fever. Emphasis must be on prevention rather than treatment of streptococcal infections because recurrent rheumatic fever is frequently preceded by asymptomatic streptococcal infection. Additionally, preventing recurrent attacks after the onset of infection is often difficult.

Heart valves with congenital malformations or acquired deformity are particularly vulnerable to infection, or endocarditis, from systemic infections or even from the transient septicemia associated with minor surgical procedures (e.g., dental extractions). Appropriate prophylactic antibiotic coverage during substantiated or potential systemic infection is critical to prevent further valvular deterioration. Once valvular damage has been sustained, the course of the disease and medical therapy vary according to the site and severity of the lesion.

Mitral valve disease produces symptoms earlier than aortic valve disease because the diseased mitral valve imposes a burden primarily on the left atrium, whereas the diseased aortic valve burdens the left ventricle. The thin-walled left atrium is poorly suited to maintain its pump-ing capability in the face of an ever-increasing pressure or volume load. Additionally, because no true valves separate the pulmonary veins from the left atrium, left atrial congestion is readily transmitted retrograde to the lungs, producing pulmonary symptoms. With aortic valve disease, the left ventricle compensates well for a long period, resulting in a long asymptomatic phase. The left atrium is protected from the left ventricular strain, as long as the mitral valve remains competent and the left ventricular pumping capability is sustained.

Medical Therapy
Mitral Valve Disease

The clinical progression of mitral valve disease is gradual and prolonged. Dyspnea is usually the most prominent and disabling symptom. However, symptoms are initially responsive to medical therapy consisting of (1) *diuretics* to reduce congestion; (2) *digoxin* to increase contractile force in the presence of mitral regurgitation or to reduce ventricular response to atrial fibrillation; if the ventricular rate is not slowed, a beta-adrenergic blocking agent or calcium channel blocker is added; (3) *antidysrhythmics* if atrial fibrillation occurs; (4) *vasodilator therapy* in the presence of mitral regurgitation to reduce afterload, thereby decreasing regurgitant flow and increasing forward blood flow; (5) *anticoagulants* if systemic embolization becomes a threat; (6) *antibiotics* for endocarditis prophylaxis; and (7) catheter balloon *valvotomy* (valvulotomy) in select patients. Eventually, surgical intervention is necessary to control the progressively disabling symptoms. Occasionally, surgical intervention is precipitated by an abrupt deterioration associated with dysrhythmias, embolization, or pulmonary infection.

Aortic Valve Disease

The management of aortic valve disease is in distinct contrast to that of mitral valve disease. Except for prophylaxis against endocarditis, no proven medical therapy is available for aortic stenosis. The onset of significant symptoms—angina, syncope, and failure—usually correlates with left ventricular decompensation, signaling a need to consider surgical intervention. The risk of surgery for most symptomatic patients is less than the risk of prolonged medical therapy. Approximately 75% of patients with symptomatic aortic stenosis will die 3 years after the onset of symptoms, unless the aortic valve is replaced. Once the patient is symptomatic, the course of aortic disease is progressively downhill. Severe aortic stenosis is a potentially unpredictable, lethal entity; sudden death can occur. Aortic regurgitation poses somewhat of a therapeutic dilemma; the timing of surgery is less well defined. However, evidence exists that aortic regurgitation should be corrected before the onset of permanent left ventricular damage. Close surveillance of patients with aortic valve disease is essential to detect early signs of clinical deterioration. As with patients with mitral valve disease, bacterial endocarditis prophylaxis is necessary.

Surgical Therapy
Mitral Valve Disease

Techniques for correcting deformities of the mitral valve have been expanded in recent years. Patients may have

(1) mitral valvotomy (valvulotomy), (2) mitral valve replacement, or (3) mitral valve repair.

Mitral valvotomy, or opening of the mitral valve, is considered for select patients with pure mitral stenosis when their symptoms have progressed to functional class II heart disease (i.e., symptomatic with ordinary physical exertion). A stenotic mitral valve can be dilated via a transventricular surgical approach or a percutaneous approach. The surgical transventricular procedure splits the valve leaflets at the point of fusion along the commissures. Balloon valvuloplasty involves threading either one or two balloon-tipped catheters through a peripheral vessel under fluoroscopic guidance into the right atrium, advancing the catheter across the atrial septum into the left atrium, and placing the balloon tip within the valve orifice. In a noncalcified pliable valve, inflation of the balloon should result in separation of the fused commissures. Candidates for either the percutaneous or the surgical approach are usually young patients without atrial fibrillation, mitral regurgitation, a calcified valve, or history of prior surgical commissurotomy.

Mitral valve replacement is generally considered for mitral regurgitation and for mitral stenosis when symptoms have progressed to functional class III heart disease (i.e., symptoms with less than ordinary physical exertion) despite medical therapy, although with improvements in surgical technique and valve design, surgery may be recommended earlier. Further disease progression to functional class IV is associated with higher surgical mortality and morbidity rates as a result of residual myocardial and pulmonary dysfunction. Systemic embolization or significant pulmonary hypertension are also indications for surgery. Mitral valve replacement involves excision of the valve, chordae tendineae, and papillary muscles. A prosthetic valve designed to simulate normal valve function is inserted (see later section for description of available prosthetics).

Reconstructive surgical techniques may be used to repair the mitral valve, particularly in the setting of degenerative, nonrheumatic disease. Repair of the valve, or *valvuloplasty,* can involve lengthening or shortening the chordae tendineae, repositioning the chordae, or resecting valve leaflets. A prosthetic ring is usually inserted in the valve annulus to stabilize and repair the valve orifice, a technique referred to as *annuloplasty.*

Aortic Valve Disease

Valve replacement is recommended for aortic regurgitation and calcific aortic stenosis. Percutaneous aortic valvulotomy is considered for elderly, high-risk patients with aortic stenosis or for young patients with noncalcific aortic stenosis.

Valve Prosthetics

Valves are of two basic types: mechanical valves and tissue valves. Each type has distinct advantages and disadvantages. The *mechanical valves,* although noteworthy for durability, are thrombogenic, and patients require long-term anticoagulation. Three types of *tissue valves* are available: (1) porcine heterograph, (2) bovine pericardial heterograph, and (3) homographs, or human heart valves (usually aortic or pulmonic), which have been cryopreserved. *Porcine* and *bovine valves* are nonthrombogenic but are less durable compared with mechanical valves. These valves tend to be recommended for elderly patients or when anticoagulation is contraindicated. *Homographs* are limited in supply, but over the long term, they may have both the necessary durability and the nonthrombogenic characteristics.

Figure 32-10 illustrates examples of prosthetic valves. All valves open and close in response to pressure

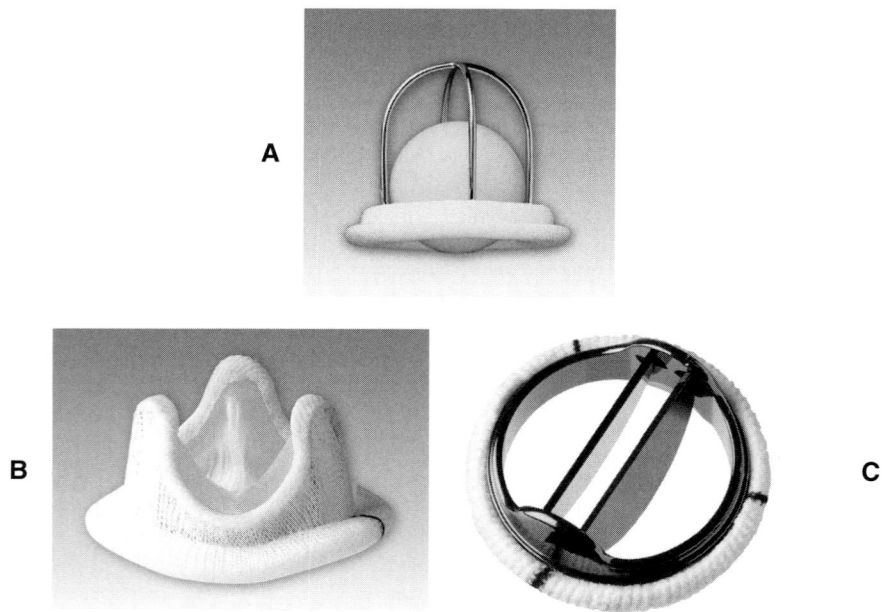

FIG. 32-10 Prosthetic valves. **A,** Starr-Edwards (caged ball) valve. **B,** Carpentier-Edwards (tissue) valve. **C,** St. Jude Medical Regent valve in open position. (**A** and **B** courtesy Edwards Lifesciences LLC, Irvine, Calif; **C** courtesy St. Jude medical, Inc., St. Paul, Minn.)

changes on either side of the valve. For example, with the disk valve in the mitral position, the disks are perpendicular to the annulus during ventricular relaxation, permitting blood flow from the atrium to the ventricle.

During ventricular contraction, as ventricular pressure exceeds atrial pressure, the disks go into a horizontal position to seal the mitral orifice, preventing backward flow.

KEY CONCEPTS

- Critical flow characteristics of normal valves are unidirectional flow and unimpeded flow.
- Two types of functional derangements caused by diseased valves are: (1) valvular stenosis and (2) valvular regurgitation.
- Valvular stenosis occurs when the valve orifice becomes restricted, impeding forward flow.
- Valvular stenosis results in an increase in pressure work, because the chamber needs to generate increased pressure to overcome the increased resistance to flow.
- Valvular regurgitation occurs when the valve leaflets fail to close securely, permitting backward flow of blood.
- Valvular regurgitation results in an increase in volume work, because the heart needs to pump the additional regurgitant volume of blood.
- Rheumatic fever has been considered the most common cause of valvular heart disease.
- Acute rheumatic fever is a sequela of a group A beta-hemolytic streptococcal pharyngitis. Both rheumatic fever and mitral stenosis remain common in developing nations.
- The eventual deformity producing valvular stenosis is characterized by cusp thickening and leaflet fusion along the commissures.
- The lesion associated with valvular regurgitation consists of shrunken, retracted cusps that inhibit cusp contact and shortened, fused chordae tendineae that restrain the AV valve leaflets.
- Functional regurgitation is valvular regurgitation that occurs secondary to chamber enlargement.
- Mitral valve prolapse is a congenital syndrome characterized by redundancy of the valve leaflets and elongation of the chordae tendineae.
- The earliest symptom of mitral stenosis is usually dyspnea on exertion, followed by susceptibility to pulmonary infection, orthopnea, and paroxysmal nocturnal dyspnea at rest.
- Atrial fibrillation frequently develops as a result of chronic atrial hypertrophy and dilation.
- Atrial fibrillation exacerbates the risk of thrombus formation and systemic embolization because of stasis of blood in the left atrium proximal to the stenotic valve.
- Mitral regurgitation permits retrograde blood flow from the left ventricle to the left atrium as a result of incomplete valve closure.
- Regurgitation creates a volume load for both the left ventricle and the left atrium.
- Early symptoms of mitral regurgitation are weakness and fatigue, exertional dyspnea, and palpitations.

- Aortic stenosis obstructs blood flow from the left ventricle into the aorta during ventricular systole.
- The left ventricle hypertrophies to generate more pressure and maintain peripheral perfusion to compensate for the restriction caused by the stenotic aortic valve.
- Critical aortic stenosis corresponds to a reduction in valvular orifice from the normal 3 to 4 cm^2 to less than 0.8 cm^2.
- The characteristic triad of symptoms associated with aortic stenosis is angina, syncope, and left ventricular failure.
- Aortic regurgitation produces a reflux of blood from the aorta into the left ventricle during ventricular relaxation.
- The pathophysiology of aortic regurgitation is left ventricular dilation, left ventricular hypertrophy, and hyperdynamic peripheral circulation.
- Indications of hyperdynamic peripheral circulation are water-hammer pulses characterized by a rapid rise and collapse of the arterial pulse; pistol-shot pulses audible on auscultation of the femoral artery; Quincke's capillary pulsation, visible as alternating flushing and paling of the nail bed capillaries; and systolic head bobbing as the collapsed neck vessels fill rapidly.
- Stenosis of the tricuspid valve restricts blood flow from the right atrium into the right ventricle during diastole.
- The pathophysiology of tricuspid stenosis is right atrial dilation, venous congestion, hepatomegaly, and systemic congestion.
- Pulmonic valve disease is usually congenital rather than rheumatic.
- Rheumatic fever and subacute bacterial endocarditis are two disease processes that can be prevented, thus reducing the incidence or severity of acquired valvular lesions.
- Treatment of acute rheumatic fever is palliative and includes antibiotics, antiinflammatory agents, analgesics, and restriction of physical activity.
- Mitral valve disease produces symptoms earlier than does aortic valve disease because the diseased mitral valve imposes a burden primarily on the left atrium, whereas the diseased aortic valve burdens the left ventricle.
- In mitral valve disease, symptoms are initially responsive to medical therapy consisting of diuretics, digoxin, antidysrhythmics, vasodilator therapy, and anticoagulants, as well as catheter balloon valvotomy in select patients.
- Techniques for correcting deformities of the mitral valve include mitral valvotomy, mitral valve replacement, or mitral valve repair.

■ Mitral valve replacement involves excision of the valve, chordae tendineae, and papillary muscles.

■ Repair of the valve, or valvuloplasty, can involve lengthening or shortening the chordae tendineae, repositioning the chordae, or resecting valve leaflets.

■ Valve replacement is recommended for aortic regurgitation and calcific aortic stenosis.

■ The two basic types of prosthetic valves are mechanical valves and tissue valves. The mechanical valves are durable but thrombogenic. The tissue valves are less durable than are mechanical valves but are nonthrombogenic.

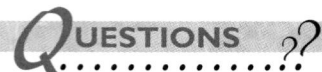

QUESTIONS ??

A sampling of review questions for this chapter appears here. Visit http://www.mosby.com/MERLIN/PriceWilson/ for additional questions.

Answer the following on a separate sheet of paper.

1. List and briefly describe five causes of valvular heart disease.
2. What is functional AV regurgitation?
3. Comment on the following statement: "Before rendering any treatment that may result in even the slightest release of bacteria into the bloodstream, one is obligated to make absolutely sure that the patient is not affected by any kind of heart deformity. If it is known or suspected that the patient has a deformity of the heart, it is absolutely necessary to administer prophylactic antibiotics."
4. What is the medical treatment for each of the following problems associated with mitral valve disease: pulmonary congestion, atrial fibrillation, and systemic emboli?
5. What is a mitral valvulotomy?
6. List the revised Jones criteria. What is their purpose? Illustrate.

Match the functional valvular disorder in column A with its effects in column B.

Column A

7. _____ Valvular regurgitation
8. _____ Valvular stenosis

Column B

a. Increased cardiac volume work
b. Increased cardiac pressure work
c. Backward flow
d. Resistance to forward flow
e. Chamber dilation
f. Muscle hypertrophy

CHAPTER

33

Cardiac Mechanical Dysfunction and Circulatory Support

MADELINE M. O'DONNELL AND PENNY FORD CARLETON

Cardiac mechanical dysfunction has a wide spectrum, ranging from mild, compensated heart failure to cardiogenic shock. This chapter provides an overview of this spectrum and an introduction to the techniques of circulatory assistance and cardiac transplantation.

Heart failure poses a surprising paradox: it is relatively straightforward as a clinical syndrome yet extremely variable and complex as a pathophysiologic state. Contributing to the complexity is the wide variety of disease entities that can cause heart failure. This discussion focuses on the common form of heart failure that occurs as a complication of ischemic heart disease.

Cardiac mechanical dysfunction and methods of circulatory support are considered relative to their effects on the three primary determinants of myocardial function: preload, contractility, and afterload. This framework is used because heart failure and the associated compensatory responses produce abnormalities in each of these determinants.

CONGESTIVE HEART FAILURE

Fundamental Concepts

Preload

Preload is the degree of myocardial fiber stretch at the end of ventricular filling or diastole. Increasing preload, up to a point, optimizes the overlap between actin and myosin filaments, increasing the force of contraction and cardiac output. This relationship is expressed by *Starling's law*; that is, stretching the myocardial fibers during diastole increases the force of contraction during systole (see Fig. 29-8). Preload is increased by elevation of ventricular diastolic volume, as occurs with fluid retention; a reduction of preload results from diuresis.

The relationship between increasing ventricular end-diastolic volume (EDV) and improved ventricular performance is illustrated in Fig. 33-1 as the *ventricular function curve*. The normal curve exhibits an initially steep, ascending limb where increments in volume and fiber stretch produce a corresponding improvement in ventricular function and cardiac output. The normal ventricle operates along the steep ascending limb where considerable reserve exists for improving ventricular function.

At the summit of the curve, a plateau or flattening is observed where additional increments in ventricular volume are not associated with improved performance. This physiologic limit results from the rise in ventricular end-diastolic pressure produced by the increased volume. Excessive pressure elevation produces pulmonary or systemic congestion and edema from fluid transudation, negating the value of further increments in volume and pressure.

The ventricular function curve characteristic of the failing ventricle is depressed and flattened (Fig. 33-2).

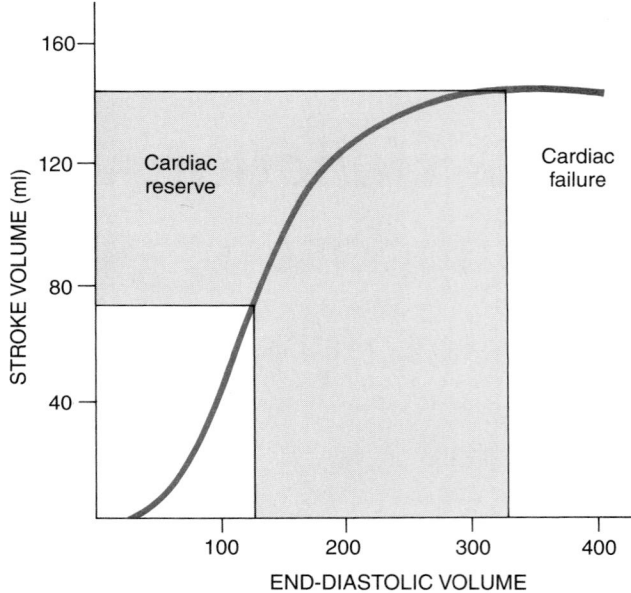

FIG. 33-1 Starling's law of the heart. As the end-diastolic volume increases, so does the force of ventricular contraction. Thus the stroke volume becomes greater, up to a critical point, after which it decreases. (From Langley LF: *Review of physiology*, ed 3, New York, 1971, McGraw-Hill.)

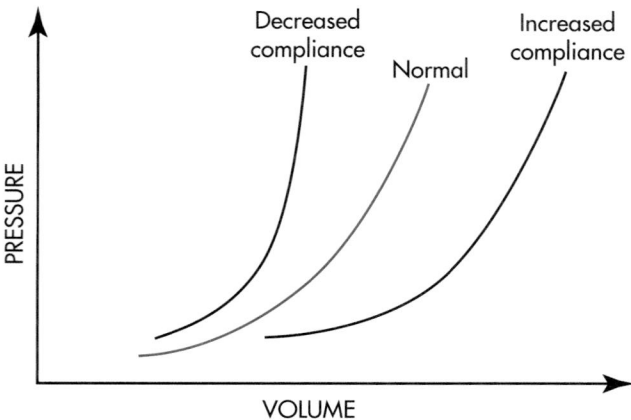

FIG. 33-3 Ventricular compliance, or the pressure-volume relationship of the ventricles. The line in the center indicates the typical relationship between pressure and volume. As volume is increased initially, only a small rise in pressure occurs. As volume increase continues, the rise in pressure is greater. The other lines indicate an alteration in pressure-volume relationships: decreased compliance on the left and increased compliance on the right. This represents a greater or lesser degree of stiffness of the ventricle in relation to the filling volume. Ventricular compliance is a dynamic phenomenon, and this property can change rapidly.

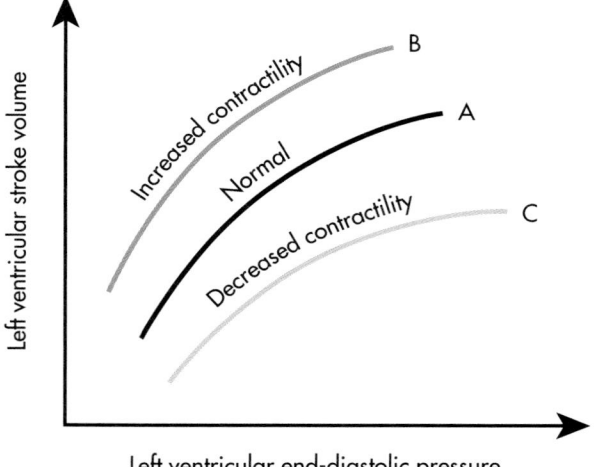

FIG. 33-2 Ventricular function curve. **A**, The solid black line represents the normal ventricular function curve. Note that increasing end-diastolic volume increases stroke volume up to a point. **B**, Displacement of the curve upward and to the left represents improved ventricular function, as would be seen with sympathetic nervous system stimulation. **C**, Displacement of the curve downward and to the right represents myocardial depression, as would be seen with acidosis or hypoxia or with cardiac failure.

lar function in the failing ventricle as would be expected in the normal ventricle.

Additionally, the pronounced flattening of the curve present with failure indicates limited cardiac reserve; after the curve flattens, no further improvement of function can be achieved with elevations of volume and pressure. The presumption is that the ventricular function curve in the failing heart flattens suddenly because the distended, hypertrophied ventricle is relatively noncompliant.

A useful analogy for understanding the effect of *chamber compliance* on the volume and pressure relationships is that of blowing up a child's balloon. Initially, balloons are extremely noncompliant and difficult to inflate; high pressures must be generated to inflate the balloon with even small volumes of air. However, after the balloon has been repeatedly inflated and deflated, it becomes increasingly compliant and easily distensible. The balloon can then be easily inflated with high volumes without exerting much pressure.

Similarly, the precise relationship between a change in intracardiac volume and the resultant change in pressure depends on the compliance or distensibility of the cardiac chambers (Fig. 33-3). An extremely compliant or distensible cardiac chamber can accommodate relatively large changes in volume without significantly increasing pressure; conversely, in the noncompliant, failing ventricle, small increases in volume result in significant pressure elevation and development of congestion and edema.

Contractility

Contractility, the second determinant of myocardial function, refers to changes in the force of contraction or inotropic state that occur independent of changes in fiber length. Changes in contractile function shift the position of the ventricular function curve (see Fig. 33-2). The ad-

Depression of the curve signifies that the failing ventricle requires higher volumes to achieve the same improvement of ventricular and cardiac output that the normal ventricle achieves with lower ventricular volumes. In other words, a given increment in ventricular volume is not associated with as great an improvement in ventricu-

ministration of positive inotropic drugs, such as catecholamines or digoxin, enhances contractility, shifting the curve upward and to the left. Factors depressing contractility, such as hypoxia and acidosis, shift the curve downward and to the right. As indicated, in most forms of heart failure, the ventricular function curve is depressed; this downward shift of the curve represents a depression of myocardial contractility.

Afterload

Afterload is the amount of wall tension the ventricle must develop during systole to eject blood. According to *Laplace's law*, three variables affect wall tension: intraventricular size or radius, intraventricular systolic pressure, and ventricular wall thickness:

$$\text{Wall tension} = \frac{\text{Intraventricular systolic pressure}}{\text{Ventricular wall thickness}} \times \text{Radius}$$

Factors that increase the pressure the ventricle must generate during systole (e.g., arterial vasoconstriction, which increases the resistance to ventricular ejection), or those that increase the ventricular radius (e.g., fluid retention) increase afterload. The failing heart is particularly sensitive to the increased workload imposed by an increase in afterload because of its limited cardiac reserve. Reduction of afterload can be achieved with interventions such as the administration of vasodilators. Ventricular hypertrophy, another consequence of heart failure, also decreases afterload according to Laplace's law. The increased muscle mass facilitates the work of ejection.

Definitions

Heart failure or *cardiac failure* is the pathophysiologic condition in which the heart as a pump is unable to meet the metabolic requirements of the tissues for blood. The critical features of this definition are (1) failure is defined relative to the metabolic needs of the body, and (2) emphasis is placed on the overall failure of the heart's pumping function. The term *myocardial failure* refers specifically to abnormalities in myocardial function; myocardial failure often leads to heart failure, but circulatory compensatory mechanisms can delay or even prevent progression to failure of the heart as a pump.

The expression *circulatory failure* is even more general than is the term *heart failure*. Circulatory failure refers to the inability of the cardiovascular system to perfuse the tissues adequately. This definition encompasses any abnormality of the circulation responsible for the inadequacy in tissue perfusion, including alterations in blood volume, vascular tone, and the heart. *Congestive heart failure* is the state of circulatory congestion resulting from heart failure and its compensatory mechanisms. Congestive heart failure is defined in contradistinction to the more general term *circulatory congestion*, which is simply circulatory overload caused by excess blood volume from cardiac failure or from noncardiac causes, such as overtransfusion or anuria.

Etiology

Heart failure is the most common complication of virtually all forms of acquired and congenital heart disease.

BOX 33-1

Causes of Overall Heart Pump Failure

A. Mechanical abnormalities
   1. Increased pressure load
      a. Central (aortic stenosis, etc.)
      b. Peripheral (systemic hypertension, etc.)
   2. Increased volume load (valvular regurgitation, shunts, increased preload, etc.)
   3. Obstruction to ventricular filling (mitral or tricuspid stenosis)
   4. Pericardial tamponade
   5. Endocardial or myocardial restriction
   6. Ventricular aneurysm
   7. Ventricular dyssynergy
B. Myocardial (muscular) abnormalities
   1. Primary
      a. Cardiomyopathy
      b. Myocarditis
      c. Metabolic abnormalities
      d. Toxicity (alcohol, cobalt)
      e. Presbycardia
   2. Secondary dysdynamic abnormalities (secondary to mechanical abnormalities)
      a. Oxygen deprivation (coronary heart disease)
      b. Metabolic abnormalities
      c. Inflammation
      d. Systemic disease
      e. Chronic obstructive lung disease
C. Altered cardiac rhythm or conduction sequence
   1. Standstill
   2. Fibrillation
   3. Extreme tachycardia or bradycardia
   4. Electrical asynchrony, conduction disturbances

From Hurst JW et al, editors: *The heart*, vol 1, ed 7, New York, 1990, McGraw-Hill.

Physiologic mechanisms producing heart failure include conditions that (1) increase preload, (2) increase afterload, or (3) reduce myocardial contractility. States that increase preload include aortic regurgitation and ventricular septal defect; afterload is increased by conditions such as aortic stenosis and systemic hypertension. Myocardial contractility can be depressed by myocardial infarction and cardiomyopathies. In addition to these three physiologic mechanisms causing heart failure, other physiologic factors can cause the heart to fail as a pump. Factors interfering with ventricular filling, such as atrioventricular (AV) valve stenosis, can produce failure. Conditions such as constrictive pericarditis and cardiac tamponade produce failure by a combination of physiologic effects, including impairment of ventricular filling and ventricular ejection. Apparently, no single physiologic mechanism or combination of mechanisms is responsible for the development of heart failure; the effectiveness of the heart as a pump can be compromised by any number of pathophysiologic states (Box 33-1). Recent studies have focused on the role of tumor necrosis factor (TNF) in the development of heart failure. The normal heart does not express TNF; however, the failing heart produces large quantities.

Similarly, no unifying biochemical explanation can be identified as the fundamental mechanism producing heart failure. The precise defect that produces the impairment in myocardial contractility is unknown. Theories suggest that an abnormality in the delivery of calcium within the sarcomere or in the synthesis or function of the contractile proteins may be responsible.

Factors that can precipitate the development of heart failure by acutely stressing the circulation include (1) dysrhythmias, (2) systemic and pulmonic infection, and (3) pulmonary embolism. Dysrhythmias interfere with the mechanical function of the heart by altering the electrical stimulus initiating the mechanical response; an effective synchronized mechanical response cannot occur without a stable cardiac rhythm. The body's response to infection stresses the heart by increasing metabolic demands on an already compromised circulation. Pulmonary embolism acutely increases the resistance to right ventricular ejection, precipitating right heart failure. Effective management of heart failure requires recognition and treatment of not only the underlying physiologic mechanism and disease state but also any factors precipitating heart failure.

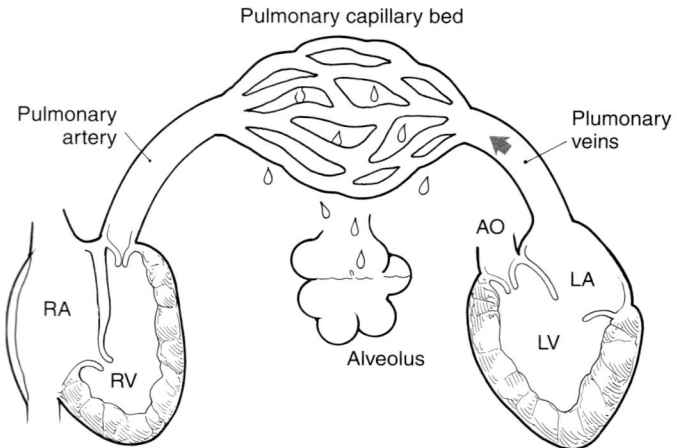

FIG. 33-4   Pulmonary edema in left heart failure. *RA*, Right atrium; *RV*, right ventricle; *AO*, aorta; *LA*, left atrium; *LV*, left ventricle. (Modified from Crawford MV, Spense MI: *Commonsense approach to coronary care*, ed 6, St Louis, 1994, Mosby.)

Pathophysiology

Basic Mechanisms

The intrinsic defect in myocardial contractility characteristic of heart failure in ischemic heart disease impairs the ability of the ventricle to empty effectively. Depressed contractility of the left ventricle reduces stroke volume and elevates residual ventricular volumes. As ventricular EDVs rise, a corresponding increase in left ventricular end-diastolic pressure (LVEDP) is produced. The degree of pressure elevation depends on the compliance of the ventricle. As LVEDP rises, a corresponding elevation of left atrial pressure (LAP) results, because the atrium and ventricle communicate directly during diastole. The increase in LAP is transmitted backward into the pulmonary vasculature, elevating pulmonary venous and pulmonary capillary pressures. If hydrostatic pressure in the pulmonary capillary bed exceeds the vascular oncotic pressure, fluid transudation into the interstitium occurs. When the rate of fluid transudation exceeds the rate of lymphatic drainage, interstitial edema results. Further elevation of pressure may cause fluid seepage into the alveoli and the development of pulmonary edema (Fig. 33-4). (See also Chapter 40 for a discussion of pulmonary edema.)

Pulmonary arterial pressure may rise in response to chronic elevation of pulmonary venous pressure. Pulmonary hypertension increases the resistance to right ventricular ejection. A sequence of events parallel to that affecting the left side of the heart can then result, culminating in systemic congestion and edema.

Development of systemic or pulmonary congestion and edema can be exacerbated by the development of functional regurgitation of the tricuspid or mitral valves, respectively. Functional regurgitation can result from dilation of the AV valve annulus or changes in the orientation of the papillary muscles and chordae tendineae secondary to chamber dilation.

Compensatory Response

In response to heart failure, three primary compensatory mechanisms are observed: (1) increased sympathetic adrenergic activity, (2) increased preload secondary to activation of the renin-angiotensin-aldosterone system, and (3) ventricular hypertrophy. All three compensatory responses represent attempts to maintain cardiac output. These mechanisms may be sufficient to maintain cardiac output at normal or near-normal levels early in the course of failure and in the resting state. Typically, however, some degree of abnormality in ventricular performance and cardiac output appears in the failing heart during exercise. As the failure progresses, compensation becomes less effective.

Increased Sympathetic Adrenergic Activity

The decrease in stroke volume with heart failure elicits a compensatory sympathetic response. The increased activity of the sympathetic adrenergic system stimulates release of catecholamines from cardiac adrenergic nerves and the adrenal medulla. Heart rate and contractile force increase to augment cardiac output. Peripheral arterial vasoconstriction occurs to stabilize arterial pressure and redistribute blood volume away from the metabolically less active organs, such as the skin and kidney, to maintain perfusion to the heart and brain. Venoconstriction increases venous return to the right side of the heart, further augmenting contractile force according to Starling's law.

As would be expected, the level of circulating catecholamines is elevated in heart failure, particularly during exercise. The heart becomes increasingly dependent on circulating catecholamines to maintain ventricular performance. Eventually, however, the myocardial response to sympathetic stimulation lessens; the catecholamines have less effect on ventricular performance. This change can best be conceptualized by referring to the ventricular function curve (see Fig. 33-2).

Normally, catecholamines produce a positive inotropic effect on the ventricle, shifting the curve upward and to the left. As the failing ventricle becomes less responsive to catecholamine stimulation, the degree of shift in response to stimulation lessens. This change may be related to the observation that the myocardial stores of norepinephrine become depleted with chronic heart failure.

Increased Preload through Activation of the Renin-Angiotensin-Aldosterone System

Activation of the renin-angiotensin-aldosterone system results in renal retention of sodium and water, increasing ventricular volume and fiber stretch. This increase in preload augments myocardial contractility according to Starling's law. The exact mechanism responsible for activation of the renin-angiotensin-aldosterone system in heart failure is unclear. However, a number of factors have been implicated, including sympathetic adrenergic stimulation of beta-receptors within the juxtaglomerular apparatus, macula densa receptor response to changes in sodium delivery to the distal tubule, and baroreceptor responses to changes in circulating blood volume and pressure.

Whatever the precise mechanism, the decrease in cardiac output with heart failure initiates the following events: (1) fall in renal blood flow and eventually of glomerular filtration rate, (2) release of renin from the juxtaglomerular apparatus, (3) renin interaction with circulating angiotensinogen to produce angiotensin I, (4) conversion of angiotensin I to angiotensin II, (5) stimulation of aldosterone secretion from the adrenal gland, and (6) retention of sodium and water in the distal tubule and collecting duct (Fig. 33-5). Angiotensin II also produces a vasoconstrictive effect that contributes to the elevation of blood pressure.

In severe heart failure, the combination of systemic venous congestion and diminished perfusion of the liver impairs hepatic metabolism of *aldosterone*, increasing circulating levels of aldosterone. *Antidiuretic hormone (ADH)* levels are also elevated in severe heart failure, which increases the absorption of water in the collecting ducts.

The role of *atrial natriuretic factor (ANF)* in heart failure is currently under investigation. ANF is a hormone synthesized in the atrial tissue. B-type natriuretic peptide (BNP) is secreted mainly by the ventricle. Natriuretic peptides are released in response to increased intracardiac volume or pressure and suppress the renin-angiotensin-aldosterone system. The plasma concentration of these peptides is higher than is normal in patients with heart failure and to a lesser extent in patients with symptomless cardiac impairment. The hormone exerts natriuretic and diuretic effects and relaxes smooth muscle. However, the natriuretic and diuretic effects are overwhelmed by the stronger compensatory factors producing retention of salt and water and vasoconstriction.

Ventricular Hypertrophy

The final compensatory response to failure is myocardial hypertrophy or increased wall thickness. Hypertrophy increases the number of sarcomeres within the myocardial cell; depending on the type of hemodynamic load producing the failure, sarcomeres develop either in parallel or in series. For example, a pressure load, as caused by aortic stenosis, is associated with increased numbers of sarcomeres arranged in parallel, producing an increase in wall thickness without increasing the internal chamber size. The myocardial response to volume loads, as in aortic regurgitation, is characterized by dilation, as well as increased wall thickness. This combination is believed to result from an increased number of sarcomeres arranged in series. These two patterns of hypertrophy are referred to as

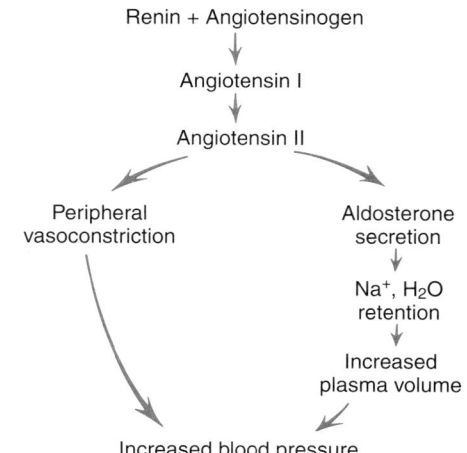

FIG. 33-5   Renin-angiotensin-aldosterone system.

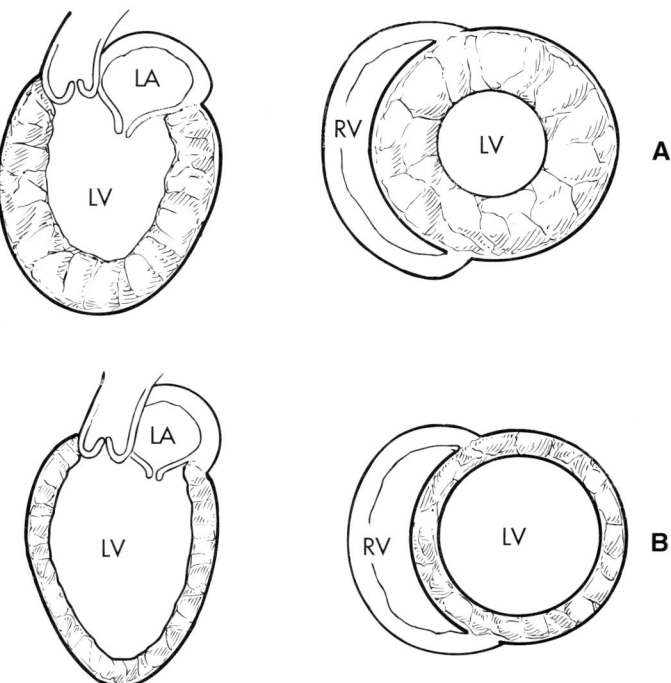

FIG. 33-6   Patterns of ventricular hypertrophy. **A**, Concentric hypertrophy secondary to a pressure load is characterized by increased wall thickness. **B**, Eccentric hypertrophy secondary to a volume load is characterized by a proportional increase in wall thickness and chamber size. *LA*, Left atrium; *LV*, left ventricle; *RV*, right ventricle. (Modified from Rushmer RF: *Cardiovascular dynamics*, ed 4, Philadelphia, 1976, Saunders.)

concentric hypertrophy and *eccentric hypertrophy* (Fig. 33-6). Whatever the precise sarcomere arrangement, myocardial hypertrophy increases the force of ventricular contraction.

Additional Compensatory Mechanisms

Additional mechanisms operate at the tissue level to facilitate the delivery of oxygen to the tissues. Plasma levels of 2, 3-diphosphoglycerate (2,3-DPG) increase, reducing the affinity of hemoglobin for oxygen. As a result, the oxygen-hemoglobin dissociation curve shifts to the right, facilitating the release and uptake of oxygen by the tissues. (See Part Seven for further discussion of the oxyhemoglobin dissociation curve.) Oxygen extraction from the blood is increased to maintain oxygen supply to the tissues in the event of a low cardiac output.

Negative Effects of Compensatory Responses

Initially, the compensatory response of the circulation is beneficial; eventually, however, the compensatory mechanisms can produce symptoms, increase cardiac work, and worsen the degree of failure. The fluid retention intended to augment contractile force causes pulmonary and systemic venous congestion and edema formation. Arterial vasoconstriction and redistribution of blood flow impair tissue perfusion in the affected vascular beds and produce signs and symptoms such as decreased urine output and weakness. Arterial vasoconstriction also increases afterload by increasing the resistance to ventricular ejection; afterload is also increased by dilation of the cardiac chambers. Consequently, cardiac work and myocardial oxygen demand or consumption ($M\dot{V}O_2$) increase. Myocardial hypertrophy and sympathetic stimulation further increase $M\dot{V}O_2$. If the increase in $M\dot{V}O_2$ cannot be met by a corresponding increase in myocardial oxygen supply, then myocardial ischemia and further myocardial compromise can result. The net result of these interrelated events is an increased myocardial burden and perpetuation of the underlying failure.

Clinical Features

Conceptual Framework

Three methods of conceptualizing failure are used in the description of clinical manifestations: (1) forward versus backward failure; (2) systolic versus diastolic failure, and (3) right heart failure versus left heart failure. *Forward failure,* "high-output failure," is characterized by a cardiac output that is above normal for the person's age, gender, and size but is still inadequate for the body's need for oxygenated blood. *Backward failure,* "low-output failure," is characterized by a cardiac output that is absolutely reduced below what is normal for a person of the same age, gender, and size. Easy fatigability, weakness, and mental confusion result from the marked decrease in cardiac output, the hallmark of forward failure, whereas pulmonary congestion and edema indicate the backup of blood resulting from the failing ventricle, the hallmark of backward failure.

Systolic and diastolic dysfunction, rather than reflecting on the hemodynamic state of the heart, reflect changes in the configuration of the ventricles. Systolic dysfunction reflects a decrease in normal emptying capacity that is associated with a compensatory increase in diastolic volume. Diastolic dysfunction is present when the filling of one or both ventricles is impaired while the emptying capacity is normal. Conceptually, systolic and diastolic dysfunction and forward and backward failure are related. Both systolic dysfunction and forward failure reflect on decrease in forward flow. Diastolic dysfunction and backward failure relate to decreased filling. With systolic dysfunction, the ventricle is frequently eccentrically hypertrophied. With diastolic dysfunction, the ventricle is frequently thick-walled and concentrically hypertrophied. The changes in ventricular configuration are called *cardiac remodeling.* These changes are molecular, cellular, and interstitial, resulting in changes in the size, shape, and function of the heart.

The terms *right heart failure* and *left heart failure* imply that the ventricles function as independent pumps. Although this distinction may be useful as a means of categorizing symptoms, the interdependence of the ventricles must be noted. The ventricles are anatomically interdependent in that they share a common wall, the *interventricular septum,* and the muscle fibers composing the ventricular walls are continuous, encircling both ventricles. Not only does anatomic interdependence exist between the ventricles but functional interdependence exists as well in that the ventricles are components of a continuous circuit, and the volume of blood ejected from each ventricle depends on the volume received by that ventricle. It is physiologically impossible for the ventricular stroke volumes to be imbalanced for a prolonged period. For example, the left ventricle cannot sustain an increase in cardiac output unless a corresponding increase occurs in cardiac output in the right ventricle. Impaired function of one ventricle eventually interferes with function of the other ventricle. In fact, left heart failure is recognized as the most common cause of right heart failure because of the phenomenon of backward failure described previously.

Because both ventricles are enclosed within the pericardium, physiologic interaction increases; extreme dilation of one ventricle progressively compresses the other ventricle within the pericardium. Additionally, the ventricles share common biochemical changes in failure; for example, the depletion of norepinephrine stores mentioned earlier does not appear to be isolated to a single chamber. In summary, the interdependence of the ventricular pumps must be recognized. However, the terms right and left heart failure may be used to refer to a complex of symptoms corresponding to failure of a particular ventricle. For example, right heart failure produces systemic venous congestion and edema (Fig. 33-7), whereas left heart failure produces pulmonary venous congestion and edema (see Fig. 33-4).

Signs and Symptoms

The clinical manifestations of heart failure should be considered relative to the degree of physical exertion associated with the appearance of symptoms. Initially, symptoms typically appear only with exertion; however, as failure progresses, exercise tolerance diminishes and symptoms are manifested earlier with lesser degrees of activity. The *New York Heart Association (NYHA) functional classification* is typically used to express the relationship between onset of symptoms and degree of physical exertion (see Box 30-1).

Dyspnea, or the sensation of difficulty in breathing, is the most common manifestation of heart failure. Dyspnea results from the increased work of breathing produced by pulmonary vascular congestion, which reduces lung compliance. Increased airway resistance also contributes to dyspnea. Just as a spectrum of pulmonary congestion exists, ranging from pulmonary venous congestion to interstitial edema and finally to alveolar edema,

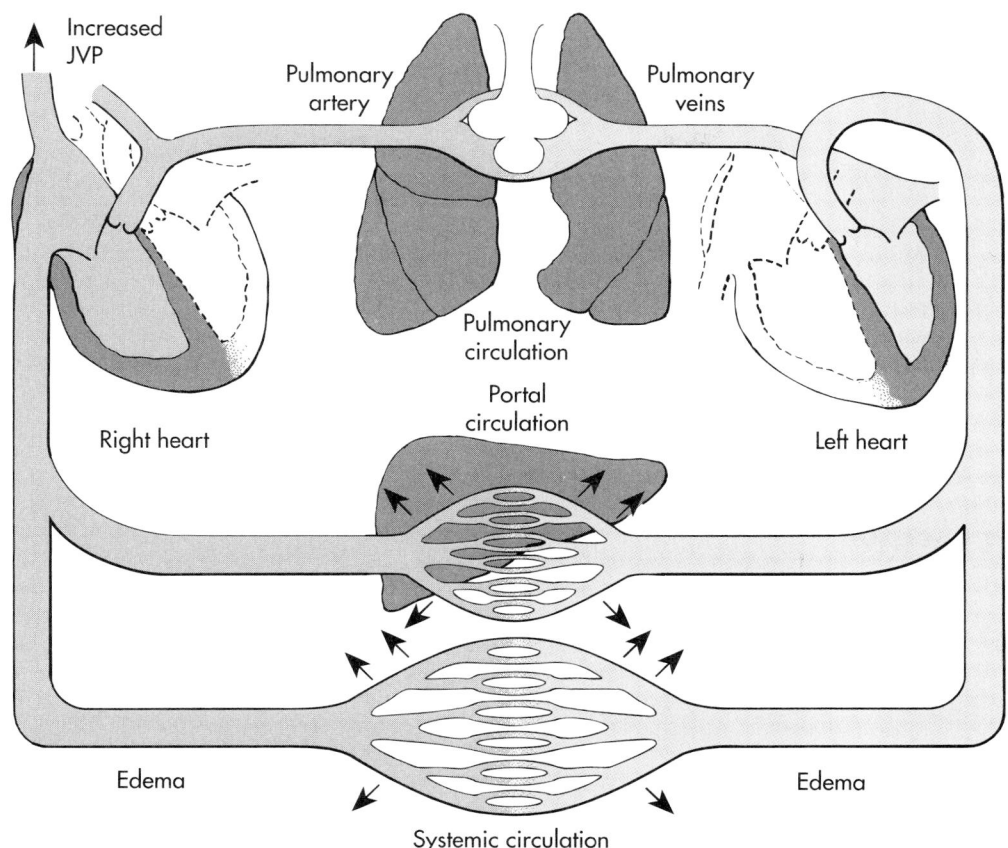

FIG. 33-7 Hemodynamic manifestations of right ventricular failure. *JVP,* Jugular venous pressure.

dyspnea presents in progressively more serious forms. *Dyspnea on exertion (DOE)* represents an early presentation of left heart failure. *Orthopnea,* or dyspnea in the recumbent position, is caused primarily by the redistribution of blood volume from the dependent portions of the body to the central circulation. Reabsorption of interstitial fluid from the lower extremities contributes further to the pulmonary vascular congestion. *Paroxysmal nocturnal dyspnea (PND),* or sudden awakening with dyspnea, is precipitated by the development of interstitial pulmonary edema. PND is a more specific manifestation of left ventricular failure than is either dyspnea or orthopnea.

A nonproductive cough may also occur secondary to the pulmonary congestion, particularly in the recumbent position. Development of *rales* as a result of pulmonary fluid transudation is characteristic of heart failure; initially, rales are audible over the lung bases because of the effects of gravity. All of these signs and symptoms may be ascribed to backward failure of the left side of the heart. *Hemoptysis* may result from bronchial vein bleeding secondary to venous distention. Distention of the left atrium or pulmonary vein may lead to esophageal compression and *dysphagia,* or difficulty swallowing.

Backward failure of the right side of the heart produces signs and symptoms of systemic venous congestion. Elevation of jugular venous pressure (JVP) is noted; the neck veins become engorged. Central venous pressure (CVP) can rise paradoxically during inspiration if the failing right heart is unable to accommodate the in-

spiratory increase in venous return to the heart. This inspiratory rise in CVP is referred to as *Kussmaul's sign.* If tricuspid valve regurgitation develops, pulsatile *v* waves may then be apparent in the jugular vein. A *positive hepatojugular reflux test* can be elicited; manual compression of the right upper quadrant of the abdomen produces jugular venous pressure elevation because, again, the failing right side of the heart is unable to accommodate the associated increase in venous return. *Hepatomegaly,* or liver enlargement, appears; liver tenderness may be noted because of the stretching of the hepatic capsule. Other *gastrointestinal (GI) symptoms,* such as anorexia, fullness, or nausea, may result from hepatic and intestinal congestion.

Peripheral edema develops secondary to fluid accumulation in the interstitial spaces. The edema is initially apparent in dependent regions of the body and is greatest at the end of the day; *nocturia,* or diuresis at night, may occur, lessening the degree of fluid retention. Nocturia results from fluid redistribution and reabsorption in the recumbent position, as well as a reduction in the degree of renal vasoconstriction at rest. Advanced failure may be associated with the development of *ascites* or *anasarca* (generalized body edema). Although the signs and symptoms of fluid accumulation in the systemic venous circuit noted earlier are classically considered as secondary to right heart failure, the earliest manifestations of systemic congestion are usually caused by fluid retention rather than overt right heart failure. All manifestations described here are typically preceded by weight gain, which simply reflects the retention of sodium and water.

Forward failure of the left ventricle produces signs of diminished organ perfusion. Because blood is shunted from nonvital organs to maintain perfusion of the heart and brain, the earliest manifestations of forward failure reflect diminished perfusion of organs such as the skin and skeletal muscles. Skin pallor and coolness result from peripheral vasoconstriction; further reductions in cardiac output associated with increased oxygen extraction and elevated levels of reduced hemoglobin produce cyanosis. The cutaneous vasoconstriction interferes with the body's ability to lose heat; therefore a low-grade fever and excessive sweating may be noted. Underperfusion of the skeletal muscles produces weakness and fatigue. These symptoms can be exacerbated by fluid and electrolyte imbalances or anorexia. Further reduction in cardiac output can be associated with changes in mental status, such as the development of insomnia, restlessness, or confusion. With severe chronic failure, progressive weight loss with poor health and malnutrition, or *cardiac cachexia*, may develop. A combination of factors may be responsible, including low cardiac output and anorexia from visceral congestion, drug toxicity, or an unappealing diet.

Examination of the arterial pulse during heart failure reveals a rapid, weak pulse. The rapid heartbeat, or *tachycardia*, represents a response to sympathetic nervous stimulation. A significant fall in stroke volume and the associated peripheral vasoconstriction reduces pulse pressure (the difference between systolic and diastolic pressure), producing a weak or thready pulse. Systolic hypotension is noted with more severe heart failure. Additionally, severe left ventricular failure may be associated with the development of *pulsus alternans*, an alteration in the strength of the arterial pulse. Pulsus alternans indicates severe mechanical dysfunction with a repetitive beat-to-beat variation in stroke volume.

Common findings on auscultation of the chest are rales, as noted earlier, and a *ventricular gallop*, or *third heart sound* (S₃). The development of an S₃ is the auscultatory hallmark of left ventricular failures. The ventricular gallop occurs during the early diastolic period and results from rapid ventricular filling of the noncompliant and distended ventricle. A *substernal heave*, or systolic lift of the sternum, may result from right ventricular enlargement. Chest radiography reveals the following: (1) pulmonary venous congestion, progressing to interstitial or alveolar edema with more severe failure; (2) vascular redistribution to the upper lobes of the lung; and (3) cardiomegaly. The electrocardiogram (ECG) frequently reveals asymptomatic ventricular premature beats and runs of nonsustained ventricular tachycardia. Bradycardic events (asystole or heart block) are usually associated with progressively worsening heart failure. The significance of these dysrhythmias is unclear, but sudden death is a common terminal event in patients with heart failure.

Characteristic changes in blood values are also apparent. For example, alterations in fluid and electrolyte concentrations are reflected in serum levels. Typically, dilutional hyponatremia is observed; potassium levels may be normal or reduced secondary to diuretic therapy. Hyperkalemia may occur late in the course of heart failure because of renal impairment. Similarly, blood urea nitrogen (BUN) and creatinine levels may be elevated secondary to changes in glomerular filtration rate. Urine is concentrated, with a high specific gravity and reduced sodium content. Abnormalities in liver function may produce minor prolongation of prothrombin time. Elevations of bilirubin and the liver enzymes aspartate aminotransferase (AST, formerly SGOT), and serum alkaline phosphatase (ALP) may be noted, particularly with acute failure.

Treatment

Heart failure is treated by instituting general measures to reduce cardiac work and by selectively manipulating the three primary determinants of myocardial function, either alone or in combination: (1) preload, (2) contractility, and (3) afterload, as well as cardiac remodeling, heart rate and rhythm. Treatment is usually initiated when symptoms appear with ordinary physical exertion (NYHA functional class II). The treatment regimen is progressively intensified until the desired clinical response is obtained. Acute exacerbations of failure or the development of severe heart failure might necessitate hospitalization and more aggressive treatment.

Reduction of Preload

Restriction of dietary salt intake reduces preload by decreasing fluid retention. If symptoms persist with moderate sodium restrictions, oral diuretics are then added to counter the retention of sodium and water. Typically the diuretic regimen is maximized before imposing extreme restrictions of sodium intake. A diet of unpalatable food can lead to loss of appetite and poor nutrition.

Vasodilation of the venous bed can also reduce preload through redistribution of blood from the central to the peripheral circulation. Venodilation produces pooling of blood in the periphery and a reduction of venous return to the heart. In extreme situations, physical removal of fluid through hemofiltration or hemodialysis may be necessary to support myocardial function.

Fig. 33-8, *A*, illustrates the improvement in ventricular function associated with a reduction in preload. As noted earlier, the failing ventricle operates on a depressed and flattened ventricular function curve. As EDV is reduced with diuretics and sodium restriction, the point on the curve corresponding to the ventricular function shift from A to B. As noted on the curve, the symptoms of congestion would be relieved as EDV falls. However, stroke volume and cardiac output would remain stable with optimal preload therapy because the shift occurs along the flat portion of the curve.

Augmentation of Contractility

Inotropic drugs increase the force of myocardial contraction. The precise mechanisms that produce this positive inotropic effect are unclear. However, the common denominator appears to be an increase in the availability of intracellular calcium to the contractile proteins, actin and myosin. As noted earlier, the calcium ion is critical to the development of cross-bridges between the contractile proteins and subsequent muscle contraction.

Two classes of inotropic drugs can be used: (1) digitalis glycosides and (2) nonglycoside agents. *Nonglycoside agents* include sympathomimetic amines, such as epinephrine and norepinephrine, and phosphodiesterase inhibitors, such as amrinone and enoximone. *Sympathomimetic amines* stimulate the adrenergic beta receptors on the myocardium, thereby directly increasing contractility. *Phosphodiesterase (PDE)* is an enzyme that causes the breakdown of a substance, cyclic adenosine monophosphate (cAMP), that promotes the movements of calcium into the cell through the slow calcium channels. Inhibition of PDE increases the level of cAMP and therefore of intracellular calcium. PDE inhibitors also cause vasodilation.

Inotropic drugs improve ventricular function by shifting the entire left ventricular function curve up and to the left (see Fig. 33-8, *B*) thus cardiac output is higher for a given EDV and pressure. Additionally, as the force of contraction increases, stroke volume increases. The increase in forward flow produces a corresponding decrease in residual ventricular volumes. As EDV decreases, an optimal point on the ventricular function curve, point C on Fig. 33-8, *B*, is reached whereby symptoms are relieved and cardiac output is maintained.

Reduction of Afterload

Two of the compensatory responses to heart failure, activation of the sympathetic nervous system and of the renin-angiotensin-aldosterone system, produce vasoconstriction and consequently increase the resistance to ventricular ejection and afterload. As afterload rises, cardiac work increases and cardiac output falls. Arterial vasodilators counter these negative effects. The common vasodilators produce dilation of the vasculature by two primary mechanisms: (1) direct dilation of vascular smooth muscle or (2) inhibition of angiotensin-converting enzyme (ACE). Direct vasodilators include drugs such as hydralazine and nitrates. For hydralazine to be effective, it must be used in combination with a nitrate. The most common combination is hydralazine-isosorbide dinitrate combination, which may be used in combination with ACE inhibitor therapy or alone when an ACE inhibitor is not tolerated.

ACE inhibitors include enalapril and captopril that block the conversion of angiotensin I to angiotensin II. This action prevents angiotensin-induced vasoconstriction and also inhibits aldosterone production and the associated retention of fluid. ACE inhibitors have demonstrated great promise in the management of all grades of overt heart failure. Consequently, therapy with oral vasodilators is now being instituted earlier in the progression of failure, for NYHA class II rather than class III or IV failure.

Arterial vasodilators reduce the resistance to ventricular ejection. As a result, the ventricle can eject more easily and more completely. In other words, cardiac work is reduced and cardiac output rises. Arterial pressure does not usually fall significantly with optimal management because the increase in cardiac output offsets the potential fall in pressure that would result from vasodilation alone.

Recent studies have shown that beta-adrenergic blockers are effective in reducing morbidity and mortality in heart failure. Carvedilol is the only beta blocker that is approved by the U.S. Food and Drug Administration for

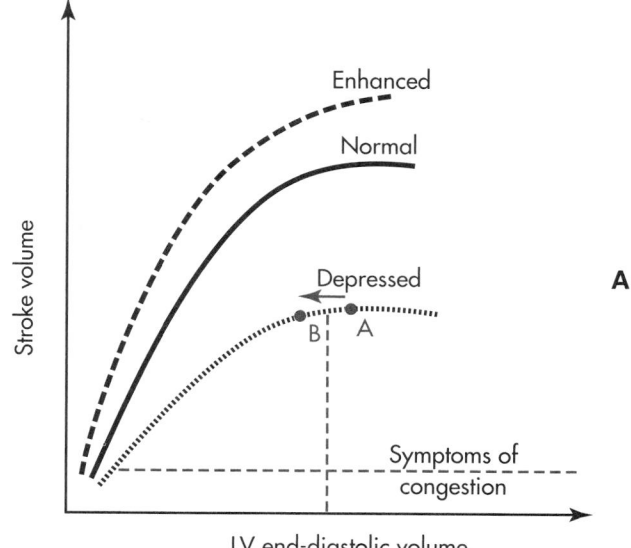

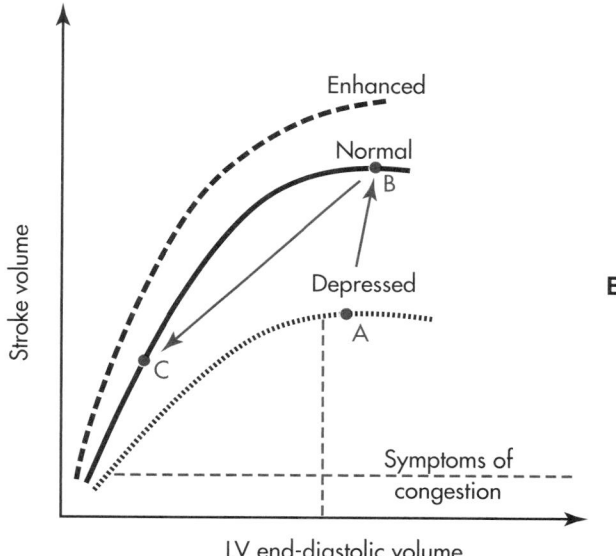

FIG. 33-8   A, Effect of preload therapy on congestive heart failure. The failing ventricle operates on a depressed and flattened ventricular function curve. As end-diastolic volume is reduced with diuretics and sodium restriction, the point on the curve corresponding to ventricular function shifts from *A* to *B*, so symptoms of congestion are relieved. Stroke volume and cardiac output remain stable, since the shift occurs on the flattened part of the curve. **B,** Effect of contractility augmentation on congestive heart failure. Inotropic drugs improve ventricular function by shifting the entire ventricular function curve upward and to the left, so cardiac output is higher for a given end-diastolic volume and pressure. In addition, as the force of contraction increases, stroke volume increases. As end-diastolic volume decreases, an optimal point *(C)* on the ventricular function curve is reached where congestive symptoms are relieved and cardiac output is maintained. *LV,* Left ventricular.

heart failure use and should probably be the beta blocker of choice in patients with symptomatic mild to moderate heart failure. Propranolol, metoprolol, or timolol may be used in asymptomatic patients with no left ventricular dysfunction following a myocardial infarction.

SHOCK

Shock does not constitute a single disease entity; it is a complex clinical syndrome encompassing a group of conditions with variable hemodynamic manifestations. However, the common denominator is the *inadequacy of tissue perfusion*. This state of hypoperfusion compromises the delivery of oxygen and nutrients and the removal of metabolites at the tissue level. Tissue hypoxia shifts metabolism from oxidative pathways to anaerobic pathways with a consequent production of lactic acid. Progressive metabolic derangements perpetuate the shock state, culminating in cellular deterioration and multisystem failure.

The nature of shock is progressive and self-perpetuating. A vicious cycle of progressive deterioration will result if shock is not treated aggressively early in its course. Shock may be characterized according to three progressively severe stages: (1) stage I, the *compensated*, or *nonprogressive*, *stage* during which compensatory responses, outlined earlier in the congestive heart failure section, stabilize the circulation, forestalling further deterioration; (2) stage II, the *progressive stage*, characterized by systemic manifestations of hypoperfusion and worsening organ function; and (3) stage III, the *refractory*, or *irreversible*, *stage* during which profound cellular derangements inevitably culminate in death.

Fundamental Concepts

The basic relationship governing the perfusion or flow of blood to the tissues is the following:

$$MAP = CO \times TPR$$

Mean arterial pressure (MAP) is the pressure head driving blood to perfuse the tissues. However, tissue perfusion can be compromised even in the face of normal arterial pressure if cardiac output (CO) is inadequate or if the resistance to blood flow is high. Most shock states are characterized by low CO and increased total peripheral resistance (TPR). However, shock can also occur with a normal, or even elevated, CO if TPR falls abruptly, as with acute vasodilation, and CO does not rise proportionally to maintain an adequate perfusion pressure. (See Chapter 29 for the fundamentals of blood flow.)

Etiology

Shock can result from a variety of conditions, which may be categorized according to four basic etiologic mechanisms: (1) cardiogenic mechanisms, (2) obstructive mechanisms, (3) alterations in circulatory volume, and (4) alterations in circulatory distribution (see Box 33-2). This section focuses on cardiogenic shock after myocardial infarction (MI) as illustrative of the shock state.

BOX 33-2

Etiologies of Shock

CARDIOGENIC SHOCK
A. Secondary to dysrhythmias
1. Bradydysrhythmias
2. Tachydysrhythmias
B. Secondary to cardiac mechanical factors
1. Regurgitant lesions
a. Acute mitral or aortic regurgitation
b. Rupture of interventricular septum
c. Massive left ventricular aneurysm
2. Obstructive lesions
a. Left ventricular outflow tract obstruction, such as congenital or acquired valvular aortic stenosis and hypertrophic obstructive cardiomyopathy
b. Left ventricular inflow tract obstruction, such as mitral stenosis, left atrial myxoma, and atrial thrombus
C. Myopathic
1. Impairment of left ventricular contractility, as in acute MI or congestive cardiomyopathy
2. Impairment of right ventricular contractility caused by right ventricular infarction
3. Impairment of left ventricular relaxation or compliance, as in restrictive or hypertrophic cardiomyopathy

OBSTRUCTIVE SHOCK*
A. Pericardial tamponade
B. Coarctation of aorta
C. Pulmonary embolism
D. Primary pulmonary hypertension

OLIGEMIC SHOCK
A. Hemorrhage
B. Fluid depletion or sequestration resulting from vomiting, diarrhea, dehydration, diabetes mellitus, diabetes insipidus, adrenocortical failure, peritonitis, pancreatitis, burns, ascites, villous adenoma, or pheochromocytoma

DISTRIBUTIVE SHOCK
A. Septicemic
1. Endotoxic
2. Secondary to specific infection, such as dengue fever
B. Metabolic or toxic
1. Renal failure
2. Hepatic failure
3. Severe acidosis or alkalosis
4. Drug overdose
5. Heavy metal intoxication
6. Toxic shock syndrome (possibly caused by a staphylococcal exotoxin)
7. Malignant hyperthermia
C. Endocrinologic
1. Uncontrolled diabetes mellitus with ketoacidosis or hyperosmolar coma
2. Adrenocortical failure
3. Hypothyroidism
4. Hyperparathyroidism or hypoparathyroidism
5. Diabetes insipidus
6. Hypoglycemia secondary to excess exogenous insulin or a beta-cell tumor
D. Microcirculatory, caused by altered blood viscosity
1. Polycythemia vera
2. Hyperviscosity syndromes, including multiple myeloma, macroglobulinemia, and cryoglobulinemia
3. Sickle cell anemia
4. Fat emboli
E. Neurogenic
1. Cerebral
2. Spinal
3. Dysautonomic
F. Anaphylactic

From Braunwald E, editor: *Heart disease: a textbook in cardiovascular medicine*, ed 2, Philadelphia, 1984, Saunders.
*Caused by factors extrinsic to cardiac valves and myocardium.

Cardiogenic shock is characterized by left ventricular dysfunction, leading to severe impairment of tissue perfusion and oxygen delivery to the tissues. Cardiogenic shock caused by acute MI is typically associated with significant left main disease and severe three-vessel disease, resulting in a loss of 40% or more of the left ventricular myocardium. In addition to massive loss of the left ventricular musculature, focal areas of necrosis may also be found throughout the ventricle. Focal necrosis is thought to result from the sustained imbalance in myocardial oxygen supply and demand. The diseased coronary vessels are unable to increase flow adequately in response to the increase in cardiac work and oxygen demand associated with compensatory responses such as sympathetic stimulation.

As a result of the infarction process, left ventricular contractility and performance may be severely impaired. The left ventricle fails as a pump and does not provide adequate CO to maintain tissue perfusion. A self-perpetuating cycle then ensues (Fig. 33-9). The cycle begins with the MI and subsequent myocardial dysfunction. Profound myocardial dysfunction leads to reduced CO and arterial hypotension. Metabolic acidosis and reduced coronary perfusion result, further impairing ventricular function and predisposing to the development of dysrhythmias. As can be deduced, this cycle of cardiogenic shock must be interrupted early in the shock state to salvage left ventricular myocardium and prevent progression to an irreversible stage, which is incompatible with survival.

Mechanical defects caused by MI can also produce significant myocardial dysfunction and shock. In the shock study (Hochman et al, 2000), mechanical defects accounted for 12% of all patients who went into cardiogenic shock. These defects include the following:

1. *Acute mitral regurgitation* caused by rupture of a necrotic papillary muscle (see Fig. 31-16). This defect produces large amounts of backward or regurgitant blood flow into the left atrium and pulmonary circuit and a corresponding reduction in forward blood flow or CO.

2. *Acquired ventricular septal defect (VSD)* resulting from rupture of an infarcted septum (see Fig. 31-17). Shunting the blood from the high-pressure left ventricle to the lower-pressure right ventricle reduces forward flow into the aorta. In the shock study (Hochman et al, 2000), ventricular septal rupture had

a mortality rate of 87.3%, the highest for any of the mechanical defects.

3. *Ventricular aneurysms* secondary to weakening and bulging of the infarcted region (see Fig. 31-19). Large left ventricular aneurysms reduce left ventricular output by becoming a reservoir for blood during ventricular ejection. The portion of ventricular volume ejected, or the ejection fraction, is reduced, compromising CO.

Pathophysiology and Systemic Effects

Cardiogenic shock may be viewed as a severe form of left ventricular failure. The pathophysiologic events and compensatory responses parallel that of failure, but they have progressed to a more severe form. The depression of cardiac contractility reduces CO and increases left ventricular volumes and end-diastolic pressure, leading to pulmonary congestion and edema.

As systemic arterial pressure falls, stimulation of the baroreceptors in the aorta and the carotid sinus occurs. Sympathoadrenal stimulation produces reflex vasoconstriction, tachycardia, and increased contractility to augment CO and stabilize blood pressure. Contractility is augmented further according to Starling's law by renal retention of sodium and water. Thus the depressed contractility of cardiogenic shock elicits compensatory responses, increasing afterload and preload. Although these protective mechanisms initially enhance arterial blood pressure and tissue perfusion, their effect on the myocardium is deleterious because of the increase in cardiac work and myocardial oxygen demand. Because coronary flow is inadequate, as evidenced by the MI, the imbalance between myocardial oxygen supply and demand increases. Further myocardial dysfunction ensues secondary to ischemia and focal necrosis, perpetuating a vicious cycle of myocardial compromise. As left ventricular performance continues to deteriorate, the shock state rapidly progresses until such profound circulatory failure exists that every major organ system is affected.

The systemic effects of the shock state contribute to its eventual irreversibility. Some organs are affected quickly and more profoundly than are others. As noted, the myocardium undergoes deleterious effects early in the shock state. In addition to the increases in myocardial work and oxygen demand, other significant changes occur. Because of the anaerobic metabolism induced by the shock state, the myocardium cannot maintain its normal level of high-energy phosphate (adenosine triphosphate) stores, and ventricular contractility is further impaired. *Hypoxia* and *acidosis* inhibit energy production and contribute to further destruction of myocardial cells. These two factors also shift the ventricular function curve downward and to the right, depressing contractility further.

Respiratory compromise develops secondary to the shock state. A potentially lethal complication is profound respiratory failure. Pulmonary congestion and intraalveolar edema lead to hypoxia and deterioration of arterial blood gases. Atelectasis and pulmonary infection may also occur. These factors predispose to the development of shock lung, now frequently referred to as adult respiratory distress syndrome (see Chapter 41). Tachypnea, dyspnea, and moist rales are noted, as well as other symptoms described earlier as manifesting backward heart failure.

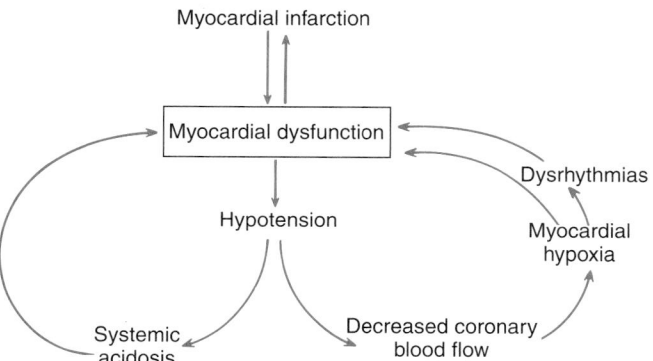

FIG. 33-9   Self-perpetuating cycle of cardiogenic shock. (From Dunkman WB et al: Clinical and hemodynamic results of IABP and surgery for cardiogenic shock, *Circulation* 46:474, 1972.)

Reduced renal perfusion results in oliguria with a urine output generally less than 20 ml/hour. With further reductions in CO, an associated fall in urine output usually occurs. Because of the compensatory retention of sodium and water, urine sodium levels are reduced. Along with the reduction in glomerular filtration rate, an increase in BUN and creatinine is noted. With prolonged, severe hypotension, acute tubular necrosis with ensuing acute renal failure may result (see Chapter 49).

Shock of prolonged duration results in *hepatic cellular dysfunction.* Cellular damage may be localized to isolated zones of hepatic necrosis, or massive hepatic necrosis may occur with profound shock. Marked derangements of liver function become apparent and are usually manifested by elevations of the liver enzymes AST and alanine aminotransferase (ALT, formerly SGPT). Hepatic hypoxia appears to be the etiologic mechanism that initiates these complications.

Prolonged *ischemia of the GI tract* typically results in hemorrhagic necrosis of the bowel. Bowel injury may exacerbate the shock state by sequestering fluid in the gut and by absorbing bacteria and endotoxins into the circulation. A decrease in GI motility is almost always noted in association with shock.

Normally, cerebral blood flow displays the property of autoregulation of flow, with dilation occurring in response to diminished flow or ischemia. Cerebral autoregulation fails to maintain adequate flow and perfusion when the MAP falls below 60 mm Hg. During profound periods of hypotension, symptoms of *neurologic deficit* may be observed. These deficits are not usually sustained if recovery from the shock state occurs, unless a concomitant cerebrovascular accident (CVA, stroke) has resulted.

During sustained shock, intravascular aggregation of cellular components of the hematologic system may occur, increasing peripheral vascular resistance further. Disseminated intravascular coagulation (DIC) may occur during the shock state, further compromising the clinical situation.

Hemodynamic Profile

Criteria for the diagnosis of cardiogenic shock have been established by the Myocardial Infarction Research Units of the National Heart, Lung, and Blood Institute. Cardiogenic shock is characterized by the following:
1. Systolic arterial pressure less than 90 mm Hg or 30 to 60 mm Hg below the previous baseline level
2. Evidence of decreased blood flow to major organ systems:
   a. Urine output less than 20 ml/hour, usually with decreased sodium content
   b. Peripheral vasoconstriction associated with cold, clammy skin
   c. Impaired mental function
3. Cardiac index* less than 2.1 L/min/m²
4. Evidence of left-sided heart failure with LVEDP/pulmonary capillary wedge pressure (PCWP) greater than 18 to 21 mm Hg

---

*Cardiac index is the CO in liters per minute per square meter of body surface area (BSA). The normal resting average is 2.8 L/min/m². Average BSA for a 150-pound man is 1.75 m².

These criteria reflect severe left-sided heart failure with evidence of forward and backward failure. The systolic hypotension and evidence of impaired tissue perfusion are characteristic of the shock state. Extreme depression of the cardiac index to less than 0.9 L/min/m² may be observed with profound cardiogenic shock.

In cardiogenic shock with acute mitral regurgitation, the regurgitant flow significantly increases LAP and PCWP. The development of severe pulmonary edema is common in the setting of acute mitral regurgitation. With the development of a ventricular septal defect (VSD), shunting and mixing of blood occur between the left and right ventricles. Consequently, the oxygen content of the blood in the right ventricle increases. Pressures of the right side of the heart also rise because of recirculation of blood through the right side of the heart and pulmonic circuit. Insertion of a pulmonary artery catheter is indicated to detect these alterations through blood sampling and pressure measurement in the right side of the heart.

Calculated systemic vascular resistance (i.e., the difference between MAP and CVP, divided by CO and multiplied by 80) is markedly increased in cardiogenic shock because of the intense peripheral vasoconstriction.

Treatment

The mortality rate from cardiogenic shock treated with conventional pharmacologic measures to optimize preload, afterload, and contractility approaches 80%. Early, aggressive intervention to interrupt the shock cycle is critical. Survival depends on the efficacy of measures to limit the extent of MI by salvaging myocardium at risk, thereby reducing the potential magnitude of ventricular dysfunction. Therapy for cardiogenic shock has evolved steadily over the last two decades as newer techniques for myocardial salvage have emerged.

In the late 1960s mechanical support of the circulation with the intraaortic balloon pump, described in the next section, was added to the standard pharmacologic regimen in an attempt to reduce cardiac work and improve coronary and peripheral perfusion. Despite an initial hemodynamic improvement during balloon pumping, however, the overall shock mortality rate did not change. Consequently, in the late 1970s emergency coronary revascularization was recommended after stabilization of the circulation with intraaortic balloon pumping. This therapeutic combination improved the shock mortality rate significantly, to approximately 50%. The advent of thrombolytic therapy and angioplasty to recanalize occluded vessels promises to further reduce the mortality rate from this lethal shock state.

Invasive monitoring of the cardiovascular system is generally performed to provide continuous information about blood pressure and intracardiac filling pressures. Placement of an indwelling arterial catheter and a Swan-Ganz pulmonary arterial catheter is usually accomplished soon after admission to an intensive care unit.

Initial measures to stabilize the circulation include the intravenous administration of agents to augment contractility, as well as efforts to reduce preload and afterload and the initiation of intraaortic balloon pumping. Definitive, aggressive treatment must be instituted within hours of the onset of the shock state, at the same time that specific diagnostic testing and definitive interventions are performed.

Positive inotropic agents, such as dobutamine and amrinone, are used to augment contractility. Preload is decreased by reduction of intravascular volume with diuretics and vascular redistribution of volume with *venodilators,* such as nitroglycerin. Nitroglycerin also exerts a positive vasodilatory effect on the coronary circulation, improving coronary blood flow. PCWP, the clinical measure of LVEDP, is used to guide the administration of diuretics and vasodilators.

Arterial vasodilators or *vasopressors* may be indicated to reduce afterload or increase arterial pressure, respectively. However, both categories of drugs must be used with caution in cardiogenic shock. Arterial vasodilators, such as sodium nitroprusside, dilate the smooth muscle of the arterial system, reducing the resistance to ventricular ejection and thereby improving CO. However, arterial pressure will fall and compromise tissue perfusion further if the increase in CO is not large enough to offset the fall in peripheral resistance with arterial vasodilation (MAP = CO × TPR).

The deleterious effects of vasopressors result from the effects of sympathetic alpha- and beta-receptor stimulation. Alpha-receptor stimulation produces vasoconstriction, which increases arterial pressure and the resistance to ventricular ejection. Beta receptor effects include augmentation of contractility. Elevation of arterial pressure and improvement in contractility are beneficial to the extent that the circulation is stabilized. However, both effects significantly increase oxygen demand, jeopardizing myocardium at risk for infarction. Agents with beta-receptor activity also are potentially dysrhythmogenic, which further hinders myocardial performance. The use of vasopressors is usually limited to those patients whose hypotension is so profound that no other means of therapy provides blood pressure support.

Vasopressor agents, such as epinephrine, norepinephrine (Levophed), and dopamine, stimulate both alpha receptors and beta receptors, although to varying degrees. Dopamine is the vasopressor of choice for cardiogenic shock. In low doses, dopamine exerts a selective vasodilatory effect on the renal vasculature.

Dysrhythmias, hypoxia, and acidosis can perpetuate the shock state. The administration of *antidysrhythmic drugs* may be indicated. Restoration of sinus rhythm generally improves CO and blood pressure. Oxygenation is supported with the administration of supplemental oxygen and the initiation of mechanical ventilation if indicated. Treatment of acute pulmonary edema involves reduction of preload with vasodilators and diuretics as described and the administration of morphine sulfate. Correction of metabolic acidosis is accomplished with adjustment of ventilation or the administration of sodium bicarbonate.

Rapid institution of the conventional measures described previously, combined with intraaortic balloon pumping, typically permits hemodynamic stabilization, allowing for cardiac catheterization and emergency revascularization or repair of mechanical defects, if indicated, under more controlled conditions. The role of thrombolytic therapy, angioplasty and early revascularization in shock therapy is currently under clinical investigation.

In some centers, *thrombolytic therapy* is initiated within hours of the MI to recanalize the affected vessel and salvage myocardium. If the thrombolytic drugs are ineffective in dissolving the clot, myocardial revascularization with either angioplasty or coronary artery bypass surgery is then considered.

The use of thrombolytic therapy in the hours immediately after infarction appears to reduce not only the mortality rate from cardiogenic shock but also the incidence of shock. The incidence of cardiogenic shock after MI has remained constant, complicating approximately 5% to 15% of MIs. Thrombolysis and early reperfusion may be most beneficial in preventing the development of shock.

The role of left heart assist devices and cardiac replacement with the artificial heart is being investigated for shock refractory to conventional measures, including intraaortic balloon pumping. Both forms of circulatory assistance are discussed in the next section.

METHODS OF CIRCULATORY ASSISTANCE

Circulatory assistance devices can be used either to support ventricular function or to replace the failing heart. Support devices include cardiopulmonary bypass, intraaortic balloon pumping, and ventricular assist devices. Alternatively, an artificial heart or transplant can be used to replace the heart.

Cardiopulmonary Bypass

Circulatory assistance was used initially for cardiopulmonary support during cardiac surgical procedures in the early 1950s. During open-heart surgery, the oxygenation and systemic circulation of blood is sustained by a heart-lung machine, referred to as *cardiopulmonary bypass* (Fig. 33-10). Catheters or cannulae are inserted into the superior vena cava and inferior vena cava to shunt venous blood away from the right side of the heart into the cardiopulmonary bypass machine. Additional blood is returned to the bypass machine by a mediastinal "sucker," which is placed in the operative field to collect blood lost during the surgical procedure. The bypass machine performs the following functions: (1) oxygenation of blood, (2) cooling of blood to induce systemic hypothermia and reduce tissue oxygen demand, and (3) filtration of blood to remove air and particulate matter. The blood is then pumped into the arterial circulation via a cannula positioned in either the aortic arch or the femoral artery. Immediately before weaning from cardiopulmonary bypass, the heat exchanger in the bypass unit rewarms the blood. *Partial cardiopulmonary bypass* can be initiated rapidly via percutaneous cannulation of the femoral vein and femoral artery. This technique has been used for resuscitation at the bedside. *Extracorporeal membrane oxygenation (ECMO)* is a form of partial cardiopulmonary bypass used for respiratory failure.

Intraaortic Balloon Pumping

The intraaortic balloon is positioned in the descending thoracic aorta immediately distal to the left subclavian

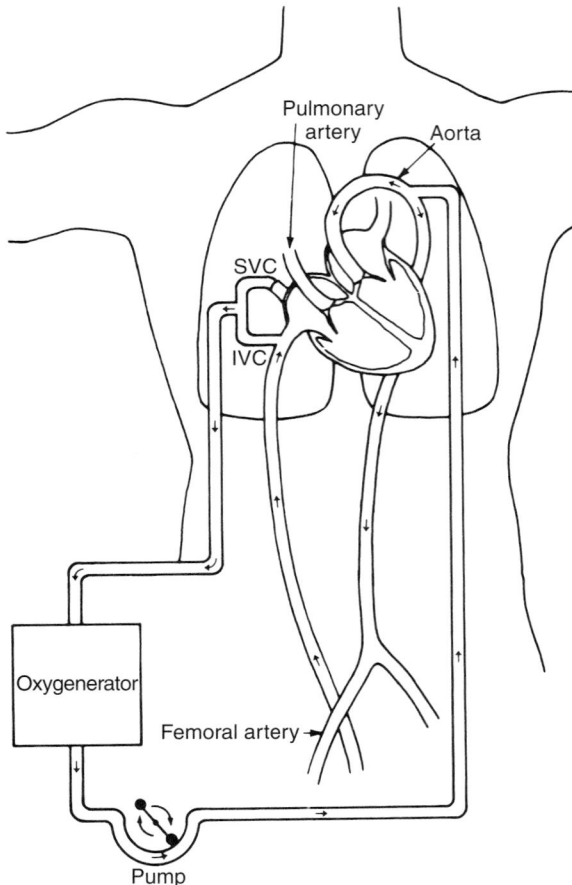

FIG. 33-10 Total cardiopulmonary bypass. Venous blood is shunted from the right atrium to the assist device via catheters inserted into the superior vena cava *(SVC)* and inferior vena cava *(IVC)*. The blood is oxygenated by the device and returned to the arterial system through a cannula in the aorta. (From Kinney M, editor: *AACN's clinical reference for critical care nurses*, New York, 1981, McGraw-Hill.)

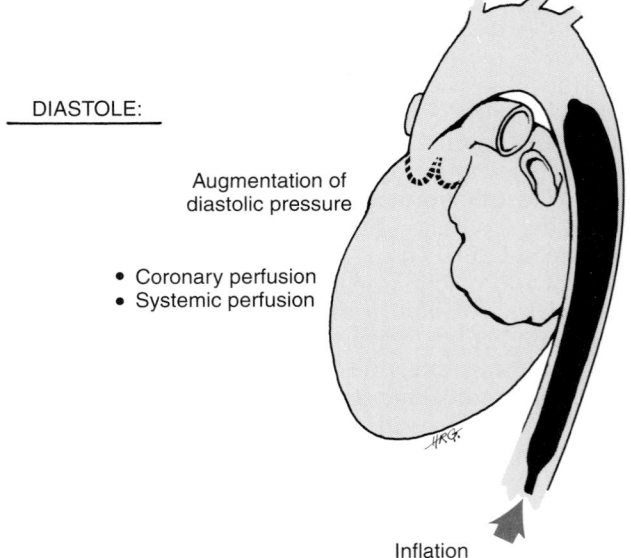

FIG. 33-11 Effect of intraaortic balloon inflation.

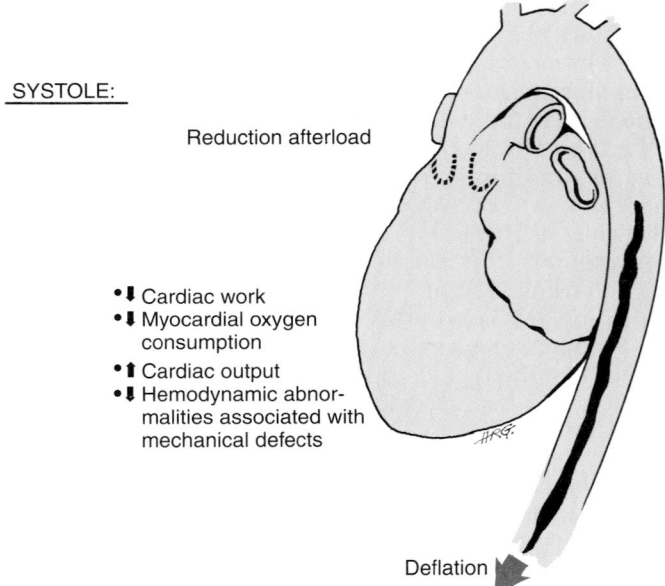

FIG. 33-12 Effect of intraaortic balloon deflation.

artery and is inserted via either a percutaneous approach or a femoral arteriotomy and threaded retrograde through the descending abdominal aorta. The balloon is inflated and deflated in synchrony with the mechanical events of the cardiac cycle. During left ventricular ejection or systole, the balloon must be deflated. During ventricular diastole the balloon is inflated.

Inflation of the balloon with gas occurs just as the aortic valve closes at the end of systole; balloon inflation raises aortic volume, elevating aortic pressure. This effect is referred to as *augmentation of diastolic pressure*. The physiologic effect of diastolic augmentation is twofold (Fig. 33-11): (1) the perfusion pressure at the coronary orifices is increased during diastole, the period of greatest coronary flow, potentially increasing coronary flow; and (2) systemic perfusion also improves through elevation of mean arterial pressure (MAP).

Balloon deflation occurs rapidly, immediately before ventricular ejection, immediately before the aortic valve opens. As gas is removed from the balloon, intraaortic volume is lowered, thereby reducing aortic pressure. This reduction lowers the resistance against which the left ventricle must eject; consequently, ventricular wall tension developed during systole is lower. In other words, balloon deflation reduces afterload. The physiologic effects are as follows (Fig. 33-12): (1) reduction in cardiac work, (2) reduction in oxygen demand and $M\dot{V}O_2$, and (3) increase in CO.

The intraaortic balloon pump is frequently used for cardiogenic shock and for failure to wean from cardiopulmonary bypass. Balloon pumping is particularly effective in the reversal of cardiogenic shock resulting from mechanical defects, such as VSD and mitral regurgitation. Initiation of balloon pumping in these patients reduces aortic pressure and resistance to ejection, thereby increasing forward flow through the aorta and reducing abnormal flow through the defect. Refractory myocardial ischemia is also responsive to balloon pumping; the intrathoracic balloon pump can influence both the supply and the demand determinants of the myocardial oxygenation balance. Coronary blood flow increases with diastolic augmentation, and myocardial oxygen demand falls as a result of the reduction of afterload. The balloon is also used to maintain organ perfusion in patients with class IV heart failure awaiting transplantation.

Ventricular Assist Devices

Ventricular assist devices (VADs) were originally used for the sole support of the left ventricle. These *left heart assist devices* bypassed the left ventricle, temporarily supporting the circulation. However, after the incidence of right heart failure, either coexistent in left heart failure or in isolation, was recognized, the design of VADs was extended to the right ventricle.

The most common indication for use of a VAD is as a bridge to transplantation. In this manner, VADs are used to stabilize and sustain a patient who would otherwise die before a heart was available. After a donor heart becomes available, VAD support is discontinued. A second indication for use of a VAD is as a bridge to recovery. The indications for use in this situation are cardiogenic shock or failure to wean from the bypass. Both conditions must be refractory to conventional pharmacologic therapy and to intraaortic balloon pumping. Ventricular assistance is intended to stabilize the circulation as the myocardium recovers. The last indication for use of a VAD is as destination therapy. In this instance, the VAD would be the final therapy. Studies that examine this use of the VAD are currently in progress.

The basic design of the current VADs shunts blood from either atrium through a pneumatic or vented electric pump into the aorta or pulmonary artery, bypassing the affected ventricle (Fig. 33-13). Alternately, a cannula may be placed in the ventricular apex for inflow into the VAD. The VAD may be internally implanted with the power source connection exiting the body, or it may be an external device with only the cannula implanted and the pump itself external to the body. Fig. 33-13 illustrates the two types of VADs. An oxygenator is not required because flow through the lungs is preserved; the device assumes only the work of pumping for the ventricle. If biventricular assist is required, separate circuits are then maintained for each ventricle.

Some electrical devices have been recently introduced that overcome the limited mobility and prolonged hospitalizations necessitated by the pneumatic devices. Figure 33-14 shows the components of the HeartMate Vented Electric (VE) Left Ventricular Assist System.

Artificial Heart

Artificial replacement of the heart has been of interest since the late 1950s. Since then, many advances have made the artificial heart clinically applicable to humans. In 1969 the artificial heart was used in Texas by Cooley for circulatory support before transplantation.

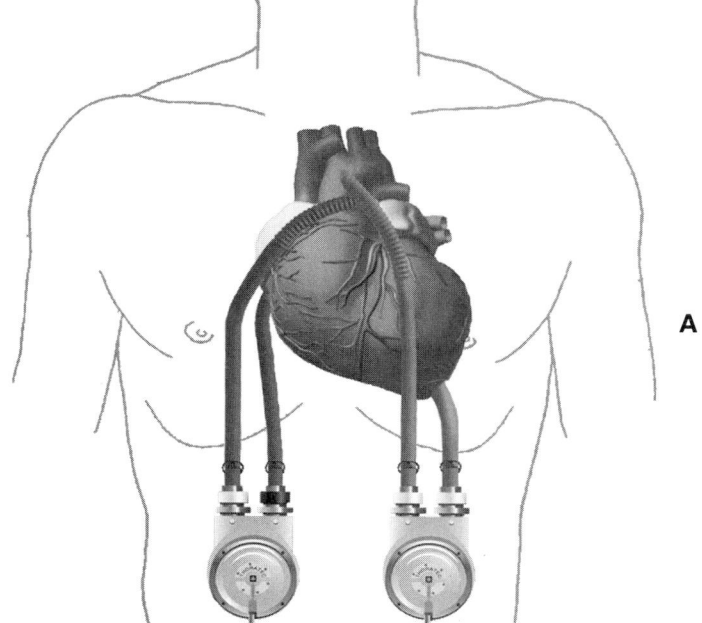

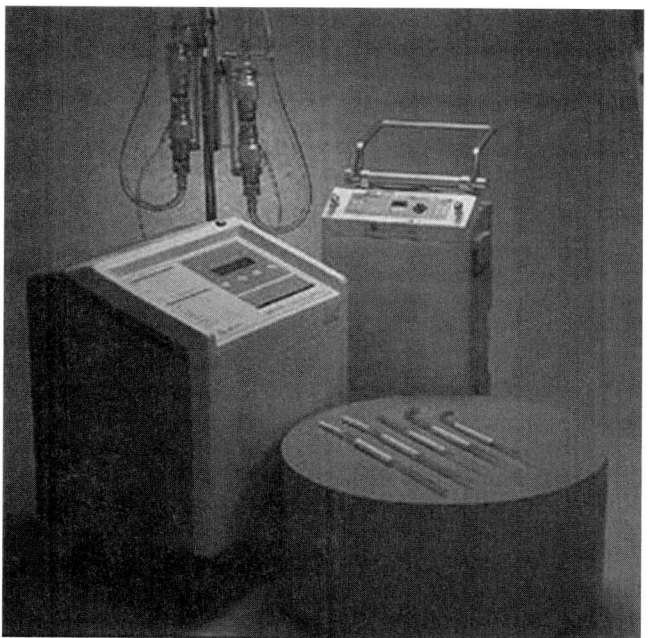

FIG. 33-13   Two examples of external ventricular assist devices. The internal component of the systems are the cannulae that exit the body and attach to blood pumps that sit outside the body; the pumps are then attached to a drive console. These devices may be used for right ventricular support, left ventricular support, or biventricular support. **A,** Thoratec Ventricular Assist Device System: placement of cannulae for biventricular support. **B,** Abiomed BVS 5000 Bi-Ventricular Support System. (**A** courtesy Thoratec Corporation, Pleasanton, Calif; **B** courtesy ABIOMED, Danvers, Mass.)

The first permanent implantation of the total artificial heart was performed in 1982 at the University of Utah for Barney Clark, DDS. Fig. 33-15 illustrates one artificial heart design, the AbioCor Replacement Heart. Development is continuing on the artificial heart to improve

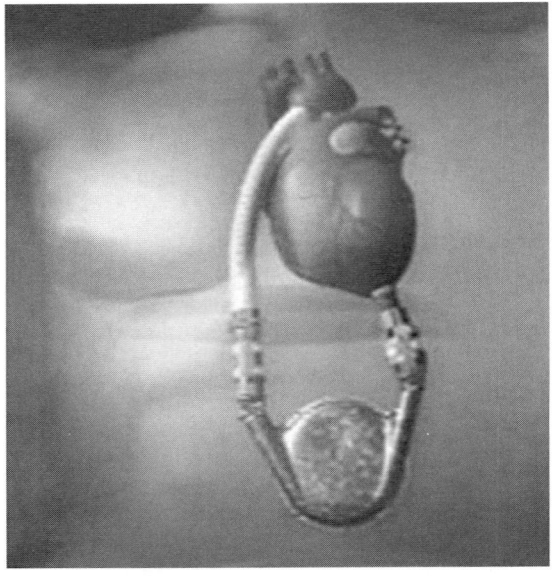

FIG. 33-14 HeartMate Vented Electric Left Ventricular Assist System: An internally implanted device with a drive line that exits the skin and attaches to a Power Base Unit or Batteries. The battery system allows the patient to return home or to work and their usual activities while awaiting a heart transplant. (Courtesy Thoratec Corporation, Pleasanton, Calif.)

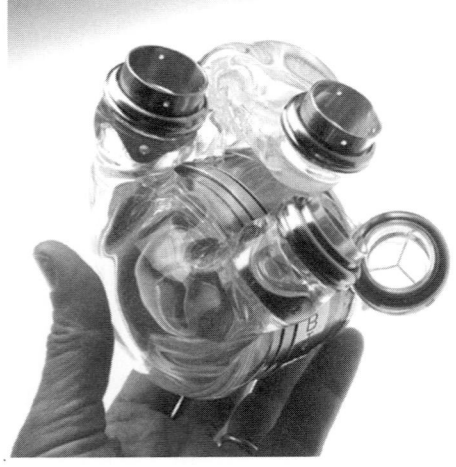

FIG. 33-15 AbioCor Replacement Heart, totally internal with no external drive lines. It was approved for clinical trials in January, 2001. (Courtesy ABIOMED, Danvers, Mass.)

long-term survival and reduce morbidity. The National Heart, Lung, and Blood Institute (NHLBI) of the National Institutes of Health (NIH) has provided funding for a permanent, tether-free, electromechanical artificial heart. Penn State and 3-M and Texas Heart Institute/Abiomed have been participating in Phase II experiments. The overall goal is to give patients a high quality of life free of percutaneous lines. The devices are electrically driven with transcutaneous electrical energy transmission systems (TEETS) with portable battery packs.

CARDIAC TRANSPLANTATION

The first human cardiac transplant was performed in 1967 by Christian Barnard in South Africa. After an initial period of enthusiastic response, interest waned because of poor long-term success. Rejection appeared to be an insurmountable problem. Over the years, refinements in immunosuppressive therapy, immunologic monitoring techniques, and organ preservation techniques have resulted in significant improvements in patient survival. Thus the procedure is no longer considered experimental. In 1986 Medicare patients became eligible for federal reimbursement for cardiac transplants.

Indications

Cardiac transplantation is considered for end-stage heart disease refractory to conventional medical and surgical therapy. Class III and IV heart failure must be evident, along with a life expectancy of less than 1 year. The two most common conditions producing such myocardial compromise are congestive cardiomyopathy and advanced coronary disease. These entities combined account for 80% to 90% of all cardiac transplants.

Coronary artery disease is discussed in Chapter 31. *Cardiomyopathies* are diseases of the heart muscle of unknown origin. The key to distinguishing cardiomyopathies from other cardiac disorders is that the underlying abnormality involves the ventricular myocardium rather than any other myocardial structure, such as the valves or coronary arteries. Cardiomyopathies may be classified according to three types of abnormalities in structure and function: (1) congestive (dilated), (2) restrictive or obliterative, or (3) hypertrophic (Fig. 33-16).

Congestive cardiomyopathy is characterized by a grossly dilated and hypodynamic ventricle. Myocardial hypertrophy may occur to a lesser degree. The hypodynamic ventricle contracts poorly, producing the predictable sequence of forward and backward failure described earlier. A noteworthy factor is that all four chambers become dilated secondary to increased volumes and pressures. Thrombus frequently develops within these chambers as a result of blood pooling and stasis; thus embolization is a threat. Typically, the onset of the disease is insidious; however, progression to end-stage refractory heart failure can result. The prognosis for refractory heart failure is extremely poor and may lead to consideration for heart transplantation. The exact cause of congestive cardiomyopathy is unknown; however, autoimmune and viral causes have been suggested. Multifactorial causation is probably the most plausible explanation.

Hypertrophic cardiomyopathy, in contrast to congestive cardiomyopathy, is characterized by a hypertrophied and hyperdynamic heart. The increase in muscle mass is not associated with significant myocardial dilation. A genetic basis is suspected. *Restrictive cardiomyopathy* represents an impairment in ventricular filling caused by reduced ventricular compliance. Endocardial or myocardial fibrosis can result in restriction to filling. The restriction reduces cavity size; progression to a more severe form of cavity restriction is referred to as *obliterative cardiomyopathy*. Although hypertrophic and restrictive cardiomyopathies can cause heart failure, congestive

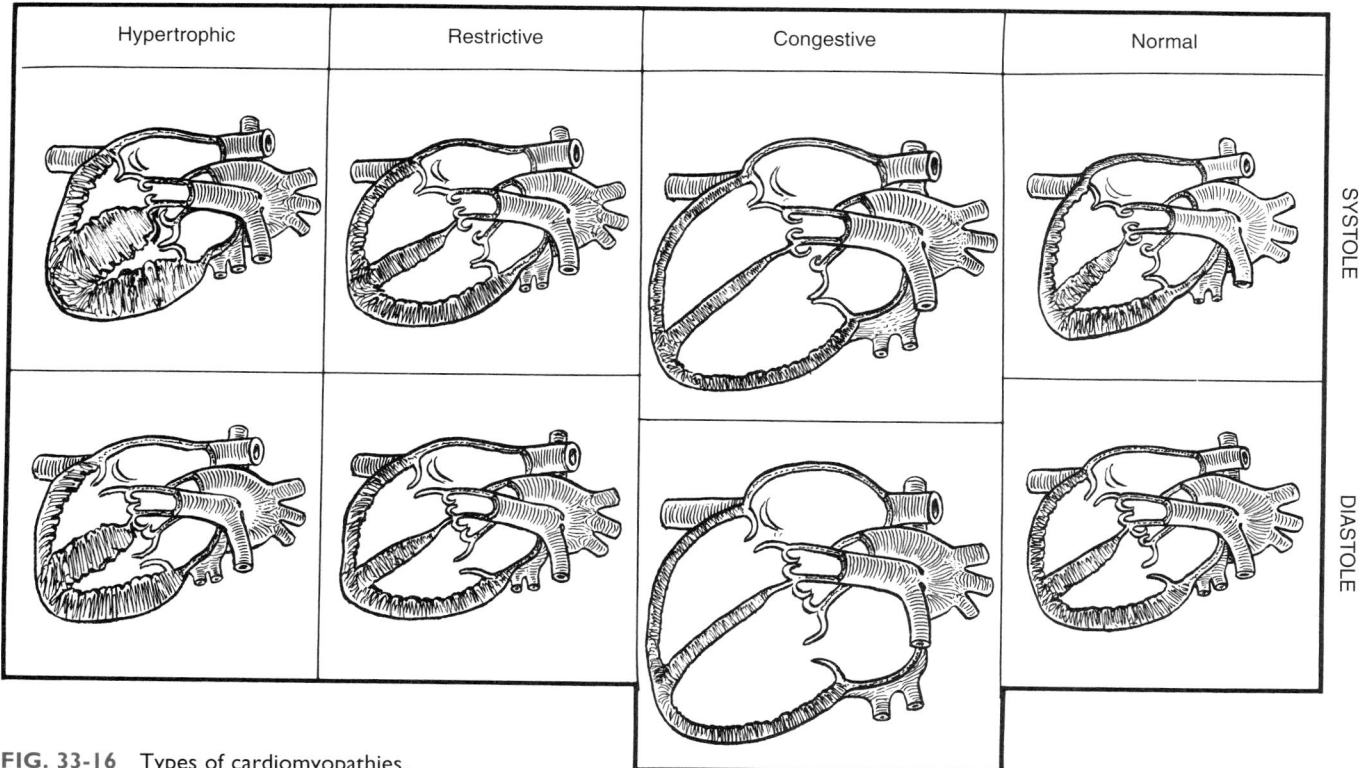

Hypertrophic	Restrictive	Congestive	Normal	
				SYSTOLE
				DIASTOLE

FIG. 33-16   Types of cardiomyopathies.

cardiomyopathy is the most significant entity relative to cardiac transplantation.

Selection Criteria

Cardiac transplant recipients who meet medical criteria for selection undergo an extensive clinical and psychosocial evaluation. As the procedure becomes better established and more widely available, decisions about which individuals are eligible for transplantation become more controversial. Donor availability continues to be a major limiting factor. Consequently, after a decision to perform a transplant has been made, establishing the individual's priority relative to others becomes a problem. Determining the relative priority of individuals with VADs and artificial hearts implanted as bridges to transplantation is a particularly complex question.

Generally, however, factors that would complicate the postoperative course or affect long-term survival must be ruled out. These factors include active systemic infection or disease, pulmonary hypertension with fixed pulmonary vascular resistance (greater than 4 Wood units),* pulmonary emboli or infarction, active peptic ulcer disease, insulin-dependent diabetes mellitus with secondary end-organ disease, irreversible liver or renal failure, obesity, and active drug addiction or alcoholism. Intangible factors, such as motivation for rehabilitation, family support structure, and psychosocial state, are also considered. As insurance coverage becomes broader, personal fi-

nancial resources become less significant to the selection process. If no contraindications are identified, then a search for a potential donor is undertaken.

Potential donors are typically young trauma victims with no evidence of cardiac damage or disease and no systemic infection. Tissue matching of the donor to the recipient includes matching of the ABO system. An appropriate size match is also important; 20% body weight difference is considered to be an acceptable discrepancy.

Procedure

The surgical technique for cardiac transplantation is relatively straightforward, as illustrated in Fig. 33-17. A portion of both atria remain in situ for anastomosis to the donor heart. The region of the right atria near the superior vena cava is left intact to preserve sinus node function. The donor heart is then sutured to the recipient's atria and to the pulmonary artery and aorta. This procedure, in which the transplant is substituted for the recipient's heart, is referred to as *orthotopic transplantation.* Additionally, this procedure is in contrast to *heterotopic,* or "piggyback," *transplantation,* which is considered in some centers if pulmonary vascular resistance is extremely high and the high afterload in the pulmonary artery is likely to lead to refractory right ventricular failure in a transplanted heart. The reasoning suggests that the native right ventricle has adapted to this high afterload state and should therefore remain in situ. Alternately, some centers are performing cardiopulmonary transplants for primary pulmonary hypertension or pulmonary vascular disease secondary to congenital heart disease.

---

*Wood units equal pulmonary vascular resistance divided by 80.

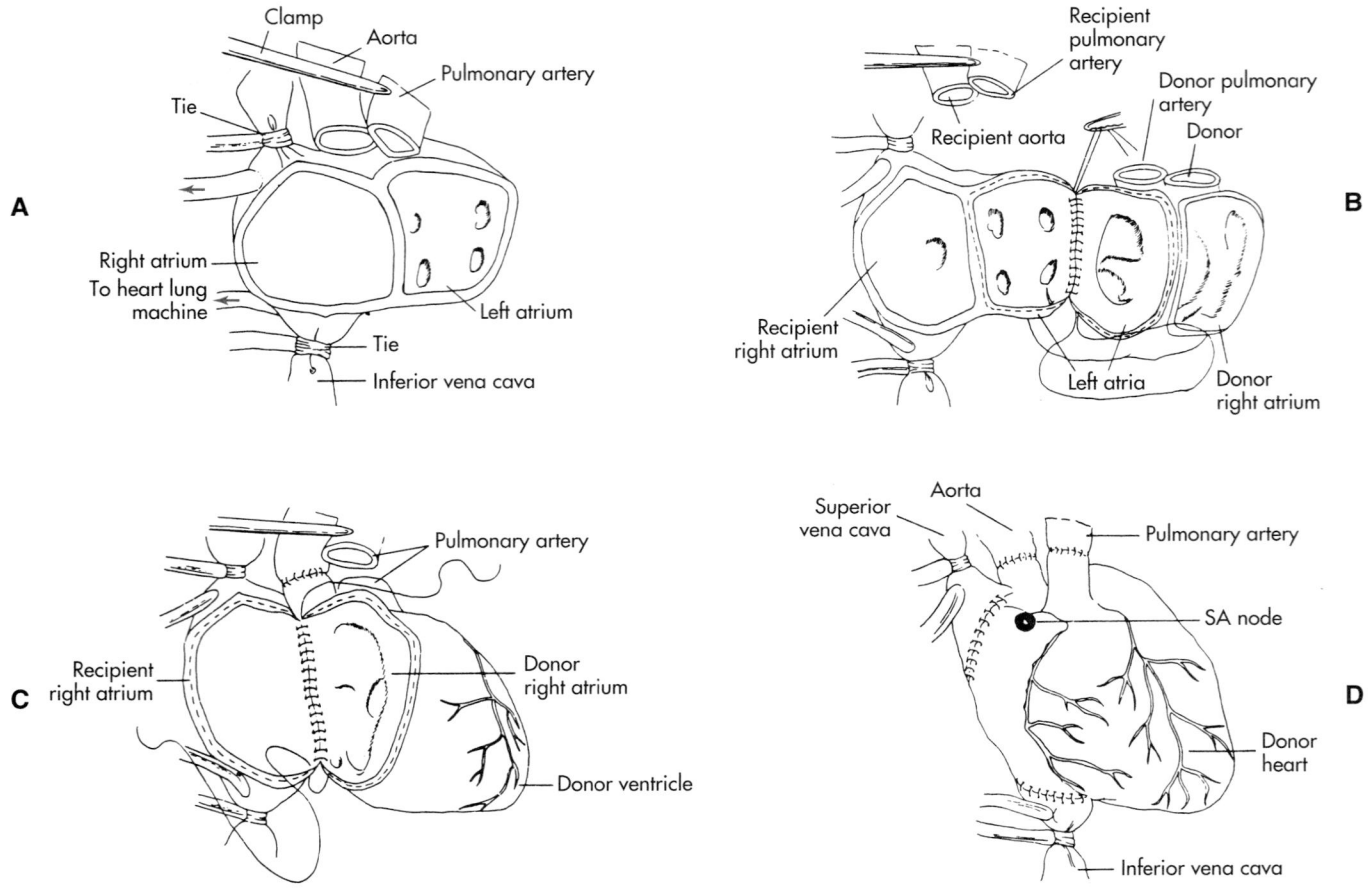

FIG. 33-17 Technique of cardiac transplantation. The procedure is performed as a conventional open-heart procedure with the usual equipment and instrumentation. It does not present any particular mechanical difficulties. The patient is routinely prepared and a median sternotomy performed. The patient is then connected to a cardiopulmonary bypass machine after systematic heparinization. The donor heart is removed after arrest is achieved by infusion of cold cardioplegia solution. It is then placed in cold saline solution for transfer to the recipient's operating room. The heart of the recipient is removed simultaneously. **A,** The aorta and pulmonary artery are divided immediately above their respective valves. Atrial walls and the interatrial septum are divided near the atrioventricular groove, leaving two large right and left atrial cuffs. **B,** Orthotopic graft is performed by anastomosing recipient and donor atrial walls and interatrial septum. **C** and **D,** Major vessels of donor and recipient. The aorta and pulmonary artery are trimmed and sutured, reestablishing anatomic continuity. The cardiac transplantation procedure is terminated as in any conventional open-heart procedure, with great care to prevent hemostasis and to eliminate entrapped air in the graft. The donor heart often starts beating spontaneously in sinus rhythm when perfusion is reestablished and rewarming is achieved. *SA,* Sinoatrial. (From Michaelson CR, editor: *Congestive heart failure,* St Louis, 1983, Mosby.)

Rejection and Infection

The greatest challenge in transplantation is the management of rejection. The body's attempt to reject foreign tissue is a fundamental biologic process. The advent of cyclosporine and monoclonal antibody preparations has significantly improved survival after transplantation. Immunosuppressive therapy with cyclosporine may be initiated preoperatively. Triple-drug immunosuppressive therapy with azothioprine, cyclosporine, and steroids is continued indefinitely after surgery. Close immunologic monitoring for signs of rejection is instituted. Transvenous endomyocardial biopsies are the "gold standard" for the detection and diagnosis of rejection. Biopsies are performed at regular intervals and as indicated. (Noninvasive methods to detect rejection, including magnetic resonance imaging and echocardiography, are under investigation.) *Endomyocardial biopsy technique* involves the insertion of a biopsy catheter, or *bioptome,* through the right jugular or subclavian vein into the right ventricle to remove several portions of the endocardium for analysis. Results are then graded by a standardized cardiac biopsy grading system. Immunosuppressive therapy can then be adjusted accordingly. Antithymocyte globulin (ATG), antilymphocyte globulin (ALG), or monoclonal OKT3 antibodies may also be added to treat rejection (see Chapter 48). In addition to potential rejection, infection is a significant problem because of immunosuppressive therapy. Infection is the leading cause of death in the first year after transplantation. Appropriate prophylactic and therapeutic measures are used.

KEY CONCEPTS

- The three primary determinants of cardiac function are preload, afterload, and contractility.
- *Starling's Law of the Heart*: as the EDV increases, the force of ventricular contraction also increases.
- *Contractility* refers to the changes in the force of contraction or inotropic state that occurs independent of changes in fiber length.
- *Afterload* is the amount of wall tension the ventricle must develop during systole to eject blood.
- *Heart failure* is the pathophysiologic condition in which the heart as a pump is unable to meet the metabolic requirements of the tissues.
- *Congestive heart failure* is the state of circulatory congestion resulting from heart failure and its compensatory mechanisms.
- Conditions that can produce heart failure are myocardial infarction (MI) and cardiomyopathies, aortic regurgitation and ventricular septal defect (VSD), aortic stenosis, and systemic hypertension.
- In response to *heart failure*, three primary compensatory mechanisms are observed: (1) increased sympathetic adrenergic activity, (2) increased preload secondary to activation of the renin-angiotensin-aldosterone system, and (3) ventricular hypertrophy.
- Over time, the compensatory mechanisms may have a negative effect resulting from increased cardiac work, thereby worsening the degree of heart failure.
- The signs of *heart failure* include: tachycardia, gallop rhythms (S_3 and S_4), tachypnea, cough, bibasilar rales, hemoptysis, increased pulmonary artery pressures, pulmonary edema, cyanosis, pulmonary hypertension, increased CVP, jugular venous distension, peripheral edema, hepatomegaly, splenomegaly.
- Symptoms of *heart failure* include: fatigue, dyspnea, orthopnea, paroxysmal nocturnal dyspnea (PND), anorexia, and indigestion.
- Goals of treatment of *heart failure*: reduce cardiac work by manipulating preload, afterload, and contractility or remodeling.
- Treatment plan for *heart failure*: restriction of salt and introduction of mild-to-moderate exercise, digitalis, diuretics, vasodilators, and beta blockers.
- *Cardiogenic shock* is a complex clinical syndrome encompassing a group of conditions with variable hemodynamic manifestations; however, the common denominator is the inadequacy of tissue perfusion.
- *Cardiogenic shock* is characterized by left ventricular dysfunction, leading to severe impairment of tissue perfusion and oxygen delivery to the tissues.
- Mechanical defects, acute mitral regurgitation, acquired VSD, and ventricular aneurysms caused by a MI can also produce shock.
- The *cardiopulmonary bypass machine* oxygenates blood, cools blood to induce systemic hypothermia and reduce tissue oxygen demand, and filtrates blood by removing air and particulate matter.
- The *intraaortic balloon pump* is inflated during ventricular diastole and deflated during left ventricular ejection or systole.
- Inflation of the intraaortic balloon pump during diastole results in augmentation of diastolic pressure leading to increased coronary and systemic perfusion.
- Deflation of the intraaortic balloon pump during systole results in decreased cardiac work, decreased myocardial oxygen consumption, increased CO, and decreased hemodynamic abnormalities associated with mechanical defects.
- The most common indication for a *ventricular assist device* is as a bridge to transplantation; however, it may also be used as a bridge to recovery or as destination therapy.
- The goal of the next generation of artificial hearts is that they can be permanent and give the patient a high quality of life free of percutaneous lines.
- Cardiac transplantation is considered for end-stage heart disease refractory to conventional medical and surgical therapy.
- The two most common conditions producing end-stage heart disease are advanced coronary artery disease and congestive cardiomyopathy.
- *Congestive cardiomyopathy* is characterized by a grossly dilated and hypodynamic ventricle.
- Infection is the leading cause of death in the first year after heart transplantation.

QUESTIONS ??

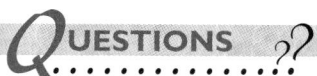

A sampling of review questions for this chapter appears here. Visit http://www.mosby.com/MERLIN/PriceWilson/ for additional questions.

Circle the correct word(s) within the parentheses or fill in the blank with the correct word or phrase for each statement.

1. Congestive heart failure is the state of (pulmonary) (circulatory) congestion resulting from failure of the heart as a (reservoir) (pump).

2. An increase in LVEDP usually causes a concomitant increase in (right atrial pressure) (left atrial pressure), which, in turn, increases (pulmonary venous) (systemic venous) pressures, which leads to (pulmonary edema) (hepatomegaly).

3. The most common mechanical complication of acquired and congenital heart disease is

   _____ _____.

4. Cardiogenic shock is typically associated with approximately _____ percent loss of ventricular myocardium.

5. During circulatory support with assist devices for the left side of the heart, venous blood is oxygenated by the (machine) (patient). Oxygenated blood flows into the left side of the heart, which acts as a (pump) (reservoir).

6. During cardiopulmonary bypass, venous blood flows through catheters placed in the _____. This venous blood is diverted to the _____, where diffusion of gases takes place. The oxygenated blood is returned to the body by a catheter placed in the _____ or_____.

7. Arrange the following events in correct chronologic order:
   _____ Renin release from the juxtaglomerular apparatus
   _____ Conversion of angiotensin I to angiotensin II
   _____ Sympathetic activation
   _____ Sodium and water retention in the distal tubule and collecting duct
   _____ Reduced renal blood flow and reduced glomerular filtration rate
   _____ Interaction of renin with circulating angiotensinogen to produce angiotensin I
   _____ Adrenal secretion of aldosterone

8. An increased pressure load, such as occurs in aortic stenosis, would result in a _____ pattern of ventricular hypertrophy, whereas an increased volume load, such as occurs in aortic regurgitation, would result in a _____ pattern of ventricular hypertrophy and chamber _____.

Match each clinical syndrome in column A with its corresponding symptoms in column B.

Column A	Column B
9. _____ Right heart failure	a. Rales
10. _____ Left heart failure	b. Dependent edema
	c. Pulmonary edema
	d. Third heart sound
	e. Increased jugular venous pressure
	f. Hepatomegaly

Match each symptom in column A with its definition in column B.

Column A	Column B
11. _____ Paroxysmal nocturnal dyspnea (PND)	a. Difficulty in breathing
	b. Sudden awakening with shortness of breath
12. _____ Cardiac asthma	
13. _____ Dyspnea on exertion (DOE)	c. Shortness of breath in the recumbent position
14. _____ Dyspnea	
15. _____ Orthopnea	d. Auscultatory findings of pulmonary congestion
16. _____ Rales	
	e. PND with wheezing
	f. Shortness of breath with physical exertion

Match the following types of cardiomyopathy in column A with their corresponding structural abnormalities in column B.

Column A	Column B
17. _____ Hypertrophic	a. Grossly enlarged, hypodynamic ventricle
18. _____ Congestive or dilated	b. Impeded ventricular filling
19. _____ Restrictive or obliterative	c. Increased ventricular muscle mass

Match the following interventions in column B with their primary physiologic effect(s) in column A.

Column A	Column B
20. _____ Reduced preload	a. Venodilators
21. _____ Reduced afterload	b. Inotropic agents
22. _____ Increased contractility	c. Intraaortic balloon pumping
23. _____ Change in vascular tone	

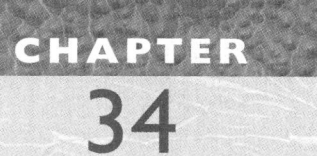

CHAPTER
34

Vascular Disease

LINDA J. DENEKAMP AND PATRICIA HENRY FOLCARELLI

𝒟isease processes can affect both the peripheral arteries and the peripheral veins, impairing either tissue perfusion or venous return to the heart. This chapter describes common arterial and venous diseases. The arterial section emphasizes atherosclerotic disease of the aorta and its major branches; occlusive and aneurysmal presentations of atherosclerosis are described in detail. Aortic dissection is also discussed. The venous section focuses on four major disease presentations: (1) superficial thrombophlebitis; (2) deep venous thrombosis, both acute and recurrent; (3) varicose veins; and (4) postthrombotic syndrome. The pathophysiology of superficial thrombophlebitis and deep venous thrombosis is considered under the broader heading of venous thromboembolic disease.

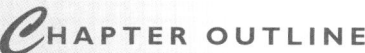

ARTERIAL DISEASE

Anatomy
Arterial Wall
The arterial wall consists of three layers: the outer layer, or adventitia; the middle layer, or media; and the inner layer, or intima. The *adventitia* contains the nerve fibers and blood vessels that supply the arterial wall and is composed of connective tissue and provides the total strength of the arterial wall. The *media* contains collagen, smooth muscle fibers, and elastin and is largely responsible for regulating the diameter of the vessel by dilation and constriction. The *intima* is a smooth layer of endothelial cells providing a nonthrombotic surface for blood flow. The intima and the media are nourished by a process of diffusion from arterial flow. The adventitia and outer portion of the media receive nutrients from the *vasa vasorum*, "vessel of vessels," whose small vessels penetrate the outer arterial wall.

Aorta and its Major Branches
The aorta traverses the thoracic and abdominal cavities, and its segments are distinguished accordingly. The *thoracic aorta* is divided into the following anatomic segments: (1) ascending thoracic aorta, (2) transverse aortic arch, and (3) descending thoracic aorta. The ascending aorta originates at the aortic valve and extends to the orifices of the vessels supplying the head, neck, and upper extremities. These vessels, collectively referred to as *brachiocephalic vessels*, arise from the aortic arch. As illustrated in Fig. 34-1, the brachiocephalic vessels include the innominate artery (brachiocephalic trunk), the left common carotid artery, and the left subclavian artery. The innominate artery divides into the right common carotid and right subclavian arteries. The axillary arteries arise from the subclavian arteries and extend to the brachial arteries, which branch into the radial and ulnar arteries. The vertebral arteries arise from the subclavian arteries bilaterally.

The descending thoracic aorta begins distal to the left subclavian artery and extends to the diaphragm. The *abdominal aorta* begins beneath the diaphragm and branches within a few centimeters to supply the abdominal organs. This portion of the aorta lies posterior to the lungs, diaphragm, duodenum, spleen, stomach, and intestines. The major visceral branches of the abdominal aorta are illustrated in Fig. 34-1 and include the celiac axis, superior mesenteric artery, and renal arteries. The inferior mesenteric artery branches off the aorta below the renal arteries. The abdominal aorta extends to the aortic bifurcation at the level of the pelvis. The *terminal aorta* is the aortic segment between the renal arteries and the

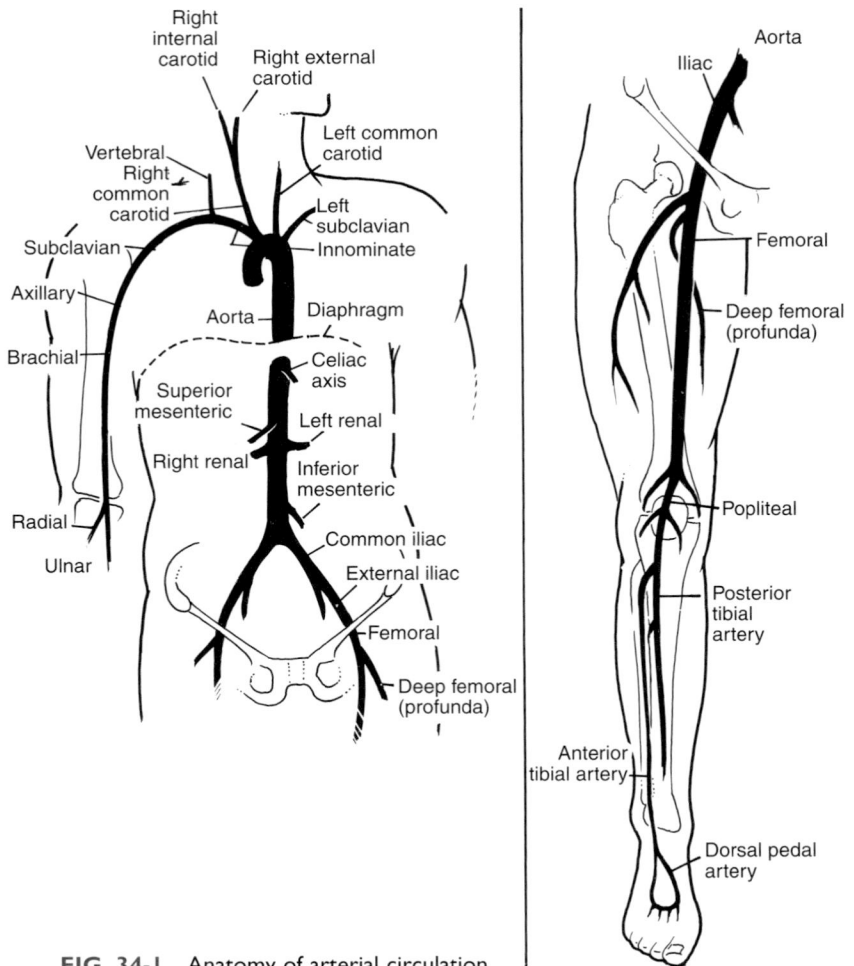

FIG. 34-1   Anatomy of arterial circulation.

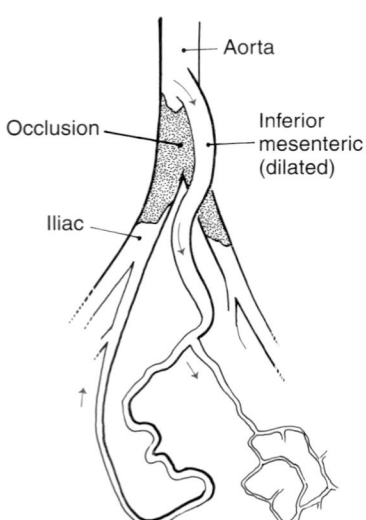

FIG. 34-2   Collateral blood flow via inferior mesenteric artery resulting from bilateral occlusion of common iliac arteries.

bifurcation; the inferior mesenteric artery is the major branch of the terminal aorta.

The aorta bifurcates into the common iliac arteries. The common iliac arteries divide into the external iliac arteries and the hypogastric or internal iliac arteries. The

external iliac arteries become the common femoral arteries. The common femoral has multiple branches, including the superficial femoral artery and the deep femoral artery, or profunda femoris. The superficial femoral artery extends to the popliteal artery, which in turn branches into the posterior tibial artery, the peroneal artery, and the anterior tibial artery. The anterior tibial artery extends to the dorsal pedal artery.

In the event of obstruction within the arterial system, important collateral networks develop to bypass the involved segment and maintain blood flow. These networks are generally enlarged, preexisting arteries that develop in the presence of stenosis or total occlusion. Collateral vessels are usually a network of smaller and more numerous vessels; however, their size and number are related to the size and the duration of the occlusion or stenosis. Arteries that are particularly important as potential routes for collateral flow to the lower extremities include the inferior mesenteric artery and the deep femoral artery. For example, the inferior mesenteric artery becomes enlarged to provide collateral flow in the setting of bilateral occlusion of the common iliac arteries (Fig. 34-2).

Etiology and Pathology
Atherosclerotic Causes

Atherosclerosis is the most common disease affecting the arterial vasculature. Atherosclerosis is characterized initially by lipid deposits in the intimal layer of the artery. Subsequently, calcification, fibrosis, thrombosis, and hemorrhage can occur, contributing to the development of a complex atherosclerotic plaque, or *atheroma.* Eventually, the media begins to degenerate. Necrosis of the fat-filled smooth muscle cells also occurs. These pathologic processes progressively occlude the vessel lumen and weaken the arterial wall. (See Chapter 31 for a discussion of theories of atherogenesis and risk factors.)

The clinical manifestations of atherosclerosis result either from *vascular occlusion* or *stenosis,* caused by intimal deposition or embolization, or from *aneurysm formation,* caused by medial degeneration. The most common course of atherosclerotic disease in the peripheral vasculature is vessel occlusion, whereas in the aorta, aneurysmal presentations are more common. Arterial occlusive and aneurysmal disease caused by atherosclerosis are discussed in subsequent sections.

Given the diffuse and progressive nature of the atherosclerotic process, however, the reader must remember that peripheral vascular disease is usually associated with cerebral and coronary disease. Management of aortic or peripheral vascular disease without regard for potential consequences resulting from vascular compromise in the coronary or cerebral beds can be catastrophic. (See Chapters 31 and 53 for discussions of coronary and cerebral atherosclerotic disease.)

Nonatherosclerotic Causes

The primary nonatherosclerotic causes of arterial disease are (1) cystic medial necrosis, (2) arterial inflammation or arteritis, (3) vasospastic disorders, and (4) fibromuscular dysplasia. Others causes include infection, trauma, and congenital anomalies.

Cystic Medial Necrosis

Cystic medial necrosis is a pathologic process that produces degenerative changes in the medial layer of the artery. The cause of this degeneration is unknown. The incidence of cystic medial necrosis is highest in younger men. Medial degeneration can lead to aneurysm formation, aortic dissection, or spontaneous arterial rupture. A variety of conditions can produce cystic medial necrosis, including *Marfan syndrome,* an inherited disorder of the connective tissue.

Arterial Inflammation

Inflammatory disorders of the aorta or peripheral arteries can result in arterial occlusion. *Thromboangiitis obliterans,* or *Buerger's disease,* is a chronic occlusive disease of the medium-size and small arteries and veins. The inflammation and subsequent healing and thrombosis of lesions produce vascular obstruction. A recurring migratory pattern of superficial thrombophlebitis is not uncommon. Smoking is directly related to the cause and course of the disease. Rest pain and ischemic ulceration are observed early. *Giant cell arteritis* most frequently involves branches of the external carotid artery but may involve the aorta and its upper branches. *Takayasu's arteritis* most commonly affects young Oriental women. Inflammation of the aorta and its branches causes stenosis and occlusion and results in both cardiovascular and neurologic symptoms. In *temporal arteritis,* occlusion and inflammation of the temporal artery may produce generalized

symptoms such as headache and malaise. The disease is usually found in women over age 50 years. Blindness secondary to ischemic optic neuritis or central retinal occlusion may occur (Graham, Ford, 1999). *Polyarteritis nodosa* is a systemic disease of unknown origin that most commonly occurs in adult men.

Vasospastic Conditions

Vasospastic conditions can also produce transient arterial occlusion. *Raynaud's syndrome* is produced by vasospasm of the small cutaneous and subcutaneous arteries and arterioles. The two forms of Raynaud's syndrome are (1) primary or idiopathic *(spastic Raynaud's)* and (2) secondary *(obstructive Raynaud's).* No identifiable cause exists for primary Raynaud's syndrome, and no vascular obstruction is present. The occurrence of vasospasm appears to relate to the local dynamics of the arterial wall. This condition is also called *Raynaud's disease.* Secondary Raynaud's syndrome results from diffuse obstructive disease caused by associated conditions, such as scleroderma.

The vasospasm of Raynaud's syndrome affects the fingers and, less often, the feet and toes. The syndrome is characterized by phasic changes in skin color, usually precipitated by exposure to cold or emotional upset. An initial phase of pallor caused by vasoconstriction is followed by a cyanotic phase and finally by a phase of rubor from reactive vasodilation. During the vasospastic episode, numbness or difficulty with fine motor movement and a sensation of coldness may be noted.

The course of primary Raynaud's syndrome is typically benign because of the intermittent nature of the vasospasm. Treatment is directed at eliminating precipitating factors, such as exposure to cold or smoking. Vasodilation with calcium channel blocking drugs, such as nifedipine, may be beneficial in select patients.

Fibromuscular Dysplasia

Fibromuscular dysplasia is characterized by abnormalities in the fibrous connective tissue of the arterial wall. This disorder most frequently affects the renal arteries of women under 40 years of age and results in renovascular hypertension (see Figs. 45-11 and 46-15). In most patients, this disorder angiographically appears as a "string of beads" caused by medial fibroplasia. This condition may be treated surgically.

Other Causes

Arterial infection typically results from septicemia. Sources of infection include bacterial endocarditis, gastroenteritis (particularly caused by *Salmonella* species), and vascular infection from intravenous drug abuse. Arterial infection tends to localize on roughened endothelial surfaces, such as atherosclerotic plaques. Vascular trauma and congenital anomalies, such as coarctation of the aorta, are also major nonatherosclerotic causes of vascular abnormality. *Compartment syndrome* is caused by increased pressure from swelling within the osteofascial compartment of the upper or lower extremities. The increased intracompartmental pressure results in decreased vascular perfusion and resultant tissue necrosis. Two common causes are revascularization and acute or chronic trauma, often as a sport injury. Treatment is fasciotomy. *Compression syndromes* are caused by arterial compression by an abnormal muscle. The most common of these are *thoracic outlet syndrome* and *popliteal artery entrapment*.

Diagnostic Procedures

Physical Examination Techniques

Physical examination yields much information relative to the degree of arterial disease. Initial visual inspection is for color, hair distribution, edema, atrophy, varicosities, ulcerations, nail condition, and skin integrity. Palpation begins by checking skin temperature at all levels. Auscultation for bruits then follows. Pulses are palpated at multiple sites for presence, strength, and equality relative to the contralateral limb. The grading of pulse strength is subjective and varies among institutions. (Three currently used systems for grading pulses are listed in Box 34-1.) Pulses may be compared before and after exercise; pulses distal to an obstructive lesion typically diminish with exercise.

Leg elevation and dependency tests are extremely useful for evaluating arterial occlusive disease because flow across obstructive lesions is pressure dependent and therefore extremely sensitive to the effects of gravity. Elevation of the extremity produces pallor, followed by redness or rubor with dependency. Elevation pallor is the result of gravitational effects, which reduce arterial pressure and consequently lower the blood volume in the capillary bed. As the extremity is lowered beneath heart level and perfusion pressure increases, color returns. Rubor results from a reactive hyperemia or maximal vascular dilation in response to tissue hypoxia.

The degree of occlusion is estimated according to the length of time required for elevation pallor and dependent rubor to occur; normally no pallor is observed during 60 seconds of leg elevation, and color returns within 10 seconds. Venous filling time in the dependent position is also determined because the veins of the dependent leg also take longer to fill because of the interference with arterial inflow. Normal venous filling time is less than 15 seconds.

Sensation, muscle strength, and skin temperature are also evaluated. Bruits and trophic changes are noted. The results of the physical examination are subjective by nature; therefore noninvasive tests may be indicated for further evaluation. A more complete discussion of signs and symptoms is included in subsequent sections.

Doppler Ultrasound

Vascular Doppler studies use ultrasound as the examination medium (see Chapter 30). A Doppler probe contains a piezoelectric crystal that transmits ultrasonic waves of a known frequency. When positioned over a segment of artery or vein, this beam strikes the red blood cells and the back-scattered or reflected wave is shifted in frequency, depending on the direction and velocity of the moving cells. This difference between the transmitted frequency and the reflected frequency is known as the *Doppler shift*. Frequency changes can be used to interpret direction of flow. Flow moving toward the probe has a higher frequency than does flow transmitted from cells moving away from the probe.

Two basic types of Doppler ultrasound are available. *Continuous-wave ultrasound* transmitters are generally small, portable units. In this type, a continuous signal is emitted from one crystal in the probe and reflected frequencies are received by another crystal within the probe. The second type, *pulsed-wave ultrasound*, is more frequently found in laboratory-based ultrasound devices. A signal crystal alternately sends and receives signals in a pulsing mode. The delay in time from emission to reception allows for sampling at specific depths, adding information to the signal. The Doppler signal can be interpreted audibly and through the technique of spectral analysis as well. A spectral analyzer visually displays all frequencies of the back-scattered signal. Time is displayed on the horizontal axis and frequency on the vertical axis. This analysis allows for less subjectivity compared with the audible-only analysis.

Duplex Scanning

The techniques of pulsed Doppler and spectral analysis have been combined with B-mode ultrasound imaging in a system called duplex scanning. *B mode*, or *brightness mode*, *ultrasound* allows for a two-dimensional image of the blood vessel in real time. The contrast between the bright vessel wall and the fluid-filled lumen of the vessel affords the examiner the ability to image vascular morphology, including irregularities in the lumen of the vessel caused by atherosclerotic plaque and aneurysmal dilation (Fig. 34-3). Both vessel wall and residual lumen can be visualized, allowing for determination of the percentage of diameter reduction or total occlusion. Duplex scanning allows the examiner to position a pulsed Doppler signal in the midstream of the visualized vessel. The received frequencies are then subjected to spectral analysis (Fig. 34-4). Color displays of the flow velocities allow for a real-time display of velocities of flow in the vessel lumen. Arterial disease produces distinctive abnormalities in flow velocity and flow patterns. *Color duplex* or *flow imaging* displays the flow of the blood vessels in color while also providing a sound waveform analysis. Flow toward the transducer is typically red; flow away from the transducer is blue. In areas of stenosis, color hue lightens. Normal arterial flow is laminar in nature, with

---

▌BOX 34-1
▌Three Pulse-Scoring Systems*

0 = Pulse absent	0 = Absent	0 = Absent
1 = Pulse present but markedly reduced	1 = Pulse present but barely palpable	1 = Pulse present but diminished
2 = Pulse present but moderately reduced	2 = Pulse normal	2 = Pulse normal
3 = Pulse present but slightly reduced	3+ = Pulse normal, easily palpable	
4 = Pulse present and normal	4+ = Abnormal pulsation (as in aneurysm)	

▌*The grading of pulses is subjective, and scoring systems to evaluate pulse strength differ among institutions.

higher-frequency (higher-velocity) flow in the midstream of the vessel and lower-frequency (lower-velocity) flow along the walls of the vessels (Fig. 34-5). In areas of narrowing, the velocity increases throughout the narrowest segment. Flow distal and proximal to the stenosed segment is turbulent, with many frequencies displayed on the spectral analysis. Frequency and turbulence increase proportionally with the degree of stenosis, whereas totally occluded vessels have no obtainable flow signal.

Computed Tomography

A tomograph is an image of a cross-sectional slice of the body. B-mode ultrasound, as described earlier, is an example of a tomograph. Computed tomographic (CT)

scanning has extended vascular imaging from two-dimensional (2-D) to three-dimensional (3-D) imaging. To construct this 3-D image, a camera rotates in a 360-degree arc around the region of interest, recording 2-D images at multiple angles. X-rays are transmitted through the body to detectors on the opposite side. Each radiographic image captures a thin anatomic slice of the region of interest. A composite 3-D image is constructed from these 2-D radiographic images by a computer. A small amount of contrast material, usually containing iodine, is injected via a peripheral site to heighten the contrast between the vessel wall and the blood.

CT scanning provides direct depiction of the vessel wall, making this diagnostic tool ideal for assessing the

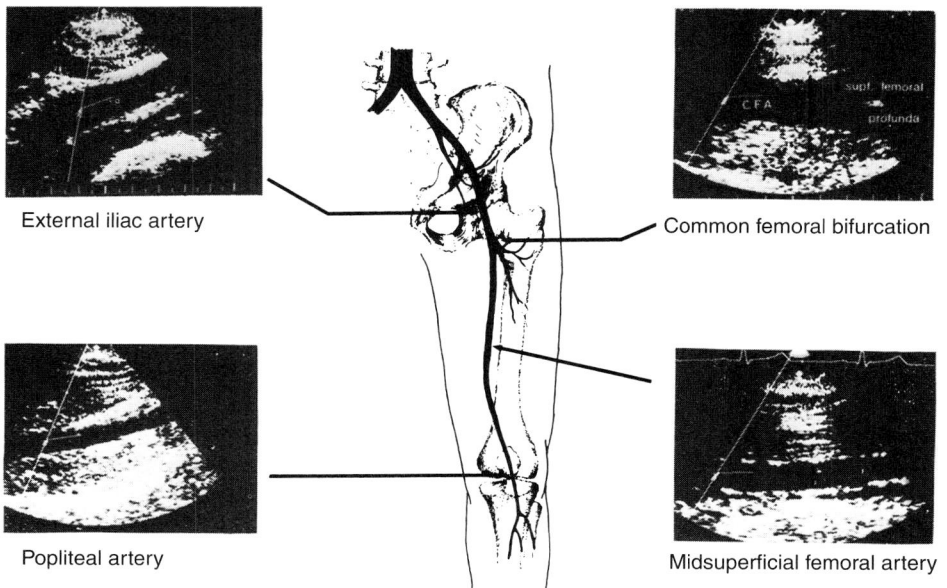

External iliac artery

Common femoral bifurcation

Popliteal artery

Midsuperficial femoral artery

FIG. 34-3 B-mode image of distal external iliac artery, common femoral artery *(CFA)* bifurcation, superficial femoral artery, and popliteal artery of a healthy volunteer. Axis of Doppler beam, angle of incidence, and a sample volume placement are displayed. (From Bernstein EF: *Vascular diagnosis,* ed 4, St Louis, 1993, Mosby.)

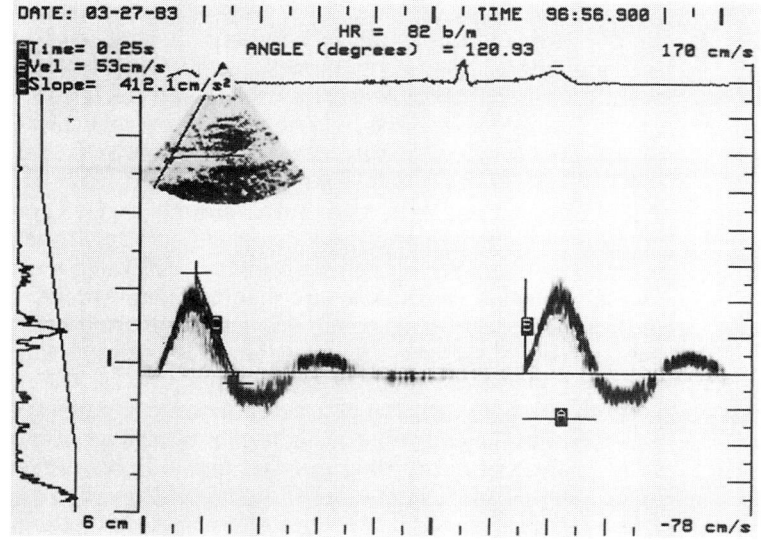

FIG. 34-4 Doppler signal is analyzed by real-time fast Fourier transform (FFT) spectrum analyzer and displayed with time on the horizontal axis, velocity (cm/sec) on vertical axis, and amplitude as shades of gray. *A,* Measurement of time: time of systolic forward flow (0.25 seconds); *B,* velocity parameters: systolic peak velocity (53 cm/sec); *C,* slope: deceleration = peak systolic velocity divided by pulse decay time = 412.1 cm/sec^2. (From Bernstein EF: *Vascular diagnosis,* ed 4, St Louis, 1993, Mosby.)

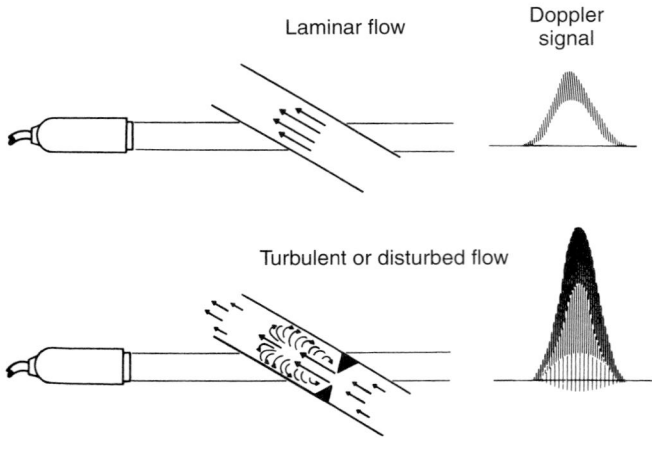

FIG. 34-5 Doppler signals recorded from laminar flow and turbulent or disturbed flow. With laminar flow, all the velocities are similar. The Doppler signal produces a relatively thin waveform with minimal spectral broadening. When blood flows across an area with a significant change in the caliber of the blood vessel, flow with multiple velocities in different directions is produced. Such disturbed flow produces a Doppler signal with multiple frequencies and marked spectral broadening. (From Feigenbaum H: *Echocardiography*, ed 4, Philadelphia, 1986, Lea & Febiger.)

size of aneurysms and the structures around vessels that indicate disease (e.g., hematoma, fluid).

Magnetic Resonance Imaging

Magnetic resonance imaging (MRI) equipment consists of a magnet that supplies the main magnetic field within the bore of a scanner, transmitter, and receiver coils, which deliver the radiofrequency pulses that excite the nuclei of the cells and receive the signals arising from the tissue nuclei. Spatial localization of the MR signal is then obtained. The MR images portray the morphologic features of the vessel and identify patterns of hemodynamically significant stenosis. *MR angiography (MRA)* is commonly used to evaluate obstructive disease from the distal abdominal aorta to the pedal vessels. MRA is often the preferred tool in visualizing the small vessels of the distal leg and foot. Because MRA is noninvasive and does not usually require administration of contrast material, it is the preferred diagnostic tool in patients with compromised renal function or who are at risk from complications related to invasive testing or contrast reactions.

Segmental Plethysmography

Segmental plethysmography measures changes in pulse volume. Pneumatic cuffs are placed around the upper thigh, lower thigh, and ankle. The cuffs are automatically or manually inflated to approximately 65 mm Hg to ensure optimal cuff contact. A transducer senses changes in cuff pressure during systole as the blood volume in the vessel fluctuates. A pulse volume recording is generated for each site, and the cuffs are deflated.

In the vascular laboratory, this technique is usually performed simultaneously with *segmental extremity pressure measurement*. First, the brachial systolic blood pressure is measured to establish a baseline. Then, a pneumatic blood pressure cuff is wrapped around the lower extremity with a stethoscope or Doppler flow probe over the arterial pulse. The pneumatic cuff is sequentially in-

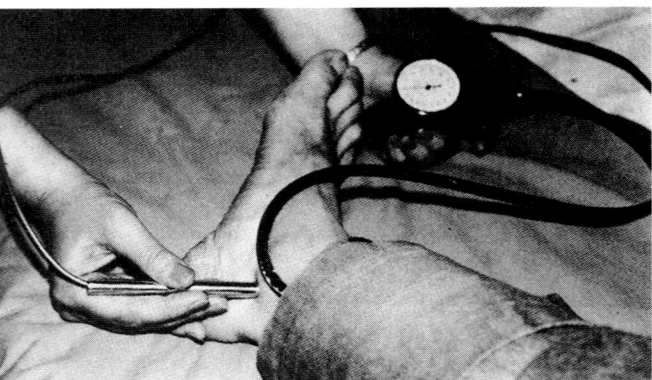

FIG. 34-6 Method of recording ankle systolic pressure. (From Yao JST: Pressure measurement in the extremity. In Bernstein EF: *Vascular diagnosis*, ed 4, St Louis, 1993, Mosby.)

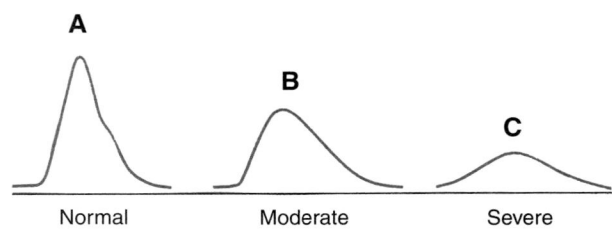

FIG. 34-7 Pulse volume recordings. **A**, Normal; **B**, moderate stenosis; **C**, severe stenosis.

flated on the ankle, upper thigh, and lower thigh to a pressure above the brachial systolic pressure and then deflated. A stethoscope or probe detects the onset of flow during systole at each site, and the corresponding cuff pressure is recorded (Fig. 34-6).

Segmental plethysmography and pressure measurements are usually performed during rest and immediately after exercise. Exercise evaluation usually involves walking on a treadmill for 5 minutes or for as long as tolerated. Flow abnormalities increase with exercise, resulting in a reduction or disappearance of pulses distal to the occlusion and an increase in pressure differences or gradients across the occlusion.

Lower-extremity pressures are compared with brachial systolic pressure and with each other. An ankle-to-arm pressure ratio is calculated. The normal ratio is equal to or slightly greater than 1 because systolic pressures at each site, including the ankle, should be equal to or greater than the brachial systolic pressure. A pressure difference greater than 30 mm Hg between segments indicates disease. Severely diseased segments may have an ankle-brachial index (ABI) of less than 4.0. These measurements are limited to patients with severe calcification of arterial walls, as is frequently found in patients with diabetes. Distal pressure in these patients may be elevated to greater than 300 mm Hg, making these pressures meaningless without concomitant segmental plethysmography. A pressure difference of 20 to 30 mm Hg between a lower-extremity site and the contralateral pulse is indicative of arterial occlusion. Analysis of pulse volume recordings and pressure relationships permits estimation of disease severity. Fig. 34-7 illustrates the abnormalities in pulse volume recordings observed with moderate and severe vascular occlusion.

Chest Radiography

Chest radiography is useful in the evaluation of aortic aneurysms and dissections. A thoracic aneurysm or aortic dissection may be detected as mediastinal widening on a chest radiograph. Anteroposterior and lateral abdominal radiographs are useful to confirm clinical suspicions of an abdominal aneurysm.

Arteriography

Arteriography, or opacification of the artery with contrast material, is rarely, if ever, necessary for diagnosis of occlusive arterial disease. However, if surgical correction is indicated, then arteriography is required to determine the precise location and extent of disease. Collateral circulation and the condition of the proximal and distal vasculature can also be evaluated.

Arteriography is performed on a selective basis for aneurysm evaluation, particularly if suprarenal extension or involvement of the visceral vessels is suggested. However, arteriography can underestimate aneurysm size because the contrast material opacifies only the blood-filled portion of the aneurysm and mural thrombi, which can occupy a significant portion of the aneurysm, will not be detected. With aortic dissections, *aortography*, or arteriography of the aorta, is indicated to determine the location and extent of dissection.

Digital Subtraction Angiography

Digital subtraction angiography (DSA) is a procedure in which a computerized technique is used to observe arterial blood circulation. In DSA, radiographic images of arterial vessels are taken both before and after the introduction of radiopaque dye. These images are converted into digital data, and a computer distinguishes or "subtracts" one set of data from another. The resulting image shows the shape of the artery. Computer manipulation of images allows for diluted contrast agents. Venous injection of contrast may be used, allowing for reduced risks from arterial puncture associated with traditional arteriography.

Occlusive Arterial Disease

Occlusive arterial disease may be acute or chronic. The term *chronic occlusive arterial disease* encompasses disorders that cause ischemia as a result of arterial obstruction. As indicated earlier, the most common cause of occlusive disease is atherosclerosis. Atherosclerotic lesions tend to develop at points of branching, bifurcation, abrupt curvature, or vascular narrowing. Turbulent flow in these regions is thought to contribute to atherogenesis, perhaps through traumatic disruption of the endothelial lining.

Lesions occur more frequently in the lower extremities than they do in the upper extremities and tend to be localized, involving segments of the artery. Common sites of involvement include (1) aortoiliac vessels, (2) femoropopliteal vessels, (3) popliteal-tibial vessels, and (4) combinations of these. The *Leriche's syndrome* is progressive occlusion of the terminal aorta, including the bifurcation and iliac arteries, from atherosclerosis and thrombosis.

Lesions may also occur in visceral branches of the abdominal aorta. Atherosclerosis of the renal artery may interfere with renal function and cause hypertension (see Chapter 46). Lesions of the celiac, inferior and superior mesenteric arteries may result in *mesenteric ischemia*. Chronic mesenteric ischemia may present as abdominal pain and weight loss and progress to bowel infarction. Surgical intervention to correct mesenteric blood flow and revascularize the intestines is most often necessary.

Pathophysiology

Chronic arterial occlusive disease progressively narrows the arterial lumen, increasing the resistance to blood flow. As the resistance to flow increases, blood flow to the tissue beyond the lesion is reduced. If the oxygen needs of the tissue exceed the vessel's ability to supply oxygen, tissue ischemia results. A single lesion must reduce the vessel lumen by approximately 50% in diameter or 75% in cross-sectional area to produce clinically significant interference with blood flow. However, multiple stenoses occurring in sequence, as frequently occurs with atherosclerosis, compound the interference with flow; in other words, in combination, less significant lesions can seriously impair flow.

The severity of ischemia distal to an obstructive lesion depends not only on the site and extent of occlusion but also on the degree of collateral flow around the lesion. Fortunately, the tendency of atherosclerotic lesions to be localized and to enlarge gradually favors the development of collateral circulation. With localized lesions, the distal artery remains patent; thus alternative routes of arterial flow can bypass the lesion to perfuse the tissue beyond. As resistance to flow increases at the site of obstruction, pressure increases proximal to the lesion with a proportionate drop in pressure distal to the lesion. This pressure gradient across the obstruction promotes flow through collateral vessels. These collateral vessels gradually enlarge. Increased velocity of flow through the collateral vessels also stimulates collateral development. Severe ischemia can result from acute occlusion because collateral networks have not had time to develop. The adequacy of collateral flow is also compromised by disease in collateral vessels.

Acute arterial occlusion is a complication primarily of another disease process. Most frequently, these occlusions occur in the lower extremities, but upper extremities can also be affected. Acute arterial occlusion can be produced by thrombosis or embolization. *Thrombosis* is the formation of a blood clot, or thrombus, within the vascular system. Arterial thrombosis usually occurs at the site of an atherosclerotic plaque or within an arterial aneurysm. Detachment of a thrombus into the bloodstream is referred to as *embolization*. The embolus is propelled downstream to lodge in the smaller branches of the arterial system, occluding the vascular lumen.

Most arterial thromboemboli originate in the left side of the heart. Mitral stenosis and atrial fibrillation interfere with left atrial emptying, predisposing to the development of atrial thrombi. Transmural myocardial infarction roughens the endothelial surface of the left ventricle, leading to the formation of mural ventricular thrombi. Embolization can also result from detachment of mural thrombi from a ventricular aneurysm. Depending on the size and destination of the clot, dislodgement of thrombi from the cardiac chambers is potentially catastrophic. Emboli tend to lodge in regions of bifurcation or branching. The term *saddle embolus* refers to acute occlusion of the aortic bifurcation and iliac arteries.

A condition referred to as *spontaneous atheroembolism* is being recognized with increasing frequency. Thrombi originating in a vascular atherosclerotic plaque may become detached and propagate distally. These emboli may contain remnants of the atheromatous plaque, as well as the thrombus. Microemboli, consisting of platelet aggregates or cholesterol fragments, can also occur, presenting as acute occlusion of a digit.

Clinical Features

The clinical manifestations of chronic arterial occlusive disease progress slowly over a period of years. The signs and symptoms result from tissue underperfusion and ischemia. The primary symptoms are *intermittent claudication* caused by muscle ischemia and ischemic rest pain. Typically, intermittent claudication occurs with exercise, when metabolic demands increase, and subsides with rest within minutes. The location of the pain correlates closely with the site of arterial disease; the arterial segment involved is always proximal to the region of ischemic muscle. For example, intermittent claudication of the hips would correlate with aortoiliac disease, whereas disease of the external iliac or common femoral vessels would be associated with thigh or calf pain. Bilateral claudication is consistent with occlusion at or above the aortic bifurcation.

Pain occurring at rest is indicative of advanced occlusive disease. Ischemic rest pain typically occurs distally in the feet and toes as a combination of aching discomfort and paresthesia. However, the pain can be severe and unremitting. Pain typically occurs in the supine position and may be particularly intense at night, awakening patients from sleep. This intensification of pain occurs because flow across the obstructive lesion is pressure dependent and therefore extremely sensitive to the effects of gravity. Venous return also improves with elevation of the legs, thereby reducing the time for oxygen extraction from the blood in the capillary beds of the lower extremities. Additionally, the reduction in sympathetic tone with sleep lowers heart rate and arterial pressure, further impairing peripheral perfusion. Leg dependency or walking may provide some relief. The increased hydrostatic pressure in the dependent position may dilate collateral vessels, increasing flow distally. Ischemic neuropathy occasionally results, particularly in patients with diabetes, producing shocklike pain in the foot and leg.

Pulses below the occlusion are diminished or absent. The change in pulses is magnified by exercise because the vasodilation induced by exercise and ischemia increases the pressure gradient across the lesion. A *bruit*, indicative of turbulent flow, may be audible over the diseased arterial segment.

Significant arterial disease of the lower extremities is characterized by *postural changes in skin color*. Elevation of the extremity produces pallor, followed by redness or rubor with dependency. The elevation pallor is the result of gravitational effects that reduce arterial pressure and consequently lower the blood volume in the capillary bed. As the extremity is lowered beneath heart level and perfusion pressure increases, color returns. The rubor results from a reactive hyperemia or maximal vascular dilation in response to tissue hypoxia. The veins of the dependent leg also take longer to fill, because of the interference with arterial inflow.

The following tissue changes result from severe, chronic ischemia of the lower extremities: (1) trophic changes of the skin and nails, with thickening of the nails and drying of the skin; (2) loss of hair, particularly on the dorsum of the feet and toes; (3) development of a temperature gradient between colder regions of poor perfusion and warmer regions of adequate perfusion; and (4) wasting of the leg muscles and soft tissues. Changes in sensation and muscle strength may be noted.

Severe ischemia culminates in ulceration and gangrene. Ischemic ulcers usually begin on the toes or heel and progress proximally. Gangrene represents tissue death or necrosis. Gangrene can be characterized as dry gangrene or wet gangrene, depending on the degree of compromise in perfusion and the resultant necrosis. *Dry gangrene* results from a total cessation of flow with necrosis of the entire region. If the obstruction is not total, areas of necrosis are then intermingled with regions of edema and inflammation, resulting in *wet gangrene.*

The constellation of clinical manifestations noted with progressive occlusion of the terminal aorta (Leriche's syndrome) includes absent or diminished femoral pulses; intermittent claudication in the buttock, hip, or thigh; and a loss of sexual potency.

Typically, the manifestations of acute occlusion, which result in sudden ischemia, differ greatly in magnitude from those of chronic ischemia. The typical manifestations are pain, pallor, pulselessness, *poikilothermia* (coolness), paresthesia, and paralysis. In some patients however, the presentation may be more gradual and less dramatic.

Treatment

Medical Therapy

Control of risk factors is important to the treatment of arterial occlusive disease. Smoking should be stopped, given its numerous harmful effects that include vasoconstriction, increased platelet aggregation and blood viscosity, and increased blood pressure. Medical therapy of associated diabetes, hypercholesterolemia, and hypertension is indicated. Dietary measures and exercise programs are stressed.

The pain of intermittent claudication usually subsides with rest. Ischemic rest pain can be relieved somewhat by dependency of the extremity or elevation of the head of the bed. Leg dependency increases perfusion pressure, thus relieving ischemia; elevation of the extremity is contraindicated because arterial flow would be further compromised. Analgesics may be necessary for pain control.

A progressive exercise program should be developed and maintained. Physical exercise appears to afford the greatest benefit in the treatment of intermittent claudication. Therapeutic response to physical exercise sustained over time is probably caused primarily by increased collateral development.

Foot care is crucial in the setting of lower-extremity vascular disease to prevent infection and traumatic ulceration. Measures include meticulous attention to cleanliness and nail care and avoidance of trauma and temperature extremes. Preventive measures to avoid injury are important because the ability to heal is retarded by the arterial insufficiency. Additionally, susceptibility to injury is increased because sensory function may be impaired. Patients with diabetes mellitus or neuropathy should be taught to inspect their feet for blisters, redness, or trauma. The wearing of properly fitting shoes at all times to avoid injury is a must.

Managing ischemic ulcers and gangrene is problematic. In addition to the measures described previously, topical antibiotic agents may be indicated. Pressure points should be padded to avoid further breakdown. Bed rest, with elevation of the head of the bed, can reduce oxygen demand and improve flow. Bed cradles are helpful to prevent bedclothes from touching the extremity. Wound infections must be treated with appropriate antibiotic therapy, often parenterally; topical wound care; and often surgical débridement. Arterial reconstruction or amputation may be necessary.

Surgical Therapy

Generally, surgery is considered for chronic occlusive disease if symptoms become disabling or threaten limb viability and are unresponsive to medical therapy. The precise indications for surgery and the choice of procedure vary according to the site of disease. Surgical intervention is discussed relative to the following anatomic sites: (1) aortoiliac disease with patent femoropopliteal arteries, (2) aortoiliac with femoropopliteal disease, (3) femoropopliteal disease, and (4) tibial-peroneal disease.

Surgery for *chronic aortoiliac disease with patent femoropopliteal vessels* is usually performed for disabling intermittent claudication and rest pain. Given the patency of the vessels distal to the site of disease, collateral networks develop around the aortoiliac vessels, preserving limb viability. Surgical correction involves either placement of a bypass graft to shunt blood around the obstruction or endarterectomy to remove atheromatous plaque (Figs. 34-8 and 34-9).

Bypass grafting with a knitted polyester (Dacron) bifurcation graft is the most common procedure; bifurcation grafts divide into two limbs to be sutured to both extremities. The proximal end of the graft is anastomosed to the side of the abdominal aorta beneath the renal arteries. The distal ends are anastomosed to either the external iliac or the common femoral arteries, depending on the extent of the disease. This aortobifemoral graft shunts blood around the diseased aortoiliac system to the lower extremities (see Fig. 34-8).

Endarterectomy consists of dissection and removal of the atheromatous plaque from the arterial lumen, as illustrated in Fig. 34-9. This procedure is performed through an arteriotomy in the vessel wall. Endarterectomy of localized disease may be performed in conjunction with aortobifemoral bypass grafting. Generally, bypass grafting is preferred to endarterectomy, because endarterectomy offers no distinct advantage and is complicated and time-consuming.

Combined aortoiliac and *femoropopliteal disease* necessitates a combination of interventions. In this instance, surgery is usually indicated for limb salvage, given the extent of disease and the severity of ischemia. The proximal aortoiliac lesion must be corrected first to ensure adequate arterial inflow into the femoropopliteal region. Aortobifemoral grafting is usually indicated. A femoral-to-femoral bypass graft to connect the two femoral arteries may be performed when one iliac artery is normal and the other is diseased or when one side of the aortobifemoral bypass has failed.

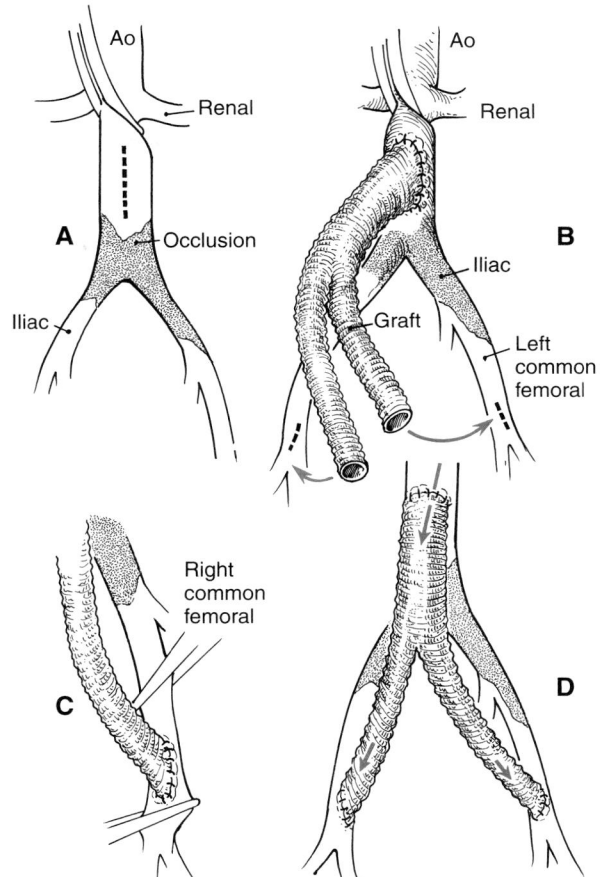

FIG. 34-8   Aortobifemoral bypass graft. **A**, Aortic incision; **B**, proximal anastomosis; **C**, distal anastomosis; **D**, completed graft. *Ao*, Aorta. (Modified from Chung E: *Quick reference to cardiovascular disease*, ed 2, Philadelphia, 1983, Lippincott.)

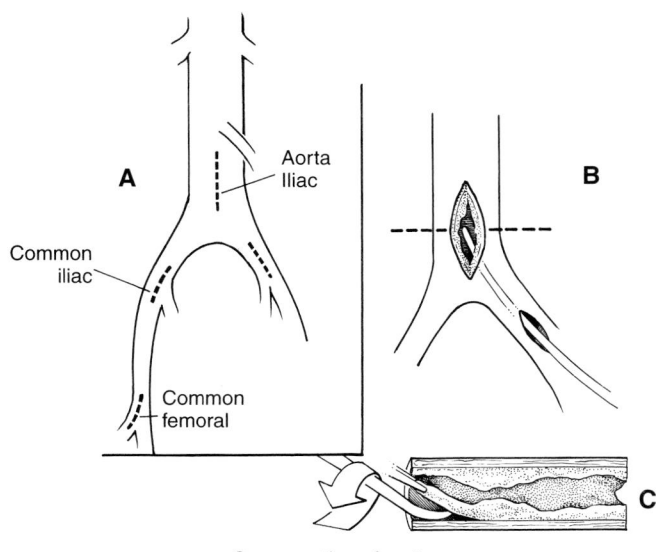

Cross section of aorta

FIG. 34-9   Endarterectomy. **A**, Arteriotomy; **B** and **C**, technique for circumferential dissection and removal of plaque. (Modified from Gaspar M, Barker W: *Peripheral arterial disease*, Philadelphia, 1981, Saunders.)

Axillary-bifemoral bypass grafting may also be performed to perfuse a diseased lower extremity. The advantage of this technique is that it avoids intraabdominal surgery. Subsequently, the distal femoropopliteal disease requires either endarterectomy or bypass grafting to obtain good flow to the distal vessels.

Despite controversy about the efficacy of *sympathectomy*, this procedure may be performed simultaneously to reduce sympathetic tone to the lower extremities and produce peripheral vasodilation. The hope is that blood flow through the grafts will thereby be improved.

In highly select patients, transluminal angioplasty may be attempted to dilate the iliac vessels. *Transluminal angioplasty* is a technique used to treat shorter segments of stenosis of the aortoiliac or femoropopliteal vessels. In some patients, angioplasty is used in conjunction with surgical treatment to dilate stenosed inflow arteries before distal reconstruction. A balloon-tipped catheter is advanced into the iliac system via the femoral artery under fluoroscopic and pressure guidance. The balloon is inflated within the diseased segment to compress the lesion and dilate the vessel. The inflated balloon causes a fracture of the intima, separation of the plaque from the media with stretching and rupture of the muscle fibers, and stretching of the adventitial layer. The damaged intimal surface heals within several hours. The role of angioplasty in vascular disease is still being defined. Angioplasty can be particularly useful if surgery is contraindicated or if the disease is restricted to short, isolated arterial segments.

Arterial reconstruction for *femoropopliteal disease* is usually performed for limb salvage. Occasionally, disabling intermittent claudication requires surgery. Bypass grafting is usually preferred over endarterectomy; however, concomitant endarterectomy may be used for localized disease. The graft of choice is the autogenous saphenous vein because of high graft failure rates with prosthetic materials such as Dacron in the lower extremity. The endothelial lining of the native vein provides an antithrombogenic surface, reducing the incidence of graft failure.

Two surgical techniques are used. With the initial technique, a segment of vein is removed from the leg and reversed before arterial anastomosis so that the venous valves do not impede flow through the vein graft. The proximal end of the reversed graft is anastomosed to the side of the common femoral artery (Fig. 34-10, *A*) and the distal end to the vessel beyond the obstruction, ideally to a branch of the popliteal artery. This approach is referred to as a *reversed saphenous vein technique*.

The *in situ* technique uses a vein segment left in place. The vein is severed from the native vessels, venous valves are removed, and the vein segment is sutured proximally and distally into the adjacent artery, replacing the diseased arterial segment. This *vein in situ technique* is preferred because trauma to the vein is minimized, thereby preserving the integrity of venous endothelium. Preoperative evaluation of the saphenous vein segment via noninvasive techniques, such as B-mode ultrasound, is essential to determine the suitability of the vessel as a vascular conduit.

A *femoral–tibial-peroneal bypass graft* may be performed when obstruction of arterial flow occurs to the tibial branches. The largest of the tibial arteries is preferred for

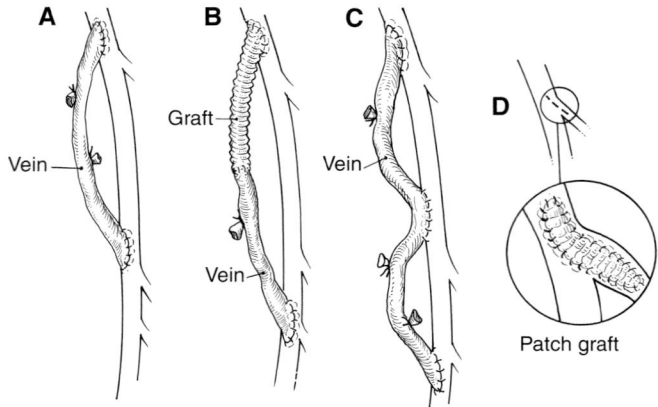

FIG. 34-10 Femoropopliteal bypass graft. **A**, Saphenous vein graft; **B**, composite graft; **C**, sequential femoropopliteal-tibial graft; **D**, profundaplasty with patch graft. (Modified from Gaspar M, Barker W: *Peripheral arterial disease,* Philadelphia, 1981, Saunders.)

anastomosis. Advances in interventional and surgical techniques have shown increased success rate of bypass grafts to the plantar and dorsalis pedis arteries, as well as the tibial arteries. When no other vessel has continuity with the foot, pedal grafting may be successfully performed for limb salvage. Although the saphenous vein remains the conduit of choice, autogenous arm veins may be used (Akbari, LoGerfo, 1999).

If the saphenous vein is not long enough to extend around the diseased segment, composite grafts of vein and prosthetic material can then be used (see Fig. 34-10, *B*). Sequential grafting may be used to provide flow at multiple points for branches of an extensively diseased segment (see Fig. 34-10, *C*).

If femoropopliteal disease involves the deep femoral artery, or profunda femoris, *profundaplasty* is then performed in conjunction with bypass grafting. This procedure usually involves endarterectomy through an arteriotomy. If necessary, a patch graft may be inserted within the vessel wall to dilate the vessel (see Fig. 34-10, *D*). Profundaplasty is important because of the profunda's importance as a collateral network for the lower extremities. In high-risk patients, profundaplasty may be performed alone under local anesthesia as a palliative procedure.

Amputation is considered in chronic occlusive disease for irreversible gangrene or uncontrolled pain. Amputation is performed as far distally as possible to minimize resultant disability.

Acute aortoiliac occlusion necessitates immediate intervention. Anticoagulation is initiated to prevent loss of collateral circulation and further propagation of emboli. Intraarterial thrombolytic agents, such as streptokinase or tissue plasminogen activator (TPA), may be administered. Patients receiving this mode of therapy require intensive care monitoring because of the serious risk of hemorrhage or repeat embolization. *Thrombectomy* via a femoral arteriotomy is another method of treatment.

Aneurysmal Arterial Disease

An *aneurysm* is a localized dilation of the arterial wall (Fig. 34-11). A *true aneurysm* results from atrophy of the

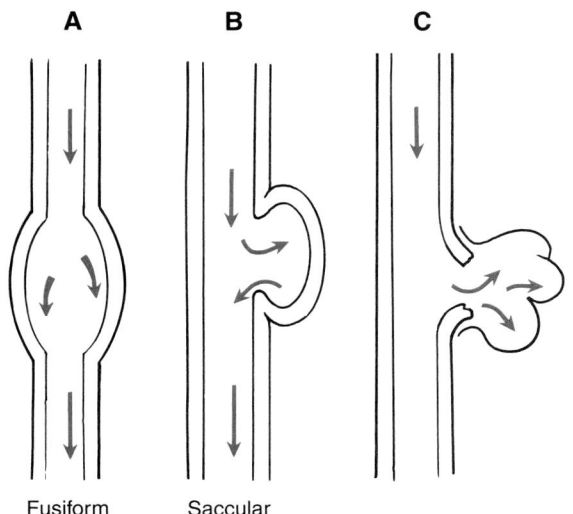

A   **B**   **C**

Fusiform   Saccular

FIG. 34-11   Aneurysm types. **A**, True fusiform aneurysm; **B**, true saccular aneurysm; **C**, false aneurysm.

medial layer of the artery. The arterial wall dilates but remains intact although distorted and composed primarily of fibrous tissue. True aneurysms can be fusiform or saccular in shape. The more common atherosclerotic *fusiform aneurysm* is a uniform, circumferential dilation, whereas the *saccular aneurysm* is a saclike outpouching connected to the arterial wall by a narrow neck. A *false aneurysm* or *pseudoaneurysm* is an extravascular accumulation of blood with disruption of all three vascular layers; the wall of the false aneurysm is thrombus and adjacent tissue. Pseudoaneurysms are most commonly the result of injury or infection or as a complication of invasive vascular procedures, such as angioplasty or arterial surgery. Aneurysms can occur anywhere in the aorta or peripheral vessels. Aortic aneurysms are classified as abdominal, thoracic, or thoracoabdominal, depending on their location. Aortic dissection is discussed in the next section.

Pathophysiology

Aneurysm formation results from degeneration and weakening of the medial layer of the artery. Medial degeneration can result from either acquired or congenital conditions, such as atherosclerosis, or Marfan syndrome. Vascular dilation can also result from the jet effect of blood streaming across an obstructive vascular plaque, creating turbulence distal to the lesion; this poststenotic dilation weakens the arterial wall.

In addition to these identifiable causes of aneurysms, the interaction of many other factors can predispose the arterial wall to aneurysm formation. Turbulence of flow at regions of bifurcation may contribute to the higher incidence of aneurysms in specific regions. Theories suggest that blood supply to the blood vessels through the vasa vasorum may become compromised with advancing age, weakening the media and predisposing the individual to aneurysm formation.

Whatever the cause, the aneurysm becomes progressively larger according to Laplace's law. Wall tension or stress is directly related to the radius of the vessel and the intraarterial pressure. As the vessel dilates and the radius enlarges, the wall tension rises, further dilating the vessel. Thus aneurysm rupture rates rise with increased size. Additionally, the vast majority of individuals with aneurysms are hypertensive, further contributing to wall stress and aneurysm enlargement.

The potential contribution of arterial size to aneurysm formation is also being considered. Individuals with large main arteries, or *arteriomegaly*, and larger body surface areas tend to have an increased incidence of aneurysms. Increased aortic blood flow may also affect the development of aneurysms.

Aneurysms typically develop layers of clot along their walls because of stagnant flow. Mural thrombi are a potential source of emboli and spontaneous aneurysm thrombosis.

Etiology and Common Sites

The most common site for aneurysm formation is the abdominal aorta. *Abdominal aortic aneurysms* typically originate beneath the renal arteries and extend to the aortic bifurcation, occasionally involving the iliac arteries. Rarely does the aneurysm extend above the renal arteries to involve the major visceral branches of the aorta. Most abdominal aneurysms are atherosclerotic in origin.

Thoracic aneurysms can affect the descending thoracic aorta beyond the left subclavian artery, the ascending aorta above the aortic valve, and the aortic arch. The descending aorta is affected most frequently. Atherosclerosis and trauma are the most common causes. Trauma to the chest, usually sustained during a motor vehicle accident, can rupture the intimal and medial layers of the descending aorta at the ligamentum arteriosus. The ligamentum arteriosus stabilizes the aorta at one point, whereas the thoracic structures move forward when the chest abruptly decelerates; this action may shear the vascular layers. Consequently, this type of injury is referred to as *deceleration trauma*. The adventitial layer may remain intact, although rupture or the development of false aneurysms may result. Disease of the arch is usually caused by atherosclerosis. Cystic medial necrosis, as in Marfan syndrome, is most severe in the ascending aorta and frequently results in aneurysm formation.

Multiple aneurysms occur frequently and may involve the peripheral and visceral arteries. The popliteal is the most frequently affected peripheral artery; visceral aneurysms are rare. Most peripheral and visceral aneurysms are atherosclerotic in origin; however, trauma and infection are also etiologic factors.

Clinical Features

Aneurysms are frequently asymptomatic. The first sign of disease may be a serious, potentially life-threatening complication, such as rupture, acute thrombosis, or embolization. Abdominal aneurysms may be detected during an abdominal examination as a palpable, expansile abdominal mass usually located in the umbilical region to the left of midline. The appearance of symptoms is usually ominous, indicating aneurysm expansion, chronic retroperitoneal bleeding, or impending rupture. Severe abdominal or back pain may be noted. Duodenal obstruction from large aneurysms may present as epigastric discomfort or difficulties with digestion. If orifices of major visceral

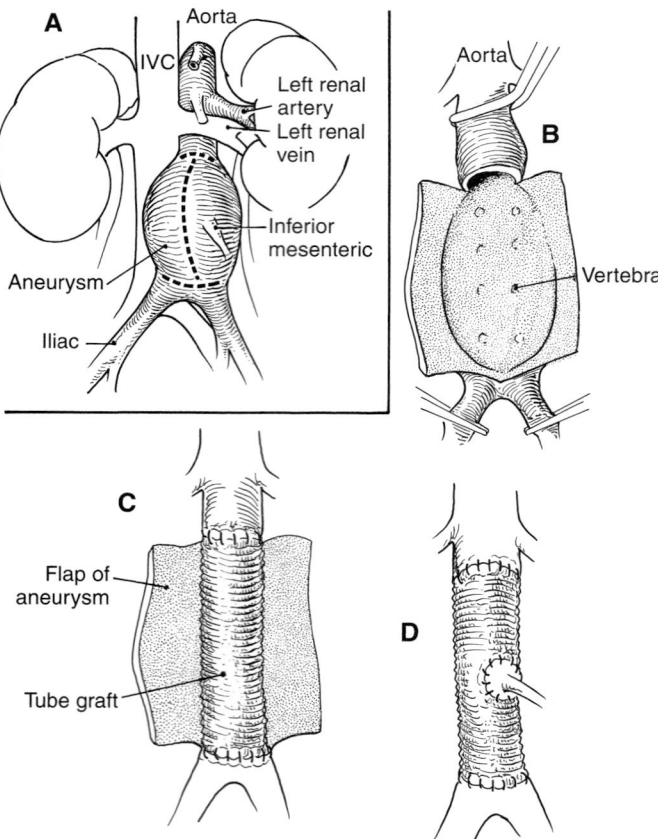

FIG. 34-12 Repair of abdominal aneurysm. **A,** Abdominal aortic aneurysm (*IVC,* inferior vena cava); **B,** preservation of external layer; **C,** insertion of tube graft; **D,** implantation of internal mesenteric artery. (Modified from Gaspar M, Barker W: *Peripheral arterial disease,* Philadelphia, 1981, Saunders.)

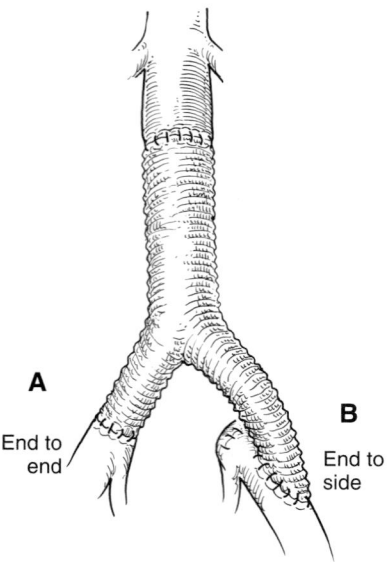

FIG. 34-13 Aortobifemoral graft. **A,** End-to-end anastomosis. **B,** End-to-side anastomosis. (Modified from Gaspar M, Barker W: *Peripheral arterial disease,* Philadelphia, 1981, Saunders.)

branches are involved, impotence may then be reported, and infrequently, visceral dysfunction may be noted. Bruits may be audible but are of little diagnostic value. Femoral pulses are diminished in some patients.

Thoracic aneurysms must be quite large to produce symptoms; consequently, aneurysms may be discovered incidentally by chest radiography. Symptoms, when they occur, are usually caused by expansion and compression of adjacent structures. Esophageal compression, although rare, produces dysphagia; recurrent laryngeal nerve compression presents as hoarseness; neck vein distention and edema of the head and arms may indicate compression of the superior vena cava. The pain associated with thoracic aneurysms occurs in the chest. Aneurysms may cause pain as a result of erosion of the vertebral column and compression of the spinal nerves.

Aneurysm rupture is catastrophic and associated with a poor prognosis. Rupture into the pericardial cavity results in exsanguination; however, rupture is usually into the retroperitoneal space, where adjacent structures exert a tamponade effect. Rupture typically presents with acute abdominal or back pain occurring in association with signs of hemorrhagic shock. A pulsatile abdominal mass may be palpable, although after rupture, detection may not be possible. Immediate surgical resection is necessary.

Treatment

Small, asymptomatic abdominal aneurysms may not warrant immediate surgical intervention. The size of these aneurysms is monitored carefully at regular intervals using palpation, abdominal radiographs, ultrasound, and CT scans. Aneurysmal enlargement to 6 cm is considered an indication for elective aneurysm resection. If the aneurysm becomes symptomatic, surgery is then considered on a more urgent basis.

The technique and type of graft used for abdominal aneurysm repair depend on the extent of the vascular involvement. If the aneurysm is confined to the aortic region below the renal arteries and above the aortic bifurcation, then a tube graft is used. The aneurysm is resected (Fig. 34-12, *A*), preserving its external layer (see Fig. 34-12, *B*); the tube graft is then anastomosed to the aorta (see Fig. 34-12, *C*). If collateral flow to the inferior mesenteric artery is inadequate, the artery is implanted into the side of the tube graft (see Fig. 34-12, *D*). The aneurysmal shell is then wrapped around the graft to minimize blood loss. If the aneurysm extends below the bifurcation or if the iliac arteries are diseased, then a bifurcation graft is used. The distal limbs of the bifurcation graft can be anastomosed end to end or end to side to the distal vessels, as shown in Fig. 34-13. Endarterectomy may be necessary.

A recently developed and exciting technique uses an *endovascular stent* to repair abdominal and aortoiliac aneurysms. The prosthetic stent is introduced via the femoral artery through the iliac artery to the aorta and anchored via hooks to the surface proximal and distal to the area of aneurysm (Kalman, 1999). Balloon expansion of the stent against the normal aortic intima excludes the aneurysm from circulation (Giesecke, 1999). This interventional approach to aneurysm repair avoids the risks and complications of major abdominal surgery and re-

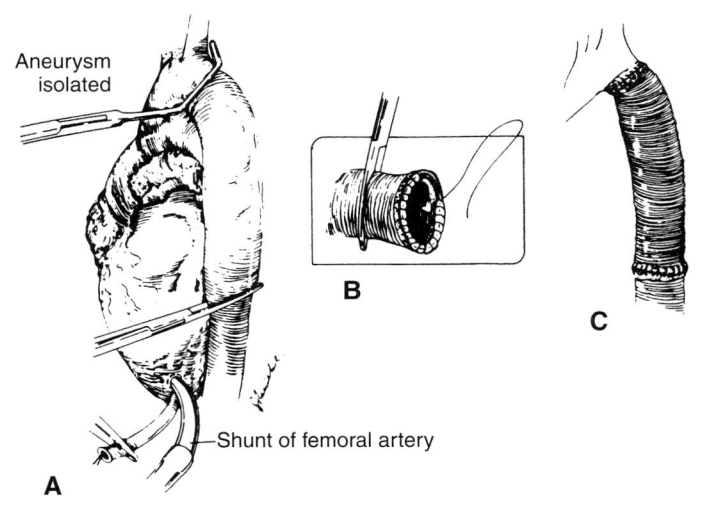

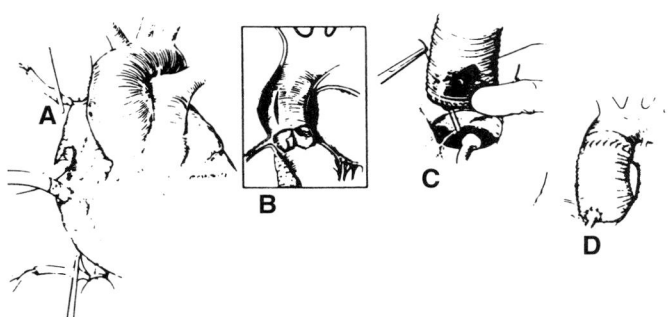

FIG. 34-14   Repair of aortic dissection. Upper panel illustrates repair of a distal aortic resection. **A,** The dissection has been isolated. A heparinized shunt extending from the apex of the left ventricle to the femoral artery is used to bypass the dissected segment and to support the circulation distal to the dissection during the repair. **B,** After resection of the dissected segment, the dissected ends of the aorta are oversewn with Teflon felt backing on the inside and outside of the aorta, both proximally and distally. **C,** A low-priority Dacron graft is sutured in the descending thoracic aorta. Lower panel illustrates the repair of a proximal aortic dissection. **A,** The patient is on total cardiopulmonary bypass. **B,** Dissection and intimal tear. **C,** Aortic valve is excised and coronary ostia is mobilized. A composite-woven Dacron graft including an attached Björk-Shiley valve is inserted because of proximal disease. **D,** The graft is sewn to the patient's aortic annulus proximally and to the distal aorta. The coronary arteries are reattached to the composite graft above the prosthetic valve. (Modified from Eagle KA et al: *The practice of cardiology,* ed 2, Boston, 1989, Little, Brown.)

covery and decreases blood loss. However, the technique is limited by the efficacy and tortuousness of the femoral and iliac arteries, as well as yet undetermined long-term effects. Complications of this approach include failure of the graft, leakage around the stent, and graft migration. Regular follow-up with CT scan as often as every 6 months is currently recommended.

Thoracic aneurysms require surgical correction. If the aneurysm is large or compressing adjacent structures, surgery is then considered on an urgent basis. The grafting technique is similar to that of abdominal aneurysm repair and involves aneurysmal resection and replacement with a tube graft placed within the aneurysmal wall. Involvement of the arch necessitates reimplantation of the brachiocephalic vessels into the graft or use of aortic patch grafts. Ascending aortic aneurysms may involve the aortic valve, requiring replacement or resuspension of the aortic valve. Peripheral perfusion is maintained during thoracic aneurysm resections by cardiopulmonary bypass, bypass of the left side of the heart, or a vascular shunt (Fig. 34-14).

Aortic Dissection

Aortic dissection is separation of the vascular layers by a column of blood (Fig. 34-15, *A*). This vascular separation creates a false arterial lumen, which communicates with the true lumen via a tear in the intima. The dissection does not extend around the circumference of the vessel; rather, it extends along the length of the vessel. This ex-

tension can partially or totally occlude any vessel in the path of the dissection by separating the vessel orifice from the true arterial lumen. Occasionally, the dissecting column of blood may reenter the true lumen or terminate; however, rapid progressive dissection is usually observed. Eventually, the false lumen may produce aneurysmal enlargement of outer vascular layers; however, aneurysm formation does not characterize the early phase of dissection. The term "dissecting aneurysm" therefore is a misnomer, even though it is used frequently as a synonym for aortic dissection.

Occasionally, an intimal tear cannot be demonstrated. In these cases, rupture of the vasa vasorum with subsequent medial hemorrhage is suspected. Consequently, the relationship between the intimal tear and the development of aortic dissection is a subject of debate. Fig. 34-16 illustrates both mechanisms for the development of aortic dissection.

Aortic dissections are characterized according to age and anatomic location. Dissections that are recognized within 2 weeks of onset are categorized as *acute dissections;* if more than 2 weeks have elapsed between onset and recognition of the aneurysm, then these are considered *chronic dissections.* Because the mortality rate of untreated aneurysms is highest in the first 2 weeks, the prognosis for chronic dissection is much better than that for acute dissection.

The DeBakey classification system is frequently used for anatomic categorization of dissections. This system distinguishes three types of dissections according to site

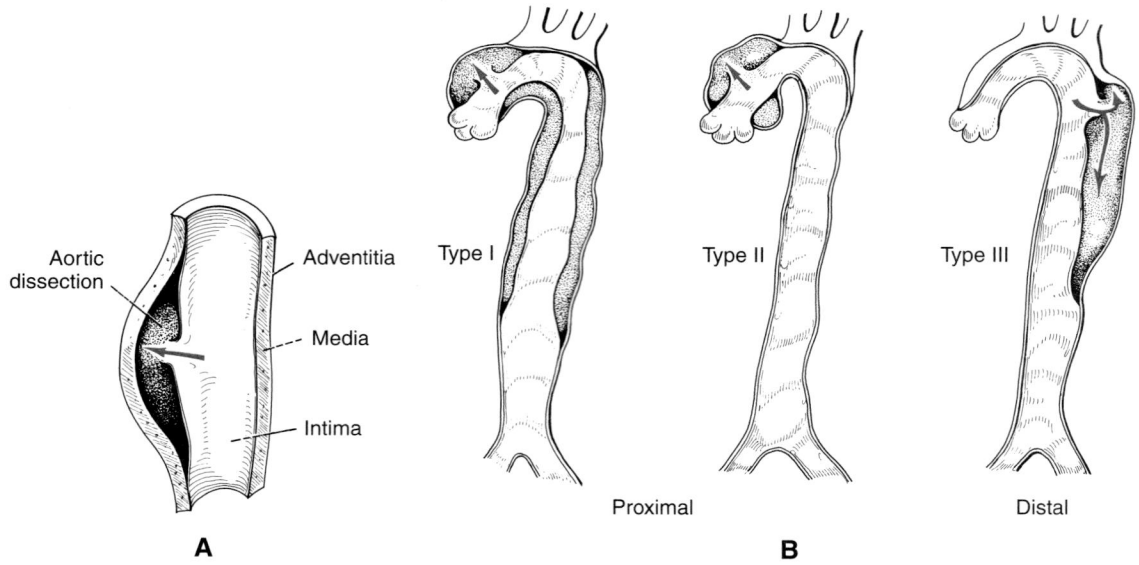

FIG. 34-15 Aortic dissection. **A**, Separation of vascular layers; **B**, classification of aortic dissection.

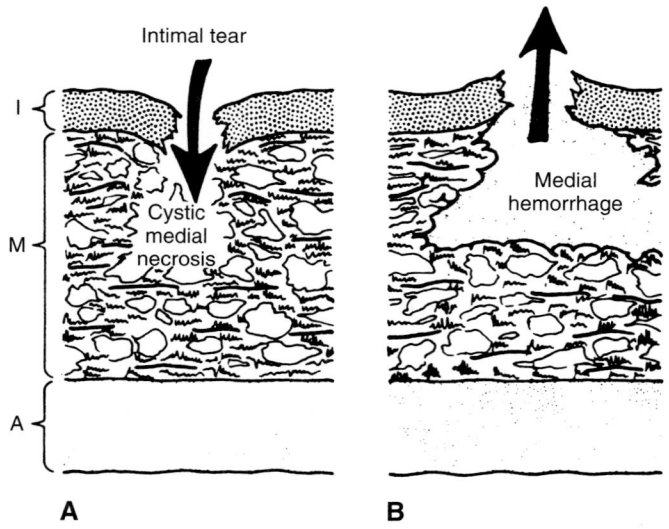

FIG. 34-16 Diagram illustrating the two possible mechanisms for the pathogenesis of aortic dissections. **A**, Primary intimal tear followed by dissection of the aorta into the media *(M)*. **B**, Primary event is hemorrhage into the aortic media followed by rupture of the overlying intima *(I)*. A, Adventitia. (From Braunwald E, Zipes DP, Libby P: *Heart disease: a textbook of cardiovascular medicine,* vol 2, ed 6, St Louis, 2001, Mosby.)

of origin and extent of dissection (see Fig. 34-15, *B*). *Type I aneurysms* originate in the ascending aorta immediately above the aortic valve and extend distally into the abdominal aorta. *Type II aneurysms* are confined to the ascending aorta. *Type III aneurysms* begin in the descending aorta immediately distal to the left subclavian artery and can extend distally to the aortic bifurcation. Another common system for anatomic classification of aneurysms simply groups type I and II aneurysms together as *proximal aneurysms* originating in the ascending aorta and distinguishes type III aneurysms as *distal aneurysms* beginning in the descending aorta.

Proximal dissections are frequently associated with cystic medial necrosis, as in Marfan syndrome. Atherosclerosis is common with distal dissections. Deceleration trauma, as mentioned earlier with aortic aneurysms, can also cause aortic dissections by disrupting the intimal and medial layers, allowing blood to enter the vessel wall.

Clinical Features

The clinical manifestations vary, depending on the site and extent of dissection; however, onset tends to be sudden and intense. Typically, severe, tearing pain is experienced. The pain can localize initially in the chest, abdomen, or back; however, as the dissection extends, the pain radiates to the back and distally toward the lower extremities. Signs of shock often develop, even though arterial pressure tends to be elevated because of underlying hypertension.

Retrograde dissection toward the aortic valve can produce aortic regurgitation manifested by a diastolic murmur and signs of congestive heart failure. As the dissection progresses, arterial branches become occluded with loss of pulses and signs of organ dysfunction; anuria may result from renal artery involvement, or lower extremity ischemia may result from iliac occlusion. Rupture is the most frequent cause of death.

Treatment

Early surgical intervention is usually indicated for proximal dissections originating in the ascending aorta and arch. Distal dissections originating in and limited to the descending aorta are usually treated medically first to control the dissection and stabilize the patient. Surgery is indicated if the dissection progresses or if complications such as arterial occlusion or hemodynamic instability arise.

Medical therapy involves the reduction of arterial pressure with drugs, such as trimethaphan camsylate (Arfonad) or sodium nitroprusside, to reduce stress on the aortic wall. The force of left ventricular contraction is reduced by administering drugs such as propranolol in an attempt to lower the velocity of ventricular ejection. Pain is controlled with analgesics and sedation. Hemodynamics and peripheral pulses are monitored carefully to detect complications. Serial chest radiography is performed to monitor the size of the dissection.

Surgical repair usually involves the resection of the involved segment and replacement with a graft. Other surgical techniques include repair and reconstruction of the aorta with sutures or patch grafts. Repair of an ascending aortic dissection may involve aortic valve replacement or annuloplasty and valve resuspension. As with aneurysm repair, the peripheral circulation can be supported with total or partial cardiopulmonary bypass or vascular shunts (see Fig. 34-14).

VENOUS DISEASE

Anatomy

In comparison with arteries, veins are thinner walled and distensible. Approximately 70% of the blood volume is contained within the venous circuit under relatively low pressure. The low-pressure, high-volume venous circuit functions as a *capacitance circuit*, in contrast to the high-pressure, low-volume resistance circuit of the arterial side. The capacity and volume of the venous circuit is an important determinant of cardiac output because the volume of blood ejected by the heart depends on its venous return.

The venous system in the lower extremities (Fig. 34-17) is divided into three subsystems: (1) the superficial venous subsystem, (2) the deep venous subsystem, and (3) the perforating (communicating) subsystem. The *superficial veins* are situated in the subcutaneous tissues of the leg and receive venous flow from smaller vessels within the skin, subcutaneous tissue, and feet. The superficial system consists of the greater saphenous vein and the lesser saphenous vein. The greater saphenous is the longest vein in the body, which extends from the malleolus of the ankle, up the inner aspect of the calf and thigh, emptying into the femoral vein immediately below the groin. The point of juncture between the two veins, the *saphenous junction*, is an important anatomic landmark. The greater saphenous vein drains the anteromedial aspects of the calf and thigh. The lesser saphenous vein extends along the lateral aspect of the calf from the ankle to the knee, draining the posterolateral aspects of the calf and emptying into the popliteal vein. The junction between the saphenous and the popliteal veins is the *saphenopopliteal junction*. Multiple anastomoses exist between the greater and lesser saphenous veins; these anastomoses are important potential routes of collateral flow in the event of venous obstruction.

The *deep venous system* carries the greater part of the venous blood in the lower extremities and is situated within the muscle compartments. The deep veins receive flow from small venules and intramuscular vessels. The deep venous system tends to parallel the arterial vessels of the lower leg, and many vessels are named accordingly. Consequently, the system includes the anterior and posterior tibial veins, peroneal vein, popliteal vein, femoral vein, profunda femoris vein, and unnamed calf

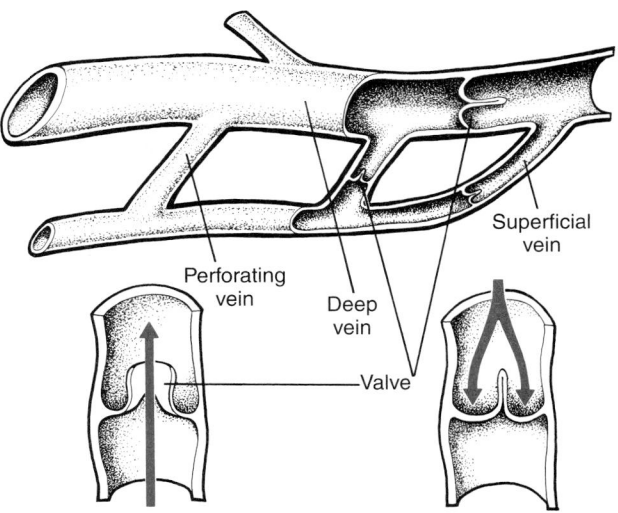

FIG. 34-17   Anatomy of the venous system of the leg.

vessels. The iliac veins are also included in the deep venous system of the lower extremity because venous drainage from the legs to the vena cava depends on the patency and integrity of these vessels. The left common iliac vein crosses beneath the right common iliac artery in its path toward the vena cava, where it has the potential to be compressed by the artery. This crossover accounts for the 2:1 preponderance of left-sided deep venous thrombosis over right-sided thrombosis.

The superficial and deep venous subsystems are connected by vascular channels referred to as *perforating veins*. The perforating veins make up the communicating subsystem of the lower extremities. Flow is normally shunted from the superficial veins to the deep veins and subsequently to the inferior vena cava.

One-way semilunar valves are distributed throughout the venous system of the lower extremities. The valves are folds of the intimal layer of the vessel and consist of endothelium and collagen. These venous valves prevent retrograde flow and direct flow proximally from the lower extremities to the vena cava and from the superficial system to the deep system via the perforators. The competency of these valves is critical because the flow of blood from the extremities to the heart is against gravity.

The physiology of venous flow against gravitational forces involves the interaction of multiple factors referred to as the *venous pump*. The venous pump is composed of peripheral and central components. The peripheral venous pump depends on compression of venous channels during muscle contraction. Muscle contraction propels flow forward within the deep venous system; the venous valves prevent retrograde flow or reflux of blood during muscle relaxation. Additionally, small valveless venous sinuses, or *venules*, located deep within the soleus and the gastrocnemius muscles function as reservoirs of blood that empty into the deep veins during muscle contraction. The contribution of these intramuscular channels is particularly important to venous return. Central forces that promote venous return include the reduction in intrathoracic pressure with inspiration and the fall in right ventricular and right atrial pressure after ventricular ejection.

Diagnostic Procedures

Because of the unreliability of clinical signs in venous disease, noninvasive and invasive methods of evaluation are of great importance. The objectives of the testing are to detect and evaluate venous obstruction or venous reflux through incompetent valves.

Physical Examination

Venous valve incompetence can be evaluated clinically by tests of venous filling time. The *Brodie-Trendelenburg test* involves emptying the saphenous vein by leg elevation and reducing arterial inflow by occlusion. With valve incompetence, rapid venous filling is noted on release of occlusion pressure and assumption of the standing position. Another technique is the *manual compression test,* which involves proximal compression of the vein as the vein is palpated distally to evaluate retrograde venous filling resulting from valve reflux.

Doppler Ultrasound

Doppler techniques are used to determine blood flow velocity and flow patterns within the superficial and deep venous systems. Venous flow can be distinguished from arterial flow because venous flow is nonpulsatile and varies with respiration. Normal venous flow patterns are characterized by an increase in flow in the lower extremities during expiration and a decrease during inspiration. With venous obstruction, these phasic respiratory variations are blunted. In veins with total obstruction of the lumen by a thrombus, the signal is absent. In partially thrombosed veins, the pitch of the signal is higher because of increased velocity of flow through the narrowed segment. Additionally, thrombosis decreases the phasicity of flow.

Doppler techniques provide a qualitative assessment of valve competence in the deep, communicating, and perforating vessels. Superficial and deep venous obstruction can be detected, although Doppler ultrasound is more sensitive to proximal vein thrombosis than it is to calf vein thrombosis. This technique is inexpensive and portable; however, a high degree of technical skill and experience is required to ensure accurate results.

Duplex Ultrasonic Scanning

The application of color flow duplex ultrasonic scanning (described earlier in the section on arterial diagnostic techniques) to venous imaging is generating much interest. With this technique, venous obstruction and valve reflux can be detected and localized, and mapping of incompetent perforating veins may be performed. While visualizing the vein in real time, the examiner samples for venous flow throughout the vessel lumen.

Venous Plethysmography

Plethysmographic techniques detect changes in the venous blood volume in the leg. Venous obstruction and valve reflux alter normal patterns of venous filling and emptying into the extremities. Common plethysmographic techniques include (1) impedance plethysmography, (2) strain gauge plethysmography, (3) air plethysmography, and (4) photoplethysmography. The techniques differ relative to the method used to detect the changes in blood volume.

In the most common technique, *impedance plethysmography (IPG)*, weak electrical currents are transmitted through the extremity, and the impedance, or resistance, to the passage of this current is measured. Because blood is a good conductor of electricity, the impedance falls when the blood volume in the extremity increases during venous filling. Electrodes on a band encircling the limb are used to measure the impedance. With *strain gauge plethysmography (SGP)*, changes in the mechanical strain on electrodes reflects changes in blood volume. *Air plethysmography* detects volume changes via corresponding changes in pressure within an air-filled cuff encircling the limb. As the venous volume increases, the pressure within the cuff increases. *Photoplethysmography (PPG)* is the newest technique and relies on the detection of reflected light from an infrared beam transmitted across the extremity. The proportion of the light reflected back to the transducer depends on the venous blood volume in the cutaneous bed.

Venography

In the setting of venous disease, venography, or *phlebography*, is the standard to which all other techniques are compared. A bolus of contrast material is injected into the venous system to opacify the veins of the lower extremity and pelvis. Descending venography with injection of contrast into the femoral vein is used to assess the extent of retrograde flow in patients with chronic venous insufficiency. Venography is considered the most reliable technique for the evaluation of the location and extent of venous disease. However, the disadvantages of invasive testing relative to noninvasive testing include greater expense, discomfort, and potential risk. Given the high correlation between combined noninvasive measures of venous obstruction—including color flow duplex scanning and plethysmography—and invasive venographic techniques, noninvasive tests are used with increasing frequency. Venography may still be used in cases of equivocal noninvasive findings or when surgical interruption of the vena cava for pulmonary embolus is planned.

Thromboembolic Venous Disease

The term *thromboembolic disease* reflects the relationship between thrombosis, the process of blood clot formation, and the ever-present risk of embolization. Frequently, the first sign of venous thrombosis is *pulmonary embolism*. Given the morbidity and mortality associated with pulmonary embolism (see Chapter 40), the primary emphasis in the treatment of deep venous thrombosis is on prevention of embolization. Consequently, the two processes are intertwined.

Historically, a distinction was made between thrombophlebitis and phlebothrombosis based on the degree of inflammation accompanying the thrombotic process. *Thrombophlebitis* was characterized by acute inflammatory signs. *Phlebothrombosis* referred to venous thrombosis without overt inflammatory signs and symptoms. The distinction was considered important in determining the risk of pulmonary embolism because inflammation was believed to increase the adherence of the clot to the vessel wall, thereby reducing the risk of pulmonary embolism. Current thinking recognizes that a clear distinction between these terms cannot be made; inflammation occurs to some degree with thrombosis. Therefore these states simply represent different degrees of an underlying process. Additionally, pulmonary embolism is always a risk, even when the presentation of venous thrombosis is silent.

The term *superficial thrombophlebitis* is the preferred term for inflammation of the superficial veins. The term *deep venous thrombosis* is preferred for thromboembolic disease of the deep veins of the lower extremity (rather than deep thrombophlebitis). The thromboembolic process in the superficial veins is more inflammatory in character and presentation than that in the deep venous system. Superficial thrombophlebitis and deep venous thrombosis are described in subsequent sections.

Pathophysiology

The precise mechanism that initiates thrombosis is poorly understood. Three categories of contributing factors, referred to as the *Virchow triad*, are usually recognized: (1) stasis of blood flow, (2) endothelial injury, and (3) hypercoagulability of blood. The relative contributions of each factor and the interrelationships among them are debated.

Stasis, or sluggish blood flow, predisposes the vein to thrombosis and appears to be a contributing factor in the setting of immobilization or prolonged limb dependency. Immobilization, such as occurs during the perioperative period or with paralysis, eliminates the effect of the peripheral venous pump, promoting stagnation and pooling of blood in the lower extremities. Theories suggest that blood stasis behind venous valve cusps may lead to platelet and fibrin deposition, precipitating the development of venous thrombosis.

Although *endothelial injury* is known to initiate thrombus formation, overt endothelial lesions cannot always be demonstrated. However, subtle endothelial changes caused by chemical changes, ischemia or anoxia, or inflammation may be implicated. Overt causes of endothelial damage include direct trauma to the vessel, such as fractures and soft tissue injury, and intravenous infusion of irritating substances, such as potassium chloride, chemotherapy, or high-dose antibiotics.

Blood hypercoagulability depends on complex interactions between a multitude of variables, including the vascular endothelium, platelets and clotting factors, and the composition and flow characteristics of blood. Additionally, the intrinsic fibrinolytic system balances the coagulation system by lysis and dissolution of clot to maintain vascular patency (see Chapter 19). Hypercoagulable states result from alterations in any of these variables. Hematologic disorders, malignancies, trauma, estrogen therapy, or a surgical event can contribute to coagulation abnormalities.

Venous thrombosis, whatever the underlying stimulus, increases the resistance to venous outflow from the lower extremities. As resistance increases, venous emptying is impaired, resulting in elevation of venous blood volume and venous pressure. Thrombosis can involve the valve pockets and disrupt valve function. Valve dysfunc-

tion or incompetence promotes stasis and pooling of blood within the extremity.

The thrombus becomes more organized and adherent to the vessel wall as it matures. Consequently, the risk of embolization is greatest in the earliest phases of thrombosis, although the tail of the clot can still be detached and embolized during the organization phase. Additionally, extension of the thrombus can produce a long, free-floating tail that can fragment and embolize into the pulmonary circulation. Progressive extension also increases the degree of venous obstruction and involves additional regions of the venous system. Ultimately, some degree of patency of the lumen may be reestablished (referred to as *recanalization*) by clot retraction and lysis via the endogenous fibrinolytic system. However, residual damage may persist. Most patients have an open lumen but scarred, unclosable valve leaflets, resulting in bidirectional venous flow.

Superficial Thrombophlebitis

Superficial thrombophlebitis involves the subcutaneous vessels of the upper and lower extremities. The most common cause of upper extremity thrombophlebitis is intravenous infusions, particularly of acidotic or hypertonic solutions. Superficial thrombophlebitis of the lower extremities is typically caused by varicose veins or trauma. If no obvious cause of superficial thrombophlebitis can be determined, then the possibility of underlying disease processes, such as Buerger's disease or malignancy, should be considered.

The course of superficial thrombophlebitis is usually benign and self-limiting. Pulmonary embolization is unusual; however, thrombus extension into the deep venous system can occur, particularly if the thrombus is close to major communicating channels or to the junctions between the saphenous veins and the popliteal or femoral veins.

Clinical Presentation

The typical presentation of superficial thrombophlebitis is acute, with aching or burning pain and superficial tenderness. Superficial thrombophlebitis is typically more painful than is deep venous thrombosis because of the proximity of the cutaneous sensory nerve endings to the inflammatory process. The skin may be erythematous and warm along the length of the vein. Slight swelling may be noted. The vein may be palpable. This firmness is sometimes called a *subcutaneous cord*. Systemic manifestations of inflammation, such as fever and malaise, may occur.

Treatment

Treatment of superficial thrombophlebitis consists of elevating the affected extremity and applying warm, moist heat. Antiinflammatory agents, such as aspirin, may help reduce discomfort and promote antithrombosis. Compression stockings or elastic bandages reduce stasis and promote venous return of the lower extremities. Any intravenous catheter in the affected area should be removed if it is a contributing factor to the superficial thrombophlebitis. If extension into a major vessel of the deep venous system is threatened, ligation or interruption of the involved superficial vein at the saphenofemoral junction may be indicated.

Acute Deep Venous Thrombosis

Deep venous thrombosis (DVT) involves the vessels of the deep venous system that affects almost 2 million Americans each year. The initial episode is referred to as *acute DVT*. A history of acute DVT predisposes to the development of *recurrent DVT*. Episodes of DVT can produce long-term disability as a result of the destruction of deep venous valves. Postthrombotic syndrome is discussed in the next section. Pulmonary embolism is a significant risk with DVT, which occurs in 30% of patients with DVT. Pulmonary embolism causes 60,000 deaths each year in the United States.

Most deep venous thrombi originate in the lower extremities; many resolve spontaneously, and others propagate or embolize. One or more veins may be involved; the calf veins are affected most frequently. Thromboses of the popliteal, superficial femoral, and iliofemoral vein segments are also common. The overwhelming majority of pulmonary emboli are caused by DVT of veins of the pelvis and lower extremity.

Major risk factors include the following: (1) marked immobility, (2) dehydration, (3) advanced malignancy, (4) blood dyscrasias, (5) history of DVT, (6) varicose veins, and (7) leg or pelvic trauma or surgery. Other predisposing factors include use of estrogen contraceptives, pregnancy, chronic congestive heart failure, and obesity.

Clinical Features

DVT is a particularly insidious problem because it is typically asymptomatic; pulmonary embolism may be the first clinical indication of thrombosis. Thrombus formation in the deep venous system may not be clinically apparent because of the large capacity of the venous system and the development of collateral circulation around obstructions. The diagnosis is particularly troublesome in that the clinical signs and symptoms associated with DVT are nonspecific, and their severity does not correlate with the extent of disease.

The most reliable signs are swelling and edema of the involved extremity. Swelling results from the increased intravascular volume caused by venous pooling of blood; edema reflects fluid seepage across the capillary membrane into the interstitium because of elevated hydrostatic pressure. The superficial veins may also be dilated because of the obstruction of flow into the deep system or shunting of blood from the deep to the superficial systems. Although unilateral swelling is typically noted, iliofemoral obstruction can produce bilateral swelling.

Pain is the most common symptom, which is typically described as aching or throbbing and may be severe. Walking may aggravate the pain. Tenderness of the involved extremity may be noted. Two techniques for eliciting limb tenderness are dorsiflexion of the foot and inflation of an air-filled cuff over the extremity. Calf tenderness on dorsiflexion of the foot is referred to as *Homans' sign* and is considered an unreliable sign of DVT; calf or thigh pain with cuff inflation is called *Lowenburg's sign*. Other signs include increased tissue turgor with swelling, increased skin temperature with dilation of superficial veins, mottling and

cyanosis caused by stagnant flow, increased oxygen extraction, and reduction of hemoglobin.

Two types of venous thrombosis are rare but bear mentioning because of their severity. The first type is *phlegmasia alba dolens*, a form of iliofemoral thrombosis. This thrombosis involves such a severe perivenous inflammatory reaction that the periarterial nerve fibers are affected, causing distal arterial spasm. The resultant decrease in arterial inflow gives the limb a pale, swollen appearance, and pulses in the arterial system are not palpable. The second type is *phlegmasia cerulea dolens* and is an even more serious iliofemoral occlusion. In this case, the sudden occlusion of venous outflow from the limb produces such rising pressure in the extremity that arterial inflow is occluded, which may lead to gangrene of the extremity. This sequela may be noted when caring for those patients who are terminally ill from a malignancy.

Treatment

Given the morbidity and mortality associated with DVT and pulmonary embolism, the therapeutic emphasis is on recognition of high-risk settings and institution of appropriate prophylaxis. When DVT is suggested, the therapeutic objective is to avoid further extension of clot and embolization.

Physical methods to minimize venous stasis are typically used for prophylaxis in high-risk settings. External support with compression stockings or elastic bandages is recommended to reduce venous stasis. However, caution must always be exercised with all types of stockings and bandages to avoid a tourniquet effect as a result of poor fit or careless application. Venous return to the heart can also be improved by active and passive leg exercises and early ambulation after surgery. Elevation of the foot of the bed above heart level and periodic elevation of the lower extremities are simple maneuvers to reduce venous hydrostatic pressure and facilitate venous emptying.

Devices are available to simulate or stimulate the mechanical pumping action of the calf muscles. *External pneumatic compression* of the lower extremities is accomplished by enclosing the calves in air-filled plastic boots, which are periodically inflated and deflated. Pneumatic boots have been used most extensively in the neurosurgical setting and postoperatively after major abdominal surgery. Anticoagulant therapy with low-dose heparin or enoxaparin, a low–molecular-weight heparin (LMWH), is advocated by some for high-risk prophylaxis.

Anticoagulant therapy with low-dose heparin is advocated by some for high-risk prophylaxis. Lower doses of heparin are thought to minimize the risk of complications while permitting adequate anticoagulation. The efficacy of this practice is controversial.

The goal of anticoagulant therapy is to prevent thrombus extension, propagation, or embolization. Anticoagulation during the acute phase may now be accomplished with intravenous heparin or subcutaneous enoxaparin (Lovenox). The use of LMWH is typically ordered for patients with DVT or pulmonary embolism who lack venous access, for those who complete anticoagulation as outpatients or for women who are pregnant. Enoxaparin is typically prescribed in doses of 1 mg/kg administered by subcutaneous injection every 12 hours. Heparin is administered as an intravenous infusion with a loading dose of 80 units/kg and then a continuous infusion of 18 units/kg adjusted accordingly. Oral anticoagulation with warfarin (Coumadin) is added before the cessation of heparin or enoxaparin. Warfarin is often added simultaneously to the intravenous or subcutaneous anticoagulants. The target for the anticoagulation therapy is to achieve an International Normalized Ratio (INR) of 2 to 3. Oral anticoagulation therapy is continued 3 to 6 months for those patients with a transient risk (after surgery) or an idiopathic cause of DVT; in patients with recurrent DVT or continued risk factors, treatment may continue for 12 months or for life.

The administration of *fibrinolytic agents,* such as streptokinase and urokinase, to dissolve clots is becoming more popular to treat DVT. These drugs are administered during the early stages of acute DVT to activate the endogenous fibrinolytic system. The fibrinolytic system is responsible for clot lysis and dissolution. Ideally, fibrinolytic therapy should be initiated within 24 to 48 hours of the onset of DVT because the mature clot is more resistant to lysis. Contraindications to fibrinolytic therapy include recent surgery or gastrointestinal bleeding.

Treatment of established DVT incorporates the physical principles noted earlier with slight modification. Bed rest is indicated initially to allow time for clot organization and adherence to the vessel wall; the hope is that bed rest will minimize the risk of pulmonary embolization. The foot of the bed should be elevated slightly to maximize venous drainage; external compression at knee or groin level from the bed or pillows should be avoided. Bed rest is typically continued until signs and symptoms, particularly edema, subside. External compression stockings or bandages may be used for treatment of edema after the first day. Progressive ambulation with external compression stockings is instituted after signs and symptoms subside.

Surgical intervention in DVT involves either venous thrombectomy or vena caval interruption to prevent pulmonary embolism. *Thrombectomy* is indicated for selected cases of massive iliofemoral DVT or extensive DVT that threatens limb survival. Thrombectomy involves insertion of a balloon-tipped Fogarty catheter through a venotomy. The balloon is then inflated, and the catheter is withdrawn, removing the clot.

In circumstances in which anticoagulant therapy cannot be used or in which it fails, venous flow through the inferior vena cava can be either totally or partially interrupted with specially designed clips (Fig. 34-18, *A*) or suturing techniques (see Fig. 34-18, *B*). With total interruption, venous return is then shunted around the obstructed vena cava via smaller collateral networks; this reduction in vessel caliber limits the potential size of an embolus reaching the heart. Vena caval clips or sutures divide the vessel into smaller compartments, preventing passage of large emboli. Devices can also be inserted transvenously to interrupt flow through the inferior vena cava. The designs of the Modin-Uddin umbrella, the Greenfield filter, and the Hunter balloon are illustrated in Fig. 34-18, *C.* The Greenfield filter is used most frequently because it has the lowest incidence of complications.

Varicose Veins

The term *varicose veins* signifies venous dilation, which is typically accompanied by vessel elongation and tortuosity (Fig. 34-19). The exact cause of varicose veins is unknown. Varicosities are distinguished as primary or secondary. The cause of *primary varicosities* appears to be inherent structural weakness in the vessel wall. Dilation can be accompanied by venous valve incompetence

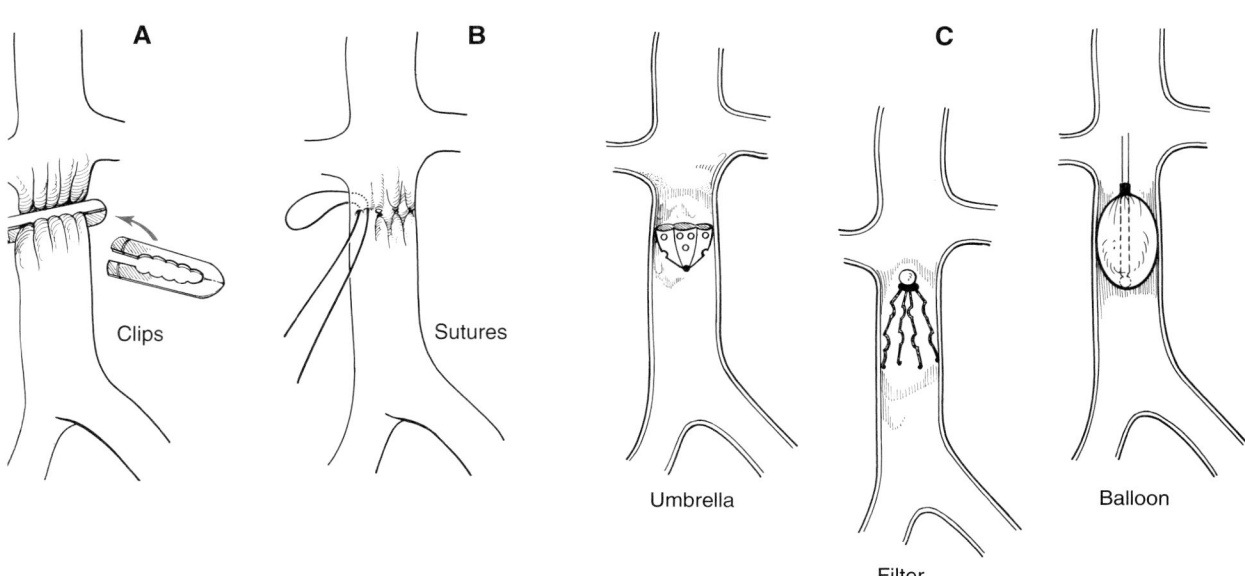

FIG. 34-18   Vena caval interruption techniques. **A**, Clipping; **B**, suturing; **C**, transvenous devices. (Modified from Moore WS: *Vascular surgery: a comprehensive review,* ed 3, Philadelphia, 1991, Sanders.)

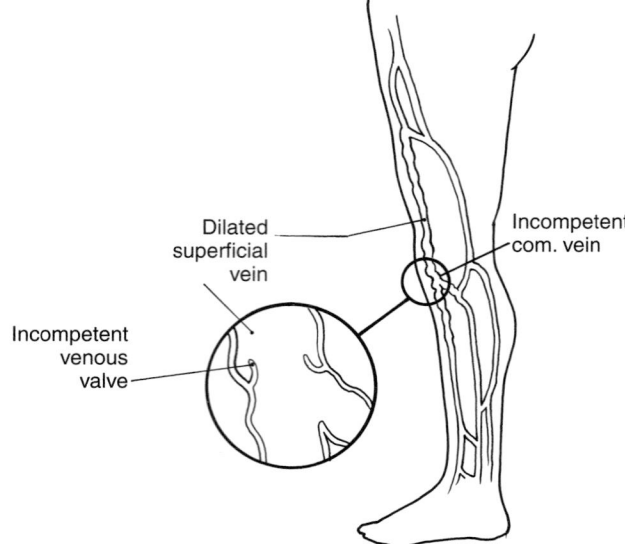

FIG. 34-19 Varicose veins. *Com*; Communicating.

because of inability of the valve cusps to overlap and prevent reflux of blood. Primary varicosities tend to involve the superficial veins because of the lack of external support or resistance within the subcutaneous tissue.

Secondary varicosities are caused by acquired or congenital pathology of the deep venous system, which produces dilation of superficial veins, perforators, or collateral channels. For example, destruction of the venous valves of the deep venous system interferes with blood return to the heart; the resultant stasis and pooling of blood result in deep venous hypertension. If the venous valves in the perforating (or communicating) vessels are incompetent, then the pressure elevation in the deep venous circuit will reverse blood flow through the perforating vessels. Venous blood will be shunted to the superficial vessels from the deep vessels, predisposing to the development of secondary varicosities in the superficial veins. In this situation, the superficial vessels function as collateral vessels for the deep venous system, shunting blood flow from the diseased region.

Predisposing Factors

A number of factors predispose the individual to the development of primary varicose veins. A familial tendency has been documented; possibly, the inherent wall weakness is inherited. Additionally, factors increasing the hydrostatic pressure and blood volume within the leg, such as prolonged standing or pregnancy, contribute to venous dilation.

Clinical Features

The most common clinical manifestation of varicose veins is *cosmetic disfigurement*. Primary varicosities may be associated with mild, dull aching of the legs, particularly pronounced at the end of the day. Discomfort is typically relieved by leg elevation and elastic support stockings. The discomfort associated with secondary varicosities

tends to be more severe. The diagnosis of varicose veins is straightforward and based on observation and palpation of dilated veins.

Complications are unusual. Superficial thrombophlebitis or hemorrhage with ecchymoses may occur. Secondary varicosities may lead to the development of edema, stasis dermatitis, or ulceration.

Treatment

Physical methods described earlier, such as elastic support, to reduce venous stasis should be used to treat varicose veins. Injection of a sclerosing agent may be considered for small, asymptomatic varices; however, sclerotherapy currently has a limited role. Surgery may be indicated to improve appearance of the lower extremity, relieve discomfort, or avoid recurrent superficial thrombophlebitis. Vein stripping surgery usually involves high ligation and stripping of the greater or lesser saphenous veins. The affected vein is ligated at either the saphenofemoral or the saphenopopliteal junction, and an intraluminal stripper is inserted to remove the entire vessel. Ambulatory phlebotomy allows the removal of smaller varicose veins through a series of tiny skin punctures under local anesthesia.

Postthrombotic Syndrome

Pathophysiology

Postthrombotic syndrome (previously called chronic venous insufficiency, or CVI) is usually produced by extensive DVT and venous valve insufficiency; it can develop months or years after the initial episode. Milder degrees of postthrombotic syndrome can develop from long-standing varicose veins with valve insufficiency. The common denominator is chronic venous stasis and elevation of venous pressures.

The chronic elevation of venous pressure produces characteristic and progressive clinical signs of venous stasis. The increased hydrostatic pressure at the capillary level results in fluid transudation into the interstitium and edema formation. Pathologic changes in the skin and subcutaneous tissue of the ankle and leg follow. Approximately 25% to 50% of patients with DVT will develop chronic venous problems.

Clinical Features

The initial presentation is persistent edema of the lower extremities. Subsequently, pathologic tissue changes produce development of a brown pigmentation because of hemosiderin deposition, induration from subcutaneous fibrosis, and dermatitis with eczematous, scaly skin. Tissue ulcerations and necrosis may occur, particularly around the medial malleolus. The extremity is swollen and painful, especially after prolonged dependency.

Treatment

As with thromboembolic venous disease, prevention is more readily accomplished than is treatment of established postthrombotic syndrome. Prevention is directed at adequate treatment of acute thrombophlebitis, DVT, and varicose veins. Control of edema is particularly important because the presence of edema indicates elevated venous pressure. The medical treatment of postthrombotic syndrome includes the physical methods described earlier, including elastic support, leg elevation, and bed rest. Additionally, the tissue is extremely vulnerable to trauma; therefore the foot should be protected whenever possible.

Antibiotic ointments may be necessary to treat the dermatitis and local inflammation or infection. Stasis ulcers are particularly difficult to treat; continual compression with the premedicated Unna's boot may be indicated. Occasionally, skin grafting is necessary in conjunction with vein ligation and stripping. Early treatment and management improve outcomes.

KEY CONCEPTS

- The arterial wall consists of three layers: the adventitia, which is the outer layer; the media, which is the middle layer; and the intima, which is the inner most layer.
- Lipid deposition in the intimal layer of the artery is the beginning of the atherosclerotic process.
- The clinical manifestations of arterial vascular disease result from stenosis or occlusion of the arterial lumen by intimal plaque, from embolization of the intimal plaque, or from aneurysm formation from degeneration of the media.
- Cystic medial necrosis, arteritis, and vasospastic disorders are nonatherosclerotic causes of arterial disease.
- Magnetic resonance angiography (MRA) is a noninvasive means of visualizing the arteries of the legs and feet without contrast material.
- The relationship of the brachial systolic pressure to the ankle systolic pressure (the ABI) is equal to slightly greater than 1.0 in a normal limb. Ratios of less than 0.4 may indicate severe arterial disease.
- To produce a significant decrease in blood flow, a single lesion or narrowing of the lumen of a blood vessel must be approximately 50% in diameter or 75% of the cross-sectional area of the artery.
- The most common sites of atherosclerotic involvement in arteries are the aortoiliac vessels, the femoropopliteal vessels, and the popliteal-tibial vessels. The atherosclerotic plaque will generally develop at points of bifurcations, curvature, or narrowing.
- Thrombus is the formation of a blood clot within the vascular system. Arterial thrombosis usually occurs at the site of an atherosclerotic plaque.
- Embolization results from the detachment of a thrombus into the blood vessel and its lodgment at a distant site.
- Intermittent claudication occurs with exercise, when metabolic demands for oxygen increase, and sub-

sides with rest within minutes. The diseased arterial segment involved is proximal to the region experiencing the claudication pain.
- The six Ps of acute arterial occlusion are pain, pallor, paresthesia, pulselessness, poikilothermia, and paralysis.
- Abdominal aortic aneurysms typically occur beneath the renal arteries and extend to the aortoiliac bifurcation; they are generally asymptomatic and palpated as part of a routine physical examination.
- A dissection of an artery is the separation of the layers of the arterial wall by a column of blood, creating a false lumen within the vessel.
- Seventy percent of the blood volume is held within the low-pressure venous system.
- The venous system in the lower extremities is divided into the deep system and the superficial system, as well as the communicating or perforating system that connects these two.
- Lower extremity venous blood flows through the superficial veins to the deep veins through the communicating veins before dumping into the inferior vena cava.
- Venous return is dependent on the venous pump— the pumping action of the muscles against the veins and on the changes in intrathoracic pressure with inspiration and expiration.
- DVT affects 2 million Americans each year, and a pulmonary embolism occurs in approximately 30% of patients with DVT.
- Virchow's triad refers to the three main factors that contribute to DVT formation: stasis of blood flow, endothelial injury, hypercoagulability of the blood.
- Approximately 25% to 50% of patients who have a DVT will eventually have symptoms of chronic venous insufficiency of the lower extremities.
- Superficial thrombophlebitis involves the subcutaneous veins of the upper and lower extremities.

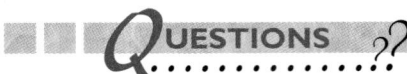

1. Label the diagrams in Fig. 34-20 by matching the number of the structure on the diagram with the appropriate term from the list.

Vessel Names

a. _____ Ascending aorta
b. _____ Aortic arch
c. _____ Aortic bifurcation
d. _____ Iliac arteries
e. _____ Descending aorta
f. _____ Popliteal arteries
g. _____ Innominate artery
h. _____ Femoral arteries

Answer the following on a separate piece of paper.

2. What are varicose veins and what causes them? Where are they generally located? What are some possible complications?

3. Which is potentially more serious, deep venous thrombosis or superficial vein thrombosis? Why? Why do the superficial veins often become dilated when deep vein thrombosis (DVT) is present?

4. List several recommendations for preventing recurrent thrombophlebitis.

5. What is an aneurysm, and what causes it? What are the dangers of an aneurysm?

6. What causes brownish pigmentation around the ankles and feet in patients with chronic venous insufficiency (CVI)?

7. List three major conditions predisposing to venous thrombosis and embolism.

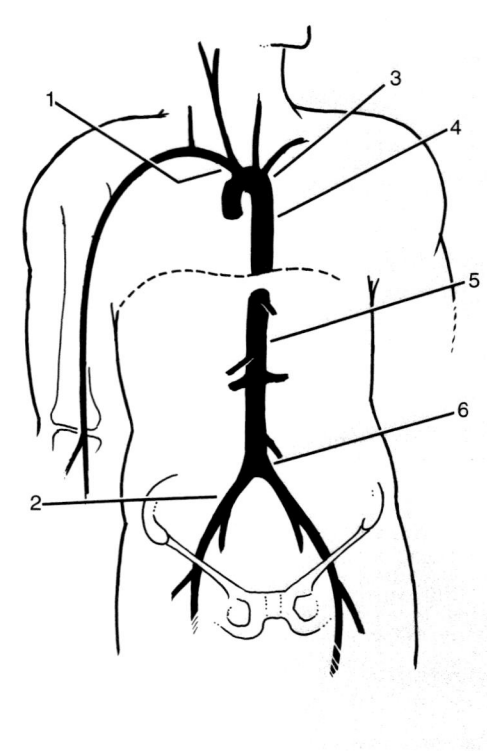
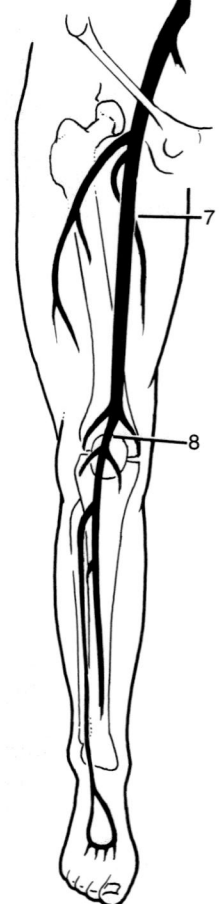

FIG. 34-20 Anatomy of arterial circulation.

Fill in the blank with the correct word.

8. _____ means inflammation of the vein accompanied by the formation of a clot; _____ means the formation of a clot in a vein in which little or no inflammation is noted.

9. An arterial disease that starts in the smaller arteries of the hands and feet and has an intense inflammatory component is _____.

Match each of the diagnostic methods in column A with the most appropriate statement in column B.

Column A

10. _____ Arteriography
11. _____ Color flow duplex scan
12. _____ Segmental plethysmography
13. _____ Radioactive fibrinogen scanning

Column B

a. Noninvasively measures the velocity of flow in a vessel
b. Visualization of arterial anatomy by injection of contrast material directly into an artery
c. Measures pulse volume
d. Injection intravenously of radioactive isotope, which is detected by a counter at the site of actively forming thrombi

Match the types of arterial dissection in column B with the appropriate category of the De-Bakey classification in column A.

Column A

14. _____ Type I
15. _____ Type II
16. _____ Type III

Column B

a. Aneurysms beginning beyond left subclavian and extending distally
b. Aneurysms confined to the ascending artery
c. Aneurysms originating in the ascending aorta above aortic valve and extending distally

*B*IBLIOGRAPHY ■ PART SIX

ACC/AHA Task Force Report: Guidelines for the evaluation and management of heart failure, *Circulation* 92:2764-2784, 1995.

Agneli G, Rossi R, Santamaria MG: Management of thromboembolism in the outpatient setting, *Sem Hematol* 37(3):23-26, 2000.

Akbari C, LoGerfo F: Diabetes and peripheral vascular disease, *J Vasc Surg* 30:373-384, 1999.

Albert NM: Manipulating survival and life quality outcomes in heart failure through disease state management, *Crit Care Nurs Clin North Am* 11:121-141, 1999.

American Heart Association: *2000 Heart and stroke statistical update*, Dallas, 1999, The Association.

American Heart Association Web Site: Statistics, available at *http://www.americanheart.org*. Accessed December 2000.

Anderson JL et al: Plasma homocysteine predicts mortality independently of traditional risk factors and C-reactive protein in patients with angiographically defined coronary artery disease, *Circulation* 102:1227-1232, 2000.

Ascher E et al: Lessons learned from a 6-year clinical experience with superior vena cava Greenfield filters, *J Vasc Surg* 32(5):881-887, 1999.

Australia-New Zealand Heart Failure Collaborative Group: Randomized placebo-controlled trial of carvedilol in patients with congestive heart failure due to ischemic heart disease, *Lancet* 349:375-380, 1997.

Batista RJV et al: Partial left ventriculectomy to improve left ventricular function in end-stage heart disease, *J Card Surg* 11:96-97, 1996.

Bauersachs J et al: Striking increase in natriuresis by low-dose spironolactone in congestive heart failure only in combination with ACE inhibition, *Circulation* 102:2325-2328, 2000.

Bays RA et al: Validation of air plethysmography, photoplethysmography, and duplex ultrasonography in the evaluation of severe venous stasis, *J Vasc Surg* 20(5):721-727, 1994.

Beattie S: Heart failure with preserved LV function: pathophysiology, clinical presentation, treatment, and nursing implications, *J Cardiovasc Nurs* 14(4):24-37, 2000.

Berne RM, Levy MN: *Cardiovascular physiology*, ed 8, Philadelphia, 2000, Mosby.

Bhatt Dl, Topol EJ: Current role of platelet glycoprotein IIb/IIIa inhibitors in acute coronary syndromes, *JAMA* 284:1549-1558, 2000.

Binder TM et al: Improved assessment of mitral valve stenosis by volumetric real-time three-dimensional echocardiography, *Am Coll of Cardiol* 36:1355-1361, 2000.

Bonow RO et al: Guidelines for the management of patients with valvular heart disease—executive summary: a report of the American College of Cardiology/American Heart Association Task Force on Practice Guidelines, *Circulation* 98:1949-1984, 1998.

Bonow RO et al: Serial long-term assessment of the natural history of asymptomatic patients with chronic aortic regurgitation and normal left ventricular systolic function, *Circulation* 84:1625-1635, 1991.

Boon A et al: Cardiac valve calcification: characteristics of patients with calcification of the mitral annulus or aortic valve, *Heart* 78:472-474, 1997.

Borer JS et al: Prediction of indications for valve replacement among asymptomatic or minimally symptomatic patients with chronic aortic regurgitation and normal left ventricular performance, *Circulation* 97:525-534, 1997.

Braunwald E: *Heart disease: a textbook of cardiovascular medicine*, vols 1 and 2, ed 5, Philadelphia, 1997, WB Saunders.

Braunwald E et al: ACC/AHA guidelines for the management of patients with unstable angina and non-ST-segment elevation myocardial infarction: executive summary and recommendations, *Circulation* 102:1193-1209, 2000.

Bridges EJ: Monitoring pulmonary artery pressures: just the facts, *Crit Care Nurs* 20:59-78, 2000.

Brown WV: Cholesterol lowering in atherosclerosis, *Am J Cardiol* 86(suppl):29H-32H, 2000.

Carabello BA, Crawford FA: Valvular heart disease, *N Engl J Med* 337:32-41, 1997.

Cheitlin MD et al: ACC/AHA guidelines for the clinical application of echocardiography: a report of the American College of Cardiology/American Heart Association Task Force on Practice Guidelines developed in collaboration with the American Society of Echocardiography, *Circulation* 95:1686-1744, 1997.

Christensen DS: The ventricular assist device, *Nurs Clin North Am* 35:945-959, 2000.

Clark RE, Zafirelis Z: Future devices and directions, *Prog Cardiovasc Dis* 1:95-100, 2000.

Cohn JN: The management of chronic heart failure, *N Engl J Med* 335:490-498, 1996.

Cohn JN, Ferrari R, Sharpe N: Cardiac remodeling-concepts from an international forum on cardiac remodeling, *J Am Coll Cardiol* 35:569-682, 2000.

Conover MB: *Understanding electrocardiology*, ed 7, St Louis, 1995, Mosby.

Cowie MR, Struthers AD, Wood DA: Value of natriuretic peptides in assessment of patients with possible new heart failure in primary care, *Lancet* 350:1349-1353, 1997.

Dajani A et al: Prevention of bacterial endocarditis: recommendations of the American Heart Association, *Circulation* 96:358-366, 1997.

Dale JB: Group A streptococcal vaccines, *Infect Dis North Am* 13:227-243, 1999.

DeWall RA, Qasim N, Carr L: Evolution of mechanical heart valves, *Ann Thorac Surg* 69:1612-1621, 2000.

Diaz MN et al: Mechanisms of disease: antioxidants and atherosclerotic heart disease, *N Engl J Med* 337:408-416, 1997.

The Digitalis Investigation Group: The effects of digoxin on mortality and morbidity in patients with heart failure, *N Engl J Med* 336:525-533, 1997.

Donovan CL, Starling MR: Role of echocardiography in the timing of surgical intervention for chronic mitral and aortic regurgitation. In Otto CM, editor: *The practice of clinical echocardiography*, Philadelphia, 1997, WB Saunders, pp. 327-354.

Doughty RN et al: Left ventricular remodeling with carvedilol in patients with congestive heart failure due to ischemic heart disease, *J Am Coll Cardiol* 29:1060-1066, 1997.

The EPIC Investigators: Use of a monoclonal antibody directed against the platelet glycoprotein IIb/IIIa receptor in high risk angioplasty, *N Engl J Med* 330:965-971, 1994.

The Epistent Investigators: Randomized placebo controlled balloon-angioplasty-controlled trial to assess safety of coronary stenting with the use of platelet glycoprotein IIb/IIIa blockade, *Lancet* 352:87-92, 1998.

Eskandari MK et al: Is color-flow duplex a good diagnostic test for detection of isolated calf vein thrombosis in high risk patients? *Angiology* 51(9):705-710, 2000.

Fahey VA: *Vascular nursing*, ed 3, Philadelphia, 1999, WB Saunders.

Faletra F, et al: Measurement of mitral valve area in mitral stenosis: four echocardiographic methods compared to direct measurement of anatomic orifices, *J Am Coll Cardiol* 28:1190-1197, 1996.

Feldman AM et al: The role of tumor necrosis factor in the pathophysiology of heart failure, *J Am Coll Cardiol* 35:537-544, 2000.

Frazier OH: Left ventricular assist, *Adv Card Surg* 9:131-148, 1997.

Garg R, Yusuf S: Overview of randomized trials of angiotensin-converting enzyme inhibitors on morbidity and mortality in patients with heart failure: Collaborative Group on ACE-Inhibitor Trials, *JAMA* 273:1450-1456, 1995.

Giesecke N: Endovascular stent repair of abdominal aortic aneurysms. *http://www.asahq.org/Newsletters/1999/03_99/TOC_0399.html*

Gilbert KB, Rogers GM: Utilization and outcomes of enoxaparin treatment for deep vein thrombosis in a tertiary care hospital, *Am J Hematol* 65(4):285-288, 2000.

Giovani G et al: Arterial abnormalities in the offspring of patients with premature myocardial infarction, *N Engl J Med* 343:840-846, 2000.

Goldstein JA et al: Multiple complex coronary plaques in patients with acute myocardial infarction, *N Engl J Med* 343:915-922, 2000.

Graham L, Ford M, Fahey VA: Arterial disease. In Fahey V, editor: *Vascular nursing*, ed 3, Philadelphia, 1999, WB Saunders.

Gronda E, Vitali E: Left ventricular assist systems: a possible alternative to heart transplantation for patients? *Eur J Heart* 4:319-325, 1999.

Guy TS: Evolution and current status of the total artificial heart: the search continues, *ASAIO J* 44:28-33, 1998.

Guyton AC, Hall JE: *Textbook of medical physiology*, ed 10, Philadelphia, 2000, WB Saunders.

Haimovici H: *Vascular surgery*, ed 4, Boston, 1996, Blackwell Science.

Hamm CW, Braunwald E: A classification of unstable angina revisited, *Circulation* 102:118-122, 2000.

Hochman JS, Buller CE, Sleeper LA, et al: Cardiogenic shock complicating acute myocardial infarction—etiologies, management and outcome: a report from the SHOCK Trial Registry, *J Am Coll Cardiol* 36:1063-1070, 2000.

Hunt SA, Frazier OH: Mechanical circulatory support and cardiac transplantation, *Circulation* 97:2079-2090, 1998.

Jaffe AS et al: It is time for a change to a troponin standard, *Circulation* 102:1216-1220, 2000.

Jaski BE et al: Left ventricular assist device as a bridge to patient and myocardial recovery, *Prog Cardiovasc Dis* 43:5-18, 2000.

Kalman P: Stent-graft repair for abdominal aortic aneurysm, *CMAJ* 11:1133, 1999.

Khand A et al: Is the prognosis for heart failure improving? *J Am Coll Cardiol* 36:2284-2286, 2000.

Konstam MA: Progress in heart failure management? Lessons from the real world, *Circulation* 102:1076-1078, 2000.

Korfer R et al: Temporary pulsatile ventricular assist devices and biventricular assist device, *Ann Thorac Surg* 68:678-683, 1999.

Kukin ML, Kalman J, Charney RH: Prospective, randomized comparison of effect of long-term treatment with metoprolol or carvedilol on symptoms, exercise, ejection fraction and oxidative stress in heart failure, *Circulation* 99:2645-2651, 1999.

Kusumoto FM: *Cardiovascular pathophysiology*, ed 1, Madison, Conn, 1999, Fence Creek Publishing.

Labugger L et al: Extensive troponin I and T modification detected in serum from patients with acute myocardial infarction, *Circulation* 102:1221-1226, 2000.

Lincoff AM et al: Management of patients with acute coronary syndromes by platelet glycoprotein IIb/IIIa inhibition, *Circulation* 102:1093-1100, 2000.

The Long Term Intervention with Pravastatin in Ischemic Disease (LIPID) Study Group: Prevention of cardiovascular events and death with pravastatin in patients with coronary heart disease and a broad range of initial cholesterol levels, *N Engl J Med* 339:1349-1357, 1998.

MacIntyre K et al: Evidence of improving prognosis in heart failure: trends in case fatality in 66,547 patients hospitalized between 1986-1995, *Circulation* 102:1126-1131, 2000.

Mahmood AK et al: Critical review of current left ventricular assist devices, *Perfusion* 15:399-420, 2000.

Marston WA et al: Healing rates and cost efficacy of outpatient compression treatment for leg ulcers associated with venous insufficiency, *J Vasc Surg* 30(3):491-498, 1999.

Marzo K, Prigent FM, Steingart RM: Interventional therapy in heart failure management, *Clin Geriatr Med* 16:549-566, 2000.

Matezky S et al: Elevated troponin I level on admission is associated with adverse outcomes of primary angioplasty in acute myocardial infarction, *Circulation* 102:1611-1616, 2000.

McCarthy PM, Hoercher K: Clinically available intracorporeal left ventricular assist devices, *Prog Cardiovasc Dis* 43:47-54, 2000.

McMurray JJ, Stewart S: Epidemiology, aetiology, and prognosis of heart failure, *Heart* 83:596-602, 2000.

Members of the Joint National Committee on Prevention, Detection, Evaluation and Treatment of High Blood Pressure: The sixth report of the Joint National Committee on Prevention, Evaluation and Treatment of High Blood Pressure, *Arch Int Med* 157:2413-2445, 1997.

Menon V et al: The clinical profile of patients with suspected cardiogenic shock due to predominant left ventricular failure: a report from the SHOCK Trial Registry, *J Am Coll Cardiol* 36:1071-1076, 2000.

Menon V et al: Outcome and profile of ventricular septal rupture with cardiogenic shock after myocardial infarction: a report from the SHOCK Trial Registry, *J Am Coll Cardiol* 36:1110-1116, 2000.

Moheler E et al: Clinical utility of troponin levels and echocardiography in the emergency room, *Am Heart J* 135:253-260, 1998.

Myer N: Using physiological and pharmacological stress testing in the evaluation of coronary artery disease, *Nurs Pract* 24:70-76, 1999.

Narula J et al, editors: *Rheumatic fever*, Washington, DC, 1999, Armed Forces Institute of Pathology, American Registry of Pathology.

National Cholesterol Education Program: *Second report of the expert panel on detection, evaluation, and treatment of high blood cholesterol levels in adults*, NIH publication No. 93-3095, Washington, DC, 1993, NIH.

Newsletter of the American College of Phlebotomy. *http://www.phlebology.com*

Nicholson A et al: Long-term follow-up of the Bird's nest IVC filter, *Clin Radiol* 54(11):759-764, 1999.

Otto CM: *Textbook of clinical echocardiology,* ed 2, Philadelphia, 1999, WB Saunders.

Otto CM: Timing of aortic valve surgery, *Heart* 84:211-218, 2000.

Otto CM et al: Association of aortic valve sclerosis with cardiovascular mortality and morbidity in the elderly, *N Engl J Med* 341:142-147, 1999.

Otto CM et al: A prospective study of asymptomatic valvular aortic stenosis: clinical echocardiographic and exercise predictors of outcome, *Circulation* 95:2262-2270, 1997.

Oxford JL et al: The comparative pathobiology of atherosclerosis and restenosis, *Am J Cardiol* 86(suppl):6H-11H, 2000.

Packer M, Bristow MR, Cohn JN, for the US Carvedilol Heart Failure Study Group: The effect of carvedilol on morbidity and mortality in patients with chronic heart failure, *N Engl J Med* 334:1349-1355, 1996.

Pagani FD et al: Extra corporeal life support to left ventricular assist device bridge to optimize survival and resource utilization, *Circulation* 19(suppl):II206-II210, 1999.

Park SJ et al: Left ventricular assist device bridge therapy for acute myocardial infarction, *Ann Thorac Surg* 69:1146-1151, 2000.

Pearson JL et al: The lipid treatment assessment project (L-TAP), *Arch Int Med* 60:459-467, 2000.

Piccione W: Mechanical circulatory assistance: changing indications and options, *J Heart Lung Transplant* 6:S25-S28, 1997.

Pietro J et al: Accuracy of exercise echocardiography to detect coronary artery disease in left bundle branch block unassociated with either acute or healed myocardial infarction, *Am J Cardiol* 85:890, 2000.

Pijls NH et al: FFR: a useful index to evaluate the influence of an epicardial coronary stenosis on myocardial blood flow, *Circulation* 92:3183, 1995.

Rhodes J, Gloviczki P: Endoscopic perforating vein surgery, *Surg Clin North Am* 79(3):667-679, 1999.

Rifkind BM: The Lipid Research Clinics Coronary Prevention Trial, *Am J Cardiol* 54(5):30C-34C, 1984.

Rogers KG: Cardiovascular shock, *Emerg Med Clin North Am* 13:793-810, 1995.

Ross R: Mechanisms of disease: atherosclerosis an inflammatory disease, *N Engl J Med* 340:115-126, 1999.

Rourke TK, Droogan MT, Ohler L: Heart transplantation: state of the art, *AACN Clin Issues* 10:185-201, 1999.

Rutherford RB, editor: *Vascular surgery,* Philadelphia, 1999, WB Saunders.

Sanborn TA et al: Impact of thrombolysis, intra-aortic balloon pump counterpulsation, and their combination in cardiogenic shock complicating acute myocardial infarction: a report from the Shock Trial Registry, *J Am Coll Cardiol* 36:1123-1129, 2000.

San Roman JA et al: Selection of the optimal stress test for the diagnosis of coronary artery disease, *Heart* 80:370, 1998.

The Scandinavian Simvastatin Survival Study Investigators: Randomized trial of cholesterol lowering in 4444 patients with coronary artery disease; the Scandinavian Simvastatin Survival Study (4S), *Lancet* 344:1383-1389, 1994.

Schindler N, Vogelzang R: Superior vena cava syndrome, *Surg Clin North Am* 79(5):683-693, 1999.

Schomig A et al: Coronary stenting plus platelet glycoprotein IIb/IIIa blockade compared with tissue plasminogen activator in acute myocardial infarction, *N Engl J Med* 343:391, 2000.

Sheffield LT et al: Recommendations for standards of instrumentation and practice in the use of ambulatory electrocardiography, *Circulation* 71:626, 1995.

Siedel HM: *Mosby's guide to physical examination,* ed 4, St Louis, 1999, Mosby.

The Sixth Report of the Joint National Committee on Detection, Evaluation and Diagnosis of High Blood Pressure (JNC VI): *Arch Int Med* 157:2413, 1997.

Spann JC, Van Meter C: Cardiac transplantation, *Surg Clin North Am* 78:679-690, 1998.

Stewart BF et al: Clinical factors associated with calcific aortic valve disease, Cardiovascular Health Study, *J Am Coll Cardiol* 29:630-634, 1997.

Stone GW et al: Improved procedural results of coronary angioplasty with intravascular ultrasound-guided balloon sizing: the Clout pilot trial, *Circulation* 95:2354, 1997.

Streif MB: Vena cava filters: a comprehensive review, *Blood* 15(12):3669-3677, 2000.

Thompson CR et al: Cardiogenic shock due to acute severe mitral regurgitation complicating acute myocardial infarction: a report from the SHOCK Trial Registry, *J Am Coll Cardiol* 36:1104-1109, 2000.

Tischler MD et al: Mitral valve replacement versus mitral valve repair: a Doppler and quantitative stress echocardiographic study, *Circulation* 89:132-137, 1994.

Torre-Amione G et al: Decreased expression of tumor necrosis factor-alpha in failing human myocytes: a potential mechanism for cardiac recovery, *Circulation* 100:1189-1193, 1999.

Tsutamoto T et al: Spironolactone inhibits the transcardiac extraction of aldosterone in patients with congestive heart failure, *J Am Coll Cardiol* 36:838-844, 2000.

Vitale N: Mechanical cardiac assistance, *Intensive Care Med* 25:543-545, 1999.

Webb JG et al: Implications of the timing of onset of cardiogenic shock after acute myocardial infarction: a report from the SHOCK Trial Registry, *J Am Coll Cardiol* 36:1084-1090, 2000.

West of Scotland Coronary Prevention Study Group: Influence of pravastatin and plasma lipids on clinical events in the West of Scotland Coronary Prevention Study (WOSCOPS), *Circulation* 97:1440-1445, 1998.

Westaby S: The artificial heart: current concepts, *Hosp Med* 60:776-777, 1999.

Westaby S: Non-transplant surgery for heart failure, *Heart* 83:603-617, 2000.

Wilson WR et al: Antibiotic treatment of adults with infective endocarditis due to streptococci, enterococci, staphylococci, and HACEK microorganisms: American Heart Association, *JAMA* 274:1706-1713, 1995.

Wong SC et al: Angiographic findings and clinical correlates in patients with cardiogenic shock complicating acute myocardial infarction: a report from the SHOCK Trial Registry, *Am Coll Cardiol* 36:1077-1083.

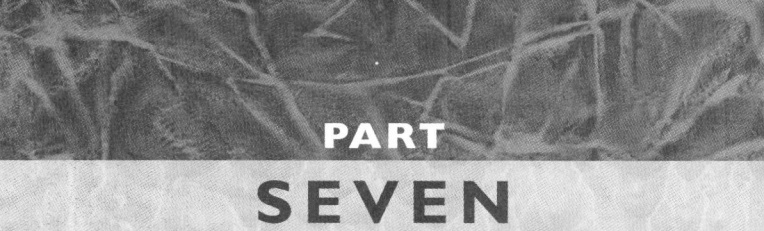

RESPIRATORY SYSTEM DISORDERS

*D*isorders of the respiratory system are a major cause of morbidity and mortality. Respiratory tract infections occur more frequently than do infections of any other organ system and range from the common cold, with its relatively mild symptoms and inconvenience, to a fulminant pneumonia. In 1999, approximately 158,900 persons died from lung cancer. Since the mid-1950s, lung cancer has been the most common cause of cancer mortality in men, and in 1987 it overtook breast cancer to become the most common cause of cancer mortality in women. Lung cancer has increased at an alarming rate and is now approximately 25 times more prevalent than it was 50 years ago. The incidence of chronic respiratory disease, notably chronic pulmonary emphysema and bronchitis, has also been increasing and is now a leading cause of chronic disability and the fourth leading cause of death. Because of the physical, social, and economic impact of respiratory diseases on the population as a whole, the prevention, diagnosis, and treatment of respiratory disorders are of paramount importance.

This part includes a brief review of respiratory tract anatomy and physiology, a discussion of the common diagnostic tests used to detect respiratory dysfunction, cardinal signs and symptoms of respiratory disease, manifestations of respiratory insufficiency and failure, and a discussion of the common respiratory diseases.

CHAPTER

35

Anatomy and Physiology of the Respiratory System

LORRAINE M. WILSON

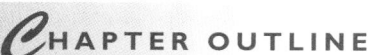
ANATOMIC CONSIDERATIONS

Respiration means literally the movement of oxygen (O_2) from the atmosphere to the cells and the return of carbon dioxide (CO_2) from the cells to the environment. O_2 consumption and CO_2 elimination are necessary for normal cellular function within the body; however, most of our billions of cells cannot exchange these gases directly with the air because they are far too distant from it. Therefore cells need special structures both for exchange and for transport.

The respiratory process consists of several steps, with the respiratory, central nervous, and cardiovascular systems playing pivotal roles. Essentially, the respiratory system consists of a series of air passages that bring outside air into contact with the *alveolocapillary membrane*, the interface between the respiratory and cardiovascular systems. The movement of air in and out of the air passages is called *ventilation* or *breathing*. The central nervous system provides the inherent rhythmic drive to breathe and reflexively stimulates the thoracic and diaphragm muscles, which provide the driving force for the movement of air. The diffusion of O_2 and CO_2 across the alveolocapillary membrane is often referred to as *external respiration*. The cardiovascular system provides the pump, conduits, and blood that are essential for the transport of gases between the lungs and cells. An adequate amount of functioning hemoglobin is essential for the transportation of gases. The final transportation phase of gas transport involves the diffusion of O_2 and CO_2 between the body capillaries and cells. *Internal respiration* refers to the intracellular chemical reactions in which O_2 is used and CO_2 is produced, as the cells metabolize carbohydrates and other substances to generate adenosine triphosphate (ATP) and release energy.

Adequate functioning of all these interrelated systems is essential for cell respiration. Malfunction of any of these components can disrupt gas exchange and transport and can seriously compromise these life processes. An understanding of the respiratory process is necessary to assess and treat clients with respiratory disorders. This chapter and Chapter 36 lay the groundwork for this understanding.

Anatomy of the Respiratory Tract

The air-conducting passages that bring air into the lungs are the nose, pharynx, larynx, trachea, bronchi, and bronchioles (Fig. 35-1). The respiratory tract from the nose to the bronchioles is lined with ciliated mucous membranes. As air enters the nasal cavity, it is filtered, warmed, and humidified. These three processes are primarily functions of the respiratory mucosa, which consists of pseudostratified, ciliated, columnar epithelium, and goblet cells (see Fig. 35-1, *B*). The epithelial surface is covered by a mucous blanket, which is secreted by both the goblet cells and the mucous glands. Coarse dust particles are filtered by hair in the nares, and fine particles are trapped in the mucous blanket. Ciliary action propels the mucous blanket posteriorly in the nasal cavity and superiorly in the lower respiratory tract toward the *pharynx*, from which it is swallowed or expectorated. The mucous blanket provides water for humidification, and a rich underlying vascular network supplies heat to the inspired air. Inspired air is thus conditioned so that it reaches the pharynx nearly dust free, at body temperature, and 100% humidified.

Air passes from the pharynx into the larynx, or voice box. The *larynx* consists of a series of cartilaginous rings

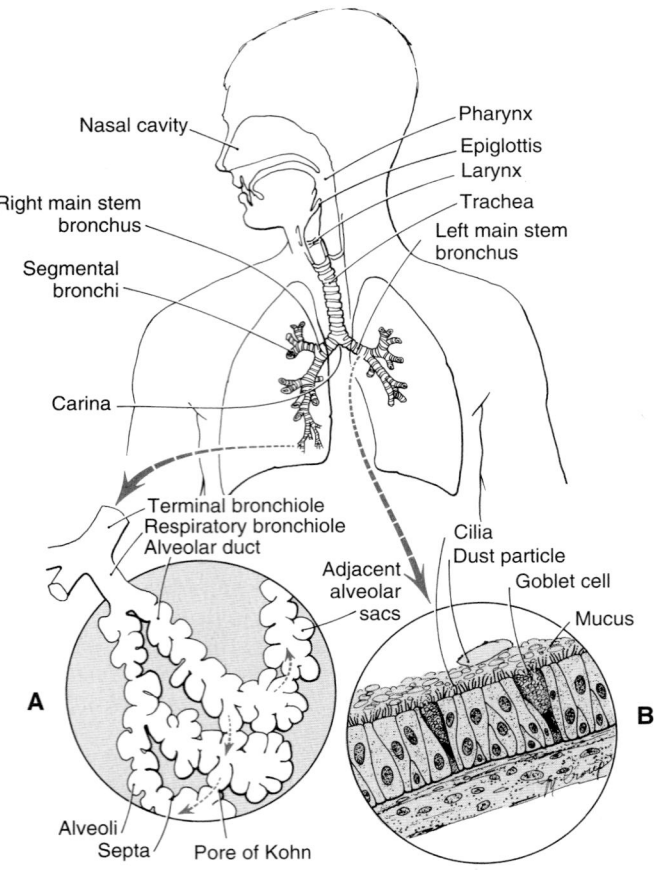

FIG. 35-1 Respiratory system. Inset **A**, Acinus, or pulmonary functional unit. Inset **B**, Ciliated mucous membrane.

united by muscles and contains the vocal cords. A triangular space between the vocal cords, the *glottis*, opens into the trachea and forms the division between the upper and lower respiratory tracts. Although the larynx has been thought of chiefly in relationship to phonation, its protective functions are much more important. During swallowing, the rising action of the larynx, the closure of the glottis, and the doorlike action of the leaf-shaped *epiglottis*, at the entrance of the larynx, all serve to guide food and fluids into the esophagus. If foreign substances do get beyond the glottis, the cough function of the larynx then assists in expelling these substances, as well as secretions from the lower respiratory tract.

The *trachea* is supported by horseshoe-shaped cartilaginous rings and is approximately 12.5 cm (5 inches) long. The structure of the trachea and bronchi is analogous to a tree and is therefore called the *tracheobronchial tree*. The posterior surface of the trachea is flattened rather than rounded because its cartilaginous rings are incomplete, and it lies immediately in front of the esophagus. Consequently, when a round, rigid endotracheal (ET) tube with inflated cuff is inserted during mechanical ventilation, erosion may occur posteriorly through the membrane to form a tracheoesophageal fistula. Anterior erosion through the cartilaginous rings may also occur but is less common. Swelling and damage to the vocal cords are also complications of ET tube use. The point at which the trachea branches into the right and left main stem

bronchi is known as the *carina*. The carina is heavily innervated and can produce severe bronchospasm and coughing when stimulated.

The right and left main stem bronchi are not symmetric (see Fig. 35-1). The *right main stem bronchus* is shorter and wider compared with the left main stem and continues from the trachea in a nearly vertical course. In contrast, the *left main stem bronchus* is longer and narrower compared with the right main stem and continues from the trachea at a more acute angle. This anatomic peculiarity has important clinical implications. An ET tube that has been placed to secure a patent airway may easily slip down into the right main stem bronchus unless well secured at the mouth or nose. If the ET tube slips, air would be unable to enter the left lung, which would collapse *(atelectasis)*. However, the more vertical course of the right bronchus makes the introduction of a catheter for deep suctioning easier. Additionally, aspirated foreign bodies are more apt to lodge in the right bronchial tree because of its vertical course.

The right and left main stem bronchi divide to become the *lobar bronchi* and then the *segmental bronchi*. This branching in ever-decreasing sizes continues down to the *terminal bronchioles*, the smallest airways that do not contain alveoli (air sacs). Terminal bronchioles are approximately 1 mm in diameter. Bronchioles are not supported by cartilaginous rings but are surrounded by smooth muscle, which allows alterations in size. All the airways down to the level of the terminal bronchioles are called *conducting airways* because their main function is to serve as air conduits to the gas-exchanging areas of the lung.

Beyond the terminal bronchiole is the *acinus*, which is the pulmonary functional unit whereby gas exchange takes place (see Fig. 35-1, *A*). The acinus consists of (1) *respiratory bronchioles*, which have occasional small air sacs or alveoli arising from their walls; (2) *alveolar ducts*, completely lined with alveoli; and (3) *terminal alveolar sacs*, the final structures of the lung. The acinus, or *primary lobule* as it is occasionally called, is approximately 0.5 to 1.0 cm ($\frac{1}{5}$ to $\frac{2}{5}$ inch) in diameter. Approximately 23 generations of branching occur from the trachea to the terminal alveolar sac. The individual alveolus (in the grapelike cluster of alveolar sacs that make up the terminal sac) is separated from its neighbor by a thin wall, or *septum*. Small openings in the septum, called the *pores of Kohn*, allow communication or airflow between terminal alveolar sacs. The alveolus has only one layer of cells, which is less than the diameter of a red blood cell in thickness. Approximately 300 million alveoli are found in each lung, with a surface area about the size of a tennis court.

There are two types of alveolar lining cells: *type I pneumocytes*, which are spread out thinly and cover more than 90% of the surface area, and *type II pneumocytes*, which are responsible for the secretion of surfactant. Fig. 35-2 shows the microscopic structure of an alveolar duct and the surrounding alveoli, which are polygonal in shape. Because the alveolus is essentially a gas bubble surrounded by a capillary network, the liquid-gas interface creates a surface tension, which tends to resist expansion on inspiration and favors collapse on expiration. The alveoli, however, are lined with a lipoprotein substance called *surfactant*, which lessens the surface tension, low-

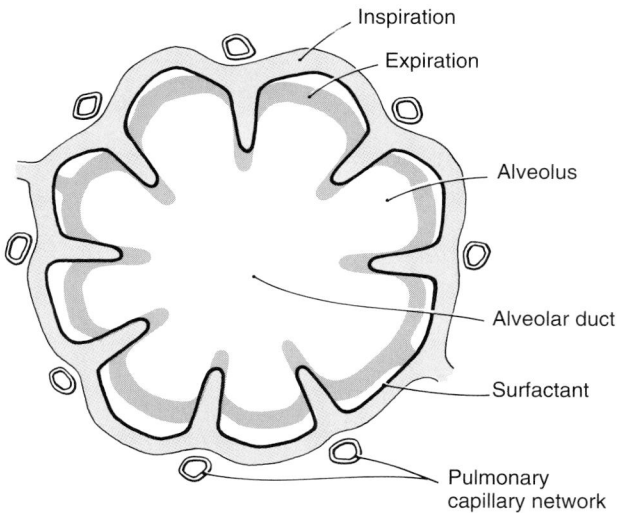

FIG. 35-2   Structural changes in the terminal alveolar sac (cross section) during the respiratory cycle. (Modified from Gluck L: Pulmonary surfactant and neonatal respiratory distress, *Hosp Pract* 6(11):45-56, 1971.)

ers the resistance to expansion on inspiration, and prevents collapse of the alveoli on expiration. The production and release of surfactant from the alveolar lining (type II) cells depend on several factors, including maturity of the alveolar cells and their biosynthetic enzyme systems, a normal surfactant turnover rate, adequate ventilation, and blood flow to the alveolar walls. Surfactant is formed relatively late in fetal life; therefore infants born with inadequate amounts (usually premature births) may develop infant respiratory distress syndrome. Surfactant is synthesized rapidly from fatty acids extracted from the blood, and its turnover rate is rapid; thus, if blood flow to an area of the lung is interrupted (e.g., by a pulmonary embolism), then the surfactant in that area may be depleted. The production of surfactant is stimulated by active ventilation, adequate tidal volumes, and periodic hyperventilation (sighing) and is inhibited by high concentrations of O_2 in the inspired air. Thus prolonged administration of high O_2 concentrations or failure to periodically deep-sigh a patient receiving mechanical ventilation will cause decreased surfactant production and subsequent alveolar collapse (atelectasis). A deficiency of surfactant is believed to be an important factor in the pathogenesis of a number of lung diseases, including acute (adult) respiratory distress syndrome (ARDS) (see Chapter 41).

Thoracic Cavity

The lungs are elastic, cone-shaped organs that lie within the thoracic cavity, or chest. The central *mediastinum*, which contains the heart and great vessels, separates the lungs (Fig. 35-3). Each lung has an apex (top of lung) and a base. Pulmonary and bronchial blood vessels, bronchi, nerves, and lymphatics enter each lung at the hilus to form the root of the lung. The *right lung* is larger, compared with the left lung, and is divided into three lobes by the interlobar fissures. The *left lung* is divided into two lobes.

Lobes are further divided into segments corresponding to the segmental bronchi. The right lung is divided into 10 segments and the left lung into 9 (see Fig. 35-3). Pathologic processes such as atelectasis and pneumonia are often localized to individual lobes and segments. Knowledge of the segmental anatomy of the lung is important not only for the radiologist, bronchoscopist, and thoracic surgeon but also for the nurse and respiratory therapist, who must know with accuracy the location of the lesion to apply their skills.

A continuous thin sheet of collagen and elastic tissue, known as the *pleura*, lines the thoracic cavity (*parietal pleura*) and encases each lung (*visceral pleura*). Between the parietal and visceral pleura is a thin film of pleural fluid that allows the two surfaces to glide over each other during respiration and prevents the separation of the thorax and lungs, as when two glass slides are stuck together with water; the slides can glide over each other, but they cannot easily be pulled apart.

The same is true of the pleural fluid between the lungs and thorax. Because no actual space separates the parietal and visceral pleurae, the so-called pleural spaces or cavities are potential spaces only. The pressure within the pleural space is less than that of the atmosphere and thus prevents the collapse of the lung. In disease, the pleura may become inflamed, or air or fluid may enter the pleural space, causing compression or collapse of the lung.

Three factors maintain this normal negative pressure. First, the *elastic tissue* of the lungs exerts a continuous force that tends to pull the lungs away from the thoracic cage; for example, the lungs tend to recoil to their smaller original size before the first expansion after birth. However, the visceral and parietal pleural surfaces in contact with each other cannot separate, thus the continuous force that tends to separate them persists. This force is popularly known as the *negative pressure* of the pleural space. Intrapleural pressures vary continuously throughout the respiratory cycle but are always negative.

The second major factor in maintaining negative intrapleural pressure is the *osmotic forces* exerted across the pleural membranes. Fluid normally moves from the capillaries in the parietal pleura into the pleural space and is then reabsorbed through the visceral pleura. The movement of the pleural fluid is believed to be governed by Starling's law of transcapillary exchange; that is, fluid movement depends on a net gradient between the hydrostatic pressure of the blood tending to push fluid out and the oncotic pressure of the plasma proteins tending to hold the fluid within. Because the net gradient for pleural fluid absorption through the visceral pleura is greater than is the net gradient for fluid formation by the parietal pleura, and because the surface area of the visceral pleura is greater than that of the parietal pleura, the pleural space normally contains only a few milliliters of fluid.

The third factor that supports a negative intrapleural pressure is the force of the *lymphatic pump.* A small amount of protein normally enters the pleural space but is removed by the lymphatics in the parietal pleura; the accumulation of protein in the intrapleural space would upset the normal osmotic balance without lymphatic removal.

These three factors therefore regulate and maintain the normal negative and intrapleural pressure. The *diaphragm*

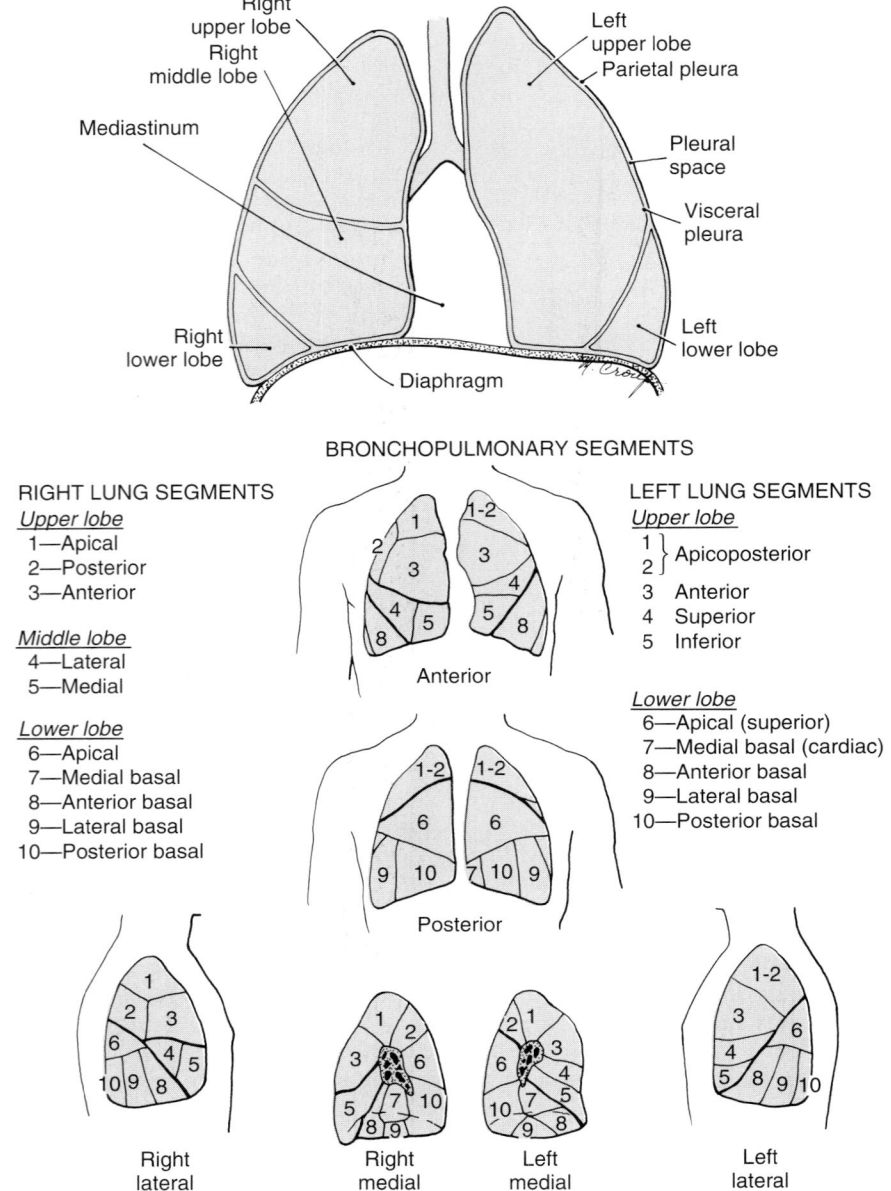

FIG. 35-3 Thoracic cavity and bronchopulmonary segments.

is a dome-shaped muscle that forms the floor of the thoracic cavity and separates it from the abdominal cavity.

Pulmonary Circulation

The blood supply to the lungs is unique in several respects. First, the lung has a dual blood supply from the bronchial and pulmonary arteries. The *bronchial circulation* provides oxygenated blood from the systemic circulation and serves to meet the metabolic needs of the lung tissue. The bronchial arteries arise from the thoracic aorta and travel along the posterior walls of the bronchi. The larger bronchial veins empty into the azygos system, which empties into the superior vena cava and returns blood to the right atrium. The smaller bronchial veins drain into the pulmonary veins. Because the bronchial

circulation does not take part in gas exchange, the unoxygenated blood accounts for a shunt, which is normally approximately 2% to 3% of cardiac output.

The *pulmonary artery* arising from the right ventricle provides mixed venous blood to the lungs, where the blood is involved in gas exchange. A vast network of *pulmonary capillaries* surrounds and envelops the alveoli, providing the intimate contact necessary for the exchange of gases between the alveoli and the blood. Oxygenated blood is then returned through the *pulmonary veins* to the left ventricle, which distributes it to the cells via the systemic circulation. Fig. 35-4 shows the functional position of the lungs in the pulmonary circulation.

Another feature of the pulmonary circulation is that it is a low-pressure, low-resistance system compared with the systemic circulation. Systemic blood pressure is ap-

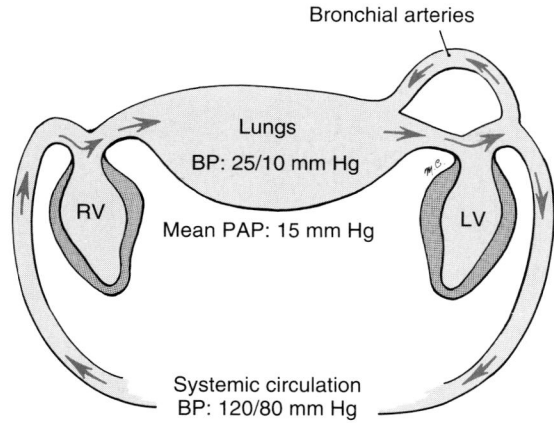

FIG. 35-4   Functional position of the lungs in the pulmonary circulation. *BP,* Blood pressure; *PAP,* pulmonary arterial pressure; *RV,* right ventricle; *LV,* left ventricle.

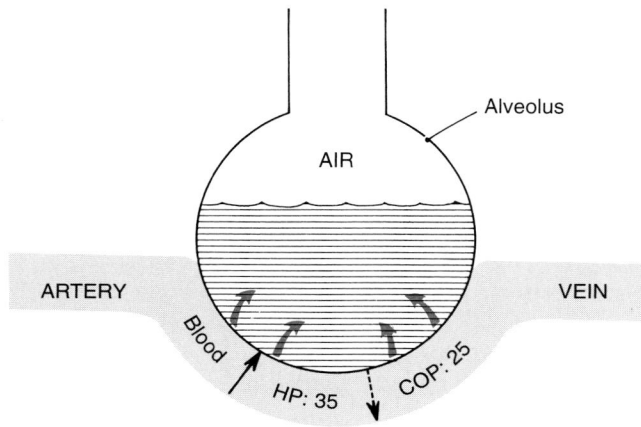

FIG. 35-5   Pathogenesis of pulmonary edema. *HP,* Hydrostatic pressure; *COP,* colloid osmotic pressure.

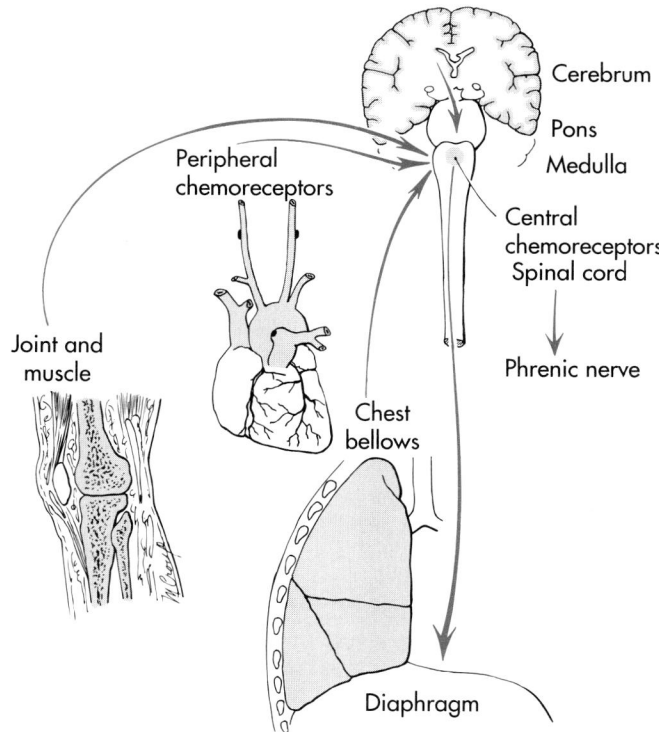

FIG. 35-6   Control of respiration.

Control of Respiration

A number of mechanisms contribute to bringing air into the lungs so that exchange of gases can occur. The mechanical function of moving air in and out of the lungs is termed *ventilation* and is accomplished by several interacting components. Of particular importance is a reciprocating pump called the *respiratory bellows.* This bellows has two volume-elastic components: the lung itself and the chest wall surrounding the lung. The chest wall consists of the skeleton and tissues of the thoracic cage, as well as the diaphragm, abdominal contents, and abdominal wall. The respiratory muscles, which are a part of the thoracic wall, provide the driving force for the operation of the bellows. The diaphragm (assisted by muscles that elevate the ribs and sternum) is the principal muscle involved in increasing the volume of the lung and thoracic cage during inspiration; expiration is a passive process during quiet breathing. The mechanics of ventilation are discussed in greater detail in Chapter 36.

The respiratory muscles are controlled by the *respiratory center,* which is composed of neurons and receptors located in the pons and medulla (Fig. 35-6). The respiratory center is the part of the nervous system that controls all aspects of breathing. The prime factor in the control of breathing is the response of the central chemoreceptors in the respiratory center to the partial pressure (or tension) of carbon dioxide ($Paco_2$) and the pH of the arterial blood. An increase in the $Paco_2$ or a decrease in the pH stimulates breathing.

A decrease of the partial pressure of oxygen in the arterial blood (Pao_2) can also stimulate ventilation. Peripheral chemoreceptors located in the carotid bodies at

proximately 120/80 mm Hg, whereas pulmonary blood pressure is approximately 25/10 mm Hg, with a mean pressure of approximately 15 mm Hg. These features of the pulmonary circulation have several important consequences. The great distensibility and low resistance of the pulmonary vascular beds allows the workload of the right ventricle to be much lighter than that of the left and allows a great increase in pulmonary blood flow during exercise without significantly increasing the pulmonary blood pressure.

As shown in Fig. 35-5, if the normal mean pulmonary hydrostatic pressure of approximately 15 mm Hg should exceed the colloid osmotic pressure of the blood of approximately 25 mm Hg, fluid would then leave the pulmonary capillaries and enter the interstitium or alveoli, causing pulmonary edema. *Pulmonary edema* interferes with gas exchange by increasing the length of the diffusion pathway between the alveolus and the capillary. Pulmonary edema is a common complication of congestive heart failure, pneumonia, and many other lung disorders.

the bifurcation of the common carotid arteries and in the aortic bodies at the aortic arch respond to decreases in Pao_2 and pH and increases in $Paco_2$. The Pao_2, however, must fall from the normal level of approximately 90 to 100 mm Hg to a level of approximately 60 mm Hg before ventilation is significantly stimulated.

Other mechanisms control the amount of air taken into the lungs. As the lung is inflated, these receptors signal the respiratory center to stop further inflation. Signals from the stretch receptors cease at the end of expiration when the lung is deflated and the respiratory center is free to initiate another inspiration. This mechanism, known as the *Hering-Breuer reflex*, was once thought to play a major role in the control of ventilation; however, more recent work shows that the reflex is largely inactive in an adult unless tidal volume exceeds 1 L, as in exercise. The reflex may be more important in newborn infants. Movements of joints and muscles (e.g., during exercise) also stimulate an increase in ventilation. Voluntary control input from the cerebrum can modify output from the respiratory centers, thus allowing interruption of the normal breathing cycle for laughing, crying, and speaking. The pattern and rhythmic control of breathing are exercised through the interaction of the respiratory centers located in the pons and medulla. Final motor output is transmitted via the spinal cord and phrenic nerve, which supplies the diaphragm, the principal muscle of ventilation. Other major nerves involved are the spinal accessory and thoracic intercostal nerves, which supply the accessory muscles of respiration and the intercostal muscles.

Neural Control of Airways

Smooth muscle is present from the trachea to the terminal bronchioles and is under the control of the autonomic nervous system. Bronchomotor tone depends on a balance between constriction and relaxation forces on the respiratory smooth muscle. *Parasympathetic (cholinergic) innervation* (via the vagus nerve) provides bronchoconstrictor tone to the airways. Parasympathetic stimulation causes bronchoconstriction and increased secretion by the mucous glands and goblet cells. *Sympathetic stimulation* by epinephrine occurs primarily via *beta$_2$-adrenergic receptors*, and causes relaxation of the bronchial smooth muscles, bronchodilation, and decreased bronchial secretions. Sympathetic innervation of the airways, however, is sparse. Recently, a third component of neural control has been described called the *noncholinergic, nonadrenergic inhibitory system* (Diamond, 1996). Stimulation of these nerve fibers located in the vagus nerve causes bronchodilation and the neurotransmitter is nitrous oxide. Airway receptors responsive to mechanical and chemical irritants provide sensory input via afferent vagal pathways and may cause bronchoconstriction, increased mucous secretion, and increased permeability of the blood vessels. An understanding of the neural control of the airways is important in understanding the pathophysiology of asthma and pharmacotherapy.

Defenses of the Respiratory Tract

The large surface area of the lung, which is separated only by a thin membrane from the circulatory system, makes a person theoretically vulnerable to invasion by foreign bodies (dust) and bacteria in the inhaled air; however, the lower respiratory tract is normally sterile. Several defense mechanisms maintain this sterility. The swallowing or gag reflex, which prevents entry of food or fluid into the trachea, and the action of the "mucociliary escalator," which traps dust and bacteria and transports them to the throat, have been mentioned. Furthermore, the mucous blanket contains factors that may be effective in defense, including immunoglobulins (Ig) (particularly IgA), polymorphonuclear leukocytes, and interferon. The cough reflex provides another, more forceful mechanism to expel secretions upward so that they may be swallowed or expectorated. The *alveolar macrophage* provides the final and most important defense against bacterial invasion of the lung. The alveolar macrophage, which is a phagocytic cell with unique migratory and enzymatic characteristics, moves freely over the alveolar surface and engulfs inert particulate matter and bacteria. After a microbial particle is engulfed, reactive O_2 metabolites, such as hydrogen peroxide within the macrophage, kill and digest the microorganism without producing any obvious inflammatory reaction. The dust particle or microorganism is then transported by the macrophage to the lymphatics or to the bronchioles, where it is removed by the mucociliary escalator. Alveolar macrophages can clear the lung of inhaled bacteria with amazing speed. Ethyl alcohol ingestion, cigarette smoking, and corticosteroid drugs interfere with this defense mechanism. Table 35-1 summarizes the defenses of the respiratory tract.

PHYSIOLOGIC CONSIDERATIONS

The physiologic process of respiration by which O_2 is transferred from the air to the tissues and CO_2 is excreted in the expired air may be divided into three main stages, as illustrated in Fig. 35-7. The first stage is *ventilation*, which is the flow of a mixture of gases into and out of the lungs. The second stage, *transportation*, must be considered from several aspects: (1) the diffusion of gases between the alveolus and pulmonary capillary (external respiration) and between the systemic blood and tissue cells, (2) the distribution of blood in the pulmonary circulation and its match with the distribution of air in the alveoli, and (3) the chemical and physical reactions of O_2 and CO_2 with the blood. Cell respiration, or internal respiration, is the final stage of respiration, during which substrates are oxidized to obtain energy and CO_2 is produced as a waste product of cell metabolism and excreted by the lungs.

Ventilation

Air moves in and out of the lungs because pressure gradients are created between the atmosphere and the alveoli by muscular mechanical means. As mentioned previously, the thoracic cage functions as a bellows. The changes in the intrapleural and intrapulmonary (airway) pressures and lung volumes during ventilation may be followed on the graph in Fig. 35-8. During inspiration, the volume of the thorax increases because of the descent of the diaphragm and the elevation of the ribs caused by the contraction of several muscles. The ster-

TABLE 35-1

Defenses of the Respiratory Tract

Respiratory Defense Mechanism	Effect
1. Air filtration	Nasal hairs filter particles >5 μm in size thus they do not reach the alveoli Air flow through the nasopharynx is very turbulent thus smaller particles (1-5 μm) tend to be deposited in nasopharyngeal secretions
2. Mucociliary clearance	Below the larynx, the mucociliary escalator entraps the smaller inhaled dust particles and bacteria that have bypassed the nose; the mucus is continuously swept toward the throat where it is expectorated or swallowed; mucus production = approximately 100 ml/day Ciliary motion is impaired by dehydration, high O_2 concentration, smoking, infections, anesthetics, and ethyl alcohol ingestion
3. Cough reflex	A protective reflex action that clears the airways by a high-pressure, high-velocity flow of air; it is a backup for mucociliary clearance when this mechanism is overwhelmed or ineffective; cough reflex ineffective below segmental level of tracheobronchial tree; mucociliary action or postural drainage necessary below this level
4. Swallowing and gag reflex	Prevents food or liquids from entering the respiratory tract
5. Reflex bronchoconstriction	Bronchoconstriction in response to the inhalation of large amounts of irritants, such as dusts or aerosols, to prevent their entry; some asthmatics have hypersensitive airways that constrict after inhaling cold air, perfumes, or other strong odors
6. Alveolar macrophages	Primary defense at the alveolar level (ciliated epithelium absent); phagocytize bacteria and fine dust particles; macrophage activity is impaired by smoke, viral infections, corticosteroids, and a number of chronic diseases
7. Collateral ventilation	Via pores of Kohn promoted by deep breathing; prevents atelectasis

nocleidomastoid muscles lift upward on the sternum, whereas the serratus, scalene, and external intercostal muscles all are involved in elevation of the ribs. The thorax enlarges in three directions: anteroposteriorly, laterally, and vertically. This increase in volume causes the intrapleural pressure to decrease from approximately –4 mm Hg (relative to atmospheric pressure) to approximately –8 mm Hg as the lungs are pulled to a more expanded position during inspiration. At the same time, intrapulmonary or airway pressure decreases to approximately –2 mm Hg (relative to atmospheric pressure) from 0 mm Hg at the beginning of inspiration. The pressure gradient between the airways and the atmosphere causes air to flow into the lungs until airway pressure at the end of inspiration is again equal to atmospheric pressure.

During quiet breathing, expiration is a passive movement produced by the elastic recoil of the chest wall and lungs. As the external intercostal muscles relax, the rib cage is lowered and the dome of the diaphragm ascends into the thoracic cavity, causing the volume of the thorax to decrease. The internal intercostal muscles may forcefully pull the ribs downward and inward during active forceful expiration, coughing, defecating, or vomiting. Additionally, the abdominal muscles may contract, increasing the intraabdominal pressure and pushing the diaphragm upward. This decrease in volume of the thorax causes both intrapleural and intrapulmonary pressures to increase. The intrapulmonary pressure now rises to approximately 1 or 2 mm Hg above that of the atmosphere. The pressure gradient between the airways and the atmosphere is now reversed, causing gas to flow out of the lungs until airway and atmospheric pressure are again equal at the end of expiration. Intrapleural pressure is always below atmospheric pressure during the respiratory cycle. Alterations in ventilation are assessed by pulmonary function tests. The alterations, their significance,

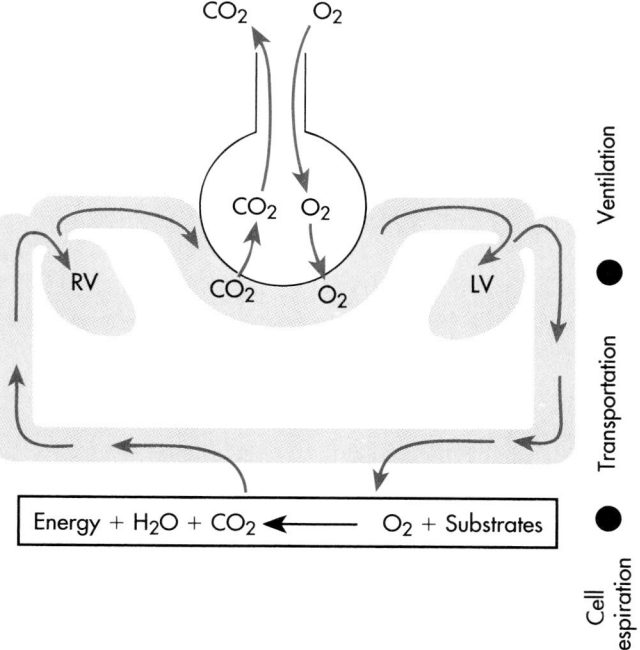

FIG. 35-7 Principal stages of the respiratory process. *RV,* Right ventricle; *LV,* left ventricle.

and additional complexities of mechanical ventilation are discussed in Chapter 36.

Transportation
Diffusion

The second stage in the respiratory process involves the diffusion of gases across the thin (less than 0.5 μm thick)

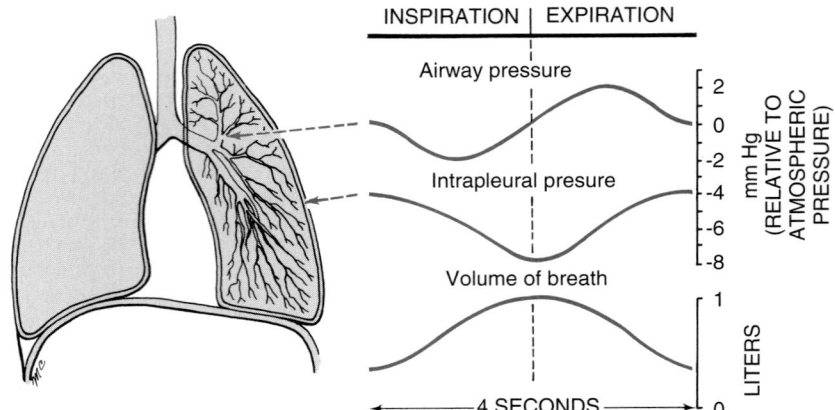

FIG. 35-8 Changes in intrapleural and intrapulmonary (airway) pressures during inspiration and expiration.

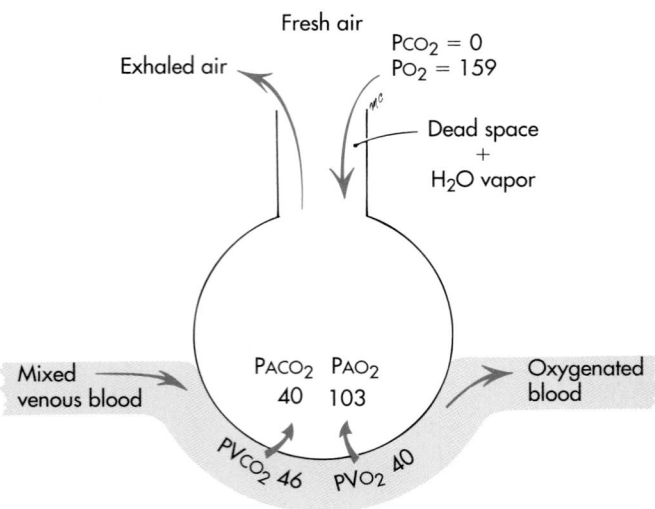

FIG. 35-9 Diffusion of gases across the alveolocapillary membrane. P_{CO_2}, P_{O_2}, Partial pressure of carbon dioxide, oxygen; P_{ACO_2}, P_{AO_2}, alveolar P_{CO_2}, P_{O_2}; P_{VCO_2}, P_{VO_2}, mixed venous P_{CO_2}, P_{O_2}.

alveolocapillary membrane interface. The driving force for this transfer is the partial pressure gradients between the blood and gas phases. The partial pressure of oxygen (P_{O_2}) in dry atmosphere at sea level is approximately 159 mm Hg (21% of 760 mm Hg). However, by the time it reaches the trachea, the P_{O_2} is reduced to 149 mm Hg because of being warmed and moisturized by the airways (760 − 47 × 0.21 = 149). The partial pressure of water vapor at body temperature is 47 mm Hg. The partial pressure of the inspired O_2 is further reduced to approximately 103 mm Hg by the time it reaches the alveoli because of being mixed with old anatomic dead space air from the conducting airways. The anatomic dead space normally holds a volume of approximately 1 ml of air per pound of ideal body weight (e.g., 150 ml per 150-pound man). Only the fresh air that reaches the alveolus is effective ventilation. As shown in Fig. 35-9, the partial pressure of oxygen in the mixed venous blood (P_{VO_2}) in the pulmonary capillary is approximately 40 mm Hg. Because the P_{O_2} in the capillary is less than that in the alveolus (P_{AO_2} = 103 mm Hg), O_2 diffuses readily into the

bloodstream. A much smaller pressure gradient (6 mm Hg) between the blood and P_{ACO_2} causes CO_2 to diffuse into the alveolus. The CO_2 is then expired into the atmosphere, where its concentration is essentially zero. The CO_2 gradient between blood and alveolus, even though small, is adequate, because it diffuses approximately 20 times more readily than does O_2 across the alveolocapillary membrane because of its greater solubility in lipid.

Under normal resting conditions, diffusion and equilibration occur between O_2 in the pulmonary capillary blood and alveolus in approximately 0.25 second of the total contact time of 0.75 second, suggesting that the normal lung has much diffusion time in reserve. In some diseases (e.g., pulmonary fibrosis), the blood-gas barrier may be thickened and diffusion slowed to the extent that equilibrium may be incomplete, particularly during exercise, when total contact time is reduced. Thus diffusion block may contribute to hypoxemia, but it is not believed to be a major factor. CO_2 elimination is thought to be unaffected by diffusion abnormalities.

Ventilation-Perfusion Relationships

The effective transfer of gas between the alveolus and pulmonary capillary bed requires an even distribution of air in the lungs and perfusion (blood flow) in the capillaries. In other words, the ventilation and perfusion of a pulmonary unit must be evenly matched. In the normal upright person at rest, ventilation and perfusion are nearly evenly matched except at the apex of the lung. The low-pressure, low-resistance pulmonary circulation results in a greater flow of blood at the base of the lung than it does at the apex as a result of the influence of gravity. Ventilation, however, is fairly evenly distributed. The mean value for the ratio of ventilation to perfusion ($\dot{V}/\dot{Q}$) is 0.8. This figure is obtained by taking the ratio of the normal rate of alveolar ventilation (4 L/min) and dividing it by the normal cardiac output (5 L/min). Fig. 35-10 illustrates the normal state of evenly matched ventilation and perfusion in the lung, which is near unity, at 0.8.

Ventilation-perfusion inequalities occur in most respiratory diseases. Fig. 35-11 illustrates three theoretic abnormal respiratory units. Fig. 35-11, *A*, depicts a *dead-space unit* in which normal ventilation occurs without perfusion, causing ventilation to be wasted ($\dot{V}/\dot{Q}$ = infinity). The second abnormal respiratory unit (see Fig. 35-11, *B*) is a *shunt*

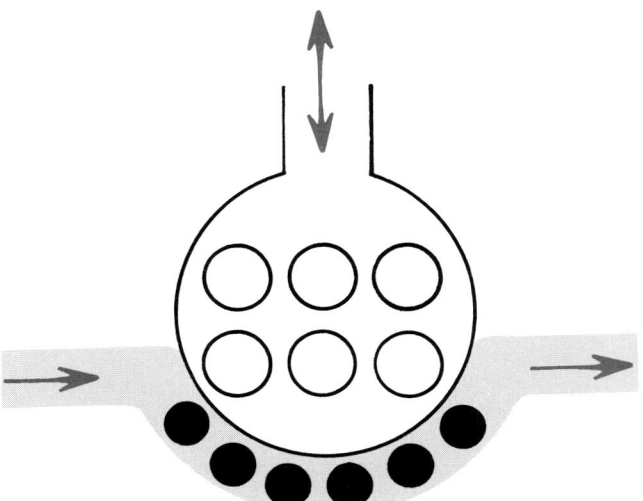

FIG. 35-10 Even match of ventilation and perfusion in an ideal respiratory unit (normal $\dot{V}/\dot{Q} = 0.8$).

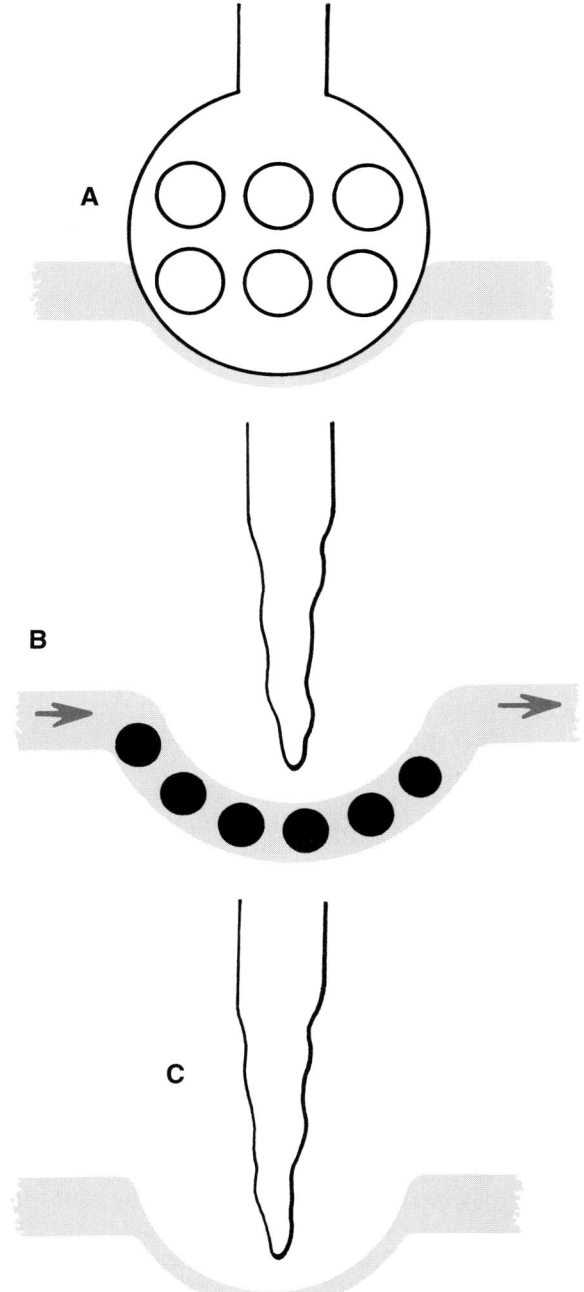

FIG. 35-11 Three theoretic respiratory units. **A,** Dead-space unit: normal ventilation but no perfusion. **B,** Shunt unit: normal perfusion but no ventilation. **C,** Silent unit: no ventilation and no perfusion.

unit in which normal perfusion occurs without ventilation, thus perfusion is wasted ($\dot{V}/\dot{Q} = 0$). The last unit (see Fig. 35-11, *C*) is a *silent unit* in which neither ventilation nor perfusion occurs. Variations occur between the three extremes depending on the overall balance between ventilation and perfusion in the lungs. Lung diseases and functional respiratory disorders may be classified physiologically according to whether they are largely shunt-producing ($\dot{V}/\dot{Q}$ less than 0.8) or dead-space–producing ($\dot{V}/\dot{Q}$ greater than 0.8) diseases.

O₂ Transport in the Blood

O_2 can be transported from the lungs to the tissues via two routes: physically dissolved in the plasma or chemically combined with hemoglobin (Hb) as *oxyhemoglobin* (HbO_2). The chemical combination of O_2 with Hb is reversible, and the actual amount carried in this form is related in a nonlinear fashion to the partial pressure of oxygen in the arterial blood (Pa_{O_2}), which is determined by the amount of O_2 physically dissolved in the blood plasma. In turn, the amount of O_2 physically dissolved in the plasma is directly related to the partial pressure of oxygen in the alveolus (PA_{O_2}). The amount of O_2 also depends on the solubility of O_2 in plasma. The amount of physically dissolved O_2 is normally very small because of its low solubility in plasma. Only approximately 1% of the total O_2 transported to the tissues is transported in this manner. This method of transport is insufficient to support life even at rest. The greatest bulk of O_2 is carried by Hb, which is located inside the red blood cells. Under certain circumstances (e.g., carbon monoxide poisoning, massive hemolysis with insufficient Hb), sufficient O_2 to support life may be transported in physical solution by subjecting the patient to O_2 under greater than atmospheric pressure *(hyperbaric oxygen chamber)*.

Fig. 35-12 illustrates the relationships involved in HbO_2 transportation. A gram of Hb can combine with 1.34 ml O_2. Because the average Hb concentration in the blood for the adult male is approximately 15 g/dl, 1 dl of blood can carry 20.1 (15×1.34) ml of O_2 when O_2 saturation (Sa_{O_2}) is 100%. However, a small amount of mixed venous blood from the bronchial circulation is added to the oxygenated blood leaving the pulmonary capillaries (see Fig. 35-9). This dilution accounts for only approximately 97% of the blood leaving the lungs being saturated and 19.5 (0.97×20.1) volume percent being carried to the tissues.

At the tissue level, O_2 dissociates from Hb into the plasma and diffuses from the plasma into the tissue cells to supply tissue needs. Although tissue needs are highly

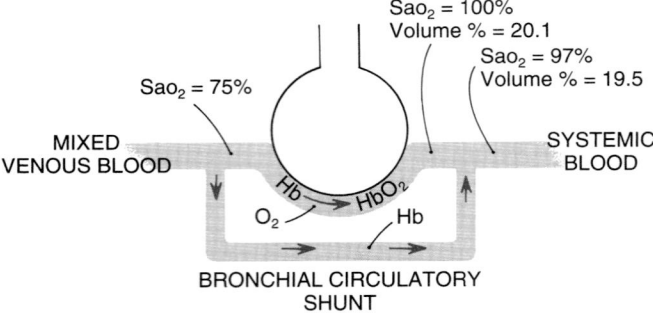

FIG. 35-12 Oxyhemoglobin *(HbO₂)* transportation. *Sao₂,* Oxygen-saturation; *Hb,* hemoglobin.

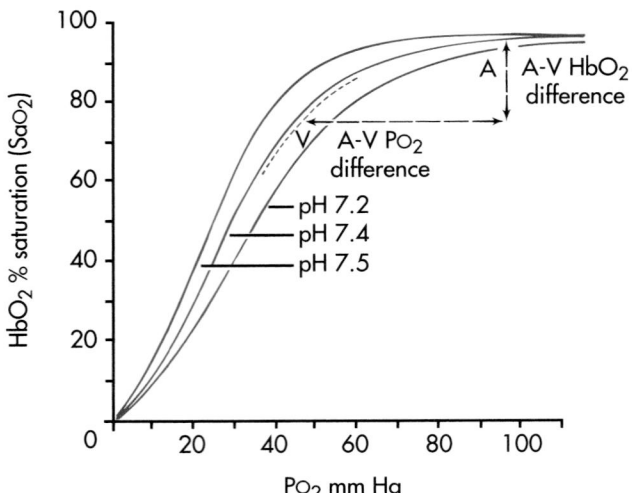

FIG. 35-13 Oxyhemoglobin *(HbO₂)* dissociation curve. *A,* Arterial; *V,* venous.

variable, approximately 75% of Hb is still normally combined with O_2 when it returns to the lungs as mixed venous blood. Thus only approximately 25% of the O_2 in the arterial blood is used to supply the tissues. Hb that has dissociated from O_2 at the tissue level is called *reduced Hb*. Reduced Hb is purple in color and accounts for the bluish color of venous blood, which is observed in the superficial veins, as in the hands, whereas HbO_2 is bright red in color and accounts for the color of arterial blood.

Oxyhemoglobin Dissociation Curve

A clear understanding of O_2 carrying capacity requires an understanding of the affinity of hemoglobin for O_2, because tissue O_2 supply and pulmonary O_2 uptake critically depend on this relationship. This knowledge is necessary to interpret blood gas measurements correctly and to apply therapeutic measures for respiratory insufficiency. If whole blood is exposed to different partial pressures of O_2 and the percentage of saturation of Hb is measured, an S-shaped curve is then obtained when these two measurements are plotted. This curve is known as the *oxyhemoglobin dissociation curve* and demonstrates the affinity of Hb for O_2 at various partial pressures. In Fig. 35-13, the middle curve represents the affinity relation between O_2 and Hb under normal conditions of body temperature (98.6° F) and a blood pH of 7.4.

TABLE 35-2 ■ ■ ■

Factors Affecting Oxyhemoglobin (HbO₂) Affinity

HbO₂ Dissociation Curve	
Shift to Left (Decreased P₅₀)	**Shift to Right (Increased P₅₀)**
1 ↑ pH	1 ↓ pH
2 ↓ Pco₂	2 ↑ Pco₂
3 ↓ Temperature	3 ↑ Temperature
4 ↓ 2,3-DPG	4 ↑ 2,3-DPG

P₅₀, Oxygen tension required to produce 50% saturation; *Pco₂,* carbon dioxide partial pressure; *2,3-DPG,* 2-3-diphosphoglycerate.

One fact of great physiologic importance to be noted about the curve is the presence of the flat upper portion, known as the *arterial portion* (A), and a lower, steeper *venous portion* (V), which is shifted slightly to the right. At the flat upper portion of the curve, large changes in Po_2 are associated with small changes in HbO_2 saturation. This factor implies that relatively constant quantities of O_2 can be supplied to the tissues even at high altitudes, where the Po_2 may be 60 mm Hg or less. Also implied is that the administration of O_2 in high concentrations (normal air = 21%) to patients with mild hypoxemia (Pao_2 = 60 to 75 mm Hg) is wasted because HbO_2 can be increased by only a small amount. In fact, the administration of high O_2 concentrations may be toxic to the lung tissues and may produce other harmful effects. The release of O_2 to the tissues is augmented by the relation of the Po_2 to Sao_2 on the steep venous portion of the curve, where large changes in HbO_2 saturation are associated with small changes in the Po_2. The arrows shown in Fig. 35-13 indicate the normal differences in HbO_2 saturation and Po_2 between arterial and mixed venous blood.

The affinity of Hb for O_2 is influenced by many other factors that accompany tissue metabolism and that may be modified by disease. Table 35-2 lists some of these factors and their effect on the affinity of Hb for O_2.

The HbO_2 curve is shifted to the right (see Fig. 35-13) in cases of a decrease in blood pH or a rise in the Pco_2. In this state, Hb has less affinity for O_2 at a given Po_2, thus less O_2 can be transported in the blood. Pathologic conditions that cause metabolic *acidosis*, such as shock (production of excess lactic acid from anaerobic metabolism) or the retention of CO_2 (as in many pulmonary diseases), cause a shift of the curve to the right. A slight shift of the curve to the right, represented by the venous portion of the normal curve (pH 7.38), assists the release of O_2 to the tissues. This shift is called the *Bohr effect*. The slight increase in acidity results from the effect of CO_2 being released from the tissues. Other factors that cause a shift of the curve to the right are an increase in temperature and increased 2,3-diphosphoglycerate (2,3-DPG), which is an organic phosphate in red blood cells that binds Hb and decreases its affinity for O_2. Red blood cell 2,3-DPG is increased in conditions of anemia and chronic hypoxemia. It is important to appreciate that although the O_2-carrying capability of Hb is decreased with a rightward shift of the curve, Hb release of O_2 to the tissues is facilitated. Therefore, in conditions of anemia and chronic hypoxemia, the rightward shift of the curve is compensatory. A rightward shift of the curve with a rise in temperature, reflecting increased cell metabolism and a greater need for O_2, is also adaptive and causes more O_2 to be released to the tissues for a given blood flow.

Conversely, an increase in blood pH *(alkalosis)* or a decrease in Pco_2, temperature, and 2,3-DPG causes a leftward shift in the HbO_2 dissociation curve (see Fig. 35-13). The shift to the left causes Hb to have a greater affinity for O_2. Thus increased O_2 uptake occurs in the lung with a leftward shift, but release of O_2 to the tissues is impaired. Therefore having hypoxia (insufficient tissue O_2 to meet metabolic needs) in severe conditions of alkalosis is theoretically possible, particularly if accompanied by hypoxemia. This condition might occur during mechanical overventilation with a respirator or at high altitudes as a result of hyperventilation. Because hyperventilation is also known to decrease cerebral blood flow as a result of the decrease in the $Paco_2$, cerebral ischemia might also account for symptoms of light-headedness common under such conditions. Stored blood loses 2,3-DPG activity and causes a greater affinity of Hb for O_2. Therefore patients who receive transfusions of massive amounts of stored blood may also have impaired O_2 release to the tissues because of the leftward shift in the HbO_2 dissociation curve.

The affinity of Hb is popularly defined by the Po_2 required to produce 50% saturation (P_{50}) and is readily measured in modern laboratories. Normally, P_{50} is approximately 27 mm Hg. It is evident that P_{50} will be increased with the shift of the dissociation curve to the right (decreased Hb affinity for O_2) and reduced with a shift of the curve to the left (increased Hb affinity for O_2).

Hb has an affinity for carbon monoxide (CO) that is approximately 250 times greater than that for O_2. When carbon monoxide is inhaled, it combines with Hb to form carboxyhemoglobin. When O_2 combines with carboxyhemoglobin, the reaction is irreversible, thus the amount of Hb available for O_2 transport is reduced. Additionally, a leftward shift of the remaining normal Hb occurs, resulting in deficient unloading of O_2 to the tissues.

CO_2 Transport in the Blood

CO_2 homeostasis is also a necessary aspect of respiratory sufficiency. The transportation of CO_2 from the tissues to the lungs for elimination is accomplished in three ways. Approximately 10% of the CO_2 is physically dissolved in plasma because CO_2, unlike O_2, is highly soluble in plasma. Approximately 20% of the CO_2 is combined with the amino groups on Hb (carbaminohemoglobin) in the red blood cell, and approximately 70% is transported as plasma bicarbonate (HCO_3^-). CO_2 combines with water as shown in the following reaction:

$$CO_2 + H_2O \rightleftharpoons H_2CO_3 \rightleftharpoons H^+ + HCO_3^-$$

This reaction is reversible and is known as the *bicarbonate–carbonic acid buffer equation*. The acid-base balance of the body is greatly affected by pulmonary function and CO_2 homeostasis. Generally, *hyperventilation* (alveolar ventilation in excess of metabolic needs) causes alkalosis (increases in blood pH above the normal 7.4) as a result of the excess excretion of CO_2 from the lungs; *hypoventilation* (alveolar ventilation insufficient to meet metabolic needs) causes acidosis (decrease of the blood pH below the normal 7.4) as a result of the retention of CO_2 by the lungs. The relationship is evident from examining the buffer equation that lowering the Pco_2, as in hyperventi-

lation, causes the reaction to proceed to the left, with consequent lowering of the H^+ concentration (elevated pH), and that raising the Pco_2 causes the reaction to proceed to the right, producing an increase in H^+ (decreased pH). Hypoventilation occurs in many conditions that affect the respiratory bellows. CO_2 retention is also associated with emphysema and chronic bronchitis caused by trapped air in the lungs.

Just as the amount of O_2 transported in the blood is related to the Po_2 to which the blood is exposed, thus the amount of CO_2 in the blood is related to the Pco_2. Unlike the S-shaped HbO_2 dissociation curve, the CO_2 dissociation curve is nearly linear in the physiologic range of Pco_2. (See Fig. 41-1, which compares the CO_2 and HbO_2 dissociation curves.) This relationship means that the CO_2 content of the blood is directly related to the Pco_2. Additionally, no significant barrier to CO_2 diffusion ever exists. Therefore the $Paco_2$ provides a good index of the adequacy of ventilation.

ASSESSMENT OF RESPIRATORY STATUS

An important point to stress is that knowledge of the blood gases (Po_2, Pco_2, and pH of arterial blood) alone does not provide sufficient information about the transport of O_2 and CO_2 to be sure that a patient's tissues are being oxygenated properly. Many other factors are involved in the transport process, such as the adequacy of cardiac output and tissue perfusion, as well as diffusion of gases at the tissue level. For example, in shock, tissue perfusion may be inadequate as a result of shunting of blood past the tissue cells, stagnation of blood caused by pooling, and inadequate cardiac output. Tissue edema may also interfere with the diffusion pathway at the tissue level. Consequently, the detection of tissue hypoxia must always involve clinical observations and the interpretation of blood gases.

Other important information needed for the assessment of a patient's respiratory status is the Hb concentration, as well as the percentage of saturation of Hb. The correlation among Pao_2, Sao_2, and HbO_2 in volume percentage for a patient with anemia (Hb = 10 g/dl), one with a normal Hb of 15 g/dl, and another with polycythemia (Hb = 20 g/dl) is shown in Fig. 35-14. All the information illustrated is necessary for a proper assessment of O_2 transport. Note that the percent saturation of Hb is independent of the Hb concentration, whereas the O_2 content in volume percent is directly related to Hb concentration. The volume percent reveals how much O_2 can be delivered to the tissues at a given Pao_2. For example, at a Pao_2 of 100 mm Hg and 100% saturation of Hb with O_2, the patient with polycythemia can transport 26.8 ml of O_2 in every 100 ml blood (O_2 content = 26.8 vol %), whereas the anemic patient can deliver only 13.4 ml at the same Pao_2 and Sao_2. This is a two-fold variation and illustrates that knowledge of the blood gases alone is insufficient information for respiratory assessment. Hb concentration, Sao_2, and cardiac status are also vital data.

It is evident from the previous discussion of the structure and function of the respiratory system that adequate respiration can be inhibited on a number of levels. For

FIG. 35-14 Relationship of hemoglobin *(Hb)* content (g/dl) to oxygen content of blood at various arterial oxygen tensions *(Pao₂)*. (From Slonim NB, Hamilton LH: *Respiratory physiology,* ed 3, St Louis, 1976, Mosby.)

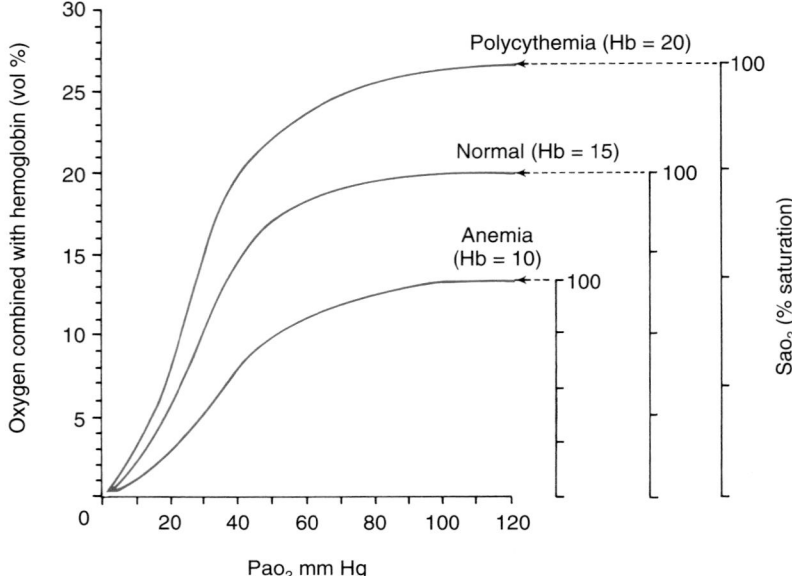

example, brain injury or barbiturate overdose in an attempted suicide may interfere with control by the respiratory centers in the central nervous system. A decrease in the P_{O_2} of inspired air as a result of high altitudes or airway obstruction interferes with respiration. Neuromuscular diseases and skeletal deformities of the chest result in inadequate bellows performance. Respiratory difficulty occurs at the alveolocapillary interface when thickening of the diffusion pathway occurs, as in pulmonary fibrosis or edema. Transport of gases in the blood may be interfered with in many respects, including the limiting factor of the amount of Hb. The pulmonary, cardiovascular, and hematologic systems are thus intimately associated with tissue oxygenation.

KEY CONCEPTS

- The term *respiration* refers to the movement of O_2 from the atmosphere to the cells and the return of CO_2; *external respiration* refers to the diffusion of gases across the alveolocapillary membrane, and *internal respiration* refers to the intracellular use of O_2 and production of CO_2.
- *Pulmonary ventilation* refers to the movement of air into and out of the air passages.
- The major function of the upper airways (nose, pharynx, and larynx) is to filter, warm, and humidify the air before it reaches the respiratory gas exchange zone of the lung.
- The *glottis* (triangular-shaped opening into the trachea between the vocal cords of the larynx) forms the division between the upper and lower respiratory tract; it is the critical barrier preventing aspiration (not the epiglottis). The respiratory tract below the glottis is sterile.
- The *conducting airways* (where no gas exchange takes place) include the trachea, bronchi, and bronchioles all the way down to the level of the terminal bronchioles.
- The right and left main stem bronchi are not symmetrical. The *right main stem bronchus* is shorter and larger in diameter and has a more vertical course compared with the *left main stem bronchus,* which is longer and smaller in diameter and has a more angular course because of the location of the heart. Some clin-

ical implications are: (1) aspirated foreign bodies are more apt to enter the right bronchial tree, and (2) the nurse must ensure that an endotracheal tube is secured from slipping down into the right main stem bronchus and causing collapse of the left lung.
- The mucosa of the large airways consists of pseudostratified, ciliated columnar epithelial cells. A layer of mucus produced by mucous glands and goblet cells covers the mucosa. The cilia beat rhythmically propelling inhaled dust particles or bacteria entrapped in the mucus toward the throat, where they are swallowed or expectorated. The defensive function of this *mucociliary escalator* is impaired by dehydration, infection, high O_2 concentration, anesthetics, tobacco smoke, and alcohol.
- *Airway structure* changes considerably in the distal progression through the tracheobronchial tree: cartilaginous structure is prominent in the upper airways but disappears at the level of the bronchioles; smooth muscle and elastic tissue occupy a greater proportion of wall thickness as the airways become smaller in size until it is maximal at the level of the terminal bronchioles.
- The *acinus* is the functional gas exchange unit of the lung and includes structures distal to the terminal bronchioles: respiratory bronchioles, alveolar ducts, and alveoli.

- Gas exchange takes place in the alveoli, which are surrounded by pulmonary capillaries. Approximately 300 million alveoli are found in the lungs, with a surface area equal to the size of a tennis court.
- Two types of epithelial cells line the alveoli: (1) *type I pneumocytes* cover more than 90% of the surface and are thin, allowing the passage of gases from alveoli into the blood; (2) *type II pneumocytes* produce a lipoprotein substance called *surfactant*, which coats the alveoli with a thin film. Surfactant acts like a detergent to reduce the surface tension of the alveoli, lowering resistance to expansion on inspiration, and preventing alveolar collapse on expiration. Surfactant is a major contributing factor in total lung compliance (elasticity) and its deficiency is important in the pathogenesis of a number of lung diseases (e.g., ARDS)
- The *pores of Kohn* are small openings in the alveolar septum that allow collateral ventilation between the alveoli, thus reducing the incidence of atelectasis.
- The *right lung is divided into three lobes* by fissures and 10 segments corresponding to the segmental bronchi; the *left lung is divided into two lobes* and nine segments.
- The pleura is a closed, double-walled membrane lining the thoracic cavity. The *parietal pleura* lines the chest cavity and the *visceral pleura* encases each lung. The pleural cavity is a potential space between the parietal and visceral pleura that is filled with a few milliliters of pleural fluid, which provides lubrication, allowing the layers of pleura to slide past each other during breathing. The accumulation of excess fluid within the pleural space is called *pleural effusion.*
- The pressure within the pleural space is always negative (less than atmospheric pressure). An important factor maintaining the negative intrapleural pressure is the elastic recoil of the lung from the thoracic cage while, at the same time, the visceral and parietal pleural cannot be pulled apart because of the thin layer of fluid holding them together (similar to two glass slides that cannot be pulled apart when wetted).
- The lungs have two different types of circulation: (1) the *bronchial circulation* meets the metabolic needs of the lung parenchyma, resulting in a small physiologic shunt, because a small amount of deoxygenated blood is mixed with the oxygenated blood leaving the lungs (called venous admixture); and (2) the *pulmonary circulation* is the lung circulation that takes part in gas exchange.
- The *pulmonary circulation* is a low-pressure, low-resistance circulation compared with the systemic circulation (mean pulmonary artery pressure = 15 mm Hg; mean arterial pressure = 90 mm Hg). Consequently, pulmonary blood flow can increase many times during exercise without an increase in pressure, and the workload of the right ventricle is much less than that of the left ventricle.
- The most important muscle of inspiration is the *diaphragm,* which descends during contraction, increasing the volume of the thoracic cavity. *Inspiration* is assisted by the external intercostal and parasternal muscles, which raise the rib cage upward and forward, increasing both the anteroposterior and lateral diam-

eters of the thorax. *Expiration* is passive during quiet breathing: the diaphragm muscle relaxes and the lung and chest wall recoil to their equilibrium positions. The diaphragm is innervated by the phrenic nerve coming from C3 through C5, and the intercostals are innervated by spinal nerves between T1 and T11. With spinal cord injuries at the C6 and C7 level, the function of the intercostals is lost, but the diaphragm is intact, thus these patients can breathe without the use of a ventilator. A C3 through C5 spinal cord injury causes partial or complete paralysis of the diaphragm, thus these patients may be dependent on a ventilator.
- The *respiratory center* is located in the pons and medulla and controls the rhythmic aspects of breathing modified by voluntary input from the cerebrum.
- Parasympathetic (cholinergic) stimulation of the airways cause bronchoconstriction and increased mucus secretion; sympathetic stimulation of the beta$_2$-adrenergic receptors causes bronchodilation and decreased mucus secretion. Stimulation of the noncholinergic, nonadrenergic inhibitory system also causes bronchodilation.
- The *chemical control of respiration* is effected by peripheral and central chemoreceptors that respond to changes in the Paco$_2$, pH, and Pao$_2$ and influence the respiratory center to maintain the blood gas parameters within the acceptable physiologic range. A rise in the Paco$_2$ (or a fall in the pH) is the prime factor stimulating breathing. The Pao$_2$ must fall below 60 mm Hg to stimulate breathing significantly.
- Defenses of the respiratory tract include: (1) air filtration by the nose, (2) cough reflex, (3) swallowing or gag reflex, (4) mucociliary escalator action, (5) reflex bronchoconstriction, (6) alveolar macrophages and IgA, and (7) collateral ventilation by pores of Kohn.
- *Ventilation,* or the movement of air in and out of the lungs, takes place because of pressure gradients created between the atmosphere and alveoli resulting from the bellows action of the chest cage powered by the respiratory muscles. Intrapleural pressure becomes more negative during inspiration and less negative during expiration. Air moves into the lungs during inspiration when alveolar pressure is less than atmospheric pressure and air moves out of the lungs during expiration when alveolar pressure is greater than atmospheric pressure.
- The driving force for *diffusion of gases* across the alveolocapillary membrane consists of partial pressure gradients between the blood and alveolar spaces. The partial pressure gradient for O$_2$ diffusion is relatively large: alveolar O$_2$ is approximately 100 mm Hg and approximately 40 mm Hg in the mixed venous pulmonary capillary blood. CO$_2$ diffusion from the blood to the alveolus requires a much smaller partial pressure gradient than O$_2$ because it is more soluble in lipid.
- Normally, equilibration of O$_2$ and CO$_2$ between the alveoli and the pulmonary capillary blood is complete within 0.25 seconds of the total contact time of 0.75 second. Because of this large reserve time, diffusion block is not believed to be a major factor in the causation of hypoxemia or hypercapnia.

- Ideally, optimal efficiency of gas exchanges would be provided by an even distribution of ventilation and perfusion so that ventilation and perfusion are always matched, but this is not the case, even in healthy individuals. The normal overall $\dot{V}/\dot{Q}$ is 0.8 (4 L/min ÷ 5 L/min). Because of the effects of gravity on pulmonary blood flow, $\dot{V}/\dot{Q}$ is greater than 0.8 at the apex of the lung (higher $\dot{V}$ and lower $\dot{Q}$) and $\dot{V}/\dot{Q}$ is lower than 0.8 at the base of the lung (higher $\dot{Q}$ and lower $\dot{V}$).
- $\dot{V}/\dot{Q}$ inequalities that cause hypoxemia occur in most respiratory diseases. There are three theoretical types of respiratory units: (1) *Dead-space units* ($\dot{V}/\dot{Q}$ >0.8), normal ventilation with little or no perfusion as in pulmonary embolism causing wasted ventilation; (2) *shunt units* ($\dot{V}/\dot{Q}$ <0.8), normal perfusion with little or no ventilation as in pulmonary edema or pneumonia causing wasted perfusion; and (3) silent units with no ventilation or perfusion. Clinically, $\dot{V}/\dot{Q}$ ratios can fall anywhere along the continuum between the extremes of a dead space unit and a shunt unit, and both may exist in the same lung.
- Because arterial blood gas (ABG) measurements reflect the physiologic status of the cardiopulmonary system, cardiopulmonary pathophysiology allows classification into two major categories: *dead-space–producing respiratory diseases* and *shunt-producing respiratory diseases*.
- Nearly all of the O_2 transported to the tissue in blood is bound to hemoglobin, and only a small fraction is dissolved in the plasma (because O_2 is not very soluble in plasma).
- The *HbO_2 dissociation curve* is S-shaped and expresses the amount of O_2 bound to hemoglobin in relation to the driving pressure of O_2, the Po_2. *Hemoglobin* is 90% saturated with O_2 at a Pao_2 of 60 mm Hg (where the curve flattens); thus only a relatively small amount of additional O_2 is transported at a Pao_2 above this level.
- The HbO_2 curve is shifted to the right by decreased pH, increased $Paco_2$ (acidosis), increased temperature or increased 2,3-DPG; it is shifted to the left by increased pH, decreased $Paco_2$ (alkalosis), decreased temperature, or decreased 2,3-DPG.
- Because the *CO_2 dissociation curve* (showing the relationship of the $Paco_2$ to CO_2 content in the blood), is nearly *linear in the physiologic range*, adequacy of ventilation may be assessed simply by examining the $Paco_2$ levels. $Paco_2$ levels greater than 45 mm Hg mean hypoventilation; $Paco_2$ levels less than 35 mm Hg mean hyperventilation.
- The assessment of the adequacy of tissue oxygenation, however, requires the assessment of the Pao_2 and Sao_2, as well as many other body systems involved in the delivery of O_2 from the environment to the tissues, such as optimal atmospheric conditions, intact nervous system control, intact thoracic cage (respiratory bellows), lung compliance (elasticity), alveolar-capillary membrane integrity, intact airway, cardiac output, hemoglobin level, and tissue ischemia.

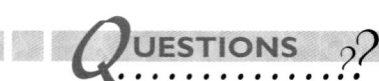

QUESTIONS ??

A sampling of review questions for this chapter appears here. Visit http://www.mosby.com/MERLIN/PriceWilson/ for additional questions.

Answer the following on a separate sheet of paper.

1. List three disorders of the respiratory system that are a major source of morbidity and mortality.
2. Define respiration.
3. Draw and label the epithelial surface of the airways, and discuss the function of the mucosal lining in respiration (see Fig. 35-1, *B*, for reference to the structure of the mucosal lining of the airways).
4. Why are foreign bodies, when aspirated, usually found in the right main stem bronchus?
5. What would happen if the pressure within the pleural space were to become equal to that of the atmosphere?
6. Sketch the position of the lungs in the circulatory system, and describe some of the unique features of blood supply to the lungs (see Fig. 35-4 for reference to the functional position of the lungs in the circulation).
7. If the mean pulmonary artery pressure is 30 mm Hg and the colloid osmotic pressure of the blood is 20 mm Hg, is pulmonary edema likely to occur? Why or why not?

Complete the following statements by filling in the blanks.

8. The structure that forms the division between the upper and lower respiratory tracts is the _____.
9. The alveoli are lined by a lipoprotein substance called _____. During inspiration, expansion is facilitated, and during expiration, collapse is prevented as this substance functions to lower the _____.
10. The movement of air in and out of the lungs is called _____. To accomplish this function, the thoracic cage and lungs have been compared with a reciprocating pump or _____. The muscle that provides the main driving force during inspiration is the _____.
11. A reflex that controls the amount of air taken into the lungs is known as the _____ reflex.
12. Centers that control the pattern and rhythmicity of breathing are located in the _____ and _____ of the brain.

13. Match the number of the structure in Fig. 35-15 with the appropriate term from the following list:
   a. Diaphragm
   b. Carina
   c. Epiglottis
   d. Mediastinum
   e. Pharynx
   f. Larynx
   g. Trachea
   h. Main stem bronchus
   i. Segmental bronchus
   j. Apex of lung
   k. Visceral pleura
   l. Parietal pleura

14. Match the number of the structure in Fig. 35-16 with the appropriate term from the following list:
   a. Pores of Kohn
   b. Alveolar duct
   c. Respiratory bronchiole
   d. Terminal bronchiole
   e. Acinus
   f. Alveolus
   g. Septum

Answer the following on a separate sheet of paper.

15. Why is the alveolar Po_2 as low as 103 mm Hg when it is 159 mm Hg in the inspired air?

16. What is the volume of a healthy individual's anatomic dead space?

17. What is the chief mechanism of gas movement in the respiratory zone of the lung? What provides the driving force?

18. Are ventilation and perfusion perfectly matched in the healthy person at rest in the upright position? Why or why not?

19. If alveolar ventilation is 3 L/min and cardiac output (perfusion) is 6 L/min, what is the $\dot{V}/\dot{Q}$ ratio? Is this value normal, or does a person with this value have dead-space–producing or shunt-producing disease?

20. What advantage would be gained, if any, by placing a patient with severe hemolytic anemia in a hyperbaric chamber?

21. If a patient is breathing fresh air at sea level, the alveolar Po_2 is approximately 103 mm Hg, the arterial blood is 97% to 98% saturated with O_2, and the O_2 content is 20 vol %, will increasing the O_2 concentration of the inspired air be advantageous? Why or why not?

22. Explain why the Po_2 can vary over a wide range and have little effect on the Hb saturation.

23. What is the Bohr effect? What is its significance in terms of tissue oxygenation?

24. When a person hyperventilates, why does the O_2 content of the arterial blood fail to increase significantly but the arterial Pco_2 decrease significantly? Explain this phenomenon in terms of the O_2 and CO_2 dissociation curves.

25. Why does an elevated arterial Pco_2 never result from impaired diffusion?

26. Does knowledge of the blood gases alone provide all the information necessary to assess accurately the respiratory status? If not, what other data are necessary?

27. Beginning with inspired air, list at least three altered mechanisms or conditions that may interfere with normal respiration.

28. The respiratory process may be divided into three stages. List and briefly describe each stage.

29. Which muscles are used during normal quiet breathing? Which muscles are used during breathing with maximum effort?

30. How many milliliters of O_2 are used by tissue cells each minute if the Hb concentration is 12.0 g/dl blood, the saturation of Hb reaches 100%, cardiac output is 5000 ml/min, and 25% of O_2 delivered is used? (1.34 ml O_2 combines with each gram of Hb. The O_2 that is transported physically dissolved in blood plasma may be ignored.)

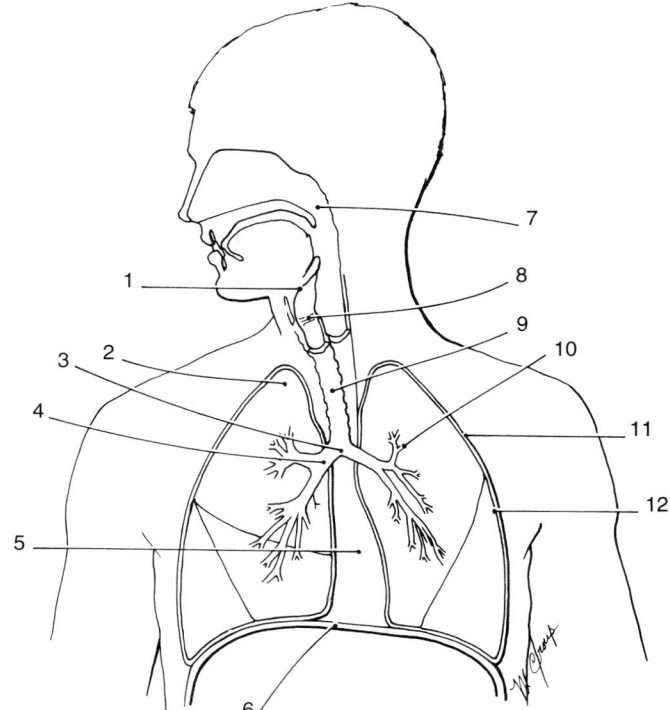

FIG. 35-15   Respiratory tract.

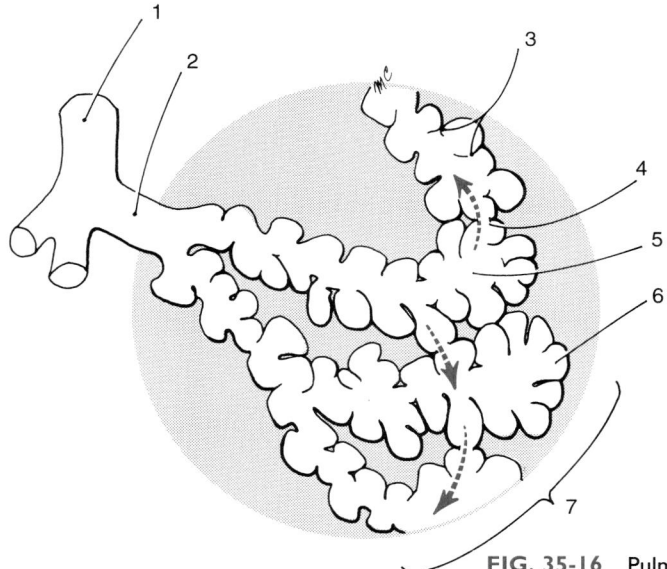

FIG. 35-16   Pulmonary functional unit.

31. Account for the fact that Hb is 100% saturated with O_2 on leaving the pulmonary capillary bed but is 97% to 98% saturated in the systemic arteries.

32. If alveolar ventilation doubles and CO_2 production remains constant, what are the effects on arterial Pco_2 and the blood pH? What happens to the HbO_2 dissociation curve, and what are the consequences?

33. What is the Po_2 in the inspired air of a climber on the summit of Mount Everest if the atmospheric pressure is 247 mm Hg and water vapor pressure at body temperature is 47 mm Hg? Could the mountain climber be able to walk very far?

Circle the word that correctly completes each sentence.

34. During inspiration, muscular contraction causes the size of the thorax to (increase) (decrease). This size change causes a(n) (increase) (decrease) in the intrapleural pressure. Because pressure in the alveoli is (less) (more) than atmospheric pressure, air moves (into) (out of) the lungs.

35. During expiration, when the diaphragm muscle relaxes, the diaphragm (ascends) (descends), thus (increasing) (decreasing) the volume of the thoracic cavity.

36. During normal quiet expiration, the size change in the thoracic cavity causes a(n) (increase) (decrease) in the intrapleural pressure. Because pressure in the alveoli is now (more) (less) than atmospheric pressure, air moves (into) (out of) the lungs.

37. A person is accidentally exposed to carbon monoxide, which combines with one half the Hb in the arterial blood. The Pao_2 will be (normal) (high) (low). The Sao_2 will be (normal) (high) (low). The arterial O_2 content will be (normal) (high) (low).

38. Generally, hyperventilation causes a(n) (increase) (decrease) in the Pco_2 and a(n) (increase) (decrease) in the blood pH, resulting in a condition of (alkalosis) (acidosis).

39. A P_{50} of 34 mm Hg means that the HbO_2 dissociation curve is shifted to the (right) (left) and the Hb affinity for O_2 is (decreased) (increased).

36

Diagnostic Procedures in Respiratory Disease

LORRAINE M. WILSON

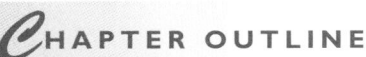
MORPHOLOGIC METHODS

Diagnostic procedures used for detecting pulmonary disease may be classified primarily as morphologic or physiologic. *Morphologic* methods include radiologic techniques, endoscopy, biopsy studies, and sputum studies. Blood gas measurements and ventilatory function tests reveal *physiologic* function.

Radiologic Techniques

The thorax is an ideal region for a radiologic examination. The aerated lung parenchyma offers little resistance to the passage of x-rays and therefore produces highly radiant shadows. The soft tissues of the chest wall, the heart and great vessels, and the diaphragm do not permit the rays to pass through as readily as does the lung parenchyma and thus appear denser on the radiograph. The bony structures of the thorax, including the ribs, sternum, and vertebrae, are even less readily penetrated, and their shadows are even denser. Radiologic methods typically used to detect pulmonary disease include routine chest radiography, computed tomography, angiography, and perfusion and ventilation lung scanning.

Routine Chest Radiography

The routine chest radiograph is taken at a standard distance after maximum inspiration and breath holding to stabilize the diaphragm. Radiographs are taken from the posteroanterior perspective and sometimes from the lateral and oblique perspectives. These radiographs provide the following information:

1. The status of the thoracic cage, including the ribs, the pleura, and the contour of the diaphragm and of the upper airway as it enters the chest
2. The size, contour, and position of the mediastinum and hilus of the lung, including the heart, aorta, lymph nodes, and root of the bronchial tree
3. The texture and degree of aeration of the lung parenchyma
4. The size, shape, number, and location of pulmonary lesions, including cavitation, fibrous markings, and zones of consolidation

The appearance of the normal chest radiograph varies somewhat according to gender and age in different subjects and to varying conditions of respiration in the same subject. Interpreting a chest radiograph is a skill that takes considerable time to acquire and is an invaluable aid to the physician when correlated with other observations.

Computed Tomography

Computed tomography (CT) is a radiographic technique by which a series of radiographs, each representing a "slice of the lung," is taken to build a detailed image. Many more shades of gray are visible with CT compared with the routine chest radiograph; additionally, less of a problem exists in detecting abnormalities because of obscuration by normal structures as with the routine chest radiograph. CT is of particular value for identifying abnormalities in configuration of the trachea or major bronchi, defining lesions and anatomy of the pleura or mediastinum (nodes, tumors, vascular structures), and generally, revealing the nature and extent of abnormal shadows in the lungs and other tissues of the thorax. Because it is noninvasive, mediastinal CT is often used for the assessment of mediastinal lymph node size in the staging of lung cancer, although it is not as accurate as is mediastinoscopy (see

Chapter 42). CT has become increasingly useful in the diagnostic evaluation of pulmonary parenchymal disease because of recent advances in technology. With high resolution CT (HRCT), the thickness of individual cross-section images are 1 to 2 mm in thickness rather than the usual 7 to 8 mm, allowing recognition of many interstitial lung or airway diseases at an early stage, such as diffuse pulmonary fibrosis or bronchiectasis.

Magnetic Resonance Imaging

Magnetic resonance imaging (MRI) uses magnetic resonance as its source of energy to take cross-sectional images of the body. MRI allows images to be constructed in any plane (transverse, sagittal, or coronal); allows distinction between normal and diseased tissues, even when they are of similar density (which would not be distinguished by CT); and allows blood vessels to be distinguished from nonvascular structures, even without the use of contrast media. However, because MRI is more expensive compared with CT, MRI is used when it can provide information not otherwise obtainable by less expensive means. MRI is particularly useful in evaluating hilar and mediastinal disease.

Ultrasound

Ultrasound is not useful in evaluating disorders of the lung parenchyma. However, ultrasound is helpful in detecting the presence of pleural fluid and is often used as a guide for needle placement for sampling of pleural fluid during a thoracentesis.

Angiography of Pulmonary Vessels

The pulmonary arterial pattern and flow can be demonstrated by injecting radiopaque fluid through a catheter inserted via an arm vein into the right atrium and right ventricle and then into the main pulmonary artery. This technique is used to locate the site of a massive embolism or to determine the extent of a pulmonary infarction. Anomalies, such as aneurysms and alterations in vascularity common in emphysema, are also detectable. However, simpler diagnostic techniques are preferred for the detection of pulmonary disease whenever possible. The major risk during angiography is the development of cardiac dysrhythmia as the catheter is passed through the heart chambers.

Lung Scan

The isotope lung scan, although a less reliable method for the detection of pulmonary embolism, is a safer procedure compared with angiography. Pulmonary perfusion and sometimes ventilation scanning are performed. A *perfusion scan* is obtained by the injection of albumin microspheres, usually labeled with technetium 99m, into a peripheral vein; these particles appear as transient emboli in the pulmonary capillaries in proportion to the active blood flow. The radioactivity distribution is counted with a scintiscanner and the image recorded with a camera. The pattern is almost always abnormal in embolism (area with absent radioactivity) but is not highly specific because abnormalities also occur in other conditions, such as emphysema and pneumonia. The *ventilation scan* uses the inhalation of a bolus of radioactive gas, usually xenon-133. The scan is usually normal in embolism but abnormal in infarction, pneumonia, and emphysema.

Another scintigraphic imaging technique, imaging with gallium 67, has been of diagnostic value in detecting and evaluating infections and inflammatory conditions affecting the lung. Gallium scanning has been used extensively for the detection of *Pneumocystis carinii* pneumonia in patients with acquired immunodeficiency syndrome (AIDS).

Bronchoscopy

Bronchoscopy is a technique that allows direct visualization of the trachea and its major subdivisions. This technique is used most frequently to confirm the diagnosis of bronchogenic carcinoma, but it can be used to remove a foreign body. The conventional bronchoscope is a hollow metal tube containing a lighted mirror-lens system, which is passed readily into the tracheobronchial tree after administration of local anesthesia. The newer *fiberoptic bronchoscope* is a flexible instrument that can transmit light and a clear image around corners. Because of its flexibility and smaller diameter, using fiberoptic bronchoscope causes much less trauma than does the conventional metal bronchoscope. The fiberoptic bronchoscope allows inspection of the smaller bronchial subdivisions and may also be passed through the nose. Tissue biopsy can be obtained by using a tiny forceps or flexible brush at the tip of the bronchoscope. Secretions for culture and cytologic studies may be obtained via suction tubes passed through the bronchoscope. The fiberoptic bronchoscopy can be performed at the bedside, although the location of choice is the operating room.

After bronchoscopy, food and fluids are withheld for 2 or 3 hours until the gag reflex returns; otherwise the patient may aspirate material into the tracheobronchial tree. Touching a cotton applicator to the back of the patient's throat is a way of testing the return of the gag reflex. When this action causes the patient to gag, swallowing may be permitted. Other complications are bleeding and pneumothorax caused by a ruptured bronchus.

Common procedures after bronchoscopy to detect these complications are the monitoring of vital signs for several hours, a chest radiograph, and the collection of all sputum for 24 hours. The nurse should also be aware that laryngeal spasm or edema may be a delayed complication and may require endotracheal intubation and the administration of oxygen.

Biopsy Studies

Tissue specimens for biopsy study may be obtained from the upper or lower airways by endoscopic techniques using either the laryngoscope or the bronchoscope. Video-assisted thoracic surgery (VATS) is a recently developed technology that is useful for both the diagnosis and the management of pleural and parenchymal diseases. This procedure involves the passage of a rigid trocar with a distal lens through a small intercostal incision into the pleura under general anesthesia. The operator can then biopsy lesions of the pleura or peripheral lung tissue or remove a peripheral lung nodule under direct vision. This procedure has largely supplanted the open-lung biopsy and thoracotomy. A cylinder of tissue can also be obtained by the newer techniques of *percutaneous needle biopsy* using an air-turbine drill. The main value of the lung biopsy is in diffuse lung disease not diagnosable by other means. Pneumothorax and bleeding are encountered in a substantial number of patients after this procedure.

Biopsy of the lymph nodes in the mediastinum is accomplished during *mediastinoscopy*. This procedure involves the insertion of a lighted mirror-lens system through an incision at the base of the anterior portion of the neck. The instrument is advanced under visual control into the mediastinum, where inspection and biopsy can be accomplished. Mediastinoscopy is the major preoperative method for pathologic evaluation of regional spread to the hilar lymph nodes in patients with lung cancer.

Sputum Studies

Gross, microscopic, and bacteriologic examinations of the sputum are important in the etiologic diagnosis of many respiratory diseases. The color, odor, and presence of blood provide valuable clues. Microscopic examination may reveal the causative organism in many bacterial pneumonias, in tuberculosis, and in some fungal infections. Exfoliative cell studies of the sputum may also be helpful in diagnosing lung carcinoma. The best time for collecting sputum is shortly after awakening because abnormal bronchial secretions tend to accumulate during sleep. Inducing sputum production by the use of a nebulizer is sometimes necessary. A popular method of obtaining tracheobronchial secretions is by bronchoalveolar lavage (BAL) through a flexible bronchoscope. Sterile saline is injected through the bronchoscope and suctioned back into a collection chamber. These bronchial washings can then be examined for malignant cells or microorganisms from the lower respiratory tract. The fluid from BAL has been used quite effectively for detecting *Pneumocystis carinii* in patients with AIDS.

PHYSIOLOGIC METHODS: PULMONARY FUNCTION TESTS

During the previous generation, numerous tests and techniques related to the study of respiratory physiology have evolved. These pulmonary function tests (PFTs) fall into two broad categories: those related to ventilatory function of the lungs and chest wall and those related to diffusion of alveolar gases. *Ventilatory* function tests include measurements of lung volumes under static and dynamic conditions, as well as pressure measurements. Tests related to diffusion of alveolar gases include analysis of gases in the expired air and in the blood. *Arterial blood gas measurements* (ABGs) typically include partial pressures (tensions) of arterial oxygen (PaO_2) and arterial carbon dioxide ($PaCO_2$) and pH and reflect cardiopulmonary physiology.

PFTs are becoming an increasingly important part of routine clinical evaluation and are taking their place among other diagnostic aids such as the chest radiograph and electrocardiogram. Important to realize, however, is that these tests show only the effects of disease on function and cannot be used to give a diagnosis on the basis of a pathologic change. Some diseases, however, have a characteristic pattern of disordered function, and distinguishing an obstructive pattern of ventilatory abnormality from a restrictive pattern is possible. *Obstructive* venti-

latory disorders affect the ability to exhale, whereas *restrictive* disorders affect the ability to inhale. Two major patterns of functional disorders that also emerge from ABGs are disorders in which increased *dead space* is present or disorders in which increased *shunting* occurs.

It is essential to realize that no single PFT can measure all possible attributes. Nevertheless, PFTs give valuable information. Ventilatory function tests give quantitative data that enable the examiner to follow the progress of a lung disease, as well as response to treatment. In cases of pulmonary disability in which surgery is planned, these tests help assess the patient's ability to tolerate anesthetics, narcotics, or removal of lung tissue and to prescribe the postoperative care needed. Because some diseases may alter only one aspect of pulmonary function, PFTs occasionally assist in establishing the diagnosis. ABGs are an invaluable aid in assessing the severity of respiratory insufficiency and guiding the appropriate therapy. This chapter focuses on the specific PFTs that are most widely used and most helpful in patient management.

Ventilatory Function Tests
Static Lung Volumes

Lung volumes and capacities are anatomic measurements that are affected by exercise and disease. There are four lung volumes and four lung capacities. Lung capacities always consist of two or more lung volumes. Fig. 36-1 shows the relationship between these measurements and the average values for a young, healthy, adult man. Table 36-1 lists the abbreviations and provides a description of the lung capacities and volumes. The following five lung capacities and volumes (designated by the abbreviations listed in the table) can be measured directly on an instrument called the spirometer: tidal volume (V_T), inspiratory reserve volume (IRV), expiratory reserve volume (ERV), vital capacity (VC), and inspiratory capacity (IC). The functional residual capacity (FRC) is measured by indirect means using helium or nitrogen washout methods

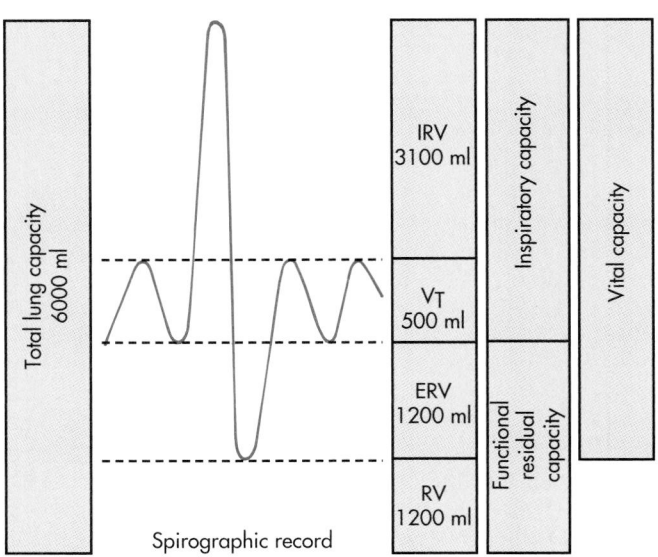

FIG. 36-1   Relationships among the lung volumes and capacities (see Table 36-1 for explanation of abbreviations).

TABLE 36-1

Lung Capacities and Volumes

Measurement	Symbol	Adult Male Average Value (ml)	Definition
Tidal volume	V_T	500	Amount of air inhaled or exhaled with each breath (value listed is for resting conditions)
Inspiratory reserve volume	IRV	3100	Amount of air that can be forcefully inhaled after a normal tidal volume inhalation
Expiratory reserve volume	ERV	1200	Amount of air that can be forcefully exhaled after a normal tidal volume exhalation
Residual volume	RV	1200	Amount of air left in the lungs after a forced exhalation
Total lung capacity	TLC	6000	Maximum amount of air that can be contained in the lungs after a maximum inspiratory effort: TLC = V_T + IRV + ERV + RV; TLC = VC + RV
Vital capacity	VC	4800	Maximum amount of air that can be expired after a maximum inspiration: VC = V_T + IRV + ERV (should be 80% TLC)
Inspiratory capacity	IC	3600	Maximum amount of air that can be inspired after a normal expiration: IC = V_T + IRV
Functional residual capacity	FRC	2400	Volume of air remaining in the lungs after a normal tidal volume expiration: FRC = ERV + RV

From Comroe JH: *The lung: clinical physiology and pulmonary function tests*, ed 2, Chicago, 1971, Mosby.

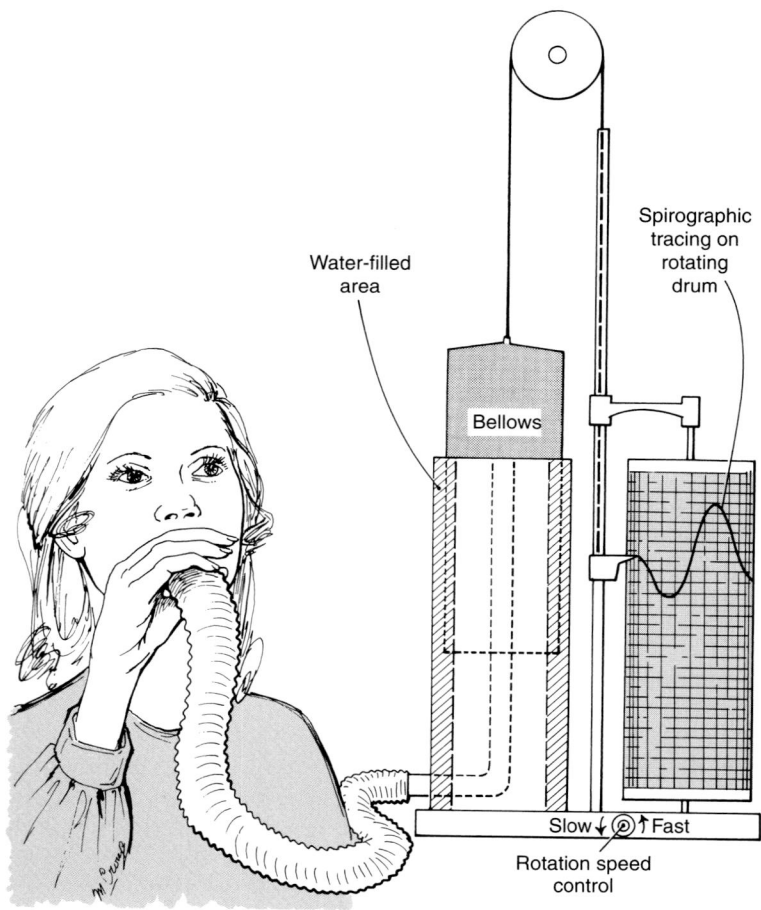

Water-filled area

Spirographic tracing on rotating drum

Bellows

Slow ↓ ⊘ ↑ Fast

Rotation speed control

FIG. 36-2   Spirometer.

or by using the body plethysmograph. The total lung capacity (TLC) and reserve volume (RV) are then derived arithmetically (i.e., TLC = FRC + IC, and RV = TLC – VC).

A *spirometer* is a simple instrument containing a bellows or bell that is displaced as the patient breathes into it through a valve and connecting tube, as shown in Fig. 36-2. As the spirometer is used, a graphic record of the measurement is made on a rotating drum with a recording pen. Computed bedside spirometry using a hand-held spirometer is also commonly performed.

TABLE 36-2

Effective Ventilation and Respiratory Pattern

Patient	V_D (ml)	V_T (ml)	f (breaths/min)	$\dot{V}_E$ ($V_T \times$ f) (L/min)	$\dot{V}_A$ [($V_T - V_D$) $\times$ f] (L/min)	V_D/V_T (%)
Patient A (rapid, shallow breathing)	150	250	40	10	4	60
Patient B (normal rate and depth)	150	500	20	10	7	30
Patient C (slow, deep breathing)	150	1000	10	10	$8^1/_2$	15

See text for abbreviations.

Measurements of the static lung volumes in practice are used to reflect the elastic properties of the lungs and thorax. The most useful measurements are the VC, TLC, FRC, and RV. Diseases that limit lung expansion (restrictive disorders) reduce these volumes. In contrast, diseases that cause airway obstruction almost always cause an increase in RV and FRC as a result of hyperinflation of the lungs. TLC may be normal or increased, and VC is often decreased. In lung diseases in which RV is increased because of air trapping, VC must decrease by an equal amount, because TLC is relatively stable (unless part of the lung is surgically removed) and because TLC = RV + VC.

Dynamic Lung Volumes and Work of Breathing

More information can be obtained about the ventilatory status if the rate of air movement into and out of the lungs is considered, as well as the work of breathing. The following definitions are useful in the discussion of effective ventilation:

- *Minute volume,* or *minute ventilation* ($\dot{V}_E$), is the volume of gas collected during expiration over a 1-minute period. $\dot{V}_E$ may be calculated by multiplying the V_T by the respiratory rate. At rest, $\dot{V}_E$ is approximately 6 or 7 L/min. The $\dot{V}_E$ is measured by collecting the expired air in a large rubber balloon and dividing the volume collected by the number of minutes taken to collect the sample. The subscript E in the symbol for minute volume means that the measurement is made during the expiratory phase of the V_T, and the dot over the V indicates that $\dot{V}_E$ is a timed measurement.
- *Respiratory frequency* (written as "f "in equations) or *rate* is the number of breaths taken per minute. At rest the respiratory rate is approximately 15 breaths per minute.
- *Tidal volume* (V_T) is the amount of air inhaled or exhaled with each breath. The V_T is approximately 500 ml at rest but may increase to 3000 ml during exercise when deep breaths are taken. V_T is obtained by dividing the $\dot{V}_E$ by the respiratory rate.
- *Physiologic dead space* (V_D) is the volume of inspired air that does not exchange with pulmonary blood; it may be regarded as wasted ventilation. V_D is composed of *anatomic dead space* (the volume of air in the conducting airways, approximately 1 ml/lb of body weight), *alveolar dead space* (alveoli being ventilated but not perfused; alveolar dead space is highly variable), and *ventilation in excess of perfusion.* In healthy individuals, V_D is only slightly greater than is the anatomic dead space,

but it may be increased if ventilated alveoli are underperfused or not perfused at all, as in pulmonary embolism. The ratio of V_D to V_T (V_D/V_T) reflects the portion of the V_T that does not exchange with pulmonary blood. In other words, V_D/V_T is a measurement of the percentage of V_T that is V_D. This ratio is calculated from data collected by measuring the carbon dioxide tension (P_{CO_2}) in the expired air and the P_{CO_2} in the arterial blood. The larger the difference between these two measurements is, the greater is the V_D. The V_D/V_T ratio does not exceed 30% to 40% in the healthy person. This ratio is frequently used to follow the course of patients receiving mechanical ventilation.

- *Alveolar ventilation* ($\dot{V}_A$) is the volume of fresh gas entering the alveoli each minute that exchanges with pulmonary blood; it is the effective ventilation. $\dot{V}_A$ is normally approximately 4.2 L/min at rest and is calculated by either of the following formulas:

$$\dot{V}_A = (V_T - V_D) \times f$$
$$\dot{V}_A = \dot{V}_E - \dot{V}_D$$

$\dot{V}_A$ is a better index of ventilation than is $\dot{V}_E$ or V_T because the measurement takes into account the volume of air wasted in ventilating the V_D. The calculations in Table 36-2 illustrate the relationship among $\dot{V}_E$, breathing pattern, and effective $\dot{V}_A$. The V_D for each of the three patients is assumed to be constant at 150 ml, but the rate and depth of breathing vary.

Several deductions can be made from the data in Table 36-2. In each case, the total amount of air entering and leaving the lungs is the same ($\dot{V}_E$), although great variation exists in the percentage of the V_T that is V_D and in the effective ventilation. The evidence suggests that rapid, shallow breathing results in less effective ventilation as more is wasted in dead-space volume. This fact becomes obvious if the formula for calculating $\dot{V}_A$ is considered. As V_T approaches V_D (150 ml), effective ventilation approaches zero, regardless of the rapidity of the respiratory rate (0 × f = 0). The percentage of the V_T that is V_D also approaches 100% as the V_T approaches the V_D. Considering that total V_D (anatomic and alveolar) can vary greatly with disease, clinical observation of ventilatory adequacy obviously has great limitations, even though some gross qualitative judgments can be made.

For air to move in and out of the lungs, the body must work to overcome the combined resistances of the thorax, lungs, and abdomen. The work (in the form of energy expenditure to move the chest bellows) is referred to as the *work of breathing*. The work of breathing can be expressed as the amount of oxygen (O_2) consumed by the respiratory muscles. In the normal person at rest, this amount is a small fraction (less than 5%) of the total body O_2 consumption, but in disease, the proportion may be significantly increased.

Expenditure of energy is required to overcome two types of resistance: elastic and nonelastic. The *elastic resistance* is the resistance to stretch caused by the elastic properties of the lungs and thorax. The elastic properties of the thorax result from the stretching properties of the tendons, muscles, and connective tissue. The elastic properties of the lungs are produced by the surface tension of fluid lining the alveoli and by the elastic fibers throughout the lung itself. *Nonelastic resistance* is the frictional resistance to airflow in the airways and, to a small degree, resistance resulting from the viscosity of the lung tissues. The work of breathing increases when an increase in either the elastic resistance (e.g., "stiff lungs" as in pulmonary fibrosis) or the nonelastic resistance (e.g., turbulent airflow in emphysema as a result of narrowing of the airways) occurs.

Compliance (written as "C" in equations) is a measure of the elastic properties (distensibility) of the lungs and thorax and is defined as the change in volume-per-unit change in pressure under static conditions. Total compliance (compliance of the lungs and thorax) or lung compliance alone can be determined. Two manometers are used to measure pressure changes: one is connected to the mouth or nostrils (to measure alveolar pressure or the total pressure exerted by the lung-thorax system) and the other to an esophageal balloon (to measure intrapleural pressure). Volume and pressure changes (ΔV, ΔP) are then measured under various degrees of lung inflation and breath holding. Compliance is estimated by calculating the slope of the pressure-volume curve, which is plotted from the data. Normal lung compliance and thoracic cage compliance over the V_T range are each

0.2 L/cm of water (H_2O), and total compliance (lungs and thoracic cage) is approximately 0.1 L/cm H_2O:

$$C = \frac{\Delta V \text{ (change in lung volume in liters)}}{\Delta P \text{ (change in pressure in centimeters of } H_2O)}$$

Compliance is reduced in restrictive patterns of pulmonary disease that increase the stiffness of the lung or thorax and limit expansion. In these patients a greater force (ΔP) than normal is required to give the same increase in volume (ΔV), causing the compliance to be smaller. Common causes of decreased lung compliance are atelectasis (collapse of alveoli), pulmonary edema, pneumonia, and pulmonary fibrosis. When pulmonary surfactant is decreased, compliance is also decreased because the lung becomes stiffer as a result of the increase in surface tension (surfactant normally reduces surface tension). Chest wall compliance is reduced in obesity, abdominal distention, and bony deformities of the chest cage such as kyphoscoliosis.

The *nonelastic airway resistance* (R_{AW}) can be measured by placing the subject in an airtight box (body plethysmograph) and measuring the pressure around the body (which reflects the change in alveolar pressure); at the same time, the rate of flow of air at the mouth is measured (Fig. 36-3). The R_{AW} reflects the nonelastic resistance of the upper airways (first to twelfth generations of the tracheobronchial tree) and is approximately 1.8 cm H_2O/L/sec of airflow. In patients with obstructive airway disease (e.g., emphysema), R_{AW} is increased and may be greater than 5 cm H_2O/L/sec.

More frequently, however, nonelastic resistance is estimated by measuring forced expiratory volumes and flow rates. This measurement is made on a spirometer or by a portable hand unit that can be used at the bedside. The volumes of air measured by the spirometer are as follows:

- *Forced vital capacity (FVC)* is the VC measurement performed with expiration as forceful and rapid as possible. This volume of air is normally approximately

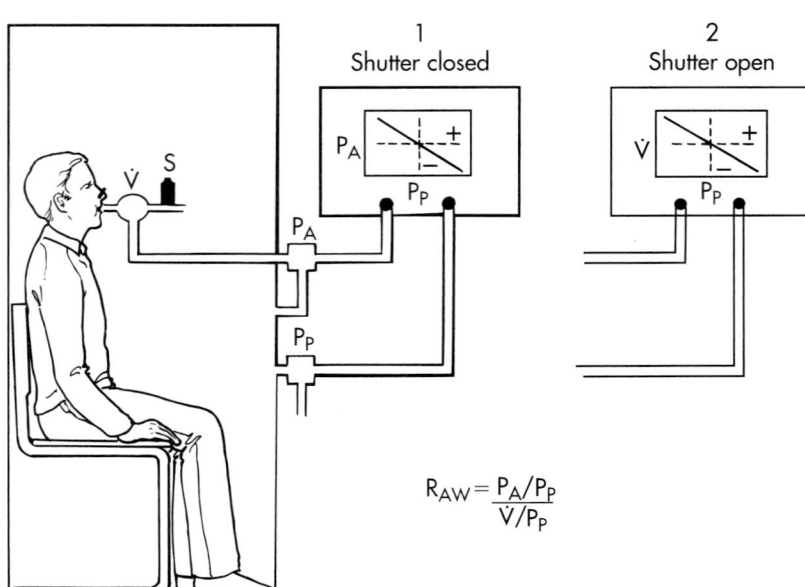

$$R_{AW} = \frac{P_A/P_P}{\dot{V}/P_P}$$

FIG. 36-3 Measurement of airway resistance (R_{AW}) in the body plethysmograph. The ratio between mouth pressure (P_A) (identical to alveolar pressure) and the box pressure (P_P) is determined with the shutter (S) closed. Then the relationship between P_P and airflow ($\dot{V}$) is estimated while the patient pants through the unobstructed pneumotachograph. Now $R_{AW} = P_A/\dot{V}$. (Redrawn from Cherniack RM: *Pulmonary function testing*, Philadelphia, 1992, WB Saunders.)

equal to the VC but may be significantly reduced in patients with airway obstruction because of premature closure of the small airways and the consequent trapping of air.

- *Forced expiratory volume* (FEV) is the volume of air that can be exhaled in a standard time period during the FVC maneuver. Usually, the FEV is measured during the first second of the forced exhalation; this is termed FEV_1. The FEV is a useful index of the impairment of ventilatory capacity, and values of less than 1 L during the first second indicate severe impairment of ventilatory function.

The FEV should always be related to the FVC or VC. Healthy individuals can expire approximately 80% of their VC in 1 second, expressed as the FEV_1/FVC ratio. Whether the FVC or VC is used for the ratio makes little difference; the result is approximately the same. This ratio is of great value in differentiating between diseases that cause airway obstruction and those that cause restriction of lung expansion. In obstructive diseases, such as chronic bronchitis and emphysema, the reduction in FEV_1 is greater than is in VC (VC may be normal); thus the FEV_1/FVC ratio is less than 80%. In a restrictive disease of the lung parenchyma, such as sarcoidosis, both the FEV_1 and the FVC or VC are reduced in approximately the same proportion, and the FEV_1/FVC ratio remains at approximately 80% or more.

The *maximum midexpiratory flow rate (MMFR)* is an important index of airway obstruction, which may be derived from a forced expiration. MMFR is the flow rate for the middle two quarters of the FVC. The MMFR appears to be independent of effort and thus may be a more sensitive index of airway obstruction in early chronic obstructive lung disease than is the FEV_1 (Fig. 36-4).

An important factor to understand is that these routine PFTs can detect only moderate to advanced obstructive disease involving the large airways, which account for 80% of the resistance. PFTs are not sensitive enough to detect obstruction of the small peripheral airways (bronchioles less than 1 mm in diameter) because these airways contribute only a small fraction of the resistance

(less than 20%). Obstructive respiratory disease is believed to begin in the peripheral airways. For these reasons, new techniques have been devised for detecting early airway dysfunction.

One technique is the *single-breath nitrogen test* to detect uneven distribution of gas in the lung and an increased closing volume. During this test, the subject fully exhales, takes a single VC inspiration of 100% O_2, and then slowly exhales to the RV. During the last expiration, the nitrogen (N_2) concentration in the expired air (now diluted with inspired O_2) is measured with a rapid N_2 analyzer and recorded along with the expired volume.

A number of important parameters may be derived from the N_2 curve (Fig. 36-5), including anatomic dead space, RV, VC, TLC, closing volume, closing capacity, and the slope of the alveolar plateau. *Closing volume (CV)* represents a lung volume at which the small airways in the lowest part of the lung begin to close and is usually expressed as a percentage of the expired vital capacity (CV/VC). *Closing capacity (CC)* consists of the CV plus the RV and is expressed as a percentage of total lung capacity (CC/TLC). The CV/VC ratio is age dependent and may be as low as 10% in the young healthy person and 40% at age 65 years.

An increase in the CV/VC or CC/TLC ratio suggests premature closure of the small peripheral airways, resulting from narrowing or loss of elastic recoil, as in chronic bronchitis and emphysema. An increased CV has been found in apparently healthy cigarette smokers. A rising slope of the alveolar plateau of the N_2 washout curve indicates uneven alveolar gas distribution in the lung and occurs in obstruction of the airways. Excellent and detailed descriptions of these and other PFTs may be found in Cherniack (1992) and West (1998).

The overall effects on alterations in the elastic and nonelastic properties of the lungs can be assessed by a simple test that measures the *maximum breathing capacity (MBC),* or *maximum voluntary ventilation (MVV).* The MVV (or MBC) can be estimated directly by having the patient breathe as rapidly and deeply as possible for 15 seconds and collecting the expired air in a Douglas bag. This

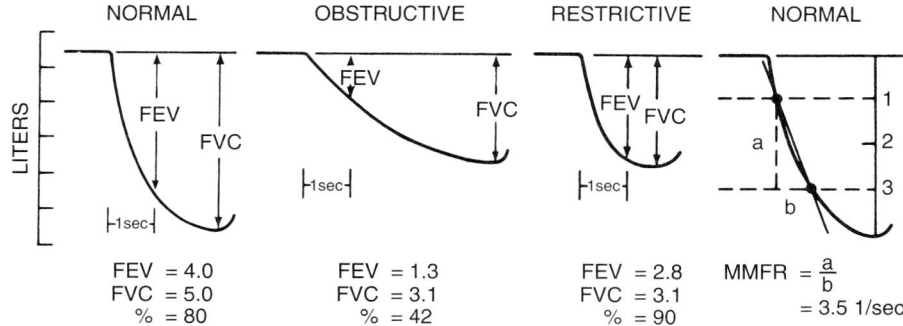

FIG. 36-4 Measurement of the forced expiratory volume *(FEV₁)* and maximum midexpiratory flow rate *(MMFR).* The patient takes a full inspiration and exhales as hard and as fast as possible. The pen moves down as the patient exhales. The FEV_1 is the volume exhaled in 1 second. The MMFR is the mean flow rate over the middle half of the forced vital capacity *(FVC).* Note the differences among the normal, obstructive, and restrictive patterns. (From Petersdorf, editor: *Harrison's principles of internal medicine,* ed 11, New York, 1987, McGraw-Hill.)

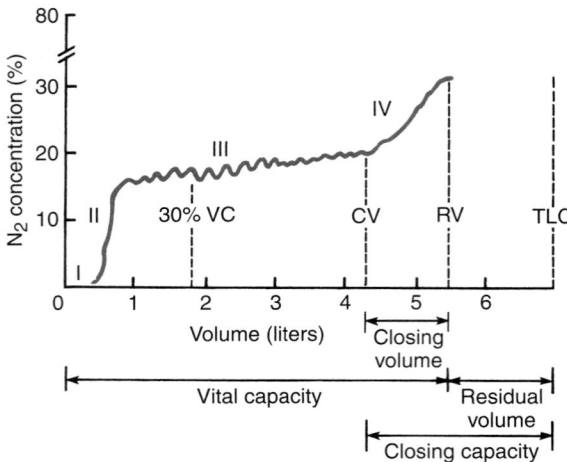

FIG. 36-5 Measurement of the closing volume (CV) by the single-breath nitrogen (N_2) method. If a vital capacity (VC) inspiration of 100% O_2 is followed by slow exhalation to residual volume (RV), four phases of the N_2 concentration measured at the lips can be recognized. Initially there is no N_2 in the expired gas because it is gas from the dead space filled with O_2 (phase I). This is followed by a rapid rise in N_2 (phase II) in which alveolar gas mixes with dead-space gas and the curve is S shaped. From then on, N_2 reaches a plateau with a gradual rise (phase III) followed by an abrupt rise (phase IV), signaling closure of the small airways in the dependent zones of the lung. Phase IV represents closing volume, and closing capacity is the volume of gas left in the lung at the point of onset of phase IV (CV + RV). (Redrawn from Cherniack RM: *Pulmonary function testing*, ed 2, Philadelphia, 1992, Saunders.)

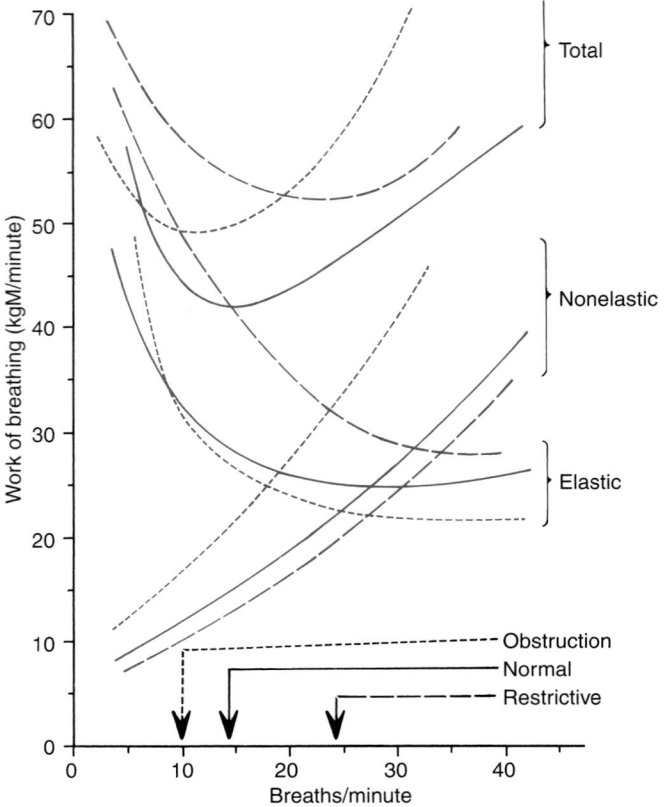

FIG. 36-6 Relationship between the mechanical work of breathing and the respiratory pattern in health and in pulmonary disease. (Modified from Cherniack M, Cherniack L: *Respiration in health and disease*, ed 3, Philadelphia, 1983, Saunders.)

volume is multiplied by 4 to determine the $\dot{V}_E$ in liters per minute. This test, used extensively for years, has been largely replaced by the FEV_1 test, which is less demanding and gives essentially the same information. The MBC may be approximated as the product of $FEV_1 \times 30$. The MBC can be affected by changes in compliance because of the increased muscular effort required. The MBC is also affected by changes in airway resistance because of the increased turbulence resulting from airway collapse when breathing at rapid rates. The healthy young male adult can move as much as 170 L air/min, compared with a $\dot{V}_E$ of approximately 6 L/min at rest. The difference represents the *pulmonary reserve*, which is large in the healthy young adult. The pulmonary reserve is reduced in restrictive and obstructive diseases but much more in the latter.

As stated previously, less than 5% of the total O_2 consumption is expended for the work of breathing in the normal person at rest. The O_2 cost of breathing is greatly increased in both obstructive and restrictive patterns of pulmonary disease. The patient with emphysema (increased airway resistance) or the person who is severely obese (restriction of chest movement) may consume 25% or more of the total inspired O_2 for the work of breathing. In severe disease, fatigue may be an important factor in the development of respiratory failure because of the increased muscular effort required for the work of breathing.

A relationship also exists between the mechanical work of breathing and the respiratory pattern (rate and depth of breathing). Respiratory physiologists have demonstrated that for any given $\dot{V}_A$, an optimal respiratory rate and V_T exists at which the total work of breath-

ing is minimal. The graphs in Fig. 36-6 show the relationship between the mechanical work of breathing, including the total work and its two components (elastic and nonelastic), expressed in kilogram-meters (kgM), and the respiratory frequency. The principle illustrated is applied to normal persons and to those with pulmonary disease. The total work is the sum of the elastic and nonelastic work. (As may be recalled, elastic work is expended to overcome the elastic resistances of the lungs and thorax and nonelastic work is expended to overcome flow resistance and tissue viscous resistance.) In the normal person at rest, at a particular $\dot{V}_A$, the total work of breathing is least at approximately 15 breaths/min (illustrated by the solid lines in Fig. 36-6). At the same $\dot{V}_A$, rapid, shallow breathing results in the least amount of work for the patient with a restrictive pulmonary disorder (increased elastic work) such as pneumonia or obesity (illustrated by the long dashed lines in Fig. 36-6). This pattern probably occurs because small increments in V_T greatly increase the elastic resistance. However, if the pattern of breathing becomes too rapid and shallow, the V_D then becomes disproportionately high. On the other hand, the person with an obstructive pulmonary disorder (increased nonelastic work), such as emphysema, adopts a slow, deep pattern of respiration (illustrated by the short dashed lines in Fig. 36-6). This pattern is adopted because a higher flow rate is likely to increase the amount of work needed to overcome resistance to airflow. In fact, if the patient with obstructive disease should voluntarily hyperventilate to blow off more CO_2, the P_{CO_2} might actually rise as a result of its increased production from the increased mechanical work of breathing.

Blood Gas Analysis

To assess respiratory function adequately, the examiner must look beyond the lung to the volume and distribution of gas transport by the circulatory system. The factors that affect gas transport and removal between the lungs and tissue cells are discussed in Chapter 35, and a systematic approach to the assessment of acid-base disorders is presented in Chapter 22. In this chapter, the technique used for the collection of blood to measure the blood gases and some general guidelines for the interpretation of measurements are presented.

Usually, a sample of arterial blood is used for the blood gas analysis. Fig. 36-7 demonstrates the correct technique for drawing a blood sample. The radial (or brachial) artery is often chosen because of its accessibility. The wrist is extended by positioning it over a rolled towel. After the skin has been sterilized, the artery is stabilized with two fingers of one hand while the arterial puncture is made with the other hand using a heparinized syringe. After 5 ml of blood has been drawn into the syringe, air is removed, and the blood is placed on ice and immediately taken to the blood gas laboratory for analysis. The intensive care nurse usually obtains the blood sample. Table 36-3 lists the normal values for the ABGs.

The Pa_{CO_2} is the best index of $\dot{V}_A$. When the Pa_{CO_2} rises, the direct cause is always generalized *alveolar hypoventilation*. Hypoventilation causes *respiratory acidosis* and a fall in the pH of the blood. Alveolar hypoventilation may occur if the V_T is decreased (the dead-space effect), as occurs in rapid, shallow breathing. Hypoventilation may also occur if the respiratory rate is decreased, as occurs in narcotic or barbiturate drug overdose. The Pa_{CO_2} may also rise to compensate for a *metabolic alkalosis*. Consequently, to interpret the Pa_{CO_2} correctly, the blood pH and bicarbonate levels must also be considered to determine whether a change is caused by a primary respiratory condition or is compensating for a metabolic condition.

The direct cause of a lowered Pa_{CO_2} is always *alveolar hyperventilation*. Hyperventilation causes *respiratory alkalosis* and a rise in the pH of the blood. Hyperventilation is common in asthma and pneumonia and represents an effort to raise the Pa_{O_2} at the expense of excreting excess carbon dioxide (CO_2) from the lungs. Brain injury or tumor, aspirin poisoning, or anxiety may also cause hyperventilation, or it may be a compensation for *metabolic acidosis*. Table 36-4 summarizes the acid-base changes in compensated acidosis and alkalosis. The thicker arrows indicate the primary disorder. The change in the bicarbonate level represents the kidneys' attempt to compensate for the respiratory acidosis or alkalosis, whereas the change in the Pa_{CO_2} in the metabolic disorders represents the lung's role in compensation. The purpose of the compensation is to return the blood pH to normal.

When the Pa_{O_2} falls below the normal value, *hypoxemia* results. Pa_{O_2} levels fall slightly with age; thus a per-

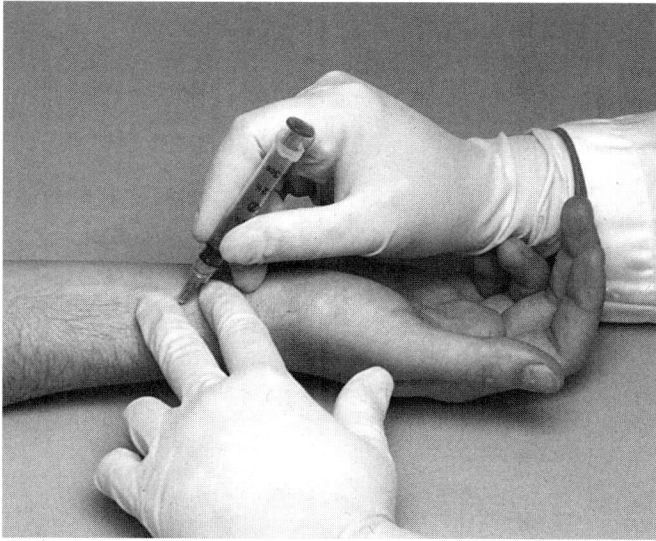

FIG. 36-7   Radial artery puncture technique for obtaining blood to test for arterial blood gas (ABG) levels. (From Potter PA, Perry AG: *Fundamentals of nursing*, ed 4, St Louis, 1997, Mosby.)

TABLE 36-3   ■ ■ ■

Normal Values for Arterial Blood Gases

Blood Gas Measurement	Abbreviation	Normal Value
CO_2 tension	Pa_{CO_2}	35-45 mm Hg (average, 40)
O_2 tension	Pa_{O_2}	80-100 mm Hg
O_2 percent saturation	Sa_{O_2}	97
Hydrogen ion concentration	pH	7.35-7.45
Bicarbonate	HCO_3^-	22-26 mEq/L

TABLE 36-4   ■ ■ ■

Acid-Base Changes in Acidosis and Alkalosis

Acid-Base Disturbance	pH	HCO_3^-	Pa_{CO_2}
Respiratory acidosis	↓	↑	↑
Respiratory alkalosis	↑	↓	↓
Metabolic acidosis	↓	↓	↓
Metabolic alkalosis	↑	↑	↑

son over age 60 years with a Pa_{O_2} as low as 70 mm Hg is normal. In severe respiratory failure the Pa_{O_2} may fall to 30 to 40 mm Hg. Hypoxemia resulting from respiratory disease is caused by one or more of the following mechanisms: (1) ventilation/perfusion imbalance (most common cause), (2) alveolar hypoventilation, (3) impaired diffusion, or (4) intrapulmonary anatomic shunts. Hypoxemia resulting from the first three abnormalities can be corrected by administering O_2. However, the intrapulmonary anatomic shunt (arteriovenous shunt) cannot be corrected by O_2 therapy.

Changes in the ABGs are critical measurements in the diagnosis of respiratory or ventilatory failure, which may

TABLE 36-5 ▪▪▪

Changes in Ventilatory Function as a Result of Pulmonary Disease

Test	Obstructive Pattern	Restrictive Pattern
RV	↑	↓
FRC	↑	↓
TLC	N or ↑	↓
VC*	N or ↓	↓
FVC	N or ↓	↓
MBC	↓	N or ↓
FEV_1†	↓	N or ↓
FEV_1/FVC	↓ (<80%)	N or ↑ (>80%)
MMFR	↓	N or ↓
CV	↑ for age or > FRC	
Compliance	N or ↑ (slight)	↓
PaO_2	↓	N (↓ ↓ exercise)
$PaCO_2$	↑	N or ↓
pH	↓ (during exacerbations)	N or ↑

Modified from Seaton A, Seaton D, Leitch A, editors: *Crofton and Douglas' respiratory diseases*, vol 1, ed 5, Oxford, 2000, Blackwell; Cherniak RM: *Pulmonary function testing*, ed 2, Philadelphia, 1992, Saunders.
N, Normal; ↓, decreased or tending to decrease; ↑, increased or tending to increase. See earlier text in chapter for test abbreviations.
*Useful test to monitor progress of restrictive lung disease.
†Most useful test to monitor progress of obstructive lung disease.

TABLE 36-6 ▪▪▪

Relationship between the PaO_2 and SaO_2 on the Normal Oxyhemoglobin Dissociation Curve

PaO_2 (mm Hg)	SaO_2 (%)
100	98
90	97
80	95
70	93
60	**89**
50	84
40	75
30	57
20	35

Note: Correspondence between PaO_2 and SaO_2 above 60 mm Hg and approximately 90%, respectively, is unreliable. A SaO_2 of at least 90% (corresponding to a PaO_2 of approximately 60 mm Hg) is considered to be in the safe range; values below these numbers mean that the patient is in trouble with oxygenation.

be insidious in onset. Respiratory insufficiency exists when the PaO_2 falls below the normal values, and respiratory failure occurs when the PaO_2 falls to 50 mm Hg. The $PaCO_2$ may be increased above or decreased below the normal values in respiratory insufficiency or failure. Respiratory failure is discussed in greater detail in Chapter 41. Table 36-5 summarizes some of the common changes in ventilatory function and ABGs in restrictive and obstructive patterns of pulmonary disease.

Pulse Oximetry

Although the measurement of ABGs is the best method of assessing gas exchange, it has the disadvantage of requiring arterial puncture to collect blood for analysis. As a result, pulse oximetry, a noninvasive method of assessing oxygenation, has come into widespread use. The pulse oximeter measures oxygen saturation of hemoglobin (SaO_2), rather than PaO_2, using a probe that is usually clipped over a finger. Two different wavelengths of light are then passed through the finger. Oxygenated and deoxygenated hemoglobin have different patterns of light absorption. Measurement of the absorption of the two wavelengths in the pulsatile arterial blood allows quantification of the two forms of hemoglobin. The amount of hemoglobin that is saturated with oxygen is calculated and displayed immediately on the device readout. The normal SaO_2 is 95% to 97%, corresponding to a PaO_2 of approximately 80 to 100 mm Hg. The usual clinical goal for oxygen saturation of hemoglobin is SaO_2 at least 90% (corresponding to a PaO_2 of approximately 60 mm Hg). Table 36-6 shows the predictable relationship between the PaO_2 and SaO_2 on the normal oxyhemoglobin dissociation curve.

Although pulse oximetry has the advantage of measuring oxygenation noninvasively, this method has certain inherent limitations. First, the clinician must be aware of the relationship between the SaO_2 and PaO_2 as shown by the oxyhemoglobin dissociation curve (see Fig. 35-13). Because the curve is relatively flat above a PaO_2 greater than 60 mm Hg (corresponding to a SaO_2 of 90%), the pulse oximeter is relatively insensitive to changes in the PaO_2 above this level. Additionally, the relationship between the PaO_2 and SaO_2 may change depending on whether the curve is shifted to the right or left by factors such as pH, temperature, and concentrations of 2,3-diphophoglycerate (2,3-DPG). Second, the device cannot distinguish between other forms of hemoglobin, such as carboxyhemoglobin or methemoglobin, when only two wavelengths are used. Third, when cardiac output is low or cutaneous vasoconstriction is present, the reading from the oximeter may be unreliable. Finally, no information is provided about pH and CO_2 elimination.

⦚EY CONCEPTS

- *Morphologic procedures* used for the diagnosis of pulmonary disease include radiologic techniques, endoscopy, biopsy, and sputum studies. Blood gas measurements, pulse oximetry, and pulmonary function tests reveal *physiologic function*.
- The *routine chest x-ray* provides information about the: (1) status of the thoracic cage and contour of the diaphragm; (2) size, contour, and position of the mediastinum and hilum of the lung, including the heart, aorta, lymph nodes, and root of the tracheobronchial tree; (3) aeration of the lung parenchyma, as well as presence of pulmonary lesions, cavitations, infiltrates, or consolidation, which appear whitish because of increased density on the dark background of the normally aerated lung parenchyma.

- The *CT scan* is superior to routine chest radiography in revealing differences in tissue density and can provide cross-section images of the lung. CT scan is an important tool used for the staging of lung cancer.
- *Ventilation and perfusion lung scans* are useful as screening methods for the detection of pulmonary thromboembolism. The gold standard for diagnosis of pulmonary thromboembolism is *pulmonary angiography.*
- The *flexible fiberoptic bronchoscope* is ideal for the diagnosis of endobronchial pathology, including tumors, bronchitis, foreign bodies, and bleeding sites. Bronchoalveolar lavage (BAL) with sterile saline can be used to detect abnormal cells or recover pathogens, such as *Pneumocystis carinii* in patients with human immunodeficiency virus (HIV) infection. Brushing or biopsy of a lesion can enhance the recovery of cellular material for the detection of neoplasms or infection. Bleeding and pneumothorax are possible complications of this procedure.
- *Video-assisted thoracic surgery (VATS)* is a recently developed technique used for biopsy of the pleura and peripheral lung tissue, as well as for the management of pleural lung disease. *Percutaneous needle biopsy* is an alternate method of obtaining a biopsy of peripheral lung tissue but has a high risk of producing pneumothorax or bleeding as complications.
- *Sputum studies* of tracheobronchial secretions can be used to detect pathogens or malignant cells but may be difficult to interpret because of contamination with oropharyngeal flora.
- *Mediastinoscopy* allows inspection and biopsy of the hilar lymph nodes and is an important diagnostic procedure for the staging of lung cancer.
- *Ventilatory or pulmonary function tests (PFTs)* provide an objective method for assessing functional changes in a patient with known or suspected pulmonary disease. Data from PFTs allow correlation of functional patterns with obstructive or restrictive patterns of pulmonary disease. Serial measurements can quantitate any deterioration or improvement in function in response to therapy. PFTs may also be used preoperatively to predict which patients are likely to have significant respiratory problems after a lung resection.
- Ventilatory function is measured under *static conditions* for determination of *lung volumes* and under *dynamic conditions* for determination of *forced expiratory flow rates.*
- Four lung volumes are particularly important: (1) Vital capacity (VC)—the volume of gas expired after a maximum inspiration (when going from TLC to RV); (2) total lung capacity (TLC)—the total volume of gas within the lungs after a maximum inspiration; (3) functional residual capacity (FRC)—the volume of gas left in the lungs at the end of expiration in the resting state during a normal tidal breathing (ERV + RV); and (4) residual volume (RV)—the volume of gas remaining in the lungs after a maximum expiration.
- *Vital capacity (VC), expiratory reserve volume (ERV),* and *inspiratory capacity (IC)* are measured by having the patient breath in and out of a spirometer, while plotting volume as a function of time.
- RV, FRC, and TLC cannot be measured with a spirometer because they include gas that is present in the lung after a maximum expiration. These lung volumes can be measured by helium or N_2 washout methods or with a body plethysmograph.
- Three measurements are commonly made during a forced expiratory maneuver: (1) Forced vital capacity (FVC)—the vital capacity measurement performed with expiration as forceful and as rapidly as possible; (2) FEV_1—the volume of air that can be expired during the first second of the forced expiration; and (3) the maximum midexpiratory flow rate (MMFR)—forced expiratory flow from 25% to 75% of the FVC or ($FEF_{25\%-75\%}$).
- Normal standards have been established for PFTs based on averages for a large number of male and female control subjects. A "normal" or predicted value is established for the patient taking a given test by entering the patient's age, height, and gender into a regression equation.
- The normal value for the FEV_1 is approximately 80% of the predicted value; values below this level indicate airway obstruction. The FEV_1/FVC ratio should be approximately 95% of the predicted ratio. The MMFR or $FEF_{25\%-75\%}$ is an even more sensitive index of airway obstruction.
- The analysis of PFTs allows abnormalities to be classified into two categories (or combinations of the two): (1) an obstructive pattern, characterized by obstruction to airflow and (2) a restrictive pattern, with evidence of decreased lung volumes but no obstruction to flow.
- An *obstructive pattern of ventilation* is present in patients with chronic obstructive pulmonary disease (chronic bronchitis and emphysema) and asthma and consists of a decrease in FEV_1, FEV_1/FVC, and MMFR. Additionally, high RV and FRC generally occur, indicating air trapping that results from premature closure of airways during forced expiration.
- A wide variety of parenchymal, pleural, neuromuscular, and chest wall disorders can cause a restrictive pattern of ventilation. A *restrictive pattern* is characterized by a reduction of lung volumes (VC, TLC, FRC, and RV), reflecting loss of lung or chest wall compliance (elasticity) while FEV_1/FVC, and MMFR are preserved.
- *Minute ventilation ($\dot{V}_E$)* is the amount of air breathed per minute and is equal to the V_T multiplied by the respiratory frequency ($V_T \times f$). $\dot{V}_E$ is normally 6 to 7 L/min under resting condition but can increase to approximately 170 L/min in a healthy young male. (The dot over a respiratory symbol means "per minute.")
- *Tidal volume (V_T)* is the volume of air inspired or expired with each breath and is normally approximately 500 ml under resting conditions.
- *Physiologic dead space (V_D)* is the volume of tidal volume that does not take part in gas exchange because it is present in the conducting airways. V_D is approximately equal to an individual's ideal body weight in pounds.
- *Alveolar ventilation ($\dot{V}_A$)* or effective ventilation is that part of the total ventilation ($\dot{V}_E$) that takes part in gas

exchange ($\dot{V}_A = [V_T - V_D] \times f$). $\dot{V}_A$ is less effective when breathing is shallow (small V_T) than it is when breathing is deep (large V_T).

- The *volume of dead space to tidal volume ratio (V_D/V_T)* is a measure of wasted V_D during the process of breathing. Normally this ratio does not exceed 30% to 40%; a value of 60% or greater indicates that the patient may need assisted ventilation because the work of breathing and moving the respiratory bellows is great to the extent that the patient will eventually tire.
- The mechanical *work of breathing (WOB)* can be expressed as the amount of O_2 consumed in moving air into and out of the lungs. Normally, 5% or less of total body O_2 consumption is expended for the WOB, but this amount can increase up to 25% in many obstructive or restrictive patterns of pulmonary disease. Fatigue in moving the respiratory bellows then becomes a factor in the development of respiratory failure.
- The WOB is composed of two resistances: (1) *elastic resistance* of the chest cage and lungs to stretch, increased in restrictive pulmonary disease during inspiration and (2) *nonelastic resistance* resulting from turbulent airflow, increased in obstructive patterns of pulmonary disease because of premature collapse of the airways during expiration.
- For any given $\dot{V}_A$, an optimal respiratory rate (f) and depth (V_T) occurs at which the WOB is minimal; this pattern will be adopted whether that person is healthy or has respiratory disease. *Nonelastic resistance is increased in patients with obstructive lung disease*, causing them to adopt a slow, deep breathing pattern to minimize the WOB. *Elastic resistance is increased in patients with restrictive respiratory disease*, causing them to adopt a rapid, shallow breathing pattern to minimize the WOB.

- The most accurate way to assess oxygenation status is by measurement of *arterial blood gases (ABGs)* but this method has the disadvantage of requiring an arterial puncture. ABGs include the measurement of the Pa_{O_2} (normal is 80 to 100 mm Hg), the Pa_{CO_2} (normal is 35 to 45 mm Hg), pH (normal is 7.35 to 7.45), and standard bicarbonate (normal is 22 to 26 mEq/L).
- The *four mechanisms causing hypoxemia* are: (1) ventilation/perfusion (V/Q) imbalance (most common), (2) alveolar hypoventilation, (3) impaired diffusion (uncommon), and (4) intrapulmonary anatomic shunting. The first three causes can be corrected by O_2 therapy but not when an anatomic shunt is present.
- Alveolar ventilation is assessed by measurement of the Pa_{CO_2}. When the Pa_{CO_2} rises above normal, the direct cause is always *alveolar hypoventilation*; when the Pa_{CO_2} falls below normal, the direct cause is always *alveolar hyperventilation*.
- *Pulse oximetry* is a noninvasive method of assessing oxygenation status (Sa_{O_2}) but suffers the following *limitations*: (1) the Sa_{O_2} is insensitive to changes in the Pa_{O_2} on the flat part of the oxyhemoglobin dissociation curve (Sa_{O_2} above 90% and Pa_{O_2} above 60 mm Hg), and the relationship between the Sa_{O_2} and **Pa_{O_2} changes** if the curve is shifted to the right or left; (2) the device cannot distinguish between the normal types of hemoglobin and methemoglobin or carboxyhemoglobin; (3) vasoconstriction or a low cardiac output causes the measurement to be inaccurate; and (4) no information about the pH and Pa_{CO_2} is provided.

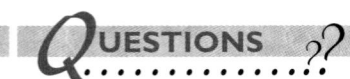

QUESTIONS ??

A sampling of review questions for this chapter appears here. Visit http://www.mosby.com/MERLIN/PriceWilson/ for additional questions.

Answer the following on a separate sheet of paper.

1. List five radiologic methods frequently used to detect pulmonary disease.

2. List four distinct features that are depicted on a routine chest radiograph.

Match each of the diagnostic tests in column A to its description in column B.

Column A
3. _____ VATS
4. _____ Angiography of pulmonary vessels
5. _____ Gallium scan
6. _____ Perfusion lung scan
7. _____ Percutaneous needle biopsy of lung
8. _____ Bronchoscopy
9. _____ Sputum studies
10. _____ CT
11. _____ Mediastinoscopy

Column B
a. Most accurate method of diagnosing pulmonary embolism
b. Method used to biopsy pleura or peripheral lung under direct visualization
c. Used to detect *Pneumocystis carinii* infection
d. Closed technique to obtain lung biopsy specimen
e. Useful technique to obtain aspiration of secretions for cytologic examination or biopsy specimen under direct visualization
f. Radiologic technique providing detailed radiographs of "slices of the lung"
g. Technique used to assess spread of lung cancer to hilar lymph nodes
h. Involves injection into a peripheral vein of albumin microspheres tagged with an isotope
i. Specimen may be obtained by aspiration of gastric contents

Answer the following on a separate sheet of paper.

12. Describe the role of ventilatory function tests and blood gas analysis in the diagnosis and treatment of pulmonary disorders. Are any of these tests specifically diagnostic?

13. Explain why alveolar ventilation is a better index of effective ventilation than is $\dot{V}_E$ or V_T.

14. Describe the procedure for the measurement of compliance of the lungs and thoracic cage. How is compliance calculated from the measurements?

15. List three common causes of decreased lung compliance and three causes of decreased chest wall compliance.

16. Why does a patient with emphysema adopt a slow, deep pattern of respiration?

17. What breathing pattern might a patient with normal airway resistance but extremely stiff lungs (low compliance) adopt? Why?

18. Describe the correct technique for the collection of blood in the measurement of ABGs.

19. List three causes of alveolar hyperventilation and hypoventilation.

20. List four causes of hypoxemia. Which one is *not* corrected by O_2 administration?

Complete the table as directed.

21. Indicate the common changes in ventilatory function and blood gases in restrictive and obstructive patterns of pulmonary disease by filling in the blanks in the table. Use the following key: N = normal, ↓ = decreased, ↑ = increased.

Changes in Ventilatory Function as a Result of Pulmonary Disease

Test	Obstructive Pattern	Restrictive Pattern
RV		
FRC		
TLC		
VC		
FVC		
MBC		
FEV_1		
FEV_1/FVC		
Compliance		
Pa_{O_2}		
Pa_{CO_2}		
pH		

Cardinal Signs and Symptoms of Respiratory Disease

LORRAINE M. WILSON

𝒫ulmonary diseases may give rise to both respiratory and general signs and symptoms. Respiratory signs and symptoms include cough, excessive or abnormal sputum, hemoptysis, dyspnea, and chest pain. General signs and symptoms include cyanosis, digital clubbing and hypertrophic osteoarthropathy, and other manifestations related to inadequate gas exchange. The reader is referred to other textbooks for a discussion of adventitious chest sounds and systematic assessment of the respiratory status.

COUGH

Coughing is a protective reflex that is caused by irritation of the tracheobronchial tree. The ability to cough is an important mechanism in clearing the lower airways, and many adults normally cough a few times on first arising to clear the trachea and pharynx of secretions that have accumulated during sleep. Coughing is also the most common symptom of respiratory disease. Any cough persisting for longer than 3 weeks should be investigated to determine the cause.

Stimuli that typically produce a cough are mechanical, chemical, and inflammatory. Inhalation of smoke, dust, and small foreign bodies is the most common cause of cough. Smokers often have a chronic cough as a result of inhaling foreign bodies (smoke) and chronic inflammation of the airways. Mechanical stimulation from tumors, either extrinsic or intrinsic to the airways, is another cause of cough (the most common tumor that causes cough is bronchogenic carcinoma). Any inflammatory process of the airways, with or without exudate, may produce a cough. Chronic bronchitis, asthma, tuberculosis, and pneumonia typically have coughing as a prominent symptom. A cough may be productive, hacking and nonproductive, brassy (as with pressure on the trachea), frequent, infrequent, or paroxysmal (intermittent coughing episodes).

SPUTUM

The normal adult produces about 100 ml of mucus in the respiratory tract per day. This mucus is transported to the pharynx by the normal cleansing actions of the cilia that line the airways. When excess mucus is formed, the normal process of removal may be ineffective and may result in the accumulation of mucus. When this buildup occurs, the mucous membrane is stimulated, and the mucus is coughed up as sputum. Excess mucus production may be caused by physical, chemical, or infective insults to the mucous membrane.

Whenever a patient produces sputum, assessing its source, color, volume, and consistency is important. Sputum produced by clearing the throat is most likely to have originated in the sinuses or nasal passages rather than in the lower respiratory tract. Profuse purulent sputum suggests the presence of a suppurative process such as lung abscess, whereas sputum production that gradually increases over a period of years suggests chronic bronchitis or bronchiectasis.

The color of sputum is also important. Yellow sputum indicates an infection. Green sputum is indicative of stagnant pus. The green color is produced by the presence of verdoperoxidase, which is liberated from polymorphonuclear neutrophils (PMNs) in the sputum. Green sputum is common in bronchiectasis because of the stagnation of sputum in dilated, infected bronchioles. Many patients with lower respiratory tract infection report having green sputum early in the morning, which becomes yellow as the day progresses. This phenomenon is probably caused by the accumulation of purulent sputum during the night, with the consequent release of verdoperoxidase.

The character and consistency of sputum also yield useful information. Pink, frothy sputum is characteristic of acute pulmonary edema. Sputum may be mucoid, sticky, and gray or white in chronic bronchitis. A foul odor to the sputum may indicate a lung abscess or bronchiectasis.

HEMOPTYSIS

Varying amounts of blood may be mixed with sputum, or blood may comprise the entire expectoration. *Hemoptysis* is the term applied to the expectoration of both pure blood and blood-streaked sputum. Any process resulting in interruption of the continuity of the pulmonary blood vessels may result in bleeding. The expectoration of pure blood is a serious symptom and may be the first manifestation of active tuberculosis. Other common causes of hemoptysis are bronchogenic carcinoma, pulmonary infarction, bronchiectasis, and lung abscess. Blood-streaked sputum (which may be rust colored) is a common feature of pneumococcal pneumonia. Sputum may have the appearance of currant-jelly (brick red) in *Klebsiella* pneumonia. Table 37-1 summarizes some of the gross characteristics of sputum in some pulmonary disorders. When blood or blood-streaked sputum is expectorated, an important factor to determine is whether the source is actually the lower respiratory tract rather than the nasal passages or gastrointestinal (GI) tract. Blood originating in the GI tract *(hematemesis)* is usually dark, similar to coffee grounds, from partial digestion and is associated with nausea, vomiting, and anemia; blood originating in the lower airways (below the glottis) is usually bright red, frothy, and associated with a history of cough with or without anemia. Blood originating in the upper air passages (e.g., nosebleed, bleeding after a tonsillectomy) is often associated with frequent swallowing and may have the appearance of partially digested blood when vomited.

DYSPNEA

Dyspnea, or *breathlessness*, is the subjective sensation of difficulty in breathing and is a cardinal symptom of car-

diopulmonary disease. A patient with dyspnea is likely to complain of shortness of breath or a sensation of suffocation. Objective signs of breathlessness include the use of accessory muscles of respiration (sternocleidomastoid, scalene, trapezius, pectoralis major), nasal flaring, tachypnea, and hyperinflation. Dyspnea is by no means always an indication of disease; the normal person usually experiences this sensation after varying degrees of physical exertion.

Distinguishing dyspnea from other signs and symptoms that may have an entirely different clinical significance is important. *Tachypnea* refers to a rapid respiratory rate greater than the normal 12 to 20 breaths per minute that may be present with or without dyspnea. *Hyperventilation* refers to ventilation that is greater than the amount required to maintain normal carbon dioxide (CO_2) elimination; it is identified by observing an arterial CO_2 partial pressure, or tension ($Paco_2$), that is less than the normal 40 mm Hg. Dyspnea is a common complaint in the *hyperventilation syndrome* in otherwise healthy individuals who are emotionally stressed (see Chapter 22). Finally, the symptom of *exertional fatigue* must be distinguished from dyspnea. The healthy person experiences exertional fatigue after varying degrees of physical exertion, and this symptom may also be experienced with cardiovascular, neuromuscular, and other nonpulmonary diseases.

In recent years, scientific interest in the measurement and neurophysiologic mechanisms of dyspnea has surged. However, no totally satisfactory explanation for dyspnea under all circumstances is yet available. The proposed sources of dyspnea include: (1) the mechanical receptors in the respiratory muscles, lung, and chest wall; according to the *length-tension theory*, sensory elements, particularly muscle spindles, play a central role in comparing the tension in the muscles with the degree of stretch; dyspnea is experienced when the tension is inappropriately large for a particular muscle length (volume of breath achieved); (2) chemoreceptors for CO_2 and oxygen (O_2) tensions (Pco_2 and Po_2) *(oxygen-debt theory)*; (3) increased work of breathing with the consequent sensation of increased effort; and (4) an imbalance between respiratory work and the capacity to ventilate. The length-tension inappropriateness mechanism is the most widely accepted theory because it explains most of the cases of clinical dyspnea. The key factor that appears to determine whether dyspnea is experienced is whether the level of ventilation or effort is appropriate to the degree of activity. However, the stimuli, sensory receptors, and nerve pathways by which the appropriateness is recognized have not been established with certainty.

TABLE 37-1

Characteristics of Sputum Seen in Various Pulmonary Disorders

Appearance	Likely Cause
Mucoid, translucent, grayish white	Atypical pneumonia, asthma
Currant-jelly (brick red)	*Klebsiella pneumoniae*
Rusty (prune juice color)	Pneumococcal pneumonia
Pink, frothy	Pulmonary edema
Salmon colored or creamy yellow	Staphylococcal pneumonia
Mucopurulent sputum: yellow, greenish, or dirty gray	Bacterial pneumonia; acute or chronic bronchitis
Purulent and foul smelling	Oral anaerobes (aspiration), lung abscess, bronchiectasis

TABLE 37-2 ■ ■ ■

Dyspnea Scale

Grade	Degree	Criteria
0	None	Is not troubled with breathlessness except with strenuous activity
1	Slight	Is troubled by shortness of breath when hurrying on the level or walking up a slight hill
2	Moderate	Walks slower than most people of the same age because of breathlessness or has to stop for breath when walking at own pace on the level
3	Severe	Stops for breath after walking 100 yards or after a few minutes walking on level ground
4	Very severe	Too breathless to leave the house or breathless when dressing or undressing

Data from Brooks SM, chairman: *ATS News* 8:12–16, 1982.

The amount of exertion sufficient to induce dyspnea varies with age, gender, altitude, state of physical fitness, and emotional involvement in the task. Dyspnea in a patient must be correlated with the minimal level of activity sufficient for its induction, that is, to determine whether dyspnea is experienced after strenuous or moderate activity or while at rest. Table 37-2 outlines a dyspnea scale developed by the American Thoracic Society that may be appropriate for the clinical assessment of chronic dyspnea. Additionally, some variations exist of the general symptom of dyspnea. *Orthopnea* is shortness of breath on assuming the recumbent position and is usually quantified by describing the number of pillows or angle of elevation required to prevent the sensation. A common cause of orthopnea is congestive heart failure resulting from the increased blood volume in the central vasculature on assuming the recumbent position. Orthopnea is also a common symptom in many respiratory disorders. *Paroxysmal nocturnal dyspnea* refers to the onset of dyspnea during the night with the urgent need to sit up to breathe. Paroxysmal nocturnal dyspnea differs from orthopnea in that the onset usually occurs after several hours of recumbency. The cause is the same as in the orthopnea of congestive heart failure, and the delayed onset is related to the mobilization of peripheral edema fluid and its addition to the central intravascular volume.

Patients who have dyspnea as a principal symptom usually have one of the following conditions: (1) cardiovascular disease, (2) pulmonary emboli, (3) interstitial or alveolar disease of the lung, (4) disorders of the chest wall or muscles, (5) obstructive disease of lung, or (6) anxiety. Dyspnea is a prominent symptom of pulmonary edema, congestive heart failure, and valvular heart disease. Pulmonary embolism is characterized by the sudden onset of dyspnea. Dyspnea is a prevalent symptom in diseases that affect the tracheobronchial tree, lung parenchyma, and pleural space. Dyspnea is frequently associated with restrictive diseases in which respiratory work is increased as a result of increased elastic resistance of the lung (e.g., pneumonia, atelectasis, congestion) or chest wall (e.g., obesity, kyphoscoliosis) or in obstructive airways disease with increased bronchial nonelastic resistance (e.g., emphysema, bronchitis, asthma). When the work of breathing is increased chronically, however, the patient may adapt to the new level and not experience dyspnea. Dyspnea may also be experienced if the respiratory muscles are weak (e.g., myasthenia gravis), paralyzed (e.g., poliomyelitis, Guillain-Barré syndrome), fatigued as a result of increased work of breathing, or less able to perform mechanical work (e.g., severe emphysema, obesity). Finally, individuals with hyperventilation syndrome secondary to anxiety or emotional stress often complain of dyspnea. The breathing pattern for this group is frequently strange, with irregularities in both frequency and tidal volume. At other times, the pattern is one of such sustained hyperventilation that the patient complains of tingling in the extremities and even a feeling of faintness (see discussion on respiratory alkalosis in Chapter 22). If the abnormal breathing pattern disappears during sleep, psychogenic causes should then be suspected.

CHEST PAIN

Chest pain has many causes, but the most characteristic pain of lung disease is that resulting from inflammation of the pleura *(pleurisy)*. Only the parietal layer of the pleura is a source of pain, because the visceral pleura and the lung parenchyma are regarded as insensitive organs.

Typically, pleurisy is usually abrupt in onset but may develop gradually. The pain occurs at the site of inflammation and is usually well localized. The pain is cutting and sharp in character and is aggravated by coughing, sneezing, and deep breathing; thus the patient often adopts a pattern of rapid, shallow breathing and avoids unnecessary movement. The pain may be somewhat relieved by applying pressure (splinting) over the involved area. The most common causes of pleuritic pain are pulmonary infection or infarction, although these conditions may be present without pain. Patients with pneumothorax or massive atelectasis may occasionally experience chest pain that is thought to be caused by traction on the parietal pleura by adhesions attached to the visceral pleura. Pleuritic pain must be differentiated from other causes of chest pain, such as myocardial ischemia, pericarditis, costochondritis, and herpes zoster (caused by involvement of the intercostal nerves).

DIGITAL CLUBBING AND HYPERTROPHIC OSTEOARTHROPATHY

Digital clubbing is a peculiar change in the shape of the tips of the fingers and toes characterized by a bulbous appearance. This physical sign is significant because it is associated with a number of serious conditions. Pulmonary disease (e.g., bronchogenic carcinoma, bronchiectasis, lung abscess, pulmonary tuberculosis) is the most common cause of digital clubbing (70% to 80% of cases). Cardiovascular disease (e.g., congenital intracardiac shunting, infective endocarditis) ranks second (10% to 15% of cases); and 5% to 10% of the cases of digital club-

Conditions Associated with Digital Clubbing

A. Pulmonary disease
  1. Pulmonary neoplasms (5%-10%)
    a. Bronchogenic carcinoma
    b. Mesothelioma
    c. Hodgkin's disease
  2. Infections
    a. Lung abscess
    b. Bronchiectasis
    c. Cystic fibrosis
    d. Empyema
    e. Tuberculosis with cavitation
B. Cardiovascular disease
  1. Cyanotic congenital heart disease
  2. Infective endocarditis
  3. Infected vascular prosthesis
C. GI disease
  1. Cirrhosis of the liver
  2. Inflammatory bowel disease
    a. Ulcerative colitis
    b. Crohn's disease
  3. Sprue
  4. Familial polyposis
  5. Neoplasms of the esophagus, liver, or small and large bowels
D. Miscellaneous
  1. Primary hereditary finger clubbing
  2. Graves' disease

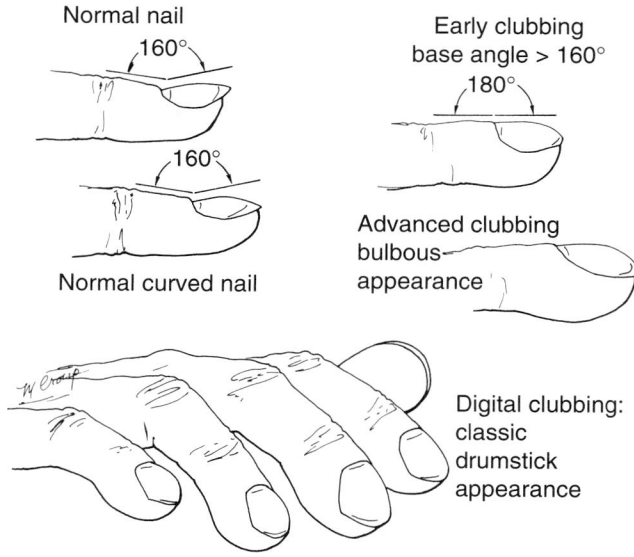

FIG. 37-1   Digital clubbing.

bing are associated with chronic diseases of the GI tract, including the liver. Bronchogenic carcinoma is the single leading cause of digital clubbing and hypertrophic osteoarthropathy. Box 37-1 lists some conditions that are typically associated with digital clubbing.

Digital clubbing must be detected as early as possible because of its diagnostic significance. The earliest sign is a loss of the angle between the nail and the dorsum of the terminal phalanx; this angle is normally 160 degrees. Fig. 37-1 illustrates the normal variations and early and advanced clubbing. In early clubbing the skin at the base of the nail may have a shiny appearance, and gentle pressure on the nail root reveals a spongy feeling (floating nail). Normally, the nail plate rests firmly against the bone. Early clubbing must be differentiated from the normal curved nail that is common in African Americans. If the normal curved nail is viewed from the side, the base angle is still approximately 160 degrees. In early clubbing, the base angle of the nail becomes greater than 160 degrees. As the condition progresses, the tissue at the root of the nail becomes heaped up, and the curvature of the nail becomes pronounced, until the soft tissue of the digit tip becomes bulbous, producing the classic drumstick appearance.

A condition closely related to digital clubbing is *hypertrophic osteoarthropathy (HOA)*, which is characterized by digital clubbing, periosteal new bone formation, and arthritis. HOA occurs most frequently in bronchogenic carcinoma and may be confused with arthritis. HOA may precede the radiographic appearance of lung cancer by many months. Patients may experience severe skeletal pain before the appearance of clubbing or HOA. Other joints besides the digits may be affected by HOA.

The pathogenic mechanism of digital clubbing and HOA is poorly understood. A popular hypothesis ascribes clubbing to hypoxia, but this premise fails to explain its presence in many conditions in which hypoxia is absent or in conditions in which hypoxia is present but clubbing is absent. For example, the devolvement of clubbing and HOA often develops early in bronchogenic carcinoma and is not associated with arterial desaturation. Curiously, the chronic hypoxia of chronic obstructive pulmonary disease (COPD) is rarely associated with clubbing; but the chronic hypoxia of tetralogy of Fallot is often associated with severe clubbing. One theory by Martinez-Lavin (1987) suggests that digital clubbing and HOA develop because of a growth factor present in the circulation that is normally inactivated by the lungs. This presence occurs because a fraction of the blood bypasses the lungs in cases of congenital heart malformations and to a lesser degree in lung cancer and cirrhosis of the liver. Subsequent research supports this theory with identification of the specific platelet-derived growth factor responsible for HOA and evidence that patients with HOA have signs of platelet-endothelial cell activation.

SIGNS OF INADEQUATE GAS EXCHANGE

Cyanosis

Cyanosis is a bluish coloration of the skin and mucous membranes that develops as a result of an increase in the absolute amount of reduced hemoglobin (hemoglobin [Hb] not united with O_2). Cyanosis may be a sign of respiratory insufficiency, although this indication is highly unreliable. There are two types of cyanosis: central and peripheral. *Central cyanosis* resulting from insufficient oxygenation of Hb in the lungs is most easily observed on the face, lips, and earlobes and under the tongue. Cyanosis is generally not detected until the absolute amount of reduced Hb is 5 g/dl or more in a person with normal Hb concentration (oxygen saturation [Sao$_2$] less than 90%). The normal amount of reduced Hb in the capillary bed is 2.5 g/dl. In the person with a normal Hb concentration, Sao$_2$ is approximately 75%, and the arterial oxygen tension (Pao$_2$) is 50 mm Hg or less when cyanosis is first detected. Anemic patients (low Hb concentration) may never become cyanotic, even though they have severe tissue hypoxia, because the absolute amount of reduced Hg is not likely to reach 5 g/dl. On the other hand, a person with polycythemia (high Hb concentration) can easily have 5 g/dl of reduced Hb when only mild hypoxia occurs. Other factors that make cyanosis difficult to recognize are variations in skin thickness, pigmentation, and lighting conditions.

In addition to cyanosis caused by respiratory insufficiency (central cyanosis), *peripheral cyanosis* occurs when severely reduced blood flow causes a great reduction in the venous saturation, thereby turning an area blue. Peripheral cyanosis may result from cardiac insufficiency, obstruction of blood flow, or vasoconstriction resulting from cold temperatures.

Small amounts of circulating methemoglobin and even smaller amounts of sulfhemoglobin can produce cyanosis, although these causes occur infrequently. These variations in cause and the difficulty in recognizing cyanosis make it an unreliable sign of respiratory insufficiency.

Hypoxemia and Hypoxia

The term *hypoxemia* refers to values of Pao$_2$ that are abnormally low and is frequently associated with *hypoxia*, or inadequate tissue oxygenation. Hypoxemia is not necessarily accompanied by tissue hypoxia. A patient can have normal tissue oxygenation with hypoxemia, just as another can have a normal Pao$_2$ with tissue hypoxia (because of the abnormalities of O$_2$ delivery and utilization by the cells, discussed in Chapter 35). A relationship exists, however, between the Pao$_2$ and tissue hypoxia, although the precise Pao$_2$ at which impairment of tissue use of O$_2$ occurs is variable. All things being equal, the more rapid the onset of hypoxemia is, the more extensive the tissue abnormalities will be. Generally, Pao$_2$ values that are persistently less than 50 mm Hg are associated with tissue hypoxia and acidosis (caused by anaerobic metabolism). Because hypoxia may exist with both normal and low values of Pao$_2$, evaluation of blood gas measurements must always be correlated with clinical observation of the patient. Cyanosis is an unreliable sign of hypoxia because Sao$_2$ must be less than 75% in patients with normal Hb before it is detectable. Table 37-3 lists clinical signs and laboratory findings that indicate hypoxia.

Hypercapnia and Hypocapnia

Just as ventilation is considered adequate when O$_2$ supply is matched with O$_2$ demand, CO$_2$ elimination through the lungs must also be matched with CO$_2$ production for adequate ventilation. Because CO$_2$ is highly diffusible, the CO$_2$ tensions are equal in alveolar air and arterial blood; thus Paco$_2$ is the direct and immediate reflection of the alveolar ventilation in relation to the metabolic rate. Thus the Paco$_2$ is used to assess the adequacy of alveolar ventilation ($\dot{V}_A$) because CO$_2$ elimination by the lungs is proportional to $\dot{V}_A$ and therefore the Paco$_2$ is directly related to CO$_2$ production ($\dot{V}co_2$) and inversely related to alveolar ventilation: Paco$_2$ α $\dot{V}co_2/\dot{V}_A$. Adequate ventilation maintains the Paco$_2$ at approximately 40 mm Hg. *Hypercapnia* is defined as a rise in the Paco$_2$ above 45 mm Hg; *hypocapnia* occurs when the Paco$_2$ is less than 35 mm Hg. The direct cause of CO$_2$ retention is alveolar hypoventila-

---

TABLE 37-3　■ ■ ■

Indicators of Hypoxemia and Hypoxia

Blood Gases/System	Laboratory Findings/Clinical Signs
Arterial blood gases	Pao$_2$*: 80-100 mm Hg (normal)
	60-80 mm Hg (mild hypoxemia)
	40-60 mm Hg (moderate hypoxemia)
	<40 mm Hg (severe hypoxemia)
	Sao$_2$: 95%-97% (normal)
	<90% (may indicate hypoxemia)
	pH: 7.35-7.45 (normal)
	<7.35 (acidemia)
	>7.45 (alkalemia)
	Paco$_2$: 35-45 mm Hg (normal)
	>45 mm Hg (hypoventilation)
	<35 mm Hg (hyperventilation)
Respiratory system	Tachypnea, decreased tidal volume, dyspnea, yawning, use of accessory respiratory muscles, flared nostrils
Central nervous system	Headache (from cerebral vasodilation)
	Mental confusion, bizarre behavior, restlessness
	Agitation, anxious facial expression, sweating
	Drowsiness progressing to coma when hypoxia is severe
Cardiovascular system	Tachycardia early; bradycardia later when the heart muscle is not receiving adequate O$_2$
	Rise in blood pressure followed by a drop when hypoxia remains uncorrected; dysrhythmias
Skin	Cyanosis of lips, oral mucosa, and nailbeds

*Pao$_2$ values are for a person less than 60 years of age breathing room air; subtract 1 mm Hg for each year person is over 60 years of age to obtain lower limits of normal.

tion (ventilation inadequate to cope with CO_2 production). Hypercapnia is always accompanied by some degree of hypoxia when the patient is breathing room air.

The major causes of hypercapnia are obstructive airways disease, respiratory depressant drugs, weakness or paralysis of the respiratory muscles, chest trauma or abdominal surgery causing shallow respirations, and loss of lung tissue. Clinical signs associated with hypercapnia are mental confusion progressing to coma, headache (as a result of cerebral vasodilation), asterixis or flapping tremor of the outstretched hands, and a pulse of large volume with warm, sweaty extremities (as a result of the peripheral vasodilation caused by the hypercapnia). In chronic hypercapnia resulting from chronic pulmonary disease, the patient may become abnormally tolerant to

the high $PaCO_2$; thus the principal drive to respiration is hypoxia. Under these circumstances, if O_2 is administered at a high concentration, respiration is then diminished, and the hypercapnia is increased.

Excessive loss of CO_2 from the lungs (hypocapnia) occurs when hyperventilation occurs (ventilation in excess of metabolic need to remove CO_2). Common causes of hyperventilation are listed in Chapter 36 and include excessive mechanical ventilation, anxiety states, cerebral trauma, aspirin poisoning, and compensatory response to hypoxia. Signs and symptoms typically associated with hypocapnia include frequent sighing and yawning, dizziness, palpitations, tingling and numbness in the extremities, and muscular twitches. Severe hypocapnia ($PaCO_2$ less than 25 mm Hg) may cause convulsions.

KEY CONCEPTS

- *Cough* is a protective reflex caused by irritation of the tracheobronchial tree as a result of mechanical, chemical, or inflammatory stimuli. Coughing is a physiologic mechanism for the clearing of excess secretions and protecting the airways from food or foreign material entering the airways.
- Coughing is the most common symptom of respiratory disease; any cough persisting for longer than 3 weeks should be investigated to determine the cause.
- *Cough* is generally characterized by whether it is *productive or nonproductive* of sputum.
- The healthy person produces about 100 ml of mucus in the respiratory tract per day, which is transported to the pharynx by the ciliary clearance mechanism.
- Excessive sputum production is commonly present in respiratory diseases that cause an acute or chronic inflammation of the tracheobronchial tree, such as chronic bronchitis.
- *Yellow or green sputum* reflects the presence of numerous leukocytes and the presence of a suppurative process involving the airways or lung parenchyma, such as acute or chronic bronchitis or pneumonia.
- A foul odor to the sputum may indicate lung abscess or bronchiectasis.
- *Hemoptysis* is the coughing up of blood or blood-tinged sputum derived from the airways. Clinically, hemoptysis may be confused with blood that originates from the upper GI tract (hematemesis) and usually has a dark, coffee-ground appearance.
- Repeated expectoration of blood-streaked sputum is present in acute or chronic bronchitis, pneumonia, bronchogenic carcinoma, cystic fibrosis, tuberculosis, bronchiectasis and pulmonary embolism.
- *Dyspnea* or breathlessness is the subjective sensation of difficulty in breathing. Objective signs of breathlessness are the use of accessory muscles of respiration (sternocleidomastoids, scalenus, trapezius), nasal flaring, tachypnea, and hyperinflation.
- *Orthopnea* is the experience of dyspnea on assuming the recumbent position and is often described by the number of pillows needed to prevent the sensation.

- Increased volume of blood in the central thoracic blood vessels (normally present in the lower extremities while the patient is in the erect position) cause orthopnea.
- *Paroxysmal nocturnal dyspnea* is waking from sleep by the experience of dyspnea and is a prominent symptom of congestive heart failure. The cause is the increased central intravascular volume associated with the recumbent position and the mobilization of peripheral edema fluid into the central vasculature.
- *The American Thoracic Society dyspnea scale*, which relates the level of activity that induces the symptom, is a standard method of assessing dyspnea.
- The key factor that appears to determine whether dyspnea is experienced is whether the level of ventilation or effort is appropriate to the degree of activity.
- Common causes of dyspnea include cardiovascular disease, pulmonary emboli, interstitial or alveolar lung disease, obstructive lung disease, disorders of the chest wall or respiratory muscles, and anxiety.
- Chest *pain* as a reflection of respiratory disease originates in the chest wall, parietal pleura, large airways, or mediastinal structures because the lung parenchyma and visceral pleura are insensitive to pain.
- *Chest pain caused by pulmonary disease* is often produced by inflammation of the parietal pleura, which may be secondary to pneumonia, pulmonary embolism, tuberculosis, or a malignant tumor extending to the pleural surface. Pneumothorax commonly causes acute pleuritic pain.
- *Pleuritic pain* is a stabbing, localized pain that is exacerbated by deep inspiration and coughing and diminished by breath holding or splinting.
- *Pleuritic pain* must be differentiated from myocardial ischemia, pericarditis, involvement of the intercostal nerves by herpes zoster, and costochondritis.
- *Digital clubbing* is a change in the normal configuration of the distal phalanx and nails of the fingers and toes and is characterized by: (1) loss of the base

angle of the nail from the normal 160 degrees; (2) a spongy feeling at the nail base; and (3) a bulbous appearance of the fingertip.

- *Digital clubbing* may be associated with pulmonary disease (tuberculosis, lung abscess, or lung cancer), cardiovascular disease (tetralogy of Fallot or infective endocarditis), or chronic disease of the liver or GI tract.
- *Hypertrophic osteoarthropathy (HOA)* may accompany digital clubbing and is characterized by periosteal new bone formation, particularly in the long bones, and arthritis in several joints.
- *Bronchogenic carcinoma* is the single leading cause of *digital clubbing and HOA,* which may precede the radiologic appearance of the cancer by many months.
- The *pathogenic mechanism of digital clubbing and HOA* is poorly understood. Chronic hypoxia is not a cause because uncomplicated COPD is not associated with clubbing. One theory proposes that digital clubbing and HOA develop because of a growth factor present in the circulation that is normally inactivated by the lungs. This presence occurs because a fraction of the blood bypasses the lungs in cases of congenital heart malformations and to a lesser extent in lung cancer and liver cirrhosis.
- *Cyanosis* is a bluish discoloration of the skin (particularly under the nails) and mucous membranes as a result of an increased amount of reduced (deoxygenated) Hb in the capillaries (oxygenated hemoglobin in arterial blood is bright red; venous blood with deoxygenated Hb is bluish red).
- *Central cyanosis* results from insufficient oxygenation of Hb owing to a low PaO_2.
- *Peripheral cyanosis* results from stagnation of blood and its deoxygenation in the peripheral circulation resulting from peripheral vasoconstriction as in a cold environment, obstruction to blood flow, or low cardiac output.
- *Cyanosis* does not become perceptible until the mean concentration of reduced Hb is approximately 5 g/100 ml of blood. The total amount of Hb affects the likelihood of detecting cyanosis. Normally the tissues extract about 25% of the oxygen from Hb thus Hb is 75% saturated when it returns to the lungs to pick up another supply of O_2. A person with a normal Hb of 15 g/100 ml of blood would have only 3.75 g/100 ml (25% of 15) of reduced Hb, thus the person would not be cyanotic. An anemic person

with an Hb of 7 to 8 g/100 would be even less likely to show cyanosis, even when severely hypoxic. A person with polycythemia and hemoglobin of 20 g/100 ml would easily show cyanosis, even though the person is not hypoxic. Therefore cyanosis is an unreliable sign of respiratory insufficiency.

- *Hypoxia* is defined as inadequate O_2 at the tissue level (the area of clinical interest, even though it cannot be measured directly in clinical settings).
- *Hypoxemia* means that PaO_2 is below the normal 80 to 100 mm Hg. Hypoxemia is classified according to PaO_2 as *mild* (60 to 80 mm Hg), *moderate* (40 to 60 mm Hg), or *severe* (<40 Hg). Most medical centers classify hypoxemia with a PaO_2 of 50 mm Hg as respiratory failure because most people experience tissue hypoxia with O_2 tensions at this level.
- Signs and symptoms of hypoxemia and hypoxia are nonspecific and include tachypnea, dyspnea, headache, mental confusion, tachycardia, and cyanosis (late sign).
- Arterial blood gas measurements are the most reliable evidence of inadequate tissue oxygenation including: low PaO_2, pH <7.35 or >7.45, and SaO_2 <90%. Whenever hypoxemia and acidemia coexist, tissue hypoxia should be assumed because these two factors in combination drop oxygen content to critically low levels.
- The $PaCO_2$ is used to assess the adequacy of $\dot{V}_A$ because CO_2 elimination by the lungs is proportional to $\dot{V}_A$ and therefore the $PaCO_2$ is directly related to CO_2 production ($\dot{V}CO_2$) and inversely related to $\dot{V}_A$: $PaCO_2 \propto \dot{V}CO_2/\dot{V}_A$.
- *Hypercapnia* or respiratory acidosis is defined as a rise in the $PaCO_2$ >45 mm Hg. The direct cause is always alveolar hypoventilation (failure to eliminate CO_2 as fast as it is produced).
- Some degree of hypoxemia always accompanies hypercapnia thus separating the signs and symptoms specific to each is difficult.
- Common conditions associated with hypercapnia include COPD, respiratory center depressant drugs, weakness or paralysis of the respiratory muscles, chest trauma, or abdominal surgery causing shallow breathing.
- *Hypocapnia* or respiratory alkalosis is defined as a fall in the $PaCO_2$ <35 mm Hg. The direct cause is always alveolar hyperventilation (eliminating CO_2 faster than it is produced).

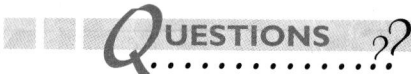

QUESTIONS ??

A sampling of review questions for this chapter appears here. Visit http://www.mosby.com/MERLIN/PriceWilson/ for additional questions.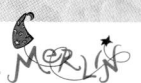

Match the signs and symptoms in column B with the possible causative factors in column A.
Each letter may be used only once.

Column A

1. _____ Interruption in the continuity of the pulmonary blood vessels
2. _____ Inflammation of the pleura
3. _____ Increase in the absolute amount of reduced hemoglobin
4. _____ Physical, chemical, or infectious insults to the mucous membrane of the respiratory tract
5. _____ Protective reflex initiated by irritation of the tracheobronchial tree
6. _____ Pathogenesis unknown; associated with early stage of bronchogenic carcinoma and with certain chronic respiratory, cardiovascular, and GI diseases
7. _____ Increased ventilatory work as correlated with the minimum level of activity sufficient for its induction

Column B

a. Cough
b. Excess sputum production
c. Hemoptysis
d. Dyspnea
e. Digital clubbing
f. Chest pain
g. Cyanosis

Answer the following questions on a separate sheet of paper.

8. What is digital clubbing? Why is it important to detect?

9. How would you detect cyanosis in an African-American patient?

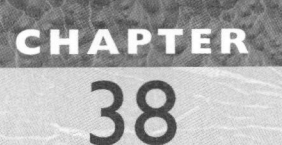

CHAPTER
38

Obstructive Patterns of Respiratory Disease

LORRAINE M. WILSON

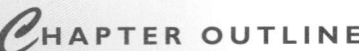

PATTERNS OF RESPIRATORY DISEASE

Respiratory diseases have been classified on the basis of etiology, anatomic site, chronicity, and changes in structure and function. None of these classifications is entirely satisfactory. The etiologic agents are unknown in some cases, whereas the same causal agent in others may affect different anatomic sites and produce different pathophysiologic effects. In this chapter and Chapter 39, respiratory diseases are classified according to ventilatory dysfunction and are divided into two categories: diseases that produce primarily an *obstructive ventilatory disorder* and those that produce a *restrictive ventilatory disorder*. This classification was chosen because spirometric and other tests of ventilatory function are carried out almost routinely, and most respiratory diseases affect ventilation. This approach has two limitations. In some respiratory disorders, the ventilatory abnormality may produce a mixed pattern (e.g., chronic emphysema with superimposed pneumonia), whereas in other disorders affecting respiration, ventilatory function may be normal (e.g., anemia, right-to-left shunt). The following pulmonary disorders, which do not readily fit into obstructive or restrictive patterns of disease, are discussed separately: cardiovascular diseases affecting the lung, respiratory insufficiency and failure, pulmonary neoplasms, and tuberculosis. Only the specific disorders that are most frequently encountered in hospital practice are considered.

CHRONIC OBSTRUCTIVE PULMONARY DISEASE

Chronic obstructive pulmonary disease (COPD) is a term often applied to a group of pulmonary diseases of long duration characterized by the main pathophysiologic feature of increased resistance to airflow. Chronic bronchitis, pulmonary emphysema, and bronchial asthma make up the entity known as COPD. An etiologic and sequential relationship appears to exist between chronic bronchitis and emphysema that does not appear to exist between these two diseases and asthma. This relationship is particularly true in regard to etiology, pathogenesis, and treatment, as discussed later in this chapter.

Chronic bronchitis is a clinical disorder characterized by excessive production of mucus in the bronchi and is manifested by a chronic cough and production of sputum for a minimum of 3 months per year for at least 2 consecutive years. This definition assumes that diseases such as bronchiectasis and tuberculosis, which also cause chronic cough and sputum production, have been excluded. The sputum produced in chronic bronchitis may be mucoid or mucopurulent.

Pulmonary emphysema is an anatomic alteration of the lung parenchyma characterized by abnormal enlargement of the alveoli and alveolar ducts and destruction of the alveolar walls. Emphysema can be diagnosed with certainty using high resolution computed tomography (CT) scanning.

Asthma is a disease characterized by hypersensitivity of the tracheobronchial tree to various stimuli and is manifested by periodic, reversible airway narrowing resulting from bronchospasm.

Worthy of note is the different bases of the definitions of the preceding diseases: chronic bronchitis is defined by clinical symptoms, pulmonary emphysema by pathologic anatomy, and asthma by clinical pathologic physiology. Although each disease may exist in its pure form, chronic bronchitis and emphysema usually exist together in the same patient. Asthma is easily separated from chronic bronchitis and emphysema on the basis of a history of paroxysmal attacks of wheezing beginning in childhood and associated with allergies. Occasionally,

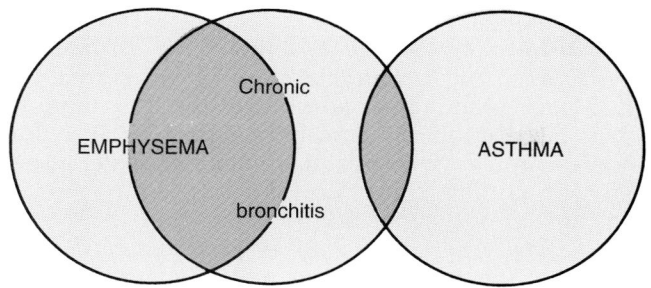

FIG. 38-1   Interrelationship between the disease entities making up COPD.

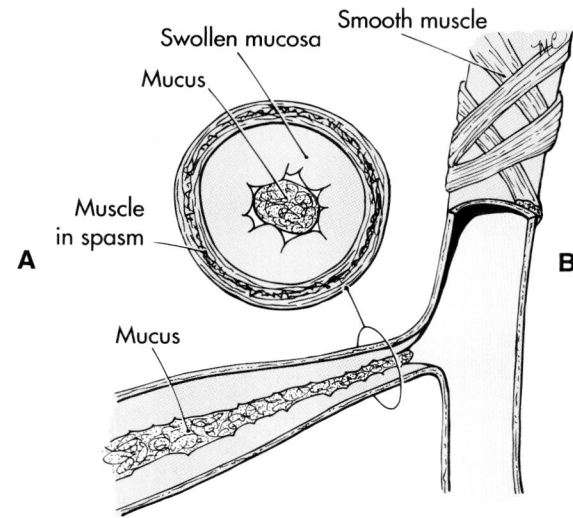

FIG. 38-2   Factors causing expiratory obstruction in bronchial asthma. **A,** Cross section of bronchiole occluded by muscle spasm, swollen mucosa, and mucus in lumen. **B,** Longitudinal section of bronchiole.

however, patients with chronic bronchitis have asthmatic features to their disease. Fig. 38-1 illustrates the interrelationship of chronic bronchitis, asthma, and emphysema. The darkly shaded areas represent individuals with features of more than one disease; the lightly shaded areas represent each disease in the predominantly pure form. For purposes of clarity, asthma is considered separately from chronic bronchitis and emphysema because asthma is more easily separated from the other two diseases. A detailed discussion of asthma is included in Chapter 10.

Asthma

The term *asthma* comes from the Greek word for *panting* and means attacks of shortness of breath. Although, in the past, this term has been used for the clinical picture of shortness of breath resulting from any cause, today asthma is confined to a condition of abnormal responsiveness of the air passages to various stimuli, causing widespread airway narrowing.

The pathologic changes involved in airway obstruction are found in the medium-sized bronchi and in bronchioles as small as 1 mm in diameter. Airway narrowing is caused by bronchospasm, mucosal edema, and hypersecretion of viscous mucus (Fig. 38-2).

Asthma can be divided into three categories. *Extrinsic*, or *allergic*, *asthma*, found in a minority of adult patients, is clearly caused by a known allergen. This form generally begins in childhood in a member of a family with a history of atopic diseases, including hay fever, eczema, and dermatitis, as well as asthma. Allergic asthma results from the sensitization of the person to an allergen, usually a protein, in the form of an inhaled pollen, animal dander, mold spores, feathers, dust, lint, or, less often, to a food such as milk or chocolate. Exposure to the allergen, even in minute quantities, produces an asthmatic attack. *Intrinsic*, or *idiopathic*, *asthma*, on the other hand, is characterized by the absence of clearly defined precipitating factors. Nonspecific factors such as the common cold, exercise, or emotion may trigger the asthmatic attack. The intrinsic type of asthma is more apt to develop after age 40 years, with the onset of attacks after infections of the nasal sinuses or tracheobronchial tree. The attacks become more frequent over time, and the condition merges into chronic bronchitis and, sometimes, emphysema. Most patients develop *mixed asthma*, which is composed of components of both extrinsic and intrinsic asthmas. Patients with intrinsic asthma often later develop the

mixed type; children who have the extrinsic type often have complete recovery at adolescence.

The pathogenesis of asthma is discussed in Chapter 10. The clinical manifestations are easy to recognize. After exposure to the causative allergen or precipitating factor, dyspnea may begin suddenly. Patients feel as though they are suffocating and must stand or sit up and devote all their energy to breathing. On the basis of the anatomic changes previously described, the apparent major difficulty is with expiration. The tracheobronchial tree widens and lengthens during inspiration, but forcing air out of the constricted, edematous, mucus-filled bronchioles, which normally contract to a certain degree during expiration, is difficult. Air is trapped distal to the obstruction, thus progressive hyperinflation of the lungs occurs. Prolonged wheezing expirations are thus characteristic as the patient struggles to force the air out. An asthmatic attack usually lasts from a few minutes to several hours, followed by a cough that is productive of considerable whitish sputum. Treatment consists of administration of bronchodilator drugs, specific long-term desensitization, avoidance of known allergens, and occasionally administration of corticosteroid drugs. Intervals between attacks are characteristically free from respiratory difficulty. Asthma is distinguished from chronic bronchitis and emphysema by its intermittent nature and the fact that destructive emphysema rarely occurs. An asthmatic attack that continues for days and is intractable to ordinary methods of treatment is called *status asthmaticus*. In these patients, ventilatory function may be so impaired as to result in cyanosis and death (see Chapter 10).

Chronic Bronchitis and Emphysema

Although chronic bronchitis and emphysema represent two distinct processes, they are often found in combination in patients with COPD. An estimated 16.2 million

Americans have chronic bronchitis or emphysema or both, which was responsible for more than 112,584 deaths in 1998. The incidence of COPD has risen 450% since 1950 and is now the fourth leading cause of death. COPD affects men twice as often as it does women, presumably because men have been heavier smokers; however, the incidence of COPD in women has increased 600% since 1950, presumably reflecting their smoking behavior.

The main pathologic findings in chronic bronchitis are hypertrophy of the bronchial mucosal glands and an increase in the number and size of goblet cells, accompanied by inflammatory cell infiltration and edema of the bronchial mucosa. The resulting increased production of mucus leads to the characteristic symptoms of cough and expectoration. The chronic cough in the presence of increased bronchial secretions appears to affect the minute bronchioles to the point of destruction and dilation of their walls. The primary etiologic factors appear to be cigarette smoking and the forms of air pollution common to the industrial environment. Continued air pollution also predisposes to recurrent infections by slowing down ciliary and phagocytic activity, causing increased mucus accumulation at the same time that defense mechanisms are weakened.

Emphysema is classified according to the pattern of involvement of the acini. Although several morphologic patterns have been described, two types are most important in relation to COPD. *Centrilobular emphysema (CLE)* selectively affects the respiratory bronchioles and alveolar ducts. Fenestrations develop in the walls, enlarge, be-

come confluent, and tend to form a single space as the walls disintegrate (Fig. 38-3). Initially, the more distal alveolar ducts and sacs and the alveoli are preserved. CLE usually affects the upper portions of the lung more severely, but distribution tends to be uneven. CLE is more prevalent in men than it is in women, is usually associated with chronic bronchitis, and is seldom found in nonsmokers.

Panlobular emphysema (PLE), or *panacinar emphysema*, is a less common morphologic pattern characterized by nearly uniform enlargement and destruction of the alveoli distal to the terminal bronchiole; both the central and the peripheral portions of the acinus are involved (see Fig. 38-3). As the disease progresses, gradual loss of all components of the acinus occurs until only a few strands of tissue remain, which are usually blood vessels. PLE is characteristically uniform in distribution throughout the lung, although the basal sections tend to be more severely affected. PLE, but not CLE, is associated with a small group of patients with primary emphysema. This form of emphysema, which is characterized by the insidious development of increased airway resistance without evidence of chronic bronchitis, has an early onset and usually produces symptoms between ages 30 and 40 years. In England, fewer than 6% of patients with COPD have *primary emphysema*, which affects women as often as it does men. The cause of this form of emphysema is unknown, but a familial type associated with a deficiency of the enzyme alpha₁-antiprotease has been described.

Alpha₁-antiprotease has been established as essential in protection of the lung against the naturally occurring

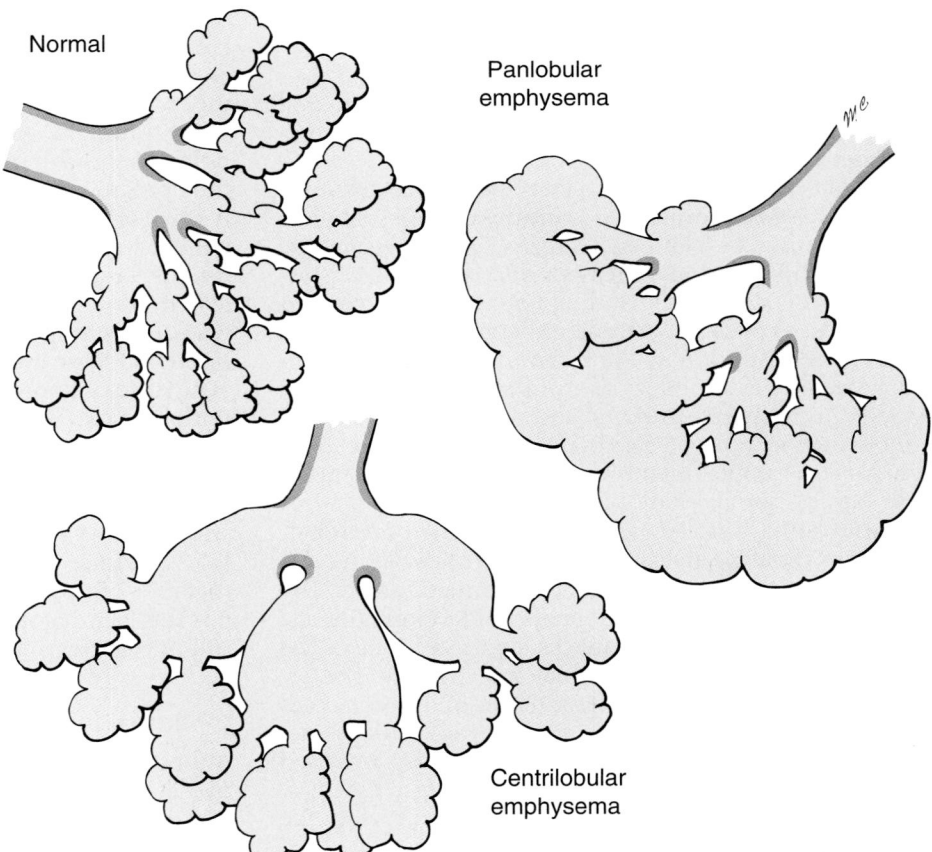

Normal

Panlobular
emphysema

Centrilobular
emphysema

FIG. 38-3 Morphologic types of emphysema. Panlobular: entire pulmonary lobule involved; destruction and distention distal to the respiratory bronchioles. Centrilobular: destruction is central, primarily involving the respiratory bronchioles.

proteases and that a deficiency of this antiprotease plays a role in the pathogenesis of emphysema. Proteases are produced by bacteria, polymorphonuclear neutrophils (PMNs), monocytes, and macrophages during the phagocytic process (see Chapter 4) and have the ability to break down the elastin and other macromolecules in lung tissue. In the healthy person, lung tissue damage is prevented by the action of antiproteases, which inhibit protease activity. This discovery was based on the study of a small group of patients with an inherited deficiency of alpha₁-antiprotease.* Genetic typing has revealed that most members of the normal population with normal levels of alpha₁-antiprotease have two M genes and are designated as type MM. Two of the most common genes associated with emphysema are the S and Z genes. Homozygous SS or ZZ individuals have serum levels of alpha₁-antiprotease that are near zero or very low and have a 70% to 80% chance of developing emphysema of the primary type (panlobular or emphysematous). Heterozygous MS or MZ individuals with one abnormal gene have intermediate levels of alpha₁-antiprotease and are believed to have an increased predisposition to develop emphysema, usually of the bronchitic type (centrilobular). In patients of the latter group, smoking can produce an inflammatory response with consequent release of proteolytic enzymes (proteases), while, at the same time, the oxidants in smoke inhibit alpha₁-antiprotease. The heterozygous state is common, with an estimated incidence of 5% to 14% of the general population affected.

PLE, although characteristic of primary emphysema, may also be associated with the emphysema of aging and with chronic bronchitis. It is believed that the deterioration of the elastic and reticular fibers of the lung, with the resultant loss of elastic recoil of the lung, leads to progressive generalized distention of the lung in the aging process. *Senile emphysema*, however, is not true emphysema because most of these older patients do not develop significant impairment of lung function. The PLE associated with chronic bronchitis is thought to be an end stage of progressive CLE because both morphologic patterns may exist in the same lung.

When the thorax of a patient who has emphysema is opened during surgery or at autopsy, the lungs are grossly enlarged; they remain filled with air and do not collapse. The lungs are whiter than normal and feel downy or billowy. Subpleural air-filled spaces called *blebs* and parenchymal air-filled spaces greater than 1 cm in diameter called *bullae* are typically observed (Fig. 38-4). Generalized dilation of the air spaces also occurs. Bullae are common in both PLE and CLE but may exist in the absence of either. Bullae generally develop because of a check-valve bronchiolar obstruction (Fig. 38-5). During inspiration, the bronchiolar lumen widens so that air is able to pass by the obstruction caused by thickening of the mucosa and excess mucus. During expiration, however, when the bronchiolar lumen normally becomes narrowed, the obstruction may prevent the egress of air. A loss of elasticity of the bronchiolar walls in emphysema may also cause premature collapse. Air is thus trapped in the affected pulmonary segment, leading to overdisten-

tion and coalescence of several alveoli. This effect is caused by fragmentation of the interalveolar elastic tissue and subsequent rupture of the attenuated interalveolar septa, resulting in a bulla. In emphysema, a single bulla or many bullae, which may or may not communicate

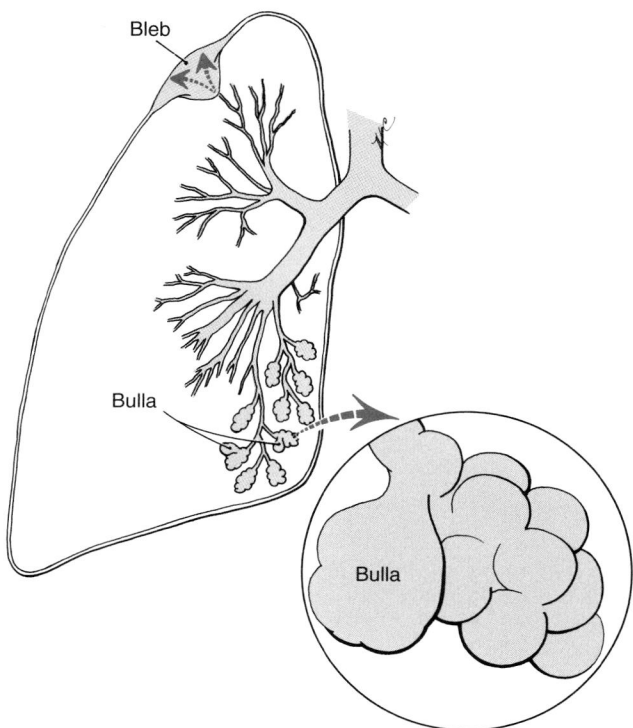

FIG. 38-4 Pulmonary blebs and bullae.

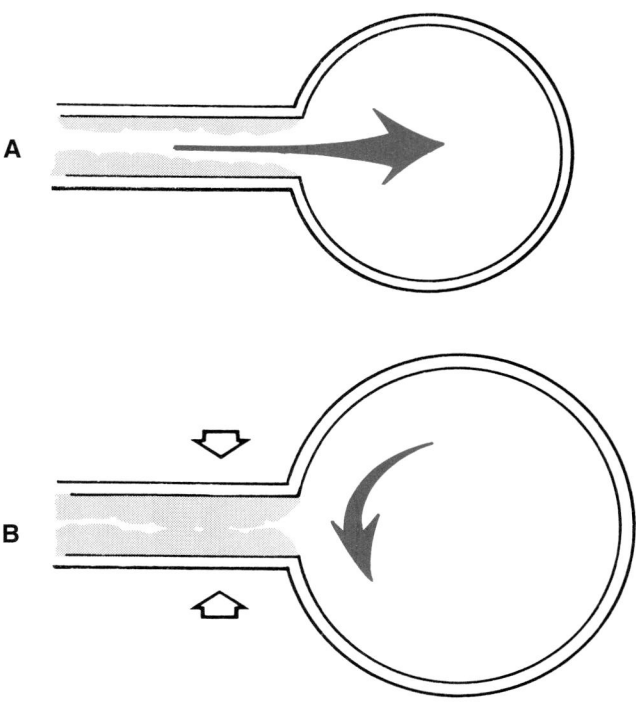

FIG. 38-5 Check-valve bronchiolar obstruction. **A,** During inspiration, lumen widens enough to allow air entry. **B,** During expiration, premature collapse and narrowed lumen prevent egress of air that becomes trapped in alveoli.

---

*Formerly known as *alpha₁-antitrypsin,* alpha₁-antiprotease is so named because it has been found to inhibit the action of other proteases, as well as trypsin.

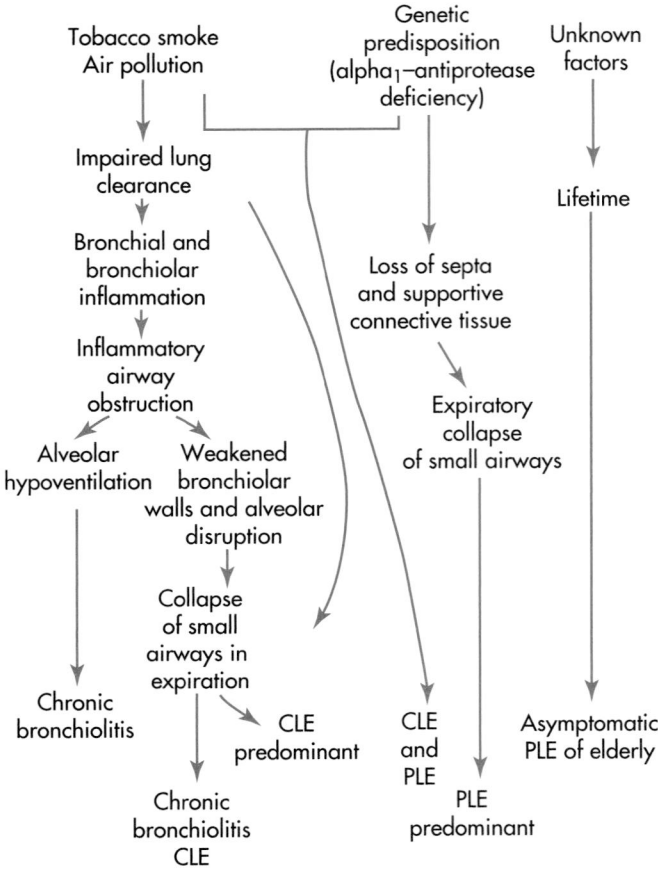

FIG. 38-6 Pathogenesis of COPD. *CLE,* Centrilobular emphysema; *PLE,* panlobular emphysema. (Modified from *Chronic obstructive pulmonary disease: a manual for physicians,* ed 3, New York, 1972, National Tuberculosis and Respiratory Disease Association.)

with each other, may be present. Blebs, which are formed by ruptured alveoli, may rupture into the pleural cavity and cause a spontaneous pneumothorax (collapse of the lung). Other changes frequently observed in the COPD lung are a reduction in the capillary bed and histologic evidence of chronic bronchiolitis (involvement of the minute bronchioles).

The flow diagram in Fig. 38-6 illustrates the pathogenesis of COPD and the morphologic types of emphysema that result. This diagram emphasizes that although a genetic predisposition may be a factor in the development of pulmonary emphysema and smoking and air pollution are the prime factors in the pathogenesis of the bronchitic type of emphysema, an interaction exists between the two. For example, people with a genetic predisposition might develop emphysema if exposed to varying degrees of air pollution. Although senile dilation of the air spaces is not considered true emphysema, normal loss of elasticity of the lung parenchyma associated with aging is a possible factor in the development of true emphysema.

The clinical course of patients with COPD ranges from what is known as the pink puffers to the blue bloaters. The clinical hallmark of *pink puffers* (associated with primary PLE) is the development of dyspnea without significant cough and sputum production. Usually, the dys-

pnea begins between ages 30 and 40 years and becomes increasingly severe. In advanced disease, the patient may be too breathless to eat and has a characteristically thin, wasted appearance. Later in the course of the disease, the pink puffer may develop secondary chronic bronchitis. The chest of the patient is barrel shaped; the diaphragm is low and moves poorly. Polycythemia and cyanosis are rare (thus the term *pink*), and cor pulmonale (heart disease resulting from pulmonary hypertension and lung disease) rarely develops until the terminal stage. Minimal ventilation/perfusion imbalance occurs; thus by hyperventilating, the pink puffer is usually able to keep blood gases within the normal range until late in the course of the disease. The lungs are usually greatly enlarged thus total lung capacity (TLC) and residual volume (RV) increase greatly.

At the other extreme of the COPD range are the *blue bloaters* (bronchitis with little evidence of obstructive emphysema). These patients usually have a productive cough and frequent respiratory infections that continue for years before functional impairment is noticeable. Eventually, however, they develop dyspnea on exertion. These patients show a diminished respiratory drive; they hypoventilate and become hypoxic and hypercapnic. The ventilation/perfusion (V/Q) ratio is also extremely distorted. The chronic hypoxia stimulates the kidney to produce erythropoietin, which, in turn, stimulates increased production of red blood cells, resulting in secondary polycythemia. Hemoglobin (Hb) levels may be 20 g/dl or higher, and cyanosis is more readily apparent because a 5 g/dl reduction of Hb readily occurs when only a small proportion of the circulating blood Hb is in the reduced form (thus the name *blue bloater*). Because these patients are not dyspneic at rest, they appear to be comfortable. A great weight loss usually does not occur, and body build is normal. The TLC may be normal, and the diaphragm is in the normal position. Death usually results from cor pulmonale (which develops early) or from respiratory failure. At autopsy, emphysema is often, although not always, present. The emphysema tends to be of the centrilobular type, although the panlobular type may also be present.

Table 38-1 contrasts the pure bronchitic (blue bloater) and emphysematous (pink puffer) types of COPD. Most patients with COPD lie somewhere between these two extremes.

The typical course of COPD is long, beginning in the patient's 20s and 30s with a "cigarette cough" or "morning cough" and the production of a small amount of mucoid sputum. Minor respiratory infections tend to persist longer than is usual in these patients. Although exercise tolerance may decrease somewhat, it is usually unnoticed as the patient becomes less energetic over time. Eventually, episodes of acute bronchitis occur more regularly, particularly in the winter, and the patient's working capacity decreases; thus work may have to be given up sometime in the patient's 50s or 60s. In patients of the predominantly emphysematous type, the course appears to be less protracted, with no previous history of a productive cough; severe debilitating dyspnea may develop within a few years. When hypercapnia, hypoxemia, and cor pulmonale develop, the prognosis is poor and death usually comes within a few years after the onset. A com-

TABLE 38-1   ▪▪▪

Differentiation of Clinical Types of COPD

Feature	Pink Puffer (Emphysematous)	Blue Bloater (Bronchitic)
Onset	30 to 40 years of age	20s and 30s: cigarette cough
Age at time of diagosis	60± years	50± years
Cause	Unknown factors	Unknown factors
	Genetic predisposition	Smoking
	Smoking	Air pollution
	Air pollution	Climate
Sputum	Minimal	Copious
Dypsnea	Relatively early	Relatively late
$\dot{V}/\dot{Q}$ ratio	Minimal $\dot{V}/\dot{Q}$ imbalance	Marked $\dot{V}/\dot{Q}$ imbalance
Body build	Thin, asthenic	Well nourished
Anteroposterior diameter of chest	Barrel chest common	Not increased
Pathologic lung anatomy	Panlobular emphysema	Centrilobular emphysema predominant
Respiratory pattern	Hyperventilation and marked dyspnea, which may occur at rest	Diminished respiratory drive
		Hypoventilation common, with resultant hypoxia and hypercapnia
Lung volume	Low FEV_1	Low FEV_1
	Increased TLC and RV	Normal TLC; moderate increase in RV
Pa_{CO_2}	Normal or low (35-40 mm Hg)	Elevated (50-60 mm Hg)
Pa_{O_2}	65-75 mm Hg	45-60 mm Hg
Sa_{O_2}	Normal	Much desaturation because of $\dot{V}/\dot{Q}$ imbalance
Hematocrit	35%-45%	50%-55%
Polycythemia	Hemoglobin and hematocrit normal until late	Elevated hemoglobin and hematocrit common
Cyanosis	Rare	Common
Cor pulmonale	Rare, except terminally	Frequent, with many episodes

$\dot{V}/\dot{Q}$, Ventilation/perfusion; Pa_{CO_2}, Pa_{O_2}, arterial carbon dioxide, oxygen tensions; Sa_{O_2}, oxygen saturation; FEV_1, forced expiratory volume in 1 second; *TLC*, total lung capacity; *RV*, residual volume.

bination of respiratory failure and heart failure precipitated by pneumonia is the usual cause of death.

Treatment of COPD

Table 38-2 summarizes the goals and modalities of treatment for patients with COPD. Therapy for the patient with chronic bronchitis and obstructive emphysema requires measures to relieve obstruction of the small airways. Although airway collapse secondary to emphysema is irreversible, many patients have some degree of bronchospasm, retention of secretions, and mucosal edema, which may be relieved by the appropriate therapy. Of paramount importance is cessation of smoking and avoidance of other forms of air pollution or allergens that may aggravate symptoms. Often the cessation of smoking alone may bring about a marked relief of symptoms and improvement of ventilation. Infection should be treated promptly, and patients who are particularly susceptible to respiratory infection may be directed to use prophylactic antibiotics. The patient is instructed to seek this medication whenever dyspnea or the amount of sputum production increases. *Streptococcus pneumoniae* and *Haemophilus influenzae* are the organisms most frequently implicated. Thus the antibiotic of choice often allows coverage of these organisms. All patients should receive pneumococcus and influenza vaccines.

Additional measures to relieve airway obstruction include provision of adequate hydration to thin bronchial secretions, use of expectorants, and use of bronchodilator drugs to relieve smooth muscle spasm. Sympathomimetic

TABLE 21-1   ▪▪▪

COPD Treatment Goals and Modalities

Goal	Modality
1. Remove bronchial irritants	Smoking cessation
2. Prevent/treat infection	Antibiotics; influenza and pneumococcus vaccines
3. Relieve bronchospasm	Bronchodilator drugs
4. Remove bronchial secretions	Percussion and postural drainage; hydration
5. Promote effective breathing	Breathing exercises
6. Prevent/delay pulmonary hypertension and cor pulmonale	Continuous low flow oxygen therapy
7. Improve exercise tolerance	Exercise program
8. Promote protease-antiprotease	α_1-antitrypsin replacement therapy
9. Improve elastic recoil of lungs	Surgical resection (selected cases)

drugs such as albuterol, terbutaline, and xanthines (e.g., aminophylline) are commonly administered. Ipratropium bromide (Atrovent), an anticholinergic agent in a metered-dose inhaler, is an effective bronchodilator in patients with chronic bronchitis. For patients with copious secretions, percussion and postural drainage are used to assist in removing obstructive secretions, which may also predispose the patient to infection. Breathing exercises may also be helpful. The patient is taught to use slow, relaxed expiration against pursed lips. This exercise prevents collapse of small bronchioles and reduces the amount of trapped air.

An important adjunct to therapy is the administration of supplemental oxygen (O_2) to patients with COPD who have significant hypoxemia (arterial O_2 [PaO_2] 55 to 60 mm Hg or less). A low flow rate of O_2 of 1 to 2 L/min given by nasal prongs delivers 24% to 28% O_2 and is effective and well tolerated. Several studies have demonstrated the beneficial effects of long-term O_2 therapy for patients with COPD. Continuous oxygen therapy was shown to be more beneficial in extending life than giving O_2 only for 12 hours at night. Some of the most important effects are the alleviation of pulmonary hypertension and cor pulmonale and improvement of exercise tolerance (hypoxemia causes pulmonary vasoconstriction, leading to pulmonary hypertension and cor pulmonale as discussed in Chapter 40). O_2 therapy also relieves the polycythemia (with hematocrit >50%) frequently present in patients with COPD. Polycythemia is a compensatory response to the chronic hypoxemia of COPD but results in increased blood viscosity and aggravation of pulmonary hypertension. An exercise program, such as walking, results in improved exercise tolerance and sense of well-being but does not improve lung function.

Replacement therapy with α_1-antitrypsin (AAT) for patients with familial AAT deficiency is currently under investigation to determine whether the disease course can be altered by this augmentation therapy. The rationale for this therapy is to replace the deficient protease inhibitor and try to inhibit or prevent unchecked proteolytic destruction of alveolar tissue. AAT is prepared from pooled human plasma and administered intravenously at weekly or monthly intervals. Initial results show that treated patients experienced a lower rate of decline in forced expiratory volume in a one-second period (FEV_1) and a lower rate of mortality compared with the untreated control group. The annual cost of AAT therapy is high and is estimated to be $25,000 to $35,000.

Two types of surgical treatment have been used experimentally to treat selected patients with severe COPD: lung volume reduction surgery and lung transplantation. *Lung volume reduction surgery* involves removing multiple regions of overdistended lung in patients with diffuse nonhomogeneous emphysema for the purpose of improving elastic recoil and improving diaphragm muscle function. The second approach to end-stage COPD is *lung transplantation,* but this option is limited because of the shortage of donor organs and the large number of patients in need.

Finally, *mechanical ventilation* may be needed to maintain acceptable blood gases when acute respiratory failure develops because of superimposed respiratory infection or progression to end-stage disease. Acute respiratory failure is discussed in Chapter 41.

BRONCHIECTASIS

Bronchiectasis is a condition characterized by chronic dilation of the medium-sized bronchi and bronchioles (about fourth to ninth generations). Two anatomic types are usually described: saccular and cylindric (Fig. 38-7). *Saccular bronchiectasis* consists of rounded cavity-like dilations, often found in dilated bronchi and typically in adults. Bronchiectasis develops when the bronchial walls

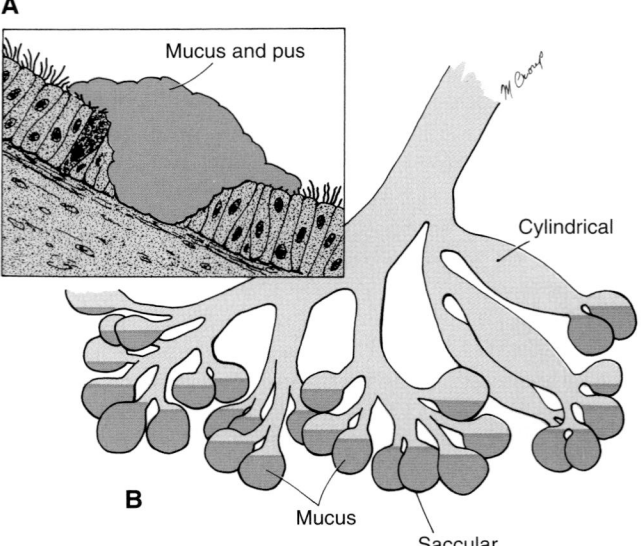

FIG. 38-7 Pathologic changes in bronchiectasis. **A,** Longitudinal section of bronchial wall: chronic infection causes damage to bronchial walls. **B,** Collection of purulent material in dilated bronchioles leading to persistent infection.

are weakened by chronic inflammatory changes involving the mucosa and muscular coat. As shown in Fig. 38-7, purulent materials collect in these dilated areas and lead to persistent infection of the affected segment or lobe. Chronic infection causes further damage to the bronchial walls, and a vicious circle is set up. No single, specific cause of bronchiectasis exists, because it is a disease based on an abnormal anatomic condition. Most often, bronchiectasis begins in childhood after repeated lower respiratory tract infections, which develop as a complication of measles, whooping cough, or influenza. Bronchial obstruction resulting from a neoplasm or an aspirated foreign body (especially if it is organic, such as a peanut) may also lead to bronchiectasis and secondary infection of the distal bronchial tree. Bronchiectasis of the upper lobes may be associated with tuberculosis, although it is frequently asymptomatic because bronchial drainage is achieved by gravity. Cystic fibrosis and Kartagener's syndrome (bronchiectasis associated with sinusitis and displacement of the heart to the right side of the thorax) are examples of congenital diseases associated with bronchiectasis.

The principal clinical feature of bronchiectasis is a chronic, loose cough productive of a large amount of mucopurulent, foul-smelling sputum. Coughing is most severe when the patient changes position. The amount of sputum varies with the stage of the disease but may be 200 ml daily in severe cases. Hemoptysis is common, usually consisting of blood streaks in the sputum. Characteristic features of advanced untreated disease are recurrent pneumonia, malnutrition, digital clubbing, cor pulmonale, and right ventricular failure.

The degree of functional disturbance depends on the extent of involvement of pulmonary tissue. Bronchiectasis localized to one or two segments of the lung may cause little impairment of pulmonary function, whereas diffuse bronchiectasis may be associated with anastomoses between the bronchial and pulmonary circulation, with resultant right-to-left shunting.

The most important feature of treatment is daily, vigorous bronchial hygiene with postural drainage, which generally must be continued for the rest of the patient's life. Bronchodilators to reduce airway obstruction and aid in the clearance of secretions are helpful in patients with hyperreactive airways. Antibiotic therapy for the control of infection is another important aspect of therapy. Before the advent of antibiotics, bronchiectasis was quite common and the prognosis was poor. Patients rarely lived beyond the age of 40 years. Bronchiectasis is much less common today and, except for the congenital forms of the disease, should be regarded as preventable. Timely vaccinations against childhood diseases frequently complicated by pneumonia, vigorous antibiotic and other appropriate treatment of pneumonia, and prompt removal of aspirated foreign bodies are all preventive measures.

CYSTIC FIBROSIS

Cystic fibrosis (CF), or *mucoviscidosis,* is a disease of genetic origin, occurring in approximately 1 in every 2500 births among Caucasians. For African Americans, the rate is 1:17,000 births, and for Asians, the rate is 1:90,000 births. The name cystic fibrosis was formulated originally to describe the pathologic changes of the lungs and pancreas in afflicted individuals. Obstruction of exocrine ducts followed by cystic dilation and fibrosis is accompanied by pancreatic insufficiency and inability to clear pulmonary secretions, which lead to the clinical hallmarks of CF, recurrent respiratory infections and malabsorption.

CF is an autosomal recessive disease. The gene responsible for CF, located on the long arm of chromosome 7, was cloned in 1989; the CF gene protein product known as the *cystic fibrosis transmembrane conductance regulator (CFTR)* was also identified (Harris, Argent, 1993). The CFTR protein is thought to be the chloride channel in epithelial cells, which explains the pathophysiologic basis of the disease: the primary abnormality is aberrant regulation of chloride transport across epithelial cells in the lungs, intestines, pancreas, and apocrine sweat glands. This defect impairs clearance of secretions in a variety of organs. The secretions of the exocrine glands that produce mucus and some other exocrine fluids produce abnormally viscid secretions. (Sweat and saliva are not particularly viscid but do contain abnormal amounts of salt.) The viscid secretions typically cause obstruction of the pancreatic and hepatic ducts and the bronchioles. The obstruction, in turn, can lead to fibrotic changes in the involved organs. Reduced chloride secretion with water following into the gut may result in meconium ileus at birth and distal intestinal obstruction later in life.

Most individuals with CF are diagnosed in the first few years of life, when recurrent respiratory infections, steatorrhea, and growth retardation prompt a *sweat chloride test.* Under standardized conditions for collection of sweat after pilocarpine administration (which stimulates sweating), more than 99% of CF patients have sweat chloride levels greater than 60 mEq/L (Denning et al, 1980). Normal chloride values range from 10 to 35 mEq/L.

The course of CF, largely determined by the degree of pulmonary involvement, varies from patient to patient. However, deterioration is inevitable, leading to debilitation and death. The prognosis has improved over the last few decades, mainly because of aggressive treatment before the onset of irreversible pulmonary changes. Median survival time has increased to 30 years from less than 2 years during the 1940s. The respiratory disease and complications that accompany CF account for more than 95% of the deaths. The sequence of events proceeds from recurrent pulmonary infections that gradually develop into bronchiectasis from retention of thick secretions to chronic pneumonia, fibrosis, V/Q imbalance, chronic hypoxemia, cor pulmonale, and respiratory failure. Pulmonary function studies invariably show an obstruction pattern, although restrictive lung volumes may be present with advanced disease. Patients with advanced disease may produce up to 200 ml of sputum per day. Finger clubbing is common.

Because pulmonary dysfunction is the overriding factor in determining survival, the management of this aspect of the disease is crucial, with removal of the obstructing bronchial secretions as the most crucial aspect of treatment. Generally, aerosol therapy is used to liquefy secretions and is followed by percussion and postural drainage. A number of agents for increasing mucus clearance are being tested. The development of an aerosolized recombinant human deoxyribonuclease (DNase) that degrades thickened mucus and allows it to be cleared more easily appears to be effective. Prevention of respiratory infection and its prompt treatment with sputum-sensitive specific antibiotics is also a central aspect of treatment.

KEY CONCEPTS

- *Obstructive patterns of pulmonary disease* include disorders of either the conducting airways or acini characterized by diminished ability to expire air. The chief causes of chronic airflow obstruction are chronic bronchitis, emphysema, chronic asthma, bronchiectasis, and cystic fibrosis.
- By common usage, the term *chronic obstructive pulmonary disease (COPD)* refers to two disorders that generally occur together—*chronic bronchitis* and *emphysema.* Although bronchial asthma can be included in this set because an asthmatic component to these two disorders frequently exists, asthma is generally discussed as a separate disease because the condition may exist independently.
- *Chronic bronchitis* is diagnosed on the basis of clinical symptoms: a chronic cough with sputum

expectoration for a minimum of 3 months per year for at least 2 years.

- *Emphysema* is a diagnosis based on pathologic anatomy: dilation and destruction of the air spaces distal to the terminal bronchiole, the alveolar ducts, and alveolar walls. A high-resolution CT scan reveals these changes.
- *Bronchial asthma* is an episodic disease characterized by hypersensitivity of the tracheobronchial tree to various stimuli manifested by reversible airway narrowing caused by bronchospasm.
- Pulmonary function tests (PFTs) indicating airways obstruction include: reduced FEV_1, FEV_1/FVC, MMFR, and RV; FRC and TLC are increased when air trapping occurs, as in emphysema.
- COPD is the fourth leading cause of death in the United States. Cigarette smoking is the most important risk factor. COPD is about twice as common in men as it is in women, but the rate in women is increasing rapidly as a result of smoking behavior.
- The main pathologic changes in *chronic bronchitis* are hypertrophy of the mucous-secreting glands and goblet cells in the trachea and bronchi, expressed as an increase in the volume of mucus.
- The pathologic changes in chronic bronchitis from smoking usually start in the smallest bronchioles, long before the advanced findings associated with chronic bronchitis and emphysema.
- Mucous plugging, mucosal edema, and muscle spasm cause airway narrowing and obstruction in chronic bronchitis.
- Generalized emphysema is permanent dilation of any part of the respiratory acinus, with destruction of tissue in the absence of scarring. Emphysema causes loss of elastic recoil of the lung tissue and decreases the force of expiration.
- The two patterns of generalized emphysema are centrilobular and panlobular.
- *Centrilobular emphysema (CLE)* affects the central part of the lobule, causing destruction of the walls and enlargement of the respiratory bronchioles. CLE is the most common form of emphysema, is unevenly distributed throughout the lung, affects the upper part of the lungs more severely, and is associated with smoking, chronic bronchitis, and inflammation of distal airways.
- The *pathogenesis of CLE* is likely related to secretion of extracellular proteases by local inflammatory cells. Cigarette smoke may also inhibit the effect of protease inhibitor alpha$_1$-antitrypsin, thereby leading to destruction.
- *Panlobular emphysema (PLE)* involves the entire respiratory lobule: respiratory bronchioles, alveolar ducts and sacs, and alveoli. PLE is commonly associated with smoking and tends to be evenly distributed throughout the lung and affects the lung bases more severely.
- The *pathogenesis of PLE*, like CLE, is related to excessive activity of extracellular proteases. Individuals with hereditary severe deficiency of alpha$_1$-antitrypsin, especially ZZ homozygotes, develop PLE at an early age.

- Patients with COPD are classified into two groups based on their clinical presentation: *predominant emphysema (pink puffers)* and *predominant bronchitis (blue bloaters)*.
- Clinical features of COPD that is *predominant emphysema* include the tendency to be thin, barrel-chested, with flat diaphragms because of air-trapping, and greatly increased TLC and RV; a long history of exertional dyspnea exists but with minimal coughing and sputum production; the term "pink puffers" is used because, early in the disease, patients are able to maintain fairly normal blood gases and color by hyperventilating. Only in the terminal stages do patients develop hypoxemia, hypercapnia, and cor pulmonale.
- Clinical features of COPD that is *predominant bronchitis* include the tendency to be overweight, but the chest anteroposterior diameter is normal or only slightly increased; a long history of cigarette smoking, frequent upper respiratory infections, cough and sputum production, particularly during the winter months, are all present; hypoxemia, hypercapnia, and compensatory polycythemia develop early in the disease, giving these patients a cyanotic appearance hence the term *blue bloaters*. Patients also develop pulmonary hypertension and cor pulmonale earlier in the disease process than do patients with predominantly emphysematous COPD. Generally, a significant $\dot{V}/\dot{Q}$ imbalance is present.
- Pneumothorax from rupture of *bullae* or *blebs* are potential complications of COPD.
- *Treatment modalities for COPD* include: smoking cessation, antibiotics for upper respiratory infections, prophylactic pneumococcal and influenza vaccines, bronchodilator drugs to relieve bronchospasm, hydration, chest physiotherapy, breathing exercises, continuous low flow rate O_2, and exercise programs. Alpha$_1$-antitrypsin augmentation therapy, as well as lung volume reduction therapy, for patients with hereditary deficiency is experimental.
- *Bronchiectasis* is a permanent, abnormal dilation of the medium-sized bronchi and bronchioles with associated inflammation and infection. Bronchiectasis usually begins in childhood following repeated lower respiratory tract infection as a complication of measles, pertussis, influenza, bronchitis, or pneumonia.
- Principal signs and symptoms of *bronchiectasis* are a chronic loose cough with production of a large amount of mucopurulent, foul-smelling sputum, malnutrition, and digital clubbing.
- Treatment for *bronchiectasis* includes antibiotic therapy and percussion and postural drainage. Prophylactic treatment includes childhood vaccination against measles and pertussis.
- *Cystic fibrosis (CF)* is the most common autosomal recessive disorder in the Caucasian population, with an incidence rate of 1:2500 newborns; 1 in 25 Caucasian adults is a heterozygous carrier.
- CF is a disease of exocrine gland function, involving multiple organs and chiefly resulting in chronic respiratory infections, pancreatic enzyme insufficiency, and associated complications.

- *CF* is caused by defects in the *cystic fibrosis transmembrane conductance regulator (CFTR) gene*, which encodes for a protein that functions as a chloride channel. CFTR mutations result in abnormalities of chloride transport across epithelial cells on the mucosal surfaces. The failure of epithelial cells to conduct chloride and associated water transport result in dry and viscid secretions in the respiratory tract, pancreas, gastrointestinal tract, sweat glands, and other exocrine tissues. Increased viscosity of these secretions makes them difficult to clear.
- Signs and symptoms of CF include meconium ileus at birth, failure to thrive, malabsorption and steator-

rhea, digital clubbing, and recurrent lung infections such as bronchiolitis, bronchitis, or pneumonia.
- The diagnosis of CF is made on the basis typical pulmonary or gastrointestinal manifestations, family history, and a positive pilocarpine-induced sweat test (sweat chloride >60 mEq/L).
- Management of CF includes chest physiotherapy, antibiotics aerosol and nebulizer treatment to liquefy mucus, oxygen therapy, and pancreatic enzymes. Nine-five percent of patients with CF die of pulmonary complications; median survival is approximately 30 years.

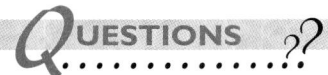

QUESTIONS ??

A sampling of review questions for this chapter appears here. Visit http://www.mosby.com/MERLIN/PriceWilson/ for additional questions.

Answer the following on a separate sheet of paper.

1. What is the ventilatory functional disorder associated with COPD?
2. Describe the interrelation of chronic bronchitis, pulmonary emphysema, and asthma.
3. Describe the symptoms of an asthmatic attack. How is it treated? What is *status asthmaticus?*
4. Contrast the two morphologic patterns of emphysema according to anatomic changes, distribution in lung, gender prevalence, type of associated COPD, and etiologic factors.

5. What are the objectives of treatment for chronic bronchitis and emphysema?
6. What are the two criteria for establishing a diagnosis of chronic bronchitis? What is the time within which these symptoms must be manifested (months per year and consecutive years)?
7. Describe the pathologic anatomic changes in the lung parenchyma in pulmonary emphysema.
8. What are subpleural air-filled spaces called? What is their cause?
9. What are parenchymal air-filled spaces more than 1 cm in diameter called? What generally causes them?

10. How does the tracheobronchial tree of the asthmatic patient respond to various stimuli? How is this manifested?
11. What anatomic changes occur in bronchiectasis? What are some possible precipitating factors, and what features tend to cause persistence and progression of the disease?
12. What are the principal clinical features of bronchiectasis?
13. Identify the mode of treatment for bronchiectasis.
14. What is the most crucial aspect of treatment of cystic fibrosis?

Match each of the diseases in column A with its basis for definition in column B.

Column A
15. _____ Chronic bronchitis
16. _____ Pulmonary emphysema
17. _____ Asthma

Column B
a. Pathologic anatomy
b. Clinical symptoms
c. Pathophysiology

Match the type of asthmatic condition in column A with the appropriate descriptive features in column B. Each item in column B may be used more than once.

Column A
18. _____ Extrinsic asthma
19. _____ Intrinsic asthma
20. _____ Mixed asthma

Column B
a. A clearly defined precipitating factor is absent.
b. The condition is clearly caused by a known allergen and usually develops in early childhood.
c. Attacks may be associated with infection of the tracheobronchial tree or of the nasal sinuses.
d. This type affects most asthmatic patients.
e. Exposure to the allergen precipitates an asthmatic attack.

Restrictive Patterns of Respiratory Disease

LORRAINE M. WILSON

$\mathscr{A}$ restrictive ventilatory disorder is characterized by increased stiffness of the lungs or thorax or both, resulting from decreased compliance and a reduction in all lung volumes, including the vital capacity. The work of breathing increases to overcome the elastic forces of the respiratory apparatus; consequently, a pattern of rapid, shallow breathing is adopted. The physiologic consequences of a restricted pattern of ventilation are alveolar hypoventilation and an inability to maintain normal blood gas tensions.

A number of diseases may contribute to pulmonary restriction through varying mechanisms. In this chapter, these diseases are divided into two classes: extrapulmonary disorders, including neurologic, neuromuscular, and thoracic cage disorders; and diseases of the pleura and lung parenchyma.

EXTRAPULMONARY DISEASE

Neurologic and Neuromuscular Disorders

In reference to extrapulmonary disorders, the term *extrapulmonary* implies that the lung tissue itself may be quite normal. The common pathophysiologic disturbance in these disorders is *alveolar hypoventilation*, although this is not entirely true in the case of kyphoscoliosis.

A number of disorders directly affecting the medullary respiratory center may cause alveolar hypoventilation.

Carbon dioxide (CO_2) retention from a variety of causes may depress rather than stimulate respiration when the arterial CO_2 partial pressure, or tension ($Paco_2$), exceeds approximately 70 mm Hg. A number of drugs are capable of depressing the respiratory center, thereby causing alveolar hypoventilation. For example, narcotic or barbiturate drug overdose is a common cause of death resulting from respiratory depression and failure. Acute "overdose" of ethanol can also cause death by depression of respiration. Anatomic damage to the respiratory center resulting from head trauma or cerebral lesions caused by a cerebrovascular accident (CVA, stroke) can also cause respiratory center depression and alveolar hypoventilation. Abnormalities of neural or neuromuscular transmission to the respiratory muscles may result in paresis or paralysis and alveolar hypoventilation. Amyotrophic lateral sclerosis, poliomyelitis, Guillain-Barré syndrome, and myasthenia gravis are neurologic disorders that may produce ventilatory insufficiency. The muscles themselves are diseased in progressive muscular dystrophy. The severity of the respiratory involvement in any of these diseases depends on the amount of anatomic involvement: vital capacity (VC) is reduced in proportion to the degree of paresis of the respiratory muscles. Although parenchymal lung disease is not primary, secondary infection is common because of ineffective coughing and limitation of respiratory excursions. Table 39-1 summarizes the extrapulmonary disorders causing alveolar hypoventilation and the mechanism responsible.

Thoracic Cage Disorders

Four major types of fixed chest wall deformities may restrict ventilation by interfering with the bellows mechanism: kyphoscoliosis, pectus excavatum, ankylosing spondylitis, and healed thoracoplasty.

Kyphosis is a term that refers to any posterior angulation of the spine (hunchback), and *scoliosis* refers to a lateral displacement of the spine. Kyphoscoliosis is therefore characterized by angulation of the spine both posteriorly and laterally. Approximately 80% of cases are idiopathic; the remaining 20% results from the aftereffects of poliomyelitis or tuberculosis of the spine (Pott's

TABLE 39-1

Extrapulmonary Disorders Causing Alveolar Hypoventilation

System or Structure	Disease or Altered Condition	Altered Mechanism
Neurologic (central nervous system, CNS)	Paco₂ >70 mm Hg Narcotics and barbiturates	Depression of the respiratory center
	Head trauma, CNS lesions	Direct anatomic damage to the respiratory center
	Poliomyelitis	Interruption of nerve transmission to respiratory muscles because of lower motor neuron lesion
	Amyotrophic lateral sclerosis	Interruption of nerve transmission to respiratory muscles because of upper motor neuron lesion
Neurologic (peripheral nervous system)	Guillain-Barré syndrome	Interruption of nerve transmission to respiratory muscles as a result of inflammation involving ganglion cells and peripheral nerves
	Myasthenia gravis	Interruption of nerve transmission to respiratory muscles because of disease involving the neuromuscular junction
Muscular	Progressive muscular dystrophy	Paresis of the respiratory muscles because of diffuse disease of the skeletal muscles
Chest cage	Kyphoscoliosis	Deformity of the chest cage causing abnormal positioning and functioning of the respiratory muscles and compression of the chest cage contents
	Closed chest wall trauma	Voluntary restriction of ventilation as a result of pain or paradoxical movement of the chest wall and thoracic contents in flail chest injury
	Pickwickian syndrome (extreme obesity)	Limitation of thoracic movement by accumulated body fat

Paco₂, Arterial carbon dioxide tension.

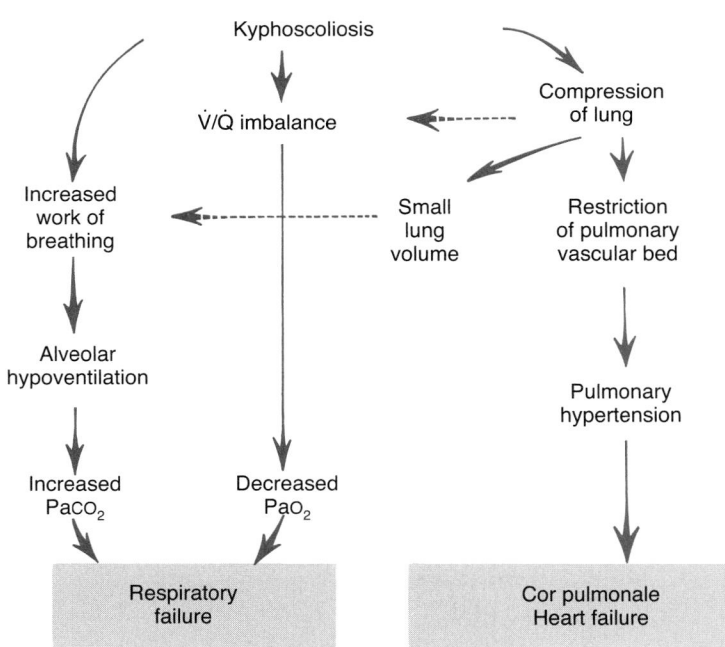

FIG. 39-1   Pathogenesis of respiratory failure and heart failure in kyphoscoliosis. $\dot{V}/\dot{Q}$, Ventilation/perfusion; *Paco₂*, arterial carbon dioxide tension; *Pao₂*, arterial oxygen tension.

disease). Kyphoscoliosis is quite common, with approximately 1% of the American population affected, although the defect is severe enough to produce cardiopulmonary symptoms in only a small proportion of these individuals. Severe kyphoscoliosis is associated with marked asymmetry of the chest and leads to abnormal functioning and positioning of the respiratory muscles and to compression of the lungs.

Fig. 39-1 shows the sequence of events that may lead to both respiratory and cardiac failure in kyphoscoliosis. In these patients, breathing entails a high work and en-

ergy cost; thus a rapid, shallow pattern is adopted, which, in turn, leads to alveolar hypoventilation by preferential ventilation of the anatomic dead space at the expense of alveolar ventilation. Additionally, compression of the lungs by the thoracic deformity causes a small lung volume and unequal distribution of ventilation and perfusion because both alveoli and pulmonary blood vessels are compressed. The consequent physiologic shunting leads to hypoxemia. When alveolar ventilation is also limited, the result is hypoxemia, hypercapnia, and respiratory acidosis. Compression of the pulmonary blood vessels and the acidosis also lead to pulmonary hypertension and cor pulmonale. The common cause of death from this chain of events is a combination of respiratory failure and heart failure.

Pectus excavatum (funnel chest) is a congenital deformity in which the lower end of the sternum is attached to the thoracic spine by fibromuscular bands, giving the lower sternal area a caved-in appearance. Compare this deformity with kyphoscoliosis in Fig. 39-2. Pectus excavatum, unlike severe kyphoscoliosis, rarely causes more than mild restriction of ventilation.

Thoracoplasty is a surgically induced depression of the thoracic cage that was once performed for the treatment of tuberculosis but is no longer common. Because this procedure is performed for an underlying lung disease, the subsequent pulmonary dysfunction is usually more closely related to the original disease than it is to the induced deformity.

Ankylosing spondylitis is a disease that causes symmetric reduction in mobility of the bony thorax as a result of the ossification of the vertebral joints and ligaments (see Chapter 75). Rib fixation and increased stiffness of the chest wall cause mild ventilatory restriction, which is not usually symptomatic.

Closed chest wall injury may also restrict ventilation. The most common chest wall injury is simple rib fracture. As a result of the pain and muscle splinting, ventilatory restriction of tidal volume (V_T) occurs, as well as an increase in respiratory frequency (f), and voluntary inhibition of the cough reflex. Healthy young people tend to tolerate these changes well, but these changes in older adults may lead to impaired clearing of secretions, respiratory tract infection, blood gas abnormalities, and even respiratory failure. Flail chest is a major defect in chest wall continuity caused by a crushing chest injury (typically observed in steering wheel injuries in motor vehicle crashes) with multiple rib fractures. The resulting instability of the chest wall causes a paradoxical movement of the chest wall accompanied by pendulum movement of the mediastinal contents during the breathing cycle. This condition may cause interference with venous return to the heart and cause dead-space air to be shunted back and forth between the lungs *(pendelluft)*, as illustrated in Fig. 39-3. A large flail segment can be temporarily stabilized with towel rolls, tape, or sandbags placed against it. Intubation and ventilator support is required for all patients with large flail segments and for any patient with underlying acute or chronic lung disease.

Pickwickian syndrome or *obesity hyperventilation syndrome* are terms used to describe a group of clinical features found in individuals who are extremely obese. These features include chronic alveolar hypoventilation, somnolence, polycythemia, hypoxemia, and hypercapnia. (The syndrome was named after the sleepy fat boy in Dickens' *Pickwick Papers*.) The somnolence common to this syndrome can be related to the CO_2 retention that depresses the central nervous system (CNS); polycythemia is the compensatory response to chronic hypoxia. In patients with pickwickian syndrome, the accumulated body fat appears to limit thoracic movement and greatly increases the work of breathing. Respiratory impairment may progress to the point of cor pulmonale and respiratory failure. Pickwickian syndrome is only one subtype of a

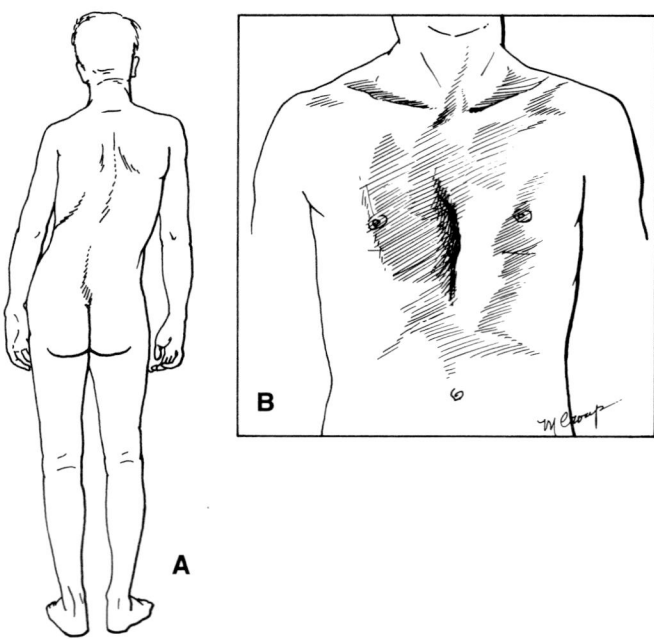

FIG. 39-2 Thoracic deformities restricting ventilation. **A,** Kyphoscoliosis. **B,** Pectus excavatum (funnel chest).

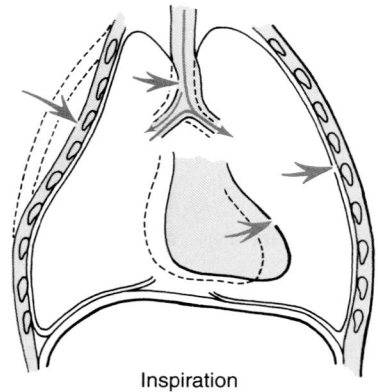
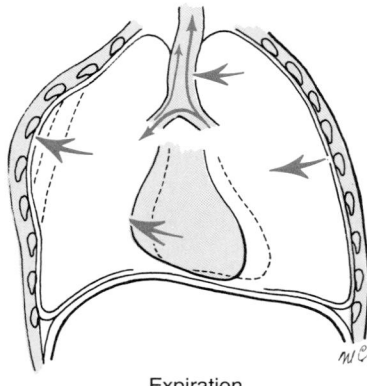

FIG. 39-3 Altered cardiopulmonary dynamics in flail chest injury. Arrows indicate the direction of motion; arrows within the trachea and bronchi indicate air being shunted back and forth between lungs during respiratory cycle (pendelluft). Note paradoxical motion of the unstable portion of the chest wall on the right side. (From Burrows B, Knudson RJ, Kettle LJ: *Respiratory insufficiency,* Chicago, 1975, Mosby.)

Inspiration   Expiration

group of disorders called *sleep apnea syndromes*, in which elements of upper airway obstruction (which results in snoring) or central hypoventilation or both may be present. Nonobese individuals may also be afflicted. It is also important to note that not all extremely obese individuals develop alveolar hypoventilation and blood gas abnormalities. Weight reduction, if successful, appears to be the most effective treatment for pickwickian syndrome and may reverse the respiratory insufficiency.

DISEASES OF THE PLEURA AND LUNG PARENCHYMA

Pleural Disorders

The pleura and pleural space are the sites of a number of disorders that may restrict the expansion of the lungs or the alveoli or both. This reaction may result from compression of the lung as a result of the accumulation of air, fluid, blood, or purulent material in the pleural cavity. Pain resulting from inflammation or fibrosis of the pleura may also cause limitation of chest expansion.

Pleural Effusion

The parietal and visceral pleura are opposed to each other and are separated by a thin layer of serous fluid. This thin layer of fluid represents a balance between transudation from the pleural capillaries and reabsorption by the visceral and parietal veins and lymphatics, as discussed in Chapter 35. *Pleural effusion* is the term applied to a collection of fluid in the pleural cavity (Fig. 39-4, *A*). Pleural effusions may be transudates or exudates. A *transudate* occurs if a rise in pulmonary venous pressure occurs, as in congestive heart failure. In these cases the balance of forces favors the passage of fluid out of the vessels. Transudation may also occur if hypoproteinemia occurs, as in liver and renal disease. The accumulation of transudate in the pleural cavity is called *hydrothorax*. The pleural fluid tends to accumulate at the base of the lungs as a result of the force of gravity. The accumulation of an *exudate* is secondary to involvement of the pleura by inflammation or malignant growth and results from increased capillary permeability or impaired lymphatic absorption. An exudate is differentiated from a transudate by the protein content and specific gravity of the pleural fluid. Transudates have a specific gravity of less than 1.015 and a protein content of less than 3%; exudates have a higher

specific gravity and protein content because of their cellular content.

When the pleural effusion contains pus, the condition is termed *empyema*. Empyema is the result of extension of infection from contiguous structures and may be a complication of pneumonia, lung abscess, or perforation of a carcinoma into the pleural cavity. Empyema that is not adequately treated by drainage may have disastrous effects on the thoracic cage. The inflammatory exudate becomes organized, and fibrous adhesions weld the parietal and visceral pleura together. This condition is termed *fibrothorax* (see Fig. 39-4). If the fibrothorax is extensive, it may cause serious mechanical restriction of the underlying tissue. Surgical peeling, called *decortication*, is sometimes necessary to separate the pleural membranes.

The term *hemothorax* is used to designate frank bleeding into the pleural cavity and does not designate a hemorrhagic pleural effusion. Trauma is the most common cause of hemothorax. The trauma may be classified as *penetrating* (e.g., knife wound) or *nonpenetrating* (e.g., fractured rib, which, in turn, lacerates the lung or an intercostal blood vessel). The thoracic duct can also drain lymph into the pleural cavity as a result of trauma or malignant tumor, a condition termed *chylothorax*.

Pneumothorax

The presence of air in the pleural cavity caused by a breach in the pleura is termed *pneumothorax*. A pneumothorax may be classified according to cause as traumatic or spontaneous; it may also be classified according to the sequence of events that follow the breach in the pleura as open, closed, or tension pneumothorax.

A penetrating wound to the chest is a common cause of *traumatic pneumothorax*. As the air enters the pleural space, which is normally subatmospheric in pressure, the lung collapses to a variable extent. If the communication is open, then a massive collapse occurs until the pressure in the pleural cavity is equal to that of the atmosphere (see *open pneumothorax*, Fig. 39-4, *B*). The mediastinum shifts in the direction of the collapsed lung and may shift to and fro during the respiratory cycle as air moves in and out of the pleural cavity. Emergency treatment of a penetrating chest wound consists of applying an airtight seal immediately over the wound. The patient should then be observed for signs of tension pneumothorax and, if present, the seal should be removed. If the defect that causes the communication between the pleural space and the

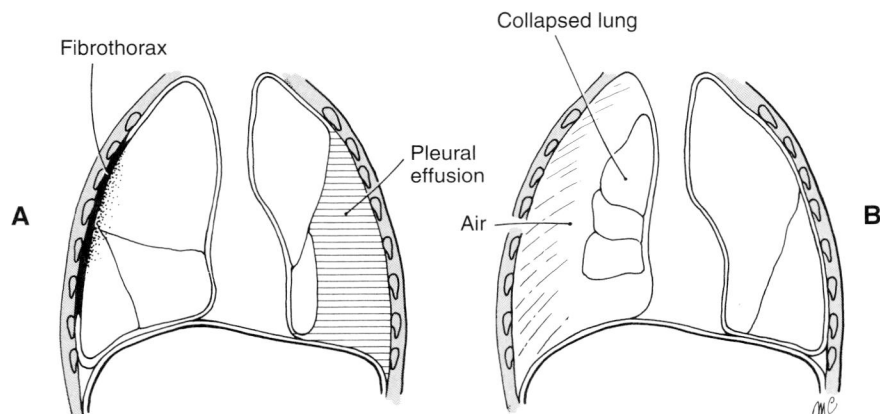

FIG. 39-4 Disorders of the pleura. **A,** Fibrothorax resulting from organization of inflammatory exudate and pleural effusion. **B,** Collapse of lung because of open pneumothorax.

atmosphere seals itself off, it is called a *closed pneumothorax*. On the other hand, if the defect remains open during inspiration and closes during expiration (check-valve effect), a large volume of air may collect in the pleural space; as a result, pressure builds up above that of the atmosphere, causing complete collapse of the lung. This is termed *tension pneumothorax*. Tension pneumothorax is a serious emergency that must be treated immediately by aspiration of air from the pleural cavity.

Spontaneous pneumothorax is the term used to designate a sudden, unexpected pneumothorax, which may occur with or without underlying pulmonary disease. Common pulmonary diseases that may cause a spontaneous secondary pneumothorax include emphysema (rupture of blebs or bullae), pneumonia, and neoplasms. A pneumothorax occurs when there is communication between a bronchus or alveolus and the pleural cavity; it causes air to gain access to the pleural cavity through the defect, which may result in an open, closed, or tension pneumothorax. A spontaneous pneumothorax may occur in apparently healthy young individuals, usually between ages 20 and 40 years, and is termed *primary* or *idiopathic spontaneous pneumothorax*. The usual cause is rupture of a subpleural bleb at the surface of the lung or localized bullous disease (see Fig. 38-4). The cause of such a bleb or bulla in otherwise healthy individuals is unknown, but a familial predisposition has sometimes been reported.

Both pleural effusion and pneumothorax limit function by restricting the expansion of the underlying lung. The degree of functional impairment and disability depends on the size and the rapidity of development. If fluid accumulates slowly, as is usually the case in pleural effusion, then a large amount of fluid may be accommodated with little apparent distress. On the other hand, rapid decompression of a lung from a massive pneumothorax may be accompanied by rapid development of shock. Table 39-2 summarizes the signs and symptoms of pleural effusion and pneumothorax. The presence of both conditions is confirmed by radiography.

TABLE 39-2

Signs and Symptoms of Pleural Effusion and Pneumothorax

Pleural Effusion	Pneumothorax
Dyspnea variable	Dyspnea (if large)
Pleuritic pain usually precedes effusion if secondary to pleuritic disease	Pleuritic pain severe
Trachea deviated away from the side of effusion	Trachea deviated away from the side of pneumothorax
Bulging of intercostal spaces (large effusion)	Tachycardia
	Cyanosis (if large)
Diminished and delayed chest movement on the involved side	Diminished and delayed chest movement on the involved side
Flat percussion note over the pleural effusion	Hyperresonant percussion note over pneumothorax
Egophony over compressed lung next to effusion	Flatness to percussion over collapsed lung
Decreased breath sounds over pleural effusion	Decreased or absent breath sounds on affected side
Decreased vocal and tactile fremitus	Decreased vocal and tactile fremitus

A first pneumothorax is treated by conservative observation if the collapse is 20% or less. The air is gradually absorbed through the pleural surfaces, which act as wet membranes, allowing oxygen (O_2) and CO_2 to diffuse through them. If the pneumothorax is large and dyspnea severe, a thoracotomy tube attached to water-sealed drainage will be necessary to aid reexpansion of the lung. If bloody effusion is associated with pneumothorax, it must be removed by drainage because clotting and organization lead to extensive pleural fibrosis. A pleural effusion is treated by needle aspiration *(thoracentesis)*. This treatment is particularly important if the effusion is an exudate, because fibrothorax may result. A small, noninflammatory effusion (transudate) may be resorbed into the capillaries after the cause of the effusion has been reversed.

Lung Parenchymal Disorders

A large number of diseases affecting the lung alveoli or interstitium (or both) lead either locally or diffusely to respiratory impairment of varying degrees. Damage to healthy lung tissue may result from invasion by bacteria, viruses, fungi, protozoa, or malignant cells and inhalation of irritating dust and fumes. Damage to the alveolar capillary endothelium from a variety of causes leads to interstitial, alveolar wall, and intraalveolar edema. Excess fibrotic tissue may be deposited as a sequela to a variety of diseases, usually inflammatory or allergenic in nature. The result is a reduction in lung compliance (stiff lungs) and interference with the gas diffusion pathway. A deficiency of surfactant, as in respiratory distress syndrome, may also produce the same results.

The physiologic abnormalities observed in patients with disease of the lung parenchyma vary widely and depend, to some degree, on the extent of the pathologic process. A restrictive defect with its concomitant decrease in lung volume and a rapid, shallow breathing pattern is common. Hypoxemia is the most important blood gas abnormality and is typically caused by a ventilation/perfusion imbalance, resulting in excess wasted ventilation or wasted perfusion caused by shunting. None of the physiologic abnormalities is specific, but pulmonary function tests are helpful in quantifying the degree of abnormality, guiding therapy, and assessing the results. Only selected, frequently encountered lung parenchymal diseases are discussed in this chapter.

Atelectasis

Atelectasis, although not a disease *per se*, is associated with disease of the lung parenchyma. *Atelectasis* is a term meaning *imperfect expansion*, implying that the alveoli in the affected part of the lung have become airless and collapsed. Atelectasis should not be confused with pneumothorax. Although alveolar collapse occurs in both conditions, the cause of the collapse is markedly different. Atelectasis occurs because alveoli become underinflated or uninflated, whereas pneumothorax occurs because air enters the pleural space. In most patients, pneumothorax is not preventable, but atelectasis is preventable with the proper nursing interventions. The two major causes of collapse are absorption atelectasis secondary to bronchial or bronchiolar obstruction and atelectasis caused by compression.

In *absorption atelectasis*, obstruction of the airway prevents air from entering the alveoli distal to the obstruction. The air already present in the alveoli is then absorbed gradually into the bloodstream, and the alveoli collapse. (More air pressure and work are required to reinflate an alveolus from a completely collapsed position, similar to blowing harder at the beginning when blowing up a balloon.) Absorption atelectasis may result from intrinsic or extrinsic bronchial obstruction. Intrinsic bronchial obstruction is most frequently caused by retained secretions or exudate. Extrinsic pressure on a bronchus typically results from neoplasm, lymph node enlargement, aneurysm, or scar tissue. This discussion is concerned with intrinsic obstruction resulting from retained secretions, the more common and preventable cause.

The physiologic defense mechanisms that act to keep the lower respiratory tract sterile have already been discussed. Some of these mechanisms also act to prevent atelectasis by preventing obstruction. These mechanisms include the combined action of the "ciliary escalator," which may be assisted by cough to move noxious particles and bacteria to the posterior pharynx, where they are swallowed or expectorated. Another mechanism that prevents atelectasis is collateral ventilation. Recent experimental studies of collateral ventilation, a subject of debate for the last 50 years, leave no doubt that air can pass from one lung acinus to another by other than the normal airways. It is now well-established that small pores,

called the *pores of Kohn* after their discoverer in 1873, between the alveoli provide a path for collateral ventilation.

Fig. 39-5 illustrates the way in which collateral ventilation prevents absorption atelectasis in the presence of bronchiolar obstruction by a mucous plug. Also illustrated is one of the causes of ineffective ventilation and its effect. Only deep inspiration is effective in opening the pores of Kohn and providing collateral ventilation to an adjacent obstructed alveolus. Collapse caused by absorption of gases in the obstructed alveolus is thus prevented. (Normally, gas absorption into the blood is favored because the total partial pressure of the blood gases is slightly less than is atmospheric pressure because more O_2 is absorbed into the tissues than CO_2 is excreted.) During expiration, the pores of Kohn close, and pressure builds up in the obstructed alveolus, which aids in the expulsion of the mucus plug. Even greater expiratory force may be built up if, after taking a deep breath, the glottis is closed and then suddenly opened as in the normal cough. In contrast, the pores of Kohn remain closed with shallow inspiration, so that there is no collateral ventilation to the obstructed alveolus; thus pressure adequate to expel the mucous plug is not attained. Absorption of alveolar gases into the bloodstream continues, resulting in collapse of the alveolus. As the air leaves the alveolus, edematous fluid gradually replaces it.

This discussion emphasizes the importance of coughing and deep-breathing exercises and other physical

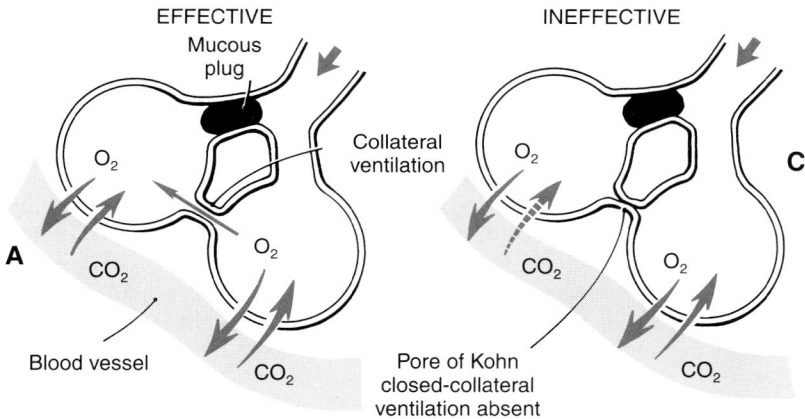

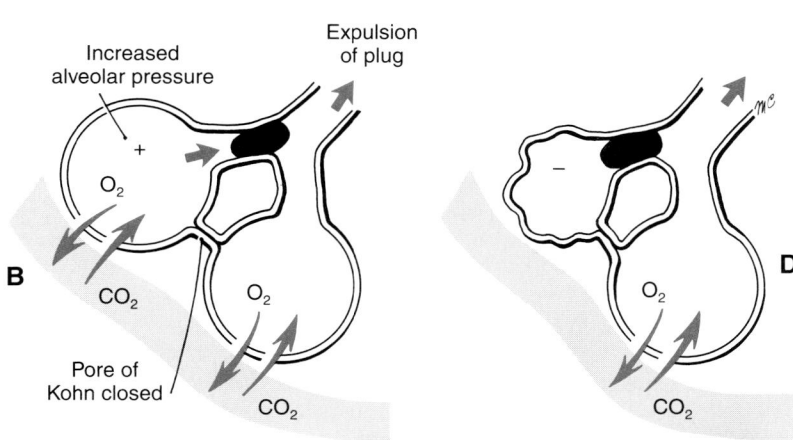

FIG. 39-5   Role of collateral alveolar ventilation in prevention of absorption atelectasis. Effective ventilation: **A**, during deep inspiration, pores of Kohn open and air enters adjacent obstructed alveolus; **B**, during expiration, pores of Kohn close; positive pressure builds up in obstructed alveolus and aids in expulsion of mucous plug. Ineffective ventilation: **C**, pores of Kohn do not open during shallow inspiration, so collateral ventilation is not provided to obstructed alveolus; **D**, obstructed alveolus collapses as alveolar gases are absorbed into bloodstream. (Modified from Kroeker EJ: *Hosp Med* 5:67-76, 1969.)

TABLE 39-3 ■■■

Lung Defense Mechanisms that Prevent Atelectasis

Protective Mechanism	Factors that Cause Interference with Mechanism
Mucus and ciliary action	General dehydration causes production of viscous mucus and scant volume.
	Inhalation of dry air increases viscosity of mucus so that crusting occurs.
	Excess mucus production (e.g., chronic bronchitis) overwhelms ciliary escalator.
	Cigarette smoke reduces or paralyzes ciliary action.
	Trauma (suctioning) reduces ciliary action.
	Anesthetics and atropine-like drugs reduce both mucus production and ciliary action.
Cough	Pain reduces expiratory force.
	Sedatives and narcotics inhibit cough initiation.
	Chronic obstructive pulmonary disease (COPD) reduces airflow rate.
Collateral ventilation	Shallow breathing is caused by pain or sedation.
	Pulmonary edema results from congestion or infection.
	Constant tidal volume respiration occurs in a patient on a mechanical respirator.
	Anesthetic gases and oxygen are rapidly absorbed, allowing less time for collateral ventilation.
Pharyngeal clearing	Unconsciousness; obtundation favors aspiration of gastric contents or upper respiratory tract secretions.

BOX 39-1

Risk Factors for Pneumonia

- Age over 65 years
- Aspiration of oropharyngeal secretions
- Viral respiratory infection
- Chronic illness and debilitation (e.g., diabetes mellitus, uremia)
- Chronic respiratory disease (e.g., COPD, asthma, cystic fibrosis)
- Cancer (particularly lung cancer)
- Prolonged bed rest
- Tracheostomy or endotracheal tube
- Abdominal or thoracic surgery
- Rib fractures
- Immunosuppressive therapy
- AIDS
- Smoking history
- Alcoholism
- Malnutrition

activity to prevent atelectasis in predisposed persons. These measures are particularly important in postoperative, bedridden, or otherwise debilitated patients because atelectasis is the prevalent cause of morbidity in this population group. Atelectasis at the lung bases is especially common in patients whose respirations are shallow as a result of pain, weakness, or abdominal distention. Retained secretions may lead to pneumonia and more extensive atelectasis.

Prolonged atelectasis may lead to the replacement of the involved lung tissue with fibrous tissue. Adequate prevention also requires familiarity with factors that interfere with normal lung defense mechanisms. Some of these factors, discussed previously, are listed in Table 39-3 for added emphasis and consideration.

Compression atelectasis results from extrinsic pressure on all or part of the lung, driving the air out and causing collapse. Common causes are pleural effusion, pneumothorax, or abdominal distention that elevates the diaphragm. Compression atelectasis is much less common than absorption atelectasis.

Loss of surfactant from the terminal air spaces leads to generalized failure of lung expansion called microatelectasis. Loss of surfactant is a prominent feature of both infant and acute (adult) respiratory distress syndrome (ARDS) discussed in Chapter 41.

Infections of the Lung Parenchyma: Pneumonias

Acute inflammation of the lung parenchyma, which is usually infectious in origin, is called *pneumonia* or *pneu-*

monitis. The first term is preferable, because the second term has frequently been used to designate a nonspecific pulmonary inflammation of unknown cause. Pneumonia is a common malady and affects approximately 1% of the American population annually. Despite the development of antibiotics, pneumonia remains the sixth leading cause of death in the United States. The emergence of nosocomial (hospital-acquired) antibiotic-resistant organisms and newly discovered organisms (e.g., *Legionella*), the increased number of immunocompromised hosts, and diseases such as acquired immunodeficiency syndrome (AIDS) have expanded the range and severity of etiologic possibilities and explains the reasons pneumonia remains as a significant health care problem. The infant and young child are particularly susceptible because of poorly developed immune responses. Pneumonia is frequently the terminal event in older patients and those debilitated by chronic diseases. Alcoholic and postoperative patients and those with chronic respiratory disease or viral infections are particularly vulnerable. As many as 60% of critically ill patients in intensive care units may develop pneumonia, and one half of these patients will die. *Pneumocystis carinii* pneumonia is currently the major terminal infection in patients with AIDS because of their immunodeficiency. Box 39-1 summarizes the risk factors for pneumonia.

Microbial agents causing pneumonia have three primary modes of transmission: (1) aspiration of secretions that contain pathogenic microorganisms that have colonized the oropharynx, (2) inhalation of infectious aerosols, and (3) hematogenous spread from an extrapulmonary site. Aspiration and inhalation of infectious agents are the two most common modes of acquiring pneumonia respectively, whereas hematogenous spread occurs infrequently. Consequently, predisposing factors include any deficiency in the defense mechanisms of the respiratory system. Colonization of the oropharynx with gram-negative bacilli and subsequent aspiration as a pathogenic mechanism of acquiring many gram-negative pneumonias have been the subjects of recent research (see later discussion).

The pathologic picture depends, to some extent, on the etiologic agent. *Bacterial pneumonia* is characterized

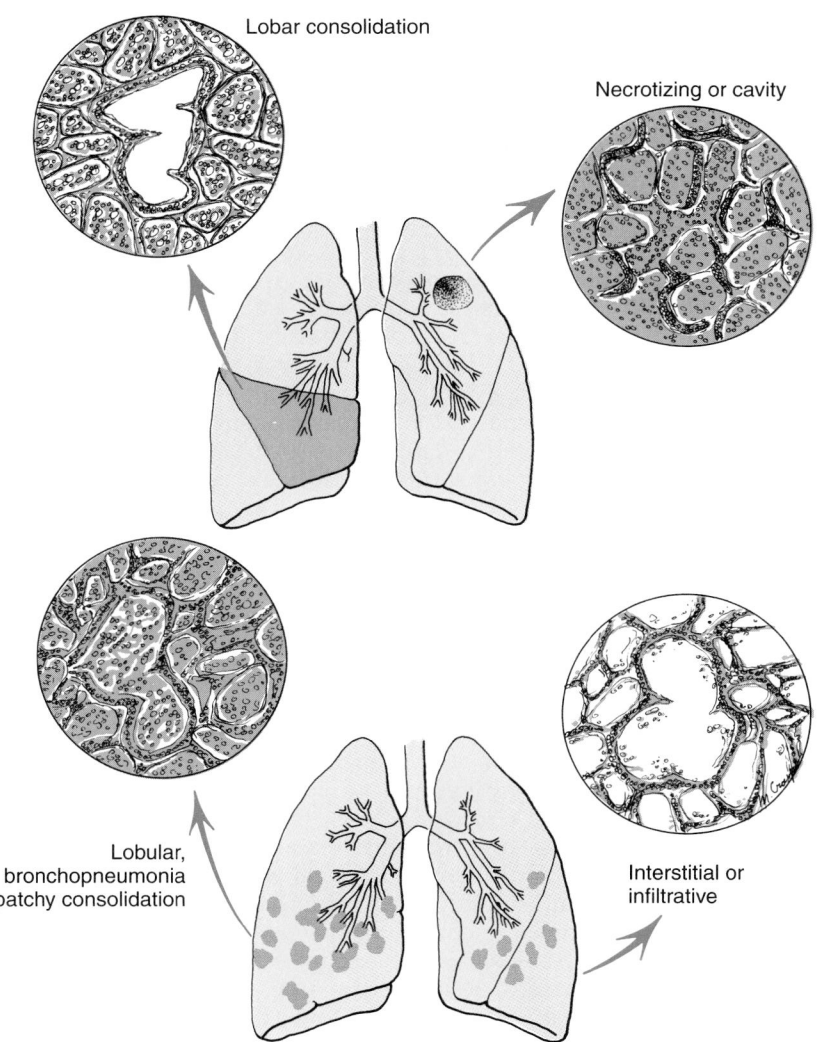

Lobar consolidation

Necrotizing or cavity

Lobular, bronchopneumonia or patchy consolidation

Interstitial or infiltrative

FIG. 39-6   Forms of pneumonia: *lobar*—entire lobe consolidated, exudate chiefly intraalveolar, *pneumococcus* and *Klebsiella* common infecting organisms; *necrotizing*—granuloma may undergo caseous necrosis and form cavity, fungi and tubercle bacillus infections are common causes; *lobular*—patchy distribution, fibrinous exudate chiefly in bronchioles, *Staphylococcus* and *Streptococcus* are common infecting organisms; *interstitial*—perivascular exudate and edema between alveoli, caused by virus or mycoplasmal infection.

by an intraalveolar suppurative exudate with consolidation. The infectious process may be classified anatomically. Consolidation of an entire lobe occurs in *lobar pneumonia*, whereas *lobular pneumonia*, or *bronchopneumonia*, refers to a patchy distribution of infectious areas approximately 3 to 4 cm in diameter surrounding and involving the bronchi. *Viral* or *Mycoplasma pneumoniae* pneumonias are characterized by an interstitial inflammation with accumulation of an infiltrate in the alveolar walls, although the alveolar spaces themselves are free of exudate and no consolidation takes place. If the infecting agent is a *fungus* or *Mycobacterium tuberculosis*, the common pathologic pattern is a patchy distribution of granulomas, which may undergo caseous necrosis with the development of cavities. Fig. 39-6 illustrates the forms of pneumonia and the common causative agent.

It is also important to differentiate between community-acquired and hospital-acquired pneumonias. The relative frequencies with which individual agents cause pneumonia are quite different in these two locations (Table 39-4). Nosocomial infections are more likely to be caused by enteric gram-negative bacteria or *Staphylococcus aureus* and less likely to be caused by pneumococci or *Mycoplasma*.

TABLE 39-4

Most Common Causes of Community-acquired and Nosocomial Pneumonias

Location of Acquisition	Causes
Community	*Streptococcus pneumoniae* *Mycoplasma pneumoniae* *Haemophilus influenzae* *Legionella pneumophila* *Chlamydia pneumoniae* Oral anaerobes (aspiration) Influenza A and B Adenovirus
Hospital	Enteric gram-negative bacilli (e.g., *Escherichia coli*, *Klebsiella pneumoniae*) *Pseudomonas aeruginosa* *Staphylococcus aureus* Oral anaerobes (aspiration)

The pattern of response also depends on the specific etiologic agent. *Streptococcus pneumoniae* (pneumococcus) is the most common cause of bacterial pneumonia, both in the community (accounting for as many as 75% of the cases) and in the hospital. Among the bacterial pneumonias, the pathogenesis of pneumococcal pneumonia has been the most extensively studied. Pneumococci usually reach the alveoli in droplets of mucus or saliva. The lower lobes of the lung are frequently involved because of the effect of gravity. After the pneumococcus is established in the alveolus, the pneumococcus elicits a typical response involving the following four successive stages*:

1. Engorgement (first 4 to 12 hours): serous exudate pours into alveoli from the dilated, leaking blood vessels.
2. Red hepatization (next 48 hours): lung assumes a red, granular appearance (*hepatization*, meaning liverlike) as red blood cells, fibrin, and polymorphonuclear leukocytes fill the alveoli.
3. Gray hepatization (3 to 8 days): lung assumes a grayish appearance as the leukocytes and fibrin consolidate in the involved alveoli.
4. Resolution (7 to 11 days): exudate is lysed and resorbed by macrophages, restoring the tissue to its original structure.

The onset of pneumococcal pneumonia is typically sudden, with chills, fever, pleuritic pain, cough, and rust-colored sputum. Rales and a friction rub may be heard over the involved tissue because of the exudate and fibrin that are in the alveoli and may be deposited on the pleural surface. Some degree of hypoxemia almost always occurs as a result of the shunting of blood through the nonventilated, consolidated area of lung; the patient may have a dusky appearance. Chest radiograph, white blood cell count, and sputum examination—including gross appearance, microscopic examination, and culture—may be helpful in making the diagnosis and following the course of the pneumonia.

The general treatment of patients with pneumonia consists of administering antibiotic drugs effective against the specific organism, providing O_2 therapy for hypoxemia, and treating complications. Complications and mortality are likely related to the specific infecting organism. Pneumococcal pneumonia generally runs an uncomplicated course, resulting in restoration of normal tissue structure. The most likely complication is a small pleural effusion. The treatment of choice is penicillin G. Before the era of antibiotics, the mortality rate for pneumococcal pneumonia was 20% to 40%, but this rate has now been reduced to 20% (Mufson, Stanek, 1999). Death is more likely to occur in older, chronically ill patients. The presence of bacteremia also affects the prognosis for pneumonia. The mortality in patients with bacteremia is approximately double that observed in the absence of bacteremia. Transient bacteremia may occur in all patients with pneumococcal pneumonia. Demonstrable bacteremia suggests ineffective localization of the pulmonary process, and not surprisingly, the mortality is higher in this group. The consequences of bacteremia may be metastatic lesions resulting in conditions such as meningitis, bacterial endocarditis, and peritonitis.

A vaccine for pneumococcal pneumonia is currently available and in adults is 80% to 90% effective against the most common pneumococcal serotypes. The vaccine is generally given to individuals at high risk of fatal outcome, for example, those with sickle cell anemia, multiple myeloma, nephrotic syndrome, or diabetes mellitus.

Other less common causes of bacterial pneumonia in the adult include streptococci other than *Streptococcus pneumoniae* and *Haemophilus influenzae* (a gram-negative bacteria). These organisms are more likely to cause infection in children. Generally, nontypical strains of *H. influenzae* are responsible for pneumonia in adults and most often affect patients with preexisting chronic obstructive pulmonary disease (COPD).

Staphylococcus aureus (a gram-positive coccus) and gram-negative aerobic bacilli, including *Pseudomonas aeruginosa*, *Klebsiella pneumoniae*, and *Escherichia coli*, are responsible for most nosocomial pneumonias. These pneumonias cause extensive damage to the lung parenchyma, and complications such as lung abscess and emphysema are common. Mortality figures for nosocomial pneumonias are as high as 33%.

Oropharyngeal and gastric colonization play a critical role in the pathogenesis of pneumonia in the hospitalized patient. The oropharynx becomes colonized by many species of gram-negative organisms within 48 hours of hospitalization. Aspiration of oropharyngeal secretions occurs during sleep and is enhanced by factors such as a nasogastric tube, altered consciousness, depressed gag reflex, or delayed gastric emptying. The role of gastric colonization has been recognized in recent years. Gastric bacterial counts rise in the presence of medications that raise the gastric pH, such as H_2 blockers (e.g., ranitidine) and antacids given to prevent stress ulceration. Sucralfate is a medication that heals ulcers without altering the gastric pH and should be used alone.

Some patients who survive *Klebsiella* (or Friedländer's) pneumonia develop a chronic pneumonia with severe progressive destruction of lung tissue that ultimately converts the patient into a respiratory cripple. A thick "red currant jelly" sputum is characteristic of this pneumonia. Most cases of *Klebsiella* pneumonia occur in middle-age or older men who are chronic alcoholics or who have some other chronic disease. Pneumonia caused by *Pseudomonas* organisms is most common in hospitalized patients who are terminally ill or who have marked suppression of immunologic body defenses (e.g., a patient with leukemia or a person who has had a renal transplant and is receiving large doses of immunosuppressive drugs). Other predisposing factors in gram-negative pneumonias include prior antimicrobial therapy, which alters the normal resident flora of the respiratory tract and allows overgrowth of certain microorganisms. Contaminated ventilatory equipment is a common source of *Pseudomonas* infection. *S. aureus* is commonly a secondary infection in hospitalized, debilitated patients and is most likely to cause a bronchopneumonia.

Viral infections typically occur in community epidemics and are generally limited to the upper respiratory tract. Although viruses are the most common cause of pneumonia in children, viral pneumonias in adults account for only approximately 10% of cases. Individuals with chronic diseases or older adults are more susceptible. Characteristic signs and symptoms include headache, fever, generalized aching of muscles, extreme fatigue, and a dry cough.

Most of these pneumonias are mild, do not require hospitalization, and leave no permanent lung damage.

---

*These stages represent the temporal course in untreated pneumococcal pneumonia. With the use of antibiotics, the course is now run in approximately 3 days.

Types A and B influenza virus and adenovirus are common infecting agents. The treatment of viral pneumonia is symptomatic and palliative because antibiotics are ineffective against viruses. Vaccination may offer protection for a limited time but does not give protection against the many other types of viruses (some unidentified) that may cause respiratory infections. Viral pneumonia may set the stage for secondary invasion by bacteria, which has already been discussed. More rarely, a fatal patchy or diffuse pneumonitis may be attributed to the virus.

Pneumonia caused by *Mycoplasma pneumoniae* is generally discussed with viral pneumonias even though the infecting organism is a bacterium. Most mycoplasmal infections are restricted to pharyngitis or bronchitis, but approximately 10% of infected patients develop pneumonia. Mycoplasmal pneumonia typically affects young adults, especially college students and military recruits, and may be implicated in as many as 50% of all cases. The clinical picture of mycoplasmal pneumonia is similar to influenza virus pneumonia with evidence of interstitial pneumonitis. Mycoplasmal pneumonia is highly contagious and, unlike viral pneumonia, responds to erythromycin, tetracycline, or doxycycline. Mycoplasmal pneumonia is often referred to as primary atypical pneumonia or "walking pneumonia."

Legionella pneumophila, a gram-negative bacteria, was first recognized as an agent in pneumonia in the late 1970s after an outbreak of disease at a convention of the American Legion. *Legionella* infections (legionnaires' disease) account for up to 7% of community-acquired pneumonias and up to 10% of nosocomial pneumonias. Legionellae thrive in aquatic environments. Diverse natural reservoirs harbor these organisms, including mud, hot streams, and stagnant lakes. Transmission to humans occurs chiefly by aspiration of contaminated water. Hot water systems, shower heads, hot tubs, humidifiers, and air-conditioning systems with stagnant water may harbor legionellae and provide a source for human infection. Infection may occur sporadically or in outbreaks. *Legionella* infections are most often observed in older adults, smokers, and others with impaired lung defenses. After an incubation period of 2 to 10 days, the illness usually begins gradually with malaise, dry cough, chills, fever, headache, confusion, diffuse myalgias, anorexia, and diarrhea. The diagnosis of *Legionella* infection may be made by culturing the organism or identifying its antigens. Chest radiographs show a patchy or lobar distribution pattern. The treatment of choice for legionnaires' disease is erythromycin or the newer macrolides (e.g., azithromycin). The overall mortality rate is 15% but is much higher in immunocompromised or untreated patients.

Chlamydia pneumoniae is now recognized as a common cause of acute respiratory tract infection and pneumonia. Serologic studies have demonstrated that this organism causes approximately 10% of community-acquired and hospital-acquired pneumonias. *C. pneumoniae* is a member of the genus *Chlamydia* but distinct from the species *C. psittaci* and *C. trachomatis*, which cause psittacosis and genital infections, respectively. *C. pneumoniae* appears to be a pathogen spread by close personal contact. The pneumonia caused by this organism is generally quite mild, with signs and symptoms resembling mycoplasmal pneumonia. As with mycoplasmal pneumonia, the infection generally responds to erythromycin or tetracycline therapy.

Pneumocystis carinii, a protozoan parasite, is the causal agent in *P. carinii* pneumonia (PCP). Recurrent PCP affects more than one half of all patients with AIDS and is a common cause of death in this population. PCP is an opportunistic infection and may also occur in other immunocompromised hosts such as patients receiving immunosuppressive therapy for cancer or organ transplantation. The three most common signs and symptoms of PCP are fever, shortness of breath, and a dry cough. The chest radiograph shows diffuse, patchy infiltrates. Trimethoprim-sulfamethoxazole or pentamidine is the treatment of choice for PCP.

Aspiration pneumonia refers to the pathologic consequences of the entry of oropharyngeal secretions, particulate matter, or gastric contents into the lower airway. Most people aspirate small amounts of oropharyngeal secretions during sleep, and the secretions are normally cleared without sequelae by the normal defense mechanisms. Three distinct aspiration syndromes may be distinguished because of the differing nature of the aspirate, signs and symptoms, and pathophysiology.

As noted previously, aspiration of pathogenic microorganisms colonizing the oropharynx is the most common mode of infecting the lower airways and causing bacterial pneumonia. *Anaerobic pneumonias* are caused by the aspiration of oropharyngeal secretions containing anaerobes such as the *Bacteroides*, *Fusobacterium*, *Peptococcus*, and *Peptostreptococcus* species common among patients with poor dental hygiene. Anaerobic pneumonia is most common in hospitalized patients and persons with chronic alcoholism with infected gums and a predisposition toward aspiration. Nearly all these pneumonias acquired in the hospital are caused by a mixture of both anaerobic and aerobic microorganisms (e.g., gram-negative bacilli, *S. aureus*). The onset of symptoms is usually gradual over 1 to 2 weeks, with fever, weight loss, anemia, leukocytosis, dyspnea, and cough productive of foul-smelling sputum. Lung abscesses form as the lung parenchyma is destroyed, and empyema may develop as the microbes make their way to the pleural surface. Most of the abscesses form in the right lung in the posterior and basilar bronchopulmonary gravity-dependent segments because of the more direct path of the right main stem bronchus. Digital clubbing is common if the abscess is chronic. Treatment consists of prolonged antibiotic therapy, usually with clindamycin or a combination of penicillin and metronidazole (Flagyl), and drainage of empyema, if present.

A second type of aspiration syndrome called *Mendelson's syndrome* is related to the regurgitation and aspiration of the acidic stomach contents. In contrast to the slow onset of anaerobic pneumonia, the resulting *chemical pneumonitis* or *aspiration pneumonitis* may develop within hours and be extremely fulminant. Massive inhalation of gastric contents may lead to sudden death from obstruction, whereas aspiration of smaller quantities of gastric contents may lead to widespread edema, tachypnea, dyspnea, tachycardia, fever, leukocytosis, and respiratory failure. The severity of the inflammatory response depends on the pH of the aspirate more than any other factor. Aspiration pneumonitis always results when the pH of the aspirate is 2.5 or less. Aspiration pneumonitis follows three common patterns: (1) rapid recovery (usually when the quantity of aspirate is small or more alkaline), (2) rapid development of acute respiratory distress syndrome (see Chapter 41), or (3) bacterial superinfection. The bacterial pneumonia that develops is partly chemical as a result of the reaction to the gastric juice and partly from the bacterial superinfection that occurs over days from organisms that may inhabit the mouth or stomach. Abscesses, bronchiectasis, and gangrene are common complications of aspiration pneumonia. The mortality rates are significantly high and have been reported as 30% to 50%. Aspiration of gastric contents is most common during or after anesthesia (especially in obstetric patients and after surgical emergencies because of the lack of surgical preparation), in infants, and in any obtunded patient with depressed gag and cough reflexes.

It is important to realize that vomiting is not a prerequisite to the entrance of gastric contents into the tracheobronchial tree, because silent regurgitation may occur in obtunded patients. Proper positioning to drain oropharyngeal secretions from the mouth is most important in the care of these patients.

A third type of aspiration syndrome is related to the aspiration of particulate matter (usually food) or nonacid fluids (e.g., near-drowning or tube feeding) causing *mechanical obstruction*. When fluid is aspirated, the trachea should be suctioned immediately to relieve the obstruction. When solid matter is aspirated, the presenting symptoms depend on the size of the object and its location in the airways. If the object is lodged high in the trachea, causing complete obstruction, apnea, aphonia, and rapid death may then ensue. If the object cannot be dislodged by means of the finger sweep or the Heimlich maneuver, an emergency tracheotomy (cricothyrotomy) may be performed. If the object (e.g., a peanut) becomes lodged in the smaller airways, the presenting signs and symptoms may include a chronic cough and recurrent infection. Therapy consists of removing the object, usually by means of bronchoscopy.

Hypostatic pneumonia is a pneumonia that develops frequently at the lung bases and is caused by shallow breathing and constantly remaining in the same position. Gravity causes blood to become congested in the dependent part of the lung, and infection aids the development of true pneumonia.

Fungi may be the cause of pneumonia, although they are a much less common cause than are bacteria. A few fungi are capable of producing a chronic granulomatous, suppurative lung disease that is often mistaken for tuberculosis. Many of these fungal infections are endemic to certain geographic regions. The most important fungal infections in the United States are *histoplasmosis* (Midwest and East), *coccidioidomycosis* (Southwest), and *blastomycosis* (Southeast). Spores of these fungi are found in the soil and are inhaled. Spores carried into the smaller divisions of the lung are phagocytized and cause an allergic reaction. After allergy develops, the reaction becomes inflammatory, with tubercle formation, central caseation, scarring, calcification, and even cavity formation. All the pathologic changes closely resemble tuberculosis to the extent that differentiation can be made only by identifi-

cation and culture of the fungus from lung tissue. Serologic and delayed hypersensitivity skin tests are not positive until a few weeks after the initial infection and may even be negative with severe disease.

It is not unusual for fungal pneumonia to complicate the final stages of terminal diseases such as cancer or leukemia. *Candida albicans*, a yeast frequently found in the sputum of healthy persons, may invade the pulmonary tissue under these conditions. Infection with *Candida* is termed *candidiasis*. Prolonged use of antibiotics may also alter the natural body flora and permit invasion of *Candida*. Amphotericin B is the drug of choice for the pulmonary fungal infections.

Pulmonary Fibrosis

Pulmonary fibrosis is not a disease entity but a pathologic term that denotes an excessive amount of connective tissue in the lung. Fibrosis results from a method of tissue repair that may follow any disease process of the lung, producing inflammation or necrosis. The most common type of pulmonary fibrosis is *localized fibrosis*, which follows localized damage to the lung parenchyma caused by conditions such as tuberculosis, pulmonary abscess, bronchiectasis, or unresolved pneumonia. Less often, pulmonary fibrosis may diffusely involve the lung parenchyma, particularly affecting the interalveolar septa. Unlike localized fibrosis, diffuse pulmonary fibrosis is a disabling and frequently fatal disorder. Diffuse pulmonary fibrosis represents end-stage lung disease from a host of known and unknown causes. A few of the more common causes of diffuse pulmonary fibrosis are listed in Box 39-2.

BOX 39-2

Common Causes of Diffuse Pulmonary Fibrosis

DISEASES OF KNOWN CAUSE
1. Pneumoconioses (occupational inhalation of dusts)
   a. Inorganic dusts
      Silica: silicosis
      Coal: "black lung"
      Iron: siderosis
      Asbestos: asbestosis
      Talc: talcosis
      Beryllium: berylliosis
   b. Organic dusts
      Cotton: byssinosis
      Sugar cane: bagassosis
      Moldy hay: "farmer's lung"
      Maple bark
2. Noxious gas inhalation of nitrogen oxides (silo filler), chlorine, sulfur oxides, or metal fumes
3. Drug sensitivity to diphenylhydantoin (phenytoin, Dilantin) or busulfan (Myleran)
4. Irradiation injury
5. Viral pneumonias
6. Chronic pulmonary edema

DISEASES OF UNKNOWN CAUSE
1. Hamman-Rich syndrome
2. Sarcoidosis
3. "Collagen diseases," progressive systemic sclerosis
4. Chronic interstitial pneumonia
5. Mucoviscidosis (cystic fibrosis)

The *pneumoconioses* are a group of diseases caused by the inhalation of certain inorganic and organic dusts. Some dusts, when inhaled in sufficient concentration into the lungs, produce a fibrous tissue reaction, whereas others are quite inert. The dust inhalation diseases are of particular interest because exposure is usually related to certain occupations, and these diseases are theoretically preventable by the institution of industrial safety standards. Only a few examples of noxious dusts or gases causing pulmonary fibrosis are listed in the box. Whether a particular dust causes disease depends on (1) the size of the particle—the most dangerous dust particle seems to be 1 to 5 μm because larger particles never reach the alveoli; (2) the concentration and length of exposure—high concentration is usually required to overcome the action of the ciliary escalator, and long exposure is usually required (e.g., coal miner's pneumoconiosis, or black lung disease, usually requires 20 years of exposure before extensive pulmonary fibrosis is noted); and (3) the nature of the dust—certain materials (particularly the organic dusts such as cotton fiber, which causes *byssinosis;* sugar cane [*bagassosis*]; and moldy hay [*farmer's lung*]) have an unusual antigenic effect and cause an allergic alveolitis. The chemical nature of inorganic dusts also influences their capacity to produce disease. Silica dust (frequently inhaled by grinders, sandblasters, and rock quarry workers), which causes *silicosis,* is particularly harmful. Theories suggest that these dust particles regularly destroy the macrophages by which they are phagocytized, resulting in the formation of fibrotic nodules. Widespread fibrosis is produced by the coalescence of the fibrotic nodules.

Asbestos is a compound of magnesium and iron silicate. Because of its unique physical characteristics (durability, heat resistance, flexibility), asbestos is widely used in industry (e.g., shipbuilding, car brake and clutch lining, air filters, insulation materials, roofing). *Asbestosis* is an interstitial process that slowly develops into a diffuse, nonnodular pulmonary fibrosis involving the terminal airways, alveoli, and pleurae. The disease is usually recognized after 20 years of exposure and tends to progress after exposure has ended. The major complications of asbestosis are bronchogenic carcinoma, malignant mesothelioma, and pleural plaques. The risk of bronchogenic carcinoma is largely confined to cigarette smokers, in whom the risk is greater than it is in smokers without asbestosis (see Chapter 42). Asbestos ex-posure occurs not only from mining and the manufacture of asbestos products but also from general community air pollution. Asbestos fibers have been found in the autopsied lungs of a high percentage of city dwellers. The potential health hazard of such low concentrations is unclear.

The inhalation of noxious gases may be associated with certain occupations. The result is a chemical pneumonitis. Of particular interest is *silo filler's disease,* which is not a pneumoconiosis but is caused by the inhalation of nitrogen oxides from fermentation of the vegetation in a freshly filled silo. The severity of reaction to noxious gases depends on the concentration of gas and length of exposure. Viral pneumonias, chronic pulmonary edema, irradiation involving the chest, and certain drugs that produce a hypersensitivity reaction (e.g., diphenylhydantoin [phenytoin], busulfan) are other known causes of diffuse pulmonary fibrosis.

Among diseases of unknown cause leading to diffuse pulmonary fibrosis is the *Hamman-Rich syndrome.* This syndrome is an unusual interstitial pneumonia that may have a rapidly fatal or a more protracted course, both with the development of severe intraalveolar and interstitial fibrosis. Other chronic interstitial pneumonias also tend to result in progressive pulmonary fibrosis, as do certain systemic diseases such as sarcoidosis, collagen diseases (especially scleroderma), and mucoviscidosis.

The systemic symptoms in the group of diseases causing pulmonary fibrosis vary widely. In the early stages, no symptoms may be present. The pulmonary symptoms, however, are strikingly similar. The primary symptom appears to be a progressive dyspnea on exertion. The common pathologic denominator is interstitial fibrosis, with the extent of fibrosis determining the effect on pulmonary function. When the fibrosis is extensive, a decrease occurs in lung elasticity, total lung capacity (TLC), VC, and residual volume (RV), which all indicate restrictive lung disease. The dyspnea reflects the poor compliance and results in a concomitant increase in the work of breathing. The term "honeycomb lung" is used to describe the appearance of the end-stage lung caused by extensive destruction of the alveoli and pulmonary vessels. These changes lead to hypoxemia and pulmonary hypertension with eventual right heart failure (cor pulmonale). In many patients, however, the symptoms do not progress beyond mild exertional dyspnea.

KEY CONCEPTS

- *Restrictive patterns of respiratory disease* are characterized by increased stiffness of the lungs or thorax or both causing decreased compliance, decreased V_T, VC, and TLC. Dysfunction is primarily with inspiration; the ratio of forced expiratory volume in a one-second period to forced vital capacity (FEV_1/FVC) is usually normal. The work of breathing is increased, and the patient adopts a pattern of rapid, shallow breathing.
- Restrictive patterns of pulmonary disease may be roughly divided into two subgroups based on the location of the pathology: extrapulmonary (usually with normal lungs) and intrapulmonary disease.

- Extrapulmonary causes of restrictive respiratory dysfunction limit thoracic cage movement, and all of the following cause alveolar hypoventilation: (1) CNS disorders that interrupt nerve impulse transmission to the respiratory muscles (e.g., depression of respiratory center by narcotics or $Paco_2$ >70 mm Hg); (2) neuromuscular disorders (e.g., muscular dystrophy, myasthenia gravis, amyotrophic lateral sclerosis, Guillain-Barré syndrome, poliomyelitis, spinal cord injury); (3) chest cage deformities (e.g., kyphoscoliosis, extreme obesity); and (4) chest cage trauma (e.g., rib fracture, flail chest).

- Intrapulmonary causes of restrictive respiratory dysfunction include (1) pleural disorders (pleural effusion or inflammation, and pneumothorax) and (2) lung parenchymal disorders (atelectasis, pneumonia, pulmonary fibrosis, and adult respiratory distress syndrome (ARDS).

- *Kyphoscoliosis* is a condition in which both posterior and lateral angulation of the spine (hunchback) occur, causing a restrictive pattern of ventilation. In severe cases, the work of breathing is greatly increased because of the abnormally stiff and distorted chest wall, causing the patient to decrease their V_T and increase their respiratory frequency, resulting in hypoventilation. Additionally, the marked chest wall distortion causes lung compression and results in ventilation/perfusion mismatch and hypoxemia. Pulmonary hypertension, cor pulmonale, and respiratory failure are the end result of the chronic hypoventilation and hypoxemia.

- *Flail chest* is the result of multiple rib fractures, usually from a steering wheel injury during a motor vehicle accident. Flail chest causes the thoracic cage to become unstable. The affected ribs cave in (flail) during inspiration as a result of the negative intrapleural pressure and during expiration the flail area bulges outward. This action compresses and restricts the underlying lung tissue and promotes atelectasis and lung collapse. Mediastinal contents may swing back and forth in the chest cavity (pendelluft). A large flail segment may be temporarily stabilized with towel rolls, tape, or sandbags placed against the segment. Intubation and ventilator support is required for all patients with large flail segments, and for any patient with underlying acute or chronic lung disease.

- *Pickwickian syndrome* or *obesity-hypoventilation syndrome* is a term used to describe a group of clinical disorders found in persons who are extremely obese. Clinical features include chronic alveolar hypoventilation, hypercapnia, hypoxemia, somnolence, and polycythemia. The Pickwickian syndrome is only one subtype of a group of disorders known as *sleep apnea syndromes* in which elements of upper airway obstruction or central depressed respiratory drive may be present. Nonobese persons may also be afflicted. Weight reduction may reverse the respiratory insufficiency.

- The accumulation of fluid in the pleural space is called *pleural effusion*, and if the fluid accumulation is extensive, compression of the lung can occur.

- Pleural fluid may be a transudate (low protein content) called *hydrothorax* and is commonly the result of high hydrostatic pressure in cardiac failure or decreased colloid osmotic pressure, as in nephrotic syndrome or liver cirrhosis.

- Pleural fluid may be an exudate (high protein fluid containing fibrinogen or fibrin). A pleural effusion containing pus is called *empyema* and may result from pneumonia, lung abscess, or a neoplasm extending into the pleural cavity. The fibrinous exudate may become organized to form fibrinous adhesions welding the parietal and visceral pleura together called *fibrothorax*. Therefore exudative pleural effusions must be treated by closed chest tube drainage.

- The presence of air in the pleural space is called pneumothorax. *Spontaneous pneumothorax* can be divided into (1) primary or idiopathic—those that occur in otherwise healthy individuals, usually a result of the rupture of a congenital subpleural bleb or (2) secondary to disease in the lungs, such as rupture of an emphysematous bulla, or as a complication of pneumonia or a malignancy.

- *Traumatic pneumothorax* may be a result of (1) a chest injury, such as a knife wound or rib fracture or (2) iatrogenic factors, such as a complication of positive pressure ventilation, subclavian cannulation, or lung biopsy.

- An *open pneumothorax (sucking chest wound)* occurs when communication takes place between the atmosphere and the pleural space via the chest wall or tear in the pleura and bronchi or alveoli with communication. During inspiration, air is "sucked" into the pleural space, causing the lung on the affected side to collapse and pushing mediastinal contents to the unaffected side; during expiration, air escapes through the chest wall, and the mediastinal contents swing back. Treatment includes placing an airtight seal over the wound and observing for tension pneumothorax and removing seal if this occurs. A communication defect that seals itself off is called a *closed pneumothorax*.

- A *tension pneumothorax* occurs when a check valve mechanism allows air into the pleural space but prevents its egress. This condition might occur in the event of a rupture of the visceral pleura, a bronchus from a fractured rib, or during mechanical ventilation with positive end-expiratory pressure. Tension pneumothorax is a medical emergency requiring immediate needle aspiration of air to prevent complete collapse of the lung and death.

- Collapse of the alveoli is called *atelectasis*. Several conditions lead to atelectasis. *Compression atelectasis* is caused by external pressure on the lung from pneumothorax, pleural effusion, or abdominal distention. *Absorption atelectasis* (most common) occurs when mucus blocks entry of air into the distal airways; the absorption of gases in the alveoli then causes alveolar collapse. Loss of normal surfactant (developmental or acquired) from terminal air spaces leads to generalized failure of lung expansion (microatelectasis).

- *Atelectasis* causes intrapulmonary shunting (perfusion without ventilation) and, if extensive, hypoxemia.

- High-risk conditions that promote *atelectasis* include (1) prolonged high fractions of inspired O_2 (Fio_2) (40% to 50%)—nitrogen is washed out, O_2 is reabsorbed, and alveoli collapse; (2) conditions associated with retained secretions, such as bronchitis, pneumonia, or postoperative status (especially after thoracic or abdominal surgery); (3) comatose condition; and (4) compounded by shallow breathing, pain, sedation, and depressed cough reflex.

- Pulmonary signs of *atelectasis* include: crackles (rales), bronchial breath sounds, egophony (E → A), dull percussion note over area of atelectasis, diminished breath sounds if the airway is closed, tracheal deviation to unaffected side, and decreased chest excursion (if area of atelectasis is large).

- Measures to prevent *atelectasis* include: deep breathing and coughing, ambulation, incentive spirometry, frequent repositioning of bedridden patients, adequate fluid intake to promote mobilization of secretions, and patient education to promote cooperation.
- *Pneumonia* (infection and inflammation of the lung parenchyma) is the sixth leading cause of death in the United States. Causative organisms include bacteria, viruses, fungi, and protozoa.
- Risk factors for *pneumonia* include age extremes (very young or very old), viral upper respiratory tract infections, cigarette smoking, ethanol abuse, COPD, cancer (especially lung cancer), chronic illness (e.g., diabetes mellitus, uremia), abdominal or thoracic surgery, prolonged bed rest, endotracheal tube or tracheostomy, rib fracture, immunosuppressive therapy, and AIDS.
- Microbial agents that cause *pneumonia* have two major *modes of transmission*: (1) aspiration of pathogenic organisms that have colonized the oropharynx and (2) inhalation of infectious aerosols. Less commonly, bacteria may reach the lung parenchyma through the bloodstream from an extrapulmonary site (especially *Staphylococcus*) or from intravenous drug use.
- Pneumonia is classified pathologically, microbiologically, and clinically.
- The *pathologic pattern of pneumonia* gives a few clues to the likely cause and severity: (1) *lobar pneumonia* occurs when organisms widely colonize the alveolar spaces, causing consolidation of the entire lobe and are often caused by pneumococcus or *Klebsiella*; patients with lobar pneumonia are extremely ill; (2) *bronchopneumonia* (patchy distribution) occurs when organisms colonize bronchi and extend into the alveoli; (3) most viral infections of the lung cause an *interstitial inflammatory response* by lymphoid cells, which is self-limiting in most cases; the common causes are the influenza and mycoplasma (viruslike bacteria) organisms; and (4) fungal or tuberculosis infections of the lung cause *necrotizing destruction of tissue or cavity formation*; fungal infections generally occur in immunosuppressed patients or rarely in healthy persons to a specific agent indigenous to a particular geographic area (histoplasmosis, coccidioidomycosis, and blastomycosis cause granulomatous inflammation of the lung and fibrosis with a pattern resembling tuberculosis).
- The *microbiologic classification of pneumonia* is based on the causative organism identified by microbiology. Causative agents of bacterial pneumonia are divided into gram-positive or gram-negative organisms. *Streptococcus pneumoniae* (or pneumococcus), a gram-positive organism, is the most common cause of bacterial pneumonia. The causative organism is not identified in more than 50% of pneumonias, and the cases are treated empirically.
- The *clinical classification of pneumonia* is based on the circumstances surrounding its development: community-acquired versus hospital-acquired (nosocomial), (2) aspiration, and (3) disease in immunosuppressed patients. The clinical classification is best suited for planning investigation and initiating therapy because knowledge of the circumstances provides a strong clue as to the likely organisms causing the infection and thus the appropriate antibiotic.
- The most common causes of *community-acquired pneumonia* are *Streptococcus pneumoniae, Mycoplasma pneumoniae, Haemophilus influenzae, Chlamydia pneumoniae,* and *Legionella pneumophila.*
- *Hospital-acquired (nosocomial) pneumonias* are caused primarily by gram-negative bacteria, such as *Escherichia coli, Klebsiella pneumoniae,* and *Pseudomonas aeruginosa* or oral anaerobes.
- Factors that predispose the patient to oropharyngeal colonization and pneumonia with gram-negative organisms include hospitalization, old age, and serious illness with compromised host defenses.
- Anaerobes found in the oropharynx are the usual cause of *aspiration pneumonia*. Organisms that cause infection are usually mixed (e.g., *Fusobacterium, Bacteroides*). *Staphylococcus aureus* and gram-negative organisms are also common causes of aspiration pneumonia in hospitalized patients. Aspiration of gastric acid causes chemical pneumonitis, which can lead to adult respiratory distress syndrome and a fulminant pneumonia. Development of lung abscess is a frequent complication of aspiration pneumonia.
- *Opportunistic infections* affect patients who are immunosuppressed and include the following: (1) protozoa—*Pneumocystis carinii*; (2) fungi—*Candida, Aspergillus*; (3) viruses—herpes simplex, cytomegalovirus; and (4) bacteria—routine bacterial pathogens responsible for community pneumonias are generally more severe, pseudomonas, or *M. tuberculosis* or atypical mycobacteria.
- Common signs and symptoms of pneumococcal pneumonia include sudden onset of fever and chills, productive cough (often with rust-colored sputum), dyspnea, pleuritic chest pain, crackles (rales), bronchial breath sounds, egophony, and dullness to percussion over affected area. Some degree of hypoxemia almost always occurs as a result of the shunting of blood through the nonventilated area of consolidation, causing the patient to have a dusky appearance. Chest x-rays (showing pulmonary infiltrates), leukocytosis, and microbiologic sputum examination may be helpful in making the diagnosis. Pneumococcal pneumonia generally heals with no residual negative effects on lung tissue.
- The hallmark of anaerobic pulmonary infection is foul-smelling, putrid sputum.
- Restrictive lung diseases cause reduced compliance of the lungs (difficult to expand with respiration). Patients who are afflicted complain of breathlessness. Diffuse alveolar wall damage causing interstitial pulmonary fibrosis is the main feature of chronic restrictive lung diseases.
- *Chronic interstitial lung disease* can be initiated by a wide range of extrinsic factors, both inhaled (industrial dust) and noninhaled (drugs, radiation), as well as intrinsic disease (sarcoidosis).
- The *pneumoconioses* are a group of diseases caused by the inhalation of certain inorganic or organic dusts, which may result in diffuse interstitial fibrosis (e.g., coal worker's pneumoconiosis), silicosis (grinders,

rock quarry workers), byssinosis (cotton mill workers), and moldy hay (farmer's lung).

■ Asbestosis predisposes to interstitial fibrosis, lung cancer, and mesothelioma of the pleura.

■ Progressive pulmonary fibrosis that is extensive causes decreased lung compliance, TLC, VC, and RV, all of which indicate restrictive lung disease. The term *honeycomb lung* is used to describe the appearance of the end-stage lung caused by extensive destruction of the alveoli and pulmonary vessels. These changes lead to hypoxemia and pulmonary hypertension with eventual right heart failure (cor pulmonale). In many patients, however, the symptoms do not progress beyond mild exertional dyspnea.

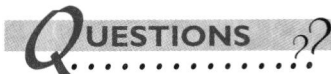

QUESTIONS

A sampling of review questions for this chapter appears here. Visit http://www.mosby.com/MERLIN/PriceWilson/ for additional questions.

Answer the following on a separate sheet of paper.

1. What are two physiologic alterations that occur as a consequence of a restricted pattern of ventilation?
2. List possible causes of traumatic and spontaneous pneumothorax.
3. Describe the emergency treatment of a penetrating chest wound.
4. Why does a pneumothorax occur when a communication exists between a bronchus or alveolus and the pleural cavity?
5. Describe the treatment for a large pneumothorax and a large pleural effusion.
6. What is a collection of fluid in the pleural cavity called?
7. When a transudate occurs, pressure increases so that the balance of forces favors the passage of fluid out of the vessels. What is this pressure called?

8. What is formed in the pleural cavity as the result of increased capillary permeability or impaired lymphatic absorption?
9. What is pleural fluid called that has a specific gravity of less than 1.015 and a protein content of less than 3%?
10. List five general disorders that may cause damage to the lung alveoli and interstitium. State the specific damage to lung tissue that each disorder causes.
11. Contrast absorption and compression atelectasis with respect to the common cause of each and the mechanism involved.
12. Why are the pores of Kohn important in maintaining collateral ventilation? Illustrate the way in which collateral ventilation prevents absorption atelectasis caused by bronchial obstruction by a mucous plug.

13. List in sequence the four stages describing the pathologic changes in the lung in untreated pneumococcal pneumonia (include name of stage, time period, and description of lung changes).
14. List three principles of treatment for patients with pneumonia.
15. List three criteria used to predict whether a particular dust will cause disease of the lung parenchyma. State the reason why each of these criteria is important.
16. List the three most important fungal infections in the United States that cause lung disease.
17. What are two consequences of pulmonary fibrosis?
18. The manifestations of extensive diffuse pulmonary fibrosis are typical of what type of pattern of ventilatory dysfunction?

Complete the following statements by filling in the blanks.

19. Pulmonary fibrosis is characterized pathologically by _____ fibrosis.
20. Pneumonia caused by gram-negative or staphylococcal organisms causes extensive damage to the lung _____. Common complications include _____ and _____. The prognosis is generally _____.

Match the type of pneumothorax in column A with the correct description in column B.

Column A
21. _____ Open
22. _____ Closed
23. _____ Tension

Column B
a. Communication between pleural cavity and atmosphere is sealed off.
b. Communication between pleural cavity and atmosphere open during inspiration and closed during expiration.
c. Communication between pleural cavity and atmosphere does not seal off.

Match each of the anatomic patterns of pneumonia in column A with its pathologic description or common causative agent in column B. More than one letter may be used for each blank in column A.

Column A
24. _____ Lobar consolidation
25. _____ Lobular consolidation
26. _____ Necrotizing or cavity formation
27. _____ Interstitial

Column B
a. Fungi or *Mycobacterium tuberculosis*
b. Viral or *Mycoplasma* pneumonia
c. *Pneumococcus*
d. *Staphylococcus* or *streptococcus*
e. Perivascular exudate and edema between the alveoli
f. May undergo caseous necrosis
g. Exudate chiefly intraalveolar
h. Fibrinous exudate chiefly in bronchioles
i. Patchy distribution of infection
j. Whole lung lobe infected

CHAPTER
40

Cardiovascular Disease and the Lung

LORRAINE M. WILSON

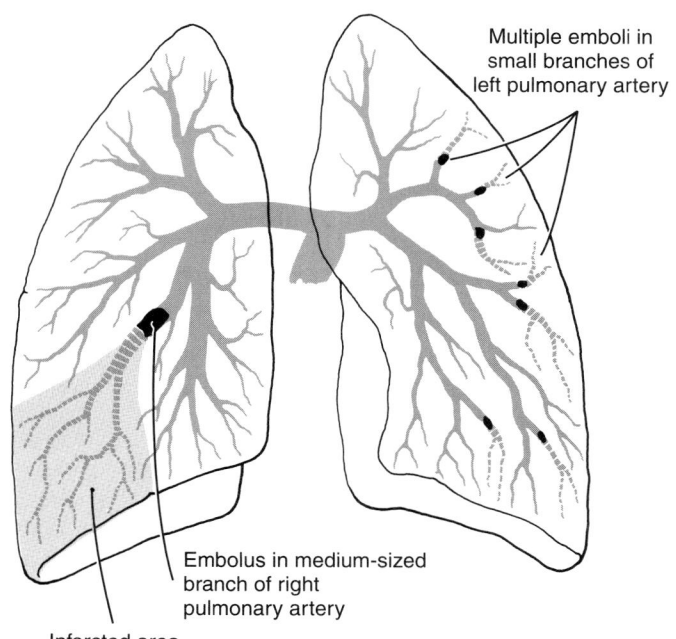

FIG. 40-1   Pulmonary embolism and infarction.

*C*hronic lung disease is an increasingly frequent cause of heart disease, and conversely, heart disease with decompensation or vascular disease may cause changes in the structure and function of the lung. This close interrelationship relates to the functional position of the lungs in the circulation (see Fig. 35-4). This chapter discusses pulmonary embolism, pulmonary edema, and cor pulmonale, all diseases demonstrating the close relationship between the heart and lungs.

PULMONARY EMBOLISM

Pulmonary embolism (PE) occurs when an embolus, usually a blood clot that breaks free from its attachment in a vein of the lower limbs, circulates through the blood vessels and the right side of the heart to become lodged in the main pulmonary artery or one of its branches. *Pulmonary infarction* is the term used to describe a local focus of necrosis resulting from the vascular obstruction (Fig. 40-1; see also Fig. 7-9).

The true incidence of PE cannot be determined because of the difficulty of the clinical diagnosis, but PE is an important cause of morbidity and mortality in a hospital population and is said to account for more than 200,000 deaths in the United States annually. Massive PE is one of the most common causes of unexpected death, being second only to coronary artery disease. Autopsy studies show that as many as 60% of patients dying in

the hospital have had a PE, but the diagnosis was missed in 70% of the cases.

Three basic factors are related to the development of venous thrombosis and subsequent PE: (1) venous stasis or slowing of the blood flow, (2) injury and inflammation to the vein wall, and (3) hypercoagulability (Box 40-1). Several diseases and activities appear to increase the risk of forming a thrombus, and patients in these states should be watched closely to detect any evidence of thrombus formation. Pregnancy, the use of oral contraceptive drugs, obesity, heart failure, varicose veins, abdominal infection, cancer, sickle cell anemia, and any prolonged inactivity such as plane, train, or bus rides increases the risk of thrombus formation. Many of these conditions are common in hospitalized patients. Venous thrombosis and PE occur predominantly in bedridden

Risk Factors for Pulmonary Embolisms

A. Conditions promoting venous stasis
1. Prolonged bedrest or immobilization
2. Postpartum status
3. Orthopedic surgery or casts
4. Obesity
5. Older age

B. Injury to the vein wall
1. Postsurgical, especially involving the thorax, abdomen, pelvis, or legs
2. Pelvic or hip fractures
3. Intravenous therapy

C. Conditions that increase blood coagulability
1. Malignancy
2. High-estrogen oral contraceptives
3. Polycythemia

D. High-risk disorders
1. Stage IV congestive heart failure
2. Postoperative status
   a. Hip surgery
   b. Extensive abdominal or pelvic surgery for malignancy
3. Postpartum status
4. History of deep venous thromboses (DVT), pulmonary embolism (PE), varicosities
5. Long-bone fractures
6. Abdominal infection
7. Diabetes mellitus
8. Sickle cell anemia
9. Chronic lung disease

patients. The single most important condition predisposing an individual to venous thrombosis is congestive heart failure; the postoperative state is next in importance. The most common site for a blood clot to form is in the iliofemoral deep veins of the legs (90%), although clots may form in the pelvic veins and in the right side of the heart. Emboli of nonthrombotic origin occur infrequently (fewer than 10% of pulmonary emboli) but include obstruction caused by air, fat, malignant cells, amniotic fluid, parasites, vegetations, and foreign material.

The signs and symptoms of a PE are extremely variable, depending on the size of the clot or clots. The clinical picture may range from no signs to sudden and almost immediate death caused by a massive saddle embolus at the bifurcation of the main pulmonary artery, resulting in blockage of the entire outflow of the right ventricle. In a patient with the signs of thrombophlebitis in leg veins, the classic syndrome associated with a moderate-sized PE consists of sudden onset of unexplained dyspnea, tachypnea, tachycardia, and restlessness. Pleuritic pain, friction rub, hemoptysis, and fever are not usually present unless infarction has occurred. Massive PE may result in a sudden shocklike state with tachycardia, hypotension, cyanosis, stupor, or syncope. Death usually follows within a few minutes. Frequently, however, the symptoms of PE are subtle, such as unexplained fever or worsening of a preexisting cardiac or cardiopulmonary condition. These subtle symptoms are likely to be associated with recurrent small, multiple pulmonary emboli and may be unnoticed until right ventricular hypertrophy and failure direct attention to the pulmonary vascular disease.

The effect of PE is to produce an area of lung that is ventilated but underperfused, thus increasing physiologic dead-space ventilation. Reflex bronchoconstriction occurs in the affected area and is thought to result from the release of histamine or serotonin from the clot. Reflex bronchoconstriction is considered to be compensatory in the occluded area, because it reduces the unevenness of ventilation and perfusion. In adjacent areas, however, reflex bronchospasm may result in considerable hypoxemia. If the pulmonary vascular bed is sufficiently reduced by a large embolus or by recurrent multiple emboli, pulmonary hypertension may then result. Estimates are that two thirds of the vascular bed must be obliterated before this event occurs.

A localized area of ischemic necrosis (infarction) is an uncommon complication of PE because of the lung's dual blood supply. Pulmonary infarction is usually associated with occlusion of a medium-sized lobar or lobular artery and insufficient collateral flow from the bronchial circulation (see Fig. 40-1). A pleural friction rub and a small pleural effusion are common signs.

Few diagnostic tests specifically distinguish a pulmonary infarction from a pulmonary infiltrate. Radioactive lung perfusion scans are abnormal in either case or in the presence of emphysema. The chest radiograph may be normal or a pleural effusion may be present in both cases. Physiologic tests and serum enzymes are similarly of little value in distinguishing an infarction from pneumonia. Additionally, the signs and symptoms of pneumonia may be similar to those of PE.

Nuclear scintigraphic ventilation/perfusion (V/Q) scanning of the lung is the single most important noninvasive diagnostic modality for detecting PE. V/Q scan results are classified as normal, high probability or nondiagnostic (intermediate or low probability) of PE. The diagnosis of PE is highly unlikely in patients with normal scans but approximately 90% certain in high probability scans. Patients with nondiagnostic V/Q scan results should have pulmonary angiography (an invasive test) because it is the most reliable method of diagnosing PE.

Prophylactic measures directed toward the prevention of initial or recurrent deep venous thrombosis (DVT) in at risk patients is important. The effectiveness of oral anticoagulants in preventing PE or DVT has been clearly shown. Low-dose heparin (3000 to 5000 units every 8 to 12 hours subcutaneously) has been a valuable prophylactic agent for hospitalized patients at risk for DVT or PE. Recently, low-molecular-weight heparins (LMWHs) have been shown to be more effective than is the standard unfractionated heparin for prophylaxis. Another prophylactic measure frequently used for high-risk patients is external compression of the lower extremities with an intermittent inflating pneumonic device. Compression stockings that provide a 30 to 40 mm Hg gradient have been proven effective in the prophylaxis of thromboembolism and are also effective in preventing progression of thrombus in patients who already have DVT or PE. The ubiquitous white stockings known as antiembolic stockings or TED hose produce a maximum compression of only 18 mm Hg and consequently are not effective in the prophylaxis or treatment of DVT or PE.

The early detection of patients with DVT (and therefore at high risk for PE) has been greatly improved by the use of three relatively new noninvasive diagnostic techniques: Doppler ultrasonic examination, impedance plethysmography, and color flow duplex scanning (see Chapter 34).

The combined approach of early detection of DVT by these improved techniques and the use of standard low-dose heparin or LMWH for patients at high risk for having DVT offers promise for the reduction of PE.

Primary therapy for acute PE consists of fibrinolytic therapy for all patients with massive or unstable PE. Fibrinolytic regimens in common use for PE include two forms of recombinant tissue plasminogen activator, t-PA (alteplase) and r-PA (reteplase) along with urokinase and streptokinase. Surgical embolectomy is reserved for cases in which the fibrinolytic therapy is contraindicated. Important adjunctive measures include pain relief with nonsteroidal antiinflammatory agents, supplemental oxygen, intensive care monitoring, and compression stockings that provide a 30 to 40 mm Hg compression gradient. Dobutamine is used to treat right heart failure and cardiogenic shock.

Primary therapy is followed by secondary prevention of PE using heparin. Heparin is essential as an anticoagulant because it inhibits clot extension but is not capable of dissolving an existing clot. Heparin augments the activity of antithrombin III and prevents the conversion of fibrinogen to fibrin. Heparin thus prevents additional thrombus formation and permits endogenous fibrinolytic mechanisms to lyse a clot that has already formed. Anticoagulation therapy alone may be sufficient when the PE is moderate-sized or small and right ventricular function is normal. A typical bolus of standard unfractionated heparin of 5,000 to 10,000 units is followed by a continuous infusion of 1000 to 1500 units/hour. A therapeutic level of heparin is indicated by an activated partial thromboplastin time (aPTT) that is at least twice the control value. The most important adverse effect of heparin is hemorrhage.

Recently, LMWHs (enoxaparin, dalteparin, and ardeparin) have been found safer and more effective than is unfractionated heparin for prophylaxis of DVT or PE. LMWH can be administered by the subcutaneous route in one or two daily doses and does not require monitoring the aPTT to adjust the dose, as does the use of the standard unfractionated heparin.

After initial anticoagulation with heparin, long-term anticoagulation is continued using warfarin. Warfarin is a vitamin-K antagonist that prevents activation of clotting factors II, VII, IX, and X. The initial dose is 7.5 to 10 mg, and thereafter the dose is lowered sufficiently to maintain an International Normalized Ratio (INR) of approximately 3.0 mg. INR is now the preferred measure for adjustment of warfarin dose rather than the prothrombin time. Anticoagulation therapy with warfarin may be continued from 6 months to 1 year or indefinitely for patients at high risk for recurrent DVT or PE. In some circumstances, prevention of recurrent PE involves placing a screen or filtering device in the lower vena cava with the goal of trapping emboli from the lower extremities en route to the pulmonary circulation.

PULMONARY EDEMA

Pulmonary edema is an excessive accumulation of serous or serosanguineous fluid in the interstitial spaces and alveoli of the lungs. If the edema is acute and extensive, death may rapidly ensue. Pulmonary edema may be pre-cipitated by an increase of hydrostatic pressure within the pulmonary capillaries, a decrease in the colloid osmotic pressure, as in nephritis, or damage to the capillary walls. Damage to the capillary walls may result from the inhalation of noxious gases, inflammation, as in pneumonia, or local interference with oxygenation. The most common cause of pulmonary edema is left ventricular failure resulting from arteriosclerotic heart disease or mitral stenosis (mitral valve obstruction). If the left side of the heart fails while the right side continues to pump blood, the pulmonary capillary pressure then rises until pulmonary edema results. The formation of pulmonary edema occurs in two stages: (1) interstitial edema, characterized by engorgement of the perivascular and peribronchial spaces and increased lymphatic flow and (2) alveolar edema, when fluid moves into the alveoli. Blood plasma is poured out into the alveoli faster than coughing or the lymphatics of the lung can clear it. This plasma interferes with diffusion of oxygen (O_2), and the consequent tissue hypoxia further increases the tendency to edema. Asphyxia may result unless measures are taken to reverse the pulmonary edema. Emergency treatment for acute pulmonary edema includes measures to reduce pulmonary hydrostatic pressure, such as placing the patient in Fowler's position with the feet dependent; rotating tourniquets; or phlebotomy (removing approximately a pint of blood). Other measures include the administration of diuretics, O_2, and digitalis to improve myocardial contractility.

In the presence of chronic passive congestion of the lungs, structural changes in the lung (e.g., pulmonary fibrosis) may result. These changes enable the lung to function for a time with the increased hydrostatic pressure without the development of pulmonary edema. The balance, however, is precarious, and the patient may have attacks of dyspnea at night (paroxysmal nocturnal dyspnea) because of the increase in pulmonary hydrostatic pressure that results from a horizontal position.

COR PULMONALE

Cor pulmonale is the condition in which hypertrophy and dilation of the right ventricle, with or without right ventricular failure, develop as a result of disease affecting the structure or function of the lung or its vasculature. By this definition, neither disease of the left side of the heart nor congenital heart disease is responsible for the pathogenesis. Cor pulmonale may be acute (e.g., massive PE) or chronic. The following discussion concerns the chronic condition.

The exact incidence of cor pulmonale is unknown, because it is often not recognized, both clinically and at autopsy. The estimated incidence of cor pulmonale is 6% to 7% of all heart disease based on studies using the criterion of postmortem ventricular wall thickness (Fishman, 1998).

Normal Function of the Pulmonary Circulation

The pulmonary circulation is interposed between the right and left ventricles for the purpose of gas exchange. Normally, flow through the pulmonary vascular bed depends not only on the right ventricle but also on the pumping action of breathing movements. Because the pulmonary circulation is a low-pressure, low-resistance circulation under normal circumstances, cardiac output can increase many times (as happens during exercise) without significant increase in pulmonary artery pressure. This condition occurs because of the enormous capacity of the pulmonary vascular bed, which is normally approximately 25% perfused at rest, and its ability to recruit more vessels during exercise.

Etiology and Pathogenesis

The etiology and pathogenesis of cor pulmonale are illustrated in Fig. 40-2. The diseases causing cor pulmonale are those in which the pulmonary vasculature is primarily involved, such as recurrent pulmonary emboli, and those in which the impediment to pulmonary blood flow is secondary to obstructive or restrictive respiratory diseases. Chronic obstructive pulmonary disease (COPD), especially the bronchitic type, is the most common cause of cor pulmonale. Restrictive respiratory diseases leading to cor pulmonale include *intrinsic* diseases, such as diffuse pulmonary fibrosis, and *extrinsic* disorders, such as extreme obesity, kyphoscoliosis, or severe neuromuscular dysfunction that affects the respiratory muscles. Finally, pulmonary vascular disease that causes obstruction to blood flow and cor pulmonale is quite rare and usually results from recurrent pulmonary emboli.

Regardless of the initiating disease, the common pathway and prerequisite for cor pulmonale is the development of increased pulmonary vascular resistance and pulmonary hypertension. Pulmonary hypertension, in turn,

increases the workload of the right ventricle, causing hypertrophy and eventual failure. The critical point in the sequence appears to be an increase in pulmonary vascular resistance through the small arteries and arterioles.

Two basic mechanisms produce an increase in pulmonary vascular resistance: (1) hypoxic vasoconstriction of pulmonary blood vessels and (2) obstruction or obliteration (or both) of the pulmonary vascular bed. The first of these two mechanisms appears to be the most critical in the pathogenesis of cor pulmonale. The hypoxemia, hypercapnia, and acidosis that characterize advanced bronchitic COPD provide an excellent example of the way in which these mechanisms operate. The *alveolar (tissue) hypoxia*, rather than the hypoxemia, provides a potent stimulus to pulmonary vasoconstriction. Additionally, chronic alveolar hypoxia promotes hypertrophy of smooth muscle in the pulmonary arterioles, which then respond more vigorously to acute hypoxia. The hypercapnic acidosis and hypoxemia act synergistically to augment the vasoconstriction. Increased blood viscosity arising from secondary polycythemia and increased cardiac output stimulated by chronic hypoxia and hypercapnia make an additional contribution to increased pulmonary artery pressure.

The second mechanism that makes a contribution to increased vascular resistance and pulmonary artery pressure is anatomic in origin. Emphysema is characterized by gradual destruction of the alveolar structure with formation of bullae and complete obliteration of nearby capillaries as well. Permanent loss of blood vessels contributes to the reduction of the cross-sectional area of the vascular bed. Additionally, pulmonary vessels are compressed externally because of the mechanical effects of the high lung volumes in obstructive disease. However,

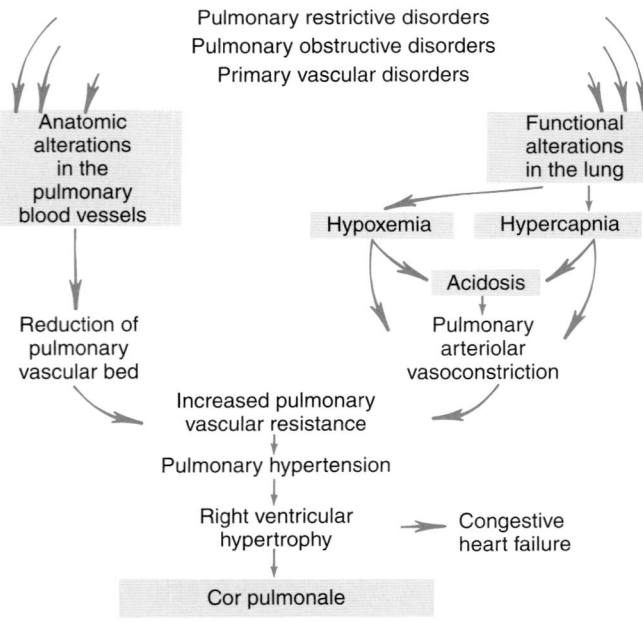

FIG. 40-2 Etiology and pathogenesis of cor pulmonale.

anatomic obstruction and obliteration of the vascular bed are believed to be less important than is hypoxic vasoconstriction in the pathogenesis of cor pulmonale. Approximately two thirds to three fourths of the vascular bed must become obstructed or destroyed before a significant rise in pulmonary artery pressure occurs. Chronic respiratory acidosis is present in a number of obstructive and respiratory diseases as a result of generalized alveolar hypoventilation or as a consequence of V/Q abnormalities. The evidence from this discussion indicates that any pulmonary disease that affects gas exchange, ventilatory mechanics, or the pulmonary vascular bed may result in cor pulmonale.

Clinical Manifestations

Diagnosis of cor pulmonale rests mainly on two criteria: (1) presence of a respiratory disease with associated pulmonary hypertension and (2) evidence of a hypertrophied right ventricle. Presence of persistent hypoxemia, hypercapnia, and acidosis or of right ventricular enlargement on radiographs should suggest the possibility of underlying lung disease. The presence of emphysema tends to obscure the diagnostic features of cor pulmonale. Dyspnea is present as a feature of emphysema whether cor pulmonale is present or not present. A sudden worsening of dyspnea or fatigue, syncope on exertion, or substernal anginal discomfort should suggest cardiac involvement. Physical signs of pulmonary hypertension include a systolic lift over the parasternal area, a loud second pulmonic sound, and murmurs resulting from functional tricuspid and pulmonic insufficiency. Gallop rhythm (S_3 and S_4 heart sounds), jugular venous distention with prominent A waves, hepatomegaly, and peripheral edema may be observed in patients with right ventricular failure.

Treatment

Treatment of cor pulmonale is aimed at correcting the alveolar hypoxia (and consequent pulmonary vasoconstriction) by the judicious administration of low-concentration O_2. Continuous use of O_2 can decrease pulmonary hypertension, polycythemia, and tachypnea; improve well-being; and reduce mortality. Bronchodilators and antibiotics help relieve airflow obstruction in patients with COPD. Fluid restriction and diuretics relieve signs attributed to right ventricular failure. Long-term anticoagulation therapy is necessary when recurrent pulmonary emboli are present.

KEY CONCEPTS

- A *pulmonary embolism (PE)* occurs when an embolus, usually a blood clot, breaks free from its attachment, circulates to the right side of the heart, and becomes lodged in the pulmonary artery or one of its branches.
- *Pulmonary infarction* (local tissue necrosis) rarely accompanies PE because the lung is protected by a dual blood supply.
- PE usually follows *deep venous thrombosis (DVT)* of the leg veins.
- *Massive PE* is one of the most common causes of unexpected death, second only to coronary thrombosis. Autopsy studies reveal that PE is a frequently missed diagnosis.
- Thrombosis in the veins is triggered by three underlying causes known as the *Virchow triad: venostasis, hypercoagulability,* and *vessel wall inflammation.* All known clinical risk factors have their basis in one or more of the triad.
- The single most important condition predisposing patients to venous thrombosis is *congestive heart failure.* Malignancy, postpartum status, postoperative status (especially orthopedic or pelvic surgery), and all patients on prolonged bedrest for a serious illness are at high risk for venous thrombosis and PE.
- The classic triad of signs and symptoms of a *moderate-sized PE* (dyspnea, chest pain, hemoptysis) are neither sensitive nor specific. The sudden onset of unexplained dyspnea, tachypnea, and tachycardia are likely the most common symptoms but hemoptysis and pleuritic pain are not usually present unless infarction has occurred.
- When *PE* involves blockage of *small peripheral vessels* by small emboli, patients may be asymptomatic. Recurrent PE over a period of many months can lead to obliteration of the vascular bed, pulmonary hypertension, and cor pulmonale.
- Shock, hypotension, tachycardia, cyanosis, stupor, or syncope are signs of a *massive embolic occlusion* of the main pulmonary artery or its major branches and usually results in sudden death.
- The main pathophysiologic consequences of embolization to the pulmonary arterial tree is an increase in the pulmonary artery pressure (which places a strain on the right side of the heart) and increased dead-space ventilation (ventilated areas not being perfused). Reflex bronchoconstriction from the release of vasoactive amines also occurs, which may result in hypoxemia.
- *Ventilation-perfusion (V/Q) scanning* is generally the first diagnostic test used to detect PE. The *gold standard* for the diagnosis of PE is *pulmonary angiography*.
- Prophylactic measures directed toward the prevention of DVT and PE in high-risk patients include low-dose standard heparin or low molecular-weight heparins (LMWHs), compression hose, and intermittent inflating pneumatic devices.
- Fibrinolysis with tissue-plasminogen activator (t-PA) to dissolve the clot is the recommended first line treatment for all patients with a large acute PE.
- Secondary treatment for acute PE involves anticoagulation with standard heparin or LMWH. Long-term anticoagulation is continued using warfarin.

- Prevention of leg vein thrombosis is the best way of preventing PE.
- *Pulmonary edema* is an excessive movement of fluid from the pulmonary vascular system, to the pulmonary interstitium, and eventually the alveolar spaces. Pulmonary edema may occur as a chronic condition or develop quickly and rapidly become fatal.
- The main cause of *pulmonary edema* is pulmonary capillary congestion resulting from *left ventricular failure*. Left ventricular failure may be caused by atherosclerotic, valvular, hypertensive or cardiomyopathic heart disease.
- Emergency treatment of *severe acute pulmonary edema* includes measures to reduce pulmonary hydrostatic pressure, such as placing the patient in high Fowler's position with the feet dependent, administration of a diuretic, O_2, and digitalis to improve myocardial contractility.
- *Cor pulmonale* is the term used to denote hypertrophy or failure of the right ventricle resulting from disorders of the lungs, pulmonary vessels, or chest wall.

- *Cor pulmonale* may be acute (secondary to a massive pulmonary embolus) or chronic and secondary to obstructive lung disease, such as COPD, restrictive lung disease, such as diffuse pulmonary fibrosis or kyphoscoliosis, or pulmonary vascular disease, such as recurrent pulmonary emboli.
- COPD is the most common cause of *cor pulmonale* with more than one half of patients developing this condition.
- The common precursor of *cor pulmonale* is increased pulmonary vascular resistance and pulmonary artery hypertension. The most important mechanism causing pulmonary hypertension is vasoconstriction of the pulmonary blood vessels resulting from hypoxia and hypoxemia. Hypercapnia augments the vasoconstriction.
- Continuous low-flow O_2 therapy to correct alveolar hypoxia and consequent pulmonary vasoconstriction can delay the development of cor pulmonale and extend the life span of patients with COPD.

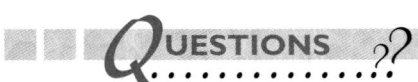

QUESTIONS ??

A sampling of review questions for this chapter appears here. Visit http://www.mosby.com/MERLIN/PriceWilson/ for additional questions.

Answer the following on a separate sheet of paper.

1. List three factors that directly relate to the development of venous thrombosis.
2. What disease is the most common cause of cor pulmonale in the United States?
3. List four conditions that may precipitate pulmonary edema.

4. What is paroxysmal nocturnal dyspnea?
5. Define cor pulmonale.
6. What is the relationship between left-sided heart failure and pulmonary edema? Is this condition the most frequent cause of pulmonary edema?
7. List three objectives in the treatment of pulmonary embolism (PE).

8. What are the two goals in the treatment of cor pulmonale?
9. Describe two mechanisms that can lead to increased pulmonary vascular resistance.

Complete the following statements by filling in the blanks.

10. A freely circulating blood clot that lodges in a blood vessel causing an obstruction is called a(n) _____.
11. A prerequisite for the development of cor pulmonale is increased pulmonary vascular resistance leading to _____ _____.

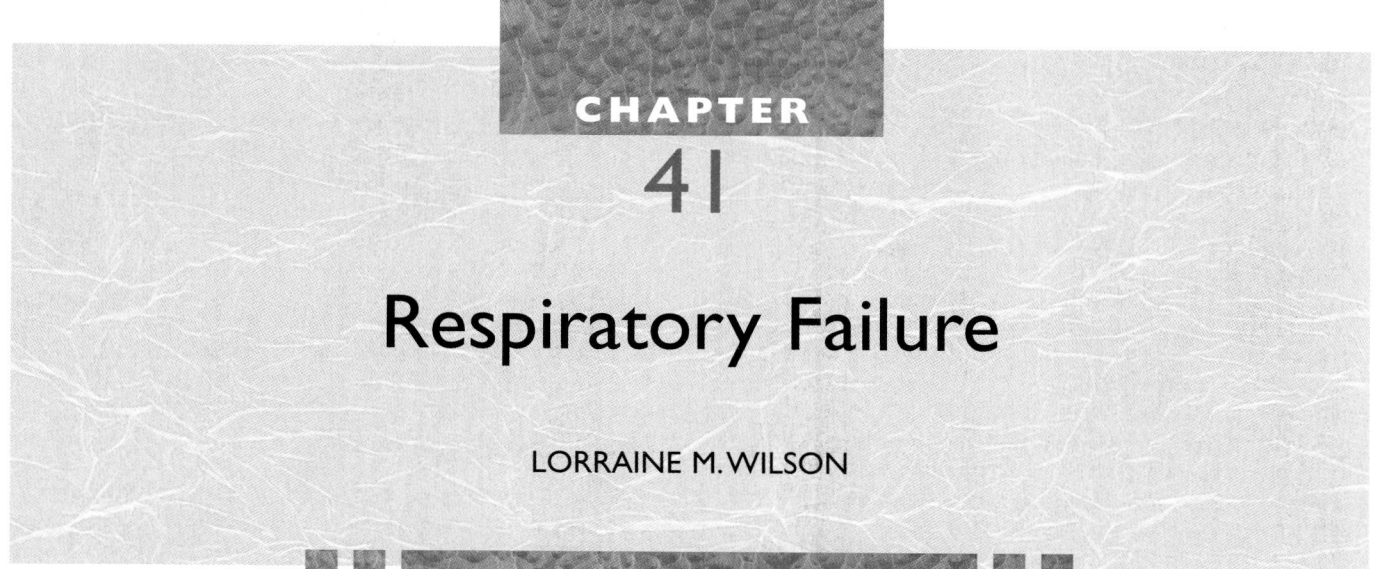

𝓡espiratory failure is a relatively common problem, which is usually, but not always, the end result of chronic disease affecting the respiratory system. Increasingly, this condition is encountered as a complication of acute trauma, septicemia, or shock.

Respiratory failure, as with the failure of any other organ system, may be characterized on the basis of clinical features or laboratory tests. The reader must remember, however, that the correlation between the clinical features and deviations of laboratory tests from the normal range is far from straightforward in respiratory failure.

Respiratory failure is said to exist when the lung cannot fulfill its primary function of gas exchange, namely, oxygenation of the arterial blood and carbon dioxide elimination. There are various grades of respiratory failure, and the condition may be acute (and possibly remittent) or chronic. *Chronic respiratory insufficiency* or *failure* refers to long-term functional impairment that persists many days or months and represents a compromise between the pathologic processes leading to failure and the compensatory processes stabilizing the situation. Blood gases may be mildly abnormal or within normal limits at rest but markedly abnormal during situations of increased demand such as exercise. Increased work of breathing (and thus decreased respiratory reserve) and reduction of physical activity are the two broad coping mechanisms in chronic respiratory insufficiency.

ACUTE RESPIRATORY FAILURE

Acute respiratory failure is numerically defined as respiratory failure with an arterial oxygen partial pressure (or tension, PaO_2) of 50 to 60 mm Hg or less with or without an arterial carbon dioxide partial pressure (or tension, $PaCO_2$) of 50 mm Hg or greater under resting conditions at sea level while breathing room air. This numeric definition based on arterial blood gases (ABGs) has been established because the line between chronic respiratory insufficiency and respiratory failure is subtle, and clinical observations alone are unreliable. On the other hand, one must understand that the definition based on ABGs is not absolute; the significance of the numbers depends on the patient's history. A previously healthy person who develops this degree of abnormality of ABGs after a near-drowning accident might be expected to be comatose, whereas many patients with chronic obstructive pulmonary disease (COPD) can function with some degree of physical activity at the same levels.

Two broad classifications of respiratory failure are based on ABG pathophysiology: (1) *hypoxemic*, or *normocapnic, respiratory failure* (hypoxemia with normal or low $PaCO_2$) and (2) *hypercapnic*, or *ventilatory*, failure (hypoxemia and hypercapnia). This chapter discusses the clinical features, causes, pathogenetic mechanisms, and management of these two types of respiratory failure.

Pathogenesis and Etiology

The successful treatment of acute respiratory failure depends not only on its recognition at an early stage but also on identification of the mechanisms at fault. Early recognition may be difficult when the onset is insidious because the clinical signs and symptoms are nonspecific. Although tissue hypoxia cannot be assessed directly, ABG measurements (one step in the long process that determines tissue oxygenation) can be helpful in drawing inferences about inadequate tissue oxygenation and the faulty mechanisms. Knowledge of the mechanisms at fault provides insight into the pathophysiology of a patient's lung disease, which, in turn, leads to appropriate treatment.

An important first step in the recognition of impending respiratory failure is awareness of the conditions and settings likely to lead to respiratory failure. Box 41-1 lists some of the common lung disorders causing respiratory failure, classified as extrinsic or intrinsic. Most of these conditions were discussed in previous chapters. *Extrinsic lung disorders* (with lungs that are normal or nearly normal) lead to ventilatory, or hypercapnic, respiratory failure through (1) depression of central respiratory drive or (2) interference with the ventilatory response. Narcotic overdose is one of the most common causes of respiratory center depression resulting in ventilatory failure. Interference with ventilatory response occurs as a result of disease or injury of the neural pathways or ventilatory muscles or mechanical dysfunction of the thoracic bellows caused by injury, pain, or deformity. Some of the possible causes of a decreased ventilatory response are listed under neuromuscular and pleural and chest wall disorders.

Although extrapulmonary, or extrinsic, lung disorders are important causes of respiratory failure, the *pulmonary*, or *intrinsic*, *lung disorders* are even more important. Chronic obstruction of the airways results in ventilatory

failure, with COPD the most common cause. Diffuse restrictive disorders of the lung parenchyma and vasculature generally cause mild hypoxemic respiratory failure; however, acute intrinsic abnormalities of the lung parenchyma such as massive pulmonary edema, atelectasis, extensive consolidated pneumonia, and acute (adult) respiratory distress syndrome (ARDS) may cause profound hypoxemia. ARDS accounts for a significant portion of the patient population of respiratory intensive care units and has a high mortality rate. This condition is discussed separately from the other causes of respiratory failure later in this chapter.

Finally, it is important to know that a number of precipitating factors can result in acute respiratory failure in patients with chronic lung disease (Box 41-2). Retained secretions, infection, and bronchospasm are the most common precipitating factors in patients with COPD causing *acute-on-chronic respiratory failure*. Important iatrogenic factors include the injudicious administration of narcotics or high fractions of inspired oxygen (FIO_2). Cor pulmonale, pulmonary embolism (especially in patients with polycythemia), and pneumothorax from an emphysematous bleb are other less common precipitating causes of respiratory failure. Some of these precipitating factors cannot be eliminated, but many of them can, which has important implications for patient education and the management of chronic respiratory disease.

Mechanisms of Hypoxemia and Hypercapnia

By definition, hypoxemia is present in respiratory failure. *Hypoxemic respiratory failure* is characterized by hypoxemia and either normocapnia or hypocapnia, whereas *ventilatory failure* is characterized by hypoxemia and hypercapnia. The treatment implications of this distinction will become evident as this discussion proceeds.

Box 41-3 lists the pathogenetic mechanisms involved in hypoxemia and hypercapnia. Only the last three mechanisms shown in the box (alveolar hypoventilation, low ventilation/perfusion [$\dot{V}/\dot{Q}$] ratio, and shunting) are important causes of hypoxemia. The primary cause of hypercapnia is alveolar hypoventilation, but $\dot{V}/\dot{Q}$ inequality generally has a trivial effect on the $PaCO_2$. It should be noted that alveolar hypoventilation causes both hypercapnia and hypoxemia, whereas $\dot{V}/\dot{Q}$ mismatch generally causes only hypoxemia.

The determination of the $PaCO_2$ with respect to the lungs is relatively simple: the $PaCO_2$ is directly related to

---

BOX 41-1

Causes of Respiratory Failure

A. Disorders extrinsic to the lungs
  1. Respiratory center depression
    a. Drug overdose (sedatives, narcotics)
    b. Cerebral trauma or infarction
    c. Bulbar poliomyelitis
    d. Encephalitis
  2. Neuromuscular disorders
    a. Cervical cord injury
    b. Guillain-Barré syndrome
    c. Amyotrophic lateral sclerosis
    d. Myasthenia gravis
    e. Muscular dystrophy
  3. Pleural and chest wall disorders
    a. Chest injury (flail chest, rib fracture)
    b. Pneumothorax
    c. Pleural effusion
    d. Kyphoscoliosis
    e. Obesity: pickwickian syndrome
B. Disorders intrinsic to the lungs
  1. Diffuse obstructive disorders
    a. Emphysema, chronic bronchitis (COPD)
    b. Asthma, status asthmaticus
    c. Cystic fibrosis
  2. Diffuse restrictive disorders
    a. Interstitial fibrosis of various causes (e.g., silica, coal dust)
    b. Sarcoidosis
    c. Scleroderma
    d. Pulmonary edema
      (1) Cardiogenic
      (2) Noncardiogenic (ARDS)
    e. Atelectasis
    f. Consolidated pneumonia
  3. Pulmonary vascular disorders
    a. Pulmonary emboli
    b. Severe emphysema

BOX 41-2

Precipitating Factors of Respiratory Failure in Chronic Lung Disease

- Infection of tracheobronchial tree, pneumonia, fever
- Change in tracheobronchial secretions (increased volume or viscosity)
- Bronchospasm (inhalation of irritants or allergens)
- Disturbance in ability to clear secretions
- Sedatives, narcotics, anesthesia
- O_2 therapy (high FIO_2)
- Trauma, including surgery
- Cardiovascular disorders (heart failure, pulmonary embolism)
- Pneumothorax

CO_2 production and nearly inversely proportional to the alveolar ventilation (West, 2000), as follows:

$$Pa_{CO_2} \propto \frac{\dot{V}_{CO_2} \text{ (production of } CO_2\text{)}}{\dot{V}_A \text{ (alveolar ventilation)}}$$

Thus if alveolar ventilation ($\dot{V}_A$) is halved, the Pa_{CO_2} will be doubled, provided CO_2 production remains constant. Conversely, if $\dot{V}_A$ should double, as in hyperventilation, the Pa_{CO_2} would be halved. Ventilatory failure with hypercapnia always involves the mechanism of alveolar hypoventilation. Pure hypoventilation, although relatively infrequent, is associated with the extrapulmonary conditions listed in Box 41-1, in which the lungs are relatively normal (with the exception of kyphoscoliosis). Alveolar hypoventilation develops in these conditions because the minute ventilation falls, as in respiratory center depression from narcotic overdose, or in the event of a disproportionately high work of breathing or total body metabolism (increased CO_2 production) for a given $\dot{V}_A$, as in obesity or chest deformity.

The hypoxemia associated with pure hypoventilation is generally mild (Pa_{O_2} = 50 to 80 mm Hg) and is directly caused by the elevation of the alveolar P_{CO_2} (Pa_{CO_2}). This fact can be explained by recalling that the partial pressure of all the alveolar or all the arterial blood gases must add up to the total (atmospheric) pressure. Thus, when Pa_{CO_2} increases, the Pa_{O_2} must decrease, and vice versa, at a constant total atmospheric pressure. The relationship between the rise in carbon dioxide tension (P_{CO_2}) and the fall in the oxygen tension (P_{O_2}) that occurs in hypoventilation can be predicted by the *alveolar gas equation* if the composition of the FI_{O_2} and the *respiratory exchange ratio* (R or RQ) is known, as follows:

$$Pa_{O_2} = FI_{O_2}(P_B - P_{H_2O}) - \frac{Pa_{CO_2}}{R}$$

where Pa_{O_2} is the partial pressure of O_2 in the alveolus; FI_{O_2} is the inspired O_2 fraction (0.21 when breathing air); P_B is the barometric pressure (760 mm Hg at sea level);

P_{H_2O} is the partial pressure of water vapor in the trachea (47 mm Hg at normal body temperature); and Pa_{CO_2} is the partial pressure of CO_2 in the arterial blood and is assumed to be equal to that in the alveolus.* R or RQ is determined by body metabolism and is equal to the volume of CO_2 produced divided by the volume of O_2 consumed ($\dot{V}_{CO_2}/\dot{V}_{O_2}$). R is 0.7 when pure fat is burned, 1.0 when pure carbohydrate is burned, and approximately 0.8 on a mixed diet. When a healthy person is breathing room air with a normal Pa_{CO_2} of 40 mm Hg and we assume that R = 0.8:

$$Pa_{O_2} = 0.21(760 - 47) - \frac{40}{0.8}$$
$$Pa_{O_2} \approx Pa_{O_2} = 100 \text{ mm Hg}$$

If a person should hypoventilate breathing room air and the normal Pa_{CO_2} should rise from 40 to 70 mm Hg, the Pa_{O_2} and Pa_{O_2} would necessarily fall from 100 mm Hg to approximately 62 mm Hg:

$$Pa_{O_2} = 0.21(760 - 47) - \frac{70}{0.8}$$
$$Pa_{O_2} \approx Pa_{O_2} = 62.23 \text{ mm Hg}$$

(NOTE: For each 10 mm Hg rise in Pa_{CO_2} above normal, the Pa_{O_2} will fall 12.5 mm Hg.)

An examination of the alveolar gas equation reveals that the hypoxemia that develops from pure hypoventilation can easily be corrected by administering O_2 and raising the FI_{O_2}. The equation also shows that if the drop in the Pa_{O_2} is greater than expected, other mechanisms causing hypoxemia must then be operating (shunting or $\dot{V}/\dot{Q}$ mismatch). Although the degree of hypoxemia that develops from pure hypoventilation in the example is not serious (because O_2 saturation is approximately 90% at a Pa_{O_2} of 62 mm Hg), this degree of Pa_{CO_2} will depress the respiratory center and cause a serious acidosis.

$\dot{V}/\dot{Q}$ inequality, or mismatch, is by far the most important mechanism causing hypoxemia in patients with chronic airway obstruction and plays a role in most other intrinsic lung disorders. $\dot{V}/\dot{Q}$ inequality refers to the *regional* imbalance of ventilation and blood flow in the pulmonary gas-exchanging units discussed in Chapter 35. Some pulmonary units have relatively high $\dot{V}/\dot{Q}$ ratios (wasted ventilation or dead space–like units), whereas others have low $\dot{V}/\dot{Q}$ ratios (wasted perfusion, physiologic shunt, venous admixture). If some alveoli receive too little ventilation in proportion to perfusion (low $\dot{V}/\dot{Q}$), there is a fall in Pa_{O_2} and a rise in Pa_{CO_2} in the blood leaving these alveoli. In effect, blood is shunted past the alveoli without adequate gas exchange taking place (venous admixture effect). Conversely, alveoli that receive too little perfusion in proportion to ventilation (high $\dot{V}/\dot{Q}$) produce high Pa_{O_2} and low Pa_{CO_2} in the blood flowing from them. The reader should recall that the healthy lung has some $\dot{V}/\dot{Q}$ inequality because of the effects of gravity (see Chapter 35), but this difference is not significant enough to cause blood gas abnormalities.

Low $\dot{V}/\dot{Q}$ ratios can cause significant hypoxemia in lung disease but generally have little effect on the $PaCO_2$. The relationship between the partial pressures and content of these two gases accounts for the difference.

Fig. 41-1 illustrates the oxyhemoglobin and CO_2 dissociation curves drawn on the same scale for comparative purposes. This figure makes the important point that the oxyhemoglobin curve has a flat portion, but the CO_2 curve does not. At a PaO_2 of approximately 60 mm Hg (when the curve starts to flatten), the O_2 content of the blood has reached more than 80% of the maximum content of approximately 19.5 vol%. A large increase in the PaO_2 (e.g., from 60 to 100 mm Hg) causes only a small increase in O_2 content. In contrast, CO_2 transport in the blood is much more efficient. Because the CO_2 curve is steep in the physiologic range of the $PaCO_2$, a small change (e.g., from 40 to 50 mm Hg) causes a large change in CO_2 content. In terms of $\dot{V}/\dot{Q}$ imbalance, this means that alveoli with high $\dot{V}/\dot{Q}$ ratios cannot fully compensate for those with low $\dot{V}/\dot{Q}$ ratios with reference to O_2 transport. The hemoglobin (Hb) from the better ventilated units, when already nearly saturated (flat part of oxyhemoglobin dissociation curve), cannot carry the excess O_2 that would be needed to compensate for the deficit caused by poorly oxygenated blood from the low $\dot{V}/\dot{Q}$ units. Because the CO_2 dissociation curve is more nearly linear in the physiologic range, the hyperventilating units with a high $\dot{V}/\dot{Q}$ ratio can compensate for hypoventilating units with a low $\dot{V}/\dot{Q}$ ratio. The result is that the mixed blood leaving the high and low $\dot{V}/\dot{Q}$ units will have a normal $PaCO_2$. However, progressive involvement of more and more of the lung by the disease process will result in more and more alveolocapillary units with low $\dot{V}/\dot{Q}$ ratios. Eventually a point is reached at which the remaining high $\dot{V}/\dot{Q}$ units cannot compensate for the low units, and hypercapnia ensues. Therefore the diseases characterized by $\dot{V}/\dot{Q}$ abnormalities (most of the intrinsic lung diseases and kyphoscoliosis) demonstrate progres-

sion through hypoxemic respiratory insufficiency and failure (which occurs first) to hypercapnic, or ventilatory, failure (which occurs later).

The important principles to remember from this discussion thus far are that (1) the factors determining oxygenation and ventilation are different and must be analyzed separately; (2) the $PaCO_2$ must be regarded as a function of the *overall* ventilation of the entire lung, without regard to local inequalities of distribution of ventilation and perfusion; (3) the PaO_2, on the other hand, depends not only on the amount of $\dot{V}_A$ but also on $\dot{V}/\dot{Q}$ matching; and (4) hypercapnia must be viewed as representing a problem not only with oxygenation but also with ventilation.

The third important mechanism causing hypoxemia is venous-to-arterial, or right-to-left, shunting of blood, which bypasses the gas-exchanging units of the lung. A true anatomic right-to-left shunt may exist in congenital heart disease, as when an opening exists between the right and left chambers of the heart or, rarely, when an arteriovenous fistula exists within the lung. A small true shunt is present in normal lungs (see Fig. 35-12) amounting to approximately 2.5% of pulmonary blood flow. In addition to these rare anatomic vascular abnormalities and the small normal shunt, shunting may also occur when alveolar spaces are nonfunctional, as when the alveoli are collapsed (atelectasis) or filled with edema fluid or with exudate, as in pulmonary edema or pneumonia. This type of shunting may be regarded as an extreme type of $\dot{V}/\dot{Q}$ mismatch in which ventilation of the involved units is zero while perfusion continues. If a large number of gas-exchange units are involved in shunting, the resulting hypoxemia can be severe. However, the $PaCO_2$ is generally normal or low because the subject can usually increase ventilation sufficiently in the remaining normal lung to blow off the CO_2 adequately. When overall hyperventilation occurs in response to severe hypoxemia, hypocapnia and respiratory alkalosis may result. Hypoxemic respiratory failure caused primarily by shunting is difficult to treat because the hypoxemia is not readily correctable by O_2 therapy.

Another type of extreme $\dot{V}/\dot{Q}$ imbalance is that exemplified by a pulmonary unit in which ventilation occurs with no perfusion (dead space). The classic example of alveolar dead-space disease is acute pulmonary embolus. Another common cause is acutely decreased pulmonary perfusion resulting from acutely decreased cardiac output or acute pulmonary hypertension with increased pulmonary vascular resistance (Shapiro, Peruzzi, Kozlowski-Templin, 1994). Destruction of the alveolar septal walls in emphysema, with replacement of several alveoli by large air spaces, results in reducing the surface area for gas exchange. The anatomic dead space can be greatly increased by a rapid, shallow breathing pattern, as illustrated in Table 36-2. The normal physiologic dead space (V_D) is 30% of the tidal volume (V_T) or V_D/V_T. If dead-space ventilation is increased significantly (wasted ventilation), overall ventilation must increase to maintain effective $\dot{V}_A$. In advanced disease the work of breathing may be so great as to cause hypercapnia and hypoxemia. When both high minute volume and high physiologic dead space is present, the condition is referred to as *high-output ventilatory failure*.

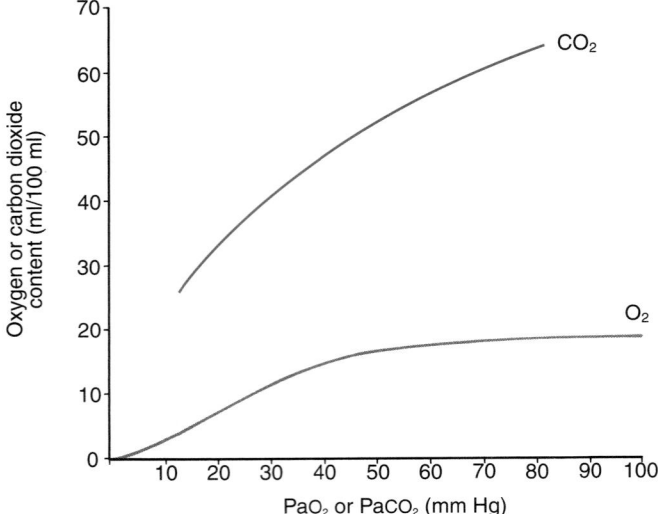

FIG. 41-1 Oxyhemoglobin and carbon dioxide dissociation curves plotted on the same scale. (Modified from Comroe JH: *The lung: clinical physiology and pulmonary function tests*, ed 2, Chicago, 1971, Mosby.)

Hypoxemia caused by high altitude can generally be ignored in the treatment of respiratory failure because it is constant for a particular locale. At sea level, P_B is 760 mm Hg. With increasing altitude, the total P_B and the P_{O_2} of inspired air decrease, although the percentage of O_2 in the air remains constant at 20.93%. For example, in Boston at sea level the P_B is 760 mm Hg and the inspired P_{O_2} is 159 mm Hg, whereas in Denver, the P_B is 632.3 mm Hg, and the inspired P_{O_2} is 132.3 mm Hg (Comroe, 1974).

Most authorities no longer consider diffusion impairment to be a significant factor in producing hypoxemia, although it may play a minor role when thickening of the alveolocapillary membrane occurs, as in pulmonary fibrosis and sarcoidosis. The normal contact time between alveolar gas and pulmonary blood is 0.75 second under resting conditions, and equilibration is normally completed in 0.25 second. Thus ample diffusion time in reserve exists. When diffusion time is somewhat reduced during exercise, the possibility exists for diffusion limitation to make a greater contribution to hypoxemia.

In summary, when hypoxemic respiratory failure is present, the principal mechanisms involved are low $\dot{V}/\dot{Q}$ ratio or shunting, either alone or in combination. Diffusion impairment may possibly make a minor contribution to the hypoxemia, although this is controversial. Hypoxemic respiratory insufficiency or failure is usually associated with restrictive or vascular diseases of the lung. Even though the work of breathing is increased in these conditions (with consequently increased CO_2 production and O_2 consumption for ventilatory work), the subject has enough strength to increase ventilation sufficiently to maintain a normal Pa_{CO_2}. Any slight rise in the Pa_{CO_2} will stimulate increased ventilation. Similarly, any fall in the Pa_{O_2} to approximately 50 to 60 mm Hg will also stimulate ventilation. Consequently, hyperventilation may result; thus the Pa_{CO_2} is decreased below normal levels (respiratory alkalosis or hypocapnia). Hyperventilation while breathing room air is generally ineffectual in correcting hypoxemia because of the sigmoid shape of the oxyhemoglobin dissociation curve. O_2 therapy is quite effective in correcting hypoxemia caused by $\dot{V}/\dot{Q}$ imbalance or diffusion impairment but ineffective if the cause is shunting.

Hypercapnic, or ventilatory, failure may be caused by hypoventilation alone or in combination with any or all of the other hypoxemic mechanisms—$\dot{V}/\dot{Q}$ imbalance, shunting, or possibly diffusion impairment. Pure ventilatory failure occurs in extrapulmonary disorders involving failure of neural or muscular control of breathing. The classic example of hypercapnic respiratory failure occurs in COPD and involves $\dot{V}/\dot{Q}$ imbalance and hypoventilation. When respiratory failure is precipitated by retained secretions and pneumonia in these patients, considerable shunting may also occur. Although obstructive disorders of the airways generally result in hypercapnic respiratory failure, reversible airway disease, as in asthma, is an exception to the rule. An acute asthmatic attack is generally characterized by hypoxemia and hypocapnia because the subjects are usually able to hyperventilate. A rise of the Pa_{CO_2} even to normal levels in a sustained asthmatic attack may be a signal that the functional status is deteriorating (see Chapter 10). The primary focus in ventilatory failure is on measures to improve ventilation and at the same time prevent serious tissue hypoxia. Methods of differentiating between the mechanisms involved in hypoxemia and hypercapnia are discussed subsequently.

Clinical Features

The manifestations of acute respiratory failure represent a combination of the clinical features of the underlying disease, the precipitating factors, and the manifestations of hypoxemia and hypercapnia. Thus the clinical picture may be quite variable because various factors may precipitate the condition. The presence or absence of preceding chronic respiratory insufficiency is another factor that modifies the clinical picture.

The signs and symptoms of hypoxemia are a direct result of tissue hypoxia. (These signs and symptoms were presented in Chapter 37 but are reviewed here.) The more frequently cited signs and symptoms do not develop until the Pa_{O_2} is in the range of 40 to 50 mm Hg. Tissues highly sensitive to O_2 depletion are principally affected, including the brain, heart, and lungs. The most prominent signs and symptoms are neurologic: headache, mental confusion, impairment of judgment, slurring of speech, asterixis, impairment of motor function, agitation, and restlessness that may progress to delirium and unconsciousness. In some cases, the neurologic signs and symptoms of hypoxic persons have been misinterpreted as alcoholic inebriation. The initial cardiovascular responses to hypoxemia are tachycardia and increased cardiac output and blood pressure. When the hypoxia persists, bradycardia, hypotension, decreased cardiac output, and dysrhythmias may occur. Hypoxemia causes vasoconstriction of the pulmonary blood vessels. The metabolic effect of tissue hypoxia is anaerobic metabolism resulting in metabolic acidosis. Although cyanosis is often regarded as a sign of hypoxia, it is unreliable (see Chapter 37). The classic symptom of dyspnea may also be absent, especially when respiratory center drive is decreased, as in the respiratory failure of narcotic overdose.

Hypercapnia while breathing room air is always accompanied by hypoxemia. Consequently, the signs and symptoms of ventilatory failure represent the effects of both hypercapnia and hypoxemia. The major effect of increases in the Pa_{CO_2} is depression of the central nervous system (CNS). For this reason, severe hypercapnia is sometimes referred to as CO_2 *narcosis*. Hypercapnia results in cerebral vasodilation, increased cerebral blood flow, and increased intracranial pressure. The resultant headache, worse on awaking in the morning (because Pa_{CO_2} increases slightly during sleep) is characteristic. Other resultant signs and symptoms include papilledema, neuromuscular irritability (asterixis), fluctuations of mood, and increased drowsiness, which may progress to frank coma. Although an increased Pa_{CO_2} is normally the most powerful stimulus to respiration, it has a depressive effect on respiration at levels greater than 70 mm Hg. Additionally, patients with COPD and chronic hypercapnia develop insensitivity to increased Pa_{CO_2} and depend on hypoxic drive. Hypercapnia causes constriction of the pulmonary blood vessels, thus aggravating any pulmonary artery hypertension that may be present. When CO_2 retention is severe, decreased myocardial contractility, systemic vasodilation, heart failure, and hypotension may ensue. Hypercapnia causes respiratory acidosis, which is often combined with metabolic acidosis when tissue hypoxia is present. This combination can cause a serious depression of the blood pH. The renal compensatory response to respiratory acidosis is reabsorption of bicarbonate to restore pH to normal. This response takes approximately 3 days; thus respiratory acidosis is much more severe when the onset is rapid.

Diagnosis

A number of situations can occur during which anyone can recognize respiratory failure. Examples are cardiac arrest, complete obstruction of the upper airways by, for example, a piece of meat, head injury serious enough to stop the breathing mechanism, or labored breathing in a person who is cyanotic. However, in many patients, the presence of respiratory failure may not be so obvious. The onset of respiratory failure is insidious in many patients with chronic respiratory insufficiency. Signs and symptoms may be nonspecific and correlate poorly with the degree of respiratory impairment until the situation is catastrophic. Great astuteness is needed to recognize every case of respiratory failure. Thus the clinician must have a high degree of suspicion and be ready to obtain measurements of ABGs when respiratory failure is suspected because this action is the only way a definitive diagnosis can be made. Generally, a $PaCO_2$ of 50 mm Hg or more or a PaO_2 of 50 to 60 mm Hg or less at sea level is accepted as indicating respiratory failure.

Assessment of Respiratory Function

Measurement of respiratory function is indispensable in the provision of adequate respiratory care, not only for accurate diagnosis, but also for evaluation of response to treatment. Measurement of ABGs provides valuable information for establishing the degree and type of respiratory failure and for identifying the mechanisms involved.

A number of bedside measurements of ventilatory function are also frequently used to assess ventilatory reserve and the need for mechanical ventilation. The ventilatory status and the acid-base status are assessed by examining the $PaCO_2$, bicarbonate (HCO_3^-), and pH.

A nomogram may be helpful in determining whether hypercapnic respiratory failure is acute or chronic or whether a mixed acid-base disorder is present. Fig. 41-2 shows the relationship between the $PaCO_2$ and pH and the alterations observed in respiratory and metabolic disorders of acid-base balance. Data that fall within a particular band usually represent the primary disorder, and data outside the band represent a mixed disorder. The following equivalences must be emphasized: (1) respiratory acidosis = hypercapnia = alveolar hypoventilation, and (2) respiratory alkalosis = hypocapnia = alveolar hyperventilation. The lettered points on the nomogram represent common values in respiratory failure. Any sudden, severe decrease in ventilation resulting in the retention of CO_2 in the blood will produce acute respiratory acidosis *(C)*. This acidosis is frequently aggravated by a coexisting metabolic acidosis from excess lactic acid produced by the tissue hypoxia that also results from decreased ventilation *(B)*. The renal compensation for a rise in the $PaCO_2$ is retention of HCO_3^- to restore blood pH to normal. This process normally takes approximately 3 days. Thus point *D* represents chronic hypercapnia, frequently observed in patients with COPD. Point *E* might represent partially compensated acute hypercapnia or a mixture of acute and chronic hypercapnia, which might occur when a patient with COPD develops a respiratory infection. Point *F* represents a mixture of chronic hypercapnia and metabolic alkalosis, which might be caused by rapid correction of the hypercapnia by artificial ventilation. When the $PaCO_2$ is lowered rapidly in a person with compensated respiratory acidosis (hypercapnia) and consequently with an increased HCO_3^-, an excess of base bicarbonate (metabolic alkalosis) is present until the kidneys can excrete the excess. Point G represents chronic hyperventilation (respiratory alkalosis), which is

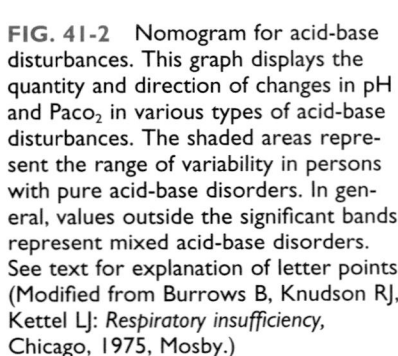

FIG. 41-2 Nomogram for acid-base disturbances. This graph displays the quantity and direction of changes in pH and $PaCO_2$ in various types of acid-base disturbances. The shaded areas represent the range of variability in persons with pure acid-base disorders. In general, values outside the significant bands represent mixed acid-base disorders. See text for explanation of letter points. (Modified from Burrows B, Knudson RJ, Kettel LJ: *Respiratory insufficiency,* Chicago, 1975, Mosby.)

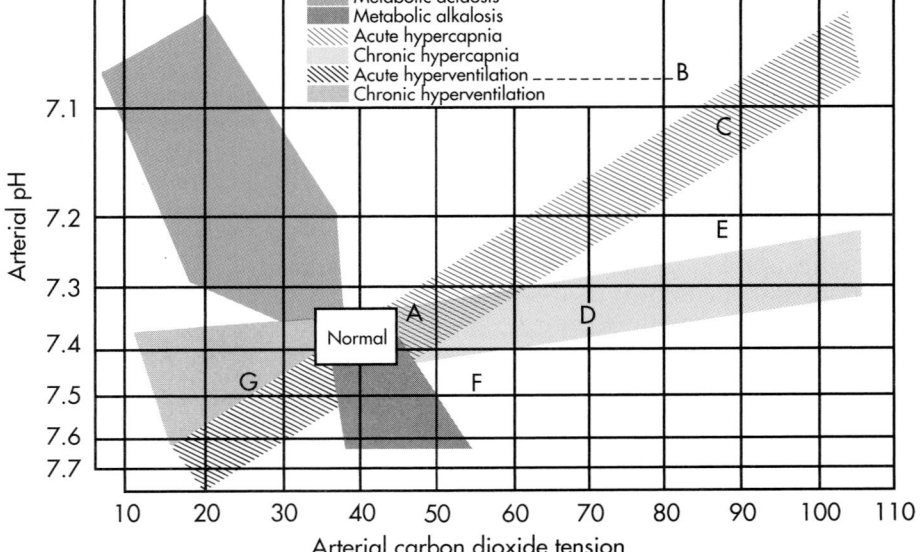

common in hypoxemic respiratory failure. Point *A* represents a mild hypercapnia. The acute and the chronic forms cannot be distinguished unless the patient's usual $Paco_2$ is known.

Evaluation of oxygenation involves examination of several parameters, including Pao_2, the alveolar-arterial O_2 difference or gradient [the $P(A - a)O_2$ or $(A-aD)O_2$], cardiac output, and Hb. The Pao_2 should be related to the $Paco_2$, pH, and HCO_3^- to determine the type of respiratory failure (hypoxemic versus hypercapnic) and the pathophysiologic mechanism. The Fio_2 must be taken into account when interpreting ABGs. Pure hypoventilation while breathing air ($Fio_2 = 0.21$) can be distinguished from the other mechanisms ($\dot{V}/\dot{Q}$ or shunt or both) by calculating the expected value of the Pao_2 for a given change in the $Paco_2$. This value can be calculated using the alveolar gas equation (see p. 611). If the change is greater than expected (e.g., $Pao_2 = 45$ mm Hg), $\dot{V}/\dot{Q}$ mismatch or shunting (or both) must also be involved.

The $P(A - a)O_2$ gradient is even more helpful in distinguishing between the pathophysiologic mechanisms. The normal $P(A - a)O_2$ gradient is approximately 10 mm Hg because of a small amount of normal shunting. Knowing that high concentrations of inspired O_2 correct hypoventilation and $\dot{V}/\dot{Q}$ imbalance (and diffusion impairment) but not absolute shunting allows the examiner to distinguish between the mechanisms, using the $P(A - a)O_2$ gradient. The $P(A - a)O_2$ gradient is normal while breathing room air if the cause of the hypoxemia is pure hypoventilation caused by an extracardiopulmonary disorder. A $P(A - a)O_2$ gradient greater than 20 mm Hg (25 in older adults) when breathing room air is considered abnormal, and the cause is a cardiopulmonary disorder. Provided that a congenital heart defect or an intracardiac (anatomic) shunt has been ruled out, the cause of the hypoxemia is a disorder within the lung. The $P(A - a)O_2$ gradient can help determine the extent to which the physiologic shunt is caused by $\dot{V}/\dot{Q}$ mismatch (venous admixture) rather than absolute intrapulmonary capillary shunting. Intrapulmonary shunting may be considered as an extreme case of low $\dot{V}/\dot{Q}$ ratio to distinguish it from venous admixture—so low that the administration of 100% O_2 no longer provides enough O_2 to the affected pulmonary capillaries to oxygenate the blood in them. The Pao_2 can be calculated by using a simplified version of the alveolar gas equation and then calculating the alveolar-arterial partial pressure difference ($Pao_2 - Pao_2$), as follows:

$$PAO_2 = Pio_2 - \frac{Paco_2}{R}$$

where: $Pio_2 = Fio_2 \times (PB - PH_2O)$

Using the figures of 760 mm Hg for P_B at sea level, 47 mm Hg for the partial pressure of H_2O at normal body temperature, and 20.93% O_2 for the Fio_2, the Pio_2 is observed to be 149.3 mm Hg ($0.2093 \times [760 - 47]$).

Making a concrete application of this formula, the following room air ($PB = 750$ mm Hg) ABG values were obtained on a 30-year-old man during an asthmatic attack: $Paco_2 = 60$ mm Hg and $Pao_2 = 40$ mm Hg. Thus $Pio_2 = 0.2093 \times (750 - 47) = 147$, and $P(A - a)O_2 = 147 - (60 \div 0.8) - 40$ mm Hg = 32 mm Hg. Because $P(A - a)O_2$ is greater than 20, alveolar hypoventilation alone

does not account for the hypoxemia, and either additional $\dot{V}/\dot{Q}$ mismatch or shunting is present.

$\dot{V}/\dot{Q}$ mismatch may be differentiated from true intrapulmonary shunting by determining the $P(A - a)O_2$ after having the patient breathe 100% O_2 for 15 minutes to wash out the nitrogen gas from the alveoli. Because $Fio_2 = 1.0$ when pure O_2 is breathed, the alveolar gas equation simplifies as follows:

$$PAO_2 = (PB - 47) - Paco_2$$

A healthy person breathing 100% O_2 at sea level would thus have a PAO_2 of 673 mm Hg ($760 - 47 - 40$). The normal Pao_2 is greater than 500 mm Hg and the $P(A - a)O_2$ gradient 30 to 50 mm Hg when 100% O_2 is breathed. $\dot{V}/\dot{Q}$ mismatch is largely corrected by administering 100% O_2; a Pao_2 less than 500 mm Hg indicates significant shunting (Cherniack, Cherniack, 1983). The $P(A - a)O_2$ gradient is also increased.

The measurement of the $P(A - a)O_2$ gradient has serious limitations in estimating the magnitude of intrapulmonary shunting, because the values change with different cardiac outputs and Fio_2 concentrations. Using a high Fio_2 will improve shunting because of venous admixture but may aggravate intrapulmonary capillary shunting by causing absorption atelectasis. For these reasons, other indexes for estimating shunt have been developed and the classic $P(A - a)O_2$ shunt determination using 100% O_2 is no longer popular. One such index is the *arterial-alveolar oxygen tension ratio* ($P[a/A]O_2$), which is not affected by supplemental O_2. An example of a normal value is the following:

$$P(a/A)O_2 = \frac{Pao_2}{PAO_2} = \frac{80 \text{ mm Hg}}{100 \text{ mm Hg}} = 0.8$$

The Pao_2 is estimated using the alveolar gas equation. The normal $P(a/A)O_2$ value is approximately 0.8, and the value decreases with increased shunting.

The $\dot{Q}_S/\dot{Q}_T$ *physiologic shunt equation* is another method of measuring shunt. This equation measures the portion of the total cardiac output ($\dot{Q}_T$) that is not oxygenated during passage through the lungs ($\dot{Q}_S$). However, this method is not always used because it requires a sample of blood from an indwelling pulmonary artery catheter. Shapiro, Peruzzi, and Kozlowski-Templin (1994) have introduced an *estimated shunt equation* that requires only measured values for Pao_2, mixed-venous O_2 tension ($P\bar{v}o_2$), O_2 saturation (Sao_2), and Hb, as follows:

$$\frac{\dot{Q}_S}{\dot{Q}_T} = \frac{C\acute{c}o_2 - Cao_2}{3.5 + (C\acute{c}o_2 - Cao_2)}$$

where $C\acute{c}o_2$ is the pulmonary capillary O_2 content; Cao_2 is the arterial O_2 content; and $C\bar{v}o_2$ is the mixed-venous O_2 content. These values are calculated by the following formulas:

$$Cao_2 = Hb \times 1.34 \times Sao_2 + (Pao_2 \times 0.0031)$$
$$C\bar{v}o_2 = Hb \times 1.34 \times S\bar{v}o_2 + (P\bar{v}o_2 \times 0.0031)$$
$$C\acute{c}o_2 = Hb \times 1.34 \times 1.0 + (Pao_2 \times 0.0031)$$

The first parts of the previous equations represent the portion of O_2 carried by Hb and the second parts the portion dissolved in the plasma. In estimating the $C\acute{c}o_2$, the assumption is made that all the available Hb is 100% saturated and that the $C\acute{c}o_2$ is equal to the Pao_2 (which is solved using the alveolar gas equation). The 3.5 constant in the equation represents arteriovenous content difference, $C(a - \bar{v})O_2$, normally 4.5 to 6.0 ml/dl in healthy adults, but assumed to be at the lower value of 3.5 in critically ill patients. The normal value for $\dot{Q}_S/\dot{Q}_T$ in a healthy person is 3% to 5%. High values indicate increased shunting.

Finally, clinicians may want to estimate the degree of shunt from the PaO_2 alone. Normally the PaO_2 should be approximately equal to $FIO_2 \times 6$. For example, while breathing 40% O_2, the PaO_2 should be approximately 240 mm Hg. When 100% O_2 is administered, the shunt is estimated by adding 5% to the shunt for every 100 mm Hg the PaO_2 is less than 700 mm Hg. Thus a PaO_2 of 300 mm Hg represents a 20% shunt, and a PaO_2 of 100 mm Hg represents a 30% shunt. A shunt of 20% or more indicates a need for ventilatory support. A 50% shunt is compatible with life only if the patient is breathing 100% O_2.

Table 41-1 lists some of the common measurements used by intensive care physicians and nurses to assess ventilatory function and oxygenation for patients in respiratory failure. The critical values listed are used as criteria of the need for mechanical ventilation. It must be emphasized that these values are only guidelines. Good clinical judgment is based on a thorough understanding of the pathophysiology of respiratory failure and involves the integration of qualitative observations with quantitative measurements.

Treatment

Priorities in the management of respiratory failure vary according to the etiologic factors, but the primary aims of treatment are the same for all patients, that is, to treat the cause of the respiratory failure and at the same time ensure adequate ventilation and clear airways.

Because the most life-threatening feature of respiratory failure is the impairment of gas exchange, the first goal of therapy is to ensure that hypoxemia, acidemia, and hypercapnia do not reach hazardous levels. A PaO_2 of 40 mm Hg or a pH of 7.2 or less is poorly tolerated by adults and can result in cerebral, kidney, and cardiac impairment and the development of cardiac dysrhythmias. A $PaCO_2$ of 60 mm Hg that has developed slowly in a patient with COPD is usually well tolerated, but rapid development to this level is not. A $PaCO_2$ of 70 mm Hg or more is usually poorly tolerated in any patient and causes CNS depression and coma.

O_2 may be delivered at a concentration of 40% to 60% to a patient with hypoxemia and a normal or low $PaCO_2$ (mask or catheter at 8 L/min with adequate humidification) to achieve a rapid correction of the hypoxemia. However, this concentration should not be continued for more than a few hours, because it has a direct toxic effect on alveolar cells, causing decreased synthesis of surfactant and decreased pulmonary compliance. Prolonged administration of O_2 (more than 24 to 48 hours) at high concentrations (greater than 50%) also causes absorption atelectasis.

TABLE 41-1

Measurements of Respiratory Function

Test	Significance	Normal Value	Critical Value
TESTS OF VENTILATORY FUNCTION			
Respiratory rate (frequency, f) per minute	Overall indicator of respiratory distress and work of breathing	12-20	>35 or <10
Tidal volume (V_T), ml	Volume of air exchanged during each breath at rest	500-700	<350
Minute ventilation ($\dot{V}_E$), L	Overall indicator of ventilation	5-10	>10
Forced vital capacity (FVC), ml/kg ideal body weight	Indicates ventilatory reserve; best indicator of need for ventilatory support	65-75	<15
Forced expiratory volume in 1 second (FEV_1), ml/kg	First-second expired volume of FVC; useful in assessing ventilatory reserve in patients with COPD as well as efficacy of measures to overcome airway obstruction	50-60	<10
Maximum inspiratory force (MIF), cm H_2O	Indicates reserve of ventilatory effort	75-100	<25
V_D/V_T	Dead space/tidal volume ratio; allows estimate of ventilation in excess of perfusion; requires collecting sample of expired air to measure $PECO_2$ and $PaCO_2$; $V_D/V_T = PaCO_2 - (PECO_2/PaCO_2)$	0.25-0.40	>0.60
$PaCO_2$, mm Hg	Reflects ability of lung to eliminate CO_2; trend should be followed in patient with chronic hypercapnia along with pH of arterial blood; serious acidemia when pH 7.2 or less	35-45	>55
TESTS OF OXYGENATION STATUS			
PaO_2 (breathing air), mm Hg	Adequacy of oxygen tension in arterial blood; expected PaO_2 can be calculated from alveolar gas equation when patient breathing higher FIO_2 than air (O_2 therapy)	80-100	<50-60
$P(A - a)O_2$ or $(A - aD)O_2$, mm Hg (breathing 100% O_2)	Alveolar-arterial oxygen tension difference; indicates oxygenation reserve	30-50	>450
$\dot{Q}_S/\dot{Q}_T$, %	Proportion of cardiac output shunted past alveoli	<5	>20
TESTS OF ACID-BASE STATUS			
$PaCO_2$, mm Hg		40 ± 5	
Arterial blood pH		7.35-7.45	
HCO_3^-, mEq/L		24 ± 3	

Values from Cherniack RM, Cherniack L: *Respiration in health and disease*, ed 3, Philadelphia, 1983, Saunders; and Bendixen HH et al: *Respiratory care*, St Louis, 1965, Mosby.

Hypoxemia with hypercapnia is always treated with low, graduated O_2 therapy, beginning with a mask that delivers 24% O_2. The concentration is increased to 28% O_2 if necessary to maintain a PaO_2 of 50 mm Hg or more. Careful monitoring of ABGs is used at all times to ensure that the O_2 therapy does not cause a deterioration in the patient's respiratory status: in the patient with COPD, attempts are made to achieve PaO_2 values that are normal for the patient (e.g., 50 to 70 mm Hg) and not those normal for the healthy adult (80 to 100 mm Hg). When achieving PaO_2 values of 50 mm Hg is not possible, artificial ventilation with a respirator may be required. (See Table 41-1 for critical values indicating need for ventilatory support.)

Table 41-2 lists the priorities and aims in the treatment of hypercapnic respiratory failure. The approach to the problem of retained lung secretions includes measures to liquefy and remove them. Liquefaction is best achieved by adequate hydration of the patient. Drugs such as potassium iodide taken orally or aerosol delivery of water may also help in the mobilization of sputum. Secretions are best removed by encouraging the patient to cough or assisting the patient's efforts by percussion, vibration, and postural drainage. When the patient is too depressed or weak to cough, secretions may be removed by aspiration via an endotracheal tube or bronchoscopy. If these methods fail, then tracheostomy may be necessary.

If bronchospasm is present in respiratory failure, bronchodilatory or corticosteroid drugs may be used. Respiratory infection, which is a common cause of hypoxemic respiratory failure, is treated with the appropriate antibiotics.

Finally, a thorough search is made for other factors that may have induced the respiratory failure, such as pulmonary embolism or left ventricular failure.

A number of excellent books dealing with the management of respiratory failure are suggested in the bibliography at the end of Part Seven for those who want to know more about this subject.

ACUTE (ADULT) RESPIRATORY DISTRESS SYNDROME

Acute respiratory distress syndrome (ARDS) is a distinct form of respiratory failure characterized by profound hypoxemia refractory to conventional treatment. Although this entity was formerly called "adult respiratory distress syndrome", the term "acute" is now preferred because this condition is not limited to adults. ARDS is preceded by a variety of serious illnesses, all of which result in a characteristic diffuse noncardiogenic pulmonary edema. Petty and Ashbaugh coined the term in 1971 after observing acute life-threatening respiratory distress in patients with no previous lung disease. Although this syndrome has been called by a variety of other names *(shock lung, wet lung, adult hyaline membrane disease, stiff lung syndrome)*, the term *adult respiratory distress syndrome* has been more widely accepted. The American Lung Association estimates that 27,000 individuals develop ARDS annually and the mortality rate remains greater than 50% despite years of research.

Etiology and Pathogenesis

ARDS develops when the lung is injured directly or indirectly by various processes. Some of the most common conditions that lead to ARDS are listed in Box 41-4.

TABLE 41-2

Priorities and Principles in Treatment of Hypercapnic Respiratory Failure

Priority	Problem	Treatment
1	Retained secretions (ineffective cough)	Adequate hydration, expectorants, aerosols; Supervised coughing; Catheter aspiration (deep suction); Bronchoscopic suction; Endotracheal tube aspiration; Tracheostomy
2	Hypoxemia	Graduated O_2 therapy with frequent monitoring of ABGs to direct therapy
3	Hypercapnia	Respiratory stimulants (drug overdose); Avoidance of sedation; Artificial ventilation via endotracheal tube or tracheostomy
4	Respiratory infection	Antibiotics
5	Bronchospasm	Bronchodilatory drugs (isoproterenol by inhalation therapy; intravenous, oral, or rectal aminophylline; corticosteroid drugs)
6	Cardiac failure	Diuretics; Digoxin (with caution if given at all)

BOX 41-4

Causes of Adult Respiratory Distress Syndrome

Shock from various causes (especially hemorrhagic, hemorrhagic acute pancreatitis, gram-negative sepsis)
Sepsis without shock, with or without disseminated intravascular coagulation (DIC)
Overwhelming viral pneumonia
Critical trauma
  Head injury
  Direct chest injury
  Multiple organ trauma with hemorrhagic shock
  Multiple fractures
    Fat embolization (associated with fracture of long bones such as the femur)
Aspiration/inhalation injury
  Aspiration of gastric contents
  Near-drowning
  Smoke inhalation
  Irritant gas inhalation (e.g., chlorine, ammonia, sulfur dioxide)
  Prolonged exposure (>48 hours) to high concentration of inhaled oxygen (FiO_2 >50%)
  Narcotic overdose
Postperfusion cardiopulmonary bypass surgery

The mechanism by which such a diversity of insults can produce a common clinical and pathophysiologic syndrome is unclear. The common denominator causing the characteristic alveolar edema appears to involve injury to the alveolocapillary membrane with the production of a capillary leak. Electron microscopy studies reveal that the air-blood barrier consists of type I pneumocytes (supporting cells) and type II pneumocytes (source of surfactant) along with basement membrane on the alveolar side; these are back to back with capillary basement membrane and endothelial cells. Additionally, the alveolus has connective tissue cells that serve as support and regulate volume. The alveolocapillary membrane is normally quite impermeable to particles. However, when injury occurs, this permeability is altered, with an influx of fluid, red blood cells, white blood cells, and blood proteins. The fluid first accumulates in the interstitium; when the capacity of the interstitium is exceeded, the fluid accumulates in the alveolus, causing congestive atelectasis. The point of vulnerability appears to be the interdigitations (small spaces approximately 60 Å in width) between the capillary endothelial cells, which become widened, allowing the influx of small particles, which then cause a shift in oncotic pressure. Thus the formation of pulmonary edema depends on the disruption of the normal relations of the Starling forces: hydrostatic pressure, oncotic pressure, and tissue pressure. Additionally, alterations in the surfactant system undoubtedly play a role in the diffuse microatelectasis. In fact, light microscopy reveals that the proteinaceous material may be organized into *hyaline membranes* lining the alveolus. The pathologic picture is similar to that of the respiratory distress syndrome occurring in the infant. The consequence of the diffuse edema and atelectasis is marked intrapulmonary shunting, which may affect more than 40% of the cardiac output.

The poor prognosis of patients with ARDS has provided considerable impetus to elucidating the mechanisms that initiate pulmonary vascular injury. These mechanisms appear to depend on the interaction of activated inflammatory cells, humoral mediators, and endothelial cells. A better understanding of these mechanisms will determine the development of effective pharmacologic interventions. Recent research has focused on the mechanisms leading to the activation of inflammatory cells (particularly the polymorphonuclear neutrophil leukocytes, PMNs), platelets, and other clotting factors, because ARDS is clearly part of an inflammation-induced systemic state that can evolve into multiple organ failure.

Clinical Features

The primary features of ARDS include a marked degree of intrapulmonary shunting with hypoxemia, a progressive loss in lung compliance, and extreme dyspnea and tachypnea resulting from both the hypoxemia and the increased work of breathing secondary to the loss of lung compliance. The normal compliance of the lungs and thorax together is approximately 100 ml/cm H_2O. In ARDS, compliance may be as low as 15 to 20 ml/cm

H_2O. Functional residual capacity is also reduced. These features are a consequence of the interstitial and alveolar edema. The result is a stiff lung that is difficult to ventilate. A hallmark of ARDS is that the hypoxemia cannot be relieved by O_2 administration during spontaneous breathing. The full-blown clinical state may become manifest 1 to 2 days after the initiating injury.

Establishing a correct diagnosis of ARDS largely depends on obtaining an accurate clinical history. The earliest laboratory finding is hypoxemia; thus measuring ABGs in the appropriate clinical setting is important. The $Paco_2$ is generally normal or low. Early chest radiographic findings may be normal despite the hypoxemia. Later, as the alveolar and interstitial fluid accumulates and the congestive atelectasis spreads, the chest radiograph shows a diffuse "whiteout" appearance. Thus another name for ARDS is *white lung*.

Treatment

The management of ARDS is aimed at correcting the accompanying shock, acidosis, and hypoxemia. Almost all patients require mechanical ventilation and high concentrations of O_2 to avoid serious tissue hypoxia. The use of positive end-expiratory pressure (PEEP) with the volume respirator is a major advance in the treatment of this condition. PEEP helps to correct the respiratory distress syndrome by reexpanding previously atelectatic areas and by reversing the flow of atelectatic edema fluid from capillaries. Another benefit of PEEP is that it allows administration of lower concentrations of Fio_2. This aspect is important because on the one hand a high Fio_2 is generally needed to achieve a minimally acceptable Pao_2, and on the other hand high O_2 concentrations are toxic to the lung and cause ARDS. The net effect of PEEP is to improve Pao_2 and allow reduction in Fio_2. Potential hazards from the use of PEEP are pneumothorax and interference with cardiac output because of high pressures. Close monitoring and attention are directed toward achieving "best PEEP," that is, ventilation at the end-expiratory pressure that results in the best lung compliance and least reduction in the Pao_2 and cardiac output.

Because sequestration of fluid in the lung is a problem, restriction of fluids and diuretic therapy are other important measures in the treatment of ARDS. Appropriate antibiotics are given to treat infection. Although the use of corticosteroids is controversial, many centers use them in the treatment of ARDS even though their benefit has not been clearly established. Another potentially promising treatment is surfactant replacement therapy for adults with the syndrome. Surfactant therapy has already been applied to infants with respiratory distress syndrome with dramatic results in reducing morbidity and mortality. Its application to ARDS awaits the results of current research. Another promising approach in the treatment of ARDS is the use of inhaled nitric oxide as a selective vasodilator of the pulmonary vasculature. Clinical studies show that inhaled nitric oxide produces vasodilation in those areas of the lung that are well-ventilated and thus promote better $\dot{V}/\dot{Q}$ matching and improved oxygenation (Anzueto et al, 1996).

KEY CONCEPTS

- Respiratory failure is said to exist when the lung cannot perform its primary function of gas exchange, namely oxygenation of the arterial blood and carbon dioxide elimination. The exact point at which gas exchange becomes adequate is somewhat arbitrary.

- The person with chronic respiratory insufficiency may be able to maintain marginal respiratory function only at the expense of considerable increased work of the cardiopulmonary system.

- Distinguishing chronic respiratory insufficiency from acute respiratory failure on the basis of signs and symptoms, which are nonspecific, may be difficult.

- In practice, acute respiratory failure (ARF) is defined on the basis of arterial blood gases as a PaO_2 value $\leq$ 50 mm Hg and a $PaCO_2$ value $\geq$ 50 mm Hg. (Some clinicians use a PaO_2 value of 60 mm Hg as the criterion.)

- The two types of acute respiratory failure are (1) *hypoxemic respiratory failure* (hypoxemia without hypercapnia) and (2) *ventilatory or hypoxemic/hypercapnic respiratory failure*.

- *Hypoxemic respiratory failure* is defined as PaO_2 $\leq$ 50 with normal or low $PaCO_2$. This is the most common type of ARF, which occurs when atelectasis is present or when alveoli fill with fluid or exudate. Examples are adult (acute) respiratory distress syndrome (ARDS) and severe pneumonia. Generally, hypoxemic respiratory failure occurs when lung disease is severe enough to interfere with O_2 exchange but the patient is capable of maintaining overall alveolar ventilation ($\dot{V}_A$).

- *Ventilatory* or *hypoxemic/hypercapnic respiratory failure* is defined as PaO_2 value $\leq$50, $PaCO_2$ $\geq$50 mm Hg. Causes of hypoxemic-hypercapnic respiratory failure include COPD (most common), chronic disorders involving the chest wall or neuromuscular disorders affecting the respiratory bellows, and CNS respiratory center depression.

- Patients with COPD may have chronic respiratory failure with blood gases that are indistinguishable from those used to define acute respiratory failure (e.g., PaO_2, 55 to 60 mm Hg; $PaCO_2$, 45 to 50 mm Hg) but may be able to maintain a blood pH that is nearly normal by renal retention of bicarbonate. The clue that these patients are in acute respiratory failure is a decrease in their arterial pH <7.35.

- A number of precipitating factors can result in what is called *acute-on-chronic respiratory failure* in patients with COPD and chronic respiratory failure, including respiratory tract infection, sedatives or narcotics, increase in volume of tracheobronchial secretions, pneumothorax, or high FIO_2.

- *Alveolar hypoventilation* is the primary pathogenetic mechanism causing hypercapnia. Alveolar hypoventilation can be caused by a decrease in the minute volume ($\dot{V}_E$) or an increase in the proportion of ventilation that is wasted as dead space ventilation (e.g., shallow breathing). $\dot{V}/\dot{Q}$ mismatch does not generally contribute to CO_2 retention as long as the patient is capable of compensating by increasing his or her total minute ventilation.

- *Alveolar hypoventilation* is also a cause of hypoxemia and the direct cause is the increased $PaCO_2$. The respiratory exchange ratio, normally 0.8, expresses the relationship between volume of CO_2 ($\dot{V}CO_2$) production and O_2 consumption ($\dot{V}O_2$). This ratio means that for every 10 mm Hg increase in the $PaCO_2$ above the normal (40 mm Hg), the PaO_2 must decrease 12 mm Hg from the normal (95 to 100 mm Hg).

- *Pure hypoventilation* alone causes only mild hypoxemia and is most common in extrapulmonary conditions and the lungs are normal.

- The three pathogenetic mechanisms causing hypoxemia are (1) alveolar hypoventilation, (2) $\dot{V}/\dot{Q}$ mismatch, and (3) shunting. (Other mechanisms play a minor role in the hypoxemia of respiratory failure: diffusion impairment and low FIO_2 [altitude].)

- $\dot{V}/\dot{Q}$ *mismatch* refers to *regional $\dot{V}/\dot{Q}$ imbalance* in gas-exchanging units, which are of two types: (1) *dead space gas exchanging units* with high $\dot{V}/\dot{Q}$ ratios (wasted ventilation) or (2) *shuntlike gas exchanging units* with low $\dot{V}/\dot{Q}$ ratios (wasted perfusion).

- High $\dot{V}/\dot{Q}$ ratio (dead space) units cannot compensate for low $\dot{V}/\dot{Q}$ ratio (shuntlike) units with respect to O_2 transport because Hb from the well-ventilated units is nearly 100% saturated; thus the result is hypoxemia. The S-shape of the oxyhemoglobin dissociation curve should be noted.

- High $\dot{V}/\dot{Q}$ units can compensate for low $\dot{V}/\dot{Q}$ units with respect to CO_2 transport; thus mixed blood leaving the high or low units will have normal $PaCO_2$. (The linear shape of the CO_2 dissociation curve should be noted.) Eventually, as a larger and larger proportion of the total lung capacity has low $\dot{V}/\dot{Q}$ ratios, the $PaCO_2$ rises. Thus diseases characterized by $\dot{V}/\dot{Q}$ imbalances progress from hypoxemic respiratory insufficiency to hypoxemic respiratory failure to hypoxemic-hypercapnic respiratory failure.

- An anatomic-like shunt (true venous admixture) may occur when the alveoli are collapsed (atelectasis), filled with exudate, or filled with edema fluid, as in ARDS or severe pneumonia. Gas units are perfused, but ventilation is absent so that gas exchange cannot take place. A large proportion of the blood being shunted through the lungs results in profound hypoxemia not correctable by O_2 therapy.

- Factors determining oxygenation and ventilation are different and must be assessed separately.

- The $PaCO_2$ must be regarded as a function of overall lung ventilation with respect to regional (local) $\dot{V}/\dot{Q}$ imbalance.

- The PaO_2 depends not only on the amount of alveolar ventilation but also on the $\dot{V}/\dot{Q}$ match.

- Hypercapnia must be regarded as a problem with both ventilation and oxygenation.

- Hyperventilation while breathing room air (FIO_2 = 21%) is generally ineffective in correcting hypoxemia because of the S-shape of the oxyhemoglobin dissociation curve.

- O_2 therapy is effective in correcting hypoxemia caused by hypoventilation, $\dot{V}/\dot{Q}$ imbalance, and diffusion defect (usually a minor problem) but not hypoxemia because of right-to-left shunting (anatomic-like shunt).
- Hypoxemic respiratory failure is generally associated with restrictive diseases of the lung. The principle mechanisms are $\dot{V}/\dot{Q}$ mismatch or anatomic-like shunt, either alone or in combination. Although the work of breathing and, consequently, CO_2 production is increased, patients generally have sufficient strength to hyperventilate and blow off CO_2 to achieve a $Paco_2$ that is normal or below normal (respiratory alkalosis).
- Hypoxemic-hypercapnic (ventilatory) failure may be caused by hypoventilation alone or in combination with any of the hypoxemic mechanisms. Pure hypoventilation generally occurs in extrapulmonary disorders involving failure of muscular or neural control of ventilation.
- Obstructive respiratory disorders generally result in hypoxemic-hypercapnic (ventilatory) failure (with the exception of asthma). COPD is a classic example of hypoventilation plus $\dot{V}/\dot{Q}$ mismatch, and considerable right-to-left shunting occurs when precipitated by retained secretions and pneumonia.
- The manifestations of acute respiratory failure represent a combination of the clinical features underlying the disease, the precipitating factors, and the manifestations of hypoxemia and hypercapnia.
- The signs and symptoms of *hypoxemia* are a direct result of tissue hypoxia. Tissues most sensitive to hypoxia are principally affected, and symptoms do not occur until the Pao_2 is approximately 40 to 50 mm Hg. The most prominent symptoms are neurologic: headache, mental confusion, impairment of judgment, slurring of speech, asterixis, impairment of motor function, agitation, and restlessness. Tachycardia, tachypnea, and dyspnea may be present. Cyanosis may be present when hypoxia is severe but is an unreliable sign.
- *Hypercapnia* while breathing room air is always accompanied by hypoxemia. Thus signs and symptoms of ventilatory failure represent the effects of both hypoxemia and hypercapnia. The major effect of an increase in the $Paco_2$ is depression of the CNS, causing increasing somnolence and, for this reason, is sometimes called *CO_2 narcosis*. Hypercapnia results in cerebral vasodilation and increased intracranial pressure resulting in headache and papilledema. $Paco_2$ levels above 70 mm Hg depress the respiratory center rather than stimulate breathing. Hypercapnia causes respiratory acidosis, which is often combined with metabolic acidosis when tissue hypoxia is present, resulting in serious depression of the blood pH that can result in cardiac dysrhythmias.
- The first goal of therapy in the treatment of patients with COPD and *acute-on-chronic respiratory failure* is to ensure that hypoxemia, acidemia, and hypercapnia do not reach hazardous levels. Patients with COPD and chronic CO_2 retention depend on a hypoxemic stimulus to breathe. Thus administering high concentrations of O_2 may cause the condition to worsen. To avoid this hazard, O_2 therapy should begin with Fio_2 of 24% (air is 21% O_2) and be gradually increased sufficiently to achieve a Pao_2 of 50 to 70 mm Hg. O_2 per nasal prongs at a flow rate of 1 to 2 L/min results in an Fio_2 of 24% to 28%. ABGs must be monitored to ensure that the O_2 therapy does not cause a deterioration of the patient's respiratory status. When achieving a Pao_2 of 50 mm Hg or more is not possible, artificial ventilation may be required. Additional goals are to treat the underlying disease and precipitating factors, such as relieving bronchospasm with bronchodilators; removing secretions by adequate hydration, aerosol therapy, and supervised coughing; or chest physical therapy. Bacterial infection is treated with antibiotics.
- *ARDS* is a distinct form of respiratory failure characterized by severe hypoxemia refractory to conventional treatment. ARDS is preceded by a variety of illnesses (e.g., sepsis, aspiration of gastric contents, critical trauma), which cause damage to the alveolocapillary membrane, resulting in increased permeability and severe noncardiogenic pulmonary edema. The pathogenesis is poorly understood.
- Pathophysiologic features of *ARDS* include marked intrapulmonary shunting and $\dot{V}/\dot{Q}$ mismatch, inactivation of surfactant, decreased lung compliance (stiff lungs), hypoxemia, and hypocapnia.
- Clinical features of *ARDS* include dyspnea, tachypnea, rales, increased $P(A-a)O_2$, decreased Pao_2, and decreased $Paco_2$. Chest x-ray shows white lung (whiteout) with diffuse congestive atelectasis.
- Management of ARDS centers on treatment of the precipitating disorder, interrupting the pathogenic sequence of events causing the capillary leak and support of gas exchange until the pulmonary process improves. No pharmacologic agents have been found that block the effect of humoral mediators on the capillary permeability defect. Almost all patients require mechanical ventilation with high concentrations of O_2 and PEEP to avoid tissue hypoxia. Mortality of patients with ARDS exceeds 50%.

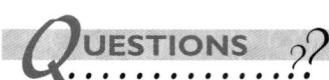

QUESTIONS ??

A sampling of review questions for this chapter appears here. Visit http://www.mosby.com/MERLIN/PriceWilson/ for additional questions.

Answer the following on a separate sheet of paper.

1. What is the relationship between respiratory insufficiency and maintaining normal ABGs?

2. What is the most common cause of chronic respiratory insufficiency?

3. List the two types of respiratory failure based on ABG changes.

4. Explain why high concentrations of O_2 must not be administered in hypercapnic respiratory failure.

5. What level of Pao_2 or $Paco_2$ would not be well tolerated in most adults?

6. List at least three measures used to treat the problem of retained secretions and pulmonary infection in hypercapnic respiratory failure.
7. What is the primary goal and first priority in the treatment of respiratory failure?
8. What are the three most common precipitating factors of acute-on-chronic respiratory failure in patients with COPD? Name two iatrogenic precipitating factors. Name as many other factors as possible.
9. Why is a patient breathing air with a $\dot{V}/\dot{Q}$ mismatch able to maintain a normal $Paco_2$ by increasing alveolar ventilation but is unable to achieve a normal Pao_2? (Explain with respect to the oxyhemoglobin and CO_2 dissociation curves.)

10. A 25-year-old male heroin addict was admitted to the hospital with severe hypoventilation because of drug overdose. The barometric pressure was 760 mm Hg. His body temperature was normal, thus the P_{H_2O} in his trachea was 47 mm Hg. On admission, his Pao_2 was 50 mm Hg and $Paco_2$ was 80 mm Hg while breathing air. Is this pure hypoventilation? Calculate the $P(A - a)O_2$ gradient to answer the question. He was given O_2 (Fio_2 = 50%). Measurement of ABGs then revealed Pao_2 = 246 mm Hg and $Paco_2$ = 80 mm Hg. What would be his expected Pao_2 when receiving 50% O_2? Is it possible that his hypoxemia was caused by pure hypoventilation? (Assume that his respiratory exchange ratio [R] is 0.8.)

11. A 60-year-old man with COPD was admitted to the hospital because of respiratory distress. He reported an increase in sputum production; the sputum was purulent, although his temperature was normal. Measurement of ABGs revealed Pao_2 of 35 mm Hg and $Paco_2$ of 55 mm Hg. Barometric pressure was 747 mm Hg. Assume R = 0.8. What was his $P(A - a)O_2$ gradient? Is his hypoxemia caused by either hypoventilation or $\dot{V}/\dot{Q}$ imbalance alone or by both these mechanisms? He was given 24% O_2. Two days later his ABGs were Pao_2 of 50 mm Hg and $Paco_2$ of 45 mm Hg. Is his condition better or worse? Calculate his $P(A - a)O_2$ to answer this question.

Match each type of respiratory disorder in column B with the type of respiratory failure it is likely to be associated with in column A.

Column A
12. _____ Hypoxemic respiratory failure
13. _____ Hypercapnic respiratory failure

Column B
a. COPD
b. Respiratory center depression
c. Asthmatic attack
d. Bacterial pneumonia
e. ARDS
f. Myasthenia gravis
g. Silicosis

Match the acid-base status in column B with the findings it fits best in column A. (Use the acid-base nomogram in Fig. 41-2 to check your answers.)

Column A
14. _____ Patient with cystic fibrosis and chronic hypercapnia
15. _____ Patient with head injury, $Paco_2$ = 40 mm Hg, HCO_3^- = 24 mEq/L, pH = 7.41
16. _____ Patient with COPD and respiratory infection, $Paco_2$ = 75 mm Hg, pH = 7.1
17. _____ COPD patient above after being on mechanical ventilator, $Paco_2$ = 55 mm Hg, pH = 7.48, HCO_3^- = 39 mEq/L
18. _____ Patient with lobar pneumonia, $Paco_2$ = 24 mm Hg, pH = 7.46, Pao_2 = 60 mm Hg
19. _____ Patient who aspirated vomitus during a cerebrovascular accident, 2 days later $Paco_2$ = 20 mm Hg, pH = 7.32, Pao_2 = 35 mm Hg

Column B
a. Normal acid-base status
b. Chronic respiratory alkalosis
c. Mixed acute and chronic respiratory acidosis
d. Mixed respiratory alkalosis and metabolic acidosis
e. Mixed chronic respiratory acidosis and metabolic alkalosis
f. Chronic respiratory acidosis

Answer the questions below related to the following case study.
A 25-year-old woman was found in her apartment by neighbors in a semicomatose condition. Paramedics brought her to the emergency room, and the physician diagnosed her condition as acute narcotic overdose. The following ABG results were obtained (breathing room air) before admission to the intensive care unit:

pH = 7.22
HCO_3^- = 34 mEq/L
Pao_2 = 39 mm Hg
Sao_2 = 62%
$Paco_2$ = 84 mm Hg
Hb = 12 g/dl

20. The Pao_2 of 39 mm Hg indicates severe _____.
21. The $Paco_2$ of 84 mm Hg indicates marked _____.
22. Calculate her $P(A - a)O_2$ using the alveolar gas equation: _____
Assume P_B = 760 mm Hg, P_{H_2O} = 47 mm Hg, and R = 0.8.
Is it normal?

23. Calculate her arterial O_2 content in ml/dl: _____.
    Is it normal?
24. The patient's hypoxemia is a result of:
    a. A problem with gas exchange intrinsic to the lungs
    b. A problem with the respiratory pump (extrinsic to the lungs) secondary to depression of the respiratory center
    c. Hyperventilation causing a left shift of the oxyhemoglobin dissociation curve and reduced Sao_2
    d. Marked left-to-right intrapulmonary shunting
25. The patient's acid-base status is best characterized as:
    a. Marked hyperventilation and metabolic acidosis
    b. Partially compensated primary respiratory acidosis
    c. Chronic respiratory alkalosis
    d. Mixed respiratory alkalosis and metabolic acidosis
26. The greatly depressed Pao_2, elevated $Paco_2$, and low pH are diagnostic of:
    a. Hypoxemic respiratory failure
    b. Hypercapnic respiratory failure
27. Acute ventilatory failure is associated with:
    a. Alveolar hypoventilation
    b. Severe hypoxemia
    c. Alveolar hyperventilation
    d. Severe hypocapnia

Pulmonary Malignant Neoplasms

LORRAINE M. WILSON

𝓜ore than 90% of primary lung tumors are malignant, and about 95% of these malignant tumors are bronchogenic carcinoma. Whenever lung cancer is mentioned, bronchogenic carcinoma is the tumor being referred to because most primary malignant tumors of the lower respiratory tract are epithelial in nature and arise from the mucosa of the bronchial tree.

Although once considered a rare form of malignant growth, the incidence of lung cancer in the industrialized countries has risen to epidemic proportions since 1930. Some of the alarming statistics were cited in the introduction to this part of the text. Cancer of the lung is now the leading cause of cancer death in both men and women. The peak incidence occurs between ages 55 and 65 years. This increase is believed to be related to increased cigarette smoking and therefore is largely preventable.

BRONCHOGENIC CARCINOMA

Etiology

Although the exact cause of bronchogenic carcinoma is unknown, three factors appear to account for the increase in incidence: smoking, industrial hazards, and air pollution. Of these factors, *smoking* appears to play the major role, accounting for 85% of the cases (Van Houtte, 2001). Massive statistical evidence indicates that a relationship exists between heavy cigarette smoking and the development of lung cancer. Three prospective studies, one involving nearly 200,000 men ages 50 to 69, followed for 44 months, revealed that the death rate from cancer of the lung per 100,000 was 3.4 in the male nonsmoker, 59.3 in those who smoked 10 to 20 cigarettes daily, and 217.3 in those who smoked 40 or more cigarettes daily. Individuals who give up smoking permanently reduce their risk to that of a nonsmoker after an abstinence of 15 years.

Great interest has arisen about the relationship of *passive smoking,* or the inhalation of other persons' smoke in an enclosed area, to the risk of developing lung cancer. Some studies have shown that nonsmokers exposed to secondhand smoke double their risk of developing lung cancer. Mortality from lung cancer is related to atmospheric pollution, but its effect is small compared with that of cigarette smoking. The death rate from cancer of the lung is twice as high in cities as it is in rural areas. Statistical evidence also shows that the disease is more common in the lowest socioeconomic classes and decreases in higher classes. This statistic may be partly explained by the fact that persons in the lowest social classes are more apt to live near their jobs, where the atmosphere may be more polluted. A *carcinogen* (cancer-producing material) that has been found in polluted air (and also in cigarette smoke) is 3,4-benzpyrene.

In certain instances, bronchogenic carcinoma appears to be an occupational disease. Of the various industrial hazards, the most important is undoubtedly *asbestos,* which is widely used in the construction industry. The risk of lung cancer in asbestos workers is about 10 times greater than that in the general population. Local benign or diffuse malignant mesotheliomas of the pleura are rare tumors that have been specifically associated with asbestos exposure. There is also increased risk in people who work with uranium, chromate, arsenic (insecticide used in agriculture), iron, and iron oxides. The risks of lung cancer from both asbestos and uranium exposure are greatly enhanced in those who also smoke cigarettes.

Two other factors that may play a role in the risk of developing lung cancer are *diet* and *familial tendency.* Several studies have shown that smokers who eat a diet low in vitamin A are at increased risk for developing lung cancer. Evidence also suggests that family members of lung cancer patients are at increased risk for developing the disease. Cytogenetic and molecular genetic studies have revealed that mutations in both protooncogenes and tumor suppressor genes are critical in the multistep development and progression of lung tumors. Typical targets include activation of oncogenes, including *K-ras* and *myc* genes and inactivation of tumor suppressor genes, including the *rb*, *p53*, and CDKN2 genes. For example, mutation of the K-*ras* gene is present in 30% of adenocarcinomas of the lung, and this mutation indicates a poorer prognosis. Studies reveal that first-degree relatives of cancer patients with inherited mutations of the p53 and rb genes have a twofold to threefold risk of developing lung cancer that is not associated with smoking.

In many tissues, chronic inflammatory changes are known to precede cancer. Evidence supports the view that chronic inflammation of the bronchial mucosa from inhaled irritants may be of greater importance than are the carcinogenic effect of any one substance. Another factor that has not received much attention is the close correspondence between the increase in the number of motor vehicles and the incidence of lung cancer.

These facts suggest that although smoking clearly plays a major part in the increasing incidence of lung cancer, it is by no means the only factor. Chronic infection; air pollution from motor vehicles and industry; occupational exposure to carcinogens; and dietary, familial, and perhaps other unknown factors may (either alone or in combination) predispose to cancer of the lung.

Pathology

Primary lung cancer is usually classified according to histologic type (Box 42-1), all of which have different natural histories and responses to treatment. Although more than a dozen types of primary lung cancer exist, bronchogenic cancer, which includes the first four cell types, makes up 95% of all lung cancer.

Bronchogenic carcinoma is usually divided into *small cell lung cancer (SCLC)* and *non–small cell lung cancer (NSCLC)* for the purposes of determining therapy. NSCLC includes the epidermoid, adenocarcinoma, large cell types, or mixtures of these. In general, SCLC is primarily managed

---

BOX 42-1

World Health Organization (WHO) Classification of Pleuropulmonary Neoplasms

BRONCHOGENIC CARCINOMAS
  I. Epidermoid (squamous) carcinomas
  II. Small cell carcinoma (includes oat cell)
  III. Adenocarcinomas (includes alveolar cell carcinoma)
  IV. Large cell carcinoma
  V. Combined epidermoid and adenocarcinoma

OTHERS
  VI. Carcinoid tumors (bronchial adenomas)
  VII. Bronchial gland tumors
  VIII. Papillary tumors of the surface epithelium
  IX. Mixed tumors and carcinosarcomas
  X. Sarcomas
  XI. Unclassified
  XII. Mesotheliomas
  XIII. Melanomas

From Kreyberg L, Liebow AA, Uehlinger EA: *Histological typing of lung tumors*, ed 2, Geneva, Switzerland, 1981, World Health Organization.

---

with chemotherapy, with or without radiation therapy, whereas NSCLC, if localized at the time of diagnosis, is treated by surgical resection. The approximate frequency of the various histologic types is as follows: epidermoid (30%), adenocarcinoma (33%), large cell carcinoma (10%), and small cell carcinoma (18%). Of the patients with bronchogenic carcinoma of all cell types, 90% are smokers, and the remaining 10% of nonsmokers who develop lung cancer usually have adenocarcinoma (Minna, 1998).

Squamous cell (epidermoid) carcinoma, a common histologic type of bronchogenic carcinoma, arises from the surface of the bronchial epithelium. Epithelial changes, including metaplasia or dysplasia from long-term smoking, typically precede the appearance of tumor. Squamous cell carcinoma is usually centrally located near the hilus and projects into the large bronchi. The tumor is seldom more than a few centimeters in diameter and tends to spread by direct extension to the hilar lymph nodes, chest wall, and mediastinum. Squamous cell carcinoma often presents with manifestations of cough and hemoptysis as a result of irritation or ulceration, pneumonia, and abscess formation from the obstruction and secondary infection. Because this type of lung cancer generally metastasizes late, early treatment improves prognosis.

Adenocarcinomas, as the name implies, show a cellular organization resembling that of bronchial glands and may contain mucus. The majority of these tumors arise in the peripheral segmental bronchi and are sometimes associated with focal lung scars and chronic interstitial fibrosis. These lesions invade blood and lymph vessels early in their development and often give rise to distant metastases before the primary lesion causes symptoms.

Bronchial alveolar cell carcinoma, a rare subtype of adenocarcinoma, arises from the epithelium of the alveoli or possibly the terminal bronchioles. The onset is generally insidious, with signs resembling pneumonia. In some cases, this neoplasm grossly resembles the uniform consolidation of lobar pneumonia. Microscopically, groups of alveoli are lined with clear mucous-secreting cells, and there is abundant expectoration of mucoid sputum. The prognosis is poor unless surgical removal of the diseased lobe is performed early. Adenocarcinoma is the only histologic type of lung cancer that does not have a clear association with smoking.

Large cell carcinomas are those with large, poorly differentiated malignant cells with abundant cytoplasm and variably sized nuclei. These carcinomas tend to develop in the peripheral lung tissue, grow rapidly, and spread to distant sites early and extensively.

Small cell carcinomas, as with the squamous cell type, are usually centrally located about the main stem bronchi. Unlike other lung cancers, this type of tumor arises from Kulchitsky's cells, a normal component of the bronchial epithelium. Microscopically, the tumor may be made up of small cells (about twice the size of lymphocytes) with dense hyperchromatic nuclei and little cytoplasm. The cells often resemble oat seeds, thus the term *oat cell carcinoma*. Small cell carcinomas have the fastest doubling time and the worst prognosis of all the bronchogenic carcinomas. Early metastasis to the mediastinal and hilar lymph nodes, as well as hematogenous spread to distant organ sites, often occurs. About 70% of patients have evidence of extensive disease (distal metastases) at the time of diagnosis, and the 5-year survival rate is less than 5%.

OTHER FORMS OF LUNG CANCER

In addition to bronchogenic carcinoma, other forms of primary lung cancer include bronchial adenomas, sarcomas, and mesotheliomas (see Box 42-1). Despite their rarity, these tumors are important because they simulate bronchogenic carcinoma and are life threatening.

Bronchial adenomas are a group of small, malignant neoplasms of low aggressiveness arising in the lower trachea or major bronchi, the most important being the bronchial carcinoid and the rarer cylindroma. *Bronchial carcinoids*, as with small cell carcinomas, are derived from Kulchitsky's cells of the bronchial mucosa. These tumors constitute about 4% of all bronchial tumors and may become apparent during the teenage to late middle age years (average age of diagnosis, 45 years), with males and females affected equally. Signs and symptoms of bronchial obstruction such as chronic cough, hemoptysis, or pneumonitis are common. Bronchial carcinoids are similar to carcinoid tumors of the intestines.* Some of these tumors secrete serotonin, 5-hydroxytryptophan, and other biologically active substances that give rise to a symptom complex known as the *carcinoid syndrome.* Symptoms include flushing, bronchoconstriction and wheezing, and diarrhea. Carcinoid tumors follow a relatively benign course, and surgical resection is usually quite successful, resulting in a 5-year survival rate of more than 90% with typical carcinoids.

Malignant mesothelioma is an uncommon tumor of the pleura associated in the great majority of patients with prior asbestos exposure. This exposure may have been brief, and the usual time between exposure and clinical onset is 25 years. Malignant mesotheliomas are highly malignant, with survival time averaging less than a year from the time of diagnosis.

Both *primary sarcoma of the lung* and *primary malignant melanoma of the lung* are very rare but highly malignant forms of lung cancer. It is more likely that either type of these lung cancers represents metastasis from an undiagnosed primary tumor rather than a primary tumor site.

Finally, it should be remembered that the lung is affected by metastatic cancer significantly more often than by a primary malignant neoplasm. The lung is a common site for secondary deposits of cancer cells originating in other organs because blood-borne microscopic tumor emboli are likely to become enmeshed in the pulmonary capillary bed. Lymph-borne tumors from the lower half of the body and abdominal cavity may also be arrested as they pass through the thoracic duct. The most common neoplasms giving rise to pulmonary metastasis in descending order of frequency are carcinomas of the breast, gastrointestinal tract, female genital tract, and kidneys; melanomas; and male genital cancer.

MANIFESTATIONS OF BRONCHOGENIC CARCINOMA

Bronchogenic carcinoma imitates a variety of other pulmonary diseases and has no typical mode of onset. Bronchogenic carcinoma often masquerades as a pneumonitis

*Carcinoid tumors are more common in the gastrointestinal tract than they are in the lungs. Although usually benign, they can be malignant.

that fails to resolve. Cough is a common symptom often ignored by the patient or attributed to smoking or bronchitis. When bronchial carcinoma develops in a patient with chronic bronchitis, cough often becomes more frequent or the volume of sputum may increase. Hemoptysis is another common sign. Initial symptoms of localized wheeze and mild dyspnea may result from varying degrees of bronchial obstruction. Chest pain may appear in various forms but is usually experienced as an ache or discomfort caused by neoplastic spread to the mediastinum. Pleuritic pain may occur when secondary involvement of the pleura occurs, resulting from neoplastic spread or pneumonia. Rapid development of digital clubbing is an important sign because it is often associated with bronchogenic carcinoma (30% of cases, usually NSCLC). General symptoms such as anorexia, fatigue, and weight loss are late symptoms.

Symptoms of intrathoracic or extrathoracic spread may also be present when the physician first examines the patient. Local extension of the tumor to the mediastinal structures may produce hoarseness as a result of involvement of the recurrent laryngeal nerve, dysphagia from involvement of the esophagus, and paralysis of the hemidiaphragm from involvement of the phrenic nerve. Compression of the superior vena cava gives rise to the *vena caval syndrome* (distention of the neck veins and edema of the face, neck, and upper limbs). Chest pain or cardiac tamponade can follow invasion of the chest wall or pericardium respectively. Tumors growing at the apex of the lungs (*Pancoast's tumor*) may involve the brachial plexus, giving rise to pain and weakness in the shoulder and arm on the affected side; the sympathetic ganglia may be similarly affected, causing a unilateral Horner's syndrome (unilateral pupil constriction and ptosis with loss of sweating on the same side of the face).

Symptoms of extrathoracic spread depend on the site of metastasis. Structures typically involved are the scalene lymph nodes (especially in peripheral lung tumors), adrenal glands (50%), liver (30%), brain (20%), bone (20%), and kidneys (15%) (see color plate 36).

Paraneoplastic syndromes are frequently associated with lung cancer. *Endocrine syndromes* are seen in 12% of patients. Oat cell tumors produce virtually any of the polypeptide hormones, such as parathyroid hormone (PTH), adrenocorticotropic hormone (ACTH), or antidiuretic hormone (ADH) giving rise to symptoms of hyperparathyroidism, Cushing's syndrome, and syndrome of inappropriate secretion of ADH (SIADH) associated with fluid retention and hyponatremia. *Skeletal connective tissue syndromes* include finger clubbing (usually in NSCLC) occurring in 30% of cases and hypertrophic osteoarthropathy (HOA) in up to 10% of cases (usually in adenocarcinomas). *Systemic symptoms* of anorexia, weight loss, and cachexia in 30% of cases are paraneoplastic syndromes of unknown origin.

DIAGNOSIS AND STAGING OF LUNG CANCER

The main tools in the diagnosis of lung cancer are radiology, bronchoscopy, and cytology. A solitary, circumscribed nodule, or *coin lesion*, on the chest radiograph is of particular importance and may be the earliest indication of bronchogenic carcinoma, although it may also occur in many other conditions. Computed tomography (CT) scan may be of further help in differentiating the suspected lesion. Bronchoscopy with biopsy is the most successful technique in the diagnosis of squamous cell carcinoma, which is generally located centrally. Scalene node biopsy is most successful in the diagnosis of those cancers inaccessible to bronchoscopy. Cytologic examination of the sputum, bronchial brushings, and examination of the pleural fluid also play an important role in the diagnosis of lung cancer.

Both the histology and the stage of disease are important to determine the prognosis, as well as the treatment plan. Distinguishing between SCLC and NSCLC is crucial. Lung cancer staging consists of two parts: (1) anatomic staging to determine the extent of the tumor and its resectability and (2) physiologic staging to determine the patient's ability to withstand various antitumor treatments.

The *TNM staging system* for lung cancer formulated by the American Joint Committee on Cancer is a widely accepted method of determining the extent of disease for NSCLC. The various T (tumor size), N (regional lymph node metastasis), and M (presence or absence of distal metastasis) factors are combined to form different stage groups (Table 42-1). Tumor size and histology are determined by radiology and examination of tissue specimen. In addition, mediastinoscopy is often useful to confirm the diagnosis and to separate operable from inoperable tumors. Tests to detect distal metastases include bone scan, brain scan, liver function studies, and gallium scan of liver, spleen, and bone.

When the TNM system was developed for bronchogenic carcinoma, the treatment of SCLC gave such poor results that it did not seem worthwhile to apply the TNM system to this variety of lung cancer. Thus a simple two-staging system is applied to SCLC. *Limited-stage disease* is defined as SCLC confined to one hemithorax and regional lymph nodes, and *extensive-stage disease* is defined as involvement more extensive than these parameters. In part, the limited-stage disease definition is related to whether the tumor can be encompassed within a tolerable radiation therapy port.

TABLE 42-1

Revised TNM International Staging System for Lung Cancer: 1997 American Joint Committee on Cancer

TNM Designation	Definition	
PRIMARY TUMOR (T) STATUS		
T0	No evidence of primary tumor	
Tx	Occult cancer seen in bronchial washing cytologies but not on radiograph or bronchoscopy	
Tis	Carcinoma in situ	
T1	Tumor ≤ 3 cm in diameter surrounded by normal lung or visceral pleura	
T2	Tumor>3 cm in diameter or any size that invades the visceral pleura or has associated atelectasis extending to hilum; must be>2 cm distal to carina	
T3	Tumor of any size with direct extension into the chest wall, diaphragm, mediastinal pleura, or pericardium without involving heart, great vessels, trachea, esophagus, or vertebral bodies; or within 2 cm of carina without involving the carina	
T4	Tumor of any size with invasion of the mediastinum or involving heart, great vessels, trachea, esophagus, vertebral bodies, or carina; or with the presence of malignant pleural effusion	
REGIONAL LYMPH NODES (N) INVOLVEMENT		
N0	No demonstrable metastasis to regional lymph nodes	
N1	Metastasis to peribronchial and/or ipsilateral hilar nodes	
N2	Metastasis to ipsilateral mediastinal or subcarinal lymph nodes	
N3	Metastasis to contralateral mediastinal or hilar lymph nodes; ipsilateral or contralateral scalene or superclavicular lymph nodes	
DISTANT METASTASIS (M)		
M0	No known distant metastasis	
M1	Distant metastasis present with site specified (e.g., brain)	
STAGE GROUPING		
Occult carcinoma	Tx, N0, M0	Sputum contains malignant cells but no other evidence of primary tumor or metastasis
Stage 0	Tis, N0, M0	Carcinoma in situ
Stage IA	T1, N0, M0	Tumor classified as T1 without evidence of metastasis to regional lymph nodes or distal site
Stage IB	T2, N0, M0	Tumor classified as T2 with evidence of metastasis to regional lymph nodes or distal site
Stage IIA	T1, N1, M0	Tumor classified as T1 with only evidence of metastasis to ipsilateral peribronchial or hilar lymph nodes; no distal metastasis
Stage IIB	T2, N1, M0 T3, N0, M0	Tumor classified as T2 or T3 with or without evidence of metastasis to ipsilateral peribronchial or hilar lymph nodes; no distal metastasis
Stage IIIA	T1-T3, N1, N2, M0	Tumor classified as T1, T2, or T3 with or without evidence of metastasis to ipsilateral peribronchial or hilar lymph nodes; no distal metastasis
Stage IIIB	Any T, N3, M0 T4, any N, M0	Any tumor classification with metastasis to contralateral hilar or mediastinal lymph nodes or to the scalene or supraclavicular lymph nodes; or any tumor classified as T4 with or without any regional lymph node metastasis; no distal metastasis
Stage IV	Any T, any N, M1	Any tumor with distal metastasis

Modified from Mountain CF: Revisions in the international system for staging lung cancer, *Chest* 111:1710-1717, 1997.

Patients with lung cancer often have cardiopulmonary and other medical conditions related to chronic obstructive pulmonary disease (COPD). Physiologic staging of these patients is necessary to predict their ability to tolerate a lobectomy or pneumonectomy. A preoperative forced expiratory volume in 1 second (FEV_1) less than 2 L may result in a FEV_1 of 0.8 L or less after pneumonectomy, a value generally considered to preclude surgery. Other major contraindications for surgery include history of recent myocardial infarction, uncontrolled major dysrhythmias, carbon dioxide (CO_2) retention, and severe pulmonary hypertension.

TREATMENT AND PROGNOSIS OF LUNG CANCER

After the histologic diagnosis and anatomic and physiologic staging procedures are completed, an overall treatment plan is formulated. The most common treatment regimens are combinations of surgery, radiation, and chemotherapy.

Surgery is the treatment of choice for patients in stages I, II, and selected stage IIIa NSCLC, unless the tumor is nonresectable or other conditions (e.g., cardiac disease) rule out surgery. Surgery may include partial or total lung removal. Approximately 30% of patients with NSCLC are considered resectable for cure. The 5-year survival rate for this resectable group is about 30%. Thus most patients initially thought to have a curable resection die of metastatic disease (usually within 2 years). The prognosis for the remaining 70% of patients who have unresectable NSCLC is even worse. *Radiation therapy* is generally recommended for stages I and II lesions if surgery is contraindicated and for stage III lesions when the disease is confined to the involved hemithorax and ipsilateral supraclavicular lymph nodes. When NSCLC is disseminated, radiation therapy may be applied to local sites for palliative purposes (e.g., spinal cord compression from metastasis to vertebrae). *Combination chemotherapy* may be prescribed for some patients with NSCLC. The median survival time for unresectable patients with NSCLC is less than 1 year, even with radiation or chemotherapy or both. A small group (6%) will survive 5 years.

The cornerstone of therapy for patients with SCLC is chemotherapy, with or without radiation therapy. Chemotherapy and chest radiotherapy may be administered to patients with limited-stage disease if they are physiologically able to withstand the treatment. Patients with extensive-stage disease are treated with chemotherapy alone. Some frequently used combination chemotherapy regimens include cyclophosphamide, doxorubicin (Adriamycin), and vincristine (CAV) and cyclophosphamide, doxorubicin, and etoposide (CAE). Combination chemotherapy increases median survival from 6 to 17 weeks, untreated, to 40 to 70 weeks. Radiation therapy is also used as prophylaxis against cerebral metastases and for the palliative management of pain, recurrent hemoptysis, effusions, or obstruction of the airways or the superior vena cava (Minna, 1998).

The overall prognosis for patients with bronchogenic carcinoma is poor (14% 5-year survival; American Cancer Society, 1995) and has improved only slightly over the past few years, despite the introduction of multiple new chemotherapeutic agents. Thus the emphasis must be placed on prevention. Health care professionals should advise people not to smoke cigarettes or live in an environment polluted by industry. Protective measures must also be taken for those who work with asbestos, uranium, chromium, and other carcinogenic materials.

KEY CONCEPTS

- Lung cancer is the leading cause of death in both men and women in the United States.
- The most important risk factor for lung cancer is cigarette smoking, and the more cigarettes that a person smokes, the greater the risk will be. Other risk factors include occupational inhalation of carcinogens, urban residence, dietary deficiency of vitamin A, chronic respiratory tract infection, and heredity.
- There are four main *histological types of lung cancer:* (1) squamous (epidermoid) cell carcinoma, (2) adenocarcinoma (with bronchoalveolar cell subtype), (3) large cell carcinoma, and (4) small cell carcinoma (includes oat cell).
- Because of differences in natural history and response to treatment, lung cancer is divided into two groups: small cell lung cancer (SCLC) and non-small cell lung cancer (NSCLC).
- Approximately 70% of cancers arise in relation to the main bronchi (central or hilar tumors), whereas 30% arise in the peripheral airways or alveoli.
- *Squamous cell carcinoma* is the most common type of cancer of the bronchus. Tumors, which are more common in men than in women, are usually central and close to the carina. These carcinomas are relatively slow growing compared with other types and may be resectable.
- *Adenocarcinomas of the lung* are usually peripheral tumors; they have an equal sex incidence and are not closely linked with cigarette smoking.
- *Bronchoalveolar carcinoma* is a special type of adenocarcinoma derived from the alveolar or distal bronchial epithelial cells. The onset is insidious with signs resembling those of pneumonia.
- *Large cell carcinoma* lacks features of differentiation by light microscopy. Lesions tend to be located peripherally (but may be central), grow rapidly, and are often widely disseminated at the time of diagnosis.
- *Small cell carcinoma* (also called *oat cell*) is the most highly malignant of lung cancers. Tumors are centrally located, grow rapidly, and have a very poor prognosis with a 5-year survival less than 5%. Because of the neuroendocrine type, this form of cancer is often associated with ectopic hormone production.

■ *Malignant mesothelioma* is an uncommon tumor of the pleura associated with prior asbestos exposure (which may have occurred 25 or more years ago). Survival time is usually less than 1 year.

■ The natural history of lung cancer allows no opportunity for screening, and it is usual for a lesion to have been growing for many years before clinical presentation.

■ The most common *symptoms of lung cancer* at presentation are usually a manifestation of locally advanced disease, including (1) persistent cough, (2) dyspnea, (3) hemoptysis, (4) pleuritic (chest) pain, (5) finger clubbing (30% of cases), and (6) less commonly, hypertrophic osteoarthropathy (HOA). Anorexia, weight loss, and fatigue are late manifestations of lung cancer.

■ Manifestations of the local spread of lung cancer can include the *vena caval syndrome, Horner's syndrome,* cardiac tamponade, *brachial plexus involvement* giving rise to pain and weakness in the shoulder and arm, compression of the recurrent laryngeal nerve giving rise to *hoarseness,* recurrent *pneumonia,* and *pleural effusion.*

■ Metastatic spread is a frequent presenting feature of lung cancer (70%). Common extrathoracic sites of lung cancer metastasis are scalene lymph nodes, adrenals, liver, brain, bone, and kidneys. The clinical effects of distal metastasis are a function of the sites of the secondary growth.

■ *Paraneoplastic syndromes* are frequently associated with lung cancer, especially oat cell carcinoma. Oat cell tumors produce virtually any of the polypeptide hormones such as PTH, ACTH, or ADH, giving rise to symptoms of hyperparathyroidism, Cushing's syndrome, and SIADH, causing fluid retention with hyponatremia.

■ Staging and histologic type determine the outcome in lung cancer.

■ For *NSCLC,* tumors are evaluated using a lung cancer specific TNM system and, on this basis, can be divided into Stages I to IV. The preferred therapy is surgical resection for patients with Stages I, II, and IIIA. For stages IIIB and IV, combinations of chemotherapy and radiation therapy offer the best option, mainly with an expectation of palliation of symptoms rather than cure. Only 30% of patients with NSCLC are considered to have resectable cancers and their 5-year-survival rate is only 30% after the surgery. The prognosis of the remaining 70% treated by chemotherapy and radiation therapy is even poorer.

■ A two-stage system is used for *SCLC: limited stage disease* refers to tumor confined to one hemithorax and regional lymph nodes; *extensive stage disease* refers to any tumor that extends beyond the definition of limited stage. Most patients with limited stage SCLC will be offered treatment with combination chemotherapy and radiation therapy to the affected side of the chest. Patients who respond may be offered prophylactic cranial irradiation in an attempt to minimize development of cranial metastasis. Most patients with extensive stage SCLC are offered combination chemotherapy and radiation therapy is generally used to treat sites of metastasis, especially to the brain or bone and for relief of vena cava obstruction.

■ The overall 5-year survival rate for lung cancer is 14%.

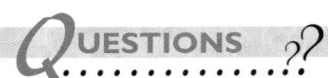

QUESTIONS ??

A sampling of review questions for this chapter appears here. Visit http://www.mosby.com/MERLIN/PriceWilson/ for additional questions.

Answer the following on a separate sheet of paper.

1. What is the carcinoid syndrome, and what type of tumor causes it?

2. What are some common signs and symptoms of bronchogenic carcinoma, and why is it difficult to diagnose on the basis of these signs and symptoms?

3. List three major diagnostic tools used for the detection of lung cancer, and describe the significant findings of each technique.

Match each histologic type of bronchogenic carcinoma in column A with its characteristics in column B.

Column A	Column B
4. _____ Squamous cell	a. Located centrally within large bronchi
5. _____ Oat cell	b. Located in peripheral lung
6. _____ Adenocarcinoma	c. Most common type
7. _____ Large cell	d. Least common type
	e. Most aggressive type, poorest prognosis
	f. Relatively slow to metastasize
	g. No clear association with smoking
	h. SCLC histologic type
	i. NSCLC histologic type
	j. Often associated with abnormal hormone secretion

Pulmonary Tuberculosis

SYLVIA A. PRICE AND MARY P. STANDRIDGE

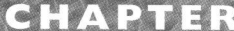

*T*uberculosis (TB) is an infectious communicable disease caused by *Mycobacterium tuberculosis.* The aerobic, acid-fast rods include both pathogenic and saprophytic organisms. Several pathogenic mycobacteria exist, but only the bovine and human strains are pathogenic to humans. The tubercle bacillus is 0.3 × 2 to 4 μm, which is smaller than a red blood cell.

PATHOGENESIS

The portals of entry for the *M. tuberculosis* organism are the respiratory tract, the gastrointestinal (GI) tract, and an open wound in the skin. Most TB infections are contracted by the airborne route, through the inhalation of droplet nuclei containing organisms of the tubercle bacillus from an infected individual. The GI tract is the usual portal of entry for the bovine strain, which is spread by contaminated milk. However, in the United States, with widespread pasteurization of milk and detection of diseased cattle, bovine TB is rare.

TB is a disease controlled by a cell-mediated immunity response. The effector cell is the macrophage, and the lymphocyte (usually T cell) is the immunoresponsive cell. This type of immunity is basically local, involving macrophages activated at the infection site by lymphocytes and their lymphokines. This response is referred to as a cellular (delayed) *hypersensitivity reaction* (see Chapter 5).

The tubercle bacilli that reach the alveolar surfaces are usually inhaled in units of one to three bacilli; larger clumps of inhaled bacilli tend to impinge on the mucociliary surfaces of the nasal passages and bronchial tree and do not cause disease. Once in the alveolar space, usually in the lower part of the upper lobe or the upper part of the lower lobe, the tubercle bacillus evokes an inflammatory reaction. Polymorphonuclear leukocytes appear on the scene and phagocytize the bacteria but do not kill the organism. After the first few days, macrophages replace the leukocytes. The involved alveoli are consolidated, and acute pneumonia develops. This cellular pneumonia may resolve itself so that no residue remains, or the process may continue, with the bacteria continuing to be phagocytized or to multiply within the cells. Lymphatic drainage of the bacilli also occurs into the regional lymph nodes. The infiltrating macrophages elongate and partially fuse to form the epithelioid cell tubercle, surrounded by lymphocytes. This reaction usually takes 10 to 20 days.

Necrosis of the central portion of the lesion results in a relatively solid, cheesy appearance called *caseous necrosis.* The area of caseous necrosis and the surrounding granulation tissue of epithelioid cells and fibroblasts evoke different responses. The granulation tissue may become more fibrous, forming collagenous scar tissue, which results in a capsule surrounding the tubercle.

The primary lesion in the lung is called the *Ghon focus,* and the combination of regional lymph node involvement and the primary lesion is termed the *Ghon complex.* A calcified Ghon complex may be seen on a routine chest radiograph of healthy persons. However, the majority of pulmonary TB infections are not apparent clinically or radiographically.

Another response that may occur at the site of the necrotic area is liquefaction, with the liquid material sloughing into a connecting bronchus and producing a cavity. The tubercular material sloughed from the walls of the cavity enters the tracheobronchial tree. The process may be repeated in other parts of the lung, or bacilli may be carried to the larynx, middle ear, or gut.

Even without therapy, small cavities close and leave a fibrous scar. As inflammation subsides, scarring may narrow or close the bronchial lumen near the junction of the cavity and the bronchus. The caseous material may thicken and be unable to flow through the communicating channel, so the cavity fills with this material and the lesion becomes similar to the unsloughed encapsulated lesion. The lesion may remain in a quiescent stage for long periods or reestablish its bronchial communication and be the site of active inflammation.

The disease may spread through the lymphatics or blood vessels. The organisms that pass through the lymph nodes reach the bloodstream in small numbers and may initiate occasional lesions in various organs. This dispersal of the organisms, referred to as *lymphohematogenous dissemination*, is usually self-limited. *Hematogenous dissemination*, an acute phenomenon, usually gives rise to miliary TB; it occurs when a necrotic focus erodes a blood vessel, allowing large numbers of organisms to enter the vascular system and be disseminated to the various organs.

EPIDEMIOLOGY

The case incidence rate of and mortality from TB declined rapidly after the advent of chemotherapy. However, from 1985 through 1992 the number of TB cases increased by 20% (Centers for Disease Control and Prevention [CDC], 2000a). Factors associated with this trend include socioeconomic and health-related problems (e.g., alcoholism, homelessness, a rise in acquired immunodeficiency syndrome [AIDS] and human immunodeficiency virus [HIV] infection), with the increased incidence noted particularly among minority group members and refugees who have entered the United States from areas where TB is endemic. Since 1993, TB morbidity has steadily declined, with the disease occurring mostly in well-defined risk groups and geographic areas that can be targeted for control efforts (CDC, 1999a).

In 1998, 18,361 new cases of TB were reported to the CDC. This statistic represents a case incidence rate of 6.8/100,000 U.S. population; 41.3% of those cases occurred in foreign-born persons (CDC, 2000d). In the United States it is estimated that 10 to 15 million persons are currently infected with TB. More than 80% of the reported new cases of TB in 1998 were in persons over 25 years of age, the majority of whom were infected in the past. Approximately 5 of 100 of the newly infected population will develop pulmonary TB 1 or 2 years after infection. Of the remaining 95%, another 5% will develop clinical disease at sometime in the future. About 10% of infected individuals will develop clinical TB during their lifetime. However, the risk is greater for immunosuppressed individuals, especially those with HIV infection. HIV destroys lymphocytes and monocytes, which are the primary defense cells against TB infection. According to the 1996 CDC data, the rate of TB disease among HIV infected tuberculin skin test positive individuals is 200 to 800 times higher than is the rate of TB for the overall U.S. population (CDC, 1998).

When considering a person's susceptibility to TB, two risk factors must be examined: the risk of acquiring the infection and the risk of developing clinically active disease after infection has occurred. The risks of acquiring the infection and of developing clinical disease depend on the infection's existence in the population, especially among persons infected with HIV; immigrants from areas of high prevalence of TB; high-risk racial and ethnic minority groups (e.g., African Americans, Native Americans, Alaskan natives, Asians, Pacific Islanders, Hispanics); and those residing in high-risk environments for the transmission of TB, such as correctional facilities, homeless shelters, hospitals, and nursing homes.

DRUG-RESISTANT TUBERCULOSIS

Drug-resistant TB occurs as the result of suboptimal treatment for TB. Drug-resistant TB is transmitted in the same manner as is drug-susceptible TB. Drug resistance is divided into two types: (1) primary resistance develops in individuals who are initially infected with resistant organisms, and (2) secondary resistance (acquired resistance), which develops during TB treatment resulting from an inadequate treatment regimen or failure to take medications appropriately.

Drug-resistance TB is a worldwide problem. Horsburgh (2000) reported that, in a recent survey of 35 countries, 12.6% of TB isolates were resistant to at least one drug, and 2.2% were resistant to both of the primary drugs, isoniazid and rifampin, used to treat TB. It is important to note that most cases of TB are drug susceptible at the time of diagnosis and only become drug resistant through suboptimal therapy.

The World Health Organization (WHO) is attempting to combat multidrug-resistant TB by focusing its efforts on a strategy of preventing the generation of new multidrug-resistant TB cases. The directly observed therapy (DOT) program has been increasingly adopted throughout the world, with 119 countries now having DOT programs. These programs have been successful in preventing increases in cases of multidrug-resistant TB in many countries especially those in which preexisting levels were low, for example, in Chile, where only 0.4% of TB cases have multidrug-resistant TB. WHO is working closely with its partners to establish effective DOT programs in every country in which TB occurs. DOT relies on the commitment of local governments using a multifaceted effort of case detection by sputum microscopy, directly observed treatment with a standard therapeutic regimen, maintenance of an uninterrupted drug supply, and monitoring outcome with a standard reporting system.

DIAGNOSIS AND CLINICAL MANIFESTATIONS

The symptoms associated with pulmonary TB are a productive, prolonged cough (duration of more than 3 weeks), chest pain, and hemoptysis. Systemic symptoms include fever, chills, night sweats, fatigue, loss of appetite, and weight loss. Individuals suspected of having TB should be referred for a physical examination, a Mantoux tuberculin test, chest radiography, and bacteriologic or histologic examination. Tuberculin skin testing should be performed in all individuals suspected of having clinically active TB, but its value is limited by false-negative reactions, particularly in immunosuppressed individuals (e.g., those with HIV infection). Individuals who have symptoms suggestive of TB, especially prolonged productive cough and hemoptysis, should receive a chest radiograph, even though they have a negative reaction to the tuberculin skin test.

According to the CDC, a case of TB is verified by a positive bacteriologic culture for the *M. tuberculosis* organism. It is imperative to query individuals suspected of having TB regarding their history of exposure and previous TB or infection. Demographic factors (e.g., country of origin, age, ethnic or racial groups) and medical conditions (e.g., HIV infection) that may increase the individual's risk for exposure to TB must also be considered.

HYPERSENSITIVITY REACTION

The pathogenicity of the bacillus does not arise from any intrinsic toxicity but from its capacity to induce a hypersensitive reaction in the host. *Tuberculoproteins* derived from the bacillus appear to induce this reaction. The tissue responses of inflammation and necrosis are the results of a cellular (delayed) hypersensitivity response of the host to the tubercle bacillus. A TB hypersensitivity reaction usually develops 3 to 10 weeks from the onset of infection. Persons who have been exposed to the tubercle bacillus develop sensitized T lymphocytes. If *purified protein derivative (PPD)* of tuberculin is injected into the skin of a person whose lymphocytes are sensitized to tuberculoprotein, the sensitized lymphocytes interact with the extract and attract macrophages to the area.

Intradermal (Mantoux) Tuberculin Test

The standard technique (Mantoux test) is the intradermal injection of 0.1 ml of PPD tuberculin containing 5 tuberculin units (TU) into the upper third of the volar aspect or dorsal surface of the forearm after the skin has been cleansed with alcohol. A disposable tuberculin syringe with a 26- to 27-gauge needle is usually preferred. The short needle is held so that the bevel faces upward, and the tip of the needle is inserted beneath the surface of the skin. A wheal 6 to 10 mm in diameter and resembling a mosquito bite should be produced when the prescribed 0.1 ml amount is accurately injected (see Fig. 9-8).

The skin reaction requires 48 to 72 hours to reach its peak after the injection, and the reaction should be read during that period, in a good light, with the subject's forearm slightly flexed. The reaction must be recorded as the diameter of the induration in millimeters, measured transversely to the long axis of the forearm. Only induration (palpable swelling), not erythema alone, is significant. Induration may be determined by inspection and by palpation (stroking the area with a finger). Absence of induration should be recorded as "0 mm," rather than negative.

The interpretation of the skin test identifies various types of reactions (Box 43-1). An indurated area measur-

BOX 43-1

Classification of Tuberculin Reaction Intradermal Mantoux Test (with TU PPD Tuberculin)

≥5 mm OF INDURATION IS CLASSIFIED AS POSITIVE IN THE FOLLOWING GROUPS:
- HIV-positive persons
- Recent contacts with a person with TB
- Persons with fibrotic changes on chest radiograph consistent with old healed TB
- Patients with organ transplants and other immunosuppressed patients (receiving the equivalent of ≥15 mg/day of prednisone for ≥1 month)

≥10 mm OF INDURATION IS CLASSIFIED AS POSITIVE IN THE FOLLOWING GROUPS:
- Recent arrivals (≤5 years) from high-prevalence countries
- Injection drug users
- Residents and employees of high-risk congregate settings: prisons and jails, nursing homes and other long-term facilities for older adults, hospitals and other health-care facilities, residential facilities for patients with AIDS, and homeless shelters
- Mycobacteriology laboratory personnel
- Persons with clinical conditions that place them at high risk
- Children <4 years of age or children and adolescents exposed to adults in high-risk categories

≥15 mm OF INDURATION IS CLASSIFIED AS POSITIVE IN THE FOLLOWING:
- Persons with no known risk factors for TB
- Targeted skin testing programs should only be conducted among high-risk groups

From Centers for Disease Control and Prevention: *Core curriculum on tuberculosis: what the clinician should know*, ed 4, Atlanta, 2000, CDC.

ing 5 mm or larger is considered a positive reaction in selected groups, reflecting sensitivity resulting from infection with the bacillus. An induration of 10 mm or larger is also classified as positive in certain groups, whereas an induration of 15 mm or greater is positive in all persons with no known risk factors for TB.

A positive reaction to the tuberculin test indicates the presence of infection but does not necessarily signify clinical disease. However, this test is an important diagnostic tool in the evaluation of an individual patient and is also useful in determining the prevalence of TB infection in a population.

Anergy Testing

Anergy is the lack of a delayed type hypersensitivity response to previously exposed antigens, such as tuberculin. Specific anergy is lack of reactivity to an individual antigen; generalized nonspecific anergy is the inability to react to any antigen (Slovis, Pittman, Haas, 2000). In immunosuppressed persons, a cellular delayed-type hypersensitivity response such as a tuberculin reaction may either decrease or disappear. The cause of anergy may result from HIV infection, severe or febrile illness, measles (or other viral infections), Hodgkin's disease, sarcoidosis, live-virus vaccination, and the administration of corticosteroids or immunosuppressive drugs. According to the CDC (2000), on average, 10% to 25% of patients with TB disease have negative reactions when tested with the tuberculin skin test at diagnosis before treatment. Approximately one third of HIV-infected persons and more than 60% of patients with AIDS may have skin test reactions of less than 5 mm, although they are infected with *M. tuberculosis*. HIV infection may suppress the skin test response because of the CD4+ T lymphocyte count, which decreases to less than 200 cells/mm³. Anergy can also occur with a relatively high CD4+ T lymphocyte count.

Anergy is detected by administering at least two other hypersensitivity antigens by the Mantoux method. The lack of standardization and outcome data limit the evaluation of the effectiveness of anergy testing. For this reason, CDC (2000a) no longer recommends anergy testing for routine TB screening among HIV-positive persons in the United States. Slovis, Pittman, and Haas (2000) contend that anergy testing is not useful in screening for asymptomatic TB in any group. The American Thoracic Society (ATS) (2000) also states that anergy testing is not recommended for use in identifying TB infection in individuals, including those infected with HIV.

Bacille Calmette-Guérin Vaccination

Bacille Calmette-Guérin (BCG), an attenuated living strain of bovine tubercle bacilli, is the most widely used vaccine in many countries. In BCG vaccination, these organisms are injected into the skin to produce a well-circumscribed, calcified, walled-off primary focus. BCG has retained its capacity to increase the immunologic resistance of animals and humans. Primary infection of BCG has the advantage over primary infection by virulent organisms because no danger exists of producing progressive disease in the host.

Vaccination with BCG usually leads to the development of tuberculin sensitivity. The degree of sensitivity is variable, depending on the strain of BCG used and the population vaccinated. Tuberculin skin testing is not contraindicated for persons who have been vaccinated with BCG. Preventive therapy should be considered for any BCG vaccinated person who has a tuberculin skin test reaction of equal to or greater than 10 mm induration, especially if any of the following circumstances are present (CDC, 1996):

1. Contact of TB case
2. From country with high TB prevalence
3. Continually exposed to populations with high TB prevalence (i.e., homeless shelters, drug treatment centers)

Despite the worldwide acceptance of BCG, vaccination is not generally recommended against TB in the United States because of the low risk of infection and the variable effectiveness of the vaccine. BCG vaccination is only 50% effective against all forms of TB. According to the CDC 1996 recommendations, BCG vaccination is rarely indicated. Health care providers considering BCG vaccination for their patients are encouraged by the CDC to discuss this with their local health department's TB control staff (CDC, 1996).

▊ RADIOLOGIC EXAMINATION

Radiologic examination often suggests the presence of TB, but it is almost impossible to make a diagnosis on this basis alone, because other diseases can mimic almost all of the manifestations of TB.

Pathologically, the earliest manifestation of TB involvement of the lung is usually a parenchymal lymph node complex. In adults, the apical and posterior segments of the upper lobe or the superior segments of the lower lobe are the usual sites of lesions, which may appear dense and homogenous. There may also be evidence of cavity formation and scattered disease, which is often bilateral. Any abnormality on the chest radiograph of an HIV-positive person may indicate TB disease. In fact, HIV–positive persons with TB disease may have a normal chest radiograph (CDC, 2000a).

▊ BACTERIOLOGIC STUDIES

Although catheterized urine, cerebrospinal fluid, and gastric contents may be microscopically examined, the most important bacteriologic study in the diagnosis of TB is examination of the sputum. The *Ziehl-Neelsen staining method* may be used. The slide is flooded with steaming carbolfuchsin and then decolorized with acid alcohol. The mixture is then counterstained with methylene blue or brilliant green. The preferred method of staining is the auramine-rhodamine technique of fluorescent staining; the auramine-rhodamine solution, once attached to the mycobacteria, resists acid-alcohol decolorization. The clinician is provided with an estimate of the number of acid-fast bacilli (AFB) detected on the slide. A positive specimen gives the clinician a preliminary indication of the diagnosis, but a negative specimen does not rule out infection with the disease.

The most accurate diagnostic method is the *culture technique*. Culture examinations should be done on all specimens. The mycobacteria are slow growing and require a complex medium. Mature colonies are cream or buff colored and warty and cauliflower-like in appearance. As few as 10 bacteria/ml of digested, concentrated material can be detected on the culture medium. The mycobacterial growth observed on the culture medium should be quantified as to the number of colonies present. The microorganism takes 6 to 12 week at 36° to 37° C to grow when using conventional biochemical tests. However, when a liquid medium is inoculated for growth such as the BACTEC radiometric system and rapid methods are used for species identification, culture results should be available within 7 to 21 days of specimen collection.

Tests are currently available that permit identification of most species of mycobacteria, and computerized programs have been developed that aid in the interpretation of data. For example, nucleic acid probes can identify the species in 2 to 8 hours. *High-performance liquid chromatography (HPLC)* detects differences in the spectrum of mycolic acids in the cell wall and is equally as rapid. Newer molecular techniques such as deoxyribonucleic acid (DNA) sequencing and polymerase chain reaction (PCR) performed on sputum or other clinical specimens to diagnose TB disease are rapidly evolving. The U.S. Food and Drug Administration (FDA) has approved the nucleic acid amplification (NAA) test. However, the NAA does not replace the need for routine AFB smear and culture (ATS, 2000).

Drug susceptibility testing should be performed on initial isolates from all patients to verify that the patient's prescribed TB drug therapy will be effective (ATS, 2000). Testing should be repeated if the patient does not improve or continues to produce culture positive sputum after two months of therapy (CDC, 2000a).

CLASSIFICATION SYSTEM FOR TUBERCULOSIS

The clinical classification system for TB is based on the pathogenesis of the disease (Table 43-1). Patients should not remain in class five for greater than 3 months.

TREATMENT

TB is treated primarily by prolonged administration of antimicrobial drugs. These drugs can also be used to prevent an infected person from developing clinical disease. The CDC (2000a) reports that new emphasis is being placed on the importance of latent TB infection (LTBI) as essential to controlling and eliminating TB in the United States.

The ATS (1994) emphasizes three principles on which treatment for TB are based: (1) regimens must include multiple drugs to which the organisms are susceptible, (2) the drugs must be taken regularly, and (3) drug therapy must continue for a sufficient time to provide the safest and most effective therapy in the shortest period. In 1994 the CDC and ATS published new guidelines for the treatment of TB disease and infection, including the following:

1. A 6-month drug regimen consisting of isoniazid (isonicotinic acid hydrazide [INH]), rifampin, and pyrazinamide given for 2 months followed by INH and rifampin for 4 months is recommended for the initial therapy of TB for patients with fully susceptible organ-

isms who adhere to treatment. Ethambutol (or streptomycin in children too young to be monitored for visual acuity) should be included in the initial regimen until the results of drug susceptibility studies are available, unless little possibility exists of drug resistance (i.e., less than 4% primary resistance to INH in the community; patient has had no previous treatment with anti-TB medications, is not from a country with a high prevalence of drug resistance, and has no known exposure to a drug-resistant case). This four-drug, 6-month regimen is effective even when the infecting organism is resistant to INH. TB treatment may need to be altered for individuals who are taking HIV protease inhibitors. Whenever possible, the case of HIV-related TB should be provided by or in consultation with experts in the management of both TB and HIV disease (CDC, 2000a).

2. A 9-month regimen of INH and rifampin is acceptable for persons who cannot or should not take pyrazinamide. Ethambutol (or streptomycin in children too young to be monitored for visual acuity) should be included in the initial regimen until the results of drug susceptibility studies are available, unless little possibility exists of drug resistance. If INH resistance is demonstrated, rifampin and ethambutol should be continued for a minimum of 12 months.

3. Treating all patients with DOT is strongly recommended.

4. Multidrug-resistant TB (MDR TB) with resistance to INH and rifampin is difficult to treat. Treatment must be individualized based on medication history and susceptibility studies. Clinicians unfamiliar with treatment of MDR TB should seek expert consultation.

5. Children should be managed in the same regimens as are adults, using adjusted doses of the drugs.

6. A 4-month regimen of INH and rifampin, preferably with pyrazinamide for the first 2 months, is recommended for adults who have active TB and who are smear and culture negative, if little possibility exists of drug resistance.

The critical factor for the successful outcome of treatment is patient adherence to the drug regimen. DOT is a

TABLE 43-1

Classification System for TB

Class	Type	Description
0	No TB exposure	No history of exposure
	Not infected	Negative reaction to tuberculin skin test
1	TB exposure	History of exposure
	No evidence of infection	Negative reaction to tuberculin skin test
2	TB infection	Positive reaction to tuberculin skin test
	No disease	Negative bacteriologic studies (if done)
		No clinical, bacteriologic, or radiographic evidence of active TB
3	TB, clinically active	*M. tuberculosis* cultured (if done)
		Clinical, bacteriologic, or radiographic evidence of current disease
4	TB	History of episode(s) of TB
	Not clinically active	or
		Abnormal but stable radiographic findings; positive reaction to the tuberculin skin test
		Negative bacteriologic studies (if done)
		and
		No clinical or radiographic evidence of current disease
5	TB suspected	Diagnosis pending

From Centers for Disease Control and Prevention: *Core curriculum on tuberculosis: what the clinician should know*, ed 4, Atlanta, 2000, CDC.

TABLE 43-2

Drugs for Treatment of Tuberculosis in Adults (Dosage in mg/kg)

Drug	Daily	Twice Weekly	Thrice Weekly	Adverse Reactions	Monitoring Reactions	Remarks
FIRST-LINE DRUGS						
Isoniazid (INH)	5 (300 mg)	15 max (900 mg)	15 max (900 mg)	Rash Hepatic enzyme level Hepatitis Peripheral neuropathy Mild central nervous system effects	Measure baseline levels of hepatic enzymes.	Pyridoxine may prevent peripheral neuropathy.
Rifampin (RIF)	10 (600 mg)	10 (600 mg)	10 (600 mg)	GI upset Drug interactions Hepatitis Bleeding problems Rash Renal failure Fever	Baseline measurements of CBC platelets and hepatic enzymes.	Significant interactions occur with methadone, contraceptives, and other drugs. RIF colors body fluids orange.
Rifabutin (RFB)	5 (300 mg)	5 (300 mg)	Not known	Rash Hepatitis Fever Thrombocytopenia	Baseline measurements of CBC, platelets, and hepatic enzymes.	RFB is contraindicated in patients taking ritonavir or delavirdine; colors body fluids orange.
Pyrazinamide (PZA)	15-30 (2 g)	50-70 (4 g)	50-70 (3 g)	Hepatitis Hyperuricemia GI upset Rash	Measure baseline levels of uric acid and hepatic enzymes.	Treat hyperuremicemia only if patient has symptoms. May make glucose control more difficult in diabetics.
Ethambutol (EMB)	15-25	50	25-30	Optic neuritis Rash	Baseline and monthly tests of visual acuity and color vision.	Other ocular effects and increased renal failure may occur.
Streptomycin (SM)	15 (1 g)	25-30 (1.5 g)	25-30 (1.5 g)	Ototoxicity Renal toxicity	Baseline and repeat tests as needed for hearing and kidney function.	Avoid or reduce dose in adults over 60 years old.
SECOND-LINE DRUGS						
Capreomycin	15-30 (1 g)	—	—	Toxicity: Auditory Vestibular Renal	Assess vestibular and hearing function. Perform BUN and creatinine tests.	Use with caution in older adults.
Ethionamide	15-20 (1 g)	—	—	GI upset Hepatotoxicity Hypersensitivity	Measure hepatic enzymes.	Start with low dosage and increase as tolerated.
Cycloserine	15-20 (1 g)	—	—	Psychosis Convulsions Headaches Drug interactions	Assess mental status. Measure serum drug levels.	Start with low dosage increase as tolerated.
Kanamycin	15-30 (1 g)	—	—	Toxicity: Auditory Vestibular Renal	Assess vestibular and hearing function. Perform BUN and creatinine tests.	After bacteriologic conversion dosage may be reduced to 2-3 times per week. Not approved by FDA.
Para-aminosalicyclic acid (PAS)	150 (12 g)	—	—	GI upset Hepatotoxicity Hypersensitivity Sodium load	Measure hepatic enzymes. Assess volume load.	Start with low dosage and increase as tolerated. Monitor cardiac patients for sodium level.

Modified from Centers for Disease Control and Prevention: *Core curriculum on tuberculosis: What the clinician should know,* ed 4, Atlanta, 2000, CDC.
BUN, Blood urea nitrogen; *CBC,* complete blood count; *GI,* gastrointestinal.

way to ensure that patients adhere to therapy. With DOT, a health care worker or designated individual observes the patient swallow each dose of TB medication. Measures such as DOT are designed to foster adherence and ensure that patients take the drugs as prescribed.

The response to anti-TB chemotherapy for patients who have positive sputum cultures is evaluated by repeated examinations of the sputum. Specimens for culture should be obtained monthly until the culture converts to negative. Patients who have converted to negative sputum cultures *after* 2 months of treatment should have at least one more sputum smear and culture at the end of the drug therapy regimen. Patients with MDR TB should have monthly cultures for the entire course of therapy. A chest radiograph at completion of the therapy provides a baseline for comparison of future films. Patients with a negative sputum *before* treatment, however, should have a chest radiograph and the clinical evaluation. The intervals for the procedure depend on the clinical circumstances and differential diagnosis.

Routine follow-up after therapy is not necessary for patients who have had a satisfactory and prompt bacteriologic response to 6- or 9-month therapy with INH and rifampin. Patients whose organisms were susceptible to the drugs administered should report any symptoms of TB, such as prolonged cough, fever, or weight loss. For patients with TB organisms resistant to INH or rifampin or both, individualized follow-up evaluations are needed.

INH is also used to treat latent TB infection (LTBI) in a dosage of 300 mg/day for adults, optimally for 9 months. Recent evidence indicates that 6 months of treatment for LTBI can also confer substantial protection against progression from TB infection (LTBI) to TB disease. Persons with HIV infections and children should always receive 9 months of therapy. It is of utmost importance that the possibility of TB disease has been ruled out before treatment for LTBI is initiated (CDC 2000a, 2000c).

All people with positive TB skin tests (see Box 43-1) are candidates for treatment of LTBI. Table 43-2 describes the antimicrobial drugs used to treat TB.

PREVENTION AND CONTROL

Public health measures are designed for early detection and treatment of cases and sources of infection. By law, all persons with class 3 or class 5 TB must be reported to the health department. Screening of high-risk groups is a significant function of state and local health departments. The purpose of early detection of persons with TB infection is to identify those individuals who would benefit from preventive therapy to stop development of clinically active TB. This preventive health measure benefits not only the infected individual but the community as well. To this end, populations at risk for developing TB must be identified, and priorities for establishing drug treatment programs must take into account the risk of therapy versus the benefit to the individual.

TB eradication involves a combination of effective chemotherapy, prompt case and contact identification and follow-up, management of persons exposed to patients with infectious TB, and chemoprophylactic therapy of high-risk population groups.

KEY CONCEPTS

- Tuberculosis (TB) is an infectious communicable disease caused by *M. tuberculosis*. Portals of entry for the *M. tuberculosis* organism are the respiratory tract, the GI tract, and an open wound in the skin.
- The majority of TB infections are contracted by the airborne route, through the inhalation of droplet nuclei containing organisms of the tubercle bacillus from an infected individual.
- TB is a disease controlled by a cell-mediated immunity response where the effector cell is the macrophage, and the lymphocyte (usually T cell) is the immunoresponsive cell. This type of immunity involves macrophages activated at the infection site by lymphocytes and their lymphokines; the response is a cellular (delayed) hypersensitivity reaction.
- The tubercle bacilli that reach the alveolar surfaces evoke an inflammatory reaction where leukocytes are replaced by macrophages. The involved alveoli are consolidated, and acute pneumonia develops, which may resolve itself so that no residue remains, or the process may continue with the bacteria continuing to be phagocytized or to multiply within the cells.
- Lymphatic drainage of the bacilli also occurs into the regional lymph nodes, and the infiltrating macrophages form the epithelioid cell tubercle, surrounded by lymphocytes.
- Necrosis of the lesion results in a cheesy appearance (caseous necrosis); the surrounding granulation tissue of epithelioid cells and fibroblasts may become more fibrous, forming collagenous scar tissue, resulting in a capsule surrounding the tubercle.
- The primary lesion in the lung is called the *Ghon focus*, and the combination of regional lymph node involvement and the primary lesion is termed the *Ghon complex*.
- A calcified Ghon complex may be seen on a routine chest radiograph of healthy persons.
- The case incidence rate of and mortality from TB declined rapidly after the advent of chemotherapy; however, from 1985 through 1993 the number of cases increased by 20%.
- Factors associated with this trend include socioeconomic and health-related problems (e.g., alcoholism, homelessness, a rise AIDS-HIV infection).
- When considering a person's susceptibility to TB, two risk factors must be examined: the risk of acquiring the infection and the risk of developing clinically active disease after infection has occurred.

- The symptoms associated with pulmonary TB are a productive, prolonged cough (duration of more than 3 weeks), chest pain, and hemoptysis. Systemic symptoms include fever, chills, night sweats, fatigue, loss of appetite, and weight loss.
- Individuals suspected of having TB should be referred for a physical examination, a Mantoux tuberculin test, chest radiography, and bacteriologic or histologic examination.
- A case of TB is verified by a positive bacteriologic culture for the *M. tuberculosis* organism.
- A positive reaction to the tuberculin test indicates the presence of infection but does not necessarily signify clinical disease. However, this test is an important diagnostic tool in the evaluation of an individual patient and is also useful in determining the prevalence of TB infection in a population.
- Drug-resistant TB occurs as the result of suboptimal treatment for TB and is a worldwide problem.
- Anergy is the lack of delayed-type hypersensitivity response to previously exposed antigens, such as tuberculin reactivity in infected individuals.
- Bacille Calmette-Guérin (BCG), an attenuated living strain of bovine tubercle bacilli, is the most widely used vaccine in many countries.

- Vaccination with BCG usually leads to the development of tuberculin sensitivity. Despite the worldwide acceptance of BCG, vaccination is not generally recommended against TB in the United States because of the low risk of infection and the variable effectiveness of the vaccine.
- Prolonged administration of antimicrobial drugs is the primary treatment for TB. These drugs can also be used to prevent an infected person from developing clinical disease.
- Three principles on which treatment for TB is based are: (1) regimens must include multiple drugs to which the organisms are susceptible, (2) the drugs must be taken regularly, and (3) drug therapy must continue for a sufficient time to provide the safest and most effective therapy in the shortest period.
- Public health measures are designed for early detection and treatment of cases and sources of infection. TB eradication involves effective chemotherapy, prompt case identification and follow-up, management of persons who have been in contact with infectious TB patients, and testing high-risk groups for TB infection.

QUESTIONS ??

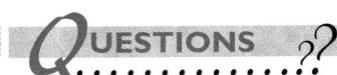

A sampling of review questions for this chapter appears here. Visit http://www.mosby.com/MERLIN/PriceWilson/ for additional questions.

Answer the following on a separate sheet of paper.

1. What groups are the most likely to develop TB once they become infected?
2. Describe the two risk factors that must be examined when a person's susceptibility to TB is considered.
3. Explain the rationale for administering at least two drugs in the treatment of TB.
4. List the three principles on which treatment for TB is based.
5. Describe the treatment for HIV-infected persons with latent TB infection (LTBI).
6. Evaluate the role of bacille Calmette-Guérin (BCG) in the control of TB in the United States.
7. What is the purpose of directly observed therapy (DOT) in the treatment of TB?
8. What are the factors most likely to be responsible for multidrug-resistant TB (MDR TB) in patients with no previous history of TB treatment?
9. What are the public health measures for prevention and control of TB in the United States?

Match the drug in column A with the associated adverse reactions in column B. Reactions may be used more than once.

Column A
10. _____ Rifampin (RIF)
11. _____ Isoniazid (INH)
12. _____ Para-aminosalicylic acid (PAS)
13. _____ Ethambutol (EMB)
14. _____ Cycloserine
15. _____ Pyrazinamide (PZA)

Column B
a. Optic neuritis
b. Hyperuricemia
c. Bleeding problems
d. Hepatotoxicity
e. Immunosuppression
f. Psychoses
g. GI upset
h. Ototoxicity
i. Nephrotoxicity
j. Hypersensitivity
k. Hepatitis
l. Drug interactions
m. Peripheral neuropathy
n. Rash

*B*IBLIOGRAPHY ■ PART SEVEN

α_1-Antitrypsin Deficiency Registry Study Group: Survival and FEV1 decline in individuals with severe α_1-antitrypsin, *Am J Respir Crit Care Med* 158(1):49-59, 1998.

American Lung Association: *Fact sheet: Adult (acute) respiratory distress syndrome (ARDS)*, January, 2001. http://www.lungusa.org

American Thoracic Society: Control of tuberculosis in the United States, *Am J Respir Crit Care Med* 146(6):1376-1395, 1992.

American Thoracic Society: Diagnostic standards and classification of tuberculosis in adults and children, *Am J Respir Crit Care Med* 161(6):1376-1395, 2000.

American Thoracic Society: Standards for diagnosis and care of patients with chronic obstructive disease, *Am J Respir Crit Care Med* 152:S78, 1995.

American Thoracic Society: Treatment of tuberculosis and tuberculosis infection in adults and children, *Am J Respir Crit Care Med* 149(5):1359-1374, 1994.

Anzueto A et al: Aerosolized surfactant in adults with sepsis-induced ARDS, *N Engl J Med* 334:1417-1421, 1996.

Bone RC: Acute respiratory failure: definition and overview. In *Pulmonary and critical care medicine*, St Louis, 1996, Mosby.

Breddin HK et al: Effects of low molecular weight heparin on thrombus regression and recurrent thromboembolism in patients with deep vein thrombosis, *N Engl J Med* 344(9):626-631, 2001.

Bryan CS: Treatment of pneumococcal pneumonia: the case for penicillin G, *Am J Med* 107(1A):63S-68S, 1999.

Centers for Disease Control and Prevention: *Core Curriculum on tuberculosis: what the clinician should know*, ed 4, Atlanta, 2000a, CDC.

Centers for Disease Control and Prevention: Essential components of a tuberculosis prevention and control program screening for tuberculosis infection in high risk populations, *MMWR* 44(RR-11):1-34, 1995.

Centers for Disease Control and Prevention: Management of persons exposed to multidrug-resistant tuberculosis, *MMWR* 41(RR-11):1-8, 1992.

Centers for Disease Control and Prevention: Notice to readers: update: nucleic acid amplification tests for tuberculosis, *MMWR* 47(RR-20):1-25, 2000b.

Centers for Disease Control and Prevention: Prevention and control of *Mycobacterium tuberculosis* in health care facilities, *MMWR* 43(RR-13):1-112, 1994.

Centers for Disease Control and Prevention: Prevention and control of tuberculosis in migrant farm workers, *MMWR* 41(RR-10):1-11, 1992.

Centers for Disease Control and Prevention: Prevention and control of tuberculosis in U.S. communities with at-risk minority populations and prevention and control of tuberculosis among homeless persons, *MMWR* 41(RR-5):1-29, 1992.

Centers for Disease Control and Prevention: The role of BCG vaccine in the prevention and control of tuberculosis in the United States, *MMWR* 45(RR-4):1-18, 1996.

Centers for Disease Control and Prevention: Targeted tuberculin testing and treatment of latent tuberculosis infection, *MMWR* 49(RR-6):1-51, 2000c.

Centers for Disease Control and Prevention: *TB Notes 2000*, No. 1, Atlanta, 2000d, CDC.

Centers for Disease Control and Prevention: Tuberculosis elimination revisited: obstacles, opportunities and a renewed commitment, *MMWR* 48(RR-9):1-13, 1999.

Cherniak NS, Altose MD, Homma I: *Rehabilitation of the patient with respiratory disease*, New York, 1999, McGraw-Hill.

Cherniak RM: *Pulmonary function testing*, ed 2, Philadelphia, 1992, WB Saunders.

Cherniak RM, Cherniak L: *Respiration in health and disease*, ed 3, Philadelphia, 1983, WB Saunders.

Comroe JH: *Physiology of respiration*, ed 2, St Louis, 1974, Mosby.

Crystal RG: α_1-antitrypsin deficiency: pathogenesis and treatment, *Hosp Pract* 2:81-94, 1991.

Crystal RG et al, editors: *The lung: scientific foundations*, ed 2, New York, 1997, Raven Press.

Denning CR: Cooperative study comparing three methods of sweat tests to diagnose cystic fibrosis, *Pediatrics* 66:752, 1980.

Diamond L, Altiere RJ: The airway nonadrenergic, noncholinergic inhibitory nervous system. In Leff AR, editor: *Pulmonary and critical pharmacology and therapeutics*, New York, 1996, McGraw-Hill.

Espinal MA et al: Standard short-term chemotherapy for drug-resistant tuberculosis, *JAMA* 283(19):2537-2545, 2000.

Feied C, Handler JA: Pulmonary embolism, *eMedicine Journal* 2(7):1-31, 2001.

Finkelmeier BA: *Cardiothoracic surgical nursing*, ed 2, Philadelphia, 2001, Lippincott–Williams & Wilkins.

Fishman AP, Elias JA, editors: *Fishman's pulmonary diseases and disorders*, ed 3, New York, 1998, McGraw-Hill.

Gerlach M, Didlier K, Gerlach H: Inhaled nitric oxide for respiratory distress syndrome, *Respir Care* 44(2):184-192, 1999.

Harris A, Argent BE: The cystic fibrosis gene and its product CFTR, *Semin Cell Biol* 4:37, 1993.

Heath CH et al: Delay in appropriate therapy of Legionella pneumonia associated with increasing mortality, *Eur J Clin Microbiol Inf Dis* 15:286, 1996.

Hirsh J, Hoak J: Management of deep vein thrombosis and pulmonary embolism: American Heart Association Medical/ Scientific Statement, *Circulation* 93:2212-2245, 1996.

Levison ME: Pneumonia, including necrotizing pulmonary infections (lung abscess). In Fauci AS et al, editors: *Harrison's principles of internal medicine*, ed 14, New York, 1998, McGraw-Hill.

Levitzky MB: *Pulmonary physiology*, ed 5, New York, 1999, McGraw-Hill.

Light RW: *Pleural diseases*, Baltimore, 1995, Williams & Wilkins.

MacIntyre N, Branson RD: *Mechanical ventilation*, Philadelphia, 2000, WB Saunders.

Manning HL, Schwartzstein RM: Pathophysiology of dyspnea, *N Engl J Med* 333:1547, 1995.

Martinez-Lavin M: Digital clubbing and hypertrophic osteoarthropathy: a unifying hypothesis, *J Rheumatol* 14:6-8, 1987.

Minna JD: Neoplasms of the lung. In Fauci AS et al, editors: *Harrison's principles of internal medicine*, ed 14, New York, 1998, McGraw-Hill.

Mountain CF: Revisions in the International System for Staging Lung Cancer, *Chest* 111(6):1710-1717, 1997.

Mufson MA, Stanek RJ: Bacteremic pneumococcal pneumonia in one American city: a 20-year longitudinal study, 1978-1997, *Am J Med* 107(1A):34S-43S, 1999.

Murray JF: *Textbook of respiratory medicine*, ed 3, Philadelphia, 2000, WB Saunders.

National Center for Health Statistics: *Health, United States, 2000*, Hyattsville, Md, 2000, NCHS.

National Heart, Lung, and Blood Institute: *Chronic obstructive pulmonary disease*, NIH Publication No 95-2020, ed 5, Washington, DC, 1995, US Department of Health and Human Service, National Institutes of Health.

Ramsey RM: Management of pulmonary disease in patients with cystic fibrosis, *N Engl J Med* 335(3):179-188, 1996.

Ruppel GL: *Manual of pulmonary function testing*, ed 9, St Louis, 1997, Mosby.

Shapiro BA, Peruzzi WT, Kozelowski-Templin R: *Clinical application of blood gases,* ed 5, St Louis, 1994, Mosby.

Silveira LH et al: A vascular endothelial growth factor and hypertrophic osteoarthropathy, *Clin Exper Rheumatol* 18:57-62, 2000.

Slovis BS, Pittman Haas DW: The case against anergy testing as a routine adjunct to tuberculin skin testing, *JAMA* 283(15):2003-2007, 2000.

Van Houtte P et al: Lung cancer. In Rubin P, editor: *Clinical oncology,* ed 8, Philadelphia, 2001, WB Saunders.

Vasquez-Abad D, Martinez-Lavin M: Macrothrombocytes in the peripheral circulation of patients with cardiogenic hypertrophic osteoarthropathy, *Clin Exper Rheumatol* 9:59-62, 1991.

Weinberger SE: *Principles of pulmonary medicine,* ed 3, Philadelphia, 1998, WB Saunders.

West JB: *Pulmonary pathophysiology,* ed 5, Philadelphia, 1998, Lippincott–Williams & Wilkins.

West JB: *Respiratory physiology—the essentials,* ed 6, Philadelphia, 2000, Lippincott–Williams & Wilkins.

World Health Organization: *Guidelines for the prevention of tuberculosis in health care facilities in resource-limited settings,* WHO/CDS/TB/99.269, Geneva, 1999, WHO.

RENAL SYSTEM DISORDERS

*T*he kidneys are vital organs that play a critical role in the maintenance of a stable internal environment. The kidneys regulate the fluid and electrolyte and acid-base balances of the body by filtering blood, selectively reabsorbing water, electrolytes, and nonelectrolytes, and excreting the excess as urine. The kidneys also excrete metabolic waste products (e.g., urea, creatinine, uric acid) and foreign chemicals. Finally, in addition to these regulatory and excretory functions, the kidneys secrete renin (important in the regulation of blood pressure), the active form of vitamin D_3 (important in the regulation of calcium), and erythropoietin (important in the synthesis of red blood cells). When the kidneys fail to perform these vital functions, a condition known as uremia or end-stage renal disease (ESRD) results. The continuing development of dialysis and renal transplants as a treatment for ESRD since the 1960s and federal financing of treatment since 1973 have provided alternatives to almost certain death.

Part Eight focuses on acute and chronic renal failure. ESRD (defined as individuals sustained by long-term dialysis or transplantation) is a major cause of morbidity and mortality in the United States. ESRD is the outcome of chronic renal disease. The incidence of ESRD has increased dramatically over the past decade so that, in 1997, one of every 3480 persons initiated long-term dialysis or received their first kidney transplant. The cause for this dramatic increase is not entirely clear. Because the incidence of ESRD rises with age, the aging of the general U.S. population may be a factor. Another factor is the rising incidence of diabetes in the United States, fueling an increase in diabetic nephropathy. Although ESRD may be caused by a host of kidney diseases, the four major causes of ESRD are diabetes (34%), hypertension (21%), glomerulonephritis (17%), and polycystic kidney disease (3.5%). In 1998 a total of 397,971 persons in the United States were treated for ESRD at a cost of $16.74 billion (public and private). Nearly 246,000 received dialysis treatment and 13,272 received a kidney transplant. In spite of advances in the treatment of ESRD over the past 40 years, mortality is high because of the prevalence of comorbidities such as diabetes and cardiovascular disease. Renal disease was the eighth leading cause of death in the United States in 1998 (U.S. Renal Data System, 2000).

Acute renal failure is a common clinical problem characterized by a relatively abrupt decline in renal function. Approximately 5% of all hospitalized patients develop acute renal failure and the majority of cases are related to surgery or trauma. Mortality for acute renal failure varies between 30% to 60%, depending on the underlying medical condition. Although many patients who develop acute renal failure may require short-term treatment with dialysis, the majority recover normal or nearly normal renal function if they survive the acute episode.

An understanding of normal renal structure and function is essential for understanding renal failure, and this is the topic of discussion in Chapter 44. Chapter 45 discusses the means of detecting renal disease. The cause and pathophysiology, consequences, and treatment of chronic renal failure are discussed in Chapters 46, 47, and 48. Finally, acute renal failure is discussed in Chapter 49. Chronic renal failure is discussed before acute renal failure because once the pathophysiology and treatment of chronic renal failure are understood, the principles of acute renal failure become easy to grasp. Another reason for this sequence is because acute-on-chronic renal failure is fairly common, although acute renal failure rarely becomes chronic.

Anatomy and Physiology
of the Kidneys and Urinary Tract

LORRAINE M. WILSON

ANATOMY OF THE KIDNEYS AND URINARY TRACT

The kidneys perform the vital function of regulating the volume and chemical composition of the blood (and the internal environment) by selectively excreting solutes and water. If both kidneys were to fail to perform this function for any reason, death would follow within 3 or 4 weeks. The kidney's vital function is accomplished by filtering the blood plasma through the glomerulus, followed by reabsorbing the appropriate amounts of solute and water along the renal tubules. Excess solutes and water are excreted in urine through the urinary collecting system to the outside of the body. This chapter reviews the gross and microscopic anatomy of the kidney and discusses its physiologic functions.

Urinary Tract

The urinary tract consists of the kidneys, which constantly manufacture urine, and the various tubes and reservoirs necessary to carry urine to the outside of the body (Fig. 44-1).

The kidneys are bean-shaped organs situated on either side of the vertebral column. The right kidney is slightly lower than the left because the liver pushes the right kidney down. The upper pole of the right kidney lies on the level of the twelfth rib. The upper pole of the left kidney lies at about the level of the eleventh rib.

The two ureters are tubes about 10 to 12 inches (25 to 30 cm) long extending from the kidneys to the bladder. Their only function is to convey urine to the bladder.

The bladder is a collapsible muscular bag located behind the symphysis pubis. There are three openings in the bladder—two from the ureters and one into the urethra. The bladder has two functions: (1) it serves as a reservoir for urine before it leaves the body, and (2) aided by the urethra, it expels urine from the body.

The urethra is a small dilatable tube leading from the bladder to the outside of the body; it is about $1\frac{1}{2}$ inches (4 cm) long in females and about 8 inches (20 cm) long in males. The opening to the outside of the body is called the *urinary meatus*.

Anatomic Relations of the Kidney

The kidneys lie at the back of the upper abdomen behind the peritoneum, in front of the last two ribs and three major muscles—the transversus abdominis, quadratus lumborum, and psoas major (Fig. 44-2). A heavy cushion of fat keeps the kidneys in position. The adrenal glands are situated over the upper pole of each kidney.

The kidneys are well protected from direct trauma—posteriorly by the ribs and overlying muscles and anteriorly by a thick cushion of intestines. When the kidneys are injured, it is almost always as a result of a force acting on the twelfth rib, which rotates inward and squeezes the kidney between it and the bodies of the lumbar vertebrae. This excellent protection from direct injury also accounts for their difficult position for palpation and surgical access. The normal-size left kidney generally is not palpable on physical examination, because the spleen overlays the upper two thirds of the anterior surface. The lower pole of the normal-size right kidney, however, may be bimanually palpated in many persons. Gross enlargement or displacement of either kidney may be detected by palpation, although this is more easily accomplished on the right.

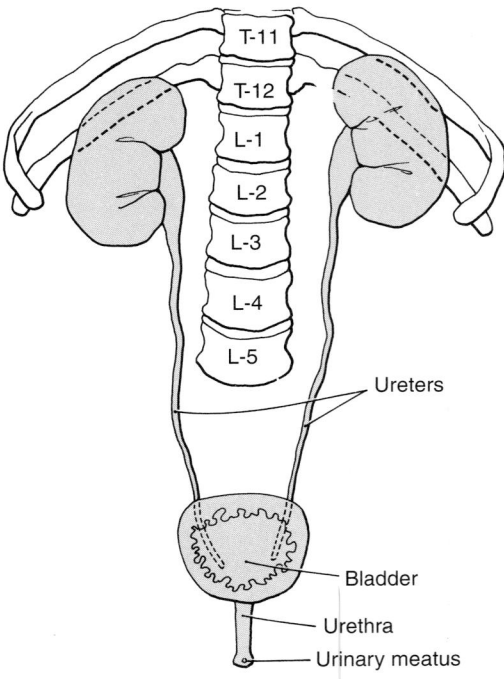

FIG. 44-1 Urinary tract, anatomic relations.

Gross Structure of the Kidney

In the adult, each kidney is about 12 to 13 cm (4.7 to 5.1 inches) in length, 6 cm (2.4 inches) wide, and 2.5 cm (1 inch) in thickness and weighs about 150 g. The size does not vary appreciably with body build. A difference of more than 1.5 cm (0.6 inch) in the pole-to-pole length of a particular kidney (compared with its mate) or a change in the shape is significant, because the majority of renal diseases are manifested by structural changes in the organ.

The anterior and posterior surfaces, upper and lower poles, and lateral margin of the kidney have a convex contour, whereas the medial margin is concave because of the presence of the hilus (Fig. 44-3, *A*). Several structures enter or leave the kidney through the hilus, including the renal artery, renal vein, nerves, lymphatics, and ureter. The kidney is encased in a thin, fibrous, glistening capsule, which is loosely adherent to the underlying tissue and can be easily stripped from the surface.

A longitudinal section of the kidney reveals two distinct regions—the outer cortex and inner medulla (see Fig. 44-3, *B*). The medulla is divided into triangular wedges called *pyramids*. The pyramids are interspersed with cortical material called the *columns of Bertin*. Pyramids have a striated appearance because they are made up of segments of the tubules and collecting ducts of the nephron. The *papilla* (apex) of each pyramid forms the papillary ducts of Bellini, which, in turn, are created by the terminal fusion of many collecting ducts. Each papillary duct is thrust into a cup-shaped terminal extension of the renal pelvis called a *minor calyx* (L. *calix*, cup). Several minor calyces unite to form major calyces, which then unite to form the pelvis of the kidney. The *renal pelvis* is the main reservoir for the renal collecting system. The ureter connects the renal pelvis to the urinary bladder.

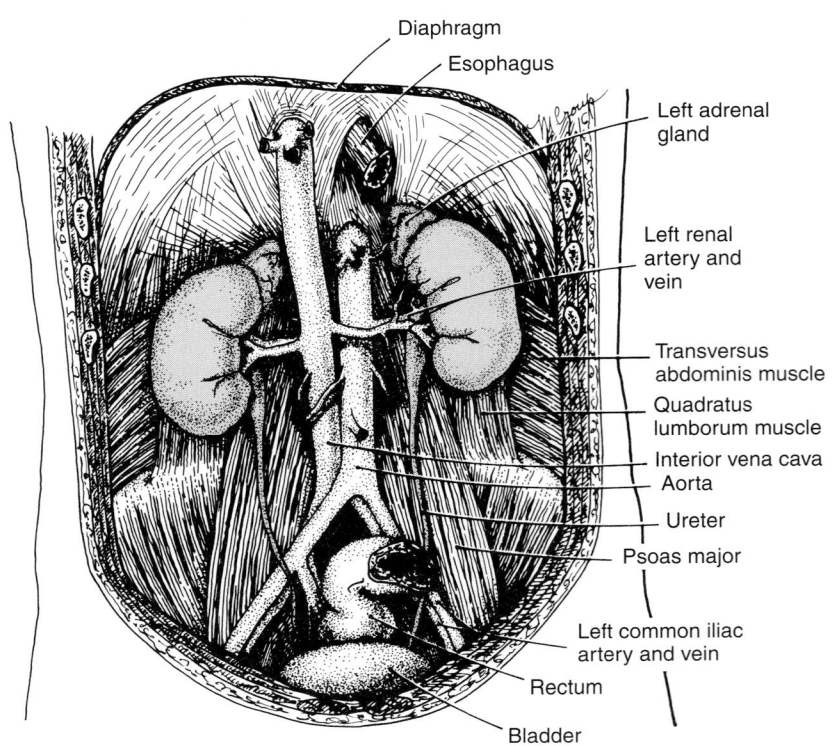

FIG. 44-2 Kidneys, anatomic relations.

Knowledge of renal anatomy is basic to understanding urine formation. Urine formation begins in the cortex and continues as the material flows through the tubules and collecting ducts. The formed urine then flows into the papillary ducts of Bellini, enters the minor calyces, major calyces, and renal pelvis, and finally exits the kidney via the ureter to the urinary bladder. The walls of the calyces, pelvis, and ureter contain smooth muscles, which contract rhythmically and help propel urine along its course by peristalsis.

Gross Vascular Supply of the Kidney

The renal arteries arise from the abdominal aorta at approximately the level of the second lumbar vertebra. Because the aorta is to the left of the midline, the right renal artery is longer than is the left (see Fig. 44-2). Each renal artery branches as it enters the hilus of each kidney.

The renal veins that drain each kidney empty into the inferior vena cava, which lies to the right of the midline. Consequently, the left renal vein is about twice as long as the right. Because of these anatomic features, the transplant surgeon generally prefers the left kidney from the donor, which is rotated and placed in the right pelvis of the recipient. Few technical difficulties are encountered with a short renal artery that is anastomosed with the internal iliac (hypogastric) artery. The renal vein, however, must be longer, because it is implanted directly into the external iliac vein (see Fig. 48-8).

As the renal artery enters the hilus, it divides into the interlobar arteries, which pass between the pyramids to form the arcuate branches, which arch over the bases of the pyramids (Fig. 44-4).

The arcuate arteries give rise to the interlobular arterioles, which form a parallel array in the cortex. These interlobular arterioles give rise to afferent arterioles.

Each *afferent arteriole* supplies blood to a tuft of capillaries called the *glomerulus* (pl., glomeruli). The capillaries of the glomerulus converge into the *efferent arteriole*, which in turn subdivides into a portal network surrounding the tubules, sometimes called the *peritubular capillaries* (not shown). The renal circulation is unusual in that it breaks into two separate capillary beds, the glomerular bed and the peritubular capillary bed arranged in series so that all the renal blood passes through both. Pressure in the first capillary bed (where filtration takes place) is rather high (40 to 50 mm Hg), while pressure in the peritubular capillaries (where tubular reabsorption is returned to the circulation) is low (5 to 10 mm Hg) and similar to capillaries elsewhere in the body. The blood passing through this portal network drains into a venous network to the interlobular, arcuate, interlobar, and renal veins to reach the inferior vena cava.

Special Features of Renal Blood Flow

The kidneys are perfused with blood, about 1200 ml/min—a volume equal to 20% to 25% of the cardiac output (5000 ml/min). This fact is quite remarkable when one considers that the combined weight of the kidneys is less than 1% of the total body weight.

More than 90% of the blood perfusing the kidney is distributed to the cortex, whereas the remainder is distributed to the medulla (the physiologic significance of this for urine concentration is discussed later).

Another special feature of renal blood flow is autoregulation of blood flow through the kidney. The afferent arterioles have an intrinsic capacity to vary their resistance

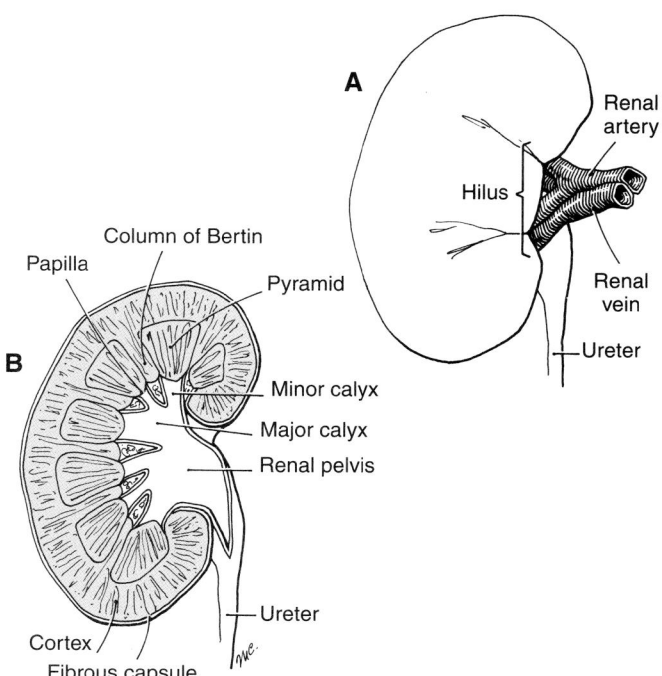

FIG. 44-3 Gross structure of the kidney. **A,** Anterior surface. **B,** Longitudinal section.

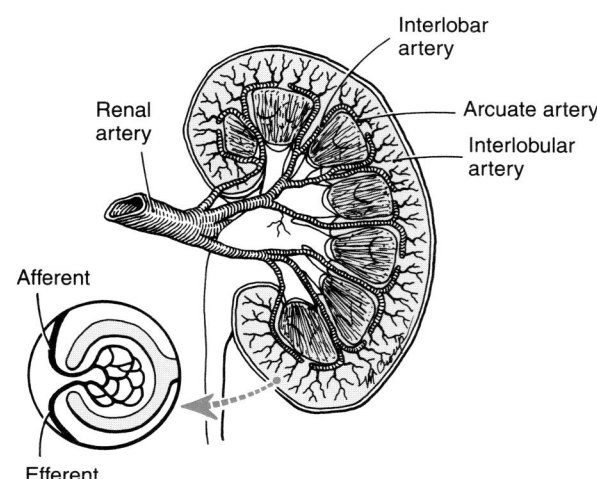

FIG. 44-4 Vascular supply to the kidney. Approximately 90% of the blood is distributed to the cortex and 10% to the medulla. *Inset* depicts the glomerular capillary tuft with afferent and efferent arterioles.

in response to changes in arterial blood pressure, thus keeping renal blood flow and glomerular filtration constant. This capability is effective over an arterial pressure range of 80 to 180 mm Hg. The result is the prevention of large changes in solute and water excretion. Autoregulation, however, can be overpowered in certain circumstances, even in the autoregulatory range. The mechanisms involved in renal autoregulation are discussed later in this chapter. Renal nerves may cause vasoconstriction in states of emergency and shunt blood away from the kidneys to the heart, brain, or skeletal muscles at the expense of the kidney. Disturbances in autoregulation and the distribution of intrarenal blood flow may be important in the pathogenesis of acute oliguric renal failure (see Chapter 49).

Variations in Renal Vascular Supply

Multiple arteries or veins can supply the kidneys (Fig. 44-5). Anomalies of the renal arteries are far more common than anomalies of the veins. In fact, about 25% or more of the population have more than one renal artery supplying a kidney. These additional arteries usually originate as small multiple branches from the aorta and supply the poles of the kidney. An arteriogram of the renal blood supply is essential in the donor before kidney transplantation is attempted because of the possibility of these variations, which may present technical difficulties for the surgeon.

Microscopic Structure of the Kidney
Nephron

The functional work unit of the kidney is called the *nephron*. There are about 1 million nephrons in each kidney, basically similar in structure and function. Thus the work of the kidneys may be considered to be the sum total of the function of all the nephrons put together. Each nephron consists of the Bowman's capsule, which surrounds the glomerular capillary tuft, the proximal convoluted tubule, the loop of Henle, and the distal convoluted tubule, which empties into the *collecting ducts* (Fig. 44-6). A normal person can survive, albeit with difficulty, with less than 20,000 nephrons, or 1% of the total nephron mass. Thus it is possible to donate one kidney for transplantation without endangering life.

Renal Corpuscle

The renal corpuscle consists of the Bowman's capsule and the glomerular capillary tuft. The term *glomerulus* is often used interchangeably with *renal corpuscle*, although it properly refers only to the capillary tuft.

Bowman's capsule is a specialized invagination of the proximal tubule (Fig. 44-7). A urine-containing space exists between the capillary tuft and Bowman's capsule called *Bowman's space*, or the *capsular space*.

Bowman's capsule is lined with epithelial cells. *Parietal epithelial cells* are flat and form the outermost part of the capsule; the much larger *visceral epithelial cells* form the innermost part of the capsule and line the outer side of the capillary tuft. Foot processes, or *podocytes*, form extensions of the visceral epithelial cells that come in contact with the basement membrane at intervals, leaving many areas free of epithelial cell contact. The area between the foot processes, usually referred to as the *slit pore*, has an average width of about 400 Å (angstrom units).

The *basement membrane* forms the middle layer of the capillary wall, sandwiched between the epithelial cells on one side and the endothelial cells on the other. The capillary basement membrane is continuous with that of the tubule and is composed of a hydrated gel of intertwined collagenous fibers. No pores are visible in the basement membrane, although it behaves as if it had pores about 70 to 100 Å in diameter.

Endothelial cells form the innermost layer of the capillary tuft. Unlike the epithelial cells, the endothelial cells are in continuous contact with the basement membrane. However, there are numerous windowlike openings called *fenestrations*, which are about 600 Å in diameter. The endothelial cells are continuous with the endothelial lining of the afferent and efferent arterioles.

The endothelial cells, basement membrane, and visceral epithelial cells are the three layers that make up the glomerular filtration membrane. The glomerular filtration membrane allows ultrafiltration of the blood by separating the formed elements of the blood and the large protein molecules from the rest of the plasma and delivering the plasma as filtrate to the urinary space of Bowman's capsule. The discriminatory nature of glomerular ultrafil-

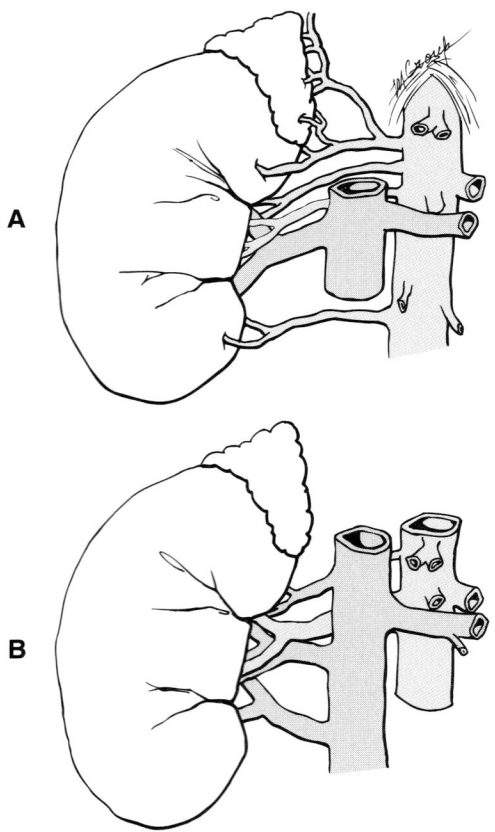

FIG. 44-5 Anomalies in renal vasculature. **A,** About 25% of the population have multiple renal arteries supplying a kidney. **B,** Multiple renal veins. (Modified from Netter FH: Kidneys, ureters, and urinary bladder. In *The Ciba collection of medical illustrations,* vol 6, West Caldwell, NJ, 1973, Ciba Medical Education Division.)

tration is a result of the unique structural arrangement and the chemical composition of the ultrafiltration barrier. The glomerular basement membrane appears to be the structure that limits the passage of solute into the urinary space on the basis of size. In addition, the filtration barrier has a negative charge owing to clusters of anion-rich macromolecules within the basement membrane and lining the epithelial and endothelial cell margins. This negative charge is why anionic albumin (which has a diameter slightly less than the smallest pore size) does not normally enter the urinary space. Larger protein molecules and blood cells do not normally appear in the filtrate and urine.

Another important component of the glomerulus is the *mesangium*, which consists of *mesangial cells* and *mesangial matrix*. Mesangial cells form a continuous network between the capillary loops of the glomerulus and are thought to function as a supporting framework. Mesangial cells are not part of the filtration membrane but do secrete the mesangial matrix. Mesangial cells have phagocytic activity and secrete prostaglandins. Because mesangial cells have contractile ability and are located adjacent to glomerular capillaries, they may have a role in influencing the glomerular filtration rate (see previous discussion) by regulating flow through the capillaries.

Mesangial cells that lie outside the glomerular tuft near the vascular pole of the glomerulus (between the afferent and efferent arterioles) are called *lacis cells* (see Fig. 44-7).

Juxtaglomerular Apparatus

The juxtaglomerular apparatus (JGA) consists of a specialized group of cells near the vascular pole of each glomerulus that has an important role in the regulation of renin release and the control of extracellular fluid (ECF) volume and blood pressure. The JGA consists of three types of cells: (1) the *juxtaglomerular (JG)* or *granular cells* (which produce and store renin) in the wall of the afferent arteriole, (2) the *macula densa* of the distal tubule, and (3) the extraglomerular mesangial or *lacis cells*. The macula densa is a group of special-staining, distal tubular epithelial cells. These cells are contiguous with both the lacis cell compartment and the renin-secreting JG cells (see Fig. 44-7).

In general, renin secretion is controlled by both extrarenal and intrarenal factors. Two important mechanisms controlling renin release involve the JG cells and the macula densa. Either decreased wall tension in the afferent arteriole or decreased salt delivery to the macula densa in the distal tubule stimulates the JG cells to release renin from granules where it is stored within the cells. The JG cells, which are specialized myoepithelial cells cuffing

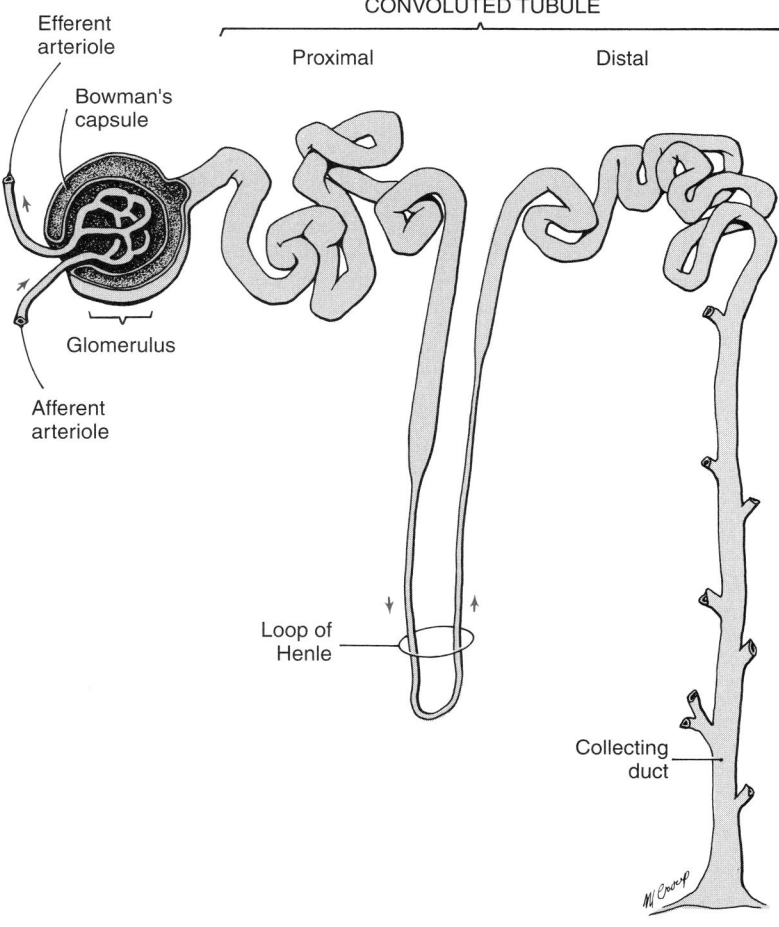

FIG. 44-6 Nephron.

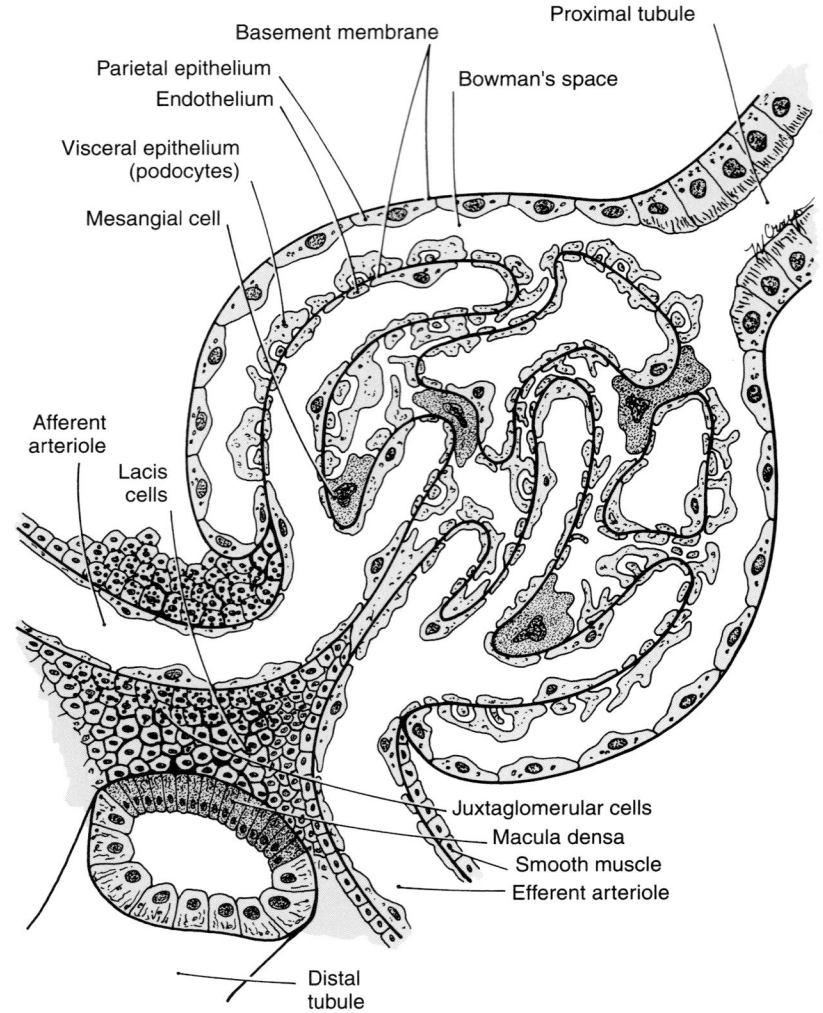

FIG. 44-7 Renal corpuscle. The glomerular capillary filter consists of three layers of cells: the endothelium, basement membrane, and visceral epithelium containing podocytes or foot processes. Mesangial cells (between the capillaries) form a supporting network for the glomerular tuft. The juxtaglomerular apparatus consists of a specialized group of cells (the macula densa and juxtaglomerular cells) near the vascular pole of the glomerulus and is important in the regulation of blood pressure. Extraglomerular mesangial cells located at the vascular pole are called *lacis cells*.

the afferent arterioles, also act as miniature pressure transducers, sensing renal perfusion pressure. A decrease in the actual ECF volume or *effective circulating volume (ECV)** results in decreased renal perfusion pressure, which is sensed as decreased stretch by the JG cells. The JG cells then release renin into the circulation, which, in turn, ac-

tivates the renin-angiotensin-aldosterone mechanism (discussed near the end of this chapter).

A second control mechanism for renin release centers in the macula densa cells, which may function as chemoreceptors, monitoring the chloride load presented to the distal tubule. Under conditions of volume contraction, less sodium chloride (NaCl) is delivered to the distal tubule (because more is absorbed in the proximal tubule); feedback from the macula densa cells to the JG cells then causes increased release of renin. The mechanism by which the chloride signal is translated into changes in renin secretion is not well understood. An increase in the ECF volume causing an increase in renal perfusion pressure and increased NaCl delivery to the distal tubule has the opposite effect of the example given of decreased ECF volume—it *suppresses* renin secretion.

*The ECV is not a measurable and distinct body fluid compartment; rather, it is related to the adequacy of tissue perfusion, that is, to the "fullness" and "pressure" within the vascular tree. ECV is made up of three components: absolute intravascular volume, cardiac output, and systemic vascular resistance. A change in any one of these three parameters without a compensatory change in the others will affect the fullness of the circulation and thus the ECV. Normally, the actual ECF and the ECV parallel each other, but under some pathologic conditions (e.g., congestive heart failure) the ECV can be reduced yet the ECF volume may be increased above normal.

Other factors influencing renin secretion include the renal sympathetic nerves, which stimulate renin release through beta$_1$-adrenergic receptors in the JGA, and angiotensin II, which inhibits renin release. Numerous other circulating factors may also alter renin secretion, including plasma electrolytes (calcium and potassium) and various hormones, including atrial natriuretic hormone, dopamine, antidiuretic hormone (ADH), adrenocorticotropic hormone (ACTH), nitric oxide (formerly known as endothelium-derived relaxing factor [EDRF]), and prostaglandins. It is probable that the JGA is a site for the integration of these diverse inputs and that renin secretion reflects the interaction of all the factors.

BASIC RENAL PHYSIOLOGY

The primary function of the kidney is to maintain the volume and composition of the ECF within normal limits. The composition and volume of the ECF are controlled by glomerular filtration and by tubular reabsorption and secretion, discussed in the following sections. Box 44-1 presents a list of renal functions that may be helpful to review at this point. These functions will be discussed again at the end of this chapter.

Glomerular Ultrafiltration

Urine formation begins with glomerular filtration of plasma. Renal blood flow (RBF) is equal to about 25% of the cardiac output, or 1200 ml/min. Assuming a normal hematocrit of 45%, renal plasma flow (RPF) is equal to 660 ml/min ($0.55 \times 1200 = 660$). Approximately one fifth of the plasma, or 125 ml/min, passes through the glomerulus into Bowman's capsule. This rate is called the *glomerular filtration rate (GFR)*. Filtration at the glomerulus is termed *glomerular ultrafiltration*, because the primary filtrate has the same composition as plasma, with the exception of the absence of proteins. Blood cells and large protein molecules or negatively charged proteins, such as albumin, are effectively restrained by the size-selective and charge-selective characteristics of the glomerular filtration membrane barrier, whereas molecules of smaller size or with a neutral or positive charge, such as water and crystalloids, are readily filtered. Calculation reveals that 173 L of fluid is filtered through the glomerulus in 1 day—an astonishing amount in organs whose combined weight is about 10 ounces. As the filtrate travels through the tubules, various substances are added to or subtracted from it so that eventually only about 1.5 L/day is excreted as urine.

The forces that account for this high GFR are entirely passive, and no metabolic energy is expended. The filtration force is a result of the pressure gradient between the glomerular capillary and Bowman's capsule. The hydrostatic pressure of the blood in the glomerular capillaries favors filtration, and this force is opposed by the hydrostatic pressure of the filtrate in Bowman's capsule and the oncotic pressure of the blood. The oncotic pressure in Bowman's capsule is essentially zero, because the filtrate is normally devoid of protein. Although never measured in humans, the glomerular capillary pressure was esti-

---

Major Functions of the Kidney

EXCRETORY FUNCTIONS
Maintains plasma osmolality near 285 mOsm by varying the excretion of water
Maintains the ECF volume and blood pressure by varying the excretion of Na^+
Maintains the plasma concentration of each individual electrolyte within normal range
Maintains the plasma pH near 7.4 by eliminating excess H^+ and regenerating HCO_3^-
Excretes the nitrogenous end-products of protein metabolism, chiefly urea, uric acid, and creatinine
Serves as excretory route for most drugs

NONEXCRETORY FUNCTIONS
Synthesizes and activates hormones
    Renin: important in the regulation of blood pressure
    Erythropoietin: stimulates red blood cell production by bone marrow
    1,25-dihydroxyvitamin D_3: final hydroxylation of vitamin D_3 to its most potent form
    Prostaglandins: most are vasodilators, act locally, and protect against renal ischemic damage
Degradation of polypeptide hormones
    Insulin, glucagon, parathormone, prolactin, growth hormone, ADH, and gastrointestinal hormones (gastrin, vasoactive intestinal polypeptide [VIP])

---

mated by Pitts (1974) to be about 50 mm Hg and intracapsular pressure to be about 10 mm Hg. These estimates are based on measurements in rats. Oncotic pressure of the blood is about 30 mm Hg. Net glomerular filtration pressure is thus about 10 mm Hg. The glomerular filtration is influenced not only by these physical forces but also by the permeability of the filtration membrane (K_f). K_f is a product of the intrinsic permeability of the glomerular capillary and the glomerular surface area for filtration. The filtration rate is much higher in the glomerular capillaries compared with other body capillaries because K_f is approximately 100 times higher (173 L/day versus approximately 2 L/day). The balance of forces involved in glomerular ultrafiltration may be summarized as follows:

$$GFR = K_f \times \left(\begin{bmatrix} \text{Intracapillary} \\ \text{hydrostatic} \\ \text{pressure} \end{bmatrix} - \begin{bmatrix} \text{Intracapsular} & \text{Intracapillary} \\ \text{hydrostatic} & + \text{oncotic} \\ \text{pressure} & \text{pressure} \end{bmatrix} \right)$$

$$\text{Net filtration pressure} = 50 - (10 + 30)$$
$$= 10 \text{ mm Hg}$$

The most accurate way to measure the GFR is to use a substance such as inulin, which is freely filtered at the glomerulus and is neither secreted nor reabsorbed by the tubules. The clearance of a substance is the volume of plasma from which that substance is completely cleared by the kidneys per unit of time. The rate of clearance of inulin is exactly equal to the GFR, measured by the administration of inulin at a constant intravenous (IV) drip rate to ensure a constant plasma concentration level. Measurement of inulin concentration in plasma (P_{in}) in mg/dl, urine (U_{in}) in mg/dl, and the volume of urine (V) in ml/min permits calculation of inulin clearance (C_{in}) in ml/min. The result must be corrected for body surface area, estimated with a nomogram that relates height and weight to body surface area. For example, if a person is passing urine at the rate of 4.2 ml/min, the U_{in} specimen is 600 mg/dl and the P_{in} is constant at 25 mg/dl, then

$$GFR = C_{in} = \frac{(U_{in})\ 600\ mg/dl \times (V)\ 4.2\ ml/min}{(P_{in})\ 25\ mg/dl}$$

$$= 100\ ml/min$$

The calculated GFR of 100 ml/min would then be normalized by correcting it to the standard normal body surface area of 1.73 m². This correction makes it is possible to compare function in persons of varying physical statures. The GFR of normal young men averages 125 ± 15 ml/min/1.73 m², and that of normal young women is 110 ± 15 ml/min/1.73 m².

Autoregulation of Renal Plasma Flow and Glomerular Filtration Rate

The GFR is not totally dependent on the physical forces operating at the glomerular membrane. The kidney has the ability to maintain the RPF and the GFR at a relatively constant level in spite of the normal daily fluctuations in systemic blood pressure and renal perfusion pressure. This phenomenon, intrinsic to the kidneys, is termed *autoregulation*. The purpose of maintaining the GFR within a narrow range is to prevent inappropriate fluctuations in salt and water excretion. Autoregulation is effective over an arterial blood pressure range of about 80 to 180 mm Hg but may be overridden even in this range under certain pathologic conditions.

Two mechanisms are largely responsible for the autoregulation of RPF and the GFR: (1) *myogenic stretch receptors* in vascular smooth muscle of the afferent arteriole and (2) *tubuloglomerular feedback (TGF)*. In addition, nor-

epinephrine, angiotensin II, and other hormones can influence autoregulation. The glomerular capillaries differ from other capillary beds in being interposed between two (afferent and efferent) arterioles. As a result, the intracapillary hydrostatic pressure (P_{gc}) is determined by three factors: (1) the systemic blood pressure and (2) and (3) the resistances at the afferent and efferent arterioles. This arrangement allows rapid regulation of the GFR by altering the resistance in the afferent or efferent arterioles. For example, a rise in systemic blood pressure and renal perfusion pressure would be expected to increase the P_{gc} and thus the rate of RPF and the GFR. However, the increased renal perfusion pressure will be sensed by the myotonic stretch receptors in the afferent arteriole, resulting in constriction of the afferent arteriole. The efferent arterioles, however, do not directly respond to changes in stretch so do not contribute to the myotonic response. The result of afferent arteriolar vasoconstriction is a reduction of RPF, P_{gc}, and GFR, thus offsetting a large increase in GFR that would be expected with the increased renal perfusion pressure (Fig. 44-8, *A*).

On the other hand, when systemic hypotension is present, the renin-angiotensin system is activated with the generation of angiotensin II. Angiotensin II causes vasoconstriction of the efferent arteriole and vasoconstriction of the afferent arteriole but to a lesser degree. The result is a reduction of renal perfusion pressure and RPF (because of increased afferent arteriolar resistance) and an increase in P_{gc} (because of increased efferent arteriolar resistance). The net result is that angiotensin II has counteracting effects on the regulation of GFR: the decrease in RPF will tend to reduce GFR, whereas the increase in P_{gc} will tend to increase GFR (see Fig. 44-8, *B*). Norepinephrine (released from the renal sympathetic nerves or from the adrenal cortex) enhances the vasocon-

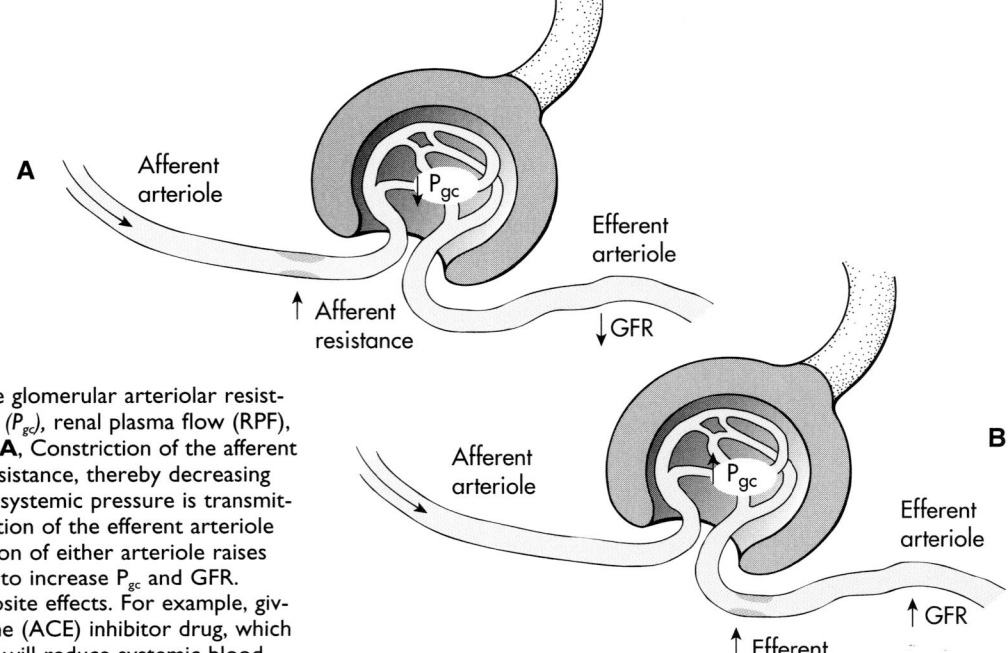

FIG. 44-8 Relationship among the glomerular arteriolar resistances, glomerular capillary pressure *(Pgc)*, renal plasma flow (RPF), and glomerular filtration rate *(GFR)*. **A,** Constriction of the afferent arteriole increases renal vascular resistance, thereby decreasing RPF, Pgc, and GFR (since less of the systemic pressure is transmitted to the glomerulus). **B,** Constriction of the efferent arteriole also decreases RPF (since constriction of either arteriole raises renal vascular resistance) but tends to increase Pgc and GFR. Arteriolar vasodilation has the opposite effects. For example, giving an angiotensin-converting enzyme (ACE) inhibitor drug, which reduces formation of angiotensin II, will reduce systemic blood pressure and Pgc.

strictive effect of angiotensin II. Angiotensin II also stimulates the release of vasodilator prostaglandins (e.g., PGI_2, PGE_2) from the glomeruli, which minimizes the likelihood of renal ischemia under conditions of systemic hypotension.

The second mechanism responsible for GFR autoregulation, TGF, refers to alterations of GFR that can be induced by changes in the flow rate of fluid in the distal tubule. TGF is mediated by the macula densa cells in the distal tubule (contiguous with the glomerular pole), which are sensitive to the chloride composition of the tubular fluid. A high rate of NaCl in the distal tubules leads to constriction of the afferent arteriole and thus a reduction in the GFR of that nephron. According to this mechanism, the nephron itself is quite literally a feedback loop. An increase in GFR leads to increased NaCl delivery to the distal nephron and hence to increased salt transfer across the macula densa cells. A reduction of the GFR follows. Conversely, if GFR is low, little salt is available for transport across the macula densa cells. The afferent arteriole dilates, and the GFR increases.

Tubular Reabsorption and Secretion

Three classes of substances are filtered at the glomerulus (Fig. 44-9): electrolytes, nonelectrolytes, and water. Some of the most important electrolytes are sodium (Na^+), potassium (K^+), calcium (Ca^{++}), magnesium (Mg^{++}), bicarbonate (HCO_3^-), chloride (Cl^-), and phosphate (HPO_4^-). Important nonelectrolytes are glucose, amino acids, and the metabolic end-products of protein metabolism: urea, uric acid, and creatinine.

The second step in urine formation after filtration is the selective reabsorption of filtered substances. Most of the substances filtered are reabsorbed through minute "pores" in the tubule, where they pass back into the peritubular capillaries that surround the tubule. In addition, some substances are secreted from the surrounding peritubular blood vessels into the tubule.

Reabsorption and secretion take place by active and passive transport mechanisms. A mechanism is active if it transports a substance against an electrochemical gradient (i.e., against a gradient of electrical potential, chemical potential, or both). Work is performed directly on the substance reabsorbed or secreted by the tubular cells, and energy is expended in the form of adenosine triphosphate (ATP) (e.g., $3Na^+/2K^+$ ATPase). A transport mechanism is passive if the substance being reabsorbed or secreted moves down an electrochemical gradient. No energy is expended in moving the substance.

Along the proximal tubule, glucose and amino acids are completely reabsorbed by active transport. Almost all the K^+ and uric acid are actively reabsorbed, and both are secreted into the distal tubule. At least two thirds of the filtered Na^+ is actively reabsorbed in the proximal tubule. Reabsorption of Na^+ continues in the loop of Henle, distal tubule, and collecting ducts, so that less than 1% of the filtered load is excreted in the urine. Most of the Ca^{++} and HPO_4^- is reabsorbed in the proximal tubule by active transport. Water, Cl^-, and urea are reabsorbed in the proximal tubule by passive transport. As large numbers of positively charged Na^+ ions leave the tubular lumen, negatively charged Cl^- ions must follow for reasons of

electrical neutrality. The exit of a large number of ions and nonelectrolytes from the proximal tubular fluids leaves it osmotically dilute, and as a result, water diffuses out of the tubule into the peritubular blood. Urea then diffuses passively down a concentration gradient established by the reabsorption of water. Hydrogen ion (H^+), organic acids such as para-amino-hippurate (PAH) and penicillin, and creatinine (an organic base) are all actively secreted in the proximal tubule. About 90% of the HCO_3^- is reabsorbed in the proximal tubule indirectly by $Na^+ - H^+$ exchange. When H^+ is secreted into the tubular lumen (in exchange for Na^+), it combines with the HCO_3^- present in the glomerular filtrate to give carbonic acid (H_2CO_3). The H_2CO_3 dissociates to water and carbon

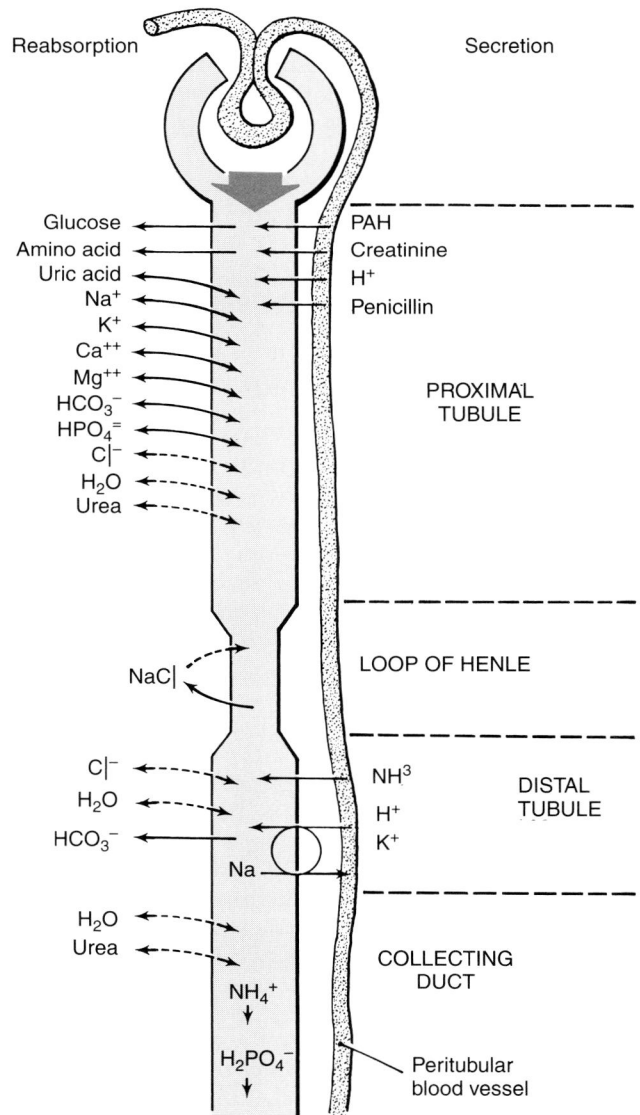

Filtration
H_2O, electrolytes, nonelectrolytes

FIG. 44-9   Tubular reabsorption and secretion along the glomerular nephron. *Solid arrows* indicate active transport, and *broken arrows* indicate passive transport.

dioxide (CO_2). Both CO_2 and H_2O diffuse out of the tubular lumen into the tubular cell. In the tubular cell, carbonic anhydrase catalyzes the reaction of CO_2 and H_2O to form H_2CO_3 once again. The dissociation of H_2CO_3 produces HCO_3^- and H^+. The H^+ is secreted, and the HCO_3^- passes into the peritubular blood along with Na^+.

In the loop of Henle, Cl^- is actively transported out of the ascending limb, followed passively by Na^+. $NaCl$ then diffuses passively into the descending limb. This process is important for urine concentration and is discussed later in this chapter.

The selective process of secretion and reabsorption is completed in the distal tubule and collecting ducts. Two important functions of the distal tubule are the final regulation of water balance and acid-base balance. If the cells are to function normally, the pH of the ECF must be maintained within the narrow range of 7.35 to 7.45. Several biologic mechanisms working in coordination contribute toward maintaining the pH within normal limits. The principal blood buffer is the bicarbonate–carbonic acid system given by the equation:

$$CO_2 + H_2O \underset{\text{anhydrase}}{\overset{\text{carbonic}}{\rightleftharpoons}} H_2CO_3 \rightleftharpoons H^+ + HCO_3^-$$

The blood pH is given by the Henderson-Hasselbalch equation:

$$pH = pK + \log \frac{[HCO_3^-] \text{ (kidneys)}}{[H_2CO_3] \text{ (lungs)}}$$

where pK is the dissociation constant of H_2CO_3. The lungs eliminate CO_2, which is produced when H^+ is buffered by HCO_3^- (left shift of the previous reaction), and thus play an important role in stabilizing the pH. The role of the kidneys in maintaining acid-base balance is the reabsorption of most of the filtered HCO_3^-. When considering disturbances in acid-base balance, it should be remembered that the serum pH is largely a function of the HCO_3^-/H_2CO_3 ratio and that the numerator is largely regulated by renal mechanisms, whereas pulmonary mechanisms regulate the denominator (through control of CO_2 elimination). A change in the numerator or denominator is followed by a unidirectional change in the other. This change, known as *compensation*, serves to protect the pH.

In addition to reabsorbing and conserving most of the HCO_3^-, the kidneys also eliminate excess H^+. About 80 mEq of acids other than H_2CO_3 is produced in the body each day. Because the lungs cannot eliminate these acids, they are called *fixed acids*. These acids are eliminated in the tubular fluid, so that it is possible for the urine to achieve a pH as low as 4.5 (a H^+ gradient that is 800 times that in the plasma). All along the tubule, H^+ is secreted into the tubular fluid. The H^+ may then be excreted by combination with filtered dibasic $HPO_4^=$ or with ammonia (NH_3). Thus H^+ is excreted as the titratable monobasic acid salt (NaH_2PO_4) or as ammonium ion (NH_4^+). NH_3 diffuses readily into the tubular lumen, but after combination with H^+ to form the charged particle NH_4^+, it is unable to diffuse back into the tubular cell. Because the minimum urine pH that can be achieved is 4.5, the amount of free H^+ that can be excreted is limited. Therefore the ammonium mechanism (and the phosphate mechanism) is important in eliminating an acid load, because NH_4^+ does not affect the urine pH. The buffering of H^+ by NH_3 or $HPO_4^=$ also has the effect of adding a new HCO_3^- to the plasma for every H^+ excreted into the urine. The H^+ that is secreted is derived from H_2CO_3 in the tubular cell, leaving HCO_3^- behind in equimolar amounts. In contrast, when HCO_3^- is reabsorbed from the tubular fluid by the mechanism previously described, HCO_3^- is merely conserved, because one H^+ is returned to the plasma for each one that is secreted into the tubular fluid. Therefore the regeneration of HCO_3^- (i.e., the de novo synthesis) by the buffering mechanism is very important in preventing acidosis.

Both uric acid and K^+ are secreted into the distal tubule, as already mentioned. Normally, about 5% of the filtered K^+ load is excreted in the urine. Water reabsorption is also completed in the distal tubule and collecting ducts.

Several hormones regulate the tubular reabsorption and secretion of solutes and water. Water reabsorption depends on the presence of ADH. Aldosterone influences Na^+ reabsorption and K^+ secretion. Increased aldosterone causes increased Na^+ reabsorption and increased K^+ secretion. A decrease in aldosterone has the opposite effect. *Atrial natriuretic peptide (ANP)*, a hormone produced and stored in the myocytes of the cardiac atria, has an opposite effect on Na^+ reabsorption to that of aldosterone. ANP is released when the atria are distended (i.e., expansion of the effective circulating volume [ECV]) and promotes Na^+ and water excretion in the collecting ducts. Parathyroid hormone (PTH) regulates Ca^{++} and $HPO_4^=$ reabsorption along the tubule. Increased PTH results in increased reabsorption of Ca^{++} and increased $HPO_4^=$ excretion. A decrease in PTH has the opposite effect.

Fig. 44-9 summarizes the major function of each part of the nephron. This selective reabsorption and secretion along the tubule enables the kidney to regulate the internal body environment in a precise manner. The following discussion examines in greater detail the role of the kidney in water metabolism.

Regulation of Water Balance

The total solute concentration of body fluids is remarkably constant in the normal person despite wide fluctuation in water and solute intake and excretion. It is through the production of urine much more concentrated or diluted than the plasma from which it is derived that the concentration of the plasma and body fluids is maintained within narrow limits. When a large volume of fluids is ingested, causing dilution of body fluids, the urine becomes dilute, and the excess water is rapidly excreted. Conversely, when water deprivation or excess solute intake causes the body fluids to become concentrated, the urine becomes highly concentrated so that solute is lost in excess of water. The water retained tends to return the body fluids to a normal solute concentration.

Before the processes involved in the regulation of body fluid balance can be understood, it is necessary to understand the concept of osmolality, a term used to express the concentration of body fluids.

Osmotic Concentration

Osmotic concentration (*osmolality*) refers to the number of particles dissolved in a solution. When a solute is added to water, the effective concentration (activity) of water is lowered relative to that of pure water. Osmotic activity is influenced only by the relative number of solute and solvent particles and is ideally independent of the nature of the solute. Solute particles that differ in mass, shape, and charge have the same effect on the osmotic activity of the solvent, provided they are equal in number. Thus six Na^+ and Cl^- ions that are completely dissociated have the same effect on the osmotic activity as do six glucose molecules in 1 kg of water even though they are quite different in mass, shape, and charge (Fig. 44-10).

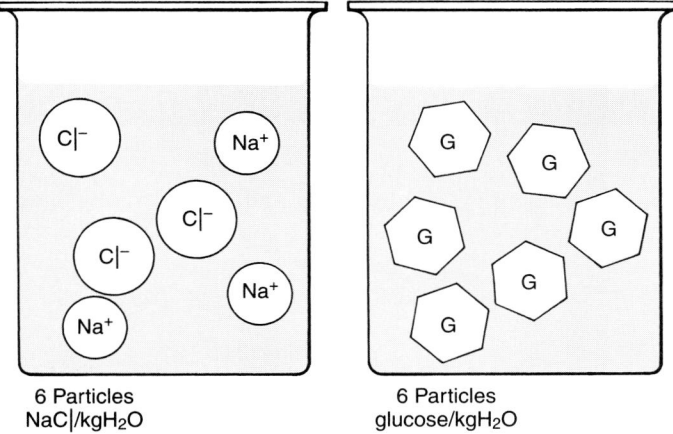

6 Particles
$NaCl/kgH_2O$

6 Particles
$glucose/kgH_2O$

FIG. 44-10   Osmotic concentration equals the number of particles per kilogram of water. It does not depend on the mass, shape, or charge of the particles in an ideal solution.

Colligative Properties of Solutions

The addition of solute particles to a solvent lowers the vapor pressure and freezing point and raises the boiling point and osmotic pressure of the solvent. These phenomena are referred to as the *colligative properties* of solutions. All these properties depend on osmotic concentration.

Fig. 44-11 illustrates the four colligative properties of solutions. The first two colligative properties are vapor pressure lowering and boiling point elevation. When particles are added to water, it is more difficult for the water to escape from the surface, because the effective concentration of water is decreased. Consequently, pure water boils at 100° C, whereas a solution of glucose and water has a boiling point higher than 100° C.

When solute particles are added to water, the osmotic pressure is increased, which is a third colligative property of a solution. Fig. 44-11 shows two glucose molecules in the left compartment and six in the right compartment separated by a semipermeable membrane. The pores in the membrane are too small to allow glucose to diffuse readily. Water, a smaller molecule, diffuses easily from the area of low osmotic concentration in the left-hand compartment to the area of higher osmotic concentration in the right-hand compartment. This process is called *osmosis*. Actually, water is moving from an area of higher water concentration (in the left compartment) to an area of lower water concentration (in the right compartment). Osmosis is thus only a special case of diffusion.

The diffusion of water from the left to the right compartment continues until osmotic equilibrium is achieved, with the result being that the fluid level is elevated in the right compartment. The force driving the water through the semipermeable membrane is called *osmotic pressure*. To prevent the water from diffusing into the right-hand

**Vapor pressure lowering
Boiling point elevation**

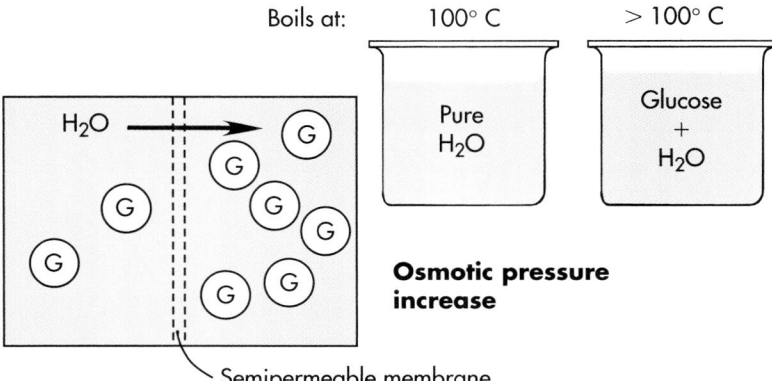

Boils at: 100° C   > 100° C

Pure H_2O

Glucose + H_2O

Osmotic pressure increase

Semipermeable membrane

Freezing point depression

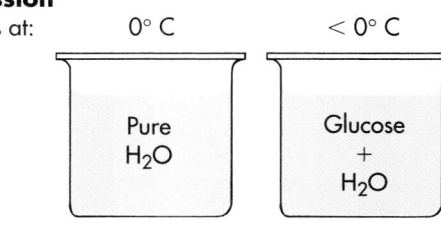

Freezes at: 0° C   < 0° C

Pure H_2O

Glucose + H_2O

FIG. 44-11   Colligative properties of solutions. G, Glucose molecule.

compartment, it would be necessary to apply physical pressure over the solution in the right-hand compartment that would be equal to the higher potential of water in the left compartment. It is common usage to speak of the osmotic pressure of a solution, although it is virtually never measured. Several other properties of solutions vary in exact proportion to the osmotic pressure and are more easily measured (e.g., depression of the freezing point and vapor pressure lowering). In fact, even the use of the term "osmotic pressure" is rather loose, because it is commonly expressed in terms of concentration rather than pressure (see following discussion).

The principle of osmosis is basic to the movement of water between compartments in the body. This principle is also applied in dialysis by putting high concentrations of glucose in the dialysis bath to facilitate the removal of excess fluid that accumulated while the kidneys were not functioning adequately.

The fourth colligative property of a solution is the freezing point depression. Particles added to water cause the solution to have a lower freezing point than that of pure water, which freezes at 0° C.

Measurement of Osmotic Concentration

Two common methods measure the osmotic concentration of body fluids. The freezing point depression as measured by the osmometer is a true measure of osmotic concentration, but the measuring procedure is complex and must be carried out in a laboratory.* This method is based on the principle that the freezing point of a solution consisting of 1 gram-molecular weight (mole or mol) of any nondissociated substance dissolved in 1 kg of water will be –1.86° C.† Such a solution is called an *osmolal solution*, and it contains 1 g-osmol of solute parti-

---

*More recently, a device to measure osmotic concentration on the basis of vapor pressure lowering has been used in some laboratories. This method is more rapid and less complicated than the osmometer method.
†One mole of any element or molecular compound contains the same number of particles (Avogadro's number: 6.02×10^{23} molecules/mol) as does any other.

cles (i.e., the number of particles needed to lower the freezing point of water by 1.86° C). The change in temperature is called the *molal freezing point constant* (K_f) and is equal to 1 osmol.

In the absence of dissociation, each molecule of solute behaves as a single particle. Therefore, because molecular size has no effect on colligative properties, 1 g-mole of albumin (mol wt 70,000) affects the freezing point of water to the same degree as does 1 g-mole of glucose (mol wt 180). If dissociation occurs, as with NaCl, for example, and two ions are formed, each molecule has the effect of two particles. In this case, then, 1 osmol is one half the molecular weight.

To calculate the osmotic concentration (osmolality) of a solution, it is necessary only to measure the lowering of the freezing point below that of pure water (ΔT). This number is then divided by K_f, the molal freezing point constant:

$$\text{Osmolality} = \frac{\Delta T}{K_f}$$

For example, blood plasma freezes at –0.53° C. When this number is divided by –1.86 (K_f), the calculated concentration is 285 mOsm (1 milliosmol = 0.001 osmol):

$$\text{Plasma concentration} = \frac{-0.53° C}{-1.86° C} \times 1000$$

$$= 285 \text{ mOsm}$$

In the healthy person, plasma concentration is 285 ± 10 mOsm/kg H_2O.

The second method of estimating concentration of body fluids is to measure the specific gravity with the urinometer (see photographs of the urinometer and osmometer in Fig. 44-12). Specific gravity is not a true measure of concentration, but because of its simplicity, specific gravity is commonly used in the clinical unit. What is actually being measured is the density (which depends on the weight of the solute particles) and not the concentration (which depends on the number of solute particles). However, estimating the concentration of urine by measuring specific gravity is fairly accurate, pro-

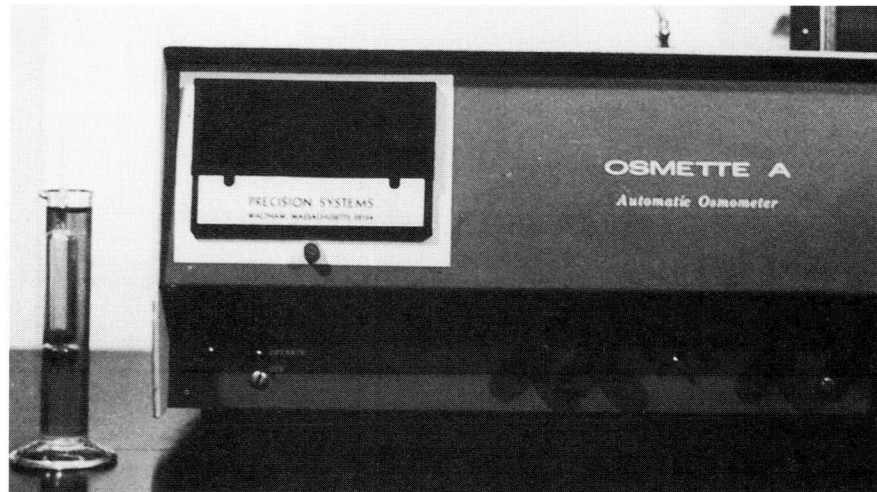

FIG. 44-12 Osmometer and urinometer. The osmometer measures the freezing point depression of a solution used to calculate osmolality. The urinometer *(left)* does not actually measure osmotic concentration but rather the density of a solution.

vided the urine has normal constituents. The correlation between the osmolal and specific gravity measurements is discussed in Chapter 45.

Osmolality versus Osmolarity

In the literature and in practice, the term osmolarity is frequently used in place of or interchangeably with the term osmolality when speaking of the concentrations of IV solutions or body fluids. This interchange often causes confusion. *Osmolality* is an expression of concentration in terms of 1000 g of water. Accordingly, neither temperature nor space taken up by the solids present in the solution has any bearing on the osmolality figure, and a direct comparison can be made of various body fluids with different water or solids content. On the other hand, such a comparison is not possible when concentration is expressed in terms of 1 L of solution (i.e., *osmolarity*). The amount of water in 1 L of solution is a function both of its temperature and the space occupied by the solids in solution. Inasmuch as colligative properties are determined only by the ratio of solute to solvent particles, the osmolarity of various body fluids is not directly comparable. The difference between osmolality and osmolarity is apparent in the diagram in Fig. 44-13. To make up a 1-osmol solution, 1 g-mole of solute particles is added to a beaker with exactly 1000 g of water. The volume of the solution is thus greater than 1 L. The 1-osmolar solution is made by first adding 1 g-mole of solute particles to the beaker and then sufficient water to reach the 1-L mark. Thus the volume of the solute is included in the solution. It is obvious that the concentrations of the two solutions are not equal. The difference between osmolality and osmolarity is negligible in the range of concentration and temperature of body fluids. It is, however, important to use osmolal units of concentration in the accurate preparation of IV solutions.

It is the function of the kidneys to keep the concentration of the body fluids constant at 285 mOsm. How this function is accomplished is explored in the following sections.

Isoosmotic Reabsorption in the Proximal Tubule

When the glomerular filtrate first enters the proximal tubule, it has the same concentration as the plasma has— 285 mOsm. The filtrate is therefore called *isoosmotic.* Along the proximal tubule, 67% to 80% of the filtrate is reabsorbed into the peritubular capillaries. This reabsorption is isoosmotic, because both water and solutes are reabsorbed in the same proportion as they exist in the filtrate. So, at the end of the proximal tubule, the concentration of the filtrate is still 285 mOsm, and about 20% of the filtrate still remains (Fig. 44-14). Even though the flow has been significantly reduced (from 125 to about 25 ml/min), urine excretion directly out of the proximal tubule would be about 1500 ml/hr. At this rate of urine excretion, death would occur within a few hours from dehydration, because a loss of 12% to 14% of the body weight in water is fatal. The next step in the process of urine formation is to greatly reduce the volume of the filtrate before it is expelled as urine.

Countercurrent Mechanism

In the kidney, there are two types of nephrons—the cortical and the juxtamedullary (next to the medulla), illustrated in Fig. 44-15. The juxtamedullary nephron has a much longer hoop of Henle than the cortical nephron, and its peritubular blood supply is in the form of hairpin loops of vessels that dip down beside the loop of Henle. These blood vessels are called the *vasa recta.* These anatomic features of the juxtamedullary nephrons largely account for the concentration of urine. In fact, the longer the hairpin loop is, the greater the concentrating ability of an animal will be. The kangaroo rat, a desert rodent, has unusually long loops and can excrete urine with an osmolality of about 6000 mOsm. In humans, about one of seven nephrons is juxtamedullary, with long loops, and the maximum concentration of urine is about 1400 mOsm.

The countercurrent mechanism, which is responsible for the conservation of water by the kidney, actually involves two basic processes: (1) the countercurrent multiplier of concentration in the loop of Henle and (2) the countercurrent exchanger in the vasa recta, which also takes the form of a hairpin loop. The loop of Henle makes the interstitial fluid in the medulla hyperosmotic

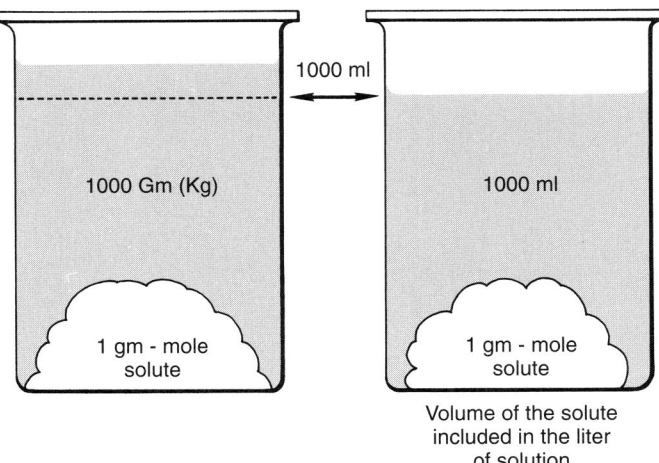

FIG. 44-13 Osmolality versus osmolarity. Osmolality *(left)* is an expression of concentration in terms of 1000 g of water. Osmolarity *(right)* is concentration expressed in terms of 1000 ml of solution. Osmolality is approximately equal to osmolarity for dilute solutions when the volume occupied by the solute is small.

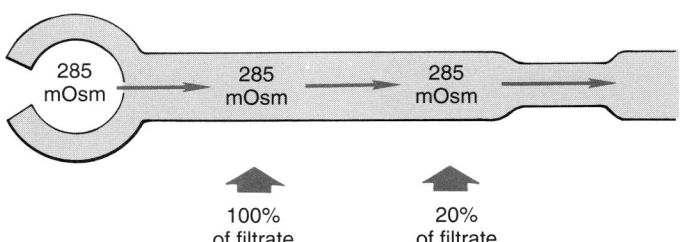

FIG. 44-14 Eighty percent isoosmotic reabsorption of the globular filtrate in the proximal tube.

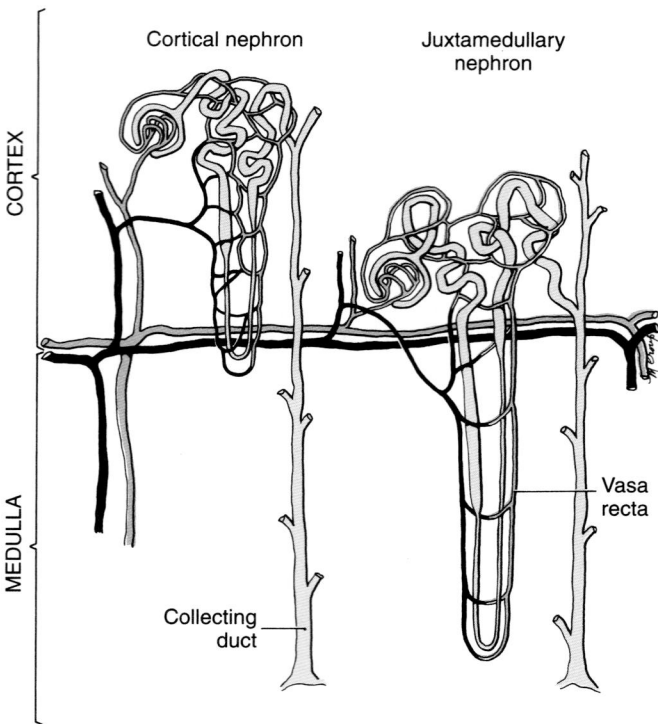

FIG. 44-15 Cortical and juxtaglomerular nephrons with vasa recta.

and the tubular fluid that emerges from it into the distal tubule hypoosmotic; these changes permit the concentration of the final urine to be modified over a wide range. The vasa recta blood vessels prevent the dissipation of the osmotic gradient in the medullary interstitial fluid that has been built up by the loop of Henle. Along the nephron, the fundamental processes involved in the production of a concentrated or dilute urine are the active reabsorption of Cl⁻ in the ascending limb of Henle and the variable permeability to the passive diffusion of water and urea along their concentration gradients.

First, the overall relationships during the production of concentrated urine is examined (Fig. 44-16). Beginning at the glomerulus, where filtration starts, the filtrate is isoosmotic with the plasma at 285 mOsm (rounded to 300 mOsm in the diagram). By the end of the proximal tubule, 80% of the filtrate has been reabsorbed, although the concentration is still 285 mOsm. As the filtrate moves down the descending limb of Henle, its concentration reaches a maximum at the tip of the loop. Then, as it moves up the ascending limb, the filtrate becomes more and more dilute until it is hypoosmotic at the top of the limb. As it proceeds along the distal tubule, the filtrate becomes more concentrated, until it is isoosmotic with the blood plasma at the top of the collecting duct. As the filtrate moves down the collecting duct, it again becomes increasingly concentrated. At the end of the collecting duct, about 99% of the water has

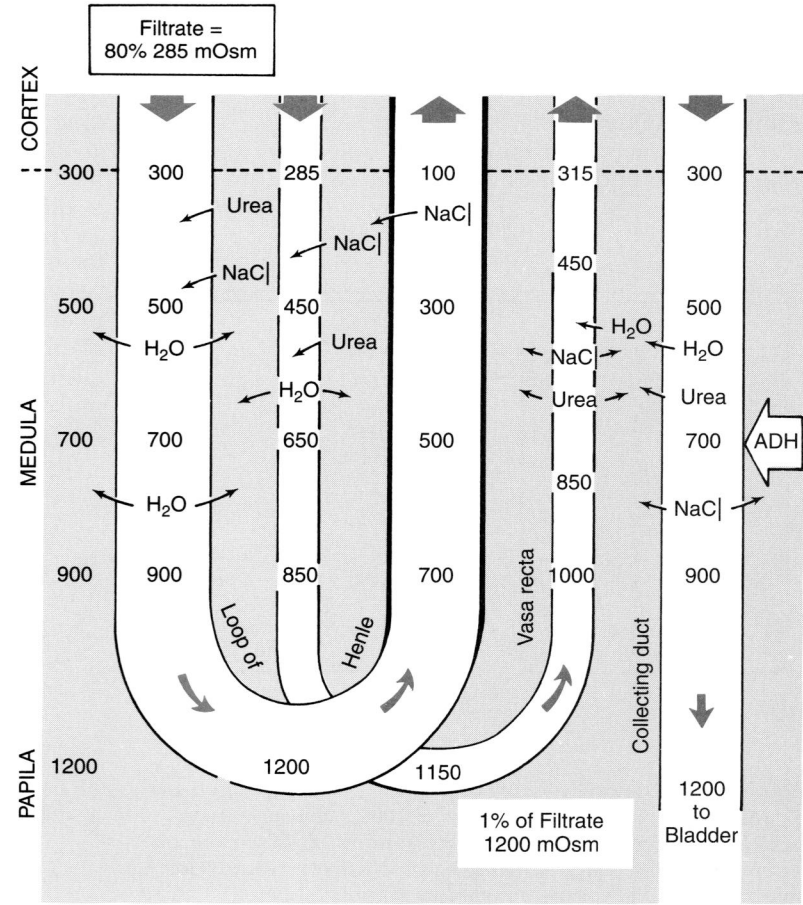

FIG. 44-16 Countercurrent mechanism. Summary of passive and active exchanges of water and ions in the nephron in the course of elaboration of hyperosmotic urine. Concentrations of tubular urine, peritubular fluid, and blood in vasa recta are in milliosmoles per liter. Boxed numbers represent proportion of glomerular filtrate within the tubule at each level. *ADH*, Antidiuretic hormone. (Modified from Netter FH: Kidneys, ureters, and urinary bladder. In *The Ciba collection of medical illustrations*, vol 6, West Caldwell, NJ, 1973, Ciba Medical Education Division.)

been reabsorbed, and about 1% of the filtrate is excreted as urine.

Of particular note on the diagram is that there is also a concentration gradient in the interstitial fluid, increasing from the cortex to the medulla. The vasa recta that dip down beside the loop of Henle also have a concentration gradient that increases as it goes down the descending limb and decreases as it moves up the ascending limb, although the decrease is much less than it is in the ascending limb of Henle. Also of note is that the limbs of the loop of Henle form parallel columns and that the filtrate flow is in opposite directions. This feature is known as *countercurrent flow* and allows the loop of Henle to function as a countercurrent multiplier, building up the concentration gradient in the interstitium. (The principle of countercurrent multiplication is reviewed in Fig. 44-17.) The entire process may now be described in greater detail.

The operation of the countercurrent multiplier in the loop of Henle is initiated by the active transport of Cl⁻ out of the ascending limb. This causes Na⁺ to passively follow down the potential gradient created by the active Cl⁻

transport. Water, however, cannot passively follow the NaCl transport, because the ascending limb is impermeable to water (indicated by the heavy lines in Fig. 44-16). Consequently, the filtrate becomes hypoosmotic as the top of the ascending limbs is approached. The interstitial fluid becomes more concentrated, setting up an osmotic gradient between the interstitial fluid and the descending limb of Henle. Water flows out of the descending limb and NaCl passively enters, causing the filtrate to become increasingly concentrated. As this process continues, a concentration gradient increasing from cortex to medulla is established in the descending limb of Henle and the interstitium until a steady state is reached.

The vasa recta, which dip down beside the loop of Henle, act as a countercurrent exchanger by passive diffusion (active transport is not involved). The blood in the vasa recta is in osmotic equilibrium with the interstitial fluid. As blood flows through the descending limb of the vasa recta, NaCl passively moves in and water moves out, causing the blood to become increasingly concentrated as it approaches the tip of the loop. In the ascending limb of

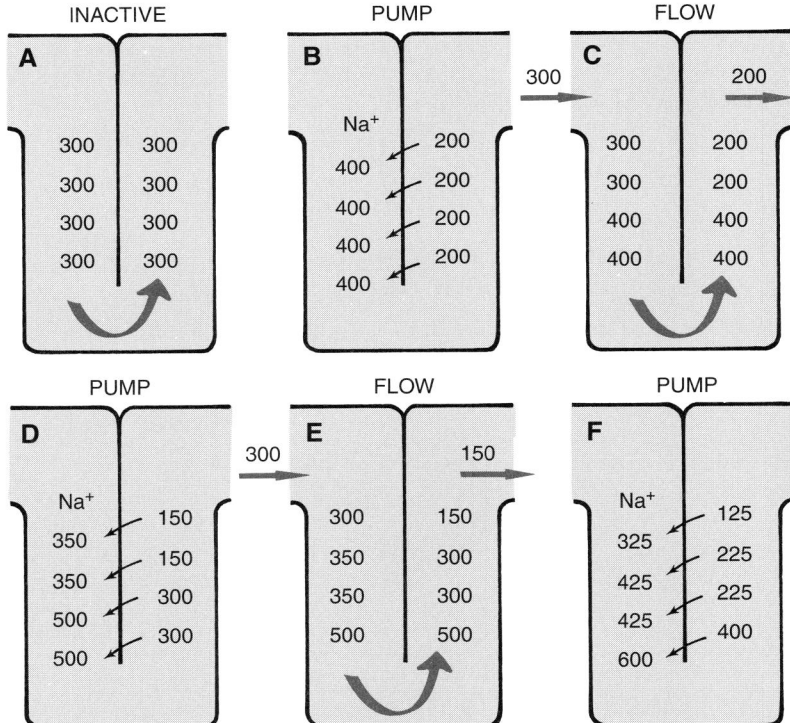

FIG. 44-17 Principle of countercurrent multiplication of concentration is based on the assumption that at any level along the loop of Henle, a gradient of 200 mOsm can be achieved between the limbs by active transport of chloride and passive diffusion of sodium ions. The changes in the concentration along the loop are illustrated in a series of discontinuous steps. *Step A:* multiplier not active, filtrate enters at 300 mOsm. *Step B:* flow stopped, ion pump activated, generating a horizontal gradient of 200 mOsm between the limbs. *Step C:* flow started, more filtrate enters at 300 mOsm, pushing some fluid around the tip from the descending to ascending limb; some fluid is ejected. *Step D:* flow stopped, ion pump activated, generating another gradient of 200 mOsm between the limbs. *Step E:* more filtrate enters at 300 mOsm, pushing filtrate around the tip from descending to ascending limb. *Step F:* flow stopped; ion pump activated, generating another gradient of 200 mOsm between the limbs; note that the concentration of the filtrate at the tip of the loop is now 600 mOsm, and there is a longitudinal gradient of 275 mOsm, whereas the ion pump was only able to generate a horizontal gradient of 200 mOsm. Continuation of this process further increases the longitudinal gradient. (Modified from Pitts RF: *Physiology of the kidney and body fluids,* ed 3, Chicago, 1974, Mosby.)

the vasa recta, opposite events occur. Na$^+$ passively diffuses out into the interstitium while water is reabsorbed into the blood vessel and is returned to the general circulation. The fact that the blood flow through the vasa recta is sluggish allows it to act as an efficient exchanger (recalling that the medulla receives only 10% of the blood supply to the kidney). If the blood flow were rapid, the NaCl that entered the descending limb would be washed away. Thus the vasa recta, acting as a countercurrent exchanger, prevent the dissipation of the concentration gradient in the interstitium built up by the loop of Henle, which acts as a countercurrent multiplier of concentration.

Along the distal tubule, Na$^+$ (Cl$^-$) is actively reabsorbed. Under conditions of antidiuresis, the hypoosmotic filtrate at the beginning of the distal tubule becomes isoosmotic by the time it reaches the top of the collecting duct. The final concentration of urine takes place in the distal tubule and collecting ducts under the control of ADH. The distal tubule and collecting ducts are permeable to water in the presence of ADH. Water diffuses out into the interstitium in response to the osmotic gradient in the medulla and then enters the ascending limb of the vasa recta and is returned to the general circulation. The final urine produced is low in volume and high in osmotic concentration.

In contrast, under conditions of diuresis and in the absence of ADH, the distal tubule and collecting ducts are virtually impermeable to water. Na$^+$ (Cl$^-$) is actively reabsorbed from the distal tubule and collecting ducts, but water does not diffuse out to maintain osmotic equilibrium. Because Na$^+$ is reabsorbed and water is left behind, a large volume of dilute urine is produced.

Urea also diffuses out of the collecting ducts into the interstitial fluid, where it contributes to the high osmotic concentration in the medulla. Some of the urea also enters the descending limb of the loop of Henle and the vasa recta and is recirculated. The effect is to trap urea in the medullary interstitium. A person on a low-protein diet is unable to concentrate urine as efficiently as would a person on a normal or high-protein diet, because urea is the end-product of protein metabolism.

Antidiuretic Hormone Mechanism for the Regulation of Plasma Osmolality

The ADH mechanism helps maintain the volume and osmolality of the ECF at a constant level by controlling the final volume and osmolality of the urine (see also Chapter 20). Deviations of the ECF volume or osmolality from normal values control the release of ADH. ADH is produced in the supraoptic nuclei of the hypothalamus and descends along nerve fibers to the posterior pituitary, where it is stored for subsequent release. ADH is controlled by a feedback mechanism with two pathways (Fig. 44-18).

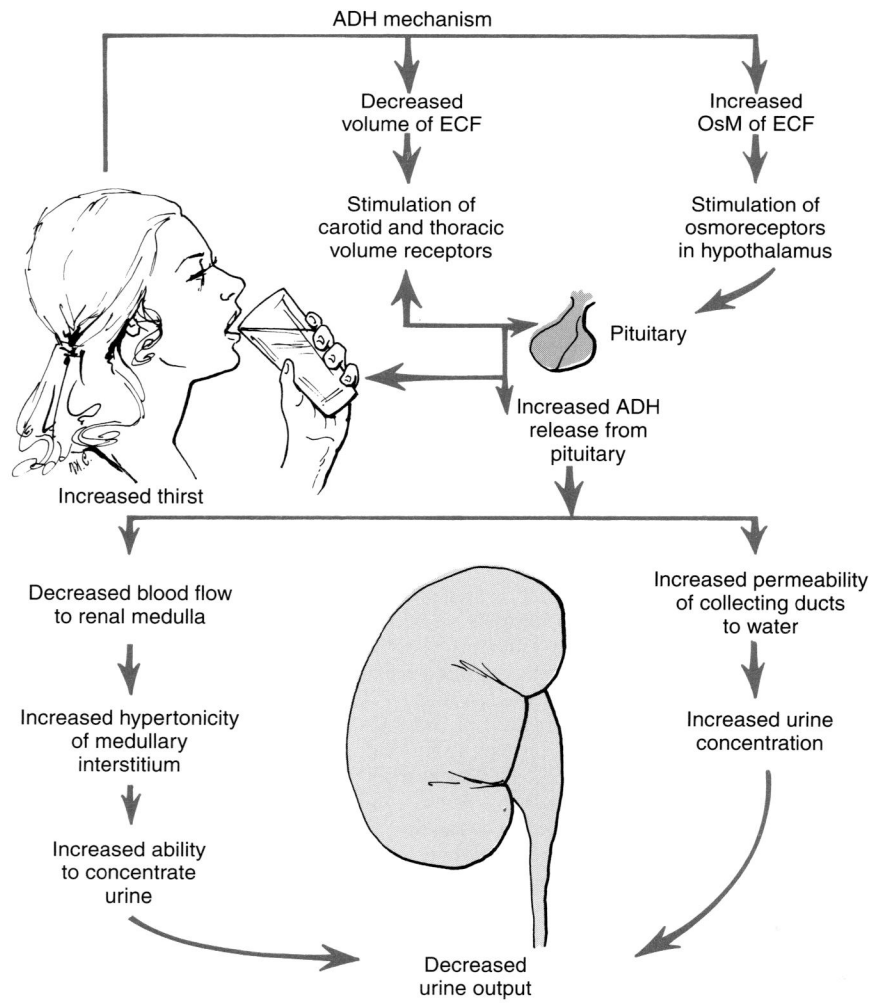

FIG. 44-18 Antidiuretic hormone *(ADH)* mechanism for the regulation of plasma osmolality. *ECF,* Extracellular fluid.

ADH release is stimulated by an increase in the ECF osmolality (from the ideal 285 mOsm) or a decrease in ECF volume. Increased osmolality or decreased ECF volume, for example, may be caused by factors such as water deprivation; fluid loss from vomiting, diarrhea, burns, or sweating; or displacement of fluid as in ascites. The subjective feeling of thirst is also stimulated by a decrease in ECF volume or an increase in ECF osmolality. For example, increased thirst is a common symptom in a person who is hemorrhaging (decreased ECF volume) or in the person who has just eaten a candy bar (increased ECF osmolality because of more glucose particles in the blood).

Osmoreceptor cells located in the hypothalamus near the supraoptic nuclei sense as little as a 1% to 2% change in the osmolality of the blood in the internal carotid circulation. Neuronal signals from the osmoreceptor then stimulate the release of ADH from the pituitary gland and simultaneously stimulate thirst. The centers that mediate thirst are located in the hypothalamus. Actions of ADH in the kidney augment the key events that occur in the loop of Henle by two related mechanisms: (1) blood flow through the vasa recta of the medulla is diminished by the presence of ADH, thus minimizing solute depletion in the interstitium; and (2) ADH increases the permeability of the collecting ducts, so that more water diffuses out to equilibrate with the hyperosmotic interstitial fluid. The net effect of these two mechanisms is increased water reabsorption and excretion of a small volume of concentrated urine. Drinking water and conservation of water by the kidneys both aid in the restoration of the ECF osmolality to normal.

When the ECF volume is reduced by about 10%, water repletion is activated as a means of restoring ECF volume regardless of ECF osmolality. In this case, baroreceptors in the arterial and venous circulations stimulate ADH release through neuronal pathways. This nonosmotic stimulation of ADH occurs independently of osmoreceptor function. Thirst is also stimulated but is probably mediated through angiotensin II (see following discussion). The ECF volume stimulus for ADH release can override the osmotic stimuli, so that significant ECF volume depletion is a cardinal cause of hyponatremia.

Conversely, low ECF osmolality or volume expansion from increased water intake activates mechanisms that counterregulate water conservation. Thirst is suppressed, and ADH release is inhibited. PGE$_2$, a prostaglandin produced in the kidney, inhibits the action of ADH on the collecting ducts. The net effect of these processes is decreased water intake and the excretion of a greater volume of dilute urine.

Even in extreme cases of a huge volume of fluid ingestion or of limited fluid intake, normal humans have amazing flexibility in maintaining the osmolality of the ECF at a constant 285 mOsm. To accomplish this task, humans are able to excrete urine as dilute as 40 mOsm or as concentrated as 1200 to 1400 mOsm. As will be shown later, the patient with renal insufficiency loses this great flexibility.

Regulation of Body Sodium Content
Renin-Angiotensin-Aldosterone System

Regulation of the effective circulating volume (ECV) or ECF volume is achieved primarily through the modification of urinary Na$^+$ excretion in contrast to the regulation of ECF osmolality, which is achieved through alterations of water balance. Na$^+$ handling is not directly involved in osmoregulation unless there are also concurrent changes in volume. Osmolality is determined by the ratio of solutes (mostly Na$^+$ and K$^+$ salts) to water, whereas the ECF volume is determined by the absolute amounts of Na$^+$ and water present. The renin-angiotensin-aldosterone mechanism plays a major role in regulation of body Na$^+$ content.

Renin is the first enzyme in the biochemical cascade of the renin-angiotensin-aldosterone system. The function of this system is maintenance of ECF volume and tissue perfusion pressure by altering vascular resistance and renal Na$^+$ and water excretion. Renal hypoperfusion, produced by hypotension and volume depletion, and increased sympathetic activity are the major stimuli to renin secretion, as shown on the top of the diagram in Fig. 44-19. Input from the JGA of the nephron, which serves as an intrarenal baroreceptor and a chemoreceptor of distal tubular NaCl delivery, was described previously. Input to the central nervous system (CNS) is provided by centrally located baroreceptors via the vagus and glossopharyngeal nerves, which, in turn, influence sympathetic outflow: baroreceptors located within the low-pressure cardiac atria and pulmonary vasculature respond primarily to the volume or fullness of the vascular tree. Increased intravascular volume distends the cardiac atria and leads to a decrease in renal sympathetic activity and the release of atrial natriuretic peptide (see later discussion), both of which increase renal Na$^+$ excretion. Decreased intravascular volume has the opposite effect. Baroreceptors located within the high-pressure aortic arch and carotid sinus respond primarily to arterial blood pressure. A decline in blood pressure produces an increase in renal sympathetic activity, leading to Na$^+$ and water retention. An increase in intravascular pressure has the opposite effect.

The release of renin from the JG cells into the circulation initiates a sequence of events that begins with cleavage of the substrate angiotensinogen (a serum glycoprotein produced by the liver) into angiotensin I. Angiotensin I is then converted into angiotensin II by angiotensin-converting enzyme (ACE) found in high concentration in the lungs but also present in a variety of sites, including the kidney. Once generated, angiotensin II has two major systemic effects: arteriolar vasoconstriction and enhanced renal Na$^+$ and water reabsorption by the distal tubules and collecting ducts. The second effect is mediated by increased aldosterone secretion by the adrenal cortex, stimulated by angiotensin II. Both of these actions will tend to correct the hypovolemia or hypotension (thus restoring tissue perfusion) that is usually responsible for the stimulation of renin secretion.

The cardiac atria possess an additional mechanism for the control of renal Na$^+$ excretion and ECF volume that is counterregulatory to the renin-angiotensin-aldosterone mechanism. The cardiac atria synthesize a hormone called *atrial natriuretic peptide (ANP)*, which is then stored in granules. ANP is released from the atrial granules in response to stretch (i.e., increased ECF volume). ANP induces Na$^+$ and water excretion by the kidneys. This diuretic effect is mediated by its vasodilatory

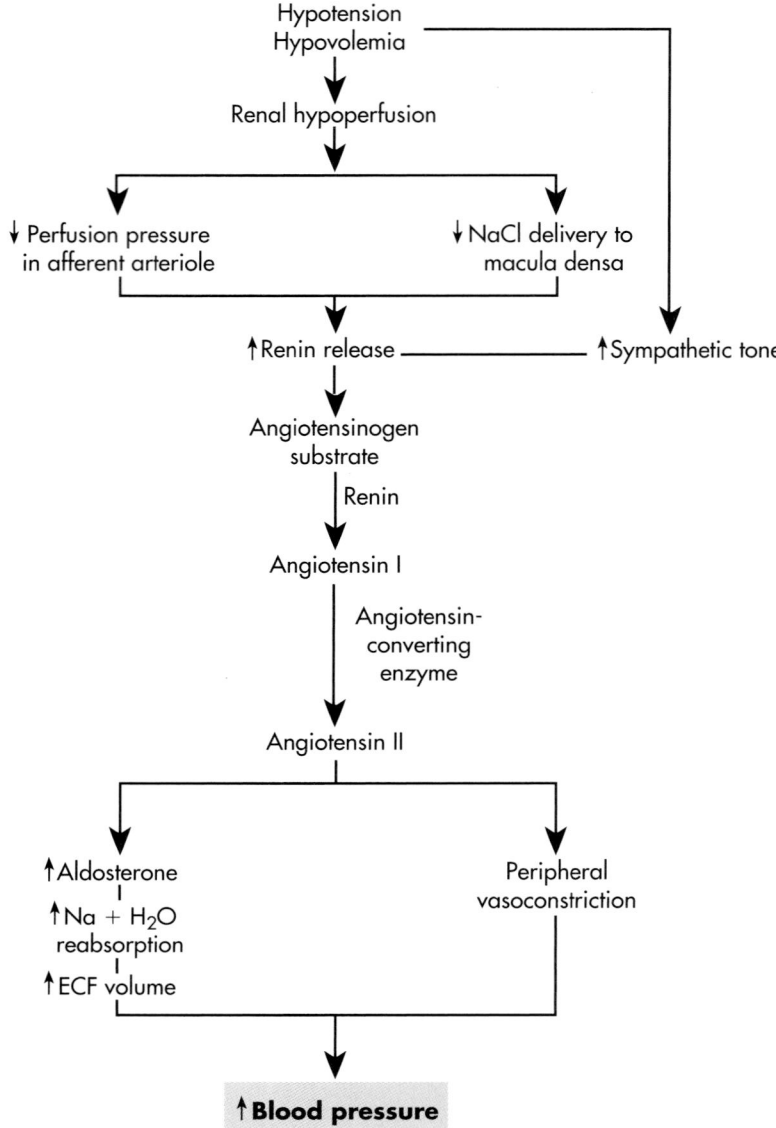

FIG. 44-19 Renin-angiotensin-aldosterone system.
ECF, Extracellular fluid.

properties, resulting in enhanced renal blood flow (RBF) and its suppressive action on aldosterone and ADH secretion.

Functions of the Kidney

The major functions of the kidneys are summarized in Box 44-1, which emphasizes their regulatory role in the body. The kidneys do excrete certain foreign chemicals (e.g., drugs), hormones, and other metabolites, but their most important function is maintaining the volume and composition of the ECF within normal limits. This task is accomplished, of course, by varying the excretion of water and solutes, and the high filtration rate allows great precision in this function. Renin and erythropoietin production and vitamin D metabolism are all important nonexcretory functions. Excessive renin secretion, which may be important in the cause of some forms of hyper-

tension, is discussed in Chapter 46. Deficiency of erythropoietin and vitamin D activation, believed to be important in the cause of anemia and bone disease in uremia, are discussed in Chapter 47.

The kidneys also play an important role in degradation of insulin and production of a group of compounds of possible endocrine significance—the prostaglandins. About 20% of the insulin produced by the pancreas is degraded by the renal tubular cells. Consequently, patients with diabetes and renal failure may require less insulin. Prostaglandins are unsaturated fatty acid hormones present in many tissues of the body. The renal medulla produces PGI and PGE_2, which are potent vasodilators. Prostaglandins may play a role in the regulation of RBF, renin release, and Na^+ reabsorption. It is also possible that prostaglandin deficiency may contribute to some forms of secondary renal hypertension, although there is insufficient evidence of this at present.

KEY CONCEPTS

- Acute and chronic renal failure are major causes of morbidity and mortality. Renal failure is the eighth leading cause of death in the United States.
- The four leading causes of ESRD are diabetes, hypertension, glomerulonephritis, and polycystic kidney disease. The annual cost of dialysis and renal transplant treatment for nearly 400,000 patients with ESRD is about $16.7 billion.
- The kidneys have a retroperitoneal position in front of the eleventh and twelfth ribs, making them vulnerable to a contusion or slicing injury in major traumatic accidents.
- Ninety percent of *renal perfusion* is distributed to the cortex and 10% to the medulla; the relative ischemia of the medulla is important for the kidney's ability to concentrate urine but also makes the interstitium vulnerable to drug toxicity.
- The functional work unit of the kidney is the *nephron*; there are about one million nephrons in each kidney. Renal reserve is large and survival with 1% of the total number of nephrons is possible.
- The *major function of the kidneys* is to regulate volume, osmolality, electrolyte, and acid-base concentrations of body fluids by excreting water and electrolytes in amounts adequate to achieve total body fluid and electrolyte balance and to maintain their normal concentrations in the extracellular fluid (ECF).
- A second function of the kidneys is the excretion of metabolic waste products including urea, uric acid, creatinine, and metabolites of various hormones and drugs.
- The kidneys have an important endocrine function of producing erythropoietin (important for the production of red blood cells), renin (important for the regulation of blood pressure), and 1,25-dihydroxyvitamin D_3 (important in the regulation of Ca^{++} metabolism).
- The kidney performs its major function by ultrafiltration of the plasma at the glomerulus, selective reabsorption and secretion of water and substances filtered along the tubules, and excretion of the excess in the urine.
- The *renin-angiotensin-aldosterone mechanism* is primarily responsible for maintaining blood pressure and tissue perfusion by regulating Na^+ homeostasis.
- The *ADH mechanism* plays a major role in regulating water metabolism and maintaining the normal osmolality of the blood by stimulating thirst and varying renal water excretion and the osmolality of urine.
- Three types of cells make up the *glomerular filtration barrier*: (1) *visceral epithelial cells* form the outer layer of the glomerular capillary and contain podocytes (foot processes) coming in contact with the basement membrane, forming slit pores 400 Å wide; (2) *basement membrane* forms the middle layer of the capillary wall and behaves as if it had pores about 70 to 100 Å in diameter; and (3) *endothelial cells* form the innermost layer of the glomerular capillary and have fenestrations about 600 Å in diameter.
- *Parietal epithelial cells* line Bowman's capsule, and *mesangial cells* (between the capillaries) form a supporting network for the glomerular capillaries and are not part of the glomerular filtration barrier.
- The main determinant of passage through the glomerular filter is molecular size. This complex "membrane" is freely permeable to water and small dissolved solutes, but retains most of the proteins and other large molecules, as well as all blood cells. Filtration also depends on ionic charge, and negatively charged proteins, such as albumin, are retained to a greater extent than would be predicted by size alone. In many renal diseases, proteinuria develops because of a loss of this charge selectivity.
- *Renal blood flow (RBF)* is about 1000 to 1200 ml/min, or 20 to 25% of cardiac output. *Renal plasma flow (RPF)* is approximately 660 ml/min. About 20% of the plasma is filtered through the glomerulus (representing the GFR) into Bowman's capsule as primary urine. All of the plasma elements are filtered, including water, electrolytes, and nonelectrolytes (ultrafiltration), except for blood cells and most of the protein.
- The GFR is an index of renal function and is directly related to the perfusion pressure of RBF. Normal GFR is about 125 ml/min in a young adult male (115 ml/min in an adult female). GFR declines at the rate of about 1 ml/min per year after the age of 30.
- Two thirds of the glomerular ultrafiltrate is reabsorbed isoosmotically in the proximal tubule, and only about 1% is excreted in the final urine.
- Transport of ions or molecules (reabsorption and secretion) along the tubules takes place by active or passive transport mechanisms. Water molecules move by osmosis when there is a concentration gradient of ions or molecules across a semipermeable membrane.
- The distal tubule actively reabsorbs Na^+ and secretes K^+ and H^+ for the regulation of acid-base and electrolyte balance.
- There are two types of nephrons in the kidney: (1) *cortical nephrons* with short loops of Henle are only capable of isoosmotic reabsorption, and (2) *juxtamedullary nephrons* with long loops of Henle (which dip down deep into the medulla) are responsible for countercurrent multiplication and formation of a concentrated urine.
- Excretion of a maximally dilute (hypoosmotic) urine depends on the ability of the kidney to lower the osmolality of the tubular fluid. Tubular fluid osmolality is lowered to about 100 mOsm/kg water in the thick ascending limb of Henle by the Na^+, K^+, Cl^- active co-transporter. Because the thick ascending limb is impermeable to water, tubular fluid becomes hypoosmotic. If the tubular fluid osmolality is 100 mOsm at the beginning of the collecting duct and no ADH is present, urine osmolality will be maintained at 100 mOsm or less as a result of additional NaCl transport in the collecting duct.

- Excretion of a maximally concentrated (hyperosmotic) urine depends on the presence of a high medullary interstitial osmolality. The loop of Henle acts as a *countercurrent multiplier* of concentration, building up a concentration gradient in the medullary interstitium driven by NaCl cotransport in the thick ascending limb. Under conditions of maximal ADH activity, the tubular fluid is able to attain a medullary osmolality of 1200 mOsm/kg water and the excretion of hyperosmotic urine. Water is reabsorbed in the collecting ducts into the vasa recta blood vessels, with hairpin loops dipping down beside the loops of Henle, which act as a *countercurrent exchanger*.
- The *juxtaglomerular apparatus (JGA)* is a compound structure consisting of three types of cells: (1) granular or JG cells are special smooth muscle cells in the walls of the afferent arteriole, which act as intrarenal baroreceptors and secrete renin; (2) macula densa cells located in the portion of the tubule at the point where it courses between the afferent and efferent arterioles of each nephron that are sensitive to Na^+ in tubular fluid and contribute to the control of renin secretion and GFR; and (3) extraglomerular mesangial (lacis) cells.
- The phenomenon whereby RBF and GFR are maintained constant (in spite of changes in the mean arterial pressure) is called *autoregulation*. Autoregulation is effective as arterial blood pressure changes between 90 and 180 mm Hg.
- The glomerular capillaries are interposed between two arterioles: the precapillary afferent arteriole and the postcapillary efferent arterioles. As a result, the capillary intraglomerular pressure (P_{gc}) (which determines GFR) is governed by the interplay of resistances between the afferent and efferent arterioles.
- Two mechanisms are responsible for autoregulation of RBF and GFR: the *myogenic mechanism* in the afferent arteriole and the flow-dependent *tubuloglomerular feedback (TGF)* mechanism.

- An increase in perfusion pressure (as in hypertension) is sensed by the baroreceptors in the afferent arteriole and causes reflex vasoconstriction, thus preventing the elevation in pressure from being transmitted to the glomerulus and thereby preventing any significant change in P_{gc} and GFR. Conversely, GFR can be preserved by vasodilation of the afferent arteriole when renal perfusion falls.
- Angiotensin II makes an important contribution when renal perfusion pressure falls, a situation in which the renin-angiotensin-aldosterone system is activated. Angiotensin II preferentially increases resistance at the efferent arteriole, thereby preventing the P_{gc} and the GFR from declining in the presence of hypotension.
- GFR is, in part, autoregulated by the rate of tubular fluid flow and Na^+ sensed by the macula densa. When GFR decreases and causes a decrease in tubular fluid flow, TGF causes vasodilation of the afferent arteriole, increased secretion of renin and vasoconstriction of the efferent arteriole. Both of these changes will tend to increase GFR, thereby raising macula densa flow toward normal.
- *Atrial natriuretic peptide (ANP)*, a hormone produced by cardiac myocytes, promotes Na^+ excretion by the collecting ducts, an effect opposite to that of the renin-angiotensin-aldosterone system.
- Much of the vasoconstrictor effects of angiotensin II and norepinephrine are counteracted by the vasodilator effects of the prostaglandins (PGE_2 and PGI) and renal resistance changes much less than would otherwise have occurred. The adaptive value of such opposing inputs is to strike a balance, on the one hand, between the need for increased total peripheral resistance, and, on the other hand, the likelihood of renal damage if renal vasoconstriction were too severe.

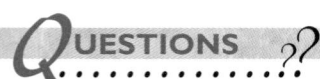

QUESTIONS ??

A sampling of review questions for this chapter appears here. Visit http://www.mosby.com/MERLIN/PriceWilson/ for additional questions.

Label the figures with the appropriate terms from each group.

1. The urinary tract (Fig. 44-20).
   Urinary meatus
   Right kidney
   Left kidney
   Ureter
   Bladder
   Urethra
2. Posterior abdominal wall, vertebrae, and ribs (Fig. 44-21).
   Eleventh rib
   Twelfth rib
   Psoas major muscle
   Transversus abdominis muscle
3. Cross section of the kidney (Fig. 44-22).
   Pyramid
   Ureter
   Renal pelvis

Papilla
Cortex
Minor calyces
Major calyx
Fibrous capsule
Medulla
Column of Bertin

4. The nephron (Fig. 44-23).
   Proximal convoluted tubule
   Distal convoluted tubule
   Collecting duct
   Loop of Henle
   Bowman's capsule
   Macula densa
   JG cells
   Afferent arteriole
   Efferent arteriole
   Glomerular capillary tuft

5. On the diagram for question 2, draw the kidneys in their correct relation to the ribs and vertebrae.
6. Trace the formation and transit of urine from the renal cortex to the bladder by lettering the following structures in sequence.
   _____ Ureter
   _____ Renal pelvis
   _____ Collecting ducts
   _____ Bowman's capsule
   _____ Proximal convoluted tubule
   _____ Bladder
   _____ Minor calyces
   _____ Distal convoluted tubule
   _____ Major calyces
   _____ Papillary ducts of Bellini

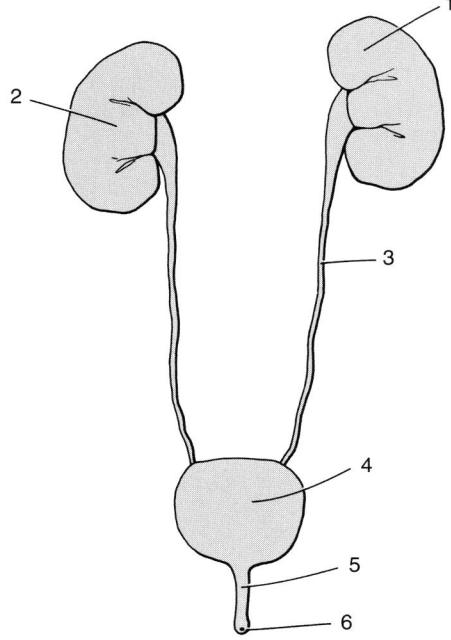

FIG. 44-20   Urinary tract.

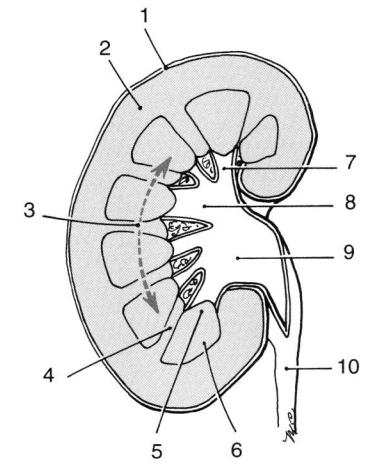

FIG. 44-22   Cross section of the kidney.

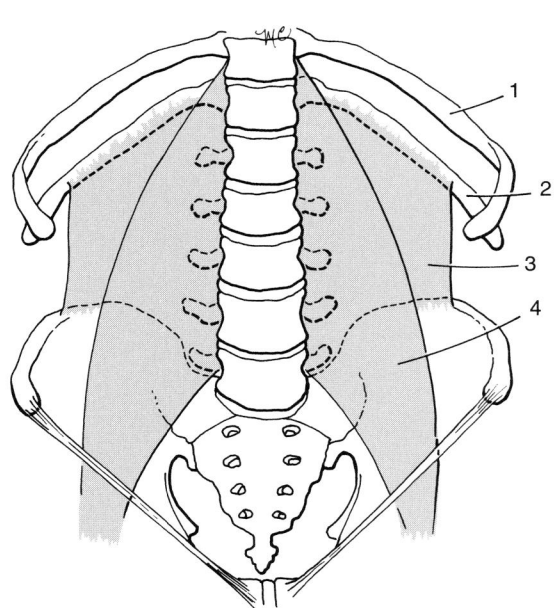

FIG. 44-21   Posterior abdominal wall, vertebrae, ribs.

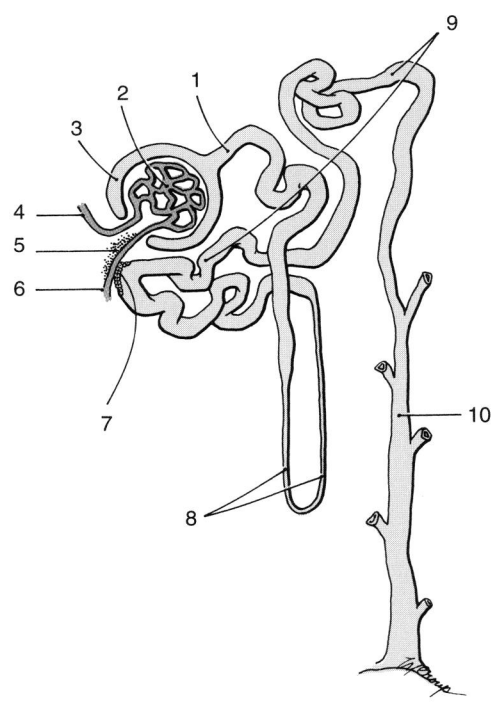

FIG. 44-23   Nephron.

7. This list contains the names of blood vessels supplying and draining the kidneys. Letter it in the correct sequence beginning with the blood vessels supplying the kidney.
_____ Renal vein
_____ Afferent arterioles
_____ Abdominal aorta
_____ Arcuate arteries
_____ Inferior vena cava
_____ Interlobar veins
_____ Glomerular capillaries
_____ Interlobular arterioles
_____ Interlobar arteries
_____ Arcuate veins
_____ Renal artery
_____ Peritubular capillaries (portal network)
_____ Interlobular veins
_____ Efferent arterioles

— — — — — — — — — — — — —

Answer the following on a separate sheet of paper.

8. Why is it especially important to obtain a renal arteriogram in a healthy person who is supplying a donor kidney for transplantation?
9. Explain how the JG cells and macula densa cells help to control blood pressure.
10. Why is a heavy blow over the twelfth rib particularly dangerous to the kidney?
11. Why is glomerular filtration called ultrafiltration?
12. How is net filtration pressure derived?
13. Define and give the normal numeric value of the GFR for men and women.

14. What kind of substance must be used to measure the GFR, and why?
15. During an inulin clearance test, the following values were obtained from a patient: P_{in} 25 mg/dl and U_{in} 500 mg/dl; urine volume 2 ml/min. Calculate this patient's GFR ignoring body surface area. Is it within normal range?
16. What are the two most important functions of the distal tubule and collecting ducts?
17. Explain how the kidneys and lungs work together in the regulation of acid-base balance in the body.

18. How do phosphate excretion and NH_3 secretion contribute to the excretion of acid by the kidney?
19. List the major functions of the kidney.
20. How are the four colligative properties of a solution affected by the addition of particles to water?
21. What does the osmometer measure? The urinometer? Which is the most accurate in estimating concentration and why?
22. Write the formula to calculate plasma osmotic concentration from the freezing point. Given that plasma freezes at

$-0.53°$ C, calculate the concentration of plasma in milliosmols.
23. Draw a cortical and juxtamedullary nephron, illustrating their position in relation to the cortex and medulla.
24. What are the vasa recta and what do they do?
25. What is the purpose of the countercurrent mechanism? What are the two basic processes involved?

Match the regulating factors in column A with the correct response in column B to a sudden decrease in the ECV secondary to the loss of 800 ml of blood.

Column A	Column B
26. _____ Renin-angiotensin	a. Increase
27. _____ Aldosterone	b. Decrease
28. _____ Atrial natriuretic peptide	
29. _____ ADH	
30. _____ PGE_2	
31. _____ Sensation of thirst	

Match the correct estimated pressures in column B with the proper glomerular filtration forces in column A.

Column A	Column B
32. _____ Glomerular hydrostatic pressure	a. 50 mm Hg
33. _____ Colloid osmotic pressure	b. 30 mm Hg
34. _____ Net filtration pressure	c. 10 mm Hg
35. _____ Hydrostatic pressure in Bowman's capsule	

Diagnostic Procedures in Renal Disease

LORRAINE M. WILSON

BIOCHEMICAL METHODS

This chapter discusses some of the commonly performed diagnostic tests for the detection of renal disease and evaluation of renal function. These tests are divided into methods that are predominantly biochemical or predominantly morphologic. These diagnostic tests are especially important in the detection of renal disease, because many serious renal diseases do not produce symptoms until renal function is significantly impaired.

Chemical Examination of Urine

Chemical testing of the urine has been greatly simplified by the introduction of impregnated paper strips that detect substances such as glucose, acetone, bilirubin, protein, and blood. A dipstick test can also measure the pH of the urine. Of particular importance in renal disease are the detection of protein or blood in the urine, the measurement of osmolality or specific gravity, and microscopic examination of the urine (discussed later under "Morphologic Methods").

Proteinuria

Healthy adults normally excrete small amounts of protein in the urine—up to 150 mg per day—consisting mainly of albumin and Tamm-Horsfall protein. The latter is secreted by the distal tubule. Proteinuria in amounts greater than 150 mg/day is considered pathologic.

Because it is easy to use, the dipstick test (Albustix, Combistix) is the most commonly used screening test for proteinuria. The end of the stick is dipped in urine and removed immediately, and the urine is shaken off by tapping the stick on the side of the container. The result is compared with the color on the label. Grading is from 0 to 4+, indicating the amount of protein in the urine (Box 45-1). Although the dipstick test is generally accurate, there are a number of pitfalls and difficulties in interpretation. Early morning samples are normally more concentrated compared with samples taken later in the day and should preferably be tested for protein. A *trace* response found in an early morning specimen is probably within normal limits, less than 150 mg/day. On the other hand, if the urine *specimen* is collected later in the day and is more dilute (e.g., specific gravity 1.006), a trace response might indicate significant proteinuria. A common cause of a false-positive result in women is contamination of the urine with vaginal secretions. All routine urine examinations should include a simple test for protein for purposes of screening. The dipstick test measurement mostly detects albumin and is insensitive to low–molecular-weight proteins. Currently dipsticks are available to measure microalbuminuria (30 to 200 mg/L), an early marker of glomerular disease. Patients with type 1 and type 2 diabetes should be periodically tested for microalbuminuria (see Chapters 47 and 48). Finally, a more accurate quantitative determination of protein should be carried out in the laboratory on a 24-hour urine specimen whenever there is significant proteinuria.

There are four major mechanisms causing proteinuria: (1) functional, (2) overflow (prerenal), (3) glomerular, and (4) tubular. *Functional proteinuria* may occur in patients with normal kidneys; it refers to a transient increase in protein excretion associated with heavy exercise, fever, or an increase in protein excretion upon assuming the upright posture (orthostatic proteinuria). Orthostatic proteinuria is a benign condition and most common in adolescents. *Overflow proteinuria* occurs with excretion of low–molecular-weight proteins when there is marked overproduction of a particular protein (almost always

Screening Test for Proteinuria

DIPSTICK GRADE	PROTEIN CONCENTRATION (MG/DL)
0	0-5
Trace	5-20
1+	30
2+	100
3+	300
4+	1000

immunoglobulin light chains in multiple myeloma). In this setting, the filtered load is increased to a level that exceeds the normal reabsorptive capacity of the proximal tubule and is increased to the point where the filtered load overwhelms the reabsorptive ability of the proximal tubule. Abnormal immunoglobulins or cryoglobulin fragments found in the urine are called Bence Jones protein and are nephrotoxic. The type of protein excreted may be identified definitively by serum or *urinary protein electrophoresis*.

Once functional and prerenal causes have been ruled out, *persistent proteinuria* implies renal disease. *Glomerular proteinuria* is associated with a number of renal diseases involving the glomerulus. Several mechanisms cause an increase in glomerular permeability, including loss of the size or charge barrier or a change in the glomerular hemodynamics (especially glomerular capillary pressure [P_{gc}]). The glomerulus filtration barrier is composed of three layers (endothelium, basement membrane, and epithelium), which have a series of pores of varying size. Normally, the glomerular membrane only allows proteins of low molecular weight to enter the filtrate (e.g., immunoglobulin light chains, amino acids) and restricts the filtration of macromolecules (e.g., albumin, immunoglobulin G [IgG]). Molecular charge is another important determinant of solute filtration. The glomerular basement membrane contains glycoproteins that are negatively charged. Thus, filtration of albumin, which is negatively charged, is limited in part by electrostatic repulsion. Low–molecular-weight proteins (such as β_2-microglobulin) or positively charged molecules are readily filtered. The renal tubules then reabsorb most of the proteins that are filtered and excrete a small amount that is undetectable on a screening test. Albuminuria is common in the various types of glomerulonephritis.

Heavy proteinuria refers to the passage of 3.5 g/day or more and is the laboratory definition of the nephrotic syndrome (discussed later). Some patients with the nephrotic syndrome may pass as much protein as 20 to 30 g/ day. *Moderate proteinuria* is associated with a broad spectrum of renal diseases; *minimal proteinuria* (less than 1 g/day) is more apt to be associated impaired tubular reabsorption of normally filtered proteins. Examples of renal disease associated with *tubular proteinuria* include a variety of tubulointerstitial diseases, such as chronic pyelonephritis (reflux nephropathy), renal tubular acidosis, Fanconi syndrome, and acute tubular necrosis (ATN).

Hematuria

The dipstick test for occult blood is an excellent screening test for hematuria. Whenever the test is positive, the urine should be examined microscopically. Hematuria is a common finding in a number of renal diseases and pathologic processes in the lower urinary tract, including infections, stones, trauma, and neoplasms. Hematuria is a prominent feature of glomerulonephritis but not of tubulointerstitial disease. The dipstick test is easy for patients to use as they check the course of hematuria during their treatment.

Hydrogen Ion Concentration

In the healthy adult, urine pH ranges widely from 4.5 to 8.0, but the average pooled specimen is quite acidic, at 6.0, because of acidic metabolites produced by the normal breakdown of body tissues and nutrients. The usual diurnal pattern consists of a rise of pH after a meal (alkaline tide) followed by a gradual fall until the next meal is ingested, whereas during normal sleeping hours, the pH reaches its minimum (nocturnal acid tide caused by hypoventilation during sleep). A diet high in animal protein tends to produce an acid urine, whereas a predominantly vegetable diet tends to produce an alkaline urine.

A persistently acidic urine may occur in respiratory or metabolic acidosis and in pyrexia (fever). A persistently alkaline urine is suggestive of urinary tract infection with urea-splitting organisms. For example, in *Proteus* infections, the urine pH is consistently at 8 or higher. Persistently alkaline urine also occurs in renal tubular acidosis (a renal disease in which there is inability to conserve bicarbonate), in potassium depletion, and in Fanconi syndrome (a renal disease in which ammonia excretion is defective).

Although random pH readings are of little diagnostic value, they are helpful in the management of certain clinical conditions in which the pH of the urine should be kept persistently high or low by diet or drugs. Alkaline urine is desirable in the treatment of patients with calculi that form in acid urine, and acid urine is desirable in patients with calculi that form in alkaline urine or those who have urinary tract infections (Table 45-1).

Common stones formed in acid urine are composed of calcium oxalate, uric acid crystals, or cystine. About two thirds of all urinary calculi are of the calcium oxalate type. Idiopathic hypercalciuria is an important predisposing factor. Thiazide diuretics decrease calcium excretion and are quite effective in preventing recurrence. Cystine stones are rare and are related to a hereditary renal tubular transport disorder involving certain amino acids. Cystine, a metabolic product of dietary methionine, is the least soluble of the naturally occurring amino acids. The excess urinary excretion of cystine (cystinuria) in an acid urine results in cystine urolithiasis. Treatment of this disorder is directed toward a reversal of risk factors by forced hydration and administration of bicarbonate or acetazolamide (Diamox) to maintain the urine pH above 7.5. A low-salt diet can reduce cystine excretion by 40% (Asplin et al, 1998). Hyperuricemia leading to uric acid crystallization is a particular hazard in patients who are receiving cytotoxic drugs for cancer or leukemia. Uric acid is formed principally as an end product of nucleoprotein metabolism. With increasing proliferation and destruction of cells, a proportional increase in uric acid occurs because of degradation of cellular nucleoproteins. The physician may order the administration of sodium bicarbonate or citrate to alkalinize the urine. It is impor-

TABLE 45-1

Factors Contributing to the Formation of Urinary Tract Calculi and Their Prevention

Urinary Stone Content	Predisposing Factors	Preventative Therapy to Achieve Desired Urine pH*
	ACID URINE	**ALKALINE URINE (PH>6)**
Calcium oxalate	Hypercalciuria	Vegetables, milk, fruit (except plums, prunes, cranberries)
Uric acid crystals	Chemotherapy, gout	Sodium bicarbonate or citrate
Cystine	Aminoaciduria	—
	ALKALINE URINE	**ACID URINE**
Triple phosphate	Urinary tract infection	Meat, breads, protein foods, cranberry juice, prunes, plums
Calcium phosphate	Hypercalciuria	Mandelamine
	Prolonged immobility	

*High fluid intake is the most important preventive measure against all calculi.

tant to encourage a high fluid intake in these patients, especially before bedtime, when the urine normally becomes more acidic, to prevent crystallization of uric acid in the renal tubules and interstitium and consequent obstruction. Some foods that help alkalinize the urine are milk, vegetables, and fruits (except prunes, plums, and cranberries).

Common stones formed in alkaline urine are composed of calcium phosphate or magnesium ammonium phosphate (triple-phosphate or struvite stones). Calcium phosphate or oxalate is often present in triple-phosphate stones. Triple-phosphate stones are often associated with urinary tract infections, especially with urea-splitting organisms. These stones occasionally grow to occupy the entire pelvicalyceal system (see Fig. 3-11). Such a stone, referred to as a "staghorn" calculus because of its shape, must be removed surgically. Because 90% of all calculi contain calcium, hypercalciuria is an important predisposing cause. Hypercalciuria is associated with hyperparathyroidism, renal tubular acidosis, and prolonged immobilization, all of which are associated with mobilization of calcium salts from bone. Meat, bread, protein foods, cranberry juice, plums, and prunes tend to produce an acid urine and thus help prevent the formation of these stones. The physician may order a drug such as methenamine mandelate (Mandelamine) to acidify the urine for persistent urinary tract infections. Probably the most important factor in the prevention of all stones regardless of composition is a high fluid intake sufficient to produce a urine output of 2.5 to 3 L/day.

The pH of the urine may be tested by using Squibb Nitrazine paper or a dipstick test. The following points should be kept in mind while performing this test: (1) only fresh urine should be used (when urine is allowed to stand, urea breaks down to ammonia and the pH becomes more alkaline); (2) the test strip should be removed promptly after being dipped in the urine to avoid washing out the test reagent; and (3) the color comparison with the standard should be made immediately in good light (daylight is preferable, and fluorescent light should be avoided).

Specific Gravity

Specific gravity is commonly measured in the clinical unit to determine the concentration of urine. Specific gravity is measured by the flotation of the hydrometer or urinometer in a cylinder of urine (Fig. 45-1). The proper

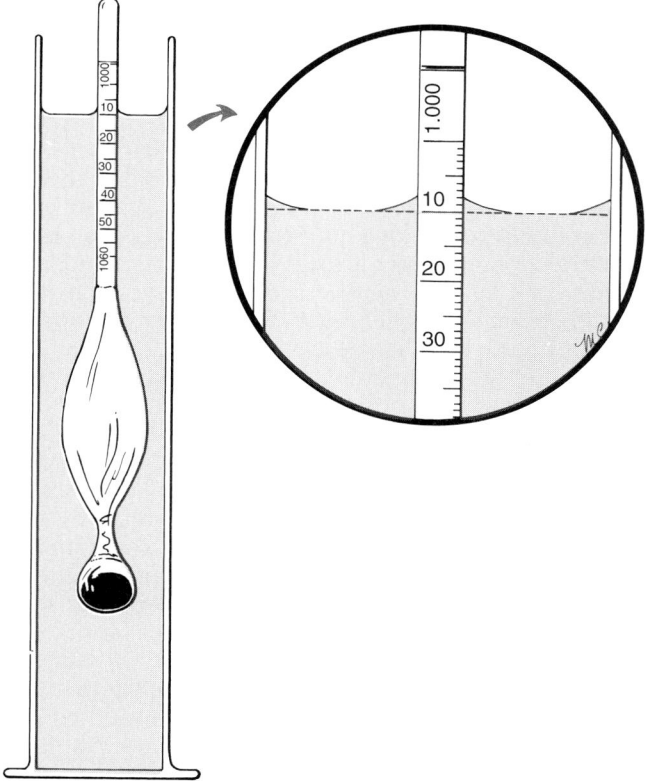

FIG. 45-1   Urinometer with scale featured.

procedure for measuring the specific gravity of urine is as follows:

1. Check the accuracy of the urinometer against distilled water to read 1.000 at its calibration temperature. Most urinometers are calibrated at a temperature of 16° C (60.8° F). This procedure is necessary because the density of water changes with temperature.
2. Fill the cylinder about three fourths full of well-mixed urine. A uniform solution is necessary because solute concentration is being measured.
3. Give the urinometer a gentle spin as it is plunged into the urine to avoid errors of surface tension at the stem and to prevent it from adhering to the sides of the cylinder.

4. Read from top to bottom. The urinometer is calibrated in units of 0.001, starting with 1.000 at the top and progressing downward to 1.060. The correct reading is at the level of the bottom of the meniscus, which should be read at eye level.
5. Correct the specific gravity reading if the temperature of the specimen deviates from the calibration temperature of the urinometer. Use a thermometer to determine the actual temperature of the urine. Add 0.001 to the reading for every 3° C (5.4° F) above the calibration temperature and subtract 0.001 for each 3° C below. For example, if a urinometer calibrated at 16° C is placed in a freshly voided urine specimen with a temperature of 31° C (88° F) and shows a reading of 1.015, then 0.005 is added to the reading.

$$31° C - 16° C = 15° C \times \frac{0.001}{3° C} = 0.005$$

The true specific gravity corrected for temperature is 1.020.

Although specific gravity measurement is simple and convenient, it is important to realize that density is being measured. The density depends on the weight, as well as on the number of solute particles in solution. The kidney's capacity to concentrate, however, is related to the concentration of particles in solution (i.e., osmolality) and not to their weight. True concentration, osmolality, is measured by freezing point depression or vapor pressure lowering, although this is more expensive and time consuming to measure.

Fortunately, when urine contains only normal constituents (mainly sodium chloride [NaCl]), the correlation between specific gravity and osmolality is sufficiently close to use specific gravity as a clinical guide to the osmolality of the urine. The relation between specific gravity and the osmolality of urine is shown in Fig. 45-2. When the urine contains normal constituents (middle line), a specific gravity of 1.010 corresponds to the osmolality of the blood at 285 mOsm. When given large amounts of water, the healthy person can excrete urine with a minimum specific gravity of 1.001 (about 40 mOsm). When deprived of fluid, maximum specific gravity is about 1.040 (1300 mOsm). If the urine should contain glucose or protein (dense particles), the specific gravity would be greater at a fixed osmolality than it would in normal urine (shifted toward the pure glucose curve); and conversely, if the urine contains much urea (a less dense molecule), the specific gravity will be lower. For example, at a concentration of 400 mOsm, the specific gravity of urine with normal constituents is about 1.013. At the same osmolality, if the urine contained a large amount of protein or glucose, the specific gravity would be about 1.030; if it contained a large amount of urea, the specific gravity would be about 1.007. These factors must be considered when the specific gravity measurement is used to estimate the ability of the kidneys to concentrate urine.

In chronic renal disease, the kidney first loses the ability to concentrate urine. Later, the ability to dilute urine is lost as well, so that the specific gravity of urine becomes fixed near 1.010 (the specific gravity of the plasma). This lost ability to dilute urine generally occurs when 80% of the nephron mass has been destroyed.

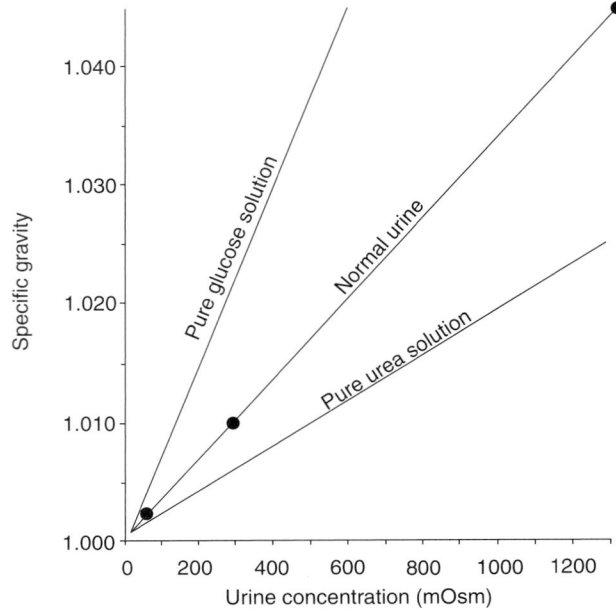

FIG. 45-2 Relationship between specific gravity and osmolality of the urine. (Modified from De Wardner HE: *The kidney*, ed 4, New York, 1973, Churchill Livingstone.)

Glomerular Filtration Rate

One of the most important indices of renal function is the glomerular filtration rate (GFR), which indicates the amount of functioning renal tissue. As noted in Chapter 44, the most accurate way to measure the GFR is by means of the inulin clearance test. However, this test is infrequently used in the clinical unit because it involves an intravenous infusion at a constant rate and timed collections of urine by catheterization. The endogenous creatinine clearance test by comparison is much simpler to carry out.

Creatinine Clearance Test

Creatinine is an end product of muscle metabolism that is liberated from the muscles at a virtually constant rate and is excreted in the urine at the same rate. The plasma (serum) level is therefore nearly constant, ranging from 0.7 to 1.5 mg/dl (the value is higher in men than it is in women because of men's greater muscle mass). Creatinine is excreted in the urine by filtration at the glomerulus, but it is not reabsorbed by the tubules. A small amount, however, is secreted by the tubules, especially when serum creatinine levels are high. Despite the small amount secreted, the creatinine clearance test is a convenient test from which to estimate the GFR in the clinical unit. To perform the creatinine clearance test, it is only necessary to collect a 24-hour urine specimen and a blood specimen during the same 24-hour period (Fig. 45-3). Creatinine clearance (C_{cr}) is then calculated from the clearance formula:

$$C_{cr} = \frac{U_{cr} \times V}{P_{cr}}$$

where U_{cr} = urine creatinine level, V = 24-hour urine volume, and P_{cr} = plasma creatinine level.

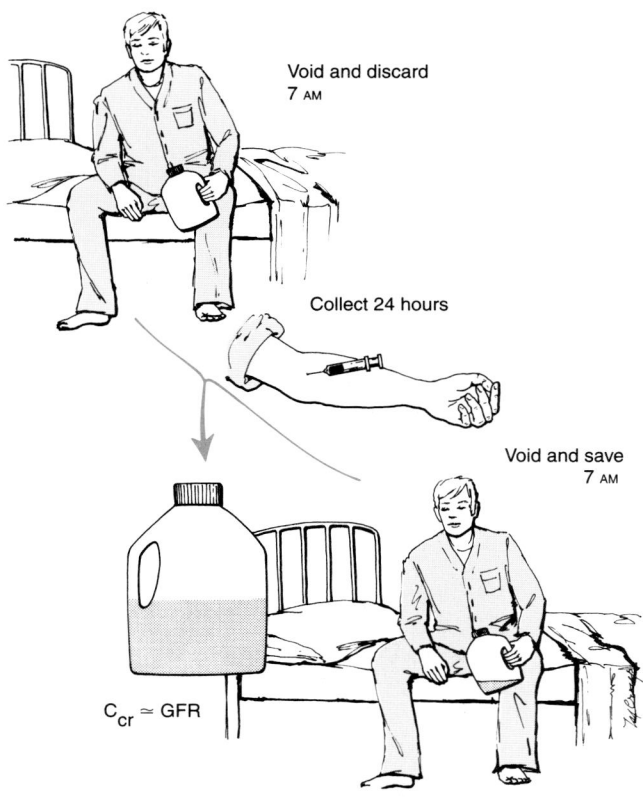

FIG. 45-3   Creatinine clearance test. C_{cr}, Creatinine clearance; *GFR*, glomerular filtration rate.

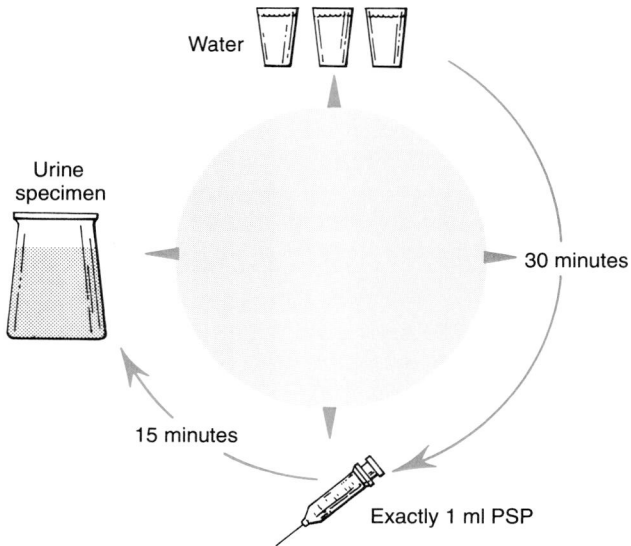

FIG. 45-4   Fifteen-minute phenolsulfonphthalein (PSP) excretion test; 28% or more of the dye normally is excreted in 15 minutes.

C_{cr} is a fairly good index of the GFR, although it is not a true measurement, because creatinine is secreted by the tubules to some extent, and the slight secretion of creatinine tends to cause overestimation of the GFR. Plasma creatinine also may be overestimated because of the difficulties inherent in the laboratory determination. Luckily, these two errors are of nearly the same magnitude and cancel each other out, so that C_{cr} approximates the GFR.

In chronic renal disease and some forms of acute renal failure, the GFR is decreased below the normal value of 125 ml/min. GFR also decreases with advancing age: every year after the age of 30, it decreases at the rate of 1 ml/min.

Plasma Creatinine and Blood Urea Nitrogen

The plasma creatinine and blood urea nitrogen (BUN) concentrations are also guides to the GFR. The normal BUN concentration is about 10 to 20 mg/dl, and plasma creatinine concentration is 0.7 to 1.5 mg/dl. Both of these substances are nitrogenous end products of protein metabolism normally excreted in the urine. When the GFR decreases, as in renal insufficiency, the plasma levels of creatinine and BUN rise. This condition is called *azotemia* (nitrogenous substances in the blood). The level of plasma creatinine as an index of the GFR is more accurate than is the BUN, because creatinine production is mainly a function of the size of the muscle mass, which changes very little. The BUN, however, is affected by the amount of protein in the diet and the catabolism of body protein. The relation of a rising plasma creatinine and BUN level to a decreasing GFR is discussed in Chapter 46.

Tubular Function Tests

A number of tests are carried out to evaluate the function and integrity of the renal tubules. The function of the tubules is selective reabsorption of the contents of the tubular fluid and secretion of substances into the tubular lumen, which are either circulating in the peritubular capillaries or are formed at the tubular cell. These processes are under the control of a wide variety of hormones, gas pressures, and plasma electrolyte concentrations. Common tests of proximal tubular function include the phenolsulfonphthalein (PSP) and para-aminohippurate (PAH) excretion tests. Distal tubular function tests include tests of concentration, dilution, acidification, and sodium conservation. The fractional excretion of sodium (FE_{Na}) is an important calculation in differentiating prerenal azotemia from acute tubular necrosis (ATN) and is discussed in Chapter 49.

PSP Excretion Test

PSP is a nontoxic dye eliminated primarily by secretion into the proximal tubule. Binding of PSP to plasma proteins is so high that only about 4% is excreted by glomerular filtration. With the usual 6 mg dose, the plasma level of the dye is only about one fifth of the tubular capacity to excrete PSP. The excretion rate of PSP is therefore usually limited by the rate of delivery to the tubules via the renal plasma flow and, in severely impaired kidneys, by proximal tubular function. The 15-minute PSP test is most commonly performed (Fig. 45-4).

Thirty minutes before the PSP dye is given, the patient is asked to drink two or three glasses of water to ensure sufficient bladder urine for urination. Exactly 1 ml (6 mg) of PSP is injected intravenously, using a tuberculin syringe for accuracy. Exactly 15 minutes after the dye is given, the patient is asked to completely empty the bladder. All the urine is then placed in a 1 L volumetric flask; 5 ml of 10% sodium hydroxide

(NaOH) is added, as well as enough water to bring the volume up to 1 L. A test tube of the pink, diluted specimen is then compared with the appropriate standards visually or by the use of a colorimeter. The person with normal renal function should excrete a minimum of 28% of the dye in 15 minutes.

The primary value of the PSP excretion test is in the detection of functional impairment early in the course of renal disease. Many physicians no longer perform this test and consider the C_{cr} test alone to be an adequate assessment of renal function. The analysis of the PSP test is so simple that it can be performed without the aid of a clinical laboratory, so it might be useful in situations where such a facility is not available.

PAH Excretion Test

Para-aminohippurate (PAH) is a substance that is filtered by the glomerulus and secreted by the proximal tubule. When given in low concentrations to humans, about 92% of PAH is cleared in one circulation through the kidneys. The PAH excretion test is therefore a fairly accurate measure of renal plasma flow (RPF). In the adult, RPF is approximately 600 ml/min. If the plasma concentration is further increased until secretory capacity is exceeded, the secretory capacity of the proximal tubule can be calculated from the filtered load and urinary excretion. Renal blood flow (RBF) can be calculated from the RPF if the hematocrit is known: RBF = RPF ÷ (1 − hematocrit).

Concentration and Dilution Tests

The measurement of urine specific gravity after water restriction is a sensitive measure of the ability of the renal tubules to reabsorb water and produce a concentrated urine. Renal function is considered normal if an early morning urine specimen has a specific gravity of 1.025 or more. When concentrating ability is doubtful, a more elaborate concentration test, such as the Fishberg concentration test, may be carried out. To ensure accuracy of results, the patient must be on a normal diet (normal salt, protein, and fluid intake) and must not be taking diuretics before the administration of the test. The patient is instructed to eat a normal evening meal at 6:00 PM and not to take food or fluids until the test is completed the next morning. Urine specimens are collected the next morning at 6:00, 7:00, and 8:00 AM. At least one of these specimens should have a specific gravity of 1.025 (800 mOsm) or more (Fig. 45-5).

The urinary dilution test is performed by having the patient drink 1 L of water within 30 minutes. Urine specimens are then collected over the next 3 hours. At least one of these specimens should have a specific gravity of 1.003 (80 mOsm) or less (see Fig. 45-5). The urinary dilution test is much less useful than the concentration test, because nonspecific factors, such as nausea or emotions, may interfere with water diuresis even in normal subjects. Diluting ability may be defective in adrenal insufficiency, hepatic disease, and cardiac failure. The ability to dilute urine is lost late in most renal diseases, whereas concentrating ability is lost early. Neither the concentration nor the dilution tests should be carried out on azotemic patients, because dehydration and water intoxication, respectively, may result.

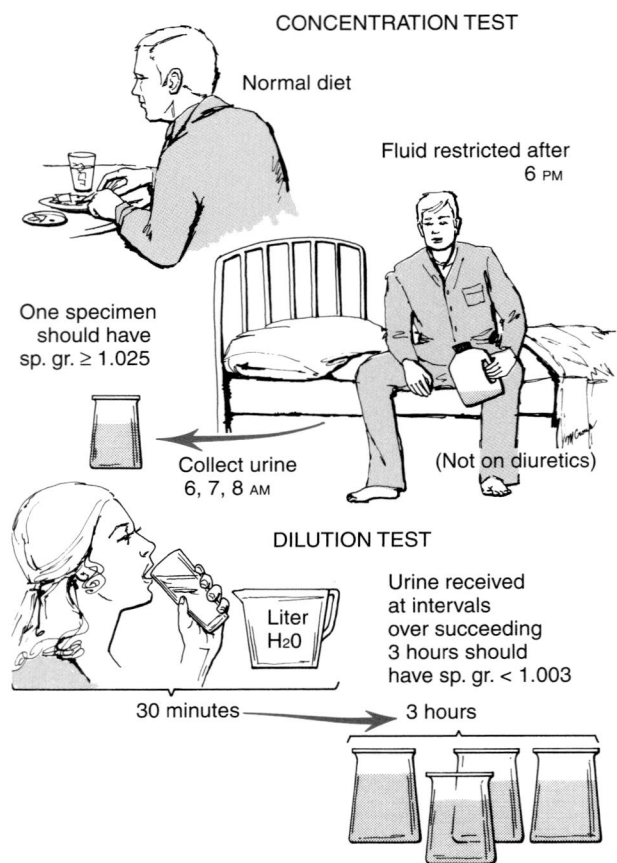

FIG. 45-5 Urine concentration and dilution tests. *sp. gr.,* Specific gravity.

Urine Acidification Test

The urine acidification test is designed to measure the maximum acid-excreting capacity of the kidney and is specific for the diagnosis of renal tubular acidosis.

In the 5-day test, control urine is collected for 2 days. The patient is then given ammonium chloride (about 12 g/day in the adult) for the next 3 days. The ammonium chloride is metabolized to urea and hydrogen chloride, producing acidosis in the patient. The urinary pH is determined daily, and on the fifth day ammonium and titratable acids are also measured. Normally, the kidney excretes the acid load and the urine pH is 5.3 or less (Fig. 45-6). In renal tubular acidosis, a hydrogen ion gradient between the tubular lumen and the plasma cannot be maintained, and a low urine pH is not achieved. Many patients with chronic renal failure can achieve a urine pH of 5.3, but excretion of ammonium and titratable acids is impaired.

Sodium Conservation Test

Healthy persons can produce urine that is virtually sodium free under conditions of dietary restriction of sodium. In renal disease, the ability to conserve sodium may be lost, and some patients suffer sodium depletion. If a person is losing more sodium than is ingested, the result is a contraction of the plasma volume, a decrease in

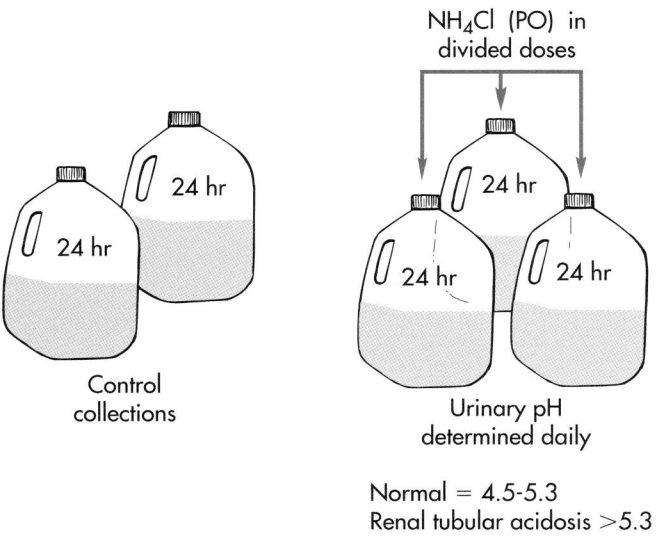

FIG. 45-6   Urine acidification test. *NH₄Cl,* Ammonium chloride; *PO,* by mouth.

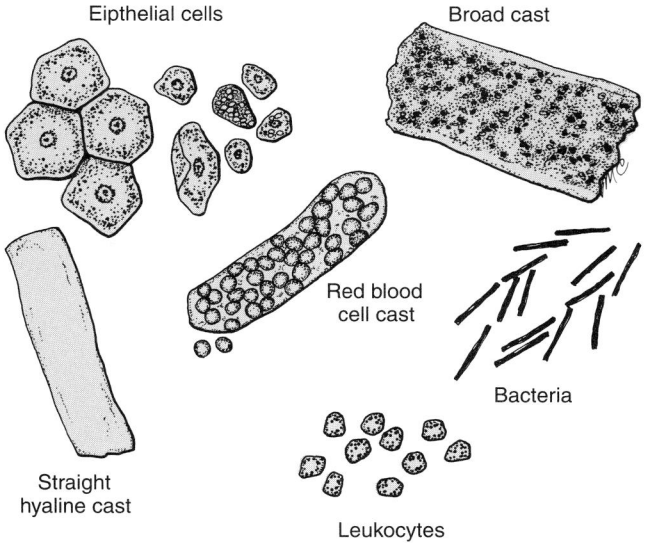

FIG. 45-7   Some formed elements in the urine sediment.

the GFR, and an accelerated course toward final renal failure. A salt-losing nephritis is more common in patients who have chronic pyelonephritis or polycystic disease. Both diseases involve primarily the renal tubules. Many patients in renal failure oscillate between states of sodium retention and depletion, so their daily intake of sodium must be defined within very narrow limits.

The sodium conservation test is sometimes used to determine how much sodium is needed in the diet of a patient with a salt-losing nephritis. The patient eats a low-sodium diet (10 mEq, or 500 mg). Sodium excretion in the urine normally falls to equal sodium intake within 1 week. In salt-losing nephritis, a large amount of sodium continues to be lost in the urine despite the restricted intake. Additional sodium may be added to the diet when the magnitude of the deficit is determined. For example, a patient who is excreting 50 mEq of sodium in urine on a 10-mEq sodium diet should be allowed an additional 40 mEq of sodium in the diet, or 50 mEq.

MORPHOLOGIC METHODS

Diagnostic methods in renal disease that are primarily morphologic include microscopic and bacteriologic examination of the urine, renal radiologic examination, and renal biopsy. These methods are discussed briefly.

Microscopic Examination of Urine

Microscopic examination of the urine is carried out on a freshly collected, centrifuged specimen, the deposit from which is suspended in 0.5 ml of urine. In healthy individuals, the urine contains a small number of cells and other elements derived from the entire length of the genitourinary tract—casts, epithelial cells from the lining of the urinary tract and vagina (females), spermatozoa (males), mucous threads, and no more than one or two

red blood cells (RBCs) and three or four white blood cells (WBCs) per high-power field.

The most common abnormal constituents of the urine are RBCs, WBCs, bacteria, and casts. All casts arise in the kidney and are thought to be "moldings" of renal tubules. Thus these casts indicate conditions exclusively within the kidneys and, for this reason, are of great diagnostic value. Casts consist of a mucoprotein matrix, the Tamm-Horsfall mucoprotein, in which cells or debris are embedded and in which a variety of serum and renal proteins may be absorbed. The Tamm-Horsfall protein is secreted by the distal tubule cells. As the protein passes down the tubule, it dehydrates and takes on the shape of the tubule. *Hyaline casts* consist of this protein and appear as clear cylinders. Cellular elements may be incorporated into hyaline casts (cellular casts) at the time of their formation. In this way, various types of casts are formed, depending on the cell type embedded in the cast (Fig. 45-7). Normally, not enough protein is present in the renal tubules to provide more than an occasional cast. *Cylindruria* (excessive excretion of casts in the urine) usually means increased proteinuria or renal excretion of cells, or both, and indicates renal disease.

Casts are classified according to shape or constituents. Cellular casts may contain RBCs, WBCs, bacteria, or tubular epithelial cells or may be mixed. RBCs and *red cell casts* are seen in active glomerulonephritis. *White cell casts* are often seen in pyelonephritis. Oval fat bodies and *fatty casts* are common in the nephrotic syndrome. Oval fat bodies are the remains of degenerated fat-filled tubular cells. *Granular casts* or *waxy casts* represent stages in the degeneration of a cellular cast, and the progression is from coarse to fine and finally to waxy. Broad granular casts are a typical finding in end-stage kidney disease. These casts are granular because of dead cells and broad because they are formed in the collecting ducts, owing to decreased urinary flow. These broad granular casts are sometimes called *renal failure casts.* Table 45-2 summarizes

TABLE 45-2   ■■■

Common Normal and Abnormal Findings in Urinalysis

Characteristic	Normal	Abnormality and Possible Significance
Appearance	Clear	Cloudy: large numbers of RBCs or WBCs as in UTI or precipitation of urate or phosphate crystals
Color	Straw yellow	Red or brown: hematuria, hemoglobinuria
		Red: beets, pyridium
		Brown: bile in jaundice, porphyrins in porphyria; melanin in melanoma
		Orange: Pyridium
Odor	Slightly aromatic	Unpleasant odor common in UTI; acetone smell in diabetic ketoacidosis; ammonia smell usual in specimen after standing because of bacterial degradation of urea
Specific gravity	1.001-1.035	Relatively constant near 1.010 in renal failure
pH	5-6.5	>7.5 suggests UTI with urea-splitting organisms
Protein	0 to trace <150 mg/day	Most renal diseases are characterized by proteinuria; nephrotic syndrome: >3.5 g/day
Glucose	Negative	Diabetes mellitus
Ketones	Negative	Diabetes mellitus; starvation
RBCs	0-2/hpf	Larger number may be seen in UTI, glomerulonephritis, neoplasm, stone, papillary necrosis, coagulopathy
WBCs	0-4/hpf	Increased numbers seen in UTI and a variety of other conditions
Epithelial cells	0-5/hpf	Excessive number of renal epithelial cells suggests renal disease
Bacteria	0	Bacteria seen in fresh unspun urine signify UTI
Oval fat bodies	0	Seen in nephrotic syndrome
Casts	0-1/hpf (hyaline)	Coagulated protein formed in renal tubules and collecting ducts; excessive number or specific types are associated with renal disease (see text)
Crystals	Many types	Cystine: abnormal aminoaciduria

hpf, High-power field; *UTI,* urinary tract infection; *RBCs,* red blood cells; *WBCs,* white blood cells.

some common normal and abnormal findings in routine urinalysis.

Bacteriologic Examination of Urine

Urine is normally sterile, and a significant number of bacteria may indicate the presence of urinary tract infection (UTI) (kidneys, bladder, or urethra) or prostatitis. Bacterial counts may be carried out by inoculating the surface of a nutrient agar plate, using a calibrated loop that delivers 0.001 ml of urine (Fig. 45-8). The agar plate is then incubated for 24 hours at 37° C, and colonies are counted. *Significant bacteriuria* is defined as more than 10^5 (100,000) colony-forming units of bacteria per milliliter of urine (CFU/ml) from a midstream clean-catch specimen. This number is based on epidemiologic studies that show that an asymptomatic individual with a count of this magnitude has an 85% chance of having a UTI. If the individual has signs or symptoms of UTI (fever, dysuria, urinary frequency), then a count lower than 10^5 CFU/ml may be significant. The bacteria may be subcultured for identification and for an antibiotic sensitivity test. This procedure is commonly referred to as a *culture and sensitivity (C & S)* test. The results of this test are a useful guide in the choice of an antibiotic for the most effective treatment.

For a bacteriologic study of the urine to have validity, the specimen must be free of contaminating bacteria from the urethra, external genitalia, and perineum. Proper techniques and precautions are therefore important in the collection of urine specimens. Collection of the urine by catheterization into a sterile container is the best way to ensure that the specimen is uncontaminated. Catheterization, however, is avoided if possible because of the danger of introducing bacteria into the urinary

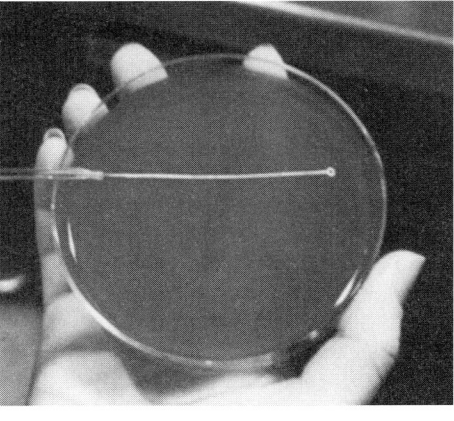

FIG. 45-8 Inoculation of the surface of a blood agar plate by means of a calibrated loop. The plate is incubated for 24 hours at 37° C. Significant bacteriuria is 10^5 (100,000) or more organisms per milliliter of urine.

tract. A "sterile-voided" specimen is generally considered adequate for a bacteriologic study. Men, and particularly women, are instructed to wash the area around the urinary meatus with soap and water. A midstream specimen is then collected in a clean or sterile specimen container. The urine is examined within 30 minutes, or a preservative is added and it is refrigerated at 4° C. Refrigeration prevents the growth of bacteria, and the preservative prevents the deterioration of casts and cells.

Although the most accurate results of bacterial counts are obtained by laboratory analysis of urine, a urinary test strip is the easiest means of diagnosing UTI qualitatively and is used frequently in primary care settings. The urinary test strip detects leukocytes and nitrites. Simultaneous detection of the two is highly suggestive of UTI. This screening test for bacteriuria relies on the ability of gram-negative bacteria to convert urinary nitrate to nitrite, which activates a chromogen. False negatives occur with infections with organisms such as enterococcus, staphylococcus saprophyticus, or other organisms that do not produce nitrite, or when urine has not been retained in the bladder long enough to change nitrate into nitrite (about 4 hours). A dip-slide method also is available for estimating urinary bacterial counts.

Radiologic Examinations

A number of radiologic procedures are available to evaluate the urinary system. The excretory urogram, or intravenous pyelogram (IVP), is the most common and important radiologic examination of the kidneys and is usually performed first. Other imaging examinations include ultrasonography, radionuclide (isotopic) imaging, computed tomography (CT), magnetic resonance imaging (MRI), voiding cystourethrography, and renal angiography.

Intravenous Pyelogram

The usual procedure for performing the IVP includes a flat-plate (plain-film) radiograph of the abdomen, followed by IV injection of contrast medium. The contrast medium circulates via the bloodstream and heart to the kidneys, where it is excreted. After injection, a radiograph is taken every minute for the first 5 minutes to visualize the cortex of the kidney. The cortex is thinned in glomerulonephritis and has a moth-eaten appearance in pyelonephritis and ischemia. Adequacy of filling of the calyces is evaluated by examination of the 3- and 5-minute radiographs. At 15 minutes, another radiograph is taken, at which time the calyces, pelvis, and ureters can be visualized. Cysts, lesions, and obstructions cause a distortion of these structures. A final radiograph is taken at 45 minutes, in which the bladder is visible. If the patient is severely azotemic (BUN >70 mg/dl), an IVP is not usually done, because this indicates that the GFR is very low. Consequently the dye will not be excreted and the pyelogram will be difficult to visualize.

Sometimes a *retrograde pyelogram* is done by passing a catheter up the ureter and injecting contrast medium directly into the kidney. The main indications for this procedure are urologic, for example, further investigation of a nonfunctioning kidney or when visualization of the IVP is not clear. This procedure is avoided if at all possible because it involves anesthesia and there is a real danger of infection.

The standard IVP, which serves many purposes, can establish the presence and position of the kidneys and evaluate their size and shape. The effect of different disease states on the kidney's ability to concentrate and excrete the dye can also be evaluated. Figure 45-9 shows some typical abnormalities revealed by the IVP. The small, atrophic kidney may be caused by unilateral renal ischemia or unilateral chronic pyelonephritis (see Fig. 45-9, *A*). Bilaterally small kidneys are common findings in chronic nephrosclerosis, pyelonephritis, and glomerulonephritis. Distortion of the renal pelvis with clubbing of the calyces is a common finding in chronic pyelonephritis (see

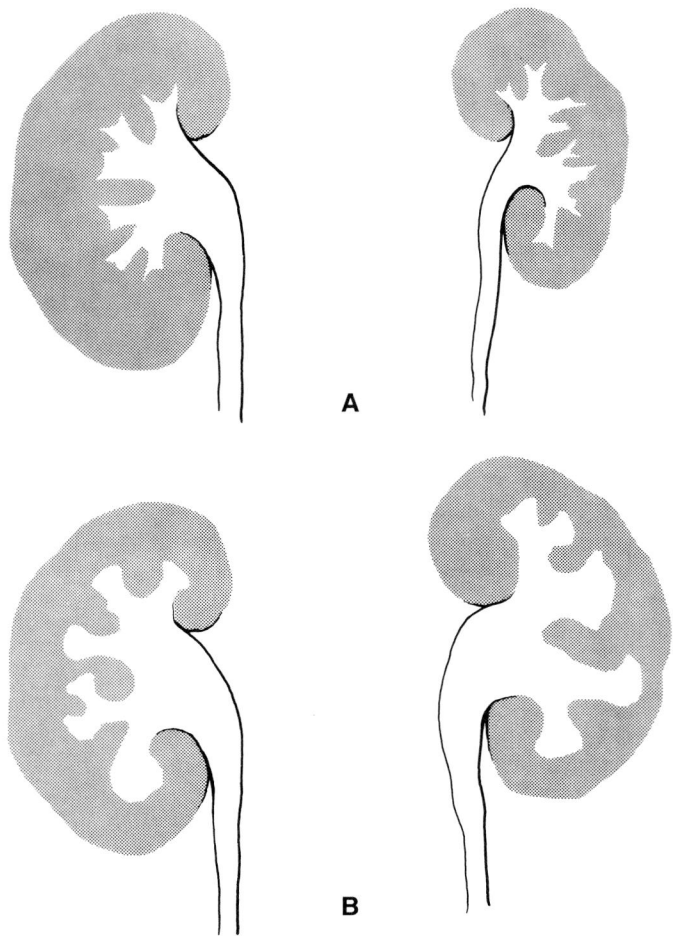

FIG. 45-9 Diagram of abnormalities viewed on the intravenous pyelogram (IVP). **A,** Small, atrophic kidney caused by unilateral renal ischemia. **B,** Clubbing of the calyces, irregularity of contour, and thinning of cortical substance may be found in chronic pyelonephritis.

Fig. 45-9, *B*). The irregular shape and the greatly thinned cortex should also be noted.

Renal Ultrasonography

High-frequency sound waves (ultrasound) directed at the abdomen are reflected from tissue surfaces of varying density. The reflected waves, or echoes, are used to construct images (sonograms) representing sections of the kidney. Ultrasonography is particularly useful in distinguishing solid tumors from fluid-filled cysts. Because ultrasound evaluation does not depend on renal function, it can be applied to patients in severe renal failure who have kidneys that cannot be visualized on the IVP. Kidney size can be determined accurately, and an obstruction can be identified. Other applications include evaluation of a unilateral nonvisualizing kidney (often caused by hydronephrosis), evaluation of renal transplants (perirenal abscess or hematoma, for example, can be differentiated from acute rejection), and renal localization for needle placement for percutaneous renal biopsy.

Renal Radionuclide Imaging

Radionuclide imaging involves the injection of a radioactive material that is subsequently detected externally by a scintillation (gamma) camera that picks up the radioactive emissions. Information is provided for the evaluation of both structure and function. The properties of a compound that bind the radioisotope determine how the kidney handles the compound—whether it is retained within the vascular system, filtered by the glomerulus, or secreted into the tubule. Three main procedures may be performed together or independently: *renal scintiangiography* uses serial imaging of the aorta and renal vasculature; *renal scintiscanning* uses imaging of the renal parenchyma using various ^{99m}Tc-labeled compounds; and *renography* is the original technique of radionuclide evaluation of the kidneys using ^{131}I hippuran, which is excreted by tubular secretion. Radionuclide imaging is used for many purposes in renal evaluation but is particularly helpful in renal transplant evaluation. Renal function may be followed, impaired diffusion detected, and acute rejection differentiated from acute tubular necrosis (ATN).

Voiding Cystourethrogram

The voiding cystourethrogram procedure involves filling the urinary bladder with contrast material via a urinary catheter. Films of the lower urinary tract are taken before, during, and after voiding. Its major diagnostic uses are to investigate abnormalities of the urethra (e.g., stenosis) and to determine whether there is vesicoureteral reflux.

Computed Tomography

CT offers far greater contrast resolution compared with conventional radiography, with detailed anatomic cross sections. CT thoroughly visualizes the entire urinary system; it plays the main role in staging renal neoplasms and has replaced the IVP in renal trauma cases. CT can show urinary calculi that are not visible by radiography. Helical CT can show arterial vessels and perfusion defects, as well as demonstrating renal vein thrombosis.

Magnetic Resonance Imaging

MRI is a noninvasive imaging technique that gives the same information as does the renal CT scan but it has the advantages of not requiring exposure to ionizing radiation nor the administration of contrast media. MRI is based on the principle that certain atoms, such as the hydrogen ion contained in the molecules and tissues of the body, act as tiny magnets. If the patient is placed in a strong magnetic field, some of the atomic nuclei align themselves in the same direction as the magnetic force. When a radiofrequency pulse is applied, some of the nuclei absorb the energy, causing them to wobble in and out of alignment (resonate) with the magnetic field. Signals emitted during the return of the magnetization vector to its equilibrium position can be analyzed to provide a detailed structural image. MRI results in more detailed images than does CT so is useful when CT is not definitive. MRI can show the renal vasculature very clearly and magnetic resonance angiography (MRA) is being evaluated as a potential replacement for conventional angiography.

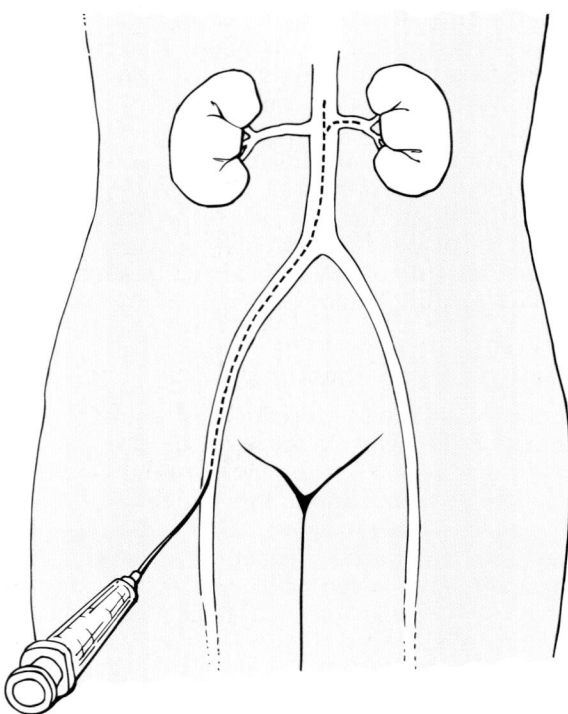

FIG. 45-10 Transfemoral approach in renal angiography.

Renal Arteriogram

The renal blood vessels may be visualized in an arteriogram. The usual procedure is to introduce a catheter via the femoral artery and abdominal aorta to the level of the renal artery. Contrast medium is injected at this level and then flows into the renal artery and its accessory branches. Additional information often can be obtained by selective renal angiography; the tip of the catheter is maneuvered into the renal artery and more contrast medium is injected (Fig. 45-10). This procedure may be used (1) to visualize renal artery stenosis, which may cause some cases of hypertension; (2) to visualize the blood vessels of a neoplasm; (3) to visualize the blood supply of the cortex, which, for example, may have a patchy appearance in chronic pyelonephritis; and (4) to ascertain the structure of the renal blood supply of a donor before renal transplantation. Fig. 45-11 is an arteriogram showing marked narrowing of the right renal artery.

Angiography is not done without discomfort and some hazard. The patient usually experiences an intense burning sensation for a few seconds as the solution enters the blood vessel. Before injection, the patient is usually tested for iodide sensitivity to avoid an anaphylactic response. Other complications following arteriogram include thrombus or embolus formation and local inflammation or hematoma at the site of entry. Although these complications are rare, vital signs are checked every 15 minutes until stable and then every 4 hours for 24 hours. Peripheral pulses are also checked for diminished strength to detect occlusion of blood flow because of a thrombus.

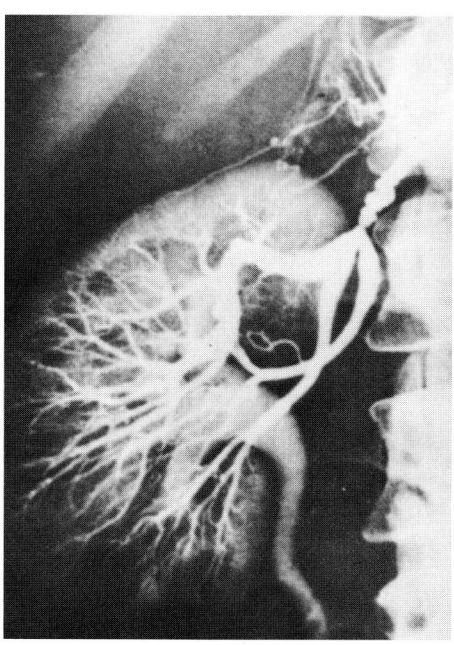

FIG. 45-11   Renal arteriogram showing stenosis of the right renal artery.

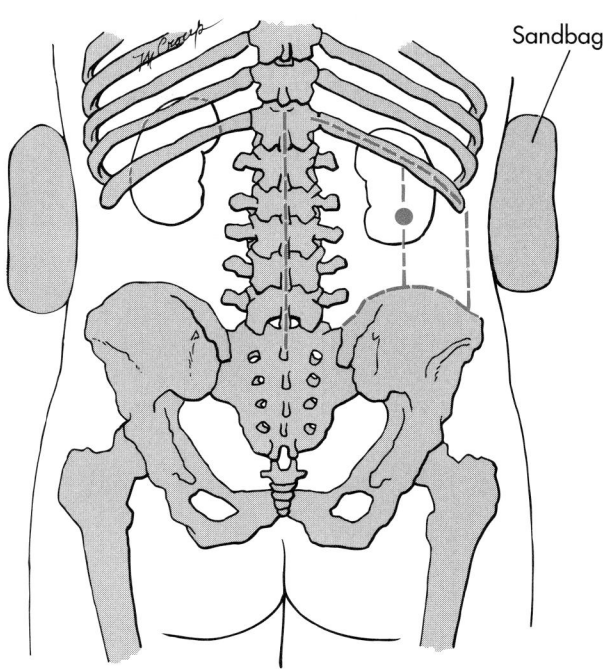

FIG. 45-12   Percutaneous renal biopsy. Site is located by radiographic reference; patient lies prone with sandbag under abdomen to fix kidney against back. Vital signs are monitored.

Renal Biopsy

Renal biopsy is one of the most important diagnostic techniques developed during the past few decades and has resulted in considerable advancement of knowledge of the natural history of renal disease. Renal biopsy is used chiefly for the diagnosis of diffuse renal disease and for following its progress.

Usually the percutaneous procedure is used for renal biopsy. The patient lies prone, with sandbags under the abdomen to fix the kidney against the back (Fig. 45-12). Local anesthesia is used. The usual site for the biopsy is over the right renal angle just below the twelfth rib. The site is located by radiographic reference. A biopsy needle is used to obtain a specimen of renal tissue. The tissue is examined, after appropriate preparation, by light microscopy, electron microscopy, and immunofluorescent microscopy. Fig. 45-13 illustrates the appearance of a normal renal biopsy by light microscopy.

Renal biopsy should be performed only by a skilled nephrologist. The procedure is dangerous in patients who are uncooperative or those who have a coagulative disorder or a solitary kidney. The most common complications are intrarenal bleeding and perirenal bleeding. Serious bleeding with gross hematuria occurs in about 5% and death in about 0.17% of cases. Arteriovenous fistula is the second most common complication.

Immediately after the biopsy, pressure is applied over the biopsy site for 10 minutes with 4 × 4-inch sponges, and the patient is kept in a prone position for 30 minutes. A pressure dressing is then applied to the biopsy site. The dressing from above and the sandbag from be-

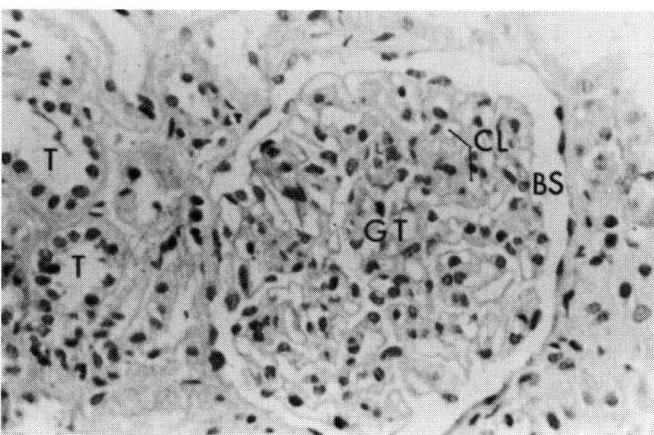

FIG. 45-13   Light microscopy of normal renal biopsy section. *BS,* Bowman's space; *GT,* glomerular tuft; *CL,* capillary lumen; *T,* tubule.

low provide pressure on the kidney and aid in the prevention of extrarenal bleeding. Lying on the sandbag is usually uncomfortable for the patient, but it immobilizes the kidney in the anteroposterior plane and is a necessary measure to ensure hemostasis. The patient should be kept in bed and as quiet as possible for the next 24 hours and should be instructed not to cough or sneeze. During this period, frequent observations of the vital signs, abdomen, and urine should be made. The patient is kept on bed rest as long as hematuria occurs.

KEY CONCEPTS

- Normal protein excretion in the urine is less than 150 mg/day.
- Significant proteinuria may be detected in a concentrated urine specimen using a dipstick test, especially if it is albumin.
- Transient proteinuria may occur in persons without kidney or systemic disease in association with fever, heavy exercise, or in association with the upright position (orthostatic proteinuria).
- Persistent proteinuria is more likely to reflect some underlying renal or systemic disorder.
- Increased excretion of low–molecular-weight proteins can occur with marked overproduction of a particular protein (almost always immunoglobulin light chains in multiple myeloma).
- The direct cause of glomerular proteinuria is an increase in glomerular permeability resulting from loss of the charge or size barrier or a change in glomerular hemodynamics.
- Tubulointerstitial disease may interfere with tubular reabsorption of proteins resulting in proteinuria.
- The nephrotic syndrome is defined as the loss of 3.5 g/day or more of protein in the urine.
- Hematuria is frequently a harbinger of renal disease (especially glomerulonephritis) or of the lower urinary tract.
- The most common type of urinary tract stone contains calcium oxalate, calcium phosphate, or both.
- Urinary stasis, infection, and indwelling catheters all promote stone formation.
- Uric acid stones form in acid urine and obstructive uropathy that results from uric acid crystallization may be a complication of cytotoxic drug therapy for cancer or leukemia.
- The most important preventive measure for urinary tract stone formation is high fluid intake.
- Measurement of the specific gravity of urine (which measures density) is used to estimate urine osmolality.
- A specific gravity of 1.010 corresponds to an osmolality of 285 mOsm/kg water, the normal osmolality of the blood. Minimum specific gravity of a dilute urine is about 1.001 (40 mOsm), and maximum urine concentration is about 1.040 (1300 mOsm).
- In progressive renal failure, the kidney first loses the ability to concentrate urine and later the ability to dilute urine is lost as well; the specific gravity becomes fixed near 1.010 (285 mOsm) in end-stage renal failure.

- The GFR is the most important index of renal function and is measured clinically by the creatinine clearance test. The normal GFR is 125 ml/min in males and 115 ml/min in women.
- The serum creatinine (normal, 0.7 to 1.5 mg/dl) and BUN (normal, 10 to 20 mg/dl) are inversely related to the GFR and may be used for the clinical assessment of renal insufficiency and failure. The BUN is less accurate compared with serum creatine because dietary protein intake and catabolic states can influence BUN.
- Renal concentrating ability is considered to be normal if the individual is able to produce urine with a specific gravity of at least 1.025 (800 mOsm) after an all-night fast.
- The urine acidification test, using ammonium chloride, is used to diagnose renal tubular acidosis.
- The most common abnormal constituents of the urine observed upon microscopic examination are RBCs, WBCs, bacteria, and casts (molded protein formed in the tubules and collecting ducts).
- Casts are named according to their embedded cellular elements (RBCs, WBCs, bacteria, tubular cells) and are of great diagnostic value because they originate in the kidney. Broad granular (renal failure) casts are associated with renal failure.
- Significant bacteriuria is defined as 10^5 (100,000) colony-forming units per ml (CFU/ml) of urine.
- Ultrasonography provides information about renal size and anatomy, including cysts or dilation of the calyces, suggesting obstruction. Doppler ultrasound can be used to assess flow in the renal arteries and veins.
- CT and MRI can be used to visualize the renal system.
- Plain radiography may reveal the renal size and detect radiopaque stones.
- Intravenous contrast will produce an IV pyelogram (IVP), showing the renal outlines and the urinary tract. The urinary tract can also be studied by injecting contrast up the ureters via the urethra and bladder (retrograde IVP).
- A voiding cystourethrogram is used to diagnose vesicoureteral reflux.
- Renal angiography can be performed using an arterial catheter inserted via the femoral artery to inject radiopaque contrast into the renal arteries to visualize them.
- Histologic diagnosis of renal disease requires renal biopsy. Percutaneous biopsy is performed with a long cutting needle through the back, usually with ultrasonic guidance.

QUESTIONS

A sampling of review questions for this chapter appears here. Visit http://www.mosby.com/MERLIN/PriceWilson/ for additional questions.

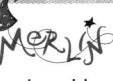

Answer the following on a separate sheet of paper.

1. Contrast the amount of protein a healthy adult and a person with nephrotic syndrome might excrete in a day. Explain the significance.

2. What is always the direct cause of glomerular proteinuria, regardless of the underlying disease process?

3. Explain why only fresh urine should be used for measuring pH.

4. Hyperuricemia leading to uric acid crystallization in the renal tubules is a particular hazard for patients receiving cytotoxic drugs. Why?

5. What are the most common factors predisposing to formation of calculi in alkaline urine? Explain.
6. What is the most important preventive measure against all calculi?
7. What are the five important points that must be considered in obtaining an accurate specific gravity measurement with the urinometer?

8. What is creatinine, and what is its normal range of values in the plasma?
9. Why is the creatinine clearance test not a true measure of GFR?
10. What effect does increasing age have on the GFR?
11. What test most accurately measures effective renal plasma flow (RPF)?

12. Which is the more accurate index of renal function, the BUN or the plasma creatinine level? Why? What is azotemia?
13. Give two examples of difficulties that may be encountered in the interpretation of the dipstick test for proteinuria.

Fill in the blanks with the correct words or numbers or circle the appropriate letter to complete the following sentences.

14. Protein excreted in the urine of the healthy adult consists mainly of _____ and _____ protein.
15. The average pooled daily urine specimen has a pH of about _____.
16. After a meal, one expects a (a) rise or (b) fall in the urine pH. This is referred to as the _____ tide.
17. During normal sleeping hours, the urine pH reaches its (a) maximum or (b) minimum because of (c) hypoventilation or (d) hyperventilation during sleep. This is referred to as the _____ tide.
18. When the urine contains normal constituents, a specific gravity of 1.010 corresponds to the normal osmolality of the blood at _____ mOsm.
19. When given large amounts of water, the healthy human being can dilute urine to a minimum specific gravity of about _____ (40 mOsm). Under conditions of water deprivation, a normal person can excrete concentrated urine with a maximum specific gravity of about _____ (1300 mOsm). What is the purpose of this great flexibility?
20. In the 15-minute PSP test the kidneys normally excrete _____% of the dye in the urine.
21. After about 14 hours of water deprivation, the urine of a person with normally functioning kidneys has a specific gravity of _____ or more. After a water load (1 L in 30 minutes), the specific gravity should be _____ or less within the next 3 hours.
22. The _____ _____ test is specific for the diagnosis of renal tubular acidosis. The urine pH should be _____ or less in the 5-day test.
23. The _____ _____ test is used to determine the proper dietary intake of sodium, especially in a patient with "salt-losing" nephritis. A negative sodium balance is most frequently found in patients with renal disorders primarily involving the (a) tubules or (b) glomerulus.

Answer the following on a separate sheet of paper.

24. Name the most common abnormal constituents of the urine sediment.
25. When is bacteriuria significant? List proper conditions of urine collection and significant bacterial count.
26. Differentiate between an IVP and a retrograde pyelogram. State the purpose of each.
27. List four reasons for performing a renal arteriogram.

28. Why is it not worthwhile to perform an IVP on a patient who is severely azotemic (BUN level greater than 70 mg/dl)?
29. Outline a plan of care for a patient after a renal arteriogram.
30. Outline a plan of care for a patient during and after a renal biopsy. What observations should be made?

Fill in the blanks with the correct words.

31. Four types of morphologic renal investigations are:
   a. _____ examination of the urine sediment
   b. _____ study of the urine
   c. Renal _____, a method that reveals the shape, size, and position of the kidneys
   d. Renal _____, a method that reveals the microscopic structure of the kidney
32. Hyaline casts are made up of coagulated _____ _____ protein secreted by the _____ tubule.
33. Excessive excretion of casts in the urine is called _____ and usually means that there is an increased glomerular permeability to _____.
34. A _____ and _____ test is sometimes done to determine the best choice of an antibiotic for treating a urinary tract infection.
35. An abnormality seen on the IVP that is diagnostic of chronic pyelonephritis is _____ of the calyces.

46

Chronic Renal Failure

LORRAINE M. WILSON

*T*his chapter gives an overview of the course of deteriorations in progressive renal failure, its general pathophysiology, and its causes.

Renal failure is usually divided into two broad categories—chronic and acute. Chronic renal failure is a progressive, slow development of renal failure, usually over a period of years, as contrasted with acute renal failure, which develops over a period of days or a few weeks. In both cases, the kidneys lose their ability to maintain normal volume and composition of the body fluids under conditions of normal dietary intake. Although the terminal functional disability is similar in the two types of renal failure, acute renal failure has some unique features and is discussed separately in Chapter 49.

Chronic renal failure follows a great number of conditions that devastate the nephron mass of the kidney. Most of these conditions involve diffuse, bilateral disease of the renal parenchyma, although obstructive lesions of the urinary tract may also lead to chronic renal failure. In the beginning, some renal diseases involve primarily the glomerulus (glomerulonephritis), whereas others involve primarily the renal tubules (pyelonephritis or polycystic kidney disease) or may interfere with blood perfusion to

the renal parenchyma (nephrosclerosis). In all cases, however, if the disease process is not halted, the entire nephron is progressively destroyed and replaced by scar tissue. The individual features of the various parenchymal renal diseases are discussed later in this chapter.

Despite the diversity of causes, the clinical features of chronic renal failure are remarkably similar, because progressive renal failure may be explained simply as a deficiency in the total number of functioning nephrons, and a fairly fixed combination of disturbances is inevitable.

OVERVIEW: CLINICAL COURSE OF CHRONIC RENAL FAILURE

An overview of the general course of chronic renal failure may be obtained by looking at the relation of the creatinine clearance and glomerular filtration rate (GFR), as a percentage of the normal, to the serum creatinine and blood urea nitrogen (BUN) levels as the nephron mass is progressively destroyed by chronic renal disease (Fig. 46-1).

The general course of progressive renal failure may be divided into three stages (designated as I, II, and III in Fig. 46-1). The first stage is called *decreased renal reserve*. During this stage, the serum creatinine and BUN levels are normal and the patient is asymptomatic. Impairment of renal function may be detected only by imposition of severe demands on the kidney, such as a prolonged urine concentration test, or by careful testing of the GFR.

The second stage in the progression is called *renal insufficiency*, when more than 75% of the functioning tissue has been destroyed (GFR is 25% of normal). At this point, the BUN level is just beginning to rise above the normal range. The rise in BUN concentration is variable, depending on the dietary intake of protein (the BUN graphs are compared for a low and normal protein intake). The serum creatinine level also begins to rise above normal during this stage. The azotemia is generally mild unless, for example, the patient is stressed by infection, heart failure, or dehydration. It is also during the stage of renal insufficiency that the symptoms of nocturia and polyuria (caused by impaired concentrating ability) begin to ap-

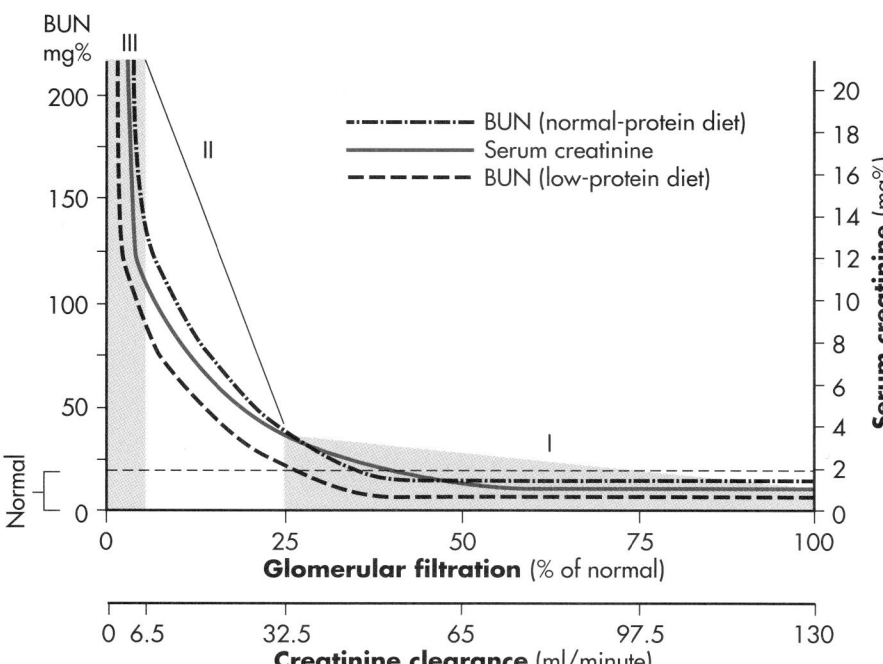

FIG. 46-1   The relationship of the blood urea nitrogen *(BUN)* and serum creatinine levels to the glomerular filtration rate during the three stages of progressive renal failure. Note that a low-protein diet delays azotemia.

pear. These symptoms occur in response to stress and sudden changes in food or fluid intake. The patient usually takes little note of these symptoms, so they may be revealed only by careful questioning. *Nocturia* (urinating at night) is defined as persistent nocturnal output of 700 ml or having to get up more than once to void during the night. Nocturia is caused by loss of the normal diurnal pattern of concentrating urine to a greater degree at night. The ratio of day to night urine is normally 3:1 or 4:1. Of course, nocturia may occasionally occur in response to anxiety or to a high fluid intake, especially of tea, coffee, or beer taken just before retiring. *Polyuria* means a persistent increase in the volume of urine. Normal urine output is about 1500 ml/day and varies considerably with fluid intake. Polyuria of renal insufficiency is usually greater in diseases that affect primarily the tubules, although it is generally moderate and rarely exceeds 3 L/day.

The third and final stage of progressive renal failure is called *end-stage renal disease (ESRD)* or *uremia.* ESRD occurs when about 90% of the nephron mass has been destroyed, or only about 200,000 nephrons remain intact. The GFR is 10% of normal, and the creatinine clearance may be 5 to 10 ml/min or even less. At this point, the serum creatinine and BUN levels rise sharply in response to small decrements in the GFR. During ESRD, the patient begins to suffer severe symptoms, as the kidneys are no longer able to maintain fluid and electrolyte homeostasis in the body. The urine becomes isoosmotic with the plasma at a fixed specific gravity of 1.010. The patient usually becomes oliguric (urine output less than 500 ml/day) because of glomerular failure, although the disease process may have initially affected the renal tubules. The complex of biochemical changes and symptoms, called the *uremic syndrome,* affects every system in the body and is discussed in detail in Chapter 47. In ESRD, unless the patient receives dialysis or renal transplantation, death will surely follow.

Although the clinical course of chronic renal disease has been divided into three stages, in practice, no sharp divisions exist between the stages. The hyperbolic shape of the graph of azotemia plotted against GFR reflects this continuous but slowly accelerating course.

GENERAL PATHOPHYSIOLOGY OF CHRONIC RENAL FAILURE

Two theoretic approaches are generally offered to account for the impaired function of the kidneys in chronic renal failure. The traditional point of view is that all the nephron units are diseased to varying degrees and that specific parts of the nephron concerned with particular functions may be destroyed or their structure altered. For example, organic lesions of the medulla disrupting the anatomic arrangement of the loop of Henle and vasa recta or the chloride pump in the ascending limb would interfere with countercurrent multiplication and exchange. The second approach, known as the *Bricker hypothesis* or *intact nephron hypothesis,* maintains that nephrons, when diseased, are totally destroyed. The remaining intact nephrons behave normally. Uremia results when the total number of nephrons is so reduced that fluid and electrolyte balance can no longer be maintained. The intact nephron hypothesis is most useful in explaining the orderly pattern of functional adaptation in progressive renal disease, that is, the ability to maintain a balance of body water and electrolytes despite a marked decrease in the GFR.

The sequence of events in the general pathophysiology of progressive renal failure may be outlined in terms of the intact nephron hypothesis. As chronic renal disease advances, the amount of solute that must be excreted by the kidney to maintain body homeostasis does not change, although there is a progressive reduction in the number of nephrons performing this function. Two important adaptations occur in the kidney in response to the threat of fluid and electrolyte imbalance. The remaining intact nephrons hypertrophy in an attempt to carry the entire workload of the kidneys (Fig. 46-2). There is an increase in filtration rate, solute load, and tubular reabsorption in each individual nephron, even though the GFR for the entire nephron mass of the kidneys is decreased below normal. This increased single-nephron GFR (SNGFR) (i.e., hyperfiltration) occurs by dilation of the glomerular afferent arterioles, resulting in enhanced single-nephron plasma flow. This adaptive mechanism is successful in maintaining body fluid and electrolyte balance down to low levels of renal function. Finally, when about 75% of the nephron mass is destroyed, the filtration rate and solute load per nephron are so high that glomerular-tubular balance (balance between increased filtration and increased tubular reabsorption) can no longer be maintained (Fig. 46-2 shows that six of the eight nephrons are destroyed). A loss of flexibility occurs in both the excretion and conservation of individual solutes and water. Modest dietary changes may upset the precarious balance, because the lower the GFR (which means fewer nephrons), the greater must be the change in excretion rate per nephron. Loss of the ability to concentrate or dilute causes the specific gravity of urine to become fixed at 1.010, or 285 mOsm (the concentration of plasma) and accounts for the symptoms of polyuria and nocturia. For example, a person on a normal diet excretes about 600 mOsm of solute each day. If this individual is incapable of concentrating urine from the normal plasma osmolality of 285 mOsm, there is an obligatory loss of 2 L of water with the 600-mOsm solute excretion

(285 mOsm/L) regardless of water intake. In response to the same solute load and water deprivation, the normal person would concentrate urine to about four times the plasma concentration and thus excrete a small volume of concentrated urine. As the GFR progresses toward zero, it becomes increasingly important to regulate the intake of water and solutes precisely to accommodate the decreased flexibility in renal function.

Several experimental observations support the intact nephron hypothesis. Bricker and Fine (1969) have shown that in patients with naturally occurring pyelonephritis and in dogs with experimental destruction of the kidney, the surviving nephrons hypertrophy and become more active than is normal. Also, when one kidney is removed in the healthy person, the remaining kidney undergoes hypertrophy, and the capacity of this kidney approaches that formerly possessed by both.

Normal kidneys under conditions of increased solute load behave much like the kidney in progressive renal failure, giving further support to the intact nephron hypothesis. The experimental data in Fig. 46-3 illustrate the concept that with progressive increases in solute load, the ability to concentrate the urine under conditions of water deprivation (upper curve) or to dilute the urine under conditions of high water intake (lower curve) is progressively lost. Both curves approach the specific gravity of 1.010 until the urine is isoosmotic with the plasma at 285 mOsm, so that a fixed specific gravity exists.

The experimental conditions just described may be induced in a normal person by giving mannitol (an osmotic diuretic). The number 10 on the x axis is arbitrarily chosen to show that the kidneys are excreting 10 times the usual solute load. At this point, each normal nephron

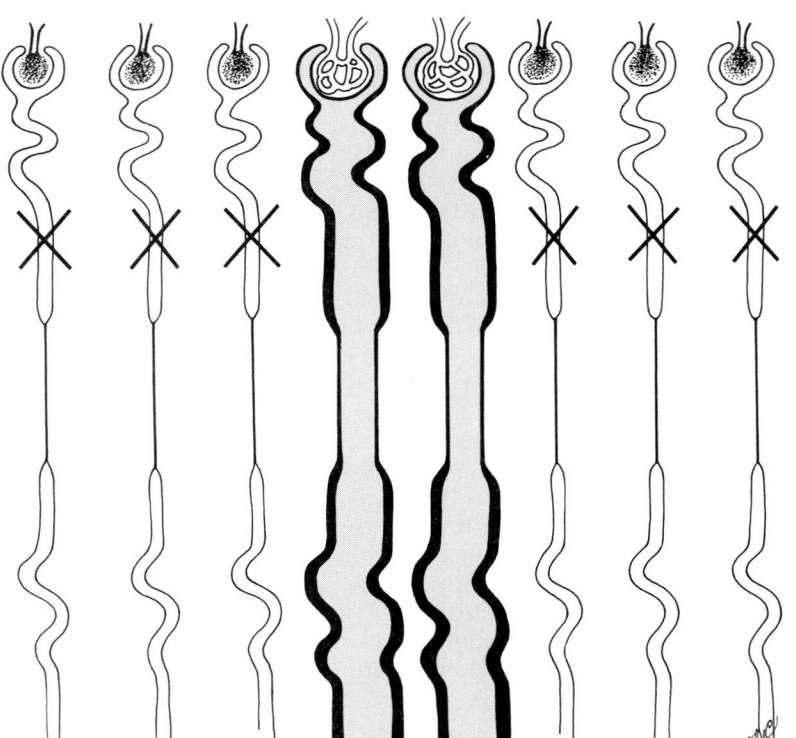

FIG. 46-2 Intact nephron hypothesis. As chronic renal disease advances and nephrons are progressively destroyed, the remaining intact nephrons hypertrophy in an attempt to carry on the entire work load of the kidney. Solute load per nephron is increased, resulting in osmotic diuresis, that is, rise in urine flow and reduction in concentration. (Modified from Netter FH: Kidneys, ureters, and urinary bladder. In *The Ciba collection of medical illustrations*, vol 6, West Caldwell, NJ, 1973, Ciba Medical Education Division.)

is undergoing an osmotic diuresis with an obligatory loss of water. The kidney has lost its flexibility to either concentrate or dilute the urine from the plasma osmolality of 285 mOsm.

Similar events probably occur in the patient with progressive renal failure. The patient with 90% destruction of nephron mass is at the same point on the graph as is the normal person with an induced solute load that is 10 times normal. The remaining 10% of the nephrons are forced to excrete 10 times the normal solute load and therefore lose their flexibility; they are unable to compensate properly by the usual changes in tubular reabsorption for excesses or deficiencies of sodium or water.

It has been noted for some time that chronic renal failure is often progressive, even when the inciting cause of injury is removed. For example, children with chronic pyelonephritis caused by vesicoureteral reflux and recurrent urinary tract infections (UTIs) develop pyelonephritic scars involving the tubules and interstitium; but when the reflux is corrected surgically and renal infection halted with antibiotics, progressive renal failure continues. These observations have led to recent major research efforts to learn the reasons for the progression of renal disease and methods to halt or slow its progression.

The most popular current explanation for progressive renal failure in the absence of active primary renal disease is the *hyperfiltration hypothesis.* According to the hyperfiltration theory, the intact nephrons are eventually injured by the increased plasma flow and GFR and increased glomerular intracapillary hydrostatic pressure (i.e., glomerular capillary pressure [P_{gc}]). Even though the increased SNGFR is adaptive in the short run, it is maladaptive in the long run.

Most of the evidence for the hyperfiltration theory of secondary injury is derived from the *remnant kidney* model in the rat. When one kidney in the rat was removed and two thirds of the other kidney destroyed, it was noted that the animal developed end-stage renal failure (ESRF) within 6 months, although a primary renal disease was not present. The rat developed protein-

uria, and renal biopsy of the remnant kidney revealed widespread glomerulosclerosis similar to lesions in many primary renal diseases. One explanation for renal lesions and progressive renal failure is based on the functional and structural changes that occur when the number of intact nephrons is reduced in an experimental animal.

Functional adaptations to a reduction of the nephron mass lead to systemic hypertension and increased SNGFR (hyperfiltration) in the remaining intact nephrons. Increased SNGFR is largely accomplished through dilation of the afferent arterioles. At the same time, the efferent arteriole constricts because of the local release of angiotensin II. Consequently, renal plasma flow (RPF) and P_{gc} increase, because most of the systemic pressure is transmitted to the glomerulus.

These functional compensations are associated with significant structural changes. The volume of the glomerular tuft increases without an increase in the number of visceral epithelial cells, resulting in a reduction of cell density within the enlarged glomerular tuft. It is believed that the combination of glomerular hypertension and hypertrophy is the significant change that causes secondary injury of the glomerular tuft and progressive destruction of nephrons. Decreased visceral epithelial density leads to fusion of the foot processes and a loss of the size-selective barrier so that increased protein is lost in the urine. The increase in permeability and intraglomerular hypertension also favors the accumulation of large proteins (e.g., fibrin, immunoglobulin M [IgM], complement) in the subendothelial space. The accumulation of these subendothelial deposits along with proliferation of mesangial matrix eventually leads to a narrowing of the capillary lumen from the compression. Other secondary injuries include microaneurysm formation from intraglomerular hypertension and thrombus formation from endothelial cell dysfunction. The aggregate effect is collapse of the glomerular capillaries and glomerulosclerosis, demonstrated by proteinuria and progressive renal failure. In addition, this sequence leads to a positive feedback loop with acceleration of the destructive process, as fewer and fewer nephrons remain intact. The structural and functional changes that lead to secondary injury of the glomerulus are summarized in Fig. 46-4 (Rose, Rennke, 1994).

Recent progress in understanding the mechanisms of progressive renal failure through the hyperfiltration hypothesis has caused clinicians to focus treatment on the prevention of secondary glomerular injury rather than to focus on the primary renal disease. Large clinical trials are now in progress with dietary protein restriction and antihypertensive therapy as a means of slowing the progress of chronic renal failure. This treatment is discussed in Chapter 48.

CAUSES OF CHRONIC RENAL FAILURE

Chronic renal failure is a clinical state of progressive, irreversible renal damage arising from many different causes. The rate of progression of these chronic renal diseases varies greatly. The course terminating in ESRD may vary from 2 to 3 months to 30 to 40 years. The most common causes of chronic renal failure may be divided into

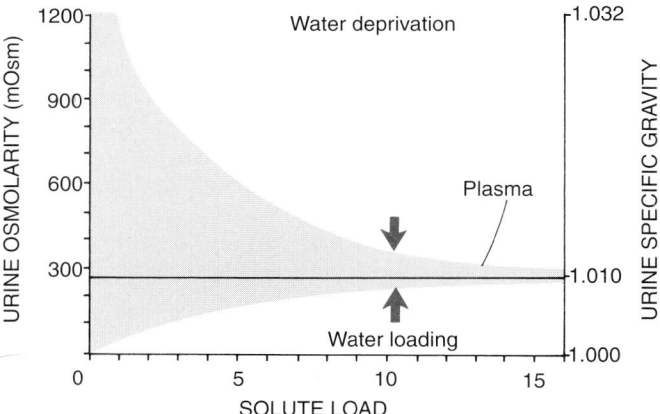

FIG. 46-3 The response of normal kidneys to an increasing solute load under conditions of water loading and deprivation. Ability to concentrate or dilute urine is progressively lost as the solute load increases. Urine specific gravity becomes fixed near 1.010 (285 mOsm). (Modified from Gordon A, Maxwell MH: Reversible uremia, *Hosp Med* 5[1]:6-18, 1969.)

FIG. 46-4 Pathogenesis of focal glomerulosclerosis in the progression of chronic renal failure. *Pgc*, Glomerular intracapillary hydrostatic pressure; Q_A, single nephron plasma flow; K_f, ultrafiltration coefficient (a measure of the number of small pores allowing filtration of water and small solutes). (Redrawn from Brevis M, Epstein FH: *Kidney Int* 26:375, 1984.)

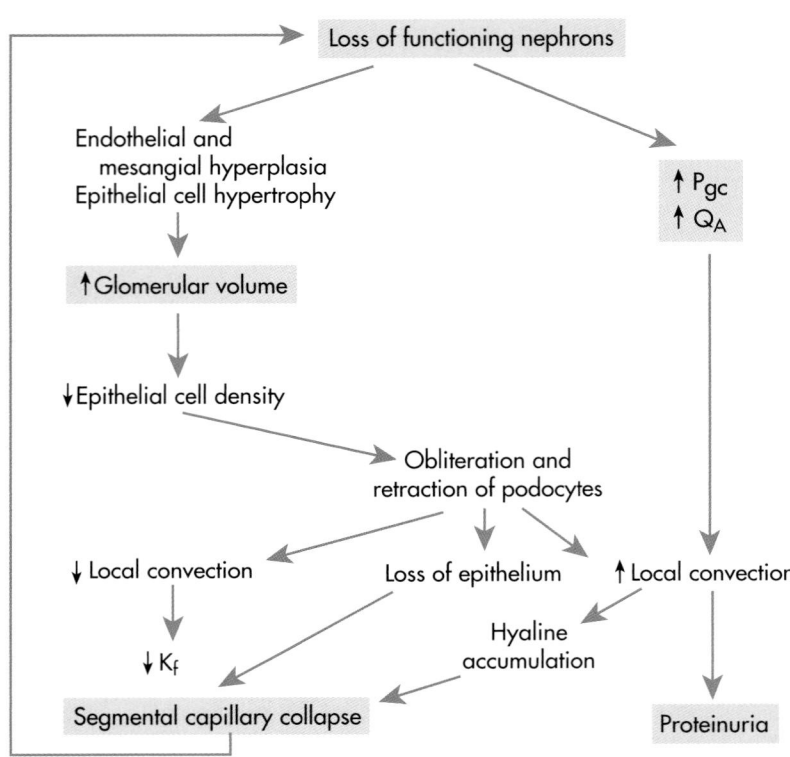

TABLE 46-1 ■■■

Classification of the Causes of Chronic Renal Failure

Disease Classifications	Disease
Infectious tubulointerstitial disease	Chronic pyelonephritis (PN) or reflux nephropathy
Inflammatory diseases	Glomerulonephritis (GN)
Hypertensive vascular disease	Benign nephrosclerosis
	Malignant nephrosclerosis
	Renal artery stenosis
Connective tissue disorders	Systemic lupus erythematosus (SLE)
	Polyarteritis nodosa
	Progressive systemic sclerosis
Congenital and hereditary disorders	Polycystic kidney disease (PKD)
	Renal tubular acidosis (RTA)
Metabolic disorders	Diabetes mellitus
	Gout
	Hyperparathyroidism
	Amyloidosis
Toxic nephropathy	Analgesic abuse
	Lead nephropathy
Obstructive nephropathy	Upper urinary tract: calculi, neoplasms, retroperitoneal fibrosis
	Lower urinary tract: prostatic hypertrophy, urethral stricture, congenital anomalies of the bladder neck and urethra

the eight classes listed in Table 46-1. No attempt is made to be all-inclusive, and only selected examples are listed under each class. These diseases are discussed in this chapter but not necessarily in the same order in which they appear in the table. It should be emphasized that although the early stages of renal disease may be quite variable, the end stages are remarkably similar and in many cases the original cause cannot be identified.

Currently, diabetes and hypertension are responsible for the largest proportion of ESRD, accounting for 34% and 21% of the total cases, respectively. Glomerulonephritis is the third most common cause of ESRD (17%). Infectious tubulointerstitial nephritis (chronic pyelonephritis or reflux nephropathy) and polycystic kidney disease (PKD) each account for 3.4% of ESRD (U.S. Renal Data System, 2000). The remaining 21% of the causes of ESRD are relatively uncommon and include obstructive uropathy, systemic lupus erythematosus (SLE), and others to be discussed in the following pages. The current distribution of the primary causes of ESRD has changed greatly from its distribution in 1967, when chronic glomerulonephritis and chronic pyelonephritis (now called *reflux nephropathy*) accounted for two thirds of the cases of ESRD. This change reflects changing practices of patient acceptance into ESRD programs, with the inclusion of a greater proportion of minorities and older patients.

The four major risk factors for the development of ESRD are age, race, gender, and family history. The incidence of diabetic renal failure increases greatly with age. ESRD caused by hypertensive nephropathy is 6.2 times more common in African Americans than it is in Caucasians. Overall, the incidence of ESRD is greater in men (56.3%) than it is in women (43.7%), although certain systemic diseases causing ESRD, such as type 2 diabetes mellitus and SLE, are more common in females. Finally, family history is a risk factor for the development of diabetes and hypertension. PKD is transmitted by autosomal dominant heredity, and there are a variety of uncommon recessive or sex-linked renal diseases.

Urinary Tract Infection, Pyelonephritis, and Reflux Nephropathy

UTIs are common and affect people throughout the life span, especially women. UTI accounts for nearly 7 million visits to physicians' offices annually in the United States (Stamm, 1998). Microbiologically, UTI exists when significant bacteriuria is present (10^5 pathogenic microorganisms/ml are detected in the urine of a properly collected midstream "clean catch" sample). The only abnormality may be colonization of the urine (asymptomatic bacteriuria), or bacteriuria may be associated with symptomatic infection of any of the structures of the urinary tract. UTI is commonly divided into two general subcategories: lower UTI (urethritis, cystitis, prostatitis) and the upper UTI (acute pyelonephritis). *Acute cystitis* (infection of the bladder) and *acute pyelonephritis* (infection of the renal pelvis and interstitium) are the most significant in terms of morbidity, but they rarely result in progressive renal failure. *Chronic pyelonephritis* (PN) refers to progressive renal injury, associated with parenchymal scarring on intravenous pyelogram (IVP), induced by recurrent or persistent infection of the kidneys. Recent evidence indicates that chronic PN occurs in patients with UTI who also have a major anatomic abnormality of the urinary tract, such as vesicoureteral reflux (VUR), obstruction, calculi, or neurogenic bladder (Kunin, 1997; Rose, Rennke, 1994). It is thought that the renal damage in chronic PN, also called *reflux nephropathy*, results from the reflux of infected urine up the ureters and then into the renal parenchyma (intrarenal reflux). Chronic PN caused by VUR is a major cause of end-stage renal failure (ESRF) in children and is theoretically preventable by the control of UTIs and correction of the structural abnormalities of the urinary tract that cause obstruction. Unfortunately, VUR may not be discovered in childhood, and the progressive renal damage may be silent until the signs and symptoms of ESRF are discovered in the adult.

Etiology and Pathogenesis

The most common infecting organism of the urinary tract is *Escherichia coli*, which accounts for more than 80% of the cases. *E. coli* is a normal inhabitant of the colon. Other gram-negative infecting organisms may include *Proteus, Klebsiella, Enterobacter,* and *Pseudomonas*. Gram-positive organisms play a lesser role in UTIs except for *Staphylococcus saprophyticus,* which accounts for 10% to 15% of UTIs in young females. In most cases, the organisms gain access to the bladder via the urethra. The infection, beginning as cystitis, may remain confined to the bladder or may ascend via the ureter to the kidney. Organisms may also reach the kidney via the bloodstream or lymphatics, but this is believed to be uncommon. The bladder and upper urethra are normally sterile, although bacteria are present in the lower urethra. The flushing action of urine flow enables the normal urinary tract to rid itself of bacteria before they have a chance to invade the mucosa. Other defense mechanisms include the antibacterial effect of the urethral mucosa, the bactericidal properties of prostatic fluid in men, and the phagocytic properties of the bladder epithelium. Despite these defenses, urinary infections may occur, and they may be related to certain predisposing factors listed in Box 46-1.

BOX 46-1

Predisposing Factors in the Development of Urinary Tract Infections and Chronic PN

Obstruction of urinary outflow (e.g., stones, prostrate disease)
Female gender
Older age
Pregnancy
Vesicoureteral reflux
Instrumentation (especially indwelling catheters)
Neurogenic bladder
Chronic analgesic abuse
Renal disease
Metabolic disturbances (diabetes, gout, urinary calculi)

PN, Pyelonephritis.

Obstruction of the urinary outflow proximal to the bladder can result in the accumulation of fluid under pressure in the renal pelvis and ureter. This buildup alone is enough to cause severe atrophy of the renal parenchyma, a condition called *hydronephrosis*. In addition, obstruction below the level of the bladder is often associated with vesicoureteral reflux (see later discussion) and infection of the kidney. Common causes of obstruction are renal or ureteral scarring, calculi, neoplasms, prostatic hypertrophy (common in men older than 60 years of age), congenital anomalies of the bladder neck and urethra, and urethral stricture.

Girls and women have a much higher incidence of UTIs and acute pyelonephritis (PN) than do boys and men, presumably because of a shorter urethra and its proximity to the anus and consequent fecal contamination. Epidemiologic studies have shown that significant bacteriuria (10^5 organisms/ml of urine) exists in 1% to 4% of school-age girls, 5% to 10% of women of childbearing age, and about 10% of women older than 60 years of age (Kunin, 1997). Only a few of these persons have clinical symptoms of UTI. Long-term follow-up studies in school-age girls reveal that girls with significant bacteriuria are more apt to have recurrent UTIs during adulthood, usually shortly after marriage or during the first pregnancy (Kunin, 1997). Although these UTIs are responsible for considerable morbidity, they rarely result in chronic PN and ESRD, except in the hidden cases with childhood damage from urologic abnormalities—mostly high grades of VUR. Infection in males is rare, and when it occurs, it is usually related to obstruction.

It has been known for some time that hydroureter and hydronephrosis, most marked on the right, always occur during pregnancy and persist for some time afterward. The dilation is attributed partly to muscular relaxation caused by the high progesterone levels and partly to obstruction of the ureters by the enlarged uterus. About 5% to 7% of the women affected have asymptomatic bacteriuria (Whalley, 1967; Norden, Kass, 1968). In a controlled study, Kass (1960) found that 42% of a placebo-treated group of women ($n = 48$) who had asymptomatic bacteriuria during early pregnancy developed PN later during the pregnancy or during the first few weeks postpartum, although none of the group treated with antibiotics for the bacteriuria ($n = 42$) developed symptomatic infection. Cystitis and PN are not more common in women with toxemia than in other women. An increased incidence of infant prematurity and mortality occurs when women develop upper UTIs during pregnancy (Stamm, 1998; Kunin, 1997).

When the renal pelvis becomes distended with newly formed urine, the smooth muscle contracts, propelling a bolus of urine into the ureter. Dilation of the ureter then initiates a peristaltic wave, which carries the urine into the bladder. Urinary flow is normally unidirectional, from the renal pelvis to the bladder, and reverse flow (reflux) is prevented by the *ureterovesicular valve* (located where the ureter is implanted into the bladder). The action of this one-way valve is vitally important in preventing backflow during the act of micturition when intravesicular pressure rises, because transmission of this pressure can damage the kidney directly. *Vesicoureteral reflux* (VUR) is defined as retrograde flow of urine from the bladder into the ureter, especially during micturition. VUR is graded from I to V, with grade I indicating reflux only into the lower ureter and grade V indicating massive reflux into the renal pelvis and calyces. VUR may be detected by injecting contrast material into the bladder through a catheter until the bladder is distended to the point at which the patient has the urge to void. Serial radiographs are taken with the bladder distended and during and after the act of voiding. The entire procedure is known as *voiding cystourethrography*. VUR has been associated with congenital malformation of the intravesicular ureter, obstruction of the bladder outlet (bladder neck or urethra), and cystitis. VUR has been demonstrated in a high proportion of patients, especially children, with recurrent UTIs and appears to be the mechanism by which organisms ascend to the kidney. It is generally believed that the reflux of infected urine into the renal parenchyma is responsible for the prominent renal scarring in humans (reflux nephropathy). The net effect is that chronic PN caused by VUR accounts for about 20% to 30% of end-stage renal failure (ESRF) in children (Rose, 1987).

Urethral and ureteric catheterization and cystoscopy commonly introduce infective organisms into the bladder or kidney. About 2% of simple, single bladder catheterizations result in infection. There is a 98% incidence of infection within 48 hours when an indwelling catheter is placed, unless meticulous attention is directed to keeping a closed drainage system. Even when the system is closed, the urine is sterile for only about 5 to 7 days. These facts indicate that catheterization is a procedure to avoid if possible.

The bladder is a distensible reservoir for urine from which the urine is evacuated at suitable intervals. The innervation of the bladder consists of a reflex arc at the S2 and S4 level of the spinal cord, the function of which is modified by sensory and motor connections to the higher centers in the brain. The act of micturition (urination) involves the coordinated contraction of the detrusor muscle (smooth muscle of the bladder wall), abdominal wall, and muscles of the pelvic floor; fixation of the chest and diaphragm; and relaxation of the internal and external sphincter muscles. Accordingly, both autonomic and voluntary activities are involved. Contraction of the detrusor muscle is reflex (stimulated when the bladder contains about 300 ml of urine), and this reflex contraction may be both inhibited and facilitated by supraspinal

portions of the nervous system under voluntary control. Interference with efferent or afferent limbs of the reflex arc or with efferent or afferent pathways connecting the sacral spinal cord to the central facilitory or inhibitory mechanisms can disrupt normal micturition; these conditions are referred to as *neurogenic bladder.*

Lapides (1976) identified five types of neurogenic bladder dysfunction, each associated with a particular neural lesion: (1) uninhibited neurogenic bladder, (2) reflex neurogenic bladder, (3) autonomous neurogenic bladder, (4) sensory paralytic neurogenic bladder, and (5) motor paralytic neurogenic bladder.

Uninhibited neurogenic bladder involves a defect of the corticoregulatory tract. This condition is common in patients who have lesions involving the cerebral cortex, as in cerebrovascular accidents or those who have disseminated cord lesions involving the corticoregulatory tracts, as in multiple sclerosis. The uninhibited neurogenic bladder resembles that of an infant. The patient is aware of a sudden desire to urinate as the bladder fills but may be unable to inhibit the desire to void even though the situation may be inappropriate. Uninhibited neurogenic bladder dysfunction is the type most frequently encountered in clinical practice. In children, the upper motor neuron dysfunction is demonstrated in persistent diurnal and nocturnal diuresis beyond the age of 2 to 3 years. Uninhibited neurogenic bladder dysfunction may be associated with recurrent UTI, especially in young girls. The patient may be able to suppress urination by voluntarily contracting the striated muscles around the urethra but is unable to control the uninhibited bladder contractions. The resultant rise in intravesicular pressure causes ischemia of the bladder wall and a lowering of local tissue immunity, with consequent infection.

Reflex neurogenic bladder results from disconnection of the sacral reflex arc from higher centers, as in cord injury or transection above the S2 level. All bladder sensation is lost, and emptying occurs through stimulation of the reflex arc whenever intravesicular pressure rises above a critical level. Emptying of the bladder is incomplete because of the lack of motor input from higher centers, and vesicoureteral reflux occurs because of the high intravesicular pressures. Both the VUR and residual urine predispose the patient with spinal cord injury to cystitis and PN.

Autonomous neurogenic bladder results from destruction of both limbs of the bladder reflex arc, as by sacral or cauda equina lesions (e.g., gunshot wound, abdominal-perineal resection surgery, neoplasia, congenital anomalies such as spina bifida and myelomeningocele). Patients with this type of lesion can neither perceive bladder fullness nor initiate urination in the normal fashion. However, these patients may learn to pass their urine by voluntarily straining and manual pressure over the suprapubic region (Credé's maneuver).

Sensory paralytic neurogenic bladder results from lesions of the sensory limb of the bladder reflex arc, as in diabetic neuropathy or multiple sclerosis. There is a gradual loss of bladder sensation, infrequent urination, and overdistention. Overdistention causes the bladder muscle to lose its tone, so that emptying is incomplete and there is residual urine.

Motor paralytic neurogenic bladder involves interruption of the motor limb of the bladder reflex arc, commonly associated with poliomyelitis, tumor, or trauma. The sensation of bladder fullness is intact, but the patient has either partial or total inability to initiate urination. Painful overdistention may result, requiring catheterization and drainage.

The pathogenic mechanisms that predisposes an individual to UTI in neurogenic bladder dysfunction include ischemia of the bladder wall from overdistention, which lessens resistance to bacterial invasion; residual urine, which provides a medium for bacterial growth; and VUR associated with increased intravesicular pressures. The use of catheters and urinary drainage is an additional predisposing factor.

Chronic analgesic abuse alone may cause chronic interstitial nephritis (see p. 699), which may be difficult to distinguish from chronic PN. In addition, recurrent UTI is common in analgesic nephropathy. Various underlying renal diseases increase susceptibility to infection and PN. Finally, metabolic disturbances such as diabetes, gout, and renal stones are often complicated by renal infection.

Acute Pyelonephritis

The clinical features of acute pyelonephritis (PN) are usually quite characteristic. In about 90% of the cases, the patient is a woman. There is an abrupt onset of fever, chills, malaise, back pain, tenderness to palpation over the costovertebral area, leukocytosis, pyuria, and bacteriuria. These signs and symptoms are often preceded by dysuria, urgency, and frequency, indicating that the infection began in the lower urinary tract. The finding of leukocyte casts indicates that the infection is in the kidney.

Fig. 46-5 illustrates the gross and microscopic appearance of the kidney in acute PN. The kidney is swollen, with multiple small abscesses on the surface. On cross section, abscesses appear as yellowish gray streaks in the pyramids and cortex. Microscopically, numerous polymorphonuclear leukocytes (PMNs) are found within the tubules (*arrow*) and in the interstitium surrounding the tubules. Segments of the tubules are destroyed, and this leukocytic material is flushed out into the urine as casts.

E. coli is the most common infecting organism in acute, uncomplicated PN. Of patients with this infection, 90% respond to antibiotic therapy and the remaining 10% may have acute recurrent infections or persistent asymptomatic bacteriuria. When acute PN is complicated by obstruction, recurrent or persistent bacteriuria occurs in 50% to 80% of patients within 2 years. It is not known with certainty how many of these patients will develop significant renal damage or how long the process might take. Treatment is directed toward appropriate antibacterial therapy, correction of predisposing factors, and careful long-term follow-up, with urine cultures at intervals to ensure that the urine is sterile.

Chronic Pyelonephritis

The identification and the causes of chronic PN are controversial. A major problem in identification is that many other inflammatory and ischemic diseases of the kidney produce segmental focalized areas of disease indistinguishable from those produced by bacterial infection. For example, nonbacterial disorders such as arteriolar nephrosclerosis and toxic nephropathies caused by analgesic abuse, lead exposure, and certain drugs (see p. 699) re-

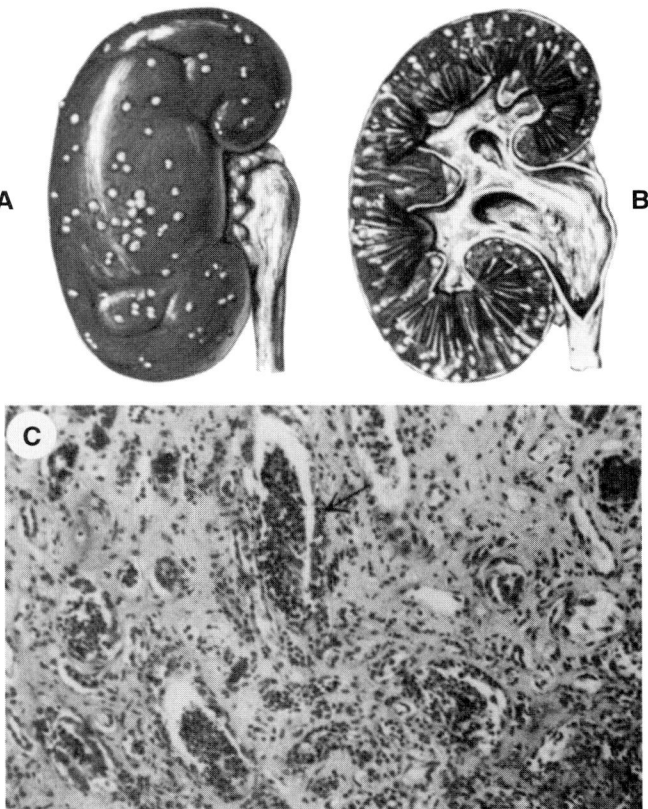

FIG. 46-5   Gross and microscopic appearance of the kidney in acute pyelonephritis. **A**, The kidney is swollen with multiple abscesses on the surface. **B**, Abscesses appear as yellowish gray streaks on the cross section. **C**, Histologically, many PMNs appear in the interstitium and within the tubules. (Illustration by Judy Simon, Department of Medical and Biological Illustrations, University of Michigan.)

sult in tubulointerstitial damage similar to that of chronic PN. It is now apparent that only a small proportion of these lesions result from infection. In the past, the diagnosis of chronic PN was almost universally applied when these tubulointerstitial abnormalities were found. The notion that a severe degree of VUR can produce the renal scarring, atrophy, and dilated calyces (reflux nephropathy) commonly diagnosed as chronic PN is now well accepted. The mechanism causing the scarring is believed to be the combined effects of (1) VUR, (2) intrarenal reflux, and (3) infection (Kunin, 1997; Tolkoff-Rubin, 2000; Rose, Rennke, 1994). The severity of the VUR is the single most important determinant of whether renal damage will occur. Most of the evidence suggests that the renal involvement in reflux nephropathy occurs early in childhood before the age of 5 to 6 years, because new scar formation rarely occurs after this age. The explanation for this observation is that intrarenal reflux ceases as the child grows older, probably because of renal growth even though VUR may continue.

In adults, VUR and reflux nephropathy may be associated with obstructive and neurologic conditions that cause obstruction of urinary drainage (as in renal calculi, or neurogenic bladder in diabetes or spinal cord injury). However, most adults with renal scarring of chronic PN developed these lesions during early childhood. Evidence to support the reflux-infection mechanism comes from animal models and the following human observations: 85% to 100% of children and 50% of adults with renal scarring have VUR, and 50% of children and 5% to 23% of adults with recurrent UTIs have VUR (Tolkoff-Rubin, 2000).

Despite the fact that the reflux neuropathy occurring in early childhood may explain the renal scarring and damage seen in many patients, the problem of how to explain progressive renal damage remains, because a sizable proportion of adults with end-stage chronic PN do not have concurrent reflux or UTI. Some patients do not even recall a history of recurrent UTI. As discussed previously in this chapter, the most popular theory explaining progressive renal failure in the presence of corrected reflux and sterile urine is the *intrarenal hemodynamic theory* or *hyperfiltration hypothesis* (Rose, Rennke, 1994). According to this theory, the initial infection-induced nephron loss leads to compensatory increases in glomerular capillary pressure (P_{gc}) and hyperperfusion in the remaining relatively normal nephrons. The intraglomerular hypertension then appears to produce glomerular injury and eventual sclerosis. An increasing body of evidence from animal and human studies support the concept of hemodynamically mediated glomerular injury. Experimental evidence shows that the control of systemic hypertension, especially by the administration of angiotensin-converting enzyme (ACE)–inhibitor drugs such as captopril or enalapril maleate, slows the decline of GFR in many patients with chronic renal failure. These drugs lower P_{gc} by opposing the action of angiotensin II and dilating the efferent arteriole. Preferential lowering of P_{gc} also occurs when dietary protein is restricted to 20 to 30 g/day, supplemented with amino acids and their keto analogues. Multiple protein-restriction studies have demonstrated marked slowing (75% to 90%) or even a cessation of the decline in GFR in many patients, although the mechanism by which protein intake affects GFR is uncertain. Moreover, this effect occurred in a wide variety of chronic renal diseases, including chronic PN and chronic glomerulonephritis.

In contrast to acute PN, the clinical features of chronic PN are quite vague. The diagnosis is often made when a patient has with symptoms of chronic renal insufficiency or hypertension, or proteinuria may be discovered in a routine examination. In some cases, there is a documented history of UTIs dating from childhood. In other cases, careful questioning may reveal a history of vague symptoms of dysuria, frequency, and sometimes loin pain. Many patients are asymptomatic until the disease is advanced. Typical findings in chronic PN include intermittent bacteriuria and white blood cells (WBCs) or white cell casts in the urine. Proteinuria is usually minimal. Because chronic PN is chiefly a medullary interstitial disease, the concentrating ability of the kidney is affected early in its course, before a significant decrease in the GFR occurs. Consequently, polyuria, nocturia, and urine with a low specific gravity are prominent early symptoms. Many patients also have a tendency to lose salt in the urine. About one half of the patients may develop hypertension. Azotemia is common in the course of chronic

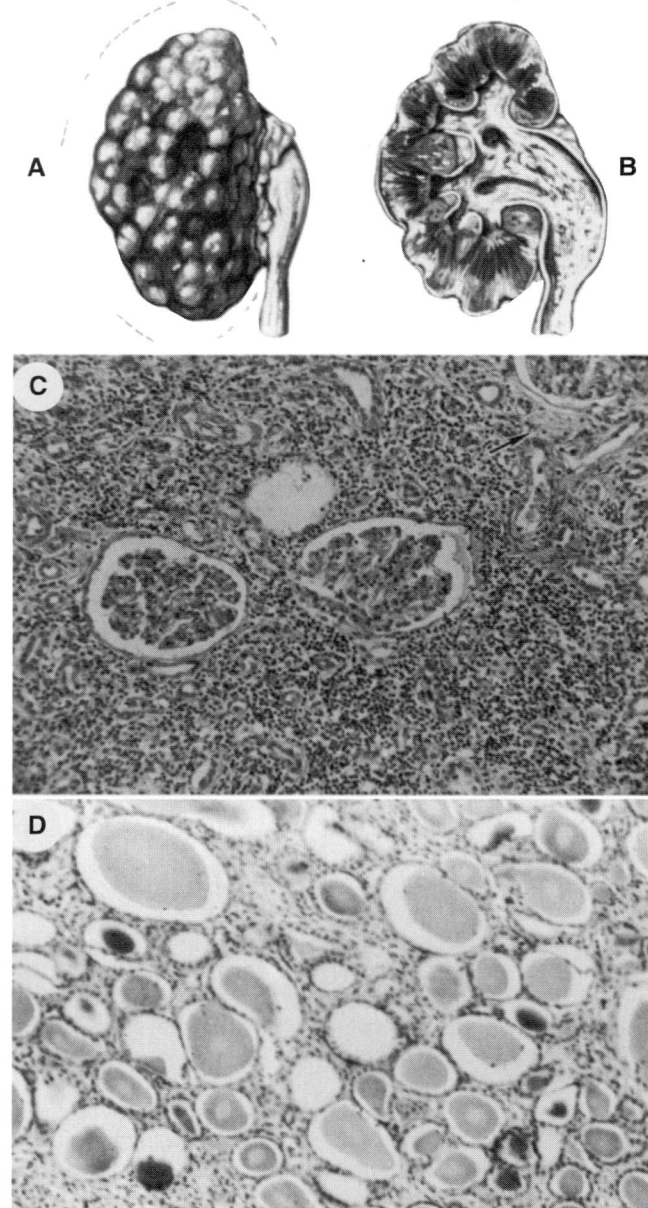

FIG. 46-6 Gross and microscopic appearance of the kidney in chronic pyelonephritis. **A,** Coarsely granular surface with U-shaped depressions. **B,** Thinning of the cortex, subcapsular scars; dilated, fibrosed pelvis; and calyces. **C,** Chronic inflammatory cells throughout interstitium; small, atrophied tubules; and an area of interstitial fibrosis *(arrows).* **D,** Thyroid-gland appearance caused by dilated tubules containing glassy-looking casts. (Illustration by Judy Simon, Department of Medical and Biological Illustrations, University of Michigan.)

PN, but advancement to renal failure usually progresses slowly.

The IVP reveals clubbing of the calyces, a thinned cortex, and small, irregular-shaped kidneys that are usually asymmetric (see Fig. 45-9, *B*). Fig. 46-6 illustrates the pathologic changes in chronic PN. The surface of the kidney is coarsely granular, with U-shaped depressions (see Fig. 46-6, *A*), subcapsular scars, and a dilated and fibrosed pelvis and calyces seen on the cross section (see Fig. 46-6, *B*). Microscopic examination of tissue sections reveals characteristic parenchymal changes: many chronic inflammatory cells consisting of plasma cells and lymphocytes (dark-staining dots) are scattered throughout the interstitium. The three glomeruli are intact but surrounded by many tubules that are small and atrophied or dilated. There is an area of interstitial fibrosis near the glomerulus (see *arrow*, Fig. 46-6, *C*). Large areas of thyroidization (having the appearance of thyroid gland tissue) are seen, consisting of dilated tubules lined with flattened epithelial cells and filled with glassy-appearing casts (see Fig. 46-6, *D*).

Glomerulonephritis

Glomerulonephritis is a bilateral inflammatory disease of the kidneys that begins in the glomerulus and is demonstrated by proteinuria or hematuria or both. Although the lesions are primarily glomerular, entire nephrons may eventually be destroyed, leading to chronic renal failure. The original disease described by Richard Bright in 1827 *(Bright's disease)* is now known to be a collection of many diseases of different causes (most of which are unknown), although immune responses seems to be implicated in several forms of glomerulonephritis.

In recent years, knowledge of the pathologic changes in renal disease has been greatly expanded by renal biopsy studies using light, immunofluorescent, and electron microscopy. As knowledge has expanded, new categories have emerged based on a greater ability to define the nature of renal lesions. Numerous attempts have been made to separate and classify the various types of glomerulonephritis by relating histologic and clinical features. Unfortunately, the various categories are not exclusive. This overlap is understandable, because the kidney has only a limited number of morphologic and functional responses. To add to this confusion, many systemic and metabolic disorders may, when there is renal involvement, have changes in the glomeruli that are indistinguishable from primary glomerulonephritis.

Table 46-2 lists the various ways in which glomerulonephritis is described and classified. This table serves as a guide for the discussion in the remainder of this chapter and should be read before proceeding. The general term *glomerulonephritis (GN)* is commonly used to refer to a number of primary renal diseases predominantly affecting the glomeruli, but it is also used to refer to glomerular lesions that may or may not be the result of the primary renal disease. For example, the renal lesion in systemic lupus erythematosus (SLE) may be referred to as proliferative glomerulonephritis (GN). The following discussion focuses on primary renal diseases that cause GN, although references are made to systemic diseases that cause similar lesions in the kidney. Systemic diseases causing renal injury are considered in more detail later in this chapter.

Acute Glomerulonephritis

The classic case of acute GN follows a streptococcal infection of the throat or sometimes of the skin after a latent period of 1 to 2 weeks. The responsible organism is usu-

ally a type 12 or 4 and 1, group A, beta-hemolytic streptococcus; rarely others. However, the streptococcus itself does not cause renal damage by infection. It is believed that antibodies are directed against a specific antigen that is a constituent of the specific streptococcal plasma membrane. An antigen-antibody complex is formed in the blood and circulates to the glomerulus, where it is mechanically trapped in the basement membrane. Complement is fixed, resulting in injury and inflammation, which attracts PMNs and platelets to the damaged site. Phagocytosis and release of lysosomal enzymes also damage the endothelium and glomerular basement membrane (GBM). As a response to injury, there is proliferation of endothelial cells and then of mesangial cells, and later, epithelial cells may increase as well. The resulting increased porosity of the glomerular capillary permits proteins and blood cells to escape into the forming urine, causing proteinuria and hematuria. It is presumed that these antigen-antibody-complement complexes appear as subepithelial nodules (or epimembranous humps) on electron microscopy and as a granular, "lumpy-bumpy" pattern on immunofluorescent microscopy; by light microscopy the glomeruli appear swollen and hypercellular, with invasion of PMNs (Fig. 46-7).

Acute poststreptococcal GN (APSGN) most frequently affects children between 3 and 7 years of age, although adolescents and young adults are also affected. The ratio of males to females is approximately 2:1.

The common presenting features of APSGN include hematuria, proteinuria, oliguria, edema, and hypertension. Common symptoms associated with the onset are fatigue, anorexia, and, sometimes, fever, headache, nausea, and vomiting. Elevation of the antistreptolysin O (ASO) titer may indicate the presence of antibodies to streptococcal organisms. Serum complement levels may be low, owing to depletion. This common finding gives further support to the hypothesis that the disease has an immune basis.

The major physiologic disturbances in APSGN are depicted on the diagram in Fig. 46-8. The GFR is usually depressed (although renal plasma flow [RPF] is generally normal). Consequently, the excretion of water, sodium, and nitrogenous substances may be decreased, resulting in edema and azotemia. Increased aldosterone may also play a role in sodium and water retention. Facial edema, particularly periorbital edema, is extremely common in the morning, although it may become more apparent in the lower extremities as the day progresses. The degree of edema usually depends on the severity of the glomerular inflammation, whether there is concomitant congestive heart failure, and how soon dietary salt is restricted.

Hypertension almost always occurs, although the rise in blood pressure may be only moderate. Whether the hypertension results from an expansion of the extracellular fluid (ECF) volume or from vasospasm is not clear.

Damage to the glomerular capillary tuft results in hematuria and albuminuria, as previously described. The urine may be grossly bloody or coffee colored. Microscopic examination of the sediment reveals cylindruria (many casts), red blood cells (RBCs), and red cell casts; the latter establishes the glomerular origin of the bleeding.

TABLE 46-2 ■ ■ ■

Classifications of Glomerulonephritis

Classification	Description
DISTRIBUTION	
Diffuse	Involves all the glomeruli; most common form results in chronic renal failure
Focal	Only a portion of the glomeruli are abnormal
Local	Only a part of the glomerular tuft is abnormal, such as a single capillary loop
BROAD CLINICAL FORMS OF DIFFUSE GLOMERULONEPHRITIS	
Acute	Classic, benign disorder that is nearly always preceded by a streptococcal infection and associated with immune-complex deposition in the GBM and proliferative cellular changes
Subacute	Rapidly progressive form of glomerulonephritis characterized by intense cellular proliferative changes that destroy the glomeruli and result in death from uremia within a few months from the onset
Chronic	Slowly progressive glomerulonephritis leading to sclerosing and obliterative changes in the glomeruli; small, contracted kidneys; and death from uremia; entire course varies from 2-40 years
PATHOGENETIC IMMUNE MECHANISM AND IMMUNOFLUORESCENT PATTERN	
Immune-complex, granular	Antibody (Ab) to either exogenous or endogenous nonglomerular antigens (Ag) is involved in the formation of circulating Ab-Ag complexes, which are passively trapped in the GBM. Complement fixation and the release of immunologic mediators result in glomerular injury; deposit is along epithelial surface and reveals a lumpy or granular pattern on immunofluorescent microscopy; associated with poststreptococcal GN, idiopathic membranous GN, and the GN of serum sickness, subacute bacterial endocarditis, malaria, and anaphylactoid purpura
Nephrotoxic (anti-GBM), linear	Antibodies form that react with the patient's own GBM as the antigen (anti-GBM or antikidney antibodies). True autoimmune disease in contrast to immune-complex GN, in which the GBM is like an innocent bystander; immune deposits are subendothelial and result in a ribbonlike linear pattern on immunofluorescence; associated with RPGN and Goodpasture's syndrome
HISTOLOGIC PATTERN	
Minimal change	Also called lipoid nephrosis or foot-process disease; glomeruli appear normal or nearly normal on light microscopy, whereas electron microscopy reveals fusion of the foot processes; only major form of GN without evidence of immunopathology; commonly presents as the nephrotic syndrome in children 1-5 years of age; responds well to corticosteroid therapy; prognosis excellent
Proliferative change	Deposition of immunoglobulin, complement, and fibrin leads to proliferation of endothelial, mesangial, and epithelial cells; latter leads to crescent formation that may encircle and obliterate the glomerular tuft—ominous sign, common in RPGN and advanced CGN
Membranous change	Epimembranous deposit of immune material along GBM causing the GBM to thicken, but there is little or no inflammation or cellular proliferation, although the capillary lumen may eventually be obliterated; most common lesion in adults with the nephrotic syndrome; responds poorly to corticosteroid and immunosuppressive therapy; generally poor prognosis and slow progression to renal failure; membranous changes are also common in systemic nephritic diseases such as diabetes mellitus and SLE
Membranoproliferative change	Also called mesangiocapillary, lobular, or hypocomplementemic GN; immune-complex material deposited between the GBM and endothelium, causing GBM thickening and proliferation of the mesangial cells and giving the glomerulus a lobular or "wire-loop" appearance on light microscopy; characterized by low serum complement level, hematuria, and the nephrotic syndrome; responds poorly to therapy, generally progresses slowly to renal failure
Focal glomerulonephritis	Proliferative or sclerosing lesions that occur at random throughout the kidneys (focal as opposed to diffuse), often affecting only part of the glomerular tuft (local); occurs during at least part of the course of SBE, SLE, polyarteritis nodosa, Goodpasture's syndrome, and purpura; idiopathic focal GN sometimes appears in children; prognosis good
CLINICAL SYNDROMES	
Acute nephritic syndrome	Acute nephritis of sudden onset, usually associated with poststreptococcal GN but can occur in many other renal diseases and as an acute exacerbation of CGN
Nephrotic syndrome	Clinical complex characterized by massive proteinuria (>3.5 g/day), hypoalbuminemia, edema, and hyperlipidemia. Occurs in many primary renal and systemic diseases; 50% of patients with CGN have it at least once
Persistent asymptomatic urine abnormalities	"Latent" stage in CGN, characterized by minimal proteinuria and/or hematuria but without symptoms; glomerular function relatively stable or may show slow progression ("silent azotemia")
Uremic syndrome	Symptomatic end-stage renal failure

AGN, Acute glomerulonephritis; *GBM,* glomerular basement membrane; *GN,* glomerulonephritis; *CRF,* chronic renal failure; *CGN,* chronic glomerulonephritis; *SLE,* systemic lupus erythematosus; *SBE,* subacute bacterial endocarditis; *RPGN,* rapidly progressive or subacute glomerulonephritis.

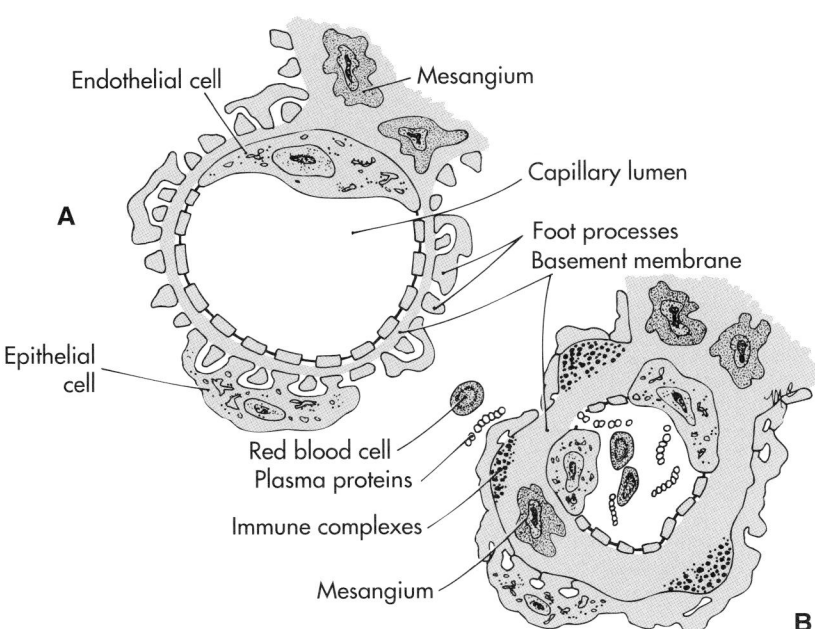

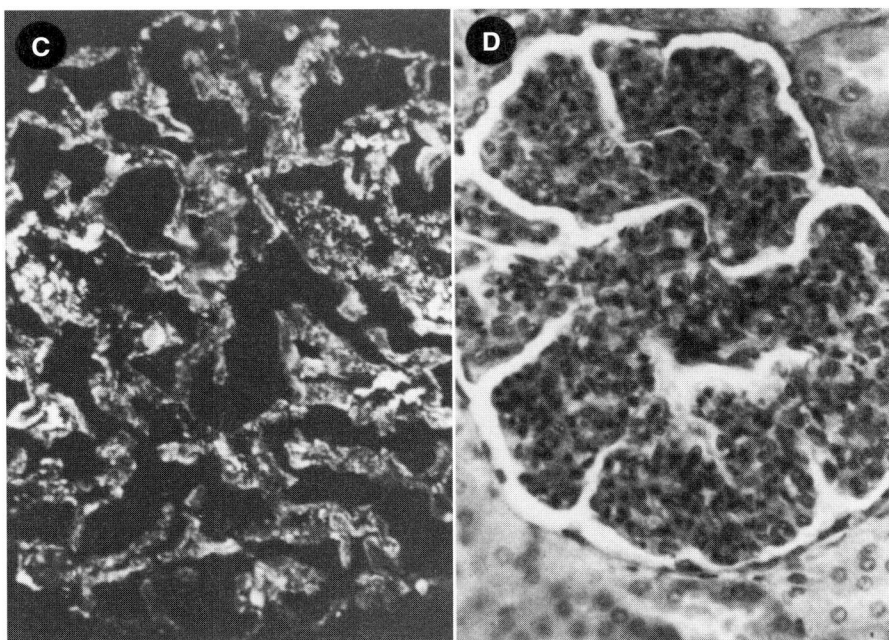

FIG. 46-7 Acute poststreptococcal glomeru-lonephritis. **A,** Diagram of electron microscopy appearance of a single capillary loop of the glomerular tuft. **B,** Diagram of electron microscopy appearance of subepithelial deposits of immune complex, thickened basement membrane, cellular proliferation, and damage to capillary. **C,** Photomicrograph of immunofluorescent preparation, showing lumpy pattern of immunoglobulin and complement deposits along glomerular capillary walls in circulating immune-complex disease. **D,** Light microscopy slide from kidney of a patient with acute poststreptococcal glomerulonephritis (APSGN), showing infiltration with polymorphonuclear leukocytes (PMNs) and hypercellularity that crowd the glomerulus filling Bowman's space. (Modified from Netter FH: Kidneys, ureter, and urinary bladder. In *The Ciba collection of medical illustrations,* vol 6, West Caldwell, NJ, 1973, Ciba Medical Education Division. Immunofluorescent micrograph courtesy Michael J. Deegan, MD, University of Michigan Medical School.)

The loss of protein is usually not great enough to cause hypoalbuminemia, and the nephrotic syndrome rarely occurs in APSGN. The urine specific gravity is usually high despite azotemia, a combination rarely occurring in renal diseases other than APSGN. This finding is explained by the fact that the acute disease has affected tubular function very little.

The usual treatment of APSGN is penicillin to eradicate any residual streptococcal infection, bed rest during the acute phase, sodium restriction in the presence of edema or signs of heart failure, and antihypertensive drugs if indicated. Corticosteroid drugs have no known beneficial effect in APSGN. Symptoms usually subside within days, although microscopic hematuria and proteinuria may

persist for months. It is estimated that more than 90% of children have a complete recovery. The prognosis is less favorable for adults (30% to 50%). Death occurs in 2% to 5% of all patients during the acute phase. In the remainder of patients, the disease may advance to a rapidly progressive GN (RPGN) or a more slowly progressive chronic GN (CGN). In RPGN, death from uremia usually occurs within a few months, whereas the entire course may vary from 2 to 40 years in CGN.

The natural history of the various forms of diffuse GN is depicted in the diagram in Fig. 46-9. Contrary to popular belief, only a small percentage of the cases of RPGN and CGN have their origin in APSGN. The precipitating factors are usually unknown.

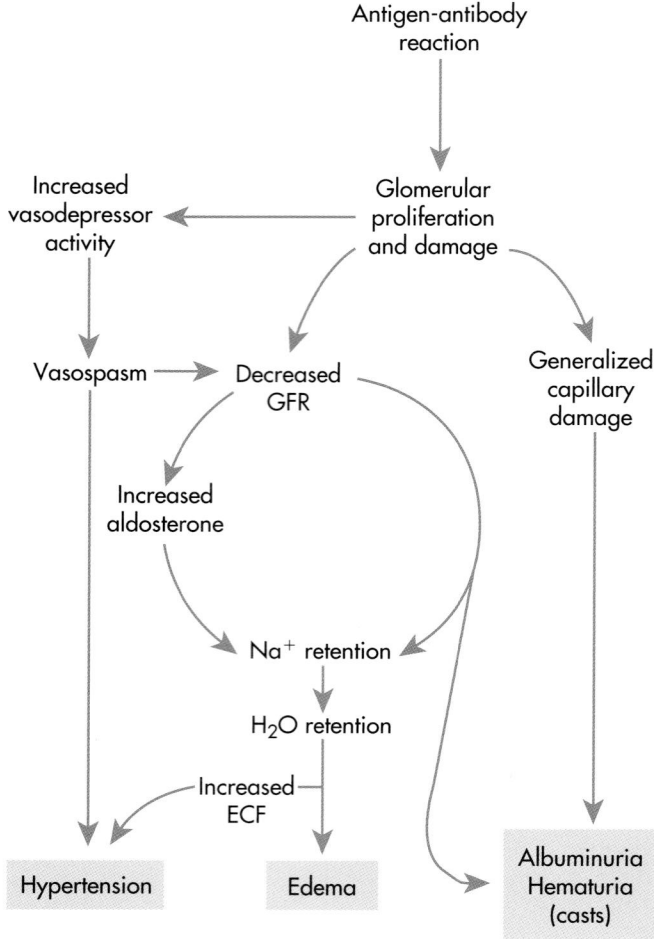

FIG. 46-8 Major disturbances in acute poststreptococcal glomerulonephritis. *GFR*, Glomerular filtration rate; *ECF*, extracellular fluid.

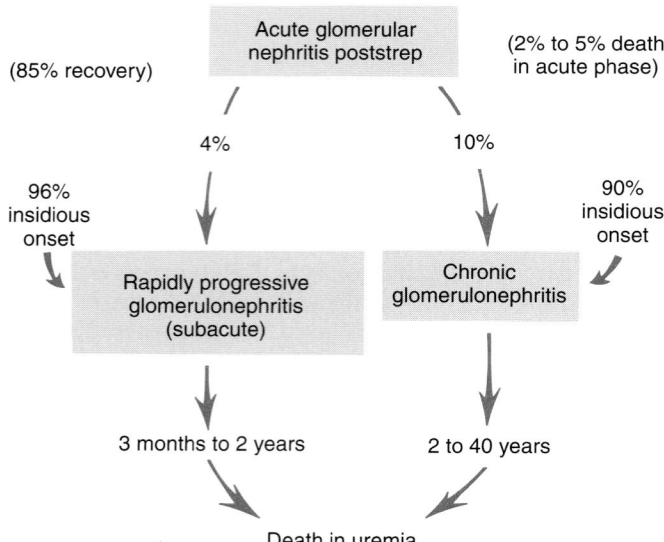

FIG. 46-9 Natural history of the various forms of diffuse glomerulonephritis.

Although APSGN has been more clearly defined, it should be noted that an acute nephritic syndrome may be associated with many other diseases affecting the kidney (e.g., subacute bacterial endocarditis [SBE], malaria, anaphylactoid purpura, the collagen diseases). An acute nephritic syndrome may also occur during the course of CGN (see Table 46-2).

Rapidly Progressive Glomerulonephritis

RPGN (formerly called *subacute GN*) is a term used to designate a fulminant renal disease with characteristic clinical and morphologic features. There is hematuria, proteinuria, and rapidly progressive azotemia, resulting in death within 2 years. At autopsy, the salient features are widespread parietal epithelial crescent formation and diffuse glomerular involvement. Goodpasture's disease or syndrome, a rare disease most common in young men, is a good example of this type of disease. The onset may be insidious or acute and is associated with lung hemorrhage and hemoptysis. There is usually no preceding illness to suggest the origin of the antibodies that develop in the patient's blood against the glomerular basement membrane (GBM). Subendothelial immune-complex material is seen with electron microscopy, and a linear pattern of immunofluorescence suggests that a nephrotoxic immune mechanism is involved in the pathogenesis (Fig. 46-10). Immunoglobulin deposits have also been found along the basement membrane in the lung alveoli. Patients who are treated aggressively early in the course of the disease with a combination of plasmapheresis (to remove anti-GBM antibodies), corticosteroids, and cytotoxic agents, such as cyclophosphamide or azathioprine, are more likely to recover. Approximately 20% of the patients regain normal renal function. The chances of recovery decrease as the number of glomeruli that are involved increases. The exact mechanism of autoantibody elimination is not known. Dialysis support may be required for patients who develop progressive renal failure. Renal transplantation may be used after the anti-GBM antibodies have disappeared. One-year renal survival approaches 90% if treatment is started early and before serum creatinine exceeds 5 mg/dl but falls to about 10% if renal failure is more advanced (Brady et al, 1998).

Chronic Glomerulonephritis

CGN is characterized by slow, progressive destruction of the glomeruli from long-standing GN. In most instances, CGN has no known relationship to APSGN and RPGN but appears to represent de novo disease. The onset tends to be insidious, and it is usually discovered late in its course when symptoms of renal insufficiency appear. According to the stage of the disease, there may be polyuria or oliguria, proteinuria of varying degrees, hypertension, progressive azotemia, and death from uremia.

In advanced CGN, the kidneys are grossly contracted, sometimes weighing as little as 50 g, and the surface is granular. These changes are caused by ischemia and the loss of nephrons. Microscopically, most of the glomeruli are altered. There may be a mixture of membranous and proliferative changes and epithelial crescent formation. Eventually, there is atrophy of the tubules, interstitial fibrosis, and thickening of the arterial walls. When marked damage to all structures has occurred, the organ is called

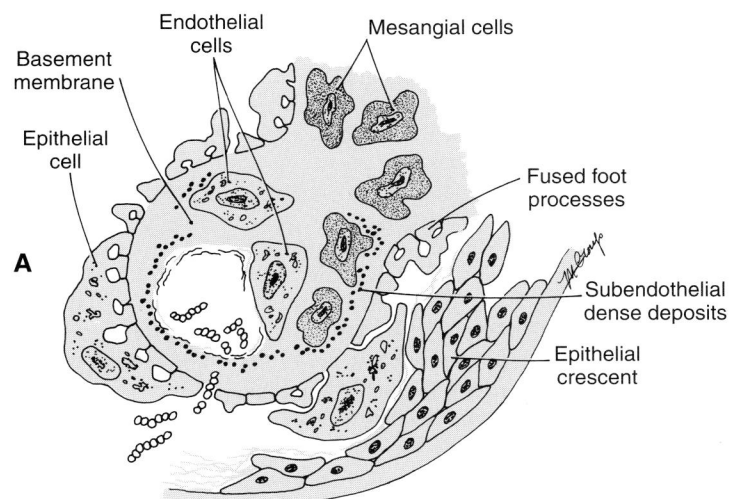

A

FIG. 46-10   Rapidly progressive glomerulonephritis. **A**, Cross section of a single capillary loop showing subendothelial dense deposits and glomerular damage. **B**, Photomicrograph of immunofluorescent preparation showing linear pattern of immune deposit typical of antiglomerular basement membrane (GBM) disease. **C**, Light microscopy slide from a patient with rapidly progressive glomerulonephritis, showing large fibroepithelial crescent *(arrows)* crowding a lobulated glomerular tuft. (A modified from Netter FH: Kidneys, ureters, and urinary bladder. In *The Ciba collection of medical illustrations,* vol 6, West Caldwell, NJ, 1973, Ciba Medical Education Division. B from Fish AJ, Michael AF, Good RA: Pathogenesis of glomerulonephritis. In Strauss MB, Welt LG, editors: *Diseases of the kidney,* ed 2, Boston, 1971, Little, Brown.)

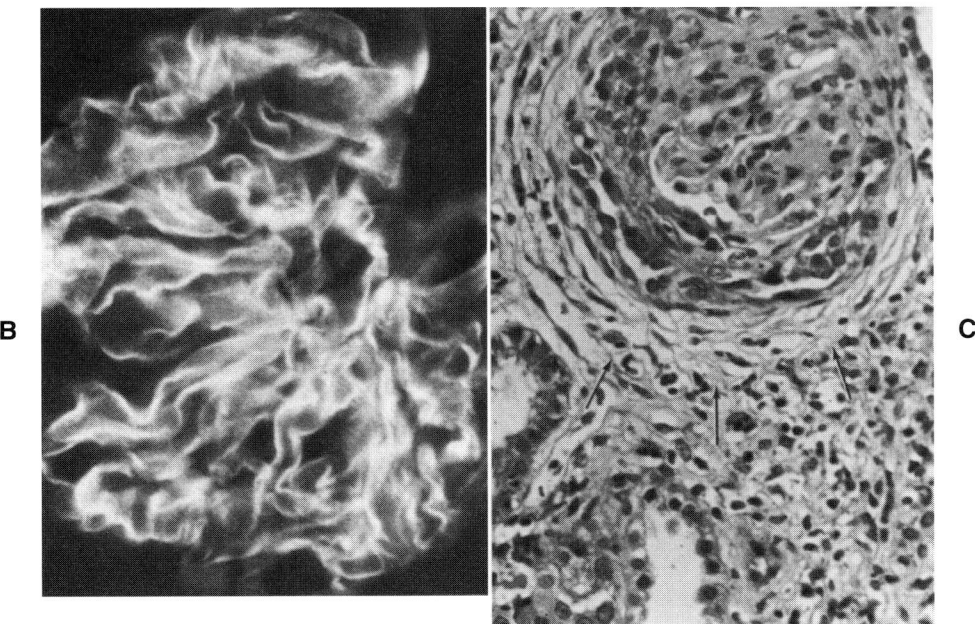

B

C

an *end-stage kidney,* and it may be difficult to determine whether the original lesion was glomerular, interstitial, or vascular (Fig. 46-11).

Nephrotic Syndrome

Although many patients with CGN have persistent, asymptomatic proteinuria throughout the course of the disease, about 50% develop the nephrotic syndrome. The nephrotic syndrome is a clinical state in which there is massive proteinuria (>3.5 g/day), hypoalbuminemia, edema, and hyperlipidemia. Usually the BUN level is normal.

The nephrotic syndrome is associated with several primary (idiopathic) glomerular diseases, or it may be associated with a large variety of systemic disorders in which the kidneys are secondarily involved. Examples of primary renal diseases associated with the nephrotic syndrome include minimal change GN, membranous GN, focal glomerulosclerosis, mesangial proliferative GN, and membranoproliferative GN (discussion follows).

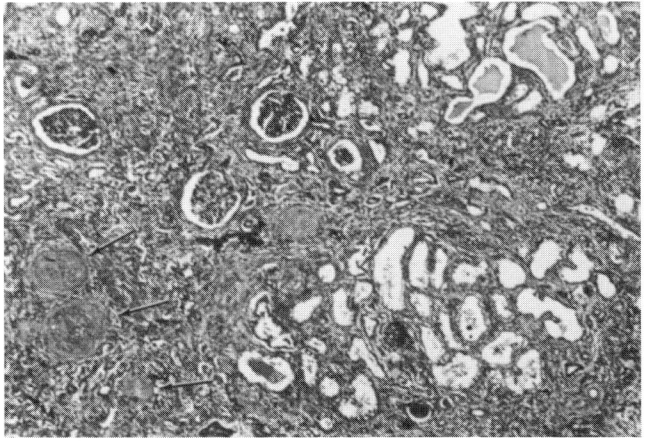

FIG. 46-11   End-stage kidney (light microscopy) from a patient with chronic pyelonephritis, showing marked distortion of the renal architecture. There is interstitial fibrosis, several glomeruli are completely hyalinized *(arrows)*, and three are spared. Marked tubular distortion and atrophy are present, and casts appear in several tubules.

Examples of systemic diseases and substances associated with the nephrotic syndrome include diabetes glomerulo-sclerosis; SLE; amyloidosis; Henoch-Schönlein purpura; drugs (e.g., gold, captopril, street heroin); other immune-complex diseases caused by chronic infection (e.g., hepatitis B, endocarditis, shunt infections); neoplasm; and acquired immunodeficiency syndrome (AIDS). Children and adults differ in the prevalence of the etiologies of the nephrotic syndrome. The cause of the nephrotic syndrome in children is predominantly primary glomerular disease, whereas it is most often associated with a systemic disorder in adults.

Minimal change GN is the typical lesion of the nephrotic syndrome in childhood (<15 years) accounting for about 70% to 80% of the cases. Older terms for this disease include *lipoid nephrosis, nil disease,* or *foot-process disease.* The last term is related to the observation that the normally discrete foot processes (podocytes) of the glomerular epithelial cells appear on electron microscopy to be fused together (Fig. 46-12). The cause is unknown, although the disease is preceded by an upper respiratory infection in about one third of the cases. Minimal change GN is the only major form of GN in which immune pathogenic mechanisms do not appear to be involved. The onset of the nephrotic syndrome is usually sudden in children ages 2 to 6 years, with a male to female ratio of 2:1. This lesion is less common in adults and accounts for only 15% to 20% of the cases of idiopathic nephrotic syndrome.

Because the etiology and pathogenesis of minimal change GN are unknown, treatment is empiric and symptomatic. More than 95% of children respond to corticosteroid therapy with complete disappearance of the proteinuria within 8 weeks. The response to corticosteroids may take longer in adults with a less favorable outcome. In the minority of patients who do not respond to steroid therapy or who have relapses, immunosuppressive drugs such as cyclophosphamide (Cytoxan) or azathioprine (Imuran) may be helpful. The small proportion of patients who do not recover generally follow a long, remitting, relapsing course ending in uremia (Siegel, 1998).

Focal glomerulosclerosis (FGS) accounts for 10% to 15% of the cases of idiopathic nephrotic syndrome in children and 10% to 20% of the cases in adults. The lesion is characterized by sclerosis and hyalinosis of some of the glomeruli (hence the term *focal*). Immunofluorescence reveals deposition of IgM and C3. The cause of the lesion is unknown. Some patients respond to corticosteroid therapy with a lasting remission, but about one half of the patients with heavy proteinuria develop end-stage renal failure (ESRF) within 10 years. If the patient receives a renal transplant, the disease commonly recurs in the transplanted organ (Brady et al, 1998).

Membranous GN is the most common cause of idiopathic nephrotic syndrome in adults, accounting for 30% to 40% of the cases, but it is rare in children (<5%). The lesions are diffusely distributed and involve all the glomeruli. The predominant histologic change seen by light microscopy is thickening of the basement membrane. IgG and C3 are seen in a granular pattern along the glomerular basement membrane (GBM). Membranous change GN follows a slowly progressive course with intermittent remissions and exacerbations. About one third of the patients develop ESRF within 5 to 10 years. Corticosteroids, sometimes in combination with cyclophosphamide, are used in an attempt to obtain a remission, but they do not appear to greatly alter the course of the disease (Brady et al, 1998).

Mesangial proliferative GN is characterized by diffuse involvement of glomeruli and proliferation of the mesangial cells and endothelial cells, representing a heterogeneous group of glomerular diseases. Immunofluorescence microscopy reveals a variety of patterns. A granular pattern of IgA and C3 deposits in the mesangium may predominate, in which case the condition is called *IgA nephropathy* or *Berger's disease.* In other cases, there may be IgG or IgM deposits in the mesangium that may represent resolving poststreptococcal GN or other systemic diseases, such as systemic lupus erythematosus (SLE) or Henoch-Schönlein purpura. This lesion is responsible for about 5% of idiopathic nephrotic syndrome in adults and 5% to 10% in children; it is more common in older children and young adults as compared with the general population. Patients who have a remission of proteinuria after corticosteroid therapy tend to do well, with less inclination to develop progressive renal failure. Progressive renal failure develops in about 20% to 30% of the patients with steroid-unresponsive nephrotic syndrome (Brady et al, 1998). Since it was first identified in 1968, IgA nephropathy is becoming the most frequently identified primary glomerular disease in the world (although, in most cases, the proteinuria is mild). The frequency of the disease varies substantially between countries. In southern Europe, Asia, and Australia, IgA nephropathy accounts for 20% to 40% of patients with primary renal disease. Japan has the highest frequency and the United States and Canada have the lowest frequencies (Julien, 1998).

Membranoproliferative GN (MPGN) is characterized both by thickening of the capillary loops and mesangial hypercellularity. MPGN, also called *mesangiocapillary* or *lobular GN,* is divided into two main subgroups (types I

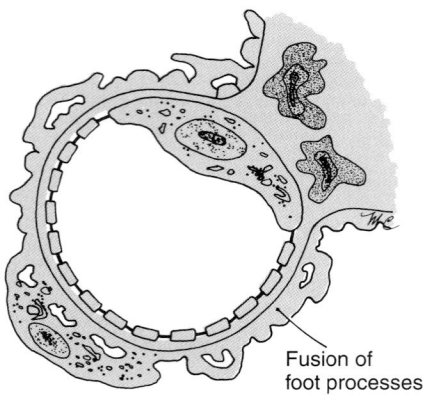

FIG. 46-12   Schema of glomerular loop showing fusion of foot processes in minimal change glomerulonephritis. (Modified from Netter FH: Kidneys, ureters, and urinary bladder. In *The Ciba collection of medical illustrations,* vol 6, West Caldwell, NJ, 1973, Ciba Medical Education Division.).

Fusion of
foot processes

and II), which have different histologies. Type I MPGN is characterized by subendothelial deposits of C3 in a granular pattern around the capillary loop. This type of pattern may also be seen in SLE. Type II MPGN is uncommon, where long segments of densely staining deposits occur within the basement membrane, causing thickening; the alternate name is *dense deposit disease*. The dense deposits may contain C3 and IgM.

MPGN is found in about 5% of cases of idiopathic nephrotic syndrome in children, especially those between the ages of 8 and 16 years, and is somewhat less common in adults. The clinical presentation is quite varied. Type I accounts for about two thirds of the cases, affecting males and females equally. Some 50% to 75% of patients present with the nephrotic syndrome. The remainder have proteinuria in the nonnephrotic range that is accompanied by hematuria. Circulating immune complexes are often present, and serum C3 levels are depressed. Type II may be associated with partial lipodystrophy with loss of subcutaneous fat in the face or other parts of the body. Low plasma C3 in type II MPGN is associated with the presence of C3-nephritic factor (C3NeF), an IgG antibody to C3-convertase, which has the effect of protecting C3-convertase from enzymatic degradation, with resultant low C3 levels.

The cause of MPGN is unknown, although, in some cases, there is a history of a preceding upper respiratory infection. Both types I and II MPGN are aggressive and progressive diseases with approximately one half of the patients dying or developing end-stage renal disease (ESRD) within 10 years. The prognosis for type II lesions is worse than it is for type I.

The major physiologic disturbances leading to edema in the nephrotic syndrome are depicted in Fig. 46-13. The initial event in most cases is an antigen-antibody reaction at the glomerulus, resulting in increased GBM permeability, massive proteinuria, and hypoalbuminemia. Patients with the nephrotic syndrome commonly pass 5 to 15 g of protein every 24 hours. Hypoalbuminemia, by decreasing colloid osmotic pressure (COP), favors the transudation of fluid out of the vascular compartment into the interstitium. This mechanism is fairly direct for the production of edema. Additionally, the hypovolemia results in a decrease of renal plasma flow (RPF) and GFR, activating the renin-angiotensin mechanism. The hypovolemia also activates volume receptors in the left atrium. The result is increased aldosterone and antidiuretic hormone (ADH) production. The kidneys retain salt and water, further aggravating the edema. By repetition of this chain of events, massive edema (anasarca) may occur. The amount of protein lost, however, does not correlate precisely with the severity of the edema, because people vary in the rate of protein synthesis to replace that which is lost. The cause of the hyperlipidemia that often accompanies the nephrotic syndrome is obscure. Serum cholesterol, phospholipids, and triglycerides are all usually increased. The mechanism of nephrotic edema differs from that of APSGN.

Complications of the nephrotic syndrome include hyperlipidemia and hypertension, which may predispose to atherosclerosis when prolonged. There is also an increased susceptibility to infection, which may be caused by loss of immunoglobulins in the urine. Thrombosis is a common complication in the nephrotic syndrome, leading to renal vein thrombosis, deep venous thrombosis in the legs, and pulmonary embolism.

The nephrotic syndrome is treated with corticosteroid and immunosuppressive drugs directed toward the nature of the lesion, a high-protein and salt-restricted diet, diuretics, sometimes intravenous infusion of albumin, and restricted activity during the acute phase. When diuretics are used, they must be used with caution because excessive diuresis will cause ECF volume depletion and increase the risk of thrombosis and renal hypoperfusion. It is also important to isolate patients from sources of infection. Patients with the nephrotic syndrome are highly susceptible to infection, and before antibiotic drugs were discovered, they often died of empyema, pneumonia, or peritonitis. Angiotensin-converting enzyme (ACE) inhibitors can reduce protein loss by reducing intraglomerular pressure and GFR. This reduction in protein loss, reduction in intraglomerular pressure, and inhibition of angiotensin II may also be helpful in reducing the fluid retention. ACE inhibitors are also the first-line drugs of choice to control systemic hypertension, which may be caused by the renal disease and may be a side effect from corticosteroid therapy. Long-term management is important, because many patients follow a course of repeated exacerbations and remissions over a period of years; however, with advancing glomerular hyalinization, proteinuria usually diminishes as azotemia progresses.

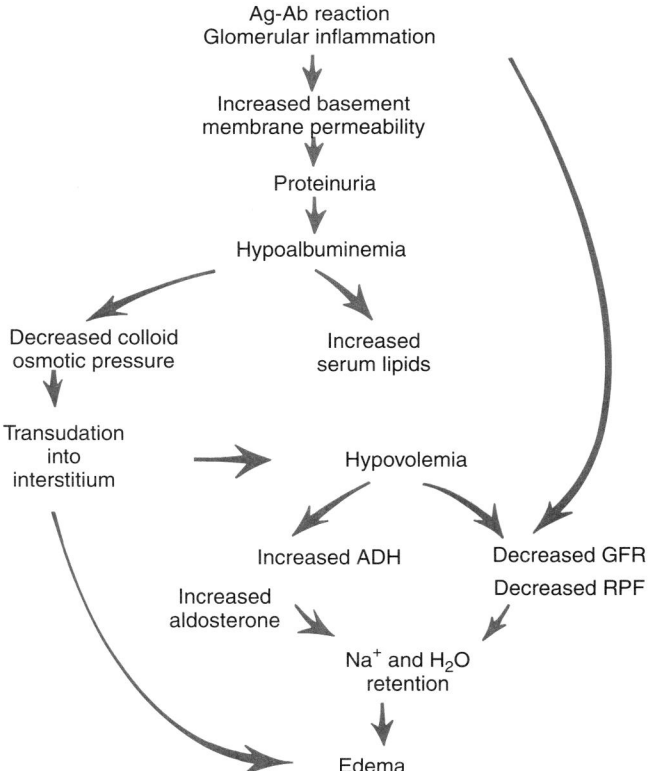

FIG. 46-13 Pathogenesis of nephrotic edema. (Modified from Schreiner FE: The nephrotic syndrome. In Strauss MB, Welt LG, editors: *Diseases of the kidney*, ed 2, Boston, 1971, Little, Brown.)

Hypertensive Nephrosclerosis

Hypertension and chronic renal failure are closely related. Hypertension may be the primary disease and damage the kidneys. Conversely, severe chronic renal disease may cause hypertension or contribute to its maintenance through the mechanism of sodium and water retention, the vasopressor effects of the renin-angiotensin system, and possibly prostaglandin deficiency. Sometimes, it is difficult for the nephrologist to determine which was the primary disease. Nephrosclerosis (hardening of the kidneys) refers to the pathologic changes in the renal blood vessels as a result of hypertension and is one of the leading causes of chronic renal failure, particularly in the non-Caucasian population.

Essential Hypertension and the Kidneys

Hypertension is defined as a sustained elevation of blood pressure above the accepted normal values of 90 mm Hg diastolic or 140 mm Hg systolic. According to this definition, about 18% of the U.S. population has hypertension. However, as many as 50% of individuals may have this disorder by the age of 65 years (Nally, 1998). The cause of hypertension is unknown in about 90% of the cases and is termed *essential hypertension* (unknown etiology and pathogenesis). The onset of essential hypertension usually occurs between the ages of 20 and 50 years, and it is more frequent in African Americans compared with the general population. Essential hypertension is classified as benign or malignant. *Benign hypertension* is slowly progressive, whereas in *malignant hypertension* there is rapid acceleration in the course of the hypertensive disease, resulting in severe organ damage.

The rate of progression of benign essential hypertension is variable, but it generally runs a slowly progressive course over a period of 20 to 30 years. Long-standing hypertension produces structural changes in the arterioles throughout the body, characterized by fibrosis and hyalinization (sclerosis) of the blood vessel walls. The chief target organs of this condition are the heart, brain, kidneys, and eyes. The usual cause of death is myocardial infarction, congestive heart failure, or cerebrovascular accident. If essential hypertension remains benign, patients are not likely to suffer renal damage sufficient to die of uremia. Most of the cases of renal insufficiency attributed to benign nephrosclerosis have underlying renal disease. Proteinuria and mild azotemia may exist for years without symptoms, and most patients who die of uremia do so as a result of the hypertension entering the malignant phase, which, occurs in less than 10% of the patients with essential hypertension.

Malignant hypertension implies severe hypertension with diastolic blood pressure greater than 120 to 130 mm Hg, grade IV retinopathy,* and renal excretory dysfunction, ranging from proteinuria to hematuria to azotemia. Malignant hypertension may occur at any time during the course of benign hypertension but usually occurs after many years. Occasionally, malignant hypertension occurs de novo, especially in African-American men in their third and fourth decades.

In the kidney, renal arteriosclerosis caused by long-standing hypertension results in *benign nephrosclerosis*. This disorder is the direct result of ischemia caused by the narrowed lumen of the intrarenal blood vessels. The kidney may be reduced in size, usually symmetrically, and has a granular, pitted surface. Histologically, the essential lesion is sclerosis of the small arteries and arterioles, which is most marked in the afferent arterioles. The closure of the arteries and arterioles leads to destruction of the glomeruli and atrophy of the tubules, so that entire nephrons are destroyed.

Malignant nephrosclerosis designates the structural renal changes often associated with the malignant phase of essential hypertension.† The kidneys may be of normal size, with minimal granularity and some petechiae from rupture of arterioles, or they may be shrunken and scarred. Histologically, there are three types of lesions: (1) proliferative endarteritis, (2) fibrinoid necrosis of arteriolar walls, and (3) fibrinoid necrosis of glomerular tufts. At first, there is marked thickening of the intima of the interlobular arteries caused by proliferation of the endothelial cells. These changes produce an appearance often referred to as "onionskin." The narrowed lumina produce ischemia of the afferent arterioles and the release of renin, and the blood pressure rises still further. Focal necrosis then occurs in the walls of the afferent arterioles, and because the necrosed areas contain fibrin, the change is called *fibrinoid necrosis*. Fibrinoid necrosis of the glomerular tufts is probably an extension of the fibrinoid necrosis of the feeding afferent arterioles. If the blood pressure remains elevated, these localized changes become widespread, with the formation of thrombi, glomerular hemorrhage, infarction of entire nephrons, and rapid death of all renal cells. Fig. 46-14 illustrates some of the above lesions. The treatment of hypertension is discussed in Chapters 31 and 48.

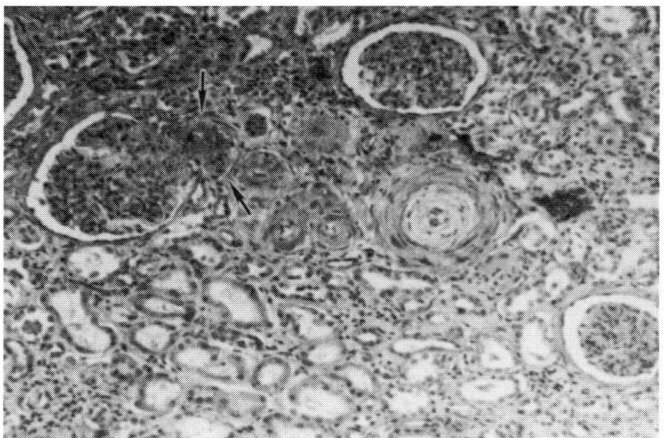

FIG. 46-14 Malignant nephrosclerosis. Light microscopy slide showing several hyalinized arterioles *(center field),* dilated tubules with atrophied lining cells *(lower center),* and an area of fibrinoid necrosis *(arrows).*

---

*Grade IV retinopathy refers to the most severe changes in the retina caused by hypertension. These changes may be viewed with the ophthalmoscope and consist of vascular sclerosis, exudates, hemorrhages, and papilledema.

†Although these gross and microscopic renal lesions are characteristic of the malignant phase of essential hypertension, they are not specific and may be superimposed on a variety of diseases associated with hypertension (e.g., chronic PN, CGN, polyarteritis nodosa).

Renal Artery Stenosis

Atherosclerotic plaques or fibromuscular dysplasia may occlude the renal artery, causing hypertension that is often of the rapidly progressive type. Atherosclerosis is found chiefly in older men and usually involves the proximal one third of the renal artery near the aorta. Fibromuscular dysplasia is characterized by excesses in fibrous connective tissue within the layers of the blood vessel and is most apt to occur in the middle and distal thirds of the renal artery, sometimes involving segmental branches. There are several histologic types of fibromuscular dysplasia, and the disorder is most common in women between the ages of 20 and 50 years.

Renal artery stenosis may be unilateral or bilateral. If the caliber of the artery is reduced by 70% or more, renal ischemia occurs. The renal ischemia activates the renin-angiotensin system, and hypertension follows. Although uncommon (about 0.5% of hypertension cases), renal artery stenosis is important because surgical correction may alleviate or markedly ameliorate the hypertensive state.

Unilateral renal artery stenosis not only causes ischemic atrophy of the involved kidney but also may eventually cause hypertensive nephrosclerosis of the contralateral kidney. The pathogenetic mechanism is depicted in Fig. 46-15. If the contralateral kidney has developed significant nephrosclerosis from the renin-induced hypertension, the function of the ischemic kidney may even be the better of the two, because the stenosed renal artery protects the occluded kidney from the full effects of the systemic hypertension.

Renal artery stenosis should be suspected when hypertension develops in persons younger than 30 years of age, when there is a truly abrupt-onset hypertension at any age, or when there is a definite worsening of previously well-controlled hypertension. Physical findings suggestive of renal artery stenosis include a continuous systolic and diastolic bruit heard over the epigastrium or the flank. Differences in carotid, brachial, or femoral pulses or blood pressure in the extremities, indicative of generalized atherosclerosis, are other nonspecific clues.

A captopril screening test is the procedure of choice for suspected renal artery stenosis, because this test has a specificity and sensitivity greater than 95% (Badr, Brenner, 1998). Rapid-sequence IVP is no longer used as a screening tool, because it has a false-positive rate of 12% in the hypertensive population. The captopril test measures the increase in plasma renin activity (PRA) in response to the administration of captopril, which is exaggerated in persons with renovascular hypertension compared with persons with essential hypertension. If the captopril test is positive, more invasive tests are administered. The most definitive diagnostic procedure is bilateral arteriography with repeated bilateral renal vein and systemic renin determinations. If the arteriogram shows unilateral renal artery stenosis, and if renal vein renin measurements from the two kidneys differ by a ratio of 1.5:1 or more, the chance of curing the hypertension by surgical reconstruction is almost 90% (Badr, Brenner, 1998). A renin ratio below 1.5:1.0 does not exclude the diagnosis of renovascular hypertension, especially if bilateral disease is present.

The aim of treatment is to control systemic blood pressure and restore perfusion to the ischemic kidney. Surgical treatment consists of revascularization of the ischemic kidney, often by means of a saphenous vein bypass graft. Alternately, percutaneous transluminal angioplasty (PCTA) or renal artery stenting may be used to enlarge the vessel lumen. Success rates with surgery or PCTA in young persons with fibromuscular dysplasia are 50% cure and 30% improvement in blood pressure; renovascular hypertension is improved in about 50% of older individuals so treated. Even if PCTA or surgery fails to

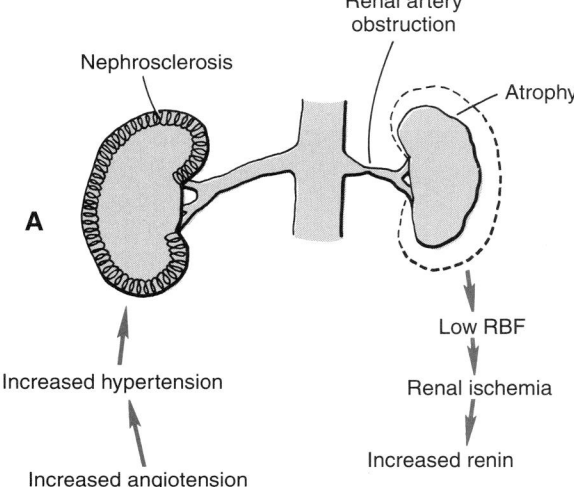
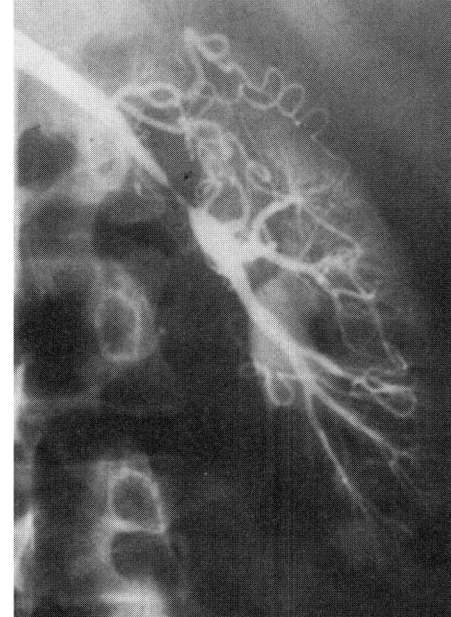

FIG. 46-15   A, Pathogenesis of nephrosclerosis in the contralateral kidney in renal artery stenosis. **B,** Renal arteriogram showing renal artery stenosis caused by fibromuscular dysplasia. *RBF,* Renal blood flow. (B from Stanley JC, Fry WF: Renovascular hypertension secondary to arterial fibrodysplasia in adults, *Arch Surg* 110:922, 1975. Copyright 1975, American Medical Association.)

normalize blood pressure, these procedures allow easier medical control of hypertension. ACE inhibitor drugs are particularly effective in treating patients with renovascular hypertension; but caution must be exercised in bilateral renal artery stenosis or stenosis of a solitary kidney, because acute renal failure may follow ACE inhibition under these circumstances. This adverse effect is presumed to be the result of the loss of angiotensin II effects on the glomerular efferent arterioles, which serve to maintain the GFR in the setting of renal hypoperfusion (see Chapters 44 and 49). It should be emphasized that, although the risk of precipitating acute renal failure is greatest with ACE inhibitor drugs, any antihypertensive drug can lead to acute renal failure if the stenosis is severe (Schrier, 1997).

Connective Tissue Disorders

The connective tissue disorders (collagen diseases) are systemic diseases, the manifestations of which are mainly attributable to the soft tissues of the body (see Part Twelve). These disorders are of particular interest in nephrology because of the high incidence of renal involvement. About two thirds of patients with SLE and progressive systemic sclerosis (scleroderma) have clinical evidence of renal involvement. The incidence is about 80% for patients with polyarteritis nodosa. Renal involvement is relatively uncommon in rheumatoid arthritis. When renal involvement does occur, it is usually a complication of therapy (gold salts, d-penicillamine) or a manifestation of secondary amyloidosis (Balow, 1998).

Systemic Lupus Erythematosus

SLE is a multisystem disease of unknown origin characterized by circulating autoantibodies to deoxyribonucleic acid (DNA). The diagnosis of SLE is confirmed by positive tests for antinuclear antibodies (ANA) (a useful screening test) and the more specific test for anti-DNA antibodies. SLE predominantly affects young women between the ages of 20 and 40 years, who account for 90% of the cases. Renal involvement is a major cause of morbidity in patients with SLE. Although renal failure is becoming less common with modern treatment, about 25% of those with SLE eventually develop renal failure.

Lupus nephritis is caused by circulating immune complexes that become trapped in the glomerular basement membrane (GBM) and cause damage. The mechanism is similar to that in APSGN, except that the source of the antigen is the body's own DNA rather than the streptococcal plasma membrane. In SLE, the body produces antibody against its own DNA. The clinical picture may be one of acute GN or of nephrotic syndrome. Although the basic cause is thought to be the same in both cases, focal, membranous, and proliferative changes in the glomeruli may all be seen. The earliest change often involves only part of the glomerular tuft (local), or only scattered glomeruli may be involved (focal). Focal GN and local GN respond quite well to corticosteroid drugs, and a complete remission may occur. The prognosis is poor for individuals who develop diffuse membranous or proliferative changes, and these patients often develop ESRD within 10 years (Fig. 46-16). A combination of corticosteroid and cytotoxic drugs is often given to patients with

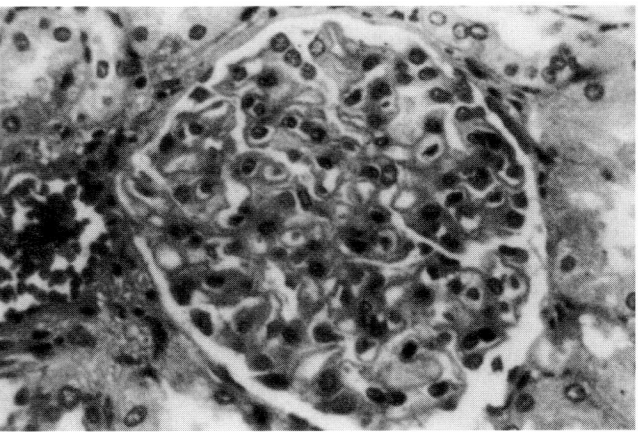

FIG. 46-16 Glomerulus from a patient with membranous lupus nephritis. Capillary walls (basement membrane) are uniformly thickened, but there is no increase in cellularity. Note the wire-loop appearance. Note the red blood cells in the lumen of the tubule *(left center)*.

active, proliferative lesions in an attempt to better preserve renal function. Patients with SLE tolerate dialysis quite well and, if transplanted, do not develop a recurrence of the renal lesions.

Polyarteritis Nodosa

Polyarteritis nodosa (PAN) is an inflammatory and necrotizing disease involving the medium-size and small arteries throughout the body, with secondary ischemia of the tissues supplied by the affected vessels. Early signs and symptoms of PAN are nonspecific, including fever, malaise, weight loss, and abdominal pain. Intractable hypertension secondary to the arteritis is often present. Men are more commonly affected than are women, and the mean age of onset is 48 years. Although the exact cause and pathogenesis are unknown, evidence suggests some form of hypersensitivity mechanism. In many cases the onset is associated with a sensitivity reaction to drugs.

Renal lesions are of two types. If the medium-size vessels within the kidney are affected, areas of renal infarction develop. If the disease is confined to the arterioles, the renal histology is that of severe focal, proliferative GN and fibrinoid necrotic changes with epithelial crescents.

The prognosis of untreated PAN is extremely poor, with a 5-year survival rate of 13%. Death commonly results from renal failure, bowel infarction, or cardiovascular or central nervous system (CNS) complications. Recently, the prognosis of PAN has been greatly improved by a therapeutic regimen consisting of corticosteroids, cytotoxic agents (cyclophosphamide or azathioprine), and plasma exchange, resulting in a 90% remission rate. Early antihypertensive therapy can lessen the morbidity and mortality associated with the renal, cardiac, and CNS complications of PAN.

Progressive Systemic Sclerosis

Progressive systemic sclerosis, or *scleroderma,* is an uncommon systemic disease characterized by diffuse sclerosis of the skin and other organs. The disease affects the vasculature of several organs, including the kidneys. Women are affected more often than are men. The onset is usually between the ages of 20 and 50 years. As in SLE, a variety of antibodies may be found in the serum, suggesting that immune mechanisms may be involved in the pathogenesis.

The interlobar arteries typically show changes resembling hypertensive nephrosclerosis. Progressive renal impairment may develop slowly over a period of years. In a few cases, hypertension and uremia may follow a malignant course, with the development of ESRF within weeks.

Although no effective therapy is available for scleroderma, aggressive antihypertensive therapy with ACE inhibitors may significantly prolong life and forestall the development of renal failure. Dialysis may also prolong life, but most patients will eventually die from extrarenal disease, especially myocardial failure or pulmonary fibrosis.

Congenital and Hereditary Disorders

Renal tubular acidosis and polycystic disease of the kidneys are hereditary disorders affecting primarily the renal tubules and may terminate in renal failure, although this is more common in polycystic disease. Both diseases have an infantile and an adult form, the manifestations of which may be quite distinct.

Polycystic Kidney Disease

Polycystic kidney disease (PKD) is characterized by bilateral, multiple, expanding cysts that gradually encroach on and destroy the normal renal parenchyma by compression. The kidney may be enlarged (sometimes as large as a football) and filled with grapelike clusters of cysts (Fig. 46-17). The cysts are filled with clear or hemorrhagic fluid.

Autosomal recessive polycystic kidney disease (ARPKD) is a rare genetic disease (1:6,000 to 1:40,000) involving a mutation localized to chromosome 6. The majority of cases are diagnosed with ultrasound in the first year of life, prompted by the finding of bilateral abdominal masses. Both liver and renal involvement are common. The kidneys are enlarged and the distal tubules and collecting ducts are dilated into elongated cysts. The time course to ESRD is variable, although many children maintain adequate renal function for years. Recent studies have shown a better prognosis than was previously reported. Of the children who survive the first month of life, 78% survive beyond 15 years. Early diagnosis and aggressive treatment of hypertension may improve the diagnosis of these children. Dialysis and renal transplant are appropriate therapies when renal failure occurs. A few children have undergone simultaneous renal and liver transplantation successfully.

Autosomal dominant polycystic kidney disease (ADPKD) is the most common inherited kidney disorder. The prevalence is about 1:500 and it is more common in Caucasian than it is in African-American populations. ADPKD is the fourth leading cause of renal failure requiring dialysis or transplantation. There are three forms of ADPKD:

- ADPKD-1 accounts for 90% of cases, and the mutated gene has been localized to the short arm of chromosome 16.
- The gene for ADPKD-2 has been localized to the short arm of chromosome 4, and progression to ESRD occurs more slowly than for ADPKD-1.

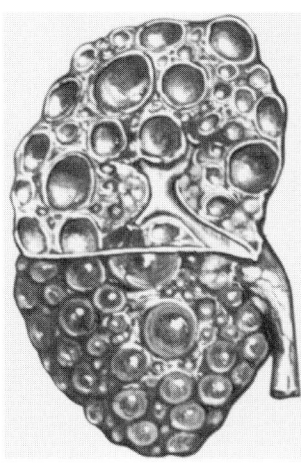

FIG. 46-17   Polycystic kidney. (Illustration by Judy Simon, Department of Medical and Biological Illustrations, University of Michigan.)

- A third form of ADPKD has been identified, but the responsible gene has not yet been localized.

The key clinical features are multiple cysts in the kidneys, which can be visualized by ultrasonography, computed tomography (CT), or magnetic resonance imaging (MRI). The cysts arise in utero and slowly destroy the surrounding normal tissue as they grow throughout adult life. Cysts arise from any part of the nephron or collecting ducts. The cysts are fluid-filled and prone to complications such as recurrent infection, bleeding, and renal stones. Flank pain, hematuria, polyuria, and palpably enlarged, "knobby" kidneys are often the presenting signs and symptoms. Hypertension and renal salt-wasting are common. Slow progressive decline in renal function is common with approximately 50% developing ESRD by age 60 years.

Treatment for patients with ADPKD is aimed at preventing complications and preserving renal function. Patients and family members should be educated about the inheritance and manifestations of the disease. Therapy is directed toward the control of hypertension and the early treatment of UTI. Patients with ADPKD have a tendency to be salt losers, so dehydration and inadequate salt intake should be avoided. The disease progresses to ESRD in about 25% of patients by the age of 50 years and in about 50% by the age of 60 years. Some patients may have a normal life span and die of nonrenal causes. ESRD is managed by dialysis or renal transplantation. Bilateral nephrectomy may be necessary before transplantation in patients with greatly enlarged kidneys.

Renal Tubular Acidosis

Renal tubular acidosis (RTA) refers to a group of disorders in which defective renal hydrogen ion (H^+) tubular excretion or loss of bicarbonate (HCO_3^-) in the urine, despite preservation of an adequate GFR. The result is a sustained metabolic acidosis. There are three subtypes of RTA: *Type 1 RTA* is characterized by defective H^+ secretion in the distal tubule, *Type 2 RTA* is characterized by defective HCO_3^- reabsorptive capacity in the proximal tubule, and *Type 4 RTA* (also called hyperkalemic distal RTA) is associated with either hypoaldosteronism or tubular resistance to aldosterone activity. Types 1 and 2 RTA may be hereditary or acquired and Type 4 RTA is acquired. Type 3 RTA was formerly used to define distal RTA in children with bicarbonate wasting; however, this condition resolves with age so the term is no longer used.

Classic *type 1*, or *distal*, RTA is characterized by the inability to maximally acidify the urine to less than pH 5.3 even in the presence of acidemia. The patient is unable to excrete the daily metabolic acid load, resulting in a progressive systemic acidemia with a plasma HCO_3^- that may be less than 10 mEq/L.

Distal RTA may occur as a primary isolated defect or in association with other diseases and disorders. The primary disorder is the most common form in childhood and is transmitted by autosomal dominant inheritance with a variable degree of expression. Females are affected more than are males. Autoimmune diseases, such as Sjögren's syndrome, are probably the major cause of this rare condition in adults. Although the exact nature of the defect responsible for the abnormalities of acidification in distal RTA is unclear, proposed mechanisms include (1) failure to transport H^+ against a steep pH gradient between the tubular lumen and peritubular fluid or (2) excessive back diffusion of H^+ from lumen to blood (Asplin, Coe, 1998).

The classic feature of distal RTA is the presence of a normal–anion gap hyperchloremic metabolic acidosis with a urine pH that is persistently above 5.3. Urine osmotic concentration and potassium (K^+) conservation are usually impaired, resulting in hypokalemia and polyuria. Bone disease, renal calculi, and nephrocalcinosis are other common manifestations of distal RTA caused by disturbed calcium (Ca^{++}) metabolism. The chronic acidosis results in mobilization of Ca^{++} salts from the bone and hypercalciuria. Bone resorption is manifested as osteomalacia in adults and as rickets and stunted growth in children. Ca^{++} salts may precipitate diffusely in the renal parenchyma (nephrocalcinosis) or within the collecting system, causing calculi. Precipitation of calcium phosphate ($CaHPO_4$) in the kidney is favored by low urinary citrate (which normally inhibits crystallization) and the elevated urine pH. Renal failure may be secondary to these complications.

The diagnosis of distal RTA is confirmed by the ammonia chloride (NH_4Cl) loading test (see Chapter 45). NH_4Cl is metabolized in the liver to hydrogen chloride (HCl). The excess H^+ normally excreted in urine causes the urine pH to fall below 5.3, but the urine pH remains above 5.3 in the person with distal RTA.

The acidemia in distal RTA may be corrected by the administration of sodium or potassium bicarbonate or citrate (metabolized into HCO_3^- in the body). The usual dose is 1 to 3 mEq/kg/day. Infants and children respond well to this therapy, and the condition is usually completely reversed. In some adults, the calcium deposits are reabsorbed after prolonged alkali therapy, whereas in others, the nephrocalcinosis is permanent. The prognosis depends on the extent of renal damage before treatment is initiated.

Type 2, or *proximal*, RTA is characterized by an alkaline urine pH and bicarbonaturia at mildly or moderately reduced plasma HCO_3^- levels. In contrast to distal RTA, the

urine pH can fall below 5.3 if the patient is sufficiently acidotic, indicating that distal acidification is intact. The basic mechanism causing proximal RTA is defective reabsorption of HCO_3^- in the proximal tubule. Normally, about 85% of the filtered HCO_3^- is reabsorbed in the proximal tubule at normal plasma concentrations. A large quantity of HCO_3^- is thus shunted to the distal tubule. Because the distal tubule has a limited capacity to reclaim HCO_3^-, an HCO_3^- diuresis occurs.

The loss of large quantities of HCO_3^- in the urine produces hyperchloremic metabolic acidosis. The severe progressive acidosis characteristic of distal RTA does not occur in proximal RTA, and the plasma HCO_3^- is usually stabilized at a moderate level between 13 and 20 mEq/L. The bicarbonaturia induces renal losses of Na^+ and K^+; therefore, ECF volume depletion and hypokalemia also occur. In contrast to distal RTA, nephrocalcinosis and nephrolithiasis do not usually occur.

As with distal RTA, proximal RTA may be inherited or acquired. When inherited, proximal RTA is often associated with Fanconi syndrome, a generalized tubular defect associated with inadequate absorption of glucose, phosphate, amino acids, and uric acid. Failure to thrive and stunting of growth, as in distal RTA, are regular features in growing children. Acquired proximal RTA in adults may be associated with multiple myeloma, Sjögren's syndrome, or amyloidosis.

Proximal RTA cannot be diagnosed by the NH_4Cl test, because these patients can acidify the urine when presented with an acid load. Rather, the diagnosis is made by the HCO_3^- infusion test. In this test, sufficient HCO_3^- is infused to raise the serum HCO_3^- level to just below the normal range (20 to 22 mEq/L), and then the urine pH and the fraction of the filtered HCO_3^- that is excreted are measured. In proximal RTA, the urine pH rises above 7, and the fractional excretion of HCO_3^- exceeds 15% (because the reabsorptive threshold for HCO_3^- has been exceeded). However, in distal RTA, the urine pH remains unchanged, and the fractional excretion of HCO_3^- is less than 3% (Asplin, Coe, 1998).

Treatment of proximal RTA may not be necessary in adults if the patient is asymptomatic and if the acidemia is mild. In children, treatment is always indicated, because even mild acidemia may retard growth. Proximal RTA is generally more difficult to treat than distal RTA. Larger doses of alkali may be necessary (10 to 15 mEq/kg/day) to keep plasma HCO_3^- in the normal range, and a K^+ supplement is usually needed because therapy causes increased losses in the urine. Thus a combination of potassium and sodium citrate (Polycitra) is the drug of choice.

Metabolic Disorders

Metabolic disorders that may lead to chronic renal failure include diabetes mellitus, gout, primary hyperparathyroidism, and amyloidosis.

Diabetes Mellitus

Diabetic nephropathy (renal disease in patients with diabetes) is one of the most important causes of death in long-standing diabetes mellitus. More than one third of all new patients entering ESRD programs have diabetic renal failure. It has been estimated that about 35% to 40% of patients with type 1 diabetes develop chronic renal failure within 15 to 25 years after the onset of diabetes. Fewer individuals with type 2 diabetes develop chronic renal failure (about 10% to 20%) with the exception of Pima Indians where the incidence is nearly 50%. Native Americans and African Americans have a particularly high risk of developing diabetic renal failure.

Diabetes mellitus affects the structure and function of the kidney in many ways. *Diabetic nephropathy* is a term that encompasses all of the lesions occurring in the kidney in diabetes mellitus. Glomerulosclerosis is the most characteristic lesion and may be diffuse or nodular. *Diffuse diabetic glomerulosclerosis*, the most common lesion, consists of diffuse thickening of the mesangial matrix* with eosinophilic material accompanied by thickening of the capillary basement membrane. *Nodular diabetic glomerulosclerosis* (also known as the *Kimmelstiel-Wilson lesion*) is less common but very specific for this disease; it consists of rounded, nodular accumulations of eosinophilic material that are usually located in the periphery of the glomerulus within the core of the capillary lobule (Fig. 46-18). Nonglomerular abnormalities in diabetic nephropathy include chronic tubulointerstitial nephritis, papillary necrosis, hyalinosis of the efferent and afferent arterioles, and ischemia. Diabetic glomerulosclerosis is nearly always preceded by diabetic retinopathy, characterized by microaneurysms around the macula.

The natural history of diabetic nephropathy from onset to ESRD may be divided into five phases or stages (Box 46-2). Recent research has demonstrated that some of the long-term complications of diabetes, such as diabetic retinopathy, neuropathy, and nephropathy, can be prevented or delayed by strict control of blood glucose and hypertension and dietary protein restriction (see Chapter 48).

Stage 1, or the phase of *early functional changes*, is characterized by renal hypertrophy and hyperfiltration. Stage 1 findings are present in virtually all patients at the diagnosis of type 1 diabetes mellitus (insulin-dependent) and develop at the onset of the disease. An elevation of the GFR commonly occurs, up to 40% above normal. This elevation is multifactorial in origin, with contributing factors including high blood glucose levels and abnormalities in glucagon, growth hormone, renin, angiotensin II, and prostaglandin effect. The kidneys exhibiting the increased GFR are larger than is normal, and individual glomeruli are larger with increased surface area. It is believed, as discussed earlier in this chapter, that these changes may lead to focal glomerulosclerosis.

Stage 2, or the phase of *early structural changes*, is characterized by thickening of the glomerular capillary basement membrane and gradual accumulation of mesangial matrix material. This stage is present at approximately 5 years from the onset of type 1 diabetes and appears to develop in all patients with diabetes mellitus. The severity of mesangial thickening or expansion observed in stage 2 is positively correlated with the future develop-

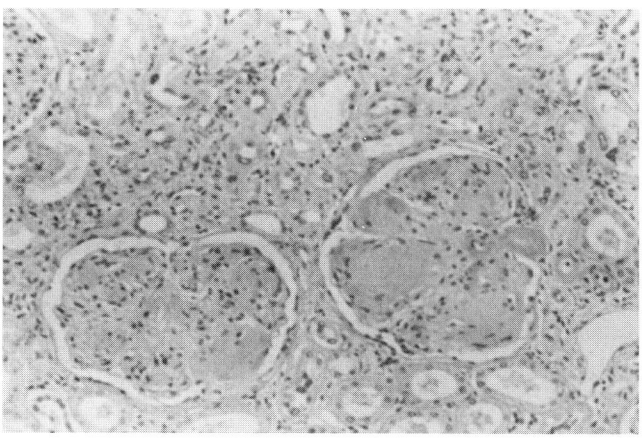

FIG. 46-18   Diabetic nephropathy (light microscopy) showing the typical nodular lesion in the two central glomeruli. Nodular appearance is caused by the deposit of mesangial matrix within the core of the peripheral capillary lobules. Initially the capillary lumina are patent, but they are gradually obliterated as the disease progresses. Note also the thickening of the basement membrane of the tubules in the lower central field.

BOX 46-2

Stages of Diabetic Nephropathy

STAGE 1 (EARLY FUNCTIONAL CHANGES)
Renal hypertrophy
Increased glomerular capillary surface area
Increased GFR

STAGE 2 (EARLY STRUCTURAL CHANGES)
Thickening of the glomerular capillary basement membrane
Normal or slightly elevated GFR

STAGE 3 (INCIPIENT NEPHROPATHY)
Microalbuminuria (30-300 mg/24 hr)
Elevated blood pressure

STAGE 4 (ESTABLISHED OR CLINICAL NEPHROPATHY)
Proteinuria (> 300 mg/24 hr)
Decreased GFR

STAGE 5 (PROGRESSIVE RENAL INSUFFICIENCY OR FAILURE)
Rapidly declining GFR (–1 ml/month)
Kidney loses up to 3% of function every month

From Dunfee TP: The changing management of diabetic nephropathy, *Hosp Med* 30(5):45, 1995.

---

ment of proteinuria and decline in renal function. The accumulation of mesangial matrix may impinge on the glomerular capillary lumina, causing ischemia and decreased surface area for filtration, but the GFR is usually still in the high-normal range (reduced from the greatly elevated GFR during stage 1). Urinary albumin excretion is generally normal during stage 2, except for bouts of reversible microalbuminuria.

Persistent hyperglycemia seems to be the most important factor in the pathogenesis of the diabetic glomerulosclerosis and involves several mechanisms, including (1) vasodilation with increased permeability of the microcirculation allowing increased leakage of solutes into

---

*The mesangial matrix is a spongy network of basement membranelike trabeculae at the center of the glomerular lobule surrounding the mesangial cells; it merges with the capillary basement membrane.

the vascular walls and surrounding tissues; (2) glucose disposal via the polyol pathway (independent of insulin), leading to accumulation of polyols and decreased levels of vital cellular components, including the glomeruli; and (3) glycosylation of glomerular structural proteins. In hyperglycemia, glucose reacts with circulating and structural proteins nonenzymatically (e.g., the glycosylation of hemoglobin produces hemoglobin A_{1c}). Glycosylation of basement membrane and mesangial proteins may be the major factor responsible for the increase in mesangial matrix and the alterations in membrane permeability leading to proteinuria.

Stage 3 diabetic nephropathy is referred to as the phase of *incipient nephropathy* and typically develops about 10 years after the onset of diabetes. The hallmark of this stage is persistent microalbuminuria (urinary albumin excretion between 30 and 300 mg/24 hr) detectable only by radioimmunoassay or other sensitive laboratory methods. Normal urinary albumin excretion is below 30 mg/24 hr, whereas albumin excretion above 300 mg/24 hr is referred to as *overt* proteinuria to distinguish it from microalbuminuria. Persistent microalbuminuria is documented with three or more separate urine collections over a 3- to 6-month period. Persistent microalbuminuria can be detected in 25% to 40% of patients, and the likelihood of progressing to stages 4 and 5 nephropathy is high in those who develop it and low in those who do not. Normal to high-normal levels of GFR and increasing blood pressure are also important features of stage 3 diabetic nephropathy.

Stage 4, or the phase of *established* or *clinical diabetic nephropathy*, is characterized by dipstick-positive proteinuria (>300 mg/24 hr) with a progressive decrease in the GFR. Diabetic retinopathy, as well as hypertension, is almost always present with stage 4 diabetic nephropathy. This stage is present approximately 15 years after the onset of type 1 diabetes and leads to ESRD in most cases. However, many patients never reach ESRD because of premature death from atherosclerotic heart disease or stroke.

Stage 5, or the phase of *progressive renal insufficiency or failure,* is characterized by azotemia (elevated BUN and serum creatinine) caused by a rapid decline in the GFR, leading to the eventual development of ESRD and the need for dialysis or renal transplantation. The average time required to reach stage 5 from the onset of type 1 diabetes is 20 years. The rate of decline in the GFR averages 1 ml/month, so ESRD occurs in approximately 5 to 10 years after the onset of proteinuria. The rate of progression may be retarded by appropriate interventions (see later discussion). The advanced diabetic nephropathy of stage 5 is generally accompanied by retinopathy, peripheral neuropathy, and hypertension (Dunfee, 1995; Schrier, 1997).

The results of a number of studies, including the 1993 Diabetes Control and Complications Trial with 1441 patients, have shown that precise regulation of blood glucose (achieved through meticulous attention to diet, exercise, self-monitoring of blood glucose, and multidose daily insulin) can slow the rate of nephropathy, retinopathy, and neuropathy significantly, especially if the therapy is begun during the third or microalbuminuria stage. Dietary protein restriction and lowering the blood pressure with ACE inhibitors decrease albumin excretion and

slow progression of diabetic nephropathy. ACE inhibitors are effective in slowing progression to renal failure because they are the only antihypertensive drugs that act by dilating the efferent arterioles, thus lowering intraglomerular pressure. By contrast, calcium antagonists (e.g., verapamil) cause dilation of the afferent arterioles in the kidney, which may increase intraglomerular pressure rather than lowering it.

Renal replacement therapy should be introduced at a much earlier stage than it is with patients without diabetes, because uremia is associated with acceleration of other diabetic complications (e.g., retinopathy). Continuous ambulatory peritoneal dialysis is the treatment of choice. Generally, mortality among patients with diabetes on long-term dialysis is about three times higher than it is among patients of comparable age without diabetes. Renal transplantation may be successful in younger patients with diabetes compared with older patients.

Uric Acid Kidney Disease

Uric acid, an end product of purine metabolism, can precipitate within the renal medullary interstitium, tubules or collecting system, leading to three types of renal disease: (1) acute uric acid nephropathy, (2) uric acid nephrolithiasis, and (3) chronic urate nephropathy.

Acute uric acid nephropathy is caused by the precipitation of uric acid crystals in the renal tubules leading to obstruction and the development of acute renal failure. Uric acid nephropathy occurs in association with chemotherapy-responsive tumors such as leukemias and lymphomas. The drugs increase the destruction of neoplastic nuclei with production of uric acid. Precipitation of uric acid is favored by the acidic pH in the distal tubules and collecting ducts. It is important to anticipate the development of this complication and initiate preventive therapy, including vigorous hydration and prophylactic use of allopurinol both before and during antineoplastic therapy.

Uric acid nephrolithiasis is common in patients with hyperuricemia, such as gout, and with malignancies with rapid cell turnover, such as the leukemia. Uric acid is also commonly present in calcium oxalate stones in patients who are not hyperuricemic. In this group, it is believed that an unexplained tendency to excrete highly acidic urine (pH <5.5) may predispose to uric acid stone formation. Uric acid may act as a nidus on which calcium oxalate can precipitate.

Chronic urate nephropathy, or *gouty nephropathy*, occurs in patients with gout and protracted hyperuricemia (>7 mg/dl). Gout may be primary or secondary (see Chapter 74). Primary gout is the direct result of the body's overproduction of uric acid or decreased excretion of uric acid. Secondary gout occurs when the overproduction or decreased excretion is secondary to another disease process or medication. The deposition and crystallization of urate in the fluids and tissues of the body is the principle cause of the major lesions of gout. The joints and kidneys are the prime targets. In chronic gout, deposit of urate crystals in the renal medullary interstitium causes interstitial nephritis, nephrosclerosis, and slowly progressive renal failure. Before the advent of antihyperuricemic drugs and aggressive treatment for asymptomatic hypertension, renal failure was the cause of death in up to 25% of patients with gout. At present, chronic urate nephropathy is believed to be a rare cause of renal failure. Gouty arthritis occurs in less than 1% of patients with renal failure, despite the invariable hyperuricemia. A possible explanation is that the elevated uric acid has not been present long enough to accumulate the necessary urate load. There is some evidence that chronic lead intoxication may play a role in some hyperuricemic patients with chronic renal failure, because lead interferes with uric acid excretion and also produces interstitial nephritis and progressive renal damage (Black, 1996).

Hyperparathyroidism

Primary hyperparathyroidism, resulting in hypersecretion of parathyroid hormone, is a relatively rare disease that can result in nephrocalcinosis and subsequent renal failure. The usual cause is adenoma of the parathyroid glands. Secondary hyperparathyroidism is a common complication of chronic renal failure. Whether the disease is primary or secondary, the manifestations are similar. These are discussed in detail in Chapters 21 and 47.

Amyloidosis

Amyloidosis is a metabolic condition in which there is a deposition, in many tissues, of an abnormal extracellular fibrillar protein, termed amyloid. Amyloid deposition can damage the kidney, liver, spleen, heart, tongue, and nervous system. The major causes of death are heart failure and renal failure. Amyloid is detected histologically as a bright-pink hyaline material; it also takes up certain special stains, such as Congo red. Amyloid can be classified according to the nature of the precursor protein and according to whether the amyloid deposits are systemic (involving many organs) or localized to one organ or tissue. A common example of localized amyloid deposit is found in patients with Alzheimer's disease. The amyloid is derived from a normal neuronal membrane protein called *Alzheimer's precursor protein (APP)*. Despite the uncertainty about the reasons amyloid is formed, well-established associations exist between amyloid deposition and particular diseases. In each case, there is an accumulation of a precursor peptide, which is processed into an amyloid protein.

Renal involvement occurs in 90% of patients with either primary or secondary amyloidosis. The fibrils in *primary amyloidosis* consist of fragments of monoclonal light chains (also called *light chain* or *AL amyloidosis*). Primary amyloidosis is associated with multiple myeloma (less than 20% of cases) and the light chains are derived from the monoclonal proliferation of B lymphocytes or plasma cells that produce an abnormal immunoglobulin. Progressive renal failure generally occurs in primary amyloidosis. Patients with multiple myeloma do very poorly with a mean survival rate less than 1 year. The major causes of death are cardiac or renal failure, infection and progression of the myeloma. The treatment of primary amyloidosis has been unsatisfactory, although reversal of amyloid deposits with intensive therapy using steroids and cytotoxic agents (melphalan) has been described.

Secondary amyloidosis (also called *reactive*, or *acquired, amyloidosis [AA]*) occurs most frequently as a complication of chronic inflammatory disease. Diseases that lead to this type of secondary amyloid include rheumatoid arthritis, tuberculosis, bronchiectasis, Crohn's disease, chronic osteomyelitis, and decubitus ulcer. AA may also be associated with *heredofamilial Mediterranean fever*, an autosomal dominant disorder. In secondary amyloidosis, the precursor of the amyloid is a circulating acute phase reactant known as *serum amyloid A (SAA)*, which is overproduced by the liver. The excess SAA is taken up by monocytes or macrophages; it is cleaved into smaller fragments, called AA protein, that can then be deposited in tissues. Secondary amyloidosis can lead to end-stage renal failure (ESRF), especially in patients with persistently high levels of SAA. Amyloid may be deposited in renal blood vessels, tubules and in the glomerulus (producing nodules resembling those of diabetic glomerulosclerosis). Usually, the clinical diagnosis is not made until the disease is far advanced. Proteinuria in the nephrotic range (>3.5 g/day) and edema are common presenting signs. Successful treatment of the underlying inflammatory disease using colchicine can sometimes lead to resolution or amelioration of the proteinuria and amyloid deposits. Patients who progress to ESRF can be treated with dialysis or renal transplantation (Sipe, Cohen, 1998).

A type of amyloid composed of β_2-microglobulin is unique to long-term dialysis patients. β_2-microglobulin is a protein of small molecular weight normally excreted in the urine but is poorly dialyzed and therefore accumulates in the blood of patients with ESRD. This protein is then deposited in bones, joints, and periarticular structures of the shoulders, neck, hands, wrists, and elsewhere, causing pain and limitation of motion. The majority of patients on dialysis for greater than 10 years will have amyloidosis. Presenting features include bone cysts, pathologic fractures, arthritis, and carpal tunnel syndrome from amyloid deposition in the wrists entrapping the median nerve. The symptoms may be eased with nonsteroidal antiinflammatory drugs (NSAIDs) or prevented by early renal transplantation.

Toxic Nephropathy

The kidney is especially vulnerable to the toxic effects of drugs and chemicals for the following reasons: (1) it receives 25% of the cardiac output, therefore it may be readily exposed to large amounts of a chemical; (2) the hyperosmotic interstitium allows chemicals to be concentrated in a relatively hypovascular region; and (3) the kidney is an obligatory excretory route for most drugs, so renal insufficiency results in drug accumulation and increased concentration in the tubular fluid. The most frequently encountered nephrotoxins result in acute renal failure and are discussed in Chapter 49. Chronic renal failure may result from analgesic abuse and exposure to lead.

Analgesic Abuse

It is generally accepted that chronic abuse of analgesics can cause renal injury. Chronic renal failure associated with excessive consumption of analgesics is a worldwide problem and perhaps the most preventable form of renal disease. The incidence of abuse varies, depending on regional differences in analgesic intake. Overall, analgesic nephropathy accounts for 9%, 3%, and less than 1% of patients undergoing dialysis in Australia, Europe, and the United States, respectively (USRDS, 1995). The responsible ingredient causing nephropathy was first thought to be phenacetin, a common pain reliever. However, subsequent evidence indicated that the combination of aspirin and phenacetin causes renal damage, because renal insufficiency was rarely a problem when aspirin or phenacetin alone was taken. The aspirin, phenacetin, and caffeine (APC) tablet was outlawed from the U.S. market in late 1983. In most countries, restriction of analgesic mixtures has greatly reduced the incidence of analgesic nephropathy but by no means eliminated it. Other over-the-counter nonphenacetin mixtures are available. The National Kidney Foundation has recommended in a recent position paper that analgesic mixtures should be available only by prescription. Some recent studies also suggest that habitual acetaminophen (Tylenol) use alone increases the risk of renal disease, but it is somewhat less than it is with the mixture of aspirin and phenacetin (Perneger et al, 1994). Acetaminophen is a primary metabolite of phenacetin (Buckalew, 1998).

Clinically evident renal disease requires the ingestion of 2 to 3 kg each of aspirin and phenacetin over time to produce significant renal damage (Murray, Goldberg, 1978). This amount is equivalent to taking 6 to 8 APC tablets per day for 5 to 8 years. Middle-aged women with a history of chronic headache or backache are the most frequent analgesic abusers. The mechanism by which these agents combine to produce renal damage is incompletely understood. One theory is that aspirin potentiates the toxic effect of phenacetin metabolites on the kidney in the following two ways (Bennett, 1989):

1. Aspirin causes medullary ischemia by inhibiting the local production of prostaglandins; PGE_2 and PGI_2 are potent renal vasodilator hormones, thus enhancing the toxic effect of phenacetin metabolites and slowing down their removal.

2. Aspirin interferes with the hexose monophosphate shunt, thereby lowering the concentration of glutathione, which normally inactivates phenacetin metabolites.

The characteristic renal lesion is papillary necrosis and chronic tubulointerstitial nephritis. The papillary tips may slough off completely and be excreted in the urine. Because the distal tubule bears the brunt of the disease, urine concentration and acidification tend to be severely impaired, and a salt-losing state may also develop. Common clinical features are hematuria (in cases of papillary necrosis), renal colic (flank pain), and UTI. Frequently, the disease progresses insidiously, so the patient may have advanced chronic renal failure and hypertension at the time of diagnosis. Early diagnosis is particularly important in analgesic nephropathy, because progressive renal injury may be halted by cessation of analgesic intake.

Lead Nephropathy

Exposure to lead occurs in a number of occupations, and lead may be ingested in illicitly distilled whiskey. Lead intoxication is still a problem in the United States, although not as great as it was when lead-based paints were used. Lead is incorporated chiefly into the bone and gradually released over a period of years; it is also incorporated into renal tubular cells. Patients with lead nephropathy typically have hyperuricemia. Acute gouty arthritis occurs in about one half of the patients with lead nephropathy, in contrast to other forms of renal failure in which gout is rare. Hypertension is also common. The basic renal lesion is interstitial nephritis, and there is slowly progressive renal failure.

KEY CONCEPTS

- Total renal failure is divided into two syndromes: (1) *chronic renal failure* occurs with slow progressive destruction of individual nephrons over a long period and is irreversible; (2) *acute renal failure* is commonly associated with a critical illness, develops rapidly over a period of days to weeks, and is generally reversible if the patient survives the critical illness.

- The clinical course of *chronic renal failure* is divided into three stages: (1) *decreased renal reserve*, during which the patient is asymptomatic, but GFR may be reduced to 25% of normal; (2) *renal insufficiency*, during which the patient may be experiencing polyuria and nocturia, GFR is 10% to 25% of normal, and the serum creatinine and BUN is mildly elevated above normal; and (3) *uremic syndrome* or *end-stage renal disease (ESRD)*, characterized by GFR under 5 to 10 ml/min, a sharp rise in the serum creatinine and BUN, and a complex of symptoms and biochemical changes.

- The *intact nephron hypothesis* is useful in explaining the orderly pattern of functional adaptation in progressive renal disease. As chronic renal disease advances and nephrons are progressively destroyed, the remaining intact nephrons experience hypertrophy. Single-nephron GFR (SNGFR) is increased in the remaining intact nephrons, enabling them to

- maintain fluid and electrolyte balance until more than 90% of the nephrons are destroyed.

- The *hyperfiltration theory* explains why glomerular injury and progressive renal failure continues when active renal disease no longer exists.

- The *four leading causes of ESRD* are *diabetes, hypertension, glomerulonephritis (GN)*, and *polycystic kidney disease (PKD)*.

- The most common uropathogen causing urinary tract infections (UTIs) is: *E. coli* (80%). Other strains are less common, including *Proteus mirabilis, Klebsiella*, and a few gram-positive microbes, such as *Staphylococcus saprophyticus*.

- The hallmark of UTI is *significant bacteriuria* ($\geq 10^5$ CFU/ml). Dipstick tests that detect pyuria by the leukocyte esterase test and nitrate help to confirm the diagnosis.

- Uncomplicated UTIs rarely cause ESRD.

- *Lower UTIs* are more common in women because of their short urethra. In men, lower UTIs are usually associated with structural abnormalities and stasis resulting from obstruction.

- *Predisposing factors in the development of UTIs* include female gender, pregnancy, advanced age, indwelling catheters, vesicoureteral reflux, urinary tract obstruction, neurogenic bladder, chronic analgesic abuse, and metabolic disorders, such as diabetes, gout, and calculi.

- *Acute pyelonephritis (PN)* is a well-defined clinical syndrome consisting of the acute onset of fever, flank pain, and costovertebral angle tenderness associated with leukocytosis, leukocyte casts, and bacteria in the urine. Ascending infection from the lower urinary tract is the most common cause.
- *Chronic PN* is a chronic tubulointerstitial disease in which chronic tubulointerstitial inflammation and scarring are associated with pathologic involvement of the renal pelvis and calyces.
- *Vesicoureteral reflux (VUR)* and *intrarenal reflux* are usually the underlying lesions causing chronic pyelonephritic scarring. Renal involvement in VUR occurs early in childhood as a result of super-imposition of a UTI on congenital VUR and intrarenal reflux. VUR may be unilateral or bilateral.
- *Chronic PN* caused by VUR is a major cause of ESRD in children and preventable by correction of the structural abnormalities of the urinary tract causing the obstruction.
- The glomerulus is the target of many primary and secondary disease processes, leading to temporary or permanent impairment of function. Glomerular disease is classified according to the histologic pattern of damage seen on renal biopsy.
- The *glomerulus* has a limited set of *histologic responses to damage*, including (1) proliferation of endothelial cells (reducing glomerular flow), (2) proliferation of mesangial cells (leading to glomerulosclerosis, as in diabetes), (3) thickening of the basement membrane, (4) capillary wall (fibrinoid) necrosis (as in hypertension), and (5) crescent formation resulting from proliferation of epithelial cells lining Bowman's capsule (as in rapidly progressive glomerulonephritis [RPGN]).
- Glomerular disease may not affect all of the glomeruli in a uniform manner: (1) in *diffuse GN*, all of the glomeruli are affected; (2) in *focal GN*, only some glomeruli are affected; and (3) in *segmental or local GN*, only a part of the glomerulus is affected.
- *Glomerular diseases produce five clinical syndromes* resulting from different combinations of the possible effects of glomerular injury: (1) *asymptomatic* hematuria and proteinuria from mild glomerular damage; (2) *acute GN* or *acute nephritic syndrome* with hematuria, acute decrease in GFR, sodium and water retention, and hypertension (e.g., poststreptococcal GN), *chronic GN* (slow, progressive glomerular damage with proteinuria and hypertension); (3) *rapidly progressive GN* to ESRF (e.g., Goodpasture's syndrome); (4) *nephrotic syndrome* (heavy proteinuria, >3.5 g/day) leading to hypoalbuminemia and edema; and (5) *uremic syndrome* or symptomatic ESRD.
- *Immune mechanisms* underlie most cases of primary GN and many of the secondary glomerular involvements.
- Two types of immune mechanisms responsible for antibody-associated glomerular injury have been established: (1) *anti-GBM nephritis*, in which antibodies are directed against the glomerular basement membrane (GBM) (e.g., Goodpasture's syndrome, characterized by linear pattern of immune deposits

visible by immunofluorescence staining, crescent formation and rapidly progressive GN); and (2) *circulating immune-complex nephritis* caused by the trapping of circulating antibody-antigen complexes within the glomeruli visible as granular subendothelial deposits (e.g., GN associated with systemic lupus erythematosus [SLE]).
- *IgA nephropathy (Berger's disease)* is the most common primary glomerular disease worldwide. Nearly one third of patients eventually develop ESRD and recurrence can occur after renal transplantation.
- The *nephrotic syndrome* is characterized by massive proteinuria (>3.5 g/day), hypoalbuminemia, generalized edema, and hyperlipidemia.
- The main causes of the nephrotic syndrome in adults include diabetes, SLE, amyloidosis, and membranous GN.
- The main cause of the nephrotic syndrome in children is *minimal change GN* (foot process disease; lipoid nephrosis). The most important feature of the nephrotic syndrome caused by minimal change GN is its dramatic response to corticosteroid therapy.
- *Renal artery stenosis* causes renal ischemia and may result in secondary hypertension. Renal artery stenosis may be caused by renal artery occlusion from atherosclerosis or fibromuscular dysplasia.
- Hypertension is intimately linked with the kidney, because renal disease may be both the cause and consequence of increased blood pressure. *Hypertensive nephrosclerosis* is the second leading cause of ESRD.
- *Benign nephrosclerosis* is the term used to describe lesions characterized by sclerosis of the small renal arteries and arterioles leading to ischemic destruction of entire nephrons. Eventually, sufficient numbers of nephrons become nonfunctioning for the patient to develop chronic renal failure. Patients with more severe hypertension, African Americans, and patients with diabetes are at greater risk of developing ESRD.
- *Malignant nephrosclerosis* is the form of renal disease associated with the accelerated phase of hypertension resulting in severe damage to the renal parenchyma and the rapid development of renal failure.
- Immunologic damage to glomeruli occurs in systemic connective tissue diseases, the most important of which is SLE (*lupus nephritis*).
- *Polyarteritis nodosa*, an inflammatory and necrotizing disease affecting medium-sized arteries, affects renal arterioles and the glomerular tuft, producing infarction of entire glomeruli or nephrons resulting in ESRD.
- *Progressive systemic sclerosis (scleroderma)* may be associated with fibrinoid necrosis of afferent arterioles and small renal arteries and show onion-skin thickening of the intima similar to that observed in malignant hypertension.
- Several cystic diseases of the kidney produce chronic renal failure, the most common of which is *autosomal dominant polycystic kidney disease (ADPKD)*. Of those individuals who inherit the mutant gene, 50% eventually require dialysis or renal transplantation.
- *Renal tubular acidosis (RTA)* occurs because the kidney is unable to excrete acid resulting in chronic metabolic acidosis.

- *Diabetes* is the most common single cause of ESRD and accounts for 30% to 40% of all cases.
- The development of *diabetic nephropathy* and ESRD occurs in five stages over a period of about 20 years: (1) early functional changes (renal hypertrophy and hyperfiltration), (2) early structural changes, (3) incipient nephropathy with microalbuminuria and hypertension, (4) established nephropathy with gross proteinuria and decreased GFR, and (5) progressive renal insufficiency with rapidly declining GFR.
- The Diabetic Control and Complications Trial showed that good glycemic control slows the rate at which proteinuria develops and progresses.

- Renal biopsy features of diabetic nephropathy include diffuse basement membrane thickening followed by proliferation of mesangial cells and nodular glomerulosclerosis (Kimmelstiel-Wilson lesion) consisting of deposition of glycoprotein material in a nodular fashion.
- *Analgesic nephropathy* is a form of tubulointerstitial disease caused by administration of analgesic agents, particularly phenacetin and NSAIDs; it is also associated with papillary necrosis. After long-term exposure to the causative agent, patients develop renal tubular failure with polyuria and eventually chronic renal failure.

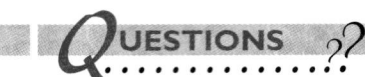

QUESTIONS ??

A sampling of review questions for this chapter appears here. Visit http://www.mosby.com/MERLIN/PriceWilson/ for additional questions. MERLIN

Answer the following on a separate sheet of paper.

1. What is the major difference between acute and chronic renal failure, and what happens to the function of the kidneys in both categories?
2. Name the three stages in the natural history of progressive renal failure in order. What percentage of nephrons is destroyed in each stage?
3. Indicate whether the laboratory values of BUN and plasma creatinine would be normal, rising just above normal, or rising sharply in each of the three stages of renal failure.
4. What happens to the creatinine clearance in progressive renal failure?
5. What is the difference between polyuria and oliguria? Define *nocturia*.

6. Explain why polyuria and oliguria occur as more and more functioning nephrons are destroyed in chronic renal failure. Explain how renal lesions could cause these symptoms.
7. Explain how the normal kidney responds to an increasing solute load, how this condition might be induced, and how the evidence supports the intact nephron hypothesis.
8. What happens to the remaining functioning nephrons in progressive renal failure (size, filtration rate, tubular reabsorption, and solute load)?
9. Explain why the original cause of chronic renal failure may be difficult to identify in some cases.
10. Discuss several predisposing factors in the development of UTI and chronic

tubulointerstitial nephritis (chronic pyelonephritis [PN]).
11. What is the significance of asymptomatic bacteriuria in school-aged children?
12. Name the three mechanisms believed to be responsible for reflux nephropathy.
13. Explain the intrarenal hemodynamic theory of progressive renal failure. How well does this theory explain silent (asymptomatic) chronic PN in patients who may be unaware of any renal disease until symptomatic end-stage renal failure (ESRF) occurs? What are the treatment implications of this theory?
14. Name three types of glomerulonephritis (GN) based on clinical classification. What is the prognosis of each type, generally speaking? Describe their natural history and relationship.

Match the descriptions in column B with the terms in column A that refer to the distribution of glomerular lesions.

Column A	Column B
15. _____ Diffuse	a. Only a portion of the glomeruli are involved
16. _____ Local	b. Part of the glomerulus is involved
17. _____ Focal	c. All the glomeruli are affected

Match the descriptive characteristics in column B with the appropriate pathogenic immune mechanism in column A.

Column A	Column B
18. _____ Circulating immune complex	a. Associated with Goodpasture's syndrome
19. _____ Anti-GBM	b. Associated with acute poststreptococcal glomerulonephritis (APSGN) and systemic lupus erythematosus (SLE)
	c. Immunoglobulin is deposited subepithelially
	d. Immunoglobulin is deposited subendothelially
	e. Autoimmune mechanism
	f. Linear or ribbonlike pattern of deposit on immunofluorescent biopsy slide
	g. Ag-Ab complexes are mechanically trapped in the filtration membrane
	h. Results in more serious injury to the glomerulus

Match the appropriate description in column B with the histologic type of GN in column A. Letters may be used more than once.

Column A
20. _____ Minimal change GN
21. _____ Membranous GN
22. _____ Proliferative GN

Column B
a. Primary change in the glomerulus is an increase in endothelial, mesangial, or epithelial cells
b. Predominant change is thickening of the basement membrane
c. Only morphologic change is fusion of the foot processes
d. Most common lesion in children associated with the nephrotic syndrome
e. Nephrotic patients with these lesions often progress to renal failure

Match the descriptive phrases in column B with the terms in column A to which they apply. Letters may be used more than once.

Column A
23. _____ PKD (adult form ADPKD)
24. _____ PKD (infantile form ARPKD)
25. _____ Distal RTA
26. _____ Proximal RTA
27. _____ Kimmelstiel-Wilson disease
28. _____ Gout
29. _____ Hyperparathyroidism
30. _____ Amyloidosis

Column B
a. Characteristic lesion of diabetic nephropathy
b. May be a hereditary disorder
c. Commonly presents as failure to thrive
d. Nephrocalcinosis is a common complication
e. Deposits in kidney common in rheumatoid arthritis, paraplegia, and multiple myeloma
f. Cysts communicate with tubules
g. Less common type of PKD
h. Urate crystals may be deposited in the renal tubules or interstitium
i. Treated with sodium HCO_3^- or sodium and potassium citrate
j. Urine acidification test may aid in diagnosis

Fill in the blanks with the correct words.
31. In acute pyelonephritis (PN), _____ (inflammatory cells) are usually found throughout the cortex and medulla and segments of the _____ are destroyed, whereas in chronic PN, in the interstitium there are many _____ and _____ cells.
32. Label Fig. 46-19 by matching the letters with the renal histologic findings from the list below.
_____ Normal tubule
_____ Area of interstitial fibrosis
_____ Hypertrophied tubule with atrophy of epithelial cells
_____ Atrophied tubule containing cast
_____ Inflammatory cells (PMNs)

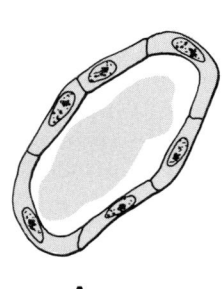
A

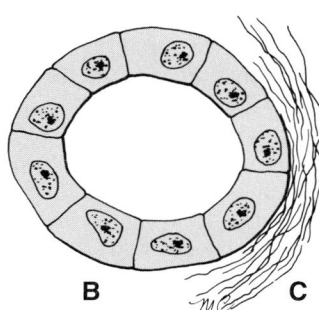
B   **C**

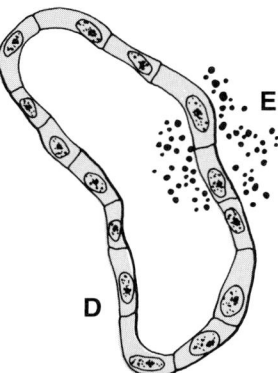
D   **E**

FIG. 46-19   Histologic findings in chronic pyelonephritis.

End-Stage Renal Disease: Uremic Syndrome

LORRAINE M. WILSON

*E*ach of the principal kidney diseases that lead to chronic progressive renal failure has unique features that relate to the cause, pathogenesis, and morphology. These differences are discussed in Chapter 46. It was also pointed out that these diseases produce many similar morphologic changes. This is particularly true when the terminal stage of chronic renal disease is reached, when it may be difficult to determine the cause of the chronic renal failure by examining the end-stage kidney.

As also explained in Chapter 46, from a functional point of view, regardless of cause, there is a common sequence of changes in renal function caused by the progressive destruction of nephrons. The rate of destruction can vary greatly, with quiescent periods and exacerbations, and the duration from beginning to end may vary from months to as long as 40 years. However, once the glomerular filtration rate (GFR) begins to fall and the blood urea nitrogen (BUN) and creatinine levels rise, there is a tendency toward rapid progression to end-stage renal failure. Because of these common functional patterns, it is possible to consider the events in the pathophysiology of chronic renal failure as a single phenomenon rather than discuss the changes in function on a disease-by-disease basis.

The common sequence of changes has this effect on the patient: when the GFR falls to 5% to 10% of normal and progresses toward zero, the patient develops what is called the *uremic syndrome*. The uremic syndrome is a symptom complex that results from or is associated with retention of nitrogenous metabolites because of renal failure. In advanced uremia, some functions of virtually every organ system in the body may become abnormal.

Two groups of clinical symptoms are present in the uremic syndrome. First, symptoms referable to deranged regulatory and excretory functions are prominent: fluid volume and electrolyte abnormalities, acid-base imbalance, retention of nitrogenous and other metabolites, and anemia caused by renal secretory deficiency. A second group of clinical features includes a constellation of cardiovascular, neuromuscular, gastrointestinal, and other abnormalities. Surprisingly, little is known about the basis of these multiple-system abnormalities, though diligent research is now being conducted to uncover these mysteries. Table 47-1 lists some of the common manifestations of the uremic syndrome discussed in this chapter.

BIOCHEMICAL DISTURBANCES

Metabolic Acidosis

Renal failure is characterized by a wide variety of biochemical disturbances. One of the constant abnormalities exhibited by the uremic patient is metabolic acidosis. On a normal diet, the kidney has to excrete 40 to 60 mEq of hydrogen ion (H^+) daily to prevent acidosis. In renal

TABLE 47-1

Manifestations of the Uremic Syndrome

Body System	Manifestations	Body System	Manifestations
Biochemical	Metabolic acidosis (serum HCO$_3$ 18-20 mEq/L)	Gastrointestinal	Anorexia, nausea, vomiting, leading to weight loss
	Azotemia (decreased GFR, leading to increased BUN, creatinine)		Ammoniacal odor to breath
	Hyperkalemia		Metallic taste, dry mouth
	Sodium retention or wasting		Stomatitis, parotitis
	Hypermagnesemia		Gastritis, enteritis
	Hyperuricemia		GI bleeding
Genitourinary	Polyuria, progressing to oliguria, progressing to anuria		Diarrhea
		Intermediary metabolism	Protein—intolerance, abnormal synthesis
	Nocturia, reversal of diurnal rhythm		Carbohydrate—hyperglycemia, decreased insulin need
	Fixed urine sp gr 1.010		Fat—increased levels of triglycerides
	Proteinuria; casts		Easy fatigability
	Loss of libido, amenorrhea, impotence, sterility	Neuromuscular	Muscle wasting, weakness
Cardiovascular	Hypertension		Central nervous system
	Hypertensive retinopathy, encephalopathy		Decreased mental acuity
	Circulatory overload		Poor concentration
	Edema		Apathy
	Congestive heart failure		Lethargy/restlessness, insomnia
	Pericarditis (friction rub)		Mental confusion
	Dysrhythmias		Coma
Respiratory	Kussmaul's breathing, dyspnea		Muscle twitching, asterixis, convulsions
	Pulmonary edema		Peripheral neuropathy
	Pneumonitis		Slowed nerve conduction, "restless leg" syndrome
Hematologic	Anemia leading to fatigue		Sensory changes in the extremities—paresthesias
	Hemolysis		Motor changes—foot drop progressing to paraplegia
	Bleeding tendency	Calcium and skeletal disorders	Hyperphosphatemia, hypocalcemia
	Decreased resistance to infection (urinary tract infection, pneumonia, septicemia)		Secondary hyperparathyroidism
Cutaneous	Pallor, pigmentation		Renal osteodystrophy
	Hair and nail changes (nails brittle, thin, ridged, alternating red and light bands associated with protein wasting)		Pathologic fractures (demineralization of bones)
	Pruritus		Calcium salts deposited in soft tissue (around joints, blood vessels, heart, lungs)
	Uremic "frost"		Conjunctivitis (uremic red eye)
	Dry skin		
	Bruises		

HCO$_3$, Bicarbonate; GFR, glomerular filtration rate; BUN, blood urea nitrogen; sp gr, specific gravity; GI, gastrointestinal.

failure, impaired ability of the kidney to excrete H$^+$ results in a systemic acidosis, with a decrease in the plasma pH and bicarbonate (HCO$_3$) concentration. The HCO$_3$ level decreases because it is used up in buffering H$^+$. Ammonium ion (NH$_4^+$) excretion is the kidney's most important mechanism for the excretion of H$^+$ and the regeneration of HCO$_3$ (because it allows de novo addition of new HCO$_3$ rather than just reabsorption of the filtered HCO$_3$ to the extracellular fluid). Total NH$_4^+$ excretion is decreased in renal failure because of the diminished number of nephrons. Phosphate excretion provides another mechanism for the excretion of H$^+$ as titratable acid (i.e., phosphate-buffered H$^+$). The rate of phosphate excretion, however, is determined by the need to maintain phosphate balance rather than acid-base balance. Phosphate tends to be retained in renal failure because of the diminished nephron mass and factors related to calcium metabolism, which are discussed later. The retention of sulfate and other organic anions also contributes to the depletion of HCO$_3$.

The serum HCO$_3$ level usually stabilizes at about 18 to 20 mEq/L (moderate acidosis) and rarely drops below this level. The most likely explanation for this lack of progression in the presence of a positive H$^+$ balance is that H$^+$ is being buffered by calcium carbonate from the bone.

It is possible that the symptoms of anorexia, nausea, and lethargy common in the uremic patient may be partly because of the acidosis. One symptom that is undoubtedly caused by acidosis is Kussmaul's respiration, although this symptom may be less prominent in chronic acidosis. *Kussmaul's respiration* is the deep, sighing respiration that occurs because of the need to increase carbon dioxide excretion and thus reduce the severity of the acidosis.

Potassium Imbalance

Potassium (K$^+$) imbalance is one of the serious disturbances that may occur in renal failure, because only a narrow plasma concentration range is compatible with life (normal = 3.5 to 5.5 mEq/L). About 90% of the normal daily intake of 50 to 150 mEq is excreted in the urine. Hypokalemia may be associated with the polyuria of early chronic renal failure, particularly in tubular diseases such as chronic pyelonephritis. However, as the patient becomes oliguric in end-stage renal failure, hyperkalemia invariably develops.

The systemic acidosis also contributes to the hyperkalemia by causing K^+ to shift from the cells to the extracellular fluid. The major life-threatening effect of hyperkalemia is its influence on the electrical conduction of the heart. Fatal dysrhythmias or cardiac standstill may occur when serum K^+ levels reach 7 to 8 mEq/L.

Sodium Imbalance

The average American diet contains 2 to 10 g sodium (Na^+) (or 5 to 25 g sodium chloride [NaCl])/day. In most normal persons, there is great flexibility in the kidney's ability to vary excretion of Na^+ in response to a variable intake. Salt excretion may vary from nearly 0 to more than 20 g daily. Patients with chronic renal failure lose this great flexibility and may be "poised on a razor's edge" with respect to the ability to vary Na^+ output. In early renal insufficiency when polyuria is present, Na^+ wasting may occur because of the increased solute load of each intact nephron. The osmotic diuresis results in obligatory Na^+ losses. This Na^+-losing tendency is more common in chronic pyelonephritis and polycystic kidneys, which affect primarily the tubules.

When oliguria supervenes in terminal renal failure, the patient is more likely to retain Na^+. The retention of Na^+ and water may result in circulatory overload, edema, hypertension, and congestive heart failure. The development of congestive heart failure secondary to the hypertension and the increased aldosterone levels present in uremic patients may also play a major role in Na^+ retention.

Hypermagnesemia

Like K^+, magnesium (Mg^{++}) is chiefly an intracellular cation and is excreted chiefly by the kidneys. The normal serum level is 1.5 to 2.3 mEq/L. The ability to excrete Mg^{++} is reduced in the uremic patient. However, hypermagnesemia is generally not a serious problem, because intake of Mg^{++} is usually reduced because of anorexia, reduced protein intake, and decreased absorption from the gastrointestinal (GI) tract. A sudden load of Mg^{++} from the ingestion of laxatives such as milk of magnesia or magnesium citrate may cause death by depressing neuromuscular activity.

Azotemia

As previously discussed, a sharp rise in the plasma urea and creatinine levels generally signals the onset of terminal renal failure and accompanies uremic symptoms. There is much evidence, however, that urea itself is not responsible for the symptoms and metabolic defects found in uremia. Some of the substances found in the blood of uremic patients that might act as toxins are the guanidines, phenols, amines, urate, creatinine, aromatic hydroxy acids, and indican. Some of these compounds act as potent enzyme inhibitors. It is likely that a combination of factors such as the acidosis and other electrolyte disturbances, hormonal disturbances, and retained toxins produce the metabolic defects and the multiple-system involvement. Present research postulates that the uremic toxins may lie in the middle molecular range in size (urea is a small molecule; albumin is a large molecule), and this has led to the *middle molecular hypothesis* and research into more efficient re-

moval of these molecules. For example, high-efficiency, high-flux (HEHF) hemodialysis using more biocompatible dialysis membranes of high permeability not only shortens dialysis time, but it is also superior in the removal of potential uremic toxins that fall in the middle molecular size (see Chapter 48).

Hyperuricemia

The intimate association of gout and the kidney was alluded to in Chapter 46. A rise in serum uric acid concentration and the formation of obstructive crystals in the kidney can cause chronic or acute renal failure. On the other hand, the serum uric acid level generally rises early in the course of chronic renal failure because of excretory impairment of the kidneys. The kidneys normally account for about 75% of the excreted uric acid. A rise in serum uric acid concentration above the normal 4 to 6 mg/dl may or may not be associated with symptoms. It is not uncommon, however, for uremic patients to have attacks of gouty arthritis from the deposition of urate salts in the joints and soft tissues.

GENITOURINARY DISTURBANCES

Urinary symptoms in uremia are intimately associated with water metabolism; these findings have been discussed in previous chapters. Polyuria caused by osmotic diuresis gradually gives way to oliguria and even anuria as the nephron mass is gradually destroyed. Nocturia and a reversal of the normal diurnal pattern of urine excretion, resulting in a relatively constant rate of urine formation throughout the day and night, is another important symptom caused by the osmotic diuresis. A constant urine specific gravity near 1.010 (285 mOsm) in the uremic patient reflects loss of the ability to concentrate or dilute the urine from the plasma concentration. These changes make the uremic patient vulnerable to acute changes in water balance. Diarrhea or vomiting may quickly cause dehydration (with subsequent hypovolemia, decreased GFR, and further deterioration of renal function), and excess water intake may cause circulatory overload, edema, and congestive heart failure.

As the nephron mass and the GFR decrease, proteinuria, which may have been prominent earlier in the chronic renal disease, may become insignificant or may disappear altogether. Broad granular casts may occasionally be found in the urine sediment and are characteristic of advanced renal failure.

Young uremic women cease to menstruate, and the men are generally impotent and sterile when the GFR falls to 5 ml/min. Both genders experience a loss of libido as the uremia becomes more severe. Sexual and reproductive function may return after renal transplantation or a regular hemodialysis program. Most physicians, however, advise women not to become pregnant when advanced renal insufficiency is present.

CARDIOVASCULAR ABNORMALITIES

Hypertension and congestive heart failure often accompany the uremic syndrome. About 90% of the hypertension is volume dependent and related to Na$^+$ and water retention, whereas probably less than 10% is renin dependent. The combination of hypertension, anemia, and circulatory overload caused by Na$^+$ and water retention contributes to the increased propensity to congestive heart failure. Other side effects of severe hypertension include retinopathy and encephalopathy. The symptoms of these disorders are the same as in nonuremic patients.

Pericarditis, once a frequent complication of chronic renal failure, is now infrequent because of the early initiation of dialysis. Retained metabolic toxins are believed to be the cause of the pericarditis. The clinical presentation of patients with uremic pericarditis is similar to that of other causes. The patient may complain of pain on deep inspiration or when lying down, but about two thirds of the patients are asymptomatic. A to-and-fro friction rub may be heard over the precordium with auscultation. The chest radiograph may reveal an enlarged cardiac silhouette when a pericardial effusion is present. Occasionally the patient with uremic pericarditis may develop a massive hemorrhagic effusion and cardiac tamponade, especially when anticoagulants are used during hemodialysis. In the event of this emergency, prompt aspiration of the fluid by the physician may be lifesaving.

Finally, it must be remembered that cardiac dysrhythmias commonly associated with K$^+$ imbalance in renal failure are also affected by imbalances in Na$^+$, H$^+$, calcium (Ca^{++}), and Mg^{++}.

RESPIRATORY CHANGES

The deep, sighing (Kussmaul's) respiration of severe acidosis has already been mentioned. However, the patient with moderate acidosis of chronic renal insufficiency is more apt to complain of dyspnea on exertion, and the increased depth of breathing is overlooked except by an experienced observer.

Other respiratory complications of renal failure are the "uremic lung" and pneumonitis. Chest radiographs of the uremic lung reveal a bilateral butterfly-shaped infiltration of the lungs (Fig. 47-1). The condition is actually pulmonary edema and is inevitably associated with fluid overload caused by Na$^+$ and water retention or left ventricular failure or both. The butterfly configuration of the pulmonary edema is the result of increased permeability of the alveolar capillary membrane around the hilus of the lung. Bilateral infection causing a pneumonitis may be superimposed on the chronically wet lung. Pulmonary congestion disappears with the reduction of body fluids by salt restriction and hemodialysis.

HEMATOLOGIC PROBLEMS

A characteristically normochromic, normocytic anemia is an inevitable feature of the uremic syndrome. Usually the hematocrit falls to the 20% to 30% range and parallels the degree of azotemia. The primary cause of the anemia is decreased red blood cell (RBC) formation. Decreased RBC formation is caused by deficient production of erythropoietin by the failing kidney. There is also some evidence that uremic toxins may inactivate erythropoietin or suppress the response of the bone marrow to its action. A

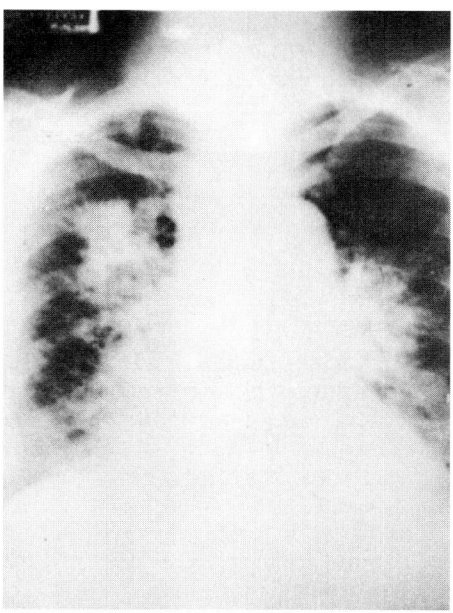

FIG. 47-1 Uremic lung, showing marked central distribution of pulmonary edema. (From Bailey GL: *Hemodialysis*, New York, 1972, Academic Press.)

second factor contributing to the anemia is that the life span of the RBC in a patient with renal failure is about one half that in the normal person. The increased hemolysis of RBCs appears to be caused by the abnormal chemical environment in the plasma and not by a defect in the cells themselves. In addition to the deficient erythropoiesis and hemolytic tendency, blood loss in the GI tract may further aggravate the anemia. Other factors contributing to the anemia include iatrogenic blood loss and iron and folic acid deficiency. The blood loss caused by frequent sampling for laboratory tests and loss in the hemodialysis tubing may be considerable (average loss is 4.6 L/yr in one study). Iron deficiency may result from blood loss and from poor GI absorption (antacids taken for hyperphosphatemia also bind iron in the gut). Folic acid deficiency is associated with uremia, and if the patient is receiving hemodialysis treatment, water-soluble vitamins are lost through the dialysis membrane. The bleeding tendency of uremia is apparently caused by a qualitative defect in the platelets and consequently results in defective adhesion. Inhibition of certain coagulation factors may also play a role.

Pallor as a result of persistent anemia is characteristic of the uremic patient. The anemia undoubtedly contributes to the symptoms of fatigue. Dyspnea on exertion may be experienced when the hemoglobin is 8 g/dl or less. Bruising, nosebleeds, and GI bleeding may be manifestations of the coagulation defect.

Infection is a fairly common complication of patients with advanced renal insufficiency. The white blood cell (WBC) count is usually normal in end-stage renal disease (ESRD), but there is evidence of defective granulocyte, lymphocyte, and monocyte-macrophage function. Decreased chemotaxis causes impairment of the acute inflammatory response and decreased delayed hypersensitivity. Uremic patients also tend to have less fever in response to an infection. The cause of the hypothermia is believed to be due, in part, to inhibition of the Na-K pump, located in cell membranes, by uremic toxins (Bailey, Mitch, 2000). Poor nutrition, pulmonary edema, and the use of cannulas and indwelling catheters may be predisposing factors in the increased susceptibility to infection. The use of large doses of corticosteroid and other immunosuppressive drugs after renal transplant to suppress tissue rejection makes these patients unusually susceptible to severe infection that may result in death.

CUTANEOUS CHANGES

The accumulation of urinary pigments (principally urochrome) combined with anemia in advanced renal insufficiency gives the skin of the light-skinned person a peculiar waxy yellow cast. In the brown-skinned person, this is observed as a yellowish brown coloration, and in the black-skinned person, as an ashen gray color with yellow tones, particularly on the palmar and plantar surfaces. The skin may be dry and scaly, and the hair may be brittle and may change color. The nails may be thin, brittle, and ridged and show alternating light and reddish bands. These nail changes are characteristic of chronic protein wasting (Muehrcke lines). Pruritus is common in the uremic patient and is considered to be a manifestation of increased parathyroid gland function and deposition of Ca^{++} in the skin. Uremic pruritus is usually quite resistant to dialysis treatment as well as to topical agents. When the BUN level is very high, fine white crystals of urea may appear on areas of the skin where there is heavy perspiration. This condition is called *uremic frost*. Multiple bruises caused by minor trauma are often seen on the skin of the uremic patient because of increased capillary fragility.

GASTROINTESTINAL SIGNS AND SYMPTOMS

The GI manifestations of uremia can cause the patient great distress. Anorexia, nausea, and vomiting are common in uremia and are often the first symptoms of disease. These symptoms are responsible, in part, for the extensive weight loss in chronic renal failure. The entire GI tract itself becomes affected in uremia. Patients often complain of a metallic taste in the mouth, and there may be an odor of ammonia to the breath. The mouth may become inflamed and ulcerated (stomatitis), and the tongue may be dry and coated. Occasionally, parotitis (inflammation of the parotid gland) occurs. The normal flora of the mouth contains organisms (tooth calculus bacteria) that can split urea in the saliva to produce ammonia. This action accounts for the uriniferous odor to the breath and the altered sense of taste and predisposes the tissue to the inflammation and infection. Mucosal ulcerations may occur in the stomach and the small or large intestine and may result in profuse bleeding. The effect of GI hemorrhage is extremely serious, because the fall in blood pressure lowers the GFR even further and the digestion of the blood causes a precipitous rise in the BUN level. Diarrhea occurs at times and may cause serious dehydration.

Although hepatitis B (HBV) infection was a significant problem in the past, it is less so today because of the implementation of universal precautions and availability of HBV vaccine. Hepatitis C (HCV) infection, like HBV, is transmitted through percutaneous exposure to blood. HCV is a problem, especially for patients who subsequently undergo renal transplantation, because it has a strong association with chronic active hepatitis and the development of primary liver cancer or cirrhosis (see Chapter 27).

INTERMEDIARY METABOLISM ABNORMALITIES

Abnormalities of intermediary metabolism are characteristic of the uremic syndrome, although the physiologic mechanisms are poorly understood.

Protein

Whatever other elements are responsible for uremic symptoms, the breakdown products of protein metabolism are of prime importance. The dietary restriction of protein generally relieves somewhat the symptoms of lassitude, nausea, and anorexia, and increasing evidence exists that it may retard the progression of renal deterioration (see Chapter 48). The patient tends to decrease protein intake voluntarily as azotemia progresses, because the appetite for protein foods generally is lost. Another reason for protein restriction in uremia is that H^+, K^+, and phosphates are derived chiefly from protein foods and must be restricted to prevent their accumulation in the blood. Abnormal protein synthesis in uremia is demonstrated by elevation or depression of selected amino acids. The significance of this phenomenon is not known.

Carbohydrates and Fats

Defective carbohydrate metabolism is commonly associated with uremia. Fasting blood sugar levels are elevated in more than 50% of uremic patients but not usually over 200 mg/dl. Insensitivity of the peripheral tissues to insulin is the possible cause. On the other hand, insulin-dependent diabetic patients who develop uremia may improve their carbohydrate metabolism and require a lower dose of insulin, in apparent contradiction to the glucose intolerance of nondiabetic patients. A possible explanation is an elevated serum insulin level because of a prolonged half-life (the kidney normally inactivates about 20% of the insulin) in uremia. Carbohydrate metabolism generally becomes normal with regular hemodialysis.

Abnormal fat metabolism is characterized by high serum triglyceride levels in uremic patients, even in those who regularly undergo dialysis. Contributing factors in the elevated triglycerides may include the elevated glucose and insulin levels and the acetate used in the dialysate. The abnormal carbohydrate and fat metabolism undoubtedly contributes to the accelerated atherosclerosis in chronic dialysis patients.

NEUROMUSCULAR ABNORMALITIES

Involvement of the neuromuscular system is a nearly universal complication of uremia. Both the central and the peripheral nervous systems are involved, with diverse consequences. Muscles may be involved partly because of the peripheral neuropathy and partly because of muscle wasting.

Central Nervous System

The degree of cerebral disturbance roughly parallels the degree of azotemia. Early symptoms are decreased mental acuity and ability to concentrate, apathy, and lethargy. The patient complains of feeling weak and tired and may be unable to perform a normal day's work without frequent rest periods. Lethargy may alternate with periods of restlessness and insomnia. The untreated patient will eventually become confused and comatose. If convulsions occur, they are usually associated with hypertensive encephalopathy. Involuntary jerking and twitching of muscles reflect this neuromuscular irritability. *Asterixis* (flapping tremor of the hands) may sometimes be present and is a manifestation of cerebral toxicity. The physical sign is induced by having the patient raise both arms with forearms fixed and fingers extended; this will result in alterations of flexion and extension at the wrist (flapping tremor).

Dialysis disequilibrium syndrome is a condition characterized by nonlocalizing neurologic symptoms, such as headache, nausea and vomiting, twitching, hypertension, and blurred vision. The condition may progress to confusion or seizures. Dialysis disequilibrium most often occurs during or within the first 12 hours of the initial dialysis treatment, the cause of which is believed to be cerebral edema. The pathogenesis is attributed to the rapid dialysis-induced changes in pH and osmolality between the extracellular and intracellular fluid compartments. *Dialysis dementia* is a progressive and frequently fatal neurologic disorder occurring in patients after many years on dialysis. Initial symptoms include slurring of speech, dysarthria which later progresses to personality changes, seizures, and eventually dementia and death. Although the pathogenesis is uncertain, aluminum toxicity to the brain, resulting from the ingestion of aluminum-containing antacids or high aluminum levels in the dialysis water, is believed to be a major factor.

Peripheral Neuropathy

Affliction of the peripheral nervous system follows a characteristic course. The earliest sign of peripheral neuropathy is the slowing of nerve conduction, which is generally tested on the peroneal nerve in the leg. A decreased velocity of nerve conduction may begin before the onset of clinical symptoms. The *restless leg syndrome* may sometimes be an early symptom. The patient may describe this symptom as a peculiar feeling that is relieved by walking or moving the legs. The second stage in the development of peripheral neuropathy is the advent of sensory changes in the extremities. The patient experiences burning pain, numbness, or tingling (paresthesias) of the toes and feet, which progresses up the leg in a stockinglike fashion. Later, paresthesias may occur in the fingers and hands. Finally, motor nerves are involved. Motor involvement usually begins as a foot drop and may progress to paraplegia. Pathologically, there is a patchy loss of myelin and damage to the peripheral nerves, possibly caused by uremic toxins and electrolyte imbalance.

Hemodialysis may halt the progress of peripheral neuropathy, but once these changes occur, they are poorly reversible (sensory) or are irreversible (motor). Therefore hemodialysis (or transplantation preparations) should be started before clinical signs and symptoms occur.

CALCIUM AND SKELETAL DISORDERS (RENAL OSTEODYSTROPHY)

If a patient with chronic renal failure survives long enough, Ca^{++} and phosphate imbalances with skeletal involvement are inevitable. The skeletal disorders called *renal osteodystrophy* comprise three lesions.

Osteomalacia is the most common bone disorder and is seen in about 60% of all patients with chronic renal failure. Osteomalacia consists of defective mineralization of bone and is caused by a deficiency of 1,25-dihydroxycholecalciferol ($1,25[OH]_2D_3$) or *calcitriol*, the most active form of vitamin D metabolized by the kidneys. The deficiency of the most active form of vitamin D leads to severely impaired absorption of Ca^{++} from the gut. In the bone, osteoblasts continue to manufacture osteoid tissue (the framework on which Ca^{++} salts are laid down to produce bone), but the low serum Ca^{++} level and ineffective action of vitamin D on the bone do not allow mineralization. Osteoid tissue eventually replaces normal bone, producing osteomalacia in adults and rickets in children. Osteoid is structurally weak and may fracture or deform under stress. On radiographs, osteomalacia presents as a generalized decrease in bone density, especially of the hands, skull, ribs, and spine.

Osteitis fibrosa, occurring in more than 30% of patients, is characterized by osteoclastic resorption of bone and replacement by fibrous tissue. The bone demineralization may be localized and may present as cystlike lesions (osteitis fibrosa cystica) or may appear on a radiograph as a generalized decrease in bone density. Increased levels of parathyroid hormone (PTH) (secondary hyperparathyroidism) that are observed in chronic renal failure cause osteitis fibrosa. The classic radiographic appearance of osteitis fibrosa is often seen in the fingers as subperiosteal bone resorption and in the skull as a patchy loss of bone density (Fig. 47-2).

Osteosclerosis, the third, less common bone disorder, is often manifested as a banded or striped appearance of the vertebrae ("rugger jersey spine") on radiographs. Osteosclerosis is caused by alternate bands of decreased and increased bone density.

Any of the lesions just described may occur alone, but a combination is more common. Hemodialysis alone does not prevent renal osteodystrophy. Only within the past few years has research uncovered some of the complex relationships in the pathogenesis of renal osteodystrophy so that effective treatment is possible. The principal factors are decreased renal function, secondary hyperparathyroidism, and vitamin D deficiency or resistance.

In addition to the classical three types of lesions comprising renal osteodystrophy (osteomalacia, osteitis fibrosa cystica, and osteosclerosis), there are three other types of bone and skeletal disorders seen in patients with ESRD detectable by bone biopsy. Vitamin D–resistant *aluminum-induced osteomalacia* consists of the

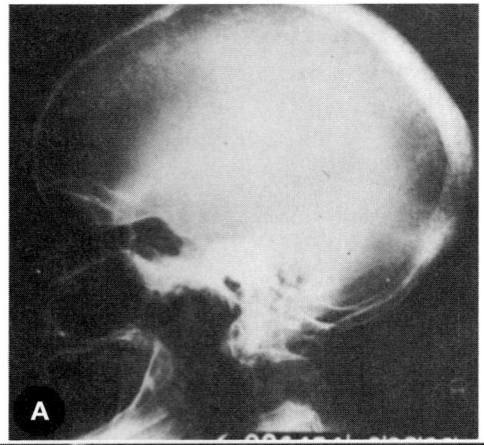

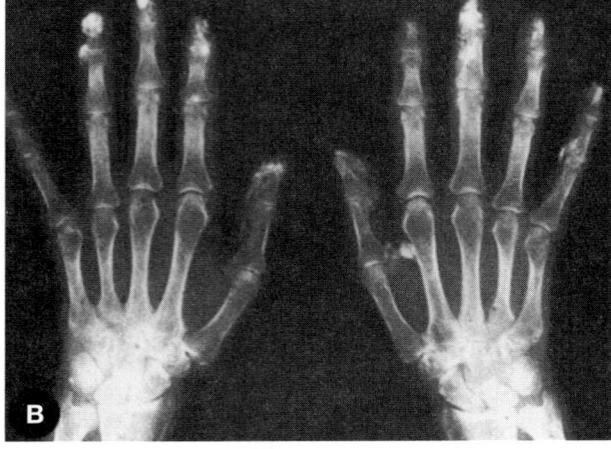

FIG. 47-2   Renal osteodystrophy. **A**, Skull radiograph shows spotty demineralization of bone, producing a "moth-eaten" appearance. **B**, Subperiosteal resorption is present in all the phalanges but is seen best on the middle phalanx of both the right and left hands, producing a jagged appearance. (Courtesy DE Schteingart.)

accumulation of aluminum metabolites in the bone, predisposing the patient to pathologic fractures, especially hip (femoral neck) fracture. The sources are aluminum hydroxide antacids commonly used as dietary phosphate-binding agents. Aluminum is also common in the community water and may be transferred to the patient during dialysis (if not first deionized).

Adynamic, or *aplastic, bone disease* is a recently described condition characterized by decreased bone mineralization but normal amounts of osteoid. Adynamic bone disease is more common in older adults, in patients with diabetes, and in those treated with peritoneal dialysis. Causal factors have been attributed to aluminum toxicity in some cases and to overzealous suppression of PTH levels that are normally elevated in ESRD (Delmez, 1998).

Dialysis-related amyloidosis is the result of the deposition of β_2 microglobulin-derived fibrils in bones and joints because of the insufficient elimination of this protein by dialysis in ESRD (see Chapter 46). Bone cysts, arthropathy, and carpal tunnel syndrome are the most common

clinical manifestations. Bone pain and pathologic fractures are common in all three of these conditions.

Pathogenesis of Renal Osteodystrophy

The sequence of events leading to secondary hyperparathyroidism and renal osteodystrophy is most easily followed in Fig. 47-3 (also see Chapter 21).

Normally, the serum Ca^{++} and phosphate are in equilibrium with solid-phase Ca^{++} and phosphate in the bones. The absorption from the gut, excretion by the kidneys, and deposition and resorption from the bone of these minerals are primarily controlled by PTH and $1,25[OH_2]D_3$. Moreover, serum Ca^{++} and phosphate levels have a reciprocal relationship; that is, when serum Ca^{++} levels go up, serum phosphate levels go down and vice versa. This interrelation serves the purpose of keeping the serum calcium-phosphate cross product constant so that calcium phosphate is not precipitated in the vascular system. For example, the normal serum Ca^{++} level is 9.0 to 11.0 mg/dl, and the normal phosphate level is 3.0 to 4.5 mg/dl. The normal cross product value in milligrams per deciliter of Ca^{++} and phosphate is thus 3 to 4.5 × 9 to 11 = 27.0 to 49.5. Precipitation of calcium phosphate salts in the soft tissues is believed to occur when their cross product exceeds 60 to 70 mg/dl.

As renal disease advances, calcium-phosphate interrelations become progressively disrupted. When the GFR falls to about 25% of normal, the kidneys retain phosphate. Phosphate retention causes the depression of serum Ca^{++} levels. The azotemic state also interferes with vitamin D_3 activation by the kidney, which is necessary for the absorption of Ca^{++} from the gut. Both these factors tend to cause hypocalcemia. Hypocalcemia stimulates the parathyroid glands to put out more PTH, which causes bone resorption of Ca^{++} and phosphate, increased excretion of phosphate, and activation of vitamin D_3 by the kidneys. Serum Ca^{++} and phosphate levels thus tend to be restored to normal. As the GFR continues to decrease, however, the low serum Ca^{++} and high phosphate levels increasingly stimulate parathyroid activity. The parathyroid glands may show hyperplasia of the secretory cells, with apparent independence of physiologic controls. The result is increasing demineralization of the bony skeleton. A rise in the serum alkaline phosphatase level is evidence that this process is occurring. The calcium-phosphate cross product may become exceedingly high, resulting in the precipitation of calcium-phosphate salts in the soft tissues of the body.

Common sites for the deposition of Ca^{++} salts are in and around joints, resulting in painful arthritis; in the kidney (nephrocalcinosis), resulting in obstruction; in the blood vessels, which may have the appearance of an arteriogram on radiographs; in the heart and lung, leading to dysrhythmias, cardiomyopathy, and pulmonary fibrosis; and in the eyes. The deposition of Ca^{++} salts in the conjunctiva and cornea of the eye is called *band keratopathy.* Band keratopathy appears as grayish or whitish granular opacities in the form of a crescent on the nasal or temporal side of the limbus (where cornea and sclera meet at colored and white parts of the eye) (Fig. 47-4). Precipitation of calcium-phosphate salts occurs on the surface of the eye because here the pH is high and favors

FIG. 47-3   Pathogenesis of renal osteodystrophy. *1,25(OH)₂D₃*, 1,25-Dihydroxycholecalciferol; *GFR*, glomerular filtration rate; *PTH*, parathyroid hormone; *Ca⁺⁺*, calcium.

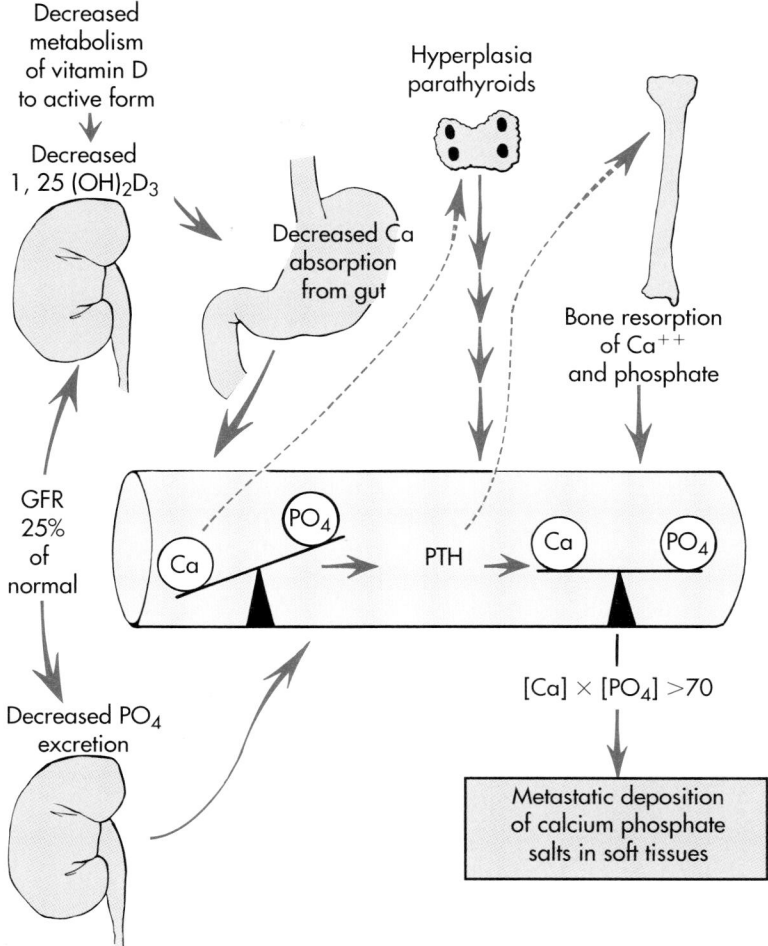

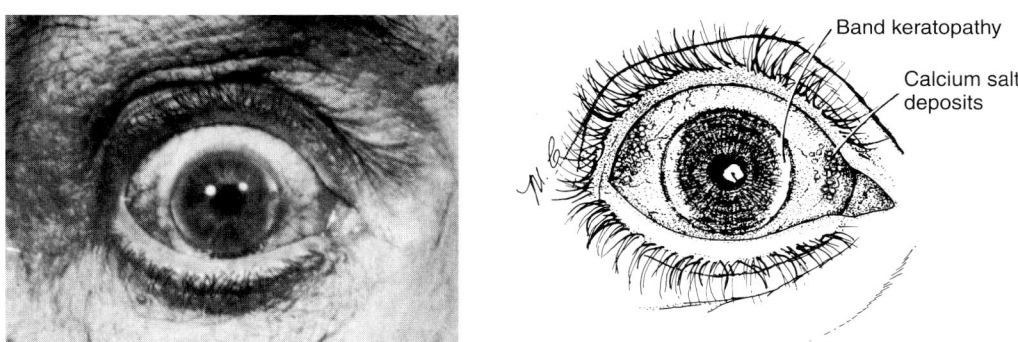

FIG. 47-4   Band keratopathy caused by deposit of calcium salts in the eye. Conjunctival deposits of calcium salts are also present. Diagram of abnormalities seen in photograph. (Photograph from Maxwell MH, Kleeman CR, editors: *Clinical disorders of fluid and electrolyte metabolism*, ed 2, New York, 1972, McGraw-Hill.)

precipitation. These deposits can be seen with the naked eye but are most easily outlined by slit lamp examination. The conjunctival deposits sometimes cause intense irritation with redness and watering of the eyes ("uremic red eye").

This discussion completes the description of the syndrome called *uremia*. Not all components are present in every patient, and the dominant features may vary from one patient to another. The prevention and treatment of these complications are considered in Chapter 48.

KEY CONCEPTS

- The *uremic syndrome* is the constellation of signs and symptoms that become apparent as renal insufficiency progresses and the GFR falls below 10 ml/min (<10% of normal) culminating in ESRD. At this point, the remaining intact nephrons are no longer able to compensate to maintain normal renal function.

- Clinical manifestations of the *uremic syndrome* may be divided into those referable to (1) *deranged regulatory* and *excretory functions*, such as fluid volume and electrolyte imbalances, acid-base imbalances, retention of nitrogenous and other metabolites, and hormonal disturbances and (2) *multiple body system abnormalities* (virtually all of them), the basis of which is poorly understood.

- *Azotemia* (nitrogenous substances in the blood) is indicated by a sharp rise in the serum creatinine and BUN above normal values and generally signals the onset of ESRD or the uremic syndrome.

- Much evidence indicates that neither the elevated *urea* nor the elevated *creatinine* are responsible for the symptoms and metabolic defects in uremia.

- The *middle molecular hypothesis* postulates that retained uremic toxins, middle-sized molecules (100 to 5000 daltons), may be responsible for many of the metabolic and body system abnormalities in the uremic syndrome. Although they are not yet identified with certainty, some possible uremic toxins are postulated to be byproducts of protein and amino acid metabolism, such as guanines, phenols, and urates.

- *Metabolic acidosis* in uremia occurs because the failing kidneys are no longer able to excrete the daily acid load resulting from fewer functioning intact nephrons. Despite a positive acid balance, the serum HCO_3^- rarely falls below 15 mEq/L because of buffering of the excess H^+ by bone salts (contributing to the demineralization of bone seen in renal osteodystrophy).

- *Hyperkalemia* develops in ESRD because of renal excretory failure (the main route of excretion) and an intracellular fluid (ICF) to extracellular fluid (ECF) shift resulting from the metabolic acidosis. A rise in the serum K^+ to 7 or 8 mEq/L may result in a fatal cardiac dysrhythmia.

- Patients with ESRD lose the normal flexibility to vary Na^+ excretion according to Na^+ intake so that excess dietary Na^+ intake results in ECF volume excess and hypertension, while a too severe restriction of dietary Na^+ intake results in ECF volume deficit and a further decrease in the GFR.

- Na^+ and water retention is the usual problem in oliguric ESRD; salt-wasting nephritis is more common in tubulointerstitial diseases, such as polycystic kidney or chronic pyelonephritis.

- Serious *hypermagnesemia* is generally not a problem in ESRD unless the patient ingests Mg^{++}-containing antacids, laxatives, or salt substitutes.

- The hyperuricemia of ESRD may lead to attacks of gouty arthritis or may be asymptomatic.

- The *polyuria* and *nocturia* associated with renal insufficiency generally gives way to *oliguria* and anuria in ESRD; the urine becomes isoosmotic with the plasma (near 285 mOsm or specific gravity of 1.010), as renal ability to concentrate or dilute urine is lost.

- Loss of libido, sterility, impotence, and amenorrhea are common reproductive system disturbances in the uremic syndrome.

- *Hypertension* is common in ESRD and may be a result of the release of renin or the increased ECF volume secondary to abnormal handling of salt and water. The hypertension produces cardiac hypertrophy and, on occasion, congestive heart failure.

- *Uremic pericarditis*, believed to be caused by uremic toxins, is now infrequent because of the early initiation of dialysis; a major complication is *cardiac tamponade* resulting from hemorrhaging into the pericardial sac, especially with the use of heparin during initial hemodialysis treatment.

- A normocytic, normochromic *anemia* typically occurs in ESRD resulting primarily from decreased production of erythropoietin (EPO). Contributing factors include decreased life span of RBCs, iron and folic acid deficiency, poor nutrition, bleeding tendency, and iatrogenic blood loss. The hematocrit is typically about 20 in untreated ESRD.

- Disturbances in blood coagulation, most often demonstrated as nosebleeds and GI bleeding, may occur as a result of impaired *platelet aggregation* in ESRD.

- There is a *blunting of the immune response* in most patients with ESRD, characterized by decreased delayed hypersensitivity and impairment of the acute inflammatory response. Although leukocyte count may be normal, leukocyte function is abnormal, resulting in increased risk of infection.

- *Infection* may be difficult to detect because uremic patients tend to have less fever in response to infection. The cause of uremic *hypothermia* is believed to be a result of inhibition of the Na-K pump.

- *Uremic pneumonitis* with characteristic butterfly-shaped infiltrates on chest x-ray represents pulmonary edema caused, at least in part, by increased permeability of the alveolar capillary membrane around the hilus of the lung. ECF volume excess may also result in pulmonary edema.

- *Cutaneous manifestations* of the uremic syndrome include: (1) a *yellow, waxy appearance of the skin* caused by a combination of retention of urochrome pigments and anemic pallor, (2) *pruritus* resulting from the deposit of Ca^{++} salts or high levels of PTH, (3) hair color changes, and (4) whitish deposits of urea called *uremic frost*.

- *GI manifestations* of uremia include nausea, vomiting, anorexia, and weight loss. Altered taste and an odor of ammonia to the breath may be present. Stomatitis, parotitis, gastritis, diarrhea, and GI bleeding may occur.

- Internal metabolism of proteins, carbohydrates, and fats are all abnormal in ESRD.
- A variety of *metabolic* and *endocrine disturbances* accompany the uremic syndrome, including glucose intolerance and insulin resistance, hyperlipidemia, PTH excess, and calcitriol and EPO deficiency.
- *Disturbances in mentation*, as well as *peripheral sensory* and *motor neuropathy*, are common in uremia. Histologically, demyelinization is observed in the distal portions of peripheral nerves.
- Enlargement of the parathyroid glands resulting from diffuse nodular hyperplasia with elevated levels of PTH is observed in ESRD. This *secondary hyperparathyroidism* is brought about by renal retention of phosphate and decreased absorption of Ca^{++} from the gut caused by impaired renal conversion of vitamin D to its active form, $1,25[OH]_2D_3$ (calcitriol).
- Histologic evidence of bone disease is found in 90% of patients with chronic renal failure; the process be-gins during the stage of renal insufficiency and long before ESRD is reached.
- The bone lesions comprising *renal osteodystrophy* include: (1) *osteitis fibrosa cystica* characterized by subperiosteal bone reabsorption in the clavicles, long bones, and phalanges caused by secondary hyperparathyroidism; (2) *osteomalacia* (renal rickets), characterized by defective mineralization of bone resulting from calcitriol deficiency; and (3) *osteosclerosis*, evidenced by "rugger jersey" spine, wherein bone density is augmented in the upper and lower margins of vertebral bodies. The toxic effects of aluminum and amyloid deposits also cause bone lesions.
- Hyperparathyroidism can predispose to the development of *metastatic calcification* or deposition of Ca^{++} salts in the soft tissues of the body; precipitation can occur if the serum concentrations of Ca^{++} and phosphate should both rise simultaneously so that their cross product ($Ca \times PO_4$) in mg/dl exceeds 60 to 70.

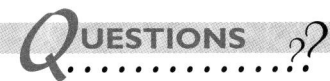

QUESTIONS ??

A sampling of review questions for this chapter appears here. Visit http://www.mosby.com/MERLIN/PriceWilson/ for additional questions. MERLIN

Answer the following on a separate sheet of paper.

1. What is meant by uremic syndrome?
2. What are the two groups of clinical symptoms present in the uremic syndrome? How does the middle molecular hypothesis account for some of these symptoms? What are the implications of this theory?
3. Explain why total NH_4^+ excretion is decreased in renal failure.
4. Why does the acidosis of chronic renal failure generally stabilize at a moderate level when there is a positive H^+ balance? What relation might the acidosis of renal failure have to the bone abnormality?
5. Why is salt-wasting associated with polyuria in early renal insufficiency?
6. Name two common laxatives that, if administered to the uremic patient, might result in death.

7. Explain the meaning of a constant finding of urine specific gravity at 1.010.
8. How are sexual and reproductive functions affected in terminal renal failure? (Explain the effects in men and women.)
9. Name four factors that contribute to the development of infection in the uremic patient.
10. Describe skin color changes in uremic patients who are white skinned, brown skinned, and black skinned.
11. Illustrate the mechanisms by which GI bleeding, vomiting, or diarrhea might cause the deterioration of renal function. (Draw flow diagrams.)
12. List several changes that might be expected in the mental, emotional, and neuromuscular status and rest pattern of a patient who is developing uremia.

13. List the stages in the development of peripheral neuropathy and the signs and symptoms that would be expected in the patient with renal failure.
14. Illustrate the radiographic appearance of the phalanges when there is subperiosteal bone resorption in renal osteodystrophy.
15. Draw a flow diagram of the pathogenesis of secondary hyperparathyroidism, and list several examples of the consequences of this condition.
16. A uremic patient has a serum phosphate level of 8 mg/dl and a Ca^{++} level of 10 mg/dl. Would metastatic calcification be expected in the soft tissues of the body? Explain.
17. What is band keratopathy? Illustrate. What causes uremic red eye?

Match the abnormality found in uremia in column A with the most likely complication resulting from that abnormality in column B. More than one letter may be used for each condition in column A.

Column A	Column B
18. _____ Pericarditis	a. Pneumonia
19. _____ Circulatory overload	b. Retinopathy
20. _____ Hypertension	c. Cardiac tamponade
	d. Pulmonary edema
	e. Encephalopathy

Treatment of Chronic Renal Failure

LORRAINE M. WILSON

*T*he treatment of chronic renal failure can be divided into two stages. The first stage consists of conservative measures designed to temper or delay the progressive deterioration of renal function. Conservative measures are begun when the patient becomes azotemic. The physician makes every effort to determine the primary cause of the renal failure and search out any reversible factors such as the following:

1. Extracellular fluid (ECF) volume depletion caused by the overzealous use of diuretics or a salt restriction that is too stringent
2. Urinary tract obstruction from calculi, prostatic enlargement, or retroperitoneal fibrosis
3. Infection, especially of the urinary tract
4. Drugs that aggravate renal disease: aminoglycosides, antitumor agents, nonsteroidal antiinflammatory drugs (NSAIDs), radiocontrast media
5. Severe or malignant hypertension

These factors are likely causes of a sudden deterioration of renal function in a patient with chronic renal failure (Schrier, 1997). Treatment of reversible factors may stabilize and prevent any further deterioration of renal function. In addition to the correction of reversible factors, methods of retarding the progression of chronic renal failure caused by secondary glomerular injury from hyperfil-

tration in intact nephrons are currently under intensive investigation. Dietary protein restriction and antihypertensive therapy (especially with the use of angiotensin-converting enzyme [ACE] inhibitors) are the two major interventions being investigated.

The second stage of treatment begins when conservative measures are no longer effective in sustaining life. End-stage renal disease (ESRD) or terminal renal failure exists at this point (glomerular filtration rate [GFR] is usually less than 2 ml/min), and the only effective treatment is either intermittent dialysis or renal transplantation. However, before this point is reached, a number of physiologic alterations occur, many of which are detrimental. Therefore dialysis is usually begun before true ESRD is reached. Box 48-1 summarizes the principles of management of chronic renal failure discussed in this chapter.

CONSERVATIVE MANAGEMENT

The basic principles of conservative management are quite simple and are based on an understanding of the range of excretion that can be achieved by the failing kidney. Dietary regulation of individual solutes and fluid is then adjusted to the limitations. Additionally, therapy is directed toward prevention and treatment of complications as they occur.

Dietary Regulation of Protein

Dietary regulation is of primary importance in the treatment of chronic renal failure. It is customary to restrict the protein intake of the azotemic patient, although there is controversy about how severe this restriction should be. The restriction of protein not only reduces the blood urea nitrogen (BUN) level and perhaps other poorly defined toxic products of protein metabolism but also reduces the intake of potassium, phosphate, and the hydrogen-ion production that stem from protein. Symptoms of nausea, vomiting, and fatigue may be ameliorated. More importantly, recent studies have demonstrated that abnormal intrarenal hemodynamics contribute to the progression of chronic renal failure in several modes of renal disease (see Chapter 46). Restriction of dietary protein intake has been demonstrated to normalize these aberrations and retard progression to renal failure. The probable mechanism is related to the fact that a low-protein intake reduces the excretory load, thus reducing glomerular hyperfiltration, intraglomerular pressure, and secondary injury of the intact nephrons.

Recall from the discussion in Chapter 46 that once the kidneys have sustained a substantial degree of damage, progressive deterioration of renal function takes place because of the deleterious effects of glomerular hypertension within the intact nephrons. When renal failure is progressive, the GFR tends to decline in a linear fashion over time so that plotting serial measurements of GFR allows prediction of the time to ESRD when dialysis treat-

ment will be necessary. However, the measurement of GFR at low levels is inaccurate. A common method of assessing the results of protein restriction in retarding the progression of chronic renal disease to ESRD is to plot the reciprocal of the plasma creatinine concentration ($1/P_{cr}$) versus time instead of the GFR. The reader should recall that

$$GFR \approx \text{Creatinine clearance} = \frac{U_{cr}V}{P_{cr}}$$

where U_{cr} is the urine creatinine concentration, V is the urine flow rate, and P_{cr} is the plasma creatinine concentration. If body muscle mass is stable, production and excretion rates of creatinine per unit time ($U_{cr}V$) will be relatively constant; thus

$$GFR \approx \frac{\text{Constant}}{P_{cr}} \propto \frac{1}{P_{cr}}$$

Therefore $1/P_{cr}$ can be used to track changes in the GFR. The approximate time until ESRD is reached can be predicted by extrapolation of the $1/P_{cr}$ versus time relationship. Changes in the slope of $1/P_{cr}$ plotted against time can be used to indicate the rate of progression of renal failure. A decrease in slope would mean that progression to ESRD is slower than expected and is the expected result of effective therapy (Fig. 48-1).

Several studies have demonstrated the possibility of retarding the rate of progression of renal failure by reducing protein intake. Using a diet containing the minimum daily requirement (MDR) of protein (0.6 g/kg) versus an unrestricted protein diet (average protein intake in the United States is 1.2 to 1.6 g/kg), Oldrizzi and associates (1985) showed that the rate of increase in creatinine was 11 times lower in the protein-restricted group of patients with chronic glomerulonephritis and 19 times lower in the protein-restricted group of patients with chronic pyelonephritis than they were in the control

---

BOX 48-1

Management of Chronic Renal Failure

CONSERVATIVE MANAGEMENT
Determination and treatment of the cause
Optimization and maintenance of salt and water balance
Correction of any urinary tract obstruction
Early detection and treatment of infection
Control of hypertension
Low-protein, high-calorie diet
Control of electrolyte balance
Prevention and treatment of renal bone disease
Modification of drug therapy with alterations in renal function
Detection and treatment of complications

RENAL REPLACEMENT THERAPY
Hemodialysis
Peritoneal dialysis
Renal transplantation

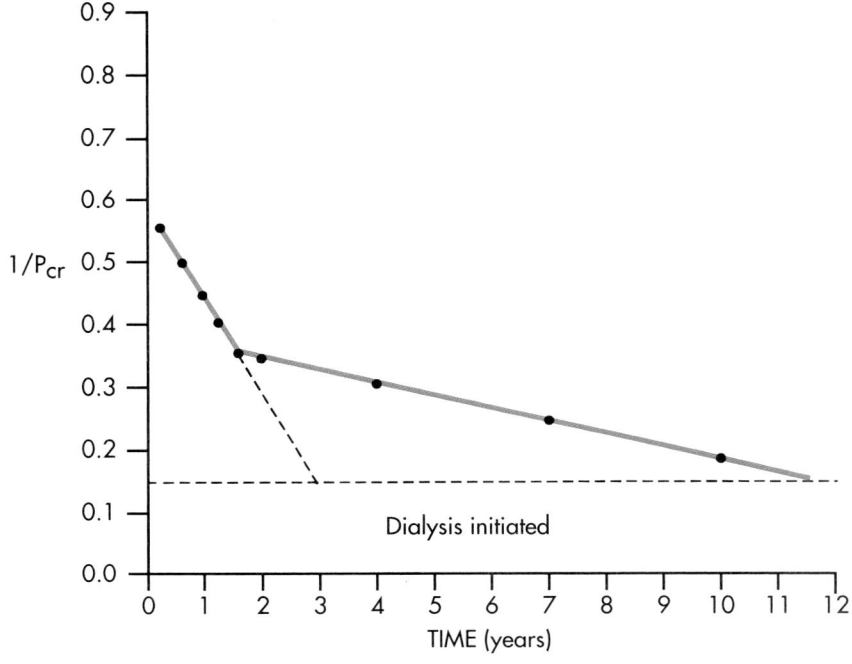

FIG. 48-1   Effect of dietary protein restriction on the rate of decline of glomerular filtration rate (GFR) in a hypothetical diabetic patient. The serum creatinine was measured every 6 months for 2 years and the reciprocal plotted. If you assume that dialysis will be necessary when the serum creatinine reaches 8 mg/dl, corresponding to a $1/P_{cr}$ of about 0.125, extrapolation of the steep slope shows that this point of deterioration will be reached in about 3 years. However, if a protein-restricted diet slowed the rate of disease progression by 75%, dialysis would not be necessary until 12 years, indicated by the more shallow slope. $1/P_{cr}$, Plasma creatinine concentration.

groups. In another study in which protein intake was less than the MDR, Giordano (1981) noted that the average time to reach ESRD was 16 months in the noncompliant group but increased to 7.6 years in the protein-restricted group. Results of studies in patients with diabetic nephropathy showed that the rate of progression was reduced by 75% in protein-restricted groups (Diabetes Control and Complications Trial Research Group, 1993).

The long-term effects of severely restricted protein diets (i.e., less than the MDR) on nutritional status are of obvious concern. It is possible to maintain nitrogen balance on a 20-g protein diet, provided the protein is of highest biologic value (i.e., contains all the essential amino acids as do milk and eggs) and adequate calories are provided in the form of fats and carbohydrates to prevent the breakdown of body protein to satisfy caloric requirements. One approach to this problem is to supplement very low–protein diets by using either a mixture of essential amino acids (EAA) or combinations of EAAs and alpha-keto or alpha-hydroxy analogues of amino acids (KA). This approach allows more variety in the diet and therefore may be more acceptable to some patients. Carbohydrate supplements may be given to ensure adequate calories to prevent breakdown of body protein. Mitch (1991) found that this therapy minimizes uremic symptoms, secondary hyperparathyroidism, and metabolic acidosis. Vitamin B complex, pyridoxine, and ascorbic acid supplements should be given with these regimens.

Finally, the Modification of Diet in Renal Disease (MDRD) multicenter study did show a beneficial effect of protein restriction in slowing the progression of renal failure in both diabetic and nondiabetic patients with moderate (GFR, 25 to 55 ml/min) and severe (GFR, 13 to 24 ml/min) renal failure. The MDRD study also demonstrated that the control of hypertension was as important as protein restriction in slowing the progression of renal failure (Klahr et al, 1994; Pedrini et al, 1996). The current clinical recommendation of protein allowance is 0.6 g/kg/day for stable, predialysis patients with severe renal failure (GFR <24 ml/min). The patient's nutritional status should be monitored to ensure that body weight and other indicators such as serum albumin remain stable (≥3 g/dL). The protein allowance may be liberalized to 1 g/kg/day when the patient is receiving regular dialysis.

Dietary Regulation of Potassium

Hyperkalemia generally becomes a problem in advanced renal failure, and it becomes necessary also to restrict dietary intake of potassium. The typical dietary allowance is 40 to 80 mEq/day. Care must be taken not to administer foods or drugs that are high in potassium. These foods or drugs include salt substitutes (which contain ammonium chloride and potassium chloride), expectorants, potassium citrate, and foods such as soups, dates, bananas, and pure fruit juices. Inadvertent administration of food or drugs high in potassium may cause a serious hyperkalemia.

Dietary Regulation of Sodium and Fluids

The dietary regulation of sodium is important in renal failure. The typical sodium allowance is 40 to 90 mEq/ day (1 to 2 g of sodium), but the optimal sodium intake must be determined individually for each patient to maintain good hydration. An intake that is too liberal can lead to fluid retention, peripheral edema, pulmonary edema, hypertension, and congestive heart failure. Sodium retention is generally a problem in glomerular disease and in advanced renal failure. On the other hand, if sodium is restricted to the point of negative sodium balance, hypovolemia, decreased GFR, and a deterioration of renal function will ensue. Sodium depletion is more common in tubulointerstitial disease and may be precipitated by vomiting or diarrhea. It is therefore important to determine the optimum sodium intake for each patient. The sodium conservation test and a careful observation of the daily weight, signs of edema, and other complications may all be helpful.

In the sodium conservation test the patient eats a low-sodium diet for 5 days (e.g., 10 mEq/day). The normal person will conserve sodium and come into balance during this period. On the fifth day, 24-hour urine samples are collected and the sodium is measured. The sodium lost in the urine at this time represents an obligatory loss and thus the "sodium floor." For example, a patient on a 10 mEq sodium diet who loses 50 mEq in the urine on the fifth day has a negative sodium balance of 40 mEq (50 − 10 = 40); 40 mEq of sodium must be added to the diet. The "sodium ceiling" is determined by observing weight, blood pressure, and other signs of ECF excess. As stated previously, the range between sodium deficit and sodium excess can be very narrow.

The intake of fluids requires careful regulation in advanced renal failure, because the patient's thirst is an unreliable guide to the state of hydration. Daily weight is the critical parameter to follow, in addition to accurate intake and output records. An intake that is too liberal may result in circulatory overload, edema, and water intoxication, and less than optimal intake will result in dehydration, hypotension, and a deterioration in renal function. The general rule for fluid intake is urine output during past 24 hours + 500 ml, the 500 ml representing insensible loss. For example, if the patient's urine output during the last 24 hours was 400 ml, the total intake per day should be 500 + 400 ml = 900 ml. Anephric patients are allowed 800 ml/day, and patients in dialysis are given sufficient fluid to allow a 2- to 3-pound weight gain between treatments. Obviously, both sodium and fluid intake must be manipulated to achieve fluid balance.

Prevention and Treatment of Complications

The second category of conservative measures used in the treatment of renal failure is composed of those directed toward the prevention and treatment of complications.

Hypertension

Renal function deteriorates more rapidly if severe hypertension develops. Additionally, extrarenal complications such as retinopathy and encephalopathy may develop. Hypertension can usually be controlled effectively by sodium and fluid restriction and by ultrafiltration when the patient is on hemodialysis, because more than 90% of hypertension is volume dependent. In some cases, an antihypertensive drug (with or without a diuretic) may be given to achieve blood pressure control. A prudent clinical strategy to prevent or retard progressive renal disease is to attain a goal mean arterial pressure (MAP) of 91 mm Hg (125/75 mm Hg). Recent evidence suggests that ACE inhibitors (e.g., captopril) may be particularly beneficial for patients with either essential hypertension or insulin-dependent diabetes mellitus (Krobin et al, 1997; Agodoa et al, 2001). In addition to lowering systemic blood pressure, these drugs directly lower the intraglomerular pressure by selectively dilating the efferent arteriole (see Chapter 46). ACE inhibitor drugs also reduce proteinuria. Because ACE inhibitor drugs lower the intraglomerular pressure and slow the progression of chronic renal failure, treatment with these drugs has been advocated even for patients with type 1 diabetes who are normotensive. When the patient is receiving hemodialysis, it is important to withhold the antihypertensive drug before treatment to prevent hypotension and shock that may result as intravascular fluid is removed through ultrafiltration if the drug blocks the normal vascular vasoconstrictive reaction. In a small number of cases (<10%) the hypertension may be renin dependent and refractory to sodium-volume control or control with a mild antihypertensive. The addition of another antihypertensive drug such as a calcium-channel blocker or minoxidil (Loniten) can usually bring the blood pressure under control. Bilateral nephrectomy may be considered as a last resort when all other methods have failed. Bilateral nephrectomy causes the anemia to become more severe, because even the end-stage kidney produces some erythropoietin.

Great care is taken to lower the blood pressure gradually, thus the patient does not become hypotensive, with consequent lowering of GFR and further deterioration of renal function. Hypertension in the majority of uremic patients is caused by fluid overload and is most effectively restored to normal by regulation of sodium and fluid intake and intermittent dialysis.

Hyperkalemia

One of the most serious complications in the uremic patient is the development of hyperkalemia. When serum potassium (K^+) reaches a level of about 7 mEq/L, serious dysrhythmias and cardiac arrest may occur (see Chapter 21). Additionally, hypocalcemia, hyponatremia, and acidosis intensify the deleterious effects of hyperkalemia. For this reason, the patient's heart may be monitored to detect the effect of the hyperkalemia (and the effects of all the other ions) on cardiac conduction.

Acute hyperkalemia may be treated by the administration of intravenous (IV) glucose and insulin, which drives K^+ into the cells, or by the careful (IV) administration of 10% calcium gluconate, with continuous electrocardiogram (ECG) monitoring if the patient is hypotensive with widening of the QRS complex. The effect of these measures is only temporary, and the hyperkalemia must be subsequently corrected by dialysis. When it is not possible to lower K^+ by dialysis, the cation exchange resin sodium polystyrene sulfonate (Kayexalate) may be used. Each gram of the resin binds 1 mEq of K^+. Kayexalate may be given by mouth or by rectal instillation. When given rectally, 50 to 100 g is mixed with 200 to 300 ml of water. To facilitate the K^+ exchange, 25 to 30 ml of 70% sorbitol (a poorly absorbed, osmotically active alcohol that has a laxative effect) is added. Obviously, orange juice (high K^+ content) should not be given to disguise the taste when Kayexalate is administered orally.

Anemia

Anemia is a nearly universal finding in patients with advanced renal disease, and hematocrits of 18% to 20% are common. The cause of the anemia is multifactorial, including deficiency of erythropoietin production, circulating factors that appear to inhibit erythropoietin, shortened red blood cell (RBC) life span, increased gastrointestinal (GI) blood loss caused by platelet abnormalities, iron and folic acid deficiency, and blood losses from hemodialysis or from frequent samples for laboratory tests. Although all of the listed factors may contribute to the anemia of chronic renal failure, it appears that erythropoietin deficiency is the major cause of the anemia, because patients respond so well to replacement of this hormone. In 1985 the human erythropoietin gene was isolated and cloned, facilitating unlimited amounts of the hormone. The recent widespread availability of recombinant human erythropoietin (EPO) has revolutionized the management of the anemia of chronic renal failure (CRF). A 6% to 10% increase in the hematocrit and a reduction of the anemia-related symptoms of weakness and fatigue can be expected. EPO is commonly administered as a subcutaneous injection (25 to 125 U/kg of body weight) three times per week. The major complication of EPO therapy is hypertension, which occurs in about one half of the patients. The rise in blood pressure caused by EPO therapy has been attributed to an increase in blood viscosity and the reversal of the anemia-induced peripheral vasodilation. Aiming for a subnormal hematocrit of 30% to 35% can ameliorate the risk of hypertension (Black, 1996).

In addition to EPO therapy, other measures to alleviate anemia in patients with CRF include minimizing blood losses and giving vitamins and blood transfusions. Taking the smallest blood sample possible for laboratory tests and minimizing residual blood left in the tubing in hemodialysis treatment can reduce iatrogenic blood loss. A multivitamin and a folic acid preparation are usually given each day, because dialysis depletes water-soluble vitamins. Oral iron or dextran iron complex (Imferon) may be given parenterally, because iron deficiency may result from blood loss and binding by antacids. Until recently, blood transfusions of packed RBCs were commonly used to treat anemia in patients with CRF but are now generally restricted to patients with hematocrits less than 24%.

Acidosis

The mild chronic metabolic acidosis of the uremic patient usually stabilizes at a plasma bicarbonate level of 16 to 20 mEq/L. Acidosis does not usually progress beyond this point, because hydrogen ion (H^+) production is balanced by bone buffering. Decreased protein intake may improve the acidosis, but when serum bicarbonate levels fall below 15 mEq/L, some nephrologists order alkali therapy, either sodium bicarbonate or citrate at a dosage of 1 mEq/kg/day orally, to alleviate the ill effects of metabolic acidosis, including excessive bone loss. The renal acidosis is not usually treated unless the plasma bicarbonate (HCO_3^-) falls below 15 mEq/L, when symptoms of acidosis may appear. The superimposition of an acute acidosis on the mild chronic acidosis may precipitate severe acidosis, which might occur, for example, in profuse diarrhea with its HCO_3^- loss. When severe acidosis is corrected by the parenteral administration of sodium bicarbonate ($NaHCO_3$), it is important to be aware of the hazard involved. Overcorrection of blood pH may precipitate tetany, convulsions, and death. It should be remembered that patients with chronic renal failure are usually hypocalcemic. A mild degree of induced alkalosis may reduce the ionized fraction of serum calcium (Ca^{++}) (usually in an acidic environment) to the point of severe hypocalcemia. The most logical mode of treatment, finally, is dialysis.

Renal Osteodystrophy

One of the most crucial therapeutic measures used to prevent the development of secondary hyperparathyroidism and its consequences is a low-phosphate diet along with the administration of agents that bind phosphate in the bowel. The prevention and correction of hyperphosphatemia preclude the sequence of events leading to Ca^{++} and bone disorders discussed in Chapter 47. A low-protein diet is also low in phosphate. The treatment should begin early in the course of progressive renal failure, when the GFR is down to one third of normal. The phosphate-binding agent of choice is currently calcium carbonate or calcium acetate. In the past, most nephrologists prescribed aluminum antacid gels (Amphogel or Basojel) as phosphate binders. However, it is now known that this regimen creates a new problem of aluminum intoxication caused by the gradual accumulation of aluminum in tissues. The major manifestations of aluminum toxicity occur in bone and skeletal muscle, leading to vitamin D–resistant osteomalacia and muscle pain. Calcium carbonate (1 to 2 g) should be taken with each meal to ensure maximum effectiveness in binding dietary phosphate and thus preventing its absorption. The goal of therapy is to maintain the serum phosphate at about 4.5 mg/dl and the Ca^{++} at about 10 mg/dl. Studies in patients with CRF show that correction of hyperphosphatemia can at least partially correct the hypocalcemia, 1,25-dihydroxycholecalciferol ($1,25[OH]_2D_3$) deficiency, and excess parathyroid hormone (PTH) secretion.

Magnesium-containing antacids should never be substituted as phosphate binders, because patients with CRF have reduced ability to excrete this ion and may develop a serious hypermagnesemia. The major complication in patients taking calcium carbonate as a phosphate binder is the occasional development of hypercalcemia from increased intestinal absorption of Ca^{++}. One approach to preventing this complication is to lower the Ca^{++} in the dialysate from the standard 3.25 to 3.50 mEq/L to 2.5 mEq/L. Both serum Ca^{++} and phosphate levels should be monitored at least monthly to ensure that the calcium-phosphate cross product is in the normal range (<60) to avoid metastatic calcification.

If severe skeletal involvement occurs for lack of or despite preventive therapy with phosphate-binding agents, subtotal parathyroidectomy or vitamin D therapy may be indicated. Severe bone demineralization, hypercalcemia, or intractable pruritus is considered an indication for parathyroidectomy. When the predominant lesion is osteomalacia, the nephrologist must begin vitamin D therapy with great care. This treatment may be quite hazardous. Not only may Ca^{++} absorption be increased, but it may also in fact lead to progressive soft tissue calcification when bone resorption and hyperphosphatemia continue unabated.

Hyperuricemia

Allopurinol is usually the drug of choice for treating the hyperuricemia of advanced renal disease. This drug reduces uric acid levels by blocking the biosynthesis of some part of the total uric acid produced by the body. Colchicine (antiinflammatory drug for gout) may be given for the relief of symptoms of gouty arthritis.

Peripheral Neuropathy

Usually, symptomatic peripheral neuropathy does not occur until renal failure is far advanced. There is no known treatment for these changes except dialysis, which stops their progression. Therefore the development of sensory neuritis is a signal that dialysis should not be delayed any longer. Motor neuropathy may be irreversible. Nerve conduction velocity tests are commonly performed every 6 months to monitor the progress of peripheral neuropathy.

Prompt Treatment of Infection

Patients with chronic renal failure have an increased susceptibility to infection, particularly urinary tract infection. Because infection of any sort may accentuate the catabolic process and impair adequate nutrition and fluid and electrolyte balance, infections should be treated promptly to prevent further deterioration of renal function. However, the detection of infection in a patient with ESRD requires a high degree of suspicion and attention to less specific indicators such as tachycardia, fatigue, or a slight rise in temperature. This caution is warranted because hypothermia is one of the clinical features of the uremic syndrome and because many patients with ESRD do not exhibit the expected rise in body temperature or white blood cell (WBC) count when an infection is present (Lewis, 1992).

Cautious Drug Administration

Because the kidney excretes many drugs, they must be cautiously administered to the uremic patient. The half-life of drugs excreted by the kidney is greatly prolonged in uremia, thus toxic serum levels may occur and the doses of these drugs must therefore be reduced. The nephrologist chooses antibiotics (nonnephrotoxic) and their doses with these facts in mind. Particular caution is necessary when digitalis drugs are ordered for the treatment of intrinsic cardiac disease in the uremic patient. In fact, cautious drug administration to the uremic patient should be the rule.

In progressive renal failure, conservative therapeutic measures finally become inadequate. Dialysis or renal transplantation is then the only means of preserving life. Continuation of many of the conservative measures may be necessary, particularly with dialysis.

DIALYSIS AND RENAL TRANSPLANTATION

The treatment of end-stage renal failure has been transformed by the development of techniques for dialysis and renal transplantation during the last 35 years. In the past, patients with renal failure were doomed to die when all conservative methods failed. Now their lives may be prolonged many years with maintenance dialysis or renal transplantation.

There is an intimate relation between these two techniques, and closely paralleled advances in both have been made. For example, the uremic patient may choose to undergo renal transplantation with a related or cadaver donor rather than be maintained on chronic intermittent dialysis. Nevertheless, dialysis will undoubtedly play an important role in the treatment. Dialysis may be used to maintain the patient in an optimal clinical state until the donor kidney is available. In the case of a cadaver renal transplant, the patient may have to wait many months. There are several choices of treatment, depending on the resources available. The initial treatment will be carried out in the medical center hemodialysis unit. The patient may then undergo home dialysis training to permit self-administration of the procedure at home until the donor kidney is available; or more commonly, treatment may be given in a satellite (out-of-hospital) or mobile hemodialysis unit near the patient's home. Dialysis may sustain the renal transplant patient through periods of postoperative oliguria, and it provides an alternative if the transplanted kidney should fail because of rejection or other complications. Renal transplantation and chronic maintenance dialysis offer about the same prognosis in regard to longevity. Each mode of treatment has its own unique problems. Renal transplantation, if successful, probably offers a better quality of life because it is less restrictive: there are usually no dietary restrictions, and it is not necessary to commit large blocks of time several times each week for dialysis.

Preparation of the Patient

It is important that the patient be prepared for the transition from conservative management to more definitive therapy long before the need arises for maintenance dialysis or renal transplantation. Not only does this approach give the patient hope, but it also allows time for indoctrination of the patient in preparation for the treatment and makes it possible for the treatment to start at the proper time.

Originally, extremely rigid criteria were used to select patients for either renal transplantation or maintenance dialysis, especially because of limited facilities and the high cost of treatment. The increase in facilities, financial support by the federal government, improvements in techniques, and success in treating some children, older individuals, diabetic persons, and patients with systemic lupus erythematosus are all factors that have helped liberalize the criteria to enable a greater number of patients to be helped.

When to Begin Treatment

There are no clear-cut guidelines in terms of measurable blood levels of creatinine or BUN to determine when definitive therapy should begin. Most nephrologists' decisions are based on the well being of the patient, who is followed closely as an outpatient. Therapy is generally begun when the patient is no longer able to work full-time, develops peripheral neuropathy, or shows other signs of clinical deterioration. The serum creatinine level is generally above 6 mg/dl in males (4 mg/dl in females), and the GFR is below 4 ml/min. In no case should the patient be allowed to become bedridden or so sick that usual activities are impossible.

Sometimes, despite being carefully followed, the patient may deteriorate rapidly over a period of a few days, usually in response to an infectious disease. Sometimes, one or two peritoneal dialyses will restabilize the patient. If this approach is not successful, intermittent hemodialysis may be initiated. If a decision for a renal transplant has been made, transplantation may be done on an elective basis at a later date.

Dialysis

Dialysis is a process by which solutes and water are diffused through a passive, porous membrane from one fluid compartment to another. Hemodialysis and peritoneal dialysis are the two major techniques used in dialysis, and the basic principles involved are the same for both—diffusion of solutes and water from the plasma to the dialysis solution in response to a concentration or pressure gradient.

Fig. 48-2 illustrates the basic principles of diffusion and osmotic and hydrostatic pressure gradients involved in dialysis. Given a semipermeable membrane with the patient's blood on one side and a solution of known composition on the other side (the *dialysate*, or dialysis bath), substances to which the membrane is permeable will move from where their concentration is high to where it is low. If the blood K^+ level is high and the K^+ level in the dialysis bath is low *(round dots)*, the net movement of K^+ will be out of the blood into the dialysis bath *(long arrows indicate direction of net diffusion)*. The *black squares* represent solutes that are in higher concentration in the dialysate (e.g., HCO_3^-), so that net diffusion is from the bath solution to the blood. Ultrafiltration (water removal) may be achieved by two methods: (1) creating a hydrostatic pressure gradient (e.g., by mechanically increasing the positive pressure in the blood compartment) and (2) creating an osmotic pressure gradient by increasing the concentration of glucose in the dialysis bath. The resulting osmotic and hydrostatic pressure gradients cause a net movement of water from the blood to the dialysis bath.* The positive pressure in the blood compartment also speeds up the diffusion of both solutes and water. Ultrafiltration in hemodialysis is achieved primarily by using the first method, whereas peritoneal dialysis uses the second method. The reader should note that protein, blood cells, and bacteria are too large to pass through the pores in the dialysis membrane.

---

*Some glucose does diffuse from the dialysis bath into the blood, but because water diffuses much more rapidly than does glucose, the major shift will be that of water from blood to bath.

FIG. 48-2 Basic principles of diffusion and osmotic and hydrostatic pressures involved in dialysis. *RBC,* Red blood cell; *WBC,* white blood cell; *G,* glucose.

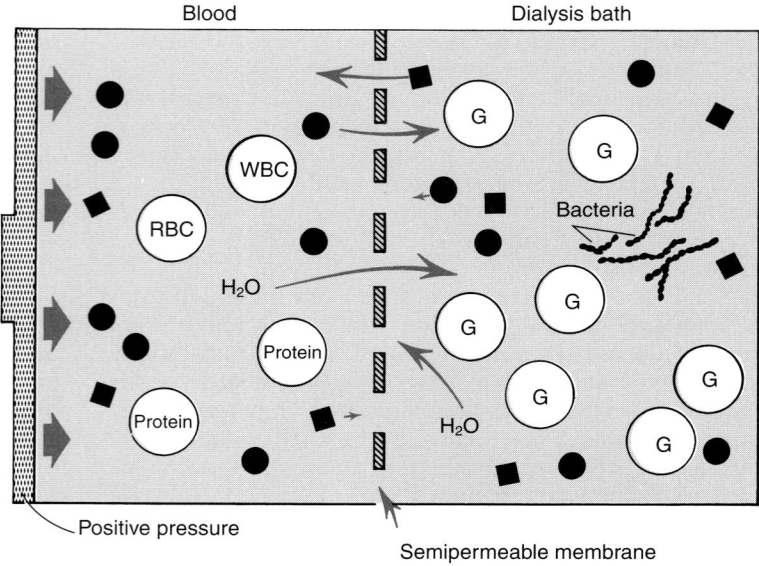

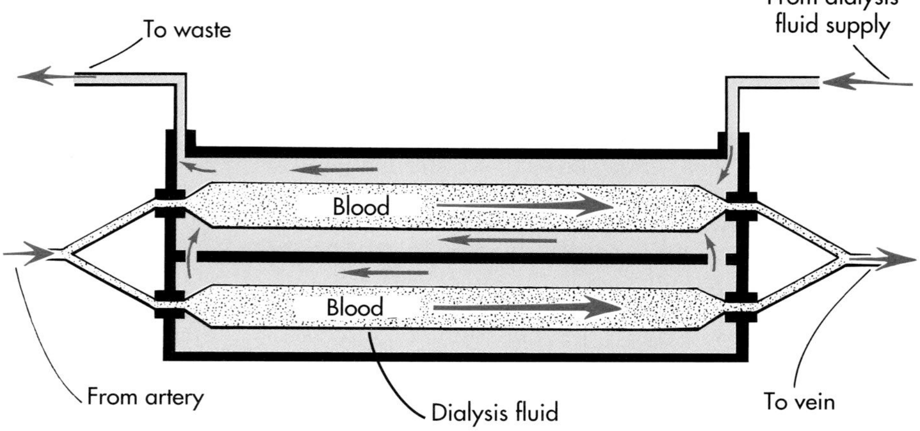

FIG. 48-3 Parallel plate dialyzer.

By using a dialysis solution that contains the important electrolytes in normal concentrations, the concentration of these electrolytes can be corrected in the blood of the patient with renal failure. The basic practical problem in dialysis is to bring enough blood into contact with enough dialysis solution across a semipermeable membrane of adequate area. This task may be accomplished inside the patient's body, using the peritoneum as the semipermeable membrane (peritoneal dialysis), or outside the body, using an "artificial kidney" and Cuprophane or Polysulfone as the semipermeable membrane (hemodialysis).

Hemodialysis

An artificial kidney machine, or hemodialyzer, consists simply of a semipermeable membrane with blood on one side and dialysis fluid on the other. Two principal types of dialyzers are in use today. The less commonly used *parallel plate dialyzer* consists of two Cuprophane sheets sandwiched between two rigid supports to form an envelope. Two or more envelopes are arranged in parallel. Blood flows between the membrane layers, and dialysis fluid may flow in the same direction as the blood or in the opposite direction (countercurrent), as shown in Fig. 48-3. The more commonly used *hollow fiber* or *capillary dialyzer* consists of thousands of tiny capillary fibers arranged in parallel (Fig. 48-4). Each fiber has a wall thickness of 30 μm, an inside diameter of 200 μm, and a length of 21 cm. (For comparative purposes, an RBC has a diameter of 7 μm.) Blood flows down the center of these tiny tubes, and dialysis fluid bathes the outside. The flow of the dialysis fluid is opposite (countercurrent) to that of the blood. This dialyzer is small and compact because of the large surface area provided by the many capillary tubes. The total internal surface area of all the fibers is about 0.5 to 2.0 m². Fig. 48-5 is a diagrammatic representation of a hemodialysis system using a hollow fiber dialyzer.

A dialysis system consists of two circuits—one for the blood and one for the dialysis fluid. When the system is in operation, blood flows from the patient through plastic tubing (arterial line), through the hollow fibers of the dialyzer, and back to the patient through the venous line. The dialysis fluid forms the second circuit. Tap water is filtered and heated to body temperature and is then mixed with a concentrate by a proportioning pump to

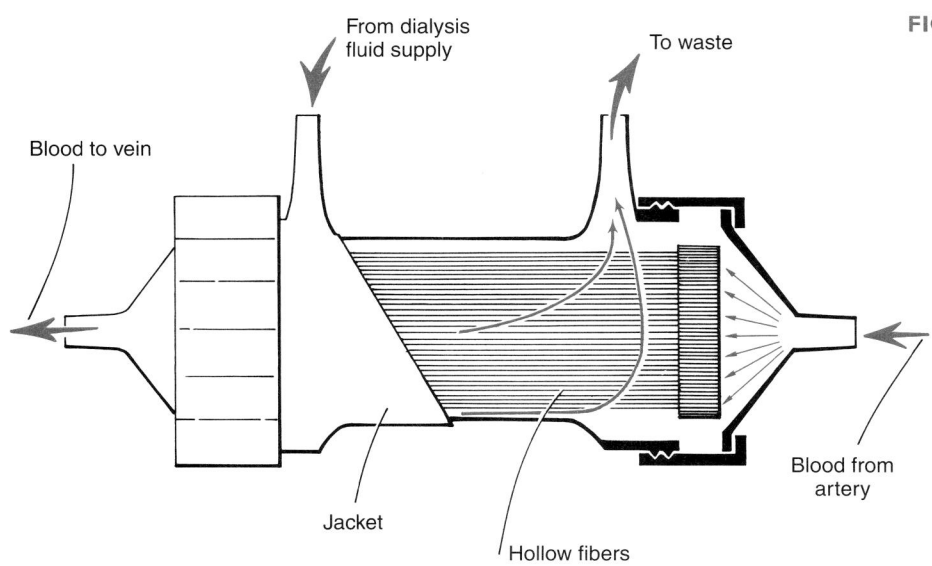

FIG. 48-4 Hollow fiber or capillary dialyzer.

Blood to vein

From dialysis
fluid supply

To waste

Blood from
artery

Jacket

Hollow fibers

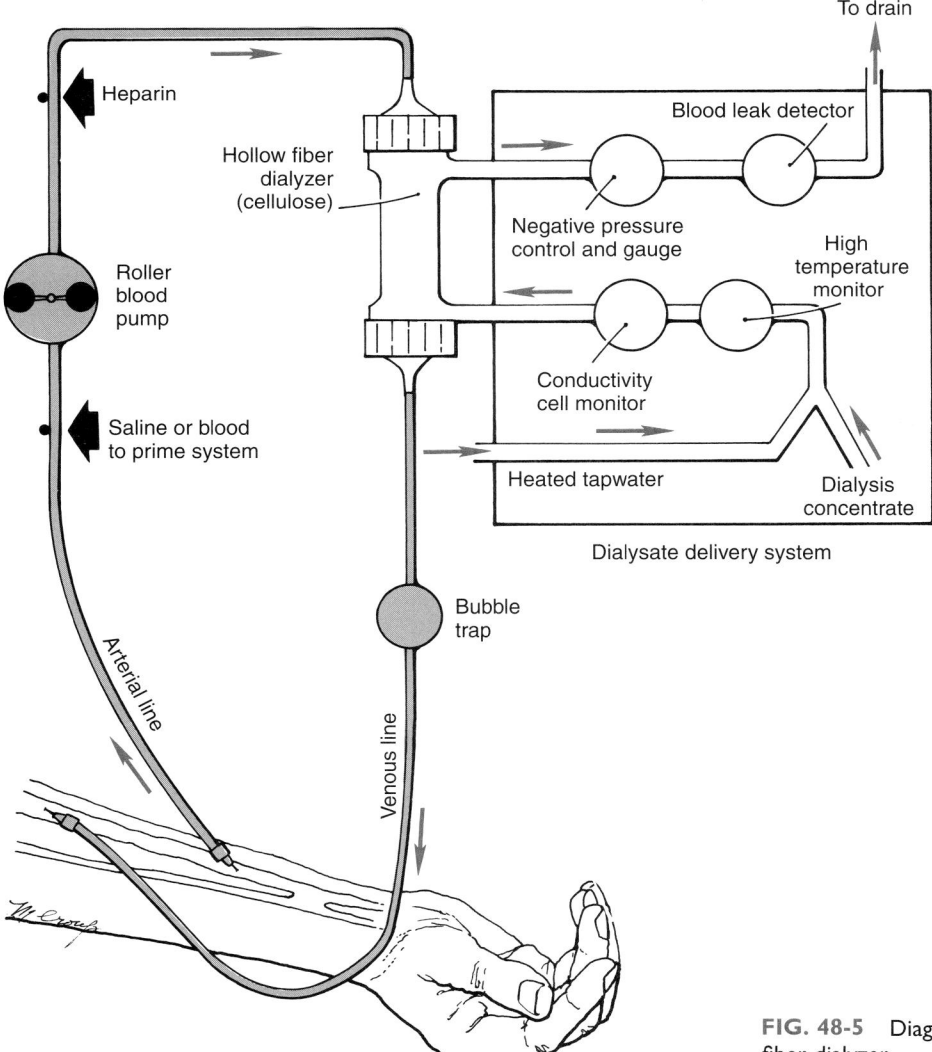

To drain

Heparin

Hollow fiber
dialyzer
(cellulose)

Blood leak detector

Roller
blood
pump

Negative pressure
control and gauge

High
temperature
monitor

Conductivity
cell monitor

Saline or blood
to prime system

Heated tapwater

Dialysis
concentrate

Dialysate delivery system

Bubble
trap

Arterial line

Venous line

FIG. 48-5 Diagram of a hemodialysis system using hollow
fiber dialyzer.

make the dialysate, or bath. The bath is then delivered to the dialyzer, where it flows on the outside of the hollow fibers before exiting to a drain. Equilibrium between the blood and the dialysate takes place across the dialyzing membrane by the processes of diffusion, osmosis, and ultrafiltration described in Fig. 48-1.

The composition of the dialysis bath is designed to approximate the ionic composition of normal blood, modified slightly to correct the common fluid and electrolyte disorders that accompany renal failure (Box 48-2). The usual components are sodium (Na^+), K^+, Ca^{++}, magnesium (Mg^{++}), chloride (Cl^-), acetate, and glucose. Urea, creatinine, uric acid, and phosphate diffuse readily from the blood to the dialysis fluid, because they are not present in the dialysis fluid. Sodium acetate, which is in higher concentration in the dialysis bath, diffuses into the blood. The purpose of adding the acetate is to correct the uremic patient's acidosis. Acetate is metabolized into HCO_3^- in the patient's body. The reason for using acetate rather than HCO_3^- is to avoid the problem of calcium bicarbonate precipitation when Ca^{++} and HCO_3^- are added to the same dialysis fluid. Recently, machines have been developed that can use two separate dialysates—one with Ca^{++} and the other with HCO_3^-, which avoids the problem of precipitation. A low concentration of glucose (200 mg/dl) is added to the dialysis bath to prevent glucose diffusion into the dialysis bath with the consequent loss of calories. In hemodialysis a high concentration of glucose is not necessary, because fluid removal may be achieved by effecting a hydrostatic pressure gradient between the blood and dialysis fluid. The hydrostatic pressure gradient is achieved by increasing the positive pressure within the dialyzer blood compartment by increasing resistance to venous outflow (not shown) or by exerting a vacuum effect in the dialysis fluid compartment by manipulating the negative pressure control. The hydrostatic pressure gradient across the dialyzing membrane also increases the diffusion rate of the solutes.

The blood circuit of the dialysis system is initially primed with saline or blood before connection to the circulation of the patient. The blood pressure of the patient may be adequate to propel the blood through the extracorporeal circuit, or a blood pump may be used to assist the flow (about 200 to 400 ml/min is a desirable flow rate). Heparin is continuously delivered to the arterial line by a slow infusion pump to prevent clotting. A clot and bubble trap in the venous line prevents air or blood clots from returning to the patient. To ensure patient safety, monitors with alarms for various parameters are included in modern hemodialyzers. A conductivity cell monitors the chemical composition of the dialysis fluid. Dialysis fluid at body temperature increases the rate of diffusion, but a temperature that is too high would cause hemolysis of RBCs, with possible death to the patient. Any tear in the dialysis membrane causing either a minor or a massive leak is detected by a photocell in the dialysate outflow.

Maintenance hemodialysis is usually performed three times per week, and the length of a single treatment varies from 3 to 5 hours, depending on the type of dialysis system used and the condition of the patient.

Vascular Access for Hemodialysis

Long-term intermittent hemodialysis requires reliable access to the vascular system. Blood must exit and return to the patient at the rate of 200 to 400 ml/min. Box 48-3 lists the major vascular access techniques classified as external (usually temporary) and internal (permanent). Vascular access remains the most vulnerable aspect of hemodialysis because of the many complications and failures. Thus numerous methods of vascular access have been developed over the years. The common denominator in most of these vascular access techniques is access to the arterial circulation and return to the venous circulation.

External (Temporary) Vascular Access

The *external arteriovenous (AV) shunt* or *cannula system* is created by placing Teflon cannula tips in an artery (usually the radial or posterior tibial) and a nearby vein (Fig. 48-6, *A*). The cannula tips are then connected by silicone rubber tubing and a Teflon bridge to complete the shunt. At the time of dialysis, the external shunt tubing is separated, and connection is made to the dialyzer. Blood then flows from the arterial line, through the dialyzer, and then back to the vein. The cannula system was devised in 1960 (Quinton et al, 1960) and made chronic intermittent hemodialysis possible for the first time. The main problem with the external AV shunt is its short life span because of clotting and infection (average life, 9 months). The external AV shunt has been largely supplanted by other means of angioaccess (see later discussion) and is mainly of historic interest. Occasionally, however, the external AV shunt is used when dialytic therapy is required for short periods, as in dialysis for drug overdose or poisoning, acute renal failure, and the initial phase of dialytic treatment for CRF.

Femoral and subclavian vein catheters are used most often in cases of acute renal failure when temporary angioaccess is required or when other means of vascular access are temporarily nonfunctional in chronic dialysis

---

BOX 48-2

Dialysate Composition

Component	mEq/L
Sodium	138-145
Potassium	0-4.0
Chloride	100-107
Calcium	2.5-3.5
Magnesium	0.4-1.0
Acetate	30-37
Glucose*	100-250*

*Glucose concentration in milligrams per deciliter.

BOX 48-3

Major Techniques of Vascular Access for Hemodialysis

External (temporary)
  Arteriovenous (AV) shunt or cannula system
  Femoral vein catheters (Shaldon and double lumen)
  Subclavian vein catheters
Internal (permanent)
  AV fistula
  AV graft

patients. Both types of catheters may be inserted at the bedside by an experienced physician.

There are two types of femoral dialysis catheters. The Shaldon catheter is a single-lumen catheter that requires a second access. If two Shaldon catheters are used, they may be placed bilaterally or in the same vein with the outflow catheter placed distally to the inflow catheter. The newer type of femoral catheter has a double lumen—one for blood outflow to the dialyzer and one for blood return to the patient. Complications associated with femoral vein catheters include laceration of the femoral artery, hemorrhage, thrombosis, embolus, hematoma, and infection.

Subclavian vein catheters are gaining wide acceptance as a temporary means of angioaccess because insertion is easier and there are fewer complications than with femoral vein catheters. The subclavian vein catheter also has a double lumen with inflow and outflow lines. Subclavian catheters may be used for as long as 4 weeks, but femoral vein catheters are usually removed 1 to 2 days after insertion.

Catheters left in place between dialysis treatments are filled with a saline-heparin solution or irrigated periodically with a saline-heparin solution to prevent clotting. If catheters are removed at the end of dialysis, pressure must be applied to the entry site until complete clotting occurs and the site must be observed for several hours thereafter to detect any recurrent bleeding.

Complications associated with subclavian vein catheterization are similar to those with femoral vein catheterization, including pneumothorax, laceration of the subclavian artery, hemorrhage, thrombosis, embolus, hematoma, and infection.

Internal (Permanent) Vascular Access

The *AV fistula* was developed by Cimino and Brescia (1962) in response to the many complications with the AV shunt. An AV fistula is constructed by anastomosing an artery directly to a vein (usually the radial artery and the cephalic vein at the wrist) in the nondominant arm (see Fig. 48-6, *B*). Blood is shunted from the artery to the vein, causing the vein to enlarge ("ripening") after a few weeks. Venipuncture with large-bore needles becomes easy and gives access to blood flowing under arterial pressure. Connection with the dialysis system is made by placing one needle distally (arterial line) and the other needle proximally (venous line) in the arterialized vein. The average life of the AV fistula is 4 years, and there are far fewer complications than with the AV shunt. The main problems are painful venipuncture, formation of aneurysms, thrombosis, difficult postdialytic hemostasis, and ischemia of the hand *(steal syndrome)*.

In some cases, it is not possible to create a fistula from the patient's own blood vessels because of disease, damage from previous procedures, or small size. An *AV graft* may then be anastomosed between an artery and vein (usually in the arm), where it serves as a conduit for the flow of blood and the site for needle puncture during dialysis. The graft creates a raised area just under the skin and looks like a raised vein. An AV graft is a prosthetic tube device made out of biologic materials (bovine carotid artery, human umbilical cord artery) or a synthetic material (Gore-Tex, or polytetrafluoroethylene, a material similar to Teflon). A segment of Gore-Tex may also be used to patch AV fistulas that have stenosed or formed aneurysms. AV graft complications are similar to those of the AV fistula, including thrombosis, infection, aneurysm, and hand ischemia caused by the shunting of blood through the prosthesis and away from the distal circulation (steal syndrome).

Peritoneal Dialysis

Peritoneal dialysis is an alternative to hemodialysis for the treatment of acute and chronic renal failure. Although peritoneal dialysis existed 20 years before hemodialysis, it was not commonly used for long-term

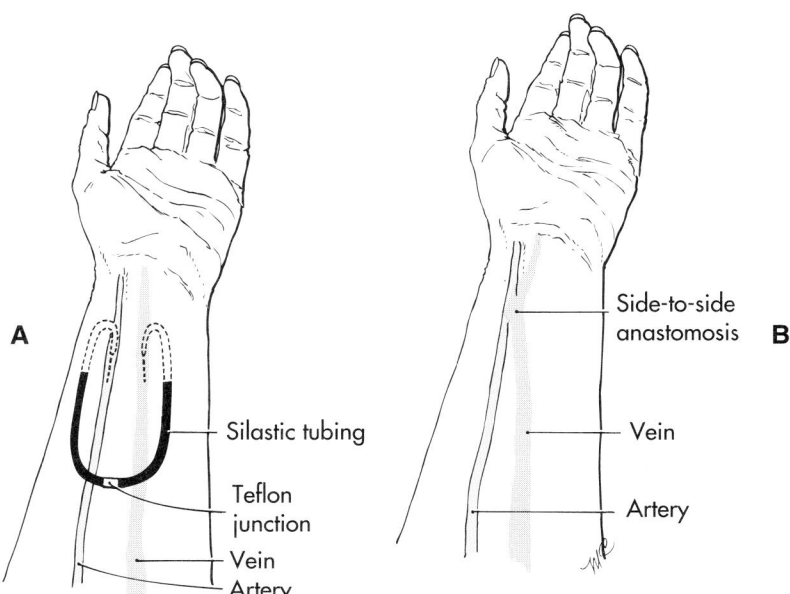

FIG. 48-6 Access to the circulation. **A,** External arteriovenous (AV) shunt or cannula system. **B,** Internal AV fistula.

treatment. However, recent engineering and medical developments have led to peritoneal dialysis becoming an alternative to hemodialysis as a treatment for chronic renal failure. Approximately 9% of ESRD patients undergo some type of peritoneal dialysis (U.S. Renal Data System, 2001).

Peritoneal dialysis is very similar to hemodialysis, except that the peritoneum functions as the semipermeable membrane. Access to the peritoneal cavity is achieved by paracentesis using either a straight, rigid trocar for acute peritoneal dialysis or the more permanent, soft Tenckhoff catheter for chronic peritoneal dialysis. Peritoneal dialysis is performed by infusing 1 to 2 L of dialysis solution into the abdomen through the catheter (Fig. 48-7). The dialysate stays in the abdomen for a variable period of time (dwell time) and then is drained off by gravity into a container placed below the patient. After the drainage is complete, new dialysate is infused and a new cycle begins. Solute removal is accomplished by diffusion, whereas ultrafiltration (water removal) is accomplished by osmosis rather than by hydrostatic pressure gradients, as in hemodialysis. Glucose is added to the dialysate to make it slightly hyperosmotic. Ultrafiltration can be enhanced by raising the glucose concentration and therefore the osmolality of the dialysate (1.5%, 2.5%, and 4.5% glucose concentrations are available).

The following are four modes of peritoneal dialysis in current use, one for acute and three for chronic dialysis:
1. Manual intermittent peritoneal dialysis
2. Continuous ambulatory peritoneal dialysis (CAPD)
3. Continuous cycler-assisted peritoneal dialysis (CCPD)
4. Automated intermittent peritoneal dialysis (IPD)

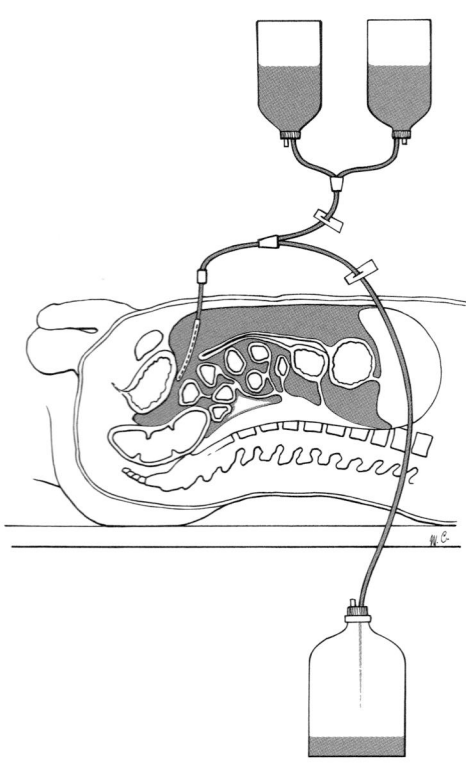

FIG. 48-7 Peritoneal dialysis.

Until 15 years ago, *manual intermittent peritoneal dialysis* was the most common method of performing peritoneal dialysis. A catheter is placed in the peritoneal cavity by paracentesis. In the adult, 2 L of sterile dialysis solution is allowed to run into the peritoneal cavity through the catheter for 10 to 20 minutes. Equilibrium between the dialysis fluid and the highly vascular peritoneal semipermeable membrane then takes place during the dwell time, usually 30 minutes. The fluid is then allowed to drain by gravity into a closed, sterile collecting system. The cycles (each lasting about 1 hour) are repeated over a period of 1 to 2 days. In acute renal failure, one or two such treatments each week usually provide acceptable control of fluid and electrolytes and azotemia.

The main advantages of the manual method of IPD are its simplicity (it does not require highly skilled personnel nor sophisticated equipment) and that it does not require access to the bloodstream. Disadvantages of this method include the large nursing time commitment, confinement during the procedure, and the relatively high risk of peritonitis. The manual method of IPD is less efficient than is hemodialysis, requiring about six times as long to achieve the same results.

CAPD is a self-dialysis technique using 2-L exchanges of dialysate four times per day, with the last exchange performed at bedtime and allowed to dwell in the peritoneal cavity overnight. The empty bag and tubing are continually attached to the catheter and concealed beneath the clothing during the 4-hour dwell time. After the dwell time, the bag is lowered to the floor and allowed to fill by gravity. CAPD was devised in the late 1970s and is the most popular method of peritoneal dialysis used today for the treatment of chronic renal failure.

Advantages of CAPD include greater freedom for the ESRD patient because it can be performed anywhere, absence of peaks and valleys in blood chemistry levels characteristic of intermittent hemodialysis, simplicity, and ease of learning. The primary disadvantage of CAPD is the risk of peritonitis, which occurs on the average of once every 40 patient weeks. Various methods have been designed to reduce the risk of contamination. One such device is an ultraviolet light used to sterilize the catheter spike and outlet port of the dialysis bag. Other disadvantages of CAPD include catheter tunnel infection, moderate protein loss, hypercholesterolemia, hypertriglyceridemia, obesity (excess calories from absorption of the glucose), and inguinal and abdominal hernias. Lower cost is not an advantage of peritoneal dialysis as originally expected because of the cost of dialysate and of hospitalization related to peritonitis. The cost to each patient receiving dialysis (whether hemodialysis or peritoneal dialysis) is estimated to be about $35,000 per year. Finally, many patients are unwilling to make the continuous time commitment of 3 to 4 hours each day to perform the exchanges.

CCPD is a variation of CAPD in which an automatic cycler machine delivers multiple overnight exchanges and an additional exchange in the morning. The dialysate then remains in the abdomen during the day for one long cycle. Both CAPD and CCPD require the abdomen to be full on a continuous basis. CCPD may be more acceptable to some patients but must be performed either at home or at a dialysis center, whereas CAPD can be performed anywhere.

An alternate to CAPD and CCPD is automated *IPD*, which allows for "dry periods" when the abdomen is empty. IPD is typically performed nightly with the aid of automated (cycler-assisted) equipment, and the peritoneal cavity remains empty during the day.

Newer Approaches to Solute Removal

The type and surface area of the dialysis membrane are important determinants of ultrafiltration and solute clearance and the immunologic response of the patient. Conventional dialysis, using a conventional low flux dialysis membrane, continues to be the primary treatment mode for CRF. Traditional dialysis membranes, composed of Cuprophan (Cupra-ammonium cellophane) or cellulose acetate have small pores (low flux). These membranes have low diffusive and ultrafiltration capabilities and are less biocompatible. Consequently, dialysis treatment is less efficient, requiring about 12 hours per week and larger molecules (some of which may be uremic toxins) are not removed. Many patients continue to manifest various disturbed metabolic functions despite vigorous hemodialysis that maintains the concentrations of classic uremic metabolites (e.g., urea, creatinine, phosphate) at near normal levels. These observations have led investigators to postulate that there are uremic toxins intermediate in molecular weight between the classic small molecules such as urea (<500 daltons) and plasma proteins (>50,000 daltons) that may partially account for the clinical abnormalities (middle molecular hypothesis). Box 48-4 summarizes some of these newer methods for the treatment of renal failure. Some of these methods are more efficient and superior in removing molecules in the middle molecular range. Some are used primarily for the treatment of acute renal failure or to remove toxins in the case of acute poisoning.

High flux, high efficiency (HFHE) dialysis uses some of the newer synthetic membranes, such as polysulphone, polymethylmethacrylate (PMMA), or polyacrylonitrile (PAN), which are not only more biocompatible than are cellulose-derived membranes but also more permeable to solutes and water. Artificial kidneys made out of these materials (HFHE dialyzers) have been used to shorten dialysis time; they also provide enhanced clearances of small molecules (e.g., urea), middle molecules (e.g., β_2 microglobin) and faster removal of fluid than conventional dialysis. HFHE dialysis membranes are used in conjunction with higher than traditional rates of flow for the blood entering and exiting the dialyzer (500 to 800 ml/min) and for rapid dialysate flow (800 ml/min). HFHE dialyzers are expensive, and not every unit has the capability of performing this type of dialysis, thus it is not a routine method.

Hemofiltration (HF), or *continuous arteriovenous hemofiltration (CAVH)*, is another form of extracorporeal therapy that may be used at the bedside in the intensive care unit to treat acute renal failure. The HF technique is based on the principle of *convection* rather than diffusion and is more analogous to function of the glomerulus than is conventional hemodialysis. HF does not use dialysate fluid; hemofilters have an inlet and outlet for blood and a single outlet for the ultrafiltrate compartment. There is no concentration gradient with convection, thus only fil-

tration of fluid takes place, and electrolytes are eliminated as they are pulled along and removed by the fluid. A high flux (large pore) membrane is used in the hemofilter. The resulting ultrafiltrate contains unwanted solutes and is discarded. Replacement fluid is then administered IV to approximately replace the large volume of fluid removed by the hemofilter. The process of hemofiltration is continuous and slow, making it particularly suitable for patients with an unstable cardiovascular status. HF may be performed by accessing the blood through an artery and returning it to a vein (CAVH) with the driving force provided by the systemic circulation; alternately, blood may be accessed from a vein and returned to another vein (*continuous venovenous hemofiltration [CVVH]*) with a blood pump providing the driving force.

Hemodiafiltration (HDF), or *continuous arteriovenous hemodiafiltration (CAVHD)* has many of the features of CAVH, but it includes the advantage of a concentration gradient to facilitate more rapid removal of urea because a dialysate is used with this procedure. Thus HDF is a combination of hemofiltration (removing fluid and solutes by convection) and hemodialysis (removing solutes by diffusion). As with HF, the extracorporeal circulation may be performed using an arteriovenous circuit (CAVHD) or a venovenous circuit (continuous venove-

---

BOX 48-4

Types of Extracorporeal Treatment Methods for Renal Failure

HEMODIALYSIS (HD)
1. Conventional hemodialysis—hemodialysis (HD) primarily by diffusion using a low flux (small pore) membrane
2. High flux and high efficiency hemodialysis (HFHE)—HD, using a high flux (large pore), more biocompatible membrane with a larger surface area and higher rates of flow than conventional dialysis

HEMOFILTRATION (HF)
1. Continuous arteriovenous hemofiltration (CAVH)—removal of water from the blood by ultrafiltration without dialysis. A volume of water with its solutes is removed by convective transfer. Primarily used to treat acute renal failure (ARF) in an intensive care setting.
2. Continuous venovenous hemofiltration (CVVH)—similar to CAVH, except that blood is accessed through a vein and returned to another vein

HEMODIAFILTRATION (HDF)
1. Continuous arteriovenous hemodiafiltration (CAVHD)—a combination of hemofiltration and hemodialysis. The blood circuit is from an artery to the dialysis machine and to a vein. Solutes are removed by convection using a high-flux membrane and dialysis fluid flows continuously through the dialysis compartment to enhance solute removal by diffusion; primarily used to treat ARF.
2. Continuous venovenous hemodiafiltration (CVVHD)—similar to CAVHD, except that blood is accessed through a vein and returned to another vein with the help of a blood pump

HEMOPERFUSION (HP)
Removal of drugs or poisons by adsorption to activated charcoal or resin; primarily used to treat acute poisoning.

nous hemodiafiltration [CVVHD]) using a double-lumen catheter. Like HF, HDF is primarily used to treat acute renal failure in the United States, although these two procedures may be used intermittently to treat chronic renal failure in Europe and Japan.

Major advantages of HF and HDF are they do not cause rapid fluid shifts, they do not require dialysis machines or dialysis staff to carry out the procedures, and they can be initiated quickly in an intensive care unit. Access to the vascular system for these procedures may be through a previously established internal fistula used for hemodialysis or by cannulation of the femoral artery or femoral vein, or a dual lumen central venous catheter may be used. *Hemoperfusion (HP)* is used for the removal of poisons or noxious substances from the blood. In HP, blood is pumped through a cartridge containing activated charcoal, which is coated with a biocompatible substance and then returned to the patient. The charcoal binds most drugs and poisons. HP is primarily used to treat acute poisoning.

Renal Transplantation

A successful renal transplant is the preferred method of treatment for patients in end-stage renal failure, although some patients may elect self-dialysis in their own home after being taught the procedure by a home-training nurse.

The first successful renal transplant was performed on identical twins in 1954 by Murray, Merrill, and Harrison in Boston. In 1998, 13,272 kidney transplants were performed in the United States. This number is small compared with the 47,210 on the waiting lists at the 251 transplant centers. Renal transplantation costs about $40,000 to $50,000. However, after a successful transplantation, the cost of care falls to less than $10,000 per year, making renal transplantation the most cost-effective treatment for ESRD patients (U.S. Renal Data System, 2001). Dialysis, by comparison, costs about $35,000 per year, and the quality of life is less compared with successful transplantation. However, the demand for renal transplantation far exceeds the number of available living-related and cadaver kidneys, limiting transplantation as a treatment option.

The surgical technique involved in renal transplantation is relatively simple and is generally performed by a surgeon with a background in urologic, vascular, or general surgery. It is standard procedure to rotate the donor kidney and place it in the contralateral iliac fossa of the recipient. The ureter then lies anterior to the renal vessels and is more readily anastomosed or implanted into the recipient bladder. The renal artery is anastomosed end-to-end to the internal iliac artery, and the renal vein is anastomosed to the external or common iliac vein (Fig. 48-8).

Tissue Typing and Immunogenetics

An *autograft* (transfer of an individual's own tissue) from one part of the body to another (e.g., skin) is always accepted. A *syngenetic graft* is a transfer of tissue between genetically identical individuals (i.e., identical twins) and usually "takes" permanently. A *xenograft* is the transfer of tissue between different species (e.g., baboon to human)

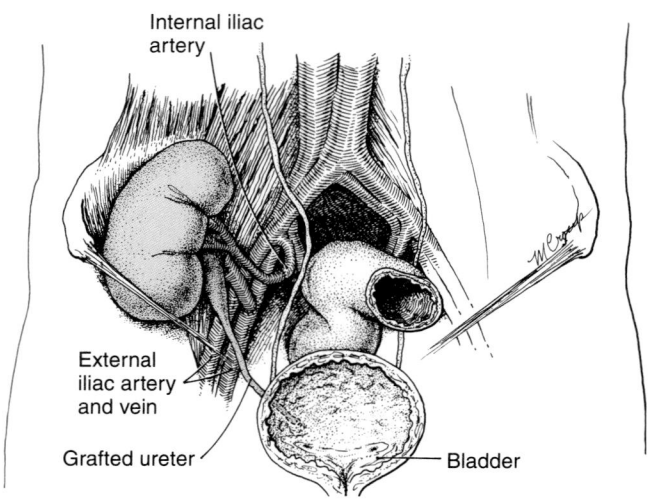

FIG. 48-8 Renal transplantation.

and is always rejected by an immunocompetent recipient. An *allograft* is a graft between genetically different members of the same species (from one human to another) and is the most common type of tissue transplantation. The major limiting factor in this procedure is the body's immunologic response that leads to rejection of the transplanted kidney. Rejection may be cell mediated or humoral. Cell-mediated rejection involves T lymphocytes produced in response to antigens in the donor kidney that are recognized as foreign cells. These lymphocytes invade the foreign donor kidney and contribute to its destruction. Humoral rejection involves the production of antibodies against antigens in the donor kidney, which the recipient's plasma cells recognize as foreign. Rejection can occur within hours or several years after transplantation.

Tissue typing or histocompatibility testing to ensure the closest possible tissue match between donor and recipient and suppressing the immune response with drugs are the two general approaches used to promote successful renal transplant and prevent rejection. Two major antigenic groups have been identified as important in determining histocompatibility: the ABO blood group system and human leukocyte antigens (HLA).

ABO Blood Group Antigens

ABO antigens are present in most tissues of the body, as well as on RBCs. The ABO antigens determine blood type and are identified serologically. Type A blood has the A antigen; type B blood has the B antigen; type AB blood has both the A and B antigens; and type O blood has neither. Naturally occurring antibodies are present in the blood serum when a particular antigen is lacking on the cells. Anti-A antibodies are found in persons who do not have the A antigen (blood types B and O), and anti-B antibodies are found in persons without the B antigen (blood types A and O). Individuals with type AB blood have neither antibody, because they have both antigens. The same general rules apply to renal transplants with respect to ABO compatibility as with blood transfusions (Table 48-1). An O kidney can be transplanted into any recipient, whereas an A kidney can be given only to an A

TABLE 48-1 ■■■

The ABO Blood Group System

Type	Antigen	Distribution in Population		Potential Donor
A	A	C	40%	A, O
		AfA	27%	
		AI	16%	
		AsA	28%	
B	B	C	11%	B, O
		AfA	20%	
		AI	4%	
		AsA	27%	
AB	A and B	C	4%	AB, A, B, O
		AfA	4%	
		AI	1%	
		AsA	5%	
O	None	C	45%	O
		AfA	49%	
		AI	79%	
		AsA	40%	

Data from Vengelen-Tyler V, ed: *Technical manual*, ed 13, Bethesda, Maryland, 1999, American Association of Blood Banks; Mourant AE, et al: *The distribution of the human blood groups and other polymorphisms*, ed 2, 1976, Oxford University Press; Bloodbook.com, 2000-2001. *http://www.bloodbook.com*
C, Caucasian; *AfA*, African American; *AI*, American Indian; *AsA*, Asian American.

TABLE 48-2 ■■■

Potential HLA Antigens by Locus

		Class I Antigens			Class II Antigens
LOCUS	A	B		C	DR
	A1	B5	B49	CW1	DR1
	A2	B7	BW50	CW2	DR2
	A3	B8	B51	CW3	DR3
	A9	B12	BW52	CW4	DR4
	A10	B13	BW53	CW5	DR5
	A11	B14	BW54	CW6	DRW6
	AW19	B15	BW56	CW7	DR7
	A23	B16	BW57	CW8	DRW8
	A24	B17	BW58	CW9	DRW9
	A25	B18	BW59	CW10	DRW10
	A26	B21	BW60	CW11	DRW11
	A27	BW22	BW61		DRW12
	A29	B27	BW62		DRW13
	A30	B35	BW63		DRW14
	A31	B37	BW65		DRW15
	A32	B38	BW67		DRW16
	AW33	B39	BW70		DRW17
	AW34	B40	BW71		DRW18
	AW36	BW41	BW72		DRW52
	AW43	BW42	BW73		DRW53
	AW66	B44	BW75		
	AW68	B45	BW76		
	AW69	BW46	BW4		
	AW74	BW47	BW6		
		BW48			

From Roitt I, Brostoff J, Male D, editors: *Immunology*, ed 3, St Louis, 1993, Mosby.

or AB recipient. Unlike blood transfusions, the rhesus (Rh) factor is not a concern with organ transplantation, because Rh antigens are not found on vascular endothelial tissues (the principal target tissue in rejection). ABO typing is always performed before blood transfusions and organ transplantation. Transplantation between ABO-incompatible persons is not done, because it generally leads to immediate hyperacute rejection.

Human Leukocyte Antigen System

The second antigen system important in organ transplantation is the major histocompatibility complex (MHC) discussed in Chapter 5. This antigen system is called the human leukocyte antigen (HLA) system in humans, because the antigens were first discovered on WBCs. The genes that code for the HLA antigens are located on the short arm of chromosome 6. Four major HLA sites or loci important for transplantation, designated A, B, C, and DR, have been identified in this region. Each sublocus controls a series of antigenic factors, and more than 100 have been identified (Table 48-2). Three of these genes (HLA-A, HLA-B, and HLA-C) code for *class I antigens*. Class I antigens are found on the surface of all nucleated cells in the body and on RBCs and platelets. Class I antigens are recognized by CD8 lymphocytes, which are the cytotoxic or "killer" T cells. Class I antigens present the major target for T cell and antibody reactions to transplanted grafts. Three genes at the D sublocus code for *class II antigens* (HLA-DR, HLA-DQ, and HLA-DP), but only the HLA-DR (D-related) gene is important in transplanted organ rejection. Class II antigens have a more limited distribution in the body than class I antigens and are present on the surface of antigen-presenting cells (e.g., B cells, activated macrophages, some activated T cells, and vascular endothelial cells) (Hutchinson, 1993). CD4 cells (helper T cells) recognize class II antigens. Helper T cell activity depends on *both* the recognition of

the foreign antigen on antigen presenting cells (APCs) and the presence on these cells of "self" class II HLA antigens. The reader should note that T cells recognize antigens only when the antigens are presented on the surface of cells (in association with either class I or II HLA self antigens). B cells do not have this requirement and can recognize antigens in plasma with their surface monomer, immunoglobulin M (IgM), acting as the antigen receptor.

In addition to the major antigens encoded by the HLA genes, an unknown number of *minor antigens* are encoded by genes at sites other than that of the HLA locus. These minor antigens can induce a weak immune response that can cause slow rejection of a graft. However, these antigens are not tested for, because laboratory tests do not exist for minor antigens.

Haplotype Inheritance of the HLA Antigens

The complex of the four histocompatibility genes (A, B, C, and DR) important in transplantation is known as a haplotype and is codominantly expressed. Because chromosomes are paired, an individual has a total of eight HLA genes (two pairs on each of the two chromosomes). Each of the chromosome sets is called a haplotype and is inherited as a set. The genotype of an individual consists of two haplotypes. In other words, each individual inherits two half-sets (haplotypes)—one set from each parent. Within a single family, only four genotypes can be present. For example, if the HLA genotype of the mother is PQ and that of the father is RS, four possible

FIG. 48-9 Pattern of inheritance of human leukocyte antigen (HLA) antigens. All children have a one-haplotype mismatch with each parent. Children 1 and 5 are HLA-identical siblings; the rest of the siblings have a one-haplotype mismatch. Some siblings have a two-haplotype mismatch or no antigens in common.

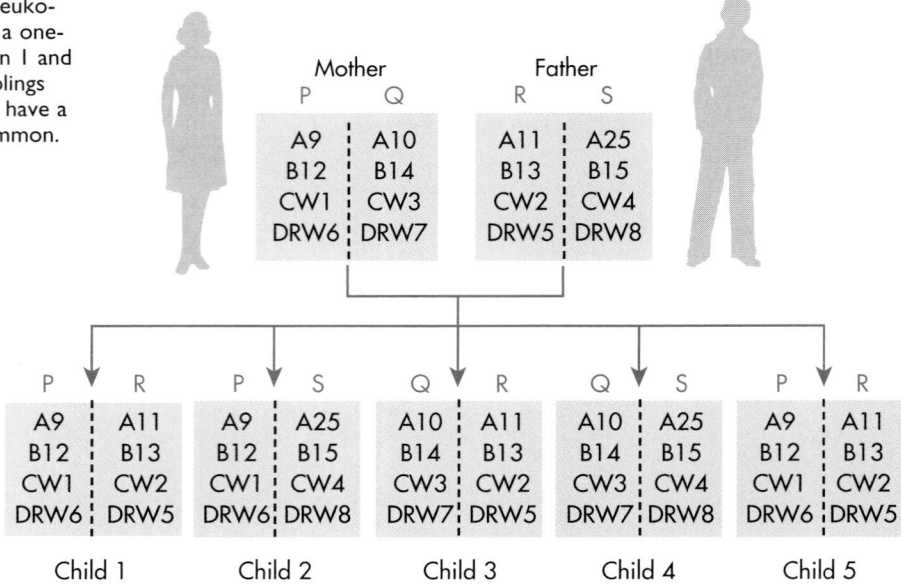

combinations exist for the children: PR, PS, QR, and QS. By the laws of simple Mendelian inheritance, 25% of the children will be HLA-identical, 50% will have one haplotype in common, and 25% will have a two-haplotype mismatch (Fig. 48-9).

In general, the closer the genetic similarity is between donor and recipient, the greater the chance of a successful transplant will be. When the donor and recipient are identical twins or HLA-identical siblings, more than 95% of the kidneys survive at the end of one year and the subsequent half-life is 25 years. A renal transplant of a one-haplotype match from a family member has a 1-year graft survival of about 91% with an 11- to 12-year half-life. With increasing numbers of mismatches for cadaver donors, 1-year kidney graft survival declines to about 81% and the half-life declines to about 7 years (U.S. Renal Data System, 2001).

Prevention of Rejection by HLA Matching

Obviously, the ideal donor for an organ transplant is a monozygotic (identical) twin, one who can provide a perfect genetic match for the recipient. Unfortunately, this circumstance rarely occurs. One way to overcome rejection of transplanted tissue is by tissue matching for histocompatibility antigens. The antigens expressed by the cells vary with different tissues, and some cells do not have antigens that present antigens for processing. For example, corneas are easily grafted because they are avascular, and the lymphatic supply of the eye prevents many antigens from triggering an immune response, thus the proportion of successful corneal transplants is very high. Bone marrow has the greatest capability of inducing rejection, followed by the skin, heart, kidney, and liver. HLA matching is not used for the liver, which seems to tolerate HLA antigen differences quite well.

Tissue typing is a technique developed to predict the outcome of organ transplantation based on a particular match of antigens between donor and recipient. The overriding consideration for organ allograft rejection is whether the donor graft carries any antigens that are not present in the recipient—called the *host-versus-graft reaction principle.** Several types of tests of the HLA system antigens are commonly performed before renal transplantations: (1) tissue typing by serology (lymphocytotoxicity test) or by deoxyribonucleic acid (DNA) or molecular techniques; (2) WBC crossmatching; and (3) antibody detection or screening.

In the *lymphocytotoxicity test,* lymphocytes are added to the sera, which may or may not have antibodies directed to HLA antigens. If the serum contains an antibody specific to HLA Class I (A, B, and C) or II (D) antigens on the lymphocytes, the antibody will bind to this HLA antigen. Complement is then added. The complement binds only to positive cells (i.e., where the antibody has bound) and, in so doing, causes membrane damage. The uptake of vital stains such as eosin by the damaged cells allows microscopic identification and indicates the presence of a specific HLA antibody. The most important use of this test is to detect specific donor-reactive antibodies present in a potential recipient before transplantation. Testing of HLA-A, HLB-B (Class I), and HLA-DR (Class II) antigens is mandatory because these antigens are most significant with respect to predicting graft survival. Testing for other HLA antigens is optional. Historically, this test has long been used to type for HLA Class I and Class II antigens, using antisera of known specificity. However, the problems of cross-reactivity and nonavailability of certain antibodies has led to the introduction of DNA-based methods. Currently, many laboratories have changed to molecular genetic methods for HLA Class typing, especially for the HLA-D antigens.

---

*The major exception to this principle is graft-versus-host disease, which can be a major complication of bone marrow transplantation. This reaction occurs because grafted immunocompetent T cells proliferate in the irradiated, immunocompromised host and "reject" cells with class II proteins, resulting in severe organ dysfunction, especially in the skin, liver, and GI tract.

Molecular genetic techniques for HLA Class typing include *restriction fragment length polymorphism (RFLP)* and *polymerase chain reaction (PCR)*. RFLP methods rely on the ability of certain enzymes to recognize exact DNA sequences and to cut the DNA at these points. Thus the frequency of a particular sequence will determine the lengths of the DNA produced by cutting with a particular enzyme. PCR is a revolutionary new system for investigating the DNA nucleotide of a particular region of interest using very small amounts of DNA as a starting point then making multiple copies. The selected portion of the DNA can then be isolated on a gel and then sequenced or typed for the presence of specific DNA sequences of HLA genes.

After the HLA tissue typing is completed and a potential donor is identified, a *WBC crossmatch* test is performed to determine if there is specific immune reactivity between the donor and recipient. The crossmatch is performed by mixing a very small amount of the patient's serum with the potential donor's white blood cells. If the patient has antibodies that react to the donor's HLA, the donor's cells will be injured. This finding is referred to as a *positive crossmatch* and is a contraindication for transplantation because the result signifies that the patient's immune system has the ability to attack the donor's cells and most likely would attack the donor's transplanted kidney. A negative crossmatch indicates that the patient does not have antibodies against the donor's HLA, and a transplant can be performed.

Lastly, a test called *antibody screening* determines whether the patient has antibodies to other HLAs. Repetitive antibody testing is beneficial for ongoing screening for patients waiting for a kidney transplant. Approximately once a month, the sera of the potential recipient are crossmatched against a pool of lymphocyte samples from random donors. The percentage of samples to which the recipient reacts is known as the *percent reactive antibody (PRA)* (Smith, 1990). The percentage is viewed as the risk of reaction with a random donor. The PRA is determined by testing the patient's serum to a panel of 60 different types of HLA. If, for example, the patient's serum reacts with 30 out of 60 HLA, then the patient's PRA is 50% ($^1/_2$ of 60). Obviously, the lower the PRA, the greater the chance of finding a compatible cadaver donor. The PRA is calculated for each monthly serum sample and after any blood transfusion. In addition to determining how much or how little PRA a patient has, HLA-antibody specificity is also determined. For example, if the patient has received a blood transfusion from a donor with HLA-A2, he or she may specifically develop antibody to A2. Some patients have one or two antibody specificities, whereas others have numerous specificities.

All patients awaiting an organ transplant must have these tests done. If the patient is awaiting a cadaveric transplant, the information related to HLA will be entered into the national transplant database managed by the United Network of Organ Sharing (UNOS). Kidneys are allocated based on the UNOS point system, designed to balance equity with efficiency. When information on a cadaveric kidney donor becomes available, all active patients on the UNOS list who have an ABO blood type that are compatible with that of the donor are assigned

TABLE 48-3

Effect of HLA-A, B, and DR Mismatching on Kidney Transplant Survival*

Donor Mismatches	Half-Life of Graft Survival	10-Year Survival
LIVING RELATED DONOR		
HLA-identical sib = 0 mismatch	24 years	74%
1 haplotype = 3 mismatches	12 years	54%
LIVING UNRELATED DONOR		
Average = 4 mismatches	12 years	54%
Cadaver (overall)	9 years	40%
0 mismatches for 6 antigens	20 years	65%
1 to 2 mismatches	10.4 years	45%
3 to 4 mismatches	8.4 years	38%
5 to 6 mismatches	7.7 years	34%

*HLA antigens are codominantly inherited; each person has two A, two B, and two DR antigens for a total of six that require mandatory testing since they are most important in predicting graft survival.

points. Efficiency dictates that kidneys be given to the patients who are likely to benefit the most, which is usually the patients in whom the longest graph survival can be expected. The fewer the mismatches of HLA-A, HLA-B, and HLA-DR antigens are, the greater is the likelihood of graft survival and longevity (Table 48-3).

Renal Transplant Rejection

The nature of the body's immunologic defense against entry of foreign proteins is such that almost all organ transplantation from another person (with the possible exception of an identical twin) is followed by an attempt on the part of the recipient to reject that organ. There are three types of rejection.

Hyperacute rejection, which occurs within minutes or hours after completion of the transplant and inevitably leads to organ loss, is caused by ABO incompatibility or previous exposure to transfused WBCs or platelets from another person whose tissues contain the same antigens as the kidney donor. The recipient has preformed circulating antibodies, and such grafts undergo rejection via the humoral immune system, in which the B cell mechanism predominates. The antibodies are deposited along the kidney vascular endothelium, and complement is activated with consequent tissue damage. The end result is diffuse vascular thrombosis and cortical necrosis (Black, 1996). Hyperacute rejection is rarely encountered today because of ABO typing and improved WBC crossmatching techniques before transplantation. There is no effective treatment for hyperacute rejection.

Acute rejection usually occurs within the first 12 weeks after transplantation. Acute rejection episodes may recur at any time after the initial one, but the incidence decreases with time. The greater the HLA antigenic disparity between donor and host (including an unrelated cadaver donor) is, the greater the likelihood of severe acute rejection episodes will be. Preformed antidonor antibodies are not present in acute rejection (as in the hyperacute case).

The overall scheme in the development of effector mechanisms in allograft rejection is illustrated in Fig. 48-10. In response to the allograft, cytotoxic (CD8) T cells recognize the class I HLA (A, B, C) antigens on the surface of the foreign cells. Helper (CD4) T cells recognize the foreign class II HLA-DR antigens on certain antigen presenting cells (APCs), such as the macrophage, in the graft. The activated T helper (CD4+) cell then releases cytokines, which are required as growth and differentiation factors for other cells involved in the rejection reaction. Interleukin-2 (IL-2) and interferon-gamma (IFN γ) stimulate the cytotoxic T cells to form a clone of cells. These cytotoxic *killer* T cells then attack the cells in the allograft. IL-2, IL-4, and IL-5 are involved in B cell activation; lymphotoxin (tumor necrosis factor beta [TNF-β]) in concert with IFN γ causes activation of macrophages. In addition to direct killing of graft cells by cytotoxic T cells, the cells can be killed by a combination of antibody and phagocytic cells called *antibody-dependent cellular cytotoxicity (ADCC)*. In this process, antibody bound to the surface of the foreign graft cell is recognized by phagocytic cells (e.g., macrophages or natural killer [NK] cells) and the cell is killed. B cell activation leading to the production of antigraft IgG antibodies and complement activation can also cause damage to the vascular endothelium. The result is platelet aggregation within the vessel, thrombosis, hemorrhage, and damage to the parenchymal cells of the allograft, as well as the release of inflammatory mediators (Roitt et al, 1993; Carpenter, Lazarus, 1998). In summary, CD4+ T cells play a central role in initiating the rejection response by binding to class II HLA-DR antigens and subsequently enhancing the effector phase of the immune reaction by stimulating cytotoxic (CD8+) T cell, B cell, and macrophage mechanisms of allograft destruction.

Histologic evidence in the rejected kidney indicates that the critical targets for destruction are the vascular endothelium of the microvasculature and the renal tubules. There is perivascular accumulation of monocytes and varying degrees of vascular injury and tubular necrosis. Immunofluorescent micrographs of the vascular epithelium show deposits of fibrin, complement, and IgG, indicating involvement of the humoral immune system in the organ rejection (Carpenter, Lazarus, 1998).

The first rejection episode commonly occurs about 2 weeks after transplantation and is characterized by renal insufficiency (rising BUN and serum creatinine), oliguria, and sometimes swelling of the graft and fever. A biopsy of the graft may be necessary to make the diagnosis and determine the extent of the lesion. Acute rejection is often reversible with appropriate drug therapy, which is aimed primarily at suppressing T cells (see later discussion). Recovery usually takes 2 to 4 weeks, and during this time, the patient requires dialysis.

Chronic rejection occurs months to years after the initial transplant and is characterized by hypertension, proteinuria, and slow loss of renal function. The cause is poorly understood but may be caused by non-HLA minor antigens, a low-grade cell-mediated rejection, or the deposition of antigen-antibody complexes in the graft. Histologically, the primary changes are in the renal arteries and glomeruli and resemble a recurrence of the primary renal disease. Unlike acute rejection, this type of rejection responds poorly to drugs and has a poor prognosis (Black, 1996).

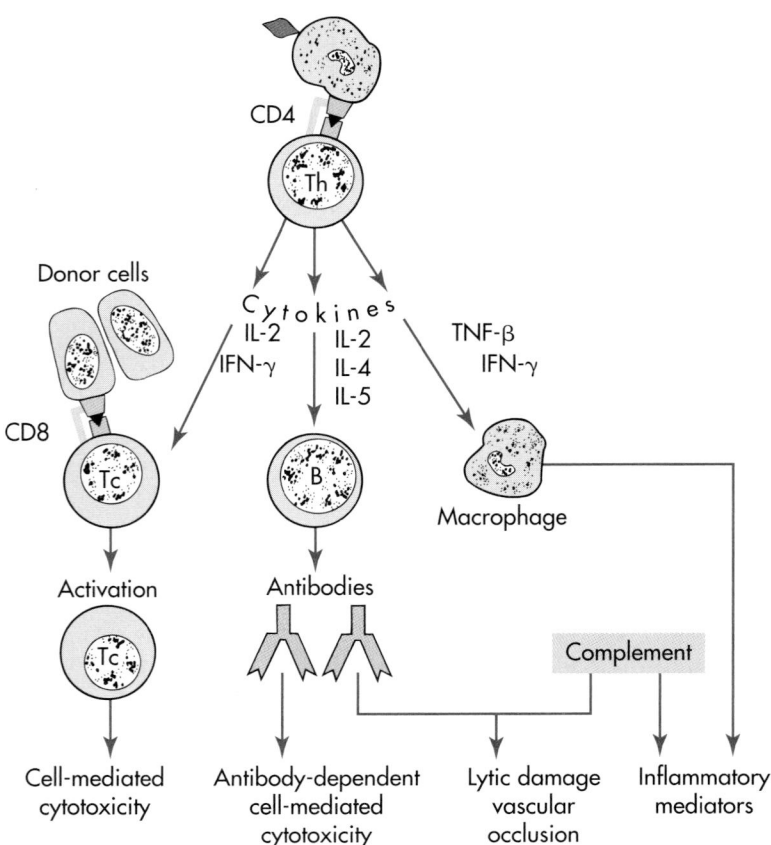

FIG. 48-10 Immunologic components of allograft rejection. *IFN-γ*, Interferon gamma; *TNF-β*, tumor necrosis factor beta. (Modified from Roitt I, Brostoff J, Male D: *Immunology*, ed 3, St Louis, 1993, Mosby.)

Immunosuppressive Treatment

The survival of the transplanted kidney depends on minimizing the body's defense mechanisms. The major immunosuppressive drugs used to prevent rejection are azathioprine, corticosteroids, and cyclosporine, and in some centers, antilymphocyte globulin (ALG) or antithymocyte globulin (ATG), and monoclonal antibodies.

Azathioprine (Imuran [PO or IV]) and corticosteroids (prednisone [PO] or Solu-Medrol [IV]) are the standard drugs ordered. Azathioprine, an antimetabolite, is a derivative of 6-mercaptopurine. Azathioprine inhibits the proliferation of lymphocytes by interfering with nucleic acid synthesis. Corticosteroids also suppress T cell proliferation by interfering with the release of IL-2 from monocytes. These drugs make the patient more susceptible to infection. Consequently, overwhelming infection is a major complication in a renal transplant recipient and the principal cause of death. To minimize the danger of both infection and rejection, the general approach is to increase the dose of corticosteroids for a limited time during the initial transplant period and to treat rejection episodes while keeping the maintenance dose low at other times.

Cyclosporine is a potent fungal metabolite and a specific immunosuppressant that prevents the replication of T cells by inhibiting the production of IL-2. Since its approval by the U.S. Food and Drug Administration (FDA) in 1983, cyclosporine has revolutionized organ transplantation. In the United States, 1-year cadaver graft survival now rivals the 80% graft survival from HLA-identical related donors (Carpenter, Lazarus, 1998). Opelz (1991) reported the results of a large international collaborative transplant study involving cadaveric renal transplants between 1982 and 1989. Cyclosporine was given to virtually all of the 30,000 transplant recipients. This study showed that although the 1-year cadaver graft survival was high, long-term graft survival at 5 years after transplant was not improved. Five-year cadaver graft survival ranged between 45% and 65%, depending on the number of mismatches for HLA-A, -B, and -DR antigens. Thus the major advantage of cyclosporine over azathioprine is during the first 1 or 2 years after cadaveric transplant and not in the rate of graft loss thereafter.

Cyclosporine may be given in combination with azathioprine and corticosteroids. The usefulness of this drug is limited by its adverse side effects, most notably its nephrotoxicity. Hypertension, hirsutism, gum hyperplasia, and increased susceptibility to infection are other side effects. The incidence of malignancy (especially lymphoma) is increased, especially when cyclosporine is used in combination with other immunosuppressants.

Antilymphocyte globulin (ALG) and antithymocyte globulin (ATG) are produced by injecting human lymphocytes (ALG) or thymocytes (ATG) into animals, which then make antibodies against them. These antibodies are then injected into the transplant patient to prevent or treat rejection. The major effect of ALG or ATG is to deplete T cells. Side effects include susceptibility to infection and to the foreign protein that can lead to fever, chills, and anaphylaxis.

Monoclonal OKT3 antibodies are administered IV and cause suppression of T cells. The drug acts by opsonization of the T3 molecule present in the cell membrane of all peripheral T cells, thus rendering them incapable of an immunologic response. OKT3 antibody is highly effective in the treatment of acute rejection (Black, 1996).

Additional immunosuppressive drugs recently introduced to prevent or treat rejection include tacrolimus (FK506, Prograf), rapamycin (sirolimus, Rapamune) mycophenolate mofetil (CellCept), and basiliximab (Simulect). Although many of the immunosuppressive drugs have greatly increased graft survival, many of these drugs have undesirable side effects. Therefore the search for agents that specifically target immune cells goes on.

A final consideration is that there is a limited choice in opting for renal transplantation as a treatment modality. The number of patients developing ESRD has increased dramatically over the last 10 years while the supply of kidneys suitable for transplantation has not. The steepest rise has been in African Americans, diabetic patients, and older adults. Consequently, the majority of patients (about 72%) will receive dialysis as a chronic form of treatment. However, the recent significant advances in tissue typing and improved immunosuppression offer hope for greater success in those patients receiving cadaver transplants (the commonest source of organs).

*K*EY CONCEPTS

- The treatment of chronic renal failure (CRF) is divided into two stages: conservative management when azotemia occurs and renal replacement therapy (dialysis or renal transplantation or both) when conservative management fails.
- The conservative management of CRF consists of measures to delay the progression of renal failure, stabilize the patient's condition, and treat any reversible factors.
- Restriction of dietary protein and control of hypertension, especially using ACE inhibitors, are two interventions that may slow the progression to end-stage renal failure in patients with CRF.
- Reversible factors in CRF include ECF volume depletion, urinary tract obstruction, infection, and severe hypertension.
- Hyperkalemia is generally a problem in end-stage renal disease (ESRD), and dietary K^+ is typically restricted to about 60 mEq/day.
- Severe hyperkalemia (>7.5 mEq/L), or if ECG changes are present with $K^+ >6.0$ mEq/L is a medical emergency and may be treated with (a) 10% IV

calcium gluconate with ECG monitoring or (b) IV glucose and insulin to drive K^+ into the cells for temporary correction followed by administration of an ion exchange resin (Kayexalate) or dialysis for more lasting lowering of the serum K^+.

■ Na^+ (and water) retention is generally a problem in ESRD, requiring regulation of dietary Na^+ and fluid allowance.

■ The Na^+ conservation test and careful observation of the daily weight and other signs of ECF volume excess (e.g., pulmonary and peripheral edema) may be helpful because the range between Na^+ deficit and excess may be very narrow in ESRD.

■ A rule of thumb for fluid allowance is 24-hour urine output + 500 ml (for insensible losses) and sufficient fluid to allow a 2- to 3-pound weight gain between treatments when the patient is on dialysis.

■ More than 90% of hypertension in ESRD is volume-dependent and can usually be controlled effectively by Na^+ and fluid restriction and by ultrafiltration when the patient is on hemodialysis.

■ Ace inhibitor antihypertensive medications slow the progression of renal failure by lowering systemic blood pressure and lowering intraglomerular pressure by selective dilation of the efferent arteriole.

■ Antihypertensive medications must be held before hemodialysis treatment to prevent hypotension and shock during the treatment.

■ The anemia of ESRD is effectively treated with erythropoietin (EPO); the risk of hypertension as a side effect can be ameliorated by aiming for a subnormal hematocrit of about 35%.

■ Before dialysis treatment, the chronic metabolic acidosis of renal failure is not generally treated, unless the serum HCO_3^- falls below 15 mEq/L.

■ The metabolic acidosis of chronic renal failure may be treated with alkali therapy.

■ Treatment must begin in the early stages of renal insufficiency (GFR <50 ml/min) when parathyroid hormone (PTH) levels begin to rise above normal to prevent secondary hyperparathyroidism and renal osteodystrophy.

■ An effective strategy to prevent secondary hyperparathyroidism must manage PTH, calcium, phosphate, and calcitriol $(1,25[OH]_2D_3)$ simultaneously.

■ Dietary phosphate restriction and administration of phosphate-binding antacids (usually calcium carbonate) with the goal of maintaining serum phosphate to <5.0 mg/dl is an important therapy for the prevention of secondary hyperparathyroidism and renal osteodystrophy.

■ If the $Ca \times PO_4$ cross-product (in mg/dl) should exceed 60, precipitation of calcium salts into the soft tissues of the body may occur (metastatic calcification).

■ Allopurinol is used to treat the hyperuricemia of renal failure; colchicine may be used to treat gouty arthritis.

■ The slowing of nerve conduction velocity may be the first indication of peripheral neuropathy in the patient with CRF.

■ Adequate dialysis may stop the progression of sensory peripheral neuropathy but motor neuropathy is poorly reversible.

■ Detection of infection in the uremic patient requires a high degree of suspicion and attention to less specific indicators, such as tachycardia, fatigue, or a slight rise in body temperature, because hypothermia and a failure of leukocytosis are common features of the uremic syndrome.

■ Careful drug administration is imperative in the treatment of patients with ESRD because the half-life is prolonged because of renal excretory failure; thus doses must be reduced.

■ Some indications for the elective initiation of dialysis treatment may include neurologic manifestations of uremia, such as encephalopathy and peripheral neuropathy; fluid overload not responding to diuretic therapy; excessively high serum creatinine (4 to 6 mg/dl), or the patient is bedridden or is so fatigued that he or she is not able to carry on activities of daily living.

■ *Hemodialysis* is a diffusion based mass transfer process between blood and dialysis fluid separated by a semipermeable membrane.

■ Solutes move in a direction according to their concentration gradients; in most instances, the direction of solute movement is from blood to dialysis fluid.

■ Ultrafiltration in hemodialysis is created by a hydrostatic pressure gradient across the semipermeable membrane.

■ Dialysis simulates the excretory and volume regulatory functions of the kidney but does not correct for the loss of endocrine and metabolic functions of the kidney.

■ Methods of vascular access for hemodialysis include the external AV shunt, internal AV fistula, internal AV graft, Sheldon catheter, and double-lumen catheters for the subclavian, jugular, or femoral veins.

■ Complications of vascular access include thrombosis, infection, high output failure, aneurysm formation, carpal tunnel syndrome, and distal ischemia.

■ Extracorporeal circulation of blood during hemodialysis requires anticoagulation accomplished by the infusion of heparin into the arterial line after the injection of a loading dose; the rate of infusion is adjusted depending on the activated clotting time.

■ Some notable complications of dialysis include hypotension, disequilibrium syndrome, dialysis dementia, hepatitis, infection, blood loss, electrolyte and acid-base abnormalities, muscle cramps, and nausea and vomiting.

■ Most patients in maintenance hemodialysis programs undergo treatment for 4 to 6 hours three times per week.

■ *Peritoneal dialysis*, like hemodialysis, uses the process of diffusion as a means of removing solutes and uremic toxins from the blood.

■ The peritoneal membrane, the analogue of the cellophane membrane in the hemodialyzer, is less effective as a barrier to diffusion of larger molecular weight solutes than are hemodialysis membranes; solutes as large as albumin may therefore pass through the peritoneal membrane and are lost from the body.

■ Intermittent peritoneal dialysis consists of placing 2 L of dialysate into the abdominal cavity, leaving it there for 20 minutes and then draining it out; this process is repeated for 8 to 10 hours, 3 to 4 days per week and may be done with the use of automated equipment in the dialysis unit or in the patient's home.

- With continuous ambulatory peritoneal dialysis (CAPD), the dialysis solution is left in the abdominal cavity 4 to 6 hours, then drained; this process is repeated 4 to 5 times/day, 7 days per week.
- Ultrafiltration is accomplished in peritoneal dialysis by creating an osmotic gradient between the blood and dialysate by means of increasing the glucose concentration of the dialysate.
- Middle molecules with a molecular weight between 500 and 5000 daltons, responsible for some uremic manifestations such as peripheral neuropathy, are better removed by peritoneal dialysis.
- Advantages of peritoneal dialysis compared with hemodialysis: simpler to perform, no anticoagulation, easier access, better removal of middle molecules, better fluid and electrolyte balance, better control of blood pressure, and fewer problems with hypotension and disequilibrium.
- Disadvantages of peritoneal dialysis compared with hemodialysis: less efficient, time consuming, and higher incidence of peritonitis.
- *Hemofiltration (HF)* is a continuous form of extracorporeal therapy primarily used to treat acute renal failure and is based on the principle of convection; blood may be accessed through an artery and returned to a vein (CAVH) or accessed from a vein and returned to another vein (CVVH); a dialysate is not used.
- *Hemodiafiltration (HDF)*, also used primarily to treat acute renal failure, is based both on the principle of convection and on diffusion (as in conventional dialysis).
- *High flux, high efficiency hemodialysis (HFHE)* uses more biocompatible high-flux (larger pores) membranes and is therefore better at removing uremic toxins in the middle molecular range; it is more efficient because of higher flow rates of blood and dialysis fluid.
- *Hemoperfusion (HP)* is an extracorporeal treatment primarily used for the removal of drugs or poisons by adsorption to activated charcoal or resins.

- Renal transplantation from living donors (related or unrelated) or cadaveric donors is the preferred method of treating ESRD but is limited by the shortage of suitable or available donors.
- *Tissue typing* of the donor and recipient before kidney transplantation consists of (1) ABO blood group compatibility required, (2) Rh not important, and (3) major histocompatibility antigens: Type I and Type II HLA-antigen matching for a better outcome.
- The 1-year graft survival is greater than 85% for cadaveric kidneys and greater than 95% for HLA matched living related transplants.
- After the first year, there is a continuous attrition of functioning kidney grafts; the mean graft half-life of a cadaver transplant is 7.7 years and 24 years for a HLA-identical sibling.
- Complications of renal transplantation include hyperacute, acute, or chronic rejection; infections; malignancies; cyclosporine toxicity; and recurrent renal disease.
- Immunologic mechanisms of *allograft rejection* include cell-mediated cytotoxicity and antibody-dependent cell-mediated cytotoxicity.
- In *hyperacute (vascular, humoral) rejection*, preformed antibodies bind to the graft endothelium and activate complement and coagulation cascades, resulting in thrombosis and loss of transplant within minutes after completion of the surgery.
- *Hyperacute rejection* can be prevented by ABO typing, careful screening for cytotoxic antibodies while the patient is on the waiting list, and a final cytotoxic crossmatch immediately before transplant.
- *Acute rejection* usually occurs within the first 12 weeks after transplantation and is caused by the appearance of newly formed cytotoxic T cells sensitized against the new graft.
- The prevention of cytotoxic T cell proliferation is achieved by using high doses of glucocorticoids and antilymphocyte preparations (monoclonal or polyclonal) for 7 to 10 days after transplantation, followed by varied combinations of prednisone, cyclosporine (IL-2 antagonist) and azathioprine (antiproliferative agent), with gradual reduction of doses for life-long maintenance levels.

QUESTIONS ??

A sampling of review questions for this chapter appears here. Visit http://www.mosby.com/MERLIN/PriceWilson/ for additional questions.

Answer the following on a separate sheet of paper.

1. When are conservative measures of treatment begun for the patient with chronic renal failure (CRF)? What are the basic principles of conservative treatment? Name four causes of sudden deterioration of renal function in the answer.

2. When conservative therapeutic measures are no longer adequate in the treatment of the uremic patient, what are the alternatives?

3. Mr. Walker, who is oliguric and uremic, had a total urine output of 500 ml during the last 24 hours. What should his approximate fluid intake be for the next day?

4. What are the two modalities of treatment for the patient with end-stage renal failure and how are they related?

5. Define dialysis.

6. Differentiate between an external and an internal shunt.

Match the uremic complications in column A with the common therapies for the prevention or treatment of the condition in column B. Conditions may have more than one treatment.

Column A
7. _____ Hyperkalemia
8. _____ Hyperparathyroidism
9. _____ Hypertension
10. _____ Osteomalacia
11. _____ Hyperuricemia
12. _____ Peripheral neuropathy
13. _____ Gouty arthritis

Column B
a. Cardiac monitor
b. Kayexalate
c. Colchicine
d. IV glucose + insulin
e. ACE inhibitor drugs
f. Allopurinol
g. Calcium carbonate
h. Vitamin D
i. IV calcium gluconate
j. Progress halted only by dialysis
k. Na^+ restriction

Match the histocompatibility test in column A with the antigens or antibodies it detects in column B.

Column A
14. _____ RBC type and crossmatch
15. _____ Lymphocytotoxicity test
16. _____ Percent reactive antibody (PRA)
17. _____ WBC crossmatch

Column B
a. Class I and Class II HLA antigens
b. ABO antigens
c. Lymphocyte antibodies
d. Risk of reaction with a random donor

Answer the following on a separate sheet of paper.
18. Name two new developments that have greatly increased survival of cadaver kidney transplants.
19. Name several newer approaches to the removal of uremic solutes. How are they related to the middle molecular hypothesis?

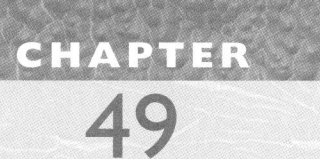

CHAPTER
49

Acute Renal Failure

LORRAINE M. WILSON

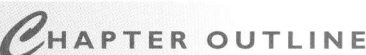

*A*cute renal failure (ARF) is a clinical syndrome characterized by a rapid decline in renal function (usually within a few days) leading to rapidly progressive azotemia. The rapid decline in glomerular filtration rate (GFR) causes the serum creatinine to rise as much as 0.5 mg/dl/ day and the blood urea nitrogen (BUN) as much as 10 mg/dl/day over several days. Acute renal failure (ARF) is usually associated with oliguria (urine output <400 ml/day). This criterion of oliguria is not arbitrary but is related to the fact that the average American diet contains about 600 mOsm of solute. If the maximal urine-concentrating ability is 1200 mOsm/L water, there is an obligatory loss of about 500 ml of water per day in the urine. Thus, when urine output falls below 400 ml/day, the solute load cannot be eliminated and the BUN and creatinine rise. However, oliguria is not a necessary feature of ARF. Recent evidence suggests that in one third to one half of ARF cases, urine output exceeds 400 ml/day and may be as high as 2 L/day. This form of ARF is called *nonoliguric*, or *high-output ARF*. ARF results in signs and symptoms similar to those of the uremic syndrome in chronic renal failure, reflecting failure of the kidney's regulatory, excretory, and endocrine functions. However, anemia and renal osteodystrophy are not usually features of ARF because of its acute onset.

ARF is a very common clinical syndrome, occurring in approximately 5% of hospitalized patients and as many as 30% of patients admitted to intensive care units. A wide variety of diseases, drugs, pregnancy-related complications, trauma, and surgical procedures may lead to ARF. In contrast to chronic renal failure, the majority of patients who develop ARF usually have prior normal renal function, and the condition is generally reversible. Despite these facts, mortality from ARF is very high (about 50%), even with the availability of dialysis treatment, perhaps reflecting the critical illnesses with which it is usually associated.

CAUSES OF ACUTE RENAL FAILURE

The causes of ARF are generally considered under three diagnostic categories: prerenal azotemia, postrenal azotemia, and intrinsic ARF (Box 49-1). This classification stresses that only in the third category (renal) is renal parenchymal damage sufficient to cause functional failure in itself. If prolonged, prerenal and postrenal factors are likely to lead to intrinsic renal failure, but with proper diagnosis, they are readily reversible. The most common intrinsic renal disease that leads to ARF is *acute tubular necrosis* (ATN), which describes a renal lesion in response to prolonged ischemia or exposure to a nephrotoxin. The diagnosis of ATN is made on the basis of excluding prerenal and postrenal causes of azotemia followed by exclusion of other causes of intrinsic renal failure (glomerular, vascular, and tubulointerstitial renal diseases).

Prerenal azotemia is the single most frequent cause of acute azotemia (>50% of cases), which may lead to ATN-type ARF. The common denominator of the prerenal causes of ARF is *prolonged renal ischemia* from decreased renal perfusion. Renal hypoperfusion is associated with a large variety of conditions resulting in intravascular volume depletion, decreased effective arterial circulating volume, or, rarely, renal vascular obstruction. Some of the most common prerenal conditions with increased risk of ARF are abdominal aortic surgery, open-heart surgery, cardiogenic shock, extensive burns, and septic shock. Most of these conditions are associated

■ Common Causes of Acute Renal Failure

PRERENAL AZOTEMIA (DECREASED RENAL PERFUSION)
1. Absolute extracellular fluid (ECF) volume depletion
   a. Hemorrhage: major surgery*; trauma, postpartum
   b. Excessive diuresis
   c. Severe gastrointestinal losses: vomiting, diarrhea
   d. Third space losses: burns*; peritonitis; pancreatitis
2. Decreased effective arterial circulating volume
   a. Reduced cardiac output: myocardial infarction; dysrhythmias; congestive heart failure; cardiac tamponade; pulmonary embolism
   b. Peripheral vasodilation: sepsis*; anaphylaxis; drugs: anesthesia, antihypertensives, nitrates
   c. Hypoalbuminemia: nephrotic syndrome; liver failure (cirrhosis)
3. Primary renal hemodynamic alterations
   a. Prostaglandin synthesis inhibitors: aspirin and other nonsteroidal antiinflammatory drugs (NSAIDs)
   b. Vasodilation of efferent arteriole: angiotensin-converting enzyme (ACE) inhibitors (e.g., captopril)
   c. Vasoconstrictor drugs: alpha-adrenergic agents (e.g., norepinephrine); angiotensin II
   d. Hepatorenal syndrome
4. Bilateral renal vascular obstruction
   a. Renal artery stenosis, emboli, thrombosis
   b. Bilateral renal vein thrombosis

POSTRENAL AZOTEMIA (URINARY TRACT OBSTRUCTION)
1. Urethral obstruction: urethral valves; urethral stricture
2. Bladder outflow obstruction: prostatic hypertrophy*, carcinoma*
3. Bilateral ureteral obstruction (unilateral if one functional kidney)
   a. Intraureteral: calculi, blood clots, sloughed papillae
   b. Extraureteral (compression): retroperitoneal fibrosis; neoplasm of bladder, prostate, or cervix; accidental surgical ligation or injury
4. Neurogenic bladder

INTRINSIC ACUTE RENAL FAILURE
1. Acute tubular necrosis
   a. Postischemic. Shock, sepsis, open-heart surgery, aortic surgery (all causes of severe prerenal azotemia)
   b. Nephrotoxic
      (1) Exogenous nephrotoxins
         (a) Antibiotics: aminoglycosides, amphotericin B
         (b) Iodinated contrast media (especially in diabetics)
         (c) Heavy metals: cisplatin, bichloride of mercury, arsenic
         (d) Cyclosporin; tacrolimus
         (e) Solvents: carbon tetrachloride, ethylene glycol, methanol
      (2) Endogenous nephrotoxins
         (a) Intratubular pigments: hemoglobin; myoglobin
         (b) Intratubular proteins: multiple myeloma
         (c) Intratubular crystals: uric acid
2. Primary renal glomerular or vascular disease
   a. Acute poststreptococcal or rapidly progressive glomerulonephritis
   b. Malignant hypertension
   c. Acute-on-chronic renal failure related to salt or water depletion
3. Acute tubulointerstitial nephritis
   a. Allergic: beta-lactams (penicillins, cephalosporins); sulfonamides
   b. Infection (e.g., acute pyelonephritis)

*Most common causes.

with systemic hypotension with compensatory activation of the sympathetic nervous system and the renin-angiotensin-aldosterone system. Angiotensin causes vasoconstriction of the renal, cutaneous, and splanchnic vascular beds, and aldosterone causes salt and water retention. This response is designed to maintain the systemic mean arterial pressure and perfusion to the vital organs. At the same time, renal autoregulatory mechanisms are activated to maintain the GFR and protect the kidney against ischemia. Angiotensin II preferentially causes constriction of the glomerular efferent arteriole (thus increasing intraglomerular pressure and GFR) and at the same time stimulates the production of vasodilator renal prostaglandins. The renal protective effect of prostaglandins can be negated by the administration of nonsteroidal antiinflammatory drugs (NSAIDs), such as aspirin, which block the production of these hormones. Thus administration of NSAIDs in the presence of renal hypoperfusion states from prerenal causes has been increasingly recognized as a precipitating cause of ischemic damage of the kidney in ARF. Angiotensin-converting enzyme (ACE) inhibitor drugs (which inhibit angiotensin II) may also precipitate ARF under conditions of renal hypoperfusion or renal vascular obstruction and so should be used with caution. The early treatment of prerenal azotemia may prevent its progression to ARF.

Postrenal causes of azotemia that may lead to ARF are less common (5%) than prerenal causes and refer to obstruction to the flow of urine at any level of the urinary tract. Prostatic enlargement (caused by cancer or benign hypertrophy) is the most common cause of bladder outlet obstruction. Cervical cancer may also cause obstruction of the urinary tract. Obstruction above the bladder (commonly caused by calculi) must be bilateral to cause urinary outflow obstruction, unless there is only one functioning kidney. It is important to realize that prolonged obstruction of urinary outflow will lead to hydronephrosis, severe damage to the renal parenchyma, and ARF. Thus the early identification and correction of urinary tract obstruction are crucial.

Acute tubular necrosis (ATN) is the most common renal lesion causing ARF (75%). ATN arises from either prolonged renal ischemia (from prerenal conditions already identified) or from exposure to nephrotoxins. Unfortunately, the terms *ATN* and *ARF* are used interchangeably in the clinical arena, although this is not correct. ATN refers to a type of lesion that is commonly but not invariably associated with ARF (see later discussion). ARF may be present without ATN. Other intrinsic renal causes of ARF without tubular necrosis include primary renal glomerular or vascular diseases such as acute poststreptococcal glomerulonephritis or malignant hypertension, respectively. Acute-on-chronic renal failure can also result from stresses such as infection or fluid loss from vomiting and diarrhea in a person with chronic renal failure and little renal reserve. Acute tubulointerstitial nephritis caused by an allergic reaction to an antibiotic or an acute pyelonephritis may likewise result in ARF. These other non-ATN causes of ARF must be ruled out before a diagnosis of ATN is made.

Nephrotoxic causes of ATN include both exogenous and endogenous nephrotoxins commonly causing the nonoliguric type of ARF. Exogenous nephrotoxins are categorized into four major groups: antibiotics, contrast media, heavy metals, and solvents.

Aminoglycoside antibiotic therapy is complicated by ARF in about 10% of the courses (e.g., gentamicin, kanamycin, tobramycin).

A variety of heavy metals are potent nephrotoxins and produce ARF with ATN. Cisplatin (platinum salt), a drug used to treat certain solid neoplasms, is the most common agent in this category. ATN caused by mercury, arsenic, chromium, or uranium is usually the result of occupational exposure, or the substance is ingested in a suicide attempt.

Both cyclosporine (used to treat transplant rejection) and contrast media can contribute to ARF by causing intrarenal vasoconstriction. Diabetics are particularly vulnerable to nephropathy from the use of contrast media. Additional risk factors for contrast media nephropathy include preexisting renal insufficiency, advanced age, volume depletion, multiple myeloma, and multiple exposures to contrast agents within a short period.

Nephrotoxic tubular injury can result from the ingestion of solvents such as ethylene glycol (antifreeze) or methanol (wood alcohol). The inhalation of fumes from carbon tetrachloride (CCl_4), a common ingredient in spot remover and other cleaning fluids, accompanied by the ingestion of ethyl alcohol (CH_3CH_2OH), is particularly dangerous because of a chemical reaction between these two compounds that forms a potent nephrotoxin. This set of circumstances (e.g., alcohol ingestion at a party and removing a clothing stain with spot remover) has resulted in ARF in a number of unsuspecting persons. For the same reasons, hobbyists using organic solvents and glues should work in well-ventilated rooms and refrain from drinking alcohol at the same time.

Endogenous nephrotoxins include hemoglobin, myoglobin, and Bence Jones protein (abnormal immunoglobulin produced in multiple myeloma). Hemolysis of red blood cells (RBCs) with the release of hemoglobin into the blood serum is usually caused by a mismatched blood transfusion. Large amounts of myoglobin are contained within muscles and may be released after a massive crush injury (rhabdomyolysis). When hemoglobin, myoglobin, or Bence Jones proteins are excreted in the urine, they have a direct toxic effect on the renal tubular cells and cause ARF. Finally, precipitation of uric acid crystals in the renal tubules, causing obstruction and ARF, may complicate certain "high turnover" malignancies (e.g., leukemia) or more commonly chemotherapy with cytotoxic agents. In both of these situations, massive cell lysis causes the release of large amounts of purine uric acid precursors. Uric acid crystallizes most readily in an acidic environment so precipitation can be prevented by administering allopurinol (inhibits uric acid synthesis) before chemotherapy or giving sodium bicarbonate to alkalinize the urine and forcing fluids.

PATHOLOGY OF ACUTE TUBULAR NECROSIS

The term *acute tubular necrosis (ATN)* is commonly applied to both nephrotoxic and ischemic renal injuries, although it does not reflect the nature and severity of the observed tubular changes. Two types of histologic lesions

are commonly observed in ATN: (1) necrosis of the tubular epithelium leaving the basement membrane intact, commonly resulting from the ingestion of nephrotoxic chemicals and (2) necrosis of both the tubular epithelium and the basement membrane, commonly associated with renal ischemia.

The severity of tubular damage in ATN caused by nephrotoxins is highly variable, and the prognosis varies accordingly. There may be necrosis of the proximal tubule epithelium with complete healing in 3 or 4 weeks. Bichloride of mercury and CCl_4 commonly produce this type of lesion. The prognosis is generally good with conservative management or supportive dialysis. In contrast, other poisons such as glycols may produce irreversible renal failure with infarction of the entire nephron, termed *acute cortical necrosis*. The prognosis in this case is poor. Calcification commonly occurs in the area of cortical necrosis if the patient is fortunate enough to survive.

Tubular damage caused by renal ischemia is also highly variable and depends on the extent and duration of the decreased renal blood flow and ischemia. There may be patchy or widespread destruction of the tubular epithelium and basement membrane or cortical necrosis. Many cases of acute cortical necrosis have followed complications of pregnancy, particularly premature separation of the placenta, postpartum hemorrhage, eclampsia, and septic abortion. When the basement membrane is disrupted, epithelial regeneration occurs in a random, haphazard manner, frequently leading to obstruction of the nephron at the site of necrosis. The prognosis depends on the extent of this type of change.

PATHOPHYSIOLOGY OF ACUTE RENAL FAILURE

Although there is now agreement concerning the pathology of the kidney damaged by ATN-type ARF, there is still considerable controversy over the pathogenesis of the suppression of renal function and the usually accompanying oliguria. Most modern concepts concerning possible causative factors are based on studies using animal experimental models in which nephrotoxic ARF is produced by injections of mercuric chloride, uranyl nitrate, or chromate, whereas ischemic damage is produced by injecting glycerol or clamping the renal arteries. Several pathologic processes have been proposed to explain the moderate reduction in renal blood flow and reduction in GFR observed in both experimental animals and humans, including (1) tubular obstruction, (2) backleak of tubular fluid, (3) decreased glomerular permeability, (4) vasomotor dysfunction, and (5) tubuloglomerular feedback. None of the proposed mechanisms can account for all the variable aspects of ATN-type ARF (Schrier, 1996).

The tubular obstruction theory proposes that ATN leads to the desquamation of necrotic tubular cells and other proteinaceous materials, which then form casts and occlude the tubule lumina. Cellular swelling as a result of the initial ischemia may also contribute to the obstruction and perpetuate the ischemia. Intratubular pressure increases, so that net glomerular filtration pressure is reduced. Tubular obstruction may be an important factor in ARF caused by heavy metals, ethylene glycol, or prolonged ischemia.

The tubular backleak hypothesis proposes that glomerular filtration continues normally but that the tubular fluid "leaks" out of the lumina through the damaged tubular cells into the peritubular circulation. Disruption of the basement membrane may be seen with severe ATN, which provides an anatomic basis for this mechanism.

Although the syndrome of ATN implies an abnormality of the renal tubule, recent evidence suggests that in some circumstances the glomerular capillary endothelial cells or basement membrane cells (or both) undergo changes that reduce permeability or the surface area for filtration. The result is a reduction of glomerular ultrafiltration.

Total renal blood flow (RBF) may be reduced to as low as 30% of normal in oliguric ARF. This level of RBF can be compatible with a substantial GFR. In fact, RBF in chronic renal failure is often as low as or lower than that found in the acute form, yet reduced but adequate renal function persists. Furthermore, experimental evidence suggests that RBF must be less than 5% before renal parenchymal damage occurs (Merrill, 1971). Thus it appears that renal hypoperfusion alone cannot account for the degree of reduction in GFR and the tubular lesions found in ARF. However, there is evidence of marked changes in the intrarenal distribution of blood flow from the cortex to the medulla during acute and prolonged hypotension. It will be recalled from Chapter 44 that, in the normal kidney, about 90% of the blood is distributed to the cortex (where the glomeruli are located) and 10% goes to the medulla. This action allows the kidney to concentrate urine and perform its functions. In contrast, in ARF the ratio of renal cortical to medullary blood distribution may be reversed, so there is relative ischemia of the renal cortex. Constriction of the afferent arterioles provides a vascular basis for the marked reduction in

GFR. Renal ischemia would then activate the renin-angiotensin system and perpetuate cortical ischemia after the initiating stimulus has disappeared. The highest concentration of renin is found in the outer cortex of the kidney (the site where ischemia is greatest) in animals and humans with ARF (Schrier, 1996). Some authors have postulated a role for prostaglandins in the vasomotor dysfunction of ARF (Harter, Martin, 1982). Renal hypoxia normally stimulates the renal synthesis of prostaglandin E and prostaglandin A (PGE and PGA) (potent vasodilators), causing renal blood flow to be redistributed to the cortex with resulting diuresis. It is possible that acute severe or prolonged ischemia may block the synthesis of these renal prostaglandins. Prostaglandin inhibitors such as aspirin are known to reduce RBF in normal persons and potentiate ATN (Schrier, 1996).

Tubuloglomerular feedback (TGF) is a phenomenon in which the flow to the distal nephron is regulated by receptors in the macula densa of the distal tubule, which lies in proximity to the glomerular pole. If distal flow of tubular filtrate were inappropriately increased, the reabsorptive capacity of the distal tubule and collecting ducts can be overwhelmed and lead to extracellular fluid (ECF) volume depletion. Thus TGF is a protective mechanism. In ATN, proximal tubular damage greatly reduces the absorptive capacity of the tubules. TGF is believed to be at least partly responsible for the decrease in GFR in the presence of ATN by causing constriction of the afferent arteriole or mesangial contraction or both, which lower intraglomerular capillary pressure (P_{gc}) and permeability, respectively. Thus a decrease in GFR caused by TGF can be considered an adaptive mechanism in ATN.

Fig. 49-1 illustrates a schema in which the various factors involved in the pathogenesis of ARF are combined.

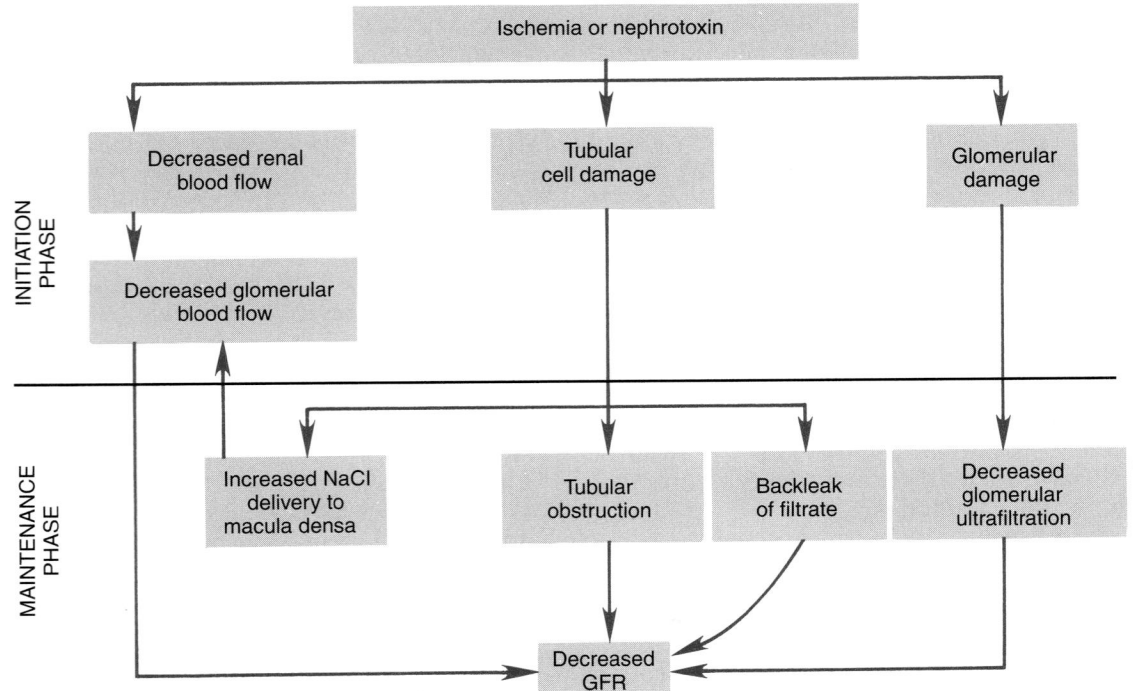

FIG. 49-1 Pathogenesis of acute renal failure. *NaCl,* Sodium chloride; *GFR,* glomerular filtration rate. (Redrawn from Harter HR, Martin KJ: Acute renal failure, *Postgrad Med* 72[6]:191, 1982).

The initiating event is generally an ischemic insult or a nephrotoxin, which damages the tubules or glomeruli or reduces RBF. ARF is then maintained through several possible mechanisms that may be present or absent and are a result of the initial injury. Each mechanism differs in the importance of its contributions to the pathogenesis according to the different theories cited. It is likely that the relative importance of these mechanisms varies with the situation and depends on the evolution of the disease process, as well as the severity of the pathologic damage. The pathophysiology of ARF is far from settled, and much more research is needed to define the relative importance of the various factors.

CLINICAL COURSE OF ACUTE RENAL FAILURE

The clinical course of ARF has been divided traditionally into three stages: oliguria, diuresis, and recovery. This tradition is followed in the following discussion while recognizing that ARF and azotemia may be present with urine output of more than 400 ml/24 hr. The clinical courses of oliguric and nonoliguric ARF are similar. However, abnormalities of blood chemistry are generally milder and the prognosis for recovery better in cases of nonoliguric ARF.

Oliguric Stage

The clinical picture is often dominated by the surgical, medical, or obstetric calamity causing the ARF. Oliguria is usually present within 24 to 48 hours after the initial injury, although this symptom may not occur until several days after exposure to nephrotoxic chemicals. Azotemia accompanies the oliguria.

It is critically important to recognize the onset of oliguria, determine the cause, and begin treatment of any reversible causes. ARF of the ATN type must be differentiated from prerenal (hypoperfusion) and postrenal (urinary tract obstruction) failure and other intrarenal disorders (e.g., acute poststreptococcal glomerulonephritis, acute pyelonephritis, acute-on-chronic renal failure). The diagnosis of ARF is made only after the other causes are excluded.

Oliguria caused by acute-on-chronic renal failure is usually evident from the history. Because patients with chronic renal failure have a limited ability to adjust fluid and electrolyte balance, they may be easily thrown into ARF by relatively minor upsets. Examples are the patient with chronic glomerulonephritis who has a gastrointestinal upset with vomiting or diarrhea or the patient with chronic pyelonephritis who gets a superimposed acute renal infection. Occasionally, a patient with undiagnosed chronic renal insufficiency may present in ARF. A history of long-standing nocturia, hypertension, systemic diseases such as systemic lupus erythematosus or diabetes mellitus, radiographic evidence of small, contracted kidneys, and signs of long-standing renal disease such as renal osteodystrophy are suggestive of chronic renal insufficiency. The patient can usually be restored to the previous state of health by treatment of the infection, correction of the fluid and electrolyte imbalance, and treatment by peritoneal dialysis if necessary.

Postrenal obstruction must be ruled out, especially if the cause of the renal failure is not apparent. The presence of anuria or of periods of anuria alternating with periods of normal urine flow suggests obstruction. Urethral and bladder neck obstruction can be evaluated by catheterization and determining residual urine in the bladder after an attempt at complete voiding. If outlet obstruction is ruled out but bilateral obstruction proximal to the bladder is suggested, ultrasound or radioisotope renal scan and retrograde pyelography may be performed.

Ultrasonography reveals renal size and may show evidence of obstructing calculi in the renal pelves or ureters. Radioisotope scans may be used to evaluate the integrity of the major renal vessels and are useful when occlusion of the renal artery or vein by an embolus or thrombus is suspected. Retrograde pyelography is used in selected cases of obstructive uropathy and may be therapeutic as well as diagnostic. Potential causes of obstruction are listed in Box 49-1. Prolonged obstruction will lead to intrinsic and often irreversible renal failure. Treatment involves immediate removal of the obstruction. Finally, prerenal oliguria is the most common antecedent situation leading to ARF and must be distinguished from ATN.

Prerenal Oliguria versus Acute Tubular Necrosis

Prerenal oliguria and azotemia are physiologic and potentially reversible; they result from shock, decreased plasma volume, and consequent decrease in RBF and GFR. Prerenal oliguria may result from any of the prerenal causes of ARF previously discussed. If left uncorrected, prerenal oliguria may progress to ATN. Serial determinations of the urine output, BUN level, creatinine level, and electrolytes should therefore be made after any major surgery, trauma, serious infection, or obstetric complication.

A few simple tests on the sediment and chemical constituents of the urine are helpful in distinguishing prerenal oliguria or azotemia from the true ARF of the ATN type (Table 49-1).

TABLE 49-1

Renal Indices in Prerenal Azotemia and Acute Renal Failure

Laboratory Test	Prerenal Azotemia	Acute Tubular Necrosis
Urinary Na+ concentration	<10 mEq/L	>20 mEq/L
Urine/plasma creatinine ratio	> 40:1	< 20:1
Urine/plasma urea ratio	> 8:1	< 3:1
FE_Na (%)*	< 1	> 1
BUN/creatinine ratio	>10:1	About 10:1
Urine osmolality	> 500 mOsm	Near 287 mOsm (fixed)
Urine/plasma osmolality ratio	> 2:1	< 1.1:1
Urine specific gravity	> 1.015	Near 1.010 (fixed)
Urinary sediment	Normal	Casts, cellular, debris

Na+, Sodium; FE_Na, fractional excretion of sodium; BUN, blood urea nitrogen.
*Most reliable index.

In prerenal oliguria, when there is not yet any damage to the renal parenchyma, the response of the kidney to decreased perfusion is to conserve salt and water. In contrast, intrinsic renal tubular damage is associated with impaired ability to conserve sodium. Consequently, urine sodium concentration is low in prerenal oliguria (<10 mEq/L) and high in ATN (>20 mEq/L).

Water reabsorption by the kidney is assessed by the concentration of a nonreabsorbable solute, such as creatinine, usually expressed as the ratio of the concentration of creatinine in urine to that of plasma (U/P creatinine). A U/P creatinine ratio of 2.0 indicates that 50% of the filtered water is reabsorbed, whereas a U/P creatinine ratio of 100 indicates that 1% of the filtered water is reabsorbed. Thus, in prerenal azotemia, the U/P creatinine ratio is high (>40), whereas it is low in the presence of intrinsic tubular renal disease (<20).

The U/P urea ratio is more than 8 in prerenal oliguria and less than 3 in established ATN. The U/P urea ratio is somewhat lower than the creatinine ratio, because there is some back diffusion of urea but not of creatinine. Thus the U/P creatinine ratio is a truer estimate of water reabsorption across the nephron.

The normal ratio of BUN to creatinine is 10:1. In prerenal azotemia this ratio is greater than 10:1 and may be 20:1 or greater. The high ratio of BUN to serum creatinine indicates the disproportionate rise of the blood levels of urea. Blood urea levels rise faster than creatinine levels because of the greater back reabsorption (its molecule is smaller than that of creatinine) in the situation of reduced renal perfusion. The production of urea may also increase markedly and contribute to the disproportionate increase in the BUN, because a catabolic state is often present in the acute illness and trauma associated with the development of prerenal azotemia.

Urine osmolality, specific gravity, and U/P osmolality ratio are additional indices of water handling by the kidney. In prerenal oliguria, urine osmolality is more than 500 mOsm (specific gravity >1.015) but decreases to about 287 mOsm (specific gravity 1.010) in established ATN as ability to concentrate is lost. The U/P osmolality progresses toward 1:1 in established ARF, indicating that the urine is isoosmotic with the plasma.

The urinary sodium concentration and U/P creatinine are the most reliable indices in distinguishing prerenal azotemia from ATN. When these indices are combined, the fractional excretion of sodium (FE_{Na}) can be calculated. The FE_{Na} is less than 1% in prerenal azotemia and is usually greater than this in established ATN. The FE_{Na} is a sensitive index in differentiating prerenal azotemia from established ARF. Fractional excretion of sodium is calculated by the following formula (Brady, Brenner, 1998).

$$FE_{Na} = \frac{U_{Na}}{P_{Na}} \times \frac{P_{Cr}}{U_{Cr}} \times 100\%$$

where U_{Na} = urinary concentration of sodium in mEq/L, P_{Na} = plasma concentration of sodium in mEq/L, U_{Cr} = urinary concentration of creatinine in mg/dl, and P_{Cr} = plasma concentration of creatinine in mg/dl.

Misleading results are occasionally obtained when (1) residual urine that has remained in the bladder for several hours is used, (2) a diuretic has been administered, (3) there is preexisting chronic renal disease, or (4) there is intermittent urinary tract obstruction.

Examination of the urine sediment may also be helpful in the differential diagnosis of ARF. In prerenal azotemia, the urine sediment is essentially normal with a few hyaline casts; brown, granular casts and many epithelial cells are likely to be present in ATN. Prerenal azotemia is fairly easy to exclude on the basis of the clinical setting and the urine chemistry. However, urine chemistry may not be helpful in differentiating postrenal obstruction from ATN and other criteria must be used.

Prevention of ATN in patients at high risk or those with prerenal azotemia or oliguria is an important therapeutic consideration. Correction of circulatory insufficiency and the resulting renal hypoperfusion is important in preventing the progression of prerenal oliguria to ATN. Blood transfusion to replace any losses and hydration with intravenous fluids may be successful in restoring circulation and increased urine output. Mannitol and furosemide have sometimes been successful in inducing diuresis and reducing the risk of oliguric ATN.

Harter and Martin (1982) suggest the following approach. After careful assessment of ECF volume and cardiac function (to exclude ECF volume excess), give 500 ml of intravenous normal saline rapidly to exclude prerenal oliguria. If urine output is unchanged, mannitol, 25 g, is given slowly intravenously (IV), followed by furosemide, 80 to 320 mg IV. If diuresis occurs (urine output >40 ml/hr), these doses may be repeated every 3 to 4 hours to maintain high urine flow rates. If this regimen is unsuccessful (urine output still <30 ml/hr), established ATN probably exists.

In established ATN, the period of oliguria may last no longer than a day or it may last as long as 6 weeks. The average duration of the oliguria is from 7 to 10 days. During the oliguric phase, the usual rise in BUN level is 25 to 30 mg/dl daily and creatinine rises at the rate of about 2.5 mg/dl daily. The retention of fluids, electrolytes, and nitrogenous substances causes the rapid development of uremic symptoms.

Diuretic Stage

The diuretic stage of ARF begins when the urine output increases to more than 400 ml/day. This stage generally lasts 2 to 3 weeks. Daily urine output rarely exceeds 4 L, provided the patient is not overhydrated. The high urine volume of the diuretic phase is caused partly by the osmotic diuresis produced by the high blood urea concentration and partly by the impaired ability of the recovering tubules to conserve filtered salts and water. During the diuretic phase, patients may develop deficits of potassium, sodium, and water. If the urinary losses are not replaced, death may end the diuresis. During the early diuretic stage, the BUN level may continue to rise, largely because urea clearance does not keep up with endogenous urea production. As the diuresis continues, however, the azotemia gradually disappears and there is great clinical improvement.

Recovery Stage

The recovery stage of ARF lasts as long as a year, during which time the anemia and concentrating ability of the kidneys gradually improve. Some patients, however, are left with a permanent reduction in the GFR. Approximately 5% of patients do not recover renal function and require long-term dialysis or renal transplantation; another 5% may have a progressive decline in renal function (Brady, Brenner, 1998).

Even though damage to tubular epithelium is theoretically reversible, ATN is a dangerous condition with a serious prognosis. The mortality is still about 50% (down from a previous rate of about 90% three decades ago) despite the most careful management of fluid and electrolyte balance and the aid of dialysis. About two thirds of patients with ATN die during the oliguric stage and about one third during the diuretic stage. Mortality is related to the causal background of the associated illnesses leading up to the acute episode. Mortality is about 60% in cases after surgery, crush injuries, and other major trauma, about 25% after incompatible blood transfusions and CCl₄ poisoning, and 10% to 15% in obstetric cases. Mortality rates are higher in older debilitated patients and in those with multiple organ failure. In general, patients with nonoliguric ARF have a better prognosis than do those with oliguric ARF: only about 25% of the former die.

TREATMENT OF ESTABLISHED ACUTE TUBULAR NECROSIS

Prevention of ischemic and nephrotoxic injury resulting in ATN requires careful attention to optimizing cardiovascular function, as well as maintaining ECF volume, especially in patients with preexisting risk factors or those taking nephrotoxic medications. Medications that reduce systemic resistance (e.g., afterload reducers) may cause renal vasoconstriction or affect the kidney's autoregulatory response (e.g., ACE inhibitors, cyclooxygenase inhibitors) and also should be used with caution. Once-daily dosing of aminoglycosides decreases the incidence of nephrotoxicity. Regular monitoring of cyclosporine blood levels can help maintain therapeutic levels and prevent nephrotoxicity. Saline infusion and hydration can reduce the incidence of nephrotoxic reactions to radiocontrast dye (Black, 1996).

After the diagnosis of ATN is established, the primary consideration is maintenance of fluid and electrolyte balance and treatment of any complications, such as infections. The same principles of conservative management in the treatment of chronic renal failure also apply to ARF. Dialysis (hemodialysis or peritoneal dialysis) replaces renal function until renal tubules regenerate and renal function is restored. Absolute indications for dialysis include signs and symptoms of the uremic syndrome, hyperkalemia, fluid retention, and severe acidosis. Continuous renal replacement may also be used in the treatment of ARF, either hemofiltration or hemodiafiltration (see Chapter 48). Generally, it is agreed that patients with multiorgan failure and hemodynamic instability benefit from a continuous mode, because it is typically less taxing on the hemodynamics. Some studies suggest that the use of biocompatible membranes, instead of the cellophane membranes used in standard hemodialysis, improve recovery rates and decrease mortality in ARF (Hakim et al, 1994). In addition to the maintenance of fluid and electrolyte balance, nutritional support improves survival. Adequate protein and caloric intake is essential, as marked increase in protein catabolism is often seen, especially in patients with shock, sepsis, or rhabdomyolysis. The risks of this catabolism include malnutrition and an impaired immune system.

Careful attention to fluid and electrolyte balance is necessary not only during the oliguric stage of ARF, but also during the diuretic stage when severe sodium, fluid, and potassium depletion may occur. The patient may lose 3 or more liters of fluid per day. There is a peculiar increased vulnerability to infection during the diuretic stage. Infections are still the leading cause of morbidity and mortality in ARF. Infection is the contributing cause of death in about 70% and the primary cause of death in 30% of patients. The presence of infection may go unrecognized because of the lack of the usual sign of fever, because hypothermia is common in renal failure. Once infection is identified, it should be treated with nonnephrotoxic antibiotics.

KEY CONCEPTS

- Acute renal failure (ARF) is a clinical syndrome characterized by a rapid decline in GFR (usually within a few days), azotemia, and perturbation of acid-base, fluid and electrolyte homeostasis.
- ARF occurs in approximately 5% of all hospitalized patients and up to 30% of patients in intensive care units and is associated with a high mortality (about 25% to 60%) depending on its cause, severity, and other factors.
- ARF may be oliguric or nonoliguric. In nonoliguric ARF, the clinical course tends to be shorter and the prognosis better (25% mortality) compared with oliguric ARF.
- In contrast to chronic renal failure, severe anemia and renal osteodystrophy are not common in ARF because of its acute onset.

- ARF is classified into three categories according to cause: prerenal, intrinsic, and postrenal. Distinguishing between the three categories is necessary to determine appropriate therapy.
- *Postrenal ARF (postrenal azotemia)*, which effectively equates with acute obstruction of urinary outflow, will cause hydronephrosis, severe damage to the renal parenchyma and intrinsic ARF if prolonged.
- The common denominator of *prerenal ARF (prerenal azotemia)* is *prolonged renal ischemia* from decreased renal perfusion; it is the most common cause of ARF.
- *Renal hypoperfusion* may occur in the setting of absolute ECF volume deficit (e.g., hemorrhage, gastrointestinal, renal or third-space fluid losses); decreased effective circulating volume (e.g., low cardiac output); bilateral renal vascular obstruction; and

renal hypoperfusion with impairment of renal autoregulatory responses (e.g., NSAIDs, ACE inhibitors, alpha-adrenergic drugs).

■ *Prerenal azotemia* is rapidly reversible upon restoration of renal blood flow (RBF) and glomerular ultrafiltration pressure.

■ *Acute tubular necrosis (ATN)* is a clinicopathologic entity characterized by the *destruction of tubular epithelial cells* and acute suppression of renal function. ATN is the most common cause of intrinsic ARF.

■ The diagnosis of ATN is made on the basis of excluding prerenal and postrenal causes of azotemia and other causes of intrarenal ARF (glomerular, vascular, and tubulointerstitial renal disease).

■ ATN arises from either prolonged renal ischemia (ischemic ATN) or from exposure to nephrotoxins (nephrotoxic ATN).

■ *Nephrotoxic causes of ATN* include exogenous (e.g., CCl_4, mercury, cyclosporine, contrast media) and endogenous nephrotoxins (e.g., hemoglobin, myoglobin, uric acid, Bence-Jones protein).

■ Clinical situations that carry a high risk of developing ischemic ATN are major surgery, severe burns, hemorrhage, and causes of severe hypotension and shock.

■ In addition to renal hypoperfusion, *pathogenic mechanisms causing ATN* include intrarenal vasoconstriction, especially of afferent arterioles; leakage of tubular fluid across the tubular basement membrane; obstruction of the tubules by casts; and tubuloglomerular feedback.

■ *Tubuloglomerular feedback* is a process leading to secondary changes in glomerular flow in ATN: (1) inadequate reabsorption of sodium chloride (NaCl) in the damaged proximal tubules leads to increased NaCl delivery to the distal tubules; (2) increased NaCl in the distal tubules is sensed by the macula densa; (3) the macula densa, in turn, causes constriction of the afferent arterioles further compromising glomerular perfusion in a vicious cycle.

■ The initiating phase of ARF is dominated by the inciting medical, surgical, or obstetric event in the ischemic form of ATN. Although this initial phase lacks specific signs and symptoms, clinicians should make every effort to recognize prerenal azotemia because effective intervention may reverse the azotemia and prevent the development of established renal disease.

■ *Urinary indices of established ATN* include high sodium excretion ($FE_{Na} > 1\%$) because sodium reabsorption is impaired, isoosmotic urine caused by impairment of concentrating ability by damaged tubules, and numerous granular and cellular casts or soughed tubular epithelial cells.

■ The clinical course of established ATN is characterized by three stages: (1) oliguric stage, (2) diuretic stage; and (3) recovery stage.

■ The *oliguric stage of ATN* (typically lasting 7 to 10 days) is characterized by sustained decreases in urine output, progressive azotemia, hypervolemia, hyperkalemia, metabolic acidosis, and other manifestations of the uremic syndrome.

■ The patient may be carried through the oliguric stage with appropriate management of fluid and electrolyte balance often with the help of dialysis treatment.

■ During the diuretic stage of ATN, usually lasting 2 to 3 weeks, urine volume increases but tubular function is still impaired so that the patient may develop deficits of potassium, sodium, and water.

■ Infections are the leading cause of morbidity and mortality in ARF, and there is a peculiar vulnerability to infection during the diuretic stage.

■ During the recovery stage of ATN, which may last up to one year, renal tubules are regenerating and the serum BUN and creatinine are normalized.

$\mathcal{Q}$UESTIONS ??

A sampling of review questions for this chapter appears here. Visit http://www.mosby.com/MERLIN/PriceWilson/ for additional questions. MERLIN

Answer the following on a separate sheet of paper.

1. Why is it particularly hazardous to use organic solvents (containing CCl_4) and drink an alcoholic beverage at the same time?

2. List the two major mechanisms of renal injury in acute intrinsic renal failure.

3. What is meant by acute-on-chronic renal failure? What are the precipitating causes?

4. What is the difference between the two types of histologic lesion commonly observed in ATN? What is the common cause?

5. What is acute cortical necrosis? List the common causes, complications, and prognosis.

6. What is the most common complication resulting in death in ARF?

7. What is the advantage of considering the causes of ARF under the prerenal, postrenal, and renal diagnostic categories?

8. List examples of common conditions causing obstructive uropathy at the level of the bladder outlet, ureters, and kidneys.

9. Name one penicillin and three aminoglycoside antibiotics that are frequently the cause of nephrotoxic ARF. What are the characteristics of patients at high risk?

10. Name and briefly describe five factors suggested as contributing to the pathogenesis of ARF.

11. What is the most sensitive laboratory test in differentiating prerenal azotemia from established ARF? By what formula is it calculated? Name some circumstances that may cause misleading laboratory test results.

12. Name two drugs commonly given in an attempt to correct prerenal oliguria and prevent progression to established ARF.

*B*IBLIOGRAPHY ■ PART EIGHT

Akash N: Dialysis-related amyloidosis: Pathogenesis and promoting factors: a review, *Dialysis and Transplantation* 29(6):325-329, 2000.

Asplin JR, Coe FL, Favus MJ: Nephrolithiasis. In Fauci AS et al, editors: *Harrison's principles of internal medicine*, ed 14, New York, 1998, McGraw-Hill.

Asplin JR, Coe FL, Favus MJ: Hereditary tubular disorders. In Fauci AS et al, editors: *Harrison's principles of internal medicine*, ed 14, New York, 1998, McGraw-Hill.

Astle SM: A new direction for dialysis, *RN* 64(7):56-60, 2001.

Badr KF, Brenner BM: Vascular injury to the kidney. In Fauci AS et al, editors: *Harrison's principles of internal medicine*, ed 14, New York, 1998, McGraw-Hill.

Bailey JL, Mitch WE: Pathophysiology of uremia. In Brenner BM, Rector FC, editors: *The kidney*, Vol. I and II, ed 6, Philadelphia, 2000, WB Saunders.

Balow JE: Renal manifestations of systemic lupus erythematosus and other rheumatic disorders. In Greenberg A, editor: *Primer on kidney diseases*, ed 2, New York, 1998, Academic Press.

Bennett WM, DeBrow ME: Analgesic nephropathy—a preventable renal disease, *N Engl J Med* 320(19):1269-1271, 1989.

Black RM: *Rose & Black's clinical problems in nephrology*, Boston, 1996, Little, Brown.

Brady HR, Brenner BM: Acute renal failure. In Fauci AS et al, editors: *Harrison's principles of internal medicine*, ed 14, New York, 1998, McGraw-Hill.

Brady HR, O'Meara YM, Brenner BM: The major glomerulopathies. In Fauci AS et al, editors: *Harrison's principles of internal medicine*, ed 14, New York, 1998, McGraw-Hill.

Brenner BM, Rector FC: *The kidney*, Vol. I and II, ed 6, Philadelphia, 2000, WB Saunders.

Bricker NS, Fine LG: On the meaning of the intact nephron hypothesis, *Am J Med* 46:1, 1969.

Buckalew VM: Nonsteroidal anti-inflammatory drugs and the kidney. In Greenberg A, editor: *Primer on kidney diseases*, ed 2, New York, 1998, Academic Press.

Carpenter CB, Lazarus JM: Dialysis and transplantation in the treatment of renal failure. In Fauci AS et al, editors: *Harrison's principles of internal medicine*, ed 14, New York, 1998, McGraw-Hill.

Cimino JE, Brescia MJ: Simple venipuncture for hemodialysis, *N Engl J Med* 267:608, 1962.

Delmez JA: Renal osteodystrophy and other musculoskeletal complications of chronic renal failure. In Greenberg A, editor: *Primer on kidney diseases*, ed 2, New York, 1998, Academic Press.

Diabetic Control and Complications Trial Research Group: Effects of intensive treatment on the development and progression of long-term complications in diabetes mellitus, *N Engl J Med* 329:977, 1993.

Dunfee TP: The changing management of diabetic nephropathy, *Hosp Med* 30(5):45-55, 1995.

Giordana C: Early diet to slow the course of chronic renal failure. Presented at Eighth International Congess of Nephrology. In Zurukzoglu W, editor: *Advances in basic and clinical nephrology*, Basal, Switzerland, Sept 1981.

Greenberg A, editor: *Primer on kidney diseases*, ed 2, New York, 1998, Academic Press.

Gutch CF, Stoner MH, Corea AL: *Hemodialysis for nurses and dialysis personnel*, ed 6, St Louis, 1999, Mosby.

Harter HR, Martin KJ: Acute renal failure, *Postgrad Med* 72(6):175-197, 1982.

Hassan A: Renal disease in the elderly, *Postgrad Med* 100(6):12-20, 1996.

Hening WA: Restless leg syndrome: diagnosis and treatment, *Hosp Med* 33(11):54-75, 1997.

Hutchinson I: Transplantation and rejection. In Riott I, Brostoff J, Male D, editors: *Immunology*, ed 3, St Louis, 1993, Mosby.

Julien BA: IgA nephropathy and related disorders. In Greenberg A, editor: *Primer on kidney diseases*, ed 2, New York, 1998, Academic Press.

Kass EH: Bacteriuria and pyelonephritis of pregnancy, *Arch Int Med* 105:194, 1960.

Klahr S et al: The effects of dietary protein restriction and blood pressure control on the progression of chronic renal disease: modification of diet in renal disease study group, *N Engl J Med* 330:877, 1994.

Kobrin S, Aradhye S: Preventing progression and complications in renal disease, *Hosp Med* 33(11):11-40, 1997.

Kunin CM: *Urinary tract infections*, ed 5, Baltimore, 1997, Williams & Wilkins.

Lapides J: *Fundamentals of urology*, Philadelphia, 1976, WB Saunders.

Lewis SL: Fever: thermal regulation and alterations in end-stage renal disease patients, *ANNA J* 19(1):13-18, 1992.

Merrill JP: Acute renal failure. In Strauss MB, Welt MB, editors: *Diseases of the kidney*, ed 2, Boston, 1971, Little, Brown.

Mitch WE: Dietary protein restriction in patients with chronic renal failure, *Kidney Int* 40:326-341, 1991.

Murray TG, Goldberg M: Analgesic-associated nephropathy in the USA: epidemiological, clinical, and pathogenetic features, *Kidney Int* 13:64, 1978.

Nally JV: Essential hypertension. In Greenberg A, editor: *Primer on kidney diseases*, ed 2, New York, 1998, Academic Press.

Norden CW, Kass EH: Bacteriuria of pregnancy—a critical appraisal, *Ann Rev Med* 19:431-70, 1968.

O'Callaghan CA, Brenner BM: *The kidney at a glance*, Malden, Mass, 2000, Blackwell Science.

Oldrizzi L, Rugiu C, Valvo E: The progression of renal failure in patients with renal disease of diverse etiology on protein-restricted diet, *Kidney Int* 27:553-557, 1985.

Opetz G: HLA matching should be utilized for improving kidney transplant success rates, *Transplant Proc* 23:46, 1991.

Pedrini MT et al: The effect of dietary protein restriction on the progression of diabetic and nondiabetic renal diseases: a meta-analysis, *Ann Int Med* 124:627, 1996.

Perneger TV, Whelton PK, Kag MJ: Risk of kidney failure associated with the use of acetaminophen, aspirin and NSAIDS, *N Engl J Med* 331:1675-1679, 1994.

Phillips BA: Restless legs syndrome: What is it? *Hosp Prac* 36(5):53-55, 2001.

Rose BD: *The pathophysiology of renal failure*, ed 2, New York, 1987, McGraw-Hill.

Rose BD, Rennke HG: *Renal pathophysiology: the essentials*, Baltimore, 1994, Williams & Wilkins.

Sanders PW: Dysproteinemias and amyloidosis. In Greenberg A, editor: *Primer on kidney diseases*, ed 2, New York, 1998, Academic Press.

Savage COS: Goodpasture's syndrome and anti-GBM disease. In Greenberg A, editor: *Primer on kidney diseases*, ed 2, New York, 1998, Academic Press.

Schrier RW: *Renal and electrolyte disorders*, ed 5, Philadelphia, 1997, Lippincott-Raven.

Schrier RW, Gottschalk CW: Acute renal failure. In *Diseases of the kidney*, ed 6, Philadelphia, 1996, Lippincott–Williams & Wilkins.

Siegel NJ: Minimal change nephropathy. In Greenberg A, editor: *Primer on kidney diseases*, ed 2, New York, 1998, Academic Press.

Sipe JD, Cohen AS: Amyloidosis. In Fauci AS et al, editors: *Harrison's principles of internal medicine*, ed 14, New York, 1998, McGraw-Hill.

Smith SL: *Tissue and organ transplantation: implications for professional nursing practice*, St Louis, 1990, Mosby.

Stamm WE, Hooten TM: Management of urinary tract infections in adults, *N Engl J Med*, 329:1328, 1993.

Svetkey LP: Renovascular hypertension. In Greenberg A, editor: *Primer on kidney diseases*, ed 2, New York, 1998, Academic Press.

Tolkoff-Rubin NE, Cotran RS, Rubin RH: Urinary tract infection, pyelonephritis, and reflux nephropathy. In Brenner BM, Rector FC, editors: *The kidney*, ed 6, Philadelphia, 2000, WB Saunders.

U.S. Renal Data System: *USRDS 2001 Annual Report*, Bethesda, Md, 2000, National Institute of Diabetes, and Digestive and Kidney Diseases, National Institutes of Health (NIH), DHHS. *http://www.usrds.org*

U.S. Renal Data System: *Incidence and causes of treated ESRD*, USRDS 1995 Annual Report, Bethesda, Md: National Institute of Diabetes, and Digestive and Kidney Diseases, National Institutes of Health (NIH), DHHS, *Am J Kidney Dis* 26(suppl 2):S39-S50, 1995.

Wehle MJ, Segura JW: Acute ureteral stones: clues to the diagnosis and initial treatment, *Hosp Med* 34(5):47-55, 1998.

Whalley P: Bacteriuria in pregnancy, *Am J Obstet Gynecol* 97:723-738, 1967.

PART
NINE

NEUROLOGIC SYSTEM DISORDERS

*M*ore than 200 clinical syndromes associated with dysfunction, disease, and injury of the nervous system are recognized. The clinical manifestations of disease involving the nervous system are perhaps the most complex and intriguing in all of medicine. Furthermore, many pathologies originating in other organ systems cause early neurologic symptoms, because of impairment of neuron function by adverse factors such as decreased blood flow or the presence of toxic metabolites. Signs and symptoms of these diseases vary in type and range from relatively simple, objective, and easily elicited signs to complex and highly individualized signs.

Only a select number of neurologic disorders are presented in this part of the text. This section begins with a concise overview of neuroanatomy, because an understanding of structure is essential to interpreting the signs and symptoms that can result from lesions within this complex body system. Organization of the nervous system is intricate but logical, and knowledge of certain core neuroanatomic relationships enables one to deduce many others by reasoning. Such a working knowledge of neuroanatomy is essential to selecting nursing assessments and to planning and evaluating care.

Anatomy and Physiology of the Nervous System

MARY S. HARTWIG AND LORRAINE M. WILSON

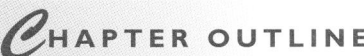

The human nervous system is a complex, highly specialized, interconnected network of neural tissue. It coordinates, interprets, and controls the interactions between the individual and the surrounding environment. This important body system also regulates the activities of most of the other body systems. The body is able to function as a harmonious unit because of the neural regulation of communications among the various systems. The phenomena of consciousness, thought, memory, language, sensation, and movement all originate within this system. Thus the ability to comprehend, learn, and respond to stimuli is a result of the integrated functioning of the nervous system, which culminates in the personality and behavior of the individual.

OVERVIEW OF THE HUMAN NERVOUS SYSTEM

This chapter provides a brief overview of selected anatomic and physiologic concepts concerning neural tissue. The constraints and the focus of this textbook do not permit an extensive coverage of this material. Readers are urged to seek the references given at the end of Part Nine to review and expand their knowledge of the nervous system.

The nervous system consists of nerve cells (neurons) and supporting cells (neuroglia and Schwann cells) so correlated and integrated that they function as a single unit. *Neurons*, with their processes, axons, and dendrites, are the basic building blocks of the nervous system; they are the specialized excitable cells of the nervous system that receive the *sensory*, or *afferent*, input from specialized endings of the peripheral nerves or sensory receptor organs and transmit the *motor*, or *efferent*, output to muscles and glands, the effector organs. Certain neurons, called *interneurons*, have the sole function of receiving and transmitting neural data to other neurons (Fig. 50-1). These interneurons, also called *association neurons*, are especially numerous in the gray matter of the spinal cord, where their interconnections are responsible for the many integrative functions of the spinal cord. *Neuroglia* provide support, protection, and nutrients for the neurons of the brain and spinal cord. *Schwann cells* protect and support the other neurons and neuronal processes outside the central nervous system.

The nervous system is divided into the central nervous system (CNS) and the peripheral nervous system (PNS).

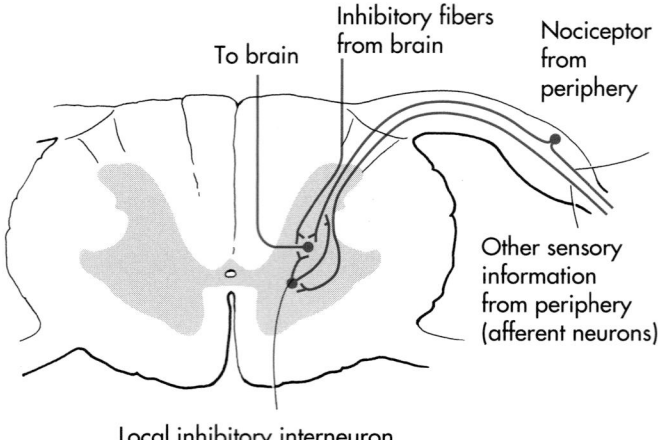

FIG. 50-1 An example of an inhibitory interneuron within the dorsal horn of the spinal cord. The interneuron (also called association neuron) transmits information from an incoming sensory neuron that modifies (in this case inhibits) the intensity of the incoming pain sensation from a nociceptor (pain receptor).

BOX 50-1
The Five Major Subdivisions of the Brain*

Telencephalon (endbrain)
  Cerebral hemispheres
    Cerebral cortex
    Rhinencephalon ("nosebrain"); limbic system
    Basal ganglia
      Caudate
      Lenticular (putamen, globus pallidus)
      Claustrum
      Amygdala
Diencephalon (interbrain)
  Epithalamus
  Thalamus
  Subthalamus
  Hypothalamus
Mesencephalon (midbrain)
  Corpus quadrigemina
    Superior colliculus
    Inferior colliculus
  Tegmentum
    Red nucleus
    Substantia nigra
  Cerebral peduncles
Metencephalon (afterbrain)
  Pons
  Cerebellum
Myelencephalon (marrow brain)
  Medulla oblongata

*The *prosencephalon* (forebrain) = telencephalon + diencephalon; the *rhombencephalon* = metencephalon + myelencephalon.

The brain and spinal cord constitute the CNS. The PNS is composed of the afferent and efferent neurons of the somatic nervous system and neurons of the autonomic (or visceral) nervous system.

The CNS is encased by the bones of the skull and vertebral column and is further protected by suspension in cerebrospinal fluid (CSF), which is produced within the ventricles (cavities) of the brain. The CNS is also covered by three layers of tissue collectively referred to as the *meninges* (dura mater, arachnoid, and pia mater).

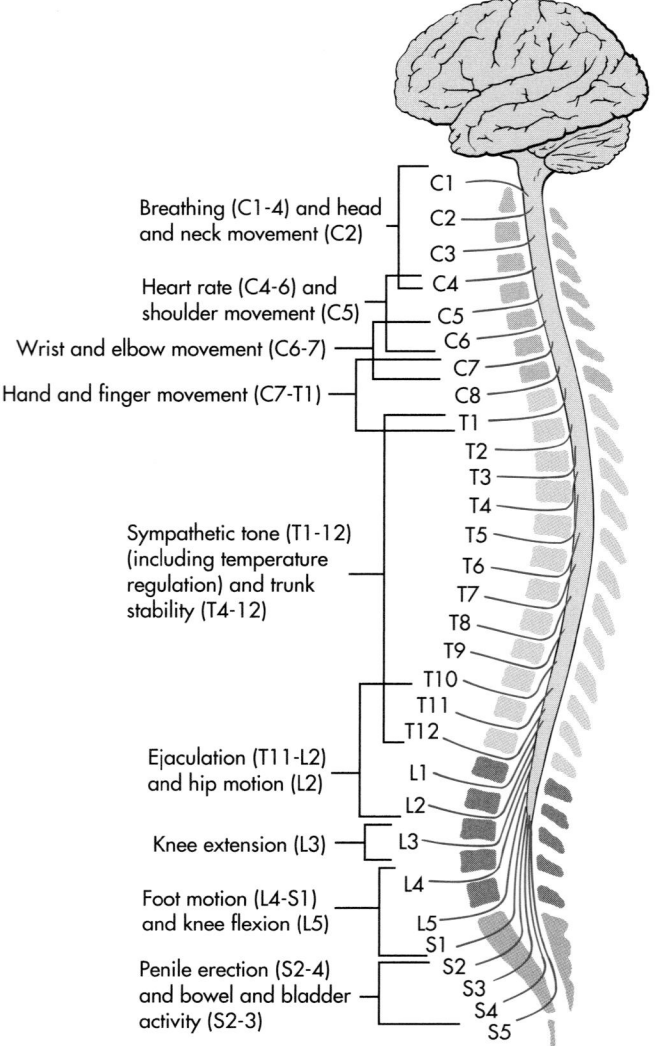

FIG. 50-2 Lateral view of the central nervous system.

The brain is divided into the forebrain, midbrain, and hindbrain on the basis of embryologic development. These categories are further subdivided on the basis of anatomic organization of the mature brain (Box 50-1). The midbrain, pons, and medulla oblongata together are called the *brainstem.*

The spinal cord is a single continuous structure that extends from the medulla oblongata through the foramen magnum of the skull and down the vertebral column to the lower level of the first lumbar vertebra (L1) in adults. The spinal cord is divided into 31 segments, from which originate the 31 pairs of spinal nerves. These segments are named after the vertebrae corresponding to the exit site for the associated nerve roots, thus giving rise to the cervical, thoracic, lumbar, and sacral divisions of the spinal cord (Fig. 50-2).

The PNS is divided anatomically into 31 pairs of spinal nerves and 12 pairs of cranial nerves. A *peripheral nerve* may consist of neurons relaying afferent (sensory) neural messages toward the CNS or relaying efferent (motor) neural messages from the CNS or both. The spinal nerves carry both afferent and efferent neural messages and are thus called *mixed nerves*. The cranial nerves

TABLE 50-1

Autonomic Effects on Various Organs

Effector Organ	Effect of Sympathetic Stimulation	Effect of Parasympathetic Stimulation
EYE		
Pupil	Dilation (mydriasis)	Contraction (miosis)
Ciliary muscle	Relaxation (far vision)	Contraction (near vision)
GLANDS OF HEAD		
Lacrimal	Decreased secretion	Stimulation of secretion
Nasopharyngeal	Decreased secretion	Stimulation of secretion
Salivary	Scanty, viscous secretion	Profuse, watery secretion
Heart	Increased rate	Decreased rate
	Increased conduction velocity	Decreased conduction velocity
	Increased force of beat	Decreased force of beat
BLOOD VESSELS*		
Coronary	Vasodilation	Minimal
Skeletal muscle	Vasodilation	Minimal
Abdominal viscera	Vasoconstriction	Minimal
Cutaneous	Vasoconstriction	Minimal
BLOOD		
Coagulation	Increased	
Glucose	Increased	
Free fatty acids	Increased	
Lungs	Bronchodilation	Bronchoconstriction
GUT		
Lumen	Decreased peristalsis and tone	Increased peristalsis and tone
Sphincters	Increased tone (usually contraction)	Decreased tone (usually relaxation)
Secretions	Possible inhibition	Stimulation
Liver	Glycogenolysis	
Gallbladder and ducts	Inhibition of contraction	Stimulation of contraction
Adrenal medulla	Secretion of epinephrine and norepinephrine	
Bladder muscle	Relaxation (usually)	Contraction
Sex organs	Ejaculation	Erection
Sweat glands	Stimulation of certain sweat glands	
Pilomotor muscles	Contraction	
Adipose tissue	Lipolysis	

*Effects of sympathetic stimulation depend on whether alpha$_1$-adrenergic receptors (vasoconstriction) or beta$_2$-adrenergic receptors (vasodilation) are stimulated.

arise from the surface of the brain; five pairs are motor, three pairs are sensory, and four pairs are mixed nerves. Functionally, the PNS is divided into the somatic nervous system and the autonomic nervous system.

The *somatic nervous system* (SNS) is composed of mixed nerves. The afferents convey conscious and unconscious sensory information (e.g., pain, temperature, touch, conscious and unconscious proprioception, vision, taste, hearing, smell) from the head, body wall, and extremities. The efferents are involved primarily with the skeletal musculature of the body. The SNS is concerned with interaction and response to the external environment.

The *autonomic nervous system (ANS)* is a mixed nervous system; its afferent fibers carry input from visceral organs (concerning the regulation of heart rate, blood vessel diameter, respiration, digestion, hunger, nausea, and elimination). The motor efferents of the ANS innervate smooth muscle, cardiac muscle, and glands of the viscera. The ANS regulates primarily visceral functions and interactions with the internal environment.

The two divisions of the ANS are the parasympathetic autonomic nervous system (PANS) and the sympathetic autonomic nervous system (SANS). The *sympathetic divi-*sion leaves the CNS from the thoracic and lumbar (thoracolumbar) regions of the spinal cord; the *parasympathetic division* leaves from the brain (via components of cranial nerves) and the sacral portion (craniosacral) of the spinal cord. The SANS increases heart and respiratory rates and decreases activity of the gastrointestinal (GI) tract. The primary focus of the SANS is to prepare the body for stress, the so-called fight-or-flight responses. In contrast, the PANS decreases heart and respiratory rates and increases GI motility as needed for digestion and elimination; it aids in conservation and homeostasis of body functions. Table 50-1 lists some of the important functions of the sympathetic and parasympathetic divisions of the ANS.

NEURAL TISSUE

Neuroglia, Schwann Cells, and Myelin

Neuroglia are the supporting cells for the neurons of the CNS, whereas Schwann cells have this function in the PNS. The neuroglia comprise about 40% of the volume

FIG. 50-3 Diagrammatic representation of the different types of neuroglial cells of the central nervous system. **A,** Fibrous astrocyte are found mainly in white matter; note glial foot processes in association with a capillary. **B,** Protoplasmic astrocytes are found in gray matter. **C,** Oligodendrocyte. **D,** Microglial cell. **E,** Ependymal cells. (Redrawn from Willis WD Jr, Grossman RG: *Medical neurobiology: neuroanatomical and neurophysical principles basic to clinical neuroscience,* ed 3, St Louis, 1981, Mosby.)

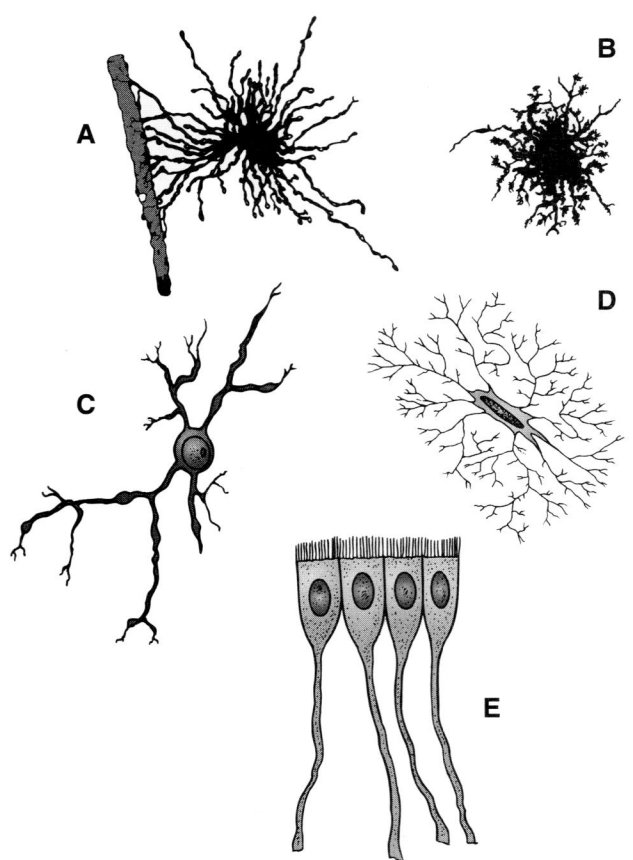

of the brain and spinal cord, and they outnumber the neurons approximately 10:1. Four distinct neuroglial cell types have been identified: microglia, and three types of macroglia (ependymal cells, astroglia, and oligodendroglia) (Fig. 50-3).

Microglia have phagocytic properties; when nervous tissue is damaged, these cells ingest and digest tissue debris. Microglia cells are found throughout the CNS and also have a role in fighting infection. These cells have properties similar to those of histiocytes (macrophages) found in peripheral connective tissue.

Ependymal cells (or *ependymocytes*) are involved in the production of CSF. These cells are the neuroglia that line the ventricular system of the CNS and provide the epithelial lining (ependyma) of the choroid plexus of the cerebral ventricles.

Astroglia (or *astrocytes*) provide essential nutrients to neurons and assist neurons in maintaining the proper bioelectrical potentials for impulse conduction and synaptic transmission. Astroglia have star-shaped cell bodies with multiple processes.

Because many of the astrocyte processes terminate on blood vessels as perivascular "feet" or foot processes, they are involved in a system of rapid transport of metabolites and also in preventing certain substances from passing from the blood vessels to neural tissue. Thus the pericapillary foot processes of astrocytes form one of the three interfaces among the blood, brain, and CSF. Together these three interfaces are collectively called the *blood-brain barrier* (Adams et al, 1997). The other two interfaces are the endothelium of the choroidal and brain capillaries that are bound together by "tight junctions" and the plasma membrane and adventitia of these vessels. The barrier formed by the capillary endothelium prevents larger molecules such as albumin (and molecules such as bilirubin bound to albumin) from entering the CSF. This anatomic barrier explains why certain dyes such as aniline, if injected into the blood, will not penetrate nervous tissues. However, the dyes will penetrate if injected into the subarachnoid space, because the blood-brain barrier systems are bypassed (Fig. 50-4). Smaller molecules are blocked from access to the brain tissue by the capillary plasma membrane and the astrocyte foot processes.

In general, the interfaces between the blood and the CSF and brain interstitial fluid are highly permeable to lipophilic substances, such as alcohol and most anesthetics, and to water, carbon dioxide, and oxygen. The blood-brain barrier is only slightly permeable to sodium, chloride, potassium, and bicarbonate ions and nearly impermeable to plasma proteins and most large organic molecules, which are not lipid soluble. Though

these barriers protect the CSF and brain tissue from foreign substances, they often make it impossible to achieve effective concentrations of therapeutic drugs in the CSF or cells of the brain tissue.

Another important barrier to passage of substances into the brain is the *blood-CSF barrier,* which exists because of the secretory function of the choroid plexus. The blood-CSF barrier is formed by tight junctions between the cuboidal epithelial cells of the choroid plexus in the ventricles, which actively secrete CSF (Fig. 50-5), and not at the choroid capillaries, which are fenestrated. The ependymal lining of the ventricles and the pia-glial surface of the brain do not impede exchanges between CSF and the brain. Thus the CSF may serve as a channel for intracerebral transport.

The primary role of the blood-brain and blood-CSF barriers is to provide control systems that regulate and maintain an optimal, stable chemical environment for the neurons of the CNS. In general, the barriers are highly permeable to water, oxygen (O_2), carbon dioxide (CO_2), glucose, and essential amino acids and are less permeable to electrolytes such as sodium (Na^+), chloride (Cl^-), hydrogen (H^+), and potassium (K^+) ions. The barriers are relatively impermeable to macromolecules such as proteins, hexoses other than glucose, free fatty acids, many drugs, and toxic substances.

In newborns, when these barriers are not fully developed, toxic substances such as bilirubin can readily enter the CNS, causing a condition called *kernicterus* (see Chapter 27). Any injury to the brain, whether from trauma, inflammation, or toxins, causes a breakdown of the blood-brain barrier, allowing free diffusion of large molecules into the nervous tissue.

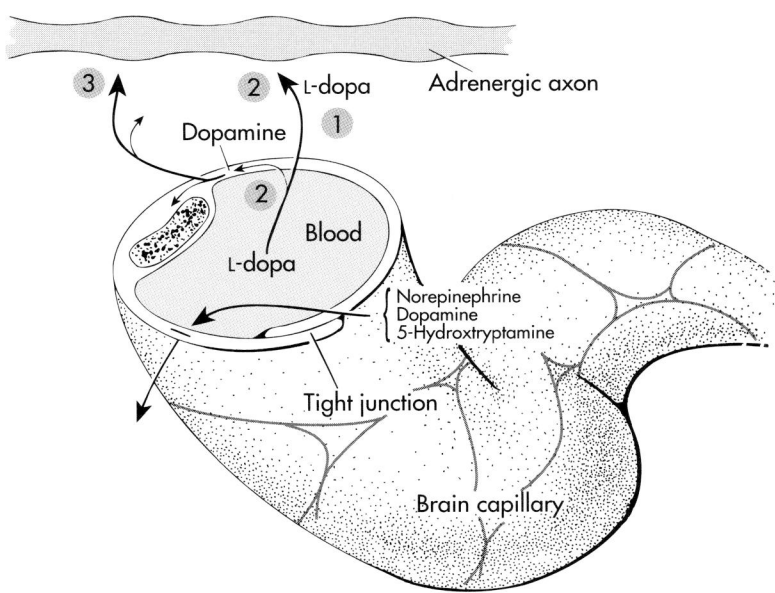

FIG. 50-4 Diagram of a brain capillary demonstrating a tight junction between endothelial cells that constitute the blood-brain barrier. The endothelial cells of brain capillaries contain enzymes that regulate the specific transport of brain biogenic amines (norepinephrine; dopamine; 5-hydroxytryptamine [5-HT], or serotonin; amino acids). Levodopa (l-dopa), an amino acid precursor of dopamine used in the treatment of Parkinson's disease, passes the blood-brain barrier *(1)*, is decarboxylated in the capillary endothelium *(2)*, and enters neural tissue *(3)*, where it is degraded by monoamine oxidase. Decarboxylation of L-dopa to dopamine *(2)* also takes place after its incorporation into axonal varicosities of aminergic neurons. (Redrawn from Carpenter MB: *Core text of neuroanatomy,* ed 4, Baltimore, 1991, Williams & Wilkins.)

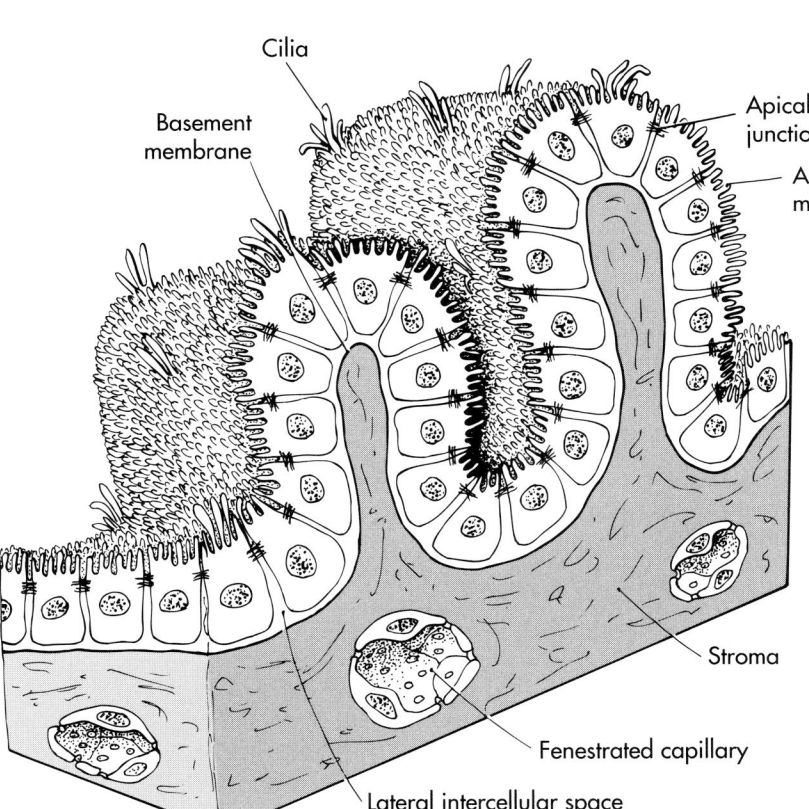

FIG. 50-5 Blood–cerebrospinal fluid (CSF) interface. Diagram of a choroid plexus villus covered by a single layer of cuboidal epithelium, with apical microvilli protruding into the CSF of the ventricles. The blood-CSF barrier is formed by the apical tight junctions between the epithelial cells. The choroid capillaries in the underlying connective tissue are fenestrated. (Redrawn from Carpenter MB: *Core text of neuroanatomy,* ed 4, Baltimore, 1991, Williams & Wilkins.)

When neurons die as a result of injury, astrocytes proliferate and fill in the space formerly occupied by the nerve cell body and its processes, an activity known as *replacement gliosis* (see the following comments on nerve cell damage). When extensive destruction of CNS tissue occurs, a cavity may be formed that becomes lined with astrocytes.

Oligodendroglia (or *oligodendrocytes*) are the glial cells responsible for myelin production within the CNS. Each oligodendrocyte surrounds several neurons, and its

plasma membrane wraps around the neuronal processes to form the myelin sheath. The Schwann cells form the myelin in the PNS.

Tumors of the neuroglia are referred to as *gliomas* and account for 40% to 50% of intracranial tumors (see Chapter 57).

Myelin is a white lipid-protein complex that insulates the nerve process. When present, myelin almost completely prevents the flow of Na$^+$ and K$^+$ ions across the neuronal membrane. Myelin is not continuous along the nerve processes, and the intervals where it is absent are called the *nodes of Ranvier* (Fig. 50-6). Nerve processes in the CNS and PNS may or may not be myelinated. Nerve fibers with myelin sheaths are called *myelinated fibers* and within the CNS are called *white matter*. Fibers that have no myelin are called *nonmyelinated fibers* and are present within the *gray matter* of the CNS. Transmission of nerve impulses along myelinated fibers is faster than it is along nonmyelinated fibers, because the impulses travel, or "jump," from node to node along the myelin sheath; this is known as *saltatory conduction*.

Schwann cells form the myelin and the neurilemma of peripheral nerves (see Fig. 50-6). The plasma membrane of Schwann cells concentrically wraps around nerve processes of the neurons in the PNS to form the myelin sheath. Not all neurons of the PNS are myelinated. The *neurilemma* is a delicate cytoplasmic membrane formed by Schwann cells that wraps around all PNS neurons (myelinated and nonmyelinated). The neurilemma provides structural support and protection for the nerve processes.

When there is damage to a nerve cell process in the PNS, a potential exists for regeneration of the nerve fiber. A complex series of degenerative and regenerative changes occurs along the damaged area as long as the cell body is still viable. When possible, the neurilemma regenerates along its original course, and a new process sprouts and grows within the neurilemma from the cell body of the damaged neuron.

No neurilemma exists in the CNS; and thus little or no regenerative potential exists for damaged central neuronal processes. The damaged areas of the CNS neurons are filled with glial cells (primarily astrocytes) through the process of replacement gliosis. A gliotic scar after brain injury may result in focal epilepsy (see Chapter 55).

Neurons

A *neuron* is a nerve cell and is the basic anatomic and functional unit of the nervous system (see Fig. 50-6). Neurons are similar to other cells in the body in several ways: they have a nucleus that contains genes, contain organelles such as mitochondria, and perform basic cellular processes such as energy production and protein synthesis. Neurons also differ from other cells in the human body in that they have specialized extensions or processes called *axons* and *dendrites*, communicate with each other through electrical and chemical processes, and contain some unique specialized structures (e.g., neurotransmitter vesicles called quanta and functional gaps between transmitting and receiving cells called synapses). Each neuron has a cell body that gives rise to one or more processes. *Dendrites* are processes that conduct information toward the cell body. The single long process that

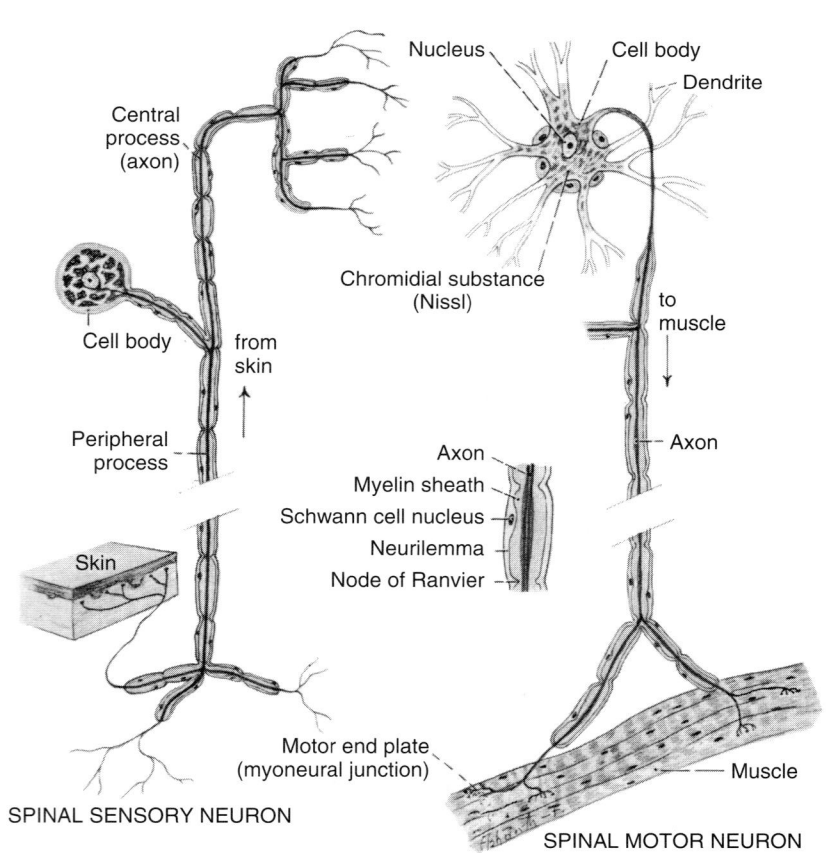

FIG. 50-6 Motor and sensory neurons. (From Jacob SW, Francone CA, Lossow WJ: *Structure and function in man*, ed 5, Philadelphia, 1982, Saunders.)

conducts information away from the cell body is called an *axon.* Dendrites and axons are often referred to, collectively, as *nerve fibers* or *nerve processes.* The ability to receive, convey, and transmit neural messages is a result of the specialized neuronal cell membrane properties of excitability and electrical-chemical conductivity. The human nervous system is composed of approximately 10^{11} (100 billion) neurons, as many (it is estimated) as there are stars in our galaxy. Neurons vary in size, shape, and length of processes. A distinction is also made according to the direction of flow of neural impulses. Thus there are afferent (sensory) neurons, efferent (motor) neurons, and internuncial (associational) neurons.

Neurons are classified as unipolar, bipolar, or multipolar according to the number and pattern of processes arising from the cell body. *Unipolar neurons* have a single process that divides into two branches a short distance from the cell body. One branch is directed toward the periphery, and the other branch travels toward the CNS. An example of a unipolar neuron is the sensory neuron of a spinal nerve (see Fig. 50-6). *Bipolar neurons* have two processes: one axon and one dendrite. Retinal rod and cone cells are bipolar neurons. *Multipolar neurons* have several dendrites and one axon, which may undergo extensive branching. Most neurons of the CNS are multipolar; for example, the motor neurons arising in the ventral horn of the spinal cord have axons that extend to skeletal muscle (see Fig. 50-6).

Neurons are also classified by the length of their processes. *Golgi type I* neurons have a long axon that may extend more than a meter in length, for example, a motor neuron from the sacral spinal cord that extends to the tips of the toes. The long fiber tracts of the brain and spinal cord and the nerve fibers of the PNS are composed of axons of this type of neuron. *Golgi type II* neurons have short axons that terminate close to the cell body. The dendrites are also short and are clustered around the cell body. Golgi type II neurons are numerous in the brain and spinal cord and are much more common than type I neurons.

A neuron, or nerve cell, shares in the biochemical machinery of all other living cells. In addition to production of energy to maintain and repair themselves, the metabolically active nerve cells make and release chemicals called neurotransmitters. Neurons primarily use glucose as a metabolic fuel but are essentially restricted to oxidative metabolism.

Most neuronal intracellular organelles are present in the cell body cytoplasm, although some are present within the cell processes. Cellular organelles and inclusions include protein-synthesizing *Nissl substance* composed of rough endoplasmic reticulum; protein-storing and protein-processing Golgi bodies; and energy-producing mitochondria, neurofibrils, microfilaments, and microtubules involved in intracellular transport. The cell body and dendritic cytoplasm are about equivalent in the types of organelles present, but the axons notably lack Nissl substance. The region of the axon known as the *axon terminal* (see following discussion) is metabolically active and contains a high concentration of intracellular organelles, especially mitochondria. The nucleus and the prominent nucleolus are located in the cell body. The centrosome may be seen in neurons prenatally and during the first few months of postnatal life, when mitosis is still possi-

ble. Centrosomes are generally absent from mature neurons, however, because these cells are incapable of dividing and increasing their numbers.

Dendrites may be long neuronal processes and branch only at their ends, or they may be short and have multiple branches. Dendrites usually transmit neural impulses toward the cell body and may be considered as extensions of the cell body to increase the receptive area for neural messages. Dendrites undergo terminal branching, and the terminal branches are called *dendritic spines.*

Each neuron has only one axon, which may be short, long, or of an intermediate length, depending on the function of the given neuron. Axons within the human nervous system can be less than 1 mm or more than 1 m in length. Axons usually arise from the cell body in an area called the *axon hillock.* The axon may give rise to a branch along its course, called an *axon collateral.* Close to the site of termination, axons branch profusely. The terminal branches, called *telodendria,* are slightly enlarged at the distal ends. The enlargements are called *synaptic boutons* or *knobs.* The diameters of axons vary from neuron to neuron and are related to the function of the neuron: the larger the diameter, the faster the conduction of the impulse. The conduction of a neural impulse along an axon is also affected by whether myelin is present, because conduction along myelinated fibers is faster.

Neurotransmitters are chemicals synthesized in the neurons, stored in synaptic vesicles in the axon terminals, and released from the axon terminal by *exocytosis.* Once released at the presynaptic junction, neurotransmitters bind with their receptors on the postsynaptic cell, causing transmission of the action potential and a cascade of chemical changes within the second cell. The neurotransmitter remaining within the synaptic cleft is then removed from the junction, which enables the postsynaptic cell membrane to repolarize and a new potential to be transmitted. Removal of the neurotransmitter molecules can be achieved by three major mechanisms: (1) removal from the synaptic cleft via diffusion or action of glial cells, (2) enzymatic degradation (deactivation) so that the structure of the neurotransmitter is no longer recognized by its receptor (acetylcholine is removed by this mechanism), and (3) reuptake, whereby the whole neurotransmitter molecule is taken back into the axon terminal that released it (norepinephrine and serotonin both are removed by this mechanism) (Fig. 50-7). Preventing any of the three removal processes will prolong the time the neurotransmitter stays in the synaptic cleft and thereby prolong its action on the postsynaptic cell. Thus, for example, medications that selectively inhibit reuptake of a neurotransmitter by its presynaptic cell effectively enhance the action of that neurotransmitter on the postsynaptic cell. Typical of this type of agent is a group of serotonin agonist medications called serotonin-specific reuptake inhibitors (SSRIs). Examples are fluoxetine (Prozac), sertraline (Zoloft), and paroxetine (Paxil). Until recently, it was thought that a neuron produced and released only one type of transmitter, called "Dale's law." However, there is now evidence that neurons can contain and release more than one kind of neurotransmitter. These chemicals change the cell permeability of a neuron, making it more or less able to conduct an impulse, depending on the neuron and the transmitter. There are about 30 known or suspected neurotransmitters, including norepinephrine, acetylcholine, dopamine, serotonin, gamma-aminobutyric acid (GABA), and glycine.

Neurons conduct neural signals throughout the body, using electrical conduction within individual neurons and chemical conduction between neurons. Neurons are not anatomically continuous with one another. The areas where neurons come in contact with other neurons or effector organs are called *synapses*. The synapse is the only location where an impulse can pass from one neuron to another or to an effector. The space between one neuron and the next neuron (or effector organ) is called the *synaptic cleft*. The neuron bringing the nerve impulse toward the synapse is called the *presynaptic neuron;* the one leaving is the *postsynaptic neuron.* An estimated 10^{14} synapses exist in the human nervous system. Synapses can be between an axon and a dendrite *(axodendritic synapse),* between an axon and a cell body *(axosomatic synapse),* between axons *(axoaxonic synapse),* and between dendrites *(dendrodendritic synapse).* One neuron can make synaptic contact with many neurons *(divergence)* and may receive synaptic contact from many neurons *(convergence)* (Fig. 50-8).

The electrical component of neural transmission deals with the transmission of the neural impulses along the length of the neuron. Neurons have cell membranes with a variable selective permeability to Na^+ and K^+ ions that is affected by chemical and electrical changes in the neuron, most notably neurotransmitters and receptor organ stimuli, respectively. In the resting state the cell membrane permeability creates a high intracellular K^+ concentration and a low intracellular Na^+ concentration, even in the presence of a high extracellular Na^+ concentration. Electrical impulses are generated by the separation of charges caused by the intracellular and extracellular ion concentration differences across the cell membrane.

If the stimuli causing electrical changes in the neuronal cell membrane cause an increased permeability to K^+ ions, the neuron becomes *hyperpolarized* and inhibited. Hyperpolarized neurons are unable to carry a nerve impulse. When the stimulus causing the electrical changes results in an increased permeability to Na^+ ions, the neuron becomes excited or *depolarized.* If the membrane is depolarized to a critical level, called the *excitation threshold,* a change of membrane permeability occurs, with sudden influx of Na^+, rapid depolarization, and generation of an action potential at the point of stimulation.

An *action potential* is transmitted along the axon as an all-or-none phenomenon rather than as a graded response. When the action potential reaches the axon ter-

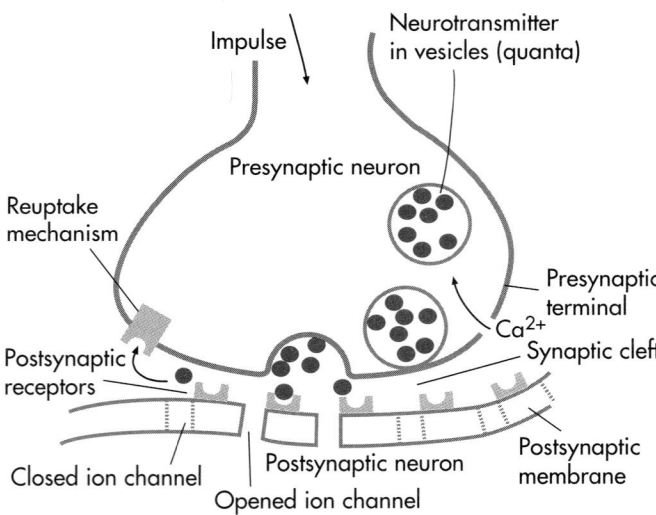

FIG. 50-7 Neurotransmitter release, binding, and reuptake at the site of a synapse between two neurons. The neurotransmitter (black circles) is synthesized within the presynaptic terminal and released within small vesicle packets called quanta. An action potential arriving at the presynaptic terminal causes fusion of the vesicle to the terminal membrane, resulting in release of the neurotransmitter into the synaptic cleft. When the neurotransmitter binds to its specialized receptors on the postsynaptic membrane, a chain reaction of chemical and electrical changes occur within the postsynaptic neuron. The neurotransmitter activity is then halted by its removal from the synaptic cleft by another mechanism that carries it back into the presynaptic terminal, where it is reused or degraded into its precursor molecules. For example, the enzyme monoamine oxidase (MAO) degrades serotonin and norepinephrine. Antidepressants called MAO inhibitors prevent such degradation. Newer antidepressant drugs block reuptake of the neurotransmitter from the synaptic cleft, allowing it to remain in the synaptic cleft for a longer period of time. As a result, the functional activity of the neurotransmitter is increased. Serotonin-specific reuptake inhibitors (SSRIs) such as Prozac and Paxil work by that mechanism.

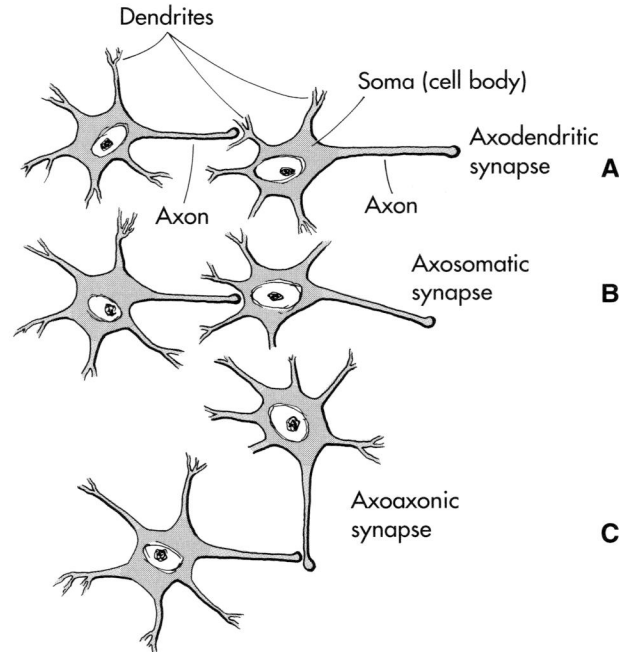

FIG. 50-8 Types of synapses. **A,** Axodendritic synapse; **B,** axosomatic synapse; **C,** axoaxonic synapse. The manner in which an axon terminates varies in different parts of the nervous system. A single axon may terminate on a single neuron; or single axon may synapse with multiple neurons (divergence); or a single neuron may receive synaptic contact from many neurons (convergence). The arrangement of these synapses will determine the means by which a neuron can be stimulated or inhibited. Convergence and divergence are important neural mechanisms of processing and integrating information.

minal, it causes a release of the neurotransmitter from synaptic vesicles by exocytosis into the synaptic cleft. The transmitter attaches itself to a receptor site on the postsynaptic neuronal or effector membrane and may or may not initiate an action potential in the postsynaptic membrane. Each neuron is covered with many synapses. The balance of the excitatory and inhibitory impulses the neuron receives at that time from all its synaptic connections determines whether an action potential will develop. This action is another demonstration of the diversity and extensive intercommunication that exists in the nervous system.

Nerves

A *nerve* is a group or bundle of nerve cell fibers surrounded by a connective tissue sheath outside the CNS. (Nerves do not exist in the CNS. The proper term for a group of fibers conducting impulses within the CNS is *fiber tract.*) The peripheral nerves are the cranial and spinal nerves and their branches. Nerves of the autonomic branch of the PNS are associated with both cranial and spinal nerves. The cranial nerves carry information directly between the brain and different parts of the head without passing through the spinal cord.

A peripheral nerve is composed of a bundle of nerve fibers surrounded by connective tissue layers thought to be continuous with CNS meningeal layers (Fig. 50-9). *Endoneurium* surrounds the individual nerve fibers adjacent to the myelin (if present) and the neurilemma and is continuous with the pia. Bundles of nerve fibers (also called *fasciculi*) are wrapped in *perineurium*, which is continuous with the arachnoid. The *epineurium* contains blood vessels and fat cells, surrounds the various fasciculi of a peripheral nerve, and is continuous with the dura.

COVERINGS OF THE BRAIN AND SPINAL CORD

The gelatinous tissue of the brain and spinal cord is protected by bone (skull and vertebral column) and by three connective tissue layers: the pia mater, the arachnoid, and the dura mater. Each layer is a separate, continuous sheet; connections between the pia and arachnoid are called *trabeculae*. The dura is also called the *pachymeninx;* the pia mater and arachnoid are collectively referred to as the *leptomeninges* (Fig. 50-10).

The *pia mater* is directly continuous with brain and spinal tissue and follows the contour of their external structure. The pia mater is a vascular layer through which blood vessels pass to the internal CNS structures to nourish the neural tissue. The pia extends below the spinal cord, which, as previously mentioned, ends at about the lower level of L1. The end of the spinal cord is cone shaped and is called the *conus medullaris*. A slender filament of pia called the *filum terminale* extends from the conus medullaris.

The *arachnoid* is a thin, fine, avascular, fibrous membrane; it hugs the brain and spinal cord but does not follow every contour as does the pia mater. The area between the arachnoid and pia mater is called the *subarachnoid space* and contains cerebral arteries, veins, arachnoid trabeculae, and the CSF that bathes the CNS. Enlargements in the subarachnoid space are called *cisterns*. One notable enlargement is the lumbar cistern in the lumbar region of the vertebral column. The lower lumbar region (usually between L3 and L4 or L4 and L5) is the area where spinal taps are performed to obtain CSF for examination.

The *dura mater* is a tough, inelastic, leatherlike tissue composed of two layers: the outer endosteal dura and the inner meningeal dura. The *endosteal* layer forms the inner periosteum of the skull and is continuous with the pe-

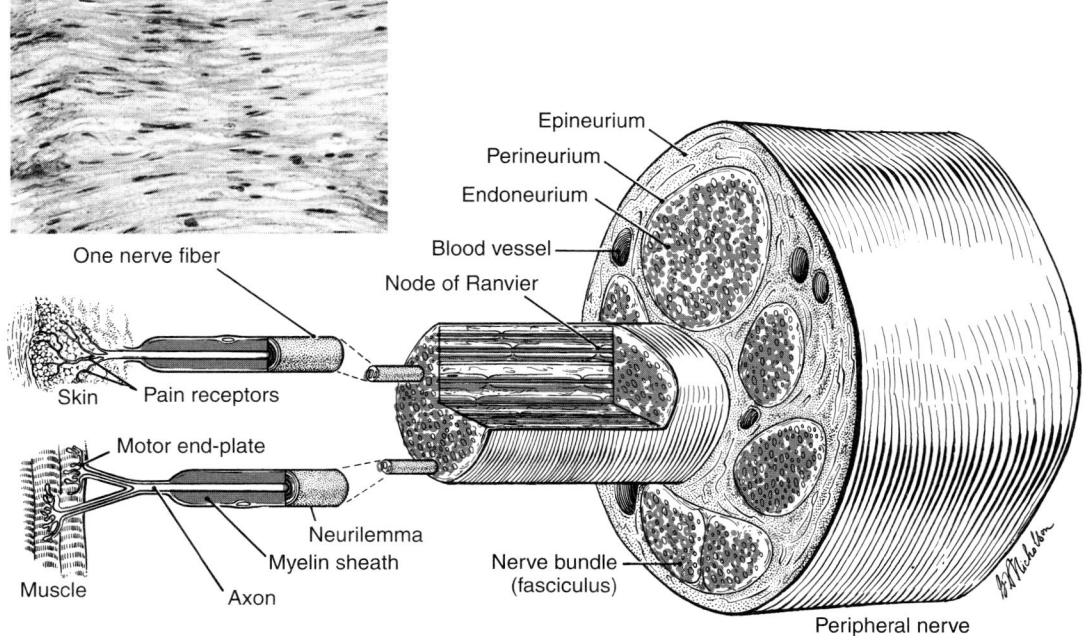

FIG. 50-9   Peripheral nerve in cross section. (From Langley LL, Telford JR, Christensen JB: *Dynamic anatomy and physiology*, ed 4, New York, 1974, McGraw-Hill.)

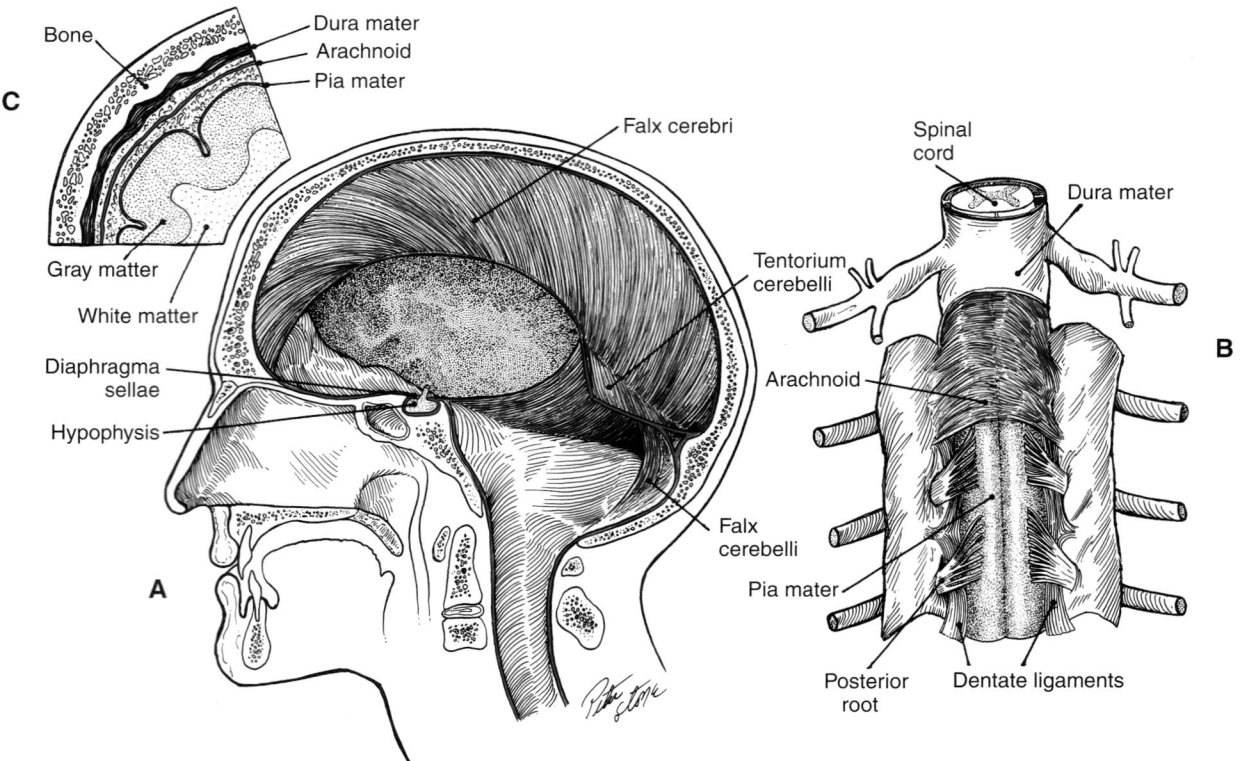

FIG. 50-10 Meninges. **A**, Extensions of the dura mater in the cranial cavity, sagittal view. **B**, Dura and arachnoid sheathe spinal nerves at their origin. The dentate ligament separates dorsal from ventral roots and adheres to the dura. **C**, A vertical section through a portion of the calvaria (cranium) and cortex. (From Langley LL, Telford JR, Christensen JB: *Dynamic anatomy and physiology*, ed 5, New York, 1980, McGraw-Hill.)

riosteal lining of the vertebral canal of the spinal cord. The inner *meningeal* dura is a thick membrane that covers the brain and dips in between brain tissues to provide support and protection. The layer becomes continuous with the spinal dura mater. The spinal dura continues to the level of the second sacral vertebra (S2), where it fuses with the filum terminale and forms the coccygeal ligament. This structure extends to the coccyx, where it becomes continuous with the periosteum and anchors the spinal cord in the vertebral canal.

The spinal cord is stabilized along the length of the vertebral canal by a series of 20 to 22 paired longitudinal ligaments referred to as the *dentate* or *denticulate ligaments*. These ligaments, which are attached to the dura at intervals, are lateral extensions of collagenous pial tissue separating the dorsal and ventral roots.

Four major sheaths of the meningeal dura extend into the cranial cavity (see Fig. 50-10, *A*). The *falx cerebelli* separate the two cerebellar hemispheres. The left and right cerebral hemispheres are separated along the longitudinal fissure of the *falx cerebri*. The *tentorium cerebelli* separates the cerebrum from the cerebellum. Finally, overlying the pituitary and penetrated by the hypothalamohypophysial portal system is the *diaphragma sellae*.

The venous sinuses are located between the two layers of dura mater where they separate. Venous sinuses are valveless channels for the drainage of cerebral blood and CSF. No vascular tissue exists in these sinuses; they are composed of dura mater with an endothelial lining.

When damage occurs to the vasculature of the brain, there may be bleeding into the *extradural* or *epidural space* (between the bone of the skull and the endosteal dura), the *subdural space* (between the meningeal dura and the arachnoid), the *subarachnoid space* (between the arachnoid and pia mater), or beneath the pia mater into the brain itself. The inner table of the skull contains grooves in which lie the anterior, middle, and posterior meningeal arteries. A fracture line running through any of these grooves may damage the contained artery and is the most common cause of *extradural* or *epidural hematoma*. A blow to the head over the parietotemporal region damaging the middle meningeal artery is the most frequent cause of extradural hematoma. *Subdural hematoma* is often caused by damage to the venous vasculature traversing the subdural space. A ruptured aneurysm of the arteries supplying the base of the brain results in *subarachnoid hemorrhage*. *Intracerebral hemorrhage* occurs when the vessels that penetrate brain tissue are involved so that blood enters the brain tissue itself.

The scalp is an additional structure that must be included in considering the coverings of the CNS. Overlying the skull, to which it is attached by the frontalis and occipitalis muscles, is a freely movable, dense fibrous tissue called the *galea aponeurotica* (Latin, *galea*, meaning "helmet"). The galea helps absorb the force of external trauma, especially glancing blows; without the protection of the scalp, the skull would be much more readily fractured. Overlying the galea is a membranous layer containing large blood vessels, a fatty layer, skin, and the hair of the scalp. When severed, the blood vessels constrict poorly and may cause severe bleeding that, however, can be controlled by digital pressure. Between the galea and the outer table of the skull is a potential space called the *subaponeurotic space*. The *diploic* and *emissary veins* (see Fig. 56-5) penetrate the skull from the dural sinuses into the subaponeurotic space and act as a safety feature (pressure valve) in case of increased intracranial pressure. These veins are also potential access sites for intracranial infection from a pyogenic focus in the scalp or sinuses or in cases of traumatic laceration of the galea. Thus meticulous removal of foreign particles, careful débridement, and flushing with normal saline and sometimes with a bactericidal agent are essential to reduce this hazard whenever the galea has been lacerated.

VASCULAR SUPPLY OF THE BRAIN AND SPINAL CORD

The CNS, as with all body tissue, depends on an adequate blood supply for its nutrients and for removal of metabolic waste products. The arterial supply of blood to the brain is a branching network of vessels that is highly interconnected to ensure adequate blood supply to the cells. This blood supply is provided via two pairs of arteries, the vertebral arteries and the internal carotid arteries, branches of which anastomose to form the cerebral arterial circle of Willis (Figs. 50-11 and 50-12).

The venous brain drainage does not closely parallel the arterial supply; it leaves the brain through the large dural sinuses and returns to the general circulation via the internal jugular veins.

The spinal cord arterial and venous systems are quite close parallels of each other and have extensive branching interconnections to adequately supply the tissue.

Carotid Arterial Supply

The *internal* and *external carotid arteries* branch from the common carotid arteries at about the level of the thyroid cartilage. The left common carotid artery stems directly from the aortic arch, but the right common carotid artery is derived from the innominate or brachiocephalic artery (a 1-inch remnant of the right aortic arch). The external carotid arteries supply the face, thyroid, tongue, and pharynx. A branch from the external carotid arteries, the *middle meningeal artery*, supplies the deep structures of the face and sends a large branch to the dura mater. A slight dilation in the internal carotid arteries just past the bifurcation is called the *carotid sinus*. Specialized nerve endings within the carotid sinuses respond to changes in arterial blood pressure to reflexly maintain blood supply to the brain and body.

The internal carotid arteries enter the skull and divide, at about the level of the optic chiasm, into the anterior cerebral arteries and the middle cerebral arteries. The middle cerebral arteries are direct continuations of the internal carotid arteries. Just after entering the subarachnoid space and before dividing, the internal carotid arteries give rise to the *ophthalmic arteries*, which enter the orbits and supply the eyes and other orbital contents,

portions of the nose, and air sinuses. Occlusion of this branch of the internal carotids (e.g., during a stroke) can result in monocular blindness.

The *anterior cerebral arteries* provide blood supply to structures such as the caudate and putamen nuclei of the basal ganglia, portions of the internal capsule and corpus callosum, and portions (mainly medial) of the frontal and parietal lobes of the cerebrum, including the somesthetic and motor cortices. An occlusion in the main trunk of an anterior cerebral artery results in a contralateral hemiplegia that is greater in the leg than it is in the arm (lower extremity more involved than upper extremity). Bilateral paralysis and sensory impairment result when there is total occlusion of both anterior cerebral arteries, again more severe in the lower extremities than in the upper.

The *middle cerebral arteries* supply arterial blood to portions of the temporal, parietal, and frontal lobes of the cerebral cortex and form a fanlike distribution over the lateral surfaces. This artery represents the major supply of blood to the precentral and postcentral gyri. Auditory, somesthetic, motor, and premotor cortices are supplied by the artery, as are the association cortices concerned with higher integrated functions in these central lobes. Occlusion of the middle cerebral artery near the origin of the main cortical branches (in the main trunk of the artery) results in severe aphasia when the language-dominant cerebral hemisphere is involved, contralateral sensory loss of position sense and two-point tactile discrimination, and a severe contralateral hemiplegia predominantly in the upper extremities and the face.

Vertebral-Basilar Arterial Supply

The right and left *vertebral arteries* originate from the subclavian arteries of their respective sides. The right subclavian is a branch from the innominate artery, and the left subclavian comes directly off the aorta. The vertebral arteries enter the skull via the foramen magnum, and at the level of the medullary pontine junction of the brainstem (where the medulla oblongata and the pons meet), they fuse to form the basilar artery. The *basilar artery* continues to the level of the midbrain, where it bifurcates to form the paired posterior cerebral arteries. Branches from the vertebral-basilar artery system supply the medulla, pons, cerebellum, midbrain, and part of the diencephalon. The posterior cerebral arteries and their branches supply a portion of the diencephalon, parts of the occipital and temporal lobes, the cochlear apparatus, and the vestibular organs. In the occipital lobe, the calcarine artery, which is a branch of the posterior cerebral artery, supplies the primary visual cortex. Occlusion of a calcarine artery can result in a contralateral homonymous hemianopsia (see Chapter 57). However, macular sparing may result from anastomosis of posterior and middle cerebral arteries in the occipital lobe.

Arterial Circle of Willis

Although the internal carotid arteries and the vertebral-basilar arteries are two separate arterial systems delivering blood to the brain, they are united by anastomosing vessels to form the cerebral arterial *circle of Willis* (see Fig. 50-12). The posterior communicating arteries connect the

FIG. 50-11 Arterial blood supply to the brain: internal carotid arteries and vertebral-basilar system. Note that the ophthalmic artery is a branch of the internal carotid artery.

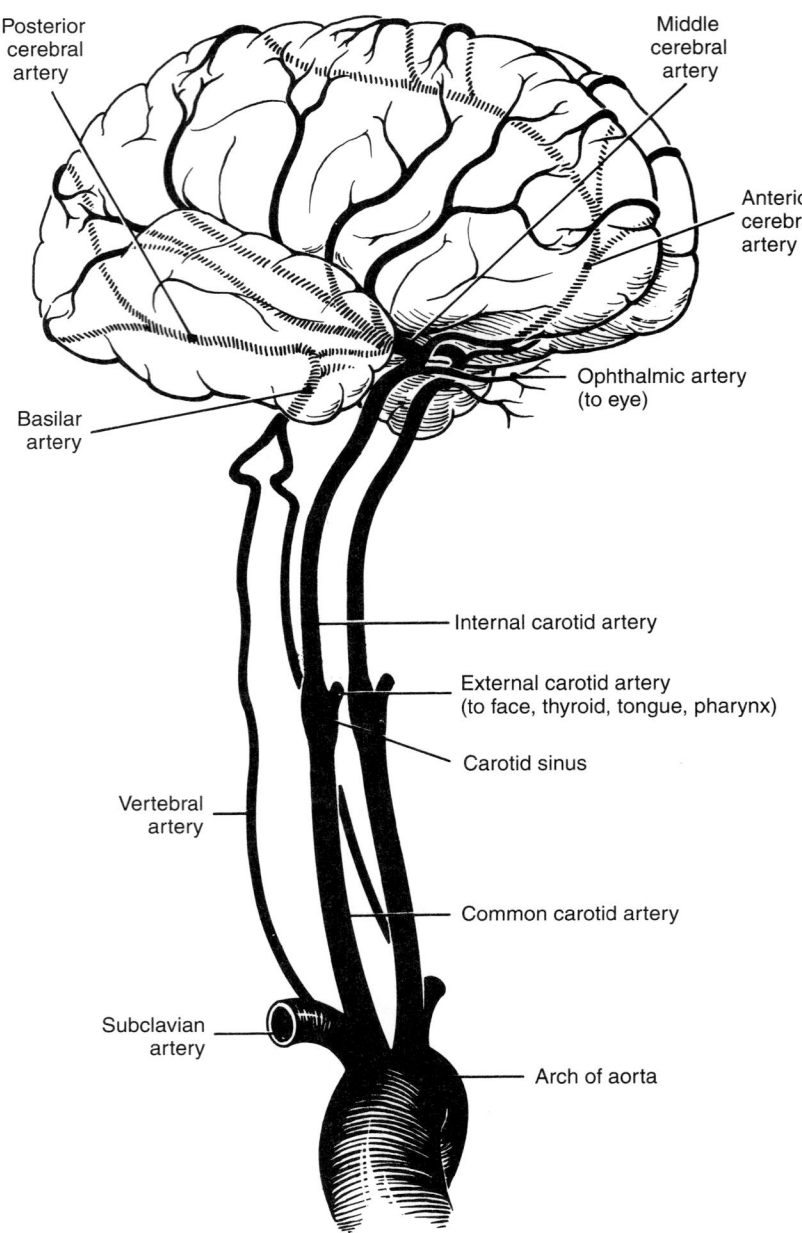

Posterior cerebral artery

Middle cerebral artery

Anterior cerebral artery

Ophthalmic artery (to eye)

Basilar artery

Internal carotid artery

External carotid artery (to face, thyroid, tongue, pharynx)

Carotid sinus

Vertebral artery

Common carotid artery

Subclavian artery

Arch of aorta

posterior cerebral arteries to the middle cerebral (and anterior cerebral arteries). The *anterior communicating arteries* connect the anterior cerebral arteries to complete the circle. There is usually only slight blood flow in the communicating arteries under normal conditions; they are a safety feature in case of dramatic changes in arterial blood pressure. The branches of the internal carotid and the vertebral-basilar systems also have anastomosing vessels.

Conducting and Penetrating Arteries

In general, cerebral arteries are either conducting or penetrating. The *conducting arteries* (the internal carotid arteries; anterior, middle, and posterior cerebral arteries; vertebral-basilar arteries; and the main branches from these arteries) form an extensive vascular network over the surface of the brain. The *penetrating arteries* are nutrient vessels derived from branches of the conducting arteries. The penetrating arteries enter the brain at right angles and

provide blood to the deep cerebral structures, such as the diencephalon, basal ganglia, internal capsule, and parts of the midbrain. For example, the *lenticulostriate (striate) arteries* are penetrating branches of the middle cerebral artery supplying the internal capsule and parts of the basal ganglia (see Figs. 53-1 and 53-3). These small arteries are often implicated in the stroke syndrome. Occlusion or rupture of the striate arteries may interrupt the motor pathways of the internal capsule and result in paralysis.

Venous Drainage of the Brain

The venous drainage for the brainstem and cerebellum closely parallels the arterial vascular distribution in those areas. Most of the venous drainage from the cerebrum occurs via the deep veins draining into superficial venous plexuses and into dural sinuses. The sinuses eventually drain into the internal jugular veins at the base of the

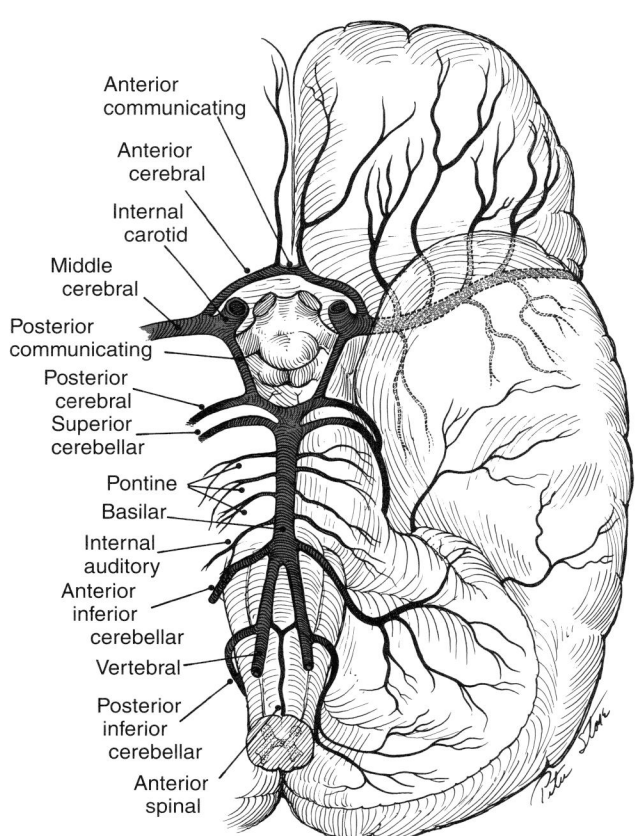

FIG. 50-12   Arteries of the brain. The circle of Willis *(center)* joins branches of the basilar and internal carotid arteries. (From Langley LL, Telford JR, Christensen JB: *Dynamic anatomy and physiology,* ed 5, New York, 1980, McGraw-Hill.)

skull, which rejoin the general circulation. The dural sinuses include the superior and inferior sagittal and the transverse (lateral) sigmoid, straight, and cavernous venous sinuses (Fig. 50-13). When a skull fracture may be present, one must consider the possibility of trauma to the cerebral venous sinuses, which may result in a subdural hematoma.

Spinal Cord Vasculature

The spinal cord receives its supply of nourishing blood via the branches of the vertebral arteries (the anterior and posterior spinal arteries and their branches) and from segmented regional vessels arising from the thoracic and abdominal aorta (the radicular arteries and their branches). From where they branch off the vertebral arteries along the surface of the medulla, the anterior and posterior spinal arteries descend into the spinal cord. The segmental arteries enter the spinal portion of the CNS through intravertebral foramina and divide into anterior and posterior vessels; they encircle the cord, forming an extensive anastomosing vascular plexus on the surface of the cord that also interconnects with the vessels from the vertebral system. Branches from this superficial vascular plexus then penetrate the cord to supply the deep tissue.

The venous drainage primarily follows the arterial distribution. Some spinal cord veins have valves, in contrast

to the valveless brain veins and venous sinuses. The vascular system of the spinal cord is directly continuous with the brain venous system. When the venous pressure is increased in the spinal cord, as in coughing or lifting heavy objects, an increase in central venous pressure may temporarily impede brain venous drainage.

VENTRICLES AND CEREBROSPINAL FLUID

The ventricles are a series of four interconnected cavities within the brain that are lined with ependymal cells (type of epithelial cell that abuts on all cavities of the brain and spinal cord) and contain CSF. There is one lateral ventricle in each cerebral hemisphere (Fig. 50-14). The third ventricle is in the diencephalon, whereas the fourth ventricle is in the pons and medulla. The lateral ventricle communicates with the third ventricle via the paired interventricular *foramina of Monro.* The third and fourth ventricles are connected via the narrow *aqueduct of Sylvius* in the midbrain. Three openings extend from the fourth ventricle: the paired lateral *foramina of Luschka* and the single medial *foramen of Magendie,* which are continuous with the subarachnoid space of the brain and spinal cord.

Within each ventricle is a specialized secretory structure known as the *choroid plexus,* which is composed of a network of blood vessels of the pia mater in intimate contact with the ependymal lining. The choroid plexus secretes the clear, colorless CSF that provides a protective fluid cushion around the CNS. The CSF contains water, electrolytes, O_2 and CO_2 gases in solution, glucose, a few leukocytes (principally lymphocytes), and a slight amount of protein. This fluid differs from other extracellular fluids in that it has higher Na^+ and Cl^- ion concentrations and its glucose and K^+ ion concentrations are lower, indicating that it is a secretion rather than a simple filtrate.

Once in the subarachnoid space, the CSF circulates around the brain and spinal cord and then exits into the vascular system (no lymph system exists in the CNS). Most of the CSF is reabsorbed into the blood through special structures called *arachnoid villi,* or *arachnoid granulations,* which project from the subarachnoid spaces into the superior sagittal venous sinus of the brain. There is constant production and reabsorption of CSF in the CNS. The total volume of CSF in the entire cerebrospinal cavity is about 125 ml, and the rate of choroidal secretion is about 500 to 750 ml/day. The CSF pressure is a function of the rate of fluid formation and the resistance to reabsorption of the arachnoid villi. The CSF pressure is commonly measured during a lumbar puncture procedure and normally averages about 130 mm water (13 mm Hg) in the recumbent position.

Hydrocephalus

Excessive CSF in the cerebrospinal cavity may elevate the pressure sufficiently to damage nervous tissue. This condition is called *hydrocephalus,* a term meaning "excess water in the cranial vault." Hydrocephalus may result from excess formation of fluid by the choroid plexuses, inadequate absorption, or obstruction to flow out of one or more of the

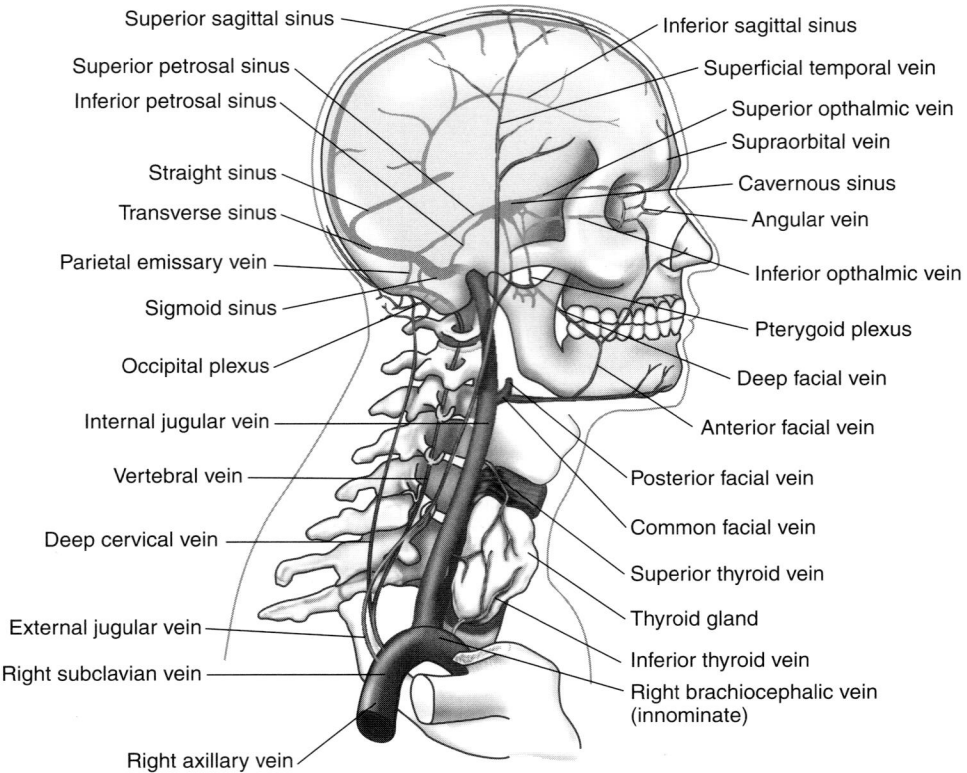

FIG. 50-13 Venous (dural) sinuses of the head. Superficial veins of the face empty into the cavernous sinus. The sinuses eventually drain into the internal jugular veins, which rejoin the general circulation. (Redrawn from Jacob SW, Francone CA, Lossow WJ: *Structure and function in man*, ed 5, Philadelphia, 1982, Saunders.)

ventricles. There are two types of hydrocephalus: noncommunicating, in which the flow of fluid from the ventricular system into the subarachnoid space is obstructed, and communicating, in which no such obstruction exists.

Noncommunicating hydrocephalus is the most common pediatric neurosurgical problem and usually has its onset in the immediate postnatal period. This type of hydrocephalus is usually caused by a congenital narrowing of the aqueduct of Sylvius; thus as fluid is formed by the choroid plexuses of the two lateral and third ventricles, the volumes of these three ventricles increase greatly. This condition flattens the brain into a thin shell against the skull. The increased pressure also causes the whole head to swell in the newborn. Obstructive hydrocephalus is also frequently associated with *meningomyelocele*, a congenital condition in which fusion of the neural tube fails to occur and thus the spinal cord is open, with cord, nerves, dura, and the more superficial coverings of the cord completely disarranged. Most children with meningomyelocele develop hydrocephalus, especially after surgical repair of the meningomyelocele. In adults, obstructive hydrocephalus is most often caused by a posterior fossa tumor with deformity of the aqueduct of Sylvius or fourth ventricle.

Communicating hydrocephalus may be caused by overdevelopment of the choroid plexuses in the newborn, thus much more fluid is formed than can be reabsorbed by the arachnoid villi. Fluid therefore collects inside the ventricles and on the outside of the brain, causing the head to swell tremendously and severely damaging the brain. Communicating hydrocephalus, however, is more frequently caused by interference with reabsorption of the CSF. This situation is usually secondary to meningitis or an irritant that occludes, obliterates, or scars the subarachnoid CSF spaces. The resultant increased volume of unabsorbed CSF causes gradual enlargement of the lateral ventricles, which, in turn, creates destructive pressure on the surrounding cerebral tissue. Because the ventricles become enlarged, the pressure within them usually is normal or decreased despite their increased volume. Therefore this form of communicating hydrocephalus is often called *low-pressure* or *normal-pressure hydrocephalus (NPH)*. This form is by far the most common in the adult. Because of the irritating effect of blood in the subarachnoid space, communicating hydrocephalus can follow subarachnoid hemorrhage by several weeks. The presenting symptoms include difficulty with walking, followed rapidly by dementia, lassitude, and eventual urinary incontinence. It is important to recognize the syndrome of low-pressure hydrocephalus, because it is a treatable form of dementing disease. All types of hydrocephalus can be treated by shunting the CSF to the extracranial venous system.

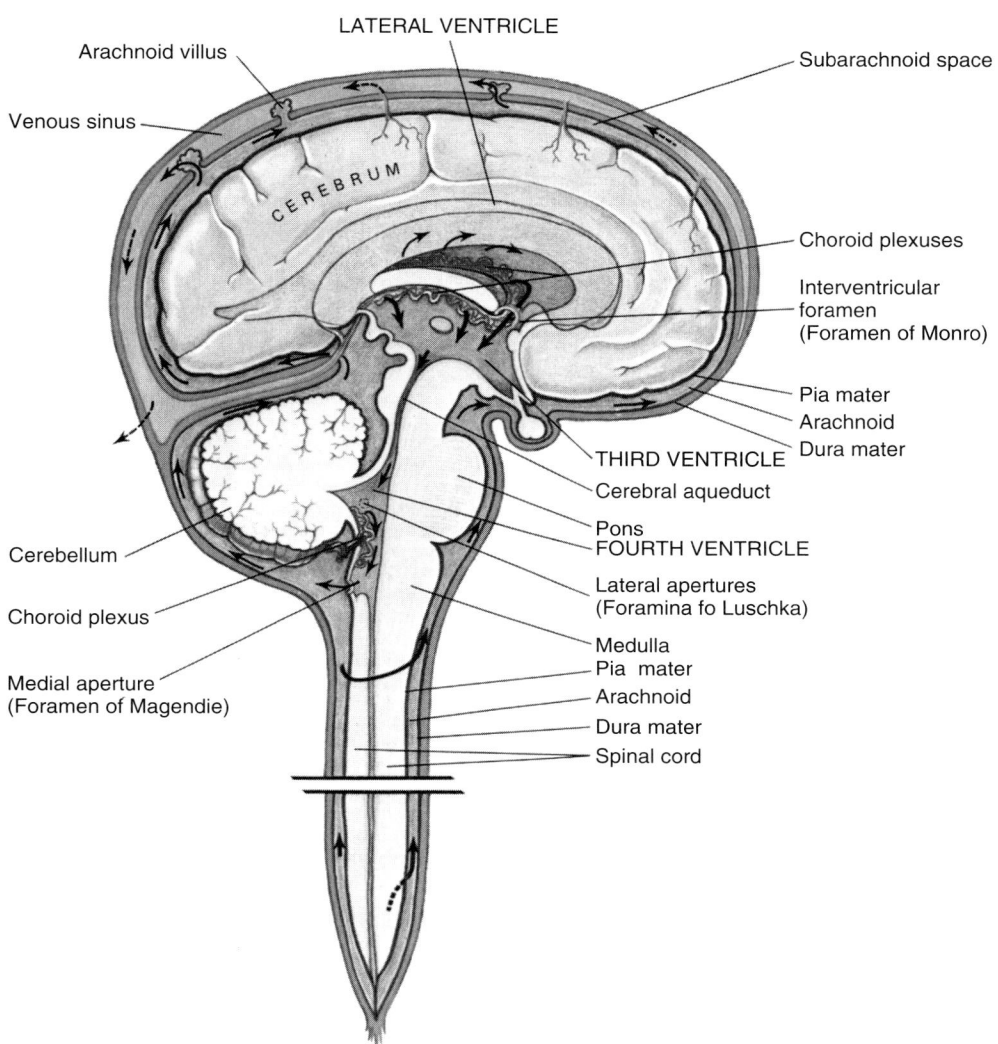

FIG. 50-14 Circulation of cerebrospinal fluid (CSF). CSF is formed in the choroid plexuses and circulates within the ventricles and subarachnoid space. It is reabsorbed by arachnoid villi into the dural sinuses. Direction of circulation (indicated by the *arrows*) is lateral ventricles → interventricular foramen (foramen of Monro) → third ventricle → cerebral aqueduct (Sylvius) → fourth ventricle → one foramen of Magendie and two foramina of Luschka → subarachnoid space → arachnoid villi. (From Guyton AC: *Basic neuroscience: anatomy and physiology,* Philadelphia, 1987, Saunders.)

BRAIN

The brain accounts for approximately 2% of the total body weight of an adult (about 3 pounds). The brain receives approximately 20% of the cardiac output, demands 20% of the body's O_2 use, and requires about 400 kcal of energy daily. The brain is the most energy-consuming tissue in the entire body and is primarily sustained by the oxidative metabolism of glucose. The tissue is fragile, and the demand for O_2 and glucose via the blood supply is constant. Brain metabolism is steady and continuous, with no rest periods. Consciousness may be lost in as little as 10 seconds once blood flow has ceased, and a lapse of even a few minutes may cause irreversible damage. Sustained hypoglycemia may also damage brain tissue. The ceaseless activity of the brain is related to its crucial func-

tion as an integration and coordination center between the sense organs and peripheral effector systems of the body, serving to organize incoming information, stored experiences, outgoing impulses, and behavior. The following discussion briefly considers the structure and function of selected parts of the brain.

Brainstem

The brain stem is continuous with the spinal cord caudally and with higher brain centers rostrally. The parts of the brainstem from below upward are the medulla oblongata, pons, and midbrain (Fig. 50-15). Many ascending and descending tracts exist throughout the brainstem. The brainstem is also an important relay and reflex center of the CNS.

Except for the olfactory and optic nerves, the nuclei of the cranial nerves are located in the brainstem. One or more of the cranial nerves are often involved in brainstem lesions, and location and expansion of such lesions can be detected by testing cranial nerve function. Cranial nerves I (olfactory) and II (optic) are actually *CNS tracts*, because they are the axons of the secondary sensory neurons carrying signals from primary sensory neurons in the nasal epithelium and the retina, respectively. As a CNS tract, the optic nerve is subject to CNS diseases (e.g., multiple sclerosis) and tumors.

The *medulla oblongata* is an important reflex center for cardiac, vasoconstrictor, respiratory, sneezing, coughing, swallowing, salivation, and vomiting reflexes. All the ascending and descending tracts of the cord are represented. On its anterior surface are two enlargements called the *pyramids*, which contain mainly voluntary motor fibers. Posteriorly, the medulla also has two enlargements that are the fasciculi of the dorsal columns' ascending tracts: the *fasciculus gracilis* and *fasciculus cuneatus*. These tracts carry pressure, conscious muscle proprioception, vibratory sensations, and two-point tactile discrimination. The medulla contains nuclei of the last four cranial nerves, IX through XII.

The *pons* (Latin for "bridge") consists of a bridge of fibers that connects the halves of the cerebellum and joins the midbrain above with the medulla below. The pons forms an important connecting link in the corticocerebellar path by which the cerebral hemispheres and the cerebellum are united. The lower portion of the pons has a role in respiratory regulation. Nuclei of the trigeminal (cranial nerve V), abducens (VI), facial (VII), and vestibulocochlear or auditory (VIII) nerves are located here.

The *midbrain* is the short part of the brainstem that lies above the pons and consists of (1) a posterior part, the *tectum*, containing the superior and inferior colliculi, and (2) an anterior part, the cerebral peduncles. The *superior colliculi* are involved in visual reflexes and in the coordination of visual tracking movements. Auditory reflexes, such as turning one's head toward a sound, are mediated through the *inferior colliculi*. The *cerebral peduncles* (or the basis pedunculi) are composed of bundles of descending motor fibers from the cerebrum. Two cranial nerves arise from the midbrain: the oculomotor (III) and the trochlear (IV). The trochlear nerves are the only ones of the 12 sets of cranial nerves that exit the brainstem on its posterior surface and cross to the opposite side. Therefore the superior oblique muscle is innervated by the contralateral trochlear nucleus. Because of its long intracranial course and its position just inferior to the free edge of the tentorium cerebelli, the trochlear nerve is at risk during surgical procedures of the midbrain. The substantia nigra and red nucleus, located in the midbrain, are part of the extrapyramidal or "involuntary" motor pathways. The *substantia nigra* has many connections, including those to the cerebral cortex, basal ganglia, red nucleus, and reticular formation. The substantia nigra is believed to have a complex inhibitory role in the areas to which it has interconnections. Lesions of the substantia nigra produce muscular rigidity, fine tremor at rest, slow and shuffling gait, and a masklike facies. Parkinson's disease involves the substantia nigra and its neurotransmitter, dopamine (see Chapter 54). The *red nucleus* has connections with the cerebellum, cerebral

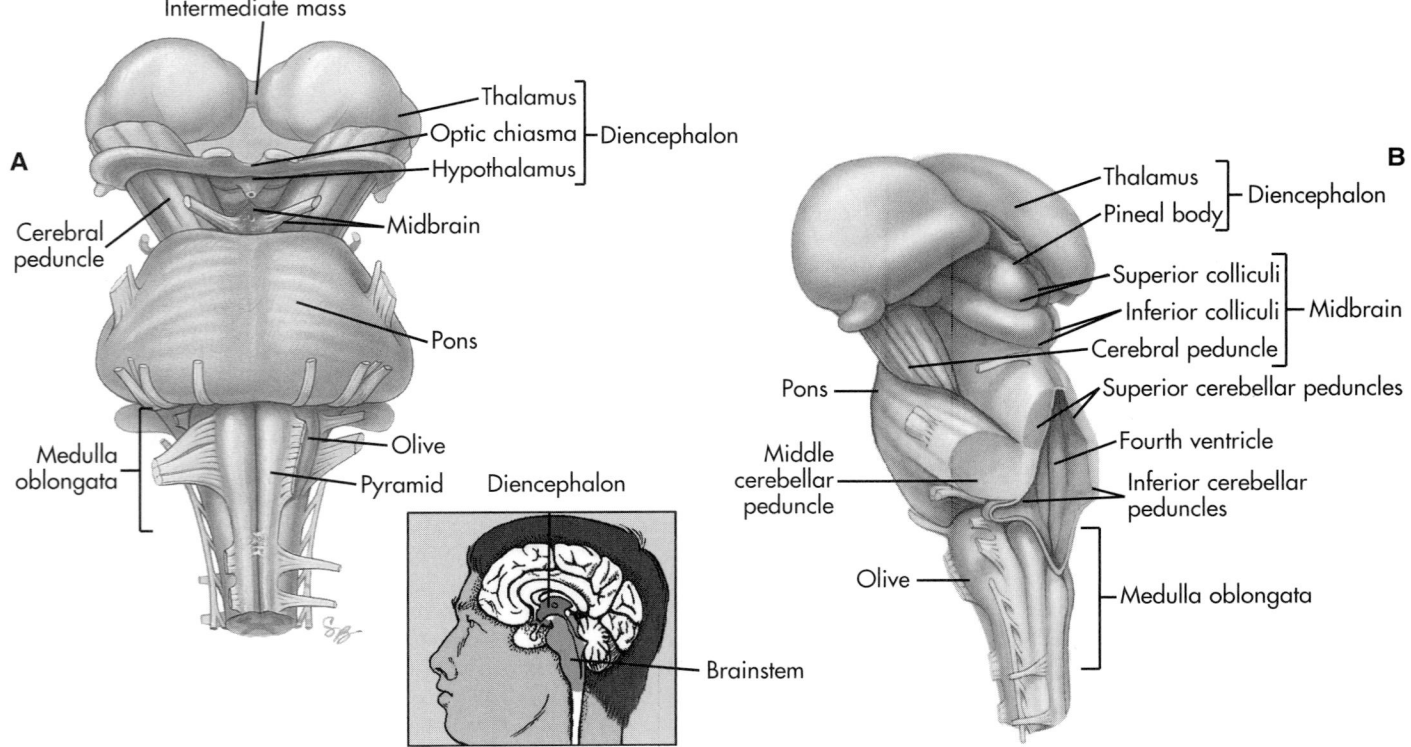

FIG. 50-15 Diencephalon and brain stem. **A,** Anterior aspect. **B,** Posterior aspect. (From Thibodeau GA, Patton KT: *Anatomy and physiology,* ed 4, St Louis, 1999, Mosby.)

cortex, substantia nigra, basal ganglia, reticular formation, and subthalamic nucleus. The role of the red nucleus involves postural reflexes and righting reflexes dealing with the orientation of the head in space.

Cerebellum

The cerebellum lies in the posterior cranial fossa, covered by the tentlike roof of dura mater, the *tentorium*, which separates it from the posterior part of the cerebrum; it is composed of a middle portion, the *vermis*, and two lateral hemispheres. The cerebellum is connected to the brainstem by three bands of fibers called *peduncles*. The *superior cerebellar peduncle* establishes connections with the midbrain; the *middle cerebellar peduncle* connects the two cerebellar hemispheres; and the *inferior cerebellar peduncle* contains fibers of the dorsal spinocerebellar tracts and connects with the medulla. All activities of the cerebellum are below the level of consciousness. Its main function is that of a reflex center through which coordination and refinement of muscular movements are affected and changes in tone and strength of contraction are related to maintaining posture and equilibrium.

Diencephalon

Diencephalon is a term used to designate structures surrounding the third ventricle and forming the inner core of the cerebrum. The diencephalon is commonly divided into four areas: thalamus, hypothalamus, subthalamus, and epithalamus. The diencephalon processes sensory stimuli and helps initiate or modify the body's reaction to these stimuli.

The *thalamus* is composed of two large ovoid structures, each with a complex of nuclei that are interconnected with the ipsilateral cerebral cortex, cerebellum, and many subcortical nuclear complexes, such as those in the hypothalamus, brainstem reticular formation, basal ganglia, and possibly substantia nigra. The thalamus is an important relay station in the brain and an important subcortical integrator as well. All the main sensory pathways (except the olfactory system) form synapses with thalamic nuclei on their way to the cerebral cortex. Evidence indicates that the thalamus acts as a center of primitive, uncritical sensation through which the individual becomes vaguely conscious of pain, pressure, simple touch, vibratory sense, and extremes of temperature. For example, pain can be felt but it cannot be localized. The finer sensory discriminations require cortical resolution. Emotional responses to the sensory stimuli, however, are possible at the thalamic level of integration. In addition to its role as a primitive sensory center, the thalamus also plays a key role in the integration of motor expressions because of its functional relation to the major motor centers in the cerebral motor cortex, cerebellum, and basal ganglia.

The *hypothalamus* lies beneath the thalamus. It regulates peripheral autonomic nervous system discharges accompanying behavior and emotional expression. The hypothalamus also plays an important role in hormonal regulation. Antidiuretic hormone and oxytocin are synthesized in nuclei located in the hypothalamus and transported via axons to the posterior pituitary, where they are stored and released. The release of anterior pituitary hormones is also regulated by hypothalamic releasing and inhibiting factors. Regulation of body water and electrolyte composition, body temperature, the endocrine functions of normal sexual and reproductive behavior, and the expression of calm or rage, hunger, and thirst are among the many functions of the hypothalamus.

The *subthalamus* is an important extrapyramidal motor nucleus of the diencephalon; it has connections with the red nucleus, substantia nigra, and globus pallidus of the basal ganglia. The function of the subthalamus is not entirely understood, but a lesion here produces the dramatic dyskinesia known as *hemiballismus*, which is characterized by violent flinging movements of the limbs on one side of the body. The involuntary movement is usually more marked in the arm than it is in the leg.

The *epithalamus* is a narrow band of neural tissue that forms the roof portion of the diencephalon. The major structures of this area are the habenular nuclei and commissure, posterior commissure, striae medullaris, and pineal body. The epithalamus has connections with the limbic system and appears to play a role in some of the basic emotional drives and in the integration of olfactory information. The pineal body secretes melatonin and helps regulate the circadian rhythms of the body and inhibit gonadotropic hormones. In young boys, destruction of the pineal gland by a tumor may result in precocious puberty.

Limbic System

The term *limbic* means "border" or "fringe" and was introduced by Broca in 1878 to refer to two gyri forming a limbus or border around the diencephalon. The "limbic system" is a functional concept and has no universally accepted definition (Fig. 50-16). The principal cortical structures include the cingulate and hippocampal gyri and the hippocampus. Subcortical portions include the amygdala, olfactory bulb and pathway, and septum. Some authors include the hypothalamus and part of the thalamus in the limbic system because of their close functional relationship. In the lower vertebrates, the limbic system is involved primarily with the sense of smell; in humans, its primary function is related to experiences and expressions of mood, feeling, and emotion, especially the reactions of fear, rage, and emotions related to sexual behavior. The limbic system is reciprocally connected to numerous central neural structures at several levels of integration, including the neocortex, hypothalamus, and the reticular activating system of the brainstem. The system is influenced by input from all sensory systems, which integrates and expresses it as a behavioral pattern via the hypothalamus, which coordinates the autonomic, somatic, and endocrine responses. The limbic system is also believed to play a role in memory, because lesions of the hippocampus may result in the loss of recent memory. Psychomotor epilepsy begins with and may be confined to the limbic structures so involved in the processes of mood, feeling, and emotion. Perceptual distortions, especially memory recall, emotional crises, and alterations in relatedness to other persons and objects characteristic of psychomotor epilepsy, may be accounted for by involvement of limbic structures (see Chapter 55).

Cerebrum

The cerebrum is the largest and most prominent part of the brain. Nerve centers governing all sensory and motor activities, as well as reason, memory, and intelligence, are located here. The cerebrum is divided into right and left hemispheres by a deep groove or furrow called the great *longitudinal fissure*. The cerebral hemispheres have an outer covering of gray matter called the *cerebral cortex* spread over an inner core of white matter termed the *medullary center*. The two hemispheres are joined by a broad band of fibers called the *corpus callosum*, and gray masses called the *basal ganglia* are embedded in the white matter (see discussion of cerebral fiber tracts). Centers for sensory and motor activities are duplicated in each hemisphere and usually are associated with the opposite side of the body; that is, the right cerebral hemisphere controls the left side of the body and the left cerebral hemisphere controls the right side of the body. This functional concept is called *contralateral control*.

Cerebral Cortex

The cerebral cortex, or gray mantle, of the cerebrum is thrown into numerous folds called *convolutions* or *gyri* (singular, gyrus). This arrangement enables a large surface area (estimated to be about 350 in²) to be contained within the narrow confines of the cranial vault. Furrows or grooves called *sulci* (singular, sulcus) created by the folds divide each hemisphere into distinct areas known as the frontal, parietal, temporal, and occipital lobes (Fig. 50-17). If the furrow is deep, it may be called a *fissure* rather than a sulcus. The *central sulcus* (fissure of Rolando) separates frontal and parietal lobes. The *lateral sulcus* (fissure of Sylvius) separates the temporal lobe below from the frontal and parietal lobes. The *parietooccipi-*

tal sulcus marks the boundaries of the occipital lobe. An additional subdivision of the cerebrum, the *insula*, lies within the lateral sulcus and is not visible on the surface.

Cerebral Fiber Tracts

The white matter of the cerebrum consists of neuron fiber tracts that may be grouped into three divisions: (1) association tracts, (2) commissural tracts, and (3) projection tracts.

The *association tracts* connect adjacent and distant cortical convolutions of the same hemisphere. *Commissural tracts*, the most prominent of which is a broad band of fibers called the *corpus callosum*, link the two hemispheres. These tracts correlate the action of the two halves of the brain as, for example, in coordinating the actions of the two arms and hands in tossing and catching a ball. *Projection tracts* connect the cerebral cortex with other parts of the brain and spinal cord, for example, basal ganglia, diencephalon, and brainstem. The *internal capsule* is a large band of ascending and descending fibers (visible on coronal section as a white irregular mass) bounded by the thalamus and caudate on one side and lenticular nuclei on the other side. The internal capsule is the main pathway for sensory input and motor output between the cerebral cortex and the brainstem. The *corona radiata* is a mass of the fibers that leave the internal capsule in a fanlike radiation to go to various parts of the cerebral cortex.

Functional Areas of the Cerebral Cortex

Certain areas of the cerebral cortex are primarily concerned with specific functions. In 1909 Brodmann, a German neuropsychiatrist, mapped the cerebral cortex into 47 areas on the basis of cellular structure *(cytoarchitecture)*.

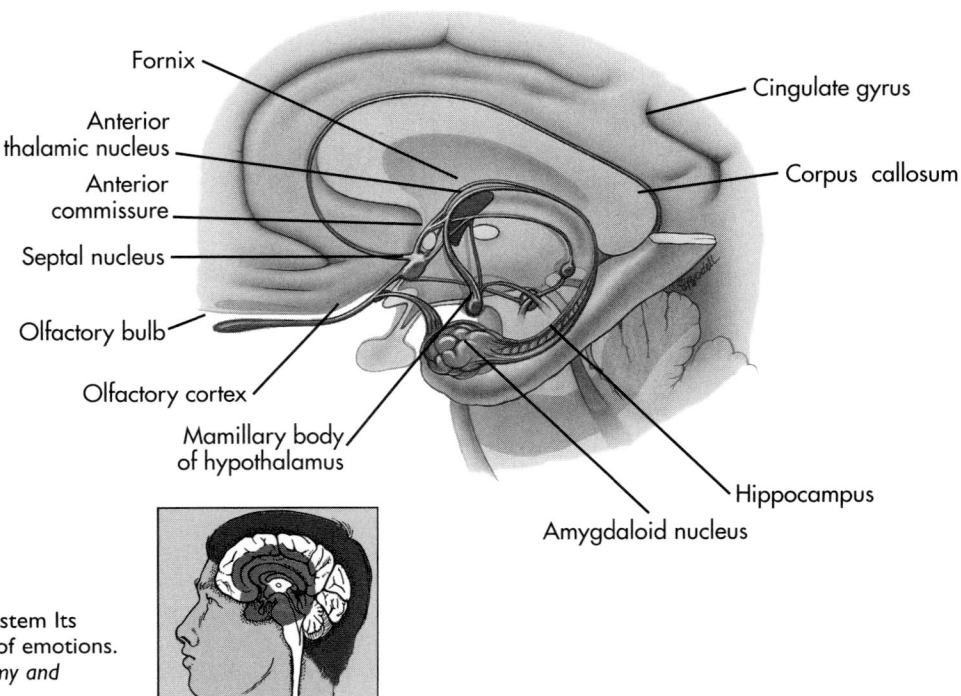

FIG. 50-16 Structures of the limbic system Its principal function appears to be arousal of emotions. (From Thibodeau GA, Patton KT: *Anatomy and physiology*, ed 4, St Louis, 1999, Mosby.)

Many attempts have been made to ascribe specific functional importance to these areas. In many cases, however, specific functions may overlap several areas. Despite these limitations, the Brodmann map is a useful general guide for the discussion of cortical functions (Fig. 50-18).

The cerebral cortex can be viewed as having primary and association areas for certain functions. The primary area is that in which the perception or the movement occurs, but the association areas are necessary for integration and higher levels of behavior and intellect. The following discussion considers the highlights of frontal, parietal, temporal, and occipital cortical functions.

The frontal cortex contains the *primary motor area*, Brodmann area 4 (Fig. 50-19), which is responsible for voluntary movements. The primary motor area is located along the *precentral gyrus* (in front of the central sulcus) and is somatotopically organized. A lesion in area 4 results in a contralateral hemiplegia. The premotor cortex, area 6, is responsible for learned skilled movements such as writing, driving, or typing. A lesion in area 6 on the dominant side may result in loss of the ability to write, or *agraphia*.

Brodmann area 8 is called the *frontal eye field* and, in conjunction with area 6, is responsible for the voluntary scanning movements of the eyes and conjugate deviation of the eyes and the head. Voluntary eye movements have input from areas 4, 6, 8, 9, and 46.

Brodmann areas 44 and 45 are known as *Broca's motor speech area;* they are responsible for the motor execution of speech. Damage to this area results in difficulty in articulation (*motor,* or *expressive, aphasia*) when the lesion involves the dominant hemisphere. The dominant hemisphere controlling speech is the left in most adults, regardless of whether they are right-handed or left-handed.

The *prefrontal cortex*, areas 9 to 12, is associated with the personality of the individual. Complex intellectual activities, some memory functions, sense of responsibil-

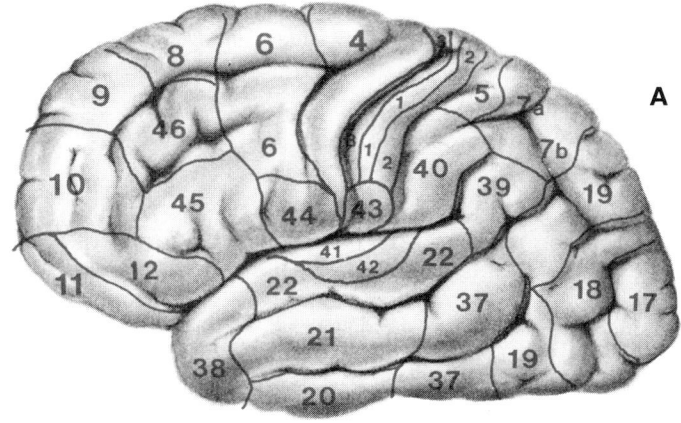

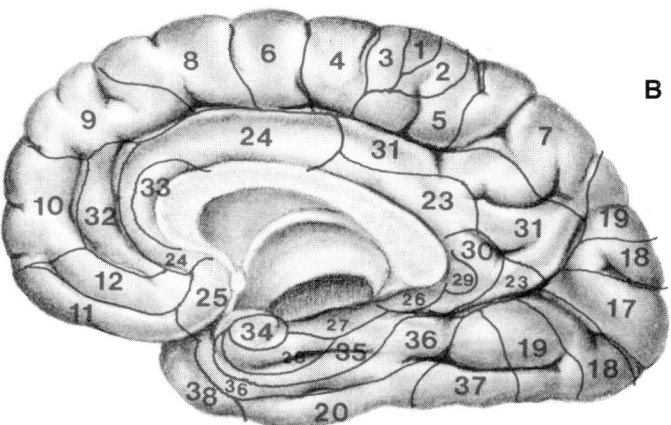

G.J.Wassilchenko

FIG. 50-18   Cytoarchitectural map of **(A)** the lateral and **(B)** the medial surface of the brain. Numbers represent the Brodmann areas. (From Thelan LA et al: *Critical Care Nursing: diagnosis and management*, ed 3, St Louis, 1998, Mosby.)

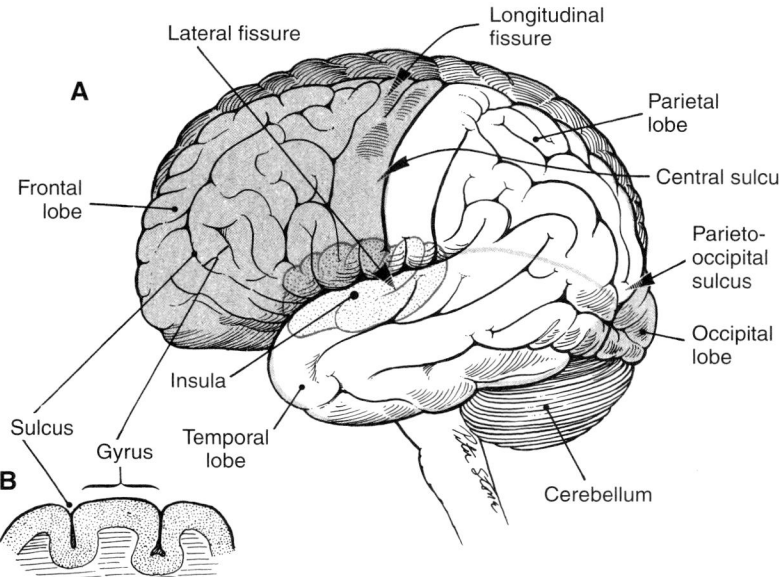

FIG. 50-17   **A**, Lateral view of the cerebrum. Note the line that demarcates the parietal and temporal lobes. **B**, Portion of the cortex in cross section. (From Langley LL, Telford JR, Christensen JB: *Dynamic anatomy and physiology*, ed 5, New York, 1980, McGraw-Hill.)

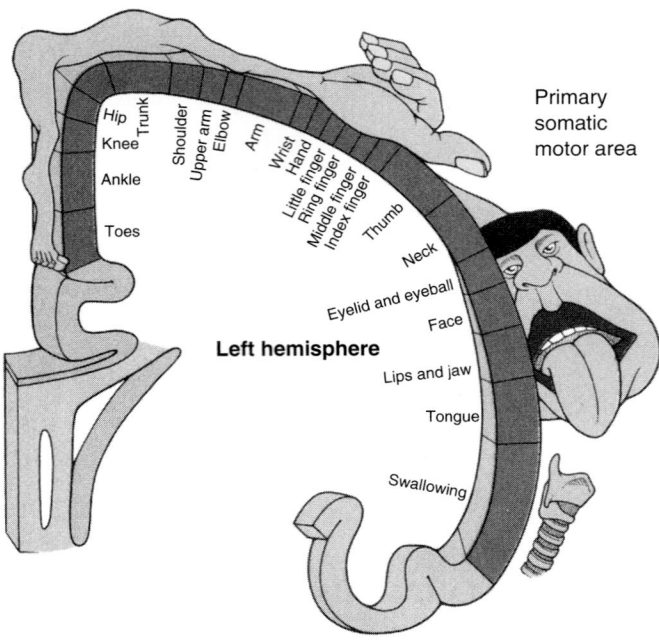

Primary somatic motor area

Left hemisphere

FIG. 50-19 Motor homunculus, showing the somatotopic organization of the primary motor cortex along the precentral gyrus of the frontal lobe. The primary sensory cortex is located on the postcentral gyrus of the parietal lobe with a similar somatotopic organization as the motor strip. (From Thibodeau GA, Patton KT: *Anatomy and physiology,* ed 4, St Louis, 1999, Mosby.)

ity for socially acceptable behavior, ideation, creative thought, judgments, and foresight are all primarily functions of the prefrontal cortex.

The parietal cortex has a major role in the higher level processing and integration of sensory information. The *primary somesthetic area* (areas 1 to 3) is located on the postcentral gyrus parallel to the motor cortex and posterior to the central sulcus. The parietal cortex is also somatotopically organized in a fashion resembling, but not identical to, the primary motor cortex. Sensations from all parts of the body are received in the primary sensory cortex, and it is here that they reach consciousness. These general sensations include pain, temperature, touch, pressure, and proprioception. The fine discrimination and more subtle aspects of sensory awareness are made possible by the primary sensory cortex. A lesion here produces contralateral sensory deficits.

The *somesthetic association area* (Brodmann areas 5 and 7) occupies the superior parietal lobe, extending to the medial surface of the hemisphere. This area has many connections with other sensory areas of the cortex. The sensory association cortex receives and integrates different sensory modalities, for example, identifying a quarter placed in the hand without looking at it. The qualities of shape, form, texture, weight, and temperature are related to past sensory experiences so that the information may be interpreted and recognition can occur. Awareness of body image, of location of body parts and body posture, and of the self are also functions of this area. Language is a diffuse function that is located throughout many areas of the cortex. A lesion of the *an-*

gular gyrus (area 39) in the dominant hemisphere results in *alexia* (inability to understand written language) and agraphia, although the individual may be able to speak normally. A lesion of the *supramarginal gyrus* (area 40) of the parietal cortex results in *astereognosis* (inability to recognize objects by touch). A lesion in this area, such as may occur after a cerebrovascular accident (CVA), or stroke, may also result in a defect in body awareness on the side contralateral to the lesion. For example, the affected person may be unaware of the arm on one side or fail to wash one half of the face.

The temporal lobe is the sensory receptive area for auditory impulses. The *primary auditory cortex* (areas 41 and 42) functions in the reception of sound, whereas the *auditory association cortex* (primarily area 22, although other parts of the temporal lobe are also included) is necessary for its comprehension. Brodmann area 22 is known as *Wernicke's area.* The temporal lobe and the nearby hippocampus also have a role in certain memory processes. The auditory association cortex is essential for the understanding of spoken language, and damage (especially on the dominant side) may result in a severe deficit in which language comprehension, naming objects, and repeating things heard are severely impaired (*sensory,* or *Wernicke's, aphasia*). In Wernicke's aphasia, speech may be grammatically or phonetically correct, but the words chosen are inappropriate or consist of nonsensical syllables. This impairment contrasts with *motor,* or *Broca's, aphasia,* in which comprehension may be unimpaired but expression is difficult. Both Wernicke and Broca's areas (and many other areas of the brain) are necessary for normal speech communication, and these two areas are connected by a bundle of fiber tracts called the *arcuate fasciculus.*

The occipital lobe contains the *primary visual cortex,* area 17, where visual information is received and sense of colors becomes conscious. Damage to area 17 results in visual field defects (see Chapter 57). The primary visual cortex is surrounded by the visual association cortex (areas 18 and 19), where visual information becomes meaningful. This area also has a role in the reflex movement of the eyes when fixing on or following an object. Damage to areas 18 and 19 on the dominant side can result in a lack of recognition of objects and their purpose even though faces may continue to be recognized. A lesion on the nondominant side may result in a failure to recognize faces *(prosopagnosia)* and to distinguish between forms of life (e.g., a cat versus a dog). The visual association cortex is adjacent to area 39 of the temporal lobe, and both are related to understanding the symbolism of language. Damage to this area results in *sensory alexia,* or inability to read with understanding.

Functional Specialization of the Cerebral Hemispheres

A characteristic of the brain with respect to sensation and motor control is that each half of the brain is concerned mainly with the opposite side of the body. Because the brain initially appears to be bilaterally symmetric, one might also assume that the two halves of the brain are functionally equivalent. However, this assumption is false. It has been known for some time that certain learned behaviors such as handedness, language percep-

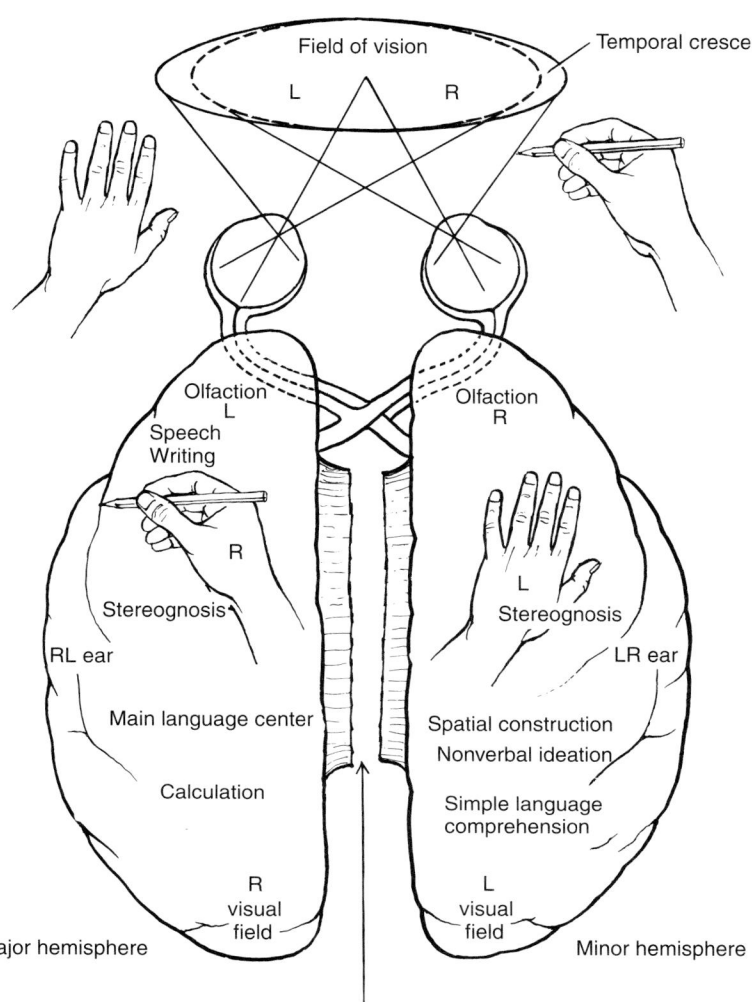

FIG. 50-20   Some of the specialized functions of the cerebral hemispheres as established by split-brain studies. RL and LR indicate that hearing is largely projected to the contralateral cortex. Olfaction is ipsilateral, whereas stereognosis is definitely contralateral. (From Noback CR, Demarest RJ: *The human nervous system,* ed 3, New York, 1981, McGraw-Hill.)

tion, speech performance, and spatial relations are predominantly a function of one or the other hemisphere. About 90% of the population is right-handed, a trait controlled by the left side of the brain. It has been determined, from observations of patients with strokes and other brain lesions, that linguistic abilities (e.g., speech, reading, writing) are predominantly functions of the left side of the brain in about 96% of the population. Moreover, recent findings reveal anatomic asymmetry of the hemispheres. The Broca and Wernicke's speech areas are generally larger in most persons. These observations led to the concept of *cerebral dominance,* with the left hemisphere considered dominant over the right.

In recent years, the concept of cerebral dominance has been giving way to the newer concept of *cerebral specialization* and integration of thought processes, because it has become apparent that each hemisphere develops a specialization in many functions. The presence of massive fiber tracts connecting the two halves of the brain suggests that communication and integration of impulses into an overall pattern of action may be an important mode of brain functioning.

The evidence for cerebral specialization has been observed in patients who have undergone a cerebral *commis-*

surotomy, a surgical procedure in which the corpus callosum and other commissures joining the two hemispheres are severed for the relief of intractable epileptic seizures. Studies of these "split-brain persons" have provided increasingly detailed information on the separated hemispheres (Fig. 50-20). The behavior of such split-brain persons appears normal on casual observation. However, careful laboratory testing, in which it is possible to ensure that sensory information reaches only one hemisphere at a time and the motor response comes from only one hemisphere, reveals that the two hemispheres are almost completely independent with respect to perception, learning, memory, and ideation. The major hemisphere (usually the left) is specialized in language and mathematic calculation and is limited in spatial tasks. The minor hemisphere (usually the right) is specialized for grasping whole concepts and perceiving abstract visual patterns, music, and spatial locations, but it is unable to communicate through verbal language, although communication can take place through gestures and emotional activities. These observations of hemispheric specialization in split-brain persons have led to the notion of two modes of thought: the *rational-analytic* associated with the left side of the brain and the *gestalt-synthetic* associated with the right.

The former mode of thought is believed to play an essential role in science, whereas the latter has an essential role in the creative arts, such as music, poetry, and imaginative expressions. Supposedly, some persons have left-hemisphere dominance and others are dominated by the right hemisphere. However, the specialization observed in the isolated hemispheres in split-brain experiments should not be overstated. Little is known about how the hemispheres interact in normal behavior, but the presence of the commissures suggests that there must be interaction.

Reticular Formation

The reticular formation is a complex network of cell bodies and interlacing fibers that form the central core of the brainstem. The network is continuous with the interneurons from the spinal cord below and extends upward into the diencephalon and telencephalon. The chief function of this diffuse reticular system is the integration of a large variety of cortical and subcortical processes, including determination of the state of consciousness and arousal, modulation of the transmission of sensory information to higher centers, modulation of motor activity, control of autonomic responses, and control of the sleep-wake cycle. This system is also the site of origin of most of the monoamines distributed throughout the CNS. The brainstem reticular formation is strategically located in the midst of ascending and descending neural pathways between the brain and spinal cord, enabling it to monitor traffic and participate in all brainstem-hemispheric transactions. The reticular formation, which is diffusely receiving and diffusely projecting, receives input from the cerebral cortex, basal ganglia, hypothalamus and limbic system, cerebellum, spinal cord, and all sensory systems. The efferent fibers of the reticular formation are distributed to the spinal cord, cerebellum, hypothalamus and limbic system, and thalamus, which, in turn, project to the cerebral cortex and basal ganglia. In addition, an important group of monoamine fibers is distributed widely in ascending paths to subcortical and cortical structures and in descending paths to the spinal cord. Many synaptic endings also exist in the brainstem, thus the reticular formation acts on itself. The reticular formation therefore influences and is influenced by all areas of the CNS.

One of the important functional components of the reticular formation is termed the *reticular activating system (RAS)*. The RAS performs a general arousal function in which it activates the cerebral cortex to become receptive to stimuli from other parts of the body. The RAS is essential to maintain the waking state and the waking electroencephalogram (EEG). Damage to certain portions of the reticular formation may result in a coma from which the individual cannot be awakened. In addition to controlling the general state of arousal, the RAS performs a screening function with respect to stimuli so that arousal and attention are selective. The RAS also is believed to play a role in habituation, that is, decreased response to a monotonous stimulus, such as the background ticking of a clock. Certain stimuli that are significant to an individual may receive selective attention, whereas others are ignored. This characteristic may explain why restaurant signs attract our attention when we are driving on the highway and are hungry or why a mother may sleep through a loud thunderstorm yet awaken to the faintest cry of her baby. Input from the cerebral cortex itself to the RAS, which, in turn, projects the impulses back to the cortex, may further increase cortical activity and arousal. This feature accounts for such states as a high degree of intellectual activity, worry, or anxiety possibly increasing cortical activity.

Several CNS monoamines, including dopamine, norepinephrine, and serotonin, play an important role in states of sleep and wakefulness. These monoamines are presumably produced in the cell bodies of neurons and distributed in vesicles via axoplasmic flow to nerve terminals. It has been demonstrated by histofluorescent staining techniques that the entire monoamine distribution system in the CNS originates in cell bodies located in the brainstem. Norepinephrine and serotonin pathways project upward to various parts of the brain and downward into the spinal cord, whereas dopamine pathways project only upward. The norepinephrine pathways, as well as those of dopamine, are believed to stimulate conscious wakefulness. Norepinephrine tracts are also responsible for rapid eye movement (REM) sleep. Destruction of the locus ceruleus (cell bodies that contain norepinephrine) in the brainstem can suppress REM sleep. Serotonin pathways arising from the raphe nuclei of the brainstem inhibit RAS arousal and promote both REM and non-REM sleep. Destruction of these nuclei produces insomnia. Certain pharmacologic agents that stimulate or inhibit the monoamines can alter sleep and arousal. For example, amphetamine, a drug that stimulates increased synthesis of norepinephrine, decreases total sleep time and REM sleep. The administration of *p*-chlorophenylalanine, a drug that blocks serotonin synthesis, results in insomnia, whereas the administration of 5-OH-tryptophan (a precursor of serotonin) restores normal sleep.

Another important function of the CNS monoamines is the regulation of emotional behavior through pathways that project to the hypothalamus and limbic system. The mechanisms effecting this control are poorly understood. The major tranquilizing drugs causing alteration in mood are believed to act on CNS monoamine neuronal systems.

CRANIAL NERVES

The cranial nerves arise directly from the brain and exit the skull via openings in the bone called *foramina* (singular, foramen). The 12 pairs of cranial nerves, designated by a name or Roman numeral, are olfactory (I), optic (II), oculomotor (III), trochlear (IV), trigeminal (V), abducens (VI), facial (VII), vestibulocochlear (VIII), glossopharyngeal (IX), vagus (X), accessory (XI), and hypoglossal (XII). Cranial nerves I, II, and VIII are purely sensory; III, IV, VI, XI, and XII are mainly motor but do carry proprioceptive fibers from the muscles they innervate; V, VII, IX, and X are mixed. Cranial nerves III, VII, and X also carry some nerve fibers of the parasympathetic branch of the ANS. The cranial nerves are discussed at length in Chapter 51. Table 50-2 is a summary of the major functions of the cranial nerves.

SPINAL NERVES

The spinal cord is composed of 31 segments of nervous tissue, each bearing a pair of spinal nerves that emerge from the vertebral canal through the intervertebral foramina (openings between the vertebral bones). The spinal nerves are named according to the intervertebral foramina

TABLE 50-2

Summary of Cranial Nerve (CN) Functions

Cranial Nerve	Nerve Component	Function
I Olfactory	Sensory	Smell
II Optic	Sensory	Vision
III Oculomotor	Motor	Elevation of upper lid Pupillary constriction Most extraocular movements
IV Trochlear	Motor	Downward inward movement of eye
VI Abducens	Motor	Lateral deviation of eye
V Trigeminal	Motor	Temporal and masseter muscles (jaw clenching, chewing); lateral movement of the jaw
	Sensory	Skin of face and anterior two thirds of scalp; mucosa of eyes; mucosa of nasal and oral cavities, tongue, and teeth Corneal or blink reflex: sensory limb carried in CN V, motor response in CN VII
VII Facial	Motor	Muscles of facial expression, including those of forehead and around eyes and mouth Lacrimation and salivation
	Sensory	Taste on anterior two thirds of tongue (sweet, sour, salty)
VIII Vestibulocochlear		
Vestibular branch	Sensory	Equilibrium
Cochlear branch	Sensory	Hearing
IX Glossopharyngeal	Motor	Pharynx: swallowing, gag reflex Parotid: salivation
	Sensory	Pharynx, posterior tongue, including taste (bitter)
X Vagus	Motor	Pharynx, larynx: swallowing, gag reflex, phonation; abdominal viscera
	Sensory	Pharynx, larynx: gag reflex; neck thoracic, and abdominal viscera
XI Accessory	Motor	Sternocleidomastoid and upper portion of trapezius: head and shoulder movements
XII Hypoglossal	Motor	Tongue movements

through which they exit, except for the first cervical nerve pair, which exits between the occipital bone and the first cervical vertebra (C1). Thus there are 8 cervical nerve pairs (and only 7 cervical vertebrae), 12 thoracic nerve pairs, 5 lumbar nerve pairs, 5 sacral nerve pairs, and 1 coccygeal nerve pair (Fig. 50-21; see Fig. 50-2). When localizing a spinal lesion according to cord level rather than vertebral level, it is important to note that the two levels do not correspond. The disparity between the length of the spinal cord and that of the vertebral canal increases the distance between the attachment of the various nerve roots and the intervertebral foramina; therefore the nerve roots arising from the lumbar and sacral segments have to pass for some distance before making their exit.

The spinal nerve is attached to the lateral surface of the spinal cord by two roots: a *dorsal*, or *posterior (sensory)*, *root*; and a *ventral*, or *anterior (motor)*, *root* (Fig. 50-22). The dorsal root shows an enlargement, the *dorsal root ganglion*, composed of the cell bodies of afferent or sensory neurons. The cell bodies of all afferent neurons of the cord are in these ganglia. The dorsal root fibers are the processes of sensory neurons that bring impulses in from the periphery to the cord. The cell bodies of motor or efferent neurons are inside the cord in anterior and lateral columns of gray matter; their axons form the ventral root fibers that pass to muscles and glands. The two roots emerge from the intervertebral foramen and join beyond it to form the spinal nerve, or nerve trunk. Thus all spinal nerves are mixed nerves; that is, they contain both sensory and motor fibers. After a short course, the nerve trunk divides into dorsal and ventral divisions, or *rami* (singular, ramus). (There are also two more divisions: a meningeal branch, supplying the spinal cord meninges and ligaments; and a visceral branch, which has two portions, the white and gray rami, and belongs to the ANS.)

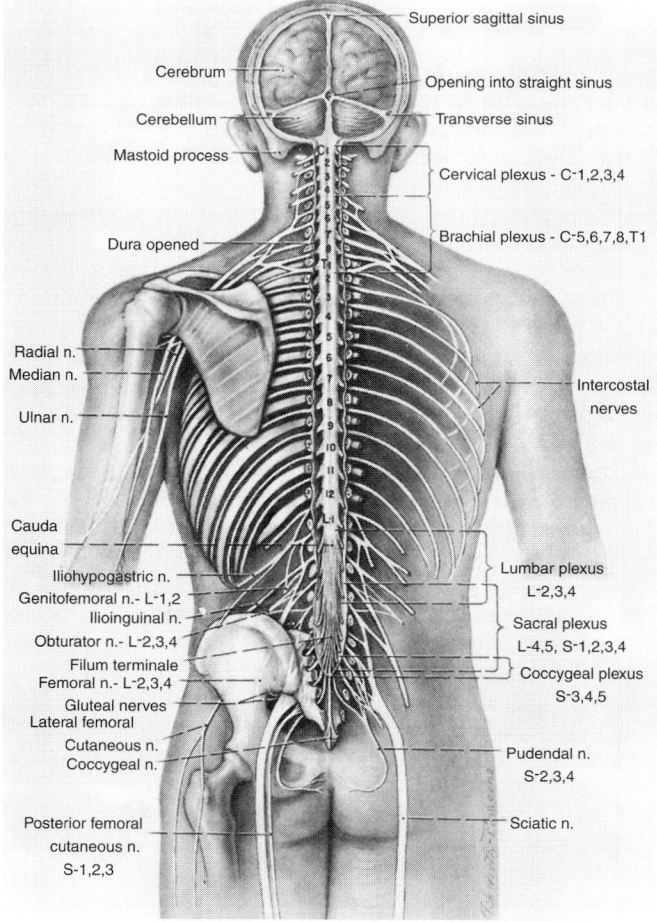

FIG. 50-21 Spinal nerves and plexuses. (From Jacob SW, Francone CA: *Elements of anatomy and physiology*, ed 2, Philadelphia, 1989, Saunders.)

POSTERIOR

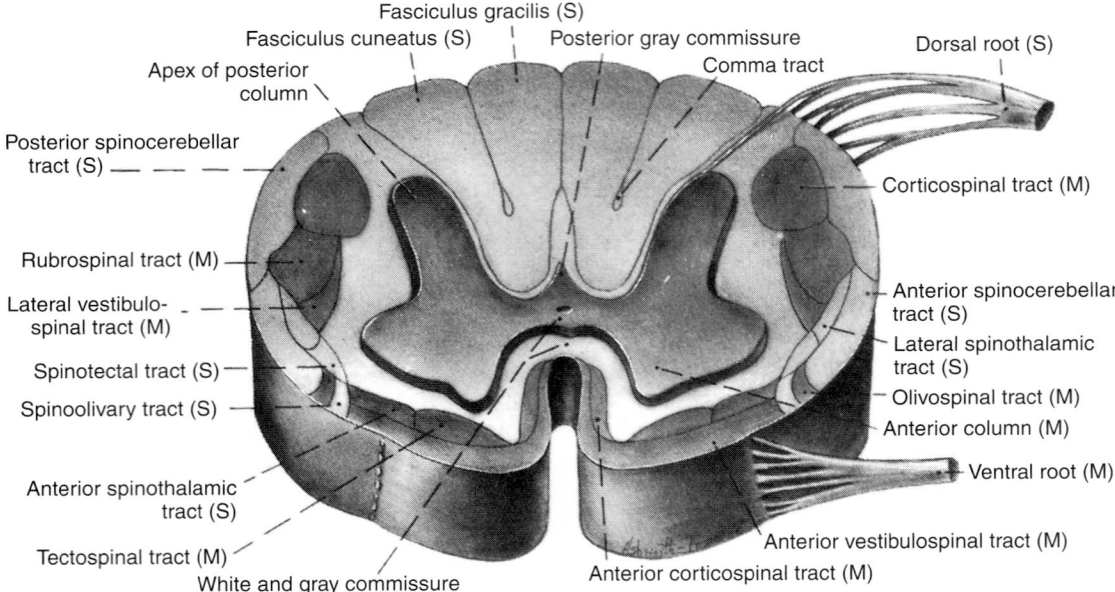

FIG. 50-22 Cross section of the spinal cord showing the major ascending sensory *(S)* and descending motor *(M)* tracts. (From Jacob SW, Francone CA: *Elements of anatomy and physiology,* ed 2, Philadelphia, 1989, Saunders.)

In general, the *dorsal division* of the spinal nerves supplies the intrinsic muscles of the back and specific segments of the skin overlying them called dermatomes (see following discussion). The *ventral division* is large and forms the main part of the spinal nerve. The ventral division supplies the muscles and skin of neck, chest, abdomen, and extremities.

In all regions except the thoracic, the ventral divisions of the spinal nerves interlace to form networks of nerves called *plexuses.* The plexuses thus formed are the cervical, brachial, lumbar, sacral, and coccygeal. In each instance, branches are given off from the plexus to the parts supplied. These branches are the peripheral nerves and have specific names.

The first four cervical nerves (C1 to C4) form the *cervical plexus,* which innervates the neck and the back of the head. One important branch is the phrenic nerve, which supplies the diaphragm.

The *brachial plexus* is formed from C5 through T1 or T2. This plexus supplies the upper extremity. Important branches are the radial, median, and ulnar nerves of the arm. The thoracic nerves (T3 through T11) do not form a plexus but pass out in the intercostal spaces as the intercostal nerves. These nerves supply intercostal muscles, upper abdominal muscles, and the skin areas of the chest and abdomen.

The *lumbar plexus* is derived from spinal segments T12 through L4, the *sacral plexus* from L4 through S4, and the *coccygeal plexus* from S4 through the coccygeal nerve. L4 and S4 contribute branches to both the lumbar and sacral plexuses. Nerves from the lumbar plexus innervate muscles and skin in the lower trunk and lower extremities. The major nerves from this plexus are the *femoral* and *ob-*

turator. The major nerve from the sacral plexus is the *sciatic,* the largest nerve in the body. The sciatic nerve pierces the buttocks and runs down the back of the thigh. The many branches of the sciatic nerve supply the posterior thigh muscles, leg and foot muscles, and nearly all the skin of the leg. Nerves from the lower sacral levels and from the coccygeal plexus supply the perineum.

Each of the spinal nerves is distributed to specific segments of the body. The area of skin supplied by the dorsal root of each spinal nerve, and therefore a single segment of the spinal cord, is called a *dermatome.* Although the dermatomes overlap, knowledge of the segmental innervation of the skin enables simple clinical evaluation, using a pin or wisp of cotton to determine the sensory function of a particular segment of the spinal cord or peripheral nerve (see Chapter 51).

The skeletal muscles also receive a segmental innervation from the ventral spinal roots. The segmental innervation of the biceps brachii, triceps, brachioradialis, abdominal muscles, quadriceps femoris, gastrocnemius and soleus, and plantar flexor muscles should be memorized, because it is possible to test them by eliciting simple muscle reflexes using a reflex hammer (see Chapter 51).

SPINAL CORD

The spinal cord serves as a center for spinal reflexes and as a conducting pathway for impulses traveling to and from the brain. The spinal cord is composed of *white matter* (myelinated nerve fibers) with an internal core of *gray matter* (unmyelinated neuronal tissue). The white matter serves as a conducting pathway for afferent and efferent impulses traveling between various levels of the spinal cord and the brain. The gray matter is the integrative area for the cord reflexes.

When seen on cross section, the gray matter is in the form of the capital letter H. The two projections of the H that pass toward the front of the body are called *anterior*, or *ventral horns*, and the two projecting backward are the *posterior*, or *dorsal*, *horns* (see Fig. 50-22).

The ventral horn is composed primarily of cell bodies and dendrites of the multipolar motor efferent neurons of the ventral roots and spinal nerves. The *ventral horn cell*, or *lower motor neuron*, is commonly called the *final common pathway*, because any movement, whether initiated in the cerebral motor cortex, basal ganglia, or reflexly in the sensory receptor, must be translated into action via this structure.

The dorsal horn contains cell bodies and dendrites from which arise sensory fibers that go to other levels of the CNS after synapsing with sensory fibers from sensory nerves.

The gray matter also contains internuncial, or associational, neurons, ANS afferents and efferents, and axons originating at different levels of the CNS. Internuncial neurons transmit impulses from one neuron to another within the brain and spinal cord. In the spinal cord, internuncial neurons have many interconnections, and many of them directly innervate the ventral horn cells. Only a few incoming sensory impulses to the spinal cord or motor impulses from the brain terminate directly on the ventral horn cell or lower motor neuron. Instead, most of the impulses are first transmitted through internuncial cells, where they are appropriately processed before stimulating the anterior horn cell. This arrangement allows highly organized patterns of muscle responses.

Reflex Arc

The reflex arc is the functional unit of the nervous system. Reduced to its simplest form, the reflex arc consists of two neurons: a sensory neuron leading from a sensory receptor or ending and a motor neuron that conveys impulses to a muscle or gland. More generally, the two neurons are not connected directly but have one or more internuncial neurons interposed between them. This type of mechanism is capable of response quite independent of the higher centers and is sufficient for the performance of simple acts such as withdrawing from painful stimuli. Reflexes may involve only one segmental level of the spinal cord or several levels. The impulses may spread upward or downward from the level at which they enter the cord by passing through internuncial neurons. Because of the multitude of interconnections of neurons within the cord, an almost infinite variety of responses is possible. Knowledge of the segmental levels of the reflexes and of the dermatomes is helpful in localizing lesions of the nervous system (see Chapter 51).

Pathways of Selected Spinal Cord Tracts

The white matter of the spinal cord conducts the long ascending and descending tracts by which afferent impulses from the spinal nerves reach the brain and those through which efferent impulses pass from motor centers in the brain to ventral horn cells of the cord and thus modify movement. The fibers that make up the white matter of the spinal cord are not scattered chaotically but are arranged in bundles that show a functional and an anatomic grouping.

Each lateral half of the spinal cord is divided into three longitudinal sections that run the length of the cord, called *dorsal, lateral*, and *ventral columns*. Within each of these divisions are distinct bands of fibers, called tracts, having quite definite locations. A fiber tract is a bundle of fibers, all having the same origin, termination, and function. The tracts may be ascending, descending, or associative.

Ascending tracts bring sensory information into the CNS and may travel to parts of the spinal cord and brain. The lateral spinothalamic tract is an important ascending tract that carries the fibers for the pain and temperature pathway. The fine touch, conscious proprioception, and vibratory pathways have fibers that comprise the dorsal columns of the spinal cord white matter. Impulses from various parts of the brain to the motor neurons of the brainstem and spinal cord are called *descending tracts*. The lateral and ventral corticospinal tracts represent the voluntary motor pathway in the spinal cord (see Fig. 50-22 for the location of the tracts of these pathways). *Associative tracts* are short ascending or descending tracts; for example, they may travel between a few segments of the spinal cord and are thus called *intersegmental tracts*. Table 50-3 lists some of the most important ascending and descending tracts of the spinal cord.

The spinal cord tracts are named to denote the origin and termination of their fibers. *Origin* means the location of the cell bodies of the tract, and *termination* refers to the point at which the axon forming the tract ends. Thus it is simple to determine whether a tract is an ascending sensory or descending motor tract by analyzing the name. For example, the rubrospinal tract is a descending motor tract with its cell bodies in the red nucleus of the midbrain and its axon termination in the spinal cord.

Ascending Pathways

Sensory information from peripheral receptors is transmitted through the nervous system in a series of neurons organized into an ascending pathway system. The sensory chain consists of three neurons, each having a long axon. The *first-order neuron* has its cell body in a dorsal root ganglion and conducts the impulse from the receptor to the spinal cord. (If the receptors of the first-order neuron lie in the regions supplied by cranial nerves, its axon enters the brainstem instead of the cord.) The cell body of the *second-order neuron* is located at variable levels of the gray matter of the spinal cord or brain stem and conveys the impulse within the white matter of the cord to the thalamus. The *third-order neuron* conducts impulses from the thalamus to the cerebral cortex, and its cell body lies in the thalamus. In general, the major sensory systems and their pathways are somatotopically organized and are crossed pathways. This feature means that organization according to body surface area is present in the spinal cord and thalamus, as well as the primary somesthetic cortex, and that each side of the brain registers sensations from the opposite side of the body. It is usually the second-order neuron that crosses at some point on its way to the thalamus. Only two of the ascending pathways are discussed in detail here.

TABLE 50-3 ▪▪▪

Major Ascending and Descending Tracts of the Spinal Cord

Tract	Function
ASCENDING	
Dorsal (posterior) columns	Fine touch capable of a high degree of localization of the stimulus, fine degree of discrimination of pressure and intensity (two-point discrimination, weight perception)
Fasciculus cuneatus (T6 and above, upper body)	
Fasciculus gracilis (T7 and below, lower body)	Conscious proprioception (position sense)
	Vibration (phasic sensations)
	Rapid transmission of sensory information
Spinothalamic	
Lateral spinothalamic	Pain
Ventral spinothalamic	Temperature, including warm and cold sensations
	Crude touch capable of much less localization of the stimulus and less discrimination of pressure and intensity
	Itching and tickling sensations
	Transmission of sensory information much slower than in dorsal columns
Spinocerebellar	
Dorsal spinocerebellar	Unconscious proprioception (muscle sense)
Ventral spinocerebellar	Coordination of posture and limb movement
	Sensory information transmitted originates almost entirely in the muscle spindles and Golgi tendon apparatus
	Large-tract fibers transmitting impulses faster than any other neurons in the body
DESCENDING	
Corticospinal	
Lateral corticospinal	Pyramidal tract carrying impulses for voluntary control of the muscles of the extremities
Ventral corticospinal	Pyramidal tract carrying impulses for voluntary control of the muscles of the trunk
Rubrospinal	Extrapyramidal tract concerned with unconscious integration and coordination of muscular movement adjusted to proprioceptive input
Tectospinal	Extrapyramidal tract concerned with reflex turning and scanning movements of the head and reflex movements of the arms in response to visual, auditory, or cutaneous sensation
Vestibulospinal	Extrapyramidal tract involved in equilibrium (maintaining balance) and coordination of head and eye movements

Pain and Temperature Pathway

The direct neural pathway for the sensations of pain and temperature is the lateral spinothalamic pathway (see Fig. 51-7). The sensory nerve fibers carrying impulses from stimulated pain or temperature receptors enter the dorsal root of the spinal cord, and once in the white matter, they bifurcate and ascend or descend a few segments before synapsing with the second-order neuron in the gray matter of the dorsal horn. The axon of this second-order neuron crosses over to the contralateral side, where it joins the other fibers in the lateral spinothalamic tract. These fibers proceed to the thalamus, where they synapse with a third-order neuron that relays the impulses to the sensory cortex. In the thalamus, the pain and temperature sensations come into consciousness vaguely but are not localized. The full extent of these sensations is consciously perceived and localized as the impulses are received in the primary and secondary somesthetic cortex of the parietal lobe. (Note: there is also an indirect spino-reticular thalamic pathway for pain.)

Fine Touch, Conscious Proprioception, and Vibration Pathway

The neural pathway for fine (discriminating) touch, conscious proprioception (awareness of body position and movement), and vibratory sense is called the *medial lemniscal system*. This system consists of the tracts that make up the dorsal white columns of the cord (the fasciculi cuneatus and gracilis) plus the medial lemniscus, a flat band of fibers extending through the brainstem.

General mechanoreceptors responsive to fine touch, vibration, body position, and movement conduct impulses into the cord through the dorsal root; they then ascend directly on the same side via the dorsal columns. The dorsal columns are somatotopically organized. First-order neurons in the dorsal cord transmit impulses from the lower part of the body (T7 and below) by fibers that form the tract known as the *fasciculus gracilis*. The fibers terminate in the *nucleus gracilis* of the medulla, where they synapse on the second-order neurons of the sensory pathway. Fibers transmitting impulses from the upper part of the body (T6 and above) occupy the more lateral dorsal column as the *fasciculus cuneatus*, which terminates in the *nucleus cuneatus*, also located in the medulla. The reason for this laminar organization is that the sacral and dorsal column fibers are pushed medially as fibers from higher segments are added. Thus the information for the feet is located in the midline of the cord, whereas information from the upper extremities is located on the most lateral side of the cord. (The laminar organization of the spinothalamic tract is opposite to that of the dorsal columns. Fibers from sacral and lumbar segments of the body are pushed laterally by fibers crossing the midline at successively higher levels. Thus the lamination is cervical to sacral segments represented from the medial to more lateral position. Because of this lamination, tumors arising outside the spinal cord first compress the spinothalamic fibers from sacral and lumbar areas, causing the early symptom of a loss of pain in the sacral area.)

Fibers from the second-order neurons cross to the opposite side of the medulla and ascend as a component of a tract called the *medial lemniscus.* The fibers of the medial lemniscus synapse with third-order neurons in the thalamus, which, in turn, sends fibers through the internal capsule to the somesthetic cortex of the parietal lobe. The sensory data reach the conscious level and become localized in the sensory cortex.

Descending Pathways

There are two major systems of motor pathways, classified as pyramidal and extrapyramidal. *Pyramidal tracts* (lateral and ventral corticospinal) are those whose fibers come together in the medulla to form the pyramids, thus the name. Most of the descending motor pathways involve two principal neurons—the upper and lower motor neurons. The *upper motor neuron* has its cell body in the cerebral motor cortex or in subcortical areas of the brain and brainstem, and its fibers conduct impulses from the brain to the spinal cord (or from the cerebrum to the brainstem [corticobulbar tract]). The spinal motor neuron (or cranial motor neuron) that innervates the muscle is called the *lower motor neuron.* Thus the upper motor neuron is entirely within the CNS, whereas the lower motor neuron begins in the CNS (anterior horn of the spinal cord gray matter) and sends its fibers out to innervate muscles. The lower motor neuron is thus a part of the PNS.

Voluntary Motor Pathway

The lateral and ventral corticospinal tracts are the major voluntary motor tracts of the spinal cord. These tracts are concerned primarily with controlled skilled movements of the extremities. Another important function of the upper motor neuron is to influence reflex movement by sending down facilitating or inhibiting impulses to alpha and gamma motor neurons (see Fig. 51-4).

The upper motor neurons of the corticospinal tracts originate in area 4 of the primary motor cortex, area 6 of the premotor cortex, and various portions of the parietal lobe. From here, fibers descend through the internal capsule to synapse with internuncial neurons at various levels of the spinal cord, which in turn synapse with neurons in the ventral horn gray matter. Some fibers, however, may synapse directly with lower motor neurons. It is also true that not all these fibers descend to spinal cord levels, because some may synapse with motor nuclei of cranial nerves (corticobulbar fibers) and in the reticular formation.

Approximately 85% of the descending fibers decussate (cross over) in the medulla and extend down the cord on the opposite side as part of the lateral corticospinal tract. The remaining 15% of the fibers remain uncrossed and descend on the same side of the cord as the ventral corticospinal tract. These fibers eventually cross the midline in the ventral gray column of the spinal cord segments (generally in the cervical and upper thoracic regions). Lesions of the corticospinal tracts produce Babinski's sign (see Fig. 51-6) and loss of performance of skilled voluntary movements, especially of the distal segments of the extremities.

EXTRAPYRAMIDAL SYSTEM AND BASAL GANGLIA

Precise delineation of the extrapyramidal system (all motor fibers not passing through the pyramids) is difficult anatomically. If the system is considered as an anatomic

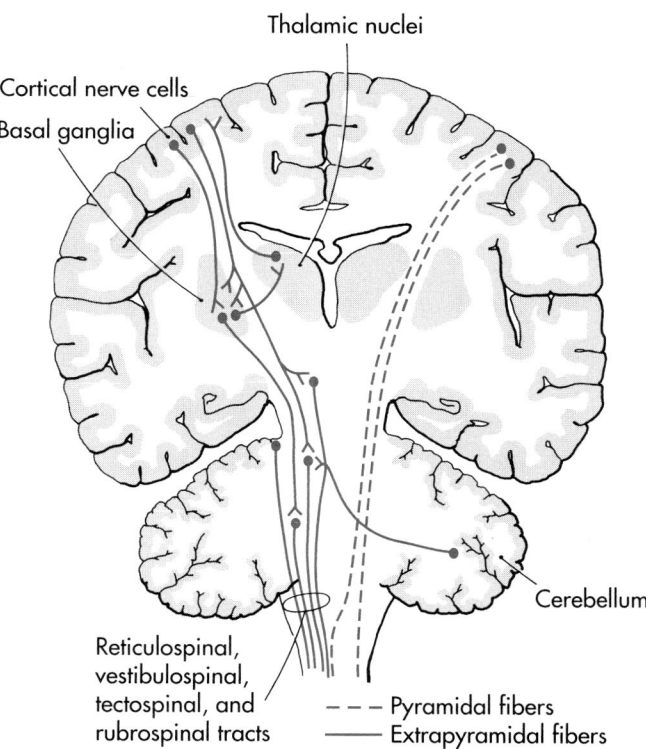

FIG. 50-23 Simplified diagram of pyramidal and extrapyramidal systems. Posture and performance of well-coordinated movements result from an integration of information received from both the cerebral cortex and the extrapyramidal systems. The cortex initiates movement, and the extrapyramidal system provides the facilitation or inhibition needed for production of purposeful, coordinated, controlled movements. Disruption of the extrapyramidal influence results in abnormal, uncontrolled movements. Components of the extrapyramidal system are the reticulospinal, vestibulospinal, tectospinal, and rubrospinal tracts.

unit, it is composed of the (1) basal ganglia and their circuits, (2) cortical areas that project to the basal ganglia, (3) cerebellar areas that project to the basal ganglia, (4) parts of the reticular formation that have connections with the basal ganglia and cerebral cortex, and (5) thalamic nuclei that connect the basal ganglia and reticular formation.

The primary function of the extrapyramidal system is to provide coarse control for voluntary muscles. (Fine control is provided by the pyramidal or corticospinal system.) The whole system works as a unit providing for integration on three levels: cortical, striatal, and tegmental. The major effect is inhibition (Fig. 50-23).

The *basal ganglia,* or *basal nuclei,* are found in each cerebral hemisphere in paired groups and are formed from the central gray matter of the telencephalon; they include the claustrum, putamen, globus pallidus, caudate, and amygdala (Fig. 50-24). The *caudate nucleus,* the most medial of the basal ganglia, is shaped like a comma with an extended tail. The *amygdaloid nucleus* lies as a knob of gray matter at the tip of the tail of the caudate. The putamen and globus pallidus together are called the *lenticular* (lens-shaped) *nucleus;* it extends from the head of the caudate. The *internal capsule* lies within borders formed by the thalamus, caudate nucleus, and lenticular nucleus. This crucial area is a passageway for all nerve fibers connecting the

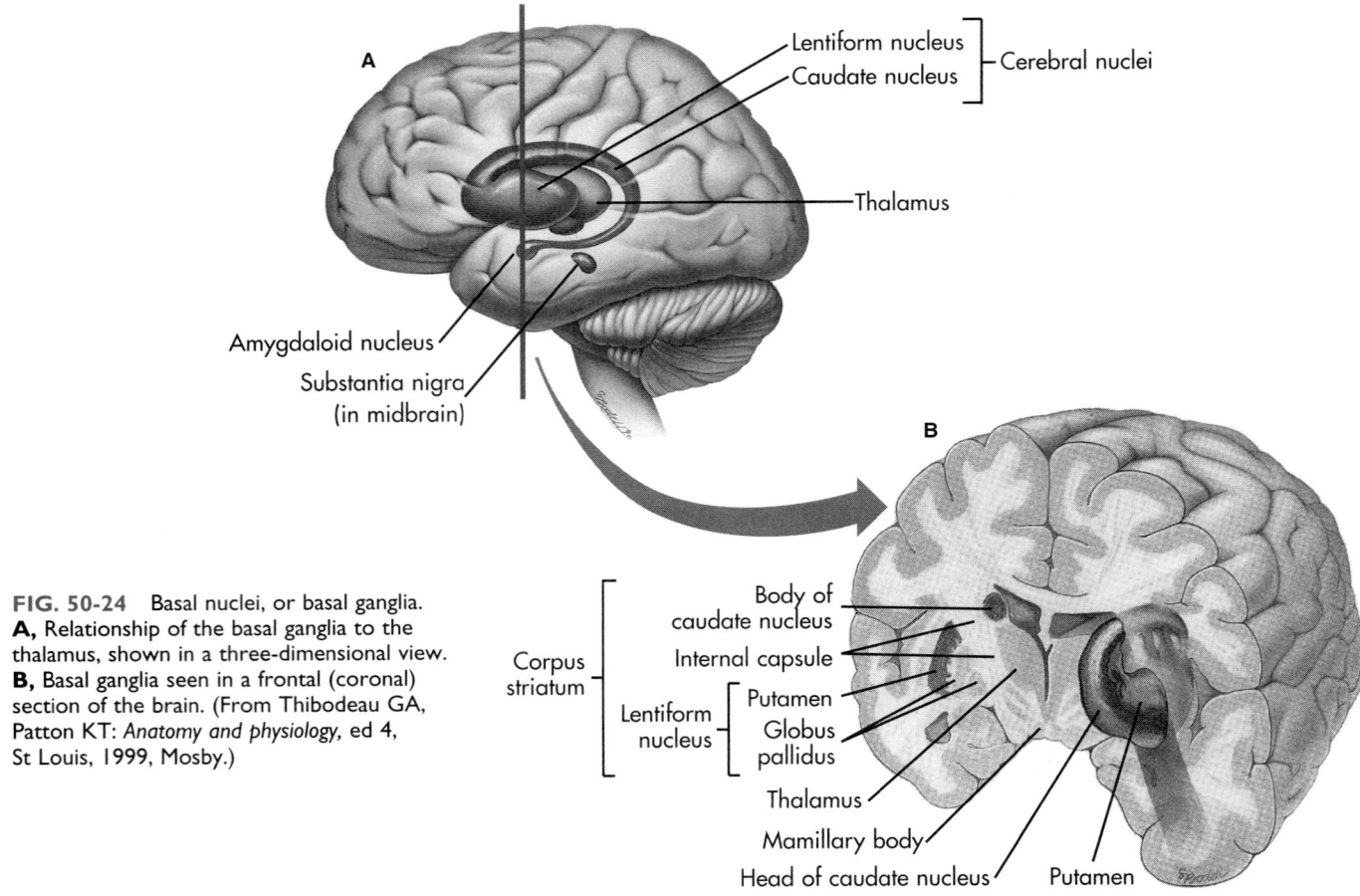

FIG. 50-24 Basal nuclei, or basal ganglia. **A,** Relationship of the basal ganglia to the thalamus, shown in a three-dimensional view. **B,** Basal ganglia seen in a frontal (coronal) section of the brain. (From Thibodeau GA, Patton KT: *Anatomy and physiology*, ed 4, St Louis, 1999, Mosby.)

cerebrum with the rest of the CNS. The caudate and lenticular nucleus, along with the adjacent part of the internal capsule, are sometimes referred to as the *corpus striatum.*

Three nuclear masses located in the upper midbrain operate in close association with the basal ganglia and are considered to be part of the extrapyramidal system: the *red nucleus;* the *substantia nigra;* and the *subthalamic nucleus,* or *corpus Luysii.*

The basal ganglia have multiple connections with other portions of the CNS, including the cerebral cortex, cerebellum, thalamus, and reticular formation. The basil ganglia are important centers of coordination, especially in the control of automatic associated movements. The corpus striatum (caudate nucleus and putamen) is responsible for the initiation and inhibition of gross intentional body movements that are unconsciously performed in the normal person; they also provide muscle tone so that exact movements can be performed, such as fine handwork requiring the coordinated effort of the entire arm and trunk for the hand to be able to perform.

A feedback system seems to operate via circular pathways from the motor cortex to the basal ganglia, thalamus, and motor cortex. Motor signals from the cerebral cortex to the pons and cerebellum are also circuitous, with the return to the cortex being through the ventrolateral nucleus of the thalamus, through which signals from the basal ganglia also pass. Because of the proximity of these circuits, it is hypothesized that basal ganglia and cerebellum feedback signals may be integrated in this area.

Broadly speaking, the basal ganglia are involved in two general activities: control of the body's motor tone and gross intentional movements. The general effect of basal ganglia excitation is of inhibitory signals to the bulboreticular facilitatory areas and of excitatory signals to the bulboreticular inhibitory areas. When the basal ganglia are not functioning adequately, the facilitatory areas become overactive and the inhibitory areas underactive, which results in rigidity throughout the body. The patient with an extrapyramidal disorder has great difficulty maintaining equilibrium while standing and posture while sitting, changing from a horizontal to a sitting position, rolling from a supine to a prone position, and walking. The righting reflex, the vestibular reflex, and proprioception are all disturbed. If the spinal cord is transected at the level of the mesencephalon, a *decerebrate rigidity* occurs, indicating that the major effect of the basal ganglia is inhibition. The tremor (abnormal movements) observed in extrapyramidal disorders is a result of excess neural activity in one area of the brain from unopposed activity in another area. This characteristic is called the *release phenomenon* and occurs often with tissue destruction in the nervous system (a lesion in *A* removes the regulatory control that *A* exerted over *B,* and consequently *B* becomes overactive).

Both the corpus striatum and the motor cortex are instrumental in the control of gross intentional movements that are normally unconscious. The control is accomplished through two pathways: (1) the globus pallidus through the thalamus to the cortex and downward via corticospinal and extracorticospinal pathways into the spinal cord and (2) downward through the globus pallidus and substantia nigra to the reticular formation and reticulospinal tracts to the cord. The globus pallidus seems to provide the background muscle tone necessary for performing exacting movements, especially with the

hands. Stimulation of the globus pallidus will stop the movement at any point and keep it locked at that point as long as the stimulation is continued.

Parkinson's syndrome and several extrapyramidal disorders of movement that involve the basal ganglia and extrapyramidal system are discussed in Chapter 54.

KEY CONCEPTS

- The nervous system is structurally divided into the *central nervous system (CNS)* (brain and spinal cord) and the *peripheral nervous system (PNS)* (somatic nervous system [SNC] and autonomic nervous system [ANS]), which make up the 31 pairs of spinal nerves and 12 pairs of cranial nerves.

- The ability to comprehend, learn and respond to stimuli is the result of integrated functioning of the nervous system.

- The cells of the nervous system are neurons and neuroglia. *Neurons* are the basic anatomic and functional unit, and *neuroglia* are support and nutrient cells.

- Two anatomic barriers regulate passage of substances from the blood into the brain: the *blood-brain barrier (BBB)* and the *blood-CSF (B-CSF) barrier*. Both barriers exist because of specialized "tight junctions" between endothelial cells of capillaries (BBB) and epithelial cells of the choroid plexus (B-CSF) barrier.

- The gelatinous tissue of the brain and spinal cord is protected by bone (skull and vertebrae) and by three layers of connective tissue called *meninges*: the *pia mater, arachnoid,* and *dura mater*. Note that the first letter of the meningeal names from innermost to outermost layer spell **PAD**, which aptly describes a major function of the meninges.

- Bleeding within the skull is described in terms of location of the bleed relative to specific meningeal layers (e.g., subdural, epidural, subarachnoid, intracranial).

- Sheaths of tough dura extend into the cranial cavity and provide important anatomic landmarks that support and divide the cerebrum and cerebellum. The *tentorium cerebelli* is located between the occipital cortex and the cerebellum, and tumors, as well as surgical procedures, are described in terms of location above or below that dural divider: supratentorial or infratentorial.

- The arterial supply of blood to the brain is a highly interconnected vascular network provided by two paired sets of arteries: *vertebral* and *internal carotid arteries*, which give rise to the *circle of Willis*.

- Venous blood drains via venous sinuses between the dural layers and returns to the general circulation via the internal jugular veins.

- Spinal cord arterial and venous systems closely parallel each other, unlike the arterial and venous systems of the brain.

- The *ventricles* are a series of four interconnecting cavities lined with ependymal cells and filled with cerebrospinal fluid (CSF). The major function of CSF is to cushion the brain within its solid vault.

- *Ventricles* communicate with each other through foramina and aqueducts. The final communicating pathway, from the fourth ventricle in the pons and medulla, is continuous with the subarachnoid space, allowing for free circulation of the CSF through the brain and spinal cord.

- *Normal CSF pressure* is approximately 9 to 14 mm Hg pressure, regulated by a constant cycle of secretion and absorption. Secretion occurs via *choroid plexuses* projecting into the ventricles, and absorption occurs via *arachnoidal villi,* which are fingerlike projections of arachnoid membrane through walls of the venous sinuses.

- The brain is the highest energy-consuming tissue in the body, receiving approximately 20% of the cardiac output.

- Because of crossover of ascending (sensory) and descending (motor) fibers, centers for sensory and motor activity are, for the most part, associated with activity on the opposite side of the body (contralateral control).

- Functional asymmetry of the two halves of the cerebral cortex currently is explained by the concepts of cerebral specialization and integration.

- The olfactory and optic nerves are actually CNS tracts, which carry signals from primary sensory neurons in the nasal epithelium and retina, respectively. The other 10 pairs of cranial nerves are located in the brainstem (medulla oblongata, pons, and midbrain). Therefore cranial nerve dysfunction is often an early indicator of brainstem lesions.

- The *reticular formation* is the central core of the brainstem, likened to a hot dog within a surrounding bun. The reticular formation determines the individual's state of arousal and consciousness, the sleepwake cycle, and modulation of all sensory, motor, and autonomic activity.

- The 31 pairs of *spinal nerves* emerge from the spinal cord through openings between vertebrae. However, because of disparity between cord length and vertebral length, the cord and vertebral levels do not correspond, especially in lumbar and sacral segments. Therefore a given vertebral level of injury will indicate a higher cord level of injury, because the nerve roots from the lumbar and sacral segments must pass for a distance before exiting the cord.

- In an arrangement inverse to that of brain tissue, the spinal cord white matter is external, and the gray matter is the internal core.

- The *anterior (ventral) horn cells* of the spinal cord contain the *lower motor neuron* or *final common pathway* for motor activity at the periphery of the body. Lesions in this area thus result in flaccid paralysis resulting from the total loss of the reflex arc.

■ The nerve pathways for pain and temperature ascend contralaterally in the spinal cord; the pathways for fine touch, proprioception and vibration ascend ipsilaterally in the cord, crossing over in the medulla. As a result, a given lateral spinal cord lesion causes different sensory losses on each side of the body below the lesion.

■ The *extrapyramidal system* provides coarse control and regulation of voluntary muscle movement. Lesions of these structures produce a "release phenomenon," or disinhibition, resulting in rigidity, abnormal postural reflexes, tremors, and bradykinesia.

■ Because the *internal capsule* is a narrowed passageway for all nerve fibers connecting the cerebrum with the rest of the CNS, lesions in that area cause more extensive neurologic deficits than do the same-sized lesions in a higher area of the cortex.

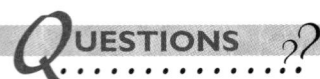

QUESTIONS

A sampling of review questions for this chapter appears here. Visit http://www.mosby.com/MERLIN/PriceWilson/ for additional questions. MERLIN

Circle "T" if the statement is true and "F" if it is false. Correct any false statements.

1. T F The nervous system is a communication system that directs and integrates all body activity.

2. T F The CNS includes the brain, spinal cord, and cranial nerves.

3. T F Interneurons relay messages between other neurons in the CNS, and large numbers may be found in the gray matter of the spinal cord, forming intersegmental tracts.

4. T F Spinal nerve trunks carry both afferent and efferent impulses to the CNS and are thus mixed nerves.

5. T F The parasympathetic branch of the ANS forms the thoracolumbar outflow from the spinal cord.

6. T F Nerve cells are not mitotic; they do not reproduce.

7. T F It is possible for a severed nerve fiber in the PNS to regenerate as long as the cell body is still viable.

8. T F Retinal rod and cone cells are examples of multipolar neurons.

9. T F The direction of a nerve impulse can be reversed.

10. T F Convergence means that a single neuron receives input from two or more neurons, and the response is the summated effect of all the different types of information.

11. T F The neurilemma is a thin membrane that envelops all nerve fibers.

12. T F Bundles of nerve fibers found in the CNS are called cranial nerves.

13. T F Lesions of the brainstem affect cranial nerves I and II (olfactory and optic).

Match the numbers in column B with the appropriate item in column A.

Column A	Column B
14. _____ Pairs of cranial nerves	a. 7
15. _____ Pairs of spinal nerves	b. 3
16. _____ Number of cervical vertebrae	c. 8
17. _____ Pairs of cervical spinal nerves	d. 12
18. _____ Oculomotor nerve (cranial nerve number)	e. 31

Match the specialized functions in column B with the cerebral hemisphere they are more likely to be associated with in column A.

Column A	Column B
19. _____ Right hemisphere	a. Mathematical calculation
20. _____ Left hemisphere	b. Speech
	c. Spatial locations
	d. Grasping of whole concepts
	e. Music
	f. Right-handedness

Answer the following on a separate sheet of paper.

21. Name and outline the components of the extrapyramidal system. What is its function? Name the basal ganglia.

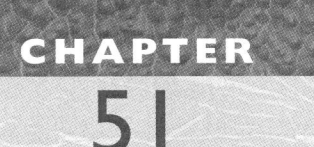

Evaluation of the Neurologic Patient

MARY S. HARTWIG

𝒯he nervous system is an intricate, vital network that shares three characteristics with the immune system. Specifically, the nervous system is: (1) a protective system that recognizes "self" from non-self and causes withdrawal from noxious stimuli; (2) a chemical factory, producing dozens of different kinds of molecules (e.g., peptides, amino acids, catecholamines) that transmit signals from one nerve cell to another or to another type of cell; and (3) a communication system that sends and receives messages sent at a distance within the body. Thus through its varied mechanisms of action, the nervous system controls not only the simplest vegetative functions of the body, such as breathing and heart rate, but it also controls the most highly complex integrative functions, such as evaluating information and problem solving.

Interference with nervous system function through disease or trauma produces specific focal or general deficits that reflect disruption of or abnormal activity in the affected areas of the central or peripheral nervous systems.

Clinical examination of the patient with a neurologic disorder yields valuable information. Symptoms presented by patients seeking health care include the ones derived from the primary neurologic disorder and those arising from fear, depression, weakness, and other symptoms arising from the individual patient's method of adapting. A logical, systematic, thorough examination of the patient and the presenting complaints can assist the clinician in differentiating and analyzing the complex clinical picture presented by most patients with a neurologic deficit. A complete and careful history and physical examination provides the final diagnosis in about 80% of patients. Despite the advances in diagnostic testing procedures, nothing has been found that can replace the history and physical examination.

For the neurologic examination to yield the necessary information, it is important, whenever possible, to gain the patient's cooperation. During the process of examination, the patient is often requested to do something that may appear nonsensical or may sound ridiculous. Careful explanation before the neurologic examination should allay the patient's anxiety and clarify the importance of the examination to the diagnostic process. Explanation about the length of the examination, the procedure to be followed, and any pain that the patient can expect will help establish trust and confidence in the examiner. The patient should be requested to answer all questions as accurately as possible and follow all directions to the best of his or her ability. Time must be allotted for the patient's questions, both before and after the examination.

NEUROLOGIC EXAMINATION

Evaluation of the nervous system starts with the examiner's first contact with the patient, when the patient is not being formally "examined." Evidence of the patient's functional ability at this time should be compared with apparent functioning elicited during the formal physical examination.

The neurologic examination, which consists of the history, a summary of the patient's symptoms, and a discussion of similar or related complaints in family members, will focus the clinician's thinking, direct the physical examination, and become the keystone for diagnosis of the problem. The close association of neurologic symptoms with symptoms of other medical disease states (e.g., diabetes mellitus, severe hypoxemia, hypertension, thyroid disorders) necessitates a complete medical evaluation, even though the patient's symptoms suggest a neurologic problem. If there is a reversible secondary condition causing the neurologic symptoms, that condition must first be treated and results evaluated before subjecting the patient to invasive and expensive neurologic tests in the search for organic neuropathology. For example, an elderly person's neurologic status (sensorium, coordination, ability to communicate intelligibly) can be profoundly impaired by an acute treatable condition such as pneumonia or urinary tract infection.

The neurologic history focuses on why the patient seeks medical attention. It is important that this information be elicited and recorded in the patient's own words, not in diagnostic terms. A detailed discussion of the neurologic examination is not included here because it can be found in many standard textbooks on neurology. A brief summary of the examination is included to help review some important points.

Important information includes the past medical history, social history, family history, and onset of present symptoms. It is important to ask the patient what problems, if any, have been experienced with each major body system and part. The patient is asked specifically about dizziness, headaches, visual disturbances, bowel or bladder dysfunction, weakness, numbness, and pain. While eliciting this information, the clinician carefully observes the patient's behavior, attitudes, attention to personal appearance and grooming, ability to answer the questions appropriately, and ability to concentrate. Once this portion of the examination is completed, the clinician can substantiate suspicions and abnormal findings with further examinations and diagnostic tests. In some cases of neurologic disorder (e.g., migraine, trigeminal neuralgia), the diagnosis is made purely on the basis of the history because there are no significant physical findings.

Organization of the neurologic examination is very important. Following a particular order allows the clinician to evaluate the information and direct the later segments of the examination. The organization of the examination includes evaluation of six major elements: (1) mental status with its seven components, (2) head and neck including cranial nerves, (3) motor function, (4) sensory function, (5) muscle stretch reflexes, and (6) special reflexes such as glabellar and plantar. Information from each segment of the examination is correlated with information previously gained, leading to a localization of the disease process.

Mental Status and Function

In general, the mental status and function portion of the examination evaluates the patient's higher cortical functions, including ability to reason, use abstraction, plan ahead, and make judgments. Speech depends on more modalities than higher cortical function; but because of its close association with testing language, it will be included with discussion of a detailed mental status examination. Changes in behavior and personality may be associated with organic brain dysfunction; therefore these

changes need to be elicited from the patient or the patient's family. In evaluating the patient's mental status, the examiner must be aware of socioeconomic, ethnic, and educational status. General knowledge and intellect may be evaluated by asking the patient to name five countries or five major rivers. The patient's ability to remember past events may be evaluated by asking the patient questions about his or her own past but may be difficult to assess. Asking the patient to repeat at least six digits may assess recent memory. Normal individuals have the ability to remember and repeat seven digits forward and four backward. Important information is obtained by evaluating the patient's ability to produce abstract thoughts and generalizations from concrete statements. Asking the patient to interpret a common saying (e.g., "A rolling stone gathers no moss") is a frequently used method.

Level of Consciousness

Evaluating the patient's level of consciousness (LOC) is an essential component of the neurologic examination that should be performed thoughtfully, with meticulous attention to accuracy. Many tools are available today for categorizing LOC, using similar terms in different ways (see Glasgow Coma Scale, Chapter 56). When using any tool, the most important criterion should be consistency, and a complete understanding of all terminology is essential. It is more objective to describe the patient's behavior and responses exactly than it is to rely on catch-all terms such as *lethargic* or *stuporous*. Table 51-1 lists several terms used to describe LOC, with descriptions of behavior associated with these terms.

Cerebral Functions

Knowledge of the functions of the cerebral lobes and subsequently related symptoms associated with deficits of that particular area of the brain assists the clinician in pinpointing the neurologic deficit. Important observations about the patient's neurologic problems are made during the neurologic examination. Table 51-2 lists the cerebral lobes and some of their known functions.

Language and Speech

One of the most important functions of the dominant hemisphere is speech. The left hemisphere is dominant for speech in right-handed persons and in most left-handed persons. There are three speech disorders of neurologic origin: dysarthria, dysphonia, and aphasia.

Dysarthria is a defect in articulation, enumeration, and rhythm of speech related to a weakness in the muscles involved in speech. This abnormality is usually detected in ordinary conversation with the patient but may be confirmed by asking for repetition of a difficult word or phrase, such as "Methodist Episcopal." The causes for this weakness can be amyotrophic lateral sclerosis, pseudobulbar palsy, or myasthenia gravis.

Dysphonia is a disorder of vocalization giving a hoarse quality to the voice. The disorder can be confirmed by detecting hoarseness or a rough quality to the voice of a

TABLE 51-1

Levels of Consciousness

Term	Characteristics
Conscious	Freely aware of surroundings; oriented to person, place, and time Cooperative Can repeat several digits a few minutes after being told them
Automatism	Relatively normal behavior (e.g., capable of feeding self) Speaks in sentences but has difficulty with memory and judgment; has no recollection of events before period of unconsciousness; may ask the same questions over and over Behaves automatically without immediate or late memory of behavior Obeys simple commands
Confusion	Performs purposeful activity (e.g., feeding) with clumsy movements Disoriented as to time, place, person, or any combination (acts as if in a daze) Memory impaired; is unable to sustain thought or expression Generally difficult to arouse Becomes uncooperative
Delirium	Disoriented to time, place, and person Uncooperative Agitated, restless, resistive (may attempt to get out of bed; thrashes around in bed; pulls off dressings, intervenous line) Difficult to arouse
Stupor	Quiet; may appear to be asleep Responds to loud verbal stimuli Annoyed by light Responds appropriately to painful stimuli
Deep stupor	Mute Very difficult to arouse (some arousal to painful stimuli) Responds to pain with automatic purposeless movements
Coma	Unconscious; body flaccid No response to verbal or painful stimuli Reflexes present; gag, knee jerk, corneal
Irreversible coma and death	Reflexes disappear Pupils become fixed and dilated Cessation of respirations and heartbeat

TABLE 51-2

Cerebral Functions and Deficits

Cerebral Lobe	Functions	Deficits
Frontal	Judgment Personality traits Complex mental skills (abstraction, conceptualizing, foresight)	Impaired judgment Impaired grooming and appearance Impaired affect Impaired thought process Impaired motor functions
Temporal	Auditory memory Recent memory Primary auditory area affecting awareness	Deficits in recent memory Psychomotor seizures Deafness
Parietal		
Dominant	Speech Calculation (mathematics) Topography of both sides of body	Aphasia Agraphia Acalculia Agnosia Sensory deficits (bilateral)
Nondominant	Sensory awareness Synthesis of complex memories	Disorientation Distortion of concept of space Loss of awareness of opposite side
Occipital	Visual memory Vision	Blindness and visual deficits

patient responding to a request to say "E" and by indirect laryngoscopy. This problem has many nonneurologic causes; among the neurologic causes are injury to the recurrent laryngeal nerve and tumors of the brainstem.

Aphasia is a general term meaning loss of the ability to comprehend, elaborate, or express speech concepts. *Motor aphasia* is loss of the ability to express thoughts in speech or writing, and *sensory aphasia* is loss of the ability to comprehend spoken or written language. For evaluation, the patient may be directed to perform certain tasks by written or verbal orders, such as, "Fold this paper" and "Write your name." The most common cause of aphasia is a cerebrovascular disorder involving the middle cerebral artery, which supplies the speech and language center.

Cranial Nerve Function

Twelve pairs of cranial nerves arise from the undersurface of the brain through small foramina; they are numbered according to the order in which they emerge, from front to rear (Fig. 51-1).

The cranial nerves are composed of afferent or efferent fibers, and some, referred to as *mixed fibers*, are of both types. The cell bodies of the afferent fibers are located in ganglia outside the brainstem, whereas the cell bodies of the efferent fibers are located in various nuclei of the brainstem.

The cranial nerves are examined not in sequence but according to function. The following mnemonic helps one to remember cranial nerve function as motor (M), sensory (S), or both (B): Some(I) Say(II) Marry(III) Money(IV), But(V) My(VI) Brother(VII) Say(VIII) Bad(IX) Business(X) Marry(XI) Money(XII). The method of examination of the cranial nerves and some pathophysiologic implications are discussed in the following sections.

Olfactory Nerve (Cranial Nerve I)

The olfactory nerve conveys smells to the brain for appreciation. With the patient's eyes closed and one nostril occluded at a time, mildly aromatic substances, such as vanilla, cologne, and cloves, are offered for identification. Especially if an anterior fossa lesion is suspected, one should test the sense of smell in each nostril separately, and then determine whether odors can be discriminated. The patient is requested to indicate the moment of first detection of the odor and, if possible, to identify the substance.

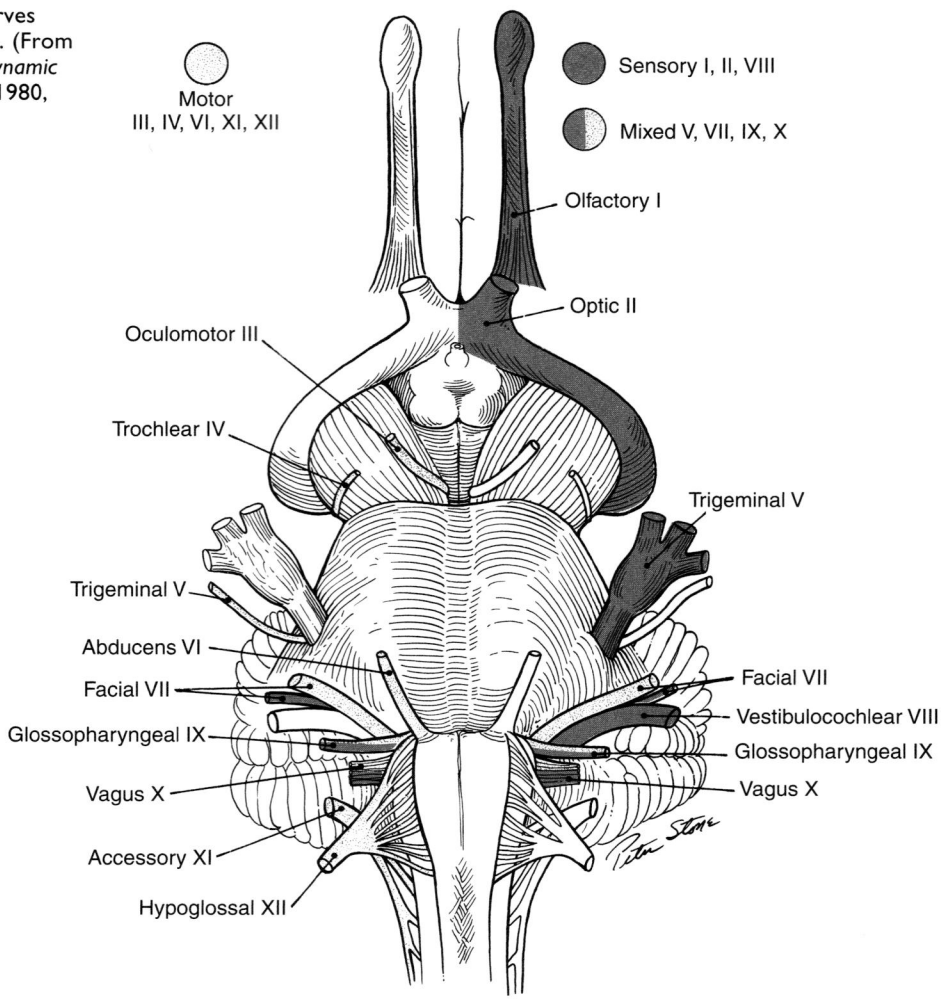

Motor
III, IV, VI, XI, XII

Sensory I, II, VIII

Mixed V, VII, IX, X

Olfactory I

Optic II

Oculomotor III

Trochlear IV

Trigeminal V

Trigeminal V

Abducens VI

Facial VII

Facial VII

Vestibulocochlear VIII

Glossopharyngeal IX

Glossopharyngeal IX

Vagus X

Vagus X

Accessory XI

Hypoglossal XII

Perception of the odor is more important than correct identification of the substance.

Nasal disorders (e.g., sinusitis, allergies, upper respiratory infections) are the most common causes of loss of smell. A tumor in the olfactory groove (olfactory groove meningioma) is a neurologic cause for the loss of smell. Any obstruction of nasal passages should be relieved by a nasal decongestant before testing.

Anosmia may also occur after meningitis, subarachnoid hemorrhage, or head injury involving the nerve fibers as they pass through the cribriform plate.

Optic Nerve (Cranial Nerve II)

The optic nerve transmits impulses from the retina to the thalamus via the optic chiasm. Higher-order visual pathways convey the information from the thalamus to the occipital cortex for recognition and interpretation. Examination of this nerve involves testing visual acuity either by using a Snellen test or, if this is not available, by asking the patient to read various sizes of newspaper print. Diseases involving the eye, optic nerve, or optic chiasm generally reduce visual acuity. Visual field examinations provide information about the optic nerve and visual pathways from the eye to the occipital cortex. For general purposes as part of a neurologic examination, visual

fields are examined by confrontation by asking the patient to cover one eye. The examiner sits directly in front of the patient, asking him or her to look straight ahead. A pencil or finger is brought into the field of vision from the four quadrants toward the uncovered eye. The patient is asked to identify when the pencil or finger first enters the visual field. This method provides a gross screening device. For a more thorough evaluation, a perimeter and tangent screen are used.

The optic disc is visualized by use of the ophthalmoscope. Neurologically, the two most significant findings are papilledema and optic atrophy. Changes in the disc occur with tumors, infections, and trauma. Other changes visualized are exudates, hemorrhages, and arteriovenous abnormalities associated with diabetes and hypertension.

Oculomotor, Trochlear, and Abducens Nerves (Cranial Nerves III, IV, and VI)

These three nerves are examined together, because they act conjugately to control the extraocular muscles (EOMs). In addition, the oculomotor nerve elevates the upper eyelid and innervates the sphincter muscle of the iris (constrictor muscle), which controls the pupil size. The innervation of the EOMs is examined by asking the patient to follow a moving finger or pencil with eyes turning

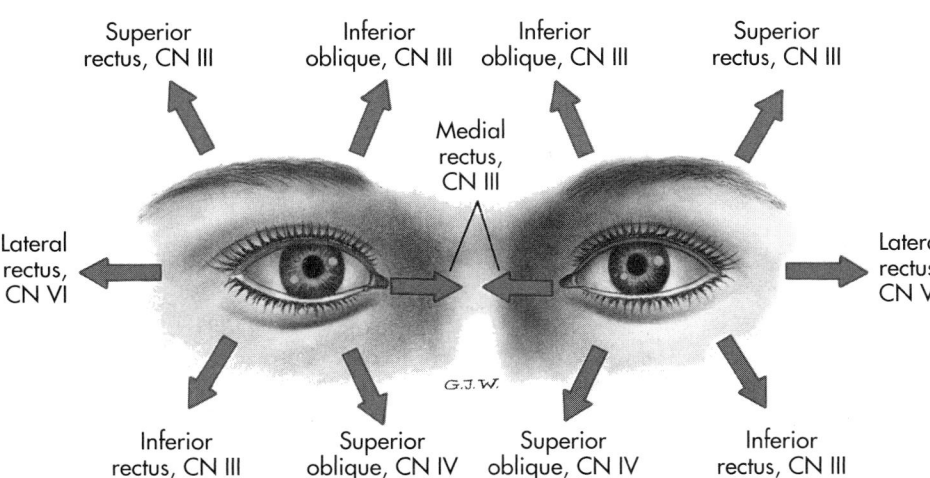

Superior
rectus, CN III

Inferior
oblique, CN III

Inferior
oblique, CN III

Superior
rectus, CN III

Medial
rectus,
CN III

Lateral
rectus,
CN VI

Lateral
rectus,
CN VI

G.J.W.

Inferior
rectus, CN III

Superior
oblique, CN IV

Superior
oblique, CN IV

Inferior
rectus, CN III

FIG. 51-2 Cranial nerves and extraocular muscles associated with the six cardinal fields of gaze. (From Seidel HM, Ball JW, Dains JE, Benedict GW: *Mosby's guide to physical examination*, ed 4, St Louis, 1999, Mosby.)

PUPIL GAUGE (mm)

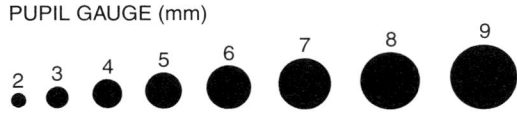

2 3 4 5 6 7 8 9

FIG. 51-3   Pupil size reference guide.

upward, downward, medially, and laterally. Weakness in muscles becomes evident when an eye cannot move in a certain direction (Fig. 51-2).

Pupils are examined in subdued light and should be round and approximately equal in size, although unequal pupils (anisocoria) are found in approximately 20% to 25% of the population. However, the difference is rarely greater than 1 mm. Both pupils should react to light directly and consensually.

In recording the size of the pupils, it is essential to use millimeters (mm) to ensure accuracy in evaluating the patient's pupillary status. This practice is particularly important when the practitioner is evaluating a patient after a head injury. Fig. 51-3 provides a pupil size reference guide.

The nuclei of the oculomotor nerves and the trochlear nerve are located in the midbrain. The nuclei of the abducens nerves lie beneath the floor of the fourth ventricle in the lower pons and are close to fibers from the facial nerve nucleus.

Myasthenia gravis is an important cause of weakness of the EOMs, causing weakness in more than one muscle and ptosis (see Chapter 54). *Horner's syndrome* consists of ptosis of the lid, constriction of the pupil, and absence of sweating on the same side of the face. These symptoms can result from vascular lesions in the brainstem, cervical spinal cord injuries and tumors, or trauma affecting the sympathetic fibers in the neck or can be a temporary side effect of cerebral angiography.

Horizontal nystagmus (rapid lateral oscillations of the eye) is an important neurologic sign; it is seen normally on extreme lateral gaze. Nystagmus can occur in any direction of gaze and can be unilateral or bilateral. Neurologic causes include multiple sclerosis, lesions of one cerebellar hemisphere, and tumor of one side of the brain. Nonneurologic causes include the use of barbiturates and tranquilizers.

Trigeminal Nerve (Cranial Nerve V)

The trigeminal nerve carries both motor and sensory fibers and supplies innervation to the temporal and masseter muscles, which are the muscles of mastication. The motor division of this nerve is examined by asking the patient to clench the teeth and move the jaw from side to side while the examiner palpates the muscles and judges the strength of contraction.

The sensory fibers of the trigeminal nerve are divided into three main branches: ophthalmic, maxillary, and mandibular (Fig. 51-4). To evaluate areas of sensory loss, each area is tested by asking the patient to respond to a touch with a piece of cotton. The corneal reflex is tested in each eye: a wisp of cotton with a fine point is touched to the cornea, causing the patient to blink.

Tumors of the posterior fossa cause loss of corneal reflex and facial numbness as early signs. The most notable disorder affecting the trigeminal nerve is *trigeminal neuralgia*, or *tic douloureux*, causing brief, excruciating pain along the maxillary or mandibular divisions of the trigeminal nerve. Myasthenia gravis and amyotrophic lateral sclerosis cause weakness and fatigue of the muscles of mastication, making chewing difficult and at times impossible.

Facial Nerve (Cranial Nerve VII)

The facial nerve has both sensory and motor function. It carries sensory fibers that mediate taste perception from the anterior tongue and motor fibers, which innervate all the muscles necessary for a variety of facial expressions, including smiling, frowning, and grimacing.

The motor division of the facial nerve is evaluated by asking the patient to perform various facial movements and observing the patient speak. Weakness of the facial muscle may be evidenced by flattening of the nasolabial fold, drooping of one side of the mouth, and sagging of the lower eyelid. The sense of taste is evaluated by asking the patient to identify sweet, sour, and salty substances, which are applied to the tongue. The ninth cranial nerve, the glossopharyngeal, carries the sensation of bitterness, which is perceived only on the posterior segment of the tongue. This point is important to remember when testing for the sensation of bitterness.

Because the nucleus of the facial nerve lies in the lateral portion of the lower pons, a lesion in the area of the

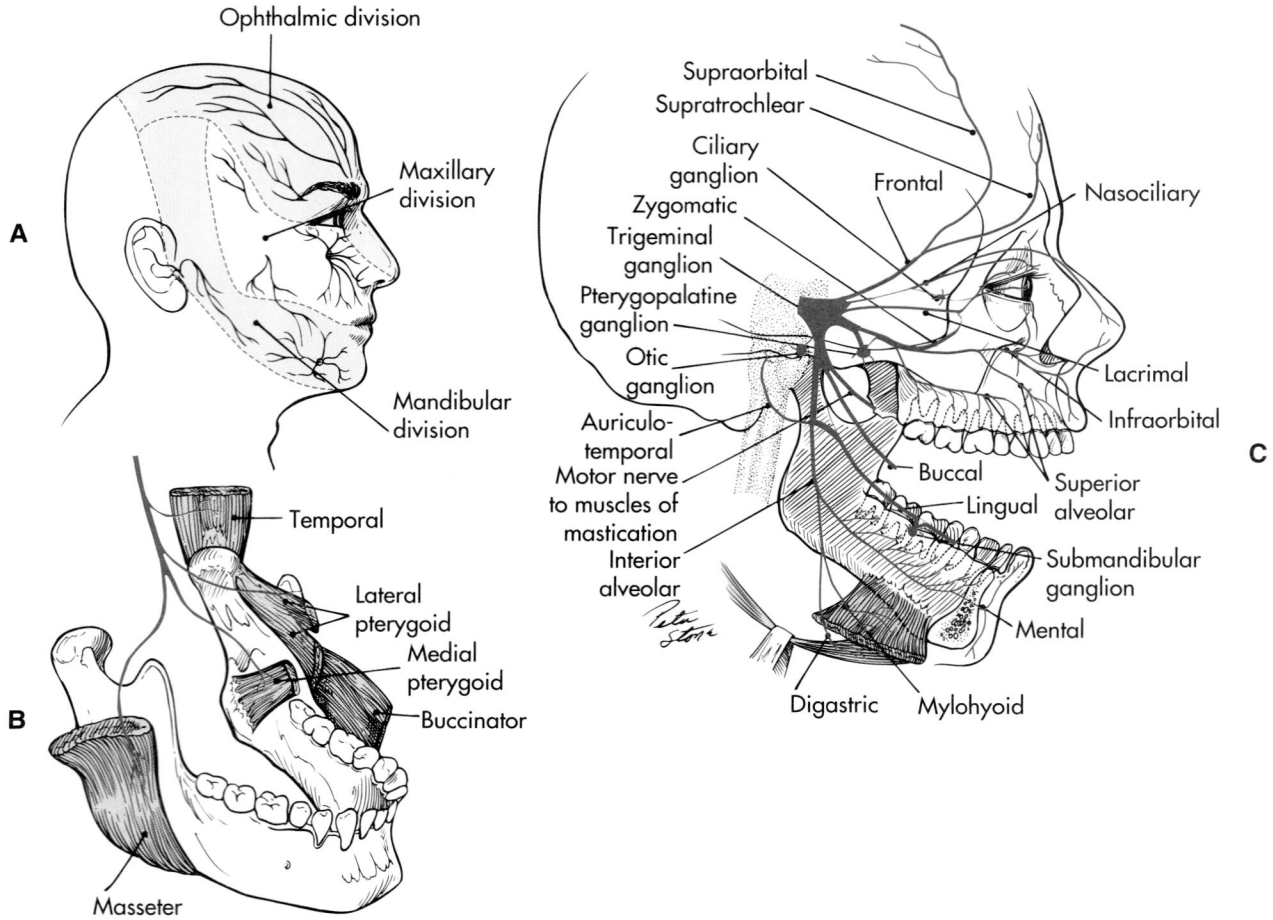

FIG. 51-4 **A**, Distribution of sensory fibers to the skin by the three branches of the trigeminal nerve. **B**, Distribution of the chief motor fibers to the muscles of mastication. **C**, Distribution of terminal branches. (From Langley LL, Telford JR, Christensen JB: *Dynamic anatomy and physiology,* ed 5, New York, 1980, McGraw-Hill.)

brainstem will often cause facial nerve dysfunction. The facial nerve enters the temporal bone and is close to the middle ear, thus it is subject to trauma from fractures of the base of the skull and the temporal bone, from surgical procedures, and from diseases of the ear. Other disorders that may result in facial nerve weakness include myasthenia gravis and Guillain-Barré syndrome. *Bell's palsy,* caused by an inflammation of the facial nerve (CN-VII), is the most common type of nerve paralysis.

Vestibulocochlear Nerve (Cranial Nerve VIII)

The vestibulocochlear nerve maintains balance and transmits impulses that allow a person to hear. Maintaining balance is the function of the vestibular division, whereas the cochlear division mediates hearing. Observing the patient's ability to hear a whisper from a distance of 2 feet can test the cochlear division. Another method of testing involves use of the tuning fork, which distinguishes between conductive hearing loss and sensorineural hearing loss. People with normal hearing will hear a tuning fork placed in the midline of the head or forehead equally well in both ears. Also, individuals will hear the tuning fork better by air conduction than they will by bone conduction. Normally, the tuning fork is heard twice as long by air conduction. The two most common tuning fork–hearing tests are the Rinne and Weber tests. In the *Rinne test* a vibrating tuning fork is placed on the mastoid process; when the patient indicates that the vibration is no longer audible, the tuning fork is placed next to the ear. If the patient again hears the vibration, air conduction (AC) is better than bone conduction (BC). This difference is normal and is arbitrarily called a "positive" Rinne. A "negative" Rinne is indicative of middle ear disease causing conductive hearing loss. In the *Weber test,* the vibrating tuning fork is placed on the top of the patient's head, in the middle of the forehead, or on the upper front teeth. The patient is asked where the sound is heard the loudest. Normally the sound is heard equally on both sides. A sound that lateralizes to one side may indicate a hearing loss. If the patient has conductive hearing loss, the sound will be heard better in the deafer ear, whereas with sensorineural loss it will be heard better in the healthy ear. If an abnormality is detected, a complete audiometer evaluation should be performed.

Acute dysfunction of the vestibular division of the vestibulocochlear nerve is manifested by vertigo, nausea, vomiting, and ataxia. The *cold caloric test* (also known as the *oculovestibular reflex* test) is used to screen for problems. This test is performed with the patient upright. Ice water (5 ml) is injected into the ear. The normal response to this stimulus is nystagmus of both eyes, vertigo, nausea, and vomiting. Little or no reaction to this stimulus indicates an abnormality of the vestibular nerve. In a comatose patient, the test is done to determine whether the brainstem is intact. With an intact brainstem and vestibular nerve, the eyes will deviate conjugately toward the irrigated ear. A negative reflex usually indicates brainstem dysfunction or a lesion involving the extraocular muscles. *Meniere's disease* involves a dilation of the endolymphatic channels in the cochlea, with eventual atrophy of the hearing mechanism resulting in vertigo, tinnitus, and hearing loss in the affected ear.

The vestibulocochlear nerve leaves the brainstem and travels along a path similar to that of the facial nerve. As with the facial nerve, the vestibulocochlear nerve is subject to damage from fractures of the base of the skull and the temporal bone. Vascular occlusions and tumors of the brainstem are other causes of damage to this nerve.

Glossopharyngeal and Vagus Nerves (Cranial Nerves IX and X)

The glossopharyngeal and vagus nerves are closely related anatomically and functionally and are evaluated together. The glossopharyngeal nerve has a sensory division, which carries taste from the posterior portion of the tongue, innervates the carotid sinus and the carotid bodies, and supplies sensation to the pharynx. The motor division innervates the posterior wall of the pharynx. The vagus nerve innervates all the thoracic and abdominal viscera and conveys impulses from the walls of the intestines, the heart, and the lungs. It is not possible clinically to examine all these functions; therefore evaluation of the vagus nerve is directed toward evaluating the motor function of the palate, pharynx, and larynx.

The first step in evaluation of the glossopharyngeal and vagus nerves is inspection of the soft palate. The soft palate should be symmetric and should not deviate to either side. When the patient says "ah," the soft palate should rise symmetrically. To induce a *gag reflex*, the posterior wall of the pharynx is touched, causing elevation of the palate and constriction of the pharyngeal muscles. The patient's *swallowing reflex* is tested by observing the reaction to drinking a glass of water. Observations are made of difficulty in swallowing or regurgitation of fluid through the nose, which would indicate weakness of the soft palate and an inability to close off the nasopharynx when swallowing. *Indirect laryngoscopy* is performed when the patient's complaint is a voice disturbance or hoarseness. The vocal cords can be observed for paresis or lesions. Bilateral lesions may cause greater difficulty in swallowing and in the ability to mobilize secretions.

The glossopharyngeal and vagus nerves leave the skull through the jugular foramen with the internal jugular vein. Therefore trauma or a tumor close to this area would affect these structures. The recurrent laryngeal nerve, a branch of the vagus that supplies the larynx, is susceptible to injury during surgery of the neck because of its proximity to the thyroid gland. Amyotrophic lateral sclerosis and myasthenia gravis frequently cause weakness in the muscles innervated by the glossopharyngeal and the vagus nerves.

Accessory Nerve (Cranial Nerve XI)

The accessory nerve is a motor nerve innervating the sternocleidomastoid muscle and the upper portion of the trapezius muscle. These two muscles flex the neck; also, the sternocleidomastoid muscle rotates the head from side to side, and the trapezius muscle rotates the scapula when the arm is raised.

The function of the accessory nerve is evaluated by observing the sternocleidomastoid and trapezius muscles for atrophy and assessing their strength. To test the sternocleidomastoid muscle, the patient is asked to turn the head toward one shoulder and to resist the examiner's attempts to move the head in the opposite direction. This test is repeated on the other side so that both the right and the left muscles are evaluated. The trapezius muscle is evaluated by asking the patient to shrug the shoulders while the examiner attempts to push downward. The patient is then asked to elevate both arms to a vertical position. A patient with weakness in the trapezius muscle will not be able to perform this action.

The accessory nerve lies close to the glossopharyngeal and vagus nerves. Tumors affecting these nerves frequently affect the accessory nerve. The cell bodies of the accessory nerve lie in the lower medulla and the upper part of the spinal cord at levels of the first through fifth cervical vertebrae and receive innervation from both cerebral hemispheres. Therefore a cerebral cortical lesion may cause little or no dysfunction in the two muscles innervated by this nerve. The most common cause for accessory nerve dysfunction is neck trauma, with direct damage to the cranial nerve cell body or axon.

Hypoglossal Nerve (Cranial Nerve XII)

The hypoglossal nerve innervates the musculature of the tongue. Normal functioning of the tongue is essential for normal speech and swallowing. Slight bilateral weakness is characterized by difficulty in enunciating consonants and difficulty in swallowing. Severe bilateral weakness causes extreme difficulty with speech and swallowing.

The tongue is examined for asymmetry, deviation to one side, and the presence of fasciculations. This examination is first performed inside the mouth with the tongue at rest and then with the tongue protruded. Strength of the muscle is evaluated by asking the patient to push out a cheek with the tongue while the examiner opposes the effort with fingers on the patient's cheek.

The nuclei of the hypoglossal nerves lie within the medulla beneath the floor of the fourth ventricle and receive innervation from both cerebral hemispheres. Injuries to the neck may cause unilateral weakness of the tongue with atrophy and fasciculations. Tumors at the base of the posterior fossa near the foramen magnum may cause ipsilateral paralysis of the tongue. Bilateral weakness can result from amyotrophic lateral sclerosis and myasthenia gravis.

Motor Function

Motor performance depends on an intact muscle, a functioning neuromuscular junction, and intact cranial and spinal nerve tracts. To understand how the nervous system functions to coordinate muscle activity, it is important first to be able to distinguish between the upper and the lower motor neurons.

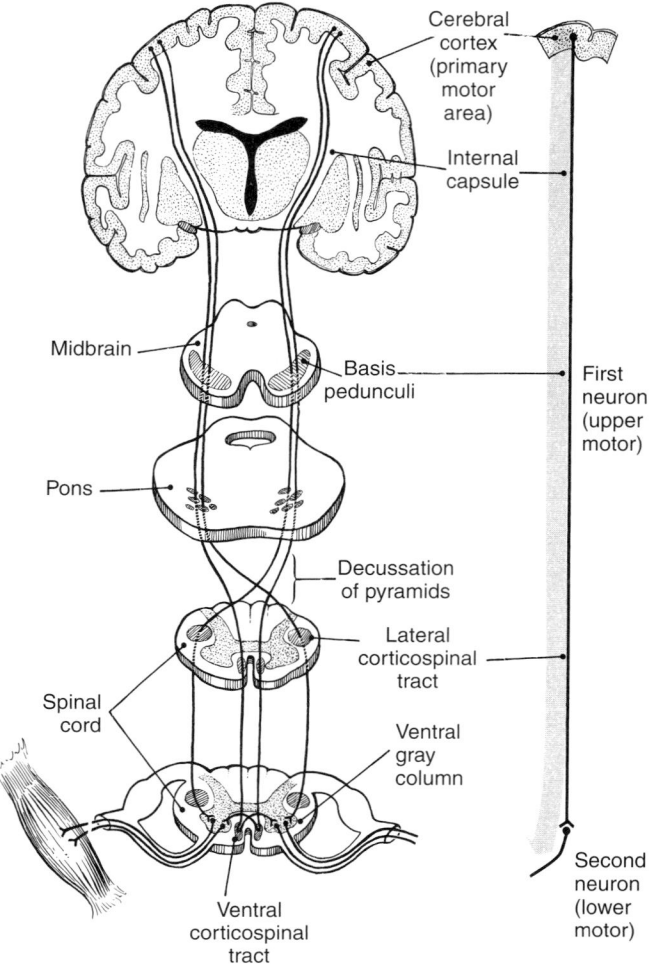

FIG. 51-5 Pyramidal motor pathways (corticospinal tracts). The tracts originate in pyramidal cells of the cortex. Fibers that cross at the medulla form the lateral corticospinal tracts, and the remaining fibers form the ventral corticospinal tracts. The basis pedunculi are part of the cerebral peduncles. (From Langley LL, Telford JR, Christensen JB: *Dynamic anatomy and physiology*, ed 5, New York, 1980, McGraw-Hill.)

The *upper motor neuron (UMN)* originates in the cerebral cortex and projects downward, one part (the corticobulbar tract) ending in the brainstem and the other (the corticospinal tract) crossing in the lower medulla and descending into the spinal cord. The cranial nerve nuclei are the end point for the corticobulbar tracts. The corticospinal tracts terminate in the region of the anterior horn of the spinal cord from the cervical to the sacral areas. The corticospinal fibers that travel through the medullary pyramids constitute the pyramidal tracts. Nerve fibers in the corticospinal tract mediate voluntary movement, particularly fine, discrete, conscious movement (Fig. 51-5).

The *lower motor neuron (LMN)* includes the motor cells of the cranial nerve nuclei and their axons, as well as the anterior horn cells of the spinal cord and their axons. The motor fibers leave through the anterior, or motor, root of the spinal column and innervate the muscles.

Lesions involving the UMN and the LMN produce characteristic changes in muscle response. Awareness of the differences in muscle weakness helps to locate the neurologic lesion. Table 51-3 summarizes this information.

TABLE 51-3

Differentiation Between Upper and Lower Motor Neuron Weakness

Characteristic	Upper Motor Neuron*	Lower Motor Neuron†
Type and distribution of weakness	Lesions in brain: "pyramidal distribution," that is, distal, especially hand muscles; weaker extensors in arm and weaker flexors in legs Lesions in cord: variable, depending on location	Depends on which lower motor neurons are involved, that is, which segments, roots, or nerves
Tone	Spasticity: greater in flexors in arms and extensors in legs	Flaccidity
Bulk	Slight atrophy of disuse only	Atrophy: may be marked
Reflexes	Accentuated, Babinski's sign present	Decreased or absent; no Babinski's sign
Fasciculations	No	Yes
Clonus	Frequently present	Absent

*Synonyms: pyramidal tract (referring to fibers in medullary pyramids), corticospinal tract, corticobulbar tract.
†Synonyms: anterior horn cell, ventral horn cell, somatic motor portions of cranial nerves, final common pathway.

Coordination and Gait

Coordination is impaired by many disorders at any level of the motor system. Incoordination is a particularly relevant sign, generally indicating problems with cerebellar function and corticospinal tract interruption. Tests that reveal a lack of coordination include tandem walking (asking the patient to walk heel to toe), ability of the patient to follow through on simple rapid movements (placing the hand on the knee alternately using the palm and back of the hand), and ability of the patient to place the heel of one foot on the opposite knee and slide it down the front of the leg. Cerebellar disease causes these movements to be slow, nonrhythmic, and inaccurate.

Gait is usually observed by asking the patient to walk. Keeping in mind that most people tend to walk slowly and carefully when observed, the examiner looks for lack of arm swing or decreased arm swing, hemiplegia, rigidity, loss of coordinated movement, tremor, apraxia (slow, shuffling steps and difficulty in lifting feet from the ground), or any combination of these characteristics. Patients with cerebellar disease walk with a wide base of support and have a tendency to stagger laterally. Slow gait, small shuffling steps, and lack of arm swing are characteristics of Parkinson's disease.

Muscle Tone and Strength

Muscle tone, which is the resistance detected by the examiner when a joint is moved through passive range of motion, is frequently altered in nervous system disorders. UMN disorders increase muscle tone, whereas LMN disorders decrease muscle tone. Table 51-4 lists some of the alterations in muscle tone frequently seen in neurologic disorders.

TABLE 51-4

Some Alterations in Motor Function Associated With Neurologic Disorders

Muscle Disorder	Clinical Findings	Neurologic Disorder
Dystonia	Persistent abnormal positions of body parts in which there is resistance to passive movement of the part	Extrapyramidal disease Wilson's disease Phenothiazine neuropathy Viral brain infection
Paratonia (gegenhalten)	Resistance to passive movement throughout the range of motion (somewhat proportional to the amount of force applied)	Frontal lobe disease
Decerebrate rigidity	Extension and pronation of the upper extremities and extension of the lower extremities	Severe brain injury above level of the pons
Hypotonia	Increased range of motion of joints (overextension and overflexion)	Cerebellar disease
Hemiballismus	Unilateral movements affecting side opposite the lesion and involving violent, flinging movements at the proximal joints	Cerebrovascular occlusions involving the subthalamic nucleus
Tremors	Involuntary rhythmic, tremulous movements Rest tremor: more pronounced at rest Intention tremor: worse when patient reaches for an object	Lesions of the cerebellar pathways

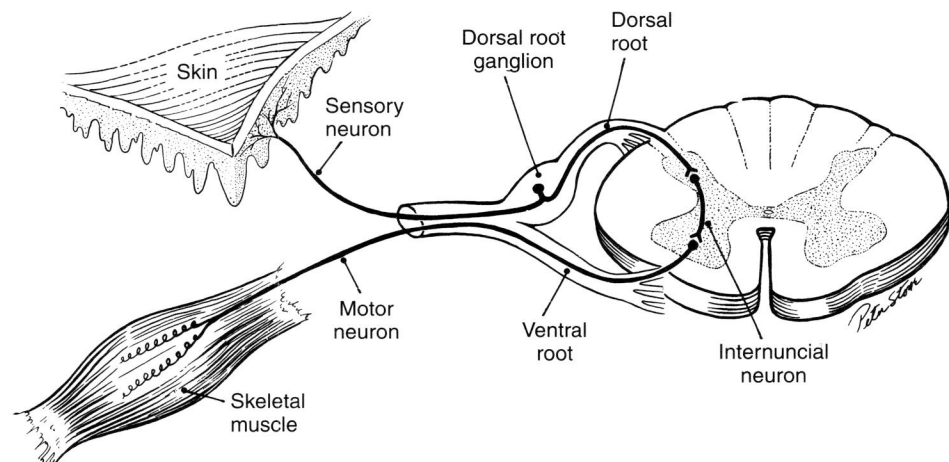

FIG. 51-6　Components of a simple reflex: a sensory, an internuncial, and a motor neuron. (From Langley LL, Telford JR, Christensen JB: *Dynamic anatomy and physiology,* ed 5, New York, 1980, McGraw-Hill.)

Major muscle groups are observed for evidence of muscle wasting, fasciculations, or contractions. Muscle strength is tested by comparing the strength of the muscles on one side of the body with those on the other side as the patient resists the examiner's counterpressure. Age, gender, and physical condition must be considered when evaluating these tests. The patient is observed for any evidence of involuntary movements, including tremors, chorea, hemiballismus, and tic.

Reflexes

A *deep tendon reflex* is elicited by a brisk tap with a reflex hammer over a partially stretched tendon. The impulse then travels along afferent fibers to the spinal cord, where it synapses with a motor, or anterior horn, neuron. After it synapses, the impulse is transmitted down the motor neuron to the anterior nerve root through the spinal nerve and then the peripheral nerve. After it is transmitted across the neuromuscular junction, the muscle is stimulated to contract. In simplest form, this action is the reflex arc (Fig. 51-6).

The deep tendon reflexes, also known as *muscle stretch reflexes,* commonly tested are the biceps reflex, the triceps reflex, the brachioradialis reflex, the patellar reflex, and the Achilles reflex. The response to reflexes is graded on a scale of 0 to +4 (Table 51-5; see also Table 57-3). It is important to compare sides when evaluating reflex responses.

Superficial reflexes are tested by stroking the skin with a firm object, such as the end of a reflex hammer or applicator, causing the muscles to contract. These reflexes include abdominal, cremasteric, plantar, and gluteal.

Assessment of reflexes gives the examiner information about the function of the reflex arc and specific spinal cord segments. Reflexes are altered in disease states involving the UMNs and LMNs.

UMN paralysis is caused by an interruption of the descending motor tracts on one side of a segment of the

TABLE 51-5 ▪▪▪

Grading of Reflexes

Grade	Significance
+4	Very brisk, suggestive of disease of the upper motor neuron, frequently associated with clonus (rhythmic oscillations between flexion and extension)
+3	Brisker than average but not necessarily indicative of disease
+2	Average or normal
+1	Somewhat diminished
0	No response

Modified from Barkauskas VH et al: *Health and physical assessment*, ed 3, St Louis, 2002, Mosby.

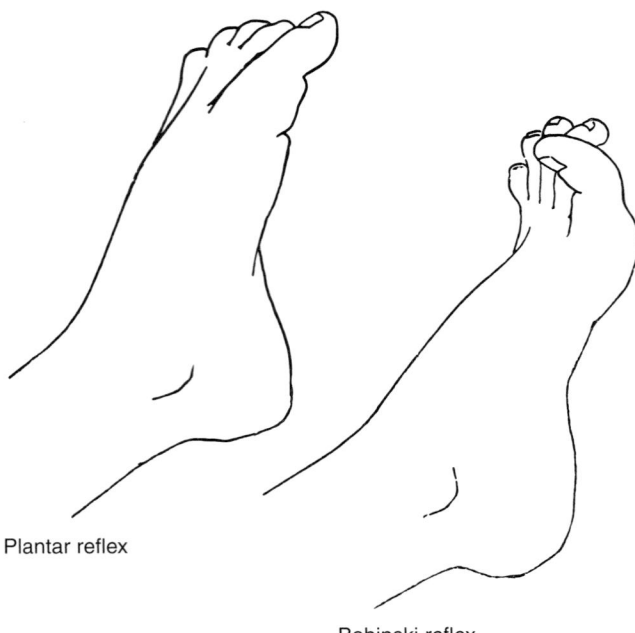

Plantar reflex

Babinski reflex

FIG. 51-7 Babinski's response. *Left,* Normal adult response to stimulation of the foot (flexion of all the toes). *Right,* Normal infant and abnormal adult response (dorsiflexion of the great toe and fanning of other toes).

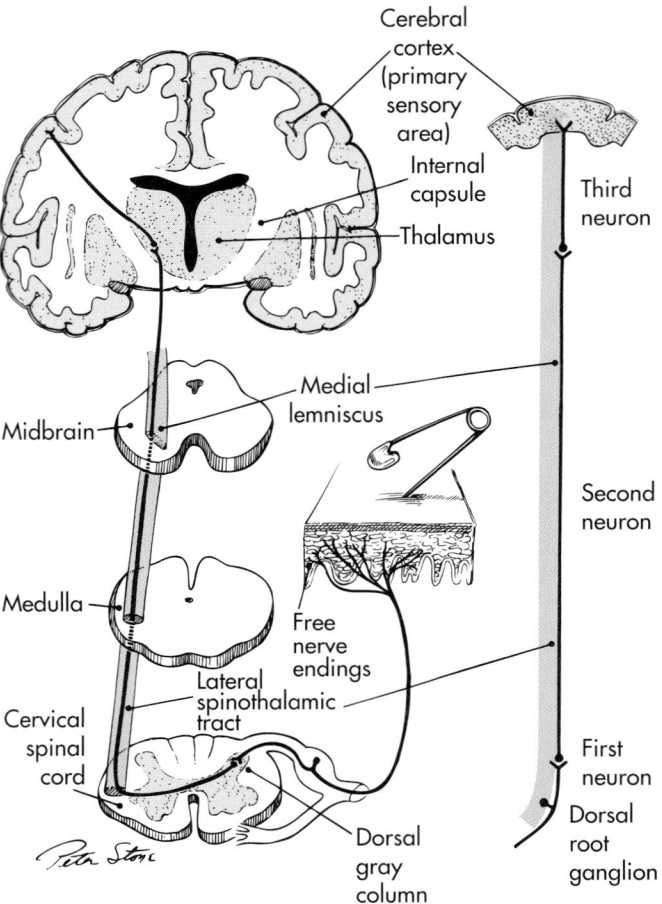

FIG. 51-8 The central pathway for impulses perceived as pain (lateral spinothalamic tract). Note that the fibers cross on entering the spinal cord. (From Langley LL, Telford JR, Christensen JB: *Dynamic anatomy and physiology*, ed 5, New York, 1980, McGraw-Hill.)

spinal cord. Immediately after the lesion occurs, the deep tendon reflexes are temporarily depressed; this condition is known as *areflexia*. In addition, the paralyzed muscles are flaccid. Several weeks or months after the lesion occurs, the deep tendon reflexes become hyperactive; the superficial reflexes are lost, and Babinski's reflex is noted.

LMN paralysis is caused by destruction of the peripheral motor nerves and the anterior horn cells. When LMN paralysis occurs, the muscles become flaccid and hypotonic and the deep tendon reflexes are lost.

The plantar reflex is elicited by stroking the lateral aspect of the sole from the heel to the ball and curving medially across the ball of the foot. The normal response to this stimulus is flexion of the toes. An abnormal response, dorsiflexion of the great toe and fanning of other toes, is known as *Babinski's reflex* and indicates UMN disease (Fig. 51-7). This reflex is seen (1) in children younger

than 2 years; (2) during periods of deep sleep, general anesthesia, and postictal (after a seizure) depression; and (3) in persons who are drunk or in moderate to severe hypoglycemic shock.

Sensory Function

The sensory system plays a vital role in conveying to the central nervous system information about the environment. When examining the sensory system, the following four areas are investigated: (1) superficial tactile sensation, including pain, temperature, and touch; (2) proprioceptive sense, which is motion or position sense; (3) vibratory sense; and (4) cortical sensory functions. Patterns of sensory loss may lead to a diagnosis of lesions of the cerebral hemisphere, brainstem, spinal cord, nerve root, and single or multiple peripheral nerves.

Perceptions of pain and temperature are carried by nerve fibers to the dorsal root ganglia where the nuclei of these nerve fibers are located. After synapsing in the dorsal horn, they cross over the midline and enter the opposite lateral spinothalamic tract. This tract ascends through the entire length of the spinal cord, medulla, pons, and midbrain and terminates in the thalamus. The thalamus,

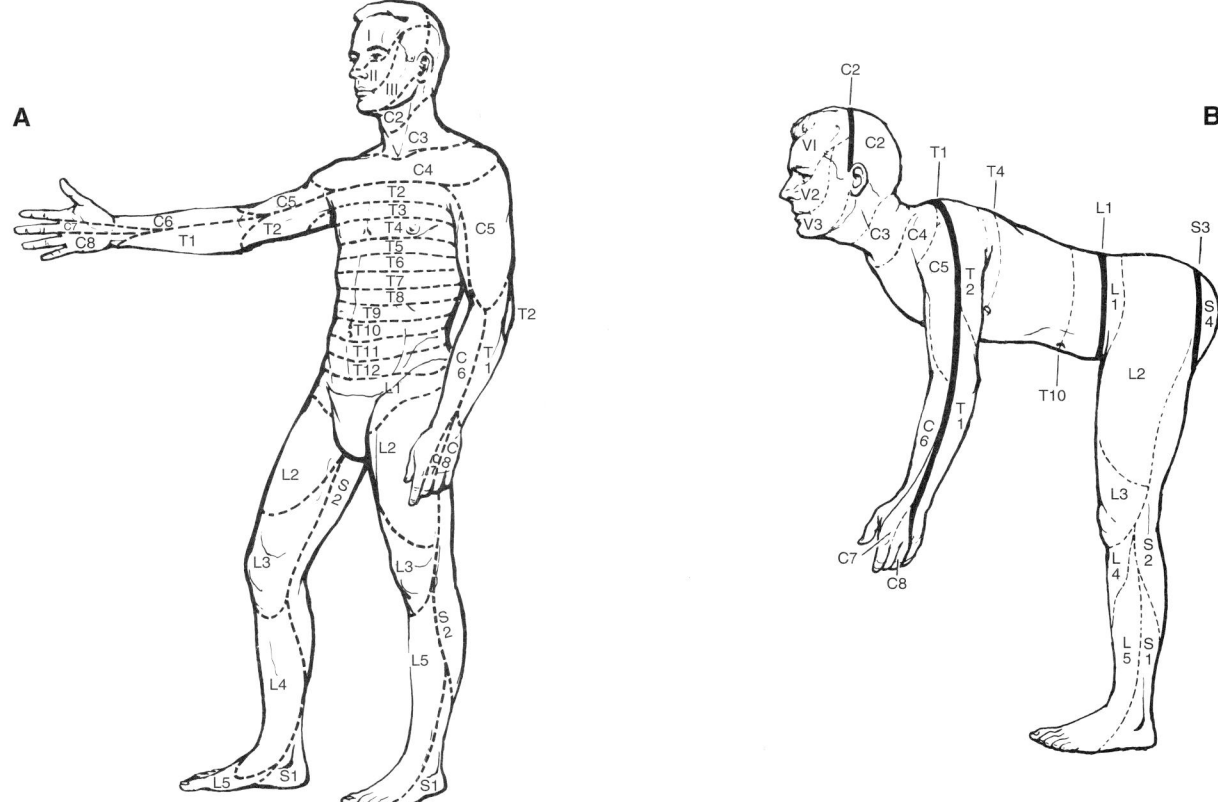

FIG. 51-9   Arrangement of the dermatomes. Each dorsal (sensory) spinal root innervates one dermatome. The first cervical nerve *(C1)* usually has no cutaneous distribution. The fifth cranial nerve *(C5)* supplies the sensory distribution to the face and anterior aspect of the head. The ophthalmic division is labeled I and VI, the maxillary division is II and V2, and the mandibular division is III and V3 in **A** and **B.**

acting as a relay station, transmits the impulse to the sensory cortex for interpretation. The ventral spinothalamic tract transmits simple touch sensation. A lesion involving the lateral spinothalamic tract will result in loss of pain and temperature sensation on the opposite side of the body below the level of the lesion. Lesions of the nerve roots and peripheral nerves impair the perception of touch (Fig. 51-8).

Fibers conducting sensations of position, vibration, and touch requiring a high degree of localization, such as stereognosis, graphesthesia, and two-point discrimination, enter the spinal column and pass into the dorsal column system. Traveling upward to the lower medulla, where they synapse and cross over, the fibers ascend as the medial lemniscus, terminating in the thalamus. The fine distinction between and perception of these sensations are carried out in the parietal cortex.

The pattern of the dermatomes is shown in Fig. 51-9. Theoretically, a lesion in the dorsal root produces loss of sensation in the area supplied by the root. However, the nerve supply overlaps considerably, which frequently confuses the clinical picture.

Sensory testing is performed with the patient's eyes closed, using a wisp of cotton to test for touch, a safety pin to test for superficial pain, and test tubes filled with hot and cold water to test for temperature.

Proprioception, position, and motion sense are first evaluated in distal joints. If proprioception is normal in the distal joint, testing the proximal joint is not necessary. A distal phalanx of one of the patient's fingers is grasped and slowly moved upward or downward, and the patient is asked to indicate the movement of the phalanx. The *Romberg test* evaluates the position sense for the legs and trunk.

Normally, an individual should be able to stand with feet together and not sway greatly or lose balance with eyes open or closed. A *Romberg sign* consists of onset of or accentuated disequilibrium with the eyes closed. This sign occurs in sensory loss because persons with proprioception abnormalities often can use visual orientation to compensate for loss of position sense but lose that compensatory factor when they close their eyes. It should be noted that the Romberg sign is not elicited in patients with cerebellar disorder, because their ataxia is independent of proprioception and therefore not compensated by visual orientation. Thus the patient will sway and lose balance with eyes open, as well as closed.

DIAGNOSTIC TESTS

In addition to the clinical history and neurologic examination, the clinical practitioner can perform several diagnostic tests to help locate and define the neurologic problem. These tests help the examiner diagnose the problem but are not a substitute for a careful and thorough neurologic examination.

Invasive Procedures

Cerebral angiography is used to identify and locate cerebrovascular abnormalities. A contrast medium is injected into the carotid, femoral, or brachial artery, and a series of cerebrovascular radiographs is taken. The contrast media most commonly used contain iodinated compounds, which have the potential to provoke severe allergic reactions; therefore all patients are carefully screened for allergies to iodine and shellfish. Attendants should be alert for any signs of allergic reaction, such as itching, palpitations, dyspnea, dizziness, or gastrointestinal disturbances, during and immediately after the procedure. Vital signs and neurologic checks are an essential part of posttest care.

Digital subtraction angiography (DSA) is a type of angiography that combines radiography and a computerized subtraction technique to visualize vessels without the interference of surrounding bone and soft tissue. A computer subtracts the interfering structures for the radiographic image. This test is used in particular for visualizing cerebral blood flow and detecting aneurysms, tumors, and hematomas. The same precautions concerning allergy to iodine apply to this procedure.

Radioisotope brain scan is useful in the diagnosis of masses, vascular lesions, and ischemic or infarcted areas of the brain. After venous injection with a radionuclide, radiographs are taken as the radioisotope passes through the brain.

Electromyography is used to differentiate muscular disease from neurologic disorders. For this test, needles are placed in the muscles and electrical signals recorded during rest and contraction. This procedure can be painful for some patients, and an analgesic may be required during the posttest period.

Nerve conduction studies complement the electromyographic (EMG) examination, helping the clinician to evaluate the presence and extent of peripheral nerve pathology. Conduction studies record the electrical response of a muscle to stimulation of its motor nerve at two or more points along its pathway to the muscle. Sensory nerve conduction studies determine the conduction velocity and amplitude of action potentials in sensory fibers by stimulating the fiber at one point and recording the response at another point along the nerve axon. Nerve conduction (NC) studies tests are particularly useful in differentiating demyelinating disorders from denervation with loss of axons and in diagnosing disorders of neuromuscular transmission. These tests can also help distinguish a mononeuropathy from a polyneuropathy.

Lumbar puncture (LP) is used to measure cerebrospinal fluid (CSF) pressure and to collect samples of the CSF for laboratory examination. Meningitis and encephalitis are the major indications for performing LP. Also, LP is routinely done in septic workups on infants and small children. Generally, an LP is contraindicated when there are signs of increased intracranial pressure, because the quick reduction of pressure from removal of CSF may cause herniation of the brain structures into the foramen magnum.

Other contraindications include an intracranial mass lesion, papilledema, uncorrected bleeding disorders, and suspected spinal cord compression. The patient lies on one side and assumes a knee-chest position. The area of the third and fourth lumbar vertebrae is cleansed with a povidone-iodine solution and anesthetized with a lidocaine solution. A spinal needle is inserted and attached to a manometer to measure the pressure; specimens are collected in numbered test tubes from the manometer stopcock. After all specimens have been obtained, the needle is removed and the puncture covered with an adhesive plaster. Patients lie flat for several hours after the procedure and are encouraged to take fluids. Headaches are common after LP. Table 51-6 lists some common CSF normal and abnormal findings.

Noninvasive Tests

Evoked potentials are produced by sensory stimulation (visual, auditory, electrical) applied to the peripheral or central nervous system and recorded from electrodes placed on the skin. Therefore evoked potentials are of very low amplitude so that they can be recorded only by averaging

---

TABLE 51-6 ■ ■ ■

Cerebrospinal Fluid Findings

Characteristics	Normal	Selected Abnormalities
Opening pressure	50 to 180 mm H_2O	Increased with intracranial mass from tumor, hemorrhage, or edema; decreased with spinal canal obstruction above LP site
Appearance	Clear, colorless	Xanthochromic (yellowish) appearance usually indicates presence of old blood or extreme elevation of protein in the CNS; cloudy appearance indicates infection (elevated WBC count, protein, microorganisms)
Cell count	0 to 5 WBCs/mm³	Increased with active disease: meningitis, acute infection, abscess, tumor, infarction, multiple sclerosis
	No RBCs	RBCs in subarachnoid hemorrhage or traumatic LP
Protein	20 to 45 mg/dl	Elevated in almost all serious pathologic CNS conditions
Glucose	40 to 70 mg/dl (normal = ²/₃ blood glucose)	Increased in systemic hyperglycemia; decreased in systemic hypoglycemia, bacterial meningitis
Microorganisms	None	Bacterial meningitis

LP, Lumbar puncture; *CNS*, central nervous system; *WBCs*, white blood cells; *RBCs*, red blood cells.

the response to a very large number of stimuli. Because different sensory stimuli travel predictable pathways and produce distinct potentials, the tests are helpful in precisely localizing a lesion. The tests are commonly used in cases of suspected multiple sclerosis and may detect subclinical lesions. They also are used frequently in intraoperative monitoring, and in assessing cranial nerve function in comatose patients. The most commonly used are somatosensory evoked potentials (SSEP), visual evoked potentials (VEP), and brainstem auditory evoked potentials (BAEP).

Computed tomography scan (CT scan) is useful in the diagnosis and monitoring of intracranial lesions or to evaluate and define the extent of a neurologic injury. A computer takes radiographs in 1-degree intervals in a 180-degree arc. Enhanced studies are performed using contrast media injected into a vascular access. Whenever contrast media are used, allergy precautions must be taken. CT scans have replaced echoencephalography and have greatly enhanced diagnostic capabilities.

Magnetic resonance imaging (MRI) uses a strong magnetic field and a radiofrequency and, when combined with the radio frequencies released by the body's tissues, produces an image that is recorded. MRI is useful in the diagnosis of tumors, infarctions, and vascular abnormalities. This procedure does not expose the patient to radiation and is painless, although patients may complain of claustrophobia and distress from the clanking metallic sounds throughout the procedure.

Electroencephalogram (EEG) measures the electrical activity of the cerebral cortex's superficial layers via electrodes placed externally on the patient's skull. Even though there are several new techniques for evaluating CNS abnormalities, the EEG is still considered indispensable because it is noninvasive and is one of the few diagnostic tests that measure real-time activity of the brain rather than preexisting anatomic changes. Wave patterns reflect the intensity and type of electrical potentials generated by neuronal activity within the brain. Normal wave patterns are labeled according to amplitude and frequency characteristics and are called *delta, theta, alpha,* and *beta.* The pattern of EEG waves is influenced by sleep state, drug use, disease, and aging. Because the EEG provides only a short sample (30 minutes to 1 hour) of brain activity, and because seizure activity and spike discharges occur only sporadically, a normal EEG does not exclude a seizure disorder.

Electronystagmogram (ENG) is an electrophysiologic test of vestibular function that may be used to diagnose disorders of the central nervous system. The test measures nystagmus (involuntary, rapid horizontal eye movements) induced by stimulation of the vestibular system. The test may cause some discomfort but is not dangerous to the patient. The ENG consists of inserting air or water at different temperatures into the external ear canals, which stimulates the semicircular canals, and recording the resulting electrical activity generated by involuntary eye muscle movements.

KEY CONCEPTS

- Many diseases of other body systems are exhibited as neurologic symptoms. Systemic problems such as hypoxia, elevated blood glucose, and hypothyroid state all profoundly affect neuronal responses and therefore can produce early and often subtle changes in nervous system function.

- Neurologic symptoms and signs are determined by history and physical examination, respectively. A neurologic examination begins with observation of the patient while the history is being obtained.

- History and physical examination are complementary; after a complete history, the examiner should know the expected deficits and determine whether and to what extent the examination findings support the history.

- Disorders of the nervous system may be stable or progressive. Either pattern may, in addition, have superimposed intermittent signs or symptoms, or intermittent signs or symptoms followed by periods of remission.

- A detailed neurologic history includes descriptions of signs and symptoms according to specific diagnostic characteristics, which one can recall by the mnemonic **TRIPLE-Q**: Timing (duration, frequency, onset, progression), Radiation, Intensity, Palliation, Location, Exacerbations or remissions, Quality.

- A thorough neurologic examination includes evaluation of six major elements: mental status (with its seven components); head and neck, including cranial nerves; motor function; sensory function; muscle stretch reflexes; and special reflexes, such as glabellar and plantar.

- It is essential that the examiner clarify with the patient what is meant by common terms used to describe symptoms. The straightforward meaning of "weakness," for example, is "loss of strength"—an indication of motor impairment. However, patients tend to use "weakness" to describe fatigue or general feelings of lack of energy (Wiederholt, 2000).

- The *upper motor neuron (UMN)* and the *lower motor neuron (LMN)* comprise the two-neuron system for voluntary muscle movement. Isolated lesions of the UMN and LMN cause specific characteristic deficits that help define the type of lesion.

- When evaluating reflexes, muscle strength, and sensory response, it is important to compare sides of the body to determine symmetry and equality of responses.

- The need for diagnostic tests is determined by a complete history and neurologic examination.

- Lumbar puncture is contraindicated in the presence of increased intracranial pressure (ICP). Collecting spinal fluid can cause a rapid decrease of "downstream" pressure, leading to brain herniation into the foramen magnum and catastrophic pressure on the brainstem.

- With evidence of head injury in a patient, the possibility of neck injury must be assumed. Any evaluation of the neck by passive or active motion must be deferred when the possibility of an acute neck injury exists.
- A voluntary motor movement requires integrated functioning of both central and peripheral nervous system structures, including the pyramidal and extrapyramidal systems, cerebellum, motor and sensory nerves, neuromuscular synapses, and muscle contractile apparatus. Thus motor abnormalities can result from impairment of any of these structures.
- In a patient who is awake, many components of neurologic testing require the patient's active participation and effort. Therefore it is important that the patient understand precisely what he or she is being asked to do through explanation or demonstration of specific tasks, such as heel-to-toe walking.
- Care must be taken to avoid suggesting to the patient the symptoms the examiner is seeking.
- In a comatose patient, if no abnormalities are detected on neurologic examination, it is unlikely that the patient's coma is the result of a structural central nervous system lesion. Conversely, intoxication or metabolic derangement must be very severe to produce abnormal findings on the neurologic examination.

QUESTIONS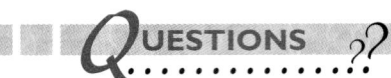

A sampling of review questions for this chapter appears here. Visit http://www.mosby.com/MERLIN/PriceWilson/ for additional questions. MERLIN

Answer the following on a separate sheet of paper.

1. What is the purpose of history taking during a neurologic examination?
2. List the six major areas of the neurologic examination.
3. List the four areas that are investigated when examining the sensory system.

Fill in the blanks with the correct word or words.

4. Interruption of the proprioceptive fibers, as in tabes dorsalis (syphilitic infection of the brain and spinal cord), may cause inability to maintain balance when standing with the eyes closed. This is called a positive _____ sign.
5. A right-sided posterolateral herniated intervertebral disk compressing the _____ spinal cord roots might be expected to produce numbness over the lateral aspect of the right foot.

Match each testing procedure in column B with the correct cranial nerve in column A.

Column A
6. _____ Optic (II)
7. _____ Trigeminal (V)
8. _____ Facial (VII)
9. _____ Vestibulocochlear (VIII)
10. _____ Oculomotor (III)
11. _____ Glossopharyngeal (IX)
12. _____ Vagus (X)
13. _____ Accessory (XI)
14. _____ Olfactory (I)

Column B
a. Occlude one nostril with digital compression; have patient indicate when odor is first detected and, if possible, identify substance.
b. Have patient say "ah" to note phonation and symmetry of the soft palate.
c. Test positional sense.
d. Cover one of the patient's eyes and bring finger into visual field.
e. Test gag reflex.
f. Have patient raise eyebrows, frown, close eyes, and tightly close eyes; observe symmetry.
g. Test for conductive versus sensorineural hearing loss.
h. Ask patient to shrug shoulders and turn head with and without resistance.
i. Have patient clench teeth; palpate masseters for tension.
j. Check for ptosis of lids, and note quality of pupils.

MARY S. HARTWIG AND LORRAINE M. WILSON

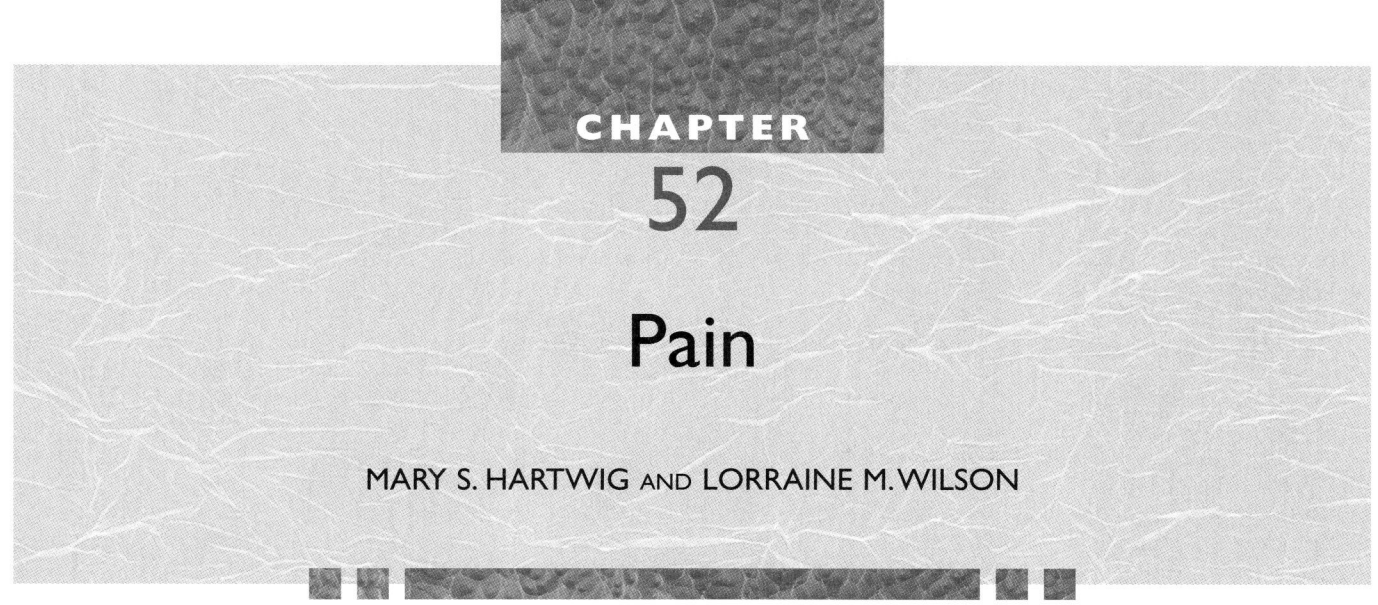

lem. No test exists to measure or confirm the pain; instead, the clinician relies almost entirely on the patient's description of the pain and its severity. Pain is the most common reason given by patients when asked why they sought medical attention. Its impact on patient well-being is becoming so widely accepted that many institutions now call pain "the fifth vital sign," grouping it with the classical signs of temperature, pulse, respiration, and blood pressure.

In most patients, the sensation of pain is produced by an injury or by stimuli that are intense enough to be potentially injurious (noxious). In the case of injury or potential injury, pain serves a protective function, eliciting a stress response with withdrawal, escape, or immobilization of a body part (e.g., removal of a finger from a hot stove). Once this protective function has been completed, however, continuing unrelieved pain can compromise the individual, because it is often accompanied by a stress response with increased anxiety, heart rate, blood pressure, and respiratory rate. Acute pain may be predictable and recurrent when there is repeated or progressive tissue injury. Examples of such situations are pain with diseases such as sickle cell anemia, cancer, and Raynaud's phenomenon. Because such conditions are typically characterized by intermittent pain-free periods, they are not representative of what is termed the "chronic pain state." That term is reserved for persons who have long-term pain without evident tissue injury or signs of persistent pain receptor (nociceptor) stimulation. In chronic pain, the pain serves no protective or other known useful biologic purpose. In addition, such a pain pattern has a strong association with psychologic states, including anxiety, depression, irritability or anger, malaise and sleep, and sense of worthlessness. A prolonged stress response promotes the breakdown of body tissue, impairs immune functioning, and increases metabolic rate, blood clotting, and water retention, thus hindering rather than helping recovery. It is important to note that many people report pain in the absence of tissue damage or any evident pathophysiologic cause. According to the IASP (2001), there is no way to distinguish their subjective experience from that resulting from tissue damage, and therefore it should be accepted as pain. A

*P*ain can be described as "an unpleasant sensory and emotional experience associated with actual or potential tissue damage, or described in terms of such damage" (International Association for the Study of Pain [IASP] Task Force, 1994, p. 210-211). This definition avoids correlating pain with a stimulus; it also emphasizes that pain is *subjective* and is both a sensation and an emotion. For clinicians, pain is a perplexing prob-

painful experience leads to physical and behavioral reactions that, if not interrupted at an appropriate and early enough stage, will lead to a chronic pain syndrome. The longer these reactions and responses are allowed to occur unabated, the more likely that a self-perpetuating cycle of pain will develop, making it more difficult for the cycle to be interrupted.

Although pain is a subjective experience with unpleasant sensory and emotional components, some objective evidence of pain exists. Watching a patient's facial expression, listening to crying or moaning, and observing changes in vital signs (e.g., blood pressure, heart rate) may give the clinician a hint of the degree of pain the patient is experiencing. These observations are highly unreliable, however, putting patients at high risk for inadequate pain relief.

During the past 30 years, intense interest and research have focused on the nature of pain and its control, resulting in an expansion of knowledge related to this complex phenomenon. The list of definitions of "pain terms" compiled by the IASP reflects the detailed study that continues to take place in the field of pain research and treatment. The list includes 24 related but distinct terms, from "allodynia" to "peripheral neuropathic pain," along with notes on specific usage (IASP Task Force, 1994). Scientists are learning that pain is a dynamic phenomenon and that the physiologic relationship between the painful stimulus and the behavioral response may be greatly modified over time. As Yan and Wu (2001) point out, much is now known about the cellular and even molecular events that cause neuropathic pain. In addition, many receptors and neurotransmitters in pain pathways have been identified and their relationships defined. This chapter first discusses the physiologic aspects of pain generation and transmission, types of pain, and assessment and treatment of pain. This overview of pain is followed by a brief discussion of two common sites for pain: headache and back pain caused by intervertebral disk disease.

NEUROPHYSIOLOGY OF PAIN

Processes: Physiologic Events

Four distinct processes are involved between the stimulus of tissue injury and the subjective experience of pain: transduction, transmission, modulation, and perception. *Pain transduction* is the process by which noxious stimuli lead to electrical activity in the pain receptors. *Pain transmission* involves the process of transmitting pain impulses from the site of transduction over peripheral sensory nerves to their terminals in the spinal cord and the network of relay neurons that ascend from the spinal cord to the brain. *Pain modulation* involves neural activity via descending neural pathways from the brain that can influence pain transmission at the level of the spinal cord. Modulation also involves the chemical factors that produce or enhance activity in the primary afferent pain receptors. Finally, *pain perception* is the subjective experience of pain that is somehow produced by the neural activity of pain transmission.

Modification of Pain Input

Woolf and Salter (2000) have identified three levels at which neural information can be modified in response to chronic pain: (1) the extent and duration of the response to the stimulus at the source can be modified; (2) chemical alterations can take place within any of the neurons or can even produce alterations in the anatomic features of these neurons or the neurons along the pain conduction pathway; and (3) prolongation of the stimulus can produce a modulation of the neurotransmitters that control the flow of information from neuron to their receptors. Yang and Wu (2001) explain that all of these alterations may lead to long-term changes in the connectivity and organization among nerve cells, leading to a "pain memory." This conclusion is supported by evidence that central neural processing may alter receptors and chemical output so that the individual may experience persistent painful sensations, though there may be diminished or even absent pain fiber stimulation (Payne, Gonzales, 1999).

Pain Receptors and Their Stimulation

The capacity of tissues to elicit pain when a noxious stimulus is applied to them depends on the presence of nociceptors. *Nociceptors* are primary afferent nerves for receiving and transmitting painful stimuli. The free nerve endings of nociceptors serve as receptors that are sensitive to painful mechanical, thermal, electrical, or chemical stimuli. The distribution of nociceptors varies throughout the body, with the largest number in the skin. Nociceptors are located in subcutaneous tissue, skeletal muscles, and joints. Pain receptors in the viscera are not located in the parenchyma of the internal organs themselves, but rather, are found in the peritoneal surfaces, pleural membranes, dura mater, and the walls of blood vessels.

A peripheral nerve consists of the axons of three different types of neurons: primary sensory or afferent neurons, motor neurons, and sympathetic postganglionic neurons. Both motor and sympathetic postganglionic fibers are efferents (carrying impulses from the spinal cord to the effector tissues and organs). The cell bodies of the primary afferent neurons are located in the dorsal (posterior) root of the spinal nerve. Once emerged from its cell body in the dorsal root ganglion (DRG), the primary afferent nerve's axon divides into two processes: one enters the dorsal horn of the spinal cord, and the other innervates tissues. Primary afferent fibers are classified according to their size, degree of myelination, and conduction velocity (Fig. 52-1). A-alpha (A-α) and A-beta (A-β) afferent fibers are largest in size and myelinated and have the fastest conduction velocity. These fibers respond to touch, pressure, and kinesthetic sense. However, the fibers do not respond to noxious stimuli and thus cannot be classified as nociceptors. In contrast, small-diameter, lightly myelinated *(A-delta [A-δ] primary afferent fibers* and unmyelinated *C primary afferent fibers* respond maximally only when noxious painful stimuli are applied to their receptive fields and thus are classified as nociceptors. Pain impulses are transmitted relatively slowly compared with sensory transmission in the large A-α and A-β fibers because of their small diameters and lack of myelin (C fibers).

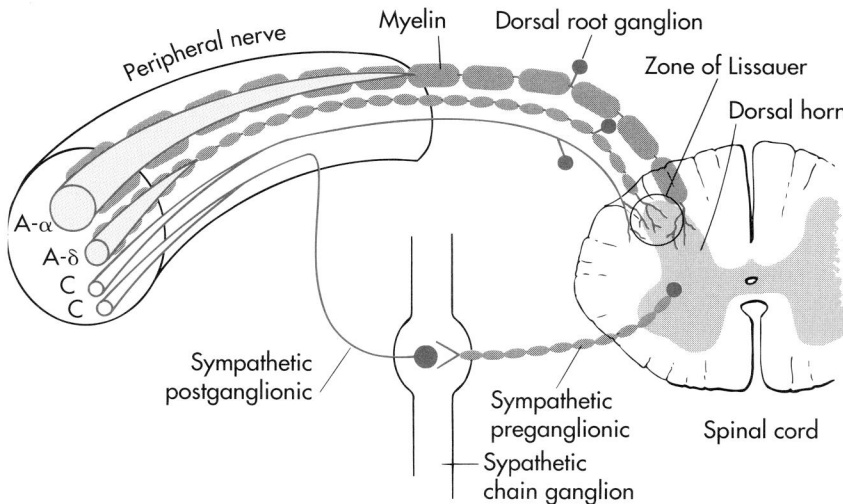

FIG. 52-1 Components of a typical cutaneous peripheral nerve. Primary afferents include (1) the large, myelinated A-alpha (A-α) fibers and A-beta (A-β) fibers (not shown) carrying impulses mediating touch, pressure, and proprioception and (2) the small, myelinated A-delta (A-δ) and unmyelinated C fibers, both of which carry impulses mediating pain. These primary afferents converge on the spinal cord dorsal horn cells, entering at the *Zone of Lissauer*. Sympathetic postganglionic fibers are efferents, composed of unmyelinated C fibers. (Modified from Fields HL: *Pain*, New York, 1987, McGraw-Hill.)

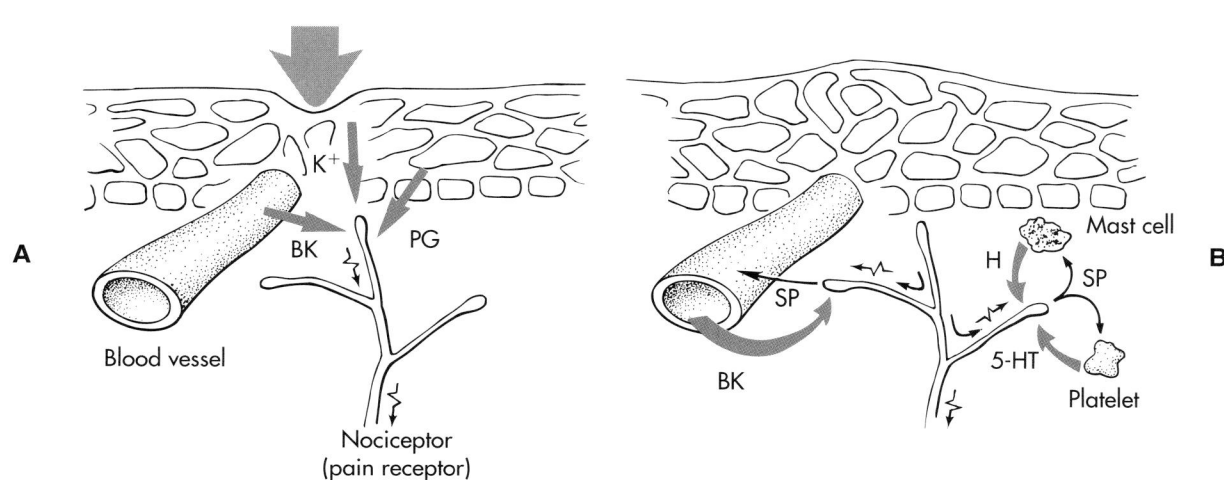

FIG. 52-2 Mechanisms of nociceptor activation and sensitization in an area of tissue injury. **A,** Direct activation by intense pressure and consequent cell damage. Cell damage leads to the release of intracellular potassium (K^+) and to synthesis of prostaglandins *(PG)* and bradykinin *(BK)*. Prostaglandins increase the sensitivity of the pain receptor to bradykinin, the most potent pain-producing chemical. **B,** Secondary activation. Impulses generated in the pain receptor are transmitted not only to the spinal cord but also into other terminal branches, where they include the release of substance P *(SP)* and other peptides. Substance P causes vasodilation and neurogenic edema with further release of bradykinin; it also causes release of histamine *(H)* from mast cells and serotonin *(5-HT)* from platelets. (Redrawn from Fields HL: *Pain*, New York, 2001, McGraw-Hill.)

A-δ and C primary afferents can be distinguished by the two types of pain they elicit, called fast pain and slow pain. *Fast pain* signals are transmitted to the spinal cord by the A-δ fibers and are felt within 0.1 second. Fast pain is generally well localized and has a prickling, sharp, or electrical quality. Fast pain is elicited in response to mechanical (e.g., cut, pinprick) or thermal stimuli on the skin surface but is not felt in deeper tissues of the body. *Slow pain* is transmitted by the C afferent fibers and is felt 1 second after a noxious stimulus. Slow pain is less well localized and has a burning, throbbing, or aching quality. Slow pain may be elicited by mechanical, thermal, or chemical stimuli in the skin or most deep tissues or organs and is usually associated with tissue damage. Be-

cause of this double system of pain innervation, tissue injury often gives rise to two distinct pain sensations: an early sharp pain (transmitted by A-δ pain fibers) followed by a dull, burning, somewhat prolonged pain (transmitted by C pain fibers).

Transduction is the process by which a noxious stimulus depolarizes a nociceptor and initiates a pain stimulus. One possible mechanism of transduction is the activation of nociceptors by pain-producing chemicals released in an area of tissue injury (Fig. 52-2). In contrast to most other sensory receptors in the body, pain receptors adapt very little or not at all. In fact, with prolonged noxious stimulation, tissue damage, or inflammation, pain receptors become increasingly sensitized, called *hyperalgesia,* with a lowering of the pain threshold. Numerous chemical substances are found in an area of injury and have varying degrees of ability to sensitize nociceptors. Many of these are released from damaged tissue cells (potassium ions, histamine), by activated mast cells (such as the potent pain stimulant, bradykinin), or by sensitized T cells and activated macrophages (multiple substances called cytokines, including the toxin, tumor necrosis factor [TNF]) (Friedman, 2000). Many other chemical agents are synthesized and released during the inflammatory process. Among these synthesized chemicals are the arachidonic acid metabolites, prostaglandins and leukotrienes. Both are produced in a chemical cascade initiated by enzyme breakdown of phospholipids that are freed from the lipid bilayer membrane of damaged cells.

In addition to substances released from damaged cells or synthesized in the area of injury, the nociceptors themselves release chemicals that enhance nociception, including substance P. *Substance P* is a neuropeptide that causes vasodilation, increased blood flow, edema with further release of bradykinin, release of serotonin from platelets, and release of histamine from mast cells.

Nociceptor activity produces several effects by this complex chain of events, including prolongation of the pain long after the stimulus has ceased and the gradual spread of hyperalgesia and tenderness (Fields, Martin, 2001). Drugs that block these chemicals, such as corticosteroids or nonsteroidal antiinflammatory drugs (NSAIDs, e.g., aspirin), which reduce inflammation and block the synthesis of prostaglandins, may reduce pain.

Pain Pathways in Central Nervous System

Ascending Pathways

The afferent A-δ and C nerve fibers transmitting pain impulses enter the spinal cord at the dorsal nerve root (Fig. 52-3). The fibers separate as they enter the cord and then reform in the dorsal (posterior) horn of the spinal cord. This area receives, transmits, and processes sensory impulses. The dorsal horn of the spinal cord is divided into cell layers called *laminae*. Two of these layers (laminae II and III), called the *substantia gelatinosa*, are particularly important in pain transmission and modulation. The substantia gelatinosa is hypothesized to be the site of the gating mechanism described in the gate control theory (see later discussion).

From the dorsal horn, the pain impulses are conveyed to neurons that transmit information to the opposite side of the spinal cord in the anterior commissure and then converge on the *anterolateral spinothalamic tract* (formerly called lateral tract), which ascends to the thalamus and other brain structures. Thus pain impulse transmission in the spinal cord is contralateral to the side of the body from which the impulses were generated. Just as two types of pain are transmitted by nociceptors (fast pain and slow pain), two parallel spinothalamic pathways transmit these impulses to the brain: the neospinothalamic tract and the paleospinothalamic tract.

The *neospinothalamic tract* is a *direct system* that carries sensory discriminative information about acute or fast pain from A-δ nociceptors to the thalamic areas. This system primarily terminates in an orderly fashion within the ventral posterolateral nucleus of the thalamus. Pain is called a *thalamic sense* because it is probably brought to consciousness in the thalamus. A neuron in the thalamus then projects its axon through the posterior limb of the internal capsule to carry the pain impulses to the primary somatosensory cortex of the postcentral gyrus. It is postulated that this organized pattern is important for the sensory-discriminative aspects of the acute pain experience, that is, its location, nature, and intensity.

The *paleospinothalamic tract*, which transmits impulses initiated in the slow-chronic type C nociceptors, is a multisynaptic, diffuse pathway that carries impulses to the brainstem reticular formation before terminating in the parafascicular and other intralaminar nuclei of the thalamus, hypothalamus, limbic system nuclei, and forebrain cortex. Because paleospinothalamic impulses are transmitted more slowly than are those in the neospinothalamic tract, the pain is associated with burning, aching, and poorly localized sensations. This system influences the expression of pain in terms of tolerance, behavior, and sympathetic autonomic responses. It is likely that visceral sensations are conveyed by this system. It is most important in chronic pain, mediating the associated autonomic responses, emotional behavior, and lowered thresholds that often occur. Thus the paleospinothalamic pathway is referred to as an *affectational and motivational nociceptor system*.

It is important to note that neither of these tracts carries pain impulses exclusively; for example, the neospinothalamic tract also conveys crude touch and pressure sensations.

Descending Pathways

Specific areas in the brain itself control or influence pain perception: the hypothalamus and limbic structures serve as the emotional center of pain perception, and the frontal cortex provides the rational interpretation and responses to pain. However, great variation exists in the way individuals perceive painful stimuli. One reason for this variation is because the central nervous system (CNS) has a variety of mechanisms for modulating or suppressing nociceptive stimuli.

Descending pathways of efferent fibers that extend from the cerebral cortex down the spinal cord can inhibit or modify incoming pain stimuli via a feedback mechanism involving the substantia gelatinosa and other layers of the dorsal horn. Consequently, descending pathways can influence pain impulses at the spinal level. One descending pathway that has been identified as important in the pain-modulating, or analgesic, system involves the following three components (Fig. 52-4; Payne, Gonzales, 1999; Guyton and Hall, 2000):

1. The first area is the *periaqueductal gray (PAG)* matter and *periventricular gray (PVG)* matter of the mesencephalon and upper pons surrounding the aqueduct of Sylvius.
2. Neurons from area 1 send impulses to the *nucleus raphe magnus (NRM)* located in the lower pons and upper medulla and the *nucleus reticularis paragigantocellularis (PGL)* in the lateral medulla.
3. Impulses are transmitted from the nuclei in 2 down the dorsolateral columns of the spinal cord to a pain inhibitory complex located in the *dorsal horns of the spinal cord*.

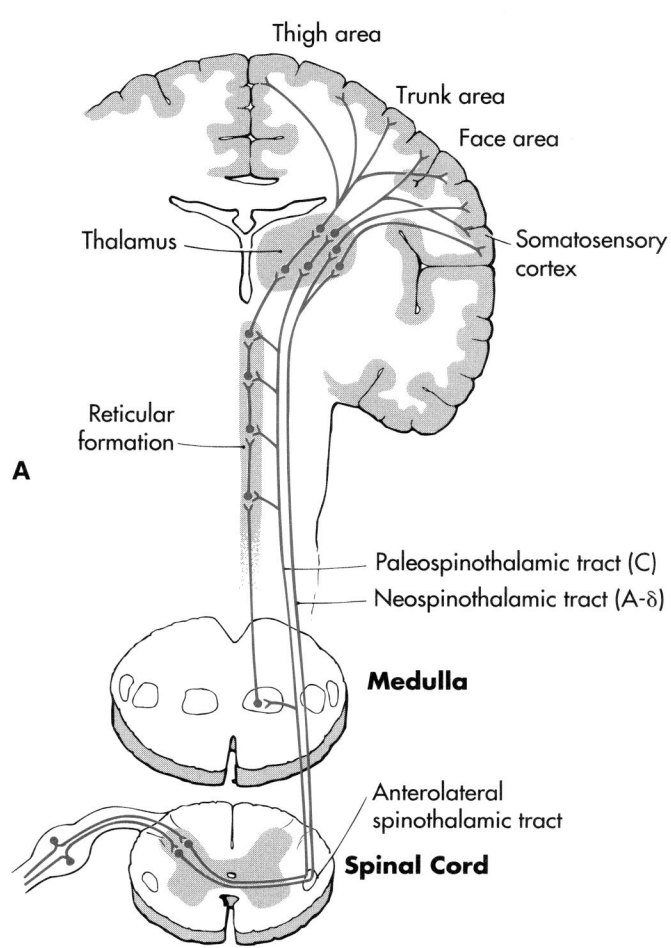

A

Thigh area

Trunk area

Face area

Thalamus

Somatosensory cortex

Reticular formation

Paleospinothalamic tract (C)

Neospinothalamic tract (A-δ)

Medulla

Anterolateral spinothalamic tract

Spinal Cord

FIG. 52-3 Ascending pain pathways. **A**, The small A-δ and C pain fibers carrying acute-sharp and slow-chronic pain impulses, respectively, synapse in the substantia gelatinosa of the dorsal horn, cross the spinal cord, and ascend to the brain in either the neospinothalamic branch or the paleospinothalamic branch of the anterolateral spinothalamic tract. The neospinothalamic tract, principally activated by A-δ peripheral afferents, synapses in the ventroposterolateral nucleus (VPN) of the thalamus and proceeds directly to the somatosensory cortex of the postcentral gyrus, where pain is perceived as sharp and well localized. The paleospinothalamic branch, principally activated by C peripheral afferents, is a diffuse pathway that sends collaterals to the brainstem reticular formation and other structures, from which further fibers project to the thalamus. These fibers influence the hypothalamus and limbic system as well as the cerebral cortex. **B**, Afferent C pain fibers synapse primarily in the substantia gelatinosa (laminae II and III) of the dorsal horn, whereas A-δ pain fibers synapse primarily in laminae I and V.

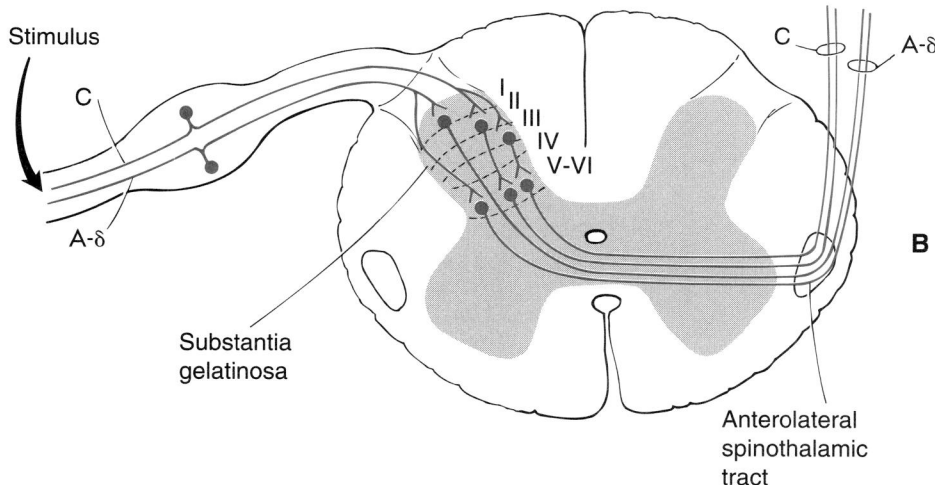

Stimulus

C

A-δ

C

A-δ

I
II
III
IV
V-VI

Substantia gelatinosa

Anterolateral spinothalamic tract

B

In animal studies, electrical stimulation of the PAG area or raphe nucleus areas can almost completely suppress strong pain signals entering via the dorsal spinal roots. A similar system may exist in humans, because stimulation of the nearby PVG area of the hypothalamus is reported to relieve clinical pain. In addition to the brainstem–to–spinal cord network, neural connections also exist from the hypothalamus and neocortex to the

PAG, allowing for pain modulation by an individual's thoughts and feelings from the higher brain centers.

Chemical substances, termed neuroregulators, may also influence sensory input to the spinal cord. These neuroregulators are known as either neurotransmitters or neuromodulators. *Neurotransmitters* are neurochemicals that inhibit or stimulate activity at postsynaptic membranes. Substance P, a neuropeptide, is a pain-specific

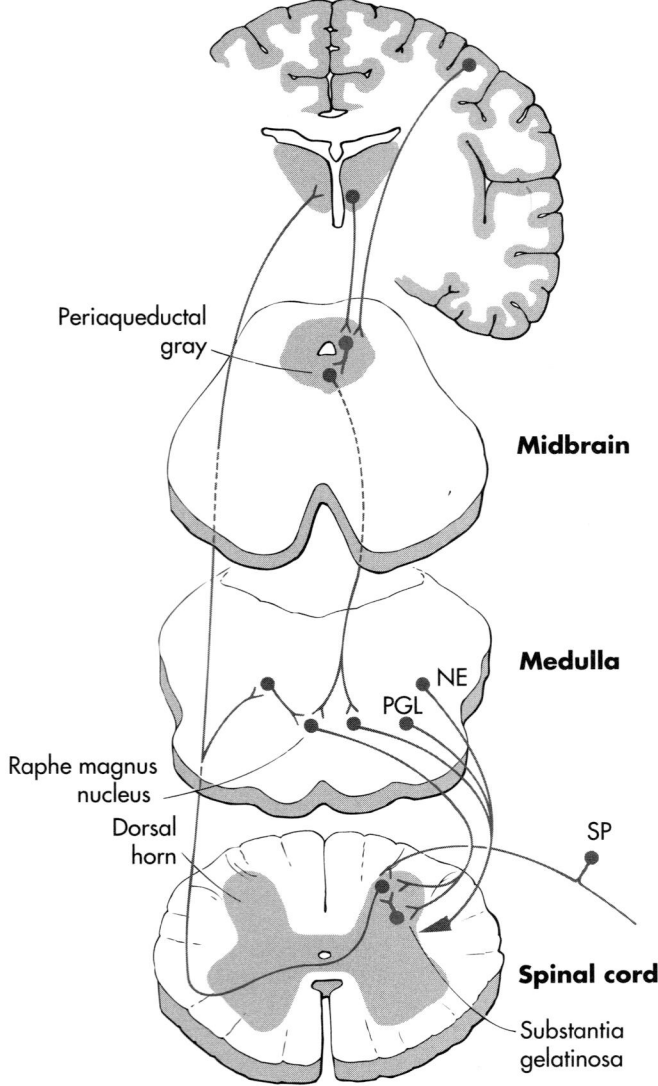

FIG. 52-4 Descending pain-modulating pathways can inhibit incoming pain signals at the spinal cord level. Endorphin-containing neurons in the periaqueductal gray and substantia gelatinosa play an active role in pain modulation. *PGL,* Nucleus reticularis paragigantocellaris; *NE,* norepinephrine cells; *SP,* substance P. (Redrawn from Fields H, Bausbaum A:Endogenous pain control mechanisms. In WallPD, Melzack R, editors:*Textbook of pain,* ed 4, New York, 2000, Churchill Livingstone.)

neurotransmitter present in the dorsal horn of the spinal cord (at the gate in the gate control theory), among other sites. Other CNS neurotransmitters involved in pain transmission include acetylcholine, norepinephrine, epinephrine, dopamine, and serotonin.

Two neurotransmitters, serotonin (5-hydroxytryptamine [5-HT]) and norepinephrine, are known to be involved in the downward inhibition of incoming pain signals (Dubner, Ren, 1999). The rostroventral medulla (RVM) contains a high percentage of serotonergic neurons that project to the spinal dorsal horn. In addition, a significant number of neurons in the dorsolateral pons contain norepinephrine and have spinal projections terminating in the dorsal horn. Pain-inhibiting (antinociceptive) signals thus originate in the cortex or the brainstem in areas

where norepinephrine or serotonin are the primary transmitters (Yang, Wu, 2001). These signals are believed to work in one of two ways: (1) the neurons carrying them may synapse on neurons that release the antinociceptive neurotransmitters γ-aminobutyric acid (GABA), serotonin, or acetylcholine, or (2) the descending signals may block pain by acting in the dorsal horn to inhibit the release of pronociceptive neurotransmitters from the incoming (afferent) sensory neurons.

Tricyclic antidepressant medications such as amitriptyline (Elavil) and the nontricyclic venlafaxine (Effexor) produce analgesia by enhancing the inhibitory action of serotonin and norepinephrine on the spinal transmission neurons. Both of these medications block presynaptic reuptake of serotonin and norepinephrine, thus enhancing their postsynaptic actions in the descending pain inhibition pathways; they are often very effective in relieving neuropathic pain. Conversely, antagonists to the two hormones can block this analgesic effect (Payne, Gonzales, 1999; Fields, Martin, 2001). Norepinephrine seems to be the more important, or at least the more potent, of the two hormonal modulators, because serotonin-specific reuptake inhibitors (SSRIs) such as fluoxetine (Prozac) or paroxetine (Paxil) have not been shown to provide pain relief. In contrast, antagonist drugs to the alpha-adrenergic receptors that release norepinephrine can partially block the antinociceptive action of descending pathways (Fields, Martin, 2001; Baumann, 1997).

There is good research evidence that descending pain inhibition pathways are immature at birth and, in animal models, have been shown not to be functionally effective until at least 10 days postnatally (Fitzgerald, Jennings, 1999). According to Fitzgerald and Beggs (2001), this delay may be the result of a deficiency of 5-HT (serotonin) and norepinephrine but may also be caused by delayed maturation of interneurons in the spinal cord. Lacking full development of their descending endogenous analgesic systems, neonates may experience exaggerated short- and long-term effects from persistent noxious sensory stimulation.

In addition to these serotonin and norepinephrine descending pain-modulating pathways, endogenous opioid peptides are present in all the regions thus far implicated in pain modulation. Moreover, connections from serotonin neurons to opioid-containing cells exist in the substantia gelatinosa. Opioid peptides, known as neuromodulators (pain reducing), are naturally occurring compounds that have morphinelike qualities. These compounds are discussed in more detail later (see also Puntillo, Casella, Reid, 1997).

PAIN THEORIES

A number of theories have been proposed to explain the neurologic mechanisms that underlie the sensation of pain, including (1) the specificity theory, (2) the pattern theory, and more recently, (3) the gate control theory and (4) the endorphin-enkephalin theory.

Specificity Theory

The specificity theory of pain, which dates back about 200 years to Descartes, proposes that pain travels from

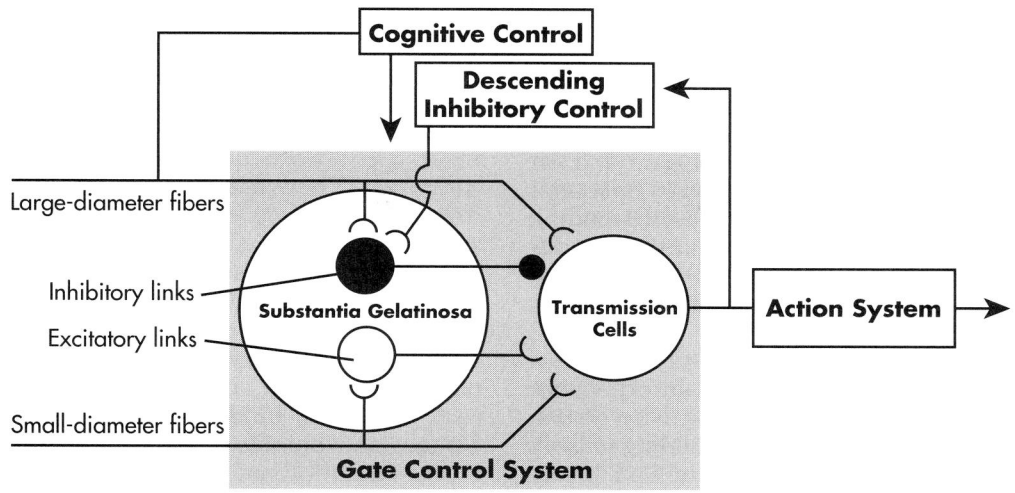

FIG. 52-5 The gate control theory of pain: Mark II. (From Melzack R, Wall PD: *The challenge of pain,* ed 3, New York, 1996, Penguin Books.)

specific pain receptors over a specific neuroanatomic pathway to a pain center in the brain and that the relationship between the pain stimulus and response is direct and invariable. Although this theory is clearly an oversimplification in the light of present knowledge, two of its principles are still valid: (1) somatosensory receptors are specialized to respond optimally to one or more specific types of stimuli, and (2) the central destination of primary afferent neurons and ascending pathways is a critical factor in distinguishing the nature of the peripheral stimulus.

Pattern, or Summation, Theory

The pattern, or summation, theory of pain was first introduced by Goldscheider in 1898. Goldscheider proposed that the summation of the skin sensory input at the dorsal horn cells produce the particular patterns of nerve impulses that evoke pain. Pain is produced by intense stimulation from nonspecific receptors, and it is the summation of the impulses that are perceived as pain. Goldscheider also identified a rapidly conducting pain fiber and a slower one. In 1943 Livingstone introduced the concept of *central summation*. One of the key concepts of the central summation theory is that nerve fiber circuits can become established in groups of spinal interneurons (a reverberating circuit) after an injury, causing ongoing pain without stimulation. This mechanism might explain phenomena such as phantom limb pain. However, procedures such as a cordotomy, which would sever the reverberating circuit, usually do not relieve pain permanently.

Gate Control Theory

Recent pain-related research has demonstrated that no single theory fully explains how pain is transmitted or perceived and that none reflects the complexity of the neuroanatomic pathways of pain transmission and modulation. To compensate for the deficiencies of the specificity and pattern theories of pain, Melzack and Wall first developed the gate control theory in 1965. Although

some of its original assumptions have been disproved, this theory provides the most comprehensive and practical model for conceptualizing pain. The discovery of endogenous opioids in the early 1970s added another dimension to the understanding of pain modulation, but no single integrated theory yet exists.

The gate control theory of pain attempts to explain the variation in pain perception of identical stimulation. Melzack and Wall combined the available facts from the clinical literature and from neurophysiology to support their theory and used a schematic model to illustrate their ideas. This theory has been the focus of intense research over the past 30 years, and the model has been modified and updated (Fig. 52-5).

The basic tenets of the gate control theory are as follows (Melzack, Wall, 1996; Wall, Melzack, 2000):

1. Both the large, myelinated sensory fibers (L) carrying information about touch and proprioception from the periphery (A-α and A-β fibers) and the small fibers (S) carrying information about pain (A-δ and C fibers) converge on the dorsal horn of the spinal cord.

2. The transmission of nerve impulses from afferent fibers to spinal cord transmission (T) cells in the dorsal horn is modulated by a gating mechanism in the substantia gelatinosa cells. If the gate is closed, the pain impulses cannot proceed. If the gate is open or partially open, pain impulses stimulate the T cells in the dorsal horn and then ascend the spinal cord to the brain, where they are perceived as pain.

3. The spinal gating mechanism is influenced by the relative amount of activity in the large-diameter (L) and small-diameter (S) primary afferent fibers. Activity in large afferents tends to inhibit pain transmission (closes the gate), whereas small-fiber activity tends to facilitate pain transmission (opens the gate). The large-diameter afferents excite the inhibitory substantia gelatinosa neurons, thereby reducing input to the T cells and consequently inhibiting pain. In contrast, activity in the small-diameter fibers inhibits the inhibitory substantia gelatinosa cells, resulting in enhancement of transmission from primary afferents to the T cells and consequently increasing pain intensity.

situation in which the pain felt in one area of the body diminishes or obliterates the pain felt in another area of

The quality, intensity, and duration of the pain are related to the nature of the surgical procedure. Any

TABLE 52-1 ■ ■ ■

Characteristics of Acute and Chronic Pain

Characteristic	Acute Pain	Chronic Pain*
Onset and duration	Abrupt onset; duration short, less than 6 months	Gradual onset; persistent, greater than 6 months
Intensity	Moderate to severe	Moderate to severe
Cause	Specific; biologically identifiable	Cause may or may not be well defined
Physiologic response	Predictable autonomic hyperactivity: increased blood pressure, pulse, and respiratory rate; dilated pupils; pallor; perspiration; nausea and/or vomiting	Normal autonomic activity
Emotional/behavioral response	Anxious; unable to concentrate; restless; distressed but optimistic about relief from pain	Depression and fatigue; immobility or physical inactivity; social withdrawal; sees no relief in sight, expects long-term pain
Response to analgesics	Effective pain relief	Often ineffective pain relief

*Chronic malignant, chronic nonmalignant, and chronic intermittent pain.

trauma, including surgical trauma, results in tissue damage. Pain-producing substances released into the injured tissue lower the pain threshold. Incisions in the upper abdomen generally cause greater postoperative pain because of respiratory movements. Muscle spasm around the area of injury may contribute to the pain. Incisional pain is generally sharp and well localized because the skin and subcutaneous tissues are well supplied with nociceptors. When deeper structures with fewer pain receptors are injured, the pain tends to be dull and poorly localized or may be referred when visceral structures are involved (see following discussion). Fear and anxiety are often part of the affective-motivational aspects of acute pain and tend to reinforce each other. Thus measures to relieve the pain also reduce the anxiety, which tends to lessen the pain. Acute postoperative pain usually disappears with healing.

When pain continues despite treatment or apparent healing and serves no biologic purpose, the pain is called chronic. *Chronic pain* may be continuous, resulting from malignant or nonmalignant causes, or may be intermittent, as in recurrent migraine headaches. Pain that persists for 6 months or longer is generally classified as chronic. Chronic pain represents a major health care problem in U.S. society. Estimates indicate that 25% of the population suffers from a chronic illness and chronic pain.

Patients with chronic pain have little or no autonomic hyperactivity but instead exhibit symptoms of irritability, lack of energy, and interference with the ability to concentrate. Chronic pain often encompasses every aspect of the person's life, creating emotional turmoil and distress, and interferes with physical and social functioning. Many factors are involved in the development of chronic pain, including organic, psychologic, social, and environmental factors (Dodd et al, 2001; Benedetti et al, 2000).

Chronic pain syndromes usually have organic causes, but the patient's personality and psychologic status influence its development. Conditions associated with chronic pain with an organic origin vary widely and include headaches, back pain, arthritis, carcinoma, and neuropathologic conditions (e.g., trigeminal neuralgia, phantom limb pain). Chronic pain syndromes are often accompanied by symptoms of anxiety, insomnia, and depression, with depression the most common. Chronic pain is a complex syndrome requiring a multidisciplinary approach for its management.

Superficial Somatic (Cutaneous) Pain

Cutaneous pain arises in the superficial structures of the skin and subcutaneous tissues. The effective stimulus for pain in the skin may be mechanical, thermal, chemical, or electrical. If the skin alone is involved, the pain is often described as tingling, sharp, cutting, or burning; but if blood vessels are contributing to the pain, it becomes throbbing in nature. The skin has many sensory nerves, and therefore damage to it is located more accurately and with greater precision than elsewhere. The area of pain may be localized along a distinct dermatome (skin segment) innervated by one dorsal (sensory) root (see Fig. 51-9). However, the dermatomes are not distinct and separate segments. Considerable overlap exists between any two adjacent dermatomes, and more so with pain and thermal senses than with tactile sensations. As a consequence, if one spinal nerve were completely nonfunctional, no area of complete anesthesia on the skin would be found, because the nerves from the two adjacent dermatomes would pick up the sensory stimuli. On the other hand, if a dorsal root of one spinal nerve were irritated, as in herpes zoster (shingles, a viral infection of a spinal ganglion), the noxious stimuli would be felt subjectively from the entire dermatome, including the overlap.

Deep Somatic Pain

Deep somatic pain refers to pain arising from muscles, tendons, ligaments, bones, joints, and arteries. These structures have fewer pain receptors, thus the pain is often poorly localized. Pain is experienced as more diffuse than cutaneous pain and tends to radiate to adjacent areas. Pain from various deep structures differs. Pain from an acute injury of a joint is well localized and usually described as sharp or burning or as throbbing. In chronic inflammation of a joint (arthritis), dull aching pains are experienced on which movement superimposes sharp, stabbing pain. Bone pain arises from stimulation of pain receptors in the periosteum and is less well localized; it is often described as a dull aching or soreness. Skeletal muscle pain is also poorly localized and is described as a dull ache or cramp. Skeletal muscle pain is particularly severe during contraction under conditions of ischemia.

Visceral Pain

Visceral pain refers to pain arising from the body organs. Visceral pain receptors are sparse compared with somatic pain receptors and are located in the smooth muscle walls of hollow organs (stomach, gallbladder, bile ducts, ureter, urinary bladder) and in the capsules of solid organs (liver, pancreas, kidney). The visceral parenchyma is relatively insensitive to cutting, heat, or pinching. The main mechanisms that generate visceral pain are abnormal stretching or distention of the wall or capsule of the organ, ischemia, and inflammation. The gut is a source of either a gnawing or a cramping pain or the intermittent pain known as *colic* when irritated by the chemical substances produced by inflammation or when distended. Other distensible structures, such as the gallbladder, bile ducts, or ureters, can cause colicky pain, often from smooth muscle spasm. Obstruction of outflow and overdistention also cause ischemia and the release of chemicals that stimulate pain receptors.

The viscera are innervated by two routes: through nerves that supply autonomic functions (the *true visceral pathway*), such as the splanchnic nerves, and through spinal nerves that supply somatic structures (the *parietal pathway*). The parietal pleura, peritoneum, and lower part of the pericardium are sensitive to pain but are supplied by spinal nerves instead of nerves of the autonomic nervous system (ANS). Pain transmitted via the true visceral pathway is poorly localized and is often referred to a *body surface area* (dermatome) distant from its origin. On the other hand, pain transmitted via the parietal pathway is felt directly over the painful area. All neurons stimulated by visceral afferent input have also been shown to receive somatic inputs. This dual innervation may be one reason for the poor localization of visceral stimuli and for the phenomenon of referred pain.

Visceral pain is transmitted through the sympathetic and parasympathetic fibers of the ANS. Visceral afferents are usually type C fibers, and the pain sensations generated usually have a dull or aching quality. Pain impulses from the thoracic and abdominal viscera are almost exclusively conducted through the sympathetic nervous system; they travel with the sympathetic nerve through the sympathetic ganglia without synapsing, and then reach the spinal nerves through the white ramus communicans and thence to the dorsal root ganglion. However, pain impulses from the pharynx, trachea, and esophagus are mediated by vagal afferents, and pain from the deep pelvic structures is transmitted in the sacral parasympathetic nerves. In the central pathways, visceral pain impulses, as well as other visceral sensations, travel the same route as do impulses from somatic structures. This factor is important in the frequent somatic referral of visceral pain.

Visceral pain is particularly unpleasant not only because of the affective component, which it shares with all pain but also because so many visceral afferents excited by the same process that causes the pain have reflex connections that initiate nausea, vomiting, sweating, blood pressure changes, and other autonomic effects.

Visceral pain, as with deep somatic pain, initiates reflex contraction of nearby skeletal muscle. This reflex spasm is usually in the abdominal wall and is most marked when visceral inflammatory processes involve the peritoneum. The anatomic details of the reflex pathways by which impulses from diseased viscera initiate skeletal muscle spasm are unclear. The spasm protects the underlying inflamed structures from inadvertent trauma. This reflex spasm is sometimes referred to as muscle "guarding."

Referred Pain

Referred pain is defined as pain originating from one site in the body that is perceived as being localized in a different site. Visceral pain is often referred to dermatomes (skin areas) innervated by the same segments of the spinal cord as the painful viscus. When visceral pain is referred to the surface of the body, it is generally localized to the dermatomal segment from which the visceral organ originated in the embryo, not necessarily where the organ is located in the adult.

Presently, the most widely accepted explanation of referred pain is the *convergence-projection theory* (Fields, Martin, 2001). According to this theory, two types of afferents entering the spinal segment (one from the skin and another from the viscera or deep muscular structures) converge onto the same sensory projection cells (e.g., spinothalamic projection cells). Because the brain has no way of knowing the actual source of the input, it mistakenly "projects" the pain sensation to the somatic site (dermatome) (Fig. 52-7). For example, myocardial ischemia results in the patient experiencing severe pain over the middle of the sternum, often radiating down the medial side of the left arm, the root of the neck, and even the jaw. The pain is assumed to be caused by the accumulation of metabolites and oxygen deficiency, which stimulate the sensory nerve endings in the myocardium. The afferent nerve fibers ascend to the CNS through the cardiac branches of the sympathetic trunk and enter the spinal cord through the dorsal roots of the upper five thoracic nerves (T1 to T5). The cardiac pain is not felt in the heart but is referred to the skin areas (dermatomes) supplied by the corresponding spinal (somatic) nerves. The skin areas supplied by the upper five intercostal nerves and by the intercostal brachial nerve (T2) are therefore affected. A certain amount of spread of the pain impulses must occur within the CNS, because the pain is sometimes felt in the neck and jaw.

Another common example of referred pain is found in the early stages of acute appendicitis. Initially, visceral pain in the appendix is produced by distention of its lumen or spasm of its muscle. The visceral afferent pain fibers enter the spinal cord at the tenth thoracic (T10) level, having ascended through the superior mesenteric plexus and the lesser splanchnic nerve. A vague aching or crampy pain is felt in the area of the umbilicus, which is innervated by the tenth (somatic) intercostal nerve. Later, the pain shifts to the lower right quadrant of the abdomen, where the inflamed appendix irritates the parietal peritoneum, which is innervated by the twelfth thoracic and first lumbar spinal nerves (T12 to L1). Here, the pain is sharp and precisely localized over the irritated peritoneum, because the impulses are transmitted directly via the spinal nerves (somatic or parietal pathway).

An understanding of the typical patterns of referred pain from visceral structures is helpful in diagnosing illness (Fig. 52-8). Table 52-2 identifies some of the dermatomes to which pain from damaged visceral structures are referred.

FIG. 52-7 The convergence-projection theory of referred pain. Afferent fibers from the viscus converge on the same pain projection neurons in the spinal cord as do afferent fibers from somatic structures (e.g., the skin). Thus visceral pain may be perceived as somatic pain.

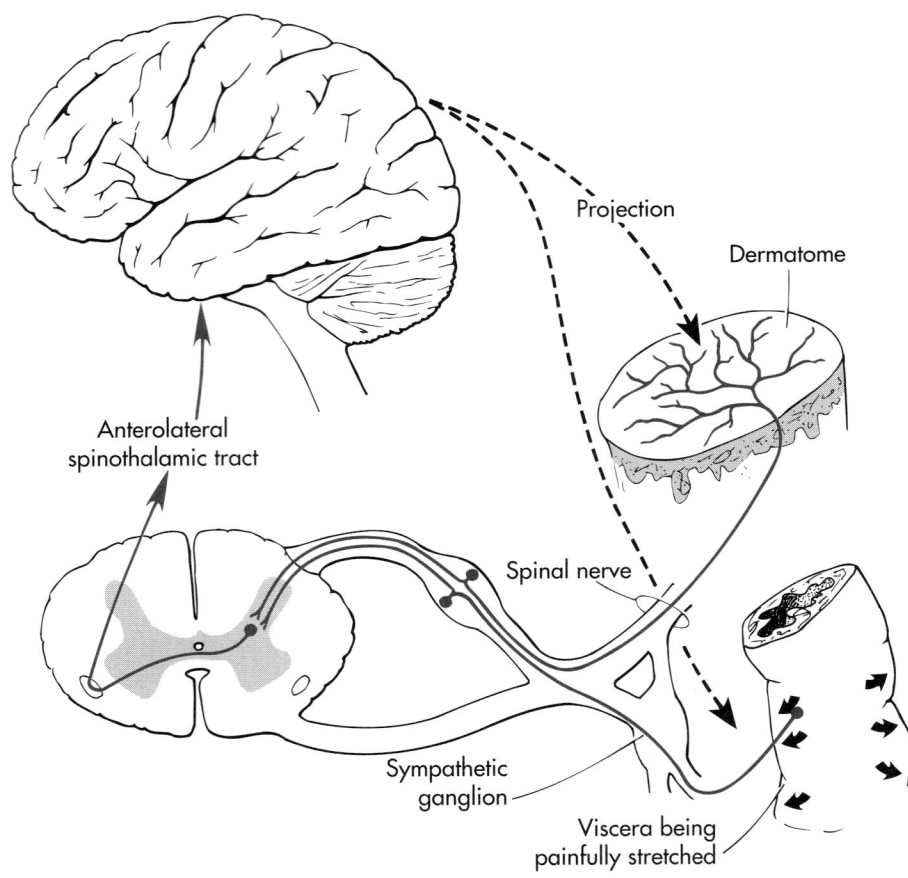

Neuropathic Pain

The nervous system normally transmits noxious stimuli from the PNS to the CNS that result in pain. Thus lesions of the PNS or CNS can result in impairment or loss of pain sensation called *hypalgesia* and *analgesia*, respectively. Paradoxically, damage or dysfunction of the CNS or peripheral nerves can cause pain. This type of pain is called neuropathic pain, or *deafferentation*. Neuropathic pain arises from the peripheral nerves along their course or from the CNS because of abnormal functioning, without involving the excitation of specific pain receptors (nociceptors).

Neuropathic pain often has a burning, tingling, or electric-shocklike quality. People with neuropathic pain suffer from instability of the ANS. Thus the pain is often made worse by emotional or physical (cold, fatigue) stress and relieved by relaxation; consequently, they may fall asleep normally despite their pain. The most characteristic feature of neuropathic pain, which is never seen in tissue damage pain, is allodynia. *Allodynia* is pain triggered by stimuli that would ordinarily be innocuous, such as a light touch or even a puff of wind. A sensory defect is typically present in the area of the pain. Neuropathic pain is often severe and refractory to treatment with opiates.

Neuropathic pain may result from lesions of the CNS *(central pain)* or damage to the peripheral nerves *(peripheral pain)*. Neuropathic central pain is a developing concept, resulting from increasing evidence that damage to peripheral nociceptive nerve endings in soft tissue, nerve plexuses, or the nerves themselves can also cause noci-

ceptive *central* pain through a process of sensitization. Such sensitization is possible because of the phenomenon of *plasticity* that is characteristic of dorsal root ganglia and dorsal horn neurons. Essentially, their responsiveness is altered over time with sustained or repetitive noxious sensory input or both. The mechanism through which sensitization occurs is believed to be molecular changes in nociceptive terminals, ectopic firing of afferent pain fibers, and physiologic changes of the N-methyl-D-aspartate (NMDA) receptor that cause chronic nociceptive pain (Schwartzman et al, 2001). The *thalamic pain syndrome* is an example of central neuropathic pain. Damage to the thalamus may be caused by a cerebrovascular accident (CVA, stroke) and results in severe burning pain in the hemiplegic side, especially in the distal limb. One theory explaining the pathogenesis of thalamic pain is the loss of central inhibition. According to this theory, damage to the neospinothalamic pathway that spares the paleospinothalamic pathway releases the latter from inhibition, resulting in summation and hyperalgesia. This action is similar to what happens when dorsal horn nociceptors excited by unmyelinated primary afferents are released from the inhibitory influence of the large, myelinated afferents, as described in the gate control theory. Activity of sympathetic efferents may also play a role in the pathogenesis of central neuropathic pain, because peripheral sympathetic blockade can sometimes relieve the pain (Fields, Martin, 2001).

Peripheral neuropathic pain occurs as a result of damage to peripheral nerves. Damage that is peripheral in ori-

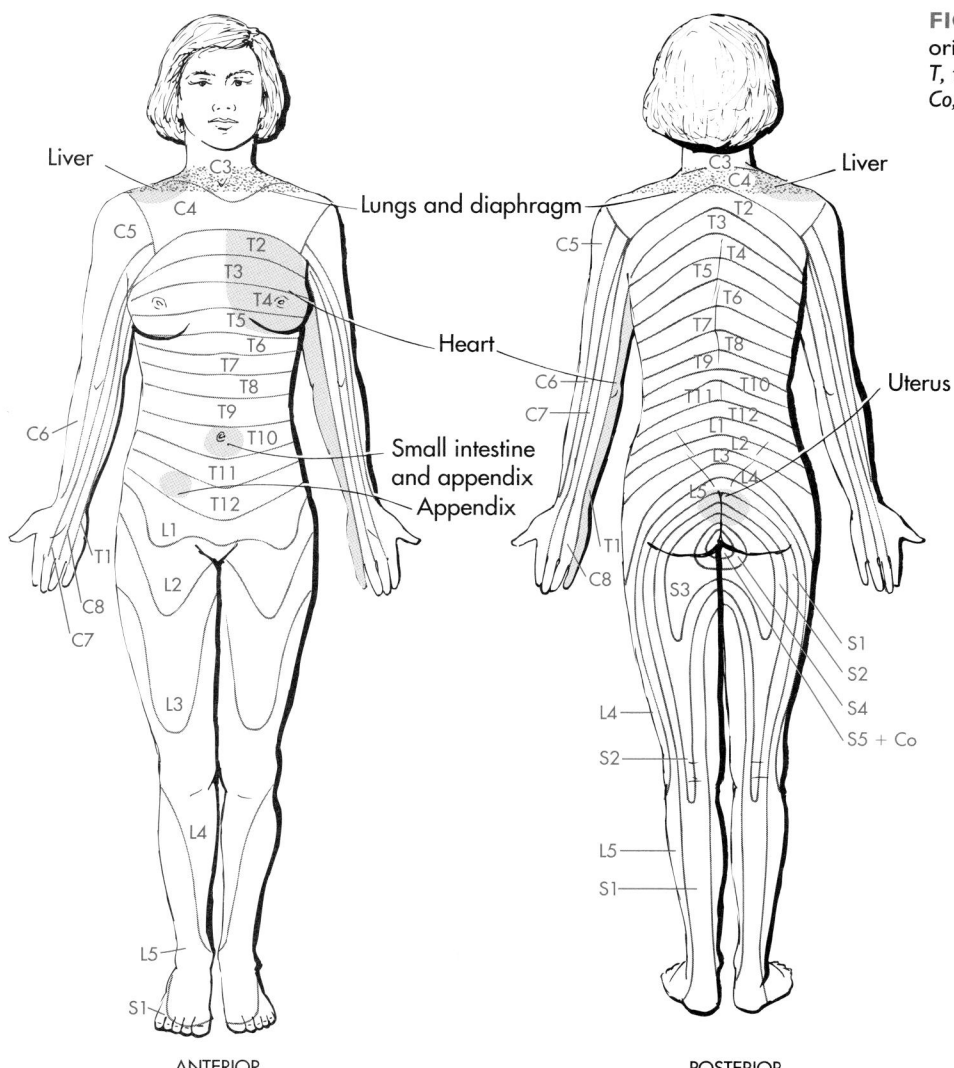

ANTERIOR   POSTERIOR

gin leads not only to spontaneous firing of the affected peripheral nerve fibers but also to spontaneous firing of the dorsal root ganglion cells of the damaged nerves. Examples of syndromes that may be present include postherpetic neuralgia, painful diabetic neuropathy, trigeminal neuralgia, causalgia, and phantom limb pain.

Postherpetic neuralgia is a dermatomal deafferentation pain that occurs as a sequela to herpes zoster (shingles). Herpes zoster is characterized by a painful vesicular rash, most often on the chest dermatomes (T3 to L3), caused by reactivation of the varicella-zoster virus (VZV). It is presumed that the virus infects the dorsal root ganglion during chickenpox and lies dormant until reactivated. Herpes zoster is most common in persons over age 50 years and in immunocompromised patients, such as those with Hodgkin's disease and non-Hodgkin's lymphoma. Persistent intractable pain occurs in the involved dermatomes months after the cutaneous lesions have healed in about 50% of older patients (postherpetic neuralgia). The exact cause is unknown, but scarring and degenerative changes in the spinal cord, ganglia, and nerve trunks may be important factors.

Diabetic neuropathy is a common complication of diabetes, especially after longstanding hyperglycemia. There is

TABLE 52-2 ■ ■ ■

Common Patterns of Referred Pain

Site of Visceral Pathology or Noxious Stimuli	Surface Areas of Referred Pain
Diaphragm	C3-C5 dermatomes: pain in ipsilateral shoulder or neck area
Heart	C3-T5 dermatomes: substernal pain radiating to back, down inner aspect of arm (usually left), and sometimes neck and jaw
Liver-gallbladder	T5-T9 dermatomes: pain in right costal margin radiating to back or right shoulder
Stomach	T7-T9 dermatomes: epigastric pain
Appendix-small intestine	T9-T11 dermatomes: periumbilical pain
Prostate	T10-T12 dermatomes: periumbilical and groin pain, sometimes radiating to scrotum and penis
Ovaries	T10 dermatome: periumbilical pain
Ureters	L1-L2 dermatomes: pain in groin and inner surface of thighs
Uterus	S1-S2 dermatomes: pain over sacrum
Rectum	S2-S4 dermatomes: low back pain radiating down posterior aspect of thigh and calf

C, Cervical; *T*, thoracic; *L*, lumbar; *S*, sacral spinal nerves.

good evidence for a strong association between impaired glucose tolerance (IGT) and neuropathy, especially painful small fiber neuropathy, described below (Vinik, 2001). IGT is a stage of abnormal response to a 2-hour oral glucose tolerance test (OGTT) in which the individual has a 2-hour OGTT result of ≥140 but less than the diagnostic level of 200 mg/dl (American Diabetes Association, 2000). IGT may affect every part of the nervous system, with the possible exception of the brain. The most common clinical picture is that of bilateral peripheral polyneuropathy that is primarily sensory. In diabetic sensory neuropathy, predominantly the small nerve fibers are affected, and these neuropathies are characteristically painful. Symptoms include numbness, paresthesias, severe hyperalgesias, and pain that is typically described as "burning." The examination may be unremarkable, with normal reflexes, normal strength, normal sensory levels, and normal electrophysiology (Vinik, 2001; Vinik et al, 2000).

Trigeminal neuralgia (tic douloureux) is a disorder that affects primarily middle aged and older adults; it consists of paroxysmal, intense stabbing pain in the distribution of the mandibular and maxillary divisions of the trigeminal nerve (fifth cranial nerve). The ophthalmic division of the nerve is rarely affected. The pain may be triggered by usually innocuous stimuli of specific areas of the face, lips or gums, as in eating, talking, yawning, shaving, tooth brushing, or by drafts of cold air. Though the pain is brief (seconds to a minute), it may be so intense that the patient winces reflexively or involuntarily (hence the term *tic*). Patients may also report a continuous facial discomfort, itching, and sensitivity. Such discomfort is generally regarded as an atypical feature of trigeminal neuralgia, though it is not infrequent. The spatial and temporal summation patterns of the pain suggest that the mechanism is an allodynia. Though most cases are idiopathic (without definable cause), some cases are secondary to another neurologic disease, such as multiple sclerosis, basilar artery aneurysm, tumor (especially of the acoustic or trigeminal nerves), or compression of the trigeminal roots by an enlarged, tortuous blood vessel (Adams et al, 1997).

Causalgia is a term used to describe the intense burning pain in an extremity that may follow partial damage to a nerve trunk, typically the median nerve above the elbow or sciatic nerve above the knee. The pain usually begins soon after the injury and, in time, becomes associated with autonomic changes and trophic changes in the extremity. Causalgia is one subtype of a group of disorders known as *reflex sympathetic dystrophies*, and all give rise to allodynia, or pain triggered by innocuous stimuli. All tissues in the extremity waste, including bones, and there is evidence of sympathetic hyperactivity, including vasomotor changes and abnormal sweating. Pain relief follows sympathetic blockage. Fields and Martin (2001) suggest that such results indicate the sympathetic nervous system can, under some conditions, be actively involved in the process of inflammation. Other mechanisms of pain generation may include loss of afferent inhibition by the large, myelinated fibers and ectopic impulse generation at the site of injury. The causes of reflex sympathetic dystrophies include nerve damage, amputations, fractures of the small bones of the hand or foot, sprains, or thrombophlebitis.

Phantom limb pain is experienced by a patient as tingling, "pins and needles" sensation (paresthesias), or less often as a burning, crushing pain in a limb that the individual no longer possesses (because it has been amputated). This sensation is possibly because some of the pain fibers have been pinched in the scar tissue of the limb stump, causing the generation of ectopic impulses. It is immaterial that the portion of the fiber attached to the receptor is missing, because a region still exists in the cerebral cortex for that portion of the extremity. All that is required is that an impulse reach the cortex for that area.

CLINICAL ASSESSMENT OF PAIN

The relief and management of pain require careful assessment to attempt to understand the patient's pain experience and identify the cause so that it can be removed, if possible. The clinician must first take a careful history, which should include the data about the pain listed in Table 52-3.

The patient can indicate the *location* of the pain by pointing to the body part or indicating the site on a drawing of a human figure. It is important to find out whether the pain is *superficial* or *deep*. Pain from a superficial lesion usually poses no problem because the cause and effect are obvious. However, exact location becomes especially important with deep pain that is referred to a dermatome when deep somatic structures or viscera are involved.

TABLE 52-3 ■ ■ ■

Essential Data to Collect for Assessment of Pain

Characteristic of Pain	Questions for Patient
Location	Where does it hurt?
	Does the pain radiate?
	Is the pain superficial or deep?
Mode of onset	When did the pain start?
	Did it begin suddenly or gradually?
	Was there any particular event that appeared to produce the pain when it began?
Pattern (timing, frequency, duration)	What time of the day does the pain occur?
	How often does it appear?
	Is it constant or intermittent?
	How long does the pain last?
Aggravating and relieving factors	What seems to trigger the pain?
	What seems to make the pain worse (e.g., movement or changes in posture, coughing or straining, eating or drinking)?
	What seems to make the pain better (e.g., rest; sleep; changes in posture such as standing, sitting, lying down, or bending; food or antacids)?
Quality	What does the pain feel like (e.g., throbbing, dull, aching, sharp, stabbing, prickling, burning)?
Intensity	How strong is your pain? (Have patient rate the pain using a verbal or visual analog scale both before and after treatment.)
Associated symptoms	Are there any problems caused by your pain (e.g., anorexia, nausea, vomiting, insomnia)?
Effects on lifestyle	Does your pain interfere with your activities at home, work, or normal social interactions?
	Has the pain affected your lifestyle in any way (e.g., eating, sleeping, sexual activity, driving)?
Methods of pain relief	What has helped control your pain in the past?
	What has not worked in relieving your pain?

The *mode of onset* is an important factor in assessing pain. A pain that has a sudden onset and reaches a peak of intensity almost immediately suggests a rupture of tissue. The pain of myocardial infarction or a ruptured peptic ulcer may develop in this manner.

The *pattern* of the pain, or the time and frequency of occurrence and duration, provides important information. Postural aches come after prolonged activity (usually late in the day) and disappear with rest, whereas arthritic pains are most severe during the first movements after prolonged inactivity (usually in the morning on awakening). Painful lesions of the bone, such as metastatic cancer, are likely to be most disturbing at night. Not all pain is constant. Intermittent pain that occurs several times a day can be equally disturbing. Attacks can last seconds, hours, or days and can affect the individual's ability to function normally (e.g., trigeminal neuralgia, migraine headache). Substernal pain lasting less than 15 minutes that is relieved by rest or nitroglycerin is characteristic of angina pectoris, but when the pain persists longer than 15 minutes, it may indicate myocardial infarction.

The *aggravating and relieving factors* of pain are more important than is the quality of the pain in providing data concerning its mechanism. Pain related to breathing, swallowing, or defecation focuses attention on the respiratory system, esophagus, and lower bowel, respectively. Pain that is brought on by activity and relieved after a few minutes of rest suggests ischemia (e.g., angina pectoris, intermittent claudication). Pain occurring several hours after meals that is relieved by food or antacid ingestion is characteristic of duodenal ulcer. Pain that is increased or altered by cutaneous stimuli may be caused by disease or injury to the sensory tracts in the PNS or CNS (e.g., causalgia, thalamic syndrome).

The *quality* of the pain may be assessed by simply asking patients to describe the pain in their own words (e.g., dull, throbbing, burning). This evaluation can also be approached using a more formal assessment, such as the *McGill Pain Questionnaire* (Fig. 52-9), which is one of the

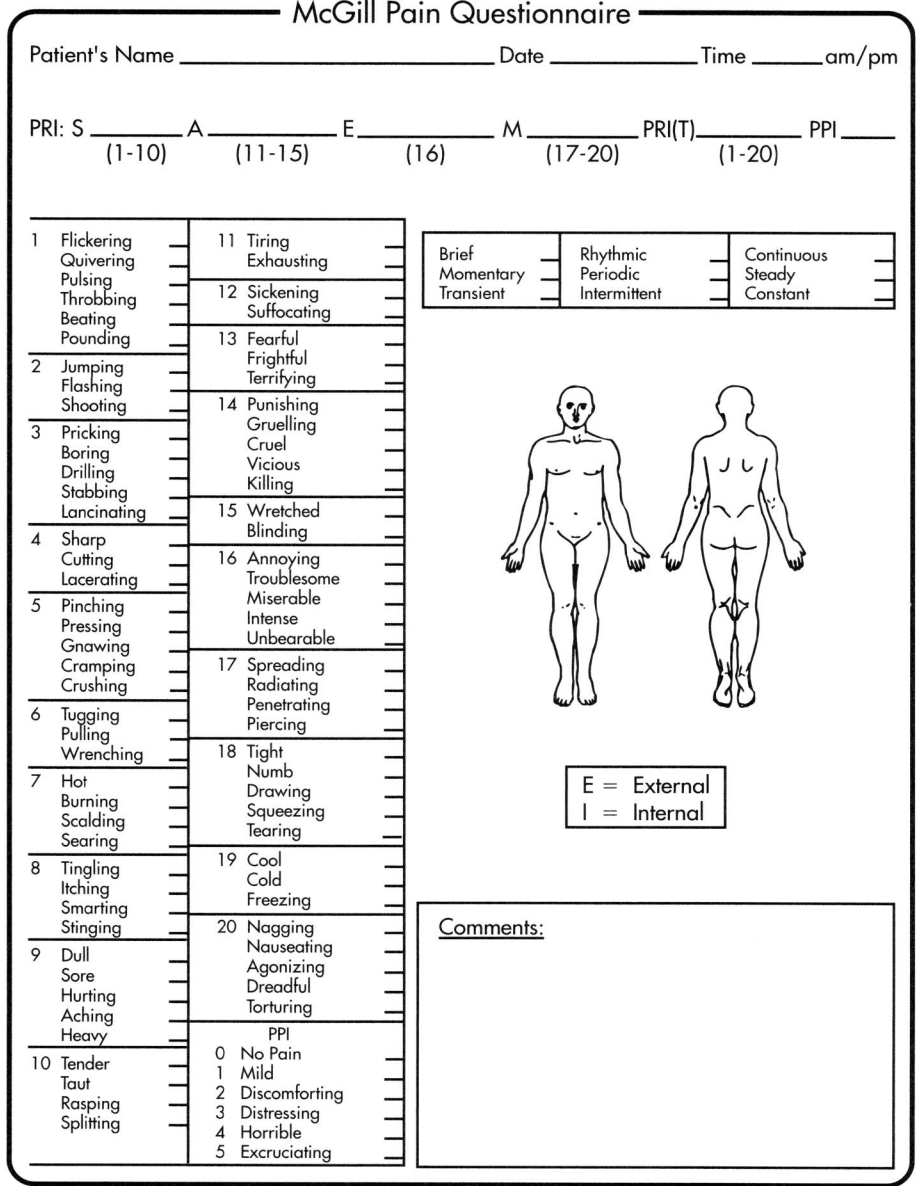

FIG. 52-9 McGill Pain Questionnaire. The pain rating index *(PRI)* is the sum of ranked values for the 20 words: *S,* subjective, 1 to 10; *A,* affective, 11 to 15; *E,* evaluative, 16; *M,* miscellaneous, 17 to 20 *PRI(T),* total PRI, (1-20); *PPI,* present pain index, a rating of pain intensity. The site of the pain is marked on the figure with an E (external) or I (internal), and the boxes above the figures are checked to describe the pattern of the pain. Comments include response to analgesics. (From Melzack R, Katz J, editors: Pain measurement in persons in pain. In Wall PD, Melzack R, editors:*Textbook of pain,* ed 4, New York, 2000, Churchill Livingstone.)

most frequently used tools for assessing pain. This tool has been validated in several languages and can be used in both acute and chronic settings, as well as for research. The questionnaire measures the physiologic and psychologic dimensions of pain and is divided into four parts. In the first part the patient indicates the location of the pain on a drawing of a human body. In the second part the patient chooses 20 words that describe the sensory, affective, evaluative, and other qualities of the pain. In the third part the patient chooses words such as *brief, rhythmic,* or *steady* to describe the pattern of the pain. In the fourth part the patient rates the intensity of the pain on a scale of 0 to 5.

The tool most often used to assess the *intensity* or *severity* of the patient's pain is some form of a *visual analog scale (VAS),* which consists of a horizontal line evenly divided into 10 segments numbered 0 to 10 (Fig. 52-10, *A*). Patients are instructed that 0 represents "no pain at all" and 10 represents the "the most severe pain they can imagine." Patients are then asked to mark the number that best describes the level of pain they are experiencing at some given point in time. A modified VAS for use with children (or with cognitively impaired adults) substitutes a continuum of smiling or crying faces for numbers (Fig. 52-10, *B*).

It is important to ask the patient about *symptoms associated* with the pain. Autonomic responses such as nausea and vomiting are common with severe, acute pain. Auras often precede migraine headaches. The examiner should provide ample opportunity to discuss what the pain means to the patient by asking about its *impact on lifestyle.* Finally, it is important to document *methods of treatment for pain* that have been used by the patient in the past and their effectiveness.

In addition to collecting subjective data about pain, direct observation of *nonverbal and verbal behavior* may provide additional clues about the patient's pain experience. Nonverbal behaviors such as facial grimacing, tearing, abnormal gait or posture, muscle tension, and guarding of parts are common indicators of pain. Verbal and emotional signals indicating pain may include crying, moaning, irritability, expressions of anger or sadness,

and changes in voice pitch or fluency. Gender and cultural differences exist in the types of displays used. As described previously, acute pain often activates a *sympathetic response,* resulting in increased heart and respiratory rates and blood pressure, pallor, flushing, sweating, and pupil dilation. Very brief and intense pain may also be followed by a rebound parasympathetic response.

Finally, the clinician should *inspect and palpate the painful area* to test range of motion of involved joints, determine if there is muscle guarding, and identify trigger points of pain and areas of decreased sensation or increased sensitivity.

MANAGEMENT OF PAIN

The overall goal in the treatment of pain is to provide the greatest relief from pain with the least possible side effects. There are two general methods for the treatment of pain: pharmacologic and nonpharmacologic. To achieve the goal of pain relief in the patient, the clinician needs to (1) use knowledge of the neuropathophysiologic aspects of pain as a basis for various interventions; (2) assess pain routinely using appropriate instruments, both before and after treatment; (3) use a variety of pharmacologic and nonpharmacologic pain-relieving methods; and (4) document the effectiveness of pain-relieving interventions. Planning is needed in consultation with the patient, and the clinician should create a relationship of warmth, empathy, and respect.

Pharmacologic Approaches

Medications are the most common form of pain control. There are three groups of pain medications: (1) nonopioid analgesics, (2) opioid analgesics, and (3) opioid antagonists and agonist-antagonists. A fourth group of medications is called *adjuvants* or *coanalgesics.* Pharmacologic management with analgesic drugs should be implemented using a stepwise approach.

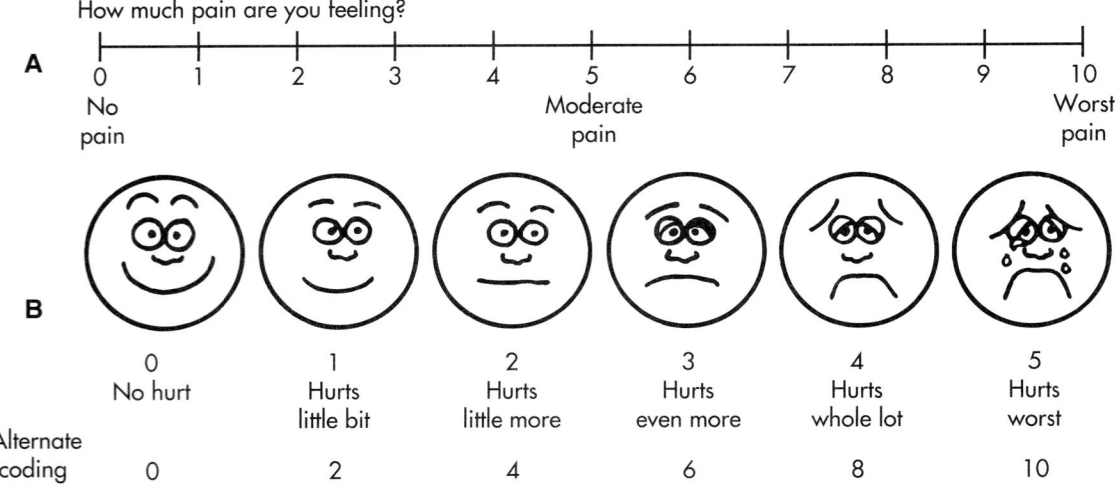

FIG. 52-10 Visual analog scales to assess intensity of pain. **A,** Numeric rating scale. **B,** Wong-Baker FACES Pain Rating Scale. Face 0 is smiling because it has no pain. Faces 1 to 5 have increasing amounts of pain (a little to the greatest imaginable) with increasingly sad expressions. (**B,** From Wong DL et al: *Whaley & Wong's nursing care of infants and children,* ed 7, St Louis, 2003, Mosby.)

Nonopioid Analgesia: Nonsteroidal Antiinflammatory Drugs (NSAIDs)

The first step, often effective for mild to moderate pain management, uses nonopioid analgesics, specifically acetaminophen (Tylenol) and the NSAIDs. A wide variety of NSAIDs are available with varying degrees of antipyretic, analgesic, and (except for acetaminophen) antiinflammatory actions; they also differ to some extent in their cost, duration of action, and side effects. Acetylsalicylic acid (aspirin) and ibuprofen (Motrin, Advil) are probably the most frequently used NSAIDs. NSAIDs are particularly effective in treating low-grade acute pain, chronic inflammatory conditions such as arthritis, and mild cancer-related pain.

NSAIDs produce analgesia by acting peripherally at the site of tissue injury by blocking the synthesis of prostaglandins from their arachidonic acid precursors. Prostaglandins (mainly PGE_1, PGE_2, and PGI_2) sensitize nociceptors and work synergistically with other inflammatory products at the site of injury, such as bradykinin and histamine, to produce hyperalgesia. Thus NSAIDs interfere with the mechanism of transduction in primary afferent nociceptors by blocking prostaglandin synthesis.

In contrast to opioids, NSAIDs do not produce physical dependence or tolerance. All share a *ceiling effect*; that is, increasing the dose above a certain level does not increase the analgesic effect. However, the ceiling dose may be higher than the recommended starting dose, thus a higher dose may be warranted. The most common complications associated with NSAIDs are GI upset, increased bleeding time (aspirin), blurring of vision, minor changes in liver function tests, and reduction in renal function.

Development of a new, more specific type of NSAID depended on an understanding of the two major classes of cyclooxygenases (COX). These enzymes comprise one of the pathways for metabolizing arachidonic acid, a breakdown product of damaged or dying human cells. One class, COX-1, is *constitutively* expressed and is necessary for normal physiologic functioning in many body systems. The second class, COX-2, is *induced* in the inflammatory state and is responsible for the production of many painful inflammatory end-products. The COX-2 inhibitors are selective in that they inhibit only the COX-2 pathway. This "sparing" of the COX-1 pathway protects the "good" prostaglandin products that are needed for physiologic functions such as protection of the gastric mucosa and adequate glomerular filtration in the kidney. Thus the COX-2 inhibitors minimize the side effects of gastric irritation and reduced renal function, while providing good antiinflammatory relief (Roberts, Morrow, 2001). Examples of COX-2 inhibitors are celecoxib (Celebrex) and rofecoxib (Vioxx).

Acetaminophen (Tylenol) is nearly as effective as is aspirin in its analgesic-antipyretic properties. However, acetaminophen has poor antiinflammatory activity, because it is only a weak inhibitor of COX in the presence of the very high concentrations of peroxides found in inflamed peripheral tissues (Roberts, Morrow, 2001). In contrast, acetaminophen does have the ability to inhibit COX in the brain, where peroxide concentration is low—thus explaining its antipyretic effect (Roberts, Morrow, 2001). The advantage of acetaminophen over aspirin as an antipyretic and analgesic is that it has no effect on the cardiovascular or respiratory systems, and produces no adverse effects on acid-base balance, platelet function, or COX-1 activity in the gastric and renal systems. If either acetaminophen or aspirin are not effective alone in relieving pain, they may be combined with a weak narcotic such as oxycodone or codeine for more effective pain relief. A major disadvantage of acetaminophen is that it can cause fatal hepatic damage in overdoses (Eaton, Klaassen, 1996). Perhaps because it is commonly perceived to be a safe household analgesic, the number of self-poisonings and suicides with acetaminophen has grown in the United States in recent years.

Opioid Analgesia

Opioids are currently the most potent analgesics available and are used in the management of moderately severe to severe pain. These drugs are the cornerstones in the treatment of postoperative and cancer-related pain. Morphine (from Morpheus, the Greek god of dreams) is an alkaloid derived from the dried juice of the opium poppy plant, and it has been used for centuries for its analgesic, sedative, and euphoric effects. Morphine is one of the most widely used drugs for the treatment of severe pain and remains the standard with which other analgesic drugs are compared.

In contrast to the NSAIDs, which act peripherally, morphine exerts its analgesic effect centrally. The actual mechanism of opioid action has become clearer since the discovery of endogenous opioid receptors in the limbic system, thalamus, PAG, substantia gelatinosa of the dorsal horn, and gut. Exogenous opioids such as morphine exert their effect by binding to opioid receptors in a manner similar to that of endogenous opioids (endorphins-enkephalins); that is, they have agonist action (enhance the receptor's action). By binding to opioid receptors in the brainstem pain-modulating nuclei, morphine exerts its effects on the descending pain-inhibiting systems. Morphine can also block the transmission of incoming nociceptor impulses at the level of the spinal cord dorsal horn by binding with opioid receptors in the substantia gelatinosa.

The action of opioids can depend on the type of receptor with which they interact. Three types of opioid receptors have been reasonably well defined: mu-, kappa-, and delta-receptors. The most important receptor type for clinical analgesia is called "mu" because of its affinity for morphine. Numerous drugs in the morphine class are mu-agonists, although they differ in potency (Baumann, 1997). Knowledge of the equianalgesic doses of opioid drugs is essential when changing medications or routes of administration. Box 52-1 lists some authoritative resources for determining dosing equivalencies for opioid analgesics and for establishing pain management programs. It should be noted that meperidine (Demerol) is no longer recommended for use in pain management because of its well-documented toxicities, especially seizure activity (American Society of Anesthesiologists [ASA], 1996; Waitman, McCaffery, 2001). See also University of Wisconsin Hospitals and Clinics' Guidelines for Meperidine Use (*http://www.wisc.edu/wcpi/prof/mguide.htm*).

Opioid drugs have a very similar pattern of side effects, including respiratory depression, nausea and vomiting, sedation, and constipation. In addition, opioids all have

BOX 52-1

Resources for Opioid Analgesic Dosing Data and for Establishing Pain Management Programs

DOSING DATA

American Society of Anesthesiologists (ASA) Task Force on Pain Management: Cancer pain section, practice guidelines for cancer pain management, *Anesthesiology* 84(5):1243-1257, 1996. Also see Template, Appendix 2, at the following address:
  http://www.asahq.org/practice/cancer/Cancer_Appendixes.html
Baumann TJ: Pain management. In DePiro JT et al, editors: *Pharmacotherapy: a pathophysiologic approach*, ed 4, Norwalk, Conn, 1999, Appleton & Lange.
Gutstein HB, Akil H: Opioid analgesics. In Hardman JG et al, editors: *The pharmacological basis of therapeutics*, ed 10, New York, 2001, McGraw-Hill.
Pasero C et al: Opioid analgesics. In McCaffery M, Pasero C: *Pain: clinical manual*, ed 2, St Louis, 1999, Mosby.
Taylor EC, Koo PJS: Pain. In Koda-Kimble MA et al, editors: *Applied therapeutics: the clinical use of drugs*, ed 7, Philadelphia, 2001, Lippincott–Williams & Wilkins.

Establishing Pain Management Programs

  http://www.jcaho.org/standard/pm.html
  Web site for Pain Standards for 2001 established by the Joint Commission on Accreditation of Healthcare Organizations (JCAHO).
Bral EE: Caring for adults with chronic cancer pain, *Amer J Nurs* 98(4):27-32, 1998.
City of Hope National Medical Center and Beckman Research Institute. Mayday Pain Resource Center (Web page). Available online at *http://www.cityofhope.org/medinfo/mayday.htm*. Accessed Dec 7, 2001.
Dahl J, Pasero C, Patterson C: Institutionalizing effective pain management practices: the implications of the new JCAHO pain assessment and management standards. Program and Abstracts of the 19th Annual Scientific Meeting of the American Pain Society; Nov 2-5, 2000; Atlanta. Symposium Abstract 302.
The Resource Center of the American Alliance of Cancer Pain Initiatives, 2000: Building an Institutional Commitment to Pain Management, the Wisconsin Resource Manual, ed 2. (The manual reviews strategies to gain support for improving pain management, a process for institutionalizing pain management, and strategies for quality improvement. Also contains sample resource tools from clinical and academic institutions throughout the United States.) Contact: The Resource Center, 4720 Medical Sciences Center, 1300 University Ave, Madison, WI 53706.

the potential to produce tolerance, dependence, and addiction. *Tolerance* is the physiologic need for higher doses to maintain the analgesic effects of the drug. Tolerance to a particular opioid develops when it is administered chronically, as for cancer-related pain. Although considerable cross-tolerance occurs between the opioid drugs, it is not complete. This characteristic provides the theoretic basis for substituting another opioid drug when a particular one becomes ineffective. Also, because of incomplete cross-tolerance, the ASA Task Force recommends that when tolerance to a particular opioid has developed, another opioid should be reduced by 25% to 50% of the calculated equianalgesic dose.* The same guidelines specify that a methadone substitution dose should be re-

duced by 75%. *Physical dependence* is also a physiologic process marked by the occurrence of a withdrawal syndrome after abrupt discontinuation of an opioid drug or after administration of an antagonist. The withdrawal syndrome is believed to result from rebound noradrenergic activity in the CNS that is depressed by chronic opioid use (Akbarian et al, 2001). *Addiction*, or *psychologic dependence*, refers to a behavioral syndrome in which there is overriding concern with the use and acquisition of the drug, resulting in drug hoarding and unapproved escalation in the dose. It is important to understand the differences among tolerance, dependence, and addiction, because evidence indicates that patients are routinely undermedicated for pain because of an exaggerated fear (by both staff and patients) of the patient becoming addicted. This fear is unfounded because addiction is extremely rare when opioids are used to treat patients in pain (McCaffery, Ferrell, Pasero, 2000). It is important to remember that patients vary in their analgesic dose requirements and the dose must be individually titrated. In recent years, tremendous progress has been made in methods of opioid administration that help to provide greater relief from unnecessary pain.

One such advance in the method of opioid administration is "around-the-clock dosing" rather than PRN "as-needed dosing" (requiring the patient to request medication from the nurse). Around-the-clock dosing has the advantage of maintaining constant blood levels of analgesic and preventing the development of severe pain, which is more difficult to alleviate after it occurs. Because the best way to treat pain is to prevent it, *patient-controlled analgesia (PCA)* systems were developed. As the name implies, the PCA apparatus delivers a preset dose of morphine (or other opioid) through an indwelling intravenous (IV) line when the patient pushes a button. The device is loaded with enough drug to cover the patient's needs for 12 to 24 hours and is usually programmed so a minimal interval of 15 to 30 minutes elapses between doses. PCA devices are most often used to control postoperative and cancer-related pain. Some of the advantages of PCA include superior pain relief with less medication, less sedation, and a decrease in the delay between request for analgesia and relief. Administration of opioids and local anesthetics via the neural axis (called neuraxial drug delivery) deposits medication directly at receptor sites. Routes of administration are epidural, subarachnoid, and intraventricular spaces. Epidural and subarachnoid drug deposition can be achieved by percutaneous catheterization, reservoir, or implantation of a catheter and pump. Advantages of direct neural delivery systems are that they (1) do not depend on systemic absorption, (2) provide analgesia with fewer side effects than systemically delivered medications, and (3) require lower doses of medication (ASA, 1996).

Opioid Antagonists and Agonist-Antagonists

Opioid antagonists are drugs that counteract the effect of opioid drugs by binding to opioid receptors and blocking their activation. Naloxone, a pure opioid antagonist, reverses both the analgesia and the side effects of opioids. Naloxone is used to counteract the effects of a narcotic overdose, the most serious of which are respiratory depression and sedation.

---

*Guidelines available at *http://www.asahq.org/practice/cancer/cancer.html*

Other opioid drugs are combinations of agonists and antagonists, such as pentazocine (Talwin) and butorphanol (Stadol). When these drugs are given to a patient dependent on narcotics, they can precipitate withdrawal symptoms. Opioid agonist-antagonists are effective analgesics when given alone and are less likely to produce undesirable side effects (e.g., respiratory depression) than pure agonist opioids.

Adjuvants or Coanalgesics

Adjuvant or coanalgesic medications are agents originally developed for purposes other than pain relief but have been found to have analgesic properties or a complementary role in the management of patients with pain. Some of these drugs are particularly effective in the control of neuropathic pain that may not respond to opioids.

Anticonvulsants, such as carbamazepine (Tegretol) or phenytoin (Dilantin), have been found to be effective for the treatment of lancinating pains associated with nerve damage. Lancinating pains (brief flashing, stabbing, or shooting) are characteristic of trigeminal neuralgia, diabetic neuropathy, and postherpetic neuralgia and often occur after laminectomy and limb amputation. Anticonvulsants are effective for neuropathic pain because they stabilize nerve cell membranes and suppress wind-up responses in nerves (McCaffery, April, 1998). Gabapentin, found to be particularly effective in lancinating pain, has an unknown mechanism of action, though it binds to a specific receptor in the brain, inhibits voltage-dependent sodium currents, and may enhance the release of GABA (Dichter, Brodie, 1996). The anticonvulsant, zonisamide (Zonegran), exerts its antiepileptic effects through sodium and calcium channel blockage, as well as through dopaminergic and serotonergic activity. In animal models, relief of pain through similar mechanisms has been found to be useful (Tomlinson et al, 2000; Malcangio, Tomlinson, 1998).

Tricyclic antidepressants, such as amitriptyline (Elavil) or imipramine (Tofranil), are very effective analgesics for neuropathic pain, as well as a broad range of other painful conditions. Some specific applications include postherpetic neuralgia, invasion of neural structures by carcinoma, postsurgical pain, and rheumatoid arthritis. In the treatment of pain, tricyclics appear to have an analgesic effect independent of their antidepressant activity. It is believed that tricyclic antidepressants relieve pain by blocking reuptake of biogenic amines in the CNS. As mentioned previously, serotonergic and adrenergic neurons in the brainstem project to and inhibit pain transmission cells in the spinal cord dorsal horn and are part of the descending pain-modulating system. Tricyclics supposedly enhance the inhibitory action of serotonin and norepinephrine on these neurons for spinal pain transmission.

Other adjuvant medications useful in the treatment of pain include hydroxyzine (Vistaril), which has analgesic effects over a range of painful conditions and an additive effect when given with morphine; muscle relaxants such as diazepam (Valium), which are used to treat muscle spasm associated with pain; and steroids such as dexamethasone (Decadron), which have been used to control the symptoms associated with spinal cord compression or bone metastasis in cancer patients.

Other adjuvants for analgesia are alpha-adrenergic receptor agonists (e.g., the alpha-2 agonist, clonidine), often given intraspinally along with opioids or local anesthetics; it also has an analgesic effect when administered systemically because it reverses the excessive sympathetic adrenergic response at central and peripheral receptors (Taylor, Koo, 2001). The alpha-1 antagonist, prazosin, has also been used in the management of sympathetically maintained pain. Major adverse effects of these agents are hypotension and potentiation of opioid-induced respiratory depression (Bral, 1998; Taylor, Koo, 2001).

Nonpharmacologic Approaches

Despite the convenience of analgesic drugs, many patients and clinicians are dissatisfied with their long-term use for nonmalignant-related pain. This situation has led to the development of a number of nonpharmacologic methods of pain management. Nonpharmacologic methods of pain control can be divided into two groups: physical therapies and modalities and cognitive-behavioral strategies. Some of these modalities can be useful alone or used as adjuncts in the management of pain.

Physical Therapies and Modalities

Physical therapies for pain relief include various forms of cutaneous stimulation (massage, transcutaneous electrical nerve stimulation, acupuncture, heat or cold applications, exercise). The rationale for cutaneous stimulation is derived from the gate control theory of pain transmission. Cutaneous stimulation stimulates the large-diameter nonnociceptive fibers to "close the gate" to pain-conducting small-diameter fibers and thus relieves pain. It has been hypothesized that cutaneous stimulation may also cause the body to secrete endorphins and other pain-inhibiting neurotransmitters.

One of the oldest and most common strategies of cutaneous stimulation is rubbing or massage. *Massage* can be accomplished using varying amounts of pressure and stimulation of various myofascial trigger points throughout the body. An oil or lotion is used to reduce friction. Massage relaxes muscle tension and increases local circulation. Back massage is particularly relaxing and, if performed by a caring person, provides an additional dimension of emotional support.

Transcutaneous electrical nerve stimulation (TENS or TNS) consists of a battery-operated device that sends weak electrical impulses via electrodes placed on the body. The electrodes are generally placed on or near the painful site. TENS units are used for the management of both acute and chronic pain: postoperative pain, low back pain, phantom limb pain, peripheral neuralgias, and rheumatoid arthritis. TENS is based on the gate control theory.

Acupuncture is an ancient Chinese technique involving the insertion of thin needles into various "acupuncture (trigger) points" throughout the body to relieve pain. An alternate, noninvasive method of stimulating the trigger points is to apply pressure with the thumbs, a technique called *acupressure*. Acupuncture is widely used in China and has even been used to perform major surgery without the use of an additional anesthetic. The use of acupuncture or acupressure techniques requires special training and has gained some popularity in the West. The gate control theory and the theory that acupuncture stimulates the release of endogenous opioids are possible explanations for its efficacy.

Range-of-motion (ROM) exercises (passive, assisted, or active) may be used to relax muscles, improve circulation, and prevent pain related to stiffness and immobility.

Heat application is a simple measure that has long been recognized as an effective method of reducing muscle spasm or pain. Heat can be delivered by conduction (hot-water bottles, electrical heating pads, lamps, hot wet compresses), convection (whirlpool, sitz bath, hot soaks), or conversion (ultrasound, diathermy). Pain from bruises, muscle spasms, and arthritis responds well to heat. Because heat dilates blood vessels and increases local blood flow, it should *not* be used after traumatic injuries when edema and inflammation are present. Because heat increases blood flow, it may relieve pain by removing the products of inflammation, such as bradykinin, histamine, and prostaglandins, that produce pain locally. Heat may also stimulate nerve fibers that close the gate, thus preventing the transmission of pain impulses up the spinal cord to the brain.

In contrast to heat therapy, which is effective for chronic pain, *cold application* is more effective for acute pain (e.g., trauma from burns, cuts, sprains). Cold may be applied in the form of cold soaks or compresses, ice bags, Aquamatic K pads, and ice massage. Cold applications reduce blood flow to an area and reduce bleeding and edema. It is believed that cold therapy produces an analgesic effect by slowing the conduction velocity of nerves so that fewer pain impulses reach the brain. Another possible mechanism is that the perception of cold predominates and reduces the perception of pain.

Cognitive-Behavioral Strategies

Cognitive-behavioral strategies are useful in changing the patient's perception of pain, altering pain behavior, and giving the patient a greater sense of control over the pain. These strategies include relaxation, imagery, hypnosis, and biofeedback. Although most cognitive-behavioral methods emphasize either relaxation or distraction, in practice, the two are almost inseparable.

With methods that emphasize *muscle relaxation,* the facilitator instructs the patient to focus on different muscle groups and voluntarily contract and relax them in sequence. Other means to induce relaxation include deep-breathing exercises, meditation, and listening to soothing music. Relaxation techniques reduce anxiety, muscle tension, and emotional stress and thus interrupt the pain-stress-pain cycle, in which pain and stress reinforce each other.

Distraction techniques reduce pain by focusing the patient's attention on another stimulus and away from the pain. Watching television, reading a book, listening to music, and engaging in a conversation are common examples of distraction. *Guided imagery* is a form of distraction in which the facilitator encourages the patient to visualize or think about a pleasant scene or desirable sensation to divert attention away from the pain. This technique is often combined with relaxation. *Hypnosis* is a cognitive method that depends on focusing the patient's attention away from the pain; it also depends on the therapist's ability to guide the patient's attention to those images that are most constructive. Distraction interventions are most effective against acute pain but can also be effective against chronic pain. The ability of distraction interventions to relieve pain is based on the theory that when two separate stimuli are presented, focusing on one will negate the other. However, the more intense the pain is, the more complex the distraction stimuli must be.

Biofeedback is a technique that depends on providing measurements of certain physiologic parameters to patients so that they may learn to control them, including skin temperature, muscle tension, heart rate, blood pressure, and brain waves. The biofeedback device transforms the physiologic parameters into visual signals viewed by the patient. The patient is first alerted to stress-related responses such as increased muscle tension, heart rate, or blood pressure and then taught how to regulate these responses through visual images, deep-breathing, or relaxation exercises. Several sessions are usually required before patients learn to control their responses. Although biofeedback has been used to manage a variety of chronic pain problems, its most common use has been to treat headaches. It is not clear how biofeedback reduces pain. Possible factors that produce the beneficial effects include muscle relaxation, reduced anxiety, distraction, and a feeling of increased control over the symptoms.

Ablative Procedures on Nociceptive Pathways

Neuroablation is the interruption of pain pathways by chemical or thermal techniques or by surgery. Thus ablation permanently blocks nerve pathways to the brain by destroying the nerves that are the source of the chronic pain. The only noncancer pain for which ablation is currently used is trigeminal neuralgia (TN), which may be cured by surgical ablation of the fifth cranial nerve (see further information at the TN web site *http://www.tna-support.org*). The ASA (1996) lists the available types of procedures for persons with chronic cancer pain and recommends that these measures should be limited to four indications: (1) when systemic therapies fail to provide adequate pain control or side effects are intolerable; (2) after failure of neuraxial drug administration; (3) when there is a focal somatic lesion, visceral or neuropathic pain with high likelihood of responsiveness to neuroablation with limited risk; or (4) when patient preference indicates appropriate neuroablation. The procedure may involve interruption at one of three levels: the peripheral nerve root (neurectomy, rhizotomy, sympathectomy), the spinal cord (cordotomy), or the brain (thalamotomy). The ASA (1996) further recommends that, except for the four specific indications, chemical, radiofrequency (thermal), and surgical neuroablation should be deferred until anticipated life expectancy is short, thereby minimizing the potential for deafferentation pain following the procedure.

⫶ MAJOR PAIN PROBLEMS

In 1985 Bristol-Meyers commissioned a large study of the prevalence and severity of pain, using a cross section of

1254 individuals older than 18 years. Findings of that study, entitled *The Nuprin Pain Report*, indicated that pain costs $55 billion and accounted for 4 billion workdays missed, making it a major health and economic problem. Fifteen years later, in October 2000, the 106th Congress of the United States passed HR 3244, which was signed into law. Title VI, Section 1603, provides for the "Decade of Pain Control and Research," which began January 1, 2001. Thus pain became the focus of the second Congressionally declared medical decade (the first was the Decade of the Brain in the 1990s).

Pain care coalitions have been hopeful that the declared "Pain Decade" will bring public attention to the problem of pain, stimulating progress in research, education, and clinical management. An early impetus for the national focus on pain was the new set of standards developed by the Joint Commission on Accreditation of Health Care Organizations (JCAHO) (*http://www.jcaho. org/*; Dahl, Pasero, Patterson, 2000). The pain standards (which were the first evidence-based standards from the JCAHO) were developed collaboratively between the JCAHO Standards Department and the University of Wisconsin (Madison) Medical School, with support from the Robert Wood Johnson Foundation. The standards reflect the intent of the clinical practice guidelines developed by the Agency for Health Care Policy and Research (AHCPR—now the Agency for Healthcare Research and Quality [AHRQ]) (*http://www.ahrq.gov*) and by the Quality Care Committee of the American Pain Society (American Pain Society, 1995). [Because of research and new technology development, the AHRQ declared the AHCPR practice guidelines themselves to be outdated and have made them available on their web site for archive purposes only.]

It is appropriate in this "Pain Decade" to examine more closely one of the most prevalent and costly types of pain in the United States: that of headache. According to the original *Nuprin Pain Report*, headache (73%) was the most common type of pain experienced by the subjects during the year studied (1985). The impact of headache, especially migraine headache, remains staggering. Lipton, Stewart, and Korff (1997) found in 1997 that migraine affects up to 30 million people in the United States and resulted in direct and indirect costs of more than $13 billion per year. In 1999 Lipton and colleagues conducted the *American Migraine Study II*, a study using identical methods to those used in their original *American Migraine Study*, a 1989 population-based survey of 20,000 U.S. households. The updated replication study showed that in the intervening decade, the prevalence and distribution of migraine remained stable. The prevalence of migraine was 18.2% among females and 6.5% among males, with 23% of households containing at least one member suffering from migraine. In addition, the number of migraineurs had increased from 23.6 million in 1989 to 27.9 million in 1999, commensurate with the growth of the population. The authors concluded that migraine is an important target for public health interventions because it is highly prevalent and disabling (Lipton et al, 2001). The authors noted that the ratio of females to males with migraine varies strongly with age: before age 12, migraine is more common in boys than it is in girls; after puberty, it becomes increas-

ingly more common in females, thus at age 20, the female-male ratio is about 2:1 (Lipton et al, 2001). In contrast to migraine headaches, cluster headaches occur with a male predominance of 80% to 90%. In the largest published study, cluster headaches had 1/25th the incidence of migraine headache (Swanson et al, 1994).

The National Center for Health Statistics (NCHS) reported in 1995 that the biggest reason for patient visits to neurologists is headache (23%), with migraines being diagnosed at 10.3% of these visits (NCHS Quarterly Fact Sheet, 1995). Interestingly, the prevalence of the problem may be similar in other societies. Bigal and colleagues (2001) studied migraine prevalence and impact among Brazilian college students. A total of 25% had migraine and experienced a 62.7% decrease in productivity while studying, validating the impact found in the United States on work performance and quality of life.

Low back pain is a remarkably common disability. The annual cost of back pain in the United States is estimated to be between $20 and $50 billion. Each year, 3% to 4% of the population is temporarily disabled, and 1% of the working-age population is totally disabled from low back problem. A common cause of back pain is degenerative intervertebral disk disease. The remainder of this chapter will discuss the two major causes of pain in the population—headache and back pain.

Headache (Cephalalgia)

The 1988 International Headache Society (IHS) Classification divides headaches into two major categories: primary and secondary (*http://www.i-h-s.org*). Primary headaches include migraine, tension-type headache, and cluster headache. Secondary headaches result from other organic disturbances, such as infection, thrombosis, metabolic disorders, tumors, or other systemic illness. After presenting some general considerations concerning headache etiology and evaluation, the remainder of the chapter will discuss the complex and often extremely disabling primary headache, migraine, as an exemplar of severe pain syndromes.

General Considerations

Pain-sensitive cranial structures that are involved in headache include all the extracranial tissues, including skin, scalp, muscles, arteries, and periosteum of the skull; cranial sinuses; intracranial venous sinuses and their tributary veins; parts of the dura at the base of the brain and the arteries within the dura; and the trigeminal, facial, vagus, and glossopharyngeal cranial nerves and the cervical nerves (C2 and C3). The brain parenchyma, much of the meningeal tissue, and the skull (except for the periosteum) are insensitive to pain. Periosteal stretch may cause local pain.

The tentorium is a sheet of dura that serves as a line of demarcation and point of reference within the cranium; it separates the posterior fossa (brainstem and cerebellum) from the anterior cerebrum (see Fig. 50-10). The posterior area (about one third of the cranial cavity) is referred to as *infratentorial*, and the anterior area (two thirds of the cranial cavity) is referred to as *supratentorial*. When head pain involves structures in the infratentorial area, it is referred to the occipital area of the head and neck by the upper cervical nerve roots. Supratentorial pain occurs in the anterior portion of the head (frontal, temporal, and parietal areas) and is mediated largely by the trigeminal nerve.

Some general mechanisms that seem to be responsible for evoking headache include the following (Lance, 2000):

- Distention or displacement of blood vessels: intracranial or extracranial
- Traction of blood vessels
- Contraction of head and neck muscles (muscular overaction)
- Stretching of periosteum (local pain)
- Degeneration of the upper cervical spine with compression of cervical nerve roots (e.g., arthritis of the cervical vertebrae)
- Deficiency of enkephalins (opiate-like brain peptides, active ingredient of endorphins)

The sympathetic nervous system is basically responsible for neural control of the cranial and extracranial blood vessels.

Assessment of the Patient with Headache

As with most conditions, competent history taking is essential to establish the correct diagnosis when the patient's complaint is headache. This concept is particularly true with headache, because positive neurologic findings are only occasionally found on physical examination. Box 52-2 presents some of the points that should be included in the history.

Patients must be rapidly assessed to rule out serious intracranial disease as a cause for the headache. Patients presenting with a "this is the worst headache of my life" scenario accompanied by vomiting, neck stiffness, photophobia, or neurologic deficits are at highest risk for serious neurologic disease. Worsening of the severity of the pain with defecating, coughing, stooping, or other maneuvers that are expected to increase intracranial pressure

(ICP) also deserve special attention (see the synopsis concerning potentially dangerous head pain syndromes by Richmond, 2000).

New-onset headache in older persons should always be taken seriously; it may reflect depression or other emotional events, but because subdural hematoma and intracranial masses are more common in older persons, these more serious causes of the headache must be ruled out.

Details regarding the speed of onset, frequency, duration, and associated symptoms are important to establish. A headache that recurs regularly over years is most likely a tension or vascular headache, whereas a severe headache with a rapid onset would suggest meningitis, intracranial hemorrhage, or infarction.

Headache location can be valuable in determining the cause. Approximately two thirds of migraine headache are unilateral, but they may vary from one side to the other with different attacks. If recurring throbbing headaches are always located on the same side, an intracranial mass or vascular malformation should be considered. Cluster headaches, trigeminal neuralgia, and focal disease of the pain-sensitive structures of the head are exceptions to this rule of thumb. Tension headaches are usually bilateral or circumferential or may be localized, depending on the muscles involved.

The clinician must listen carefully to the patient's description of the pain. A headache described as pulselike or throbbing is generally vascular in origin. Patients with cluster headaches almost always complain of extremely intense, deep, boring pain that lasts 20 to 30 minutes.

Associated symptoms reported by the patient may also help in differentiating the cause of the headache. Although nausea and vomiting frequently accompany migraine headache, they may also be seen in any disease that elevates the ICP. The distinctive ANS findings (flushing of the forehead, injection and lacrimation of the conjunctiva, nasal congestion) are helpful in diagnosing cluster headache.

Patients should be queried about factors that precipitate or aggravate the headache. Headaches that worsen with head movement, coughing, sneezing, or walking are likely to be either vascular or inflammatory. Exposure to certain foods or other triggers (e.g., changes in barometric pressure) may precede the migraine headache.

Two different instruments have been developed that allow the headache sufferer to provide an accurate description of the impact of headache on his or her life. These tools are the *Headache Impact Test (HIT)* (*http://www. headachetest.com*) (Ware et al, 2000) and the *Migraine Disability Assessment (MIDAS)* (*http://www.qolid.org*) (Stewart et al, 2001).

Once the history of the headache is obtained, the clinician should evaluate the patient with a careful and deliberate physical examination, looking for the physical findings of life-threatening conditions sometimes associated with headaches.

Migraine Headache

Migraine headache is an episodic recurrent pain syndrome that is now classified into three types: *migraine without aura* (formerly common migraine), *migraine with aura* (formerly classic migraine), and *migraine variants* (retinal migraine, ophthalmoplegic migraine, familial

---

BOX 52-2

Essential Data to Obtain in Assessing Headache

GENERAL QUESTIONS
- What, if anything, brings on the headache (precipitating factors)?
- When was the onset (number of years, medical conditions, past head injury)?
- Are there any early warnings (prodromal symptoms)?
- Does the headache occur alone or with associated features (nausea, vomiting, dizziness, photophobia, blurred vision)?
- How would you describe the headache (location, frequency, time of day, duration, quality, precipitating factors, relieving factors)?
- Does anyone else in your family have headaches or similar symptoms?

SPECIFIC DIAGNOSTIC QUESTIONS
- How do headaches interfere with your life?
- Has there been any change in your headache pattern over the last 6 months?
- How frequently do you experience headaches of any type?
- How often do you use medication to treat headaches?

hemiplegic migraine, and confusional migraine in children). Migraine headaches are approximately two to three times more common in women than in men, tend to run in families, are thought to be genetically based, and most typically are seen in young, otherwise healthy women. About 75% to 80% of migraine sufferers have a first-degree relative with headache (Russell, Olesen, 1995). Migraines are most common in women younger than 40 years, though they may occur in menopause with erratic hormonal output changes. Indeed, though migraine prevalence diminishes with age, it remains significant beyond the sixth decade of life, remains twice as prevalent in women as it is in men, and may worsen during menopause (Cady, 1999).

Migraine without Aura

Migraine without aura is by far the most common type, accounting for an estimated 80% of all persons with migraine (Headache Classification Committee of the IHS, 1988). Migraine without aura may be initiated at nociceptive neurons on blood vessels. Pain signals travel from the vessels to the primary afferent and then to the trigeminal ganglion, eventually reaching the trigeminal nucleus caudalis, an area of pain processing in the brainstem. Activated neurons within the CNS then express the gene c-fos, which is suppressed by butabarbital (Butalbital, Butisol) within the caudate nucleus (Cutrer et al, 1995).

The IHS defines migraine as at least five lifetime attacks of headache that meet the following criteria (Headache Classification Committee, 1988):
1. Duration of 4 to 72 hours if left untreated
2. Headache pain with at least two of the following four features: unilateral location, throbbing (pulsating) quality, moderate to severe intensity of pain, or pain aggravated by routine physical activity
3. During the headache, at least one of the following two features: (a) nausea or vomiting or both, (b) photophobia and phonophobia

It is important, when using IHS criteria, that the clinician remember that not all migraine attacks need to fulfill all these characteristics; for example many migraines are bilateral or nonthrobbing (Cady, 1999). It is also important to understand that the impact and disability of migraine may be a result of symptoms that in themselves can be disabling and a source of distress in addition to the pain of the migraine attack. Stang and Osterhaus (1995) and Cady (1999) point out that, during an episode of migraine, many physiologic functions are disrupted: (1) impaired sensory processing results in visual and auditory dysfunction (photophobia and phonophobia); (2) disruption of GI motility can lead to nausea and vomiting and inability to take oral antimigraine medication; (3) autonomic disruption can lead to symptoms such as diarrhea; and (4) cerebral impairment can lead to cognitive and mood changes.

Migraine with Aura

Patients who have migraine with a preceding *aura* likely experience the cascade of neurobiologic changes 24 to 48 hours before onset of the headache (Silberstein, 2000). Typically these disruptions of neurologic function begin and end before the onset of headache (Cady, 1999). The spreading quality of the typical focal neurologic symptoms suggests that the aura is similar to the cortical "spreading depression" that occurs when a wave of electrical depolarization proceeds across the cortex and stimulates excitable neurons, leading to disruption of their function and trigeminal activation (Lauritzen, 1994; Bolay et al, 2001). It is known that such spreading depression requires N-methyl-D-aspartate (NMDA) glutamate receptor activity (Silberstein, 2000). Typical aura symptoms include abnormal visual and other sensory changes such as flashing or jagged lights or abnormal taste and smell, as well as motor and speech deficits (aphasias) (Thomsen et al, 2001). Auras may also be somatosensory such as numbness in one hand or one side of the face (Cady, 1999).

The IHS diagnostic criteria for *migraine with aura* specify that at least three of the following four characteristics must be present:
1. One or more fully reversible aura symptoms indicating focal cerebral cortical or brainstem dysfunction or both
2. At least one aura symptom develops gradually over more than 4 minutes
3. No aura symptom lasts more than 60 minutes. (The duration proportionally increases if more than one aura symptom is present.)
4. Headache (as described under *migraine without aura*) follows the aura with a free interval of less than 60 minutes and may begin before or with the aura. The headache usually lasts 4 to 72 hours but may be absent (aura without headache).

Migrainous Nervous System

Studies of auditory- and visual-evoked potential have demonstrated that migraineurs have a nervous system more sensitive to environmental and internal factors than do those without migraine (Wang et al, 1996). Such sensitivity seems to predispose such individuals to other disorders. Common are vertigo, abdominal pain, and motion sickness (American Medical Association, 1998). Other comorbidities include mood disruptions such as depression, anxiety, panic disorder, epilepsy, asthma and peripheral vascular disease (Silberstein, Lipton, Goadsby, 1998). Cady (1999) recommends that persons with migraine be identified as a population at risk for other known disorders (similar to managing the care of persons with hypertension or hyperlipidemia) so that early intervention can reduce their impact.

Migraine and Stroke

There appears to be an increased risk of stroke for patients with migraine, especially women, but the relationship is complex and still controversial (Silberstein, 2000). In the past three decades, several studies have attempted to determine the nature of the stroke risk, but results have been contradictory (Collaborative Group for Study of Stroke in Young Women, 1975; Henrich, Horwitz, 1989; Tzourie et al, 1995; Buring, 1995). Both migraine and stroke are chronic neurologic disorders associated with changes in cerebral blood flow, focal neurologic deficits, and headache; their relationship seems to be bidirectional (i.e., stroke may cause headache, and a prolonged migraine aura may produce a true migrainous infarction).

Pathophysiologic Changes

Though the specific cause of migraine headache remains unknown, understanding of the mechanisms has advanced greatly since the early 1990s. Before "the Decade of the Brain," migraine was defined as a vascular disorder, presumably provoked by a triggering event that caused vasoconstriction, followed by vasodilation, inflammation, and headache (Cady, Farmer-Cady, 2000). Current understanding of migraine events is that the vascular events that do occur during the pain episodes are a secondary phenomenon reflecting neurochemical disturbances in the CNS (Cady, Farmer-Cady, 2000). Changes in neurochemicals (especially dopamine and serotonin) lead to loss of central neural regulation (Couch, 1995). Eventually, the vascular equilibrium of the cranial vessels is disrupted and the vessels dilate, extravasating plasma into the perivascular space. The trigeminal afferent that innervates these vessels reactively releases various neuropeptides, setting up a sterile inflammatory response around the blood vessel wall (Cady, 1999). Therefore research suggests that the initiation of a migraine attack involves a primary CNS dysfunction with subsequent activation of the trigeminovascular system, and the release of the peptides, in particular, the neuropeptide calcitonin gene-related peptide, probably from C fibers (Edvinsson, 2001).

Migraine "Triggers"

Many people with migraine headaches can identify one or more triggers that initiate a pain episode. Common triggers are red wine, chocolate, pungent smells, flickering lights, alcohol, caffeine, nicotine, and foods high in refined sugar. Emotional stress and irregular sleep cycle are also known to be potent migraine triggers in some individuals. Therefore protective factors such as regular sleep and awakening times, regular meals, regular exercise, and biofeedback can be helpful in prophylaxis of migraine episodes (Cady, 1999). "Menstrual migraine" is a well-known phenomenon, and estrogen withdrawal is presumed to be the trigger for the migrainous attacks (Fettes, 1997). Many headache authorities think the term "menstrual migraine" should be restricted to migraines that occur in women that experience 90% of all their attacks between the 2 days before and the last day of their menstrual periods (*http://www.achenet.org/women/menst*). The postulated cause of menstrual migraine is abnormality of neurotransmitter responses in the serotonin and opioid systems to normal cyclic changes in ovarian hormones, as well as changes in the density and sensitivity of receptors in the CNS that respond to opiate drugs (morphine, codeine, among others). In addition, changes in prostaglandin levels occur that result in sensitization of pain receptors and neurogenic inflammation (Fettes, 1997; *http://www.achenet.org/women/menst*). Because menstrual migraine is related to falling estrogen levels, treatment with percutaneous or oral estrogen is often effective in preventing and treating this kind of headache.

Pharmacotherapeutic Management

Generally, these methods are classified as abortive therapies or prophylactic therapies. Prophylactic treatment is indicated if headaches are more frequent than four headaches per month, last longer than 12 hours, or account for a significant amount of total disability per month. Many patients require both prophylactic and abortive treatments (Vaitkus, Vilionskis, 2001).

Acute Treatment

Acute treatment (symptom abortive) medications include over-the-counter (OTC) products such as Excedrin Migraine or aspirin, full doses of NSAIDs and 5-hydroxytryptamine (5-HT-1, serotonin) agonists may stop the headache event, if given early enough. Other first-line medications are vasoconstrictor substances such as ergot alkaloids (ergotamine tartrate) and Cafergot (a combination of caffeine and ergotamine taken at the onset of the headache). The triptan drugs (e.g., sumatriptan, zolmitriptan, naratriptan, and rizatriptan) are selective serotonin 1b/1d agonists. Their mechanism of action is to restore integrity to the dilated cranial vasculature and trigeminal afferent nerves so that vasodilation and ensuing extravasation and inflammation is stopped (Cady, Farmer-Cady, 2000). The advantage of triptan drugs over ergotamine is that antiemetics are usually not required, and they also have a positive effect on the nausea and photophobia that typically accompanies migraine. Cyproheptadine (Periactin), a serotonin and histamine antagonist, is sometimes very helpful in reducing the pain and frequency of headaches. Perhaps because of its sedative and mild analgesic properties, Midrin (a combination drug that includes acetaminophen) is also used. A precaution to its use is that it may cause hypertensive crisis in the presence of monoamine oxidase inhibitors (MAOIs), which are used for depression.

It is known that early pharmacologic intervention produces high efficacy, so that administration of medication at the start of symptoms results in much greater likelihood of aborting the headache. In late headache, phenothiazines given intravenously may be effective; they are sometimes combined with dihydroergotamine or other 5-HT-1 agonists. Narcotic analgesics also may be necessary in late, intractable headache management. Some refractory headaches may be so-called "drug-rebound headaches"—daily headache sustained by the daily intake of analgesic agents or headache remedies (Maizels, 2001).

Prophylactic Treatment

Prophylactic treatment is generally indicated when patients have more than two acute migraine attacks per month or whose daily activities are seriously compromised by headaches (Diamond, 2001). In addition, prophylaxis may be used when comorbidities emerge that can be treated with medications having efficacy for migraine and for the comorbid disorder as well (Cady, 1999).

Many different medications are useful in the prophylaxis of migraine. These drugs include tricyclic antidepressants and serotonin-specific reuptake inhibitors (SSRIs), beta-blockers, calcium channel blockers, and divalproex sodium. The doses for migraine prophylaxis frequently are much lower than the doses used to treat the comorbid disorder such as depression, seizures, or hypertension (*http://www.achenet.org/prevention*). Each of these medications has an efficacy rate of 50%, rather than eliminating headaches altogether (Cady, 1999). Antiepileptic (AEP) medications have also been found to be effective, because migraine and epilepsy share many clinical features and treatments (Silberstein, 2000). The only AEP medication found by the U.S. Headache Consortium (2000) to have documented benefit is valproate/divalproex sodium (Depakote). However, other AEPs used effectively in migraine prophylaxis are gabapentin (Neurontin, *http://www. achenet.org*) and topiramate (Young et al, 2001). There have also been trials using botulinum toxin type-A, which seems to interfere with action potentials that stimulate the temporal branch of the facial nerve (Smuts, Niekerk, Barnard, 2001).

The incidence and prevalence of migraine pain in the United States creates a heavy personal, social, and financial burden, with over 92% of migraineurs reporting at least some headache-related disability (Lipton et al, 2001). The large number of self-help migraine web sites and headache remedy books available for general readership evidences the public's search for effective prophylaxis and therapies. Ongoing research into its pathophysiology, especially the neural and vascular mechanisms, is needed to ease the burden of migraine disability.

Cluster Headache

Cluster headache is a distinctive and treatable neurovascular headache syndrome, although much less common than migraine. A variety of names have been used for this condition, including histamine headache, Horton's headache, migrainous headache, and paroxysmal nocturnal neuralgia. The episodic type is most common and is characterized by one to three short-lived attacks of periorbital pain per day over a 4- to 8-week period (clusters) followed by a pain-free interval that averages 1 year.

Cluster headaches occur much more frequently in men than in women. The characteristic pain is constant, severe, nonthrobbing, and unilateral and is often localized to the eye or side of the face. The onset is characteristically 2 or 3 hours after falling asleep and is apparently associated with rapid eye movement (REM) sleep. The cluster headache lasts from minutes to hours and is associated with conjunctival injection, lacrimation, blocked nostril, and sometimes flushing of the cheek on the affected side. Alcohol is often mentioned as a precipitating factor if drinking occurs during a headache-prone period. Other assorted factors include stress, changes in the climate, and attacks of hay fever. The ophthalmic and extracranial arteries and the facial and scalp capillaries are usually dilated, and the internal carotid artery is narrowed.

At the peak of the headache, the pain is intolerable and incapacitating. In contrast to the person with migraine, the individual with cluster headache paces the floor restlessly and is unable to lie down or sit still. Many persons have even contemplated suicide.

The pathogenesis of cluster headache is unknown. No consistent changes in cerebral blood flow have been shown to accompany the attacks of pain. In one theory, the basic pathophysiology is considered to be the trigeminal vascular system, the final common pathway, with pain initiated in a cyclical fashion by a disordered central pacemaker (May, 1999; Matthew, 1993). In mammals, the anterior hypothalamus contains cells that constitute the principle circadian pacemaker, and the posterior hypothalamus contains cells that control autonomic functions. Both would have to be activated to account for the symptoms (autonomic and periodic) of cluster headache. The pacemaker is modulated by serotonergic dorsal raphe projections. Thus both migraine and cluster headache may result from abnormal serotonergic neurotransmission, albeit at different locations.

Drugs useful in the prevention of cluster headache attacks include the vasoconstricting agent ergotamine tartrate, the serotonin antagonist methysergide, lithium, verapamil, and prednisone. When ergotamine is used, it should be given 1 to 2 hours before an expected attack. Inhalation of 100% oxygen for 15 minutes during an attack is effective for some patients, probably resulting from a reduction in cerebral blood flow. Sumatriptan (6 mg subcutaneously) will often shorten an attack.

Muscular Contraction Headache (Tension Headache)

Muscular contraction, or tension, headache produces pain by a sustained contraction of the scalp, forehead, and neck muscles that is accompanied by extracranial vasoconstriction. The pain is characterized by a bandlike tightness around the head and tenderness of the occipitocervical area. This type of headache is very common. The acute form is associated with conditions of temporary stress, anxiety, or fatigue generally lasting 1 or 2 days. The chronic tension headache is more common in women than it is in men and is typically bilateral, unremitting (occurring during both day and night and lasting from months to years), dull, nonpulsating, and often associated with anxiety, depression, and repressed feelings.

Ideally, nonaddictive drugs should be prescribed for the person with chronic tension headache. Aspirin and acetaminophen are practical choices. Narcotic analgesics may be abused and may lead to tolerance (renal failure occurs in some persons who abuse phenacetin; see Chapter 46). Tranquilizers are probably not beneficial and may actually increase the depression. In patients who are tense and anxious, diazepam (Valium), 5 mg three times a day for 1 month, may be effective. If the patient is also depressed, the tricyclic antidepressant drug amitriptyline (Elavil), 25 mg three times a day, is added. In some headache treatment centers, tricyclic antidepressants are being used alone and are effective in increasing cerebral norepinephrine. Biofeedback, relaxation, self-hypnosis, and other conditioning techniques have been beneficial to some patients with headache and play an increasing role in therapy, because a real danger of overmedication exists in the patient with muscular tension headache.

Traction Inflammatory Headache

Traction inflammatory headache is usually secondary to organic disease. Masses of any origin (e.g., tumor, blood clot, abscess) may cause traction on and displacement of pain-sensitive structures. Headache is the outstanding symptom of a brain tumor (primary or metastatic), and as the tumor grows, the pain becomes more frequent and severe. By the time most patients with intracranial tumors present with headache, they have other significant diagnostic findings that suggest a tumor. Headache, vertigo, and other localizing neurologic signs are the usual manifestations of chronic subdural hematoma. A rapidly expanding intracranial mass causing increased ICP may displace cerebral structures, resulting in headache.

Headache is a symptom associated with many inflammatory processes. Meningitis, encephalitis, and infection of the sinuses, teeth, nose, or eyes frequently occur with the symptom of headache. Traction on the attached parts of the brain, especially the trigeminal and hypoglossal nerves, is likely to cause headache. Headache is also a symptom in particular immunologic disorders, especially periarteritis nodosa and giant cell arteritis.

Postlumbar Puncture Headache

Headache after lumbar puncture (LP) occurs in one of four patients, usually within hours of the procedure. The headache is dramatically positional: it begins when the patient sits or stands upright and is diminished or eliminated by lying down. Head shaking worsens the headache. The pain is usually in the frontal area and has the quality of a dull ache but may be throbbing. The symptoms usually resolve over a few days but may persist for weeks.

Although the exact mechanism of spinal headache is unknown, it is postulated that leakage of CSF through a tear in the dura caused by the LP results in a loss of the brain's supportive cushion. Thus, when the patient sits upright, there is dilation and tension on the brain's anchoring structures, the pain-sensitive dural sinuses, resulting in pain. Factors associated with spinal headache include use of a large-bore needle, withdrawal of a large volume of CSF, and repeat LPs. A small number of patients have a sterile meningitis.

To reduce the risk of spinal headache, the patient should remain flat in bed for at least 3 hours after an LP. Once a headache begins, treatment consists of bedrest in a quiet, dark room and analgesics of increasing strength. An epidural blood patch, accomplished by injecting about 15 ml of the patient's own blood into the epidural space at the site of the LP, is usually an effective treatment for those who are not helped by analgesics. The blood acts as a fibrin patch to seal the hole in the dura and prevent further leakage of CSF. In some persistent cases, a short course (10 days) of steroid therapy may be helpful.

Back Pain

Back pain, especially of the lower back, is a very common problem in the adult population. The numerous causes of back pain include arthritis of the spine, herniated intervertebral disk disease, and various soft tissue problems resulting from sprains, strains, and other trauma. Physiologic origins of low back pain are usually mechanical or biochemical irritations to nociceptive endings or to nerves and nerve roots in the lumbar spine. It is essential to rule out acute disk problems in any patient with a complaint of back pain, because failure to do so may result in permanent neurologic deficits.

Herniated Intervertebral Disk Disease

One of the most common causes of back pain in the adult is *herniated nucleus pulposus* (herniated disk). Although more common in adults, disk disease can also occur in children and adolescents.

The vertebral column consists of a series of joints between the bodies of the adjacent vertebrae, the joints of the vertebral arches, the costovertebral joints, and the sacroiliac joints. Longitudinal ligaments and the intervertebral disks join the bodies of adjacent vertebrae. The *anterior longitudinal ligament*, a broad, thick band, runs longitudinally on the front of the vertebral bodies and intervertebral disks and fuses with the periosteum and annulus fibrosus. Lying within the vertebral canal on the posterior aspects of the vertebral bodies and intervertebral disks is the *posterior longitudinal ligament*.

Between the vertebral bodies, from the second cervical vertebra (C2) down to the sacral vertebrae, are the *intervertebral disks*. These disks form a resilient fibrocartilaginous joint between the vertebral bodies. The intervertebral disk consists of two basic parts: the nucleus pulposus at the center and the annulus fibrosus surrounding it. The disk is separated from the bone above and below by two thin hyaline cartilage plates (Fig. 52-11).

The *nucleus pulposus* is the semigelatinous central portion of the disk; it contains bundles of collagenous fibers,

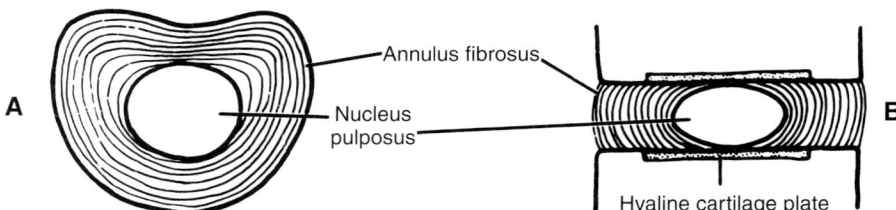

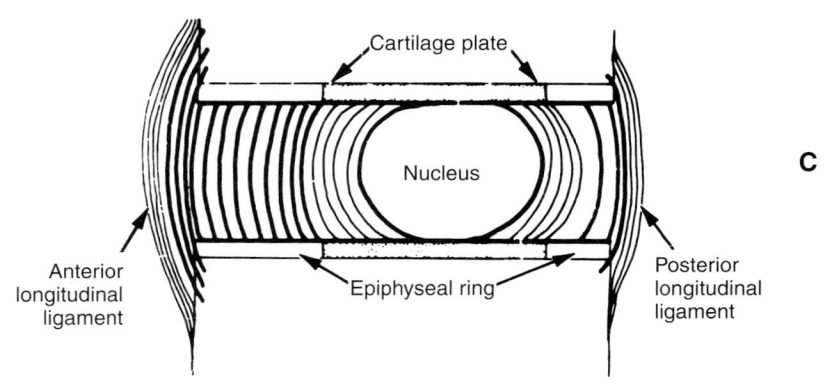

FIG. 52-11 A, Annulus fibrosus is composed of concentric fibrous rings that surround the nucleus pulposus. **B,** Nucleus pulposus abuts on the hyaline cartilage plate. **C,** Annulus fibers form three groups, with innermost fibers passing from one cartilage plate to the next, middle fibers passing between the epiphyseal rings of the vertebral bodies, and outermost fibers attaching between the vertebral bodies and the undersurface of the epiphyseal ring. Anterior fibers are more numerous and are supported by the powerful anterior longitudinal ligament, whereas the posterior longitudinal ligament gives only weak reinforcement to the less numerous posterior fibers. (From McCulloch JA, Transfeldt EE: *McNab's backache,* ed 3, Baltimore, 1997, Williams & Wilkins.)

connective tissue cells, and cartilage cells. This material functions as a shock absorber between adjacent vertebral bodies, and it also plays an important role in the exchange of fluid between the disk and the capillaries.

The *annulus fibrosus* consists of concentric fibrous rings, which surround the nucleus pulposus. The functions of the annulus fibrosus are to permit motion between the vertebral bodies (because of the spiral structure of the fibers), to retain the nucleus pulposus, and to function as a shock absorber. Thus the annulus functions similar to the hoops around a water barrel or as a coiled spring, pulling the vertebral bodies together against the elastic resistance of the nucleus pulposus, whereas the nucleus pulposus acts as a ball bearing between the vertebral bodies (Fig. 52-12).

Intervertebral disks account for approximately one fourth of the length of the vertebral column. The thinnest disks are in the thoracic region, and the thickest ones are in the lumbar region. With increasing age, the water content of the disks is reduced, and they become thinner (Schwartz, 1998).

Pathophysiology

The lumbar region is the most common area for herniation of the nucleus pulposus. The water content of the disk decreases with increasing age (from 90% in infancy to 70% in old age; Schwartz, 1998). In addition, the fibers become coarsened and hyalinized, which contributes to the changes that lead to herniation of the nucleus pulposus through the annulus with compression of the spinal nerve roots (Fig. 52-13). As a general rule, herniation is most likely to occur in regions of the vertebral column where a transition occurs from a more mobile segment to a less mobile one (lumbosacral and cervicothoracic junctions).

The vast majority of disk herniations occur in the lumbar area at the fourth to fifth lumbar (L4 to L5) or fifth lumbar to first sacral (L5 to S1) interspace. The most common direction of herniation of the nuclear material is posterolateral. Because the nerve roots at the lumbar area slant downward as they exit through the neural foramina, a disk herniation between L5 and S1 affects the S1 nerve root rather than L5 as might be expected. A herniation of the disk between L4 and L5 compresses the L5 nerve root (Fig. 52-14).

Cervical disk herniations, although less common compared with lumbar disk herniations, usually involve one of the three lower cervical roots. A cervical disk herniation is potentially serious, and spinal cord compression

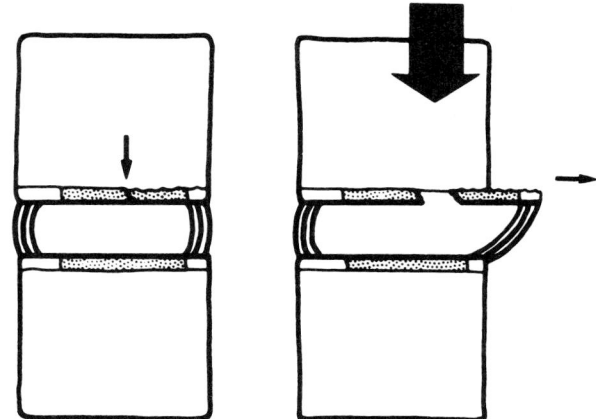

FIG. 52-13 The first morphologic change to occur in a disk rupture is a separation of the cartilage plate from the adjacent vertebral body. When a vertical compression force is then applied, the detached portion of the cartilage plate is displaced posteriorly, and the nucleus pulposus exudes through the torn fibers of the annulus. (From McCulloch JA, Transfeldt EE: *McNab's backache,* ed 3, Baltimore, 1997, Williams & Wilkins.)

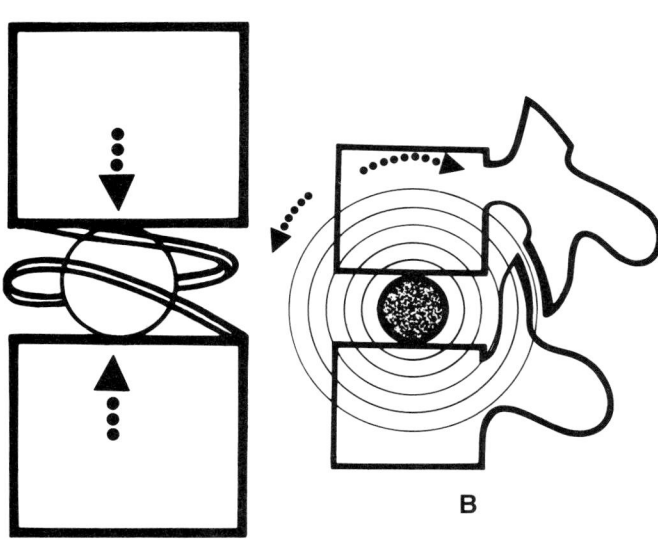

FIG. 52-12 **A,** Annulus acts as a coiled spring, pulling the vertebral bodies together against the elastic resistance of the nucleus pulposus. **B,** Nucleus pulposus acts as a ball bearing, with the vertebral bodies rolling over the incompressible gel in flexion and extension while the posterior vertebral joints guide and steady the movement. (From McCulloch JA, Transfeldt EE: *McNab's backache,* ed 3, Baltimore, 1997, Williams & Wilkins.)

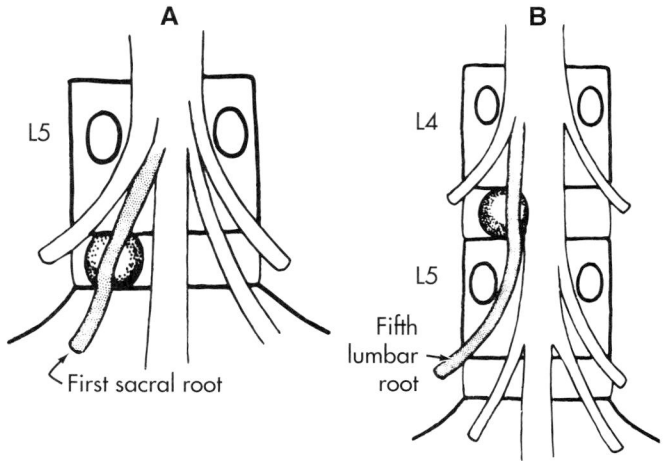

FIG. 52-14 **A,** Posterolateral herniation of the L5 to S1 disk generally compresses the S1 nerve root. **B,** Herniation of the L4 to L5 disk compresses the L5 root. (From MacNab I: *Backache,* Baltimore, 1977, Williams & Wilkins.)

is possible, depending on the direction of protrusion. A lateral herniation of a cervical disk generally compresses the root below the disk level. Thus a C5 to C6 disk compresses the C6 nerve root, and a C6 to C7 disk involves the C7 root (Schwartz, 1998).

The patient generally gives a history of transient episodes of pain and gradual loss of spinal mobility. Although the patient tends to associate the problem with a particular incident of lifting or bending, herniation is a gradual process marked by periods of nerve root compression (causing many symptoms and periods of anatomic readjustment).

Signs, Symptoms, and Diagnosis

Clinical symptoms depend on the location of the herniation and variation in the individual anatomy. Table 52-4 provides a summary of the most common signs and symptoms.

The diagnosis of herniated intervertebral disk is often made from the history alone and can be confirmed during physical examination. Evaluating maneuvers such as leg raising and walking on the toes or heels is also helpful in making the diagnosis. Radiographs may be normal or may show evidence of distorted spinal alignment (generally caused by muscle spasm); they are also helpful to rule out other causes of back pain, such as spondylolisthesis (forward slippage of the anterior portion of a vertebral segment over a lower segment, usually at L4 or L5), spinal cord tumors, or bony spurs. However, it is impossible to diagnose a herniated disk by radiography alone. Magnetic resonance imaging (MRI) or computed tomography (CT) myelogram is necessary to establish the location and type of pathology. A spine MRI or CT will show spinal canal compression by the herniated disk and a CT-myelogram defines the size and location of the disk herniation. An electromyogram (EMG) may be performed to determine the exact nerve root involved. A nerve conduction velocity test may also be performed.

Treatment

The mainstay of treatment for herniated disks is an initial short period of bedrest on a firm mattress and NSAIDs for pain followed by physical therapy. Under this regimen, over 90% of people will recover and return to normal activities. A small percentage of people may need further treatment, which may include surgery.

For people with an acute lumbar herniated disk as a result of some sort of trauma (e.g., lifting a heavy object) followed by severe pain in the back and leg, narcotic analgesics and NSAIDs will be prescribed. If there is also an element of back muscle spasm, muscle relaxants are usually given. Prolonged bedrest is not recommended because it has deleterious effects both physically and psychologically. Research shows no benefit of bedrest more than 2 days for patients with acute low back pain, nor does traction show a benefit (Malmivaara, 1995; Bigos, 1999). For people unable to do physical therapy because of pain, corticosteroid injections into the area of the herniation can be very helpful in controlling the pain for several months. For patients with cervical herniations, a soft cervical collar helps relieve the pain and muscle spasms by limiting neck motions. A rigid neck collar may occasionally be necessary to eliminate weight bearing on the cervical spine in persons with severe muscle spasms and pain.

Once low back pain has subsided, the patient begins a program of graded exercise to strengthen the back and abdominal muscles. It is important that patients limit lifting and use the proper body mechanics. Proper techniques involve keeping the spine straight, bending the knees, and keeping the weight close to the body to use the powerful leg muscles and avoid using the back muscles.

TABLE 52-4

Signs and Symptoms of Herniated Disk Disease

Location of Herniation	Nerve Root Involved	Pain	Weakness	Paresthesias	Atrophy	Reflexes
L4 to L5	L5	Over sacroiliac joint, hip, lateral aspect of thigh and calf, medial aspect of foot (pain that radiates down hip and leg is called *sciatica*)	May produce footdrop, difficulty in dorsiflexion of foot and/or great toe; difficulty walking on heels	Lateral leg, distal portion of foot, between great and second toes (see dermatome map, Fig. 52-8)	Unremarkable	Usually unremarkable; knee or ankle reflexes may be diminished.
L5 to S1	S1	Over sacroiliac joint, posterior portion of entire leg to heel, lateral aspect of foot	May produce weakness of plantar flexion, abduction of toes and hamstring muscles; difficulty walking on toes	Midcalf and lateral aspect of foot, including fourth and fifth toes (see dermatome map, Fig. 52-8)	Gastrocnemius	Ankle reflex may be absent or diminished.
C5 to C6	C6	Neck pain radiating to shoulder, arm, and forearm	Biceps	Radial aspect of forearm, thumb, and index finger	Unremarkable	Biceps reflex is diminished or absent.

L, Lumbar; *S*, sacral; *C*, cervical.

Surgery is generally reserved for patients who experience persistent intractable pain or frequent attacks of pain despite conservative therapy or have signs of a major neurologic deficit, such as progressive motor weakness from nerve root injury or bowel or bladder incontinence. The usual procedure is a partial hemilaminectomy with excision of the involved and prolapsed intervertebral disk. A spinal fusion may be performed if an unstable bony mechanism is present. Other surgical procedures include microsurgical diskectomy (removing fragments of nucleated disk through a very small incision) and chemonucleolysis. The latter procedure involves injecting chymopapain (an enzyme from the papaya tree) into the herniated disk. The chymopapain causes hydrolysis of the proteins, decreasing their water-binding capacity in the nucleus pulposus. The enzyme only attacks the nucleus pulposus and not the annulus fibrosis. This treatment relieves the pressure on the nerve root, effectively relieving pain, and provides patients with an alternative to laminectomy. Ongoing research to develop a biocompatible replacement of the nucleus pulposus offers promise for improved treatment of degenerative intervertebral disk disease. Two groups of researchers working to achieve this goal are at the University of Pennsylvania and in Europe (see *http://www.uphs.upenn.edu/ortho/link/* and *http://www.materials.drexel.edu/LBTE%20website/JT.htm*).

KEY CONCEPTS

- *Pain* is a dynamic process in which the physiologic relationship between the pain stimulus and the sensory output of pain response may be modified over time. This feature of the nervous system is called "plasticity."
- In the *neurophysiology of pain*, there are four distinct processes that occur between a noxious stimulus causing tissue injury and the subjective experience of pain: (1) pain transduction, (2) pain transmission, (3) pain modulation, and (4) pain perception.
- *Nociceptors* are primary afferent nerves for receiving and transmitting painful stimuli to the CNS.
- *Nociceptor activity* is transmitted to the spinal cord by *two types of neurons*: (1) *A-delta (A-δ)* small myelinated fibers transmit sharp, well-localized sensations (*fast pain*) felt within 0.1 second and (2) small unmyelinated *C fibers* transmit burning, aching, throbbing, poorly localized sensations felt after 1 second (*slow pain*). Because of this double innervation, tissue injury (e.g., cut on finger) gives rise to two distinct pain sensations—an early sharp pain followed by a dull, burning, and somewhat prolonged pain.
- Most *ascending pain pathways* (A-δ and C pain fibers) enter the dorsal (posterior) horn of the spinal cord, synapse with interneurons, cross over, and ascend in the opposite side of the cord. Thus unilateral loss of cord function results in decrease of pain sensation on the opposite side of the body below the lesion. Lack of crossover of some fibers at the spinal cord level may explain why pain can return after nerve resection.
- The *anterolateral spinothalamic tract* has two ascending pain pathways: (1) the *neospinothalamic tract* carries A-δ pain impulses and projects in a direct route to the thalamus and to the sensory cortex resulting in well-localized sharp pain perception, and (2) the *paleospinothalamic tract* transmits C pain impulses and follows a diffuse multisynaptic path, resulting in a poorly localized, burning, aching pain sensation (also conveys visceral pain).
- *Pain threshold* is the point at which a stimulus is perceived as painful; this is relatively predictable from individual to individual. *Pain tolerance* is the point at which the individual seeks relief from the pain; this is a very individualized phenomenon.
- Acute physiologic response to pain mimics activation of the sympathetic nervous system with increased blood pressure, respiratory rate, diaphoresis, and dilated pupils.
- The *gate control theory of pain* response stipulates that inputs from pain fibers (A-δ and C pain fibers) can be inhibited by simultaneous activation of large sensory fibers (A-α and A-β) synapsing at the same level of the spinal cord.
- The strength of a pain signal can be modified by emotional and behavioral information descending from the cerebral cortex and by other peripheral sensations.
- Chronic pain alters the strength of the response in the postsynaptic neuron, as well as the anatomic configuration of the pathway itself.
- The three major categories of pain according to origin in the nerve-conduction pathway are nociceptive, neuropathic, and psychogenic.
- *Superficial somatic (cutaneous) pain* arises from noxious stimuli to well-innervated superficial well-body structures such as the skin and subcutaneous tissues and is well-localized, tingling, cutting, burning, or sharp.
- *Deep somatic pain* arises from poorly-innervated deep structures such as blood vessels, skeletal muscles, bones and joints; it is dull, poorly localized, and often radiates to adjacent structures or produces autonomic nervous system responses including nausea, sweating, increased heart rate, and reflex contraction of nearby skeletal muscles.
- *Visceral pain* arises from the sparsely-innervated *smooth muscle walls of hollow organs* or the *capsule of solid organs* sensitive to stretching, inflammation, and ischemia; it results in pain that is diffuse, poorly localized, and often referred, as well as producing autonomic nervous system responses. The parenchyma of many organs lack pain receptors (e.g., lung, brain) thus surgical incision does not cause pain.
- The phenomenon of *referred pain* from a visceral organ to a dermatome (body surface area) can be explained

by the *convergence-projection theory*: pain impulses from the viscera travel to the CNS by a dual pathway—the *parietal (somatic) pathway* and the *true visceral pathway*; then the visceral pain is referred to the surface of the body where it is localized to the dermatomal segment from which the visceral organ originated in the embryo (e.g., the pain of early appendicitis is referred to the T10 periumbilical dermatome; however, late appendicitis caused by inflammation of the peritoneum travels via parietal [somatic] pathway alone and is localized to the right lower quadrant).

- *Neuropathic (deafferentation) pain* is caused by injury or damage to nerve fibers in the PNS or in the CNS, resulting in interruption of the ability of the nerve fibers to conduct sensory information (e.g., postherpetic neuralgia; diabetic neuropathy, tic douloureux).
- Neurotransmitters (neuromodulators) in the pain pathway can be pronociceptive (induce or increase pain or both) or antinociceptive (inhibit or decrease pain or both).
- In the postsynaptic nerve cell, a cascade of chemical events occurs that facilitates transmission of the pain and also activates certain genes. This gene activation can alter the very structure of the nerve cell involved.
- *Descending pain modulating pathways* projecting from the PAG and PVG to the *substantia gelatinosa* in the dorsal horn can inhibit pain signals at the level of the spinal cord.
- Neural information can be modified by targeting three points in the *pain signal pathway*: the peripheral extent and duration of response to the stimulus, the chemical reactions within the neurons along the pain conduction pathway, and the action of neurotransmitters that convey signals between neurons.
- In current pain control, an attempt is made to *select a pharmacologic agent based on type of pain experienced*. Examples are anticonvulsants (e.g., Neurontin) or antidepressants (e.g., amitriptyline) for neuropathic pain and antiinflammatory agents (e.g., NSAIDs) for pain associated with inflammation.
- *NSAIDS* modulate pain by inhibiting prostaglandins peripherally, thus altering nociceptor activity.
- *Acetaminophen* modulates pain by inhibiting cyclooxygenase (COX) in the brain.
- Spinal cord pain transmission can be altered by *cutaneous stimulation* (gate control theory). TENS (or rubbing a sore spot immediately after an injury) stimulates large A-α (nonnociceptor) fibers, thus closing the gate in the substantia gelatinosa to pain transmission by small nociceptors (A-δ and C fibers).
- *Opioids* (endogenous and exogenous) modulate pain by combining with opioid receptor sites distributed throughout the CNS.

- *Tricyclic antidepressants* produce analgesia by enhancing the inhibitory action of serotonin on the spinal transmission neurons.
- Epidural administration of clonidine, an *alpha-adrenergic blocking agent*, achieves an analgesic effect by blocking sympathetically mediated pain transmission.
- In chronic pain, gene therapy may eventually be used to introduce antinociceptive receptors in nerve cells, decreasing their sensitivity to pain signals.
- *Anticonvulsants* are especially helpful in decreasing neuropathic pain because they suppress ectopic sites of impulse generation in damaged peripheral nerves.
- *Pain-sensitive cranial structures* include all extracranial structures (skin, scalp, muscles, arteries, and periosteum of skull), cranial sinuses, intracranial venous sinuses, dura and arteries within at base of brain, cranial nerves V, VII, IX, X, and cervical nerves C2 and C3.
- There are two types of *migraine headache*: migraine with aura (formerly *classical* migraine) and migraine without aura (formerly *common* migraine).
- Auras occur in approximately 15% of *migraine headaches*; they are caused by a wave of electrical depolarization across the cortex, resulting in disruption of neuronal function.
- A *tension headache* is caused by sustained contraction of the scalp, forehead, and neck muscles that is accompanied by extracranial vasoconstriction.
- *Traction inflammatory headache* is secondary to organic disease, such as intracranial mass (e.g., brain tumor) or inflammatory conditions, such as meningitis, encephalitis, and sinus infection.
- To reduce the risk of *postlumbar puncture headache*, the patient should lie flat in bed for at least 3 hours after the procedure.
- *Intervertebral disks* are fibrocartilaginous disk-shaped structures between adjacent vertebral bodies that act as shock absorbers and greatly increase spinal mobility. The *nucleus pulposus* forms the semigelatinous center of the disk and acts as a ball bearing between the vertebral bodies; the nucleus pulposus is surrounded and supported by the *annulus fibrosis* similar to the hoops around a wooden water barrel.
- *Herniated disk disease* is a disorder involving rupture of annulus pulposus (disk's outer ring), allowing the nucleus pulposus to protrude (herniate) and press against spinal nerve roots, causing pain and possible neurologic deficit.
- The *majority of herniated disks* occur between L4 and L5, compressing the L5 nerve root or between L5 and S1, compressing the S1 nerve root.

 UESTIONS ??

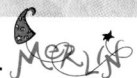

A sampling of review questions for this chapter appears here. Visit http://www.mosby.com/MERLIN/PriceWilson/ for additional questions.

Match each pain characteristic in column A with the type of pain (acute or chronic) in column B.

Column A
1. _____ Duration: 6 months or more
2. _____ Cause: may not be well defined
3. _____ Onset: abrupt
4. _____ Benefit: warns of danger
5. _____ Autonomic response: sympathetic stress response
6. _____ Emotional response: depression
7. _____ Response to analgesics: often unresponsive

Column B
a. Acute pain
b. Chronic pain

Distinguish between narcotic physical dependence, tolerance, and addiction by placing the correct letters from column B in column A.

Column A
8. _____ Higher doses required to achieve pain relief
9. _____ A common fear of patients and some health care professionals
10. _____ Drug needed for normal function
11. _____ Abrupt discontinuation of the drug causes withdrawal symptoms
12. _____ Psychologic dependence on the drug

Column B
a. Physical dependence
b. Tolerance
c. Addiction

Match the following modalities for coping with pain in column A with the most appropriate description in column B.

Column A
13. _____ Biofeedback
14. _____ Guided imagery
15. _____ Music therapy
16. _____ Cold applications
17. _____ Progressive muscle relaxation

Column B
a. A form of distraction
b. Depends on monitoring physiologic responses
c. Works best for acute pain such as a burn
d. Reduces muscle tension and stress

Answer the following on a separate sheet of paper.

18. List nine categories of subjective data relevant to pain assessment.
19. List reactive and behavioral data relevant to pain assessment.

20. What is the physiologic function of the pain sensory system? What would be the advantages and disadvantages of having a congenital insensitivity to pain?

21. List several questions you would ask a patient during history taking who complains of chronic headache.

Fill in the blanks with the appropriate word or words.

22. Headache involving supratentorial structures is referred to the _____ two thirds of the head, and the pain pathway involves the _____ nerve.
23. Headache involving infratentorial structures is referred to the _____ area and is conveyed by the _____ nerves.

Match the headache characteristics in column B with the three categories of headache in column A. Letters may be used more than once.

Column A
24. _____ Classic migraine headache
25. _____ Cluster headache
26. _____ Tension headache

Column B
a. Flushed skin
b. Preceding aura
c. Generally unilateral
d. Generally bilateral
e. Throbbing quality
f. Dull ache, constant day and night
g. Precipitated by stress, fatigue
h. Precipitated by alcohol
i. Genetic predisposition
j. Photophobia or phonophobia or both
k. Mechanism involves sustained contraction of head and neck muscles

CHAPTER

53

Cerebrovascular Disease

MARY S. HARTWIG

Diseases of the cerebrovascular system were known in the ancient world, as recorded in the Old Testament (2nd Kings, 4:18-20). This Biblical story tells of a grown boy who, while visiting his father in the field, suddenly cried, "My head, my head." He was carried to his mother and died while sitting in her lap. Neurosurgeons have cited this scene, which begins the account of a miracle by the prophet Elisha, as possibly the first written description of a subarachnoid hemorrhage. Certainly to this day, the unexpected, acute, and devastating nature of the boy's malady remains typical of that particular subset of cerebrovascular disorders, all of which are grouped under the time-worn but graphic clinical term, *stroke*.

EPIDEMIOLOGY OF STROKE

Incidence

Stroke is the third most common cause of mortality in adults in the United States. Annual mortality from new and recurrent strokes is over 200,000. The national incidence of first stroke has been estimated at 750,000 per year, with 200,000 of these representing recurrent strokes. Rates among African Americans are 60% higher than those among Caucasians (Broderick et al, 2001). This higher incidence may be related to the known increased incidence of hypertension among African Americans. Though persons may have a stroke at any age, two thirds of strokes occur in persons over the age of 65. On a worldwide basis, the statistics are even more stark: coronary heart disease and stroke are the first and second leading causes of death and rank fifth and sixth as causes of disability (Murray, Lopez, 1999). Evaluation of the

World Health Organization's (WHO) mortality data base suggests that the main factors associated with the cardiovascular disease "epidemic" are global changes in nutrition and smoking, plus urbanization and aging of populations (WHO, 1997).

In the United States women account for more than one half of all stroke deaths, more than twice the number of women dying from breast cancer (National Rural Health Association, 2001). Women also account for about 43% of strokes per year but suffer 62% of the stroke deaths. The National Stroke Association suggests the explanation is that stroke risk increases with age and that women live longer than do men. Additional risk factors also take their toll: women above the age of 30 who smoke and take oral contraceptives with higher estrogen content have a stroke risk 22 times higher than average (*http://www.stroke.org*). Because disabilities following stroke can be so devastating, and because women are more likely than are men to have the more serious disabilities following stroke, the National Stroke Association has made education about risk factors and emergency care a priority, especially for women.

Morbidity

Stroke is a major cause of disability in adults. Four million Americans have a neurologic deficit resulting from stroke; two thirds of these deficits are moderate to severe (National Stroke Association, 2001). The chance of dying from an initial stroke is 30% to 35%, and the chance of major disability for survivors is 35% to 40% (Wolf et al, 2000). About one third of all stroke survivors will have another stroke within 5 years; 5% to 14% of these will have a repeat stroke within the first year.

Until 2001, reports of stroke incidence have included only symptomatic strokes, even though "silent" strokes have been estimated to be 5 to 20 times more common, according to researchers at the University of California at Los Angeles (Leary, Saver, 2001). Modeling from large population-based studies of the prevalence of silent stroke, the researchers estimated the annual incidence to be more than 11 million persons.

Cost

In the United States the annual cost of stroke is about $30 billion. That figure includes $17 billion in direct costs of the stroke itself (hospitals, physicians, and rehabilitation) and indirect costs of $13 billion for consequences such as decreased or lost work productivity.

Geographic Distribution

There is a so-called "stroke belt" in the United States in which each area has a stroke incidence and death rate more than 10% higher than that of the remainder of the country. This belt comprises the District of Columbia and 12 contiguous states: Virginia, North Carolina, South Carolina, Georgia, Florida, Alabama, Mississippi, Louisiana, Arkansas, Tennessee, Kentucky, and Indiana. The National Stroke Association (*http://www.stroke.org*) suggests that the cause of the higher incidence and mortality rate is multifactorial, including an above-

average population of African Americans, higher percentage of older adults, and diet.

Risk Factors

The same factors that are well-known risks for atherosclerotic heart disease are also risk factors for stroke (see Box 31-2). Demographic risk factors include older age, race and ethnicity (African Americans have higher rates than do Caucasians), and family history of stroke. Modifiable risk factors include atrial fibrillation, diabetes mellitus, hypertension, sleep apnea (Qureshi et al, 1997), heavy alcohol use, and smoking. It is an important understanding in the field of public health that the major risk factor for stroke is chronic hypertension (known better by the lay term "high blood pressure"). Therefore because in most cases hypertension is treatable, and because sustained reduction of hypertension to physiologically "normal" levels prevents stroke, diagnosis and aggressive treatment of hypertension is a major focus of cerebrovascular medicine (see Chapter 31).

Obesity, which is rapidly becoming a major health problem in the United States, has only recently been demonstrated to be an independent risk factor for stroke. Using body mass index (BMI) as the independent variable, researchers found that subjects enrolled in the U.S. Physicians' Health Study with a BMI of greater than 27.8 kg/m^2 had a significantly higher risk for both ischemic and hemorrhagic strokes (Kurth et al, 2001). Thus obesity seems to be an important risk factor for stroke, not only through weight-exacerbated conditions such as hypertension, diabetes, and elevated cholesterol but also through other mechanisms as yet not identified.

Interestingly, dyslipidemia has not been shown to be associated with an increased risk of stroke, unless the individual also has coronary artery disease (CAD). For persons with CAD, there is a clear relationship between elevated lipids and the prospective risk of stroke and transient ischemic attack (TIA) for each of the following: total cholesterol, low-density lipoprotein (LDL) cholesterol, and triglycerides. With high-density lipoprotein (HDL), there is an inverse relationship (Tanne, Koren, 2001). Despite the overall lack of correlation between stroke and high lipid levels, two studies have demonstrated that administration of a lipid-lowering statin medication to persons with known CAD reduces their risk of stroke (Sacks et al, 1996; LIPID, 1998). Elevated homocysteine levels are also receiving scrutiny, because they have been found to be a risk factor for progression of aortic atherosclerotic plaques in patients with stroke and TIA (Sen, Oppenheimer, 2001).

CEREBRAL BLOOD SUPPLY

The cerebrovascular system supplies the brain with a rich flow containing the nutrients critical for normal brain function. Interruption in *cerebral blood flow (CBF)* for just a few seconds produces symptoms of cerebral dysfunction. If prolonged for several seconds, CBF deficiency results in unconsciousness and finally in cerebral ischemia. Irreversible damage to the brain will begin after 4 to 6 minutes when there is complete lack of oxygen supply

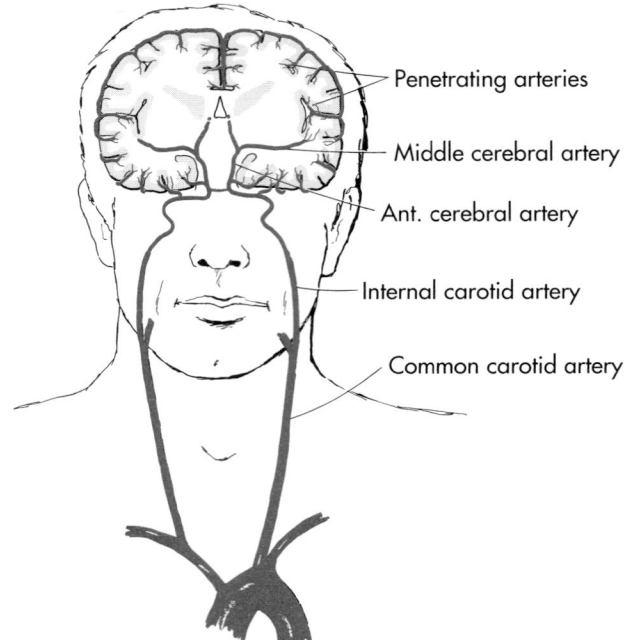

FIG. 53-1 Course of the internal carotid artery from the carotid bifurcation to its continuation as the middle cerebral artery. The penetrating lenticulostriate arteries arise from the first portion of the middle cerebral artery to supply the basal ganglia and internal capsule. These arteries are frequently implicated in a stroke syndrome. The middle cerebral artery continues to course over the cerebral hemisphere, sending short and deep penetrating arteries into the brain. The subarachnoid arterial anastomoses, which supply collateral circulation, are shown between the middle and anterior cerebral arteries.

(usually a result of cardiopulmonary arrest). Normal CBF is about 50 ml/100 grams of brain tissue/minute. In a resting state, the brain receives one sixth of the cardiac output; in terms of oxygen extraction, it uses 20% of the body's oxygen. When a cerebral vessel is occluded, the collateral circulation helps maintain some CBF to the ischemic area. The adjacent parts of the brain in which small amounts of CBF are maintained by collateral flow are called "ischemic penumbra." Study of these areas has intensified in recent years, as researchers have searched for ways to restore CBF to the ischemic penumbra and therefore reduce the amount of permanent damage.

Four large arteries supply the brain with blood: *two internal carotid arteries* and *two vertebral arteries* (which join the basilar artery to form the *vertebrobasilar system*). As described in Chapter 50, the arterial blood to the brain originates from the aortic arch. On the left side, the common carotid and subclavian arteries arise directly from the aortic arch. On the right, the brachiocephalic trunk (innominate) artery arises from the arch and then further divides into the right common carotid artery and the right subclavian artery. Further branching occurs, with the internal carotids arising from each common carotid artery and the vertebral arteries arising from the subclavian arteries. On both sides, the arterial circulation to the brain is supplied anteriorly by the two internal carotid arteries and posteriorly by the two vertebral arteries.

The internal carotid arteries divide into the anterior and middle cerebral arteries after entering the cranium through the base of the skull (Fig. 53-1). The vertebral arteries are smaller and pass through the transverse foramina of the cervical vertebrae, entering the skull through the foramen magnum; they join to form the basilar artery (the vertebrobasilar system) at the junction of the pons and medulla in the brainstem. The basilar artery, in turn, travels to the midbrain, where it branches into paired posterior cerebral arteries. The anterior circulation meets the posterior circulation to form an arterial halo called the *circle of Willis*. The circle is formed by the anterior cerebral arteries, anterior communicating artery, internal carotid arteries, posterior communicating arteries, and posterior cerebral arteries (Fig. 53-2).

In general, the cerebral arteries are either conducting or penetrating. The *conducting arteries* (carotid, middle and anterior cerebral, vertebral, basilar, and posterior cerebral) and their branches form an extensive network over the surface of the brain. In general, the carotid arteries and their branches supply the major part of the cerebral hemispheres, and the vertebral arteries supply the base of the brain and the cerebellum. The *penetrating arteries* are nutrient vessels derived from the conducting arteries. These vessels enter the brain at right angles and provide blood to structures below the cortical level (thalamus, hypothalamus, internal capsule, and basal ganglia). Circulation to the two hemispheres is generally symmetric, with each side retaining its own separate blood supply. However, anomalies of the classic distribution are common and generally insignificant. When a problem arises, these anomalies can cause confusion when an attempt is made to correlate clinical findings with pathophysiologic phenomena.

Collateral Circulation

Collateral circulation may gradually develop when normal flow to a part is decreased. Most cerebral collateral circulation between major arteries is via the circle of Willis. The effect of this collateral circulation is to ensure a well-distributed blood supply to the brain, thus minimizing ischemia in the event of arterial occlusion. The brain also has other collateral circulation sites, such as that between external and internal carotid arteries via the ophthalmic artery (see Fig. 50-11). These function only when other routes are impaired. Theoretically, these communicating channels are capable of providing an adequate blood supply to all areas of the brain. Practically, this feature is often not the case. It is estimated that anomalies in the circle of Willis occur in almost one half the population and autopsy findings show that the prevalence of such variations are even higher in patients with stroke (see Fig. 53-2). A major vessel occlusion in one person will produce either no symptoms or a transient neurologic deficit. In another individual, the same occlusion site may cause a major loss of function. These differences would seem to be related to the state of the individual's collateral circulation.

Cerebral Microcirculation

Because of the much greater metabolic rate in the neuronal grey matter of the brain as compared with the white

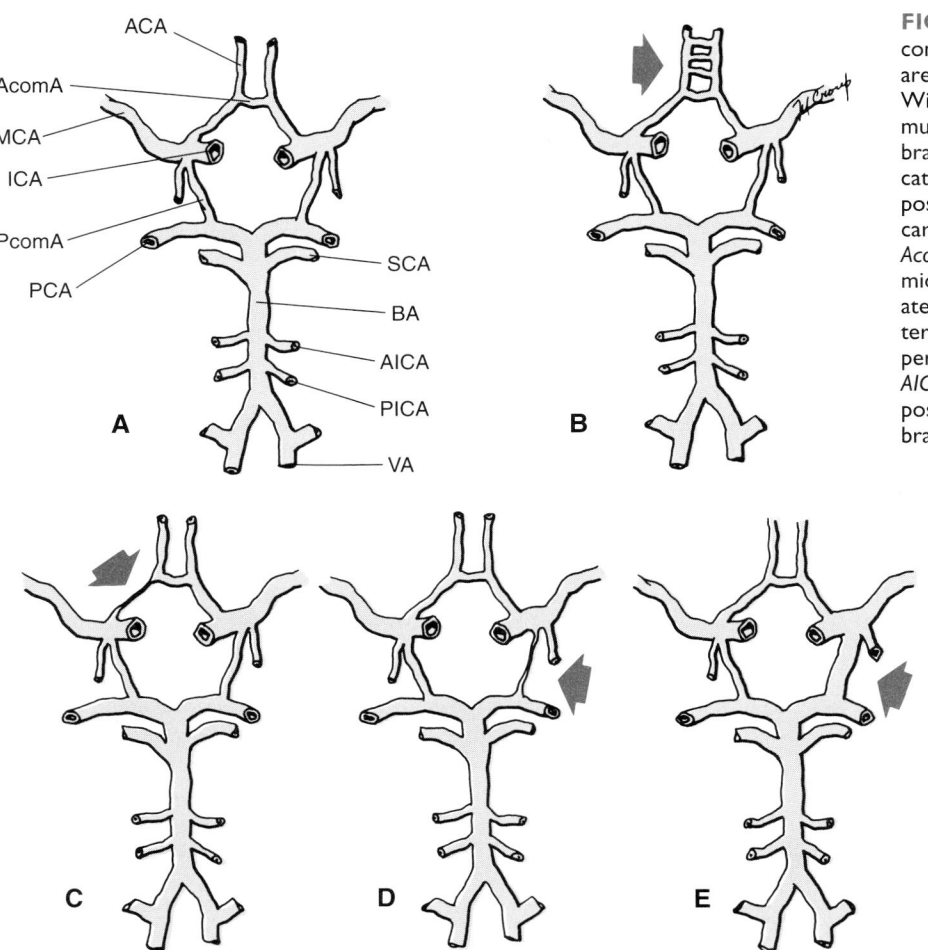

A

ACA
AcomA
MCA
ICA
PcomA
PCA
SCA
BA
AICA
PICA
VA

B

C   **D**   **E**

FIG. 53-2 The circle of Willis and some common anatomic variations. The anomalies are indicated by arrows. **A,** Normal circle of Willis. **B,** Reduplication of the anterior communicating artery. **C,** Stringlike anterior cerebral artery. **D,** Stringlike posterior communicating artery. **E,** Embryonic derivation of posterior cerebral artery from internal carotid artery. *ACA,* Anterior cerebral artery; *AcomA,* anterior communicating artery; *MCA,* middle cerebral artery; *ICA,* internal carotid atery; *PcomA,* posterior communicating artery; *PCA,* posterior cerebral artery; *SCA,* superior cerebellar artery; *BA,* basilar artery; *AICA,* anterior inferior cerebellar artery; *PICA,* posterior inferior cerebellar artery; *VA,* vertebral artery.

matter, the number of capillaries and blood flow are correspondingly about four times as great (Guyton, Hall, 2000). The capillaries of the brain are much less permeable than are almost all other capillaries in the body. The reason is that the spaces between endothelial cells are characterized by "tight junctions" that prevent leakage of capillary fluid. The result is the so-called *blood-brain barrier.* These "tight junctions" are also a feature of the interface between the blood and the cerebrospinal fluid (CSF)—the *blood-CSF barrier.* Another important protective feature of the brain capillaries is that they are supported on all sides by glial feet or pseudopods. These structures are projections from the supportive glial cells that fit against the outer surfaces of the capillaries and provide support that prevents excessive stretching and rupture in the event of exposure to high intraluminal pressure. Ischemic damage from stroke may cause disruption of the blood-brain and blood-CSF barriers, as well as increased vascular permeability and cerebral edema.

Regulation of Cerebral Blood Flow

Cerebral autoregulation is the ability of the normal functioning brain to regulate the volume of its own blood supply under conditions of constantly changing pressure in the supplying arteries. This action is accomplished by altering the size of the resistance vessels to maintain

blood flow pressure to the brain within a physiologic range of 60 to 160 mm Hg of mean arterial pressure (MAP). In persons with hypertension, this autoregulatory range increases to as high as 180 to 200 mm Hg (Guyton, 2000). When mean systemic arterial pressure decreases suddenly to a lower pressure within the physiologic range, arterioles dilate to decrease resistance and thereby maintain constant blood flow to the cerebral tissues. Conversely, when systemic arterial pressure increases suddenly within the physiologic range, arterioles constrict to maintain steady volume of flow into the cerebral capillaries, even in the face of much greater arterial driving pressure.

As just explained, autoregulation is an extremely important property of healthy brain circulation that functions to protect the brain from sudden decreases or increases in arterial blood pressure. Without this pressure regulation, sudden pressure changes may produce brain ischemia or, at the other extreme, capillary damage from high unsustained pressure. Unfortunately, with extremes of pressure change beyond the physiologic range of 60 to 160 mm Hg, the protective autoregulatory mechanism may fail, thus blood flow to the brain passively follows the pressure level in the systemic circulation. Obviously, this event can be a physiologic catastrophe under extremes of low or high MAP. Therefore protecting the brain's autoregulatory mechanism becomes a very important goal in treating patients with any cerebral insult. The means by which this goal is accomplished include strict titrating of intravenous medication to control MAP, assuring adequate oxygenation and ventilation so that the blood pH is kept within normal range, keeping serum electrolytes within normal range.

Three well-known metabolic factors influence CBF (Guyton, Hall, 2000). In situations where increased intracranial pressure (ICP) is a clinical problem, it is important that these factors be maintained within physiologic limits to maintain sufficient CBF, while preventing a rise in ICP. These factors are carbon dioxide (CO_2) concentration ($PaCO_2$), hydrogen ion concentration or blood acidity (pH), and oxygen (O_2) concentration (PaO_2). Hypercapnia (increased $PaCO_2$), acidemia (decreased pH), and hypoxemia (deficient PaO_2) alone or in combination with one or more of the other metabolic factors cause cerebral vasodilation and thus increase blood flow through cerebral vessels. Increased CBF, in turn, can cause elevated pressure within the cranium when there is brain injury and swelling. Conversely, hypocapnia (decreased $PaCO_2$) and alkalemia (increased pH) cause cerebral vasoconstriction. Therefore therapeutic measures include regulating the blood flow within physiologic parameters through manipulating the $PaCO_2$ and PaO_2 levels and the acid-base balance.

Several other factors influence CBF: blood volume and viscosity, perfusion pressure, and ICP. According to the Monro-Kellie doctrine, any factor that increases one of the three space-occupying components within the bony skull (brain tissue, CSF, and blood) will eventually cause an increase in ICP (See Chapter 56).

STROKE: GENERAL CONSIDERATIONS

Definition of Stroke

The term, *stroke* or cerebrovascular disease, refers to any sudden neurologic insult that results from restriction or cessation of flow through the arterial supply system of the brain. The term stroke is generally used specifically to mean cerebral infarction. An older, still frequently used, term is *cerebrovascular accident (CVA)*. However, this term is no longer defensible scientifically, because the underlying pathology is usually well established or easily identifiable or both. As a result, the processes by which many pathologic disorders (e.g., hypertension) lead to stroke are predictable, reproducible, and even modifiable. Therefore the occurrence of stroke is not an "accident" in any sense of the word. Another term often used in public information efforts is *brain attack*. The intent is to teach the public that morbidity and mortality in stroke are as serious as they are with heart attacks, and prompt intervention when it occurs is as important. "Stroke" is still the most widely used term among providers of health care and the public alike and will be used in this text.

Major Classifications of Stroke

Older classification systems typically divided strokes into three categories by causation: thrombotic, embolic, and

TABLE 53-1	▪▪▪

Major Classifications of Stroke

Cerebral Ischemia-Infarction (80%-85%)	Intracranial Hemorrhage (15%-20%)

Thrombotic occlusion
  Lacunar
Embolic occlusion
  Cardiogenic
  Artery-to-artery
	Intracerebral (parenchymal)
	Subarachnoid (SAH)
	Subdural (usually traumatic)
	Epidural (traumatic)

hemorrhagic. These events were often diagnosed based on the history of the development and evolution of symptoms. With newer imaging techniques such as computed tomography (CT) scan and magnetic resonance imaging (MRI), it is now possible to diagnose subarachnoid and intracerebral hemorrhage with a high degree of certainty. Differentiating between thrombi or emboli as the cause of an ischemic stroke is still not clear-cut, and therefore they are currently included in the same classification group—"ischemic stroke." Thus the two basic categories of circulatory impairment leading to stroke are ischemia-infarction and intracranial hemorrhage, comprising 80% to 85% and 15% to 20% of all strokes respectively (Table 53-1).

Ischemic cerebrovascular disease is divided into two broad categories: thrombotic and embolic occlusion. The precise cause of the ischemia often cannot be determined. Lacunar strokes involve the small, deep penetrating arteries of the brain, such as the lenticulostriate arteries branching from the middle cerebral artery. These arteries branch at 90 degrees from the major conducting arteries of the circle of Willis and are usually end-arteries with poor collateral circulation. About 15% of ischemic strokes are the result of lacunar infarcts. Cerebral ischemia is caused by a reduction of blood flow that lasts for a few seconds to a few minutes; if prolonged more than a few minutes, infarction of brain tissue occurs.

Intracranial hemorrhage may occur into the brain tissue itself (parenchyma), subarachnoid space, or the subdural or epidural space. Subdural and epidural hematomas are usually the result of trauma and are discussed in Chapter 56. The majority of intracerebral hemorrhages are associated with hypertension. Subarachnoid hemorrhage is usually the result of a saccular (Berry) aneurysm, or less commonly, an arteriovenous malformation (AVM).

General Pathophysiologic Mechanisms

Interference with the brain's blood flow supply can occur anywhere within the arteries that form the circle of Willis: the internal carotids and the vertebrobasilar system or any of their branches (Fig. 53-3). In general, if blood supply to brain tissue is cut off for 10 to 20 minutes, infarction or death of the tissue will occur. It is important to remember that occlusion of any particular artery does not necessarily cause infarction in the area of the brain perfused by that artery. The reason is that there may be adequate collateral circulation to the artery's perfusion territory. The underlying pathologic event may be one of a

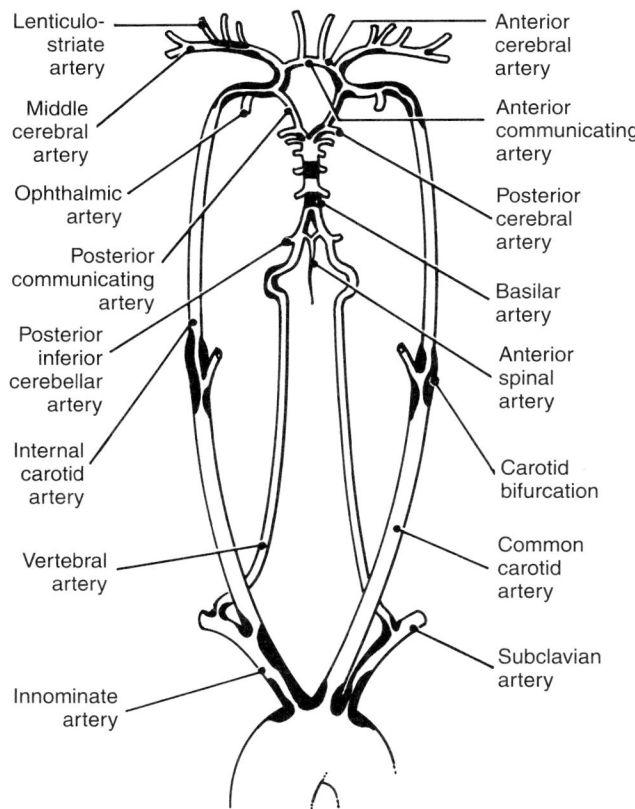

Lenticulo-striate artery

Middle cerebral artery

Ophthalmic artery

Posterior communicating artery

Posterior inferior cerebellar artery

Internal carotid artery

Vertebral artery

Innominate artery

Anterior cerebral artery

Anterior communicating artery

Posterior cerebral artery

Basilar artery

Anterior spinal artery

Carotid bifurcation

Common carotid artery

Subclavian artery

FIG. 53-3 Extracranial and intracranial arteries supplying blood to the brain. The circle of Willis and its principal branches are also shown. The sites of atherosclerosis of the cerebral blood vessels are designated *(dark areas)*, the main locations being the carotid bifurcation and the takeoff of the branches from the aorta, innominate, and subclavian arteries. These are the sites that are amenable to surgery.

variety of processes that occur within the blood vessels supplying the brain. The pathology may be (1) a *disease state of the vessel itself*, as in atherosclerosis and subsequent thrombosis, vascular wall dissection, or inflammation; (2) decreased perfusion from *impaired flow states*, such as shock or blood hyperviscosity; (3) blood flow interruption caused by a clot or infectious *embolus* originating in the heart or an extracranial vessel; or (4) and *vascular rupture* within cerebral tissue or the subarachnoid space.

Transient Ischemic Attack

A stroke may be preceded by a *transient ischemic attack (TIA)* similar to angina in a heart attack. TIAs are sudden, brief episodes of neurologic deficits caused by focal cerebral ischemia that tend to resolve with various degrees of rapidity and completeness but usually within 24 hours. The term is a clinical one and does not imply the cause. These attacks produce various kinds of symptoms, depending on the location of the affected cerebral tissue, and are caused by the same kinds of vascular impairments that cause a stroke. TIAs are important because they constitute an advance warning of future cere-

bral infarction. TIAs precede thrombotic strokes in 50% to 75% of affected patients. Therefore the individual who develops a TIA requires a full medical and neurologic workup. This measure is essential in prevention of stroke, because treatable causes, such as atrial fibrillation, often can be found. The simplest clinical workup includes complete blood count (CBC), basic metabolic panel, coagulation factors, electrocardiogram (ECG), and carotid Doppler (noninvasive) studies. A term now falling into disuse is Reversible Ischemic Neurologic Deficit (RIND). Sometimes called a "small stroke," an RIND describes a TIA with signs that last for longer than 24 hours. Typically, the cause is atherosclerotic stenosis of a carotid artery. A patient with an obvious carotid bruit (pronounced **broo**-ee) on the affected side should have carotid Doppler studies and angiography. These studies are essential to diagnosing a surgically correctable lesion. Even without a bruit present, the diagnostic procedures should be performed if symptoms of deficits in the carotid (anterior) circulation are present, especially if accompanied by emboli in the retinal arterioles (Wiederholt, 2000).

It is not always easy to identify the cerebral territory affected in a TIA. However, the occurrence of monocular blindness with or without contralateral weakness or numbness always points to the carotid system, as does receptive or sensory aphasia. The transient dimness or loss of vision in one eye (*amaurosis fugax*) is caused by arrest of blood flow through the ophthalmic artery (which branches off the internal carotid) that provides flow to the retinal arteries. Carotid stenosis caused by an atherosclerotic plaque, microemboli from atherosclerotic plaques, or a decrease in cardiac output can cause inadequate cerebral perfusion to the brain, which produces these symptoms. The hallmarks of vertebral-basilar involvement are bilateral weakness, vision loss, dizziness, falling attacks, numbness or any combination (i.e., a disturbance in the long motor or sensory tracks bilaterally). The attacks may all take approximately the same pattern, or they may vary considerably in detail, although maintaining the same basic pattern. The greater the frequency of TIAs, the greater the probability of a future stroke.

The *subclavian steal syndrome*, a form of TIA, is the classic example of obstruction in an extracranial artery that impairs flow through the vertebral-basilar arterial system. If the subclavian artery is occluded near its origin, the flow of blood in the vertebral artery may be reversed so that blood is drained away (stolen) from the basilar artery and circle of Willis to supply the arm at the expense of the cerebral circulation (Fig. 53-4). The most common site of the obstruction (usually caused by atherosclerosis) is in the left subclavian artery, near the origin of the left vertebral artery. When the left arm is exercised, blood is diverted from the right vertebral artery to the left vertebral artery where the flow is retrograde, thus causing cerebral ischemia. This "subclavian steal" may cause vertebral-basilar TIAs (with clinical manifestations as previously described) but rarely causes stroke. A difference in pulse amplitude and blood pressure (>20 mm Hg) between arms may be noted on physical examination. The diagnosis is confirmed by angiography and the condition may be corrected surgically by endarterectomy or bypass graft.

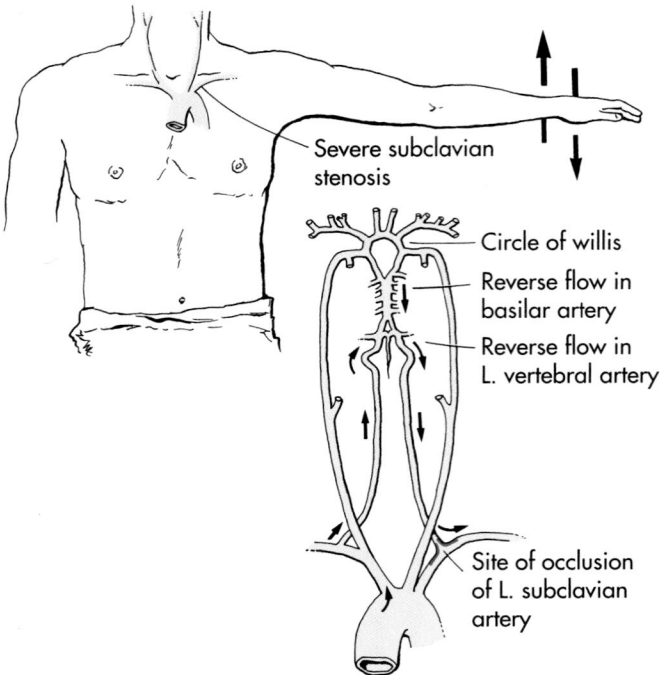

FIG. 53-4 Pathophysiologic mechanism producing intermittent cerebrovascular insufficiency in the subclavian steal syndrome. Cerebral ischemia is produced by the retrograde flow of blood from the brain to supply the arm. The abnormal flow is greatest during exercise of the arm supplied by the occluded subclavian artery. Signs and symptoms referable to portions of the brain supplied by the vertebral-basilar arteries are manifested, such as dizziness, ataxia, falling or visual disturbances (patients often complain of a "curtain" descending over the visual fields).

ISCHEMIC STROKE

About 80% to 85% of strokes are *ischemic strokes*, resulting from obstruction or clotting in one or more of the major arteries of the cerebral circulation. The obstruction can result from clots (thrombi) formed either within a vessel of the brain, or within a distal vessel or organ. In a distal vascular thrombus, clots may break off, or they may form within an organ such as the heart, and then be carried in the arterial system to the brain as an embolus. There are many different causes of primary thrombotic and embolic stroke, including atherosclerosis, arteritis, hypercoagulable state, and structural heart disease. However, thrombosis complicating atherosclerosis underlies most cases of thrombotic stroke, and emboli from a large vessel or cardiac source accounts for most cases of embolic stroke (Smith et al, 2001). Box 53-1 lists some of the causes of ischemic stroke.

Blockage of flow in the internal carotid artery is a common cause of stroke in older adults, who frequently develop atherosclerotic plaques in blood vessels, causing areas of narrowing or stenosis. The origin of the internal carotid artery (where the common carotid branches into the internal carotid and external carotid) is the most common site of the atherosclerosis. Less commonly, atherosclerosis of the middle or anterior cerebral arteries may be the site of atherosclerosis. Blood is driven

---

BOX 53-1

Some Causes of Ischemic Stroke

THROMBOSIS
Atherosclerosis (most common)
Vasculitis: temporal arteritis, polyarteritis nodosa
Arterial dissection: carotid, vertebral (spontaneous or traumatic)
Hematologic disorders: polycythemia, hemoglobinopathies (sickle cell disease)

EMBOLISM
Cardiac source: atrial fibrillation (most common), myocardial infarction, rheumatic heart disease, valvular heart disease, prosthetic valves, ischemic cardiomyopathy
Atherosclerotic thromboembolic arterial source: common carotid bifurcation, distal vertebral artery
Hypercoagulation states: oral contraceptives, carcinoma

VASOCONSTRICTION
Cerebral vasospasm following SAH

SAH, Subarachnoid hemorrhage.

---

through the vascular system by pressure gradients, but in a stenosed vessel, the more rapid flow of blood through a narrower lumen decreases the pressure gradient across the constriction. When a critical degree of stenosis is reached, the increased turbulence around the blockage results in a sharp drop in flow rate. Clinically, critical stenosis in human beings is 80% to 85% of the luminal cross-sectional area (Hademenos, 1997). Another cause of ischemic stroke is vasospasm, which is often a reactive vascular response to bleeding into the space between the arachnoid and pia mater layers of the meninges. Most ischemic stroke is not painful, because the brain substance is insensitive to pain. However, the large vessels in the neck and in the brainstem are highly innervated with pain receptors, and injury to these vessels during an ischemic episode can cause a headache. Therefore, with a clinical picture of headache in the presence of an ischemic stroke, it is important to perform diagnostic tests that can detect injuries such as dissecting aneurysms in the neck and brainstem vessels.

Subtypes of Ischemic Stroke

There are four basic subtypes of ischemic stroke according to cause: lacunar, large vessel thrombosis with low flow, embolic, and cryptogenic. Cryptogenic strokes are ischemic strokes resulting from sudden occlusion of a large intracranial vessel but with no apparent cause.

Lacunar Strokes

Lacunar infarcts are the result of hypertensive small-vessel disease and cause stroke syndromes that typically evolve over several hours or sometimes longer. Lacunar infarcts represent infarction following atherothrombotic or hyaline-lipid occlusion of one of the penetrating branches of the circle of Willis, middle cerebral artery stem, or vertebral and basilar arteries (Smith et al, 2001). Each of these branches is very small (30 to 100 μm in diameter) and penetrates deep into the gray and white matter of the cerebrum and the brainstem. The branches are susceptible to thrombosis either from atherothrombotic disease or by the development of lipohyalinotic thickening. Thrombosis occurring within these vessels causes small softened, infarcted areas that are referred to as *lacunes* (Greek, small lakes). The symptoms may be very severe, though isolated and discrete, depending on the affected vessel's depth of tissue penetration before thrombosis occurred.

There are four common lacunar syndromes: (1) pure motor hemiparesis from infarction of the posterior internal capsule, (2) pure motor hemiparesis from infarction of the anterior limb of the internal capsule, (3) pure sensory stroke from a thalamic infarct, and (4) ataxic hemiparesis or dysarthria and clumsy hand or arm caused by basal pons infarct. More than 30 lacunar syndromes have been identified, and the intravascular pathology is usually lipohyalinosis or microatheromas with clotting inside the vascular lumen. These vessel changes are almost always the result of endothelial dysfunction caused by persistent hypertensive disease (Smith, 2001). Both lacunar stroke and deep intracerebral hemorrhage seem to be associated with arterial pathology of the small penetrating brain vessels. Differentiation of the two causes of stroke can be difficult. In general, patients with lacunar infarcts are more likely to be older, have higher cholesterol, and have diabetes than are those with deep intracerebral hemorrhage (Labovitz, 2001).

Large Vessel Thrombotic Strokes

Large vessel thrombosis with low flow is the second subtype of ischemic stroke. A majority of these strokes occur during sleep, when the individual is relatively dehydrated and circulatory dynamics are decreased. The signs and symptoms resulting from such an ischemic stroke depend on the location of the occlusion and the extent of the intact collateral flow to the affected brain tissue. These strokes are often associated with a narrow, stenotic, atherosclerotic lesion of the internal carotid artery, or less commonly in the middle cerebral artery stem or at the junction of the vertebral and basilar artery. Unlike coronary artery thrombosis, in which vascular occlusion tends to be sudden and complete, thrombosis of cerebral vessels tend to be gradual in onset, even evolving over several days. This pattern has given rise to the term, "stroke-in-evolution." Many of these evolving strokes are actually the result of distal embolization, particularly when the source of the thrombus is the carotid arteries.

Thrombotic strokes may, from a clinical point of view, appear to "stutter," with symptoms appearing and disappearing in rapid succession. These individuals may have experienced several lacunar-type TIAs before finally experiencing a stroke. Particularly ominous are so-called "crescendo TIAs," in which the patient experiences increasing number and frequency of TIAs. The likelihood of these evolving to a thrombotic stroke is very high.

Another mechanism of low flow in partially thrombosed arteries is *perfusion deficit* that can occur with sudden reduction in cardiac output or systemic blood pressure. Blood flow may be dependent on high intravascular pressure to maintain blood flow across a stenotic intraarterial lesion. Sudden reduction of that pressure can lead to generalized reduction in CBF, brain ischemia, and stroke. Therefore nonsymptomatic hypertension, especially in older adults, must be treated carefully and cautiously, because sudden blood pressure reduction can precipitate stroke or coronary artery ischemia or both. This characteristic is the reason outpatient treatment of high blood pressure with rapid-acting agents such as nifedipine (Procardia) under the tongue is contraindicated (JNC VI, 1997). If this type of severe hypertension is symptomatic, it should be treated in a controlled inpatient environment using intravenous agents that can be titrated to the patient's clinical condition. For the same reason, persons who have stenotic lesions of their carotids must be cautioned about orthostatic hypotension that can occur with the introduction of potent antihypertensive agents. These medications can produce cerebral ischemia if they cause a sudden drop in blood pressure. The reduced pressure may be sufficient to impair perfusion via arteries that depend on a minimal perfusion pressure to maintain CBF.

Embolic Strokes

Embolic strokes are classified by the artery involved (e.g., vertebral artery stroke) or by the origin of the embolism. The origin of an embolic stroke can be either a distal artery or the heart (cardioembolic stroke). Cardiac mural thrombi are the most common sources: myocardial infarct, atrial fibrillation, diseased heart valves, artificial heart valves, and ischemic cardiomyopathy (Smith, Hauser, Easton, 2000). Of these, atrial fibrillation by far is the most common cause. Next in importance are thromboemboli arising in arteries, most often over an atheromatous plaque in the carotid arteries.

Strokes resulting from embolism usually produce sudden neurologic deficits with their maximal effect at the onset. Typically, the attack occurs during waking activities. These embolic thrombi commonly lodge at a stenotic vessel site. Cardioembolic strokes, the most frequent kind of embolic stroke, are diagnosed when there is a known cardiac cause such as atrial fibrillation or when recent myocardial infarction precedes a sudden large-vessel occlusion in the brain. The emboli originate from thrombotic material formed on a wall of a heart chamber or on the mitral valves. Because embolic fragments from the heart are typically very small clots, they reach the brain through the carotid or vertebral arteries. Thus the clinical symptoms they produce are dependent on which part of the circulation is obstructed and how deeply into the arterial tree the clot traveled before it lodged.

In addition, an embolism can break down and move farther along in the vasculature, causing symptoms to clear. However, the fragments later lodge farther downstream and produce other focal symptoms. Unfortunately, persons with cardioembolic strokes have a higher risk of suffering a hemorrhagic stroke later, when petechial bleeding or outright hemorrhage occurs into the infarcted tissue hours or even days after the initial embolic event. The reason for the hemorrhage is that the arterial wall structures distal to the original embolic occlusion are weakened or friable caused by lack of perfusion. Therefore restoration of perfusion pressure can lead to arteriole or capillary bleeding in affected vessels.

Cryptogenic Strokes

Though cardioembolism presents a dramatic, nearly pathognomonic clinical picture, some patients develop sudden occlusion of a large intracranial vessel for which no cause can be found. These are called cryptogenic strokes because the source is "hidden," even after extensive diagnostic tests and clinical evaluation. It can happen that the cause remains obscure for months or years, when new, similar symptoms develop for which the cause can be found. The majority of strokes with no determinable cause, however, occur in patients with clinical profiles indistinguishable from those with atherothrombosis.

Other Causes of Ischemic Stroke

Some less frequent causes of stroke are fibromuscular dysplasia, arteritis (e.g., temporal arteritis, polyarteritis nodosa), and hypercoagulable disorders. Although they generally fall into the classification of thrombotic strokes, each has features of some of the other subtypes of stroke etiology as well. Fibromuscular dysplasia occurs in the cervical arteries and is seen almost exclusively in women. On Doppler examination, there are numerous areas of sausagelike appearance in the artery, with stenotic narrowing alternating with areas of dilation.

Temporal (giant cell) arteritis is an affliction occurring primarily in older adults in which the external carotids, and especially the temporal arteries, are the site of a granulomatous inflammation with giant cells. Temporal arteritis is included here because it is encountered relatively frequently. Temporal arteritis can cause severe, focal, nonreversible deficits, and it is highly treatable if detected early. Early signs are nonspecific and vague, which typically leads to delay in diagnosis. Therefore health care providers need to be aware of the disease and act on the patient's risk profile, signs, and symptoms to intervene effectively. Temporal arteritis is rare in patients under the age of 50 and affects men more than women. Early symptoms are nonspecific and include weight loss, anorexia, general muscular aches, and fatigue. The signature laboratory finding is a very elevated erythrocyte sedimentation rate (ESR). An elevated ESR in an at-risk patient should be followed by a temporal artery biopsy to locate the typical causative granulomatous lesion. If the inflammation is not treated promptly, the neurologic complication of blindness can occur quickly resulting from ischemic optic neuritis (although it rarely causes stroke). Unfortunately, this blindness often is not reversible. The treatment consists of prednisone in moderately high doses (Wiederholt, 2000).

Ischemic Cascade and Secondary Injury

During the 1990s, the so-called "decade of the brain," researchers made great progress in discovering why neuronal cells die during ischemic stroke. Most strokes culminate in a core area of cell death (infarction) in which blood flow is so drastically reduced that the cells usually cannot recover. This perfusion threshold usually occurs when CBF is 20% of normal or less. Normal CBF is about 50 ml/100 g brain tissue/minute. The National Stroke Association (2001) has summarized the following mechanisms of cell injury from a stroke.

1. Without neuroprotective agents, nerve cells exposed to ischemia that is 80% or greater (CBF of 10 ml/100 g brain tissue/minute) will be irreversibly damaged within a few minutes. This area is called the *ischemic core* (Fig. 53-5). Surrounding the ischemic core is another area of tissue called the *ischemic penumbra* or "transitional zone" in which CBF is between 20% and 50% of normal (10 to 25 ml/100 g brain tissue/min). Neuronal cells in this area are endangered but not yet irreversibly damaged. There is evidence that the time window for the development of the penumbra in stroke can vary from 12 to 24 hours.

2. Rapidly within the core infarction, and over time within the ischemic penumbra, brain cell injury and death progress as follows:

   - Without adequate blood supply, brain cells lose their ability to produce energy—particularly adenosine triphosphate (ATP).
   - When this energy failure occurs, the cellular sodium-potassium pump fails, resulting in neuronal swelling.
   - One of the ways brain cells respond to energy failure is by elevating the concentration of intracellular calcium. Worsening that problem, and driving the concentrations to dangerous levels, is the process of *excitotoxicity* in which brain cells release excessive amounts of the excitatory neurotransmitter *glutamate*. Released glutamate stimulates chemical and electrical activities in other brain cells by attaching to a molecule on other neurons, the N-methyl-D-aspartate (NMDA) receptor. This receptor binding triggers the activation of the enzyme nitric oxide synthase (NOS), which leads to the production of

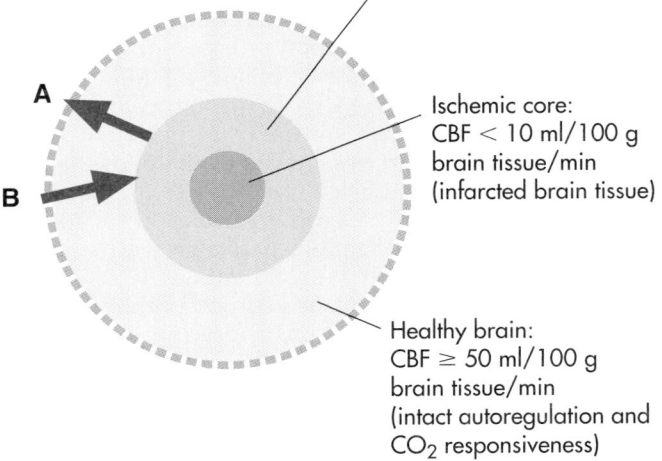

Ischemic penumbra: CBF = 10-25 ml/100 g brain tissue/min (loss of autoregulation and CO_2 responsiveness)

Ischemic core: CBF < 10 ml/100 g brain tissue/min (infarcted brain tissue)

Healthy brain: CBF ≥ 50 ml/100 g brain tissue/min (intact autoregulation and CO_2 responsiveness)

FIG. 53-5 Effects of autoregulation and chemoregulation on cerebral blood flow (CBF) to the ischemic penumbra. **A,** A decrease in systemic blood pressure or an increase in the $PaCO_2$ causes vasodilation in the healthy (hyperemic zone) brain vessels stealing blood away from the ischemic penumbra. **B,** Conversely, an increase in systemic blood pressure or a decrease in the $PaCO_2$ causes vasoconstriction in the healthy brain vessels so that more blood is provided to the ischemic penumbra.

the gas molecule, nitric oxide (NO). Production of NO can occur rapidly in large volumes, causing the degradation and destruction of vital cellular structures. This process occurs through weakening the deoxyribonucleic acid (DNA) of neurons, which, in turn, activates the enzyme, poly (adenosine diphosphate– [ADP-] ribose) polymerase (PARP). PARP is a nuclear enzyme that recognizes DNA strand breaks and is instrumental in DNA repair (Mandir et al, 2001). However, PARP is thought to cause and accelerate excitotoxicity following cerebral ischemia, leading to severe cellular energy depletion and cell death (apoptosis).

- NO occurs naturally in the body and promotes many physiologic functions that depend on vasodilation, such as penile erection; it also is the active chemical in potent vasodilating medications such as sodium nitroprusside (Nipride). However, in excessive amounts, NO can lead to damage and death of neurons. Medications that can block NOS and the production of NO or inhibit action of the PARP enzyme may ultimately be useful in reducing brain damage from stroke.
- Brain cells ultimately die as a result of the actions of calcium-activated proteases (enzymes that digest cell proteins), lipases (enzymes that digest cell membranes), and free radicals formed as a result of the ischemic cascade.
- Finally, infarcted brain tissue swells and can cause pressure and distortion and crushing of the brainstem.

Mechanical and chemical factors cause secondary damage after the initial ischemic episode. The most injurious of these factors are (1) disruption of the blood-brain and blood-CSF barriers from exposure to toxic substances, (2) cerebral interstitial edema caused by increased vascular permeability in affected arteries, (3) *hyperperfusion zones* surrounding ischemic tissue that can steal blood flow and hasten infarction of ischemic neurons (see Fig. 53-5), and (4) loss of cerebral autoregulation thus CBF becomes unresponsive to pressure differentials and metabolic needs.

Loss of autoregulation is a grave complication of stroke that can initiate a vicious cycle of increased cerebral edema, increased ICP, and steadily increasing neuronal damage. With autoregulation gone, the arterioles are no longer capable of regulating CBF according to metabolic demand. Nor are they capable of protecting the cerebral capillaries from sudden increases or decreases in pressure. Instead, flow to the brain now is controlled solely by the mean systemic arterial pressure (MAP). With severe hypotension, cerebral perfusion pressure falls, leading to ischemia. Ultimately, given the chemical changes that ischemia induces within the cell, damage from increasing cerebral edema will occur, further reducing flow to the brain in a low-flow system. Unfortunately, with loss of autoregulation, uncontrolled systemic arterial hypertension can produce the same outcome. Similar to extremely low-pressure states, in high-pressure states, CBF follows the systemic MAP. Therefore CBF becomes elevated, even in spite of increased ICP, and the brain capillaries become distended and permeable. This event, of course, sets up a different type of vicious cycle, with loss of oncotic pressure in the cerebral capillaries and interstitial brain edema occurring.

Signs and Symptoms of Stroke

It is important to recognize that stroke is a medical emergency, because early intervention can halt and even reverse damage to neurons from impaired perfusion. The herald event of stroke or cerebrovascular accident (CVA) is abrupt onset of one or more focal neurologic deficits. There may be rapid improvement of the deficits, progressive worsening of the deficit, or they may be fixed. Seizure activity is not usually a feature of stroke. General symptoms include sudden numbness or weakness of the face, arm, or leg, particularly on one side of the body; visual disturbance such as double vision or trouble seeing in one or both eyes; sudden confusion; stumbling while walking, dizziness, loss of balance or coordination; and sudden severe headache with no known cause.

Points of bifurcation or angulation of major vessels are most vulnerable to impaired flow resulting from stenosis. Major clinical features associated with arterial insufficiency to the brain may be focal and temporary, or the dysfunction may be permanent, with actual tissue death and neurologic deficit. It is difficult to establish a close correlation between symptoms associated with a particular vessel and actual clinical manifestations in a particular patient because of the following factors:

1. There is individual variation of collateral circulation with regard to the circle of Willis (see Fig. 53-2). Total occlusion of a carotid artery may produce no symptoms if the left anterior cerebral and left middle cerebral arteries receive adequate blood from the anterior communicating artery. If this blood supply is not adequate, symptoms may include confusion, contralateral monoparesis or hemiparesis, and incontinence.
2. Leptomeningeal anastomoses are significant over the cerebral cortex between the anterior, middle, and posterior cerebral arteries. Anastomoses also exist between the anterior cerebral arteries of the two hemispheres across the corpus callosum.
3. Each of the cerebral arteries has a central area to supply with blood and a peripheral supply area, or border area, which it may share with another artery. Anastomoses exist between external and internal carotid arteries, as around the orbit, with blood from external carotid vessels going to the ophthalmic artery.
4. Various systemic and metabolic factors are significant in determining the symptoms that a particular pathologic process will produce. For example, a stenosed vessel may produce no symptoms as long as systemic blood pressure is 190/110 mm Hg; but if it is reduced to 120/70 mm Hg, variable symptoms may result, depending on the location of the stenotic area. Hyponatremia and hyperthermia are metabolic factors that promote development of neurologic deficits in the presence of stenotic blood vessels. Hyponatremia causes neuronal swelling caused by osmotic shift of fluid from a hypotonic extracellular fluid (ECF) compartment into a relatively hypertonic intracellular fluid (ICF) compartment. Hyperthermia increases the metabolic activity and oxygen need of cells that may not be able to receive the needed oxygen because of stenosed supplying arteries.

Neurovascular Syndromes

Major clinical features associated with arterial insufficiency to the brain may be associated with the following groupings of signs and symptoms listed below called *neurovascular syndromes*. The following descriptions apply particularly to ischemia and infarction resulting from thrombosis or embolism. Although hemorrhage within these vascular territories may give rise to many of the same effects, the total clinical picture is apt to differ because, in its deep extension, the hemorrhage may involve the territory of more than one vessel. Additionally, it displaces tissues and causes an increase in ICP.

1. *Internal carotid artery* (anterior circulation: symptoms usually unilateral). Most common location of lesion is the bifurcation of the common carotid into the internal and external carotids. Branches of the internal carotid are the ophthalmic, posterior communicating, anterior choroidal, anterior cerebral, and middle cerebral. Variable syndromes may develop. The pattern depends on the amount of collateral circulation.
   a. Monocular blindness (episodic and called "amaurosis fugax") on the side of the involved carotid may occur, caused by retinal artery insufficiency.
   b. Sensory and motor symptoms involve contralateral extremities because of middle cerebral artery insufficiency.
   c. Lesion may occur in the area between the anterior and middle cerebral arteries or the middle cerebral artery. Symptoms initially develop in upper extremities (e.g., weak, numb hand) and may involve the face (supranuclear-type weakness). If the lesion is in the dominant hemisphere, expressive aphasia occurs because of involvement of Broca's motor-speech area.
2. *Middle cerebral artery* (most common)
   a. Contralateral monoparesis or hemiparesis (usually affecting an arm)
   b. Occasional contralateral hemianopsia (blindness)
   c. Global aphasia (if dominant hemisphere is involved): disturbance of all functions involving speech and communication
   d. Dysphasia
3. *Anterior cerebral artery* (confusion is primary symptom)
   a. Contralateral weakness greater in the leg: proximal arm also possibly involved; voluntary movement of that leg is impaired.
   b. Contralateral sensory deficits
   c. Dementia, grasp, pathologic reflexes (frontal lobe dysfunction)
4. *Vertebral-basilar* (posterior circulation: manifestations usually bilateral)
   a. Weakness in one to four extremities
   b. Increased tendon reflexes
   c. Ataxia
   d. Bilateral Babinski's sign
   e. Cerebellar signs such as intention tremor, vertigo
   f. Dysphagia
   g. Dysarthria
   h. Syncope, stupor, coma, dizziness, memory disturbances, disorientation
   i. Visual disturbances (diplopia, nystagmus, ptosis, paralysis of single eye movements, homonymous hemianopsia)
   j. Tinnitus, hearing loss
   k. Facial, mouth, or tongue numbness
5. *Posterior cerebral artery* (in lobe of midbrain or thalamus)
   a. Coma
   b. Contralateral hemiparesis
   c. Visual aphasia or word blindness (alexia)
   d. Third cranial nerve palsy: hemianopsia, choreoathetosis

Because of the anatomic locations of neurons that control the numerous discrete motor and sensory modalities in the cerebral cortex, specific symptoms of CVA can vary widely, depending on location and size of cerebral vessels involved and location and number of neurons injured. As previously indicated, several clinical syndromes have been defined, based on the deficits that occur from occlusion of the artery after which the syndrome is named. An example is middle cerebral artery syndrome (contralateral paralysis of the face, arm, and leg; motor aphasia; and homonymous hemianopsia).

A good history of the symptoms surrounding a stroke event can help identify whether the flow disruption was in the anterior circulation of the brain (internal carotid artery distribution) or in the posterior circulation (vertebral-basilar artery distribution). Certain symptoms are typical of disruption to circulation in the anterior part of the circle of Willis. These symptoms are transient monocular blindness (*amaurosis fugax*) and aphasia (Wiederholt, 2000). Typical signs of circulatory impairment in the posterior part of the circle of Willis include *diplopia* (double vision), *homonymous hemianopsias* (see Fig. 57-1, specific visual field losses), ataxia, vertigo, and cranial nerve palsies (Wiederholt, 2000).

When the pathologic events and ensuing chemical cascade have ceased, the patient is said to have a "completed" stroke. The result is a fixed neurologic deficit that has developed quickly or over time. That is, diagnostic tests may be abnormal or normal immediately after the initial symptoms began. Similarly, focal electroencephalogram (EEG) changes may not be evident early or may not be demonstrated until more than 24 hours after an acute brain infarction. As discussed previously, it may be impossible to distinguish between a hemorrhagic and an ischemic infarct by clinical criteria. Making the diagnosis early is important, because anticoagulation is contraindicated in hemorrhagic infarct but can prevent further spread of damage in ischemic infarct. CT scan has been found to be very useful in detecting hemorrhage and should be done as soon as possible to detect whether hemorrhage is present.

HEMORRHAGIC STROKES

Hemorrhagic strokes, accounting for about 15% to 20% of all strokes, may occur when intracerebral vascular lesions rupture, causing bleeding into the subarachnoid space or directly into brain tissue. Some vascular lesions that can lead to subarachnoid hemorrhage (SAH) are saccular (Berry) aneurysms and arteriovenous malformations (AVMs). Another mechanism of hemorrhagic stroke is recent cocaine or amphetamine use, because these substances can cause severe hypertension and intracerebral or subarachnoid bleeding.

Hemorrhage can rapidly produce neurologic symptoms because of pressure on neural structures within the bony skull. Ischemia can be a secondary consequence of either spontaneous or traumatic hemorrhage. The mechanism of such ischemia is twofold: (1) pressure on blood vessels resulting from extravasation of blood into the fixed volume of the skull and (2) reactive vasospasm of blood vessels exposed to free bleeding into the space between the arachnoid and pia mater layers of the meninges. Typically, hemorrhagic strokes lead to rapid loss of brain function and unconsciousness. However, if the bleed evolves more slowly, the affected individual is likely to have a severe headache, which is the typical scenario with subarachnoid hemorrhage (SAH). The main preventive measures for cerebral hemorrhage are to prevent head injuries and control high blood pressure.

Hemorrhagic Stroke Subtypes

It is possible for hemorrhage to occur anywhere within the central nervous system. In general, bleeding events within the skull are classified by location in relation to the cerebral tissue and the meninges and by the type of vascular lesions present. Bleeding into the outermost layers of the meninges, such as subdural and epidural hemorrhage, is most often associated with trauma. The types of bleeds underlying hemorrhagic stroke are intracerebral (parenchymal), intraventricular, and SAH (Smith, 2001). In addition to anatomic vascular lesions, causes of hemorrhagic strokes are hypertension, bleeding disorders, overly aggressive anticoagulation (especially in older adults), and amphetamine and intranasal cocaine use. Box 53-2 lists some common causes of intracerebral hemorrhage.

Hypertensive Intracerebral (Parenchymal) Hemorrhage

Intracerebral hemorrhage into the brain tissue (parenchyma) is most often the result of hypertension-induced vascular injury and from rupture of one of the many small arteries that penetrate deep into the brain substance. If hemorrhage occurs in persons without underlying hypertension, then workup needs to be done for other causes such as bleeding disorders, arteriovenous malformations, and eroding tumors. Strokes caused by intracerebral hemorrhage most commonly occur while the patient is awake and active, thus they are often witnessed. Because of their location near the deep terminal arteries, the basal ganglia and the internal capsule frequently receive the brunt of the pressure and ischemia

---

BOX 53-2

Some Causes of Intracerebral Hemorrhage

Hypertensive intracerebral hemorrhage
Subarachnoid hemorrhage (SAH)
    Ruptured saccular (Berry) aneurysm
    Ruptured arteriovenous malformation (AVM)
    Trauma (see Chapter 56)
Cocaine, amphetamine abuse
Bleeding from brain tumors
Hemorrhagic infarction
Systemic bleeding disorders including anticoagulation
    therapy

---

caused by this type of stroke. Recalling that the basal ganglia modulate voluntary motor function and that all the afferent and efferent nerve fibers in one half of the cortex are compacted together to enter and leave the internal capsule, one can see that a stroke in either of these regions would be expected to produce devastating deficits. Typically, bleeding deep within the brain produces abrupt onset of focal neurologic deficits that worsen progressively over minutes to less than 2 hours. Hemiparesis on the side opposite the bleed is the typical first sign of internal capsule involvement.

Cerebral infarction following embolism to a cerebral artery may be a result of hemorrhage rather than to blockage by the embolism itself. The reason is that, when an embolism resolves or is cleared from the artery, the vascular wall beyond the site of the occlusion is weakened for the first several days following the occlusion. Therefore, during that time, leaking or hemorrhage from the fragile vessel wall can occur. For that reason, good control of hypertension is essential in preventing further damage in the early weeks following embolic stroke.

The mortality rate for hypertensive intracerebral hemorrhage is very high—nearly 50%. Hemorrhages occurring in the supratentorial space (above the tentorium cerebelli) have a good prognosis if the volume of the bleed is small. However, bleeds into the infratentorial space in the pontine or cerebellar areas have much poorer prognoses by comparison because of the rapid pressure on vital brainstem structures (Smith, 2001). The main treatment for hemorrhagic stroke is to lower the blood pressure if hypertension is the cause and to counteract anticoagulation if an endogenous or drug-induced bleeding disorder is the cause. Little can be done about the hemorrhage that has already occurred. As discussed under ischemic stroke, reducing the blood pressure too rapidly or too drastically can lead to decreased perfusion and extension of the ischemia. Monitoring for and treating ICP elevation and clot evacuation if the level of consciousness deteriorates are the only interventions that are likely to have a positive impact on the prognosis. In persons under the age of 40, cocaine use is an important cause of stroke caused by intracerebral hemorrhage. The precise relationship between cocaine and vascular bleeding is controversial, though it is known that cocaine enhances sympathetic nervous system activity and thereby may cause sudden extreme elevations of blood pressure. The bleed may occur in intracerebral or subarachnoid vessels; in the latter case, a vascular aneurysm is usually present.

Hemorrhage directly into the ventricles of the brain is uncommon. More commonly, hemorrhage within the brain parenchyma dissects into the ventricular system, leaving little evidence of the origin of the bleed. As with ischemia, the main neurologic deficits reflect damage to a particular area of the brain. Therefore, visual field loss occurs with occipital hemorrhage, and weakness or paralysis with frontal damage to the motor cortex.

Subarachnoid Hemorrhage

SAH has two major causes: rupture of a vascular aneurysm and head trauma. Fig. 53-6 shows the common sites of *saccular (berry) aneurysms*, most of which occur in the circle of Willis (see color plate 37). Because bleeds can be massive and extravasation of blood into the subarach-

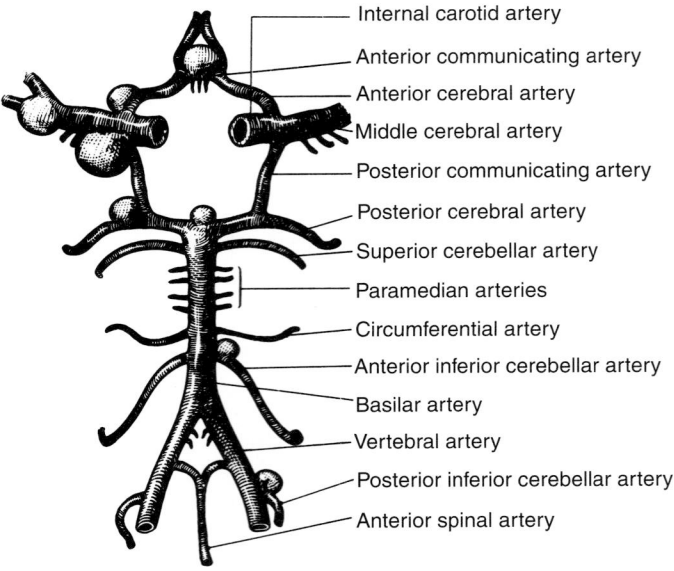

- Internal carotid artery
- Anterior communicating artery
- Anterior cerebral artery
- Middle cerebral artery
- Posterior communicating artery
- Posterior cerebral artery
- Superior cerebellar artery
- Paramedian arteries
- Circumferential artery
- Anterior inferior cerebellar artery
- Basilar artery
- Vertebral artery
- Posterior inferior cerebellar artery
- Anterior spinal artery

FIG. 53-6 The common sites of saccular (berry) aneurysms. Each is drawn in direct proportion to the frequency at that site. (Modified from Goldman L, Bennett J: *Cecil textbook of medicine,* ed 21, Philadelphia, 2000, Saunders.)

noid meningeal layer rapid, mortality is extremely high—about 50% in the first month after a bleed. The reason for the high mortality is that four major complications can cause ischemia of the brain and delayed morbidity and mortality long after the bleed is controlled. These complications are (1) reactive vasospasm with infarction, (2) rerupture, (3) hyponatremia, and (4) hydrocephalus. For patients who survive the initial bleed, rerupture or rebleeding is the most dangerous complication in the immediate postbleed period (Adams et al, 1997). Vasospasm is a complication that occurs 3 to 12 days following the initial bleed. The extent to which the arterial spasm causes ischemia and infarction depends on the severity and distribution of the involved vessels.

A widely used tool for classifying severity of SAH is the Hunt and Hess Classification Grading Scale (Hunt, Hess, 1968). The five-point scale (Table 53-2) is widely used clinically and in research. A modification of the Hunt and Hess Scale (New York Department of Neurosurgery, 1996) includes seven grades of severity, numbered 0 to 5. An unruptured aneurysm is grade 0, and the original grade 2 is subdivided into grades 1a and 2. This more recent seven-point scale is included in the Brain Attack Coalition's (2001) web site listing of five different stroke scales, all of which are used to evaluate stroke patients. Except for the Hunt and Hess scale, which is used to assess immediate degree of dysfunction, the other scales are used during stroke recovery to assess degree of disability, level of functioning, and progress in rehabilitation. These scales are available at the Brain Attack Coalition site (2001): *http://www.stroke-site.org*

Arteriovenous malformations (AVMs) are congenitally malformed capillary beds and are a less common cause of SAH. Normally, a capillary bed consists of blood vessels that are only 8/1000 mm in diameter. Because of their minute size, the tiny arterioles have high vascular resistance that slows the flow of blood so that oxygen and

TABLE 53-2

Hunt and Hess Scale for Grading SAH

Grade	Neurologic Status
I	Asymptomatic; or minimal headache and slight nuchal rigidity
II	Moderate-to-severe headache; nuchal rigidity; no neurologic deficit except cranial nerve palsy
III	Drowsy; minimal neurologic deficit
IV	Stuporous; moderate to severe hemiparesis; possibly early decerebrate rigidity and vegetative disturbances
V	Deep coma; decerebrate rigidity; moribund appearance

Hunt WE, Hess RM: Surgical risk as related to time of intervention in the repair of intracranial aneurysms, *J Neurosurg* 28:14-20, 1968.

nutrients can diffuse into the brain tissue. In an AVM, the vessels are enlarged and allow blood to be shunted between the high-pressure arterial and the low-pressure venous systems. Eventually, venule walls weaken, and blood can extravasate rapidly into the cerebral tissues. In most of these patients, the hemorrhage is mainly intraparenchymal with spillage into the subarachnoid space. Hemorrhages may be massive, leading to death, or may be as small as 1 cm in diameter.

EVALUATION OF STROKE ETIOLOGY

History of Signs and Symptoms

The patient's clinical condition, symptoms and history of evolution of symptoms, and deficits are essential and can guide the clinician in determining the most likely cause of the stroke. History from a reliable historian should include:

1. Description of the onset and initial symptoms. Seizure at onset is indicative of embolic stroke.
2. Progression of symptoms or patient complaints or both
3. History of TIAs
4. Risk factors, particularly hypertension, atrial fibrillation, diabetes, smoking, and alcohol use
5. Drug use, especially cocaine
6. Current medications, including ones recently discontinued. For example, sudden discontinuation of the antihypertensive medication clonidine (Catapres) can cause severe rebound hypertension. Additionally, abrupt discontinuation of phenytoin (Dilantin) or phenobarbital for seizure disorder can precipitate status epilepticus as long as weeks after the discontinuation.

Initial Clinical Evaluation

The patient should receive a thorough physical examination focusing on each of the following systems:

1. Peripheral vascular system. Auscultate carotid arteries for bruits and blood pressure in both arms for comparison.
2. Heart. A thorough cardiac workup is essential, starting with careful auscultation and a 12-lead ECG. It is especially important to check for murmurs and dysrhythmias, because persons with atrial fibrillation, acute myocardial infarction, or valvular heart disease may develop further obstructive emboli.

3. Retina. Look for cupping of optic disk, retinal hemorrhages, diabetic changes.
4. Extremities. Evaluate for cyanosis and infarcts as signs of peripheral emboli.
5. Neurologic examination. Nature of intactness is necessary to determine site and extent of a stroke.

Imaging Techniques

Advances in both CT and MRI technologies have greatly enhanced the accurate diagnosis of acute ischemic stroke. When combined perfusion CT and CT angiography are performed within 24 hours of stroke onset, there is improved accuracy of early infarct localization, vascular localization, and diagnosis of etiology (Ezzedine et al, 2001). It remains difficult to differentiate between embolic and thrombotic causes of ischemic strokes.

A refinement of MRI technology is *diffusion-weighted imaging (DWI)*, which is based on detecting random movements of protons in water molecules. This movement is restricted within cells but is unrestricted in the extracellular space. In stroke, when neural tissue is ischemic, cellular membrane integrity is disrupted, affecting the freedom of water molecules to move about. As a result of the alteration in molecular movement, injured neural tissue can be detected by DWI, which shows infarcted areas as bright white. This technique is extremely sensitive, revealing perfusion abnormalities in more than 95% of patients with demonstrated strokes (Szabo et al (2001). It is especially helpful in early identification of acute lesions, making possible determination of number, size, location, and vascular territory of brain lesions. There is good evidence that DWI is also helpful in diagnosing late secondary stroke injury that may not show imaging abnormalities in the first few hours after a clinically definite acute cerebral ischemic episode (Kidwell, Saver, Mattiello, 2001).

Perfusion-weighted imaging (PWI) involves sequential scans over 30 seconds following injection of gadolinium. Brain areas that are underperfused have delayed appearance of injected contrast dye, with low blood flow appearing as white. Serial scans may reveal three different types of patterns: early reperfusion, delayed reperfusion, and persistent perfusion deficit (Ryan, 2000).

Standard laboratory analysis includes urinalysis, CBC, erythrocyte sedimentation rate (ESR), basic metabolic panel (sodium, potassium, chloride, bicarbonate, glucose, blood urea nitrogen, and creatinine), serum lipid profile, and serology for syphilis. In patients with suspected ischemic stroke, it is standard care to obtain a laboratory panel that evaluates for hypercoagulable states. The usual tests are prothrombin with international normalized ratio (INR), partial thromboplastin time, and platelet count. Other tests that may be done are anticardiolipin antibodies, protein C and S, antithrombin III, plasminogen, Leiden V factor, and activated protein C resistance.

Techniques for Diagnosing and Evaluating Stroke Syndromes

Chest x-ray examination is a standard procedure because it may detect an enlarged heart (cardiomegaly) and any lung infiltrates associated with congestive heart failure.

Lumbar puncture involves examination of the CSF that will frequently give valuable clues to the cause of a stroke, especially when the patient arrives unresponsive and can give no history. For example, there may be blood in the CSF in hemorrhagic strokes, especially with subarachnoid hemorrhage. The information to be gained must be weighed against the risks of performing a lumbar puncture on a comatose patient. That is, with increased ICP, sudden reduction of CSF pressure at the low spinal level might precipitate downward movement of the cranial contents, with herniation into the brainstem and sudden death.

Carotid ultrasonography of the carotid arteries is standard evaluation to detect impaired carotid blood flow and the possibility of correcting the cause of the stroke.

Cerebral angiography can provide valuable information in diagnosing cause and location of stroke. Specifically, cerebral angiography can reveal ulcerative lesions, stenosis, fibromuscular dysplasia, arteriovenous fistula, vasculitis, and thrombus formation within major vessels. Currently, cerebral angiography is considered the most accurate means of identifying and measuring stenosis of the cerebral arteries; however, its usefulness is somewhat offset by complications that occur in up to 12% of individuals who have a suspected stroke. Principal risks from the procedure are dissection of the aortic or carotid artery and embolization from large vessels to the intracranial vessels. Therefore the advantages of gaining important diagnostic information must be weighed against the possibility of extending the stroke when the injected contrast medium displaces the blood flow. In general, angiography is usually reserved for patients with TIAs in the anterior part of the circle of Willis, because the problem may be surgically correctable. However, angiography is not done for patients with signs and symptoms of posterior circulation lesions, because these lesions are not surgically accessible (Wiederholt, 2000).

Transcranial Doppler, which is ultrasonography that combines imaging and sound, enables the assessment of flow within arteries and can identify stenosis that is impeding flow to the brain. This type of technology, called transcranial Doppler (TCD), can also be used to assess collateral blood flow and total CBF across the anterior and posterior aspects of the circle of Willis. The advantage of this procedure is that it can be performed at the bedside, is noninvasive, and is less costly; it also can be done serially to assess for changes in CBF pattern. The latter capability is especially crucial in monitoring onset and resolution of arterial vasospasm following intracranial bleeds.

Positron emission tomography (PET) scanning may be helpful because it can identify the extent to which areas of the brain are receiving and metabolizing glucose and the extent of injury. Thus areas of decreased perfusion can be identified.

Transesophageal echocardiogram (TEE) is especially sensitive in detecting potential cardioembolic sources (Narayanan et al, 2000). Echocardiograms have become a routine component of ischemic stroke evaluations when cardioembolic causes of stroke are suspected but atrial fibrillation has been ruled out as an explanatory cause of embolization. Structural defects revealed by TEE, and associated with cardiac thrombi and subsequent embolization, are mitral or aortic valve vegetations, atrial septal defect, patent foramen ovale, protruding aortic plaque, and abnormal mitral valve.

ACUTE STROKE THERAPY

Because of the cascade of metabolic changes that produce neuronal damage for variable periods after the actual cessation of flow to a brain area, stroke is an evolving event. Therefore rapid intervention is essential to reduce morbidity and mortality. One of the most important tasks of clinicians in the face of acute focal, nonconvulsive neurologic deficit is to determine whether its cause is hemorrhage or ischemia-infarction. The emergency treatment differs for the two types of stroke, because treatment for thrombus formation can exacerbate the bleed with a hemorrhagic CVA. The approaches to emergency treatment involve three goals: (1) prevent acute brain injury by restoring perfusion to noninfarcted ischemic areas, (2) reverse neuronal injury to the extent possible, and (3) prevent future neurologic injury by protecting cells in the ischemic penumbral area from further damage by the glutamate cascade.

Therapies that have demonstrated effectiveness in preserving brain function and minimizing neuronal damage after ischemic stroke are (1) aspirin administered within 48 hours, (2) thrombolytic therapy administered within 3 hours, and (3) intensive care in specialized stroke units. In these units, carotid stenting has been fairly successful in restoring perfusion to affected brain areas when atherosclerosis with thrombosis is the precipitating cause of low flow. Because acute strokes commonly are associated with cardiac dysfunction and arrhythmia, ECG monitoring is initiated on admission to the acute care setting. It has been shown that, in moderate to large ischemic or hemorrhagic stroke, the QT interval is frequently prolonged, a finding that is known to be associated with fatal dysrhythmias. Therefore the use of medications that increase the QT interval are contraindicated in persons with acute stroke (Afsar, 2001).

The optimal approach to management of intracerebral hemorrhage is still debatable. Early expansion of the hemorrhage is a major contributor to death and disability, and there are no reliable interventions to prevent it. After the acute period of the stroke, chronic antihypertensive medication should be started.

Medical Treatment

Neuroprotection

In acute ischemic stroke, much of the neuronal tissue injury may be reversible within a certain window of time. Preserving the function of the tissue is the goal of so-called *neuroprotective* strategies. Hypothermia is a long-used effective neuroprotective therapy in cases of brain trauma and continues to be studied in stroke. The mode of action is to lower the metabolic activity and thereby the oxygen requirements of neuronal cells. Neurons are thereby protected from further damage resulting from continued hypoxia or the excitotoxicity that may result from the glutamine cascade that typically follows neuronal cell injury. The Cleveland Clinic has studied use of cooling blankets and ice water baths within 8 hours of symptom onset and maintaining hypothermia to 89.6° F

for 12 to 72 hours while the patient is on life support. During rehabilitation, patients given hypothermic treatment tended to have less disability (Rankin scale) and smaller infarcted areas compared with a control group (Abou-Chebl et al, 2001).

Another approach to tissue preservation is the use of neuroprotective medications. A great deal of stroke research has tested medications that can lower the metabolism of neurons, prevent the release of toxic substances from damaged neurons, or minimize the damaging hyperexcitatory response of neurons in the ischemic penumbra surrounding the infarcted area of a stroke. Expanding knowledge regarding the pathophysiology of ischemic brain cell injury has led researchers to focus on the development of calcium antagonists, glutamate antagonists, antioxidants, and other types of neuroprotective agents. The challenge in attempting postinsult neuroprotection is to find an agent that is selective for ischemic neurons, that is, with a good therapeutic index (lethal dose ÷ therapeutic dose) (Salazar, Fulmor, Srinivas, 2000). Various agents have been tested, including a nitroxide (Leker et al, 2000). A promising neuroprotective agent, cerebrolysin (CERE) has effects on neuronal calcium metabolism and also exhibits neurotrophic effects (Ladurner, 2001). Many different kinds of drugs and compounds are in various stages of development for the prevention and acute interventional treatment of stroke. Given the multidimensional and sequential nature of ischemic brain cell injury, it is likely that no single drug will be able to completely protect the brain during stroke; most likely, a combination of agents will be necessary for full recovery potential.

Anticoagulation

The European Stroke Initiative (2000) recommends that oral anticoagulation (INR 2.0 to 3.0) is indicated after stroke caused by atrial fibrillation. A higher level of anticoagulation (INR 3.0 to 4.0) is required for stroke patients who have mechanical prosthetic valves. For patients who are not candidates for warfarin (Coumadin) therapy, aspirin alone or an aspirin-dipyridamole combination may be used as initial antithrombotic therapy for stroke prophylaxis.

Intravenous Thrombolysis

The only drug that has received approval from the U.S. Food and Drug Administration (FDA) for acute ischemic stroke treatment is a recombinant form of tissue plasminogen activator (TPA). With its approval in June 1996, TPA became possible to abort brain injury, and the age-adjusted national death rate for stroke declined 1.1% from 1995 (Peters et al, 1998). This success resulted in intense efforts to educate the public and health care professionals that stroke is an emergency and that acute stroke symptoms should be treated with the same urgency as a gunshot wound to the head. Thus treatment with intravenous TPA continues to be the standard of care for acute stroke within the first three hours after symptom onset (National Institutes of Health [NIH], 1995). However, only 1% to 2% of patients currently receive therapy, usually because they present to emergency care too late to be treated within the recommended 3-hour time window. The greatest risk of using thrombolytic treatment is intracerebral hemorrhage. Therefore the therapy must be used only on patients who have been carefully screened and who meet none of the following exclusion criteria:

- CT evidence of intracranial bleeding an expanding mass
- Angiogram that is negative for presence of a clot
- Elevated prothrombin time/INR, indicating bleeding tendencies
- Presence of partially-healed wounds and vessels from recent surgery or trauma
- Very high diastolic blood pressure; loss of autoregulation is a major risk

In addition, persons with a history of recent cocaine or amphetamine use often are excluded because of the risk of bleeding from cerebral vessels under high pressure.

Intraarterial Thrombolysis

The use of intraarterial thrombolysis for patients with acute ischemic stroke is undergoing study, though it is not currently approved by the FDA (Furlan et al, 1999). Patients with a greater risk of hemorrhage from this therapy are those with higher National Institute of Health Stroke Scale (NIHSS) scores, longer times to vessel recanalization, higher serum glucose levels, and lower platelet counts (Kidwell et al, 2001).

Perfusion Therapy

Similar to efforts used to restore cerebral circulation in the case of vasospasm during recovery from subarachnoid hemorrhage, induced hypertension has been tried in an attempt to elevate mean arterial blood pressure and thereby increase cerebral perfusion (Hillis et al, 2001).

Control of Edema and General Medical Therapy

Cerebral edema occurs in most ischemic cerebral infarctions, especially with large vessel involvement in the territory of the middle cerebral artery. Conservative therapy consists of keeping the patient slightly dehydrated, with a normal or slightly elevated serum sodium.

Surgical Treatment

Surgical decompression is a drastic intervention that is still undergoing clinical trials and is reserved for the most massive strokes. In this procedure, one side of the skull is removed (a hemicraniectomy), allowing infarcted, edematous brain tissue to expand without being confined within the rigid bony structure of the skull. Thus the procedure prevents pressure on and distortion of vital surviving tissue and brainstem structures.

More conservative surgical procedures are routinely used in patients with CVA. The proper selection of the individual who will most benefit from surgery remains a difficult task. Improving CBF is the primary goal of surgical intervention. *Carotid endarterectomy (CEA)* is performed to improve cerebral circulation (Fig. 53-7). Patients undergoing this procedure frequently have other complicating problems, such as hypertension, diabetes mellitus, and widespread cardiovascular disease. The procedure is performed with the patient under general anesthesia so that good airway and ventilatory control can be maintained. A temporary shunt is used to minimize ischemia to the brain. It is essential to maintain a normal or slightly high arterial blood pressure to maintain adequate cerebral circulation, because regional blood flow in these

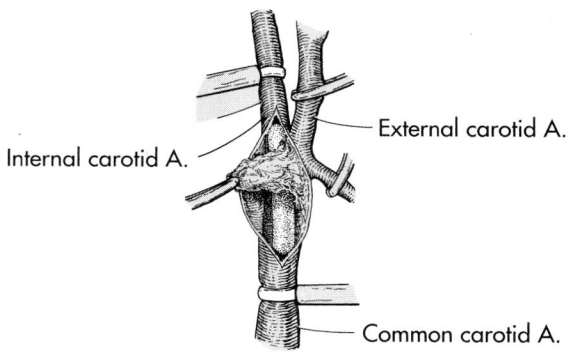

FIG. 53-7 Diagram of a carotid endarterectomy. A bypass tube is used during the removal of an atherosclerotic lesion at the carotid bifurcation.

patients is directly proportional to the systemic arterial pressure. *Revascularization procedures* are performed to increase regional blood flow to areas where circulation is compromised. Revascularization is primarily a prophylactic procedure and is most likely to benefit patients with TIAs or those who are at an early stage in the course of a thrombosis-in-evolution. Patients with fixed neurologic deficits can expect no benefit from these procedures and are not considered appropriate candidates.

Surgical intervention in the case of aneurysms is directed toward prevention of a recurrence of the hemorrhage. Ligation of the common carotid artery in the neck is the most conservative treatment of aneurysm. *Intracranial procedures*, such as clipping or ligating the neck of the aneurysm, necessitate major neurosurgical intervention. Aneurysms can also be painted with a physiologic glue, which provides an elastic cap and keeps them from rupturing. Before surgery can be undertaken, arteriograms are necessary. Arteriograms are a serious threat to the patient because (1) the dye, as with the original free blood, can cause vasospasm because of irritation, and (2) the pressure necessary to insert the dye may cause rebleeding in the newly ruptured area. The patient must be stabilized before surgery. The vasospasm must be resolved or minimized. Toward this end, the patient is placed on an aneurysm protocol, which may include the following precautions adapted to the individual patient:

1. Darkened room. No rectal temperatures are taken, because this may stimulate the vagus nerve and elevate blood pressure.
2. Phenobarbital given intravenously decreases possibility of seizures.
3. Dexamethasone (Decadron) for its diuretic effect. Dexamethasone also seems to protect the brain by stabilizing cerebral membranes and decreasing cerebral edema.
4. A H2-receptor blocker or proton-pump inhibitor to prevent the gastrointestinal irritation that may be a side effect of dexamethasone administration.
5. Aminocaproic acid (Amicar) to prevent lysis of the clot. Aminocaproic acid levels, streptokinase levels, and clot lysis times are monitored daily.
6. Hydralazine hydrochloride (Apresoline), for blood pressure stabilization, if blood pressure is greater than 140 mm Hg systolic.
7. Fluid restriction based on serum osmolality; may be as severe as 800 to 1200 ml/24 hours.

Various shunt procedures may be performed (ventriculoatrial shunt) if obstructive hydrocephalus is present. Free blood in the subarachnoid space may obstruct CSF circulation and cause acute hydrocephalus. Shunts are used more frequently than they were in the past and generally have replaced the decompression craniotomies formerly done to reduce the symptoms of increased ICP. Research continues on therapies that may save vital brain tissue that is compromised during the ischemic or hemorrhagic event. These therapies include calcium channel blocker medications, platelet inhibitors, thrombolytic agents, free-radical scavengers, and hemodilution.

STROKE RECOVERY

Phenomenon of Brain Plasticity

Many studies have divided the process of recovery from stroke into stages. Initially, there is a reperfusion of ischemic tissue accompanied by cessation of the glutamine-induced inflammatory changes that can lead to further neuronal injury. Functional loss should regress as neurons in the former ischemic penumbra start to recover. Then, in the days and weeks after an acute stroke, the brain begins the laborious process of recouping lost functions (Azari, Seitz, 2000). This process of relearning function depends on the amazing ability of the brain to reorganize itself (a phenomenon called "*plasticity*") in learning a task or during recovery from injury. Plasticity is a unique capacity that distinguishes the nervous system from all other tissues in the body, because neuronal tissue does not have the ability of other tissues to regenerate. The brain's plasticity is greatest from infancy through early adolescence, during which time many of the neural pathways to be used for language and motor skills are formed.

Ongoing ability to learn new languages and skills in adulthood indicates that the brain retains some plasticity throughout a person's lifetime (Azari, Seitz, 2000). Learning in the uninjured brain involves what is called "neural networks" that are organized for specialized tasks and that are normally located in the same discrete area of the brain. A familiar example is the motor cortex (concerned with voluntary muscle control), which is predictably located just anterior to the central sulcus in the frontal lobe. Similarly, the neuronal center for vision is located in the occipital cortex. Because of the phenomenon of plasticity, these specialized regions may develop to various degrees in different individuals, largely through interactions with the person's environment; their basic locations on the "cortical map," however, remain predictable from person to person (see Fig. 50-18).

Role of Brain Plasticity in Recovery from Stroke

Remarkably, brains that have experienced neuronal damage appear to exhibit an alternative form of functional reorganization called "*adaptive plasticity*" (Azari, Seitz, 2000). The recruitment mechanism has been demonstrated in persons with neuronal damage resulting from chronic degenerative changes, as well as in persons following acute injury such as stroke and head trauma. Thus researchers have discovered through the use of positron emission tomography (PET) scanning that adults with aphasia caused by stroke in Broca's area of the left hemisphere can use mirror-image areas in the right hemisphere to initiate language (Heiss et al, 1999). This type of plasticity involves recruitment of cortex that is within the same system as the damaged brain area. It may also involve the use of compensatory pathways from the newly recruited area to the spinal cord. Azari and Seitz (2000) have also discovered that some persons with stroke injury recruit neural networks in regions of the brain that normally are not involved in motor function. For example, persons with stroke-induced paresis (weakness) were found to use parts of the occipital (visual) cortex, as well as additional parts of the motor cortex, when they attempted to perform a motor task such as finger movement. This adaptation is an apparent compensatory mechanism in which the brain can allocate functions such as speech and movement outside their primary anatomic boundaries in the cerebral cortex. Neuroscientists refer to this process of recruiting nonprimary cortex in recovery from stroke dysfunction as "*cross-modal plasticity*" (Cohen et al, 1999).

The process of recruiting neurons within the same system as the damaged area seems to occur more readily than the process of cross-modal plasticity. Therefore, in less damaged brain areas, the process of functional recovery occurs more quickly, even within a few weeks. However, in areas with actual neuronal infarction, it may take the damaged areas much longer to recruit new brain areas and then to relearn a task. Hence further recovery can occur long after the actual stroke event occurred.

The development of functional imaging techniques has made it possible to pinpoint sites of neural activity in the intact living brain when a person is performing specific tasks. The most widely used of these techniques in research and clinical studies are *PET* and *functional MRI (fMRI)*. PET techniques make use of a property of radioactive tracers, which is to emit positrons. The positron particles are localized and measured by a detection device that is positioned around the subject's head. In contrast, fMRI derives its images from the differing responses of oxygenated and deoxygenated hemoglobin to magnetic fields. Both PET and fMRI yield data that are translated into images of cross-sectional slices of the brain taken at several different levels. Computer techniques then combine the data contained in the slices to produce three-dimensional images of the brain. In addition to studying functional neuronal areas in uninjured brains, fMRI and PET have been used to identify areas of cortical injury and disease. Another, newer, application of the technology is to reveal areas that are active during task completion by persons who have had a stroke. This new technique explains how scientists have learned about the phenomenon of plasticity and the progressive recruitment of functioning brain areas during particular tasks. It is possible that fMRIs may prove useful in helping to evaluate stages of recovery and the efficacy of rehabilitation measures in effecting functional recovery.

GRADING STROKE SEVERITY

Neurorehabilitative Protocols

The neuromuscular spasticity following stroke results in major impaired functional ability. Many different kinds of treatments have been used to alleviate spasticity, including physical therapy, medications, electrical stimulation, and surgery. Researchers have attempted to evaluate strokes in terms of whether tissue is salvageable with therapeutic interventions (Evans, 2000). An innovative attempt to provide precise diagnostic criteria and guidance for therapy compares the defect size detected by *magnetic resonance diffusion-weighted imaging (MR DWI)* with defect size revealed by *MR perfusion-weighted imaging (MR PWI)*. The comparison is based on the theory that DWI measures infarcted tissue, and PWI defects indicate blood flow deficits. If the area of abnormality on DWI is smaller than that on PWI (DWI <PWI), the cerebral tissue is at risk for infarction because of an energy deficit. That is, a larger area of tissue has poor perfusion and is dysfunctional than is infarcted. In this case, the tissue may be salvageable via therapeutic interventions to restore perfusion.

If blood flow is not reestablished, the final infarct size will be larger. DWI less than PWI has been found to be the predominant pattern in acute stroke, with the mismatch declining over the initial 24 hours poststroke. However, if DWI is larger than PWI, partial or complete reperfusion may have occurred, with flow already reestablished to the remaining viable tissue. With matched defects (DWI = PWI), the likelihood of improvement is poor also, because all of the tissue that has been underperfused has infarcted. In summary, unless the area of infarct (DWI) is smaller than the area of perfusion deficit (PWI), the opportunity to limit and prevent extension of infarct size is minimal.

Recently, characteristics of these imaging techniques have been found to be useful in evaluating the effectiveness of stroke therapy and even in making prognoses about recovery. Baird and colleagues (2001) have developed and tested a "Stroke Recovery Scale" that uses three predictors: National Institute of Health Stroke Scale (NIHSS) score, time between stroke onset and MR DWI, and the volume of ischemic brain tissue measured on MR DWI. The quantitative results of two predictors (NIHSS score and time from onset to imaging) are grouped into three groups, and one predictor (DWI lesion volume) is dichotomized into two groups. Points are then assigned to each category, with zero the lowest possible total score and 7 the highest. The scoring is interpreted as follows: 1 to 3, low likelihood of good recovery; 3 to 4 medium likelihood; 5 to 7, high likelihood of good recovery. At 3 to 6 months post-CVA, the standard against which the Stroke Recovery Scale was tested was the Barthel score, an assessment of 10 activities of daily living. Tested sensitivity is only 77%, and specificity is 70%. Therefore, although further refinement and testing of the new scale is needed, its development illustrates the potential usefulness of imaging techniques as early predictors of eventual stroke recovery.

STROKE PREVENTION

Primary Prevention of Stroke

The approach in primary prevention is prevention and treatment of modifiable risk factors. Hypertension is the most prevalent of these, and it has been shown that its re-

duction has an extremely high impact on the risk of stroke. Recent attention has focused on the importance of isolated systolic hypertension (ISH), which is now considered a major risk factor for stroke (Domanski et al, 1999). It has been found that active treatment of ISH significantly reduces the risk of stroke, particularly in older adults. In one randomized clinical trial, persons with ISH taking the calcium channel blocker nitrendipine (Cardif, Nitrepin) showed a 42% reduction in fatal and nonfatal stroke over an average 2-year interval (JNC VI, 1997; Staessen et al, 1997).

The European Stroke Initiative (ESI, 2000) has published recommendations for stroke management that reflect current practice. The most detailed and well-studied primary prevention recommendation is that oral anticoagulation should be used as primary prophylaxis for all patients with atrial fibrillation who are at high risk for stroke—persons with hypertension, age older than 75, systemic embolism, or decreased left ventricular function. The ESI recommended a target INR of 2.5 for anticoagulation. The INR target is lower (2.0) for persons older than age 75, who have a higher risk of cerebral hemorrhage. Because atrial fibrillation increases the risk of having a stroke nearly fivefold, anticoagulation in this population is extremely important. A second important primary prevention approach is to consider carotid endarterectomy (CEA) in symptomatic patients with carotid bruits, especially with stenosis of 60% to 90%.

Good diabetic management is another important factor in primary stroke prevention. Prolonged elevated glucose levels are associated strongly with endothelial cell dysfunction, which, in turn, triggers eventual development of atherosclerosis (Laight et al, 1999). In addition, a newly recognized component of the metabolic abnormalities in diabetes mellitus is a so-called prothrombic state in which there are elevated levels of plasminogen activator inhibitor-1 (PAI-1) (Bastard et al, 2000). The tendency to abnormal clot production is further accelerated by insulin resistance, resulting in heightened tendency to intravascular coagulation (Laakso, 1999).

There are two major approaches to stroke prevention: (1) public health or population strategy and (2) the high-risk strategy. The population strategy is based on legislation and fiscal and educational programs targeting reduction of risky behaviors in the entire population. The high-risk strategy directs efforts at persons who have an above-average risk of a stroke event. To be most cost effective, the high-risk approach must be based on a person's baseline (absolute) risk of an event rather than based on age alone or a consideration of the relative risk associated with a single risk factor. In all age groups and in all risk categories, women have a lower absolute risk than men.

Secondary Prevention of Stroke

Secondary prevention refers to strategies to prevent recurrence of stroke. The main approaches are control of hypertension, CEA, and the use of antiplatelet antiaggregant medications. Studies such as the European Stroke Prevention Study of antiplatelet antiaggregant drugs (Diener, 1996) and numerous meta-analyses of glycoprotein IIb/IIIa inhibitor medications clearly show the efficacy of platelet antiaggregant medications in preventing recurrent stroke (Albers et al, 2001). Aggrenox is the only combination of aspirin and dipyridamole that has been demonstrated to be effective for secondary stroke prevention.

STROKE RESEARCH

A promising area of basic stroke research is the area of stem cell transplants to promote recovery from cerebrovascular damage. Stem cells—found primarily in bone marrow and in embryonic tissue—have the ability to develop into any of the body's organ cells, including neurons. Neuroscience investigators refer to cells with this potential as being "omnipotential" or "pluripotential"—that is, possessing the ability to develop into a variety of different cells, depending on stimulus and nurturing environment. Thus rat research has shown that stem cells transplanted into both healthy and stroke-injured adult rats develop into neurons. These stem cells grew in the area of stroke damage and formed connections with adjacent cells in as little as 3 to 6 weeks (Gupta et al, 2001). Further research will depend on whether there is sufficient support at the national levels to support research programs on the use of stem cells or any fetal tissue.

𝒦EY CONCEPTS

- *Cerebrovascular disease* (stroke) is the third leading cause of death (after heart disease and cancer) in the United States; it is also a leading cause of neurologic disability.
- The same risk factors for atherosclerotic heart disease are also *risk factors for stroke*.
- The *most important modifiable risk factor* for both *ischemic* and *hemorrhagic stroke* is hypertension.
- The brain requires a constant supply of glucose and oxygen, which is delivered by the circulation and requires 15% of the cardiac output and 20% of the body's total oxygen consumption.
- The *normal adult cerebral blood flow (CBF)* is about 50 ml/100 mg of brain tissue per minute and remains constant over a wide range of blood pressure and intracranial pressure (ICP) because of autoregulation of cerebral vascular resistance.
- Four large arteries supply the brain with blood: *two internal carotid arteries* and *two vertebral arteries* (which join the basilar artery to form the *vertebrobasilar system*).
- The carotid arteries provide the major part of the blood supply to the cerebral hemispheres; the main vessels supplying the brainstem and cerebellum are derived from the vertebrobasilar system.
- The *penetrating cerebral arteries*, derived from the conducting cerebral arteries, enter the brain at right angles and supply blood to the deep structures of the brain, such as the internal capsule and basal ganglia.
- The anatomy of the *circle of Willis* plays an important role in modulating the size and location of ischemic lesions because the circle, via its communicating arteries, helps to provide a well-distributed collateral circulation to the brain in the event of the occlusion of one of the carotid arteries.
- *Anatomic variations in the circle of Willis* are common—only about 50% of the population have "normal" circles of Willis, and the prevalence of such variations are even more common in patients who have had a stroke.
- The *ophthalmic artery* provides a route for collateral circulation between the external and internal carotid arteries.
- The degree of metabolic activity in the brain is more or less constant and consequently the *CBF* needs to be regulated within relatively narrow limits (about 50 ml/100 g brain tissue/min).
- *Irreversible brain damage* occurs when cerebral perfusion drops below a certain critical level, when there is insufficient oxygen in the blood or when there is a combination of both these factors.
- *Autoregulation* maintains CBF at near normal levels despite a wide variation in mean arterial pressure (MAP). Both pressure-related and metabolic factors contribute to autoregulation.
- When MAP drops, the cerebral arterioles dilate, ensuring adequate CBF despite low arterial pressures. Conversely, cerebral arterioles constrict with high distending pressures, thereby preventing the delivery of high systemic arterial pressure to brain tissue. This *autoregulatory response* is effective over a MAP range between 60 and 160 mm Hg.
- *Cerebral arterioles* also change their caliber in response to pH and blood gas levels. *Hypercapnia, acidemia,* and *hypoxemia* lead to vasodilation and thus to an increase in CBF and ICP; *hypocapnia* and *alkalosis* cause vasoconstriction and a decrease in CBF and ICP.
- *Autoregulation of CBF* may fail as a result of brain injury or extremes of blood pressure (as may occur in stroke); when this failure occurs, vasomotor tone diminishes and CBF becomes passively dependent on changes in the systemic blood pressure.
- *Autoregulation* within the cerebral circulation is mediated by changes in arteriolar resistance for the purpose of maintaining CBF within the normal range and protecting the brain against sudden increases or decreases in systemic blood pressure.
- *Stroke* refers to any sudden neurologic insult that results from restriction or cessation of CBF; cerebral infarction is the specific meaning. *Cerebral vascular accident (CVA)* and *brain attack* are frequently used synonyms for stroke.
- There are two basic categories of circulatory impairment leading to stroke—ischemia-infarction and intracranial hemorrhage—accounting for about 85% and 15% of strokes respectively.
- Four *general pathophysiologic mechanisms of stroke* are (1) disease state of the blood vessel itself (e.g., atherosclerosis with thrombus formation), (2) decreased

perfusion from impaired flow states, (3) blood flow occlusion by an embolus, and (4) vascular rupture.

- *Transient ischemic attacks (TIAs)* are distinguished from full-blown strokes in that the focal neurologic deficits occurring are fully reversible and usually last no more than a few minutes (but occasionally may last up to 24 hours).

- *TIAs* are important as a warning sign of impending stroke because they precede thrombotic strokes in 50% to 75% of affected patients.

- *Subclavian steal* may cause a vertebrobasilar TIA if the subclavian artery is obstructed (usually by an atherosclerotic plaque). Exercise of the left arm may draw blood in a retrograde fashion down the left vertebral artery to the distal subclavian artery, thus causing cerebral ischemia.

- *Lacunar strokes* are caused by thrombosis and occlusion of the *small penetrating arteries of the brain* that supply the basal ganglia and hemispheric white matter, as well as the brainstem; hypertension and diabetes are major risk factors.

- Lacunar infarction is common in the distribution of *lenticulostriate branches* of the middle cerebral artery.

- Lacunar infarcts are generally very small (< 1 cm in diameter) and may or may not result in fixed focal neurologic deficits.

- The majority of *thrombotic strokes* are caused by thrombosis complicating atherosclerosis; the most common sites of involvement are at the carotid bifurcation, origin of the middle cerebral artery, and at either end of the basilar artery.

- A majority of *thrombotic strokes* occur during sleep and the evolution of signs and symptoms tends to be gradual over several days from the onset.

- *Sudden, severe reduction in systemic blood pressure* can reduce CBF and precipitate a stroke, especially in patients with a stenotic atherosclerotic lesion and compensatory hypertension.

- Most *emboli* causing a stroke are derived from thrombi; the most common origin is the heart or from an atherosclerotic lesion.

- The territory of distribution of the *middle cerebral artery* is the brain region most commonly affected by embolic infarction.

- *Embolic strokes* typically occur during waking activities and produce sudden neurologic deficits with their maximum effects at the onset.

- In ischemic stroke there is a loss of autoregulation and chemoregulation in the *ischemic penumbra* surrounding the ischemic core (area of focal infarct) so that CBF to the penumbra varies with systemic blood pressure. Consequently, a decrease in MAP or an elevation of the Pa_{CO_2} (acidosis) will cause blood to be stolen away from the ischemic area to surrounding normal brain tissue resulting in enlargement of the infarcted area.

- The *ischemic cascade in stroke* resulting in focal infarction is triggered by anaerobic metabolism, which leads to cellular acidosis, decreased ATP formation, sodium-potassium pump failure, intracellular accumulation of Ca^{++}, Na^+, Cl^-, and water, causing cellular edema.

- *Excitotoxicity* results from the excess release of the neurotransmitter *glutamate*, which, in turn, activates NMDA receptors, increasing intracellular levels of Ca^{++} and activation of enzymes and mediators that ultimately cause neuronal death.

- The signs and symptoms of an *ischemic stroke* vary depending on the location of the artery occluded and the extent of the spared collateral flow.

- In ischemic strokes involving the *carotid system, unilateral signs predominate*—hemiparesis or hemiplegia, hemihypesthesia, hemianopsia, aphasia, and agnosia; when the *vertebrobasilar system* is involved, *bilateral signs* are more commonly found—motor or sensory (or both)—in combination with a disturbance of cranial nerves, cerebellum, or other structures in or related to the brainstem.

- *Episodic blindness in one eye (amaurosis fugax)* is a common manifestation of ipsilateral occlusion of the *carotid artery* and the ophthalmic artery branch to the retina in a TIA.

- The hallmark presentation of an *ischemic stroke* involving the *middle cerebral artery* is the abrupt onset of a contralateral hemiparesis or monoparesis (usually affecting the arm), contralateral hemianesthesia, global aphasia if the dominant hemisphere is involved, dysphasia, and homonymous hemianopsia; when collateral circulation limits the ischemia to a part of the territory, only some of the signs and symptoms are present.

- Occlusion of the *vertebrobasilar artery* circulation results in weakness in one to four extremities, increased tendon reflexes, bilateral Babinski's signs, ataxia, dizziness, syncope, dysphagia, dysarthria, and visual disturbances (e.g., dimming of vision, diplopia, ptosis, nystagmus).

- Spontaneous intracranial hemorrhage resulting in a stroke is caused by *intracerebral (parenchymal) hemorrhage* and *subarachnoid hemorrhage (SAH)*.

- The most common cause of *intracerebral (parenchymal) hemorrhage* is hypertensive vascular damage.

- Subarachnoid hemorrhage is most often caused by a ruptured *Berry aneurysm* or head trauma and less commonly by an *arteriovenous malformation (AVM)*.

- Cocaine and amphetamines are usually associated with hemorrhagic stroke in the younger adult.

- A *careful history and physical examination* with a thorough search for contributing conditions are basic to the evaluation of cerebrovascular disease.

- Therapy in ischemic stroke is aided by a precise diagnosis that determines the primary vascular pathology and the extent and location of the stroke; CT scans, MRI, angiography, and ultrasonography are important brain imaging technologies.

- *Stroke* signs and symptoms should be *treated with the same urgency as a gunshot wound to the head.*

- The first priority of clinicians in the *acute management of stroke* is to determine whether its cause is ischemia-infarction or hemorrhage; a CT scan can accomplish this task. Thrombolytic therapy with TPA within a 3-hour time window from onset may abort brain injury in the case of a thromboembolitic cause but would exacerbate bleeding if the cause is hemorrhagic.

- The use of *medications that increase the QT interval are contraindicated* in persons with acute stroke because prolongation of the QT interval is associated with fatal dysrhythmias.
- *In the acute management of ischemic stroke, hypotension must be avoided* at all costs. Blood flow to the ischemic penumbra is dependent on systemic arterial blood pressure because of the loss of autoregulation.
- Recovery from stroke is aided in large measure by the phenomenon of brain "plasticity"—the process of neuronal reorganization that allows the brain to learn or relearn tasks.
- Good diabetic management is a crucial factor in primary stroke prevention.
- With a clinical picture of headache in the presence of an ischemic stroke, diagnostic tests are needed to de-

tect possible dissecting aneurysms in the neck and brainstem vessels.

- *Atrial fibrillation* can lead to microthrombi formation in the atria, producing the *risk of embolic stroke.* Therefore atrial fibrillation must be treated urgently and prophylactic anticoagulation initiated.
- The Hunt and Hess scale is a tool used widely in clinical care and research to classify the severity of SAH. Other stroke scales are available that assess the degree of disability, level of functioning, and progress in rehabilitation.
- A "Stroke Recovery Scale" uses a clinical evaluation score, time elapsed since symptoms onset, and MRI results to evaluate effectiveness of stroke treatment and to make prognoses about recovery.

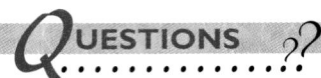

QUESTIONS ??

A sampling of review questions for this chapter appears here. Visit http://www.mosby.com/MERLIN/PriceWilson/ for additional questions. MERLIN

Answer the following on a separate piece of paper.

1. What is a stroke?
2. Differentiate between a thrombotic stroke and an embolic stroke with respect to clinical features.
3. What are the clinical features of a lacunar stroke?
4. What are the clinical features of a hemorrhagic stroke?
5. What is the role of antiplatelet agents in cerebrovascular disease?
6. What is the role of anticoagulation in cerebrovascular disease?
7. What is the role of endarterectomy in cerebrovascular disease?
8. What is the major purpose of clipping the neck of a Berry aneurysm located on the anterior communicating artery of the brain?

Neurologic Disorders
with Generalized Symptomatology

MARY S. HARTWIG

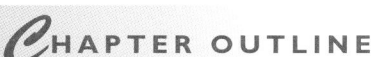

*D*iseases of the nervous system caused by primary pathology of the neuron unit traditionally have been classified as *degenerative,* implying a progressive downhill course. However, such use of that descriptor is neither precise nor exclusive. The term is not precise because some potentially devastating neuronal injuries such as those found in Guillain-Barré syndrome may resolve completely; it is not exclusive because some apparently degenerative diseases such as normal pressure hydrocephalus and multiinfarct dementia actually are caused by neuronal injury from long-standing secondary rather than primary causes (i.e., pressure and impaired blood supply). In addition, for many primary neurologic de-

fects, the cause is unknown or is under investigation. Therefore primary pathologic processes of the nervous system are classified here according to specific impairment of neurologic function. As a group, these diseases are described as neurologic disorders with generalized symptomatology.

DEMENTIAS

Primary Dementia: Alzheimer's Disease

The most common form of dementia, Alzheimer's disease (AD) is a degenerative, progressive disease of the brain that causes specific defects in neurons, resulting in impaired memory, thinking, and behavior. In normal aging, nerve cells in the brain are not lost in large numbers. In contrast, AD disrupts three key processes—nerve cell communication, metabolism, and repair. This disruption ultimately causes many nerve cells to stop functioning, lose connections with other nerve cells, and die. Initially, AD destroys neurons in parts of the brain that control memory, especially the hippocampus and related structures. As hippocampal nerve cells stop functioning properly, short-term memory fails, along with a person's ability to do easy and familiar tasks. AD also attacks the cerebral cortex, particularly the areas responsible for language and reasoning. Loss of language skills, decreased ability to make judgments, and personality changes occur. Emotional outbursts and disturbed behavior, such as wandering and agitation, begin to occur and become more and more frequent as the disease runs its course. Eventually, many other areas of the brain are involved, the regions atrophy, and the AD patient becomes bedridden, incontinent, unable to interact with others, and totally dependent on others to perform the most basic personal tasks, such as feeding, bathing, and toileting.

The rate of deterioration in functioning varies greatly from person to person. Life expectancy from the onset of symptoms until death ranges from 3 to 20 years, with an average of 8 years. Though it can occur as early as the fourth decade of life, AD primarily affects persons older than age 65 years. Current estimates are that 1 in 10 persons over age 65 and nearly one half of those over age 85 have AD. With the rapid expansion of the older population, it is estimated that 14 million persons will have AD by 2050. Costs to the U.S. economy are enormous: estimates of annual cost vary from $50 billion to at least $100 billion (*http://www.alz.org, 2001*). These cost estimates include lost business productivity as a result of caregiving by employees, costs of stress-related health problems for family members, and long-term care. Nursing homes already have felt the impact, with 50% of residents having AD or a related disorder.

AD is the most common dementing disorder, accounting for roughly 60% to 80% of all dementia patients in the United States. Vascular dementia (VaD), dementia with Lewy bodies (DLB), and frontotemporal dementia (FTD) together account for 15% to 20% of dementias, with other disorders (e.g., hydrocephalus; vitamin B_{12} deficiency) accounting for about 5% (Morris, 2000). The non-AD disorders may mimic AD or may coexist with AD or both (Box 54-1). However, current diagnostic measures do not provide a good means of discriminating among VaD, DLB, and FTD and AD.

Pathology and Pathogenesis

Macroscopically, the brain changes in AD involve a severe loss of hippocampal and cortical neurons, as well as amyloid depositions in intracranial blood vessels. Microscopically, there are morphologic (structural) and biochemical changes in neurons. *Morphologic changes* comprise two characteristic lesions that ultimately progress to degeneration of the soma (body) and/or the axons and dendrites of neurons (Fig. 54-1). One hallmark lesion in AD is the *neurofibrillary tangle*, an abnormal intracellular structure consisting of twisted, tangled threads composed chiefly of a protein called "tau." Within the central nervous system (CNS), tau proteins have been most widely studied as the structural building block that binds and stabilizes microtubules, which are essential components of the cytoskeleton (internal support framework) of the neuronal cell. Inside the neurons, microtubules form structures that guide nutrients and other molecules from the cell body to the ends of the axon, thus forming a communicating bridge with other neurons. In neurons of persons affected by AD, abnormal phosphorylation of the tau protein occurs, producing chemically changed tau that can no longer bind the microtubules together. (Ishihara et al, 1999). The abnormal tau twists into paired helical filaments that are wound around each other. With collapse of the internal transport system, intercellular communication malfunctions first, and cell death eventually follows. Formation of tangles and loss of neurons progress together as AD progresses.

The other characteristic lesion is *senile plaque*, composed mainly of amyloid-beta (A-beta) that forms in the tissue fluid surrounding neurons rather than inside the neuronal cell. A-beta is a fragment of a larger protein called amyloid precursor protein (APP), which is normally imbedded in the neuronal membrane and plays a role in the growth and survival of neurons. APP is cut into fragments by proteases, and one of the fragments is a "sticky" A-beta that evolves into poorly soluble clumps. The clumps eventually become mixed with portions of neurons and glial cells (especially microglia and astro-

---

BOX 54-1
Cause of Dementia

INFECTIONS
Neurosyphilis
Tuberculosis
Viral diseases

METABOLIC DISORDERS
Hypothyroidism
Electrolyte imbalance

NUTRITIONAL DEFICIENCIES
Vitamin B_{12} deficiency
Niacin deficiency
Korsakoff's deficiency (thiamine)

SPACE-OCCUPYING LESIONS
Subdural hematoma
Tumor
Abscess

BRAIN INFARCTS

TOXIC SUBSTANCES
Drugs
Alcohol
Arsenic

VASCULAR DISORDERS
Cerebral embolus
Cerebral vasculitis

MISCELLANEOUS
Parkinson's disease
Wilson's disease
Huntington's disease (chorea)
Depression
Previous head injuries

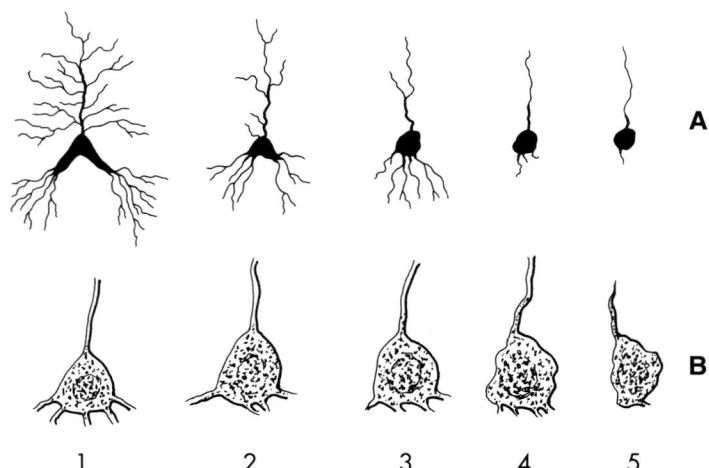

FIG. 54-1 Diagrammatic sketches of the progressive degenerative changes in neurons in Alzheimer's disease. The cell body and its processes become swollen and misshapen, and there is gradual loss of dendrites. **A,** Progressive loss of axonal and dendritic processes, and **B,** increasingly abnormal pathologic inclusions in cell bodies, distortion of the nucleus, and choking of the cytoplasmic space.

cytes). Over time, the A-beta mixture solidifies into fibrils that form mature, compact, insoluble plaques believed to be toxic to intact neurons. In addition, A-beta disrupts intercellular connections, reducing responsiveness of blood vessels, thus making neurons more susceptible to stressors such as ischemia. The presence of microglia in the plaque suggests that ongoing inflammation is involved in causing neuronal damage (Medscape, 2000). Another possibility is that A-beta generates free radicals (a type of molecule that easily reacts with other molecules, producing toxic chemical changes that damage other cells). Though tangles and plaques are not unique to AD, their abundance and widespread distribution in the brain are the hallmarks of this type of dementia.

Biochemical changes in the CNS are the other characteristic microscopic finding in AD. The cortex of the human brain contains large numbers of cholinergic axons that release acetylcholine, a key neurotransmitter in cognitive functioning. Because they heavily populate the cortex and hippocampus, cholinergic neurons are lost extensively in the degenerative changes that take place in AD. Neurochemically, the earliest and most prevalent abnormality in the brains of patients with AD is the depletion of cholinergic markers, such as choline acetyltransferase. Somatostatin may also be decreased, frequently to 50% of normal levels. Two currently approved medications for AD (tacrine (Cognex) and donepezil hydrochloride (Aricept) act by inhibiting acetylcholinesterase, an enzyme that normally breaks down acetylcholine. These drugs do not stop or reverse the progression of AD and appear to help only some patients with AD for a short period (months to 2 years).

There are two types of AD: *familial AD (FAD)*, which follows a specific inheritance pattern, and *sporadic AD*, in which there is no apparent inheritance pattern. AD is also described as early onset (symptoms first appear before age 65, most commonly in the age range of 30 to 60 years) and late onset (first symptoms at age 65 and older). *Early-onset AD* is rare (approximately 5% to 10% of cases), tends to run in families, and involves autosomal dominant, or inherited, mutations that are believed to be the actual cause of the disease. So far, three early onset genes with AD-causing mutations have been identified on three different chromosomes. These are mutations in the APP gene on chromosome 21, mutations (presenilin 1) in a gene on chromosome 14, and mutations (presenilin 2) in a gene on chromosome 1. If just one of these mutations is present in only one of the two genes inherited from the parent, the person will develop that form of early-onset AD. The *presenilin mutations* may cause neuronal degeneration by modifying beta-amyloid production or by stimulating the process of apoptosis, a process in which cells are genetically programmed to die.

There is no current evidence that the presenilin or APP mutations play a major role in the more common nonfamilial form of *late-onset AD*. This form of AD is associated with inheritance of at least one copy of the apolipoprotein E epsilon 4 (APOE ϵ4) allele on chromosome 19. Scientists have long suspected that more than one gene may be involved in increasing an individual's risk of developing late-onset AD. It is important to note, however, that the inheritance of APOE ϵ4 alleles is not a certain predictor of AD. In addition, some studies have shown that carrying an APOE ϵ4 allele is a greater predictor of AD in Caucasians than it is in Hispanics or African Americans (Tang et al, 1998; Reiman et al, 1996). Some reports have shown evidence of a risk factor gene on a region of chromosome 12, and international investigators are searching intensively for other genetic markers that might play a role in AD.

There are some parallels between AD and other neurologic disorders that also involve deposits of abnormal proteins in the brain. Among these disorders are prion diseases, frontotemporal dementia (FTD), Parkinson's disease, and Huntington's disease. *Prions*, infectious types of protein substances, have been demonstrated to be the pathologic trigger in diseases such as bovine spongiform encephalopathy ("mad cow" disease) in animals and Creutzfeldt-Jakob disease in humans. Both AD and prion diseases are characterized by formation of insoluble amyloid fibrils, though from different proteins. Investigators have found that in both Parkinson's and Huntington's disease, abnormal proteins and fibrils are formed that are similar to the varieties of fibrils found in AD and prion disease.

Researchers have explored numerous other factors implicated in triggering or sustaining the progression of AD. Such factors, believed to play a long-term role in brain and cognitive health, may be more amenable to disease modification than are genetic factors. One such factor is oxidative stress, caused by molecules called "free radicals" that are produced through normal metabolic mechanisms. *Free radicals* are highly reactive substances that can modify other molecules, such as deoxyribonucleic acid (DNA) and the phospholipids in cell membranes. The new molecule, in turn, becomes reactive and can release additional free radicals that further damage neurons. The neuronal toxicity may lead to AD through mechanisms such as alteration of protein structure in the cell wall and damage to the cell membrane that regulates flow of molecules between the extracellular fluid (ECF) and intracellular fluid (ICF).

Another factor implicated in AD is inflammation (Willare et al, 1999). Particularly intriguing is the evidence from the Baltimore Longitudinal Study of Aging that long-term use of nonsteroidal antiinflammatory drugs (NSAIDs) is associated with decreased prevalence of AD. A role for inflammatory processes is also suggested by the presence of microglia in the characteristic plaque and by a 1998 study (Griffin et al) that demonstrates how glia and neurons can interact in a vicious cycle to cause the neuronal changes seen in AD.

Closely related to the theories of oxidative stress and inflammation is that of long-term neuronal damage from brain infarction, areas of brain injury caused by interrupted blood supply to neurons. Snowdon and colleagues (1997) have conducted a longitudinal study of elderly nuns from the School Sisters of Notre Dame, including yearly physical and cognitive examinations and brain dissection after death. The study suggests that nuns with infarctions in specific brain areas had greater clinical dementia than would be expected from the extent of plaques and tangles in their cerebral tissue. A related avenue of investigation is whether other diseases (such as atherosclerosis and arteriosclerosis) that potentially decrease blood supply to the brain also influence the development of AD.

Even after intensive laboratory and clinical investigation of the disease, conclusive diagnosis of AD still depends on postmortem autopsy, in which characteristic plaques and tangles are found in specific regions of the brain. However, clinicians use several validated instruments to clinically diagnose "probable AD" in patients. These instruments include brain scans and tests that measure memory, language, and other cognitive skills, such as computation.

Clinical Features

Patients with the symptoms of dementia should be tested to detect potentially reversible nutritional, endocrine, and infectious causes for their symptoms. In addition to a complete physical and an extensive neurologic examination, diagnostic tests frequently ordered include complete blood count (CBC) and blood studies for syphilis, serum electrolytes, and vitamin B_{12}, as well as thyroid function tests. A computed tomography (CT) scan may show ventricular widening and cortical atrophy and confirms the absence of brain tumor, brain abscess, or chronic subdural hematoma, which are treatable. Other treatable causes of dementia must also be ruled out. Box 54-1 lists causes of dementia other than AD.

During the early stages of AD, the patient remains somewhat independent but experiences diminished problem-solving capacity, diminished ability to cope with complex situations and think abstractly, emotional lability, forgetfulness, apathy, and loss of recent memory. As the disease progresses, the patient's behavior becomes more erratic and bizarre, with a tendency toward wandering and violent outbursts. Family members must remain constantly vigilant to protect the person from harm. Deterioration is predictable and occurs over a 3- to 10-year period. During the later stages of the disease, patients become incontinent and are unable to attend to any of their basic needs or to recognize family members. Death is usually the result of malnutrition or infection.

Management of the patient with AD involves both the patient and the family. Tranquilizers and antidepressants may be useful in managing the patient's behavior. Experimental drugs are being used in some medical centers in an attempt to slow brain deterioration, but no approved drug therapy has been developed. Family support groups are essential to help families cope. Adult day-care centers, home health aides, and extended care facilities become indispensable to the family as the patient's condition deteriorates and total care is necessary. The challenge in the future will be to meet the needs of increasing numbers of these patients.

Secondary Dementias: Nutritional Degenerative Disease

Lack or deficiency of particular nutrients is known to have a deleterious effect on the brain. Several vitamins in particular are known to be essential for normal brain metabolism. Deficiencies of the B vitamins B_1, B_6, B_{12}, niacin, and pantothenic acid are associated with various neurologic disorders. Despite continued research, much remains unknown about the role of nutrition on the development of the nervous system and its healthy maintenance.

Alcoholism is a major problem in the United States. The alcoholic person is frequently the victim of severe nutritional deficiencies caused by decreased appetite, abusive drinking, and the presence of chronic illnesses, untreated infections, and anemia.

Wernicke-Korsakoff syndrome is associated with extensive alcohol abuse and nutritional deprivation (as in gastric carcinoma, thyrotoxicosis, and hyperemesis gravidarum). The term *cerebral beriberi* is used in reference to this disease. Pathologic changes involve necrosis of nerve cells and myelinated structures. Symptoms are related to the involved brain structures. Paralysis of gaze, nystagmus, and ataxia are caused by lesions in the midbrain, the cerebellar vermis, and the floor of the fourth ventricle. The psychologic symptoms, dull mentation, impairment of recent memory, and amnesia are generally caused by lesions of the thalamic nuclei and the hypothalamus. In addition, these patients have postural hypotension, dyspnea, tachycardia, cirrhosis of the liver, and anemia.

Thiamine is the therapy of choice for patients with Wernicke-Korsakoff syndrome. Improvement of symptoms varies; the disorders of mentation (apathy, inattentiveness, and listlessness) improve rapidly, whereas ataxia and nystagmus demonstrate slow but gradual improvement. Unfortunately, amnesia does not improve significantly.

CENTRAL MOTOR SYSTEM DISORDERS WITH MIXED SYMPTOMATOLOGY

Huntington's Disease

Huntington's disease (HD) is an uncommon inherited disease named for the American physician George Huntington, who first wrote about the illness in 1872. An earlier name for the disease was Huntington's "chorea," a Greek word for "dance." Chorea describes the constant, uncontrollable, writhing, twisting, and turning movements that progressively worsen throughout the course of the disease. However, some persons with adult-onset HD have severe rigidity and inability to move rather than chorea, thus the predominant symptom is akinesia. Patients experience a long, progressively debilitating course (10 to 25 years), eventually becoming completely bedridden, totally dependent for basic needs, and exhibiting socially problematic behaviors. The National Institute of Neurological Disorders and Stroke (NINDS, 2000) estimates that more than 30,000 persons in the United States have HD, or 1 in 10,000 persons.

HD results from genetically programmed neurodegeneration in regions of the *basal ganglia*. These structures lie deep within the brain and are more accurately called "nuclei," which is the term for clusters of neurons within the CNS. The basal ganglia, in addition to manufacturing neurotransmitters such as dopamine and acetylcholine, also fine-tune, control, and coordinate voluntary movement. Within the basal ganglia, HD especially targets neurons of the *striatum*, particularly those in the *caudate nuclei*, the *putamen* and the *globus pallidus*. Also affected is the brain's outer surface, or *cortex*, which controls thought, perception, and memory. One known biochemical derangement is a deficiency of gamma-aminobutyric acid (GABA), caused by a deficiency in glutamic acid decarboxylase and choline in the basal ganglia. Current research is focused on four lines of investigation: excitotoxicity, or cell stimulation by the brain's natural chemicals; defective energy metabolism; oxidative stress, whereby normal brain activity produces toxic compounds called free radicals that damage neurons; and trophic factors in the body that cause cell death rather than normal cell growth and repair.

HD is linked to a defect on chromosome 4, one of the 22 nonsex-linked, or "autosomal" pairs of chromosomes. Thus males and females are at equal risk for acquiring HD. The specific genetic defect underlying HD is a small sequence of DNA on chromosome 4 in which several base pairs are repeated several times. The normal gene has three DNA bases, composed of the sequence CAG. In people with HD, the sequence abnormally repeats itself dozens of times. With each successive generation, the number of CAG repeats may expand further. Discovery of the HD gene in 1993 has made possible a genetic test to diagnose HD in persons with characteristic symptoms or to detect the disease in offspring of affected individuals. The blood test analyzes DNA for the HD mutation by counting the number of repeats in the HD gene region of chromosome 4. Generally, persons free of the disease have 28 or fewer CAG repeats; individuals with HD usually have 40 or more repeats. Intermediate numbers indicate that the individual may not develop HD but that future generations are at risk.

HD is an autosomal-dominant disorder, because only one copy of the defective gene needs to be inherited from one affected parent to cause the disease. Each child of an HD parent has a 50-50 chance of inheriting the HD gene, thus a person who inherits the HD gene, and lives to adulthood, will sooner or later develop the disease. However, if an offspring does not inherit the gene, he or she will not develop the disease and cannot pass it to future generations. A very small number of cases of HD are *sporadic*, occurring without a family history of the disorder. Such cases are usually related to a new genetic mutation that occurs during sperm development, increasing the number of CAG repeats to pathologic levels. Diagnosis is based on the genetic test plus extensive medical and family histories, including genealogy, and a thorough medical examination. Diagnosticians will also prescribe CT and magnetic resonance imaging (MRI) to view brain structures. Typically, persons with HD have shrinkage of the paired caudate nuclei and putamen, along with enlargement of the lateral ventricles. However, these changes are not specific to HD and thus are diagnostic only in conjunction with a thorough history and physical evaluation. The cerebral cortex is ultimately affected also, leading to deterioration of memory and perception.

The onset of HD is insidious and generally begins with some chorea-like movements, emotional lability, intellectual deterioration, lack of attention to appearance, and forgetfulness. As the disease progresses, the symptoms become more debilitating and obvious to family and friends. Gradually, the patient is unable to concentrate or attend to the activities of daily living and is subject to violent outbursts and combativeness.

No known definitive treatment or cure exists for HD. Symptomatic treatment consists of administering haloperidol and chlorpromazine to minimize the chorea-like movements. As the disease progresses, family members can no longer cope with the constant attention required by these patients and confinement to an institution is necessary. Families require much emotional support to cope with the long-term and debilitating nature of the disease. It is also appropriate to offer genetic counseling and a thorough explanation of the disease because of its hereditary transmittal.

Amyotrophic Lateral Sclerosis–Motor Neuron Disease

Amyotrophic lateral sclerosis (ALS) is a progressive neurologic disease that affects persons in the 40- to 70-year age groups. *ALS* is the term used in the United States; *motor neuron disease (MND)* is used in Europe. Another name commonly used in the United States is Lou Gehrig's disease, after the Yankee's baseball player who died of the disease in 1941. Incidence worldwide is 2/100,000 population; prevalence is 6/100,000 (International Alliance of ALS/MND Associations, 2000). Although 90% of cases are sporadic, with no known cause, 10% are familial. Approximately 20% of familial cases have a mutation in the superoxide dismutase (SOD_1) gene on chromosome 21, and some persons with sporadic ALS-MND also have the SOD_1 gene mutation. Other theories of causation include (1) a slow latent viral infection (e.g., mutated poliovirus) or (2) an autoimmune disorder.

Pathologic changes involve the anterior horn cells of the spinal cord and the lower brainstem and the motor neurons of the cerebral cortex that give rise to the corticospinal tract. Deterioration of these neurons cause neurogenic atrophy of the musculature they innervate. Sensory neurons are unaffected. This neuronal deterioration causes loss of fine motor control and muscle atrophy—the first symptoms noted by the patient. Atrophic weakness usually follows a proximal to distal pattern, which progresses to involve the neck, tongue, pharyngeal, and laryngeal muscles and later the trunk and lower extremities. However, many patients have weaknesses beginning in the legs. Intellectual capacity and memory remain unaffected, and patients generally remain in control of bowel and bladder functions. The average patient survives 2 to 6 years after diagnosis, although some patients live 10 years or longer. Death is generally caused by respiratory failure, although long-term ventilatory therapy can prolong life. Treatment is supportive and symptomatic, and attention must be given to family members who are caring for a chronically ill, progressively deteriorating loved one.

Extrapyramidal Syndromes

Extrapyramidal syndromes are disorders concerned with movement that result from lesions involving those parts of the brain other than the corticospinal pathways, principally the basal ganglia (see Chapter 50). More data are available about the clinical aspects of extrapyramidal dysfunction compared with its pathophysiologic basis. Neurochemical changes seem to be involved in some cases.

Tremor

Tremor is an involuntary movement that results from an excess of neuronal activity in one area as a result of unopposed activity in another area. The tremor is most marked peripherally; it may be suppressed by will or with vigorous activity. In general, there are alternating contractions of the flexor and extensor muscle groups, so movement is at right angles to the axis of the limb. The tremor of parkinsonism occurs at rest and temporarily disappears during voluntary activity. In contrast, a tremor caused by cerebellar deficiency is an *intention tremor* and is increased with purposeful activity.

Rigidity

Rigidity is characteristic of Parkinson's disease and classically shows a relatively constant resistance to muscle stretching. Rigidity must be differentiated from *spasticity*, which occurs with pyramidal tract disorders (upper motor neuron lesions). In spasticity, resistance at first increases as the stretching or pulling force increases because more motor units are brought into play. Additional force will finally cause a sudden loss of resistance ("clasp knife" effect). In contrast, rigidity produces a smooth, constant resistance to forceful stretching because, although the stretching causes some motor units to fire, motor units fall out as readily as others are recruited by the external force.

Chorea

Chorea refers to movements that are sudden, random, and involuntary. Fragments of purposeful movement are apparent, but normal progression is lacking and the movements are disorganized. Chorea may be generalized, as in HD, or lateralized.

A *lateralized chorea* is seen with lesions in the ventrolateral thalamus or subthalamic nucleus. Occlusion of a penetrating branch of the posterior cerebral artery results in an infarct of the thalamic area and is often the basis of the hemichorea.

Chorea may involve proximal or distal extremities, face, head, and trunk. In some patients, speech and mastication are affected. The involuntary movements in the limbs may make walking and purposeful movement of the hands difficult. Choreiform movements tend to be aggravated by physical activity and environmental stimuli but may disappear during sleep.

The pathology in chorea involves extensive areas of the nervous system, most notably degeneration of the corpus striatum and the cerebral cortex. The pathophysiology in chorea may be related to an increased (or altered) response of striatal dopamine receptors. This hypersensitivity hypothesis is supported by biochemical and pharmacologic data. Levodopa (L-dopa) can cause an increase or exacerbation of chorea; neuroleptic drugs can decrease or ameliorate the abnormal movements, supposedly by competing with dopamine at the receptor sites.

Athetosis

Athetosis is marked by involuntary movements combined with instability of posture. It is evidenced by slow, rhythmic, writhing, wormlike movements that usually occur in the peripheral parts of the upper extremities, especially the fingers and hands. The face, neck, tongue, lips, and lower extremities may be affected. Attempts to perform a voluntary activity and emotional stimuli cause an exaggeration of the abnormal movements. Coordinated activity is not possible in the affected muscle groups.

The globus pallidus, putamen, and possibly the corpus striatum are involved in the pathology of athetosis. Hypoxia at birth is a causative factor in some cases; others are related to kernicterus, in which the unconjugated bilirubin is taken up by lipid-rich brain tissue (especially the basal ganglia, thalamus, cerebellum, and cerebral gray matter) and causes damage (see Chapter 27). Four types of *cerebral palsy* (a popular term referring to a motor dysfunction that is congenital or acquired during infancy) are identified: cerebral spastic diplegia (legs affected more than arms), the hemiplegic variety, double athetosis *(choreoathetosis)*, and ataxic. Clinical manifestations often overlap. Cerebral palsy may be, but is not always, associated with mental retardation, disorders of perception and higher sensory function, and seizure disorders.

Dystonia

Dystonia differs from athetosis in that the larger axial muscles rather than the appendicular muscles are involved. As a group, the dystonias are characterized by sustained muscle contractions, causing abnormal postures and involuntary twisting and other repetitive movements. The movements may be very painful, affecting the whole body, groups of muscles, or a single muscle. Many of the nonparkinsonian dystonias are inherited, and recently a gene (DYT1) abnormality has been identified in early-onset dystonia. Bizarre or grotesque postures of the limbs or trunk from excessive muscle tone are noted. Voluntary movement is seriously impaired, and sometimes the entire musculature of the body may be thrown into spasm by an effort to move an arm or leg or to speak. The pathology seems to involve the putamen and thalamus. Surgical lesions made in the ventrolateral thalamus may produce improvement. Some early-onset dystonias are responsive to levodopa.

Hemiballismus

Hemiballismus is the involuntary, violent movement of a large body area (entire leg, shoulder, pelvic girdle). Usually, only one side of the body is involved. Attempting a normal activity may invoke a ballistic movement instead. This syndrome is believed to be caused by extensive lesions of the subthalamic nuclei, usually secondary to hemorrhage or, less often, an infarct or a tumor. Death occurs in 4 to 6 weeks in 60% of patients and is generally the result of exhaustion, pneumonia, or congestive heart failure. The recent use of neuroleptics (dopamine antagonists), such as haloperidol and chlorpromazine, has improved the survival rate.

Dyskinesias

A more general term to describe abnormal involuntary movements, *dyskinesia,* refers to writhing, grotesque movements, and can include dystonic movements. These movements can be a sign of the disease process in Huntington's chorea, Tourette syndrome, Parkinson's disease (PD), and the dystonias. Secondary disease (e.g., tardive dyskinesia) is associated with use of neuroleptic drugs, such as haloperidol and the phenothiazines. Paradoxically, dyskinesias can also be a delayed adverse effect of the antiparkinson medications such as L-dopa.

Parkinsonism

Parkinsonism is a syndrome characterized by rhythmic tremors, bradykinesia, rigidity of muscles, and loss of postural reflexes. The movement disorder results primarily from a defect in the dopaminergic (dopamine-producing) pathway that connects the substantia nigra to the corpus striatum (caudate and lenticular nuclei). (See basal ganglia in Fig. 50-24.) The basal ganglia are part of the extrapyramidal system; influence the initiation, modulation, and completion of movement; and regulate automatic movements.

Parkinsonism is the most common disorder involving the extrapyramidal system, and several causes exist. The vast majority of cases are considered to be of unknown cause or idiopathic. *Idiopathic parkinsonism* is referred to as *Parkinson's disease (PD)* or *paralysis agitans.* PD affects nearly 1 million Americans and is a leading cause of disability; it is a slowly progressive disease of middle or late life, with onset typically after 60 years of age. There is no apparent genetic cause and no known cure.

Parkinsonian symptoms, to a greater or lesser degree, accompany several other conditions that structurally damage the nigrostriatal pathway or interfere with the action of dopamine within the basal ganglia. *Postencephalic parkinsonism* was a common sequelae of an encephalitis (von Economo's disease) that occurred between 1918 and 1925; studies indicate that an influenza A virus may have been responsible. *Drug-induced parkinsonism* may be a side effect of certain antipsychotic drugs, such as phenothiazines and butyrophenones (postsynaptic dopamine-receptor blockers). Another type of dopamine-receptor blocker, metoclopramide (useful for gastrointestinal disturbances), can also precipitate parkinsonism. Reserpine (an antihypertensive drug) is a presynaptic dopamine depleter that occasionally induces parkinsonism. Drug-induced parkinsonism is usually reversible when the drugs are discontinued, although some patients remain symptomatic for weeks to years. The use of an illicit designer drug, 1-methyl-4-phenyl-1,2,3,6-tetrahydropine (MPTP), induces parkinsonism by selectively destroying dopaminergic neurons of the substantia nigra. Parkinsonism is also associated with poisoning by heavy metals (lead, manganese, mercury) and carbon monoxide.

Major pathologic changes in PD involve the loss of dopamine-containing neurons in the substantia nigra and other pigmented nuclei. Many of the remaining neurons contain Lewy bodies (eosinophilic cytoplasmic inclusions). The loss of dopamine-containing neurons in the substantia nigra leads to a severe reduction of dopamine in nerve terminals of the nigrostriatal tract. The reduction of dopamine in the corpus striatum upsets the normal balance between dopamine (inhibitory) and acetylcholine (excitatory) neurotransmitters and underlies most of the symptoms in PD.

Although these pathologic changes are well known, the basic question concerning what triggers the nigrostriatal pathologic changes and concomitant neurochemical alterations remains unanswered. No convincing evidence supports a viral pathogenesis. The finding that MPTP, a meperidine derivative, produces parkinsonism that is clinically indistinguishable from idiopathic PD has generated renewed interest in exogenous toxins. Possible toxic agents, such as cyanide in well water and agricultural pesticides, have been proposed but not yet confirmed. Genetic influences may also play a role, as suggested by identification during the 1980s of a common gene mutation called "alpha synuclein" in several affected members of an Italian family. That finding was not supported by a 1990s study of twin males who were registered into the U.S. military in World War II. However, it is strongly suspected that heredity influences the development of PD, especially in younger persons (Parkinson's Institute, 2000).

Clinical Manifestations

The cardinal signs of parkinsonism are rigidity, tremor (especially at rest), akinesia or bradykinesia, and loss of postural reflexes. The dysfunction is chronic and progressive but with wide variation of symptoms among patients.

Rigidity may be isolated to one muscle group and primarily unilateral or may be widespread and bilateral. Parkinsonism decreases muscle strength and speed and is a major factor in the deformities associated with the syndrome. Passive movement of the involved limbs or trunk meets with a taffylike resistance that is relatively constant throughout the range of motion. Parkinsonism has been compared with bending a lead pipe and is sometimes called *lead-pipe rigidity.* "Catches" often occur during passive movement, giving a cogwheel or rachetlike character to the rigidity called *cogwheel rigidity.* Both flexor and extensor muscles are tightly contracted *(increased tonus),* indicating impaired control of opposing muscle groups.

When the rigidity involves the trunk, it is largely responsible for the gait and postural problems associated with parkinsonism. Patients stoop when they stand so that the chin is farther forward than the toes. They walk in shuffling, hasty, accelerating steps, as if stumbling forward and trying to hurry the feet back under them *(festinating gait).*

The tremor associated with parkinsonism occurs at rest and is called a *rest tremor.* When muscles are tensed to perform a purposeful act, the tremor usually stops. (About one third of patients have intention tremor along with rest tremor, but, as noted, intention tremors are generally associated with cerebellar dysfunction.) Tremors involving the hands are described as *pill rolling* and are the result of rhythmic movement of the thumb and first two fingers. Tremors are the result of regular alternating contractions (4 to 6 cycles per second) in antagonistic muscles. Tremors are likely to be worse when the patient is tired, under emotional stress, or focusing attention on the tremor. The basis for the tremor is not clear. Degeneration of the basal ganglia results in loss of inhibitory influence, and the increased feedback in various circuits may result in oscillation. Not every patient has an obvious tremor. If the patient incidentally has a cerebrovascular accident (CVA, stroke) and hemiplegia occurs, the tremor disappears on the paralyzed side.

Patients may experience either akinesia or bradykinesia. *Akinesia* is characterized by a decrease in spontaneous movement and difficulty in initiating spontaneous or new movements. *Bradykinesia* is characterized by an abnormal slowness in deliberate movement. Either symptom is very disabling and obvious when the patient attempts any voluntary activity such as walking, talking, or writing. Loss of associated movement is noted, for example, when the patient does not swing the arms while walking. The face is expressionless, and the voice is low and monotonous. Writing becomes progressively cramped and may reflect the tremor. *Micrographia* is the small handwriting that eventually trails off and cannot be deciphered. When automatic movement (normally unconscious) is performed consciously, much more work and energy are necessary. Thus patients with parkinsonism frequently complain of fatigue and muscle pain.

Secondary signs include gait disturbances, postural problems, and autonomic nervous system (ANS) disorders. Gait disturbances are characterized by increasing impairment of postural and righting reflexes. The patient cannot stop and turn quickly but turns *en bloc* rather than sequentially as a healthy person would. Because balance is poor, patients hurry along, trying to keep up with the center of gravity; they have difficulty in making adjustments to changes in position and tend to fall. Wheeled walkers may help prevent falls in some patients, although the conventional ones tend to roll away. A special autostop walker is currently available and is proving useful.

Autonomic manifestations of parkinsonism include sweating, oily skin accompanied frequently by seborrheic dermatitis, drooling, swallowing difficulties that lead to choking and gradually interfere with the ability to tolerate any oral feedings, constipation, and bladder problems, which are aggravated by anticholinergic drugs and prostatic hypertrophy.

Additional features of parkinsonism include the following:

- Oculomotor disorders: blurring convergence resulting from inability to sustain contraction of the ocular muscles. This symptom is often indistinguishable from an early symptom of a distinct and rare neurodegenerative movement disorder called progressive supranuclear palsy (PSP). The term derives from the characteristic diagnostic symptom of the inability to voluntarily gaze downward. To add to the diagnostic problem, persons with PSP often will show some response to the antiparkinson drug, carbidopa/levodopa (Sinemet). However, the prognosis is poorer, and the PSP patient ultimately develops symptoms of brainstem involvement, such as speech problems (dysarthria) and swallowing difficulty (dysphagia).
- Oculogyric crisis: spasms of the conjugate eye muscles, in which the eyes are fixed, usually in an upward gaze, for minutes to hours; associated with parkinsonism of exogenous origin, such as drug induced or postencephalitic
- Extreme fatigue and muscle pain from muscles exhausted by rigidity
- Postural hypotension related to medication side effects, as well as interference with blood pressure control mediated by the ANS
- Impaired respiratory function related to hypoventilation, inactivity, aspiration of food or saliva, and reduced airway clearance

Diagnosis

Diagnosis of parkinsonism is based on clinical findings. The key to making a diagnosis of true PD is a therapeutic response to levodopa (L-dopa). Other forms of parkinsonism involve degeneration of the neurons that formerly received the dopaminergic input and thus do not respond to L-dopa. Table 54-1 lists major neurologic features of the disease.

TABLE 54-1 ∎∎∎

Major Neurologic Findings in Parkinson's Disease

Neurologic Finding	Comment
Rest tremor*	Pill-rolling movement of fingers characteristic; tremor decreased with voluntary movement and during sleep
Bradykinesia*	Slowness in initiating and maintaining movement
Cogwheel rigidity*	Motion interrupted by "catches"; resistance relatively constant throughout range of motion
Postural and gait* abnormalities	Stooped, shuffling, festinating gait; unable to turn quickly, turns en bloc
Micrographia	Small handwriting that trails off; tremor may be obvious when drawing concentric circles
Masklike facies	Wide-eyed, unblinking, staring expression; blinks two or three times/minute (normal blinking, 12 to 20 times/min)
Monotone	Expressionless speech
Hyperactive glabellar (blink) reflex	Exaggerated sensitivity to finger tapping over glabella (between eyebrows) causes the patient to blink with each tap (it takes effort for a normal person to blink); early sign of Parkinson's disease

*Major or cardinal symptoms of PD.

Treatment

Dopaminergic drugs are used to try to restore the balance between dopamine and acetylcholine. Dopamine does not cross the blood-brain barrier, but L-dopa, a metabolic precursor of dopamine, does cross it (see Fig. 50-4). However, L-dopa is largely decarboxylated in the periphery (stomach, liver, heart, kidneys), and only a small amount reaches the basal ganglia. Large doses are necessary to achieve results. To improve the efficiency of L-dopa, the drug was combined with a decarboxylase inhibitor that will not cross the blood-brain barrier. There is less breakdown of the drug in the peripheral tissues, thus more is available to the brain and side effects are reduced. carbidopa/levodopa (Sinemet), approved in 1974, is available in the ratio of 1 part carbidopa to 10 parts levodopa. Therapy with these drugs is begun with small doses, which are gradually increased until symptoms disappear or side effects appear.

All patients on these drugs experience some side effects, including gastrointestinal (GI) effects such as nausea and vomiting (80% to 90% of patients lose weight). Administering the drug to patients after they have just eaten can reduce this side effect. Cardiac dysrhythmias, postural hypotension, and CNS symptoms (nightmares, confusion, insomnia, hallucinations, depression) may also occur. Abnormal involuntary movements (dyskinesias) are bothersome and increase with long-term use of these drugs. These effects are dose related, but decreasing the dose often results in the return of the parkinsonism symptoms.

Despite progression of the disease, these drugs have maintained improvement in most patients for 5 to 10 years. Before these drugs were discovered, the average patient was totally disabled in about 9 years. After about 5 to 10 years, patients begin to experience an on-off phenomenon (sudden variation in response to drugs), which is believed to be related to a decrease of dopamine production that is outstripping the drug's replacement capacity.

Other drugs used in the treatment of parkinsonism include anticholinergics, antihistamines (which also have an anticholinergic action), and amantadine (a synthetic antiviral compound with dopaminergic effects used in the treatment of Asian influenza). These drugs are often used in combination with carbidopa/levodopa (Sinemet). The belladonna alkaloids atropine and scopolamine were the first centrally active anticholinergics used to treat parkinsonism but have been largely replaced by synthetic anticholinergics such as trihexyphenidyl (Artane) and benztropine (Cogentin). These drugs are used to block acetylcholine-stimulated nerve impulses, which lead to tremors, bradykinesia, and rigidity. Adverse effects include dry mouth, constipation, and urinary retention. The use of diphenhydramine (Benadryl) and other antihistamines is based on their central cholinergic blocking action. Dopamine agonists, such as bromocriptine (Parlodel), stimulate dopamine receptors left inactive when dopamine is in short supply. This drug works best early in treatment. Side effects include nausea, vomiting, headache, fatigue, light-headedness, confusion, vertigo, and hypotension. The monamine oxidase B (MAO-B) inhibitor, selegiline (Eldepryl), is thought to block the activity of the brain enzyme MAO-B, which terminates the action of dopamine at synapses in the brain. In clinical trials, this drug was found to prolong the effectiveness of L-dopa therapy in some patients; when given to patients with early symptoms, it appears to delay the onset of more disabling symptoms. Vitamin E therapy is also under investigation. Some evidence suggests that it may slow the biochemical oxidative activity that is toxic to brain cells in PD.

Surgical lesions (using stereotaxic techniques) made in the globus pallidus or ventrolateral thalamus may be a successful treatment in selected patients with parkinsonism. Rigidity may decrease, but there is no effect on the akinesia. Many patients do not benefit from surgery; this treatment is best reserved for those who do not respond to drug treatment, who have unilateral involvement and normal blood pressure, and who are relatively young. Experimental fetal tissue implantation into the mesencephalon (midbrain) shows promise, but the technique and the research are plagued by ethical considerations. A current therapy undergoing study is deep brain stimulation.

These therapies, along with physical and occupational therapy, help maintain function for a longer period than was previously possible. One must remember, however, that parkinsonism is a chronic, progressive disease that gradually causes severe disability.

Demyelinating Diseases

A large number of neurologic diseases are termed *demyelinating diseases* because their common pathologic feature is focal areas of destruction involving the myelin sheath of nerve fibers in the CNS. The axon often is damaged as well, but destruction of myelin is the primary change. Multiple sclerosis is the primary demyelinating disease and is the focus of this discussion.

Acute Disseminated Encephalomyelitis

Acute disseminated encephalomyelitis (postvaccinial or postinfectious), although rare, is a demyelinating disorder that deserves mention because it is essentially preventable. This is an acute encephalitic or myelitic process of variable course characterized by symptoms that indicate damage to the white matter of the brain or spinal cord. The pathologic findings consist of numerous circumscribed areas of perivascular demyelinization. About 1 week after measles and 10 days to 2 weeks after vaccination for rabies or smallpox, neurologic symptoms develop rapidly. These symptoms consist of headache, drowsiness, stupor, ocular palsies, and often a flaccid paralysis of all four limbs caused by a transverse cord lesion. Variations in severity are common.

Postvaccination encephalomyelitis may occur after rabies vaccination, presumably from sensitization to vaccine-containing brain tissue. This type is essentially allergic encephalitis and does not occur with the use of the newer duck embryo vaccines, which are free of nerve tissue. Encephalomyelitis may also follow smallpox vaccination, especially the primary vaccination, but the source of the material used for the vaccination seems to have little bearing on its occurrence. The incidence is estimated to be 1 in 5000 vaccinations. The recent decision not to include smallpox vaccination as part of the routine pediatric immunization program in the United States should decrease the incidence of this complication.

Postinfectious encephalomyelitis that develops after a viral infection, especially measles, occurs in about 1 in 1000 cases. The mortality rate is 10% to 20%, and about 50% of those who survive are left with some neurologic damage. The use of measles vaccine in the United States has greatly reduced the occurrence of encephalomyelitis. Some evidence indicates that the measles virus may play a role in the cause of multiple sclerosis.

Multiple Sclerosis

Multiple sclerosis (MS) is one of the most common neurologic disorders affecting young people. In the United States an estimated 250,000 to 350,000 people are affected—1 in 1000 or less than one tenth of 1% (Reingold, 2000). Women are affected at twice the rate of men, although in later-onset MS, the female-male ratio is much lower. Symptoms rarely occur before age 15 or after age 60. The mean age of occurrence is 30 years, with a range between 18 and 40 in most patients. MS is characterized by the widespread occurrence of patches of myelin destruction followed by gliosis in the white matter of the CNS. The hard yellow plaques found on autopsy are responsible for its being so named. The characteristic course of MS is a series of isolated attacks that affect different parts of the CNS. Each attack subsequently shows some degree of remission, but the overall picture is one of deterioration.

Etiology and Pathology

The fundamental nature of the disturbance that leads to MS is not known with certainty. Recent evidence supports the theory that MS is an autoimmune disease, perhaps linked to an undetermined environmental trigger such as a viral infection. This hypothesis derives from the observation that viral infections usually cause inflammation involving the production of gamma interferon, a chemical known to worsen MS. The illness is more common in temperate climates (northern Europe, northern United States), with an incidence of 10 per 100,000 population, and it is rare in the tropics; in Japan, however, MS occurs infrequently at any latitude. There is also a slightly higher familial incidence of the disease: it is about eight times more common in close relatives of a person with MS than it is in the general population. Whether this increased familial occurrence is caused by a genetic predisposition (a hereditary pattern does not exist) or whether there is common exposure to an infectious agent (probably viral) during childhood, which in some way may lead to MS during early adulthood, is unknown. Migration studies reveal that if adults move from a high-risk to a low-risk area, they retain the high risk for developing MS. However, a person who emigrates before the age of 15 years acquires the low risk of the second residence. These data are consistent with a possible viral cause with a long latency period between initial exposure and clinical onset of disease. The mechanism of action may be that of an autoimmune reaction attacking myelin.

A number of viruses have been proposed as possible causative agents in MS. Some investigators suspect the measles (rubeola) virus. Various measles antibodies have been found in the serum and cerebrospinal fluid (CSF) of patients with MS, and evidence suggests that these antibodies are produced in the brain. If the measles virus is involved, it probably invades the subject in early life, lies dormant for a number of years, and then stimulates an autoimmune response. More recently, the strain of reactivated herpes virus (herpes virus-6 [HHV-6]) that causes a common childhood illness, roseola, was implicated and was found to cause a heightened immune response in more than 70% of patients with the relapsing-remitting form of MS (Soldan et al, 1997). Another theory suggests that certain genetic factors render some people more susceptible to CNS invasion by various "slow" viruses. Slow viruses have long incubation periods and possibly develop only in conjunction with an abnormal or deficient immune status. Certain histocompatibility antigens (HLA-A3, HLA-A7) have been found to be more common in MS patients compared with control subjects. The presence of these antigens may be related to a deficient immunologic defense against viral infection. What does seem certain is that an abnormal inflammatory response of the immune system occurs and precipitates the characteristic destruction of myelin. Because the disease varies greatly in its clinical, radiologic, and pathologic findings, it is likely that the cause is multifactorial, with a variety of genetic and environmental factors contributing to MS susceptibility. Finding a single cause that can be reliably demonstrated to exist in all cases has been a frustrating endeavor. Current best evidence supports the following etiologic mechanisms: direct toxins, including biologic agents; cell-mediated and humorally mediated immune mechanisms; and a primary oligodendrogliopathy that results in demyelination and axonal injury (Wingerchuk et al, 2001).

Several events are generally considered to be precipitating factors, among them pregnancy, infection (especially with fever), emotional stress, and injury. Complete recovery is usual after the first attack. Remission usually occurs within 1 to 3 months with successive attacks.

Eventually, however, recovery is not complete, and patients are left with additional permanent damage after each bout.

The lesions of MS occur only in the white matter of the CNS. Autopsy examination shows that the lesions are most prominent in the pyramidal tracts and posterior columns of the cord, around the ventricles of the brain, in the optic nerve and tract, in the brainstem and cerebellar peduncles, and around large veins. In the acute phase, the involved area is edematous, inflamed, and pinkish in color. The size may vary from a few millimeters to several centimeters in diameter. Macrophages remove the areas of degenerating myelin, and as the acute phase subsides, a reactive gliosis develops. The end result is a shrunken area of demyelination called a *plaque*. The axon cylinders and cell bodies are not destroyed, although the scar is capable of damaging the underlying axon fiber so that nerve fiber conduction is disrupted. The symptoms of MS caused by the demyelinization become irreversible as the condition progresses.

Clinical Features

The location of the lesions determines the clinical manifestations of MS. Any combination of the following signs and symptoms may coexist:

1. *Sensory disorders.* Paresthesias (numbness, tingling, "dead" feeling, "pins and needles") may vary in degree from one day to the next. If there is a lesion of the posterior columns of the cervical cord, flexion of the neck causes shocklike sensations to run down the cord (Lhermitte's sign). Proprioceptive disorders often give rise to sensory ataxia and incoordination of the arms. Vibration sense is often diminished. Because sensory disorders cannot be demonstrated objectively, these symptoms may be thought to be hysterical.

2. *Visual complaints.* Many patients experience visual problems as an initial symptom. Diplopia (double vision) is often reported, as well as blurred vision, red-green color distortion, and abnormal visual fields with blind spots (scotomas) in one or both eyes. Vision may be totally lost in one eye for several hours to days. An optic neuritis is the basis for these visual disturbances. Diplopia from brainstem lesions affecting the nuclei or fiber tracts of the extraocular muscles and nystagmus are other common complaints.

3. *Spastic weakness of the limbs.* Weakness of a limb on one side of the body or an asymmetric distribution in all four limbs is a common complaint. The patient may complain of tiredness and heaviness in one leg and noticeably drags that foot and has poor control. The patient may complain that the leg jumps spontaneously, especially when in bed. More profound spasticity is accompanied by painful spasm of the muscles. The tendon reflexes may be hyperactive and abdominal reflexes absent; the plantar responses are extensor (Babinski's sign). These signs indicate involvement of the corticospinal pathways.

4. *Cerebellar signs.* Nystagmus (rapid oscillation of the eyeball horizontally or vertically) and cerebellar ataxia are other common symptoms and indicate

involvement of the cerebellar and corticospinal tracts. Uncoordinated voluntary movements, intention tremors, balance disturbances, and dysarthria (scanning speech with words broken into syllables and pauses between syllables) are characteristics of cerebellar ataxia.

5. *Bladder dysfunction.* Lesions in the corticospinal tracts often cause disorders of sphincter control; hesitancy, urgency, and frequency are common and indicate a reduced-capacity spastic bladder. Acute retention and incontinence also occur.

6. *Disorders of mood.* Many patients develop euphoria—an unrealistic feeling of well-being. This feeling is believed to be caused by involvement of the white matter of the frontal lobes. Other signs of cerebral impairment may include loss of memory and dementia.

Diagnosis, Prognosis, and Treatment

There is no single test or single set of symptoms that conclusively diagnoses MS. Diagnosis of MS is usually made on the basis of a history of neurologic episodes that cannot be related to a single lesion of the CNS and are characterized by relapses and remissions. Plaques may sometimes be visualized by MRI. Use of the contrast agent gadolinium can help distinguish new and old plaques. A new tool, magnetic resonance spectroscopy (MRS) may prove to be even more useful in that it reveals information about early biochemical alterations in the brain rather than later anatomic changes. Analysis of the CSF can be helpful: MS is often associated with elevated leukocytes and protein (particularly myelin basic protein and the antibody immunoglobulin G). A laboratory procedure called electrophoresis separates and graphs these proteins, often identifying the presence of a characteristic pattern in MS called "oligoclonal bands."

Progression of MS is extremely variable. The classic and most common picture is one of intermittent relapses followed by more or less complete remission. Remission is less complete with each ensuing exacerbation, and thus within 10 to 20 years, the patient is significantly disabled. This state is called relapsing-remitting (RR) MS. There are three other, less common, patterns of MS. The first is primary-progressive (PP), characterized by a steady, gradual decline of function with no clear-cut periods of remission. There may be temporary plateaus during which the patient's status remains stable. The second alternative course of the illness pattern is secondary-progressive (SP) MS. The patient experiences an RR pattern, followed by a more rapid PP course. The most infrequently seen pattern is an aggressive form called progressive-relapsing (PR) MS. The disease takes a rapidly progressive course, with intermittent acute attacks that cause rapid, severe loss of function with no remission. These three less-common patterns are distinguishable only over time, and PP, SP, and PR are often included together in a category called chronic progressive MS.

Treatment of MS is symptomatic. During an acute relapse the patient rests, although complete bedrest is avoided. Adrenocorticotropic hormone (ACTH) or glucocorticoids are used during the acute phase to hasten remission. The benefits of drug therapy are difficult to evaluate because of the episodic nature of the disease and are probably nonspecific or based on their antiinflammatory action. Immunosuppressive agents and plasmapheresis have been reported to be helpful in stabilizing patients and slowing deterioration. Patients experience alterations in all functions: vision, mobility and coordination, nutrition, elimination, and communication. Care of the patient with MS requires a total health care team approach.

MOTOR SYSTEM DISORDERS WITH PREDOMINANT LOWER MOTOR NEURON SIGNS

Myasthenia Gravis

Myasthenia gravis, meaning "grave muscle weakness," is the only neuromuscular disease that incorporates both rapid fatigue of voluntary muscle and prolonged recovery time (recovery may actually take 10 to 20 times longer than normal). Mortality rates in the past have been as high as 90%. The death rate has been reduced drastically since medications and respiratory care units have become available.

The clinical syndrome was first described in 1600. In the late 1800s myasthenia gravis (MG) was distinguished from muscle weakness caused by true bulbar palsy. In the 1920s a physician with MG noticed an improvement after taking ephedrine for menstrual cramps. Finally, in 1934, another physician from England (Mary Walker) noted the similarity of symptoms in MG and curare poisoning. She used the curare antagonist physostigmine for MG and observed marked improvement.

The prevalence of MG is estimated to be 14 per 100,000 population, with 36,000 cases in the United States. The peak age of onset is 20 years, with the ratio of women to men being 3:1. A second peak, although lower than the first, occurs in older men in their seventh and eighth decades of life.

Mortality generally results from respiratory insufficiency, although with improvements in respiratory intensive care, this complication is becoming more manageable. Spontaneous remission may occur in 10% to 20% of patients and can be induced in selected patients by elective thymectomy. Young women who are in the early stages of the disease (first 5 years after onset) and who do not respond well to drug therapy benefit most from this procedure.

Pathophysiology

Skeletal or striated muscles are innervated by large myelinated nerves that originate in the anterior horn cells of the spinal cord and the brainstem. These nerves send their axons out in the spinal or cranial nerves to the periphery. Individual nerves branch many times and are capable of stimulating up to 2000 skeletal muscle fibers. The combination of the motor nerve and the muscle fibers it innervates is called a *motor unit.* Although each motor neuron innervates many muscle fibers, each muscle fiber is innervated by a single motor neuron.

The area of specialized contact between the motor nerve and the muscle fiber is called the *neuromuscular synapse* or *junction* (Fig. 54-2). The neuromuscular junction is a chemical synapse between a nerve and muscle consisting of three basic components: a presynaptic element, a postsynaptic element, and a synaptic cleft about 200 Å wide between two elements. The presynaptic element consists of the axon terminal, which contains synaptic vesicles filled with the neurotransmitter acetylcholine. Acetylcholine is synthesized and stored in the axon terminal (bouton). The plasma membrane of the axon terminal is called the *presynaptic membrane*. The postsynaptic element consists of the *postsynaptic membrane* (postjunctional membrane), or *motor end-plate*, of the muscle fiber. The postsynaptic membrane is formed by an invagination, called the *synaptic gutter* or *trough*, of the muscle membrane or sarcolemma into which the axon terminal protrudes. The postsynaptic membrane has many folds (subneural clefts), which greatly increase the surface area. The postsynaptic membrane also contains acetylcholine receptors and is capable of generating an end-plate potential, which, in turn, can generate a muscle action potential. Acetylcholinesterase, an enzyme that destroys acetylcholine, is also located in the postsynaptic membrane. The *synaptic cleft* refers to the space between the presynaptic and postsynaptic membranes. The space is filled with a gelatinous material through which extracellular fluid (ECF) may diffuse.

When a nerve impulse reaches the neuromuscular junction, the presynaptic axon terminal membrane is depolarized, causing the release of acetylcholine into the synaptic cleft. The acetylcholine diffuses across the synaptic gap and unites with the acetylcholine receptor sites in the postsynaptic membrane. This combination causes a change in permeability to both sodium and potassium in the postsynaptic membrane. The sudden influx of sodium ions and efflux of potassium ions lead to depolarization of the end-plate, known as the *end-plate potential (EPP)*. When the EPP reaches threshold, it generates an action potential in the nonjunctional muscle membrane, which is propagated along the sarcolemma. This action potential sets off a series of reactions, resulting in the contraction of the muscle fiber. Once transmission across the neuromuscular junction has occurred, acetylcholine is destroyed by the enzyme acetylcholinesterase. In normal persons, the amount of acetylcholine released is more than sufficient to result in an action potential.

In MG, neuromuscular conduction is impaired. The number of normal acetylcholine receptors is reduced, which is thought to be the result of an autoimmune injury. Antibodies to the acetylcholine receptor protein have been found in the serum of many MG patients. Determining whether this is a primary or secondary consequence of receptor damage caused by an unknown primary agent will be of great value in determining the exact pathogenesis of MG. Fig. 54-3 illustrates the probable defect in MG (Drachman, 1994).

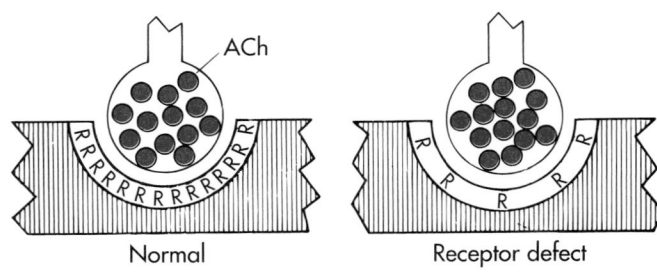

FIG. 54-3 Defect in myasthenia gravis. Schematic representation of normal neuromuscular junction and one with a receptor deficit seen in myasthenia gravis. Circles indicate ACh-containing vesicles within nerve endings. *ACh*, Acetylcholine; *R*, acetylcholine receptors.

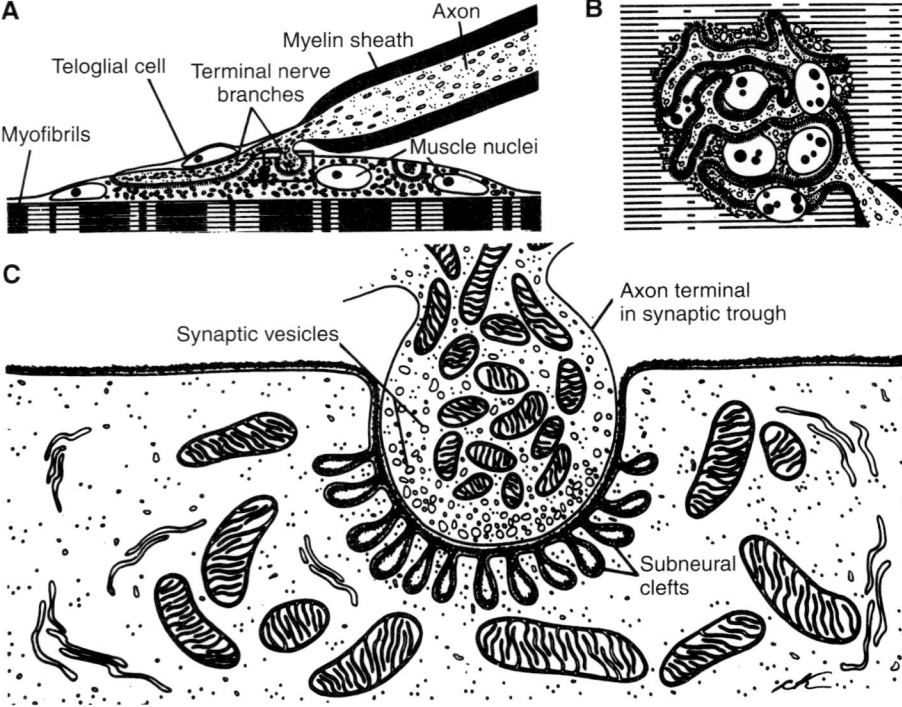

FIG. 54-2 Muscle and neuromuscular junction. Schematic representation of the motor end-plate as seen by light and electron microscopy. **A**, End-plate as seen in histologic sections in the long axis of the muscle fiber; **B**, as seen in surface view with the light microscope; **C**, as seen in an electron micrograph of an area such as that in the rectangle in **A**. (From Curtis B, Jacobson S, Marcus E: *An introduction to the neurosciences*, Philadelphia, 1972, Saunders.)

In patients with MG, the muscles appear normal macroscopically, although disuse atrophy may be present. Atrophy present results from disuse. Microscopically, in some patients lymphocytic infiltrates may be found within the muscle and other organs but no consistent abnormality is found in the skeletal muscle.

Clinical Manifestations

As mentioned previously, it is currently hypothesized that MG is an autoimmune disorder that impairs acetylcholine receptor functioning and decreases the efficiency of the neuromuscular junction. MG most frequently presents as an insidious, progressive disease characterized by muscle weakness and fatigability. However, the condition may remain localized to a specific group of muscles. Because the course is so variable from one patient to another, it is difficult to determine the prognosis. Box 54-2 presents the hallmarks of the disease.

In 90% of patients, the initial symptoms involve the ocular muscles, causing ptosis and diplopia. The diagnosis can be established by attention to the levator palpebrae muscles of the eyelids. If the disease remains confined to the eye muscles, the course is very mild and is not associated with increased mortality.

The facial, laryngeal, and pharyngeal muscles are also frequently involved in MG. This involvement may result in regurgitation through the nose when swallowing is attempted (palatal muscles); abnormal, nasal speech; and failure of the mouth to close, which is termed the *hanging jaw sign*. With facial muscle involvement, a snarl-like appearance may be present when the individual attempts to smile.

Respiratory muscle involvement is evidenced by a weak cough, eventual attacks of dyspnea, and inability to clear mucus from the tracheobronchial tree. The shoulder and pelvic girdles may become involved in advanced cases; generalized weakness of any skeletal muscles may occur. Standing, walking, or even holding the arms above the head, as to comb the hair, may become difficult.

Generally, rest and anticholinesterase agents can relieve symptoms of MG. Symptoms are aggravated or exacerbated by (1) alterations in hormonal balance, as during pregnancy, fluctuations in the menstrual cycle, or disturbances in thyroid function; (2) concurrent illness, especially upper respiratory tract infections and those associated with diarrhea and fever; (3) emotional upsets—most patients experience more muscular weakness when they are upset; and (4) alcohol (especially with tonic water, which contains quinine, a drug promoting muscle weakness) and other drugs.

Diagnosis

A diagnosis can be made on the basis of the patient's history and the physical examination. One must acknowledge the reality of MG. Many patients have been bluntly told to see a psychiatrist because their symptoms have a psychologic basis only. Asking the subject to perform a repetitive action until tiredness is evident can help establish a diagnosis. Electromyography (EMG) reveals a characteristic falling off in the amplitude of motor unit potential with continued use. A specific test for MG is the presence of serum antibodies to the acetylcholine receptor. At least 80% of patients with MG have abnormally high serum levels of the antibodies, but patients with mild or isolated ocular forms of MG may have false negative results. The diagnosis is confirmed by the *Tensilon test*. Edrophonium chloride (Tensilon), a cholinesterase inhibitor drug, is given intravenously. In MG patients, there is a marked improvement of muscle strength within 30 seconds. When a positive result is obtained, it is important to make a differential diagnosis between true MG and myasthenic syndrome. Patients with *myasthenia syndrome* have the same symptoms as those with true MG, but the cause is related to other pathologic processes, such as diabetes, thyroid abnormalities, and widespread malignancy. The age of onset of the two conditions is an important distinguishing factor. Patients with true MG are usually young, whereas those with myasthenic syndrome tend to be older. Symptoms in the myasthenic syndrome usually disappear if the basic disease can be controlled.

Abnormalities of the thymus gland occur in MG. Even when too small to be radiologically observable, the thymus glands of most patients are histologically abnormal. The tendency is for younger women to have thymic hyperplasia, whereas older men have thymic neoplasms.

Treatment

If the patient survives for 10 years, the disease usually remains benign, and death from MG itself would be rare. These patients must learn to live within the limits prescribed by their disease: they need 10 hours of sleep at night to awaken refreshed, and they need to alternate work and rest periods; they must also avoid precipitating factors and must take their medications on time.

Medical treatment with *anticholinesterase drugs* is the treatment of choice to counteract the symptoms of MG. Neostigmine inactivates or destroys cholinesterase, thus the acetylcholine is not destroyed immediately. The effect is restoration to almost normal muscular activity, at least 80% to 90% of former strength and endurance. Besides neostigmine (Prostigmin), pyridostigmine (Mestinon), and ambenonium (Mytelase), other synthetic analogs of the originally used drug, physostigmine (Eserine), are used. Disagreeable side effects in the GI tract (cramping, diarrhea) are called *muscarinic side effects*. It is important for the patient to realize that these symptoms can indicate too much medication has been taken on a particular day and that the next dose must be decreased accordingly to avoid a cholinergic crisis. Because neostigmine is the most apt to cause muscarinic effects, it may be prescribed initially so that the patient is made aware of the exact nature of this side effect. Pyridostigmine is available in a time span form and is often used at bedtime so that the patient can sleep through the night without having to awaken to take medication.

For long-term, more lasting effect on controlling MG, the patient has two basic treatment choices. The first of these choices is immunosuppressive drugs, all of which have a low therapeutic index (ratio of toxic dose to therapeutic dose). Corticosteroid therapy is associated with clinical improvement in many patients, although many serious side effects are associated with long-term use. Some patients respond well to a combined regimen of corticosteroids and pyridostigmine. Azathioprine, an immunosuppressive drug, is being used with good results; side effects are minor when compared with those associated with corticosteroids and consist mainly of GI upset, liver enzyme elevation, and leukopenia. Plasma exchange may be effective in myasthenic crisis because of its ability to remove antibodies to the acetylcholine receptors, but it is not useful in the chronic management of the disease.

The second long-term treatment option is major chest surgery to remove the thymus gland (thymectomy). Approximately 15% of patients with MG have a tumor or hyperplasia of the thymus gland called a *thymoma*. Because the thymus is involved in the development of the immune system, removal of the gland is curative in some patients. Decision to perform thymectomy is made on an individual basis, because its benefit in reducing symptoms is not as great in older patients or in persons who have had MG for more than 5 years. Approximately 30% of patients with MG without a thymoma who undergo thymectomy eventually experience medication-free remission. Another 50% of patients experience noticeable improvement (Keesey, Sonshine, 1997).

Crisis in Myasthenia Gravis

When unable to swallow, clear secretions, or breathe adequately without artificial assistance, the myasthenic patient is in crisis. The two types of crises are (1) *myasthenic crisis*, a condition in which the patient needs more anticholinesterase drugs, and (2) *cholinergic crisis*, a condition caused by an excess of anticholinesterase drugs. In either situation, ventilation and an adequate airway must be maintained. Edrophonium chloride (Tensilon) (2 to 5 mg) is given intravenously as a test to differentiate between the types of crises. The drug produces a temporary improvement in myasthenic crisis and no improvement or worsening of symptoms in cholinergic crisis.

If in myasthenic crisis, the patient is maintained on the respirator. Anticholinesterase drugs are withheld because they increase respiratory secretions and may precipitate a cholinergic crisis. Medicines are restarted gradually, and often the dose can be lowered after a crisis.

In a cholinergic crisis, the patient may have taken an excess of medication by mistake or the dose may have been excessive because of a spontaneous remission. Many patients who develop this type of crisis are called *brittle myasthenics*. These episodes are difficult to control with medication and have a narrowed therapeutic range between underdose and overdose. The response to drugs is often only partial. In cholinergic crisis, the patient is maintained on artificial ventilation, anticholinergic drugs are with-

held, and 1 mg of atropine may be given intravenously and repeated if necessary. When atropine is administered, the patient must be carefully observed because respiratory secretions can thicken, making suctioning difficult, or a mucous plug can occlude a bronchus, causing atelectasis.

Guillain-Barré Syndrome

Guillain-Barré syndrome (GBS, pronounced *ghee-yan bah-ray*) is an acute demyelinating polyneuropathy that is known by several other names: idiopathic polyneuritis, Landry's ascending paralysis, and acute inflammatory polyneuropathy. The principle feature of GBS is a primarily ascending motor paralysis with variable disturbances of sensory function. GBS is a lower motor neuron disorder in that the peripheral nerve, the final common pathway for motor movement, is involved. The syndrome, which is seen throughout the world, occurs in all seasons, similar to an endemic disease, and affects both genders and all age-groups. The incidence is approximately 1 to 2 cases per 100,000 persons per year (0.001 to 0.002% of the population). Attempts to isolate a causative infectious agent have been unsuccessful, and its cause remains unknown. However, it is known that GBS is neither hereditary nor contagious (NINDS, 2000). The syndrome became well publicized in the United States in 1976 when an outbreak of more than 500 cases occurred during the national vaccination campaign against the swine influenza virus. Although there may be no known precipitating event, a careful patient history often reveals an unremarkable viral illness that occurred 1 to 3 weeks before the onset of motor weakness. Other typical preceding events are a mild respiratory or GI infection, surgery, immunizations, Hodgkin's disease or other lymphomas, and lupus erythematosus. The most frequently reported precipitating event is infection with *Campylobacter jejuni*, which typically causes a self-limited GI illness characterized by diarrhea, abdominal pain, and fever. Approximately 1 in 2000 *C. jejuni* infections are complicated by GBS, which affects approximately 1% of the U.S. population each year (Allos et al, 1998).

The most likely sequence of events in the pathologic cascade is that the precipitating event (e.g., a virus or inflammatory process) changes the cells in the nervous system so that the immune system "recognizes" them as nonself or foreign cells. Subsequently, sensitized T lymphocytes and macrophages attack myelin. In addition, the T lymphocytes induce B lymphocytes to produce antibodies against certain constituents of the myelin sheath, contributing to myelin destruction (NINDS, 2000).

The result is mild to severe demyelinating injury that interferes with impulse conduction in the affected peripheral nerves. (In contrast, the demyelination in MS is confined to the CNS.) Pathologic changes follow a consistent pattern: lymphocytic infiltrations occur in the perivascular spaces adjacent to the nerve and become the foci of myelin degeneration. In some cases, the nerve axons themselves show evidence of wallerian degeneration, indicating a more proximal axonal lesion that has led to degeneration of the axon and myelin distal to it. The anterior horn cells of the spinal cord and the motor nuclei of the cranial nerves may become affected as the inflammation extends proximally from the peripheral nerve axons. If the nerve cell body is not destroyed, peripheral nerve regeneration may take place, with recovery of motor function. However, if the cell body of the lower motor neuron dies because of an aggressive inflammatory response, nerve regeneration cannot take place, affected muscles atrophy, and recovery is less complete.

Demyelination of peripheral nerve axons causes both positive and negative symptoms. The positive symptoms are pain and paresthesias arising from either abnormal impulse activity in sensory fibers or electrical "cross-talk" between damaged, abnormal axons. The negative symptoms are muscle weakness or paralysis, loss of tendon reflexes, and decreased sensation. The first two negative symptoms are caused by *motor* axon damage; the last results from *sensory* fiber damage. Conduction block, slowed conduction, and impaired ability to conduct impulses underlie the negative symptoms. Most people experience the greatest weakness within the first 2 weeks after onset of symptoms; by the third week, 90% of all patients are at their weakest level (NINDS, 2000). The recovery period varies greatly: from a few weeks or as much as a few years. Approximately 30% of GBS patients have some residual weakness after 3 years. A few persons (about 3%) may have an unpredictable relapse of muscle weakness and paresthesias many years after the acute attack.

In GBS, sensory symptoms tend to be mild and may consist of pain, tingling, and numbness, as well as abnormalities in vibratory and position sense. However, the polyneuropathy is predominantly motor, and clinical findings may vary from mild muscular weakness to paralysis of the respiratory muscles requiring ventilatory management. Skeletal muscle weakness is often so acute that atrophy is not present, but loss of muscle tone and areflexia are readily detectable. Tenderness is usually elicited by deep pressure or squeezing of muscles. The arms may be spared, or their muscles may be less weakened than the leg muscles. Autonomic symptoms include postural hypotension, sinus tachycardia, and lack of ability to sweat. If cranial nerves are involved, paralysis of affected facial, ocular, and oropharyngeal muscles usually follows arm involvement. Cranial nerve symptoms include facial palsy and speech difficulties, visual disturbances, and swallowing difficulties. The term *bulbar palsy* is sometimes used to refer specifically to paralysis of the jaw, pharynx, and tongue musculature caused by damage to cranial nerves IX, X, and XI, which arise from the medulla oblongata, originally called the *bulb*.

Patient history and clinical findings of paralysis and paresthesias are especially important in diagnosing GBS. Typically, history will reveal that the symptoms are bilateral and appeared relatively quickly, over days or weeks rather than months. Principal diagnostic tests are EMG, nerve conduction velocity, and lumbar puncture to examine the CSF. The CSF is under normal pressure and is acellular, although, later in the course of the disease, high protein levels may be found. Body temperature is usually normal, and spleen and lymph node enlargement are not typical of this disease. Initial therapeutic management is supportive, with focus on support of ventilation, blood pressure, and cardiac function. If mechanical ventilation is required, patients under 60 years of age without preexisting lung disease can usually be weaned within 2 weeks. A Mayo Clinic study found that mechanical ventilation

was required in 81% of GBS patients with a poor outcome and that mortality was 20% in patients ventilated for GBS. However, ventilated patients who survived did well, with 79% eventually regaining independent ambulation. Nineteen percent of patients improved at least one functional grade beyond 1 year. Predictors of poor maximal recovery in ventilated GBS patients were increased age, upper limb paralysis, duration of ventilation, and delay of more than 2 days to transfer to a tertiary center (Fletcher et al, 2000). Early plasmapheresis has been found to decrease the severity of symptoms. Intravenous administration of a high-dose immunoglobulin has also been beneficial, but glucocorticoid therapy has fallen into disuse because of lack of evidence of its efficacy. As soon as voluntary movement returns to skeletal muscles, intensive physiotherapy is initiated to prevent muscle and joint contractures.

Postpolio Syndrome

Postpolio syndrome (PPS), or postpoliomyelitis neuromuscular atrophy, is a progressive muscle weakness usually beginning 20 to 30 years after recovery from viral poliomyelitis infection that attacked the anterior horn cells of the spinal cord, as well as cranial nerve nuclei. The estimated total incidence is about 25% of the polio survivor population, which The Easter Seal Society most recently estimated at 1,600,000 in the United States (NINDS, 2000).

The classic triad of symptoms includes unusual fatigue, new muscle weakness with or without muscle atrophy, and muscle pain that is often accompanied by muscle twitching (International Polio Network, 1999). Other symptoms are typical of a lower motor neuron paresis or paralysis: muscle pain, fasciculations, and muscle weakness that may reach a plateau or progress to muscle atrophy. The limbs are affected most often. However, the respiratory muscles may be involved, as well as head and neck muscles innervated by cranial nerves IX, X, and XI (bulbar paralysis). The result may be respiratory failure, severe sleep apnea, difficulty swallowing, episodes of choking, or aspiration.

The following general criteria must be met for a diagnosis to be made: prior episode of paralytic polio; period of functional stability; gradual or abrupt new weakness usually accompanied by several of the listed symptoms; and exclusion of other medical, orthopedic, and neurologic conditions that may cause the symptoms. Diagnosis is made through a thorough history, neurologic examination, and laboratory studies, including MRI, electrophysiologic studies, muscle biopsy, and CSF analysis.

The cause of the long latent PPS is controversial but is usually believed to involve an abnormality of surviving lower motor neurons, accompanied by a progressive slow disintegration of peripheral nerve axons. The most widely accepted explanation of the weakness is a dysfunction of the motor unit, with loss of individual nerve terminals in the motor units that remain after the initial polio attack.

Treatment is supportive and directed toward maintaining respiratory function, alleviating symptoms, and preventing complications. Currently, there is no treatment that prevents or cures PPS. Drugs such as pyridostigmine and selegiline, which work at the neuromuscular junction, have been used with some success for symptomatic treatment.

CNS INFECTIOUS AND INFLAMMATORY DISORDERS

Infections of the CNS constitute a serious medical problem requiring immediate recognition and treatment to minimize serious neurologic sequelae and ensure patient survival.

CNS infection by viruses occurs relatively infrequently but can be serious. Generally, viruses invade the CNS via the blood, although certain infections such as rabies and varicella-zoster invade the CNS via the peripheral nerves.

Signs and symptoms of viral CNS infections vary greatly according to the susceptibility of the different CNS cells to the virus. Infections limited to the meninges produce symptoms suggestive of meningitis (nuchal rigidity, headache, fever), whereas if the brain parenchyma is involved, the patient shows a decreased level of consciousness, seizures, focal neurologic deficits, and increased intracranial pressure (ICP).

Viral Meningitis and Encephalitis

Viral meningitis is an infection involving the meninges; it tends to be benign and self-limiting. *Viral encephalitis* involves the brain parenchyma and is more serious. Various viruses are known to cause meningitis and encephalitis (Box 54-3).

Viruses generally replicate themselves at the original site of infection (e.g., nasopharyngeal or GI systems) and then spread to the CNS via the vascular system. Contrary to previous thinking, the blood-brain barrier does not provide complete protection against the invasion of viruses. Encephalitis involves an inflammatory reaction of the brain parenchyma, causing degeneration and phagocytosis of neural cells.

Patients with viral meningitis present with abrupt onset of headache, fever, and nuchal rigidity; they may also experience malaise, sore throat, nausea, vomiting, and abdominal pain. In addition, viral meningitis caused by the enteroviruses is associated with rashes; mumps meningitis is associated with parotitis as well as oophoritis and pancreatitis. Type 2 herpes simplex meningitis may coincide with eruption of genital herpes lesions.

In addition to the meningeal signs, viral encephalitis presents with decreasing levels of consciousness, seizures, and focal symptoms, depending on the area of brain involved. Patients with herpes simplex encephalitis may show bizarre behavior and hallucinations.

In evaluating the patient with the signs and symptoms of viral meningitis and encephalitis, it is important to differentiate these diseases from other more treatable infections, such as subacute bacterial endocarditis or brain abscess. CSF pressure may be normal or elevated and may contain protein in small or large quantities; the electroencephalogram (EEG) may show changes, especially in encephalitis. Virologic studies can specifically identify the virus; this identification has become more important because herpes simplex encephalitis is currently treated with adenine arabinoside.

Other specific antiviral agents are not currently used, and patients are treated supportively. The prognosis is good for patients with meningitis but poorer for patients with encephalitis. Mortality rates vary from 50% in herpes simplex encephalitis to less than 1% in specific types of arbovirus encephalitis. Sequelae such as seizures, hydrocephalus, and other neurologic deficits are common.

Reye's Syndrome

Reye's syndrome is a rare, acute multiorgan dysfunction that produces its most lethal effects on the brain (encephalitis) and liver (fatty degeneration). Seen in children and young adolescents, the Reye's syndrome peak occurs in January through March, when influenza is most common. Reye's syndrome is often called a two-phase illness, because it almost invariably follows a previous infection with influenza, varicella, adenovirus, coxsackievirus, echovirus, or parainfluenza virus, with apparent recovery from the original viral infection. It is now well accepted that a strong association exists between Reye's syndrome and the use of salicylates (aspirin) in children or adolescents with viral infections. The asymptomatic or recovery period in postviral infections varies from hours to days. Vomiting and convulsions followed by delirium and coma ensue after this apparent recovery. Fever is not usually present.

Pathologically, the brain swells with injury to the neuronal mitochondria. Fatty infiltration of the liver occurs, spreading rapidly through the parenchyma. Fat deposits can also be found in the myocardium and renal tubules. The relationship between the viral infection and the encephalopathy and liver damage is unknown.

Coma and decerebrate posturing from increased ICP are often seen. Electrolyte imbalances, especially hyponatremia, hypokalemia, and high serum ammonia levels, are serious problems. Treatment is nonspecific and is directed toward reducing ICP and correcting metabolic and electrolyte abnormalities.

Hypertonic glucose solutions are used for hydration to maintain a blood sugar of 200 to 300 mg/dl, because low blood sugar leads to increased production of ammonia and fatty acids. Peritoneal dialysis has been used in some patients to reduce elevated blood ammonia levels.

BOX 54-3

Viruses Causing Central Nervous System Infections

ENTEROVIRUSES
Poliovirus
Coxsackie virus (coxsackievirus) types A and B
Echovirus (ECHO virus)

HERPESVIRUSES
Herpes simplex virus types 1 and 2
Cytomegalovirus

MYXOVIRUSES
Measles virus
Mumps virus
Influenza virus

Some children who recover have residual neurologic deficits, including impaired mental capacity, seizures, and hemiplegia. Mortality rates ranges from 25% to 50%, depending on factors such as age, severity of symptoms, and time of diagnosis and treatment.

Bacterial Infections

Bacterial infections of the CNS present a challenging problem. A variety of bacteria infect the meninges and brain parenchyma. The most common infecting bacteria are *Staphylococcus aureus, Streptococcus pneumoniae,* and *Haemophilus influenzae.* Isolation of the specific agent involved is essential in the treatment of bacterial CNS infections.

Bacteria enter the CNS by several different routes. The ears, sinus, mastoid, and face are the most common sites of the original infection. Bacteria are able to travel from the site of origin to the CNS because of the high vascularity of the face and neck and the anatomic structuring of the venous sinuses within the brain. Early and conscientious treatment of these primary infections significantly reduces the incidence of secondary CNS infections.

Brain Abscess

Brain abscess is an infective process involving the brain parenchyma; it is caused primarily by the spread of an infection from adjacent foci or through the vascular system. A previous history of otitis media, mastoiditis, suppurative sinusitis, or infection of the face, scalp, or skull is common. Bronchiectasis, lung abscess, empyema, and bacterial endocarditis are also known to lead to brain abscess.

Infection may invade the brain several different ways. In otitis media the infection may extend through the tympanic cavity or through the mastoid and meninges to reach the brain tissue. The infection extends via the veins of the inner ear, causing the veins to thrombose. This thrombosis impairs cerebral circulation, leading to ischemia and infarction, which facilitate the development of a local infection. Any tear in the dura caused by trauma is a potential source of infection of the brain.

Generally, abscesses are localized near the original site of infection. However, abscesses resulting from retrograde venous propagation are located at some distance from the primary site in the distribution of the nearest venous sinus. Metastatic abscesses are generally located along the middle cerebral artery. Early in the course of the disease, the infected tissue is edematous and infiltrated with leukocytes. Gradually, the outer portion becomes thickened because of the presence of collagen in the abscess wall. In the center of the abscess, liquefaction necrosis occurs. Abscess cavities can spread through the white matter, penetrating the walls of the ventricles or into the meninges.

Brain abscess most frequently occurs between the ages of 20 and 50 but has been found in all age groups. The patient presents with headache and focal neurologic signs that vary with the location of the abscess (Table 54-2). Signs of increased ICP (especially nausea, vomiting, and decreasing level of consciousness) are the most common findings.

Generally, a CT scan identifies and localizes the major abscess and surrounding smaller abscesses. Because of the danger of brain herniation, lumbar puncture is usually avoided when the presence of a large mass is suspected. Early diagnosis and prompt antibiotic therapy are essential if the patient is to survive. Residual neurologic deficits, especially convulsions, are common.

TABLE 54-2

Focal Symptoms Seen in Brain Abscess

Lobe	Symptoms
Frontal	Drowsiness, inattentiveness, disturbed judgment, impaired intelligence, occasionally convulsions
Temporal	Inability to name objects; inability to read, write, or understand spoken words; hemianopia
Parietal	Impaired position sense and stereognostic perception, focal seizures, homonymous hemianopia, dysphasia, acalculia, agraphia
Cerebellar	Suboccipital headache, stiff neck, impaired coordination, nystagmus, impaired gait, intention tremor

KEY CONCEPTS

- It is vital to determine whether a *dementia* is secondary to a treatable cause.
- For most dementias, there is no known cause and no definitive treatment.
- Specific pathologic findings in *dementias of the Alzheimer's type (DAT)* are neuronal degeneration, intracellular neurofibrillatory tangles, diminished and deformed cell processes, and extracellular amyloid plaques.
- Factors associated with increased risk of DAT are decreased estrogen levels and presence of beta protein.
- Primary pathologic processes of the nervous system are classified as neurologic disorders with generalized symptomatology.

- The most common form of dementia, *Alzheimer's disease (AD)*, is characterized by structural and biochemical changes in neurons.
- Brain diseases resulting in progressive degeneration of neurons are usually multifactorial in origin, with genetic, environmental, and physiologic events all playing a role.
- Parkinsonism is a basal ganglia disorder that may be idiopathic (e.g., *Parkinson's disease [PD]*) or the result of various drug toxicities.
- *Extrapyramidal syndrome (EPS)* refers to a constellation of signs caused by a loss of fine-tuned regulation of the voluntary motor pathways by the basal ganglia. The resultant difficulty in controlling and

initiating movement underlie the cardinal symptoms: akinesia, tremors at rest, rigidity, and loss of postural reflexes.

- *Huntington's disease (HD)* is an autosomal dominant inherited disorder that involves neuronal degeneration in the caudate nucleus and putamen of the basal ganglia; it progresses slowly, resulting in severe choreiform movements and gradual intellectual deterioration.

- *Amyotrophic lateral sclerosis (ALS)*, or *Lou Gehrig's disease*, is a progressive degenerative disorder involving motor neurons in the cortex, lower brainstem, and spinal cord. The result is atrophy of innervated muscles, the most devastating of which involves the muscles that control swallowing and respiration.

- *Multiple sclerosis (MS)* is a demyelinating disease of the brain and spinal cord that affects young adults, especially women.

- In MS, the loss of myelin and subsequent scarring of the white matter of nerve tracts can occur anywhere in the CNS but especially affects cranial nerves II and III (optic and oculomotor nerves), cerebellum, and spinal tracts. The results are characteristic of impaired nerve conduction in these fibers: diplopia, scotomas, and decreased visual acuity, loss of coordination, muscular weakness, and sensory impairment.

- *Myasthenia gravis (MG)* is an autoimmune disease affecting receptors at the neuromuscular endplate and resulting in early muscular fatigue, weakness, and slow recovery of skeletal muscle function.

- *Reye's syndrome*, a rare acute multiorgan dysfunction that includes encephalitis, is strongly associated with the use of aspirin in children or young adults with viral infections.

QUESTIONS ??

A sampling of review questions for this chapter appears here. Visit http://www.mosby.com/MERLIN/PriceWilson/ for additional questions. MERLIN

Answer the following on a separate sheet of paper.

1. Name the sites in the brain that are affected in Parkinson's disease (PD). How are these areas of the brain affected? Where are these areas located in the brain?

2. Name the type of fiber tract involved in PD. What is the general function of this fiber tract?

3. Define Parkinson's syndrome and name three types.

4. Discuss the role of dopamine in parkinsonism.

5. Name and briefly describe five movement disorders of the extrapyramidal motor tracts.

6. Name two drugs known to cause extrapyramidal dysfunction and parkinsonian signs and symptoms.

7. Name several neurologic findings (include one reflex) common in patients with PD.

8. What serious demyelinating disorder may follow measles or vaccination for rabies? Why does this complication now occur rarely?

9. Describe the pathology in multiple sclerosis (MS). What are the most likely symptoms that would cause you to suspect MS in a patient?

10. Discuss the two major morphologic changes and the major biochemical change that occurs in the brain affected by Alzheimer's disease (AD).

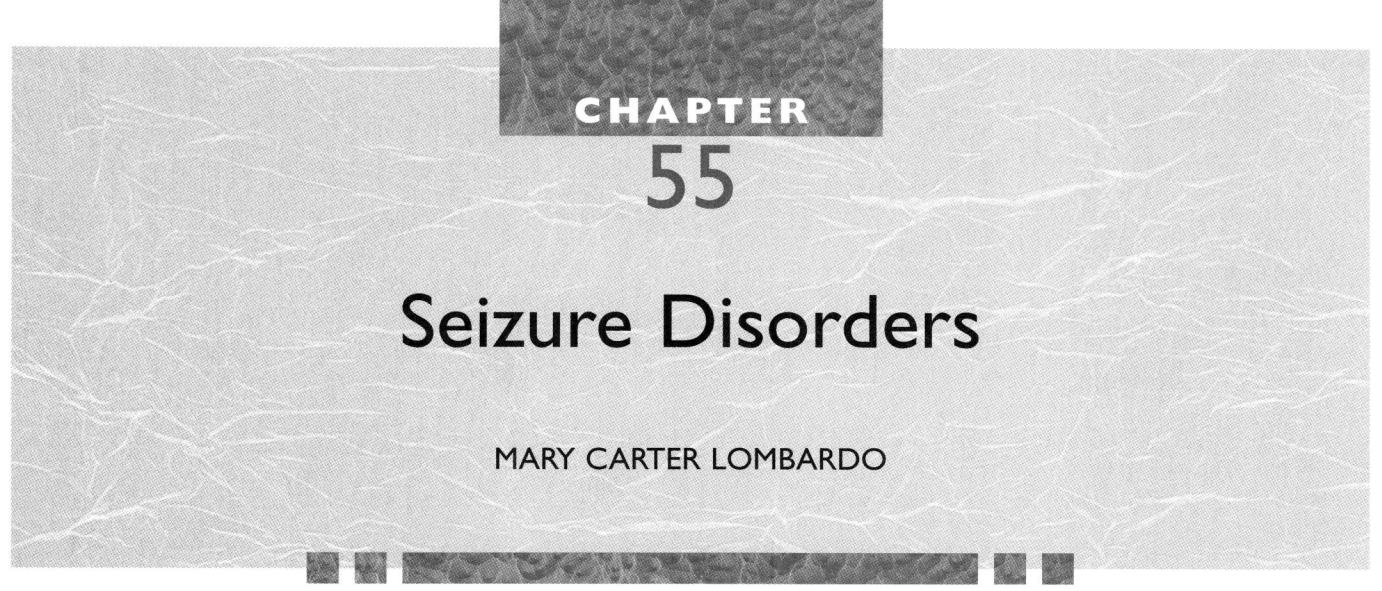

CHAPTER
55

Seizure Disorders

MARY CARTER LOMBARDO

Seizures are a relatively common neurologic problem. The estimate is that 1 in 10 persons will experience a seizure sometime during their lifetime. The two peak times for the incidence of seizures are during the first decade of life and after age 60 years. Seizures are the result of excessive paroxysmal discharge from a hyperexcitable population of neurons (the seizure focus) that interfere with the normal functioning of the brain. However, seizures also arise from normal brain tissue under certain pathologic conditions, such as changes in acid-base or electrolyte balance. The seizure itself, if short lived, is rarely damaging, but it can be a manifestation of a threatening underlying disorder, such as metabolic derangement, intracranial infections, drug withdrawal, drug intoxication, or hypertensive encephalopathy. Depending on the location of these hyperexcitable neurons, the seizure exhibits itself as any combination of altered level of consciousness and disturbances in motor, sensory, or autonomic functions. The term "seizure" is generic, and other specific descriptions are applicable according to the characteristics observed. Seizures may be isolated or repetitive. Recurrent, spontaneous, nonmetabolically-induced seizures occurring over a span of years are termed *epilepsy*. Generalized motor seizures involving loss of consciousness and some combination of tonic-clonic muscle contractions are often called *convulsions*. Convulsive seizures typically produce severe, involuntary, skeletal muscle activity that may progress from one body part to the entire body or may occur suddenly with whole body involvement. *Status epilepticus* is a prolonged continuous seizure or a series of repetitive seizures without interictal consciousness.

Data on seizure incidence are somewhat difficult to uncover. It is estimated that 10% of persons will have at least one seizure in their lifetime and approximately 0.3% to 0.5% will be diagnosed with epilepsy (based on the criterion of two or more unprovoked seizures). Gender-specific reports indicate slightly higher rates for males than for females. Age-specific incidence shows a consistent pattern of the highest rate in the first year of life, a rapid decline toward adolescence, and a gradual leveling off during the middle years with another peak after age 60. More than 75% of patients with epilepsy have their first seizure before age 20; when the first seizure occurs after age 20, seizure disorder is usually secondary. Epilepsy may be classified as idiopathic or symptomatic. In the *idiopathic* or *essential epilepsy*, no known central lesion can be demonstrated. In *symptomatic* or *secondary epilepsy*, a cerebral abnormality promotes the seizure response. Among the many conditions that may be responsible for secondary epilepsy are head injuries (including those before and after birth), metabolic and nutritional disorders (hypoglycemia, phenylketonuria, vitamin B_6 deficiency), toxic factors (alcohol intoxication, narcotic withdrawal, uremia), encephalitis, hypoxia, circulatory disturbances, electrolyte imbalances (especially hyponatremia and hypocalcemia), and neoplasms.

PATHOPHYSIOLOGY

Seizures result from excessive paroxysmal discharge either from a seizure focus or from normal tissue under assault from a pathologic condition. The seizure activity depends partly on the location of the excessive discharge. Lesions in the midbrain, thalamus, and cerebral cortex are most likely to be epileptogenic, whereas lesions in the cerebellum and brainstem do not generally evoke seizures.

At the cell membrane level, certain biochemical phenomena characterize the seizure focus, including the following:

- Instability of the nerve cell membrane, allowing the cell to be more susceptible to activation
- Hypersensitive neurons with lowered thresholds for firing and firing excessively

- Polarization abnormalities (excessive polarization, hypopolarization, or lapses in repolarization) caused by an excess of acetylcholine or a deficiency of gamma-aminobyuric acid (GABA)
- Ionic imbalances altering the acid-base or electrolyte balance, which alter the neuronal chemical homeostasis, interfering with neuronal depolarization. This altered balance leads to excess in excitatory neurotransmitters or depletion in inhibitory neurotransmitters.

The metabolic changes that occur during and immediately after a seizure are caused, in part, by increased energy needs from the neuronal hyperactivity. Metabolic needs are drastically increased during seizures; the electrical discharges of motor nerve cells may be increased to 1000 per second. Cerebral blood flow is increased, as is tissue respiration and glycolysis. Acetylcholine appears in cerebrospinal fluid (CSF) during and after seizures. Glutamic acid may be depleted during seizure activity.

Generally, no gross change is found at autopsy. Histopathologic evidence supports the hypothesis that the lesion is neurochemical rather than structural. No consistent pathologic factor has been identified. Focal abnormalities in the metabolism of potassium and acetylcholine are found to be present between seizures. Seizure foci seem especially sensitive to acetylcholine, a facilitatory transmitter; they are slow to bind and remove the acetylcholine.

TYPES OF SEIZURES

Each major clinical center for epilepsy uses the classification that works best for its purposes. Table 55-1 shows the classification (modified) adopted by the International League Against Epilepsy. Electroencephalographic study, MRI, clinical assessment, and history are used to identify the type of seizure.

Seizures are classified as partial or generalized based on whether consciousness is lost or preserved. Seizures in which consciousness is preserved are known as *partial seizures*. Partial seizures are further divided into *simple partial* (consciousness is preserved) and *complex partial* (consciousness is altered but not lost).

Partial seizures begin in a specific area of the brain, usually the cerebral cortex. The symptoms of these seizures depend on the location of the focus in the brain. For instance, if the focus is in the motor cortex, muscle jerks may be the primary symptoms; whereas, if the focus is the sensory cortex, the patients experience sensory symptoms including numbness, crawling sensations or a feeling of "pins and needles." Usually some clonic movements are associated with the sensory seizure, because some motor representation exists in the sensory cortex. Autonomic symptoms include pallor, flushing, sweating, and vomiting. Distortions of memory, dysphagia, and déjà vu are examples of psychic symptoms of partial seizures. It is extremely important to observe where the seizure began, because this may offer a clue as to the location of the lesion. Some patients may experience progression to the opposite hemisphere with a loss of consciousness.

The seizure discharge in complex partial seizures (previously known as psychomotor or temporal lobe seizures) often arises from the medial temporal or inferior frontal lobe and involves disturbances in higher level cerebral function and thought processes, as well as complex motor behavior. These seizures can be precipitated by music, blinking lights, or other stimuli and are frequently accompanied by coordinated involuntary, repetitive motor activities known as automatic behaviors. Examples of these behaviors include picking at clothes, fumbling with objects, clapping hands, lip smacking, or repetitive chewing. Patients may experience a clouded, "dreamy" feeling of unreality. The patient is conscious during the attack but generally does not recall what happened. Complex partial seizures may spread and become generalized seizures.

Generalized seizures involve the entire cerebral cortex and diencephalon and are characterized by the onset of bilateral, symmetric seizure activity that occurs in both hemispheres without evidence of a localized start. Patients are unconscious and are unaware of their surroundings during these seizures. These seizures generally start without an aura or warning. There are several types of generalized seizures (see Table 55-1).

TABLE 55-1

Classification of Seizures

Classification	Characteristics
PARTIAL	Consciousness preserved although may be altered; focused in one area but may spread to others
Simple Partial	• Can be motor (abnormal, unilateral movements), sensory (abnormal smells, sounds, sensations), autonomic (tachycardia, bradycardia, tachypnea, flushing, epigastric discomfort), psychic (dysphagia, memory distortions) • Usually lasts less than 1 minute
Complex Partial	Beginning as simple partial seizures; progressing to altered consciousness accompanied by: • Motor symptoms, sensory symptoms, automatisms (lip smacking, chewing, picking at clothes) • Some complex partial seizures may progress to generalized seizure • Usually last 1-3 minutes
GENERALIZED	Loss of consciousness; no focal onset, bilateral and symmetric; no aura
Tonic-Clonic	Tonic-clonic spasms of muscles; bowel and bladder incontinence; tongue biting, postictal phase
Absence	Commonly misdiagnosed as daydreaming: • Vacant stare, slight droop to head, fluttering of eyelids, or rapid blinking; no loss of postural tone • Lasts a few seconds
Myoclonic	Sudden shocklike contractions localized to a few muscles or limb; tends to be brief
Atonic	Sudden loss of muscle tone with loss of body posture (drop attacks)
Clonic	Slow single or multiple sharp, repetitive, jerking movements of arms, legs, or torso
Tonic	Sudden increase in muscle tone (stiffening, contraction) of face and upper body; flexion of arms and extension of legs • Eyes and head may deviate to one side • May cause respiratory arrest

TABLE 55-2

Physiologic Effects of Seizures

Early (Less than 15 Minutes)	Late (15-30 Minutes)	Prolonged (Longer than 1 Hour)
Elevated heart rate	Decrease in blood pressure	Hypotension with decrease in cerebral blood flow causing cerebral hypotension
Elevated blood pressure	Decrease in blood sugar	Disruption in the blood-brain barrier leading to cerebral edema
Elevated glucose level	Dysrhythmias	
Elevated core body temperature	Noncardiac pulmonary edema	
Elevation in white blood cells		

Absence seizures (formerly called petit mal) are characterized by short lapses of consciousness, rarely lasting more than a few seconds. For example, there may be a brief pause in conversation, a vacant look, or a rapid blinking of the eyes. The patient may experience one or two seizures a month or several a day. Absence seizures occur almost exclusively in children; onset is rare after 20 years of age. These episodes may disappear after puberty or be replaced by other seizures, especially tonic-clonic seizure.

Tonic-clonic seizure (formerly called grand mal) is the classic seizure of epilepsy. The tonic-clonic seizure starts with a rapid loss of consciousness. A cry may be uttered, from the forced expiration caused by thoracic or abnormal spasms. The patient experiences loss of upright position, tonic then clonic movements, and bladder or bowel incontinence (or both), along with other autonomic dysfunctions. In the tonic phase, muscles contract and body position may be distorted. This phase lasts for a few seconds. The clonic phase involves opposing muscle groups contracting and relaxing, giving a jerking movement. The contractions gradually decrease in number but not in strength. The tongue may be bitten; this occurs in approximately half the patients (spasms of the jaw and tongue). The entire seizure lasts from 3 to 5 minutes and is followed by a period of unconsciousness that may last from a few minutes to as long as 30 minutes. The patient regaining consciousness may appear confused, stuporous, or dull. This stage is referred to as the *postictal period.* Generally, the patient has no recollection of the seizure.

The physiologic effects of tonic-clonic seizures are dependent on the length of time the seizure persists. Prolonged tonic-clonic seizures lead to severe neurologic and cardiorespiratory effects. The early effects are caused by an increase in circulating catecholamines. If the seizure continues beyond 15 minutes, catecholamine depletion occurs resulting in secondary or later effects. Seizures lasting beyond 30 minutes may result in respiratory and cardiac arrest (Table 55-2).

Febrile tonic-clonic seizures, frequently referred to as *fever convulsions,* are most common in children under 5 years of age. Theories suggest that these seizures are caused by a rapid onset of hyperthermia related to a viral or bacterial infection. These seizures are generally of short duration, and there may be a familial predisposition. In some instances, the seizures may continue beyond early childhood and the child may experience nonfebrile seizures later in life.

In addition to these common types of generalized seizures, some may be considered secondary. *Head injuries* continue to be the most common cause of acquired

seizures. The incidence varies depending on the type and severity of the initial injury. Regardless of the mechanism, dura penetration is a significant risk factor for seizure development. With regard to seizure pathophysiology, two major factors are considered. The primary injury results from traumatic mechanical forces that shear dendrite processes, destroy capillaries, and disrupt the extracellular environment. The secondary injury is produced by cerebral edema. Accumulation of toxic metabolic products and ischemia from systemic hypotension, hypoxia, and hypercarbia contribute to the cerebral edema. The pathophysiologic mechanisms for the occurrence of seizures after head trauma include ischemia resulting from an altered vascular supply, the mechanical effects of scarring, the destruction of dendrite inhibitory controls, defects in the blood-brain barrier, and changes in the extracellular ionic buffering systems.

A clinical controversy continues to exist regarding the prophylactic treatment of head-injured patients for seizures following brain injury. Seizures occur most often within the first 30 to 90 days following head injury. Most institutions treat patients prophylactically who are considered high risk. Characteristics of the high-risk patients include a score of less than 10 on the Glasgow Coma Scale, presence of intracranial hemorrhage, penetration injury of the dura, or depressed skull fracture, or any combination. Phenytoin (Dilantin) is the drug of choice for prophylactic treatment.

Seizures may result from the acute phase or a sequela of a *central nervous system (CNS) infection* involving bacterial, viral, and parasitic organisms. It is noteworthy that seizures are typically the first clinical sign of a cerebral abscess. Infection accounts for about 3% of cases of acquired epilepsy.

Metabolic abnormalities, as an underlying cause of seizures, include hyponatremia, hypernatremia, hypoglycemia, hyperosmolar states, hypocalcemia, hypomagnesemia, hypoxia, and uremia. The neurologic symptoms of serum sodium alterations result from an increase or decrease in neuronal intracellular fluid volume and correlate with absolute levels of less than 125 mEq/L or greater than 150 mEq/L but, more importantly, correlate with the rapidity of the change. Advances in cardiopulmonary resuscitation (CPR) have contributed to an increased incidence of survival for patients experiencing cerebral hypoxia and its sequela, anoxic encephalopathy, causing it to become a more common cause of acquired seizure disorder.

Brain tumors are an additional cause of acquired seizures, particularly in patients 35 to 55 years of age. Seizure can be a presenting sign in certain brain tumors, especially meningioma, glioblastoma, and astrocytoma. Whether a cerebral neoplasm produces seizures depends on its type, rate of growth, and location. Tumors that are supratentorial and involve the cortex are most likely to be associated with a seizure. The highest incidence occurs with tumors along the central sulcus with involvement of the motor strip. The farther the tumor is from this area, the less likely it is to cause seizures.

Arteriosclerotic cerebrovascular insufficiency and *cerebral infarctions* are the predominant causes of seizures in patients with vascular disorders, and these appear to be increasing as the older population increases. Large infarctions and deep infarctions extending to deep subcortical structures are more likely to cause recurrent seizures.

Numerous *toxic substances and drugs* are associated with seizures. With some therapeutic medications, seizures are manifested as a toxic effect. Drugs with this potential include aminophylline, antidiabetic medications, lidocaine, phenothiazines, physostigmine, and tricyclics. Abuse of substances such as alcohol and cocaine may also lead to seizures.

STATUS EPILEPTICUS

Status epilepticus is defined as a state of continuous or intermittent seizure activity lasting 20 minutes or longer during which the patient does not regain consciousness. Status epilepticus should be considered a neurologic emergency. Significant neuronal damage can result from the continuous abnormal electrical activity. Mortality remains high, about 22% to 25%, for status epilepticus despite aggressive drug therapy. Seizure activities lasting longer than 60 minutes and older age are factors that contribute to a poorer prognosis. Death in status epilepticus is caused by hyperpyrexia, increased bronchial secretions causing airway and ventilatory obstruction, aspiration of vomitus, and failure of compensatory and regulatory mechanisms.

Two types of status epilepticus are possible: *convulsive status epilepticus* and *nonconvulsive status epilepticus*. The tonic-clonic seizure of *convulsive status epilepticus* alerts clinicians to the continuation of the seizure activity. This is not the case with *nonconvulsive status epilepticus*. These patients may account for as many as 10% of the status epilepticus patients in the intensive care unit. No overt clinical signs of seizures characterize this type of status epilepticus, however, the patient remains obtunded or unconscious longer than 30 minutes after the overt tonic-clonic seizures have ended. This comatose state is often attributed to the sedative effects of drugs administered during the overt seizure state. The only tool to diagnose nonconvulsive status epilepticus is an electroencephalogram. Because of frequent misdiagnosis, mortality is extremely high. Death is caused by decompensation and collapse of cardiovascular function, leading to lethal dysrhythmias and deterioration of autonomic functions. In status epilepticus, both convulsive and nonconvulsive, the treatment goal is rapid termination of the seizure activity. Aggressive management is required. Pharmacologic agents frequently used include benzodiazepines, fosphenytoin (which can be given without regard to serum phenytoin levels), and phenobarbital. The American Academy of Neurology recommends that all status epilepticus patients also receive thiamine (vitamin B_1) and 50% dextrose. All patients with intractable seizures require intubation and ventilatory support. If all else fails, clinicians may consider deep sedation with a midazolam (Versed) infusion or barbiturate coma.

DIAGNOSTIC TOOLS

The electrical activity of the cortex is of extremely low voltage; it is amplified and recorded by an electroencephalograph. The record is called an *electroencephalogram (EEG)*.

Brain waves are individualized and vary with activity (e.g., intense mental activity = low amplitude, high frequency; slow-wave sleep = low frequency, amplitude increased). Spikes indicate an irritative focus. Brain waves are slowed with hypoxia, anesthesia, sedatives, low carbon dioxide (CO_2), deep sleep, and relaxation; they are accelerated with increased CO_2 levels, sensory stimulation, light anesthesia, and drugs such as methylprednisolone (Medrol).

The superficial layers of cortex are responsible for the electrical activity recorded on EEGs. Masses of dendrites forming a dense network are thought to be the source. The cerebellum has a similar network, and a similar pattern can be recorded from that area.

EEGs should be used in conjunction with careful clinical evaluations. The EEG is a physiologic recording and does not distinguish one entity from another; for example, EEG cannot distinguish a tumor from a thrombosis. Ten percent of patients with seizures have normal EEGs. In addition, an abnormal record is not always definitely diagnostic. In fact, even in patients with diagnosed epilepsy, seizure activity is often nonclinical.

The EEG is only one test, not a conclusive diagnostic determination. Caution should be used in the interpretation of EEG tracings. For example, scalp electrodes frequently may not perceive the electrical activity from the inferior aspect of the frontal and temporal and occipital lobes.

Certain activating techniques, such as hyperventilation and strobe light stimulation, are used to initiate abnormal electrical patterns in some patients. Even after multiple EEGs, the results may be negative in as many as 20% of patients. A normal EEG is common in children with tonic-clonic seizures.

The gold standard for epilepsy diagnosis is simultaneous video-EEG monitoring, which links EEG findings to a verified attack. Patients are monitored on a 24-hour basis with radiotelemetry. Electrodes are implanted and attached to a telemetry pack that is secured to the patient's head. The EEG recording is used to identify specific areas of the brain involved in abnormal discharges, and this data is correlated with the video recording. Additional testing includes neuroimaging with computed tomography (CT) and magnetic resonance imaging (MRI) to reveal focal neuropathy. MRI is preferred because it detects small lesions (such as tiny tumors, vessel malformations or scar tissue) in the temporal lobe. Mesial temporal sclerosis, a common cause of temporal epilepsy, is visible with MRI but not with CT.

TREATMENT

The primary management mode for the seizure patient is drug therapy to prevent the occurrence of seizures or to reduce their frequency, allowing the patient to lead an essentially normal life. Approximately 70% to 80% of patients benefit from anticonvulsant drug therapy. The drug selected is determined by the type of seizure and the side effect profile. Doses are individualized. Table 55-3 lists some of the common drugs used to treat epilepsy and their side effects.

It is important to remember that not every seizure patient requires drug therapy and the choice to use medications is based on a variety of factors. Some questions that the clinician must consider include the following. Is this an isolated seizure? Is the cause of the seizure the result of a reversible condition (e.g., electrolyte imbalance, elevated serum osmolality, hypoglycemia)? Is this seizure

TABLE 55-3

Pharmacologic Agents for Treatment of Seizures

Drug	Therapeutic Use	Dose/Blood Level	Adverse Effects
Phenytoin (Dilantin)	Generalized seizures (tonic-clonic)	300-400 mg/day Therapeutic level: 10-20 μg/ml	Hirsutism, hypertrophic gums, gastric distress, blurred vision, vertigo, hyperglycemia, macrocytic anemia (with long-term use)
Fosphenytoin (Cerebyx)	Status epilepticus	15-20 mg PE/kg	Toxic level 30-50 μg/ml Blood dyscrasias, hypotension, nephritis, ventricular fibrillation
Carbamazepine (Tegretol)	Complex partial seizures Generalized seizure (tonic-clonic)	600-1600 mg/day Therapeutic level: 4-12 μg/ml	Bone marrow depression, gastric distress, sedation, blurred vision, constipation, skin rash
Phenobarbital (Luminal)	Generalized (tonic-clonic)	90-180 mg/day Therapeutic level: 20-40 μg/ml	Sedation, gastric distress
Diazepam (Valium)	Status epilepticus	Adult: 5-10 mg (up to 30 mg) Child: 1 mg every 2-5 min to a total dose of 10 mg	Sedation, cardiac and respiratory depression
Lorazepam (Ativan)	Status epilepticus	Adult: 2-10 mg Child: 0.1 mg/kg, max dose 4 mg	Dizziness, drowsiness, tachycardia, hypotension
Midazolam (Versed)	Status epilepticus (still under investigation) Infusion (intubated, ventilated patients only)	Infuse slowly using infusion pump to desired result	Hypotension, apnea, bronchospasm, laryngospasm
Clonazepam (Klonopin)	Myoclonic	Adult: 1.5-20.0 mg/day Child: 0.01-0.02 mg/kg/day Therapeutic level: 0.02-0.10 μg/ml	Drowsiness, confusion, headache, vertigo, syncope
Ethosuximide (Zarontin)	Absence	Adult: 20-40 mg/kg/day Child: 20 mg/kg/day Therapeutic level: 40-90 μg/ml	Nausea, vomiting, weight loss, constipation, diarrhea, sleep disturbances, blood dyscrasias
Valproic acid (Depakote, Depakene)	Generalized (tonic-clonic), myoclonic, absence, partial seizures	750-3000 mg/day Therapeutic level: 50-150 μg/ml	Nausea, hepatotoxicity
Felbamate (Felbatol)	Lennox-Gastaut syndrome, partial seizures	Adult: 1.2 g/day Used in polypharmacologic therapy	GI upset, anorexia, weight loss, headache, insomnia, hepatotoxicity
Gabapentin (Neurontin)	Partial seizures (Note: Also used in pain syndromes)	Adult: 900-1800 mg/day Therapeutic level: not established	Leukopenia, dry mouth, blurred vision, myalgia, weight gain, fatigue
Lamotrigine (Lamictal)	Partial seizures, Lennox-Gastaut syndrome	Adult: 100-500 mg/day Child: 15 mg/kg/day Used in polypharmacologic therapy Therapeutic level: not established	Hepatotoxicity, rash, Stevens-Johnson syndrome, headache, dizziness, blurred vision
Oxcarbazepine (Trileptal)	Partial seizures (Note: Also used in pain syndromes)	Adult: 1200-2400 mg/day Therapeutic level: not established	GI upset, sedation, diplopia, hyponatremia, skin rash
Tiagabine (Gabitril)	Partial seizures	Adult/child: 4-56 mg/day Therapeutic level: not established	Dry mouth, dizziness, sedation, unsteady gait, headache, exacerbation of generalized seizures
Topiramate (Topamax)	Partial seizures	Adult: 400 mg/day Therapeutic level: not established	Pharyngitis, insomnia, weight loss, constipation, dry mouth, sedation, anorexia
Zonisamide (Zonegran)	Partial seizures	100-400 mg/day Therapeutic level: 20 μg/ml	Adults (>16 years): Somnolence, ataxia, fatigue, anorexia, dizziness, renal stones, leukopenia

related to alcohol use or abuse? Is the patient pregnant and the cause of the seizure could be eclampsia? Generally, the patient must have at least two seizures before the diagnosis of epilepsy is considered. Seizures must be distinguished from other conditions that mimic them. These conditions include migraine headaches, stroke, vertigo, sleep disorders, and pseudoseizures.

Historically, a combination of drugs was used on the premise that lower doses could be prescribed, thereby reducing the incidence of side effects. Currently, a monopharmacologic approach is preferred, which minimizes the number of drugs used and the resultant side effects and synergistic effects. Physicians generally give patients two trials on single drug therapy before adding combination drug therapies.

There is some clinical controversy regarding the routine treatment of childhood epilepsy with drug therapy. Children experiencing the first single seizure are generally not treated pharmacologically. Children with few or with minor seizures may not require drug treatment. Some pediatric neurologists believe that drugs are palliative only and that most children with seizures should receive antiepileptic drug therapy only when the impact of the seizures outweighs the adverse effects of the medications.

Whichever approach is used, careful clinical assessment and frequent monitoring of drug levels are critical in patient management. Assessing drug levels allows individualization of drug dose to the patient's need. Patients metabolize drugs at varying rates. Factors such as serum protein levels and ability of the liver enzymes to biodegrade drugs influence the dose requirements and serum drug levels.

In the past, diet and surgery were also treatments for seizures, and these methods are still used occasionally today. A ketogenic diet was popular in the 1920s. A variation of the ketogenic diet, the *medium-chain triglyceride diet*, was reintroduced in the early 1970s. This high-fat, low-carbohydrate diet altered body chemistry by producing ketones. The resulting acidotic state seems to have an anticonvulsant effect on some children with myoclonic seizures.

Acetazolamide (Diamox), used in conjunction with anticonvulsant agents, produces a relative acidosis similar to a ketogenic diet. This state seems to create a climate that decreases the likelihood of producing seizure activity. Dehydration states also seem to decrease seizure activity, as does physical activity (possibly related to the production of lactic acid).

Approximately 20% to 30% of patients with seizures are refractory to medical management. Some of these patients are candidates for surgical treatment in an attempt to better control the seizure activity and, in some instances, eliminate them entirely. Surgical intervention is not for all patients and most neurosurgical facilities have stringent patient selection criteria. Patients with partial seizure disorders are most amenable to surgical treatment. Although success rates vary, and results may take up to 2 years, 60% of patients experience a total elimination of seizures, and 20% of patients experience a 90% reduction in the frequency of seizures.

Diagnostic evaluation of potential candidates is done to localize the seizure focus and determine the ability to

TABLE 55-4 ■ ■ ■

Surgical Treatments for Seizure Disorders

Surgical Procedure	Comments
Lesionectomy	Removal of a specific lesion Good results
Temporal resection	Removal of temporal lobe, includes removal of hippocampus and amygdala If done in dominant hemisphere, causes temporary speech deficit Good-to-excellent results
Extratemporal resection	Most involve the frontal lobe; parietal and occipital resections done rarely More than one half of patients improve
Hemispherectomy	Used in Rasmussen's epilepsy Good-to-excellent results Better outcomes with young patients

safely resect the affected portion of the brain. Included in the extensive presurgical evaluation are CT scans, MRI, positron emission tomography (PET), and single-photon emission computerized tomography (SPECT). Mapping of cortical function is critical to ensure optimal results. In addition to these specialized diagnostic tests, the evaluation includes EEG evaluation, neuropsychologic testing, and psychosocial assessment. It is essential that the patient be a motivated candidate for rehabilitation and understands the realistic expectations of the surgery. Diagnostic surgical options are available if noninvasive diagnostic tests are inconclusive.

The surgical goal is to remove the smallest amount of brain tissue that will lead to an elimination of seizure activity or a significant reduction in the seizure activity. Table 55-4 summarizes some of the surgical options available.

Additional options under investigation include the use of a *vagal nerve stimulator*. With this technique, a neurocybernetic prosthesis is implanted around the left vagus nerve. It is theorized that stimulation of the vagus nerve desynchronizes cerebral electrical activity, giving an antiepileptic effect. A limited number of these devices have been used, and the results have been less than ideal, with less than 50% of patients experiencing a reduction in seizure activity.

Maintaining a patent airway and preventing injury are the two critical objectives in the care of the person experiencing a seizure. Maintaining the patient in a side-lying position reduces the risk of aspirating stomach contents and saliva and prevents the tongue from obstructing the airway. Protecting the head during the seizure and removing any objects that may cause harm can prevent injury.

The importance of the holistic approach in managing the person with a seizure disorder cannot be overstated. Patients and family need to understand the medication regimen and dosage and side effects, appropriate care for a person experiencing a seizure, the psychologic problems associated with seizures, and the public's attitude toward persons with seizures.

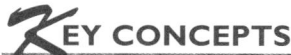

EY CONCEPTS

- A *seizure* is a paroxysmal event caused by abnormal hypersynchronous discharges from an aggregate of CNS neurons. Depending on the location of these hyperexcitable neurons, the seizure exhibits itself as any combination of altered level of consciousness, as well as disturbances in motor, sensory, or autonomic functions.

- The term *seizure* needs to be carefully distinguished from that of epilepsy. *Epilepsy* describes a condition in which a person has *recurrent*, nonmetabolically-induced seizures caused by a chronic underlying process.

- Seizures are a relatively common neurologic problem. Approximately 10% of the population will have at least one seizure during their lifetime, with the highest incidence occurring in early childhood and late adulthood (after age 60 years), and 0.3% to 0.5% will be diagnosed with epilepsy (based on the criterion of two or more unprovoked seizures).

- Epilepsy may be classified as idiopathic or symptomatic. In *idiopathic or essential epilepsy*, no known central lesion can be demonstrated. In *symptomatic or secondary epilepsy*, a cerebral abnormality promotes the seizure response. Conditions associated with secondary epilepsy include head injuries, metabolic and nutritional disorders (hypoglycemia, phenylketonuria, vitamin B_6 deficiency), toxic factors (uremia, alcohol intoxication, narcotic withdrawal), encephalitis, stroke, cerebral hypoxia or neoplasms, and electrolyte disturbances, especially hyponatremia and hypocalcemia.

- The main characteristic that distinguishes the different categories of seizures is whether the seizure is *partial* (with preservation of consciousness) or *generalized* (with loss of consciousness).

- *Partial seizures* occur within discrete areas of the brain and are typically associated with structural abnormalities of the brain.

- *Simple partial seizures* cause motor, sensory, autonomic or psychic symptoms without an obvious alteration in consciousness during the seizure, which usually lasts less than 1 minute. The symptoms depend on the location of the hyperactive neurons in the brain.

- *Complex partial seizures* are characterized by focal seizure activity and an alteration in consciousness that impairs the patient's ability to maintain contact with their environment. Symptoms vary but usually include purposeless behavior, such as picking at clothes, clapping hands, lip smacking, or chewing motions, which last 1 to 3 minutes. The patient is conscious but has no memory of his actions during the seizure. This type of seizure focus often arises from the medial temporal or inferior frontal lobe.

- *Generalized seizures* involve diffuse areas of the brain simultaneously in a bilaterally symmetric fashion. These seizures generally start without an aura, and patients are unconscious and unaware of their surroundings during the seizures. There are several types of generalized seizures.

- *Absence seizures (petit mal)* are characterized by sudden, brief lapses of consciousness without loss of postural control and typically last a few seconds. Typical manifestations are a vacant stare and rapid eye blinking with a rapid return of consciousness with no postictal confusion. Absence seizures are often misdiagnosed as "daydreaming." Absence seizures almost always begin in childhood and may disappear by adolescence or are replaced by another type of seizure, especially tonic-clonic.

- Generalized motor seizures involving loss of consciousness and tonic-clonic muscle contractions are often called *convulsions*.

- *Generalized tonic-clonic (grand mal) seizures* arise from both cerebral hemispheres simultaneously and are the classic seizure of epilepsy. These seizures typically begin with a loud cry precipitated by air rushing from the lungs through the vocal cords. The patient falls to the ground, losing consciousness. The body stiffens (tonic phase) and then alternates between episodes of muscle spasm (tonic phase) and relaxation (clonic phase). Contraction of the jaw muscles may cause the patient to bite his or her tongue, and the patient may be incontinent of urine and feces. Respirations are impaired and secretions may pool in the oropharynx causing partial airway obstruction. The seizure lasts 3 to 5 minutes and is followed by a *postictal period* of unconsciousness that may last up to 30 minutes. The patient is typically confused as consciousness returns and has no recollection of the seizure.

- The *physiologic effects of tonic-clonic seizures* depend on the length of time the seizure persists. Early effects (tachycardia, hyperpyrexia, hypertension, and hyperglycemia) are caused by the release of catecholamines. Prolonged seizures (> 30 min) cause depletion of catecholamines and hypotension, hypoglycemia, dysrhythmias, decrease in cerebral perfusion and cerebral edema, and possible cardiac or respiratory arrest.

- *Status epilepticus* refers to continuous or intermittent seizure activity lasting 20 minutes or longer, during which the patient does not regain consciousness. Status epilepticus is a medical emergency because cardiorespiratory dysfunction, hyperthermia, irreversible neuronal damage, and death may occur as a consequence of prolonged seizures. *Generalized convulsive status epilepticus* is obvious when the patient is having convulsions, but if the patient remains unconscious longer than 30 minutes following the seizure, *nonconvulsive status epilepticus* is possible. In these cases, the EEG may be the only method of establishing the diagnosis. The first step in the management of status epilepticus is to attend to any acute cardiorespiratory problems or hyperthermia and to begin anticonvulsant drug therapy without delay to terminate seizure activity. Benzodiazepines (e.g., Ativan, Valium) and fosphenytoin are commonly used to treat status epilepticus. Thiamine and 50% dextrose is also recommended.

- *Febrile convulsions* associated with viral or bacterial infection are most common in children under the age of 5 years. Simple febrile seizures are not associated with an increased risk of developing epilepsy. In some instances, patients who have a family history of febrile seizures or epilepsy are at greater risk for developing nonfebrile seizures later in life.
- *Diagnostic tools used to evaluate seizures* include the EEG, CT scanning, and MRI. The gold standard for epilepsy diagnosis is simultaneous video-EEG monitoring.
- Many conditions can mimic seizures and the differential diagnosis includes syncope, migraine attacks, transient ischemic attacks, stroke, and metabolic disturbances, such as alcoholic blackouts, delirium tremens, hypoxia or hypoglycemia, and psychogenic or pseudoseizures.
- *Treatment plans for a seizure disorder* must be individualized, given the many different types and causes of seizures, as well as the differences in efficacy and toxicity of antiepileptic medications.
- If the sole cause of the seizure is a metabolic disturbance, such as an abnormality of serum glucose or electrolytes, then treatment is aimed at reversing the metabolic problem and preventing its recurrence.

- *Antiepileptic drug therapy* is the mainstay of treatment for most patients with epilepsy. The overall goal is to prevent seizures without causing any untoward side effects, preferably with a single medication that is easy for the patient to follow. Seizure classification is an important element in designing the treatment plan, because some antiepileptic drugs have different activities against various seizure types.
- Noncompliance and abruptly stopping anticonvulsant medication therapy may precipitate seizures.
- Surgical resection of the temporal lobe or other parts of the brain may be carried out for a select group of patients with refractory seizures (not controlled with medication) after a careful presurgical evaluation.
- Maintaining a patent airway and preventing injury are the two critical objectives in the care of a patient experiencing a seizure. Maintaining the patient in a side-lying position reduces the risk of aspirating stomach contents and saliva and prevents the tongue from obstructing the airway. Objects that may cause injury should be removed from the bed. The onset, duration, and description of the seizure (e.g., level of consciousness, motor activity) should be carefully documented.

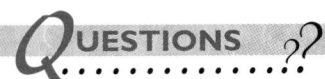

QUESTIONS

A sampling of review questions for this chapter appears here. Visit http://www.mosby.com/MERLIN/PriceWilson/ for additional questions. MERLIN

Answer the following on a separate sheet of paper.

1. Define epilepsy.
2. What is the incidence of epilepsy in the general population of the United States? What is the incidence for the offspring of epileptic persons?
3. What conditions may cause seizures?
4. List the areas of the brain associated with lesions that are likely to be epileptogenic.
5. Describe the factors that play an instrumental role in precipitating seizures.
6. Describe the metabolic changes that can occur during and immediately after a seizure.
7. Discuss the clinical difference between convulsive and nonconvulsive status epilepticus.

CHAPTER
56

Central Nervous System Injury

MARY CARTER LOMBARDO

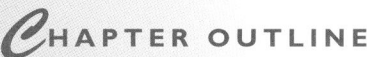

INCREASED INTRACRANIAL PRESSURE

Increased intracranial pressure (ICP) is defined as an increase in the pressure exerted within the cranial cavity. Normally the cranial cavity is occupied by brain tissue, blood, and cerebrospinal fluid (CSF). Each portion occupies a specific volume, giving a normal ICP of 50 to 200 mm water or 4 to 15 mm Hg. ICP is normally influenced by everyday activities and rises temporarily to levels much higher than is normal. A few of these activities are deep abdominal breathing, coughing, and straining. Temporary increases in ICP present no difficulty, but sustained increased pressure has a detrimental effect on living brain tissue.

The cranial cavity is a rigid compartment filled to capacity with incompressible substances: the brain (1400 g), CSF (approximately 75 ml), and blood (approximately 75 ml). An increase in the volume of any of these three major substances results in encroachment of the space occupied by the others and increased ICP. The *Monro-Kellie hypothesis* provides a conceptual model for understanding increased ICP. The theory states that because the bony skull cannot expand, if one of the three intracranial compartments expands, the other two must compensate by decreasing in volume, if the ICP is to remain constant. These compensatory mechanisms within the cranium are limited, but interruption of neural function can be severe when they fail. Compensation consists of increased drainage of CSF into the spinal canal and adaptation of the brain to increased pressure without increasing ICP. Compensatory mechanisms with potentially lethal consequences are reduction of blood flow to the brain and displacement of the brain downward or horizontally (herniation) when ICP becomes increasingly elevated. These last two compensatory mechanisms can have dire consequences for neural function. When the increase in ICP is serious and sustained, compensatory mechanisms are ineffective, and the pressure elevation can cause neuronal death (Fig. 56-1).

Brain tumors, brain injury, cerebral edema, and obstruction in CSF flow all contribute to increased ICP. Cerebral edema, perhaps the most common cause of increased ICP, has many causes, including an increase in intracellular fluid, hypoxia, fluid and electrolyte imbalances, cerebral ischemia, meningitis, and injury. Regardless of the cause, the effects are basically the same.

ICP generally increases gradually. After head injury, edema formation may take 36 to 48 hours to reach its maximum. A rise in ICP to 33 mm Hg (450 mm water) significantly reduces cerebral blood flow (CBF). The resulting ischemia stimulates the vasomotor centers, and the systemic blood pressure rises. Stimulation of the cardioinhibitory center produces bradycardia, and respiration is slowed. This compensatory mechanism, known as *Cushing's reflex*, helps to maintain CBF. (The decreasing respiration, however, leads to carbon dioxide [CO_2] retention and resultant cerebral vasodilation, which contribute to increasing ICP.) Systemic blood pressure will continue to rise proportionately to the increasing ICP, although eventually a point is reached when the ICP exceeds the arterial pressure and cerebral circulation ceases, with resultant brain death. Generally, this event is heralded by a rapidly decreasing arterial blood pressure.

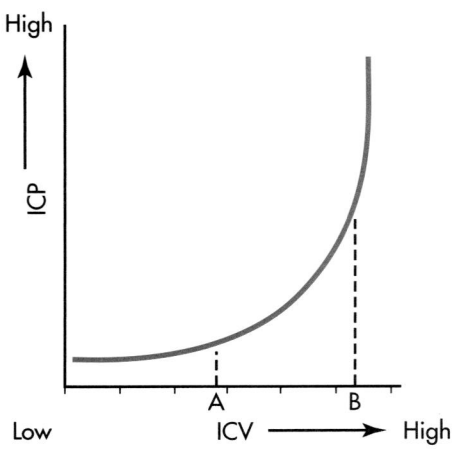

FIG. 56-1 The relationship of intracranial volume *(ICV)* to intracranial pressure *(ICP)*. Compensatory mechanisms are effective up to point *A* with expanding ICV, and ICP does not increase above the normal range. However, as the ICV continues to increase, a critical point *B* is reached where a small increase in ICV causes a large increase in ICP.

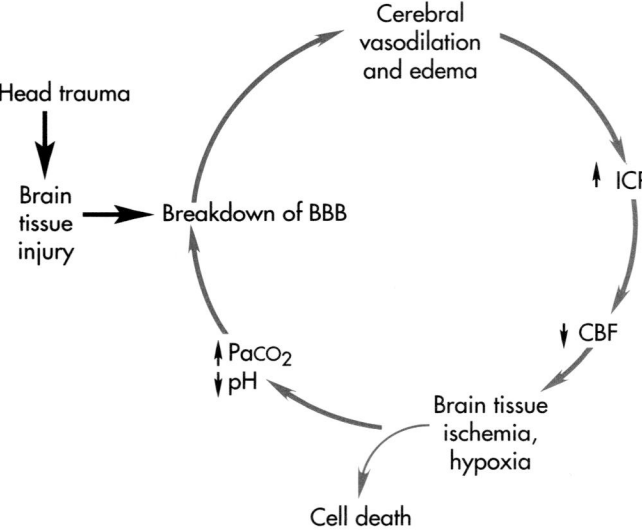

FIG. 56-2 The cycle of progressive neurologic deficit associated with an expanding intracranial mass lesion. *BBB*, Blood-brain barrier; *ICP*, intracranial pressure; *CBF*, cerebral blood flow; *Paco₂*, arterial carbon dioxide tension.

The cycle of progressive neurologic deficit associated with cerebral contusion and edema (or any expanding intracranial mass lesion) is illustrated in Fig. 56-2. Brain trauma causes tissue fragmentation and contusion, resulting in a breakdown of the blood-brain barrier (BBB), with vasodilation and exudation of fluid, causing edema. Edema leads to an increase in tissue pressure and an eventual increase in ICP, which, in turn, leads to decreased CBF, ischemia, hypoxia, acidosis (decreased pH and increased arterial carbon dioxide tension [$Paco_2$]), and further breakdown of the BBB. This cycle continues so that cell death and edema formation increase progressively unless intervention occurs.

Clinical Manifestations and Assessment

Clinical manifestations of increased ICP are numerous and varied and may be subtle. Alteration of the patient's level of consciousness (LOC) is the most sensitive indicator of all the signs of intracranial hypertension. The clinical triad of symptoms is headache, caused by stretching of the dura and blood vessels; papilledema, caused by pressure and swelling of the optic disc; and vomiting, which is frequently projectile. The presence of widened pulse pressure and decreased pulse and respiratory rates signals brain decompensation and impending death. Other signs of increased ICP include hyperthermia, motor and sensory changes, altered speech, and seizures.

Decerebrate posturing is a condition that develops when a brain lesion or the consequences of increased ICP interrupt signals from higher structures to the pons and medulla and to the lower structures. The result is blockage of strong excitatory input from the cerebral cortex, red nuclei, and basal ganglia to the medullary inhibitor system. The pontine excitatory system becomes dominant, leading to generalized rigidity of upper and lower extremities (total extensor rigidity of the antigravity muscles of the neck, trunk, and legs, as shown in Fig. 56-3, *A*). This type of abnormal posturing is spastic as well as rigid, because the pontine antigravity signals preferentially excite the gamma motor neurons in the spinal cord, tightening muscle spindles and activating stretch reflexes. The brain lesion may be bilateral or unilateral, with muscular rigidity on the side opposite the brain lesion. Decerebrate posturing has a particularly serious prognosis because it indicates severe damage to the cerebral hemisphere and imminent brainstem involvement, leading to interference with respiratory and cardiac centers in the medulla.

Decorticate posturing is another form of abnormal motor response with brain injury that suggests a higher cortical lesion, with less severe damage to one or both of the cerebral hemispheres. Typically, the arm, wrist, and fingers are flexed and the upper extremity is adducted and internally rotated. In contrast, the lower extremity is either in extensor rigidity or unresponsive (see Fig. 56-3, *B*).

The *Glasgow Coma Scale (GCS)* is the most widely used scale to assess the patient's arousability and reaction to a stimulus. This scale grades the patient's best response in three categories: eye opening, verbal responses, and motor responses. A deteriorating score indicates a worsening of the patient's neurologic status (Table 56-1).

Two general types of pathologic processes lead to coma with severely increased ICP: those that cause global ischemia of the cerebral hemispheres and those that depress or destroy brainstem-activating mechanisms. Coma occurs only when both cerebral hemispheres or when brainstem divisions are dysfunctional. The major catastrophe of coma is death from brain herniation. The two main paths of herniation are through the tentorial notch and through the foramen magnum. *Uncal herniation* involves displacement of the median aspect of the temporal lobe (uncus) through the tentorial notch, thus compressing the upper brainstem, the third cranial nerve (CN III), and the posterior cerebral artery (Fig. 56-4). *Central herniation* involves downward displacement of the diencephalon through the tentorial opening in the midline, which compresses the midbrain. In both cases, there is a progression of rostral-to-caudal compression of

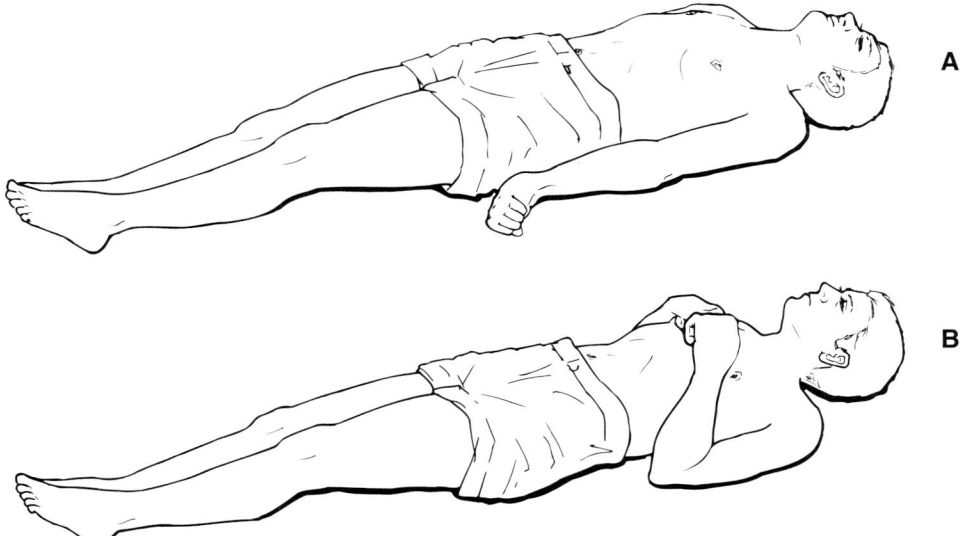

FIG. 56-3 Abnormal posturing. **A**, *Decerebrate posture* results from damage to the brain and brainstem. The jaws are clenched and the neck extended. The arms are adducted and stiffly extended at the elbows, with forearms pronated and wrists and fingers flexed. The legs are stiffly extended at the knees, with plantar flexion of the feet. **B**, *Decorticate posture* results from damage to one or both corticospinal tracts within or very near the cerebral hemispheres. In this posture the upper arms are held tightly to the sides, with elbows, wrists, and fingers flexed. The legs are stiffly extended and internally rotated, with plantar flexion of the feet.

TABLE 56-1 ▪▪▪

Glasgow Coma Scale

Parameter/Response	Score	Parameter/Response	Score
EYE OPENING (E)		**BEST MOTOR RESPONSE (M)**	
Spontaneous: eyes open to approach	4	Obeys commands: for example, "raise your arm; hold up two fingers"	6
To speech: eyes open to name or command	3	Localizes pain: does not obey but locates and tries to remove painful stimulus	5
To pain: eyes open to digital pressure over proximal nailbed	2	Flexion withdrawal: flexes arm in response to pain with no purposeful attempt to stop stimulus and without abnormal flexion posture	4
None: does not open eyes to any stimulus	1		
BEST VERBAL RESPONSE (V)		Abnormal flexion to pain: flexes arms at elbow and pronates, making a fist (decorticate posturing)	3
Oriented: converses; knows who and where he or she is and month and year	5	Abnormal extension to pain: extends arms at elbow, usually adducts and internally rotates arm at shoulder (decerebrate posturing)	2
Confused: converses but disoriented in one or more spheres	4	None: no response to pain; flaccid	1
Inappropriate words: no sustained conversation; words disorganized or inappropriate	3		
Incomprehensible: makes sounds (e.g., moans) but no recognizable words	2		
None: no sounds even with painful stimuli	1		

Modified from Ropper AH: In Fauci AS, editor: *Harrison's principles of internal medicine*, ed 14, New York, 1998, McGraw-Hill.
Coma score = E + V + M: 15 = fully alert; <8 = comatose. After head injury a score >11 indicates an 85% chance of a good recovery or moderate disability, whereas a score of 3 or 4 indicates an 85% chance of dying or remaining vegetative. Intermediate scores correlate with proportional chances of recovery.

first the midbrain, then the pons, and finally the medulla, leading to the appearance of neurologic signs and progressively diminished LOC.

Although the GCS scores the best response, it does not consider localized signs. The brainstem contains several intrinsic reflexes that are convenient to examine. When brainstem reflexes are normal, the cause of coma is generally diffuse cerebral dysfunction.

Normal pupillary symmetry, size, shape, and reaction to light indicate intact functioning of the midbrain and CN III. Equal, round, and reactive pupils (2.5 to 5.0 mm) (see Fig. 51-3) usually exclude midbrain damage as a cause of coma. An enlarged (greater than 5.0 mm) and poorly reactive pupil can result from transtentorial herniation and compression of the midbrain and CN III. Bilaterally dilated and unreactive pupils indicate severe

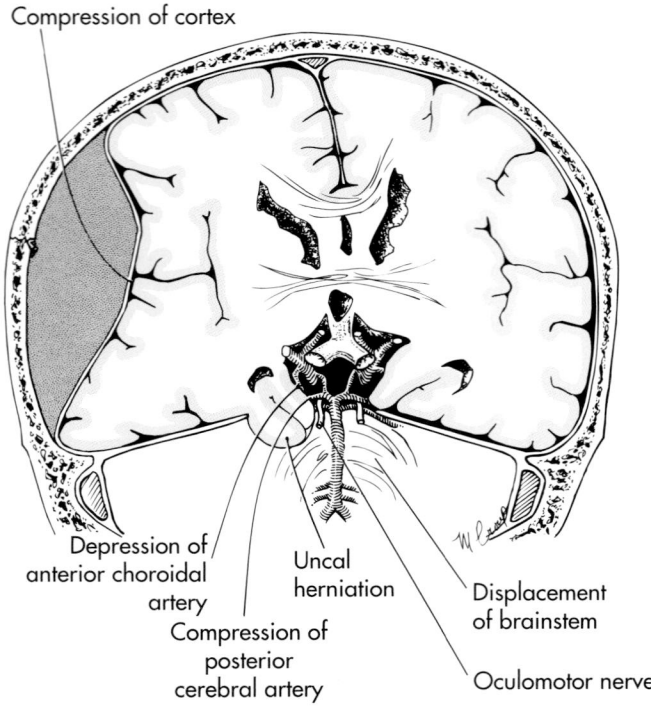

Compression of cortex

Depression of anterior choroidal artery

Uncal herniation

Compression of posterior cerebral artery

Displacement of brainstem

Oculomotor nerve

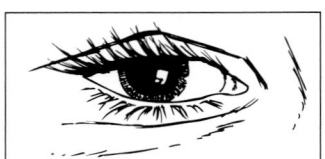

FIG. 56-4 Mechanisms of signs and symptoms of an expanding intracranial hematoma over the parietotemporal region. The expanding hematoma compresses the cortex, pushing the brain to the opposite side and displacing the brainstem, cranial nerves, and vessels. The extreme medial portion of the temporal lobe (uncus) becomes herniated under the edge of the tentorium cerebelli. Compression of the oculomotor nerve by the herniated uncus may lead to ipsilateral pupil dilation, ptosis, and eventual pupil fixation. Compression of the cerebral cortex and distortion of the brainstem result in depression of consciousness. In the brainstem the reticular activating system is involved. The arterial supply and venous return to the brainstem may be compromised by pressure. Interference with the cardiorespiratory centers is evidenced by irregularity or slowing of pulse; elevation of blood pressure; and abnormalities of respiratory rate, depth, and rhythm. Pressure on the corticospinal and associated pathways may result in a contralateral Babinski's sign and contralateral weakness or paralysis.

midbrain damage. Oval-shaped pupils are often associated with early midbrain–CN III compression.

Evaluation of brainstem functioning includes spontaneous motion of each eye and the oculocephalic and oculovestibular tests. The resting position of eyes may be conjugate (both eyes in the same position), disconjugate (eyes in different positions), or skewed (vertical disconjugate position). An adducted eye at rest indicates paresis of the lateral rectus muscle resulting from a CN VI lesion, whereas abduction indicates paresis of the medial rectus muscle from a CN III lesion. A skewed deviation results from a lesion of the pons. A note of caution: moving the

head of a comatose patient to check for brainstem reflexes must be done only after cervical fracture has been ruled out.

The *oculocephalic reflex* is tested by briskly turning the head from side to side while holding the eyes open. With an intact brainstem, the eyes deviate conjugately in the direction opposite to the head turning (*doll's eyes present*). With a brainstem lesion, the eyes move in the same direction as the head is turned (*doll's eyes absent*). CN III (nuclei in midbrain) and CN VI (nuclei in pons) are responsible for eye movements, thus this procedure is a good test to evaluate brainstem function. The *oculovestibular reflex* is tested by slowly injecting ice water into the external auditory canal until eye deviation or nystagmus occurs. This test, called the *ice-water caloric test*, is more powerful in eliciting eye reflexes, is used as an adjunct to testing the oculocephalic reflex, and has the same significance in the evaluation of brainstem pathways. The response of a comatose person with an intact brainstem is slow conjugate deviation of the eyes toward the irrigated ear, where they remain for 30 to 120 seconds. An extremely abnormal movement, such as skewing or jerky movements, usually indicates a brainstem lesion.

The *corneal reflex* is tested by touching a wisp of cotton to the cornea. The normal response is bilateral lid closure, which depends on the integrity of pontine pathways involving CN V and CN VII.

Finally, medullary function may be assessed by testing the *gag reflex* by touching a tongue blade to both sides of the posterior pharynx. The nuclei of CN IX and CN X mediating pharyngeal responses are located in the medulla.

The outcome of many neurologic conditions can be altered by the early recognition and treatment of increased ICP. ICP may be monitored directly by the use of epidural, subarachnoid, or intraventricular sensors. ICP monitoring is most often indicated after head injuries or brain surgery. A detailed discussion of ICP monitoring techniques, assessment, and treatment may be found in neurologic intensive care nursing textbooks.

HEAD INJURY

Anatomy

The brain is protected from injury by the hair, skin, and bones that surround it. Without this protection, the delicate brain, which makes people what they are, would be extremely susceptible to injury and destruction. Moreover, a neuron once destroyed does not regenerate. Head injury can have catastrophic implications. Some problems are caused directly by the injury; many others are secondary to the injury. The medical team must work to prevent and detect the early effects of brain injury to avoid the sequence of events that leads to mental and physical deficit and even death.

Just above the skull lies the *galea aponeurotica*, a freely moveable, dense, fibrous tissue that aids in absorbing the force from external trauma. Between the galea and the skin are a fatty layer and a deep membranous layer that contains large vessels. When severed, these vessels constrict poorly and may cause significant blood loss in a patient with a scalp laceration. Directly beneath the galea is

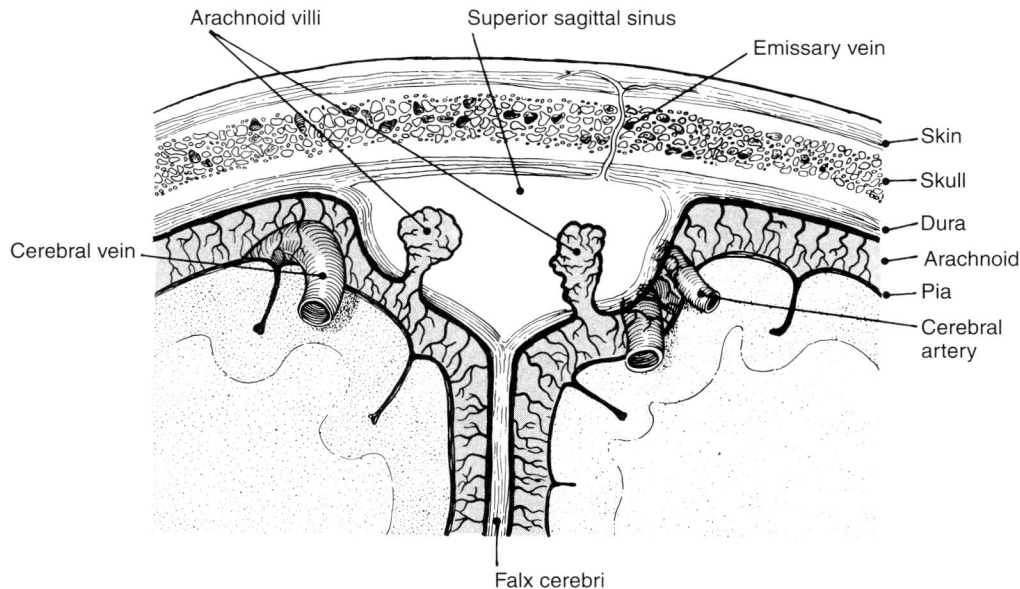

FIG. 56-5   Meninges in greater detail. Coronal section through the superior sagittal sinus. Emissary vein shown connecting scalp with superior sagittal sinus. The subarachnoid space is filled with cerebrospinal fluid. It enters the sinus through the arachnoid villi. (From Langley LL, Telford JR, Christensen JB: *Dynamic anatomy and physiology*, ed 5, New York, 1980, McGraw-Hill.)

the subaponeurotic space, which contains the *emissary* and *diploic veins*. These vessels may carry infection from the scalp to deep within the skull, which underscores the extreme importance of thorough cleansing and débridement of the scalp whenever the galea has been torn.

In the adult, the skull is a rigid compartment that does not allow for expansion of intracranial contents. The bone is actually composed of two walls or tables separated by cancellous bone. The outer wall is called the *outer table*, and the inner wall is called the *inner table*. This structure provides for increased strength and insulation with less weight. The inner table contains grooves in which lie the anterior, middle, and posterior meningeal arteries. When fracture of the skull involves tearing of one of these arteries, the resultant arterial bleeding, which accumulates in the epidural space, may lead to a fatal outcome unless it is detected and treated immediately. This condition constitutes one of the true neurosurgical emergencies, demanding immediate surgical intervention.

Covering the brain and providing added protection are the meninges. The three layers of the meninges are the dura mater, the arachnoid, and the pia mater. Each has a separate function and differs from the other two in structure (Fig. 56-5) (see Chapter 50).

The *dura* is the tough, semitranslucent, inelastic outer membrane that (1) protects the brain, (2) encloses the venous sinuses (which are composed of dura mater and endothelial lining only—no vascular tissue), and (3) forms the periosteum of the inner table. The dura is closely attached to the interior surface of the skull. Because of the problems that arise when a tear in the dura is not completely repaired and made airtight, its most important function may be protection. The fracture may expand instead of healing, and chronic leakage of CSF may occur, which may lead to the development of meningocerebral cicatrix, causing focal epilepsy. In some

instances, however, the dura is purposely left open. These situations include cerebral edema (to allow for decompression of the bulging brain), drainage of CSF, or after exploratory trepanning (to allow for inspection and evacuation of clots).

The dura has a rich blood supply. The middle and posterior areas are supplied by the middle meningeal artery, which branches off the internal carotid and vertebral arteries. The anterior and ethmoid vessels are also branches of the internal carotid and supply the anterior fossa. A branch of the occipital artery, the posterior meningeal, supplies blood to the posterior fossa.

Lying close to the dura but not attached to it is the fine, fibrous, elastic membrane known as the *arachnoid*. This membrane is not attached to the dura mater. However, the space between the two membranes—the subdural space—is a potential space. Bleeding between the dura and the arachnoid spreads freely, limited only by the barriers of the falx cerebri and tentorium. The cerebral veins passing through this space have little support except that provided by the dura and the arachnoid and therefore are susceptible to injury and rupture in head (cerebral) trauma.

Between the arachnoid and the pia mater (which lies directly beneath the arachnoid) is the *subarachnoid space*. This space widens and deepens in places and allows for circulation of CSF. In the superior sagittal and transverse sinuses, the arachnoid forms villous projections (pacchionian bodies), which serve as a pathway for the emptying of CSF into the venous system.

The *pia mater* is a delicate membrane that is richly supplied with minute blood vessels and is the only meningeal layer that dips into all the sulci and blankets the ridges of the gyri; the other two layers bridge the sulci. In some of the fissures and sulci on the medial side of the hemispheres, the pia forms a barrier between the ventricles of the brain and the sulcus or fissure. This barrier provides a structural support for the choroid plexus of each of the ventricles.

The brain damage seen in head trauma can be caused in two different ways: (1) by the immediate effects of the trauma on the functioning brain and (2) by the later effects of the brain cells' response to the trauma.

Immediate neurologic damage is caused by the penetration and laceration of brain tissue by an object or piece of bone, by the effects of force or energy transmitted to the brain, and by the effects of acceleration-deceleration on the brain, which is confined in a rigid compartment.

The degree of damage caused by these problems can depend on the force applied: the greater the force, the greater the damage. Two kinds of force are applied in two ways, causing two different effects. First, local injury is caused by a sharp object with low velocity and little force. Disruption of neurologic functioning occurs in a localized area and is caused by penetration of the dura at the point of impact by the object or fragments of bone. Second, generalized injury occurs, which is more often seen in blunt trauma to the head and after motor vehicle crashes. The damage occurs as the energy or force is transmitted to the brain. The protective layers of hair, scalp, and skull absorb much of the energy or force; with violent trauma, however, these structures cannot protect the brain. The remaining energy is transmitted to the brain, causing damage and disruption along the way as delicate tissues are subjected to the force. If the head is moving and is suddenly and violently stopped, as in a motor vehicle crash, damage is caused not only by local injury to tissue, but also by acceleration and deceleration. The force of acceleration and deceleration causes the contents within the rigid skull to move, thereby forcing the brain against the inner surface of the skull on the side opposite the impact. This type of injury is also called *contrecoup injury*. As has been noted, some areas within the cranial vault are rough, and as the brain moves across them (e.g., the sphenoid ridge), they tear and lacerate the tissues. The damage is intensified when trauma also causes rotation of the skull. The areas of the brain likely to receive the greatest amount of damage include the anterior portion of the frontal and temporal lobes, the posterior sections of the occipital lobes, and the upper portion of the midbrain.

The secondary damage to the brain is caused by a cycle of cerebral swelling and ischemia resulting in a cascade of effects, which has a deleterious effect on the brain. Secondary injury occurs from minutes to hours following the initial injury. Whenever neural tissue is injured it responds in a predictable manner, causing alterations in the intracellular and extracellular compartments. Some of these alterations include an excessive release of glutamine, calcium flow abnormalities, production of lactate, the damaging effect of free radicals, and sodium pump alterations at the cellular wall, which contribute to additional damage and swelling of brain tissue.

The neurons, the functional cells within the brain, depend from minute to minute on a constant supply of nutrients in the form of glucose and oxygen and are very susceptible to metabolic injury when supplies are cut off. As a result of injury, the cerebral circulation may lose its ability to regulate the available circulating blood volume, causing ischemia of certain areas within the brain.

Treatment Principles

The injured brain is extremely sensitive to deviations in its physiologic environment. Even brief episodes of hypotension, hypoxia, or increased ICP can be catastrophic to the injured brain. The initial care of the head-injured patient is directed toward securing the airway and providing adequate oxygenation and ventilation. Hypotension is harmful to the head-injured patient because it compromises cerebral perfusion pressure and contributes to cerebral edema and cerebral ischemia.

A computed tomography (CT) scan of the head is the radiologic method of choice for evaluating head-injured patients. The criteria for surgical intervention include rapid deterioration in neurologic status, a midline shift of 5 mm or more, and the need to restore a watertight dural barrier (Valadka, 2001). Medical management focuses on the maintenance of physiologic parameters as close to normal as is possible and intervening immediately when they deviate. Goals of medical management include (1) maintaining a mean arterial pressure (MAP) of 80 mm Hg or more, (2) aggressively treating fever, (3) maintaining an ideal oxygen saturation (Sao_2) of 100%, (4) avoiding hyperventilation, (5) preventing negative nitrogen balance by enteral feeding or hyperalimentation, and (6) aggressive management of increased ICP.

Measures to reduce increased ICP include induced drainage of CSF via ventriculostomy, analgesia, and sedation. Mannitol is administered in bolus doses of 0.25 to 1.0 g/kg of body weight. Some trauma centers are investigating the use of hypertonic saline as a substitute for mannitol. Hypothermia is used as a method of decreasing increased ICP in some centers, but clinical trials have failed to demonstrate a significant benefit.

Epidural Hematoma

Epidural hematoma is a serious sequela to head injury and carries a mortality rate of approximately 50%. Epidural hematoma occurs most frequently in the parietotemporal area from a tear in the middle meningeal artery (Fig. 56-6, B). In the frontal and occipital areas, hematomas are frequently not suspected and produce poorly localizing signs. When epidural hematoma is not associated with additional brain injuries, early treatment is generally followed by recovery with little or no neurologic deficit.

Presenting signs and symptoms vary, but the typical patient with epidural hematoma gives a history of head injury followed by a short period of unconsciousness, which is followed by a lucid period. It is important to note, however, that this lucid interval is not reliably diagnostic of epidural hematoma. First, the lucid interval may go unobserved, especially if it does not last long. Second, the patient with additional serious brain injury may remain stuporous.

An expanding hematoma in the temporal area causes the temporal lobe to be forced downward and inward. This pressure causes the medial portion of the lobe (the uncus and part of the hippocampal gyrus) to herniate under the edge of the tentorium, causing the neurologic signs observed by the medical team (see Fig. 56-4).

The pressure of the herniation of the uncus on the arterial circulation to the reticular formation of the medulla

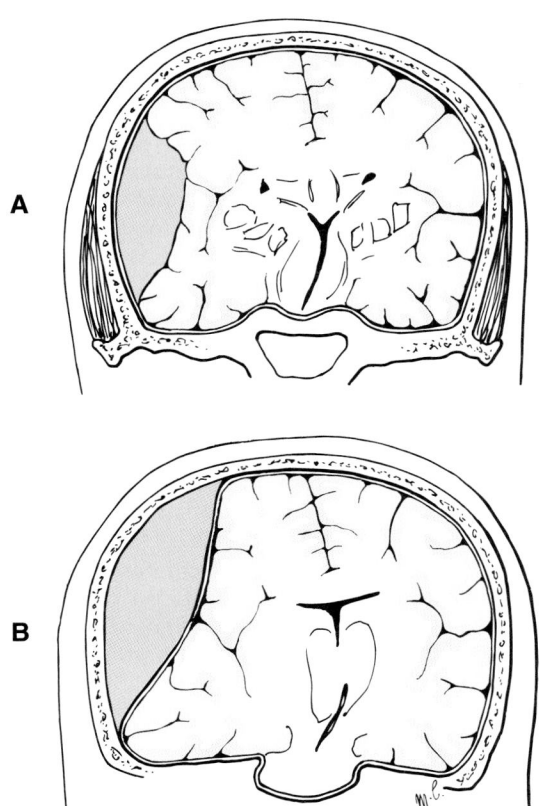

A

B

FIG. 56-6   **A**, Subdural hematoma, usually a result of laceration of the subdural vein. **B**, Epidural hematoma in the temporal fossa, usually a result of laceration of the middle meningeal artery.

causes unconsciousness. Also located in this area are the nuclei to CN III (oculomotor). Compression of this nerve produces dilation of the pupil and ptosis of the eyelid. Compression of the corticospinal pathways ascending in this area causes weakness in motor responses contralaterally (i.e., side opposite the hematoma), brisk or hyperactive reflexes, and Babinski's sign.

As the developing hematoma enlarges, it pushes the entire brain toward the opposite side, causing severe ICP. Late signs of increased ICP develop, including decerebrate rigidity and disturbances in vital signs and respiratory functioning.

Epidural hemorrhage is diagnosed from clinical signs and symptoms, as well as by carotid arteriogram, echoencephalogram, and CT scan. Treatment is by surgical evacuation of the hematoma and control of the bleeding from the lacerated middle meningeal artery. Surgical intervention must take place early, before serious compression of brain tissue causes brain damage. Mortality remains high, even when the condition is diagnosed and treated early because of the associated severe brain trauma and sequelae.

Subdural Hematoma

Whereas an epidural hematoma is generally arterial in origin, a subdural hematoma is venous (Fig. 56-6, *A*). It is caused by rupture of the veins in the subdural space.

Subdural hematomas are divided into types that differ in symptoms and prognosis: acute, subacute, and chronic.

Acute Subdural Hematoma

Acute subdural hematomas cause serious and significant neurologic symptoms within 24 to 48 hours after injury. Frequently associated with serious brain trauma, these hematomas are also associated with a high mortality rate. Acute subdural hematomas are seen in patients taking anticoagulants who sustain what seems to be minor head trauma. This injury is often associated with deceleration injuries from motor vehicle crashes.

Progressive neurologic deficit results from compression of brain tissue with herniation of the brainstem into the foramen magnum, leading to compression of the brainstem. This condition quickly leads to cessation of respiration and loss of control of pulse and blood pressure.

Diagnosis is made with a carotid arteriogram and echoencephalogram or a CT scan. Acute subdural hematoma should always be considered in patients who have suffered severe neurologic trauma and show signs of deteriorating neurologic status. Because more than half of these hematomas are bilateral, it is extremely important to consider the type of injury incurred and to use appropriate diagnostic measures (e.g., bilateral arteriograms) to rule out the possibility of bilateral hematomas.

Treatment consists mainly of removal of the hematoma, decompression by removal of areas of skull and portions of the frontal or temporal lobes if necessary, and relaxation of the compressing dura. Even with prompt diagnosis and surgical intervention, mortality rates are about 60%, with most related to the severe brain trauma and major organ failure that accompanies severe trauma.

Subacute Subdural Hematoma

Subacute subdural hematoma causes significant neurologic deficit more than 48 hours but less than 2 weeks after injury. As with acute subdural hematoma, subacute subdural hematoma is caused by venous bleeding into the subdural space.

The typical clinical history of a patient with a subacute subdural hematoma shows head trauma causing unconsciousness with subsequent gradual improvement in neurologic status. Over time, the patient demonstrates signs of deteriorating neurologic status. The LOC begins to decrease gradually over a period of hours. As the ICP increases from the accumulating hematoma, the patient may become difficult to arouse and nonresponsive to verbal and painful stimuli. As with acute subdural hematoma, the shift of intracranial contents and the increasing ICP caused by the accumulation of blood lead to uncal or central herniation and give rise to neurologic signs of brainstem compression.

Treatment, as in the treatment for acute subdural hematoma, is the early and prompt removal of the clot. This goal can be accomplished by various means, according to the patient's clinical condition. Because many of these clots are bilateral, both subdural spaces should be evaluated and, if indicated, surgically explored.

Chronic Subdural Hematoma

Chronic subdural hematoma presents an interesting clinical history. The cerebral trauma responsible for it may be trivial or even nonexistent or forgotten and is often the result of low-impact injury. The onset of symptoms is usually delayed for weeks, months, and possibly years after the initial injury. Common symptoms include headache, lethargy, and confusion. In older adults, these symptoms may be mistaken for early signs of dementia.

The initial trauma ruptures one of the veins transversing the subdural space. Slow bleeding thus occurs into the subdural space. Within 7 to 10 days after bleeding has occurred, a fibrous membrane surrounds the blood. As breakdown of blood cells within the hematoma occurs, an osmotic pressure gradient is built up, pulling fluid into the hematoma. This increase in the size of the hematoma may cause further bleeding by tearing the surrounding membrane or vessels, increasing the size and pressure of the hematoma. If allowed to follow its natural course, the contents of the subdural hematoma undergo characteristic changes (Table 56-2).

Chronic subdural hematoma has frequently been nicknamed "the imitator" because the signs and symptoms are generally nonspecific and nonlocalizing and may be caused by many different disease processes. Some patients complain of a headache. The most typical signs and symptoms include progressive alteration in LOC, including apathy, lethargy, and decreased attention span, and decreased ability to use higher cognitive skills. Hemianopsia, hemiparesis, and pupillary abnormalities are observed in fewer than 50% of patients. The CSF is rarely helpful in confirming a diagnosis and may be nonspecifically abnormal, with increased protein content and xanthochromia, or may contain a few red blood cells; the pressure is generally normal. When aphasia is present, it is usually an *anomic* type, which is characterized by well-articulated speech and normal grammar that conveys little or no information. The ability to understand the spoken word (comprehension) and the ability to repeat sentences and phrases remain unchanged.

Diagnosis is best made by arteriography. CT scan may demonstrate a hematoma, thereby avoiding the necessity of an arteriogram, but a negative CT scan does not necessarily rule out a diagnosis of subdural hematoma.

Small hematomas resolve spontaneously if allowed to follow their natural course. In patients with small hematomas with no neurologic signs, the best medical course is probably close monitoring. For the patient with progressive neurologic deficit and debilitating symptoms, however, the best course is surgical removal because the greatest danger in chronic subdural hematoma is that it may cause herniation of the temporal uncus and death.

Mild Traumatic Brain Injury (Concussion)

Concussion is often thought to be a benign event, but, in reality, it can have significant life-long sequelae. Patients with a history of head injury and a GCS score of 15 are frequently underdiagnosed. Concussion is suspected when the mechanism of injury involves a blow to the head, acceleration-deceleration injury or a shaking incident, which are common following a sports or playground injury.

Clinical signs and symptoms of concussion vary according to the severity, but memory gaps or amnesia involving the accident is the hallmark sign. The patient is usually confused at the time of the incident, and the confusion persists for a period after the injury. There are no focal neurologic signs characteristic of a more severe head injury.

Most patients recover from concussion with no serious sequelae, but some may experience *postconcussion syndrome*. Cognitive dysfunction, persistent dizziness, and headaches characterize the syndrome; other characteristics may include sleep disturbances, speech disorders, and behavioral problems, which can be subtle or dramatic. These symptoms may persist for days, weeks, or longer following the concussion.

SPINAL CORD INJURY

Approximately 10,000 new spinal cord injuries occur in the United States each year, primarily to young, single men. The cost of these injuries in terms of disability and rehabilitation is tremendous. The cause of spinal cord injuries is primarily automobile crashes, followed by falls and sports injuries. Contact sports and diving accidents are the primary sports causes of quadriplegia.

The acute management of the patient with a spinal cord injury begins at the moment the injury is suspected and focuses on the primary goals of treatment, which include maximizing neurologic recovery, restoring normal alignment, and preventing secondary complications. These goals can be accomplished only by the combined efforts of a multidisciplinary team.

Mechanisms of Injury

The vertebral column is constructed with a circumferential bony ring that provides ideal protection for low-velocity penetrating injuries and contusions, but the intervertebral articulations are weak points for flexion, extension, or rotational stress. Dislocations and fractures that do not break the vertebral ring allow the vertebrae above and below the area of injury to act as fulcrums for

TABLE 56-2 ■ ■ ■

Stages in the Natural History of Nonlethal Subdural Hematoma

Stage	Description
Stage I	Dark blood spreads widely over the brain surface beneath the dura.
Stage II	Blood congeals and becomes darker, thicker, and gelatinous (2 to 4 days).
Stage III	Clot breaks down and after about 2 weeks has color and consistency of crankcase oil.
Stage IV	Organization begins with formation of encasing membranes: an outer thick, tough membrane derived from dura and a thin inner one from arachnoid. The contained fluid becomes xanthochromic.
Stage V	Organization is completed. Clot may become calcified or even ossified (or may resorb).

Modified from Jackson FE: *CIBA Clin Symp* 18(3):67-93, 1966.

other vertebrae and their attached soft tissue to undergo concussion, stretching, and contusion and thus disrupt the spinal cord.

The stresses of flexion, extension, and rotation, along with the relative weakness of the articulations of the vertebrae, cause fractures and dislocations to occur most often at points where a relatively mobile portion of the vertebral column meets a relatively fixed segment, that is, between the lower cervical area and the upper thoracic segment, between the lower thoracic and upper lumbar segments, and between the lower lumbar segment and the sacrum.

Most of the damage in spinal cord injury occurs at the time of initial injury. This additional insult is followed by a series of deleterious events leading to secondary damage and additional injury. Sources of secondary injury include bone fragments projecting into the spinal canal, stretching or shearing of both the cord and surrounding vascular tissue, and ligaments and muscle spasm, resulting in cord compression. Mechanical instability contributes to compression of both the cord and its blood supply leading to further structural damage. Systemic factors, including blood pressure and pulmonary function, which profoundly affect oxygenation and perfusion, will profoundly influence the amount of secondary injury.

Research has demonstrated the ischemia that occurs following the initial spinal cord insult resulting in a cascade of damaging events, which are significantly worsened by systemic hypotension and hypoxia. Locally, the injury causes loss of autoregulation of blood flow, petechial hemorrhages, inflammation and edema. These changes are particularly damaging to the gray matter because of its higher susceptibility to trauma and its higher metabolic demands.

The core zone of irreparably damaged tissue is surrounded by a zone of ischemic but potentially salvageable tissue that remains viable for a period of time (Amar, 1999). The focus of initial medical and surgical interventions is directed toward reversing the ischemia in this area and preventing extension of the infarcted zone. Preservation of even a small amount of this ischemic tissue has significant implications for neurologic recovery.

Reduction of secondary injury is the role of methylprednisolone therapy, approved by the U.S. Food and Drug Administration (FDA) for spinal cord injury in 1990. It is postulated that methylprednisolone, a synthetic steroid, suppresses the inflammatory response at the injury site, reducing edema formation. In addition, methylprednisolone blocks the formation of free radicals that contribute to secondary injury because of their ability to disrupt the cell walls and contribute further to edema and cord ischemia.

Following spinal cord trauma, release of neurotransmitters becomes excessive, causing an overexcitement of nerve cells. Glutamate is the neurotransmitter used by nerve cells to activate one another. Excessive glutamate accumulation leads to damage of nerve cells in two ways: (1) It allows high levels of calcium to enter the cells, which, in turn, inappropriately activates cellular proteases causing damage to many cellular processes, in-cluding cell membrane damage, and mitochondrial damage contributing to further development of free radicals, and (2) it alters sodium exchange at the cell membrane, allowing water to enter the neuronal cell, which contributes, to further edema formation (Amar, 1999).

Spinal Shock

Spinal shock is a temporary physiologic disorganization of spinal cord function that occurs immediately after the injury and may last from hours to weeks. In the acute stage, there is complete or nearly complete loss of reflex activity below the level of the cord injury. Flaccid paralysis, loss of deep tendon reflexes, loss of temperature control and vasomotor tone, and bowel and bladder paralysis that result in urinary retention and paralytic ileus are all frequently seen in these patients. Spinal shock is not a cardiovascular problem; it may coexist with neurogenic shock and hemorrhagic shock. Neurogenic shock results from an impairment of descending sympathetic innervation to the vasculature, dilating the blood vessels and causing hypotension and bradycardia. It is essential to exclude hemorrhage as the source of hypotension in the patient with a spinal cord injury.

Under normal conditions, axons descending from the supraspinal portions of the nervous system deliver low-frequency impulses to the neurons to maintain the neuron in a state of excitability or readiness. When the injury removes the "background tone," the resting excitability of the spinal cord is greatly reduced. Spinal shock also occurs in partial transection of the cord.

Transection of the spinal cord produces widespread alterations in visceral functions. Immediately after transection of the spinal cord, there is complete atony of the smooth muscle of the bladder wall. At the same time, constrictor tone of the sphincter muscle increases, probably because of loss of an inhibitory influence. With recovery of somatic reflexes, which may occur in 25 to 30 days after cord section, tone returns to the bladder muscles and reflex emptying of the bladder occurs. This process is produced by simultaneous contraction of the smooth muscle walls and, to a certain extent, relaxation of the tone of the sphincter. After reflex emptying of the bladder, a considerable residual volume is left. Cutaneous stimulation to the abdomen, perineum, or lower extremities greatly facilitates reflex emptying.

In the intestinal tract, it appears as if digestion and absorption proceed normally. Great difficulty is encountered in the evacuation of feces from the lower bowel and rectum. Normally, the presence of fecal matter in the lower bowel and rectum, which passively stretches the walls, produces active contraction and peristalsis; this, combined with relaxation of the sphincter, causes defecation. This mechanism is depressed during spinal shock. The sphincter ani muscles relax only slightly in response to passive dilation; therefore retention of fecal material occurs. With the recovery of reflex excitability, reflex evacuation of the bowel occurs, which is facilitated by tactile stimulus of the skin areas of the sacral segments and by manual dilation of the sphincter ani muscle.

Reflex actions on the peripheral vessels and organs innervated by the autonomic nervous system are profoundly affected by spinal shock. Transection of the spinal cord causes an immediate and profound fall in arterial pressure. This reduction is the result of elimination of the bulbar vasoconstrictor mechanism; when spinal nerves are separated from the medullary centers, the important coordination between the state of the blood vessels and subsidiary centers in the spinal cord is lacking. In the person with an intact spinal cord, the spinal centers are regarded as subordinated to the higher vasoconstrictor center in the medulla. The hypotension persists for some time after transection. Spinal neurons innervating peripheral effectors concerned with body temperature control are permanently severed from the descending influences of the thermoregulatory center.

Treatment for spinal shock revolves around maintaining normal hemodynamic parameters with aggressive fluid resuscitation, vasopressors, and measures to maintain a heart rate greater than or equal to 60 bpm. Careful monitoring of urine output, right atrial or pulmonary artery pressures, hemoglobin, and hematocrit is essential. Over a period of weeks, reflex function begins to return with the occurrence of brisk tendon reflexes; in addition, the bladder and bowel regain some reflex function.

Cervical Spinal Cord Injury

High cervical spine injuries are associated with multiple problems. Initial trauma care, including cervical spine immobilization and airway management, has contributed to the survivability of this devastating injury.

Injuries at the first cervical vertebra (C1) level account for 3% to 13% of all cervical spine fractures. Severe deficits at the C1 level are usually fatal. Diagnosis of high cervical fractures can be difficult, and these injuries are frequently associated with concurrent injuries, including vertebral artery injury. These patients have little or no motor control of the head and are ventilator dependent.

A C2- or C3-injured patient has some neck control, which allows the patient to develop tolerance for the upright position. Because innervation to the respiratory accessory muscles (sternocleidomastoid and scalenus muscles) is partially preserved, the patient is dependent on a ventilator; however, the patient may be able to spend some time off the ventilator. These patients are termed *respiratory quadriplegics.*

The spinal respiratory center is located primarily at the C4 level. The phrenic nerve root must be intact if the patient is to develop any voluntary control of ventilation. Ventilatory capacity will not be normal in these patients, but depending on other factors, they may progress to a life without a ventilator that offers some measure of control and freedom.

Patients with a C5 injury retain control of their head, neck, shoulders, and diaphragm and may have partial control of the elbow. Partial control of the wrist is preserved after a C6 injury; in C7 injury, the patient has full elbow extension, wrist flexion, and some finger control; in C8 to first thoracic vertebra (T1) injury, the patient has reasonably good finger control, allowing independence with respect to many of the activities of daily living.

Autonomic Dysreflexia

Autonomic dysreflexia *(hyperreflexia)* is a potentially life-threatening reaction that can occur any time after the individual with complete or partial cord transection recovers from spinal shock. Dysreflexia is characterized by a generalized, undampened cardiovascular response to discharge from the sympathetic nervous system, which emerges from the thoracic and lumbar sections of the spinal cord. The abnormal mass reflex occurs because the spinal cord lesion interrupts normal spinothalamic pathways, carrying impulses to the brain from sensory receptors below the cord lesion. The result is reflex sympathetic outflow from the thoracolumbar section of the spinal cord below the lesion. In turn, the autonomic motor pathways that carry efferent impulses back to the peripheral blood vessels and viscera are interrupted by the lesion. Thus the higher the lesion (T6 or above), the more likely an individual will develop autonomic dysreflexia.

The response is usually initiated by one or more noxious sensory impulses, such as a distended bladder, full rectum, shearing force against partially denervated skin, or exposed decubitus ulcer. Interruption of the ascending impulses triggers sympathetic outflow, causing intense arteriolar spasm and blood pressure elevation. The hypertension is sensed in the aortic and carotid sinus receptors and transmitted to the medulla oblongata via CN IX and the carotid sinus nerve. Parasympathetic stimulation causes the heart rate to decrease compensatorily, but the blood pressure remains elevated and even continues to climb because the cord lesion interrupts the descending autonomic responses, which normally provide negative feedback to the sympathetic outflow from the cord. Signs of autonomic hyperreflexia are sudden hypertension to levels greater than 200 mm Hg systolic; bradycardia as low as 30 to 40 bpm; severe, pounding headache; flushed skin and sweating above the level of the lesion; and pallor and "goose bumps" from pilomotor spasm below the level of the lesion. The patient may also complain of nausea and nasal congestion.

Because of the severe hypertension, immediate action must be taken to prevent a cerebrovascular accident (CVA, stroke). Elevating the head of the bed will often lower the blood pressure because of the venous pooling that occurs with high spinal cord injury. The source of the noxious stimulus must be removed; emptying a full bladder or bowel will produce relief. Similarly, careful attention to bowel and bladder regimens will dramatically reduce the incidence of dysreflexia. Anesthetic cream applied to the anus often prevents triggering dysreflexia when enemas or suppositories are administered. Intravenous antihypertensive medications such as trimethaphan camsylate (Arfonad), a ganglionic blocker, may be necessary if the hypertension is not relieved effectively by conservative measures.

Thoracic-Lumbar-Sacral Spinal Cord Injury

Patients with injuries of the thoracic (T), lumbar (L), and sacral (S) spine are considered paraplegic. The mechanism of injury in this area is typically a flexion injury caused by a fall onto the buttocks or a hyperextension injury, both of which cause compression fractures. A heavy direct blow is needed to fracture the midthoracic vertebral bodies unless they have been previously softened by osteoporosis or neoplasm.

The paraplegic patient is capable of achieving an independent lifestyle with respect to the activities of daily living. Patients with a T2 to T12 injury retain full upper extremity control and a limited amount of trunk control. In an L1 to L5 injury the patient may have full trunk control and, depending on the level of injury, hip, knee, ankle, and some foot control, which allows these patients to walk with braces. In a S1 to S5 injury the patient has some foot control but experiences bowel and bladder dysfunction.

Treatment of Spinal Cord Injuries

The early handling and treatment of patients with spinal cord injuries are critical for the prevention of further neurologic damage. Prehospital management should assume that trauma victims are spinal cord injured. It is estimated that 10% to 25% of patients suffer additional spinal cord injury resulting from inadequate stabilization following injury (Amar, 2001). The types of trauma most likely to result in spinal cord injury include motor vehicle crashes (including all-terrain vehicles and motorcycles), gunshot wounds, diving accidents, and falls.

Initial management of the suspected spinal cord injury addresses airway, ventilation and oxygenation, and circulatory support before neurologic evaluation and resuscitation. Patients with an injury at the C4 level or higher cannot breathe spontaneously. The jaw thrust maneuver is designed to minimize movement of the neck during resuscitation. Establishing an effective airway is the initial priority. Controversy exists as to the methods used to secure the airway. Acceptable methods include cricothyrotomy and oral intubation. The key factor is "in line" stabilization of the neck (manually maintaining the neck in a neutral position) during the endotracheal intubation procedure. It is essential that hypoxia be eliminated as soon as possible because hypoxia significantly contributes to the secondary injury accompanying spinal cord trauma. Maintenance of a MAP of 100 mm Hg permits spinal cord perfusion. It is critical to determine whether the cause of the hypotension is neurogenic shock or hypovolemic shock (Table 56-3). The objective is to restore the MAP to normotensive levels while avoiding fluid overload and hypertension. The patient is monitored carefully to prevent fluid overload, which puts the patient at risk for heart failure and pulmonary edema. Hypotension is also treated with vasopressors, such as dobutamine and dopamine, which have positive inotro-

pic and chronotropic effects. Patients with injuries above the T6 level are at increased risk for circulatory complications caused by sympathetic nervous system disruption. As a consequence, on rare occasions, deep suctioning will stimulate a vasovagal response, leading to cardiac standstill.

The methylprednisolone protocol is a standard for the treatment of spinal cord injury. The drug is administered within the first 3 hours after the injury occurs. Patients benefit from treatment that is given up to 8 hours after the injury.

The primary treatment for cervical injury is reduction and stabilization of the fracture, most effectively achieved by skeletal traction with tongs or wires inserted in the skull to achieve and maintain reduction. Stabilization is achieved by anatomic reduction and by tension of the spinal ligaments and soft tissue of the cervical area. Slight extension of the neck creates tension in the anterior spinal ligament.

Reduction of fracture dislocations of the thoracic and lumbar spines is no longer recommended. At present, treatment consists of bedrest until pain subsides. Single compression fractures of the body of a vertebra, with flexion angulation of the spine without spinal cord deficit, may be treated by positioning on a specially designed frame (e.g., Stryker, Bradford, Foster), using extension to stretch the anterior spinal ligament and expand the vertebral body.

A controversial therapy is decompression of the spinal cord. There are two schools of thought on early surgical decompression. Some neurosurgeons believe (1) that severe injury to the cord can rarely be reversed, (2) that the damage that occurs in spinal cord injury occurs early in the injury, during which surgical intervention would seriously jeopardize the patient's life with little or no chance of improving postoperative functioning, and (3) that because function returns gradually over a period of up to 2 years, the risk of surgery is not warranted. Others believe that the postinjury edema and swelling of the spinal cord increase the neurologic deficit; therefore laminectomy with decompression always has some potential value. All surgeons agree that patients showing progressive deficit in neurologic function and those with open fractures benefit from surgical decompression.

The management of spinal cord injury remains controversial. As scientists understand more about the underlying molecular events associated with spinal cord injury, more effective treatment strategies can be devised. Several new areas of research hold promise for the future. One important area of research is neural regeneration of the damaged spinal cord. Some promising results are being obtained in animal studies. Cografting of several types of animal cells (animal fetal brain tissue and animal adult peripheral nerve tissue) onto the damaged spinal cord of rats has shown evidence of regeneration.

The research is a long way from being applied to humans, but it holds significant promise for the future. Additional experiments involve the transplant of Schwann cells (normally found in the peripheral nervous system) to the area of spinal cord injury. It is thought that these cells can induce the injured spinal cord axons to regrow.

TABLE 56-3   ■ ■ ■

Neurogenic versus Hypovolemic Shock

Parameter	Neurogenic	Hypovolemic
Blood pressure	Low	Low
Pulse	Bradycardia: slow, bounding	Tachycardia: rapid, weak, thready
Skin	Warm, dry	Cold, clammy

KEY CONCEPTS

- The initial care of the neurologically injured patient is directed toward securing the airway and providing adequate ventilation and oxygenation.
- *Level of consciousness* is the most sensitive indicator of increased intracranial pressure.
- *Decorticate posturing* indicates that the lesion or injury is above the brainstem; decerebrate posturing indicates brain stem involvement.
- Conditions that increase ICP include acidosis, hypotonic intravenous solutions, decreased protein intake, and position changes that involve hip or knee flexion.
- *Oculocephalic reflex* (doll's eyes) indicates brainstem integrity.
- An *epidural hematoma* is caused by arterial bleeding (middle meningeal artery); a subdural hematoma is caused by venous bleeding.
- Fixed, dilated pupils result from compression of CN III (oculomotor).

- *Postconcussion syndrome* is associated with persistent headaches, dizziness, and cognitive and behavioral changes.
- *Spinal shock* is a temporary condition that involves loss of autonomic nervous control, areflexia, loss of sensation, and flaccid paralysis.
- Return of reflexes below the level of the injury is a sign of spinal shock resolution.
- Hypotension, bradycardia, and warm periphery characterize *neurogenic shock*.
- To achieve maximum therapeutic results, methylprednisolone is administered within 3 hours of spinal cord injury.
- Pounding headache, hypertension, and bradycardia are signs of *autonomic dysreflexia*, which is most often caused by a distended bladder or a full rectum.
- *Vertebral fractures* occur most commonly in areas in which a mobile portion of the vertebral column meets a more rigid section.

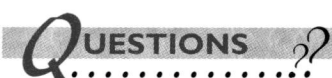
QUESTIONS ??

A sampling of review questions for this chapter appears here. Visit http://www.mosby.com/MERLIN/PriceWilson/ for additional questions. MERLIN

Answer the following on a separate sheet of paper.

1. What is normal intracranial pressure (ICP) in mm Hg? What causes increased ICP, and why is it dangerous?
2. Explain the mechanisms that account for the following signs and symptoms of intracranial hematoma: hemiparesis, seizures, mental dysfunction, depression of consciousness, changes in vital signs (increased systolic blood pressure, bradycardia), decerebrate rigidity, and dilated ipsilateral pupil.
3. What two general mechanisms account for brain damage in head trauma?
4. What is a contrecoup injury? What areas of the brain are most likely to be injured in a deceleration automobile accident?
5. List the three most common sites of spinal cord injury.
6. What is the foremost rule in the treatment of spinal cord injury?
7. Contrast the mechanisms for posttraumatic epidural and subdural hematomas.

Match each meningeal structure in column A with the appropriate statements from column B.

Column A
8. _____ Dura mater
9. _____ Arachnoid
10. _____ Pia mater

Column B
a. Fine, fibrous middle layer of the meninges
b. Inner meningeal layer closely applied to the brain and spinal cord
c. Encloses the venous sinuses and separates the brain into compartments
d. Circulation of CSF in a space directly under this layer
e. Middle and posterior portions supplied by the middle meningeal artery

CHAPTER 57

Central Nervous System Tumors

MARY CARTER LOMBARDO

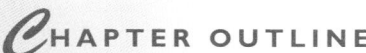
BRAIN TUMORS

Intracranial tumors include space-occupying lesions, both benign and malignant, that develop in the brain, meninges, and skull. Brain tumors derive from neuronal tissue, supportive brain tissue, the reticuloendothelial system (RES), brain coverings, and residual developmental tissues, or they metastasize from systemic carcinomas. Brain metastases are caused by systemic malignancies from the lung, breast, melanoma, lymphoma, and colon cancer. Brain tumors can occur at any age; they may occur in children under age 10 but are most frequently found in adults during the fifth and sixth decades of life. Patient survival from malignant brain tumors has not changed much during the last 20 years.

There are many classifications of brain tumors. Perhaps the one easiest to understand is the *Kernahan and Sayre classification,* in which the tumor is named for the cells present in the adult nervous system, in vascular tissue, and in developmental defects and the degree of malignancy is graded I to IV (IV being the most malignant) (Table 57-1).

Because patients with brain tumors have diverse and confusing symptoms, diagnosis may be difficult. Symptomatology of brain tumor depends on size, location, and invasiveness of the tumor.

Certain tumors occur more frequently in a particular age group. During infancy and childhood, posterior fossa tumors are much more common than are supratentorial lesions (middle or anterior fossa), which are more common in adults. The brain tumor of a child is likely to be a malignant astrocytoma of the cerebellum of grades I or II. In the middle-aged or older person, the most common brain tumor is a glioblastoma multiforme, the most malignant glioma, characterized by a rapid growth rate.

Research into the genetic component of brain tumors is beginning to show promise; the discovery of mutations of the TP53 (Li-Fraumeni syndrome), P16 (melanoma-glioma syndrome), and MMAC1 (mutated in multiple advanced cancers) genes in patients with brain tumors will have significant impact on the future. Presence of these genetic abnormalities might be used in the future as genetic markers and may help in developing gene therapy strategies for the treatment of brain tumors (Fueyo, 1999).

Gliomas

Gliomas account for approximately 40% to 50% of brain tumors. Gliomas are classified based on embryologic origin. In the adult, the neuroglia of the central nervous system (CNS) provide for the repair, support, and protection of the delicate nerve cells. Gliomas consist of connective tissue and supporting cells. The neuroglia possess the potential to continue to divide throughout life. Glial cells congregate to form dense cicatricial scars in regions of brain where neurons disappear because of injury or disease. Glial tumors account for nearly one half of all childhood brain tumors. Most pediatric glial tumors are low-grade tumors most commonly located in the posterior fossa and diencephalic region (Smith, 1998).

TABLE 57-1 ■ ■ ■

Brain Tumors

Tumor	Percent of All Brain Tumors
Gliomas	40-50
Astrocytoma grade I	5-10
Astrocytoma grade II	2-5
Astrocytoma grades III and IV (glioblastoma multiforme)	20-30
Medulloblastoma	3-5
Oligodendroglioma	1-4
Ependymoma grades I to IV	1-3
Meningioma	12-20
Pituitary tumors	5-15
Neurilemmomas (mainly cranial nerve VIII)	3-10
Metastatic tumors	5-10
Blood vessel tumors	
Arteriovenous malformations, hemangioblastomas, endotheliomas	0.5-1
Tumors of developmental defects	2-3
Dermoids, epidermoids, teratomas, chordomas, paraphyseal cysts	
Craniopharyngiomas	3-8
Pinealomas	0.5-0.8
Miscellaneous	
Sarcomas, papillomas of the choroid plexus, lipomas, unclassified	1-3

From Schwartz SI, editor: *Principles of surgery,* ed 7, New York, 1999, McGraw-Hill.

There are three types of glial cells: microglia, oligodendroglia, and astrocytes. The *microglia* are of mesodermal embryologic origin and therefore are generally not classified as true glial cells. The microglia enter the CNS through the vascular system and function as phagocytes, clearing away the debris and combating infection.

The oligodendroglia and the astrocytes are true neuroglia and, as with neurons, arise from the ectoderm. *Oligodendroglia* are involved in myelin formation. The function of astrocytes is still under investigation; evidence shows that they may play some role in impulse conduction and synaptic transmission of neurons and may serve as conduits between blood vessels and neurons.

Astrocytomas infiltrate the brain and are frequently associated with cysts of various sizes. Although astrocytomas infiltrate the brain tissue, the effect on brain functioning is minimal early in the illness. Generally, astrocytomas are nonmalignant, although they may undergo a malignant change to a glioblastoma, a highly malignant astrocytoma. These tumors are generally slow growing; therefore the patient frequently does not seek medical attention for several years, until debilitating symptoms occur, such as seizures or headaches. Complete surgical excision is generally not possible because of the invasive nature of the tumor, but it is sensitive to radiation.

The *glioblastoma multiforme* is the most malignant of the gliomas. This tumor has a rapid growth rate, and complete surgical excision is impossible. Life expectancy is usually about 12 months. The tumor may occur anywhere but most often involves the cerebral hemisphere and often spreads to the opposite side via the corpus callosum.

The *oligodendroglioma* is a slow-growing lesion similar to the astrocytoma but is composed of oligodendroglial cells.

The oligodendroglioma is relatively avascular and is prone to calcification; it is usually found in the cerebral hemisphere of young people. These tumors may present as a partial seizure disorder that is present for up to 10 years, or they may be clinically aggressive and cause significant symptomatology related to increased intracranial pressure.

Oligodendrogliomas are the most chemosensitive of all human solid malignancies. The most commonly used chemotherapy regimens include melphalan, thiotepa, temozolomide, paclitaxel (Taxol), and platinum-based regimens. It is postulated that the neoplastic cells originating from the oligodendroglia are susceptible to the alkylating effects of cytotoxic chemotherapy. A fuller explanation awaits the results of more generic research (Cairncross, 1998).

Ependymoma is a rare malignant tumor arising in close relationship to the ependymal covering of the ventricle; it most commonly occurs in the posterior fossa but can occur in any part of the ventricular fossa. The tumor is more commonly found in children than in adults. Two major factors influencing successful resection of the tumor and long-term survival include age and anatomic location of the tumor. The younger the patient, the poorer the prognosis, which is especially apparent when the child is younger than 7 years of age. The reason for the poorer prognosis is not clear. It is postulated that embryonal tumors in children are different from the more mature adult tumors and that the more immature neural tissue in children results in more aggressive tumor behavior, which negatively affects outcomes (Spagnoli, 2000). Patients with tumors located in the floor or roof of the ventricle have a higher survival rate after surgical resection than do patients with tumors of the lateral process. This difference is because floor and roof tumors can be completely resected, whereas lateral tumors tend to infiltrate the cerebellar peduncle and pontine structure making complete removal impossible. Radiation treatment is used postoperatively except for children younger than 3 years who receive chemotherapy.

Meningeal Tumors

The *meningioma* is the most important tumor arising from the meninges, the mesothelial lining cells, and the connective tissue cells of the arachnoid and the dura. Most meningeal tumors are benign and encapsulated and do not infiltrate adjacent tissue but rather compress the underlying structures. Older adult patients are most frequently affected and women more often than are men. These tumors are often quite vascular and therefore take up radioactive isotopes during a brain scan. Complete surgical excision is possible, especially if the tumor is not in a critical area and diagnosis is made early. Meningiomas of the area around the brainstem and the base of the skull are often not accessible for complete excision. Because of the slow growth of this tumor, symptoms may be overlooked and the diagnosis missed completely. Symptoms include idiopathic epilepsy, hemiparesis, and aphasia.

Pituitary Tumors

Pituitary tumors arise from the chromophobe, eosinophil, or basophil cells of the anterior pituitary. These tu-

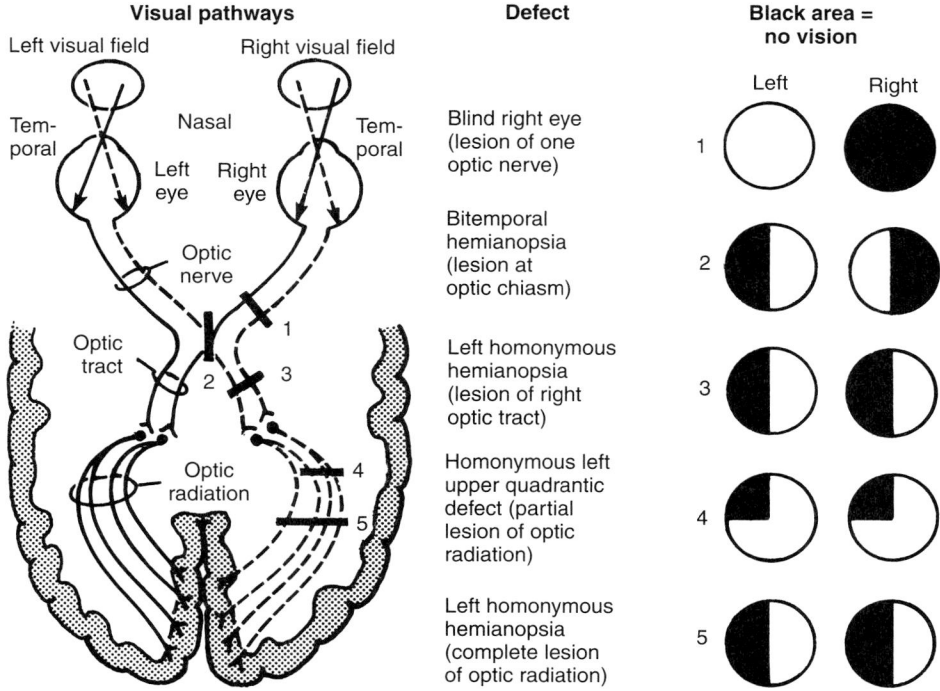

FIG. 57-1 Visual field defects produced by selected lesions in the visual pathways. (Modified from *Programmed practice in anatomy and physiology of the nervous system*, Englewood Cliffs, NJ, 1972, Prentice-Hall.)

mors cause headache, bitemporal hemianopsia (from pressure on the optic chiasm), and signs of abnormal secretion of hormones from the anterior pituitary. Fig. 57-1 illustrates the various visual field defects that typically occur when lesions involve the optic tract.

Chromophobe tumors are nonsecretory tumors that compress the pituitary gland, the optic chiasm, and the hypothalamus. Symptoms of this brain tumor include depression of sexual function, secondary hypothyroidism, and adrenal hypofunction (amenorrhea, impotence, loss of hair, weakness, hypotension, low basal metabolism, hypoglycemia, and electrolyte disturbances).

Eosinophilic adenomas are generally smaller and slower-growing tumors than are chromophobe tumors. The symptoms include acromegaly in adults and gigantism in children, headache, sweating disturbance, paresthesias, muscular pain, and loss of libido. Disturbances in visual fields (bitemporal hemianopsia) are rare.

Basophil adenomas are generally small. These tumors are associated with the symptoms of Cushing's syndrome (obesity, muscle wasting, skin atrophy, osteoporosis, plethora, hypertension, salt and water retention, hypertrichosis, diabetes mellitus).

Neurilemmomas (Auditory Nerve Tumors)

Auditory nerve tumors constitute 3% to 10% of intracranial tumors; they probably arise from the Schwann cells of the nerve sheath. The nerve fibers in the eighth cranial nerve (CN VIII) are eventually destroyed. Bilateral auditory neurilemmoma may occur in von Recklinghausen's disease. Generally benign, these tumors occasionally undergo malignant change.

Symptoms of auditory neurilemmoma include first deafness, tinnitus, loss of caloric vestibular reactivity, and vertigo, followed by suboccipital discomfort, staggering gait, involvement of adjacent cranial nerves, and signs of increased intracranial pressure (ICP). Nystagmus, especially horizontal, is usually present. Treatment consists of complete removal of the tumor, if possible, because incomplete removal is generally accompanied by recurrence of the tumor. Surgery leaves the patient with facial paralysis and deafness.

Metastatic Tumors

Metastatic lesions, which account for approximately 5% to 10% of brain tumors, may originate from any primary site. The most common primary tumors are those of the lung and breast, but neoplasms from the genitourinary tract, gastrointestinal (GI) tract, bone, and thyroid may also metastasize to the brain. The metastatic lesion may be single or multiple and may be a late stage in the metastatic process or the first sign of a previously unrecognized primary tumor. Single lesions may be surgically excised to extend life or to reduce symptoms. The edema surrounding these lesions is responsive to corticosteroid therapy.

Blood Vessel Tumors

These tumors include the angiomas, hemangioblastomas, and endotheliomas and make up a small percentage of brain tumors. *Angiomas* are congenital arteriovenous (AV) malformations, present from birth, which slowly enlarge. These tumors may compress surrounding brain tissue and bleed intracerebrally or into the subarachnoid space. *Hemangioblastomas* are neoplasms composed of embryologic vascular elements most often found in the cerebellum. The von Hippel-Lindau syndrome is a combination of cerebellar hemangioblastoma, angiomatosis of the retina, and cysts of the kidney and pancreas.

Tumors of Developmental Defects (Congenital)

Rare congenital tumors include *chordomas,* which are composed of cells derived from the embryonic notochord remnants and are found at the base of the skull. These tumors grow slowly but are highly invasive, making complete surgical removal impossible. *Dermoids* and *teratomas* may occur anywhere in the CNS. *Teratomas* frequently occur in the ventricular system and obstruct the third ventricle, the aqueduct, or the fourth ventricle. *Craniopharyngiomas* arise from remnants of the embryonic craniopharyngeal duct (Rathke's pouch) and are usually located posterior to the sella turcica. Symptoms of congenital tumors generally exhibit themselves early in a child's life but may be silent for many years. The symptoms include defects in visual fields, generally irregular, and hypothalamic and pituitary dysfunctions.

Pinealomas (Adnexal Tumors)

Pinealomas account for a small number of intracranial lesions and include tumors that originate within the pineal body *(pinealoma)*, as well as those from the surrounding choroid plexus *(choroid papilloma)*. Pinealomas compress the aqueduct, causing obstructive hydrocephalus, and the hypothalamus, giving rise to precocious puberty and diabetes insipidus. Choroid papilloma causes intraventricular bleeding and also obstructs the ventricular system.

Pathophysiology of Brain Tumors

Brain tumors give rise to progressive neurologic deficit. The symptoms occur on a continuum, which underscores the importance of the history when examining the patient. Symptoms should be discussed within a time perspective. When did the symptom develop? Was it associated with anything? How long have you had this?

The neurologic deficit in brain tumors is generally thought to be caused by two factors: the focal disturbances caused by the tumor and the increased ICP.

Focal disturbances occur when there is compression of brain tissue and infiltration or direct invasion of brain parenchyma with destruction of neural tissue. Dysfunction is greatest with the fastest-growing infiltrating tumors (e.g., glioblastoma multiforme).

Alteration in blood supply because of compression from the growing tumor causes necrosis of brain tissue. Interference with arterial blood supply is usually characterized by an acute loss of function and may be confused with primary cerebrovascular disorders.

Seizures as a manifestation of altered neuronal excitability are related to the compression, invasion, and alteration in the blood supply to the brain tissue. Some tumors form cysts, which also compress the surrounding brain parenchyma, increasing the focal neurologic deficit.

The increased ICP may result from several factors: an increase in the mass within the skull, edema formation around the tumor, and alteration in cerebrospinal fluid (CSF) circulation. The tumor's growth causes an increase in mass because it occupies space within the relatively fixed volume of the rigid compartment of the skull. Malignant tumors produce edema in the surrounding brain tissue. Although the mechanism is not completely understood, it is thought that an osmotic gradient causes absorption of fluid by the tumor. Some tumors may cause hemorrhage. Venous obstruction and edema caused by breakdown of the blood-brain barrier cause an increase in intracranial volume and ICP. Obstruction of CSF circulation from the lateral ventricles to the subarachnoid space causes hydrocephalus.

Increased ICP becomes life threatening when any of the previously discussed causes develops rapidly. Compensatory mechanisms require days or months to be effective and therefore are not useful when increased ICP develops rapidly. These mechanisms include decreased intracranial blood volume, decreased CSF volume, decreased intracellular fluid contents, and decreased parenchymal cell numbers. Untreated, increased ICP causes herniation of the uncus or the cerebellum. Uncal herniation is caused when the medial gyrus of the temporal lobe is displaced inferiorly through the tentorial notch by a mass in the cerebral hemisphere. This action compresses the midbrain, causing loss of consciousness and compression of the third cranial nerve (CN III). The cerebellar tonsils are displaced downward through the foramen magnum by a posterior mass in cerebellar herniation. Compression of the medulla and respiratory arrest rapidly ensue. Other physiologic changes that occur with rapidly developing increased ICP include progressive bradycardia, systemic hypertension with a widening pulse pressure, and respiratory failure (see Chapter 56).

Clinical Manifestations

The classic triad of symptoms in brain tumor consists of headache, vomiting, and papilledema. However, there is great variety in symptoms, depending on the site of the lesion and the rapidity of growth.

Headache

Headache is perhaps the most common symptom found in patients with brain tumors. The pain may be described as deep, aching, steady, dull, and sometimes agonizingly severe. The pain is most severe in the morning and is aggravated by activities that normally increase ICP, such as stooping, coughing, or straining at stool. The headache is somewhat relieved by aspirin and application of cold packs to the site.

The headache associated with brain tumor is caused by traction and displacement of pain-sensitive structures within the intracranial cavity. These pain-sensitive structures include the arteries, veins, venous sinuses, and cranial nerves.

The headache has a localizing value in that one third of headaches overlie the tumor site, and the other two thirds are near or above the tumor. Occipital headache is the first symptom in tumors of the posterior fossa. Approximately one third of supratentorial lesions give rise to a frontal headache. A complaint of a generalized headache has little localizing value and usually indicates extensive displacement of intracranial contents with increased ICP.

Nausea and Vomiting

Nausea and vomiting occur as a result of stimulation of the emetic center in the medulla. Vomiting is most frequent in children and in association with increased ICP with brainstem displacement. Vomiting may occur without preceding nausea and may be projectile.

Papilledema

Papilledema is caused by venous stasis, which leads to engorgement and swelling of the optic disc. When seen by funduscopy, papilledema suggests increased ICP. Using this sign as diagnostic of brain tumor is often difficult because the fundi in some persons may not show papilledema, even with very high ICP.

In association with the papilledema, some disturbances in vision may occur. These disturbances include enlargement of the blind spot and *amaurosis fugax* (fleeting moments of dimmed vision).

Localizing Symptoms

Other signs and symptoms of brain tumor tend to have an increased localizing value. Tumors of the frontal lobe give symptoms of mental changes, hemiparesis, ataxia, and disturbances of speech. Mental changes are exhibited by subtle changes in personality. Some patients experience periods of depression, confusion, or bizarre behavior. The most common changes involve higher level reasoning and judgment skills. Hemiparesis is caused by pressure on the neighboring motor areas and pathways. If the motor area is involved, jacksonian seizures and obvious motor weakness may occur. Tumors involving the lower end of the precentral cortex cause weakness of the face, tongue, and thumb, whereas tumors of the paracentral lobule produce weakness in the foot and lower extremity. Tumors of the frontal lobe may cause unsteadiness in the gait, often imitating cerebellar ataxia. When the left or dominant frontal lobe is affected, aphasia and apraxia may be evident.

Tumors of the occipital lobe may give rise to convulsive seizures preceded by an aura. With involvement of the occipital cortex, contralateral homonymous hemianopsia occurs (see Fig. 57-1). There may be visual agnosia, difficulty in judging distances, and a tendency to become lost in familiar surroundings.

Temporal lobe tumors cause tinnitus and auditory hallucinations, probably from irritation of the temporal auditory receptive or adjacent cortex. Varying degrees of sensory aphasia appear, beginning with difficulty in naming objects, when the temporal lobe of the dominant hemisphere becomes involved. Mental symptoms similar to those that develop with frontal lobe tumors may occur. Pressure from a growing tumor on the frontal cortex may result in facial weaknesses. Lesions of the anterior temporal pole cause a superior quadrantanopsia, which may progress to a complete hemianopsia.

Tumors in the parietal sensory cortex cause loss of cortical sensory function and impairment of sensory localization, two-point discrimination, graphesthesia, position sense, and stereognosis. Visual defects from parietal or

TABLE 57-2   ◼◼◼

Disorders of Movement Seen in Cerebellar Tumors

Disorder	Description
Intention tremor	Oscillating tremor most marked at the end of fine movements
Asynergia	Lack of cooperation between muscles, for example, failure of the wrist extensors during flexion of the fingers, allowing the wrist to flex
Decomposition of movement	Performance of actions in successive parts rather than as a whole, for example, touching the nose by first flexing the forearm, then the arm, and lastly adjusting the wrist and forearm
Dysmetria	Errors in the range of movement, for example, in touching a point, stopping the action before reaching the point or moving past it
Deviation from line of movement	Example: carrying food to the ear instead of the mouth
Adiadochokinesia	Inability to perform alternating movements, for example, tapping quickly and smoothly
Nystagmus	Rapid oscillation of the eyes while fixing the gaze on region and object

parietooccipital tumors usually involve inferior homonymous quadrants.

Cerebellar tumors cause early papilledema and frequently produce nuchal headache. Cerebellar lesions also cause disorders of movement, varying according to the size and specific location of the tumor within the cerebellum. Table 57-2 lists the most common of these disorders. Less conspicuous but equally characteristic of cerebellar tumor is *hypotonia* (absence of normal resistance to stretch or to displacement of a limb from a given posture) and hyperextensibility of joints. In speech, the patient tends to decompose words into separate syllables pronounced in a staccato rhythm called *scanning speech.*

Tumors of the ventricles and hypothalamus produce varied deficits. Invasive lesions of the third ventricle and the hypothalamus produce somnolence, diabetes insipidus, obesity, and disturbances of temperature regulation. A small tumor in the third ventricle, on the other hand, causes steady headache and papilledema with few localizing signs. Tumors involving the fourth ventricle give rise to rapid development of increased ICP with papilledema and cerebellar symptoms.

Diagnosis

Any patient suspected of having an intracranial lesion should undergo a complete medical evaluation with special attention to the neurologic examination. Specific diagnostic studies are undertaken after the neurologic examination and proceed from the noninvasive procedures that cause the least risk to those that use more dangerous, invasive techniques.

Skull radiographs give valuable information about bone structure, thickening, and calcifications; the position of the calcified pineal gland; and the position of the sella turcica. The electroencephalogram (EEG) gives information about the altered excitability of the neurons.

A shift of intracerebral contents can be seen on the echoencephalogram. A radioactive brain scan will show areas of abnormal accumulation of radioactive substances. Brain tumors and vascular occlusion, infection, and trauma cause breakdown of the blood-brain barrier, causing an abnormal accumulation of the radioactive substance.

Cerebral angiography is an invasive procedure that aids in the final diagnosis and helps the physician determine appropriate treatment.

Diagnosis of brain tumors has been aided considerably by the use of magnetic resonance imaging (MRI) and computed tomography (CT) scans. These procedures are now widely available and have become the diagnostic procedures of choice, replacing invasive techniques.

Treatment

Surgical treatment of brain tumors primarily revolves around surgical resection, chemotherapy, and radiation therapy. Improvements in surgical techniques and the advent of lasers and computer-assisted devices allow for precise resections in patients with surgically accessible brain tumors. Surgical resection remains a mainstay of therapy because it both kills and removes the tumor. In addition, surgical resection permits histologic evaluation and accurate grading of the tumor while allowing the patient to return to a functionally active life while undergoing additional therapies.

Radiation treatment 20 to 30 years ago involved whole brain radiation; currently, advances in radiotherapy technique allow more precise radiation therapy. Stereotactic techniques allow accurate placement of iodine seeds directly into the tumor area. Conformal radiation therapy (narrowing the beam to the size and shape of the tumor) reduces exposure of the surrounding tissue to radiation.

Chemotherapy is delivered in a variety of ways, including systemically, intraarterially, or via impregnated polymer wafers that deliver the chemotherapy agent directly to the tumor tissue. Major problems with bone marrow depression, pulmonary, and hepatic complications continue to be major complicating factors in chemotherapy. The blood-brain barrier also complicates the administration of chemotherapy agents. Research into the forcible opening of the blood-brain barrier using hyperosmotic mannitol has been disappointing. Research into the use of dexamethasone for closing the blood-tumor barrier and the effect of antiepileptic drugs on chemotherapy drug metabolism is ongoing and is beginning to show promise.

Genetic research will provide future practitioners with genetic information that will be translated into the identification of potential targets for antitumor drug development. The knowledge base concerning these genetic factors that lead to histologic cancers grows daily. The genetic involvement in gliomas, astrocytomas, and medulloblastomas is beginning to show promise. Areas of research include the use of a gene-directed enzyme prodrug ("a suicide gene"), gene therapy to enhance the immune system activity against cancer cells, and the transfer of tumor suppressor genes into the cancer cells (Engelhard, 2000). The future discovery and development of new therapies holds great promise for a more precise, more effective and less toxic treatment than current therapies.

SPINAL CORD TUMORS

Spinal tumors develop in the spine or its contents and generally produce symptoms by involvement of the spinal cord or nerve roots. Primary cord tumors are about one sixth as common as are brain tumors and have a better prognosis because about 60% are benign. The spinal cord undergoes not only actual tumor growth but also compression caused by an encroaching tumor. Spinal tumors occur in all age groups but are rarely encountered before the age of 10 years.

The spinal column is a site for metastasis in about 5% of cancer patients; about 20% of these patients develop symptomatic spinal cord compression. Metastasis to the spinal column occurs most commonly with breast, lung, prostate, and kidney cancers. A major factor that influences metastasis to the spinal column is the vascular drainage of the tumor and the epidural venous system that allows retrograde movement of the tumor emboli.

Primary spinal tumors are classified according to the location of the tumor in relation to the dura and the spinal cord. The major classification divides tumors into extradural and intradural. Intradural tumors are then subdivided into extramedullary and intramedullary.

Extradural tumors generally arise from the bone of the spinal column or within the extradural space. Ninety percent of extradural tumors are malignant. The most common tumor affecting the spinal vertebral column is a metastatic carcinoma. Extradural neoplasms within the extradural space are typically metastatic carcinomas and lymphomas.

Intradural extramedullary tumors lie between the dura mater and the spinal cord (Fig. 57-2). The most common tumors in this area are benign neurofibromas and meningiomas. These tumors compress the spinal cord and can be surgically removed.

Intradural intramedullary tumors arise from within the spinal cord itself. The same tumors that affect the brain also affect the spinal cord. Ependymomas are the most common, followed by astrocytomas, glioblastomas, and oligodendrogliomas.

The spinal cord accommodates to compression that occurs slowly, as seen in meningiomas and neurofibromas, producing few signs and symptoms, especially in the early stages. Acute compression of the cord, such as that occurring with metastatic lesions, causes rapid, progressive neurologic deficit. Resulting symptoms depend largely on the area affected, as well as the location of the lesion within the spinal column.

Because of the anatomic organization within the cord, compression from lesions outside the cord generally produces symptoms well below the site of the lesion, with the level of sensory impairment gradually ascending as the compression increases and affects areas deeper within the cord. Lesions located deep within the cord may spare superficially arranged fibers and give rise to sensory dissociation, with loss of pain and temperature senses and preservation of the sense of touch. By disturbing position sense, cord compression may also result in ataxia.

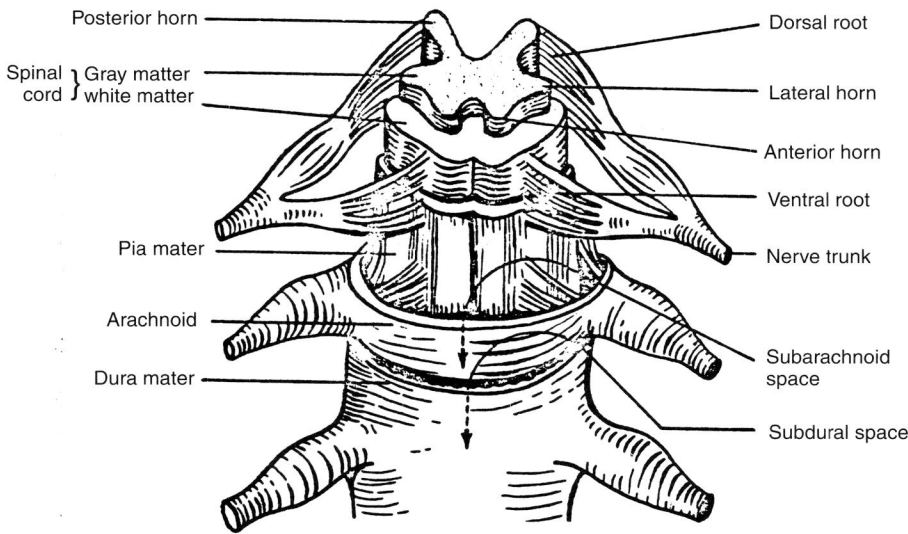

FIG. 57-2   Structure of the spinal cord. (From *Programmed practice in anatomy and physiology of the nervous system,* Englewood Cliffs, NJ, 1972, Prentice-Hall.)

TABLE 57-3   ▪ ▪ ▪

Symptoms and Signs of Common Vertebral Root Lesions

Root	Location of Pain	Sensory Loss	Reflex Loss	Weakness and Atrophy
C5	Lower neck, tip of shoulder, arm	Deltoid area (inconsistent)	Biceps	Shoulder abductors, biceps
C6	Lower neck, medial scapula, arm, radial side of forearm	Radial side of hand, thumb, index finger	Biceps	Biceps
C7	Lower neck, medial scapula, precordium, arm, forearm	Index finger, middle finger	Triceps	Triceps
C8	Lower neck; medial arm and forearm, ulnar side of hand; fourth and fifth fingers	Ulnar side of hand, fourth and fifth fingers		Intrinsic hand muscles
L4	Low back, anterior and medial thigh	Anterior thigh	Quadriceps	Quadriceps
L5	Low back, lateral thigh, lateral leg, dorsum of foot, great toe	Great toe, medial side of dorsum of foot, lateral leg and thigh		Toe extensors, ankle dorsiflexors and evertors
S1	Low back, posterior thigh, posterior leg, lateral side of foot, heel	Lateral foot, heel, posterior leg	Achilles	Ankle dorsiflexion, plantar flexion

From Simpson J, Magee K: *Clinical evaluation of the nervous system,* Boston, 1973, Little, Brown.
C, Cervical; *L,* lumbar; *S,* sacral vertebrae.

Spinal Cord Compression at Different Levels

Tumors of the Foramen Magnum

Tumors of the foramen magnum are most commonly meningiomas, accounting for 60% to 70% of these tumors. These tumors arise from the dura of the craniocervical junction. Symptoms are unusual, bizarre, confusing, and slowly progressing, causing difficulty in diagnosis. The initial and most common symptom is posterior cervical pain accompanied by hyperesthesia in the second cervical vertebral (C2) dermatome.

Nodding or any activity that increases ICP, such as coughing, straining, lifting or sneezing, aggravates the pain. Additional symptoms include motor and sensory deficits in the hands, which the patient reports as difficulty in writing or buttoning clothes. Extension of the tumor leads to spastic quadriplegia and marked loss of sensation. Other symptoms include dizziness, dysarthria, dysphagia, nystagmus, respiratory difficulties, nausea and vomiting,

and atrophy of the sternocleidomastoid and trapezius muscles. Neurologic findings are not always present but include hyperreflexia, nuchal rigidity, spastic gait, palsies of CN IX to XI, and weakness of the extremities.

Tumors of the Cervical Region

Cervical lesions produce radicular-like motor and sensory signs that involve the shoulders and arms and may involve the hands. Involvement of the hands from an upper cervical lesion (i.e., above C4) is thought to result from compression of the descending blood supply to the anterior horns via the anterior spinal artery. The patient generally has weakness and atrophy involving the shoulder girdle and arms. Lower cervical tumors (C5, C6, C7) may cause the loss of upper extremity tendon reflexes (biceps, brachioradialis, triceps). Sensory loss extends along the radial border of the forearm and thumb in a C6 compression and involves the middle and index fingers in lesions at C7; C7 lesions cause sensory loss of the index and middle fingers (Table 57-3).

Tumors of the Thoracic Region

Patients with lesions of the thoracic area often present with insidious spastic weakness in the lower extremities and later paresthesias. Patients may complain of pain and a tight, binding feeling across the chest and abdomen, which may be confused with pain from intrathoracic and intraabdominal disorders. Patients with lower thoracic lesions may have loss of lower abdominal reflexes and Beevor's sign (the umbilicus elevates when the patient, in the supine position, raises the head against resistance).

Tumors of the Lumbar-Sacral Region

A complex diagnostic situation exists in the case of a tumor involving the lumbar and sacral regions because of the proximity of the lower lumbar and sacral segments and the descending nerve roots from higher levels of the cord. Upper lumbar cord compression spares the abdominal reflexes, abolishes the cremasteric reflexes, and may produce weakness of hip flexion and spasticity of the lower legs. Patients have loss of the knee jerk reflex with brisk ankle reflexes and bilateral Babinski's signs. Pain is usually referred to the groin. Lesions involving the lower lumbar and upper sacral segments cause weakness and atrophy of perineal, calf, and foot muscles and loss of the ankle jerk reflex. Loss of sensation in the perianal and genital area and impairment of bowel and bladder control are characteristic signs of lesions involving the lower sacral area.

Tumors of the Cauda Equina

Lesions of the cauda equina cause early sphincteric symptoms and impotence. Other characteristic signs include dull, aching pain in the sacrum or perineum, sometimes radiating to the legs. Flaccid paralysis corresponds to the nerve roots involved and is sometimes asymmetric.

Symptoms are produced not only by the anatomic location of the spinal cord but also by its position within the spinal canal. The pathology of extradural and intradural tumors is discussed next.

Extradural Tumors

Extradural tumors are primarily metastases from a primary lesion in the breast, prostate, thyroid, lungs, kidney, or stomach (see color plate 36). Pain is generally the first symptom, which is described as being dull, constant, and localized over the area of the tumor, followed by pain radiating along the dermatome pattern. The localized pain is most severe at night and is aggravated by movements of the spine and bedrest. The radicular pain is intensified by coughing and straining. Pain may be present for weeks or months before spinal cord involvement.

The common clinical course of extradural tumors is rapid compression of the spinal cord from encroachment of the tumor on the cord, collapse of the vertebral column, or hemorrhage from within the metastasis. Once symptoms of spinal cord compression develop, they rapidly cause total loss of spinal cord function. Spastic weakness and loss of vibration and joint position senses below the level of the lesion are the first signs of cord compression. Without prompt surgical decompression, paresthesias and sensory loss progress quickly to irreversible paraplegia.

Extradural spinal cord tumors can be diagnosed by radiography of the spine. Most patients with tumors demonstrate osteoporosis or obvious bone destruction of the vertebral body and pedicles. A myelogram definitively localizes the tumor, although high-resolution CT scans are proving equal to myelograms in diagnostic accuracy. The CSF shows elevated protein and normal glucose levels.

Treatment depends on the nature of the lesion; extradural metastasis requires urgent management. Modalities include analgesics, corticosteroids, radiation therapy, chemotherapy, and hormonal therapy. Symptoms of cord compression require surgical decompression if medical management does not quickly relieve the symptoms. Prognosis is dependent on the cause and severity of the compression.

Intradural Tumors

Intradural tumors, in contrast to extradural tumors, are generally benign. The clinical course is much slower by comparison and may extend over months to years. Intradural tumors are divided into two types: extramedullary and intramedullary.

Extramedullary Tumors

Approximately 65% of all intradural tumors are extramedullary; they may be either neurofibromas or meningiomas.

Neurofibromas arise from the dorsal nerve roots. These tumors sometimes form a dumbbell-like or hourglass-like growth extending into the extradural space. A small percentage of neurofibromas undergo sarcomatous changes and become invasive or metastasize.

Meningiomas are usually loosely attached to the dura, arising probably from the arachnoid membrane, and approximately 90% are found in the thoracic region. These tumors are more frequent in middle-aged women. The posterolateral aspect of the cord is the most common site for these tumors.

Extramedullary cord lesions cause compression of the spinal cord and the nerve roots at the affected segment. The *Brown-Séquard syndrome* may result from lateral compression of the cord. This syndrome, caused by damage to one half of the cord, is characterized by ipsilateral signs of dysfunction of the corticospinal tract and the posterior column below the level of the lesion and contralateral reduction in pain and temperature perception below the level of the lesion. The patient complains of pain, first in the back and then along the spinal roots. As with extradural tumors, pain is aggravated by movement, coughing, sneezing, or straining and is most severe at night. The nocturnal aggravation of pain is caused by traction on the diseased nerve roots when the spine elongates with removal of the shortening effect of gravity. The sensory loss is vague at first and located below the level of the lesion (because of dermatome overlap). The loss gradually rises to below the segmented spinal cord level. Tumors of the posterior aspect may be exhibited by paresthesias and later by proprioceptive sensory loss, adding ataxia to the weakness. Anteriorly situated tumors may cause little sensory loss but may cause severe motor disability.

With extramedullary tumors, CSF protein is almost always elevated. Spinal radiographs may show enlargement of a foramen and thinning of the adjacent pedicle. As with extradural tumors, myelograms, CT scans, and MRI are essential for precise localization. Early surgical removal is essential for a complete recovery.

Intramedullary Tumors

The histologic structure of intramedullary tumors is essentially the same as that of intracranial tumors. More than 95% of these tumors are gliomas. In contrast to intracranial tumors, intramedullary tumors tend to be more benign histologically and have a more benign course. Approximately 50% of intramedullary tumors are ependymomas, 45% are astrocytomas, and the rest are oligodendrogliomas and hemangioblastomas.

Ependymomas arise at all levels of the spinal cord but are found most often in the conus medullaris of the cauda equina. All other intramedullary tumors occur equally frequently in all areas of the spinal cord.

Intramedullary tumors grow into the central part of the spinal cord and destroy crossing fibers and neurons of the gray matter. The destruction of crossing fibers results in bilateral sensory loss of pain and temperature sense extending throughout the segments involved in the lesion, leading to damage to peripheral skin areas. The senses of touch, motion, position, and vibration are usually preserved unless the lesion is large. The loss of pain and temperature sensation with preservation of the other senses is known as *dissociated sensory loss.* Alteration in the function of muscle stretch reflexes results from damage to the anterior horn cells. Weakness, with atrophy and fasciculations, is caused by involvement of the lower motor neurons.

Intramedullary tumors may extend through several segments of the spinal cord. As the lesion progresses, involvement of the corticospinal and spinothalamic tracts causes loss of pain and temperature sense, and upper motor neuron signs extend below the level of the lesion. Table 51-3 lists some differentiating features between upper and lower motor neuron lesions.

Other signs and symptoms include dull, aching pain localized to the level of the lesion, impotence in males, and sphincter disturbances in both genders.

Radiography reveals visible widening of the spinal canal and erosion of the pedicles. On myelogram, CT scan, or MRI, the spinal cord appears enlarged.

Surgical removal is sometimes possible with intramedullary tumors, especially ependymomas and hemangioblastomas, but recurrences are not uncommon. Again, early diagnosis is imperative to ensure a good prognosis.

KEY CONCEPTS

- *Malignant brain tumors* can be primary or represent a metastasis from another site.
- *Gliomas* (malignant tumor) are the most common type of brain tumor.
- Brain tumors are classified according to location and type of developmental tissue involved.
- General symptoms indicative of a brain tumor include seizures, increased ICP, headache, nausea and vomiting, and papilledema.
- Local symptoms of brain tumors are caused by compression of tissue in a particular area of the brain.
- Neurologic deficits associated with brain tumors are caused by increased ICP and compression or infiltration of brain tissue.
- Diagnosis of brain tumors is often difficult because of the vague and confusing nature of the symptoms that are frequently attributed to other causes.
- Primary spinal cord tumors are more likely to be benign than brain tumors.
- Spinal cord tumors are classified according to location of tumor in relation to the dura and spinal cord.
- Symptoms of spinal cord tumors result from spinal cord compression and include pain, changes in reflexes, and altered sensation and motor function.
- Pain associated with spinal cord tumor results from referred pain based on the nerve root involved.

QUESTIONS

A sampling of review questions for this chapter appears here. Visit http://www.mosby.com/MERLIN/PriceWilson/ for additional questions.

Match the type of glioma in column A with its characteristic in column B.

Column A
1. _____ Glioblastoma multiforme
2. _____ Medulloblastoma
3. _____ Oligodendroglioma
4. _____ Ependymoma

Column B
a. Often contains calcium
b. Most malignant
c. Typically arises in the fourth ventricle in children
d. Radiosensitive posterior fossa tumor of childhood

Match the localizing symptoms of brain tumors in column A with their probable location in column B.

Column A
5. _____ Homonymous hemianopsia
6. _____ Impairment of sensory localization, two-point discrimination
7. _____ Superior quadrantanopsia progressing to hemianopsia
8. _____ Disturbances of judgment; jacksonian seizures; ataxia and tremor
9. _____ Obesity and disturbance of temperature regulation

Column B
a. Frontal lobe
b. Temporal lobe
c. Occipital lobe
d. Parietal lobe
e. Hypothalamus

Answer the following on a separate sheet of paper.

10. What makes the diagnosis of a brain tumor so difficult? What are the most common general signs and symptoms?

Match the site of spinal cord pathology in column A with the signs and symptoms in column B. Letters may be used more than once.

Column A
11. _____ Pain increased by coughing or sneezing
12. _____ Loss of vibratory and position sense
13. _____ Babinski's sign
14. _____ Fasciculations
15. _____ Spasticity
16. _____ Ataxia

Column B
a. Posterior (dorsal) root
b. Posterior column (major ascending tract)
c. Corticospinal tract (major descending tract)
d. Anterior horn cells

BIBLIOGRAPHY ■ PART NINE

Abou-Chebl A, De Georgia MA, Krieger DW: Cooling for acute ischemic brain damage (COOL AID): preliminary efficacy data of moderate hypothermia for acute ischemic stroke, *Stroke* 32:336, 2001, abstract.

Adam C, Baulac M, Saint-Hilaire J, et al: Value of magnetic resonance imaging-based measurements of hippocampal formations in patients with partial epilepsy, *Arch Neurol* 51:130-143, 1994.

Adams RD, Victor M, Ropper AH: *Principles of neurology*, ed 6, New York, 1997, McGraw-Hill.

Afsar N, Fak AS, Metzger J, et al: Acute stroke increases QT dispersion in patients without cardiac disease. Program and abstracts of 125th Annual Meeting of the American Neurological Association, October 15-18, 2000, Boston, abstract 12.

Akbarian S, Bates B, Liu RJ, et al: Neurotrophin-3 modulates noradrenergic neuron function and opiate withdrawal, *Mol Psychiatry* 6(4):593-604, 2001.

Albers GW, Amarenco P, Easton JD, et al: Antithrombotic and thrombolytic therapy for ischemic stroke, *Chest* 119 (suppl 1):300S-320S, 2001.

Allos BM, Lippy FT, Carlsen A, et al: *Campylobacter jejuni* strains from patients with Guillain-Barré syndrome, *Centers for Disease Control: Emer Infect Dis* 4(2):263-268, 1998.

Alvaro M, Kumar D, Julka IS: Transcutaneous electrostimulation: emerging treatment for diabetic neuropathic pain, *Diabetes Technol Ther* 1(1):77-80, 1999.

Amar A, Levy M: Contemporary management of spinal cord injury, *Contemp Neurosurg* 23:1-10, 2001.

Amar A, Levy M: Surgical controversies in the management of spinal cord injury. *J Am Coll Surg* 188:550, 1999.

American Diabetes Association: Clinical practice recommendations, 2000, *Diabetes Care* 23(suppl 1): S1-S116, 2000.

American Heart Association: *Heart and stroke: 2001 statistics*, Dallas, 2001, AHA. *http://www.americanheart.org/statistics/*

American Medical Association: *Migraine and other headaches*, Chicago, 1998, AMA.

American Pain Society Quality of Care Committee: Quality improvement guidelines for the treatment of acute pain and cancer pain, *JAMA* 274:1874-1880, 1998.

American Society of Anesthesiologists: Task Force on Pain Management: Practice guidelines for cancer pain management, *Anesthesiology* 84(5):1243-57, 1996.

Anderson G, Miller J: The newer antiepileptic drugs: their collective role and defining characteristics, *Formulary* 32:114-132, 2001.

Arnautovic K, Al-Mefty O: Foramen magnum meningiomas, *Contemp Neurosurg* 22:1-6, Nov 15, 2000.

Asbury AK: Approach to the patient with peripheral neuropathy. In Braunwald E, et al, editors: *Harrison's principles of internal medicine*, ed 15, New York, 2001, McGraw-Hill.

Azari NP, Rüdiger JS: Brain plasticity and recovery from stroke, *Am Sci* 88(5):426-431, 2000.

Baird AD, Dambrosia J, Janket S, et al: A three-item scale for the early prediction of stroke recovery, *Lancet* 357:2095-2099, 2001.

Barami K, Rengachary S: Atlas fractures, *Contemp Neurosurg* 22:1-5, 2000.

Bastard JP, Pieroni L, Hainque B: Relationship between plasma plasminogen activator inhibitor I and insulin resistance, *Diabetes Metab Res Rev* 16:192-201, 2000.

Baumann TJ: Pain management. In DePiro JT, Talbert RL, Yee GC, et al, editors: *Pharmacotherapy: a pathophysiologic approach*, ed 4, Norwalk, Conn, 1999, Appleton & Lange.

Benedetti C, Brock C, Cleeland C, et al: National Comprehensive Cancer Network, NCCN practice guidelines for cancer pain, *Oncology* 14(11A):135-150, 2000.

Berne RM, Levy MW: *Principles of physiology*, ed 3, St Louis, 2000, Mosby.

Bigal ME, Bigal JM, Betti M, et al: Evaluation of the impact of migraine and episodic tension-type headache on the quality of life and performance of a university student population, *Headache* 41(7):710-719, 2001.

Bigos SJ: Perils, pitfalls, and accomplishments of guidelines for treatment of back problems, *Neurol Clin North Am* 17(1):179, 1999.

Bolay H, Reuter U, Dunn A, et al: Meningeal and central trigeminovascular activation following cortical spreading depression, *Cephalalgia* 21:526, 2001, abstract LB-2.

Brain Attack Coalition (2001). *http://www.stroke-site.org*

Brain Resources and Information Network (BRAIN) (2000): *Guillain-Barré syndrome fact sheet*, National Institute of Neurological Disorders and Stroke, PO Box 13050, Silver Spring, MD 20911.

Brain Trauma Foundation: Guidelines for the management and prognosis of severe traumatic brain injury, ed 2, 2000, Brain Trauma Foundation. *http://www.braintrauma.org/guidelines.nss*

Bral EE: Caring for adults with chronic cancer pain, *Am J Nurs* 98(4):27-32, 1998.

Broderick JP, Miller Ro, Khoury JC, et al: Incidence rates of stroke for blacks and whites: preliminary results from the greater Cincinnati/Northern Kentucky stroke study, *Stroke* 32:320, 2001, abstract.

Brookmeyer R, Gray S, Kawas C: Projections of Alzheimer's disease in the United States and the public health impact of delaying disease onset, *Am J Public Health* 88(9):1337-1342, 1998.

Buring JE, Hebert P, Romero J, et al: Migraine and subsequent risk of stroke in the Physicians' Health Study, *Arch Neurol* 52:129-134, 1995.

Cady RK: Focus on primary care female population with migraine, *Obstetr Gynecol Survey* 54(12):S7, 1999.

Cady RK, Farmer-Cady K: Migraine: changing perspectives on pathophysiology and treatment, *Consultant*, Sept 15, S13-S19, 2000.

Carpenter MB: *Core text of neuroanatomy*, ed 4, Baltimore, 1991, Williams & Wilkins.

Cham BM, Kormanik P: Salvage chemotherapy with paclitaxel for recurrent oligodendrogliomas, *J Clin Oncol* 15:3427-3432, 1997.

Chiu JH, Chen WS, Chen CH, et al: Effect of transcutaneous electrical nerve stimulation for pain relief on patients undergoing hemorrhoidectomy: prospective, randomized, controlled trial, *Dis Colon Rectum* 42(2):180-5, 1999.

Cohen LG, Weeks RA, Sadato N, et al: Period of susceptibility for cross-modal plasticity in the blind, *Ann Neurol* 45(4):451-460, 1999.

Collaborative Group for the Study of Stroke in Young Women: Oral contraceptives and stroke in young women, *JAMA* 231:718-722, 1975.

Consensus statement: Medical management of epilepsy, *Neurology* 51(suppl 4):S15-20, 1998.

Cotran RS, Kumar V, Collins ST: *Pathological basis of disease*, ed 6, Philadelphia, 1999, WB Saunders.

Couch JR: Complexities of presentation and pathogenesis of migraine headache. In Cady RK, Fox AW, editors: *Treating the headache patient*, New York, 1995, Marcel Dekker.

Crossman AR, Neary D: *Neuroanatomy: an illustrated color text*, ed 2, New York, 2000, Churchill Livingstone.

Cutrer FM, Limmroth V, Ayata G, et al: Attenuation by valproate of c-fos immunoreactivity in trigeminal nucleus caudalis induced by intracisternal capsaicin, *Br J Pharmacol* 116:3199-3204, 1994.

Dahl J, Pasero C, Patterson C: *Institutionalizing effective pain management practices: the implications of the new JCAHO pain assessment and management standards.* Program and Abstracts of the 19th Annual Scientific Meeting of the American Pain Society, November 2-5, 2000, Atlanta, symposium, abstract 302.

Davis KL, Mohs RC, Marin D, et al: Cholinergic markers in elderly patients with early signs of Alzheimer disease, *JAMA* 281(15):1433-1434, 1999.

Dewji NN, Singer SJ: Specific intercellular binding of the beta-amyloid precursor protein to the presenilis induces intercellular signaling: its significance for Alzheimer's disease, *Proc Natl Acad Sci USA* 95(25):15055-15060, 1998.

Diamond S: A fresh look at migraine therapy: new treatments promise improved management, *Postgrad Med* 109(1):49-54, 57-60, 2001.

Dichter MA, Brodie MJ: New antiepileptic drugs, *N Engl J Med* 334(24):1583-1950, 1996.

Diener HC, Cunha L, Forbes C, et al: European stroke prevention study, 2: dipyridamole and acetylsalicylic acid in the secondary prevention of stroke, *J Neurol Sci* 143:1-13, 1996.

Dodd M, Janson S, Facione N, et al: Advancing the science of symptom management, *J Adv Nurs* 33(5):668-676, 2001.

Domanski MJ, Davis BR, Pfeffer MA, et al: Isolated systolic hypertension: prognostic information provided by pulse pressure, *Hypertension* 34:375-380, 1999.

Drachman DB: Myasthenia gravis and other diseases of the neuromuscular junction. In Braunwald E et al, editors: *Harrison's principles of internal medicine*, ed 15, New York, 2001, McGraw-Hill.

Dubner R, Ren K: Endogenous mechanisms of sensory modulation, *Pain* 6:S45-54, 1999.

Eaton DL, Klaassen CD: Principles of toxicology. In Klaassen CD, editor: *Casarett and Doull's toxicology: the basic science of poisons*, ed 5, New York, 1996, McGraw-Hill.

Edvinsson L: Aspects on the pathophysiology of migraine and cluster headache, *Pharmacol Toxicol* 89(2):65-73, 2001.

Englehard H: Gene therapy for brain tumors, *Surg Neurol* 54:3-9, 2000.

European Stroke Initiative: European stroke initiative recommendations for stroke management, *Cerebrovasc Dis* 10:335-351, 2000.

Evans R: *Technology advances our understanding of cerebrovascular events.* 125th annual meeting of the American Neurological Association, October 15, 2000. *http://www.medscape.com*

Ezzedine MA, Lev MH, McDonald CT, et al: Impact of contrast CT angiography and whole brain contrast CT perfusion study on the accuracy of cerebrovascular diagnosis in patients presenting with a major stroke-like syndrome, *Stroke* 32:325, 2001, abstract.

Fedorov EM: Critical care extra: helping patients with aphasia, *Am J Nurs* 101(1):24GG-24JJ, 2001.

Ferrell B: Pain observed: the experience of pain from the family caregiver's perspective, *Clin Geriatr Med* 17(3):595-609, viii-ix, 2001.

Fettes I: Menstrual migraine, *Postgrad Med* 101:67-77, 1997.

Fields HL, Martin JB: Pain: pathophysiology and management. In Braunwald E et al, editors: *Harrison's principles of internal medicine*, ed 15, New York, 2001, McGraw-Hill.

Fitzgerald M, Beggs S: The neurobiology of pain: developmental aspects, *Neuroscientist* 7(3):246-257, 2001.

Fitzgerald M, Jennings E: The postnatal development of spinal sensory processing, *Proc Natl Acad Sci USA* 96:7719-7722, 1999.

Fletcher DD, Lawn ND, Wolter TD, et al: Long-term outcome in patients with Guillain-Barré syndrome requiring mechanical ventilation, *Neurology* 54:2311-2315, 2000.

Fountain N et al: Migraine, epilepsy, MS, *Patient Care* 33:150-168, 1999.

Fountain N, Dreifus F: Seizure disorders, *Cur Pract Med* 2(5):724-728, 1999.

Friedman R: Pain at the cellular level: the role of the cytokine tumor necrosis factor-alpha, *Reg Anesth Pain Med* 25(2):110-112, 2000.

Fueyo J, Gomez-Manzano C, Yung C, Kyritsis A: Targeting in gene therapy for gliomas, *Arch Neurol* 56:445-448, 1999.

Fuller G: *Neurological examination made easy*, New York, 1994, Churchill Livingstone.

Furlan A, Higashida R, Wechsler L, et al: Intra-arterial prourokinase for acute ischemic stroke: the PROACT II study: a randomized controlled trial, *JAMA* 282:2003-2011, 1999.

Goldman L, Bennett JC: *Cecil textbook of medicine*, ed 21, Philadelphia, 2001, WB Saunders.

Gould D: Wound management and pain control, *Nurs Stand* 14(6):47-54, 1999.

Griffin WS et al: Glial-Neuronal Interactions in Alzheimer's disease: the potential role of a "cytokine cycle" in disease progression, *Brain Pathol* 8(1):65-72, 1998.

Grimson W et al: Image-guided surgery, *Sci Am* 286(6):62-69, 1999.

Gupta G et al: Neural progenitor cells proliferate and differentiate when transplanted into ischemic brain or retina, *Stroke* 32:333, 2001, abstract.

Guyton AC: *Basic neuroscience: anatomy and physiology*, Philadelphia, 1987, WB Saunders.

Guyton AC, Hall JE: *Textbook of medical physiology*, ed 10, Philadelphia, 2000, WB Saunders.

Hademenos GJ: The biophysics of stroke, *Am Sci* 85(3):226-235, 1997.

Haerer AF: *De Jong's the neurological examination*, Philadelphia, 1994, Lippincott–Williams & Wilkins.

Hamza MA et al: Effect of the frequency of transcutaneous electrical nerve stimulation on the postoperative opioid analgesic requirement and recovery profile, *Anesthesiology* 91(5):1232-1238, 1999.

Hardman JG et al, editors: *Goodman and Gilman's the pharmacological basis of therapeutics*, ed 10, New York, 2001, McGraw-Hill.

Haroun, V et al: Neurofibrillary tangles in non-demented elderly subjects and mild Alzheimer disease, *Arch Neurol* 56(6):713-718, 1999.

Hauser SL, Goodkin DE: Multiple sclerosis and other demyelinating diseases. In Braunwald E et al, editors: *Harrison's principles of internal medicine*, ed 15, New York, 2001, McGraw-Hill.

Headache Classification Committee of the International Headache Society: Classification and diagnostic criteria for headache disorders, cranial neuralgias and facial pain, *Cephalalgia* 8(suppl 7):1-96, 1988.

Heiss WD et al: Differential capacity of left and right hemispheric areas for compensation of poststroke aphasia, *Ann Neurol* 45:430-438, 1999.

Henrich JB, Horwitz RI: A controlled study of ischemic stroke risk in migraine patients, *J Clin Epidemiol* 42:773-780, 1989.

Hill JR et al: Molecular genetics of brain tumors, *Arch Neurol* 56:439-441, 1999.

Hillis AE et al: Improved function and perfusion with pharmacological blood pressure elevation, *Stroke* 32:319, 2001, abstract.

Hoff JT, Boland MF: Neurosurgery. In Schwartz SI, editor: *Principles of surgery*, ed 6, New York, 1994, McGraw-Hill.

Hunt WE, Hess RM: Surgical risk as related to time of intervention in the repair of intracranial aneurysms, *J Neurosurg* 28:14-20, 1968.

IASP Task Force on Taxonomy. In Merskey H, Bogduk N, editors: *Classification of chronic pain*, ed 2, Seattle, 1994, IASP Press.

International Polio Network (IPN): *Handbook on the late effects of poliomyelitis for physicians and survivors*, Gazette International Networking Institute (GINI), 4207 Lindell Boulevard, #110, St Louis, Mo. 63108-2915, 1999.

Ishihara T et al: Age-dependent emergence and progression of a tauopathy in transgenic mice over-express the shortest human tau isoform, *Neuron* 24(1-20):751-762, 1999. (Accompanied by a mini-review, "Neurodegenerative Tauopathies: Human Disease and Transgenic Mouse Models," pp. 507-510.)

JNC VI: The sixth report of the Joint National Committee on Prevention, Detection, Evaluation, and Treatment of High Blood Pressure, *Arch Intern Med* 157:2413-2447, 1997.

Jacob SW, Francone CA, Lossow WJ: *Structure and function in man*, ed 5, Philadelphia, 1982, WB Saunders.

Juarez G, Ferrell B, Borneman T: Cultural considerations in education for cancer pain management, *J Cancer Educ* 14(3):1688-1673, 1999.

Keesey JC, Sonshine R: *A practical guide to myasthenia gravis*, The Myasthenia Gravis Foundation of America, 1997.

Kerns RD et al: Readiness to adopt a self-management approach to chronic pain: the pain stages of change questionnaire, *Pain* 72:227-234, 1997.

Kidwell CS et al: Predictors of hemorrhagic transformation following intra-arterial thrombolysis, *Stroke* 32:319, 2001, abstract.

Kurth T et al: Body mass index and the risk of stroke in men, program and abstracts of the 53rd Annual Meeting of the American Academy of Neurology, *Neurology* 56(suppl 3):A227, 2001.

Laakso M: Benefits of strict glucose and blood pressure control in type 2 diabetes: lessons from the UK Prospective Diabetes Study, *Circulation* 99:561-562, 1999.

Labovitz DL, Sacco RL: Determinants of lacunar infarct versus deep intracerebral hemorrhage in a multiethnic population-based incidence cohort. Program and abstracts of the 53rd Annual Meeting of the American Academy of Neurology, May 5-11, Philadelphia, 2001.

Ladurner G: Neuroprotection in acute ischemic stroke, *Stroke* 32:323, 2001, abstract.

Laight DW, Carrier MJ, Anggard EE: Endothelial cell dysfunction and the pathogenesis of diabetic macroangiopathy, *Diabetes Metab Res Rev* 15:274-282, 1999.

Lance JW: *Mechanism and management of headache*, ed 6, Boston, 2000, Butterworth.

Lauritzen M: Pathophysiology of the migraine aura: the spreading depression theory, *Brain* 117:199-210, 1994.

Leary MC, Saver JL: Incidence of silent stroke in the United States, *Stroke* 32:363, 2001, abstract.

Leker RR, Lavie G, Teichner A, et al: The nitroxide antioxidant tempol is cerebroprotective in a model of focal cerebral ischemia, *Eur J Neurol* 7(suppl 3):SC-34, 2000.

Levin V: Chemotherapy for brain tumors of astrocytic and oligodendroglial lineage. The past decade and where we are heading, *Neuro-oncol* 1:68-79, 1999.

Lipton RB, Stewart WF, Diamond S, et al: Prevalence and burden of migraine in the United States: data from the American migraine Study II, *Headache* 41(7):646-657, 2001.

Lipton RB, Stewart WF, Reed M, Diamond S: Migraine's impact today. Burden of illness, patterns of care, *Postgrad Med* 109(1):38-40, 43-45, 2001.

Lipton RB, Stewart WF, von Korff M: Burden of migraine: societal costs and therapeutic opportunities, *Neurology* 48(suppl 3):S4-S9, 1997.

The Long-Term Intervention with Pravastatin in Ischemic Disease (LIPID) Study Group: Prevention of cardiovascular events and death with pravastatin in patients with coronary heart disease and a broad range of initial cholesterol levels, *N Engl J Med* 339:1349-1357, 1998.

Lynch M: Pain: the fifth vital sign, *Adv Nurs Pract* 9(11):28-36, 2001.

Maizels M: Headache evaluation and treatment of primary care physicians in an emergency department in the era of triptans, *Arch Intern Med* 161(16):1969-1973, 2001.

Malcangio M, Tomlinson DR: A pharmacologic analysis of mechanical hyperalgesia in streptozotocin/diabetic rats, *Pain* 76:151-157, 1998.

Malmivaara A et al: The treatment of acute low back pain—bed rest, exercise or ordinary activity? *N Engl J Med* 332:351, 1995.

Mandir AS, Poitras MF, Berliner AR, et al: NMDA but not non-NMDA excitotoxicity is mediated by poly (ADP-ribose) polymerase, *J Neurosci* 20(21):8005-8011, 2000.

Matthew NT: Cluster headache, *Neurology* 42(suppl 3):22-31, 1992.

May A et al: Hypothalamic activation in cluster headache attacks, *Lancet* 352:275, 1998.

McCaffery M: Gabapentin for lancinating neuropathic pain, *Am J Nurs* 98(4):12, 1998.

McCaffery M: How to make the most of nonopioid analgesics, *Nursing* 28(8):54-55, 1998.

McCaffery M, Ferrell B, Pasero C: No justified use of placebos for pain, *J Nurs Scholarship* 32(2):114-115, 2000.

Melzack R, Wall PD: *The challenge of pain*, New York, 1996, Penguin Books.

Montes-Sandoval L: An analysis of the concept of pain, *J Adv Nurs* 29(4):935-941, 1999.

Mouton PR, Martin LJ, Calhoun ME, et al: Cognitive decline strongly correlates with cortical atrophy in Alzheimer's dementia, *Neurobiol Aging* 19(5):371-377, 1998.

Murray CJL, Lopez AD: *Global burden of disease*, Cambridge, Mass, 1996, Harvard University Press.

Narayanan JT, Recht LD: Which patients should undergo transesophageal echocardiography as part of their stroke work-up? Program and abstracts of 125th Annual Meeting of the American Neurological Association; Boston, (October 15-18, 2000), abstract 147.

National Center for Health Statistics Quarterly Fact Sheet. Spotlight on: Office Visits to Neurologists, December, 1995. *http://www.cdc.gov/nchs/releases/95facts/fs_dec95.htm*

National Institute of Neurological Disorders and Stroke (NINDS): Guillain-Barré Syndrome Information, 2000.

National Institute of Neurological Disorders and Stroke, t-PA Stroke Study Group: Tissue plasminogen activator for acute ischemic stroke, *N Engl J Med* 333:1581-1587, 1995.

National Rural Health Association: More women die from stroke, *Rural Clin Q* 11(2):1-6, 2001.

NYU Department of Neurosurgery (1996). *http://mcns10.med.nyu.edu*

Payne R, Gonzales GR: Management of pain. In Derek D, Geoffrey WC, et al, editors: *Oxford textbook of palliative medicine*, ed 2, New York, 1999, Oxford University Press.

Pellock J: Treatment of epilepsy in the new millennium, *Pharmacology 2000* 20:129S-138S, 2000.

Peters KD, Kochanek KD, Murphy SL: Deaths: final data for 1996, *Natl Vital Stat Rep* 47:1-100, 1998.

Puntillo K, Casella V, Reid M: Opioid and benzodiazepine tolerance and dependence: application of theory to critical care practice, *Heart Lung* 26(4):317-324, 1997.

Qureshi A, Giles WH, Croft JB, Bliwise DL: Habitual sleep patterns and risk for stroke and coronary heart disease: a 10-year followup from NHANES I, *Neurol* 48(4):904-911, 1997.

Reiman EM, Caselli RJ, Yun LS, et al: Preclinical evidence of Alzheimer's disease in persons homozygous for the epsilon 4 allele for apolipoprotein E, *N Engl J Med* 334(12):752-758, 1996.

Reingold SC: *Research directions in multiple sclerosis*, National Multiple Sclerosis Society, 2000.

Richman E: When a headache isn't just a headache, *Clin Trends News in Neurol* 8(11), 2000. *http://www.neurologyreviews.com/nov00/nr_nov00_headache.html*

Roberts LJ, Morrow JD: Analgesic-antipyretic and antiinflammatory agents and drugs employed in the treatment of gout. In Hardman JG, Limbird LE, Gilman AG, editors: *Goodman & Gilman's the pharmacological basis of therapeutics*, ed 10, New York, 2001, McGraw-Hill.

Robertson C, Valadka A, et al: Prevention of secondary ischemic insults after severe head injury, *Crit Care Med* 27:2086, 1999.

Ropper AH: Trauma of the head and spine. In Braunwald E et al, editors: *Harrison's principles of internal medicine*, ed 15, New York, 2001, McGraw-Hill.

Russell MB, Olesen J: Increased familial risk and evidence of genetic factor in migraine, *BMJ* 311:541-544, 1995.

Ryan EW: American Heart Association Scientific Sessions 2000: AHA Plenary Session VII: Stroke in the New Millennium, 2000.

Sacks FM, Pfeffer MA, Moye LA, et al: The effect of pravastatin on coronary events after myocardial infarction in patients with average cholesterol levels. Cholesterol and recurrent events trial investigators, *N Engl J Med* 335:1001-1009, 1996.

Salanova V, Markland O, Worth R: Clinical characteristics and predictive factors in 98 patients with complex partial seizures treated with temporal resection, *Arch Neurol* 51:1008-1013, 1994.

Salazar DE, Fulmor IE, Srinivas N, et al: BMS-204352-a novel maxi-K potassium channel opener for the treatment of stoke: safety and clinical pharmacology in healthy subjects, *Eur J Neurol* 7(suppl 3):SC-40, 2000.

Schwab M, Bartholdi D: Degeneration and regeneration of axons in the lesioned spinal cord, *Physiol Rev* 76:319-370, 1996.

Schwartz SIires GT, Spencer FC, Galloway AC: *Principles of surgery*, ed 7, New York, 1998, McGraw-Hill.

Schwartzman RJ, Grothusen J, Kiefer TR, Rohr P: Neuropathic central pain: epidemiology, etiology, and treatment options, *Arch Neurol* 58(10):1547-1550, 2001.

Schwartzman RJ, Maleki J: Postinjury neuropathic pain syndromes, *Med Clin North Am* 83:597-626, 1999.

Sen S, Oppenheimer SM: Hyperhomocysteinemia is a risk factor for progression of aortic atheroma in stroke/TIA patients, *Stroke* 32:332, 2001, abstract.

Shapiro W: Current therapies for brain tumors, *Arch Neurol* 56:429-432, 1999.

Silberstein SD: *Migraine, cluster, trigeminal neuralgia, and mood disorders: common ground for treatment*, AACME activity, 2000, Jefferson Medical College of Thomas Jefferson University & Medscape, Inc. *http://medscape.com/viewprogram/315*

Silberstein SD: Update on migraine headache: Report from IHC 2001: The 10th Congress of the International Headache Society, Medscape Neurology, 2001. *http://www.medscape.com/viewprogram/315*

Silberstein SD, Lipton RB, Goadsby PJ: *Headache in clinical practice*, Oxford, UK, 1998, Isis Media.

Simon R, Aminoff M, Greenberg D: *Clinical neurology*, New York, 1999, Lange Medical Books–McGraw-Hill.

Smith M, Freidlin B, Reis L, Simon R: Trends in reported incidence of primary malignant brain tumors in children in the United States, *J Natl Cancer Inst* 90:1269-1277, 1998.

Smith WS, Hauser SL, Easton JD: Cerebrovascular disease. In Braunwald E et al, editors: *Harrison's principles of internal medicine*, ed 15, New York, 2001, McGraw-Hill.

Smuts JA, Van Niekerk M, Barnard PWA: Decrease in migraine attack frequency correlated with frontalis muscle denervation pattern following botulinum toxin type A injection. Program and abstracts of the 17th World Congress of Neurology, June 17-22, London, UK, *J Neurol Sci* 187(suppl 1):S75, 2001, abstract 195.

Snowdon DA, Greiner LH, Mortimer JA, et al: Brain infarction and the clinical expression of Alzheimer disease: the Nun Study, *JAMA* 277(10):813-817, 1997.

Soldan SS, Berti R, Salem N, et al: Association of human herpes virus 6 (HHV-6) with multiple sclerosis: increased IgM response to HHV-6 early antigen and detection of serum HHV-6 DNA, *Nat Med* 3(12):s1394-1397, 1997.

Spagnoli D et al: Combined treatment of fourth ventricle ependymomas: report of 26 cases, *Surg Neurol* 54:19-26, 2000.

Staessen JA, Fagard R, Thijs L, et al: Randomised double-blind comparison of placebo and active treatment for older patients with isolated systolic hypertension. The Systolic Hypertension in Europe (Syst-Eur) Trial, *Lancet* 350:757-764, 1997.

Stang P, Osterhaus JT: Epidemiology of migraine. In Cady RK, Fox AW, editors: *Treating the headache patient*, New York, 1995, Marcel Dekker.

Stewart WF, Kawas C, Corrada M, Metter EJ: Risk of Alzheimer's disease and duration of NSAID use, *Neurology* 48:626-632, 1997.

Stewart W, Lipton R, Dowson AJ, Sawyer J: Development and testing of the Migraine Disability Assessment (MIDAS) Questionnaire to assess headache-related disability, *Neurology* 56(6 Suppl 1):S20-S28, 2001.

Stillwell S: When you suspect epidural hematoma, *Am J Nurs* 100(9):68-74, 2000.

Swanson JW, Yanagihara T, Stang PE, et al: Incidence of cluster headaches: a population-based study in Olmsted County, Minnesota, *Neurology* 44(3, pt. 1):433-437, 1994.

Szabo K, Behrens S, Hirsch J: Subgroup analysis of patients with severe acute neurological ischemic syndromes without diffusion weighted magnetic resonance imaging abnormalities, *Stroke* 32:318, 2001, abstract.

Tang MX, Stern Y, Marder K, et al: The APOE-epsilon4 allele and the risk of Alzheimer disease among African Americans, Whites, and Hispanics, *JAMA* 279:751-755, 1998.

Tanne D, Koren N: Blood lipids are important independent risk factors for ischemic stroke or TIA: a prospective follow-up of over 11,000 patients in the BIP registry, *Stroke* 32:32, 2001, abstract.

Taylor EC, Koo PJS: Pain. In Koda-Kimble MA et al, editors: *Applied therapeutics: the clinical use of drugs*, ed 7, Philadelphia, 2001, Lippincott–Williams & Wilkins.

Thibodeau GA, Patton KT: *Anatomy and physiology*, ed 4, St Louis, 1999, Mosby.

Thomsen LL, Eriksen MK, Olesen J, Russell MB: Clinical characteristics of Danish families with familial hemiplegic migraine, *Cephalalgia* 21:301, 2001, abstract P1-G10.

Tomlinson DR, Malcangio M, Patel J, et al: *Effects of zonisamide on mechanically-induced nociception in rats with streptozocin-diabetes. Program of the Worldwide Pain Conference 2000, July 15-21*, San Francisco, 2000.

Tripathy M, Kaushik S: Carbamazepine for pain management in Guillain-Barré syndrome patients in the intensive care unit, *Crit Care Med* 28(3):655-658, 2000.

Tzourio C, Tehindrazanarivelo A, Iglesias S, et al: Case-control study of migraine and risk of ischemic stroke in young women, *BMJ* 310:830-833, 1995.

U.S. Headache Consortium: Evidence-based guidelines for migraine headache: overview of program description and methodology, *Neurology* 54:1553, 2000.

Urba S, Weinstein SM: National Comprehensive Cancer Network: NCCN practice guidelines for cancer pain, *Oncology* 14(11A):135-150, 2000.

Vaitkus A, Vilionskis A: Analysis of use of medications for migraine. Program and abstracts of the 17th World Congress of Neurology, June 17-22, 2001; London, UK, *J Neurol Sci* 187(suppl 1):S74, 2001, abstract P0191.

Valadka A, Gopinath S: Current issues in the management of severe head injury, *Contemp Neurosurg* 23(1):1-8, 2001.

Van der Spank JT, Cambier DC, De Paepe HM, et al: Pain relief in labour by transcutaneous electrical nerve stimulation (TENS), *Arch Gynecol Obstet* 264(3):131-136, 2000.

Vastag B: Not so fast: research on infectious links to MS questioned, *JAMA* 285(3):279-281, 2001.

Vieweg U et al: Differential treatment in acute upper cervical spine injuries, *Surg Neurol* 54:203-211, 2000.

Vinik AI: Diabetic neuropathy: a small-fiber disease. 61st Scientific Sessions of the American Diabetes Association, June 2001.

Vinik AI, Park TS, Stanbury KB, Pittenger GL: Diabetic neuropathies, *Diabetologia* 43(8):957-973, 2000.

Waitman J, McCaffery M: Meperidine—a liability, *Am J Nurs* 101(1):57-58, 2001.

Wall PD, Melzack R, editors: *Textbook of pain*, ed 4 , New York, 2000, Churchill Livingstone.

Want W, Timsit-Berthier M, Schoenen J: Intensity dependence of auditory evoked potentials is pronounced in migraine: an indication of cortical potentiation and low serotonergic neurotransmissions? *Neurology* 46:1404-1409, 1996.

Ware JE, Bjorner JB, Kosinski M: Practical implications of item response (IRT) and computer adaptive testing, *Med Care* 38(suppl 2):73-82, 2000.

WHO: Geneva WHO mortality database. *http://www3.who.ch/whosis/menu.cfm?path=whosis,whsa*

Wiederholt WC: *Neurology for non-neurologists*, ed 4, Philadelphia, 2000, WB Saunders.

Willare LB, Hauss-Wegryzniak B, Wenk GL: Pathological and biochemical consequences of acute and chronic neuroinflammation within the basal forebrain cholinergic system of rats, *Neuroscience* 88(1):193-200, 1999.

Wingerchuk DM, Lucchinetti CF, Noseworthy JH: Multiple sclerosis: current pathophysiological concepts, *Lab Invest* 81(3):263-281, 2001.

Wolf PA, Albers G, Higashida RT, Grotta J: Plenary session VII: stroke in the new millennium. 73rd Scientific Sessions of the American Heart Association, New Orleans, Louisiana, November 12-15, 2000.

Woolf CJ, Salter MW: Neuronal plasticity: increasing the gain in pain, *Science* 288:1765-1768, 2000.

Yang J, Wu CL: Gene therapy for pain, *Am Sci* 89(2):126-135, 2001.

Young MA, Hoffberg H: Poststroke rehabilitation: improving patient functionality. *Clin Advisor*, Feb, 25-32, 2001.

Young WB, Shechter AL, Hopkins MM: Topiramate: a case series study in migraine prophylaxis, *Cephalalgia* 21:370-371, 2001, abstract P2-17.

Zaki PA, Bilsky EJ, Vanderah TW, et al: Opioid receptor types and subtypes: the delta receptor as a model, *Ann Rev Pharmacol Toxicol* 36:379-401, 1996.

ENDOCRINE SYSTEM AND METABOLIC DISORDERS

*T*his part discusses basic concepts in endocrinology and metabolism. These concepts should help the reader acquire an understanding of clinical problems associated with endocrine diseases. This part examines general physiologic concepts, including structure and mechanism of action of hormones, principles of neurohypothalamic control of pituitary function, circadian rhythms, feedback control of endocrine function, and mechanisms that control blood glucose.

The following clinical entities have been selected for discussion: Cushing's syndrome, Addison's disease, primary and secondary aldosteronism, hirsutism, panhypopituitarism, acromegaly, diabetes mellitus, hyperthyroidism, hypothyroidism, goiter, carcinoma of the thyroid, and pheochromocytoma.

Principles of Endocrine and Metabolic Control Mechanisms

DAVID E. SCHTEINGART

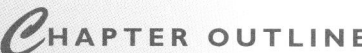HAPTER OUTLINE

*A*s living organisms develop complex structure and function, integration of their various components becomes essential to their survival. This integration is effected by two systems: (1) the central nervous system (CNS) and (2) the endocrine system. These two systems are related from the embryologic, anatomic, and functional standpoints. For example, many of the endocrine glands originate from the neuroectoderm, an embryonic layer that also gives origin to the CNS. In addition, there are anatomic connections between the developed CNS and the endocrine system, primarily through the hypothalamus. As a consequence, stimuli that disturb the CNS frequently alter the function of the endocrine system as well. Conversely, a change in the function of the endocrine system may affect the function of the CNS. The integrated operation of the neuroendocrine system helps maximize the response of the organism to internal and external stimuli.

FUNCTIONS OF THE ENDOCRINE SYSTEM

The endocrine system is made up of hormone-secreting glands that help maintain and regulate vital functions such as (1) response to stress and injury, (2) growth and development, (3) reproduction, (4) ionic homeostasis, (5) energy metabolism, and (6) immune response.

When injury or stress occurs, the endocrine system triggers a series of responses aimed at maintaining blood pressure and preserving life. The hypothalamic-pituitary-adrenal axis is chiefly involved in this response.

Without a properly functioning neuroendocrine system, there is failure to grow and reach maturity; infertility also occurs. The hypothalamic-pituitary-gonadal axis is chiefly involved in this function.

The endocrine system is important in maintenance of ionic homeostasis. Mammalian organisms live in an external environment that changes constantly. However, tissues and cells live in an internal environment that must remain constant. The endocrine system participates in the regulation of this internal environment through maintenance of sodium, potassium, water, and acid-base balance. Aldosterone and antidiuretic hormone (ADH) are responsible for this function. Endocrine function also controls the calcium concentration. Calcium is required for regulation of many biochemical reactions in living cells and for normal neural activation of muscle cell function. The parathyroid glands regulate calcium homeostasis.

The endocrine system acts as a regulator of energy metabolism. The basal metabolic rate is increased by thyroid hormone, and energy is made available to cells through the integrated action of gastrointestinal and pancreatic hormones.

There is interaction between the neuroendocrine system and the immune response. Cortisol modulates and release of cytokines involved in cell-mediated immunity and cytokines such as interleukin 6 (IL-6) can stimulate adrenocorticotropic hormone (ACTH) and cortisol secretion.

HORMONES

The endocrine system is made up of glands that synthesize and secrete substances called *hormones*. Hormones cause the physiologic and biochemical changes that mediate the types of regulation described earlier. Once they are released into the bloodstream, hormones are transported to target tissues where they exert their effects. These effects frequently involve the regulation of ongoing enzymatic reactions. Hormones are generally secreted in very low concentrations. For instance, hormones are present in blood at a concentration of 10^{-6} to 10^{-12} molar. In contrast, another blood component, sodium, is usually present at a concentration of 10^{-1} molar. Despite these low concentrations, hormones exert marked metabolic and biochemical effects on their target tissues.

Hormones fall into two main classes: (1) steroids and thyronines, which are lipid soluble, and (2) polypeptides and catecholamines, which are water soluble. In addition, some hormones are in the category of glycoprotein, a combination of a sugar portion and a protein. The main characteristic of steroid hormones is the presence of a multicyclic structure, the cycloperhydrophenanthrene nucleus (Fig. 58-1). Examples of steroid hormones are the adrenocortical hormones and the hormones produced by the gonads. Polypeptides hormones are made up of chains of specific amino acids that vary in length, molecular weight, and constituent amino acids. Some polypeptide hormones, such as insulin, have a more complex structure with two amino acid chains linked together by disulfide linkages. The molecular structure of insulin is illustrated in Fig. 58-2. Other polypeptide hormones are parathormone or parathyroid hormone (PTH), the tropic hormones of the pituitary gland (with the exception of thyroid-stimulating hormone [TSH], or thyrotropin, and gonadotropins), vasopressin, and glucagon. Examples of glycoprotein hormones are TSH and gonadotropins (e.g., luteinizing hormone [LH] and follicle-stimulating hormone [FSH]). Most hormones are synthesized as higher–molecular-weight precursors and are designated in their initial stages as prohormones. For example, insulin is synthesized as proinsulin, a continuous peptide, which—after

losing a portion of the molecule, the C peptid—becomes a two-chain structure. Adrenocorticotropic hormone (ACTH) is derived from proopiomelanocortin (POMC), a 31,000–molecular-weight glycoprotein, which, by sequential enzyme catalyzed cleavages, generates a series of peptides, including opiates and the 39-amino-acid peptide ACTH.

In addition to the classic hormones, which are produced by specific endocrine glands and act on specific target organs, a number of substances generated by hormone action act directly on cells and promote growth. Some of these substances have insulinlike activity, whereas others mediate the action of hormones, such as growth hormone. Insulin-like growth factor-1 (IGF-1) is a well-recognized growth factor, generated in tissues under the effect of growth hormone, which is capable of promoting tissue growth. There are also compounds that are hormonelike in their mechanism of action but are produced in the blood itself. An example is angiotensin II, a polypeptide hormone that stimulates the adrenal cortex to secrete aldosterone. Angiotensin I is synthesized in the blood from renin substrate (a hepatic protein) under the catalytic effect of renin, an enzyme secreted by renal cells. Angiotensin II is then generated from angiotensin I in the lung by the loss of two amino acids, a reaction that is catalyzed by angiotensin-converting enzyme (ACE).

Although most hormones are synthesized by distinct endocrine glands, organs not classically considered endocrine glands contain groups of cells capable of synthesizing hormones. Many of these cells are derived from the neural crest and have the capacity to take up amine precursors and decarboxylate them for synthesis of hormones. These cells have been described as being part of the amine precursor uptake and decarboxylation (APUD) system. Tumors derived from these cells may acquire the capacity to secrete hormones that, because of their origin in cells outside the classic endocrine glands, are called *ectopic hormones.*

Much is known about the way hormones work on their target tissues or cells. Hormones influence cellular metabolic processes either directly or indirectly by first interacting with specific cell receptors. The combination of the hormone with its receptor may bring about changes within the cell by one of two mechanisms: (1) generation of a second messenger within the cell or (2) translocation of the hormone-receptor complex into

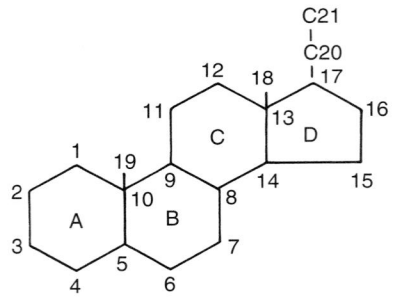

FIG. 58-1 A steroid nucleus. It has four rings: A, B, C, and D. The numbers designate the carbons within the molecule. Groups attached to different carbons are recognized by the respective numbers. For example, 17-hydroxy steroids have a hydroxyl group attached to the carbon in the 17 position.

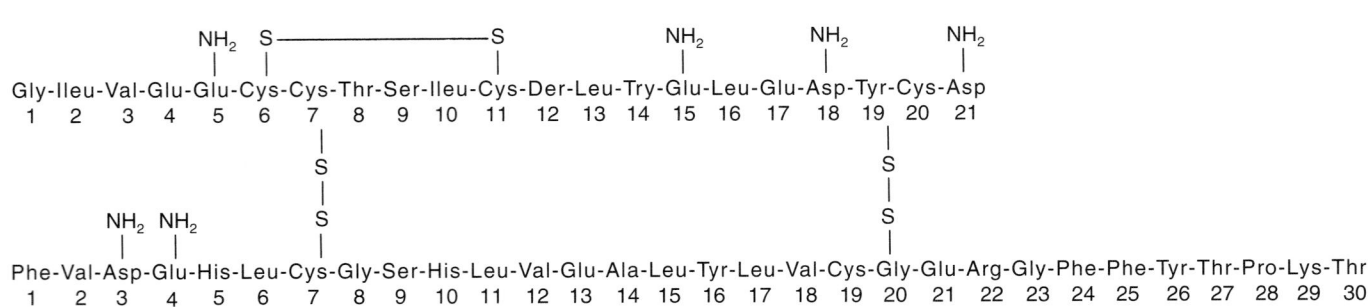

FIG. 58-2 Molecular structure of insulin, a polypeptide hormone. The hormone has two chains, A and B. The A chain has 21 amino acids, and the B chain has 30 amino acids. The two chains are linked to each other by disulfide linkages.

the nucleus, where the complex induces or inhibits protein synthesis by the cell.

Polypeptide hormones and catecholamines appear to act via a second messenger mechanism, whereas steroid hormones are freely permeable to the cell membrane and exert their effects directly on the cell nucleus. More specifically, polypeptide hormones act by first interacting with a specific cell membrane receptor, and as a result of this interaction, a membrane-bound enzyme, adenylate cyclase, is activated and adenosine triphosphate (ATP) is converted to adenosine 3′,5′-monophosphate (cyclic AMP). The latter then binds to the regulatory subunit of a protein kinase, thereby liberating a catalytic subunit of this enzyme. This action, in turn, initiates the phosphorylation of certain key enzymes that specifically either activate or inactivate the biologic potency of these enzymes (Fig. 58-3).

Different polypeptide hormones activate different specific enzyme mechanisms, which mediate hormone action. For example, glucagon activates the enzyme phosphorylase by the process described, which brings about the enzymatic cleavage of glycogen to glucose-1-phosphate. ACTH increases steroidogenesis by activating one or several enzymes of the steroidogenic pathway. Insulin binds to the alpha subunit of the insulin receptor, a heterotetrameric glycoprotein in the cell membrane, and stimulates tyrosine phosphorylation of the beta subunit. A phosphorylation cascade then initiates a signal for the transport of glucose and the flux of certain ions across the cell membrane. In contrast to the way peptide hormones exert their effects, steroid hormones work directly inside the cell by entering the cell across the cell membrane and binding to cytosol receptor proteins. The steroid-receptor complex then is translocated to the nucleus of the cell, where it

binds specifically to its locus on the deoxyribonucleic acid (DNA) and alters transcription, leading to the synthesis of one or several specific messenger ribonucleic acids (mRNAs). These products leave the nucleus and travel to the ribosome, where they direct the synthesis of proteins. By changing mRNA, steroids can modify the way protein is synthesized (Fig. 58-4).

In summary, hormonal action involves the combination of the hormone with its specific receptors in cells that are the targets of hormone action. The physiologic action of the hormone and the specificity of such action are intimately linked to the interaction of the hormone with its specific receptor.

PHYSIOLOGY OF THE ENDOCRINE SYSTEM

The CNS is connected to the pituitary through the hypothalamus; this is the most clearly established link between the CNS and the endocrine system. The two systems are interrelated by both neural and vascular connections.

As demonstrated in Fig. 58-5, the pituitary is divided into an anterior and a posterior lobe. In rodents, there is also an intermediate lobe, but, in humans, the intermediate lobe is vestigial and not clearly separated from the anterior lobe. Blood vessels link the hypothalamus with the cells of the anterior pituitary gland. These blood vessels end in capillaries at both ends and, for this reason, are known as a *portal system*. In this particular case, the system connects the hypothalamus with the pituitary gland (hypophysis) and is called the *hypothalamic-hypophyseal* portal system. The portal system is an important vascular channel because it allows for the movement

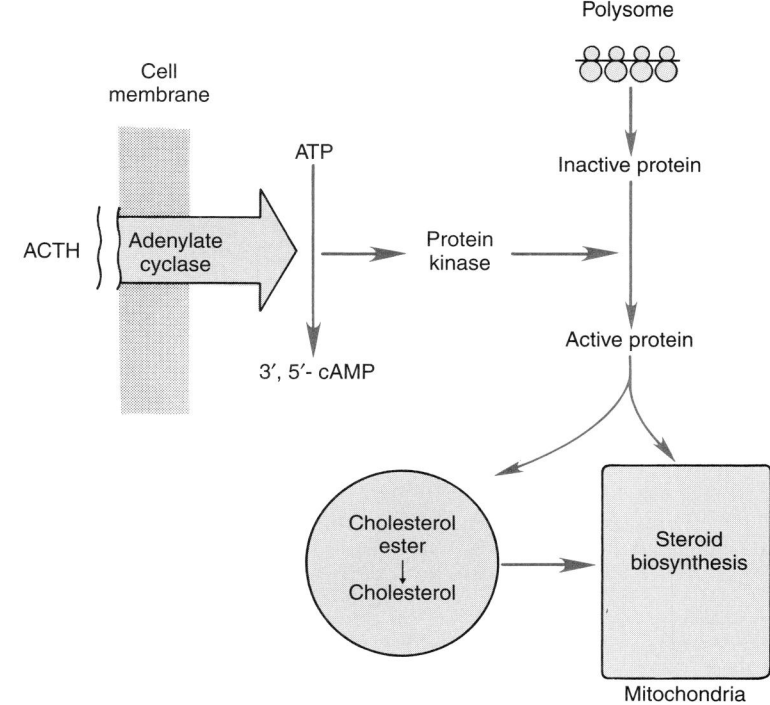

FIG. 58-3   Mechanism of action of adrenocorticotropic hormone *(ACTH)*, a protein hormone. ACTH activates adenylate cyclase, increasing the synthesis of 3′, 5′-cyclic adenosine monophosphate *(cAMP)*. In turn, cAMP stimulates a protein kinase, which activates a rapid turnover protein. This protein causes increased release of cholesterol for use in steroid biosynthesis and stimulation of conversion of cholesterol to pregnenolone in the cell mitochondria. *ATP*, Adenosine triphosphate.

FIG. 58-4 Mechanism of action of steroid hormones. These hormones bind to intracellular receptor proteins, which subsequently carry the steroid molecule to the cell nucleus. In the nucleus the steroid modifies the formation of messenger ribonucleic acid *(mRNA)* and protein synthesis. *DNA,* Deoxyribonucleic acid; *St,* steroid hormone; *R,* receptor protein.

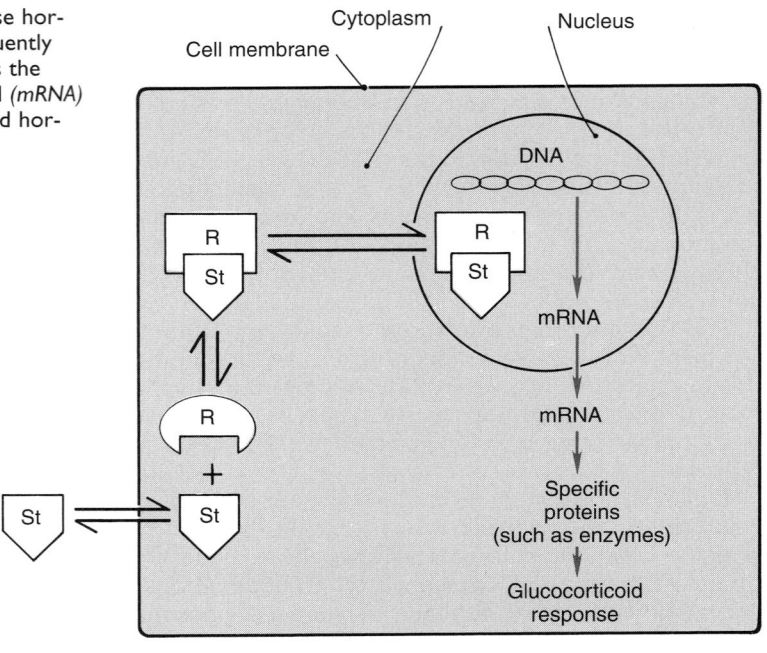

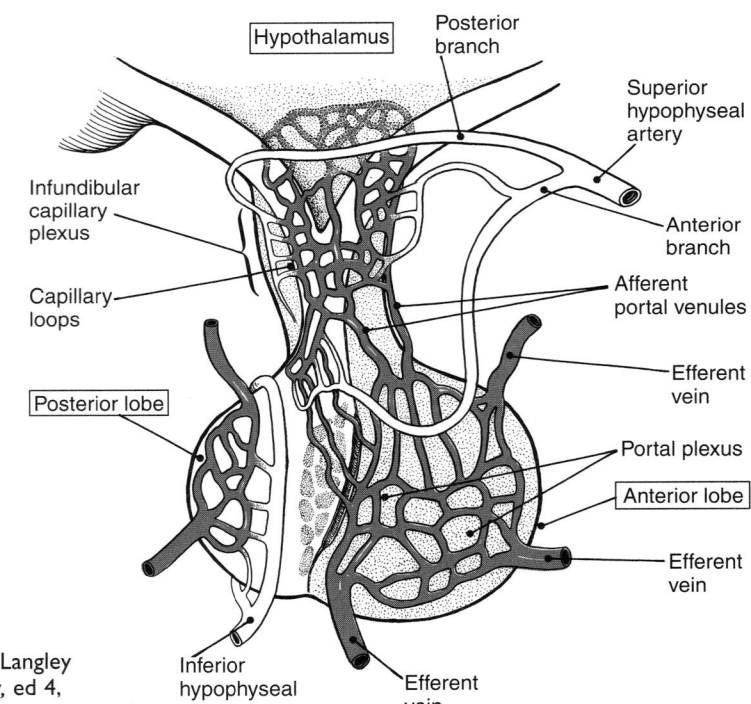

FIG. 58-5 Hypothalamic-hypophyseal portal system. (From Langley LL, Telford JR, Christensen JB: *Dynamic anatomy and physiology,* ed 4, New York, 1980, McGraw-Hill.)

of releasing hormones from the hypothalamus to the pituitary gland, enabling the hypothalamus to modulate pituitary function. Stimuli originating in the brain activate neurons in the hypothalamic nuclei, which synthesize and secrete low–molecular-weight proteins. These proteins, or neurohormones, are known as *releasing and inhibiting hormones.* These hormones are discharged into the blood vessels of the portal system, through which they reach cells in the pituitary gland. The pituitary gland responds to these releasing hormones by discharging pituitary tropic hormones. In this chain of events, the hormones released by the pituitary gland travel with the blood and stimulate other glands, causing the release of target gland hormones. The target gland hormones, in turn, act on the hypothalamic and pituitary cells and modify hormone secretion.

Fig. 58-6 illustrates a modality of feedback control in which the hormonal product of the target gland inhibits

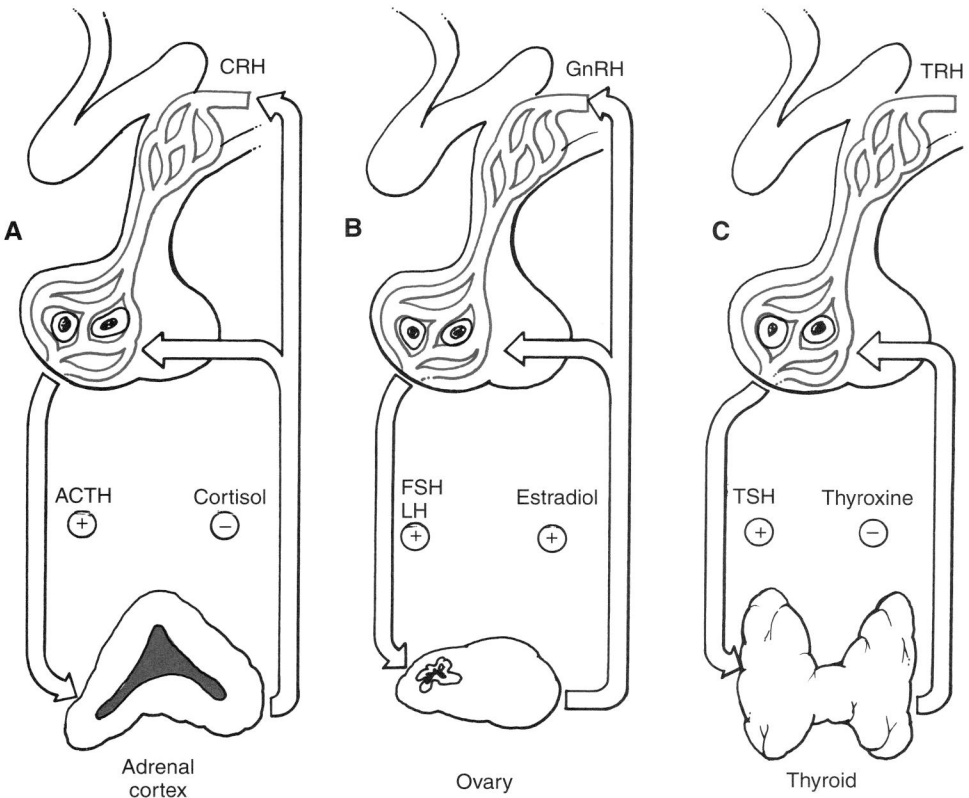

FIG. 58-6   Feedback-regulating systems where the target gland hormone feeds back to the hypothalamus. Pituitary release of the tropic hormone follows. **A**, Corticotropin-releasing hormone (*CRH*). **B**, Gonadotropin-releasing hormone *(GnRH)*. **C**, TSH-releasing hormone *(TRH)*. *ACTH*, Adrenocorticotropic hormone; *FSH*, follicle-stimulating hormone; *LH*, luteinizing hormone; *TSH*, thyroid-stimulating hormone (thyrotropin).

the release of the corresponding pituitary tropic hormone. This type of regulation of hormone secretion is known as a *negative-feedback control system*. In the hypothalamic-pituitary-adrenal system (see Fig. 58-6, *A*), corticotropin-releasing hormone (CRH) causes the pituitary to release ACTH. Then, ACTH stimulates the adrenal cortex to secrete cortisol. Cortisol, in turn, feeds back on the hypothalamic-pituitary axis and inhibits the production of CRH-ACTH. The system fluctuates, varying with the physiologic requirements for cortisol. If the system produces too much ACTH and therefore too much cortisol, the cortisol feeds back and inhibits the production of CRH and ACTH. This is a sensitive system, because an excessive production of cortisol or the administration of cortisol or other synthetic glucocorticoids can quickly inhibit the hypothalamic-pituitary axis and shut off the production of ACTH. The concept of feedback control has practical implications in patients receiving chronic corticosteroid therapy. These patients have suppressed ACTH release. If steroids are suddenly withdrawn, patients may develop adrenal insufficiency.

Another example of feedback control (see Fig. 58-6, *B*) is the action of gonadotropin-releasing hormone (GnRH), which stimulates the pituitary to secrete FSH and LH. In women, estrogens are initially produced by the ovary in small amounts; the estrogens feed back on the hypothalamus, stimulating the secretion of GnRH. This action, in turn, triggers FSH and LH release, ovulation, and secretion of estrogen and progesterone. The action of estrogens is an example of *positive feedback control*. A third example (see Fig. 58-6, *C*) of feedback control is release of thyrotropin-releasing hormone (TRH), which is secreted by the hypothalamus and causes the pituitary to secrete TSH. In turn, TSH stimulates the thyroid to secrete thyroxine. Thyroxine then feeds back and inhibits production of TRH and TSH.

Although the interaction between pituitary hormones and the target gland hormones occurs through systemic circulation (the *long-loop system*), other interactions occur between pituitary hormones and their releasing hormones through their local vascular system (the *short-loop system*).

Other systems regulate hormone production independently of the hypothalamic-pituitary axis. One example is the *renin-angiotensin-aldosterone system*. As illustrated in Fig. 58-7, the kidney has juxtaglomerular (JG) cells, which are located in the wall of the afferent arteriole of the glomerulus. These cells secrete the enzyme *renin*. The perfusion pressure in the renal arteriole influences the production of renin. Changes in the pressure of blood flowing through the afferent arteriole into the glomerulus are sensed by stretch receptors near the JG cells. This action causes changes in the secretion of renin, which, in turn, activates angiotensin II. Angiotensin II

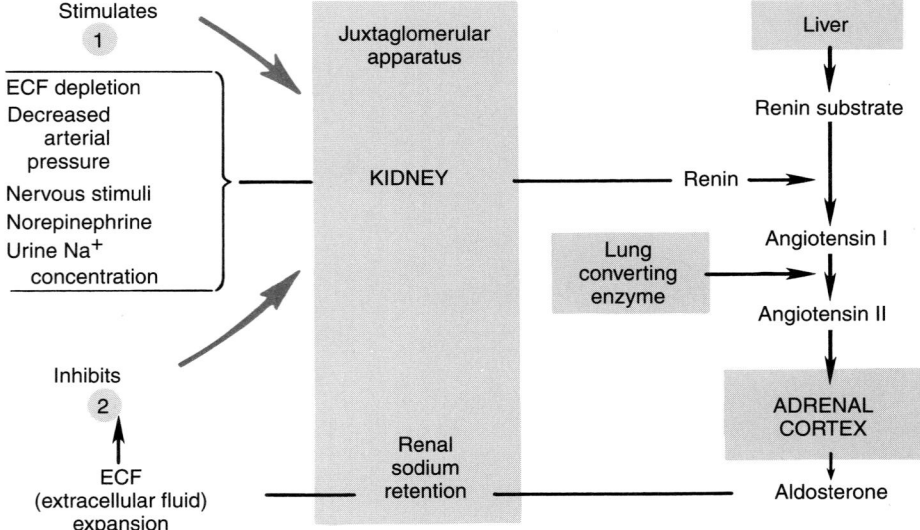

FIG. 58-7 Regulation of aldosterone secretion by the renin-angiotensin system. *1,* Extracellular fluid space *(ECF)* depletion, decreased arterial pressure, nervous stimuli, norepinephrine, and increased urinary sodium stimulate renin release. *2,* ECF expansion, by counteracting these factors, inhibits renin release.

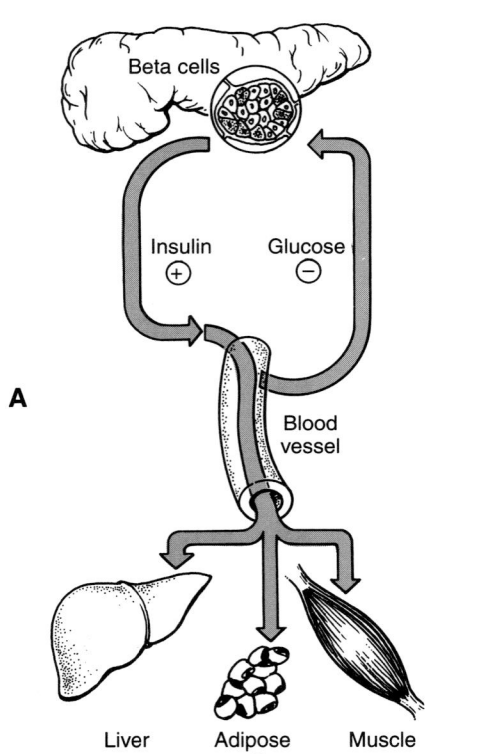

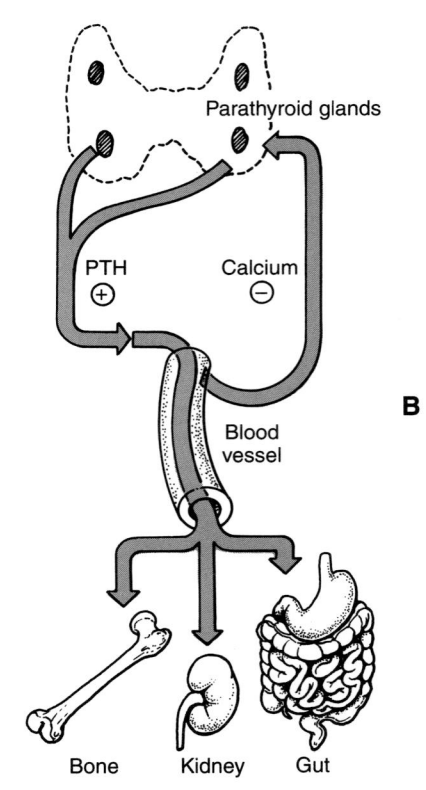

FIG. 58-8 Feedback-regulating systems where the metabolic substrate of hormone action controls the release of the hormone. *PTH,* Parathyroid hormone, or parathormone. (See text for details.)

stimulates the production of aldosterone by the adrenal cortex. Aldosterone promotes renal tubular reabsorption of sodium. As sodium is reabsorbed, volume is expanded, the pressure rises in the afferent arteriole, and renin production is shut off. Thus renin, angiotensin, and aldosterone release are determined by volume and pressure changes affecting the JG cells.

Figure 58-8 illustrates another modality of feedback control, in which the metabolic substance controlled by the hormone acts directly on its release. In Fig. 58-8, *A,* insulin and glucose are depicted. Insulin responds to changes in the level of glucose in blood. When glucose

levels increase, insulin is secreted. When glucose levels decrease, insulin is shut off. Although some of the pituitary hormones may indirectly influence insulin release, no clear evidence indicates that the pituitary gland directly and specifically controls insulin secretion.

PTH and calcium constitute another unique control system (see Fig. 58-8, *B*). A drop in calcium level stimulates PTH secretion. Conversely, an increase in calcium shuts off PTH production.

Another physiologic characteristic of the hypothalamic-pituitary axis is the presence of rhythms. *Rhythms* are a common feature of the production of many hormones,

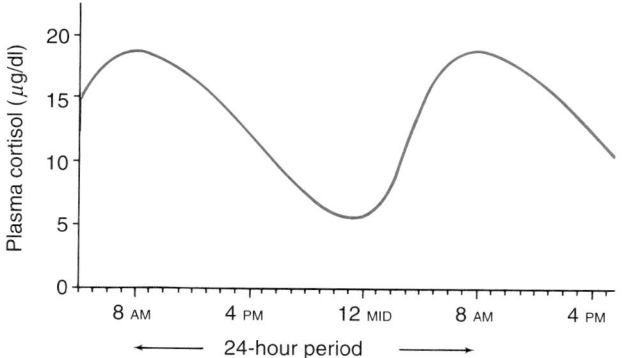

FIG. 58-9   Circadian rhythm of cortisol secretion.

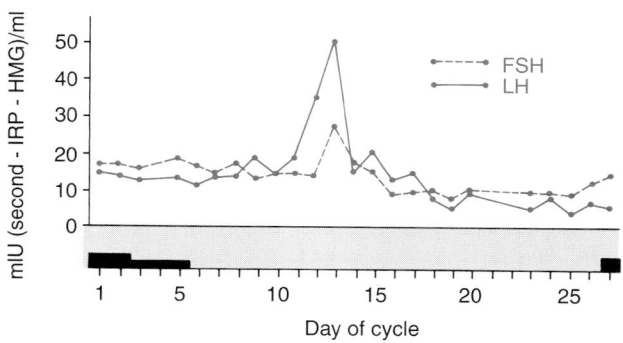

FIG. 58-10   Monthly cyclic release of gonadotropins in normal menstruating women. Depicted is the midcycle surge of follicle-stimulating hormone *(FSH)* and luteinizing hormone *(LH)*.

and they originate in brain structures. ACTH provides an excellent example of rhythmic, or cyclic, hormone release. When ACTH and cortisol levels are measured on an hourly basis for 24 hours, the levels are seen to rise early in the day, decline later, and rise again during the night to reach a peak by the next morning (Fig. 58-9). This type of rhythm is referred to as a *diurnal*, or *circadian*, *rhythm*. Because hormonal release by the pituitary gland occurs in short spurts, it is also said that there is episodic hormonal release.

Gonadotropins, the tropic hormones of the pituitary gland that controls gonadal function, are involved in a different kind of cycle or rhythm. In women, the release of gonadotropins is cyclic and occurs on a monthly basis rather than on a diurnal basis (Fig. 58-10). The presence of the normal cyclic release of gonadotropins is specific and characteristic of female reproductive endocrine function. In men, on the other hand, the release of the same gonadotropins does not have this cyclic nature, and it occurs at a constant rate. If the cyclic release of gonadotropins in a woman is abolished, cessation of normal menstrual cycles with suppression of ovulation and fertility occur.

Other hormones are not released with a spontaneous rhythm but are released in response to metabolic stimuli. For example, insulin is released in response to meals.

DISEASES OF THE ENDOCRINE SYSTEM

Hormones do not act directly on cells or tissues—they must first bind to specific receptors in the cell membrane or in the cytosol of the cell. For a metabolic event to occur, the metabolic steps distal to the interaction of the hormone and the receptor must all be intact. It thus appears that not only is the hormone concentration important for the final strength of the signal that turns on the cellular machinery, but the number and affinity of the receptors for the hormone are also critically important. As a consequence, two mechanisms for endocrine disease can be postulated: (1) disturbances in which primarily the hormone concentrations are changed and (2) disturbances in which primarily the receptor and postreceptor mechanisms are defective. Most endocrine diseases can

be understood conceptually in terms of the metabolic actions of the hormones involved, resulting from either excessive or deficient hormone production or action. Thus knowledge of the metabolic consequence of the excessive or deficient hormone secretion will help identify the clinical picture emerging from these disturbances. For example, if production of thyroxine, the thyroid hormone, is excessive, one can predict an increase in the basal metabolic rate and in heat production. In effect, patients with hyperthyroidism demonstrate a high metabolic rate, increased heat sensitivity, and weight loss. Conversely, lack of thyroxine results in the opposite metabolic effects, such as low basal metabolic rate and increased sensitivity to cold temperature. Primary disturbances at the receptor level lead to syndromes of hormone resistance. Mutations in the cortisol receptor decrease the binding of the hormone to its specific receptor and cause a syndrome of primary glucocorticoid resistance. Mutations in the thyroid hormone receptor cause a syndrome of thyroid hormone resistance. A second type of receptor-mediated disorder is Graves' disease, in which an autoimmune process forms antibodies against the TSH receptor, resulting in stimulation of thyroid function. Antibodies produced against the insulin receptor lead to syndromes of severe insulin resistance.

Treatment of Endocrine Diseases

The treatment of endocrine diseases is based on the change in hormone production underlying the specific disease. In simple terms, patients who have a disease caused by a *deficit* of hormone secretion are treated by replacement of these hormones. An example is a patient with diabetes whose pancreas is not making enough insulin. Treatment for the metabolic consequence of insulin insufficiency is the administration of insulin or an insulin secretagogue. Similarly, a patient whose thyroid is not making enough thyroid hormone becomes hypothyroid and is treated with replacement amounts of thyroxine.

The treatment of diseases of hormone *excess* is more complex, because several therapeutic alternatives are usually available. Removal of the whole gland or part of the gland that produces the hormone in excess is one such alternative. The removal of the entire gland, however, results in total deficit of hormone, necessitating hormonal replacement to restore levels to normal. The pituitary gland provides an example of the consequence of total gland removal. Because it is a gland with multiple functions—the anterior lobe secretes tropic hormones, and the posterior lobe secretes ADH, among others—removal of the pituitary gland leads to cessation of secretion of many hormones, or *panhypopituitarism*. In contrast, removing part of a gland can eliminate a hormone excess, leaving only enough hormone production to maintain normal function.

Modern surgical techniques allow for removal of only the part of the gland that is abnormal. These techniques are used when a small tumor of the pituitary gland causes excessive hormone production. The tumor can be resected by microsurgical techniques without removal of the rest of the pituitary gland. In other cases, removal of only a part of a gland is not possible. For example, if the adrenal glands are removed to treat Cushing's disease, both the adrenal cortex and the adrenal medulla must be removed. Although the body can function well without the adrenal medulla, the total capacity to secrete catecholamines may be impaired.

Another alternative for dealing with hormone excess is the administration of drugs that interfere with hormone production by either blocking or destroying the tissue that makes the hormone. For example, a patient with hyperthyroidism can be given radioactive iodine in large concentrations. The radioactive iodine concentrates in the thyroid gland and destroys the cells that make thyroxine, causing remission of the disease. Another example is adrenal hyperfunction, in which the glands can be blocked by drugs that interfere with the biosynthesis of adrenocortical hormones.

Suppression of hormone production is also illustrated by oral contraceptives. Estrogens and progestogens are given to inhibit pituitary release of gonadotropins; this, in turn, suppresses normal ovarian function and ovulation.

In summary, endocrine diseases are those of either hormone deficit or hormone excess. Replacing the deficient hormone treats the deficit state. The excessive state can be treated either by surgically removing the whole gland or part of the gland that is working excessively or by giving drugs that block or destroy the tissues making the hormone.

KEY CONCEPTS

- The endocrine system can be divided into (1) *endocrine organs* entirely devoted to the production of hormones (e.g., pituitary, adrenal, thyroid, parathyroid, (2) *endocrine components in mixed organs*, which are discrete endocrine cell clusters within organs that have another function (e.g., pancreas, ovary, testis), and (3) *diffuse endocrine* or *paracrine system*, which are scattered cells within an organ or tissue that produce hormones acting locally on adjacent cells and do not enter the bloodstream and are thus not truly endocrine cells (e.g., in the gut and bronchial mucosa).
- The *nervous and endocrine systems* are *communication systems* that regulate the basic metabolic activities of the body and thus serve an *integrative function* for complex organisms.
- The *nervous and endocrine systems* are *intimately linked* embryonically, anatomically, and functionally. The neuroectoderm in the embryo gives rise to the nervous system, as well as many endocrine glands. Both systems are anatomically linked through the hypothalamic-hypophyseal portal system. Both systems regulate basic metabolic activities of the body.
- *Functions of the endocrine system* include (1) response to stress or injury (via the hypothalamic-pituitary-adrenal axis), (2) growth and development, (3) reproduction (via the hypothalamic-pituitary-gonadal axis), (4) energy metabolism (via thyroid and pancreatic hormones), (5) fluid and electrolyte metabolism (via ADH, aldosterone, and parathyroid hormones), and (6) immune response.
- An interaction between the neuroendocrine system and the immune response exists. Cortisol modulates the release of cytokines involved in cell-mediated immunity and cytokines such as IL-6 can stimulate ACTH and cortisol secretion.

- The endocrine system is made up of glands that synthesize and secrete chemical substances called *hormones*, which are carried in the blood to target tissues where their action is exerted.
- Hormones are either protein derivatives (glycoproteins, polypeptides, or amines) or cholesterol derivatives (steroids).
- *General characteristics of hormones*: (1) secreted in minute amounts; (2) pulsatile release with a circadian rhythm, which must be considered in the interpretation of serum values; (3) act by altering the rate of a physiologic response; and (4) most are inactivated by the liver and excreted in the urine.
- *Hormones* can be classified into two broad categories based on their *mechanism of signaling and interaction with target cell receptors*: (1) *steroids and thyronines* (lipid soluble) diffuse across the target cell membrane and *combine with intracellular receptor sites*, ultimately signaling mRNA to synthesize some protein; (2) *polypeptides and catecholamines* (water soluble) combine with the *target cell surface receptor*, which then uses a *second messenger* (usually cyclic AMP) and ultimately changes some function of the target cell.
- *Steroid hormones* include cortisol, aldosterone, gonadal hormones, and cholecalciferol (vitamin D). Thyroxine (T_4) and triiodothyronine (T_3) are *thyronine hormones*.
- Examples of *polypeptide hormones* include the hypothalamic-releasing hormones, pituitary tropic hormones, parathyroid hormone (PTH), calcitonin, insulin, and glucagon. Epinephrine and norepinephrine are *catecholamines*.
- Regulation of hormone secretion is achieved by (1) negative feedback based on the blood level of

the hormone, (2) change in the concentration of some other plasma substance (e.g., glucose and insulin, Ca^{++} and parathormone), and (3) rhythm of secretions originating in brain (e.g., circadian rhythm of cortisol secretion, growth hormone, menstrual cycle hormones).

■ *Diseases of the endocrine system* are of three types: (1) hormone deficiency, (2) hormone excess, and (3) hormone target cell receptor resistance.

■ *Hormone deficiencies* may be caused by infections, infarction and tissue death, tumor, surgical removal, autoimmune disease, dietary deficiency, and heredity and are generally treated by replacement therapy.

■ *Hormone excess* may be caused by failure of negative feedback, ectopic site production, failure of inactivation or excretion or it may be iatrogenic; treatment is hormone suppression by total or partial gland removal or by drugs to suppress hormone production, suppress tropic hormone release, or by giving a hormone antagonist.

■ *Hormone target cell receptor resistance* may be caused by a receptor defect (e.g., type 2 diabetes), autoantibody injury or destruction, heredity, or absent target cells and is generally treated by enhancing hormone-receptor interaction (sulfonylurea drugs for type 2 diabetes).

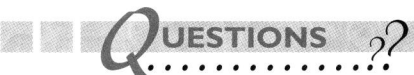 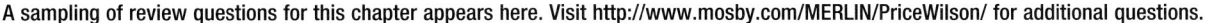 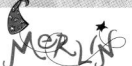

QUESTIONS ??

A sampling of review questions for this chapter appears here. Visit http://www.mosby.com/MERLIN/PriceWilson/ for additional questions.

Answer the following on a separate sheet of paper.

1. Cite two mechanisms by which hormones can work on their target cells.

2. In the table below, list the two types of hormones that are differentiated by their chemical structure. State two examples of each type and identify the location of production for each example.

Type of Hormone	Examples	Location of Production
a	1	1
	2	2
b	1	1
	2	2

3. Write a brief description of the way angiotensin II is synthesized in the blood and stimulates a peripheral gland.

4. Identify the role played by the hypothalamus in the hypothalamic-pituitary system.

5. What is the function of the hypothalamic-hypophyseal portal system?

6. Give an example of the way the feedback control mechanism operates to regulate endocrine hormone secretion.

7. Define circadian rhythm by identifying the hormonal levels (high or low) of ACTH and the time of day each level occurs.

8. Cite the two postulated mechanisms for endocrine disturbances.

9. State the rationale for providing hormone replacement or suppression as treatment for endocrine diseases caused by hormonal deficit or excess.

Disorders of the Pituitary Gland

DAVID E. SCHTEINGART

GENERAL CONCEPTS

The pituitary gland is a complex structure under the brain lying within a bony wall cavity, the *sella turcica*, in the sphenoid bone and is formed early in embryonic development from the fusion of two ectodermal hollow processes. An invagination from the roof of the primitive oral region, Rathke's pouch, extends upward toward the base of the brain and is met by an outpouching of the floor of the third ventricle, destined to become the neurohypophysis. The developed pituitary gland is thus formed by a posterior lobe, or *neurohypophysis*, in continuity with the hypothalamus and an anterior lobe, or *adenohypophysis*, connected to the hypothalamus through the pituitary stalk. A vascular structure, the hypothalamic-hypophyseal portal system, also connects the hypothalamus with the anterior pituitary gland. It is through this system that releasing hormones from the hypothalamus reach the cells of the pituitary gland to promote hormone release.

The anterior pituitary gland has multiple functions, and because of its ability to regulate the function of other endocrine glands, it is also known as the *master gland*. The anterior pituitary cells are specialized to secrete specific hormones. Seven such hormones have been well identified and their physiologic metabolic roles defined. These hormones are adrenocorticotropic hormone (ACTH), melanocyte-

stimulating hormone (MSH), thyroid-stimulating hormone (thyrotropin, TSH), follicle-stimulating hormone (FSH), luteinizing hormone (LH), growth hormone (GH), and prolactin (PRL). Some of these hormones (ACTH, MSH, GH, and prolactin) are *polypeptides,* whereas others (TSH, FSH, and LH) are *glycoproteins.* Morphologic studies indicate that a specific cell type synthesizes each hormone. In a sense, the anterior pituitary gland is a conglomeration of independent glands, all of which are under hypothalamic control.

The posterior lobe of the pituitary gland, or neurohypophysis, is concerned mainly with the regulation of fluid balance. Vasopressin or antidiuretic hormone (ADH) is synthesized primarily in the supraoptic and paraventricular nuclei of the hypothalamus and stored in the neurohypophysis.

PHYSIOLOGIC AND METABOLIC ROLES OF ANTERIOR PITUITARY HORMONES

GH, prolactin, and MSH have direct metabolic effects on target tissues. In contrast, ACTH, TSH, FSH, and LH exert their main effects through the regulation of secretion of other endocrine glands and are therefore known as *tropic hormones* (Table 59-1).

GH, or somatotropin, has major metabolic effects in children and adults. In children, GH hormone is required for somatic growth. In adults, GH may preserve normal adult organ size, and it participates in the regulation of protein synthesis and nutrient disposal. GH produces insulin-like growth factor-1 (IGF-1), which mediates its growth-promoting effect. Without IGF-1, GH cannot promote growth. Secretion of GH is regulated by a growth hormone–releasing hormone (GHRH) from the hypothalamus and by somatostatin, an inhibiting hormone. The release of GH is stimulated by hypoglycemia and by amino acids such as arginine; it is also modified by stress and by exercise.

MSH, which is a constituent of proopiomelanocortin, increases skin pigmentation by stimulating the dispersion of melanin granules in melanocytes. The secretion of MSH is regulated by corticotropin-releasing hormone

TABLE 59-1

Anterior Lobe Pituitary Hormones and Function

Hormone	Releasing Hormone	Target	Function (Stimulates)
ACTH	CRH	Adrenal cortex	Steroidogenesis
MSH	CRH	Melanocytes	Pigmentation
TSH	TRH	Thyroid follicles	T_4, T_3
LH (men)	GnRH	Leydig cells	Testosterone
FSH (men)	GnRH	Seminiferous tubules	Spermatogenesis
LH (women)	GnRH	Corpus luteum	Progesterone
FSH (women)	GnRH	Follicular cells	Estrogens
Prolactin	TRH (+)	Mammary gland	Lactation
	Dopamine (−)		
GH	GHRH (+)	Systemic	Growth
	Somatostatin (−)		

See text for meaning of abbreviations.

(CRH), and it is inhibited by a rise in cortisol. Deficient secretion of cortisol can stimulate MSH release, and high cortisol levels suppress its secretion.

Prolactin is one of a group of hormones necessary for breast development and milk secretion. The release of prolactin is under tonic inhibition by the hypothalamus through dopamine, secreted by the tuberohypophyseal dopaminergic neuron system. In its absence, increased prolactin secretion and lactation may occur. Thyrotropin-releasing hormone (TRH) stimulates prolactin secretion.

ACTH regulates the growth and function of the adrenal cortex and is especially important in the control of the production and release of cortisol. By itself, ACTH does not appear to have significant extraadrenal effects. CRH and arginine vasopressin (AVP) act synergistically to stimulate ACTH secretion.

TSH stimulates the growth and function of the thyroid gland. TSH causes thyroxine (T_4) and triiodothyronine (T_3) release, and these in turn regulate the secretion of TSH. TRH stimulates TSH secretion.

FSH and LH are also known as gonadotropins. In men, FSH maintains and stimulates spermatogenesis, and LH stimulates the secretion of testosterone by the Leydig, or interstitial, cells of the testes. FSH and LH are secreted in men in a continuous or tonic fashion. In contrast, in women, FSH stimulates follicular development and the secretion of estrogens by the follicular cells. LH induces ovulation and maintains and stimulates the secretion of progesterone by the corpus luteum, which develops from the follicle after ovulation has occurred. The release of FSH and LH in women follows a cyclic pattern so that the levels of these two hormones rise at midcycle and slowly decline toward the end of the cycle, when menstruation occurs. FSH and LH secretion is modulated by the pulsatile pattern of secretion (amplitude and frequency) of gonadotropin-releasing hormone (GnRH).

The clinical consequences of deficiencies in ACTH and TSH release are adrenal insufficiency and hypothyroidism, respectively. Absence of gonadotropin release leads to hypogonadism. Conversely, excessive secretion of ACTH leads to adrenocortical hyperfunction, or Cushing's syndrome. Syndromes of excessive TSH or gonadotropin release are more rare.

A clinical diagnosis of a pituitary disorder requires biochemical confirmation by specific tests that reveal the abnormality of pituitary function characteristic of the suspected condition. The pituitary hormones described, ACTH, MSH, TSH, FSH, LH, GH, and prolactin, can all be measured in serum or plasma.

CLINICAL DISORDERS OF THE PITUITARY GLAND

Clinical syndromes associated with abnormal function of the pituitary gland include disorders of hormone deficit and hormone excess.

Hypopituitarism

Pituitary insufficiency typically affects all the hormones normally secreted by the anterior pituitary gland. The clinical manifestations of *panhypopituitarism* are therefore a composite of the metabolic effects caused by the deficient secretion of each one of the pituitary hormones.

Several pathologic processes may result in pituitary insufficiency by destroying the normal pituitary cells: (1) pituitary tumors, (2) vascular thrombosis leading to necrosis of the normal pituitary gland, (3) infiltrative granulomatous diseases, and (4) idiopathic or possible autoimmune disease.

The clinical syndrome resulting from panhypopituitarism differs in children and in adults. In children, interference with somatic growth is caused by deficiency of GH release. *Pituitary dwarfism* develops as a consequence of this deficiency. As the child reaches adolescence, secondary sexual characteristics and the external genitalia fail to develop (Fig. 59-1). In addition, patients may present with various degrees of adrenal insufficiency and hypothyroidism; they may have difficulty in school and exhibit slow intellectual development; and their skin is usually pale because of the absence of MSH.

When hypopituitarism develops in adults, loss of pituitary function frequently has the following chronology: GH deficiency, hypogonadism, hypothyroidism, and adrenal insufficiency. Because the adult has already completed somatic growth, adult patients with hypopituitarism are of normal height. Manifestations of GH deficiency may be expressed by unusual sensitivity to insulin and by fasting hypoglycemia. With the development

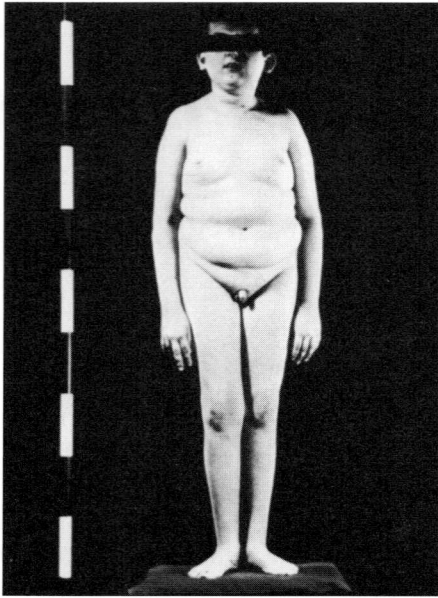

FIG. 59-1 Short stature and absence of secondary sexual characteristics in a patient with panhypopituitarism developing during childhood.

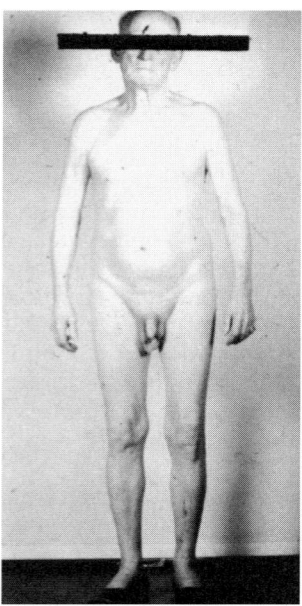

FIG. 59-2 Panhypopituitarism in the adult. There is pallor and a loss of body hair growth.

of *hypogonadism*, men exhibit a decrease in libido, impotence, and a progressive decrease in body hair growth, beard, and muscular development (Fig. 59-2). In women, cessation of menstrual periods, or *amenorrhea*, is one of the early manifestations of pituitary failure. This is accompanied by atrophy of the breasts and the external genitalia. Both men and women show various degrees of hypothyroidism (see Chapter 60) and adrenal insufficiency (see Chapter 62). Deficiency of MSH causes a sallow or pale appearance in these patients.

Occasionally, patients exhibit isolated pituitary hormone failure. Under these circumstances, the cause of the deficiency is likely to be in the hypothalamus and involve the corresponding releasing hormone.

In patients with panhypopituitarism, the baseline level of these tropic hormones is low, as is the level of hormones produced by the target glands controlled by these hormones.

Patients with hypopituitarism have, in addition to low basal hormone levels, a blunted or absent response to the administration of hormone secretagogues. Combined pituitary function tests can be performed on these patients by injecting (1) insulin to produce hypoglycemia, (2) CRH, (3) TRH, and (4) GnRH. Hypoglycemia, with a serum glucose level of less than 40 mg/dl, normally causes the release of GH, ACTH, and cortisol; CRH stimulates ACTH and cortisol release; TRH stimulates TSH and prolactin release; and GnRH stimulates the release of FSH and LH. Patients with panhypopituitarism fail to respond to any of these four secretagogues. In addition to the biochemical studies, radiographic examination of the pituitary gland is mandatory in patients with suspected pituitary disease, because pituitary tumors are a common cause of these disorders.

The treatment of hypopituitarism involves the replacement of the deficient hormones. Human GH, the only one effective in humans, is produced by recombinant deoxyribonucleic acid (DNA) techniques and is available to physician specialists for the treatment of patients with GH deficiency. When administered to children with pituitary dwarfism, human GH may cause significant increase in height. Recombinant human GH is also available for hormone replacement of adult patients with panhypopituitarism. Pituitary hormones can be administered only by injection. Thus, for long-term daily replacement therapy, the hormones of the target glands affected by the pituitary deficiency are administered instead. For example, adrenal insufficiency caused by deficiency of ACTH secretion is treated by giving hydrocortisone orally. Giving thyroxine orally treats hypothyroidism caused by TSH deficiency. Administering androgens and estrogens can treat gonadotropin deficiency. However, induction of ovulation necessitates the administration of gonadotropins. GH deficiency requires daily GH injections.

Giantism and Acromegaly

Giantism and acromegaly are caused by excessive secretion of GH, which can result from a pituitary tumor that secretes GH or from a hypothalamic abnormality that leads to increased GH release. Some patients develop acromegaly in response to extrapituitary neoplasia that secretes GHRH ectopically. These patients have hyperplasia of pituitary somatotropes and hypersecretion of GH.

When GH excess occurs during childhood and adolescence, the patient experiences rapid longitudinal growth and becomes a giant. After somatic growth is completed, GH hypersecretion will cause not giantism but thickening of bones and soft tissue. This condition is termed *acromegaly*, and patients with acromegaly exhibit enlargement of hands and feet. Hands become not only larger, but also more square (spadelike), and the fingers become more round and stubby (Fig. 59-3). Patients may relate

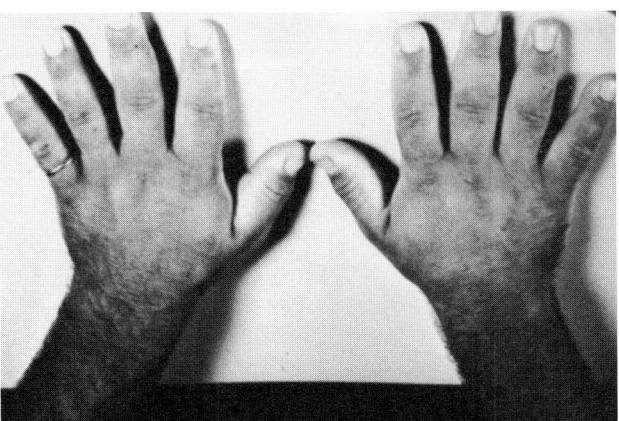

FIG. 59-3   Hands of a patient with acromegaly.

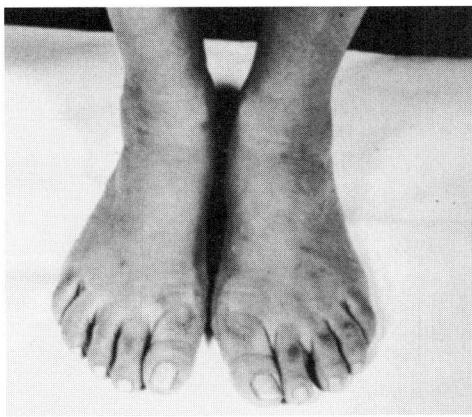

FIG. 59-4   Feet of a patient with acromegaly.

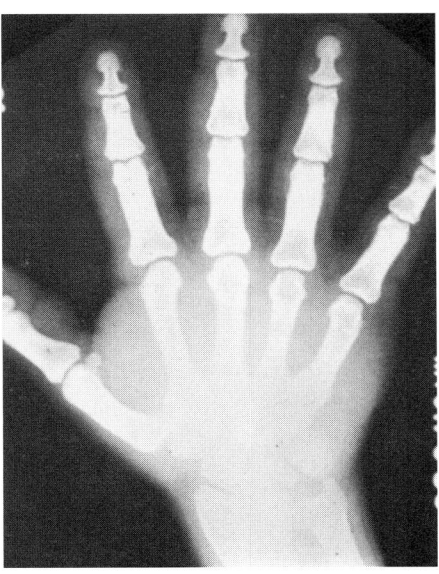

FIG. 59-5   Radiographic appearance of the hand of an acromegalic patient. There are increases in the soft tissues and in the density of the bones, squaring off the phalanges, and increased tufting of the terminal phalanges.

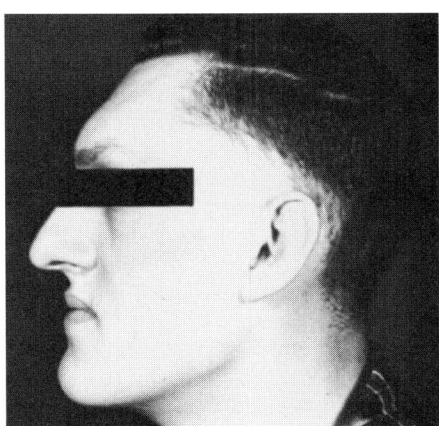

FIG. 59-6   Profile of a patient with acromegaly. There is prominence of the supraorbital ridges and of the nose and coarsening of facial features. Note the mandibular enlargement with prognathism.

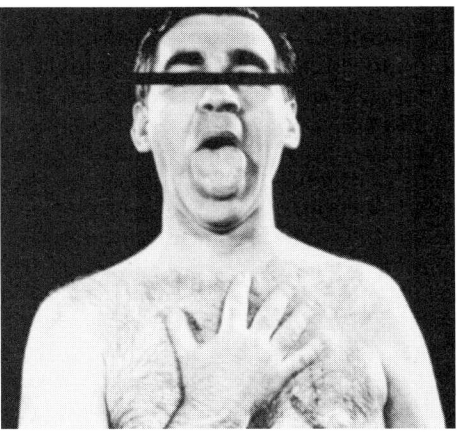

FIG. 59-7   Enlargement of the tongue in a patient with acromegaly. Note also acromegalic hand.

the need for a larger size of glove. The feet also become larger and wider, and patients describe changes in shoe size (Fig. 59-4). The enlargement is usually caused by growth and thickening of bones and by increased growth of soft tissue (Fig. 59-5).

In addition, changes in facial features help diagnose the condition on simple observation. Facial features become coarse, and there is enlargement of the paranasal and frontal sinuses. Frontal bossing, prominence of the supraorbital ridges, and deformity of the mandible with development of prognathism and underbite (Fig. 59-6) also occur. Enlargement of the mandible causes the teeth to spread apart. Enlargement of the tongue occurs, which causes difficulty with speech (Fig. 59-7). The voice becomes deeper as a result of thickening of the vocal chords.

Deformities of the spine, caused by overgrowth of bone, lead to back pain and changes in the physiologic curvature of the spine. The radiographic examination of the skull in acromegaly shows typical changes, including enlargement of paranasal sinuses, thickening of the calvaria, deformity of the mandible (which resembles a boomerang), and most importantly, enlargement and destruction of the sella turcica, suggesting a pituitary tumor (Fig. 59-8).

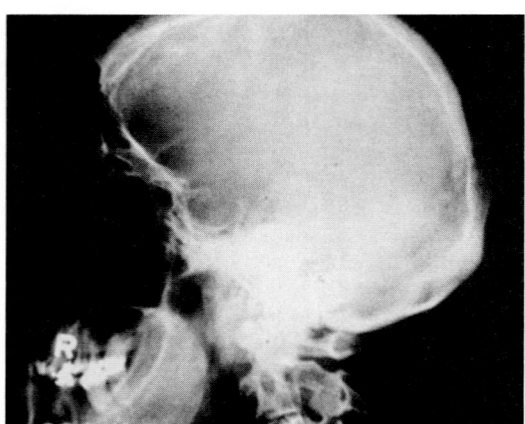

FIG. 59-8 Radiographic appearance of the skull of a patient with acromegaly. There is marked enlargement and destruction of the sella turcica and suggestion of intrasellar calcification. The calvaria is thick, and there is marked prominence of the frontal and paranasal sinuses. The angle of the mandible is rounded. There is also evidence of underbite.

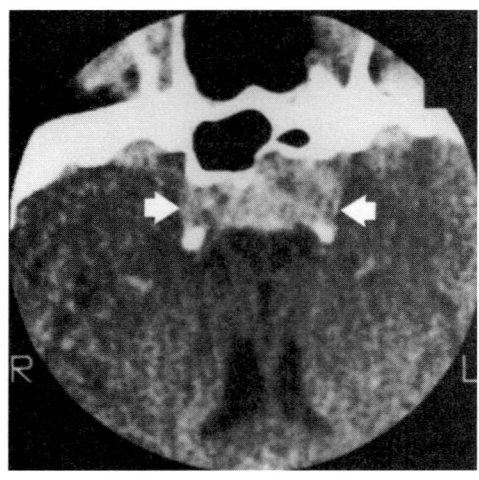

FIG. 59-9 Coronal cut of the sella turcica as shown on this computed tomography (CT) scan of a patient with a large prolactin-secreting macroadenoma. The enhancing intrasellar mass extends superiorly and laterally beyond the confines of the sella turcica. Also, there is destruction of the floor of the sella, which, instead of a straight horizontal contour, has an irregular appearance.

When acromegaly is associated with a pituitary tumor, the patients may exhibit bitemporal headaches and visual disturbance with bitemporal hemianopsia resulting from suprasellar extension of the tumor and compression of the optic chiasma.

Patients with acromegaly exhibit high basal GH and IGF-1 levels and can be tested further by the administration of oral glucose. In normal subjects, the induction of hyperglycemia by oral glucose suppresses GH levels. In contrast, patients with acromegaly or giantism fail to suppress GH levels.

Computed tomography (CT) scanning and magnetic resonance imaging (MRI) of the sella turcica demonstrate pituitary microadenomas, as well as macroadenomas with extrasellar extension involving the suprasellar cistern, the parasellar regions, or the sphenoid sinus (Fig. 59-9).

Treatment of acromegaly or giantism is rather complex. Pituitary irradiation, surgery to the pituitary gland to resect a pituitary tumor, or combinations of these procedures may result in amelioration or remission of the disease. Medical treatment using octreotide, a somatostatin analog, is also available. Octreotide can induce sustained suppression of GH and IGF-1 levels, decrease in tumor size, and marked clinical improvements.

Prolactin-Secreting Pituitary Tumors

The combination of persistent milk discharge and absent menses—*galactorrhea-amenorrhea*—is a relatively common endocrine syndrome in women and is associated with increased prolactin secretion.

The presence of galactorrhea is usually demonstrated by manual expression of the nipple, although it may occur spontaneously and range from mild to severe. The elevated prolactin levels probably cause the associated amenorrhea. Prolactin is believed to inhibit the secretion of gonadotropic hormones by interfering with the hypo-

thalamic secretion of GnRH. In addition, prolactin may block the effect of gonadotropins on the gonad.

Approximately 20% of patients with galactorrhea exhibit a prolactin-secreting pituitary adenoma. In many instances, the adenoma is small and barely detectable by radiographic visualization of the sella turcica. In other instances, larger pituitary adenomas have been described. Normal prolactin levels range from 2 to 25 ng/ml. In patients with prolactin-secreting pituitary adenomas, levels may range from 100 ng/ml for small tumors to greater than 1000 ng/ml for large pituitary tumors.

Other patients may have galactorrhea and elevated prolactin levels without detectable pituitary adenomas; they may have undergone interruption of the normal tonic inhibition of prolactin release by the hypothalamus. Galactorrhea can be observed with (1) hypothalamic lesions that interrupt the release of dopamine, (2) drugs with effects on the central nervous system (phenothiazines, antidepressants, haloperidol, alpha-methyldopa), (3) oral contraceptives and estrogens, (4) endocrine disorders such as hypothyroidism and hyperthyroidism, (5) local neurogenic factors, (6) breast stimulation, (7) chest wall injury, and (8) spinal cord lesions.

In the presence of the galactorrhea-amenorrhea syndrome, it is necessary to obtain a basal serum prolactin level. If the prolactin level is elevated above normal, radiographic examination of the sella turcica should be performed, including CT with coronal cuts and MRI of the pituitary gland. These studies may demonstrate the presence of abnormalities suggestive of a pituitary microadenoma.

When the diagnosis of a prolactin-secreting pituitary tumor is confirmed, two forms of treatment are usually available: (1) transsphenoidal resection of the prolactin-secreting pituitary tumor and (2) suppression of prolactin secretion by the administration of bromocriptine, or pergolide, an ergot derivative with potent dopamine receptor agonist activity. Treatment of hyperprolactinemia by the methods described frequently leads to disappearance of galactorrhea and restoration of normal menstrual cycles and fertility.

Prolactin-secreting pituitary tumors also occur in men, in whom the hyperprolactinemia is associated with hypogonadism and oligospermia. These tumors are frequently large and extend beyond the confines of the sella turcica. The management of prolactin-secreting pituitary microadenomas in men is similar to that described for women. In patients with large prolactin-secreting macroadenomas, bromocriptine may result in rapid and dramatic decrease in tumor size, without the need for surgical resection.

Disorders of Vasopressin Secretion

Arginine vasopressin (AVP) is an antidiuretic hormone (ADH) synthesized in the supraoptic and paraventricular nuclei of the hypothalamus together with its binding protein, *neurophysin II*. AVP is then transported from the neuronal bodies, where it is produced, along the axons to nerve terminals in the posterior pituitary gland, where it is stored. AVP and its inactive neurophysin are then secreted in response to specific stimuli. The secretion of AVP is regulated by stimuli that arise in osmotic and volume receptors. An increase in extracellular fluid osmolality or a decrease in intravascular volume stimulates AVP secretion. AVP then binds to a receptor, AVPR 2, in the renal tubule through which it activates *adenylate cyclase* and increases the generation of cyclic adenosine monophosphate (cAMP). This action, in turn, increases the permeability of the renal collecting duct epithelium to water. In addition, vasopressin regulates a water channel, aquaporin (AqP2) through which water is reabsorbed. As a result, urine concentration increases and serum osmolality decreases to normal. Serum osmolality is usually kept constant within narrow limits between 280 and 296 mOsm/kg water (H_2O). With normal renal function, maximal renal concentration is associated with a urine osmolality of 1200 mOsm/kg H_2O.

Disturbances of AVP secretion include *diabetes insipidus (DI)* and the *syndrome of inappropriate ADH secretion (SIADH)* (also see Chapter 21). In patients with DI, the disorder may be secondary to a destruction of the hypothalamic nuclei where vasopressin is synthesized (*central* DI) or the result of unresponsiveness of the renal tubules to vasopressin (*nephrogenic* DI) in spite of very high levels of this hormone.

Several conditions may result in DI, including tumors of the hypothalamus, large pituitary tumors that extend above the sella turcica and destroy the hypothalamic nuclei, head trauma, surgical injury of the hypothalamus, intracerebral vascular occlusions, and granulomatous diseases. In many cases a lesion is not detectable by available imaging techniques. Nephrogenic DI can be inherited through mutations in the vasopressin receptor or in AqP2, the water channel, and is manifested in children less than 2 years of age. In the adult, nephrogenic DI is usually acquired as a result of a variety of renal and systemic diseases that involve the kidney, including multiple myeloma, sickle cell anemia, hypercalcemia, and hypokalemia. Lithium therapy

for bipolar disorder can also cause unresponsiveness to vasopressin.

Patients with DI have *polydipsia* and *polyuria* with urine volumes between 5 and 10 L/day. These large renal losses of water are compensated for by increased water intake. If unable to keep up oral intake of water, patients become dehydrated, experience weight loss, and have dry skin and mucous membranes. Because of the ingestion of large quantities of water required to maintain hydration, these patients also complain of epigastric fullness and anorexia. The thirst and urination usually continue during the night, and patients have interrupted sleep with frequent nocturia. Patients usually prefer the ingestion of ice cold water. Serum osmolality is increased with values frequently greater than 300 mOsm/kg H_2O. Concomitantly, urine osmolality is low, between 100 and 200 mOsm/kg H_2O. Because patients are dehydrated, renal function may be impaired and blood urea nitrogen (BUN) and serum creatinine may be increased. When patients with suspected DI are asked to withhold fluids for 18 hours, their urine specific gravity fails to increase and urine osmolality remains low. When patients adhere strictly to water deprivation during this test, thirst may become intense and they may develop orthostatic hypotension and experience significant weight loss. The subcutaneous administration of aqueous vasopressin to patients with central DI is associated with antidiuresis. Urine volume decreases and the specific gravity increases immediately after the administration of vasopressin. These patients have a deficiency of vasopressin but have normal renal responses to the hormone. In contrast, patients with nephrogenic DI fail to respond to AVP.

Central DI is treated with AVP. The most frequently used preparation is 1-desamino-8D-arginine vasopressin (DDAVP), which is administered intranasally or orally and has a duration of action of 12 to 24 hours. AVP is not effective in patients with nephrogenic DI. Nephrogenic DI is managed with fluid replacement, treatment of the underlying renal disease and discontinuation of lithium therapy if possible. Treatment with a combination of hydrochlorothiazide and amiloride may decrease the severity of the polyuria. In children with nephrogenic DI, the condition improves with age.

SIADH is usually observed in association with diseases that affect the hypothalamus or the lungs or subsequent to drug administration. Patients develop a *hypoosmolar syndrome* with excessive and inappropriate water retention. Symptoms result from severe *hyponatremia* and involve the central nervous system (CNS) with irritability, mental confusion, seizures, and coma, especially when the serum sodium decreases below 120 mEq/L. Serum osmolality is low, and urine osmolality is high and elevated above serum osmolality. In these patients, BUN and serum creatinine levels are low and urine sodium is greater than 20 mEq/L.

Treatment of SIADH is based on water restriction to less than 1000 ml/day and the administration of 3% to 5% sodium chloride solutions together with furosemide. The diuretic induces the loss of water and sodium chloride, which is restored in a hypertonic form. Demeclocycline, a drug that directly inhibits the effect of AVP at the renal tubule level, can be used effectively to reverse the hypoosmolality associated with SIADH.

KEY CONCEPTS

- The *pituitary gland (hypophysis)* lies within a bony wall cavity, the sella turcica of the sphenoid bone, in close proximity to the optic chiasm and the cavernous sinuses. Thus tumors of the pituitary may lead to visual field defects, cranial nerve palsies, or invasion of the sphenoid sinus.

- The pituitary gland has two components: (1) the *adenohypophysis* (anterior lobe), derived from Rathke's pouch, and (2) the *neurohypophysis* (posterior lobe), an extension of the ventral portion of the hypothalamus.

- Various cell types of the anterior pituitary produce seven different hormones: adrenocorticotropic hormone (ACTH), melanocyte stimulating hormone (MSH), thyrotropin (TSH), growth hormone (GH), follicle stimulating hormone (FSH), luteinizing hormone (LH), and prolactin (PRL).

- The *anterior pituitary* is called the *master gland*, because, together with the hypothalamus, it orchestrates the complex regulatory functions of many endocrine glands in the body.

- Anterior pituitary hormones are under feedback control by target gland hormone levels; thus pituitary hormone levels in the blood rise when the target gland fails. The anterior pituitary, in turn, is under control of the hypothalamus via *hypothalamic–releasing and inhibiting hormones* transported to the pituitary via the *hypothalamic portal vessels* in the pituitary stalk.

- In addition to releasing and inhibiting hormones, the hypothalamus synthesizes two other hormones, *oxytocin* and *antidiuretic hormone (ADH)* or *vasopressin (AVP)*, which are transported to the posterior pituitary (neurohypophysis) for storage. In response to neural stimuli, these hormones are released from storage in the *posterior pituitary* gland.

- *Diseases of the anterior pituitary* may come to clinical attention because of increased or decreased secretion of hormones, designated *hyperpituitarism* or *hypopituitarism* or by *pressure from a neoplasm on adjacent structures*, such as the optic chiasm. Thus tumors of the pituitary may lead to visual field defects, cranial nerve palsies, or invasion of the sphenoid sinus.

- *Hypopituitarism* results from impaired production of one or more of the anterior pituitary hormones, which can result from diseases of the pituitary or hypothalamus.

- Pituitary insufficiency typically affects all the hormones normally secreted by the anterior pituitary and is termed *panhypopituitarism*.

- The most important *pituitary causes of panhypopituitarism* include (1) *surgical removal or radiation therapy* of a pituitary tumor, (2) obliteration of normal pituitary by a *primary benign pituitary tumor* or metastatic tumor (e.g., breast cancer), and (3) ischemic necrosis of the anterior pituitary following a severe fall in blood pressure, most commonly associated with intrapartum or postpartum hemorrhage (*Sheehan's syndrome*). Rare causes include inflammation (autoimmune hypophysitis, sarcoidosis) or trauma from skull fracture.

- Hypothalamic causes of *panhypopituitarism* include destruction of the hypothalamus by a primary brain tumor (e.g., craniopharyngioma), infarction, or inflammation (e.g., sarcoidosis).

- Clinical manifestations of *panhypopituitarism in children* include *pituitary dwarfisms* (GH deficiency), failure of normal adolescent sexual development (LH and FSH deficiency), varying degrees of adrenal insufficiency (ACTH deficiency), hypothyroidism (TSH deficiency), and pale skin (MSH deficiency).

- Clinical manifestations of *panhypopituitarism in adults* usually occur in the following sequence: loss of GH (insulin sensitivity, fasting hypoglycemia), loss of FSH and LH (impotence, decreased libido, muscle mass, beard and body hair growth in men; amenorrhea, atrophy of breasts and external genitalia in women); loss of TSH (hypothyroidism), loss of ACTH (adrenal insufficiency), and loss of MSH (causes a pale or sallow appearance).

- *Biochemical diagnosis* of pituitary insufficiency is made by demonstrating low levels of the anterior tropic hormones, as well as low levels of hormone produced by the target gland. *Stimulation tests* may be required to test pituitary reserve: GH, ACTH, cortisol responses to insulin-induced hypoglycemia; prolactin and TSH responses to injection of thyrotropin-releasing hormone (TRH); and FSH and LH responses to GnRH—patients with panhypopituitarism fail to respond to these provocative tests.

- *Pituitary CT and MRI* are important radiographic diagnostic methods, because pituitary adenomas are the most common cause of both pituitary hormone hyposecretion and hypersecretion syndromes in adults.

- *Treatment of hypopituitarism* consists of hormone replacement therapy including Human GH to children with pituitary dwarfism, target gland hormones—hydrocortisone, thyroxine, androgens, or estrogens.

- *Prolactin (PRL)* secretion differs from the other hormones of the anterior pituitary in that it is under tonic inhibitory control of the hypothalamus, mediated by dopamine.

- *Hyperprolactinemia* is the most common pituitary hypersecretion syndrome in both males and females, and a (benign) prolactin-secreting pituitary microadenoma or macroadenoma is the most common cause; other causes include pregnancy and lactation (physiologic), chest wall injury, hypothalamic lesions that interrupt the release of dopamine (e.g., craniopharyngioma), drugs that inhibit dopamine receptors (e.g., phenothiazines, antidepressants), hypothyroidism, and chronic renal failure.

- *In nonpregnant, nonpostpartum women, amenorrhea, galactorrhea (milk production), and infertility* are the hallmarks of *hyperprolactinemia*; if the tumor extends beyond the sella turcica, visual field defects may be seen from pressure on the optic chiasma.

- *Men with hyperprolactinemia* usually present with *impotence, diminished libido, infertility, or signs of central*

CNS compression, such as headache or visual field defects (e.g., hemianopsia) because their tumors are generally larger (macroadenomas).

■ *Diagnosis of hyperprolactinemia* is likely with *PRL levels above 100 μg/dL* caused by microadenomas, other sellar lesions that decrease dopamine inhibition, or other nonneoplastic conditions causing hyperprolactinemia; the finding of an elevated PRL should be followed by a pituitary CT scan or MRI, which may reveal a microadenoma or other lesion.

■ *Bromocriptine or pergolide*, potent dopamine-receptor agonists, is the *treatment of choice* for patients with hyperprolactinemia; dopamine agonists suppress PRL secretion and synthesis, as well as lactotrope cell proliferation; *transsphenoidal surgical resection* (using an endonasal approach) of large PRL-secreting tumors may be necessary when there are visual defects or inadequate response to drug treatment.

■ *Growth hormone (GH) hypersecretion* is usually the result of *somatotrope adenomas* or from a hypothalamic abnormality that leads to increased GH release; rarely, it may be caused by an extrapituitary neoplasm that releases GHRH ectopically.

■ *GH hypersecretion* during childhood and adolescence before epiphyseal closure results in *gigantism* and in adults who have completed growth—*acromegaly*.

■ *Clinical features of acromegaly* include coarse facial features with prominent supraorbital ridges, frontal bossing, enlarged mandible, thick ears and nose; enlarged, spade-shaped hands and feet; prognathism causing chewing difficulty; enlarged tongue causing speech difficulty; deep, husky voice caused by enlargement of the larynx; and deformities of the spine.

■ Bitemporal hemianopsia and headaches may present when acromegaly is associated with suprasellar extension of the pituitary adenoma with pressure on the optic chiasma.

■ *Diagnostic tests for GH hypersecretion* include serial photographs, GH suppression test with oral glucose, and CT scan and MRI of the sella turcica revealing tumor size.

■ The goals of *treatment of GH hypersecretion* are to restore GH levels to normal and to decrease symptoms referable to a pituitary mass lesion. To achieve these goals, the tumor may be removed surgically by a transsphenoidal approach or destroyed by irradiation; GH secretion can also be reduced by drug therapy with octreotide, a somatostatin analog.

■ The most common disorder of the neurohypophysis (posterior pituitary) is a deficiency of *arginine vasopressin (AVP)* or *antidiuretic hormone (ADH)* secretion producing the syndrome called *central diabetes insipidus (DI)* or of unresponsiveness of the renal tubules to ADH called *nephrogenic DI*.

■ Causes of *central DI* include head trauma, surgical injury of the pituitary or its stalk, inflammatory or neoplastic lesions of the hypothalamus or pituitary; *nephrogenic DI* results from a variety of renal diseases, lithium therapy, or systemic diseases affecting the kidney, such as multiple myeloma.

■ *DI* is characterized by polyuria, polydipsia, and hyperosmolality of the blood; central DI is treated with DDAVP, preferably by intranasal spray.

■ *Nephrogenic DI* is managed by fluid replacement, treatment of the underlying renal disease, and discontinuation of lithium therapy if possible. AVP is not effective in patients with nephrogenic DI.

■ *Syndrome of inappropriate secretion of ADH (SIADH)* is the most common cause of hypoosmolality (<275 mOsm/kg water), and it is associated with excess sodium excretion with excess water retention. (See Chapter 21.)

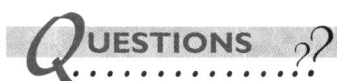

QUESTIONS

Match the statements in column A with the structures of the pituitary gland in column B.

Column A

1. _____ Derived from neural cells of the developing third ventricle
2. _____ Derived from Rathke's pouch
3. _____ Connected to the hypothalamus by the hypothalamic-hypophyseal portal system
4. _____ Confined within the sella turcica of the sphenoid bone

Column B

a. Adenohypophysis
b. Neurohypophysis
c. Both adenohypophysis and neurohypophysis

Match the hormones in column A with one of the functions in column B.

Column A
5. _____ Adrenocorticotropic hormone (ACTH)
6. _____ Growth hormone (GH)
7. _____ Luteinizing hormone (LH)
8. _____ Follicle-stimulating hormone (FSH)
9. _____ Prolactin
10. _____ Thyrotropin
11. _____ Melanocyte-stimulating hormone (MSH)
12. _____ Vasopressin

Column B
a. Stimulates spermatogenesis in men
b. Stimulates the formation and release of thyroid hormones
c. Initiates milk secretion after parturition
d. Stimulates the secretory activity of the adrenal cortex
e. Produces IGF-1
f. Decreases free water clearance
g. Stimulates the corpus luteum to secrete progesterone in women
h. Increases pigmentation of the skin

Answer the following on a separate sheet of paper.
13. Explain the medical treatment currently being tested for treatment of acromegaly or giantism.
14. How is human GH produced?
15. List four pathologic processes that may result in pituitary insufficiency.

16. What are the likely complications when patients with suspected DI are requested to withhold fluids for 18 hours? Explain the rationale for the administration of aqueous vasopressin.
17. What is the rationale for the treatment of SIADH?

Thyroid Gland Disorders

DAVID E. SCHTEINGART

GENERAL CONSIDERATIONS

The thyroid gland has two lobes joined by a thin isthmus and is located below the cricoid cartilage in the neck. Embryologically, the thyroid gland originates from an evagination of the pharyngeal epithelium, which carries with it cells from the lateral pharyngeal pouches. This evagination descends from the base of the tongue into the neck until it reaches its final anatomic location. Some thyroid tissue occasionally may be left along this track, giving rise to thyroglossal cysts, nodules, or a pyramidal thyroid lobe. The thyroid gland normally weighs between 10 and 20 g in adults. Histologically, the gland is made up of nodules composed of tiny follicles separated from each other by connective tissue (Fig. 60-1). The thyroid follicles are lined with cuboidal epithelium, and their lumen is filled with colloid. The follicular epithelial cells initiate the synthesis of thyroid hormones and activate their release into the circulation. The colloidal material, *thyroglobulin*, is where thyroid hormones are synthesized and eventually stored. The two principal hormones produced by the follicles are *thyroxine* and *triiodothyronine*. Another hormone-secreting cell within the thyroid gland is the *parafollicular cell*, or *C cell*, found in the basal portion of the follicle in contact with the follicular membrane. These cells originate in the embryologic ultimo-

branchial body and secrete *calcitonin*, a hormone that lowers serum calcium levels and thus contributes to the regulation of calcium homeostasis. The follicular thyroid hormones are derived from the iodination of tyrosyl residues in thyroglobulin. Thyroxine (T_4) contains four iodine atoms, and triiodothyronine (T_3) contains three iodine atoms (Fig. 60-2). T_4 is secreted in larger quantities than is T_3, but when compared on a milligram-per-milligram basis, T_3 is the more active of the two hormones.

Biosynthesis and Metabolism of Thyroid Hormones

The biosynthesis of thyroid hormones involves a sequence of steps regulated by specific enzymes. These steps are (1) trapping of iodide, (2) oxidation of iodide to iodine, (3) organification of iodine into monoiodotyrosine and diiodotyrosine, (4) coupling of iodinated precursors, (5) storage, and (6) hormone release (Fig. 60-3). The trapping of iodide by the thyroid follicular cells is an active, energy-requiring process. This energy is derived from oxidative metabolism within the gland. Iodide is available to the thyroid from ingested food or fluids or that released by deiodination of thyroid hormones or iodinated agents. The thyroid takes up and concentrates 20 to 30 times the amount of iodide present in plasma. Iodide is converted to iodine, catalyzed by an iodide peroxidase enzyme. Iodine is then incorporated into a tyrosine molecule, a process described as *organification of iodine*. This process takes place at the cell-colloid interphase. The resulting compounds, monoiodotyrosine and diiodotyrosine, are then coupled as follows: two molecules of diiodotyrosine make T_4, and one molecule of diiodotyrosine and one molecule of monoiodotyrosine make T_3. The coupling of these compounds and the storage of the resulting hormones take place within thyroglobulin. Hormones are released from storage by incorporation of colloid droplets into the follicular cells by a process called *pinocytosis*. Within these cells, thyroglobulin is hydrolyzed and the hormones are released into the circulation. The various steps described are stimulated by thyrotropin (thyroid-stimulating hormone [TSH]).

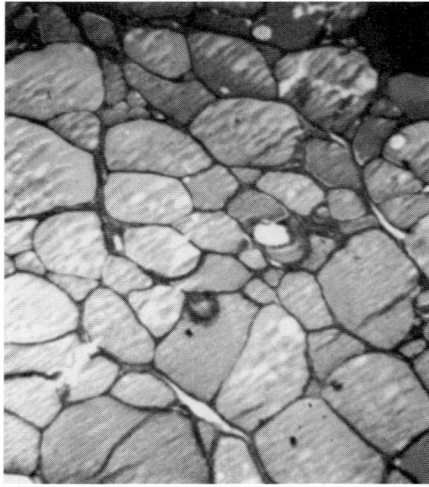

FIG. 60-1 Histology of the thyroid gland. Note colloid of filled follicles.

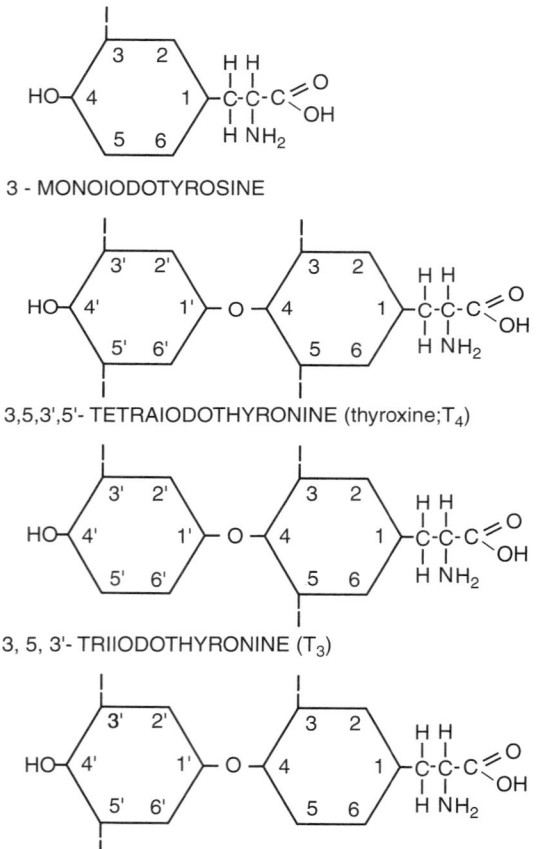

3 - MONOIODOTYROSINE

3,5,3',5'- TETRAIODOTHYRONINE (thyroxine;T_4)

3, 5, 3'- TRIIODOTHYRONINE (T_3)

3, 3', 5'- TRIIODOTHYRONINE (reverse T_3; RT_3)

FIG. 60-2 Chemical structures of thyroid hormones.

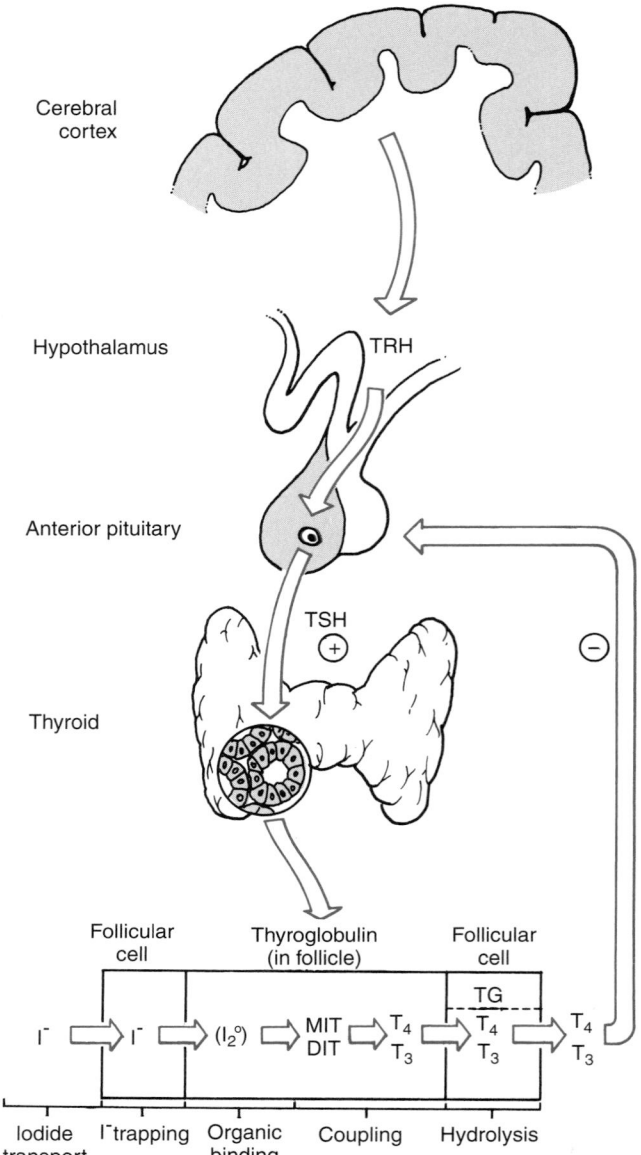

FIG. 60-3 Synthesis and secretion of thyroid hormones. The box indicates steps that occur within the thyroid gland. Thyroid function is regulated by the hypothalamic-pituitary axis. *TRH*, Thyrotropin-releasing hormone; *TSH*, thyroid-stimulating hormone (thyrotropin); *MIT*, monoiodotyrosine; *DIT*, diiodotyrosine; *TG*, thyroglobulin; T_3, triiodothyronine; T_4, thyroxine; $I_2°$, iodine; I^-, iodide. (Modified from Ezrin C et al, editors: *Systematic endocrinology*, ed 2, New York, 1979, Harper & Row.)

Thyroid hormones circulate in plasma bound to plasma proteins: (1) thyroxine-binding globulin (TBG), (2) thyroxine-binding prealbumin (TBPA), and (3) thyroxine-binding albumin (TBA). Most of the circulating hormone is bound to these proteins, and a small proportion (less than 0.05%) is free. The bound and free hormones are in a state of reversible equilibrium. The free hormone is the fraction that is metabolically active, and the larger, protein-bound fraction is not readily accessible to target tissues. Of the three binding proteins, TBG binds thyroxine most specifically. In addition, thyroxine has greater affinity than does triiodothyronine for these binding proteins. As a consequence, triiodothyronine is transferred more readily to its target tissues, a factor that accounts for its greater metabolic activity.

Thyroid hormones are chemically altered before excretion. An important alteration is *deiodination*, which accounts for the disposal of 70% of the secreted hormone.

Another 30% is lost in the stool through biliary excretion as glucuronide or sulfate conjugates. As a result of deiodination, 80% of T_4 may be converted into 3,5,3'-triiodothyronine, and the remaining 20% is converted to reverse 3,3',5'-triiodothyronine (rT_3), a metabolically inactive hormone.

Thyroid function is controlled by the pituitary glycoprotein hormone TSH, which, in turn, is regulated by thyrotropin-releasing hormone (TRH), a hypothalamic neurohormone. Thyroxine exerts negative feedback regulation of TSH secretion by acting directly on the pituitary thyrotropes.

Several drugs and conditions can alter the synthesis, release, and metabolism of thyroid hormones. Drugs such as perchlorate and thiocyanate are capable of inhibiting thyroxine synthesis. As a result, they cause a decrease in thyroxine levels and, through negative feedback stimulation, an increase in release of TSH by the pituitary gland. This condition leads to enlargement of the thyroid gland and the development of a goiter. These drugs are therefore called *goitrogens*. Other drugs, such as thiourea derivatives and mercaptoimidazoles, can be used as antithyroid drugs because they inhibit the initial oxidation of iodide, the conversion of monoiodotyrosine to diiodotyrosine, or the coupling of iodotyrosine to produce iodothyronine. These drugs are useful in the treatment of conditions caused by excessive thyroid hormone secretion. Iodine, when given acutely and in large doses, is capable of blocking the organic binding and coupling reactions. The continued administration of large doses of iodine may lead to goiter development and a hyperthyroid state. Finally, drugs such as lithium carbonate and glucocorticoids inhibit thyroid hormone release.

Changes in the concentration of TBG can also cause changes in the level of total circulating thyroxine. Increases in TBG, as seen with pregnancy, birth control pills, hepatitis, primary biliary cirrhosis, and hepatocellular carcinoma, may lead to increased levels of protein-bound thyroxine. Conversely, decreases in TBG, as seen with chronic liver disease, severe systemic illness, nephrotic syndrome, large doses of glucocorticoids, androgens, and anabolic steroids, will cause a decrease in circulating protein-bound thyroxine.

Nutritional changes, such as those observed during fasting or carbohydrate- and protein-deprived diets, can decrease the proportion of thyroxine deiodinated to T_3 and increase the less metabolically active rT_3. This alteration in the deiodination of thyroxine appears to be a mechanism for fuel conservation in states of food deprivation.

Action of Thyroid Hormones

Thyroid hormones have effects on cellular growth, development, and energy metabolism. These effects are genomic, through the regulation of gene expression, and nongenomic, through direct effects on the cell cytosol, membrane, and mitochondria. To accomplish these effects, free thyroid hormones diffuse across the cell membrane and enter the nucleus, where they specifically bind and activate the thyroid hormone receptor. The activated thyroid hormone receptor then binds to nuclear deoxyribonucleic acid (DNA) through its DNA-binding domain and increases transcription of messenger ribonucleic acid (mRNA) and protein synthesis. More than 30 genes are regulated by thyroid hormone. Specifically, both thyroxine and triiodothyronine stimulate energy-producing electron transfer processes in the respiratory enzyme system of the cell mitochondria. The stimulation by thyroid hormones of oxidative processes leads to stimulation of thermogenesis. In addition to these thermogenic effects, thyroxine and triiodothyronine potentiate the action of epinephrine by increasing the sensitivity of beta-receptors to catecholamines. Thyroid hormones also stimulate somatic growth and are involved in the normal development of the central nervous system. In the absence of these hormones, mental retardation and delayed neurologic maturation is present at birth and in infancy.

Tests of Thyroid Function

The functional status of the thyroid gland can be ascertained by means of thyroid function tests. The following tests are currently used in the diagnosis of thyroid disease:
1. Serum total thyroxine and triiodothyronine levels
2. Free thyroxine
3. Serum TSH levels
4. Radioisotope thyroid uptake

The *serum thyroxine and triiodothyronine levels* are measured by radioligand assays. The measurement includes bound and free hormone. Normal levels for thyroxine are 4 to 11 μg/dl; for triiodothyronine, they are 80 to 160 ng/dl. The serum *free thyroxine* measures the metabolically active, circulating thyroxine levels.

Plasma TSH levels can be measured by a radioimmunometric assay; normal values, by the third-generation assay, range from 0.02 to 5.0 μU/ml. The plasma TSH level is a sensitive and reliable indicator of thyroid function. Values are high in patients with primary hypothyroidism, in whom the low thyroxine levels are associated with a feedback increase in pituitary TSH release. Conversely, values are below normal in patients with autonomous increase in thyroid function (Graves' disease, hyperfunctioning thyroid nodules) or in those receiving suppressive doses of exogenous thyroid hormone. With the availability of highly sensitive TSH radioimmunometric assays, this test alone can be used in the initial evaluation of patients with suspected thyroid disease.

Some tests can measure the metabolic response to circulating thyroid hormone levels but they are not routinely used in the clinical evaluation of thyroid function. These tests include the basal metabolic rate (BMR), which measures the oxygen consumption in the resting state; the serum cholesterol level; and the characteristics of response of the Achilles tendon reflex. In patients with hypothyroidism, the BMR is decreased and the serum cholesterol level is high. The Achilles tendon reflex shows slow relaxation. Opposite findings are seen in patients with hyperthyroidism.

The *radioactive iodine (^{123}I [RAI]) uptake test* measures the ability of the thyroid gland to trap and organify iodide. The patient receives a tracer dose of RAI, which the thyroid traps and concentrates over a 24-hour period. The radioactivity present over the thyroid is then calculated. Normally, the uptake ranges from 10% to 35% of the administered dose. Values are high in hyperthyroidism and low when the thyroid gland has been suppressed.

TABLE 60-1 ■ ■ ■

Thyroid Function Tests

Test	Hyperthyroidism	Hypothyroidism
RAI uptake	Increased	Decreased
Serum thyroxine	Increased	Decreased
Free thyroxine	Increased	Decreased
Serum TSH	Decreased	Increased

RAI, Radioactive iodine; *TSH,* thyroid-stimulating hormone

Hyperthyroidism and hypothyroidism are the two major functional abnormalities for which one needs reliable laboratory tools. Few supportive laboratory investigations may be required in severe cases. However, additional tests may be necessary in the diagnosis of mild cases of thyroid dysfunction. Table 60-1 summarizes the changes in thyroid function tests observed in patients with hypothyroidism and hyperthyroidism.

DISEASES OF THE THYROID GLAND

As with other endocrine diseases, those of the thyroid gland may involve the following:
1. Excessive thyroid hormone production (hyperthyroidism)
2. Deficient hormone production (hypothyroidism)
3. Thyroid enlargement (goiter) without evidence of abnormal thyroid hormone production

In addition, patients with severe systemic illnesses may develop changes in thyroxine metabolism and in thyroid function. These findings are known as euthyroid sick syndrome or nonthyroidal illness.

Hyperthyroidism

Also known as *thyrotoxicosis,* hyperthyroidism may be defined as the response of body tissues to the metabolic effects of excessive amounts of thyroid hormone. The condition may develop spontaneously or may result from the intake of excessive amounts of thyroid hormones. The most common types of spontaneous hyperthyroidism are (1) Graves' disease and (2) toxic nodular goiter.

Graves' disease usually occurs in the third and fourth decades of life and more frequently in women than men. There is familial predisposition to Graves' disease and frequent association with other forms of autoimmune endocrinopathy. In Graves' disease, the two major groups of features are thyroidal and extrathyroidal, either of which may be absent. The thyroidal features include a goiter, caused by hyperplasia of the thyroid gland, and hyperthyroidism, which results from excessive thyroid hormone secretion. Symptoms of hyperthyroidism include manifestations of hypermetabolism and of sympathetic overactivity. Patients complain of fatigue; tremor; heat intolerance; increased sweating with warm, moist skin; weight loss, often with increased appetite; palpitations and tachycardia; diarrhea; and muscle weakness and atrophy. The extrathyroidal manifestations include ophthalmopathy and localized skin infiltrations, usually confined to the lower legs. The ophthalmopathy, present

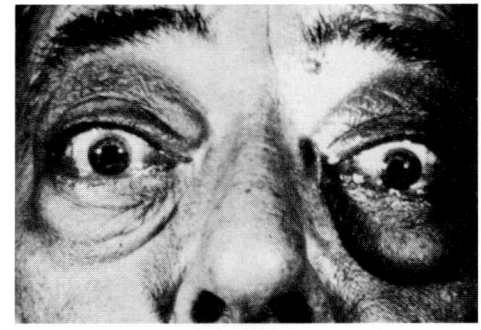

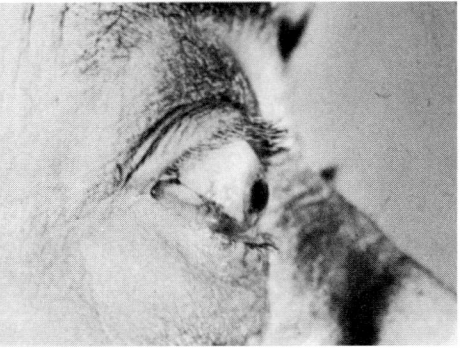

FIG. 60-4 Exophthalmos with periorbital edema in a patient with Graves' ophthalmopathy. **A,** Frontal view. **B,** Lateral view. (Courtesy James C. Sisson, MD, Department of Internal Medicine, University of Michigan.)

in 50% to 80% of these patients, is characterized by stare, widening of the palpebral fissures, decreased blinking, lid lag, and failure of convergence. The lid lag is characterized by a slower movement of the eyelid relative to the eyeball when patients are asked to slowly lower their gaze. Infiltration of the orbital tissues and ocular muscles with lymphocytes, mast cells, and plasma cells leads to exophthalmos (proptosis of the eyeballs), congestive oculopathy, and weakness of extraocular movements (Fig. 60-4, *A* and *B*). The ophthalmopathy can be quite severe, and in extreme cases, vision may be threatened. The extrathyroidal manifestations of Graves' disease may follow a clinical course that does not parallel the severity of hyperthyroidism. For example, these manifestations may be absent or may progress when the hyperthyroidism is minimal or has been controlled by treatment. Graves' disease develops as a manifestation of an autoimmune disorder. An immunoglobulin G (IgG) antibody is present in the serum of these patients. This antibody appears to react with the TSH receptor or the thyroid plasma membrane. As a result of this interaction, the antibody is capable of stimulating thyroid function independently of pituitary TSH, leading to hyperthyroidism. This thyroid-stimulating immunoglobulin (TSI) may result from an inherited abnormality of immune surveillance that permits a particular clone of lymphocytes to survive, proliferate, and secrete stimulatory immunoglobulins in response to some precipitating factor. A similar immune response appears to be responsible for the ophthalmopathy observed in these patients.

Toxic nodular goiter develops most frequently in older patients as a complication of chronic nontoxic nodular goiter. The onset of hyperthyroidism in these patients is insidious, and the clinical manifestations of hyperthyroidism are less severe than those in Graves' disease. Patients may present with dysrhythmias and heart failure resistant to digitalis therapy. Patients may also show evidence of weight loss, weakness, and muscle wasting. The multinodular goiter usually present in these patients contrasts with the diffuse thyroid enlargement seen in patients with Graves' disease. Patients with toxic nodular goiter may show eye signs (stare, widening of palpebral fissure, decreased blinking) resulting from sympathetic overactivity; however, they lack the more dramatic manifestations of infiltrative ophthalmopathy seen in Graves' disease.

Patients with severe manifestations of hyperthyroidism may develop thyroid crisis or storm. In these cases, there is a general worsening of the clinical manifestations described earlier, to the point where they become life threatening. Fever is almost always present and may be an important clue to the onset of serious complications. This crisis can be precipitated by minor trauma and stress, such as an infectious illness, surgery, or anesthesia.

In the presence of clinical manifestations of hyperthyroidism, laboratory tests show high serum total and free thyroxine and triiodothyronine levels and low serum TSH. RAI uptake by the thyroid is increased. Patients with Graves' disease also have measurable levels of TSI. Occasionally, the therapeutic misuse of thyroid hormone leads to clinical manifestations of hyperthyroidism. Some patients with psychiatric illness may take large amounts of thyroxine or triiodothyronine and become thyrotoxic. These patients may deny taking thyroid hormones and pose a real challenge to the medical personnel attempting to establish the proper diagnosis. This form of thyrotoxicosis is called *thyrotoxicosis factitia.* Characteristic of this type of thyrotoxicosis is the presence of high thyroxine and low TSH levels. However, RAI uptake is low because the thyroid gland is suppressed.

Management of hyperthyroidism includes one or several of the following procedures:

1. Prolonged treatment with antithyroid drugs such as propylthiouracil or methimazole, given for at least 1 year; these drugs block thyroxine synthesis and release.
2. Beta blockers such as propranolol given together with the antithyroid drugs. Because the clinical manifestations of hyperthyroidism are the result of sympathetic activation induced by thyroid hormones, they can be significantly ameliorated by beta blockers; they decrease tachycardia, nervousness and excessive sweating. Propranolol also inhibits the peripheral conversion of thyroxine to triiodothyronine.
3. Surgical subtotal thyroidectomy after preoperative drug therapy with propylthiouracil.
4. Treatment with radioactive iodine (RAI).

Treatment with RAI is used in most adult patients with Graves' disease but is usually contraindicated in children and pregnant women. In patients with toxic nodular goiter, antithyroid drugs and ablative therapy with RAI can also be used. However, if the goiter is large and there are no contraindications for surgery, surgical resection of the goiter should be considered. Treatment of the ophthalmopathy of Graves' disease involves correction of hyper-

thyroidism and prevention of hypothyroidism that may develop after surgical or radiation ablative therapy. In many patients, the ophthalmopathy follows a self-limiting course and no further treatment is necessary. However, in severe cases in which vision is threatened, treatment with large doses of glucocorticoids and orbital decompression procedures may be necessary to salvage the eye. Hypothyroidism is a frequent outcome in patients with hyperthyroidism receiving surgical or RAI therapy. Of patients treated with RAI, 40% to 70% may go on to develop hypothyroidism over the following 10 years.

Hypothyroidism

There are several types of hypothyroidism. Depending on the location of the initiating problem, the disease can be classified as (1) *primary,* resulting from a pathologic process that destroys the thyroid gland, or (2) *secondary,* caused by deficiency of pituitary TSH secretion. Depending on the age of onset of the hypothyroid state, the disease can be classified as (1) adult hypothyroidism, or *myxedema,* (2) juvenile hypothyroidism (onset after age 1 to 2 years), or (3) congenital hypothyroidism, or *cretinism* caused by lack of thyroid hormone before or shortly after birth.

Some patients with hypothyroidism have an atrophic or absent thyroid gland as a result of surgical or radioisotopic ablation of the gland or because of its destruction by circulating autoimmune antibodies. Developmental defects may also account for the absence of a thyroid gland in a patient with congenital hypothyroidism. Goiters are often observed in hypothyroid patients with hereditary defects in thyroid hormone biosynthesis; the concomitant increase in TSH release causes thyroid enlargement. Goiters may also be seen in patients with *Hashimoto's thyroiditis,* an autoimmune disease in which lymphocytic infiltration and destruction of the thyroid gland supervene in association with antithyroglobulin or antithyroid cell microsomal antibodies. Patients with secondary hypothyroidism may have pituitary tumors and be deficient in other pituitary tropic hormones.

The clinical manifestations of hypothyroidism in the adult and juvenile forms include fatigue; hoarseness; cold intolerance and decreased sweating; cool, dry skin; facial puffiness; and slow movements (Fig. 60-5). There is slowing of intellectual and motor activity and slow relaxation of deep tendon reflexes. Women with hypothyroidism frequently complain of hypermenorrhea.

Congenital hypothyroidism, or cretinism, may be present at birth or become evident within the first several months of life. Early manifestations of cretinism include persistent physiologic jaundice, hoarse cry, constipation, somnolence, and feeding problems. Subsequently, the child shows delay in reaching the normal milestones of development. The child with congenital hypothyroidism exhibits short stature; coarse features; a protruding tongue; broad, flat nose; widely set eyes; sparse hair; dry skin; a protuberant abdomen; and umbilical hernia.

Radiographic examination of the skeleton shows retarded bone age, epiphyseal dysgenesis, and delayed dental development. A major complication of unrecognized and untreated congenital and juvenile hypothyroidism is mental retardation, which is preventable by

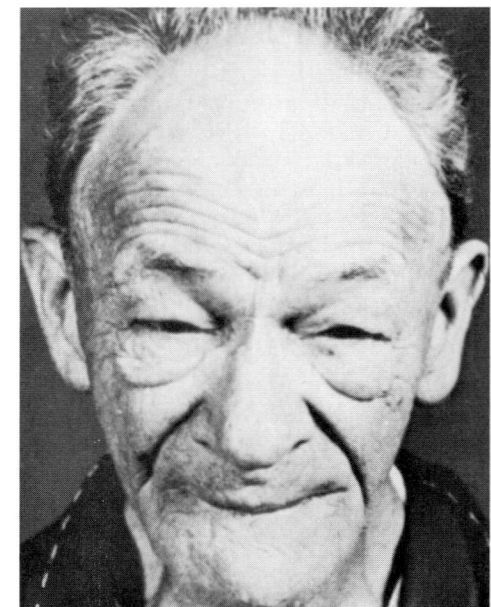
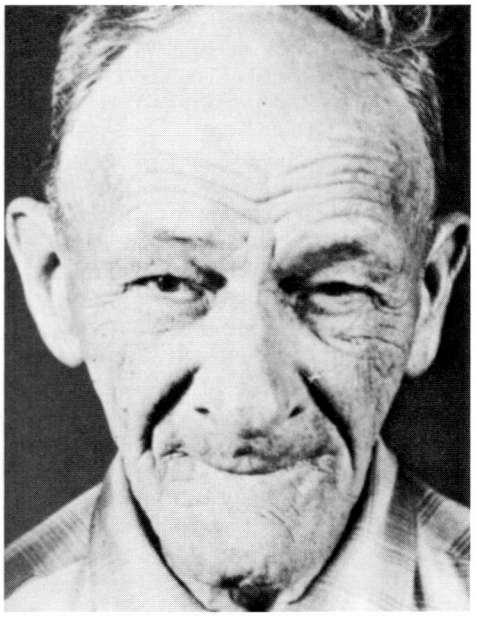

FIG. 60-5 Facial appearance of patient with myxedema. **A,** At the time of initial diagnosis. **B,** After replacement therapy with thyroxine. (Courtesy James C. Sisson, MD, Department of Internal Medicine, University of Michigan.)

early correction of hypothyroidism. Health care personnel attending newborn and small infants must be alert for this condition.

Laboratory test results that confirm the presence of hypothyroidism include low serum thyroxine and triiodothyronine levels, low BMR, and elevated serum cholesterol. Serum TSH levels may be high or low, depending on the type of hypothyroidism. In primary hypothyroidism, serum TSH levels are high, together with low thyroxine. In contrast, both measurements are low in patients with secondary hypothyroidism.

Treatment of hypothyroidism includes the administration of thyroxine, which is usually begun at low dosage levels (50 μg/day), especially in older patients or patients with severe myxedema, and gradually increased over days and weeks to a full maintenance dosage of 150 μg/day. In younger adults, a full maintenance dose can be started immediately. The measurement of TSH levels in patients with primary hypothyroidism is used to determine the adequacy of the replacement therapy. These levels should be maintained within the normal range. Adequacy of treatment in patients with secondary hypothyroidism should be determined by following the level of free thyroxine.

Nontoxic Goiters

Nontoxic, diffuse, colloid goiters and colloid nodular goiters are common disorders that affect 16% of women and 4% of men age 20 to 60, as demonstrated in a survey of Tecumseh, a community in Michigan. Patients usually have no symptoms other than the cosmetic appearance, but occasional complications may occur. The thyroid may be diffusely enlarged or contain nodules or both.

The causes of nontoxic goiter include iodine deficiency or an intrathyroidal chemical defect caused by a variety of factors. As a result of this defect, the thyroid gland has an impaired capacity to secrete thyroxine, leading to increased TSH levels and hyperplasia and hypertrophy of the thyroid follicles. The enlarged thyroid gland frequently undergoes exacerbations and remissions, with hypervolution and involution of areas of the thyroid gland. Fibrosis may alternate with hyperplasia, and nodules containing thyroid follicles may develop.

Clinically, patients may demonstrate a protuberance in the lower third of the neck. With large goiters, mechanical compression problems may develop, including displacement of the trachea and esophagus and symptoms of obstruction.

If the impairment of thyroid function is severe, the goiter may be accompanied by hypothyroidism. To ascertain the functional status of the goiter, measurements of serum free T_4 and TSH levels may be necessary. In addition, RAI or technetium pertechnetate scintiscans show whether the nodules are "cold" or "hot." Cold nodules may represent carcinoma, and hot nodules are nearly always benign. Ultrasound scanning of the thyroid gland may be used to detect cystic changes in thyroid nodules. Cystic nodules are rarely cancerous.

A direct way of determining if a thyroid nodule is benign or malignant is a fine needle aspiration biopsy and examination of the cytology of the lesion. This simple procedure can be performed in the physician's office.

Treatment of goiter involves suppression of TSH with thyroxine, which can eventually result in suppression of pituitary TSH and inhibition of thyroid function with atrophy of the thyroid gland. Surgery may be indicated for large goiters to remove the mechanical and cosmetic problems they cause. In communities where goiters develop as a consequence of iodide deficiency, the use of iodized table salt should be encouraged.

Thyroid Neoplasms

Thyroid neoplasms usually present as discrete enlargements of the thyroid gland. At times, the condition may resemble a benign nodular goiter. Thyroid nodules are clinically palpable in approximately 5% to 10% of adults in the United States. The majority of these nodules are benign, but some nodular goiters are carcinomatous. To determine whether a thyroid nodule is benign or malignant, known risk factors and the clinical characteristics of the mass should be assessed and certain laboratory studies performed.

Risk Factors

The risk of a carcinoma in a thyroid nodule is high, approximately 50%, in a child under 14 years of age. In contrast, the risk is less than 10% in adults. Men have a higher incidence of carcinomatous thyroid nodules than do women. The recent appearance of a nodule or rapid enlargement of a preexisting nodule should raise a suspicion that the nodule is malignant. Previous exposure to therapeutic radiation of the head and neck regions may also increase the risk of developing thyroid carcinoma in the future. The incidence of radiation exposure during childhood in patients under 15 years of age with thyroid carcinomas has been reported to be as high as 50%; for patients under 30 years of age, 20%. The incidence increases within the first 5 years after exposure and continues up to 30 years but then begins to decline. Certain types of thyroid cancer, such as medullary thyroid carcinoma, may occur with familial incidence. The discovery of a goiter in a patient with a positive family history for this type of carcinoma is therefore significant for the diagnosis of a thyroid malignancy.

Clinical Characteristics

A thyroid carcinoma should be suspected on clinical grounds if the nodule is single, hard on palpation, fixed to surrounding tissue, and associated with satellite lymphadenopathy.

It is generally agreed that thyroid cancer can be subdivided clinically into a large group of well-differentiated neoplasms of slow growth and high curability and a smaller group of highly anaplastic tumors with a uniformly fatal outlook. There are four main types of thyroid cancer according to morphology and biologic behavior: (1) papillary, (2) follicular, (3) medullary, and (4) anaplastic.

Papillary carcinoma is the most common type of thyroid cancer and accounts for 80% of malignant thyroid tumors in children and in adults less than 40 years of age. Papillary carcinoma is approximately twice as common in females as it is in males. These neoplasms grow slowly and spread via lymphatics to regional nodes in approximately 50% of the cases. Treatment is surgical excision of the affected lobe with removal of regional lymph nodes if they are suspected of being involved.

Follicular carcinoma composes approximately 20% of all thyroid cancers. The gender and age distributions are similar to those of papillary cancer, although the incidence is somewhat higher later in life. In its most indolent form, the tumor closely resembles normal thyroid tissue, although at times it may be rapidly progressive, spreading rapidly to distant sites. These tumors not only resemble thyroid follicles histologically but are also ca-

pable of taking up RAI. The mode of metastasis is via the bloodstream to distant sites, such as the lungs and bones. As with papillary tumors, the growth of this type of cancer is slow, with the disease evolving over many years. The treatment is total or nearly total thyroidectomy and removal of the involved lymph nodes. If metastases are present and capable of taking up RAI, ablation of the metastases with large doses of RAI can be carried out. After total thyroidectomy (by surgery or RAI), serum thyroglobulin should be undetectable. The level is elevated in patients with metastatic disease, and a rise is indicative of recurring disease.

Medullary thyroid carcinoma (MTC) is rather uncommon, comprising 5% to 10% of all cases. The cell of origin of this neoplasm is the parafollicular, or C, cell. Similar to its precursor cell, the tumor is capable of secreting calcitonin. MTC can occur as a sporadic tumor, usually involving one thyroid lobe or can be familial, occurring in members of families with multiple endocrine neoplasia (MEN) 2A and 2B. Patients with MEN 2A present with hyperparathyroidism and pheochromocytoma in addition to MTC. Patients with MEN 2B have, in addition, ganglioneuromas involving the tarsal plates of the eyelids, tongue, and lips and exhibit a marfanoid habitus. Members of these families have mutations of the RET protooncogene that can be used as a screening test to identify nonaffected members at risk for early thyroidectomy. Measuring serum calcitonin levels can follow the progression and clinical course of MTC. Although the tumor apparently grows slowly, it tends to metastasize to local lymph nodes at an early stage. Later, the tumor spreads by the bloodstream to the lungs, liver, bones, and other organs. Because of the tendency for early metastases, these types of cancer are treated with total thyroidectomy.

Anaplastic carcinomas of the thyroid are histologically undifferentiated and extremely malignant and often prove fatal in weeks or months. These carcinomas show evidence of early local invasion of structures surrounding the thyroid and of metastases, via both the lymphatics and the bloodstream. At present, this type of carcinoma is uniformly fatal regardless of the mode of treatment. Surgical resection should be attempted, followed by radiation therapy and chemotherapy.

Patients who have had resection of either papillary or follicular thyroid carcinomas should be followed for many years for evidence of recurrence or metastases. After thyroidectomy for papillary or follicular carcinoma, patients are placed on suppressive doses of levothyroxine. Periodically, patients are taken off thyroid replacement and stimulated with TSH. A large dose of RAI is administered, and the neck and the rest of the body are scanned for areas of RAI uptake. If metastases are detected in this manner, large ablative doses of RAI can be administered.

Euthyroid Sick Syndrome

Changes in thyroid function resembling hypothyroidism have been described in many hospitalized patients with severe systemic illness. In most of these patients, the level of free thyroxine is normal, and these patients are not truly hypothyroid but have euthyroid sick syndrome; they have low levels of T_3 and increased levels of rT_3; occasionally, serum T_4 levels also decrease. TSH levels are usually normal or only slightly above normal. These findings are explained by changes in T_4 conversion to T_3 and decreased binding of T_4 to binding proteins. The biochemical change that leads to these changes in thyroid function is a decrease in 5'-deiodination, which affects the conversion of T_4 to T_3 and the subsequent clearing of rT_3 to reverse T_2. A decrease in the total serum T_4 level is usually caused by a decrease in binding of T_4 to thyroxine-binding proteins. Patients with the most severe depression of serum thyroxine level have the least favorable prognosis.

KEY CONCEPTS

- The *thyroid* is a butterfly-shaped pure endocrine gland consisting of two lobes connected by an isthmus, which sits just below the cricoid cartilage in the neck.
- The *thyroid gland* secretes two different types of hormones from two cell types: (1) the *thyroid follicle cells*, which make up the bulk of the gland, produce the hormone *thyroxine (T_4)* and *triiodothyronine (T_3)*, and (2) the *parafollicular cells* or *"C cells,"* which are a minority population of cells in small clusters between the follicular cells that produce *calcitonin*, which is involved in calcium homeostasis.
- Control of thyroid hormone secretion is vested in the *hypothalamic-pituitary-thyroid axis*. Thyroid stimulating hormone (TSH), produced by the anterior pituitary, is under inhibitory negative feedback on the anterior pituitary related to levels of circulating thyroid hormone and stimulation by thyrotropin-releasing hormone (TRH) derived from the hypothalamus.
- Normal thyroid hormone secretion requires: adequate drive (TSH); adequate amounts of functioning thyroid tissue, adequate amounts of substrate (iodide), and adequate enzymes for organification and coupling. A deficiency of any one of these will lead to hypofunction of the gland.
- Thyroid hormones affect many systems. The *major effect is stimulation of cellular metabolism*. Thyroid hormones stimulate somatic growth in the child and are involved in the normal development of the central nervous system—absence of thyroid hormones at birth results in mental retardation and delayed neurologic development (*cretinism*).
- T_3 and T_4 are *transported in the blood* reversibly bound to the plasma proteins: (1) thyroxine-binding globulin (TBG) binds T_4 tightly and T_3 loosely; (2) thyroxine-binding prealbumin (TBPA); and (3) thyroxine-binding albumin (TBA). A small fraction of T_3 and T_4 are in the free metabolically active form and available to the tissues; free hormones are in reversible equilibrium with bound hormones. Any change in TBG leads to changes in the amount of circulating free T_4, producing changes in thyroid function test results.
- Eighty percent of T_3 is produced in the peripheral tissues from the deiodination of T_4; rT_3, an inactivated form of T_3, is a byproduct.
- *Rule of fours*: T_3 *is four times as strong as T_4 is in its metabolic effects; the metabolic effects of T_4 on the tissues lasts four times longer than those of T_3*; thus these two thyroid hormones balance each other quite well.
- Tests used for the diagnosis of thyroid disease include: (1) serum T_3 and T_4 levels, (2) free thyroxine, (3) serum TSH, and (4) radioisotope thyroid uptake (RAI) test. In hyperthyroidisms, all values are increased except serum TSH, which is decreased. In hypothyroidism all values are decreased except TSH, which is increased.
- The term *"goiter"* has been traditionally used to mean any *swelling of the thyroid gland*. Thyroid enlargement has many causes and may be associated with either decreased, increased (toxic goiter), or normal (nontoxic goiter) thyroid hormone output. These terms are best avoided because they are imprecise and imply no specific pathology.
- Hyperthyroidism or thyrotoxicosis may be defined as the response of the body to excessive T_3 or T_4 or both.
- The two major causes of hyperthyroidism are *Graves' disease*, occurring mainly in younger adults, and *toxic nodular goiter*, occurring mainly in older adults. Less common causes include self-administration of thyroid hormone (thyrotoxicosis factitia) or excessive production of TSH by a pituitary tumor (secondary hyperthyroidism).
- *Graves' disease* is a form of autoimmune thyroiditis that presents with symptoms of hyperthyroidism, diffuse enlargement of the thyroid gland, exophthalmos, and other signs and symptoms of hypermetabolism (heat intolerance, sweating, weight loss, tachycardia, anxiety, and restlessness).
- *Graves' disease* is caused by the presence of an IgG antibody called *long-acting thyroid stimulator (LATS)*, which acts directly on thyroid follicle cells, stimulating them to divide (causing hyperplasia) and to synthesize and secrete thyroid hormone continuously, out of control of TSH from the pituitary. The thyroid hormones are therefore synthesized and secreted irrespective of need and the normal feedback mechanism is bypassed.
- *Toxic nodular goiter* is characterized by small, discrete autonomously functioning nodules that secrete excess thyroid hormones. The onset is insidious and the clinical manifestations are less severe than those of Graves' disease. Exophthalmos is absent, but there may be staring and decreased blinking from the increased sympathetic activity.
- The *treatment* goal in the management of *hyperthyroidism* is to block the adverse effects of thyroid hormones and stop their hypersecretion by ablative therapy with RAI, surgical subtotal thyroidectomy, or prolonged treatment with propylthiouracil (blocks thyroxine synthesis). Beta blockers, such as propranolol, are given to decrease sympathetic activation, thus decreasing symptoms of nervousness, tachycardia, and excessive sweating.

- The signs and symptoms of *hypothyroidism* result from reduced output of thyroid hormone.
- *Hypothyroidism* in adults ranges from a severe disorder (*myxedema*) to one that may be much less severe and not uncommonly missed.
- Important causes of *primary hypothyroidism* include surgical or RAI ablative therapy for Graves' disease (most common) and Hashimoto's thyroiditis (an autoimmune disease, most common cause of thyroid disease in children). Other causes include living in an iodine-deficient geographic area (e.g., Michigan) and some drug therapy (e.g., lithium).
- *Secondary hypothyroidism* (rare) is caused by pituitary or hypothalamic dysfunction secondary to tumor or treatment with surgery or irradiation—there is deficiency of pituitary TSH secretion.
- *Characteristic clinical features of myxedema* include lethargy, periorbital edema and facial puffiness, hoarseness, dry, coarse, cold skin, bradycardia, slowing of intellectual and motor activity, and cold intolerance.
- *Laboratory* tests that confirm the presence of hypothyroidism include low serum T_4, low free T_3 and T_4, and elevated serum cholesterol. *TSH levels are high in primary hypothyroidism and low in secondary hypothyroidism.*
- *Treatment* of hypothyroidism includes the administration of T_4 starting at 50 μg/day and progressing to a maintenance dose of up to 150 μg/day. Adequacy of replacement therapy is determined by monitoring serum T_4, rT_3 uptake, and TSH.
- *Congenital hypothyroidism (cretinism)* may be caused by untreated maternal hypothyroidism or an inherited enzyme defect resulting in failure of normal T_3 and T_4 synthesis.
- It is important to detect *congenital hypothyroidism* (cretinism) before mental retardation and impairment of central nervous system development occurs.
- *Signs and symptoms of cretinism* that may be observed include hypoactive, somnolent infant causing feeding problems; hoarse cry; large tongue; persistent physiologic jaundice; and coarse, dry scaly skin. The diagnosis is confirmed by a radioimmunoassay showing decreased levels of T_4, T_3, and increased TSH. Treatment includes administration of Synthroid (T_4).
- *Nontoxic goiter* is defined as thyroid enlargement not associated with an inflammatory or a neoplastic process and not initially associated with hyperthyroidism or hypothyroidism.
- *Nontoxic goiter* may be caused by iodide deficiency or intrinsic defects in hormone synthesis, both of which will lead to increased output of TSH and thus to hyperplasia of the thyroid.
- Treatment of goiter involves suppression of TSH with thyroxine, surgical removal if large and causing tracheal obstruction, and iodized table salt for iodine-deficient geographic areas.
- *Euthyroid sick syndrome (ESS)* is the presence of abnormal thyroid function tests resembling hypothyroidism in patients with normal thyroid function but suffering from severe nonthyroidal systemic illness.
- The cause of ESS is believed to be decreased peripheral conversion of T_4 to T_3, increased conversion of T_4 to reverse T_3, and decreased binding of thyroid hormones to TBG; the result is decreased T_3, high rT_3, decreased serum total T_4, and normal TSH.
- A RAI scintiscan is a useful test to differentiate a benign from a malignant thyroid nodule; "hot" nodules (those taking up the isotope) are generally benign, and "cold" nodules (those that fail to take up the isotope) are more apt to be malignant (especially if hard, fixed to surrounding tissue, and accompanied by neck lymphadenopathy).
- There are three main types of malignant tumors derived from thyroid follicle cells: papillary carcinoma, follicular carcinoma, and anaplastic carcinoma of the thyroid.
- *Risk factors for thyroid cancer* include (1) thyroid nodule in a child under age 14 years (50% are malignant) and (2) irradiation exposure to the head or neck during infancy or childhood.
- *Medullary carcinoma of the thyroid* is derived from the parafollicular calcitonin-producing C cells of the thyroid. This type of thyroid cancer can be familial and associated with multiple endocrine neoplasia (MEN).

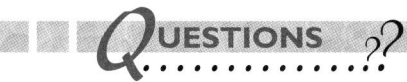

QUESTIONS ??

A sampling of review questions for this chapter appears here. Visit http://www.mosby.com/MERLIN/PriceWilson/ for additional questions.

Answer the following on a separate sheet of paper.

1. Describe the location and function of the follicular epithelial cells in the thyroid gland.

2. List the steps and describe the process of biosynthesis of thyroid hormones.

3. List the tests that are presently used in the diagnosis of thyroid disease.

4. After a total thyroidectomy, what is the significance of elevated serum thyroglobulin in patients with metastatic disease?

Fill in the blanks with the appropriate word or number.

5. The thyroid takes up and concentrates _____ to _____ times the amount of iodide present in the plasma.

6. Solitary, nonfunctioning thyroid nodules have a _____ % chance of being carcinomatous.

7. Normal levels of thyroxine _____ μg/dl; for triiodothyronine, _____ μg/dl.

8. Two types of spontaneous hyperthyroidism are _____ and _____.

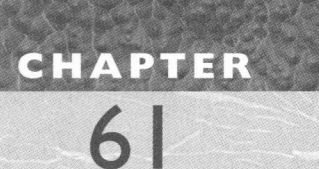

Adrenal Hypersecretion Disorders

DAVID E. SCHTEINGART

*T*his chapter focuses on three selected adrenocortical clinical entities: Cushing's syndrome, aldosteronism, and androgen excess. In addition, pheochromocytoma, a rare catecholamine-secreting tumor of the adrenal medulla, is discussed. The first discussion concentrates on situations in which the plasma concentration of cortisol increases above normal physiologic levels and results in Cushing's syndrome. Causes of spontaneously abnormal elevations of plasma cortisol are considered. The second discussion focuses on another hormone of the adrenal cortex, aldosterone, and the condition known as aldosteronism. The third discussion deals with the pathophysiology and clinical manifestations of androgen excess. The chapter includes some aspects of the pharmacology of synthetic corticosteroids and the metabolic side effects that result from their chronic administration. Finally, the discussion of pheochromocytoma is important, because it is a cause of hypertension that is usually correctable if diagnosed and treated properly.

The adrenal cortex synthesizes and secretes four types of adrenocortical hormones: (1) glucocorticoids, (2) mineralocorticoids, (3) androgens, and (4) estrogens. The glucocorticoid hormone is cortisol; the principal mineralocorticoid hormone is aldosterone. There are other compounds, either naturally occurring or synthetic, with glucocorticoid or mineralocorticoid activity.

Cushing's syndrome results from the combined metabolic effects of persistently elevated blood levels of glucocorticoids. These high levels may occur spontaneously or as a result of the administration of pharmacologic doses of glucocorticoid compounds. To better understand the clinical manifestations of Cushing's syndrome, it is useful to begin with a review of the metabolic consequences of glucocorticoid excess.

METABOLIC EFFECTS OF GLUCOCORTICOIDS

Glucocorticoid excess causes alteration in the following:
1. Protein and carbohydrate metabolism
2. Distribution of adipose tissue
3. Electrolytes
4. The immune system
5. Gastric secretion
6. Brain function
7. Erythropoiesis

In addition, glucocorticoid excess also suppresses inflammation.

Glucocorticoids have catabolic and antianabolic effects on protein, causing a decrease in the ability of protein-forming cells to synthesize protein. As a consequence, there is loss of protein from tissues such as skin, muscles, blood vessels, and bone. Clinically, the skin atrophies and breaks down easily; wounds heal slowly. Rupture of elastic fibers in the skin causes purple stretch marks, or *striae* (Fig. 61-1). Muscles also atrophy and become weak. Thinning of blood vessel walls and weakening of perivascular supporting tissue result in easy bruising (Fig. 61-2). This condition can be severe enough for petechiae or even large areas of ecchymosis to appear under the cuff when the patient's blood pressure is taken. Bone is also

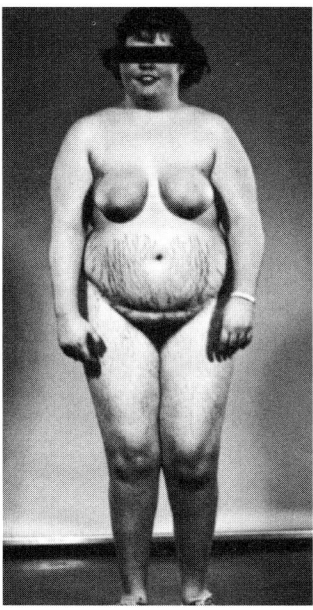

FIG. 61-1   Abdominal striae in a patient with Cushing's syndrome produced by chronic administration of large amounts of glucocorticoids.

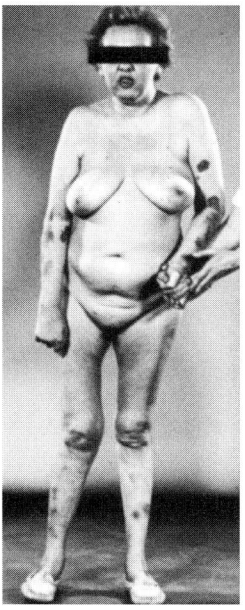

FIG. 61-2   Marked protein catabolism in a patient with Cushing's syndrome. Muscles are markedly atrophic, and multiple ecchymoses are seen on the upper and lower extremities.

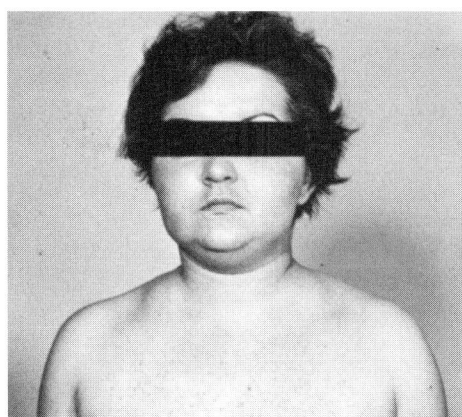

FIG. 61-3   Typical cushingoid facies with roundness of the face, double chin, prominent upper lip, and fullness of the supraclavicular fossae.

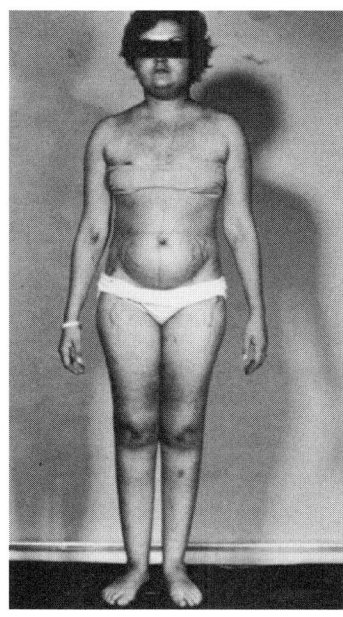

FIG. 61-4   Patient with Cushing's syndrome with acne over the chest, striae over the abdomen and upper thighs, and relatively thin upper and lower extremities. She also has pretibial edema.

affected. There is a loss of protein matrix of bone, causing a condition known as *osteoporosis*. This condition may be a serious complication of glucocorticoid excess, because it causes the bone to become brittle and develop pathologic fractures. Osteoporosis occurs most frequently in the spine, causing vertebral collapse and resultant back pain and loss of height.

Abnormally high levels of glucocorticoids also affect carbohydrate metabolism. Glucocorticoids stimulate gluconeogenesis and interfere with the action of insulin in peripheral cells. As a consequence, patients may develop hyperglycemia. In a person with an adequate insulin-secreting capacity, the effect of glucocorticoids is countered by increasing insulin secretion that subsequently normalizes glucose tolerance. In contrast, patients with diminished insulin-secreting capacity are unable to compensate, and they develop abnormal responses to glucose tolerance tests, fasting hyperglycemia, and clinical manifestations of diabetes mellitus.

Excessive glucocorticoid levels also affect the distribution of adipose tissue, which accumulates in the central areas of the body, causing development of truncal obesity, round face (moon face), supraclavicular fossa fullness, and cervicodorsal hump (buffalo hump) (Fig. 61-3). The truncal obesity and thinning of the upper and lower extremities as a result of muscle atrophy give patients the classic cushingoid appearance (Fig. 61-4).

Glucocorticoids have minimal effects on serum electrolyte levels. However, when given or produced in large concentrations, glucocorticoids may cause sodium retention and potassium waste, leading to edema, hypokalemia, and metabolic alkalosis.

Glucocorticoids can inhibit the immune response. Immune responses are of two major types: one results in production of humoral antibodies by B lymphocytes and plasma cells following antigenic stimulation; the other depends on sensitized T lymphocyte–mediated reactions. Glucocorticoids impair humoral antibody production and inhibit proliferation of germinal centers of spleen and lymphoid tissue in the primary response to antigen. Impairment of the immunologic response can occur at each of the stages of this response: (1) initial processing of antigens by cells of the monocyte-macrophage system, (2) induction and proliferation of immunocompetent lymphocytes and release of cytokines, (3) antibody production, and (4) the inflammatory reaction. Glucocorticoids also suppress delayed hypersensitivity reactions. For example, glucocorticoids may convert the skin test for tuberculosis from positive to negative. In addition, the glucocorticoid-mediated inhibition of cellular immunity is probably important in suppressing transplant rejection.

Gastric secretory activity is increased by glucocorticoids. Hydrochloric acid and pepsin secretion may be increased in certain individuals taking glucocorticoids. It has also been suggested that steroids alter mucosal protective factors and that this may contribute to ulcer formation.

Psychologic changes, which are commonly seen with glucocorticoid excess, are characterized by emotional lability, euphoria, insomnia, and episodes of transient depression. The neuropsychiatric manifestations of glucocorticoid excess occur in patients with spontaneous Cushing's syndrome and in those receiving pharmacologic doses of glucocorticoids. These changes are reversed when the patient's cortisol levels return to normal.

Glucocorticoids cause involution of lymphoid tissue, stimulation of neutrophil release, and enhancement of erythropoiesis.

The most important and clinically useful pharmacologic effect of glucocorticoids is their ability to suppress the inflammatory response. Many studies in vitro and in vivo show that glucocorticoids can inhibit hyperemia, extravasation of cells, cellular migration, and capillary permeability. They also inhibit the release of vasoactive kinins and suppress phagocytosis. By their effects on mast cells, glucocorticoids inhibit histamine synthesis and suppress the acute anaphylactic reaction based on antibody-mediated hypersensitivity. The antiinflammatory properties of glucocorticoids have placed them in the forefront of therapeutic agents available for the treatment of a variety of disorders, such as collagen vascular diseases, in which suppression of inflammation is desirable. However, there are clinical conditions in which the immune suppression and antiinflammatory effect of glucocorticoids may be a disadvantage. With acute infection, the body may be unable to defend itself appropriately while receiving pharmacologic doses of glucocorticoids.

Suppression of the Hypothalamic-Pituitary-Adrenal Axis

The administration of glucocorticoids in doses that surpass physiologic concentrations for longer than 3 weeks can significantly suppress the ability of the hypothalamic-pituitary axis to release corticotropin-releasing hormone (CRH) and adrenocorticotropic hormone (ACTH). Therefore the administration of corticoids on a long-term basis may result in adrenal insufficiency (1) when steroids are withdrawn and (2) in response to stress.

CUSHING'S SYNDROME

Cushing's syndrome may result from long-term administration of pharmacologic doses of glucocorticoids (iatrogenic) or from excessive cortisol secretion caused by a disturbance in the hypothalamic-pituitary-adrenal axis (spontaneous).

Iatrogenic Cushing's syndrome is seen in patients with conditions such as rheumatoid arthritis, asthma, lymphoma, and generalized skin disorders who receive synthetic glucocorticoids as antiinflammatory agents. In *spontaneous Cushing's syndrome*, adrenocortical hyperfunction develops either as a result of excessive stimulation by ACTH or as a consequence of adrenal pathology leading to abnormal production of cortisol.

Cushing's syndrome can be divided into two types: (1) ACTH dependent and (2) ACTH independent (Fig. 61-5). Among the ACTH-dependent types, adrenocortical hyperfunction may result from abnormal and excessive secretion of ACTH by the pituitary gland (Fig. 61-6). Because this is the type originally described by Harvey Cushing in 1932, it is also designated as Cushing's disease. Eighty percent of these patients have an ACTH-secreting pituitary adenoma. The remaining 20% have histologic evidence of pituitary corticotrope hyperplasia. It is not clear if the hyperplasia arises from a disturbed release of CRH by the neurohypothalamus. In either case, there is excessive secretion of ACTH, loss of normal circadian rhythm of ACTH, and diminished sensitivity of the feedback control system to levels of circulating cortisol. ACTH may be secreted excessively in patients who have neoplasms with the capacity to synthesize and release peptides resembling ACTH both chemically and physiologically. The excessive amount of ACTH produced under these circumstances leads to excessive stimulation of cortisol secretion by the adrenal cortex and, secondarily, to suppression of pituitary ACTH release. Thus the high ACTH levels in such a patient come from the neoplasm and not from the patient's own pituitary gland. A large number of neoplasms can cause the ectopic secretion of ACTH. These neoplasms are usually derived from tissues originating in the neuroectodermal layer during embryonic development. Oat cell carcinoma of the lung, bronchial carcinoids, thymomas, and islet cell tumors of the pancreas are among the most common. Some of these tumors are capable of ectopic CRH secretion. In this instance, ectopic CRH stimulates pituitary ACTH secretion, which causes excessive cortisol secretion by the adrenal cortex. The types of Cushing's syndrome associated with excessive ACTH secretion—pituitary or ectopic—are frequently associated with hyperpigmenta-

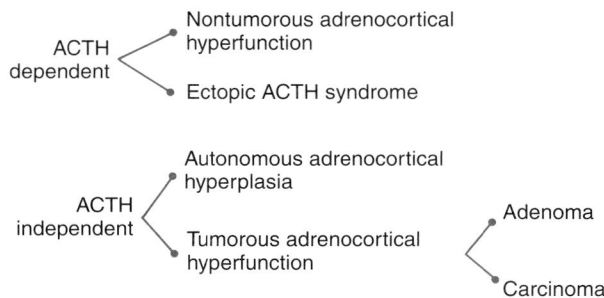

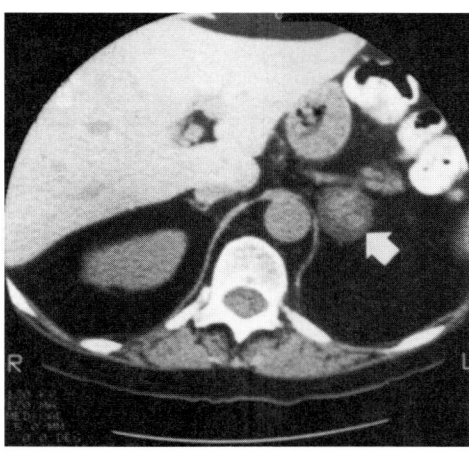

FIG. 61-5   Classification of Cushing's syndrome. *ACTH,* Adreno-corticotropic hormone.

FIG. 61-7   Computed tomography (CT) scan of the upper abdomen, demonstrating a left adrenal mass in a patient with Cushing's syndrome secondary to an adrenocortical adenoma.

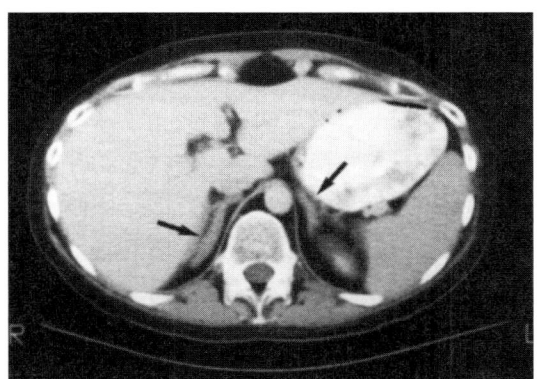

FIG. 61-6   Computed tomography (CT) scan of the upper abdomen, demonstrating bilateral adrenal enlargement in a patient with ACTH-dependent Cushing's syndrome.

tion. This hyperpigmentation is caused by the secretion of peptides related to ACTH and by breakdown fragments of ACTH that have melanotropic activity. The pigmentation is present in both skin and mucous membranes.

Adrenocortical hyperfunction can occur independently of ACTH control, such as when a tumor or bilateral, nodular adrenocortical hyperplasia with a capacity to secrete cortisol in an autonomous fashion develops in the adrenal cortex. Adrenocortical tumors leading to Cushing's syndrome may be benign (adenomas) (Fig. 61-7) or malignant (carcinomas). Adrenocortical adenomas may lead to severe Cushing's syndrome, but they usually develop slowly, and symptoms may be present for several years before the diagnosis is finally made. In contrast, adrenocortical carcinomas develop rapidly and may lead to metastasis and early death.

The presence of Cushing's syndrome can be determined on the basis of the medical history and the physical findings already described. The diagnosis is usually confirmed by the measurement of abnormally high levels of cortisol in plasma and urine. Specific tests can determine the presence or absence of a normal circadian rhythm of cortisol release and a sensitive feedback control mechanism. Absence of circadian rhythm and diminished or absent sensitivity of the feedback control system are characteristics of Cushing's syndrome.

Several diagnostic procedures can be used to establish the nature of the underlying pathology in Cushing's syn-

drome and to localize a lesion amenable to surgical management. Patients with ACTH-dependent Cushing's syndrome have high ACTH levels. In contrast, patients with ACTH-independent Cushing's syndrome have high cortisol but suppressed ACTH levels.

Physiologic testing can help distinguish pituitary from ectopic forms of Cushing's syndrome. In ectopic ACTH syndrome, the abnormal secretion of ACTH or cortisol (or both) is not likely to be altered by stimulating or suppressive maneuvers that test the presence or absence of a normal negative feedback control mechanism. Two such tests are the high-dose (8 mg) dexamethasone suppression test and the CRH stimulation test. Patients with either ectopic ACTH syndrome or primary adrenocortical disease do not suppress ACTH or cortisol levels with high doses of dexamethasone and do not stimulate these levels with the administration of ovine CRH; these features are characteristic of most patients with pituitary ACTH-dependent Cushing's syndrome.

Identification of the nature and localization of the lesion responsible for Cushing's syndrome is based on the radiographic visualization of pituitary and adrenal lesions and on nuclear scanning of the adrenal glands.

High-resolution computed tomography (CT) scanning of the pituitary gland can demonstrate areas of decreased density or enhancement consistent with a microadenoma in about 30% of these patients. Magnetic resonance imaging (MRI) with gadolinium contrast gives a positive finding in the majority of these patients. CT scanning of the adrenal glands usually shows adrenal enlargement in patients with ACTH-dependent Cushing's syndrome and adrenal masses in patients with adrenal adenoma or carcinoma.

Nuclear scanning of the adrenal glands involves the intravenous administration of radioactive cholesterol. Cholesterol labeled with ^{131}I is taken up and concentrated by the adrenal cortex. Images of the adrenal glands can be obtained by scanning techniques within 3 to 7 days after injection of the tracer (Fig. 61-8). Patterns suggestive of normal adrenal glands, adrenal hyperplasia, or adrenal adenoma or carcinoma can be obtained with adrenal photoscanning. The test is particularly useful in distin-

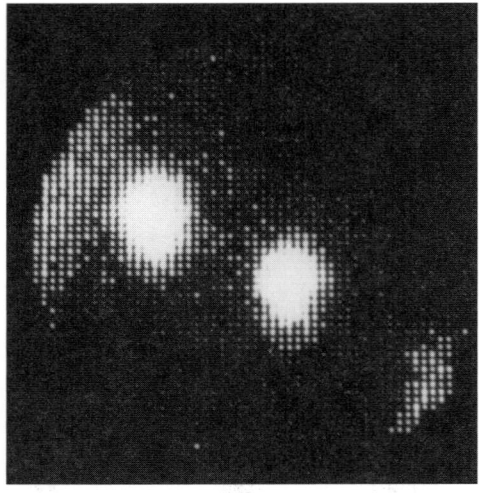

FIG. 61-8 ^{131}I 6-beta-iodomethyl-19-norcholesterol nuclear scan of the adrenal glands in a patient with ACTH-dependent Cushing's syndrome. There is bilateral increased uptake of radioactivity consistent with adrenocortical hyperfunction.

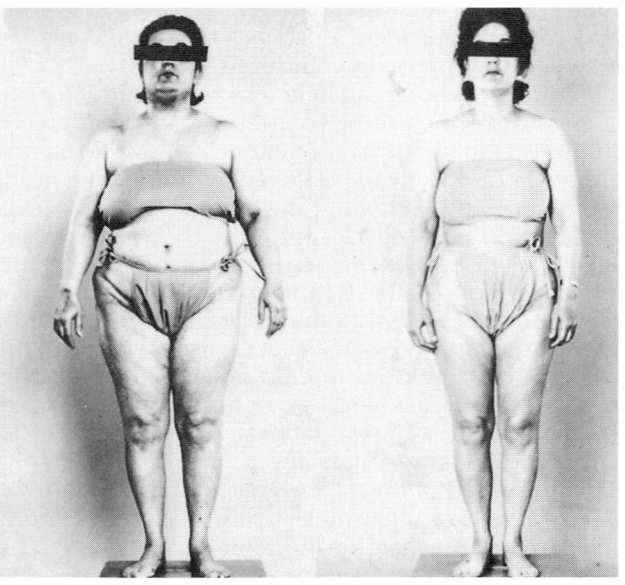

FIG. 61-9   Response to treatment of Cushing's syndrome with milotane, an adrenal inhibitor.

guishing benign from malignant adrenal masses. Benign masses take up the radioactive tracer while malignant masses do not. Ectopic ACTH-secreting tumors may be occasionally visualized with radioactive octreotide.

Treatment

Treatment of ACTH-dependent Cushing's syndrome differs, depending on whether the source of ACTH is pituitary or ectopic. Several approaches to therapy can be used in patients with pituitary hypersecretion of ACTH. If a pituitary tumor is recognized, a transsphenoidal resection of the tumor should be attempted. If there is evidence of pituitary hyperfunction but a tumor is not clearly detected, cobalt irradiation of the pituitary gland can be used in-

stead. This treatment modality is particularly effective in young people with Cushing's syndrome. Chemical agents capable of blocking (ketoconazole, aminoglutethimide) or destroying cortisol-secreting adrenocortical cells (mitotane) can also control cortisol excess. If pituitary surgery, radiation therapy, and/or medical treatment with adrenal inhibitors fail, the disease can be controlled by a total adrenalectomy and subsequent administration of physiologic doses of cortisol. When the treatment of Cushing's syndrome is successful, remission of the clinical manifestations occurs 6 to 12 months after institution of therapy (Fig. 61-9).

When adrenal neoplasms are the cause of cortisol excess, removal of the neoplasms followed by chemotherapy in patients with carcinoma is the preferred mode of treatment.

Treatment of ectopic ACTH syndrome is based on (1) resection of the neoplasm secreting ACTH or (2) adrenalectomy or chemical suppression of adrenal function, as prescribed for the patients with the pituitary ACTH-dependent type of Cushing's syndrome.

ALDOSTERONISM

Aldosteronism results from excessive production of aldosterone, the mineralocorticoid steroid hormone of the adrenal cortex. The metabolic effects of aldosterone relate to electrolyte and fluid balance. Aldosterone enhances proximal renal tubule reabsorption of sodium and causes potassium and hydrogen ion excretion. The clinical consequences of aldosterone excess are sodium and water retention, expansion of the extracellular fluid volume, and hypertension. In addition, hypernatremia, hypokalemia, and metabolic alkalosis occur.

There are two types of aldosteronism: (1) primary and (2) secondary. In *primary aldosteronism* (Conn's syndrome) the excessive production of aldosterone occurs as a result of a tumor (Fig. 61-10) or hyperplasia of the adrenal cortex. Most aldosterone-secreting tumors are benign and small—0.5 to 2.0 cm. Primary aldosteronism is a form of endocrine hypertension and probably affects 1% to 2% of patients with hypertension. Recognition of this condition can enable the cure of this type of hypertension.

Secondary aldosteronism occurs in conditions in which afferent arteriolar pressure in the renal glomerulus decreases, leading to stimulation of the renin-angiotensin system. Angiotensin stimulates aldosterone production. Secondary aldosteronism is seen in congestive heart failure, cirrhosis of the liver, and nephrotic syndrome, conditions in which edema is a prominent clinical feature. Congestive heart failure exemplifies the way secondary aldosteronism may develop. Patients in congestive heart failure cannot pump blood normally and develop a fall in cardiac output. Perfusion pressure to the afferent arteriole of the renal glomerulus decreases. The fall in pressure is sensed by stretch receptors in the juxtaglomerular apparatus, and renin is secreted in increased amounts. Renin activates angiotensin production, which, in turn, stimulates aldosterone secretion by an otherwise normal adrenal cortex. The increased production of aldosterone will, in turn, promote sodium and water reabsorption,

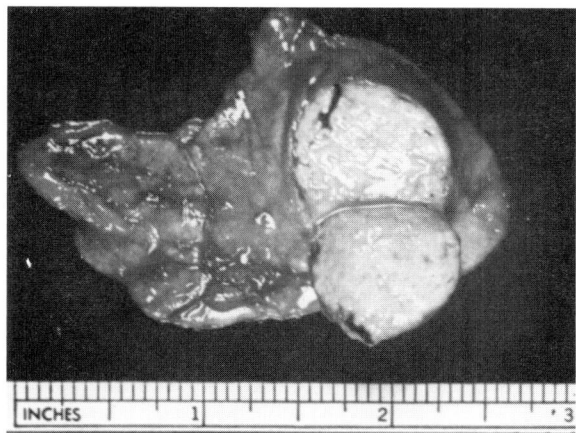

FIG. 61-10 Aldosterone-secreting adrenocortical adenoma.

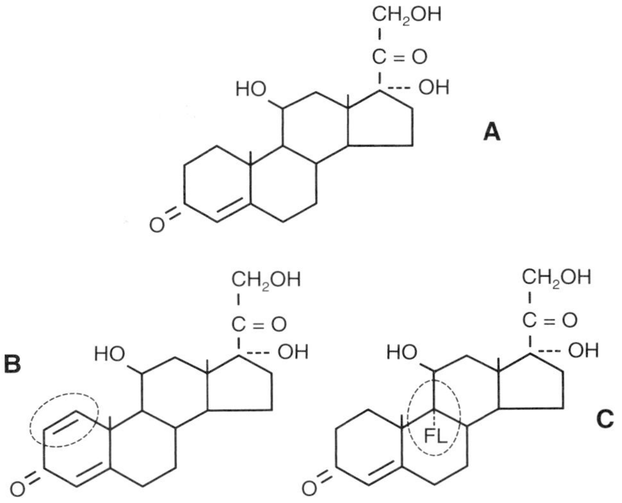

FIG. 61-11 Changes in the basic chemical structure of cortisol, leading to compounds with different pharmacologic characteristics from the parent compound. **A**, Cortisol. **B**, Prednisolone. **C**, 9Alpha-fluorocortisol.

expansion of the extracellular fluid compartment, and possibly an increase in afferent arteriolar pressure.

Secondary aldosteronism can also develop in conditions in which a partial occlusion of the renal artery occurs, leading to renal vascular hypertension (see Chapter 46).

The diagnosis of aldosteronism is based on the measurement of increased levels of aldosterone in plasma and urine and measurements of plasma renin. Plasma renin is low in primary aldosteronism and high in secondary aldosteronism.

CT scanning and nuclear photoscanning can also help detect and localize an adrenal lesion in patients with primary aldosteronism. If a tumor cannot be localized, samples of adrenal venous blood may be obtained by selective catheterization of the right and left adrenal veins. A higher concentration of aldosterone on the side suspected of harboring a tumor helps confirm the presence of the lesion.

Treatment of primary aldosteronism includes unilateral adrenalectomy through a laparoscopic approach, with resection of the aldosterone-secreting adenoma. Patients with adrenal hyperplasia are treated by the administration of aldosterone antagonists such as spironolactone.

PHARMACOLOGY AND USE OF SYNTHETIC CORTICOSTEROIDS

Synthetic analogs of cortisol with glucocorticoid and antiinflammatory activity are frequently used either topically or systemically to treat many medical conditions. For example, steroids are used topically to treat skin disorders and systemically to treat conditions such as rheumatoid arthritis, asthma, and acute allergic reactions. Although therapeutically effective, steroids also have side effects. These side effects are related to the metabolic activity and action on various organ systems, as described earlier.

Altering the basic chemical structure of cortisol, the naturally occurring glucocorticoid, makes it possible to alter the pharmacologic characteristics of this compound (Fig. 61-11). For example, if a double bond is introduced between carbons 1 and 2 in the cortisol molecule, prednisolone is produced, which has, on a milligram-per-milligram basis, less sodium-retaining and more antiin-

flammatory activity than the parent compound, cortisol. That is, 1 mg prednisolone is a much more potent antiinflammatory and immunosuppressive agent than 1 mg cortisol. Another possible structural alteration is the introduction of a fluorine atom in an alpha position on carbon 9 of the steroid nucleus. The resulting compound, 9alpha-fluorocortisol, has strong sodium-retaining properties similar to aldosterone, a naturally occurring mineralocorticoid. By this substitution, a compound with predominantly glucocorticoid activity becomes a mineralocorticoid.

Dozens of synthetic compounds have been created in the manner just described. In most cases, the objective has been the development of steroid compounds with strong antiinflammatory activity and minimal adverse metabolic effects. Although this objective has been reached to some extent, therapy with any of the currently available synthetic corticosteroid preparations, if given long enough and in sufficiently high doses, results in Cushing's syndrome and persistent suppression of endogenous hypothalamic-pituitary-adrenal function. In many instances, steroids are the only effective treatment for serious systemic diseases. Under these circumstances, the development of Cushing's syndrome may be a necessary trade-off in the control of a serious and crippling disease. The adverse effects of corticosteroid therapy can be minimized by administering a double dose of the drug on an alternate-day schedule instead of giving it daily and in divided doses. For example, if a patient needs prednisolone, 20 mg daily, instead of taking it in doses of 5 mg every 6 hours, the patient receives a 40-mg dose every other morning.

SYNDROMES OF ANDROGEN EXCESS

One of the most common problems seen by the endocrinologist among young women is hirsutism, which is usually a manifestation of androgen excess.

It is well documented that a complex relationship exists between the growth of hair in men and women and sex hormones. For example, the growth of beard; hair in the ears, nasal tip, and upper pubic triangle; and coarse hair over the trunk and limbs depend on adult male levels of circulating androgens. The growth of hair at the axilla, lower pubic region, and, in part at least, the limbs is initiated by pubertal events in both sexes and is mediated by weaker adrenal androgens. Androgen-type hair is coarse and dark. Certain hair growth appears to be independent of sex hormones. This hair is fine and light in color and includes lanugo hair, eyebrows, and eyelashes. Ethnic and genetic factors play important roles in the development of hair growth patterns.

Hirsutism is defined as excessive growth of body hair in the female in a characteristic masculine distribution over the facial, periareolar, abdominal, and sacral areas (Fig. 61-12). It may be associated with baldness (Fig. 61-13) or temporal recession of the hairline (Fig. 61-14). Hirsutism may be present alone or as part of a virilizing syndrome, which is the clinical picture observed in girls and women of all ages with signs and symptoms of defeminization and masculinization. The characteristic findings in defeminization include amenorrhea, decrease in libido, atrophy of the breasts, and loss of feminine body contour. Masculinization includes hirsutism, seborrhea, acne, deepening of the voice, increased muscular development, and enlargement of the clitoris (Fig. 61-15).

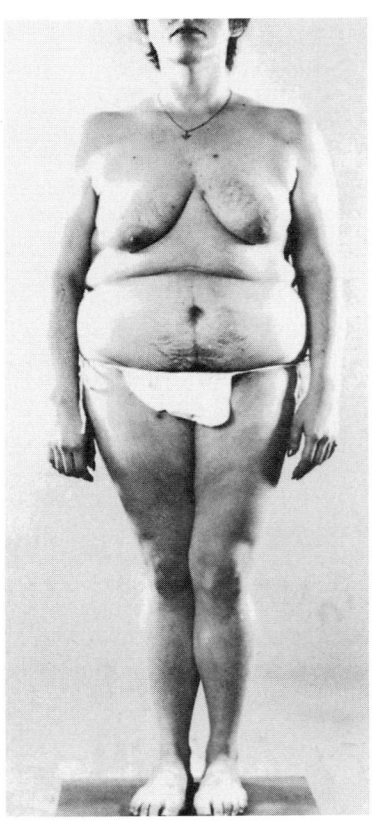

FIG. 61-12 Hirsutism in the female. Excess of body hair over the breasts, abdomen, and extremities.

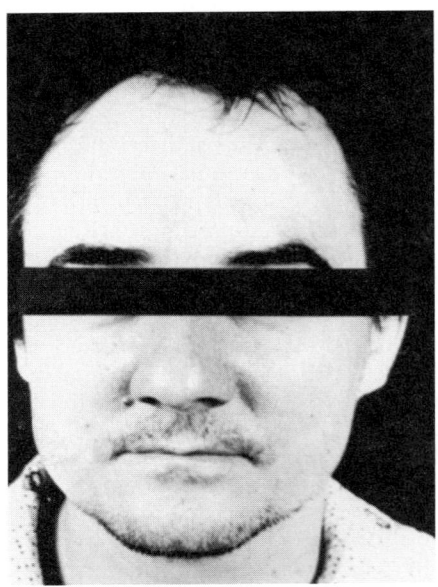

FIG. 61-14 Recession of the hairline in a woman with androgen excess. Note the excessive facial hair growth over the upper lip, chin, and sideburn areas.

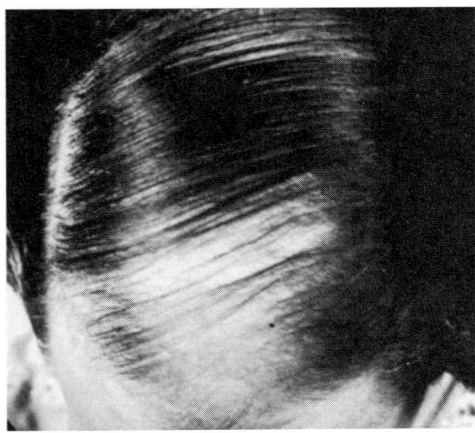

FIG. 61-13 Baldness in a woman with androgen excess.

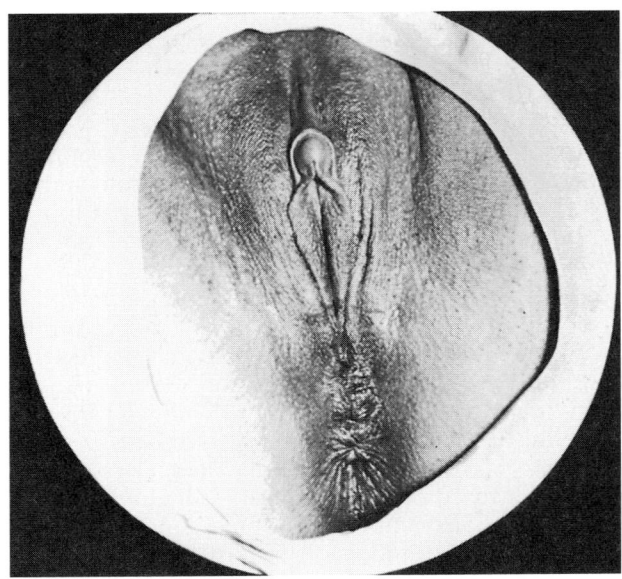

FIG. 61-15 Clitoral enlargement in a woman with androgen excess.

True virilism is currently recognized as a rare condition, almost always associated with adrenal or ovarian tumors or with the syndrome of congenital adrenal hyperplasia. In contrast, hirsutism, often without any other signs of virilism but frequently accompanied by irregular or absent menstrual periods and acne, is a common clinical entity and associated with polycystic ovary syndrome (PCOS). When hirsutism is present alone and without virilization or menstrual irregularity, women are thought to have simple or idiopathic hirsutism. No specific hormonal abnormality or etiologic mechanism has been described as the sole cause of these types of hirsutism.

Androgen Physiology

Both men and women normally secrete various androgens. The three major types of androgens are (1) dehydroepiandrosterone, (2) delta 4-androstenedione, and (3) testosterone (Fig. 61-16).

Dehydroepiandrosterone (DHEA) and its metabolite, DHEA sulfate, are generally considered to be weak androgens. The adrenal gland is the main source of this type of androgen and can be measured in the urine as 17-ketosteroids.

Delta 4-androstenedione is a stronger androgen product than DHEA but weaker than testosterone, of which it is a precursor. The adrenal cortex and the ovary also produce delta 4-androstenedione.

Testosterone is the most potent of the three androgen compounds. There are several sources of testosterone, including the adrenal cortex, the ovary, the testes, and peripheral tissues. Testosterone is metabolized to a potent androgen, dihydrotestosterone (DHT); finally, both testosterone and DHT may be converted to androstenediol in peripheral tissues and excreted as such in the urine.

Testosterone can be produced in several endocrine and peripheral tissues from precursors. Testosterone circulates in the plasma partially bound to a carrier protein (sex hormone–binding globulin [SHBG]), and it is removed through metabolic degradation in the liver and other peripheral tissues (Fig. 61-17). Testosterone levels are therefore a balance between production and metabolic clearance. Although a large portion of circulating androgens is bound to SHBG, a small fraction is unbound. The biologic effects of circulating androgens are related to the levels of free, unbound androgens in plasma. Women with hirsutism usually have abnormalities in testosterone secretion, transport and metabolism. For example, hirsute women have less testosterone binding, higher free testosterone levels, and more active metabolic clearance tests than women without hirsutism. Although in normal women testosterone is extracted and metabolized almost completely by the liver, in virilized women, 32% of secreted testosterone is extracted and metabolized by extrahepatic peripheral tissues. These tissues are then subject to greater androgenic activity than that found in normal women.

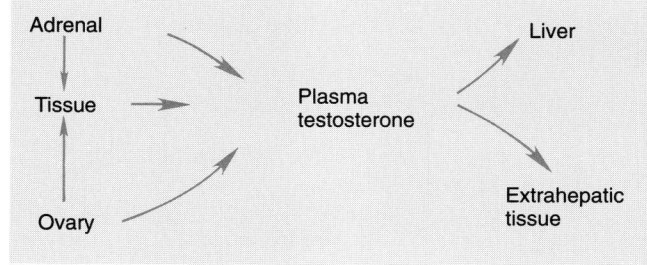

FIG. 61-17 Metabolism of plasma testosterone. The plasma level of testosterone results from a balance between the production of testosterone by adrenal, ovarian, and peripheral tissues and clearance by the liver and extrahepatic tissues.

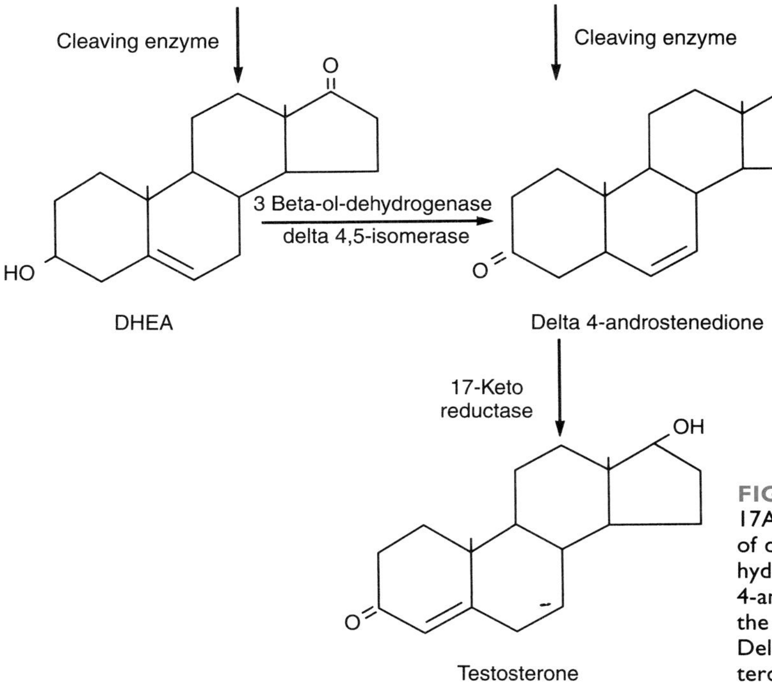

FIG. 61-16 Three major types of androgens in the female. 17Apha-hydroxypregnenolone is the immediate precursor of dehydroepiandrosterone (DHEA), whereas 17alpha-hydroxyprogesterone is the immediate precursor of delta 4-androstenedione. The transformation of the precursor to the androgen hormones is catalyzed by a cleaving enzyme. Delta 4-androstenedione can, in turn, be converted to testosterone by a step catalyzed by 17-ketoreductase.

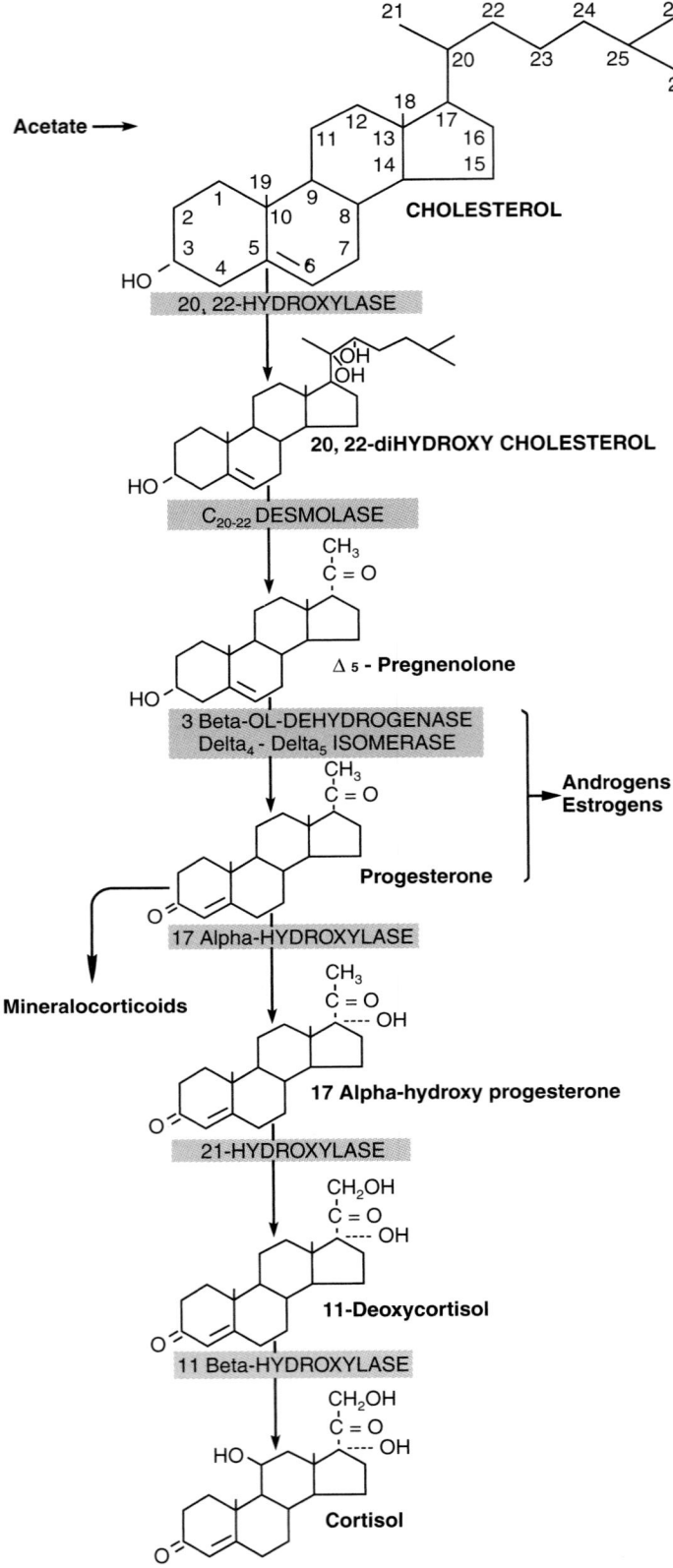

FIG. 61-18 Pathway of cortisol biosynthesis. Pregnenolone and progesterone are precursors of androgens and estrogens. Progesterone is also a precursor of mineralocorticoids. The biosynthesis of cortisol takes place in the adrenal cortex. Each step is controlled by specific enzymes. A defect in 21-hydroxylase is the cause of the most common type of congenital adrenal hyperplasia.

Androgen Excess: Differential Diagnosis

I. Androgen excess of adrenocortical origin
  A. Cortisol excess: Cushing's syndrome
  B. Androgen excess only
    1. Prenatal: congenital adrenal hyperplasia (CAH)
    2. Postnatal: prepubertal
      a. Late manifestations of CAH
      b. Carcinoma
    3. Pubertal or postpubertal
      a. Hyperplasia, with or without polycystic ovaries
      b. Carcinoma
II. Androgen excess of ovarian origin
  A. Neoplasms: arrhenoblastoma, adrenal rest cell neoplasms, hilus cell neoplasms, luteoma
  B. Hilus cell or Leydig cell hyperplasia
  C. Polycystic ovary syndrome
III. Simple or idiopathic hirsutism
IV. Miscellaneous causes
  A. Endocrine
    1. Acromegaly
    2. Pregnancy
    3. Hypothyroidism
    4. Menopause
    5. Androgen therapy
    6. Inanition
  B. Nonendocrine
    1. Immobilization
    2. Body cast
    3. Porphyria
    4. Congenital ectodermal dysplasia

Differential Diagnosis of Androgen Excess

Five major categories of conditions are associated with androgen excess: (1) polycystic ovary syndrome (PCOS), (2) adrenocortical or ovarian tumors, (3) late-onset or nonclassical adrenocortical hyperplasia, (4) simple or idiopathic hirsutism, and (5) miscellaneous states (Box 61-1).

In *polycystic ovary syndrome*, hirsutism is frequently associated with infertility, amenorrhea, obesity, and enlarged ovaries. In these patients, testosterone production rates are clearly increased and are responsible for the manifestations of androgen excess. The increased production of androgens in the PCOS may be secondary to the hyperinsulinemia that develops in association with obesity. The high insulin levels stimulate insulin-like growth factor-1 (IGF-1) concentration in the ovary and cause increased androgen secretion. Alternatively, PCOS may result from hypothalamic-pituitary abnormalities affecting the cyclic release of gonadotropins. Patients with PCOS often have sustained elevations of serum luteinizing hormone (LH). These changes in gonadotropin secretion may lead to anatomic changes in the ovary and stimulation of ovarian androgen production.

Adrenal and ovarian tumors can be associated with androgen excess. Adrenocortical carcinomas secrete androgens alone or in combination with cortisol and produce either a pure virilizing syndrome or a mixed Cushing's virilizing syndrome. Tumors of the ovary, such as arrhenoblastomas and hilus cell neoplasms, are capable of secreting large amounts of testosterone and producing virilization.

Congenital adrenal hyperplasia (CAH) is a condition in which there is an inborn defect in one of the enzymes involved in cortisol biosynthesis. The most common type is a defect in 21-hydroxylase (Fig. 61-18). As a consequence

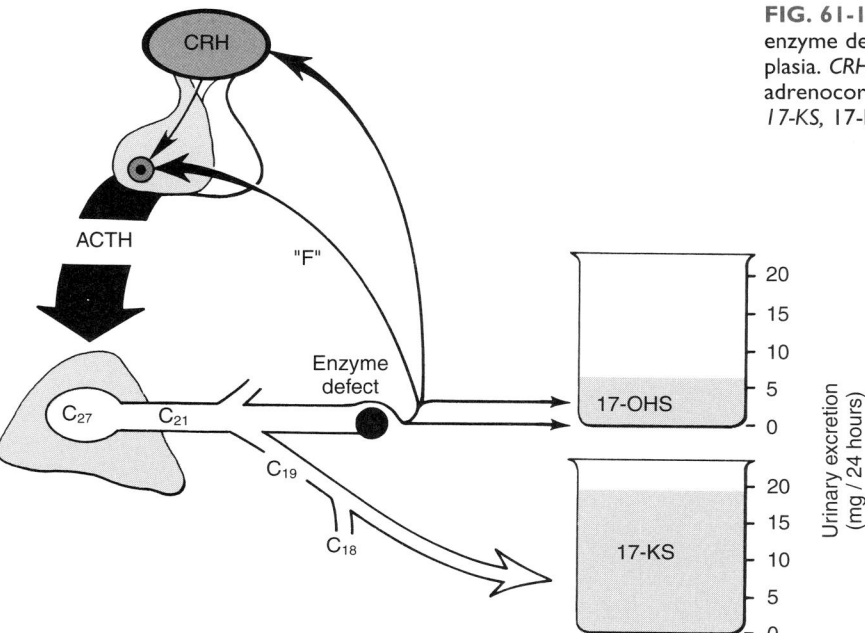

FIG. 61-19 Biochemical and physiologic consequence of enzyme deficiency in patients with congenital adrenal hyperplasia. *CRH*, Corticotropin-releasing hormone; *ACTH*, adrenocorticotropic hormone; *17-OHS*, 17-hydroxysteroids; *17-KS*, 17-ketosteroids; *F*, feedback.

of 21-hydroxylase deficiency, the adrenal cortex has an impaired capacity to secrete cortisol. The decrease in cortisol production causes an increase in ACTH secretion in response to the negative feedback activation of pituitary function. ACTH stimulates the adrenal cortex, causing the precursors of cortisol biosynthesis to be shunted to the biosynthesis of androgens (Fig. 61-19). When the fetus is exposed to increased amounts of androgen, it undergoes changes in the development of the external genitalia. For example, a female fetus with this defect develops an enlargement of the clitoris and fusion of the labia majora. The genitalia then resemble male external genitalia. At the time of birth, this ambiguity in sexual development may create difficulties in sexual identification of the newborn. The syndrome of a masculinized genetically female fetus caused by androgen excess in utero is called *female pseudohermaphroditism* (Fig. 61-20).

Manifestations of androgen excess in patients with congenital adrenal hyperplasia can also develop at puberty or after puberty. About 4% to 12% of women with hirsutism may have this condition described as *late-onset or nonclassic CAH* and is a consequence of a milder form of congenital adrenal hyperplasia with only partial defects in 21-hydroxylase, 11-beta-hydroxylase, or 3-beta-ol-dehydrogenase, delta 4,5-isomerase.

Many women have hirsutism without any other clinical manifestations of androgen excess. The problem usually begins after puberty and progresses slowly over years. The urinary 17-ketosteroid level may be slightly or moderately elevated, and the testosterone production rate moderately increased. The free testosterone level may also be elevated. The specific biochemical defect and the pathophysiology of this type of androgen excess are not well understood. However, it may be the result of increased activity of 5 alpha reductase, the enzyme that regulates the conversion of testosterone to DHT in the hair follicle, with a consequent stimulation of hair growth by DHT.

There are a number of miscellaneous causes of hirsutism. Some of these causes are of endocrine origin and

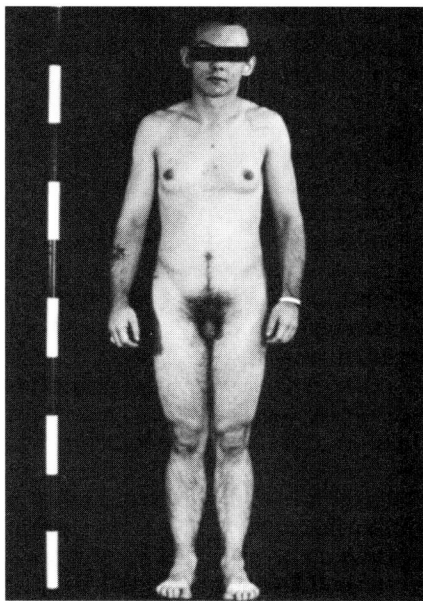

FIG. 61-20 Female pseudohermaphroditism in a patient with congenital adrenal hyperplasia caused by 21-hydroxylase deficiency. This patient had a male phenotype but was genetically a female. Note the masculine muscle development and body hair growth pattern. On casual examination the patient appeared to have a developed penis. On closer examination, however, this penis was seen to be an enlarged clitoris. The patient also had developed gynecomastia as a result of increased estrogen production accompanying the androgen excess.

include the hirsutism associated with acromegaly, pregnancy, hypothyroidism, menopause, androgen therapy, and inanition. Increased hair growth may occur without hormonal stimulation. Hirsutism is seen in disorders such as porphyria and congenital ectodermal dysplasia or in areas of the body that have been either immobilized or placed in a body cast.

Clinical and Laboratory Evaluation of Hirsute Women

If a patient presents with complaints of excessive hair growth, it is necessary to determine whether the hirsutism is present by itself or accompanied by manifestations of virilization, as described earlier. It is also important to determine whether the symptoms are those of androgen excess alone or are accompanied by symptoms of cortisol excess. A history of recent onset and rapid progression of excessive hair growth frequently suggests a malignancy as the source of excessive androgen production.

Tests to document excessive androgen production include measurement of blood levels of total and free testosterone, DHEA, and androstenedione. When PCOS is suspected, measurement of serum LH, and glucose and insulin levels is helpful. Patients suspected of non-classical CAH should have, in addition, measurement of serum17 alpha-hydroxyprogesterone and 17 alpha-hydroxypregnenolone before and after stimulation with corticotropin. In the presence of an enzyme defect, this stimulation results in an exaggerated rise of these steroid precursors and helps confirm the diagnosis. Patients suspected of an adrenal or ovarian androgen-secreting tumor should undergo a pelvic examination, as well as an abdominal and pelvic CT scan, MRI, or ultrasound.

Treatment

The treatment of androgen excess relates to the underlying pathology. If androgen excess is part of Cushing's syndrome, correction of Cushing's syndrome in the manner previously described will result in remission of the manifestations of androgen excess. CAH can be effectively suppressed by chronic suppressive therapy with corticosteroids. Patients with adrenal or ovarian tumors should undergo resection of these tumors. Patients with PCOS can be treated by androgen suppression with (1) oral contraceptives, (2) synthetic corticosteroids, (3) spironolactone, or (4) insulin sensitizers. Oral contraceptives suppress ovarian androgen production by suppressing pituitary gonadotropins; synthetic corticosteroids such as dexamethasone, given as a single 0.5-mg dose at bedtime, suppress both adrenal and ovarian androgens. Spironolactone suppresses androgen production and androgen action at the target tissue level. Insulin sensitizers such as metformin and thiazolidinedione analogs have been shown to decrease androgen production by reducing the hyperinsulinemia associated with many states of androgen excess.

▓ PHEOCHROMOCYTOMA

Pheochromocytoma, a rare cause of secondary hypertension, is an adrenal medullary or sympathetic chain (paraganglioma) tumor that releases excessive amounts of catecholamines (epinephrine, norepinephrine, and dopamine) in a sustained or intermittent manner. Pheochromocytoma affects 0.1% to 0.5 % of the hypertensive population and may have a fatal outcome if undiagnosed or untreated. Pheochromocytoma occurs equally in men and women and has a peak incidence between ages 30 and 50. About 90% of these tumors are derived from adrenal medullary chromaffin cells, and 10% are extraadrenal, located in the retroperitoneal area (organs of Zuckerkandl), celiac and mesenteric ganglia, and urinary bladder. Patients with multiple endocrine neoplasia (MEN) II, have increased secretion of catecholamines with the clinical manifestations of a pheochromocytoma from bilateral adrenal medullary hyperplasia. Pheochromocytomas are usually benign (95% of cases), but they may be malignant and present with distant metastases.

The clinical manifestations of these tumors are related to the release of catecholamines. The most prominent feature is hypertension that may be paroxysmal (45% of cases) or sustained. Patients with paroxysmal symptoms develop acute episodes of severe hypertension (250/140 mm Hg) lasting minutes to hours. The episodes may be triggered by exercise, ingestion of tyrosine-containing foods (red wine, aged cheese, yogurt), caffeine-containing foods, abdominal palpation, or induction of anesthesia. Patients remain normotensive between episodes. Together with the hypertension, patients complain of pounding headaches on the top of their head, palpitations, pallor, diaphoresis, and dysrhythmias. Patients with sustained hypertension may also show variability in their high blood pressure readings and complain of headaches and irregular heartbeat. Occasionally, patients present with symptoms of orthostatic hypotension, especially if the tumor secretes significant amounts of dopamine. The biochemical evaluation of patients suspected of a pheochromocytoma consists of measurement of plasma or urinary levels of epinephrine, norepinephrine, and their metabolites metanephrine and normetanephrine.

Because normal adrenal secretion of epinephrine and norepinephrine may vary, distinction between physiologic and pathologic hypersecretory states may be difficult with a single determination of catecholamine levels. Circulating norepinephrine is derived from sympathetic neurons, whereas epinephrine is derived chiefly from the adrenal medulla. Norepinephrine can increase with a change from the recumbent to the upright position. Catecholamines are also increased with an acute myocardial infarction, volume depletion, hypothyroidism, and other physical or emotional stress. Peripheral vasodilators, cocaine, phenoxybenzamine, phentolamine, prazosin, and theophylline can increase catecholamine release. Insulin-induced hypoglycemia can evoke major increases in epinephrine and small increases in norepinephrine. Drugs such as clonidine, reserpine, guanethidine, haloperidol, Thorazine, and alpha-methyldopa decrease plasma norepinephrine levels.

Basal plasma catecholamine levels should be obtained with the patient resting in the supine position for at least 30 minutes. Normal levels for epinephrine range from 0 to 100 pg/ml; for norepinephrine, 0 to 500 pg/ml; and for dopamine, 0 to 100 pg/ml. Markedly increased levels (epinephrine more than 500 pg/ml and norepinephrine greater than 1500 pg/ml) are virtually diagnostic of pheochromocytoma.

Basal urinary catecholamines should be collected for 12 hours during the night. Normal levels for epinephrine are 0 to 20 mg/day; for norepinephrine, 0 to 100 mg/day; for metanephrines, 0 to 300 mg/day; for normetanephrines, 50 to 800 mg/day; and for vanillylmandelic acid (VMA), 0 to 7 mg/day. Patients with pheochromocytoma have high urinary catecholamine levels.

In borderline cases, a clonidine suppression test may help differentiate normal subjects from patients with a pheochromocytoma. Clonidine, 0.3 mg, is administered orally after two baseline blood samples for epinephrine and norepinephrine are obtained; plasma epinephrine and norepinephrine samples are repeated 3 hours after clonidine administration. Patients with a pheochromocytoma fail to suppress catecholamine secretion, whereas clonidine will restore normal levels of catecholamines in other hyperadrenergic states.

Treatment consists of surgical resection of the pheochromocytoma and exploration of the retroperitoneal space for paraganglia-derived tumors. Patients' blood pressure should be stabilized preoperatively by alpha-adrenergic blocking agents, such as phenoxybenzamine, and beta blockers, such as propranolol, when needed. Phenoxybenzamine is also used as medical treatment to block catecholamine effects in patients with malignant, unresectable pheochromocytomas.

KEY CONCEPTS

- The *adrenal glands* are paired small organs sitting atop the upper poles of each kidney with two distinct endocrine components—the cortex and the medulla.
- The *adrenal medulla*, occupying the central portion of the gland, secretes the catecholamines, epinephrine and norepinephrine.
- The *adrenal cortex* synthesizes and secretes three main groups of steroid hormones originating with cholesterol: (1) *glucocorticoids* (e.g., cortisol, from the zona fasciculata), (2) mineralocorticoids (aldosterone from the zona glomerulosa), and (3) *sex steroids* (androgens and estrogens from the zona reticularis).
- Major *metabolic effects of excess cortisol* include the following: (1) protein metabolism: catabolic effect causing loss of protein from skin, muscles, and bone, resulting in striae, atrophied muscles, osteoporosis; (2) carbohydrate metabolism: stimulates gluconeogenesis and antagonizes the effects of insulin resulting in hyperglycemia; (3) fat metabolism: mobilization of fatty acids from adipose tissue and redistribution of fat to face and trunk; (4) inhibition of the inflammatory, cellular, and humoral immune responses compromising immune defense and slowing the healing process; (5) stimulates gastric secretory activity (pepsin and hydrochloric acid [HCl]), increasing risk of peptic ulcer; and (6) brain function—excess associated with emotional lability.
- Secretion of cortisol is regulated by the *hypothalamic-pituitary-adrenal axis* involving a multilevel feedback control mechanism. Hypothalamic CRH stimulates the release of ACTH from the pituitary, which, in turn, binds with receptors of the adrenal cortex leading to cortisol release.
- *Three major factors control ACTH secretion* and thus control of cortisol secretion: (1) *sleep-wake cycle* with serum cortisol levels, reaching a peak about 8:00 AM and a nadir at about 10:00 PM; (2) modulating impact of *stressors* on the hypothalamus; and (3) inhibitory effect of increased *free plasma cortisol* on ACTH release.
- The clinical syndromes of *adrenal cortical hyperfunction* are caused by overproduction of adrenal steroid hormones. The features will depend on which of the steroid groups are dominant—excess glucocorticoids (Cushing's syndrome), aldosterone (aldosteronism), or adrenal androgens (producing hirsutism and virilization in females).
- Signs and symptoms of *Cushing's syndrome* (cortisol excess) include the typical facies (moon face) with acne and hirsutism; truncal obesity with fullness of the supraclavicular fossae, buffalo hump and abdominal striae; muscle weakness and wasting; osteoporosis; skin fragility and slow wound healing; and peptic ulceration, hypertension, and emotional lability.
- The *most common cause of Cushing's syndrome* is iatrogenic—therapeutic administration of superphysiologic doses of cortisol (or related analogs) used to treat a variety of inflammatory and autoimmune disorders (e.g., rheumatoid arthritis) and prevent organ transplant rejection.
- *Cushing's syndrome* is divided into two types: (1) *ACTH-dependent type* caused by hypersecretion of ACTH (source: pituitary adenoma [80%] or pituitary corticotroph hyperplasia [20%], or ectopic ACTH secretion [e.g., oat cell lung cancer]) and (2) *ACTH-independent type* caused by hypersecretion of adrenal cortisol (source: benign or malignant adrenal tumor; autonomous adrenocortical hyperplasia) or from the prolonged therapeutic administration of cortisol.
- The diagnosis of Cushing's syndrome is based on the clinical features and demonstration of an elevated plasma cortisol level.
- Elucidation of the cause of Cushing's syndrome is through the *dexamethasone suppression test*, MRI, and CT scan visualization of the pituitary and adrenals, and through analysis of blood ACTH level (high ACTH: pituitary adenoma or ectopic ACTH source; low ACTH: primary adrenal tumor).
- *Treatment of ACTH-dependent Cushing's syndrome* consists of trans-sphenoid surgical resection of a pituitary adenoma, irradiation for pituitary hyperplasia, or surgical removal of an ACTH-producing ectopic neoplasm or chemical suppression of adrenal function with ketoconazole.
- *Treatment of ACTH-independent Cushing's syndrome* includes surgical resection of the adrenal tumor or medical ablation (e.g., metyrapone) followed by replacement therapy.
- *Aldosterone* (the chief mineralocorticoid) is the major regulator of extracellular fluid volume by causing

Na^+ (and water) retention by the distal tubule of the kidney and is controlled by the renin-angiotensin-aldosterone mechanism. It is also the major determinant of K^+ balance.

- *Primary aldosteronism* (Conn's syndrome), excessive aldosterone secretion by the adrenal gland, is almost invariably caused by an adrenal cortical adenoma (adrenal carcinoma or bilateral adrenal hyperplasia as causes are rare).
- *Secondary aldosteronism*, excessive secretion of aldosterone by an extraadrenal stimulus, occurs as a result of activation of the renin-angiotensin-aldosterone mechanism (e.g., congestive heart failure, liver cirrhosis, nephrotic syndrome) or as a result of renal artery stenosis.
- *Effects of aldosteronism* include retention of Na^+ and water, leading to systemic hypertension, and excessive urinary K^+ loss, leading to hypokalemia, metabolic alkalosis, and cardiac dysrhythmias.
- The *diagnosis of aldosteronism* is based on establishing the presence of abnormal electrolyte levels (high Na^+, low K^+, metabolic alkalosis) and is confirmed by detection of elevated plasma aldosterone levels and by visualization of an adrenal cortical adenoma by CT scan or MRI. Plasma renin level is low in primary aldosteronism and high in secondary aldosteronism.
- *Treatment of primary aldosteronism* consists of surgical excision of an adrenal adenoma or administration of spironolactone (an aldosterone antagonist) for adrenal hyperplasia.
- *Excess secretion of androgens* in females causes *virilization*—acne, deepening of the voice, enlargement of the clitoris, temporal hairline recession or baldness, oligomenorrhea or amenorrhea, and *hirsutism* (excessive growth of coarse dark hair with a masculine distribution over face, nipples, and pubic areas).
- The *three major androgens* in order of increasing potency are (1) dehydroepiandrosterone (DHEA), (2) delta-4-androstenedione, and (3) testosterone. The first two androgens are produced by the adrenals and converted to testosterone in the peripheral tissues; a small amount of testosterone is produced by the adrenals and ovaries and a large amount by the testes in males.
- Testosterone circulates partly in the free (active) form and partly bound to sex hormone–binding globulin (SHBG) and is removed by metabolic degradation in the liver and peripheral tissues.
- In males, less than 2% of androgens are derived from the adrenals, but in females, this rises to 50%. Normal women degrade almost all the testosterone in the liver, but in hirsute women 32% is metabolized in peripheral tissues, resulting in higher levels of testosterone in the free (active) form.
- Five major conditions are associated with *androgen excess*: (1) polycystic ovary syndrome (PCOS), (2) benign or malignant androgen-producing tumors of the ovary or adrenals, (3) late-onset congenital adrenal hyperplasia, (4) idiopathic hirsutism, and (5) miscellaneous.
- *Classic congenital adrenal hyperplasia (CAH)* is a condition caused by an enzyme deficiency involved in the cortisol biosynthesis pathway, most commonly *21-hydroxylase deficiency*. This deficiency leads to cortisol deficiency, increased ACTH in response to negative feedback to the pituitary, and increased androgen synthesis, leading to female pseudohermaphroditism in a female fetus.
- *Nonclassical late-onset CAH* (pubertal or postpubertal) involves a partial deficiency of an enzyme in the cortisol biosynthesis pathway resulting in a milder form of CAH.
- The causes of hirsutism can be divided into four broad categories: familial, idiopathic, drugs, and androgen excess. The first three causes are not associated with other signs of androgen excess.
- Drugs that induce a growth in body hair include phenothiazines, minoxidil, and phenytoin.
- In the female, the differential diagnosis of hirsutism and virilization is between adrenal and ovarian etiologies.
- The sudden onset of progressive hirsutism and virilization in a female suggests an adrenal or ovarian malignancy as the source of the excessive androgen.
- *Adrenal carcinoma*, the most common adrenal tumor causing virilization, is associated with markedly increased excretion of urinary 17-ketosteroids and high levels of plasma DHEA.
- The most common virilizing ovarian tumor, the *arrhenoblastoma*, is usually characterized by normal levels of 17-ketosteroids and DHEA because the tumor usually secretes the potent androgen, testosterone.
- The most common cause of excess androgen production is *PCOS*; virilization is less common than with ovarian or adrenal tumors, whereas hirsutism is quite frequent. Many patients with this condition have hyperinsulinemia, glucose intolerance, elevated levels of LH, and are obese.
- Patients with PCOS can be treated by androgen suppression: oral contraceptives, synthetic corticosteroids, spironolactone, or insulin sensitizers, such as metformin.
- *Pheochromocytoma* is the most important condition affecting the adrenal medulla—its hallmark is hypertension caused by excess release of catecholamines (epinephrine and norepinephrine) in a paroxysmal or sustained manner.
- The *paroxysmal attacks in pheochromocytoma* are characterized by a sudden, severe increase in blood pressure, severe throbbing headache, sweating (most severe over the trunk), and palpitations with or without tachycardia.
- The laboratory diagnosis of pheochromocytoma depends on demonstrating the presence of elevated serum levels of catecholamines (e.g., epinephrine, norepinephrine) or their metabolites in a 24-hour urine, vanillylmandelic acid (VMA). Measurement of catecholamines in plasma is useful if the sample can be obtained during an attack.
- Treatment of pheochromocytomas consists of preoperative stabilization of blood pressure with alpha-adrenergic blocking agents (e.g., phenoxybenzamine) and surgical excision of the tumor.

 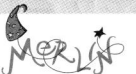

Answer the following on a separate sheet of paper.

1. Explain the statement that glucocorticoids have a catabolic effect on protein metabolism.
2. What effects do abnormally high levels of glucocorticoids have on glucose metabolism?
3. The hypothalamic-pituitary axis may be activated under stress. Explain the process by which it occurs.
4. How do the basic chemical structures of 9alpha-fluorocortisol and prednisolone differ? In relation to pharmacologic effects, what is achieved by altering the basic chemical structure of cortisol?
5. List three types of treatment for pituitary ACTH-dependent Cushing's syndrome. What is the purpose of the treatment modalities?
6. What is the preferred treatment for Cushing's syndrome that is secondary to an adrenal tumor?
7. Explain the way secondary aldosteronism develops in response to congestive heart failure.

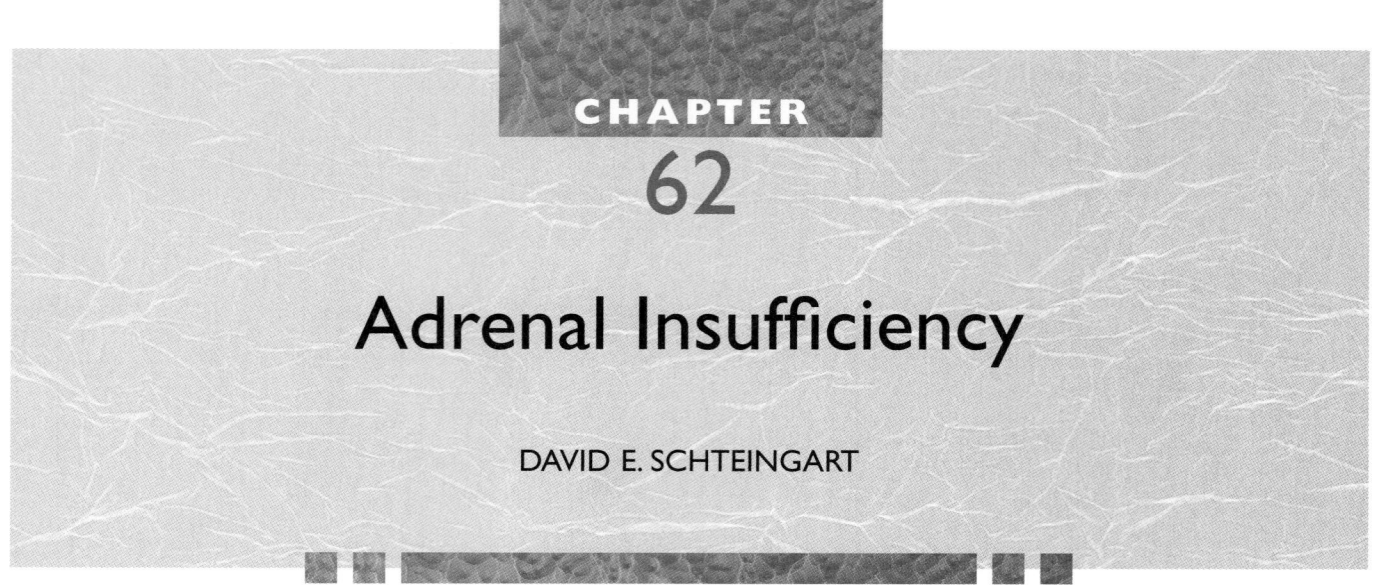

CHAPTER
62

Adrenal Insufficiency

DAVID E. SCHTEINGART

*T*he syndrome of adrenocortical insufficiency develops as a result of deficient secretion of cortisol and aldosterone. If untreated, this condition may be incompatible with life. Main causes of adrenocortical insufficiency are (1) primary disease of the adrenal cortex or (2) deficient secretion of adrenocorticotropic hormone (ACTH). Isolated corticotropin-releasing hormone (CRH) deficiency can lead to ACTH and cortisol deficiency, but it is only seen as a result of chronic exposure to pharmacologic doses of glucocorticoids or following the removal of a cortisol-secreting adrenocortical adenoma.

When the cause of adrenocortical insufficiency is a pathologic process of the adrenal cortex, the condition is known as *Addison's disease.* Patients with Addison's disease have involvement of all three zones of the cortex, resulting in deficiency of all the adrenocortical secretions: cortisol, aldosterone, and androgens. Occasionally, patients present a partial deficiency of adrenocortical hormone secretion. This deficiency is seen in cases of hyporeninemic-hypoaldosteronism, which involves only the secretion of aldosterone, or congenital adrenal hyperplasia, in which a partial enzyme defect blocks only the secretion of cortisol.

Addison's disease is rare and has a prevalence of 4 in 100,000 people; two thirds of people affected are women. The diagnosis is made between ages 20 and 50. In the past, tuberculosis was the main cause of Addison's disease. Presently, with better chemotherapy for tuberculosis, few patients with this condition develop adrenal insufficiency. Instead, destruction of the adrenal cortex is a result of an autoimmune process in more than 50% of patients with Addison's disease. Adrenal autoantibodies are found in high titers in some patients with Addison's dis-

ease. These antibodies react with antigens in the adrenal cortex, including the enzyme 21 hydroxylase and cause an inflammatory reaction that eventually destroys the adrenal gland. Usually, more than 80% of both glands must be destroyed before signs and symptoms of insufficiency develop. Addison's disease may occur concurrently with other endocrine diseases in which autoimmunity plays a role. Among these are Hashimoto's thyroiditis, certain cases of type 1 diabetes mellitus, and hypoparathyroidism. There also appears to be a familial predisposition for autoimmune endocrine disease, which is probably related to abnormal reactivity of the patient's immune system. Less common causes of Addison's disease are hemorrhage associated with the chronic use of anticoagulants, especially heparin, noncaseating granulomatous diseases, cytomegalovirus (CMV) infection in patients with acquired immunodeficiency syndrome (AIDS), and metastatic neoplasms that involve both adrenal glands. Rare cases have been described in whom primary adrenocortical insufficiency develops as a result of mutations in genes encoding for proteins that regulate adrenal development (SF-1, DAX-1) or steroidogenesis (StAR).

METABOLIC CONSEQUENCES OF CORTISOL, ALDOSTERONE, AND ANDROGEN DEFICIENCIES

The clinical picture of Addison's disease results from lack of cortisol, aldosterone, and androgens. *Cortisol insufficiency* causes diminished gluconeogenesis, decreased liver glycogen, and increased sensitivity of peripheral tissues to insulin. The combination of these changes in carbohydrate metabolism may cause inability to maintain normal blood glucose levels, leading to hypoglycemia in the fasting state. Because of low hepatic glycogen content, patients with adrenal insufficiency are unable to withstand food deprivation for a long time. Increased sensitivity to insulin as a result of cortisol deficiency may be a problem for patients with type 1 or 2 insulin-requiring diabetes mellitus who develop adrenocortical insufficiency. These patients may notice that the insulin dose that kept them under control in the past now causes hypoglycemia.

Another consequence of cortisol deficiency is a negative feedback increase in the secretion of proopiomelanocortin (POMC)-derived peptides, including ACTH, and α– and β–melanocyte-stimulating hormone (MSH). The clinical consequence is hyperpigmentation, usually found in the distal portion of the extremities over sun-exposed areas but also in areas not normally exposed to the sun. These areas include the nipples, extensor surfaces of the extremities, genitalia, buccal mucosa, tongue, palmar creases, and knuckles. The assessment of pigmentation may be more difficult in a dark-skinned person. In these patients, a history of change in pigmentation as ascertained by the patients or their relatives may be a good way of assessing the presence of hyperpigmentation. Treatment with cortisol decreases the hyperpigmentation.

Because cortisol is required for a normal stress response, patients with cortisol deficiency are unable to withstand surgical stress, anesthesia, trauma, infection, and other febrile illnesses. Under these circumstances a patient may develop life-threatening acute adrenal insufficiency.

Aldosterone deficiency is manifested by increased renal sodium loss and enhanced potassium reabsorption. Salt depletion is associated with water and volume depletion. The decrease in circulating plasma volume leads to postural hypotension. Patients with Addison's disease can have a normal blood pressure when lying down but marked hypotension and tachycardia when they stand up for several minutes. By definition, postural hypotension occurs when systolic and diastolic blood pressures drop by more than 20 mm Hg when the patient assumes the upright position. Postural tachycardia exists when the pulse rate increases by more than 20 beats per minute (bpm) under these circumstances. The decrease in blood pressure and the increase in pulse rate usually persist for more than 3 minutes after the change in position. Thus a person with Addison's disease may have a blood pressure of 120/80 mm Hg when recumbent, but blood pressure may drop to 60/40 mm Hg after the patient assumes the upright position. Likewise, the pulse rate may rise from 80 to 140 bpm with a change in position.

The decrease in intravascular volume and in renal afferent arteriolar pressure stimulates renin release and increases production of angiotensin II. However, because the adrenal cortex is destroyed, angiotensin II is not able to stimulate aldosterone production and restore its level back to baseline. High renin and low aldosterone levels are characteristic of primary aldosterone deficiency.

Androgen deficiency may affect growth of axillary and pubic hair. This effect is masked in men, in whom testicular androgens exert the major androgenic metabolic effects. In women, androgen insufficiency causes loss of axillary and pubic hair and decreased hair over the extremities.

Secondary adrenal insufficiency develops when there is ACTH or CRH deficiency. This deficiency, in turn, causes a decrease in cortisol secretion and eventually adrenal cortical atrophy. The secretion of aldosterone is less affected than cortisol because aldosterone secretion is regulated by the renin-angiotensin system. However, with prolonged ACTH deficiency and adrenal atrophy, the adrenal cortex may become less responsive to angiotensin II, and deficiency of aldosterone secretion may also develop.

The most common cause of secondary adrenal insufficiency is chronic treatment with corticosteroids. This treatment leads to suppression of CRH and ACTH secretion that persists when treatment is interrupted. A consequence is secondary adrenal insufficiency. Other causes of ACTH deficiency are large pituitary tumors with destruction of normal corticotropes, hypothalamic tumors such as craniopharyngiomas, pituitary infarction, and autoimmune panhypopituitarism. Secondary adrenal insufficiency is also a consequence of surgical hypophysectomy and some types of radiation therapy directed to the pituitary gland.

Diagnosis and Treatment

The diagnosis of Addison's disease is suspected on the basis of the clinical manifestations of cortisol, aldosterone, and androgen deficiency described previously. The diagnosis is confirmed with appropriate laboratory tests.

When symptoms develop over weeks or months, a diagnosis is made of chronic adrenal insufficiency. In contrast, symptoms may develop rapidly and lead to a diagnosis of acute adrenal insufficiency or addisonian crisis. This condition can occur when the diagnosis and treatment are delayed and symptoms progress or when patients with an established diagnosis develop an intercurrent acute illness that is not covered by stress doses of steroids. Acute adrenal insufficiency is a medical emergency. Patients present with vomiting, dehydration, hypotension, and hypoglycemia.

The diagnosis of adrenal insufficiency is made by specific laboratory tests. Patients with primary adrenal insufficiency have decreased cortisol and aldosterone but high ACTH and renin levels. In addition, the intravenous infusion of synthetic ACTH fails to elicit a rise in cortisol levels (Fig. 62-1). Because of aldosterone deficiency, electrolyte levels show hyponatremia, hyperkalemia, and metabolic acidosis. Patients with adrenal insufficiency secondary to ACTH deficiency have low levels of both cortisol and ACTH. Aldosterone levels are usually nor-

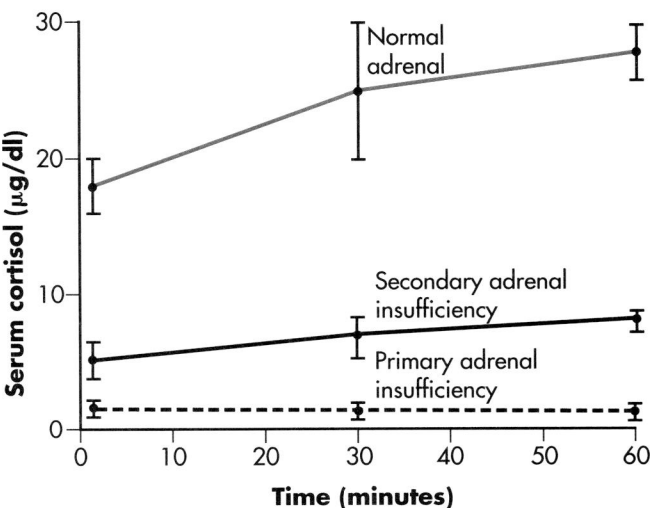

FIG. 62-1 Cortisol response to synthetic ACTH stimulation in normal subjects and in patients with adrenal insufficiency. In secondary adrenal insufficiency, baseline control levels are low but they respond slowly to ACTH. In primary adrenal insufficiency, this response is absent.

mal. An intravenous infusion with synthetic ACTH causes a rise in plasma cortisol, but the rise is subnormal. Adrenal imaging by computed tomography (CT) or magnetic resonance imaging (MRI) can also give information about the possible cause of adrenal insufficiency. Patients with ACTH deficiency or autoimmune destruction of the adrenal cortex usually exhibit small adrenals. In contrast, adrenal masses are found in patients with granulomatous disease, adrenal hematomas, or tumor metastases. The autoimmune cause of adrenal insufficiency may be confirmed by measuring high titers of adrenal autoantibodies. However, the test may become negative if the patient has had the disease for some time.

Treatment of Addison's disease involves replacement with cortisol, usually 20 to 30 mg/day in divided doses, and an aldosterone analog, 9alpha-fluorocortisol. When the dose of these steroids is properly adjusted, patients return to a normal metabolic state and are able to live a normal life. The doses of cortisol and 9alpha-fluorocortisol need to be increased two to three times under conditions of stress (e.g., febrile illness, surgery, trauma), otherwise, patients may develop acute adrenal insufficiency. Treatment of secondary adrenal insufficiency necessitates cortisol replacement only but patients should be tested to confirm their aldosterone secretion is normal.

KEY CONCEPTS

- Adrenocortical insufficiency may be primary (Addison's disease), which is characterized by high levels of ACTH, or it may be secondary, which is characterized by low levels of ACTH.
- The most common cause of primary adrenocortical insufficiency, Addison's disease, is autoimmune destruction of the adrenal glands (>50% of cases); less common causes are infection (e.g., tuberculosis, AIDS), bilateral metastatic neoplasm, adrenal hemorrhage secondary to anticoagulant therapy, and bilateral adrenalectomy.
- Secondary adrenocortical insufficiency may be caused by (1) hypothalamic-pituitary disease (e.g., panhypopituitarism), resulting in decreased ACTH, or (2) sudden withdrawal of exogenous corticosteroid drugs.
- Usually more than 80% of the adrenal glands must be destroyed before signs and symptoms of adrenocortical insufficiency are evident.
- The manifestations of Addison' disease result from cortisol, aldosterone, and androgen deficiency, including (1) progressive weakness and fatigue, (2) anorexia, (3) weight loss, (4) low blood pressure, (5) orthostatic hypotension, (6) hyperpigmentation, (7) fluid and electrolyte disturbances—hyperkalemia, hyponatremia, hypovolemia, metabolic acidosis, (8) fasting hypoglycemia, and (9) reproductive system disturbances—amenorrhea and loss of axillary and pubic hair in women.
- In Addison's disease the hyperpigmentation of body areas (like a deep tan noted on sun-exposed areas, nipples, genitals, buccal mucosa, palmar creases) is caused by increased secretion of melanocyte stimulating hormone (MSH). MSH is a part of the large ACTH molecule, which is elevated.
- Mineralocorticoid (aldosterone) deficiency in Addison's disease causes loss of Na^+ from the distal renal tubules resulting in hyponatremia. Associated water loss leads to extracellular fluid volume deficit and postural hypotension. K^+ and H^+ are retained by the renal distal tubules, resulting in hyperkalemia and metabolic acidosis.
- Glucocorticoid (cortisol) deficiency in Addison's disease may result in hypoglycemia. Because cortisol is required for a normal stress response, patients with

cortisol insufficiency may not be able to withstand the stress of trauma, infection, or surgery and may develop evidence of vascular collapse.
- Diagnostic indicators of primary adrenocortical insufficiency include (1) decreased serum cortisol, (2) decreased urinary 17-hydroxycorticosteroids (cortisol metabolites), (3) increased ACTH, (4) hyponatremia, hyperkalemia, and metabolic acidosis, (5) high serum renin, and (6) low serum aldosterone.
- Patients with primary adrenocortical insufficiency fail to increase serum cortisol levels in response to administration of ACTH (they have high ACTH levels and end-organ failure), whereas cortisol levels do rise when there is secondary adrenocortical insufficiency (they have low ACTH levels).
- Treatment of primary adrenocortical insufficiency consists of hormone replacement therapy: (1) cortisol, 20 to 30 mg/day, in divided doses with increased doses during times of stress, such as surgery, and (2) 9alpha-fluorocortisol (aldosterone analogue) 0.1 to 0.2 mg/day.
- In secondary adrenocortical insufficiency (e.g., as a result of panhypopituitarism), adrenal hypofunction is the result of a lack of ACTH stimulation. Consequently, patients are not hyperpigmented because ACTH levels are low. Patients also have relatively normal fluid and electrolytes levels because aldosterone secretion is normal.
- Patients with acute adrenal insufficiency (Addisonian crisis) present with vomiting, dehydration, hypotension, and hypoglycemia; this condition is a medical emergency.
- Iatrogenic acute adrenocortical (secondary) failure may occur when prolonged high-dose therapeutic corticosteroid therapy is abruptly stopped. Prolonged corticosteroid therapy leads to suppression of normal endogenous steroid production by the adrenal cortex, which becomes mildly atrophied. Sudden cessation of exogenous steroid therapy produces acute adrenocortical failure with hypovolemic and hypotensive shock, hypoglycemia, and risk of sudden death. Corticosteroid drug dosages must always be tapered before complete withdrawal to allow time for adrenocortical function to recover.

A sampling of review questions for this chapter appears here. Visit http://www.mosby.com/MERLIN/PriceWilson/ for additional questions.

Answer the following on a separate sheet of paper.

1. List the causes of primary and secondary adrenal insufficiency and how each affects ACTH levels.

2. Explain the physiologic basis of the following manifestations of adrenocortical insufficiency: (a) hyperpigmentation of skin; (b) orthostatic hypotension; (c) hyperkalemia and hyponatremia; (d) fasting hypoglycemia; (e) scantiness of pubic and axillary hair in a woman.

3. What is the treatment for primary adrenocortical insufficiency?

4. Explain why corticosteroid drug dose must be tapered and never abruptly withdrawn when a patient is on prolonged corticosteroid therapy.

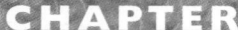

CHAPTER
63

Pancreas: Glucose Metabolism and Diabetes Mellitus

DAVID E. SCHTEINGART

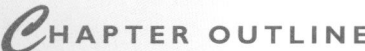

ROLE OF THE PANCREAS IN REGULATING GLUCOSE METABOLISM

Carbohydrates are present in various forms, including simple sugars, or monosaccharides, and complex chemical units, such as disaccharides and polysaccharides. After ingestion, carbohydrates are broken down into monosaccharides and are absorbed, primarily in the duodenum and proximal jejunum. After absorption, the blood glucose level rises temporarily and eventually returns to baseline. The physiologic regulation of the blood glucose level largely depends on the liver (1) extracting glucose, (2) synthesizing glycogen, and (3) performing glycogenolysis. To a lesser extent, peripheral tissues—muscles and adipocytes—extract glucose for their energy needs, thus contributing to the maintenance of normal blood glucose levels.

The liver's uptake and output of glucose and the use of glucose by peripheral tissues depend on the physiologic balance of several hormones that (1) lower blood glucose levels or (2) raise blood glucose levels. Insulin, the blood glucose–lowering hormone, is produced by the beta cells of the islets of Langerhans of the pancreas. Hormones that raise blood glucose levels include (1) glucagon, secreted by the alpha cells of the islets of Langerhans; (2) epinephrine, secreted by the adrenal medulla and other chromaffin tissues; (3) glucocorticoids, secreted by the adrenal cortex; and (4) growth hormone, secreted by the anterior pituitary gland. Glucagon, epinephrine, glucocorticoids, and growth hormone constitute a counterregulatory mechanism that prevents insulin-induced hypoglycemia (Fig. 63-1).

Tests of Glucose Tolerance

A normal fasting serum glucose level (autoanalyzer technique) is 70 to 110 mg/dl. *Hyperglycemia* is defined as a fasting glucose level more than 110 mg/dl and *hypoglycemia* as a level less than 70 mg/dl. Glucose is filtered by the renal glomerulus and is almost totally reabsorbed by the renal tubule as long as the plasma glucose concentration does not exceed 160 to 180 mg/dl. When the serum glucose concentration rises above this level, glucose appears in the urine, a condition called *glycosuria*.

An individual's ability to regulate plasma glucose levels within the normal range may be determined by testing (1) the fasting serum glucose level and (2) the serum glucose response to a glucose load.

Maintenance of normal fasting glucose levels depends on hepatic glucose production, peripheral tissue glucose uptake, and hormones that regulate glucose metabolism. Failure of these functions causes an increase or a decrease in fasting glucose levels. In patients with diabetes mellitus (a condition of relative or absolute insulin deficiency), the fasting serum glucose becomes abnormal once the disease is established. A more sensitive method for uncovering abnormalities in glucose metabolism is the measurement of glucose levels after a glucose load. A nondiabetic individual who ingests a glucose load exhibits an early transient rise in glucose levels that trigger insulin secretion and insulin-mediated glucose disposal with return of these levels to normal. The test traditionally used to evaluate glucose disposal is the *oral glucose tolerance test (OGTT)*. This test has been used for a definitive diagnosis of early diabetes, but it is not required for

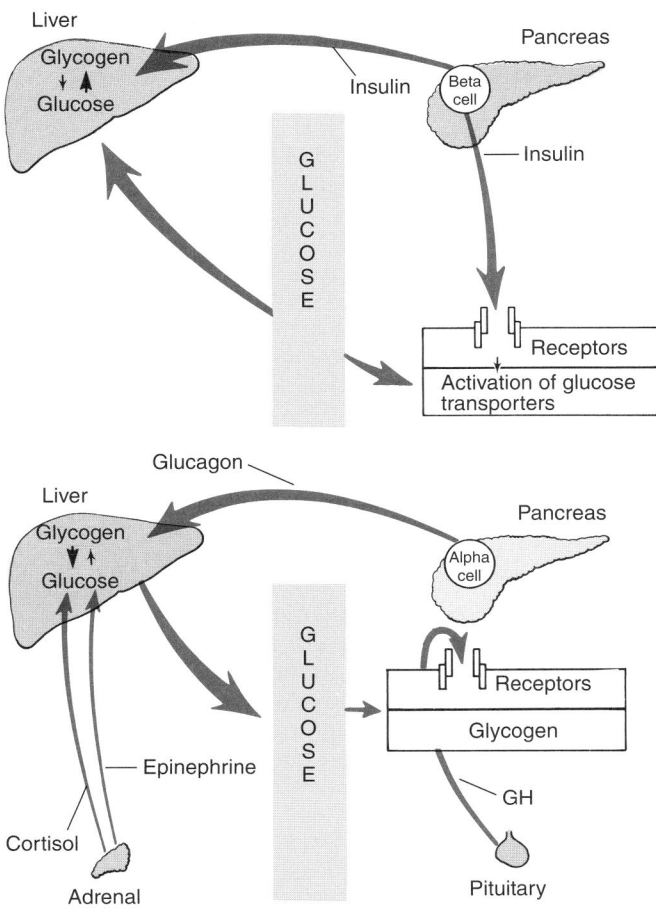

FIG. 63-1   Outline of regulation of blood glucose. *GH,* Growth hormone.

screening and should not be performed in patients with clinical manifestations of diabetes and documented hyperglycemia.

For the OGTT, serum glucose levels are measured before and after ingestion of 75 g of glucose. Glucose levels are measured at $1/_2$-hour intervals for 2 hours after the glucose load. In healthy, ambulatory people with normal glucose tolerance, the fasting glucose level is 70 to 110 mg/dl. After the ingestion of glucose, glucose levels rise initially but return to baseline within 2 hours. Normal values for the OGTT have been defined as serum glucose levels less than 200 mg/dl at $1/_2$, 1, and $1 1/_2$ hours and less than 140 mg/dl at 2 hours (National Diabetes Data Group criteria). Criteria differing slightly from these values have been proposed by other investigators and health organizations.

DIABETES MELLITUS

Definition

Diabetes mellitus is a genetically and clinically heterogeneous group of disorders of metabolism manifested ultimately by loss of carbohydrate tolerance. In its fully developed clinical expression, diabetes mellitus is characterized by fasting and postprandial hyperglycemia, atherosclerotic and microangiopathic vascular disease, and neuropathy. The clinical manifestations of hyperglycemia usually precede by many years the clinical recognition of vascular disease. Patients with only mild abnormality of glucose tolerance (impaired fasting glucose and impaired glucose tolerance) may still be at risk for the metabolic complications of diabetes.

Etiology

Evidence indicates that diabetes mellitus has diverse causes. Although different types of lesions may ultimately lead to insulin insufficiency, genetic determinants are usually critical in most patients with diabetes mellitus. *Type 1 diabetes mellitus* is in most cases a genetically determined autoimmune disease with symptoms that develop at the end of a gradual process of immune destruction of insulin-producing cells. Genetically susceptible individuals appear to respond to a triggering event, probably a viral infection, by producing autoantibodies against the beta cells, which leads to a decline of glucose-stimulated insulin secretion. Clinical manifestations of diabetes mellitus occur when more than 90% of the beta cells have been destroyed. In the more severe forms of diabetes mellitus, beta cells are completely destroyed, resulting in insulinopenia and all of the associated metabolic abnormalities caused by insulin deficiency. Evidence for the genetic determination of type 1 diabetes is its association with specific histocompatibility (human leukocyte antigen [HLA]) types. The type of histocompatibility genes associated with type 1 diabetes (DW3 and DW4) are the ones that code for proteins that play a critical role in monocyte-lymphocyte interactions. These proteins modulate T cell responses that are part of the normal immune response. When a defect occurs, the disordered T lymphocyte function plays an important role in the pathogenesis of islet cell destruction. There is also evidence of increased islet cell antibodies that are directed to specific antigenic components of the beta cell. The triggering event that determines the autoimmune process in genetically susceptible individuals may be an infection with coxsackie B4 or mumps or other viruses. Outbreaks of new-onset type 1 diabetes have been observed at certain times of the year in members of the same social groups. Certain drugs known to trigger other autoimmune diseases may also initiate the autoimmune process in patients with type 1 diabetes. Islet cell antibodies are present in a high percentage of patients with new-onset type 1 diabetes and provide strong evidence of an autoimmune mechanism in the pathogenesis of the disease. Immunologic screening and assessment of insulin secretion in persons at high risk for developing type 1 diabetes may allow early treatment with immunosuppressive therapy that could delay the onset of the clinical manifestations of insulin deficiency.

In patients with *type 2 diabetes,* the disease has a strong familial pattern of occurrence. The concordance rate for type 2 diabetes in monozygotic twins is almost 100%. The risk of developing diabetes is nearly 40% for siblings of patients with type 2 diabetes and 33% for their offspring. The genetic transmission is strongest and best characterized in *maturity-onset diabetes of the young*

(MODY), a subtype of diabetes in which the disease is transmitted in an autosomal dominant pattern. There is a 1:1 ratio of diabetic-to-nondiabetic children when one parent has type 2 diabetes, and about 90% of obligate carriers have type 2 diabetes. Type 2 diabetes is characterized by defects in insulin secretion, as well as in insulin action. The initial event appears to be the development of resistance to insulin in target cells of insulin action. Insulin initially binds itself to specific cell surface receptors. Binding activates the receptor and starts a cascade of intracellular reactions that lead to mobilization of GLUT 4 glucose transporters and increased glucose transport across the cell membrane. In patients with type 2 diabetes, a defect exists in insulin receptor binding. This defect may be caused by a decreased number of receptor sites in the cell membrane of insulin-responsive cells or by intrinsic abnormalities of the insulin receptor. As a consequence, abnormal coupling occurs between insulin receptor complexes and the glucose transport system. Postreceptor abnormalities may also impair insulin action. In the face of insulin resistance, normal glucose levels are maintained for a long time through an increase in insulin secretion. Eventually, beta cell failure occurs with a decline in the amount of circulating insulin that is no longer sufficient to maintain euglycemia. About 80% of patients with type 2 diabetes are obese. Because obesity is associated with insulin resistance, it is likely that impairment of glucose tolerance eventually develops, leading to type 2 diabetes. Weight reduction is associated with improvement in insulin sensitivity and recovery of glucose tolerance.

Classification of Diabetes

Several classifications of diabetes mellitus have been proposed, based on the modalities of clinical presentation, age of onset, and natural history of the disease. Box 63-1 describes a classification proposed by the American Diabetes Association (ADA), based on contemporary knowledge of the pathogenesis of the diabetic syndrome and disorders of glucose tolerance. This classification has been endorsed by the World Health Organization (WHO) and generally adopted. Four clinical classes of

---

BOX 63-1

ADA Classification of Diabetes and Abnormalities of Glucose Intolerance

1. Diabetes mellitus
   a. Type 1
      (1) Autoimmune
      (2) Idiopathic
   b. Type 2
2. Gestational diabetes mellitus (GDM)
3. Other specific types
   a. Genetic defects of beta cell function: MODY
   b. Genetic defects of insulin action: Severe insulin resistance syndromes
   c. Endocrinopathies: Cushing's syndrome, acromegaly
   d. Diseases of the exocrine pancreas
   e. Drug or chemically-induced
   f. Infections
4. Impaired glucose tolerance (IGT)
5. Impaired fasting glucose (IFG)

ADA, American Diabetes Association

---

disorders of glucose tolerance are described: (1) diabetes mellitus types 1 and 2, (2) gestational diabetes, and (3) other specific types. Two other categories of abnormal glucose tolerance are impaired glucose tolerance and impaired fasting glucose.

Type 1 diabetes has been termed in the past juvenile-onset type and insulin-dependent type; however, it can occur at any age. Type 1 diabetes has an incidence of 30,000 new cases per year and can be divided in two subtypes: (a) autoimmune, resulting from autoimmune dysfunction with destruction of beta cells; and (b) idiopathic, without evidence of autoimmunity and of unknown origin. This subtype occurs more frequently in individuals of African-American and Asian ethnic background.

Type 2 diabetes has been termed in the past adult or maturity-onset type and non–insulin-dependent type and has an incidence of 650,000 new cases per year. Obesity is frequently associated with this type.

Gestational diabetes (GDM) is first recognized during pregnancy and affects 4% of all pregnancies. Risk factors for its development are older age, ethnicity, obesity, multiparity, family history, and previous history of gestational diabetes. Because of the increased secretion of various hormones with metabolic effects on glucose tolerance, pregnancy is a diabetogenic condition. Patients with a genetic predisposition for diabetes may first show glucose intolerance or clinical manifestations of diabetes with pregnancy. The recommended criteria for the biochemical diagnosis of gestational diabetes are those proposed by O'Sullivan and Mahan (1973). According to these criteria, GDM is present when two or more of the following values are met or exceeded after a 75-g oral glucose challenge: fasting, 105 mg/dl; 1 hour, 190 mg/dl; 2 hours, 165 mg/dl; and 3 hours, 145 mg/dl. Recognition of GDM is important because these patients are at increased risk for perinatal morbidity and mortality and have increased frequency of viable fetal loss. Most pregnant women should be screened for diabetes during 24 to 28 weeks of gestation.

Other specific types include (a) genetic defects in the beta cell as recognized in MODY. This subtype of diabetes has strong familial prevalence and manifests itself before age 14 years. Patients are frequently obese and insulin resistant. The genetic defects have been well characterized in the form of four different mutations and phenotypes (MODY 1, MODY 2, MODY 3, and MODY 4); (b) genetic defects of insulin action, causing *severe insulin resistance syndromes* and acanthosis nigricans; (c) diseases of the exocrine pancreas causing chronic pancreatitis; (d) endocrine diseases such as Cushing's syndrome and acromegaly; (e) drugs with toxic effects on the beta cells; (f) and infections.

According to the ADA criteria for nonpregnant adults, the diagnosis of diabetes mellitus is based on the findings of (1) classic symptoms of diabetes and unequivocal hyperglycemia, (2) fasting plasma glucose levels ≥126 mg/dl (7 mmol/L) on at least two occasions, and (3) glucose levels obtained during an oral glucose tolerance test (OGTT) ≥200 mg/dl at 2 hours and at least at one other time between 0 and 2 hours after ingestion of glucose. The fasting glucose level of 126 mg/dl was chosen because it has the best concordance with the 2-hour postglucose value of 200 mg/dl and is the level at which diabetic retinopathy, a complication of diabetes, first occurs. The fasting blood glucose is the preferred method of screening for diabetes.

The diagnosis of diabetes mellitus in children is also based on the finding of classic symptoms of diabetes and random plasma glucose >200 mg/dl.

Patients with *impaired glucose tolerance (IGT)* do not meet the criteria described for diagnosis of diabetes mellitus; however, their OGTTs show abnormal values. These patients are asymptomatic. Biochemically, patients with IGT exhibit normal fasting plasma glucose levels ($\geq$110 and <126 mg/dl) but values during an OGTT are $\geq$200 mg/dl at $1/2$, 1, or $1^1/_2$ hours and 140 to 200 mg/dl at 2 hours. Some patients with IGT may have underlying conditions that may be responsible for secondary types of diabetes. In other individuals, IGT may be the expression of an early stage in the development of diabetes. These individuals are not considered to have diabetes but are recognized as being at higher risk than the general population for the development of diabetes. Some of these patients may remain in this class for many years. Many patients return to normal glucose tolerance spontaneously, but 1% to 5% of persons with IGT proceed to overt clinical diabetes annually. Although clinically significant renal and retinal microangiopathic complications of diabetes are absent in patients with IGT, many studies of such groups have shown an increased prevalence of arterial disease, electrocardiographic abnormalities, and cardiac death or increased susceptibility to atherosclerotic disease. Appropriate intervention, including caloric restriction or weight loss in obese persons with IGT, may lead to improvement in glucose tolerance and a possible change in the occurrence of these complications. *Impaired fasting glucose* is defined as values between 110 (upper limit of normal) and 126 mg/dl. Patients with impaired fasting glucose are also at increased risk of developing diabetes and the metabolic complications associated with IGT.

Epidemiology

The prevalence rate of diabetes mellitus is high. Estimates are that there are 16 million individuals with diabetes in the United States and that 600,000 new cases are diagnosed every year. Diabetes is the third leading cause of death by disease in the United States and the leading cause of blindness in adults, through the development of diabetic retinopathy. The incidence of heart attack in individuals with diabetes is at least $2^1/_2$ times that of nondiabetic individuals of a comparable age.

Seventy-five percent of diabetic patients eventually die of vascular disease. Heart attacks, kidney failure, cerebrovascular accidents (CVAs, strokes), and gangrene are the major complications. In addition, there is an increased rate of intrauterine fetal death in infants of women with poorly controlled diabetes.

The economic impact of diabetes is substantial as a result of medical expenses and lost wages in addition to the financial consequence of many of the complications such as blindness and vascular disease.

Clinical Manifestations

The clinical manifestations of diabetes mellitus are related to the metabolic consequence of insulin deficiency. Patients with insulin deficiency are unable to maintain

normal fasting plasma glucose levels or glucose tolerance after ingesting carbohydrates. If the hyperglycemia is severe and exceeds the renal threshold for this substance, glycosuria supervenes. Glycosuria leads to osmotic diuresis, which causes increased urine output *(polyuria)* and thirst *(polydipsia)*. Because of the loss of glucose through the urine, patients develop negative caloric balance and weight loss. Increased hunger *(polyphagia)* may also develop as the result of calorie loss. Patients complain of fatigue and sleepiness.

Patients with type 1 frequently exhibit an explosive onset of symptoms with polydipsia, polyuria, weight loss, polyphagia, fatigue, and somnolence occurring within a few days or weeks. Patients may become extremely ill and develop *ketoacidosis*, and they may die if treatment is not instituted promptly. Insulin therapy is usually required for metabolic control, and patients are generally sensitive to insulin. In contrast, patients with type 2 may be completely asymptomatic, and the diagnosis may be made only after a laboratory examination of their blood and performance of OGTTs. With more severe degrees of hyperglycemia, these patients may develop polydipsia, polyuria, fatigue, and somnolence. Ketoacidosis does not usually develop because patients are relatively and not absolutely insulin deficient. The amount of insulin still being secreted is sufficient to inhibit ketogenesis. If the hyperglycemia is severe and patients do not respond to diet therapy or to oral hypoglycemic drugs, insulin therapy may be required to normalize glucose levels. These patients usually exhibit diminished peripheral sensitivity to insulin. The patients' own insulin levels may be diminished, normal, or high but inadequate to maintain normal blood glucose levels. Patients are also resistant to exogenous insulin.

Assessment of Glycemic Control

A method for determining glycemic control in all types of diabetes is the measurement of *glycated hemoglobin*. Hemoglobin does not normally contain glucose when it is first released from the bone marrow. During its 120-day life span in the red blood cell, hemoglobin normally incorporates glucose. If the ambient glucose level rises above normal, the amount of glycated hemoglobin will rise accordingly. Because of the slow hemoglobin turnover, a high value indicates that blood glucose levels have been high for 4 to 8 weeks. Normal values for glycated hemoglobin depend on the method of measurement employed but ranges between 3.5% and 5.5%. It is advisable to determine the reference values for each laboratory. Table 63-1 summarizes the range of glycated hemoglobin observed in patients with diabetes. The test can be done in an ambulatory care clinic within a few min-

TABLE 63-1

Glycated Hemoglobin Levels in Diabetes

Normal/Glucose Control	Glycated Hemoglobin (%)
Normal value	3.5-5.5
Good glucose control	3.5-6.0
Fair glucose control	7.0-8.0
Poor glucose control	Greater than 8.0

utes and provides a quick and reliable indicator of the level of glycemic control in the preceding 4 to 8 weeks.

Management

The management of diabetes mellitus is based on (1) meal planning, (2) exercise and controlled physical activity, (3) hypoglycemic oral agents, (4) insulin therapy, (5) home glucose monitoring, and (6) diabetes education and self-management. Diabetes is a chronic disease, and patients need to master the treatment and learn how to make adjustments to achieve optimal metabolic control. Patients with type 1 diabetes are insulin deficient and always require insulin therapy. Patients with type 2 diabetes have insulin resistance and relative insulin deficiency and can be treated without insulin.

The meal plan of diabetic patients is aimed at controlling the number of calories and the amount of carbohydrates ingested daily. The recommended number of calories varies, depending on the need for maintaining, reducing, or increasing body weight. For example, if a patient is obese, a calorie-restricted diet may be prescribed until the patient's weight has dropped into an optimal range for that person. In contrast, young patients with type 1 diabetes may lose weight during the state of decompensation. These patients should receive sufficient calories to restore their weight and for growth. The meal plan should be developed in consultation with a registered dietitian and based on a patient's diet history, food preferences, lifestyle, cultural background, and physical activity.

To prevent excessive postprandial hyperglycemia and glycosuria, diabetic patients should avoid excessive intake of carbohydrates. Usually, carbohydrates make up 50% of the total daily calorie allowance. This carbohydrate allowance must be distributed in such a way that the intake matches the patients' requirements throughout the day. For example, larger amounts are given at times of greater physical activity. Fat intake should be limited to 30% of the total daily caloric allowance, and at least one half should be of the polyunsaturated type. One approach to meal planning is the food exchange system. This system groups together foods with similar amounts of carbohydrate, protein, and fat, and therefore calories. This system allows patients to "trade" the food on each exchange list for any other food on the same list. Other approaches to meal planning call for carbohydrate counting and matching with an appropriate dose of short-acting insulin. Patients can count either the number of carbohydrate servings or the grams of total carbohydrate. Insulin can then be taken in a ratio of 1 unit per 15 gm of total carbohydrate. This ratio can be increased upwards depending on the patient's response. Insulin-resistant patients with type 2 diabetes may require 2 to 5 units for every carbohydrate serving or 15 gm total carbohydrate.

Exercise appears to facilitate the transport of glucose into cells and to increase sensitivity to insulin. In nondiabetic individuals, insulin release decreases during exercise and hypoglycemia is avoided. However, patients who take insulin injections are unable to exert this control, and the increased glucose uptake during exercise can lead to hypoglycemia. This factor is particularly important when a patient engages in physical exercise when the insulin dose has reached its maximal or peak effect time. By appropriate timing of their physical exertion, patients may be able to improve the control of their glucose levels. For example, if patients exercise when their blood glucose level is high, they may be able to lower this level with exercise alone. Conversely, if patients need to exercise when the blood glucose level is low, they must receive additional carbohydrate to prevent hypoglycemia.

Patients with early type 2 diabetes may be able to maintain normal blood glucose levels by means of a meal plan and physical exercise. However, as the disease progresses, oral hypoglycemic drugs are indicated. These drugs include insulin sensitizers and sulfonylureas. Two types of insulin sensitizers are available, metformin and thiazolidinediones. Metformin, a biguanide, can be given as first-line monotherapy in doses of 500 to 1700 mg/day. Metformin decreases hepatic glucose production, decreases intestinal absorption of glucose, and enhances insulin sensitivity, especially in the liver. Metformin does not promote weight gain as does insulin, and it is particularly useful in obese patients. Lactic acidosis is a rare but serious complication, especially in patients with renal insufficiency and congestive heart failure. Thiazolidinediones increase peripheral insulin sensitivity and decrease hepatic glucose production. The effect of these drugs appears to be mediated through interaction with the nuclear receptor peroxisome proliferator-activated receptor gamma (PPAR-gamma). The two thiazolidinedione analogs, rosiglitazone, in doses of 4 to 8 mg/daily, and pioglitazone, in doses of 30 to 45 mg/daily, can be given as monotherapy or in combination with metformin, sulfonylureas, or insulin. These drugs can cause water retention and are not recommended in patients with congestive heart failure.

If glucose levels are not optimally controlled by the strategies described, type 2 diabetic patients with some remaining islet cell function are good candidates for the use of *sulfonylureas*. These drugs stimulate beta cell function and increase the secretion of insulin. In contrast, patients with type 1 diabetes have lost their insulin-secreting capacity, and treatment with sulfonylureas will be ineffective. There are potential adverse effects from the use of oral hypoglycemic agents (Table 63-2). However, second-generation sulfonylureas cause little or no water retention, a potential problem with some of the first-generation agents. The two sulfonylurea compounds most commonly employed are glipizide, 2.5 to 40.0 mg/daily, and glyburide, 2.5 to 25.0 mg/daily. Glyburide has a longer half-life than does glipizide, and the total daily dose can be given once daily. Combining sulfonylureas with insulin sensitizers is a common drug therapy for patients with type 2 diabetes. To decrease the postprandial rise in glucose levels in these patients, carbohydrate absorption can be decreased or delayed by the preprandial use of acarbose, an alpha glucosidase inhibitor that acts on the small intestine by blocking the digestion of complex carbohydrates.

Insulin Management

In people without diabetes, insulin secretion compensates for varying amounts of food intake and exercise. In contrast, individuals with diabetes are unable to secrete sufficient quantity of insulin to maintain euglycemia. As a

TABLE 63-2

Oral Hypoglycemic Agents

Agent	Half-Life (Hours)	Timing Dose	Initial Dose (mg)	Maintenance Dose (mg)	Toxicity	Tablet Size (mg)
Glipizide (Glucotrol)	2 to 4	Twice daily	2.5	5 to 40	Gastrointestinal Skin Hematologic	5,10
Glyburide (Micronase, DiaBeta)	10	Once or twice	5.0	2.5 to 20.0	Skin Gastrointestinal Hematologic	1.25 to 5.00
Metformin (Glucophage)	1.3 to 4.5	Three times daily	1000	1500-1700	Lactic acidosis	500, 850
Rosiglitazone		Once daily	4.0	4-8	Edema	4.0
Pioglitazone		Once daily	30	30-45	Edema	30

TABLE 63-3

Insulins

Type	Description	Effect on Blood Glucose (Hours after Administration)		
		Onset	Peak	Termination
SHORT ACTING				
Lispro	Clear	Immediate	30-90 min	3-5
Regular (crystalline zinc)	Clear	30 min	2-4 min	6-8
INTERMEDIATE ACTING				
NPH*	Cloudy: crystalline zinc insulin suspension 50% saturated with protamine	2-3	4-8	13.8
LONG ACTING				
Ultralente (UL)†	Cloudy: crystalline insulin suspension High zinc content, no protamine	6	16-18	24
Glargine	Isoelectric point 7.0; decreased solubility at physiologic pH; forms microprecipitate in subcutaneous tissue	—	None	22.8

*Delayed action of NPH is controlled by protamine content; it is prepared in sodium phosphate buffer.
†Lente insulins (semi and ultra) do not contain protamine and are prepared in sodium acetate buffer; their time of action depends on their variable zinc content and crystal size.

consequence, blood glucose rises to high levels in response to meals, and levels are high in the fasting state. Patients with severe insulin insufficiency require injections of insulin in addition to a meal plan. Several preparations of insulin are available (Table 63-3). This insulin is identical to human insulin and is prepared by recombinant deoxyribonucleic acid (DNA) techniques. Changes in the crystalline structure and amino acid sequence of the insulin molecule has resulted in preparations with different duration of action that can be used to customize the insulin treatment to patients' specific needs. Insulins are classified as *short acting, intermediate acting, or long acting*, according to the time required for the maximal plasma glucose–lowering effect to take place after injection. *Short-acting insulins* produce their maximal effect within minutes to 6 hours after injection and are used to control postprandial hyperglycemia. Short-acting insulin is also used for intravenous treatment and in the management of patients with diabetic ketoacidosis. Short-acting insulins may be used in combination with longer-acting insulins. *Intermediate-acting insulins* have their peak within 6 to 8 hours after administration and are used for the day-to-day control of the patient with diabetes. *Long-acting insulins* have a peak effect within 14 to 20 hours after administra-

tion and are rarely used in the routine management of these patients. One of the two newer insulin analogs is lispro, a very short-acting insulin analog with decreased capacity for self-association and faster absorption; it has very rapid onset of action and can be used immediately before or immediately after meals. When given after a meal, the dose can be adjusted to cover the food eaten, allowing patients flexibility in their meal choices. Another type of insulin is glargine, in which glycine has been substituted for asparagine at position 21 of the A chain, and two arginine molecules have been added at position 30 of the B chain. This insulin analog has a very long and even action without a peak and can be used to provide a basal level of insulin to patients on an intensive insulin treatment program.

Blood glucose control for insulin-requiring diabetic patients can be achieved by the use of intermediate-acting insulin administered before breakfast and supper, with the larger portion given before breakfast. Short-acting insulin is frequently combined with intermediate-acting insulin for physiologic regulation of glucose during postprandial periods, particularly in patients with type 1 diabetes. The patient can prepare this combination by mixing variable quantities of the two types of insulin or can be given as a ready mix of 70% NPH, 30% regular insulin (70/30), or 75% NPH, 25 lispro insulin (75/25). More intense insulin therapy has been achieved using more frequent insulin injections or continuous subcutaneous insulin infusion systems. When frequent insulin injections are given, short-acting regular insulin is given before each meal, and intermediate-acting NPH insulin is given at bedtime. A convenient choice for this type of treatment is insulin glargine administered once daily at bedtime combined with multiple doses of lispro at meal time. The dose of regular insulin is adjusted according to a preestablished algorithm that takes into account the prevailing glucose level and size of the meal. Patients need to purchase insulin syringes and needles for self-subcutaneous administration of insulin. Insulin pens loaded with a fixed amount of insulin are also available for convenient use by patients. The injections are usually given in the abdomen or in the limbs, making sure that the site is rotated and that insulin is not injected into a blood vessel or into a scar.

Intensive insulin therapy can be administered through a subcutaneous insulin infusion pump. Several lightweight, portable pumps are available that deliver a continuous basal infusion, as well as preprandial boluses given 30 minutes before each meal. Patients on insulin therapy must monitor their glucose level before each insulin dose. This assessment is accomplished by finger stick, which produces a drop of capillary blood. The blood is applied to a test strip and read off a glucose meter. The meter can store the glucose values in its memory, and this information can be unloaded by the health care professional for further advice on the insulin program. Intensive insulin therapy frequently results in improved glucose control.

Patients with diabetes mellitus can lead a relatively normal life if they are well informed about their disease and its management. Patients can learn to administer their own insulin, monitor their blood glucose level, and use this information to regulate their insulin dosage and plan their diet and exercise to minimize hyperglycemia and hypoglycemia. For patients with type 2 diabetes who are obese, asymptomatic, and have moderately elevated glucose levels, the treatment of choice is dietary restriction and weight reduction. However, the success rate in weight reduction among these patients is low, and they may eventually require therapy with hypoglycemic agents.

Complications

Complications of diabetes mellitus can be divided into two major categories: (1) acute metabolic complications and (2) long-term vascular complications.

Acute Metabolic Complications

The metabolic complications of diabetes result from relatively acute changes in plasma glucose concentration. The most serious metabolic complication of type 1 diabetes is *diabetic ketoacidosis (DKA)*. With severe insulin insufficiency, patients develop severe hyperglycemia and glycosuria, decreased lipogenesis, increased lipolysis, and increased oxidation of free fatty acids with production of ketone bodies (acetoacetate, hydroxybutyrate, and acetone). The increase in ketones in plasma causes ketosis.

The increased production of ketones causes an increased hydrogen ion load and metabolic acidosis. Marked glycosuria and ketonuria also lead to osmotic diuresis and resultant dehydration and loss of electrolytes. Patients may become hypotensive and develop a state of shock. Eventually, because of decreased cerebral oxygen availability, patients may become comatose and die. Coma and death from DKA are rare today, because patients and health care personnel are aware of the potential dangers of this complication, and treatment of DKA can be instituted early.

DKA is treated by (1) reversing the metabolic derangement caused by the lack of insulin, (2) restoring water and electrolyte balance, and (3) treating conditions that may have precipitated ketoacidosis. Treatment with short-acting (regular) insulin—administered as a continuous intravenous infusion or as frequent intramuscular injections—and glucose in water or saline infusions increases glucose use, decreases lipolysis and ketone body production, and restores acid-base balance. In addition, patients may need potassium replacement. Because intercurrent infections can increase insulin requirements in patients with diabetes, it is not unusual for infection to precipitate acute diabetic decompensation and DKA. Thus antibiotics may be necessary in the management of these patients.

Hyperglycemic, hyperosmolar, nonketotic coma (HHNK) is another acute metabolic complication that occurs most often in older individuals with type 2 diabetes. Because of relative but not absolute insulin deficiency, hyperglycemia develops without ketosis. Hyperglycemia is severe, with serum glucose levels greater than 600 mg/dl. Hyperglycemia causes hyperosmolality, osmotic diuresis, and profound dehydration. The patient may become unconscious and may die if the condition is not quickly reversed. The mortality rate may be as high as 50%. The treatment of HHNK consists of rehydration, electrolyte replacement, and regular insulin. The major difference between HHNK and DKA is the lack of ketosis with HHNK.

Another frequent metabolic complication of diabetes is *hypoglycemia* (insulin reaction, insulin shock), mainly a complication of insulin therapy. Insulin-dependent diabetic patients may occasionally receive insulin in amounts larger than that needed to maintain normal glucose levels with resulting hypoglycemia. Symptoms of hypoglycemia are caused by epinephrine release (sweating, shakiness, headache, palpitations) and by lack of glucose in the brain (bizarre behavior, dullness of sensorium, coma). *It must be emphasized that hypoglycemic attacks are dangerous and, if frequent or prolonged, may cause permanent brain damage or even death.* Management of hypoglycemia requires the prompt administration of carbohydrate, either orally or intravenously. Occasionally, glucagon, a glycogenolytic hormone, is administered intramuscularly to raise blood glucose levels. Insulin-induced hypoglycemia in a diabetic patient can trigger the release of counterregulatory hormones (glucagon, epinephrine, cortisol, growth hormone), which raise glucose levels frequently to a hyperglycemic range *(Somogyi effect)*. The lows and highs in glucose levels lead to poor diabetic control. Prevention of hypoglycemia by reducing the insulin dose also ameliorates subsequent hyperglycemia.

Chronic Long-Term Complications

The long-term vascular complications of diabetes involve small vessels—microangiopathy—and middle- and large-size vessels—macroangiopathy. *Microangiopathy* is a specific lesion of diabetes that affects capillaries and arterioles of the retina *(diabetic retinopathy)*, renal glomeruli *(diabetic nephropathy)*, peripheral nerves *(diabetic neuropathy)*, and muscles and skin. Histochemically, the lesions are characterized by increased accumulation of glycoprotein. In addition, because the chemical components of the basement membrane can be derived from glucose, hyperglycemia causes an increased rate of formation and thickening of basement membrane. These cells do not require insulin for glucose use. Histologic evidence of microangiopathy is already apparent in patients with IGT. However, clinical manifestations of vascular disease, retinopathy, or nephropathy usually appear 15 to 20 years after the onset of diabetes.

A strong relationship exists between hyperglycemia and the incidence and progression of retinopathy. An early manifestation of retinopathy is the presence of microaneurysms (tiny saccular dilations) of the retinal arterioles. Subsequently, hemorrhages, neovascularization, and retinal scars may lead to blindness (Fig. 63-2). The most successful treatment of retinopathy is panretinal photocoagulation. A laser beam is focused on the retina, producing a chorioretinal scar. Over the course of several sessions, an average of 1800 scars are placed throughout the posterior pole of the retina. This treatment approach appears to suppress neovascularization and subsequent hemorrhage.

Early manifestations of nephropathy are proteinuria and hypertension. As the loss of functioning nephrons progresses, patients develop renal insufficiency and uremia. At this stage, patients may require dialysis or renal transplantation. The pathogenesis of diabetic nephropathy, and current research on interventions to slow its progression are discussed in Chapters 46 and 48.

Neuropathy and cataracts result from disturbances in the polyol pathway (glucose → sorbitol → fructose) caused by lack of insulin. In the lens, there is increased accumulation of sorbitol, leading to the formation of cataracts and blindness. In nerve tissue, there is an increased accumulation of sorbitol and fructose and a decreased concentration of myoinositol, leading to neuropathy. The biochemical alteration in nerve tissue interferes with metabolic activity of the Schwann cells and causes axonal loss. Motor conduction velocity decreases early in the course of neuropathy. Subsequently, the patient has pain, paresthesias, decreased vibratory and proprioceptive sensations, and motor impairment with loss of deep tendon reflexes, muscle weakness, and atrophy. Neuropathy may involve peripheral nerves (mononeuropathy and polyneuropathy) (see color plate 38), cranial nerves, or the autonomic nervous system. Involvement of the autonomic nervous system may be accompanied by nocturnal diarrhea, delayed gastric emptying with gastroparesis, postural hypotension, and erectile dysfunction. Patients with diabetic autonomic neuropathy may suffer painless acute myocardial infarctions. They may also lose the catecholamine response to hypoglycemia and become unaware of hypoglycemic reactions.

Diabetic *macroangiopathy* has the histopathologic characteristics of atherosclerosis. A combination of biochemical disturbances caused by insulin insufficiency probably leads to this type of vascular disease. The disturbances include (1) accumulation of sorbitol in the vascular intima, (2) hyperlipoproteinemia, and (3) abnormality in blood coagulation. Diabetic macroangiopathy eventually leads to vascular occlusion. When the disturbance involves peripheral arteries, it may result in *peripheral vascular insufficiency* with intermittent claudication and *gangrene of the extremities and cerebral insufficiency and stroke.* When it involves the aorta and coronary arteries, it may lead to angina and myocardial infarction.

Diabetes also interferes with pregnancy. Women with diabetes who become pregnant are prone to spontaneous abortions, intrauterine fetal death, large fetal size, and premature infants with a high incidence of respiratory distress syndrome and fetal malformations. The outcome of pregnancy in diabetic mothers has improved with tighter blood glucose control before and during pregnancy, early delivery, and advances in the field of neonatology and in the management of complications in the newborn. The change in hormonal environment during pregnancy causes a progressive increase in insulin requirement, which reaches a peak in the third trimester, with a sharp drop in insulin requirements at delivery.

Present clinical and experimental evidence suggests that long-term diabetic complications develop because of the chronic abnormality in metabolism caused by insufficient insulin secretion. Diabetic complications can be minimized or prevented if the treatment of diabetes is effective enough to bring glucose levels, as indicated by glycated hemoglobin, to within the normal range. The importance of glucose control in ameliorating or preventing the complications of diabetes has been highlighted by the results of the Diabetes Control and Complications Trial (DCCT), conducted as a multicenter study over a 10-year period. Patients with type 1 diabetes who re-

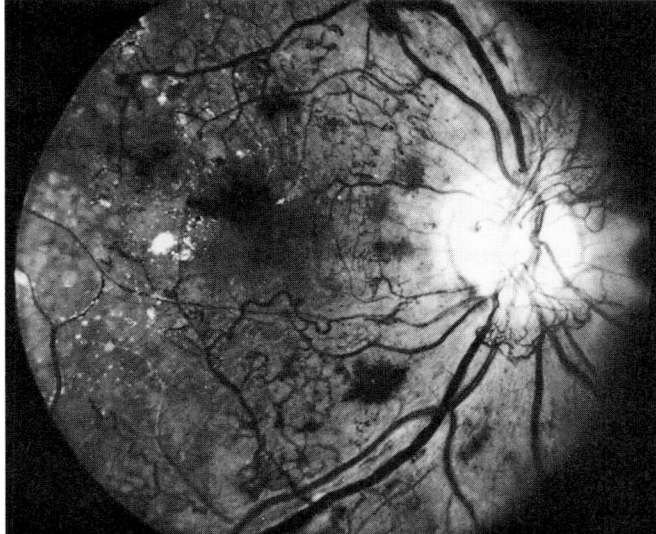

FIG. 63-2 Diabetic retinopathy. Note the hemorrhages, exudates, neovascularization, and dilation of the veins in the fundus of a patient with diabetes mellitus. (From the Ophthalmology Department, University Hospital, University of Michigan.)

ceived intensified insulin therapy and decreased their glycated hemoglobin levels to <7% experienced a 50% to 75% reduction in the major microangiopathic complications, including retinopathy, nephropathy, and neuropathy. A similar 10-year study, the United Kingdom Prospective Diabetes Study (UKPDS), showed the importance of glycemic control in risk reduction of complications in patients with type 2 diabetes.

The ultimate objective in the treatment of diabetes is *prevention*. The recognition of individuals at risk for developing type 1 diabetes may lead to early detection of the autoimmune process, causing the destruction of beta cells and treatment with specific immunosuppressive agents. Once the disease has developed, pancreatic transplantation may restore the insulin-secreting capacity. In patients with type 2 diabetes, a better understanding of the molecular mechanism of insulin resistance may lead to development of pharmacologic agents that might specifically enhance insulin action. Research in these areas is in progress.

KEY CONCEPTS

- *Metabolism* encompasses the total collection of chemical reactions in the body and reflects the ability of the body to capture and store the energy derived from foods and to make that energy available in the appropriate form when needed.
- Glucose is used by most body cells as an energy source. Some cells (e.g., brain cells) can only use glucose for energy. Fat and muscle cells require a carrier facilitated by insulin to transport glucose across the cell membrane.
- The absorptive ("eating") and postabsorptive (fasting, between meals) are the two functional states that encompass the mechanisms involved in overall body metabolism.
- During the absorptive state, glucose rises above the baseline temporarily and is the main energy provider; excess glucose not needed for energy is stored as glycogen in the liver and skeletal muscles or converted into fat to be used in the postabsorptive state.
- During the postabsorptive (fasting) state, endogenous fat stores provide the main source of energy, but a continuous supply of glucose must be available for brain and nervous system energy needs.
- The physiologic regulation of glucose largely depends on the liver. The liver's uptake and output of glucose and the use of glucose by peripheral tissues depend on the physiologic balance of several hormones that lower and raise blood glucose levels.
- *Insulin*, the *blood glucose-lowering hormone*, rises a few minutes after eating and returns to baseline within 3 hours. Insulin lowers blood glucose by increasing glucose transport into cells and by glycogenesis. Insulin plays a crucial role in regulating carbohydrate, fat, and protein metabolism.
- *Glucagon, growth hormone, epinephrine*, and *cortisol* are *counterregulatory hormones* that raise blood glucose and have an opposite effect to that of insulin. These hormones are important in preventing hypoglycemia during the fasting state and during stress.
- The *normal fasting serum glucose* is 70 to 110 mg/dl. *Hyperglycemia* is defined as a serum glucose of >110 mg/dl and *hypoglycemia* as a level <70 mg/dl.
- An individual's ability to regulate plasma glucose may be determined by testing (1) the fasting serum glucose level and (2) the serum glucose response to ingestion of a glucose load (oral glucose tolerance test [OGTT]).
- Glucose is filtered at the renal glomerulus and almost completely reabsorbed, provided its serum level does not exceed the normal renal threshold for glucose, 160 to 180 mg/dl. *Glycosuria* occurs when the renal threshold is exceeded. Excretion of glucose in the urine is accompanied by increased excretion of water and electrolytes (*osmotic diuresis*) and figure very strongly in the pathophysiology of diabetic ketoacidosis (DKA) and hyperglycemic, hyperosmolar, nonketotic coma (HHNK).
- *Diabetes mellitus* is a set of disorders characterized by either an absolute or a relative deficiency of insulin or insulin resistance (or both). In its fully developed clinical expression, diabetes mellitus is characterized by fasting and postprandial hyperglycemia, atherosclerotic and microangiopathic vascular disease, and neuropathy.
- Two main types of primary diabetes mellitus are recognized: (1) *type 1 diabetes* (formerly called juvenile-onset or insulin-dependent diabetes mellitus (IDDM) and (2) *type 2 diabetes* (formerly called adult-onset or non–insulin-dependent diabetes mellitus (NIDDM).
- *Type 1 diabetes* is characterized by an *absolute lack of endogenous insulin* caused by autoimmune destruction of the pancreatic beta cells in the islets of Langerhans, or it may be idiopathic.
- *Type 2 diabetes* is characterized by peripheral insulin resistance, impaired insulin secretion, and excessive hepatic glucose production. There is no evidence of autoimmune-mediated destruction of the pancreatic beta cells. Obesity is often associated with this type.
- *Genetic predisposition* plays an important role in susceptibility to diabetes. Most persons with type 2 diabetes have a family history of diabetes, although no reliable genetic marker has been identified.
- The major histocompatibility complex (MHC) haplotype, especially the DR3 and DR4 genes coding for class II proteins, are present in the majority of patients with type 1 diabetes.
- To diagnose any of the clinical categories of glucose intolerance, the level of *plasma glucose* (also called blood glucose or blood sugar) is measured. Measurements may be of a fasting, random, or postprandial plasma glucose or with an OGTT.
- *Normoglycemia* is defined as a fasting plasma glucose (FPG) ≤110 mg/dl or a 2-hour plasma postprandial glucose of <140 after the OGTT.

- *Three ways to diagnose diabetes* according to ADA criteria include (1) classic symptoms of diabetes (polyuria, polydipsia, and weight loss) plus random plasma glucose (RPG) ≥200 mg/dl, (2) FPG ≥126, or (3) 2-hour postprandial plasma glucose of ≥200 mg/dl during an OGTT. A diagnosis of diabetes must be confirmed, on a subsequent day, by measurement of FBG, 2-hour plasma glucose using the OGTT, or RPG (if symptoms are present).
- *Gestational diabetes (GDM)* is a disorder of glucose tolerance of variable severity with onset of first recognition during pregnancy. Women with GDM have an increased risk for the development of type 2 diabetes.
- *Impaired fasting glucose (IFG)* is defined as FPG ≥110 and <126 mg/dl, and *IGT* is defined as 2-hour plasma glucose ≥140 and <200 mg/dl. Individuals with IFG or IGT are at high risk for the subsequent development of diabetes.
- The management of diabetes is based on a diabetic regimen, including diet, exercise, drugs, diabetes education and self-management, and home glucose monitoring.
- For patients with type 1 diabetes, emphasis is on daily or more frequent injections of insulin balanced carefully with diet and exercise.
- For patients with type 2 diabetes, emphasis is on diet, weight control, and exercise. Medications, such as antidiabetic agents and insulin, are used as needed.
- *Insulin replacement therapy* is required in type 1 diabetes and in a minority of the cases of type 2 diabetes. Insulin is classified according to its onset, peak, and duration of action. A combination of insulins may be used for optimum control. Regular insulin (short-acting) and NPH insulin (intermediate-acting) are commonly used.
- *Intensive insulin therapy* is achieved by using more frequent insulin injections or by continuous subcutaneous insulin infusion systems.
- *Oral antidiabetic agents* may be successfully used in the treatment of *type 2 diabetes*. (1) *Sulfonylureas* (e.g., glipizide, glyburide) exert their effect primarily by stimulating release of endogenous insulin; (2) *metformin* (a biguanide) suppresses hepatic glucose release and enhances insulin sensitivity; (3) *thiazolidinediones* (e.g., rosiglitazone, pioglitazone) likewise share metformin's capacity to lessen insulin resistance, reducing both glucose and insulin levels with little risk of causing hypoglycemia; and (4) *acarbose* delays absorption of ingested carbohydrate, thus decreasing the postprandial rise in glucose in these patients.
- Measurement of *glycated hemoglobin* (Hb A_{1c}) is a method of assessing glycemic control in all types of diabetes. A level of 3.5% to 6.0% indicates good glucose control, fair control is 7% to 8%, and >8% is poor control.
- *Acute metabolic complications of diabetes* include DKA, hyperglycemia, HHNK, and hypoglycemia.
- *DKA* is an acute metabolic complication primarily seen in type 1 diabetes and is characterized by hyperglycemia (>300 mg/dl), metabolic acidosis caused by accumulation of ketone acids, and osmotic diuresis. Ketosis results from marked increase in free fatty acid release from adipocytes, with a resulting shift toward ketone body synthesis in the liver. DKA may be precipitated by any event that increases insulin deficit, such as acute infection or physiologic stress (e.g., surgery).
- *Treatment of DKA* consists of assessing and correcting the characteristic abnormalities: regular insulin to correct the hyperglycemia; intravenous fluids to correct the volume deficit; K^+ replacement, and treatment of the precipitating condition.
- *HHNK* is an acute metabolic complication primarily seen in type 2 diabetes and is characterized by severe hyperglycemia (>600 mg/dl), causing severe hyperosmolality, osmotic diuresis, and dehydration. HHNK is similar to DKA but with more severe hyperglycemia, volume depletion, and free water depletion. Ketosis is not present.
- Treatment of HHNK consists of rehydration, electrolyte replacement, and regular insulin.
- *Hypoglycemia* (insulin shock or reaction) is a frequent complication of insulin therapy. Hypoglycemia becomes symptomatic when insufficient glucose is available to meet the energy needs of the central nervous system (generally <50 mg/dl). Symptoms of shakiness, sweating, tachycardia, and nervousness are caused by the release of epinephrine in an attempt to raise glucose levels. The most common precipitating conditions are excessive administration of insulin or oral hypoglycemic agent, consumption of too little food, or an unusually high activity level.
- *Treatment of hypoglycemia* consists of rapid restoration of normal serum glucose levels. The specific type of intervention is based partially on the patient's level of consciousness—administration of orange juice or other sugar-containing drink if the patient is conscious and intramuscular glucagon or an ampule of 50% intravenous glucose if the patient is not conscious.
- *Hypoglycemic attacks* are dangerous and, if frequent or prolonged, may cause permanent brain damage or even death. The brain requires a continuous supply of glucose.
- The *long-term complications of diabetes* can be divided into three types: microvascular, macrovascular, and peripheral neuropathy.
- *Diabetic retinopathy* is the leading cause of blindness and is caused by an underlying microangiopathy. Early manifestations are the presence of microaneurysms of the retinal arterioles with subsequent hemorrhages, neovascularization, and retinal scars, leading to blindness.
- *Diabetic glomerulosclerosis* is the leading cause of end-stage renal disease (ESRD), accounting for 33% of the new cases. Progression of diabetic nephropathy takes place in stages (see Chapter 46): early functional and structural changes consisting of renal hypertrophy, thickening of the glomerular capillary basement membrane, and increased glomerular fil-

tration rate (GFR); microalbuminuria and hypertension; established nephropathy with proteinuria; and rapid decline of GFR to ESRD.

■ *Diabetic neuropathy* may involve the peripheral nerves, cranial nerves, or autonomic nervous system and is a common long-term complication of both type 1 and type 2 diabetes. Peripheral neuropathies primarily alter sensory perception.

■ *Peripheral neuropathy* is an important cause of *intractable ulceration of the foot* in diabetics. Loss or impairment of sensation leads to loss of pain withdrawal with skin damage from trauma and pressure from tight-fitting shoes. Vascular disease with diminished blood supply also contributes to development of the lesion, and infection is common.

■ *Macrovascular disease* refers to atherosclerosis with the development of coronary artery disease, stroke, peripheral vascular disease, and increased risk of infection. Type 2 diabetes is most associated with macrovascular disease.

■ The incidence of *myocardial infarction (MI)* in individuals with *diabetes* is at least $2\frac{1}{2}$ times that of patients without diabetes. Patients with diabetic autonomic neuropathy may suffer painless (silent) MIs.

■ *Peripheral vascular disease* (and neuropathy) leading to gangrene of the foot in diabetics is the leading cause of nontraumatic leg amputation.

■ 75% of patients with diabetes eventually die of vascular disease—MI, strokes, renal failure, and gangrene of the lower extremities.

■ *The Diabetic Control and Complications Trial (DCCT)*, a 10-year controlled study with type 1 diabetics, demonstrated that intensive insulin therapy, resulting in tighter normalization of plasma glucose, significantly reduced the development of the complications of retinopathy, nephropathy, and neuropathy.

QUESTIONS ??

A sampling of review questions for this chapter appears here. Visit http://www.mosby.com/MERLIN/PriceWilson/ for additional questions.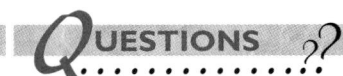

Answer the following questions on a separate sheet of paper.

1. What is the purpose of measuring the fasting blood glucose level?
2. Administration of a glucose load to a nondiabetic individual causes a rise in blood glucose. Which mechanism brings glucose back to baseline levels?
3. What is the purpose of the food exchange system?
4. What are the advantages of the second-generation oral sulfonylureas?
5. Why is it important to identify individuals who are at risk for developing diabetes mellitus?

Match the glucose level in column B with the appropriate term in column A.

	Column A	**Column B**
6.	_____ Hypoglycemia	a. 160 to 180 mg/dl
7.	_____ Normal plasma glucose	b. 210 mg/dl
8.	_____ Renal threshold for glucose	c. 40 mg/dl
9.	_____ Hyperglycemia	d. 70 to 110 mg/dl

Match each statement in column A with the appropriate condition in column B.

	Column A	**Column B**
10.	_____ Most likely to occur in an elderly person with type 2 diabetes	a. Diabetic ketoacidosis (DKA)
11.	_____ More likely to occur in a person with type 1 diabetes	b. Hyperglycemic, hyperosmolar nonketotic coma (HHNK)
12.	_____ Often caused by inadequate food or missed meals	c. Hypoglycemia
13.	_____ Kussmaul's respirations are characteristic	
14.	_____ Hyperglycemia usually more severe	
15.	_____ Reversed by administration of glucose or glucagon	
16.	_____ Confusion, restlessness, and diaphoresis	
17.	_____ Rehydration and insulin used in treatment	

*B*IBLIOGRAPHY ▪ PART TEN

Alberti KG, Zimmet PZ: Definition, diagnosis and classification of diabetes mellitus and its complications. Part 1: diagnosis and classification of diabetes mellitus provisional report of a WHO consultation, *Diabetic Med* 15:539-553, 1998.

American Diabetes Association: Standards of medical care for patients with diabetes mellitus, *Diabetes Care* 23(suppl 1):532-542, 2000.

Chase HP et al: The impact of the diabetes control and complications trial and Humalog insulin on glycohemoglobin levels and severe hypoglycemia in type 1 diabetes, *Diabetes Care* 24:430-433, 2001.

The Diabetes Control and Complications Trial Research Group: The effect of intensive treatment of diabetes on the development and progression of long-term complications in insulin-dependent diabetes mellitus, *N Engl J Med* 329:977-986, 1993.

Dimneen SF et al: Effects of changing diagnostic criteria on the risk of developing diabetes, *Diabetes Care* 21:1408-1413, 1998.

Goldstein BJ: Current views on the mechanism of action of thiazolidinedione insulin sensitizers, *Diabetes Tech & Therap* 1:267-275, 1995.

Greenspan FS, Gardner DG: *Basic and clinical endocrinology,* ed 6, Norwalk, Conn, 2000, Appleton & Lange.

Lepore M, Pampanelli S, Fanelli C: Pharmacokinetics and pharmacodynamics of subcutaneous injection of long-acting human insulin analog, glargine, NPH insulin and continuous subcutaneous infusion of insulin lispro, *Diabetes* 49:2142-2148, 2000.

Niewoehner CB: *Endocrine pathophysiology,* Malden, Mass, 1998, Blackwell Science.

Report of the Expert Committee on the Diagnosis and Classification of Diabetes Mellitus, *Diabetes Care* 20:1183-1197, 1997.

Schteingart DE: Cushing's syndrome. In Becker KL: *Principles and practice of endocrinology and metabolism,* ed 3, Philadelphia, 2001, Lippincott–Williams & Wilkins.

Schteingart DE: Disorders of the adrenal gland. In *Kelley's textbook of internal medicine,* ed 4, Philadelphia, 2000, Lippincott–Williams & Wilkins.

UK Prospective Diabetes Study Group (UKPDS): Intensive blood-glucose control with sulphonylureas or insulin compared with conventional treatment and risk of complications in patients with type 2 diabetes, *Lancet* 352:837-853, 1998.

REPRODUCTIVE SYSTEM DISORDERS

The male and female reproductive systems consist of gonads and tubular structures. The gonads produce gametes, ova, and spermatozoa, which are specialized cells that unite, male and female, to produce a new individual. The systems of both genders provide means for deposition of spermatozoa from the male reproductive system to the female reproductive system in which the gametes unite and the resultant zygote is nurtured, grows, and develops until birth. Hormones direct and regulate the development and maintenance of the structures and sexual functions.

Dysfunctions of the reproductive system can be categorized broadly into developmental, endocrinologic, infectious processes, and neoplasms. Chapter 64 discusses disorders of the female system, such as menstrual problems, endocrine malfunctions, infections, and benign and malignant conditions of the reproductive organs and breasts. Chapter 65 discusses disorders of the male system, such as hypogonadism, functional alterations, infections, and benign and malignant neoplastic changes of the reproductive organs. Chapter 66 discusses sexually transmitted diseases, such as the classic venereal diseases of syphilis and gonorrhea, as well as other epidemiologically important infections transmitted sexually.

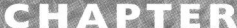

CHAPTER
64
Female Reproductive System Disorders

KATHLEEN BRANSON HILLEGAS

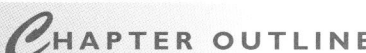

ANATOMY AND PHYSIOLOGY

Developmental Changes of the Female Reproductive System

Prenatal Development

The female has a sex chromosome configuration of XX. During the embryonic phase, the cells that develop into the reproductive system will undergo differentiation. The reproductive system of the male and female develop from the same gonadal tissue and have the potential to develop into either male or female genitalia. The müllerian duct system and the wolffian duct system are at first indistinguishable (Figs. 64-1 and 64-2). These systems develop into the gonads, the ducts from the gonads to the exterior, external genitalia, and the secondary sex glands. Differentiation of the embryo into a male or female is affected by the genetic configuration, as well as by hormones. By the end of the twelfth week of gestation, the sex of the fetus can be visually determined. In the female embryo, the internal structures (uterus, fallopian tubes, and the inner one third of the vagina) arise from the müllerian duct system, whereas the wolffian duct system regresses.

In the differentiation of the male karyotype (XY) the *SRY* gene on the Y chromosome initiates the development of the testis that then produce testosterone, which stimulates the wolffian duct system to develop into the epididymis, vas deferens, and seminal vesicles. The müllerian system is suppressed from developing. The external genitalia of the male are further developed by the presence of dihydrotestosterone. In the absence of the male factors (genes and hormones) the fetus will develop into a female. (American Academy of Pediatrics, 2000).

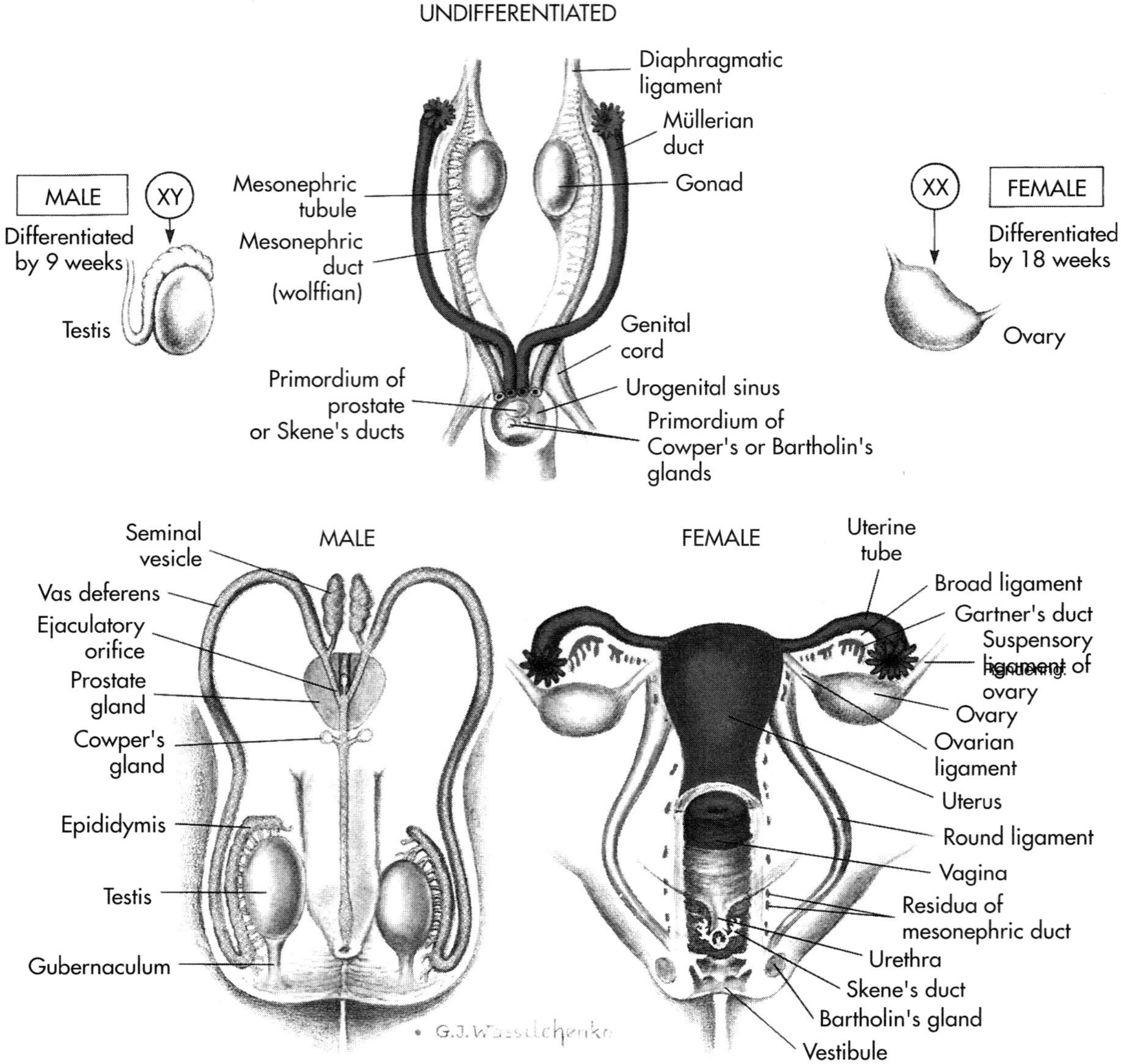

FIG. 64-1   Homologues of internal genitals. (From Lowdermilk DL, Perry SE, Bobak IM: *Maternity and women's health care*, ed 6, St. Louis, 1997, Mosby.)

Development at Puberty

At puberty, usually between age 9 to 16 years in girls, further changes in the female reproductive system take place. The primary and secondary sexual characteristics develop as a result of the hormonal influence of estrogen. The external signs of puberty are observed when the nipples and breast buds swell and the areola enlarges, axillary and pubic hair develops, hips widen, and a growth spurt occurs. The uterus and ovaries also grow and mature. There are differences in sexual maturation rates by race, with African-American girls maturing at an earlier age than do Caucasian girls. African-American girls have an average age of onset of breast development at 8.87 years as compared with an average age of 9.96 years for Caucasian girls. Pubic hair development is seen in African-American girls at 8.78 years and 10.51 years in Caucasian girls. *Menarche*, the onset of menstruation, usually occurs between 12 and 13 years of age, with a range of 9.1 to 17.7 years. African-American girls experience menarche at 12.16 years and Caucasian girls at 12.88 years (Herman–Giddons et al, 1997).

Changes with Aging

Reproductive system changes from aging usually begin to occur during the fifth decade of life. Most women have experienced menopause by their early 50s. At that time, a reduction in the hormone estrogen leads to an eventual cessation of menstruation along with typical symptoms of decreased hormone production, which include atrophy of the reproductive organs, decreased lubrication, and vasomotor instability.

Structures of the Female Reproductive System

The internal organs of the female reproductive system are two ovaries, two fallopian tubes or oviducts, the uterus, and the vagina (Fig. 64-3). The external genitalia collec-

UNDIFFERENTIATED

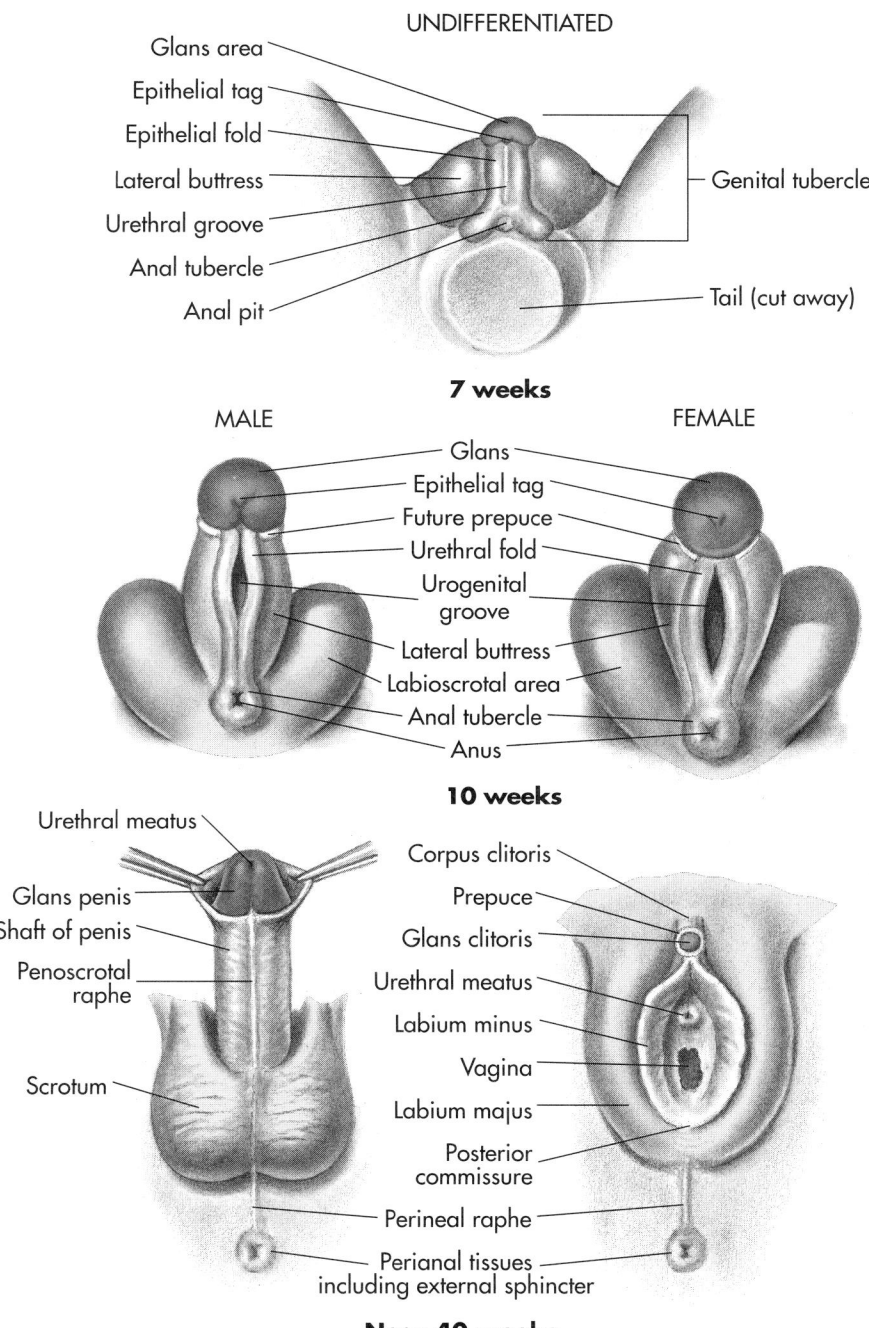

7 weeks

10 weeks

Near 40 weeks

FIG. 64-2   Homologues of external genitals. (From Lowdermilk DL, Perry SE, Bobak IM: *Maternity and women's health care*, ed 6, St. Louis, 1997, Mosby.)

tively are called the *vulva* and comprise the structures visible externally from the pubis to the perineum: the mons pubis, the labia majora, the labia minora, the clitoris, and the vestibule, an almond-shaped area inside the labia minora. The urethral meatus, the vaginal opening or introitus, and two sets of glands, Skene's glands and Bartholin's glands, open onto the vestibule (Fig. 64-4).

In the mature female, the ovaries develop and release ova (oogenesis) and produce steroid hormones: the estrogens—estrone (E_1), estradiol (E_2), and estriol (E_3)—and androgens and progesterone. Small amounts of estrogens and androgens are also secreted by the adrenal cortex. The androgens are converted to estrogens peripherally in adipose tissue. E_2 is the most potent estrogen and is secreted in the largest amounts by the ovaries.

The fallopian tubes extend from the ovaries to the uterus and open into the uterine cavity, providing a direct communication from the peritoneal cavity to the uterine cavity.

The uterus lies centrally in the pelvis and is divided structurally into the body or corpus and the cervix. The inner layer, the *endometrium,* consists of surface epithelium, glands, and connective tissue (stroma). The endometrium is shed during menstruation. At the lowest

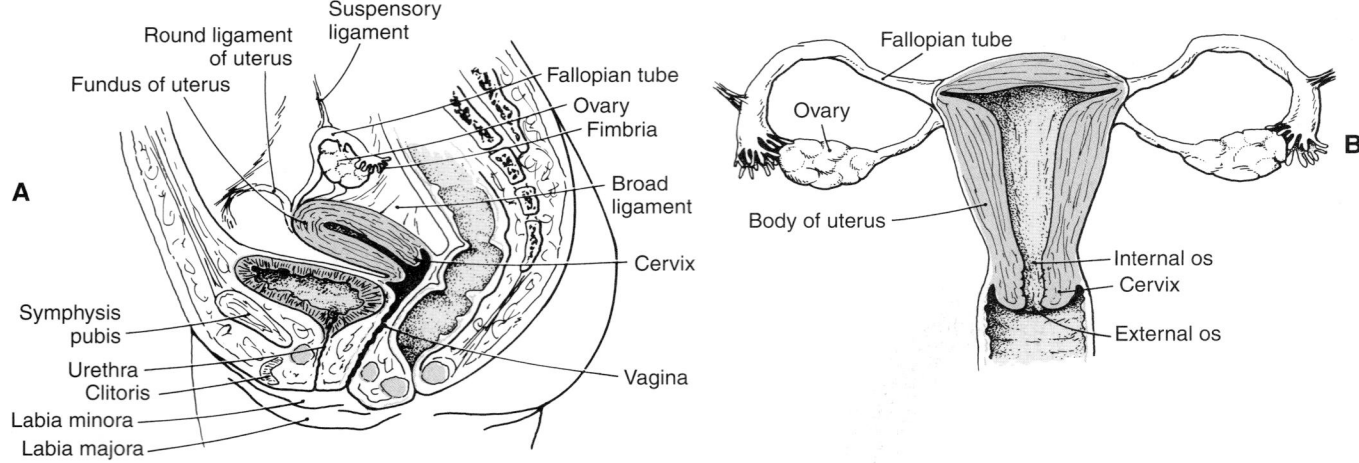

FIG. 64-3 Female internal reproductive organs. **A**, Cross section. **B**, Ovaries, fallopian tubes, and uterus.

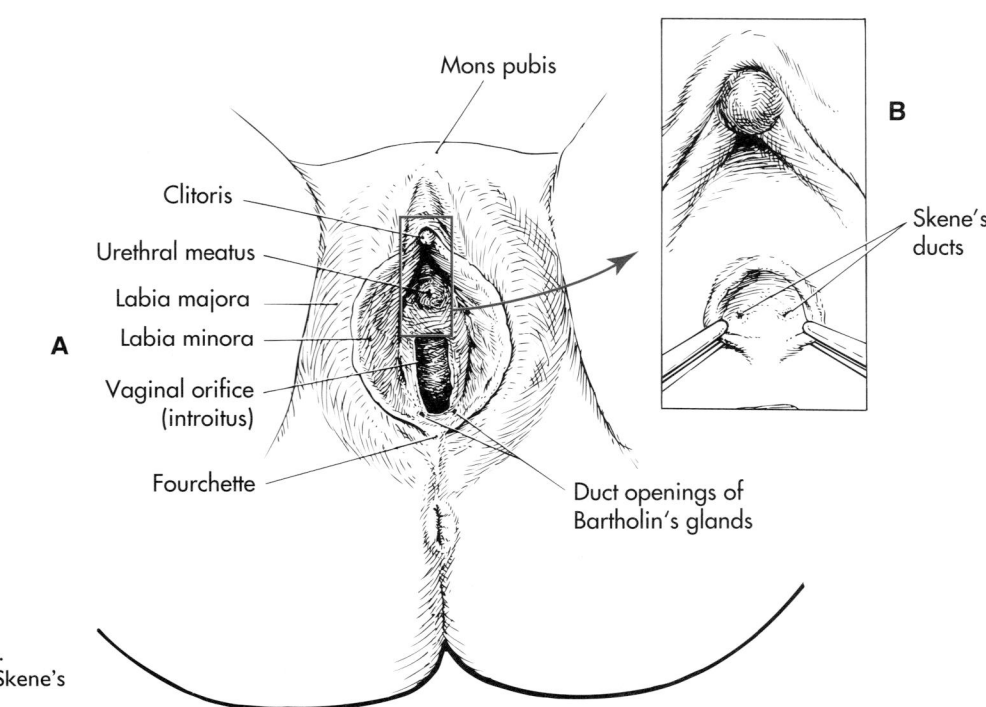

FIG. 64-4 Female external genitalia. **A**, Vulva. **B**, Paraurethral opening of Skene's glands.

portion of the corpus is the *internal os* of the cervix. The *external os* is at the lower end of the cervix. The canal of the cervix provides a direct communication from the cavity of the uterine body, through the internal os and the external os, to the vagina.

The vagina extends from the cervix of the uterus to the *introitus* on the vestibule, the border between the internal and external genital structures. Thus there is continuous communication from outside the body to the peritoneal cavity through reproductive system structures. The internal pelvic organs can be palpated through the thin walls of the upper vagina, and there is ready access surgically through the vaginal wall behind the cervix to the peritoneal cavity.

The mons pubis lies over the anterior surface of the symphysis pubis and extends downward and is continuous with the labia majora. Medial to the labia majora are the labia minora. The labia minora converge and fuse in-

feriorly to form the fourchette and superiorly to form the prepuce of the clitoris. The *clitoris* is a small body of erectile tissue above the labia minora.

FUNCTIONS OF THE FEMALE REPRODUCTIVE SYSTEM

The female reproductive system functions by means of complex hormonal interactions to produce a mature ovum cyclically and to prepare and maintain an environment for conception and gestation (Fig. 64-5).

Hormonal Functions

Cyclic hormonal changes initiate and regulate ovarian function and endometrial changes. The regular,

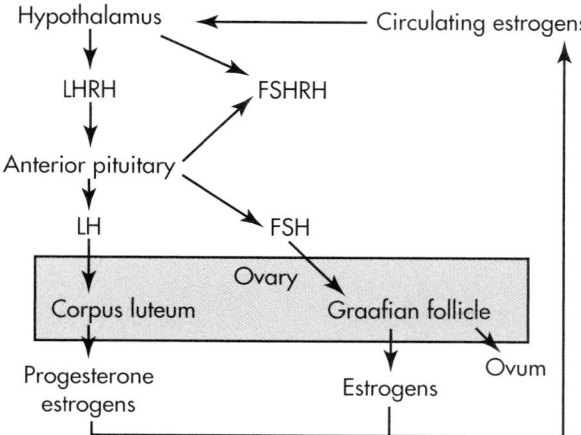

FIG. 64-5 Hypothalamic-pituitary ovarian hormone axis. *LHRH,* Luteinizing hormone–releasing hormone; *FSHRH,* follicle-stimulating hormone–releasing hormone.

monthly occurrence of a menstrual cycle depends on a series of cyclic, well-coordinated steps, which involve hormone secretion at various levels of this integrated system. The center of hormonal control of the reproductive system is the hypothalamus. The two hypothalamic gonadotropic hormone–releasing hormones (GnRH), called follicle-stimulating hormone–releasing hormone (FSHRH) and luteinizing hormone–releasing hormone (LHRH), stimulate the anterior pituitary to secrete follicle-stimulating hormone (FSH) and luteinizing hormone (LH), respectively. The series of events initiated by the secretion of FSH and LH involves production of estrogens and progesterone from the ovary that result in physiologic changes in the uterus. Estrogen and progesterone, in turn, influence the production of the specific GnRH in a feedback system that regulates gonadotropic hormone levels. These steps have been carefully studied through daily measurements of the levels of FSH and LH in the blood and levels of estradiol and progesterone in the blood and urine. The ovarian cycle, the endometrial cycle, and the changes in the levels of the hormones during a menstrual cycle are illustrated in Fig. 64-6.

Normal Menstrual Cycle

Generally, the menstrual cycle interval ranges from 15 to 45 days, with the average being 28 days. Duration of flow varies with a range of 2 to 8 days, with the average being 4 to 6 days. Menstrual blood does not clot. The amount lost each cycle ranges from 60 ml to 80 ml.

Ovarian Cycle
Follicular Phase

The cycle begins with the first day of menstrual flow, or sloughing of the endometrium. FSH induces the growth of several primordial follicles in the ovaries. Generally, only one follicle continues to grow and becomes the graafian follicle and the others degenerate. The follicle consists of an ovum and its two surrounding cell layers. The inner layer of granulosa cells synthesizes progesterone, which is secreted into the follicular fluid during

the first half of the menstrual cycle and serves as a precursor for estrogen synthesis by the surrounding layer of theca interna cells. Estrogen is synthesized in the luteinized cells of the theca interna. The pathway of estrogen biosynthesis proceeds from progesterone and pregnenolone via 17-hydroxylated derivatives to androstenedione, testosterone, and estradiol. A high content of aromatizing enzyme in these cells facilitates the conversion of androgens to estrogens. In the follicle, the primary oocyte begins to mature. At the same time, the growing follicle secretes increasing amounts of estrogen into the system. Rising estrogen levels cause LHRH to be released by a positive feedback system.

Luteal Phase

LH induces ovulation of the maturing oocyte. Just before the ovulation, the primary oocyte completes its first meiotic division. High levels of estrogen now inhibit the production of FSH. Next, estrogen levels begin to drop. After expulsion of the oocyte from the graafian follicle, the granulosa layer becomes vascularized and intensely luteinized, forming the yellow corpus luteum of the ovary. The corpus luteum continues to secrete small amounts of estrogen and increasing amounts of progesterone.

Endometrial Cycle
Proliferative Phase

Immediately after menstruation, the endometrium is thin and in a resting state. This stage lasts about 5 days. Increasing levels of estrogen from the growing follicle stimulate the endometrial stroma to begin to grow and thicken, the glands to undergo hypertrophy and proliferation, and the blood vessels to become prominent. The glands and stroma grow at about an equal pace. As the glands become longer, they maintain their straight, tubular form. The glandular epithelium is columnar with uniform eosinophilic cytoplasm and central nuclei. The stroma is fairly compact in the basal layer but looser toward the surface. Vessels follow a slightly spiraling course and are smaller. The length of the proliferative phase varies widely among individuals, ending at ovulation.

Secretory Phase

After ovulation, under the influence of increasing levels of progesterone and continuing estrogen from the corpus luteum, the endometrium becomes thick and velvetlike. There is greater and more elaborate convolution of glands and infolding of the glandular epithelium, giving a "saw tooth" appearance. The nuclei of the cells move downward, and the surface of the epithelium acquires a frayed appearance. The stroma becomes edematous. Heavy infiltration with leukocytes occurs, and the blood vessels become more and more tightly coiled and dilated. The length of the secretory phase among all women is constant at 14 ± 2 days.

Menstrual Phase

The corpus luteum functions until about the twenty third or twenty fourth day of a 28-day cycle and then begins to regress. The resulting sharp drop in progesterone and estrogen removes the stimulation to the endometrium. Ischemic changes occur in the arterioles, and menstrual flow occurs.

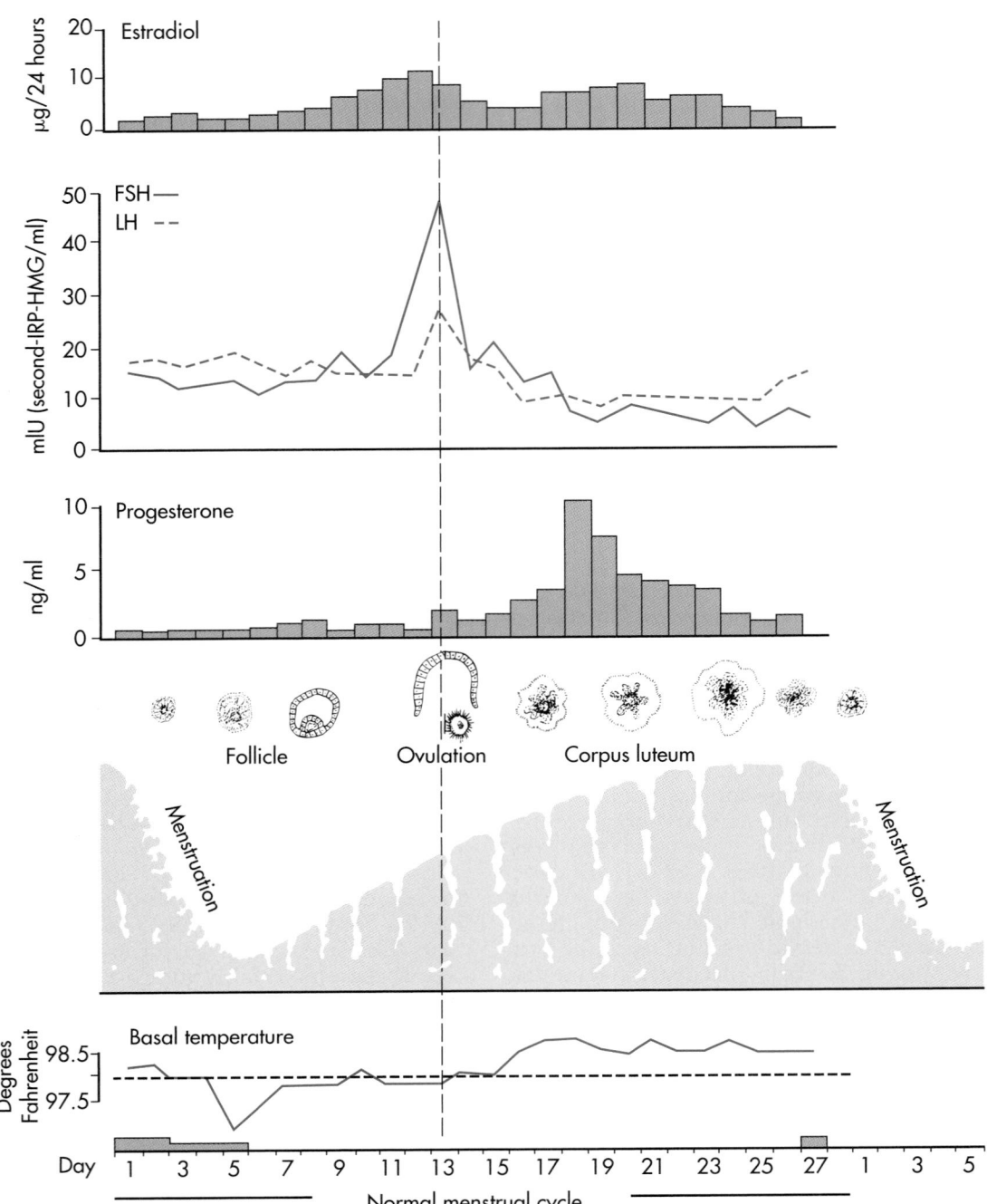

FIG. 64-6 Normal menstrual cycle. The horizontal bars on the time scale indicate the occurrence of menses. The interrupted vertical line at midcycle depicts the time of ovulation. Basal body temperature rises during the luteal phase of the cycle, coinciding with the onset of progesterone secretion. *FSH,* Follicle-stimulating hormone; *LH,* luteinizing hormone.

Sexual Response Cycle

The normal *sexual response cycle* as described by Masters and Johnson (1966) is composed of four phases: excitement, plateau, orgasm, and resolution. Sexual activity can be experienced alone or with others. These same four phases are experienced with differing kinds of sexual stimulation, masturbation, coital, and fantasy. The entire body in involved in the sexual response cycle, and the nervous system is an important part. Myotonia and vasoconstriction are two important responses. During the excitement phase, muscle tension is increased as sexual stimulation is processed through the nervous system. The blood pressure and heart rate increase, the vagina lubricates, the uterus elevates, which pulls the vagina open, the breasts swell, and nipples become erect. With orgasm, the vagina, uterus, and rectum contract at intervals. Uterine contractions are similar to labor. Increased heart rate, blood pressure, and breathing are experienced during orgasm. Resolution phase follows, when the uterus, breasts, cardiovascular system, and other bodily changes return to their normal state.

Climacteric and the Menopause

The climacteric is the physiologic phase in which regression of ovarian function takes place. Menopause, which is the cessation of regular cycle uterine bleeding, is just one event in the climacteric. Menopause usually occurs between the ages of 45 and 52 years. During the climacteric, estradiol levels decrease and the ovaries decrease in size and are virtually devoid of follicles. Microscopic examination reveals cortical thinning and a relative thickening of the medulla from increased fibrous connective tissue. Blood vessels at the hilus and medulla become progressively sclerotic. Anatomic involution of the ovaries is accompanied by a decrease in their ovulatory and endocrine functions. The decrease in circulating estradiol levels increases pituitary gonadotropin secretion by negative feedback. This increased production of FSH and LH continues for many years after the onset of menopause. Signs, symptoms, and physiologic changes associated with menopause result from decreasing circulating estrogen. Menopausal symptoms may begin before changes in the menstrual cycle occur. Regular menstrual bleeding may occur until the menopause, with cycles becoming shorter because of shorter follicular phases, or cycles may be variable and more widely spaced, with some being ovulatory and some being anovulatory. Any bleeding after 6 months of amenorrhea is abnormal, and the cause must be investigated to rule out carcinoma.

Common symptoms of menopause include hot flushes, palpitations, headache, cold hands and feet, irritability, vertigo, anxiety, nervousness, depression, insomnia, night sweats, forgetfulness, inability to concentrate, fatigue, and weight gain. The most common problem is vasomotor instability manifested by hot flushes. The typical sign of the hot flush is reddened and warm skin, principally of the head and neck, which lasts anywhere from a few seconds to 2 minutes. This event is followed by cold chills. Other associated physiologic changes are increased heart rate, peripheral vasodilation, a rise in skin temperature, and concomitant pulsatile LH release. Bilateral oophorectomy at any age after menarche results in the same symptoms.

The skin of the genitalia and the lining of the vagina and urethra become thinner and dryer, resulting in a greater potential for irritation, infection, and dyspareunia. The labia, clitoris, uterus, and ovaries decrease in size. Skin elasticity decreases. An increase in facial or body hair growth may occur as a result of the decrease in estrogen levels and the unopposed effect of circulating androgens.

Osteoporosis occurs in about 25% of postmenopausal women within 15 to 20 years after menopause. Men of the same age can also be affected with the same type of osteoporosis as a part of the aging process, but the incidence and the extent of bone loss are greater in women. Vertebral fractures, Colles' fractures, and hip fractures are the major complications. Hip fractures are responsible for a mortality as high as 15% in women older than 60 years.

Symptomatic Therapeutic Measures

Any therapy chosen during the perimenopausal and postmenopausal years must be individualized. Estrogen replacement therapy (ERT) decreases the incidence of osteoporotic fractures, prevents or reverses atrophic genital and urethral lining changes, diminishes hot flushes, and may decrease the incidence of atherosclerotic coronary disease. Hormone replacement therapy has been shown to increase the bone mineral density of frail elderly women (Villareal, 2001). ERT is absolutely contraindicated in women with, or with a history of, estrogen-dependent tumors of the breast, uterus, or kidney; genital bleeding of unknown cause; deep vein thrombosis; cerebrovascular disease; or liver disease. Estrogens are relatively contraindicated in women with hypertension, diabetes mellitus, cholecystitis and cholelithiasis, pancreatitis, congestive heart disease, past endometriosis, or retinopathy.

Estrogen and a progestin, known as hormone replacement therapy (HRT), are administered in a cyclic fashion to mimic the endometrial cycle and prevent hyperplasia of the endometrium. Several different regimens can be used. Uterine bleeding (menstrual periods) will occur in about 50% of women on replacement therapy. Estrogen alone may be administered continuously to women who have undergone a hysterectomy/salpingo-oophorectomy, although some clinicians prescribe cyclic therapy with estrogen and progestin in these women.

A thorough history and complete physical examination, including a mammogram, are mandatory before prescribing ERT. Periodic Papanicolaou (Pap) smears of the cervix (or of the vaginal cuff in a woman who has had a hysterectomy), yearly mammograms, and endometrial biopsy every 1 to 2 years or if there is breakthrough bleeding should be performed to monitor for and rule out any malignant changes of the cervix, breast, or endometrium.

Recommendations and guidelines for the use of ERT and HRT are undergoing examination and revision as current prospective randomized clinical trials answer many questions about the safety and efficacy of the use of ERT and HRT and the prevention of coronary heart disease. The American Heart Association has recently issued a guideline (Mosca et al, 2001) advising that women should not begin ERT or HRT as a secondary prevention for cardiovascular disease. It is also advised that there is not yet enough data to recommend taking HRT alone as primary prevention for cardiovascular disease.

MENSTRUAL DISORDERS

Amenorrhea

Primary amenorrhea is the absence of menarche by the age of 17 years, regardless of the presence or absence of secondary sexual development; secondary amenorrhea is the absence of menses for 3 months or longer after having established menstrual cycles. Amenorrhea is physiologic in the prepubertal girl, the pregnant woman, and the postmenopausal woman; otherwise, amenorrhea is an indication of dysfunction or abnormality somewhere in the reproductive system. Amenorrhea is a symptom and not a disease entity. The cause of amenorrhea can be physiologic, endocrinologic, organic, or developmental (Table 64-1).

Girls with no evidence of onset of puberty by age 13 years or who do not develop menses by 5 years after onset of puberty should be evaluated. Mature women who

TABLE 64-1 ▪ ▪ ▪

Causes of Amenorrhea

Developmental Stage	Pathology
PRIMARY AMENORRHEA	
Absent or arrested secondary sexual development	Hypothalamic dysfunction
	Pituitary dysfunction
	Ovarian failure or dysgenesis
Normal secondary sexual development	Hypothalamic dysfunction
	Pituitary dysfunction
	Incomplete development of müllerian system
Abnormal secondary sexual development	Hypothalamic dysfunction
	Pituitary dysfunction
	Ovarian failure or dysgenesis
	Nonphysiologic sex hormone production
	Androgen insensitivity
SECONDARY AMENORRHEA	
Postmenarche	Endometrial dysfunction
	Ovarian dysfunction
	Hypothalamic dysfunction
	Pituitary dysfunction

are amenorrheic for 3 months should also be evaluated. A thorough history and physical examination, with attention to the influence of altered hormonal states, are essential first steps to clinical evaluation. Essential information involves dietary and exercise habits, evidence for psychologic disturbances, lifestyle, environmental stresses, family history of genetic disorders, abnormal growth and development, and signs of androgen excess. The physical examination includes inspection of the genitalia and palpation of the pelvic organs and evaluation of body dimensions, body habitus, the extent and distribution of body hair, and breast development and secretions. The normal arm span is about equal to body height; in hypogonadism, arm span is more than 2 inches greater than is body height. Breast development and pubic hair are evaluated according to the Tanner developmental scale (Figs. 64-7 and 64-8). Pelvic examination and palpation of the internal organs can usually rule out anomalies of müllerian duct derivatives, such as dysgenesis of the gonads, androgen insensitivity syndrome, Turner syndrome, imperforate hymen, vaginal or uterine aplasia, or vaginal septum. Problems with the development of the gonadal tissues from the embryonic period may not be evident until puberty, when the expected course of development is altered.

Stage 2 (pubertal)

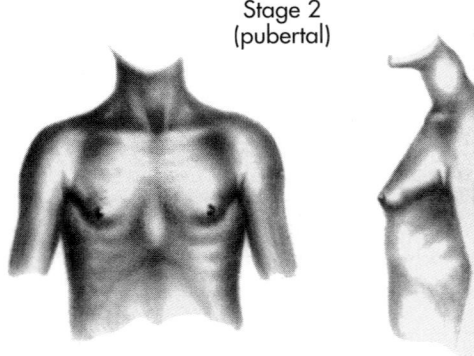

Breast bud stage—small area of elevation around papilla; enlargement of areolar diameter

Stage 4

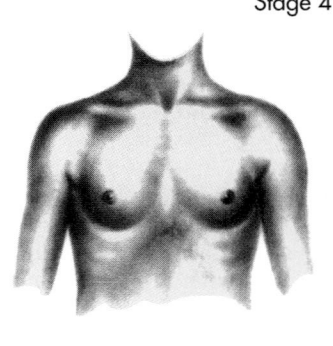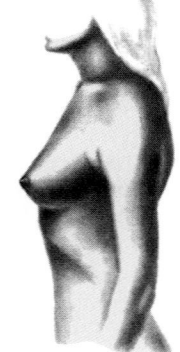

Projection of areola and papilla to form a secondary mound (may not occur in all girls)

Stage 3

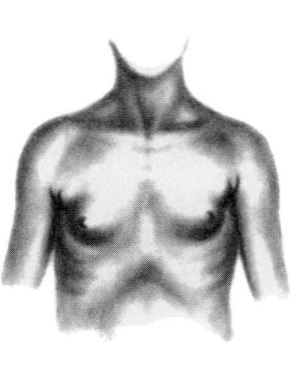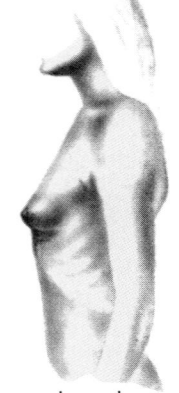

Further enlargement of breast and areola with no separation of their contours

Stage 5

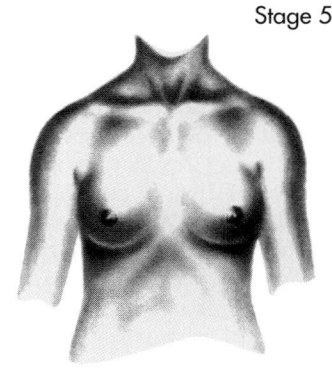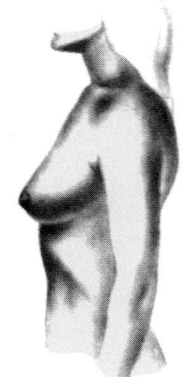

Mature configuration; projection of papilla only caused by recession of areola into general contour

FIG. 64-7 Development of breasts in girls—average age span 11-13 years. Stage 1: (prepubertal—elevation of papilla only) is not shown. (Modified from Marshall WA, Tanner JM: *Arch Dis Child* 44:291,1969; and Daniel WA, Paulshock BZ: *Patient Care*, pp. 122-124, May 13, 1979.)

Laboratory Assessment of Amenorrhea

The first step is to determine whether hormonal failure is caused by a hypothalamic-pituitary problem or by a gonadal disorder. This determination is made by measuring serum FSH. If the serum FSH is repeatedly elevated, the woman most likely has a primary ovarian failure. If the serum FSH is normal or low, the problem most likely lies in the hypothalamus or the pituitary gland. In this case, evaluation of thyroid and adrenal function may determine if the patient has isolated gonadotropin deficiency or panhypopituitarism. In the presence of galactorrhea, a serum prolactin level should be obtained. A radiograph of the pituitary fossa and computed axial tomography (CT) of the pituitary gland may help determine if the patient has a pituitary tumor with or without suprasellar extension. In patients in whom amenorrhea is associated with hirsutism, measurement of 17-ketosteroids and serum testosterone and dehydroepiandrosterone (DHEA) should be carried out. Levels are usually elevated in patients with excessive androgen secretion. More specific tests to determine the source of the excessive secretion of androgens include a pelvic examination, laparoscopy, adrenal scintiscan, and abdominal CT scan. Selective catheterization and sampling of blood from the adrenal and gonadal veins may help localize the source of androgen hypersecretion. Conditions related to androgen excess are discussed in Chapter 61.

Treatment of the Amenorrheic Patient

Treatment of amenorrhea is often based on the specific underlying pathologic condition. Women with prolactin-secreting pituitary adenomas should be treated with either transsphenoidal resection of the pituitary tumor or suppression of prolactin secretion with bromocriptine. Women with excessive androgen secretion should receive suppressive therapy with corticosteroids or oral contraceptives. Both of these preparations suppress the excessive secretion of androgens, probably by inhibiting gonadotropin release.

Women with hypothalamic-pituitary or ovarian deficiency should receive replacement therapy with estrogens and progesterone administered cyclically. Combined treatment with estrogens and progesterone helps to maintain secondary sexual characteristics and prevent vaginal and breast atrophy and osteopenia. Therapy can be continued through the expected time of menopause at age 45 to 52 years.

Women with primary gonadal disorders remain infertile. However, ovulation can be induced and fertility restored in some women with isolated gonadotropin deficiency, polycystic ovarian disease (PCOD), or excessive weight loss if weight is regained. Ovulation and fertility can be obtained with clomiphene citrate, a nonsteroidal compound that has both estrogenic and antiestrogenic properties, depending on the site of action. In responsive

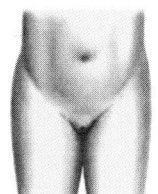

Stage 1 (prepubertal)

No pubic hair; essentially the same as during childhood; no distinction between hair on pubis and over the abdomen

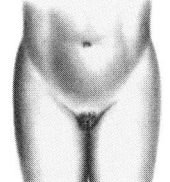

Stage 2

Sparse growth of long, straight, downy, and slightly pigmented hair extending along labia; between stages 2 and 3 begins to appear on pubis

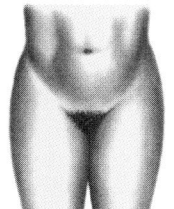

Stage 3

Hair darker, coarser, and curly and spread sparsely over entire pubis in the typical female triangle

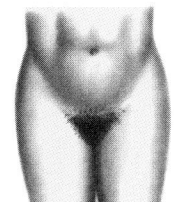

Stage 4

Pubic hair denser, curled, and adult in distribution but less abundant and restricted to the pubic area

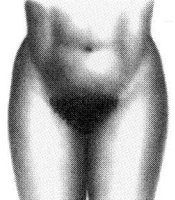

Stage 5

Hair adult in quantity, type, and pattern with spread to inner aspect of thighs

FIG. 64-8 Growth of pubic hair in girls—average age span for 2 through 5, 11 to 14 years. (Modified from Marshall WA, Tanner JM: *Arch Dis Child* 44:291,1969; and Daniel WA, Paulshock BZ: *Patient Care*, pp. 122-124, May 13, 1979.)

women, ovulation occurs 4 to 8 days and menstruation 14 to 21 days after clomiphene has been stopped. Several courses of treatment may be necessary before ovulation and fertility or normal menstrual cycles are established. An otherwise intact pituitary gland is required for a positive response to therapy.

In women with hypopituitarism or pituitary tumors, fertility can be restored by treatment with human FSH and human chorionic gonadotropin (hCG), which acts like LH. This therapy is expensive and requires careful control of dosage and estradiol response to avoid multiple pregnancies or the development of ovarian cysts.

Premenstrual Syndrome

Premenstrual syndrome (PMS) or premenstrual tension (PMT) is a constellation of physical and psychologic symptoms that occur during the luteal phase of the menstrual cycle and diminish with the onset of menses. These symptoms may be severe enough to interfere with some aspect of the person's (and her family's) life. In about 10% of women, premenstrual symptoms are severe enough that medical attention is sought. Although no specific definition of PMS is universally accepted, most experienced clinicians require three findings to make the diagnosis: (1) the symptom complex is consistent with PMS, (2) the symptoms occur exclusively during the luteal phase of ovulatory menstrual cycles, and (3) the symptoms are severe enough to disrupt the person's life. The symptoms associated with PMS are diverse, but each patient describes a unique set of multiple symptoms, all occurring during the characteristic time in the cycle. Psychologic disorders, including depression and anxiety, frequently are confused with PMS and must be ruled out before initiating therapy. At least 150 symptoms have been reported with this syndrome. Some of these symptoms are listed in Box 64-1. Estimates of the incidence of PMS symptoms range from 25% to 100% of menstruating women. For many women, the symptoms are only annoying and do not significantly interfere with their activities; for others, perhaps 5% to 10% of women with PMS, there are serious difficulties. The diagnosis of PMS is best made after the woman keeps a menstrual calendar with a daily symptom diary for 2 to 3 months. Fewer than 50% of these women are found to have a definite diagno-

sis of PMS when their records are evaluated for the cyclicity of symptomatology present with true PMS.

Symptoms may begin to occur at menarche and worsen with time; most women report that symptoms begin after childbirth and worsen after each pregnancy. Secondary psychologic difficulties such as marital discord, withdrawal from social activities, and difficulties maintaining relationships, including with their children, are often seen in women with long-standing PMS.

The cause of PMS is unknown. Theories include derangements in the amounts of estrogen and progesterone production, changes in other ovarian hormone production, altered central nervous system (CNS) effects of ovarian steroids, and changes in serotonin synthesis during the luteal phase.

The symptoms are so variable that no single therapy is effective for all women. The major goal of treatment is to provide as much relief as possible for the most significant symptoms. Simple interventions, such as exercise, alteration of diet, and avoidance of salt, alcohol, and caffeine, may result in dramatic improvement and should be given an adequate trial. Changes in lifestyle to reduce stress may also provide relief. For women in whom symptoms of anxiety predominate, a trial of anxiolytic agents administered during the luteal phase can be tried. However, the mainstay of treatment for PMS is use of agents that suppress ovarian function. Oral contraceptive pills may provide a simple and inexpensive solution. Alternatives to use for relief of symptoms for some women include GnRH agonists such as medroxyprogesterone acetate to suppress ovulation. Abnormal uterine bleeding and progestin-related adverse effects associated with this drug may limit its usefulness. Emotional support, education, and counseling for the woman and her family are also beneficial.

Dysmenorrhea

Dysmenorrhea is pain during menstruation caused by uterine muscle cramping. Primary dysmenorrhea occurs in the absence of any underlying physical disturbance and only during ovulatory cycles. The cause is the presence of excessive amounts of prostaglandin $F_{2\alpha}$ in menstrual blood, which stimulates uterine hyperactivity. The major symptom is pain that begins with the onset of menses. The pain may be sharp, dull, cyclic, or steady; it lasts for a few hours to 1 day. Occasionally, symptoms last longer than 1 day but rarely more than 72 hours. Associated systemic symptoms are nausea, diarrhea, headache, and emotional changes.

Treatment is use of nonsteroidal antiinflammatory agents, which block prostaglandin synthesis through inhibition of the enzyme cyclooxygenase. Therapy is most successful when begun before the onset of menstruation and continued until the symptoms have abated. Progesterone will also inhibit endometrial prostaglandin synthesis. Therefore treatment with oral contraceptives is also effective. These drugs reduce the amount of menstrual fluid and thus the prostaglandin concentration.

Secondary dysmenorrhea occurs because of an underlying physical problem, such as endometriosis, uterine polyps, leiomyoma, cervical stenosis, or pelvic inflammatory disease (PID). In the case of an abnormal pelvic examination, further evaluation is necessary to establish the diagnosis. Dysmenorrhea may occur in women with in-

---

BOX 64-1

Some Symptoms of Premenstrual Syndrome

Somatic Symptoms	Emotional and Mental Symptoms
Abdominal bloating	Anxiety
Acne	Change in libido
Alcohol intolerance	Depression
Breast engorgement and tenderness	Fatigue
	Food cravings
Clumsiness	Hostility
Constipation or diarrhea	Inability to concentrate
Headache	Increased appetite
Peripheral edema	Insomnia
Weight gain	Irritability
	Lethargy
	Mood swings
	Panic attacks
	Paranoia
	Withdrawal from others

creasing menometrorrhagia. A careful evaluation should be done to look for abnormalities within the uterine cavity or pelvis that may be precipitating both signs. Hysteroscopy, hysterosalpingogram (HSG), transvaginal sonogram (TVS), and laparoscopy are all procedures that may be used for evaluation. Treatment is aimed at correcting the underlying condition.

Dysfunctional Uterine Bleeding

Dysfunctional uterine bleeding is bleeding that occurs when no demonstrable organic cause is present. Most patients with dysfunctional bleeding are having anovulatory cycles. Anovulation occurs secondary to failure of any developing ovarian follicles to mature to the point of ovulation with subsequent formation of the corpus luteum. The exact cause of anovulation is not completely understood but probably results from dysfunction of the hypothalamic-pituitary-ovarian axis. This event results in continued production of estrogen by the follicles and, without a corpus luteum, no production of progesterone. This altered hormone state results in alternating periods of anovulatory bleeding, which is usually very heavy, with amenorrhea. This situation is caused by the variation in the degree of estrogen stimulation to the endometrium, as well as to the degree of estrogen withdrawal. The frequency of the periodic bleeding episodes depends on variations in the number of functioning follicles. Several follicles can be active at one time, producing high levels of estrogen. Under the influence of high estrogen levels and no progesterone, the endometrium can proliferate for weeks or months. In time, estrogen withdrawal will occur, caused either by the eventual degeneration of some follicles, causing levels to drop, or by the needs of the enlarging endometrial tissue becoming greater than the amount of estrogen produced can support. Both conditions result in estrogen breakthrough bleeding, which can vary in timing, duration, and amount.

In adolescents, irregular, prolonged, or excessive bleeding is commonly associated with the establishment of regular menstrual cycles secondary to immaturity of the hypothalamic-pituitary-ovarian axis and results in anovulatory cycles in 20% of cases. In the first 2 years after menarche, the incidence of anovulatory cycles is 75% or more and nearly 50% in the next 2 years. Forty percent of cases occur in women over 40 years of age. In this situation, premenopausal changes of the hypothalamic-pituitary-ovarian axis are occurring and result in anovulatory cycles. However, in older women, care is given to exclude pathologic causes because of the possibility of endometrial cancer. If bleeding is particularly heavy, an acute condition can develop that requires prompt intervention because hypovolemia and anemia may develop secondary to blood loss.

The diagnosis is made by history, absence of ovulatory cycle body temperature changes, and low serum progesterone levels. Diagnostic procedures are usually not necessary in young perimenarchal patients, but pelvic examination must be performed to exclude pregnancy or pathologic conditions. In the older perimenopausal woman, endometrial aspiration, curettage, or both should be done for tissue examination to clearly establish that anovulatory or dyssynchronous cycles are the cause and to rule out malignant changes.

Treatment initially is aimed at interrupting the process with use of hormonal therapy. Numerous regimens are available, including estrogens followed by progesterone, progesterone alone, or combination oral contraceptive pills. High-dose conjugated estrogens are prescribed daily until bleeding is controlled—usually 2 to 3 days; then a lower dose is prescribed daily during the remainder of the cycle. Medroxyprogesterone acetate daily is added from day 15 to day 25 of the cycle to stimulate the luteal phase. The hormones are discontinued on day 25. Menses should then occur within 3 to 4 days. Oral contraceptive pills alone at three or four times the usual dose can be effective and simpler than the sequential hormones. The dose is lowered when bleeding diminishes. Medroxyprogesterone acetate daily for 10 days can be used if biopsy examination shows proliferative endometrium. Therapy is continued for three to six cycles and then discontinued. Further evaluation is required if anovulatory cycles continue.

Abnormal Uterine Bleeding

Abnormal uterine bleeding includes bleeding caused by pregnancy, systemic disease, or cancer, as well as abnormal menstrual bleeding. Patterns of the bleeding have been defined and placed into seven categories, six of which are associated with the menstrual cycle (Table 64-2).

Evaluation of abnormal uterine bleeding requires a careful history and physical examination. Diagnostic and screening procedures include cytologic examination, endometrial biopsy, histologic examination, hysteroscopy, and dilation and curettage. Other procedures used are assay of the beta-subunit of hCG for complications of pregnancy and trophoblastic disease, pelvic ultrasonography, and laparoscopy.

Management of these abnormal conditions depends on the specific diagnosis, realizing that more than one condition can be involved. If pathologic causes are excluded, if there is no significant risk of cancer developing, and if no acute life-threatening hemorrhage is occurring, many women with abnormal menstrual bleeding can be treated with hormone therapy.

REPRODUCTIVE ORGAN INFECTIOUS PROCESSES

Infections can occur in any of the reproductive organs and structures. The anatomy of the female reproductive system allows ascent of organisms from the lower tract to the upper tract and potentially the peritoneal cavity, as well as descent from the upper tract in which there is

TABLE 64-2	■ ■ ■

Abnormal Bleeding Patterns

Terminology	Pattern
Menorrhagia	Heavy or prolonged menstrual flow
Hypomenorrhea	Unusually light menstrual flow; spotting
Metrorrhagia	Bleeding at any time between periods
Polymenorrhea	Frequent menstrual periods
Menometrorrhagia	Bleeding at irregular intervals; amount and duration vary
Oligomenorrhea	Menstrual bleeding at more than 35-day intervals; decreased amount
Contact bleeding	Bleeding after coitus; caused by erosion, cervical polyps, vaginitis, or cervicitis

hematogenous spread of the organism from a primary site elsewhere in the body.

Infections of the cervix, endometrium, and salpinx frequently occur concurrently, and they share overlapping microbial etiologies. Histopathologic studies show that 40% of women with mucopurulent cervicitis and 80% of women with acute salpingitis also have endometritis. Cervicitis and salpingitis are common infections of sexually active women during the reproductive years. These infections are a major public health concern because of the profound impact that salpingitis has on the reproductive health of women. Damage to the fallopian tubes that results from salpingitis is the major cause of tubal infertility and ectopic pregnancy. Infections of the female reproductive organs are discussed in Chapter 66.

STRUCTURAL OR DISPLACEMENT DISORDERS

Diethylstilbestrol-Exposed Vaginal and Cervical Abnormalities

Daughters of women who took diethylstilbestrol (DES) during pregnancy are at risk for a variety of uterine and vaginal disorders. DES was widely prescribed from 1938 until 1971 to prevent miscarriage and other complications of pregnancy (National Institutes of Health, 1995). In 1971 the U.S. Food and Drug Administration (FDA) withdrew approval for the use of DES in pregnancy because there was an increase in clear cell adenocarcinoma of the vagina or cervix in women who were less than 25 years of age. Studies have revealed that DES-exposed daughters have a variety of reproductive system anomalies that include adenosis; anatomic differences in the vagina, cervix, or uterus; cervical dysplasia; clear cell adenocarcinoma; pregnancy problems (premature labor, spontaneous abortion, ectopic pregnancy); and infertility.

Mothers who took DES during pregnancy are at about a 30% higher risk for developing breast cancer. Between 1946 and 1971, 2 to 3 million women took DES between the eighth and sixteenth weeks of pregnancy to prevent threatened spontaneous abortion. Women in their mid-20s whose mothers took DES are known to have sequelae that correspond with the time of fetal development during which the drug was used. DES causes development defects of the genital tract and adenoma of the vagina that may undergo malignant changes. Incidence rose sharply at 14 years, with the peak at 19 years. Some women in their 30s and 40s have developed malignant changes. Because DES was last used in 1971, the youngest of fetuses who were exposed during pregnancy would now be in their 30s.

Intersex and Ambiguous Genitalia

Errors along the pathway to genital development in the embryo can result in ambiguous genitalia or intersex conditions. Common types of intersex problems are congenital adrenal hyperplasia (CAH), Turner syndrome, androgen insensitivity syndrome (AIS), and gonadal dysgenesis. The overall incidence of intersex conditions is estimated from studies to be 1.728 per 100 live births (Fausto-Sterling, 2000).

Individuals with *CAH* have a normal 46,XX karyotype and have external genitalia that are masculinized while having an internal uterus, fallopian tubes, and upper vagina. This state is due to an autosomal recessive mutation. Genitalia of females are masculinized because the precursors to cortisol have androgenic effects on the genitalia (see Chapter 61). Most individuals with CAH have a deficiency in 21-hydroxylase, which can be determined by serum levels. The genitalia may range from a slightly enlarged clitoris all the way to a penis and a scrotum without gonads. These differences in external genitalia may appear at birth or with the onset of puberty. CAH can be life threatening because of severe changes in salt metabolism. Alteration in the synthesis of enzymes needed for the formation of cortisol results in a decrease in the levels of cortisol, which then stimulates the production of adrenocorticotropic hormone (ACTH) by the adrenal glands. Because CAH can present as a life-threatening crisis, treatment to address fluid and electrolyte balance is critical; management with cortisol is to treat adrenal insufficiency. If treated, the individual will be able to reproduce (Parker, 1998). CAH can be diagnosed early in pregnancy, and the mother can receive cortisol to prevent the development virilization of the genitalia in the 46, XX embryo (American Academy of Pediatrics, 2000).

Turner syndrome occurs with an individual that has a 45,XO karyotype; the second X is missing (see Chapter 2). Dysgenesis of the gonads occurs and the ovaries do not develop. The individual with Turner syndrome is usually short and does not develop secondary sex characteristics. The treatment for this condition is administration of estrogen and growth hormone.

Androgen insensitive syndrome (AIS) occurs with a genetic XY karyotype embryo that has the inability to respond to androgen. The presence of androgen is necessary for the development of the wolffian duct system into the penis and scrotum. The individual with AIS develops genitalia that are feminine. At puberty, breasts will develop, as well as a female body shape.

The management of intersex conditions is currently being reviewed and debated with the aim of developing recommendations. The North American Task Force on Intersex (NATFI) is revising medical nomenclature and is developing guidelines for the treatment of intersex individuals (NATFI, 2000). This task force is interdisciplinary and also includes intersex advocates, as well as surgeons, endocrinologists, psychologists, psychiatrists, geneticists, and epidemiologists. This issue has become paramount because adult individuals who were sex-assigned and surgically altered as infants have formed advocacy groups that have criticized treatment options that involved surgeries and sex assignment that proved to be inappropriate with puberty and adulthood.

Displacement Disorders of the Genital Tract

The weakening of the pelvic floor supports causes displacement disorders of the female genital tract. Factors contributing to this condition are congenital abnormalities, aging, pregnancy trauma, childbirth, surgery, infection, and subsequent scarring. The uterus can be prolapsed; that is, the ligaments that suspend the uterus can be disrupted, resulting in a uterus that slips down into the vaginal canal or completely protrudes through the vagina. Sometimes the uterus is anteflexed or is retroflexed, which

Cystocele

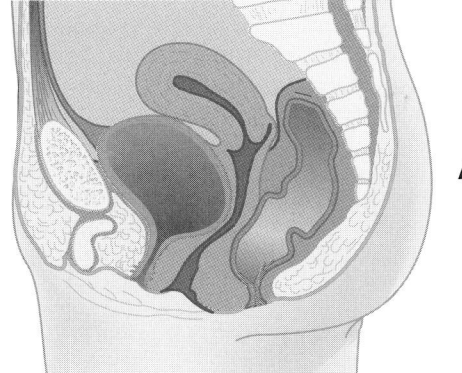

Rectocele

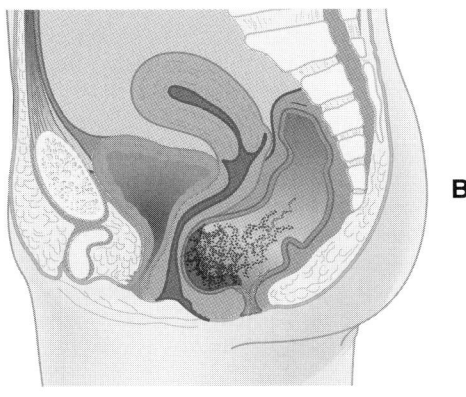

FIG. 64-9   A, Cystocele and **B,** rectocele. (From Matteson PS: *Women's health during the childbearing years: A community-based approach.* St. Louis, 2001, Mosby.)

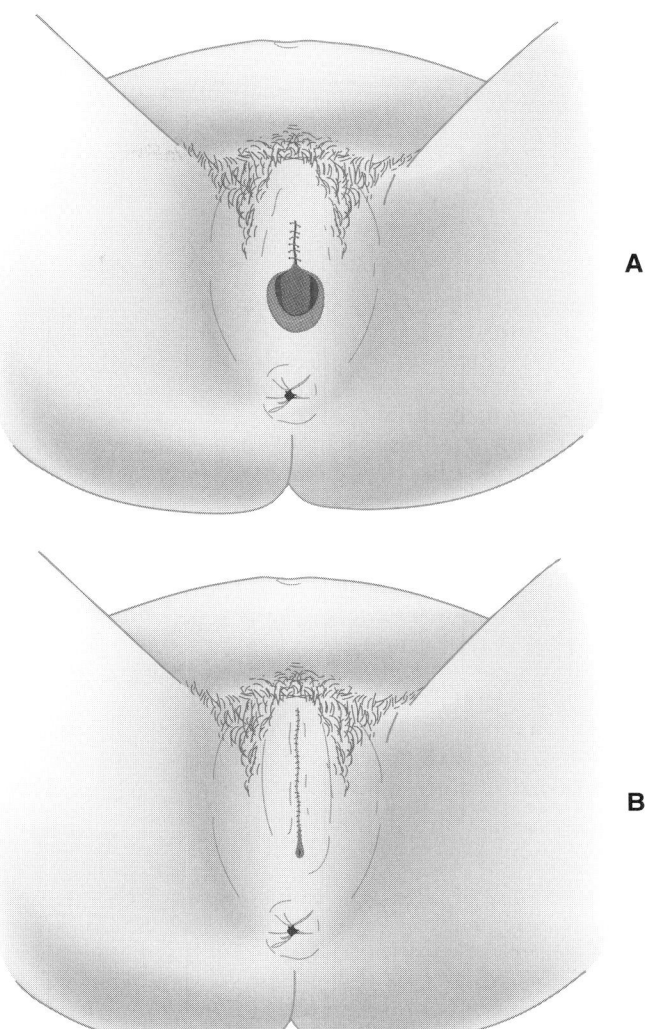

FIG. 64-10   Female genital mutilation. **A,** Type II and **B,** Type III. (From Matteson PS: *Women's health during the childbearing years: A community-based approach.* St. Louis, 2001, Mosby.)

may cause symptoms that include low backache, deep pelvic pressure, urinary tract infections, and dyspareunia. Surgical repair may be necessary to bring the uterus back up into its proper position in the abdomen. Sometimes, a pessary is used to keep the uterus in place.

A *cystocele* is a weak area in the vagina in which the bladder bulges into the vaginal canal. This situation can cause difficulties with urination and contribute to infections in the urogenital system. Surgical suspension of the bladder may be necessary to repair the problem. A cystocele can be a result of a traumatic birth or birth of a large infant. A *rectocele* is the herniation of the rectum into the vaginal canal (Fig. 64-9).

A fistula is an abnormal opening between the vaginal canal and the bowel or bladder or the rectum or colon. This abnormality is a very distressing complication that can occur as a result of infection at a surgical site following gynecologic surgery, radiation therapy, congenital anomalies, cancer, or traumatic delivery. Sometimes, small fistulas will heal with antibiotics. Surgical repair may be necessary to correct large fistulas.

Female Circumcision

In 28 African countries and some Middle Eastern cultures, *female circumcision (FC)* or *female genital mutilation (FMG)* is practiced. FC-FMG procedures are of three types

as classified by the World Health Organization. Type I FC-FMG involves removal of the prepuce and part of or the whole clitoris. Type II FC-FMG involves the removal of the prepuce, clitoris, and part of or the whole labia minora. Type III FC-FMG, the most extensive, involves the removal of the entire external genitalia and infibulation, which is the narrowing of the vaginal opening by stitching it (Fig. 64-10). Nonprofessionals usually do circumcisions with nonsterile instruments on young girls. Immediate complications include infection, bleeding, hemorrhage, pain, and urinary retention. Because it is illegal for FC-FGM to be performed in the United States on females under the age of 18, immediate complications will usually not be seen. Long-term complications will more likely be seen in the United States in immigrant women. Complications include ulceration of the skin, scaring and keloid scar formation, tenderness of the vulva and perineum, sebaceous and dermoid cysts, neuroma of the clitoral nerve, incontinence, vaginal obstruction, fistula, infections of the urinary tract and vagina, dysmenorrhea, and dyspareunia. In the woman who is infibulated, defibulation is necessary for a vaginal delivery. During pregnancy, health care professionals can begin counseling for the defibulation. Defibulation can be done during the second trimester or at the time of delivery (Toubia, 1999).

BENIGN LESIONS OF THE UTERUS AND OVARIES

Endometrial Hyperplasia and Polyps

Endometrial hyperplasia, an overgrowth of the endometrium, and *endometrial polyps,* soft pedunculated tumors, are caused by abnormal hormone production. The most common cause is anovulatory cycles, with prolonged production of estrogen and absence of progesterone. This condition is highly associated with dysfunctional uterine bleeding.

Diagnosis is made by examining tissue after dilation and curettage (D and C) of the uterus. The diagnostic D and C often corrects the problem. In postmenopausal women, if hyperplasia progresses, hysterectomy may be indicated.

Cervical polyps are benign masses, derived from the endocervix, that protrude from the cervix through the external os. These polyps are small (1 to 2 cm), nonneoplastic globular masses and probably result from chronic inflammation. These masses are seen in about 5% of women, and through erosion and ulceration, may cause intermenstrual bleeding or spotting.

Leiomyomas

A *leiomyoma* is a benign, well-circumscribed uterine tumor. Other names for this tumor include fibroid, myoma, fibroma, and fibromyoma. Approximately 20% to 25% of women over the age of 35 years have a uterine leiomyoma. These tumors are composed mostly of smooth muscle and some fibrous material.

Leiomyomas are classified according to their location. An *intramural* tumor is located in the muscle wall of the uterus and may distort the cavity, as well as protrude from the external surface. A *subserous* tumor is just beneath the serosa and projects from the external surface of the uterus. This tumor may become pedunculated and extend into the pelvic or abdominal cavity. A *submucous* tumor is just beneath the endometrium. These tumors also may become pedunculated and may protrude into the uterine cavity, through the cervical os, into the vagina, or out the vaginal opening. In this last event, infection is a complication.

The size of leiomyomas varies greatly and can be large enough to fill the pelvic and abdominal cavities. Leiomyomas are subject to degeneration with alteration in blood supply caused by growth, pregnancy, or uterine atrophy in menopause. Torsion or twisting of a pedunculated leiomyoma may occur.

Leiomyomas can sometimes be palpated abdominally; most often they are diagnosed when masses are felt on bimanual pelvic examination. Most leiomyomas do not produce symptoms, and thus treatment is not necessary. Problems that may occur, however, include frequently excessive abnormal uterine bleeding and resultant anemia; pressure on the bladder that causes urinary frequency, urgency, and potential for cystitis; pressure on the rectum that causes constipation; and pain if the tumor degenerates or if there is torsion of a pedunculated leiomyoma.

No intervention is necessary for women who are asymptomatic or near menopause or who have small tumors. Regular examination should be performed to monitor changes. During the childbearing years, myomectomy may be performed if significant symptoms are present or if infertility occurs secondary to the leiomyoma. In some cases, hysterectomy may be performed if, for example, there is intractable abnormal uterine bleeding, particularly in the perimenopausal woman.

MALIGNANT CONDITIONS OF THE REPRODUCTIVE ORGANS

Carcinomas of the reproductive organs are among the most common in women. Research has led to earlier detection, as well as to more effective treatments. Emphasis is being placed on basing treatment decisions on research findings that determine the best outcomes. Because this is a rapidly changing area and new and improved treatment protocols are available, it is imperative that health care professionals know where and how to locate the most up-to-date data. The information in this section is based on data from CancerNet, which is a service of the National Cancer Institute, a division of the National Institutes of Health (http://cancernet.nci.nih.gov). This chapter will discuss the most common sites where cancer of the female reproductive system occurs. These sites are the endometrium, cervix, ovary, vagina, and vulva.

Carcinoma of the Endometrium

Carcinoma of the endometrium is the most common female pelvic malignancy, accounting for 6% of all cancers in women. Adenocarcinomas make up 75% to 89% of the endometrial tumors. Uncommon carcinomas of the endometrium are clear cell carcinoma, squamous cell carcinoma, and mucinous cell carcinoma. Approximately 34,000 new cases are diagnosed each year, although in most cases (75%), the tumor is confined to the uterine corpus (stage I) and therefore can be cured. The 6000 yearly deaths make uterine cancer only the seventh leading cause of death in women, and the death rate has been declining significantly (−1.2% per year) in recent years (SEER, 2001).

Endometrial carcinoma is primarily a disease of postmenopausal women, although 25% occur in women less than age 50 years and 5% below age 40 years. Prolonged, unopposed estrogen therapy is associated with an increased incidence of endometrial cancer. Women taking tamoxifen for breast cancer treatment or prevention are also at somewhat increased risk. The use of estrogen and progesterone together has been shown to prevent the increase of endometrial cancer. In menopausal women who have a uterus, hormone replacement therapy (HRT) should include progesterone in addition to estrogen to prevent an increase in endometrial cancer (CancerNet, 2001). Symptoms that women experience usually include abnormal uterine bleeding and bleeding after menopause. Malignant endometrial cells may occasionally be found in a Pap smear of asymptomatic women with endometrial carcinoma. The Pap smear findings

TABLE 64-3

Staging and 5-Year Survival in Gynecologic Malignancies

Stage	Endometrial	% 5-Year Survival	Cervix	% 5-Year Survival	Ovary	% 5-Year Survival
0			Carcinoma in situ	100		
I	Confined to corpus	89	Confined to uterus	85	Confined to ovary	90
II	Involves corpus and cervix	80	Invades beyond uterus but not pelvic wall	60	Confined to pelvis	70
III	Extends outside uterus but not outside true pelvis	30	Extends to pelvic wall and/or lower third of vagina or hydronephrosis	33	Intraabdominal spread	15-20
IV	Extends outside the true pelvis or involves rectum or bladder	9	Invades mucosa of bladder or rectum or extends beyond true pelvis	7	Spread outside abdomen	1-5

must be followed up, but this is not a reliable screening or diagnostic modality to detect the disease. Risk factors for this cancer are the use of unopposed estrogen, obesity, early menarche, nulliparity, late menopause, hypertension, diabetes, and hereditary nonpolyposis colorectal cancer (HNPCC) (American Cancer Society, 2001).

Diagnosis and staging of the tumors is done with clinical evaluation and follows the guidelines set forth by the International Federation of Gynecology and Obstetrics (FIGO) and the American Joint Committee on Cancer (AJCC). Evaluation includes inspection, palpation, colposcopy, cervical curettage, hysteroscopy, cystoscopy, proctoscopy, and x-ray examination of the lungs and CT scan of the skeleton for metastasis. Diagnosis is made by examination of tissue from biopsy curettage of the endometrial cavity. Table 64-3 lists the stages and prognosis for endometrial carcinoma as well as that for cervical and ovarian cancer.

Treatment for stage I endometrial cancer is hysterectomy with bilateral salpingo-oophorectomy and removal of some pelvic lymph nodes. If the nodes are negative, no further treatment is needed. If the nodes are positive, irradiation is recommended. Treatment for stage II is the same as that for stage I with postoperative irradiation. Stage III women are treated with surgery and irradiation. If it is not possible to do surgery, then irradiation therapy may be used. Progestational drugs hydroxyprogesterone (Delalutin), medroxyprogesterone (Provera), and megestrol (Megace) may be used if the patient is unable to undergo irradiation. Stage IV women may be treated according to symptoms and site of the spread of disease. The use of progestational drugs and irradiation therapy may be used. Clients with stage IV endometrial cancers should consider experimental treatment in clinical trials because there is no standard treatment at this time.

Carcinoma of the Cervix

Carcinoma of the cervix is the second most frequent genital cancer in women and is responsible for 6% of all cancers in women in the United States (CancerNet, 2001). The majority (90%) of these cervical cancers are squamous cell carcinomas and 10% are adenocarcinomas. Other rare types include adenosquamous cell carcinoma, clear cell carcinoma, malignant melanoma, sarcoma, and malignant lymphoma.

BOX 64-2

Papanicolaou (Pap) Smear Terminology and Classifications

A. BETHESDA SYSTEM CLASSIFICATION OF PAP TESTS (CURRENT USAGE)
- **ASCUS** (atypical squamous cells of undetermined significance)
  Squamous cells are thin, flat cells that form the surface of the cervix.
- **LSIL** (low-grade [early changes in the size and shape of cells] squamous intraepithelial lesion)
  Lesion refers to an area of abnormal tissue; *intraepithelial* means that the abnormal cells are present only in the surface layer of cells.
- **HSIL** (high-grade squamous intraepithelial lesion)
  High-grade means that there are more marked changes in the size and shape of the abnormal (precancerous) cells that look different than normal cells.

B. COMPARISON OF TERMINOLOGY BETWEEN THE CURRENT BETHESDA SYSTEM AND CERVICAL INTRAEPITHELIAL NEOPLASIA (CIN) (CURRENT AND OLDER USAGE)
- Mild dysplasia may also be classified as   LSIL or CIN1
- Moderate dysplasia may also be classified as   HSIL or CIN2
- Severe dysplasia may also be classified as   HSIL or CIN3
- Carcinoma in situ may also be classified as   HSIL or CIN3

Comment: LSIL or CIN1 are associated with a small risk of progression to invasive cervical carcinoma, whereas HSIL or CIN2 or CIN3 are associated with a higher risk. (From National Cancer Institute (2001). Questions and answers about the Pap test, *Cancer Facts.* Retrieved November 30, 2001 from the World Wide Web: *http://cis.nci.nih.gov/fact/5_16.htm*).

Cervical cancer is routinely screened by the Papanicolaou (Pap) smear test. Box 64-2 presents the new Bethesda terminology for the classification of Pap test results and compares it with the older cervical intraepithelial neoplasia (CIN) classification system. The Pap test has significantly reduced mortality rates from cervical cancer in the United States—mortality rates fell 70% from 1950-1970 and 40% from 1970-1995. The current recommendations from the American College of Obstetricians and Gynecologists and the American Cancer Society are to perform pelvic examination and Pap smear screening annually for all women who are or have been sexually active or have reached the age of 18 years. After three or more consecutive satisfactory normal annual examinations, the Pap test may be done less frequently at the discretion of the physician. Although detection of cervical cancer at a very early (and curable) stage is possible with the use of the Pap smear test, many women do not get them done. It is estimated that about one third of eligible women do not have Pap smears done. Seventy percent of newly diagnosed women with invasive cervical cancer had not had a Pap test done in the past 5 years (American Cancer Society, 2001). The peak incidence of carcinoma in situ is 20 to 30 years of age in both African-American and Caucasian women. Women older than 65 years account for 25% of the invasive cervical carcinomas and have between 40% and 50% of the mortality from cervical carcinoma (CancerNet, 2001).

The major risk factor for cervical cancer is infection with the human papillomavirus (HPV)) that is transmitted sexually. Worldwide epidemiologic studies confirm that HPV infection is the principal factor in the development of cervical cancer (Bosch et al, 1995). More than 20 different types of HPV have been associated with cervical cancer. Studies show that women with HPV-16, -18, and -31 have higher rates of *cervical intraepithelial neoplasia (CIN)* (CancerNet, 2001). Recent research has demon-

strated that women with the HPV-18 strain have a mortality rate that is higher and have a poorer prognosis (Schwartz et al, 2001). Other risk factors for development of cervical cancer include sexual activity at a young age, high parity, increasing numbers of sexual partners, low socioeconomic status, and smoking (CancerNet, 2001).

Squamous cell carcinoma usually occurs at the junction of the squamous epithelium and the columnar mucous epithelium of the endocervix (*squamocolumnar junction* or *transformation zone*). Fig. 64-11 illustrates the location of the transformation zone of the cervix, and Fig. 64-12 shows the progressive cellular abnormalities eventually terminating in invasive cervical carcinoma). Cervical dysplasia and carcinoma in situ (HSIL) precede invasive carcinoma. Preinvasive carcinoma is not evident during a routine pelvic examination. The Pap smear is used as a screening test for detection of neoplastic changes. An abnormal smear is followed up with biopsy to obtain tissue for cytologic examination. Because the cervix has a normal appearance, colposcopy is used to define the abnormal area or areas for taking tissue samples. Punch biopsy of discrete areas or cone biopsy (the removal of a cone-shaped portion of tissue from the cervix that includes most or the entire transformation zone) of the whole squamocolumnar junction is performed.

Preinvasive forms of cervical dysplasia including carcinoma in situ may be removed completely by cone biopsy or eradicated by laser, cautery, or cryosurgery. Regular, frequent follow-up for recurrence of the lesion is important after these treatments.

Invasive carcinoma of the cervix occurs when the tumor invades the epithelium into the stroma of the cervix. Cervical cancer spreads by direct extension into the paracervical tissue. Continued growth results in a visible lesion that involves progressively more of the cervical tissue. Invasion may occur in several sites simultaneously as long strands of tumor cells extend deeply into the connective tissue and eventually invade lymph vessels and venules. Invasive cervical carcinoma may further invade or extend to the vaginal wall, the cardinal ligaments, and

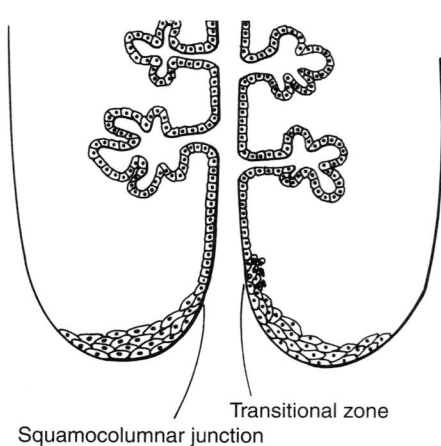

Transitional zone
Squamocolumnar junction

FIG. 64-11 Squamocolumnar junction of the uterine cervix.

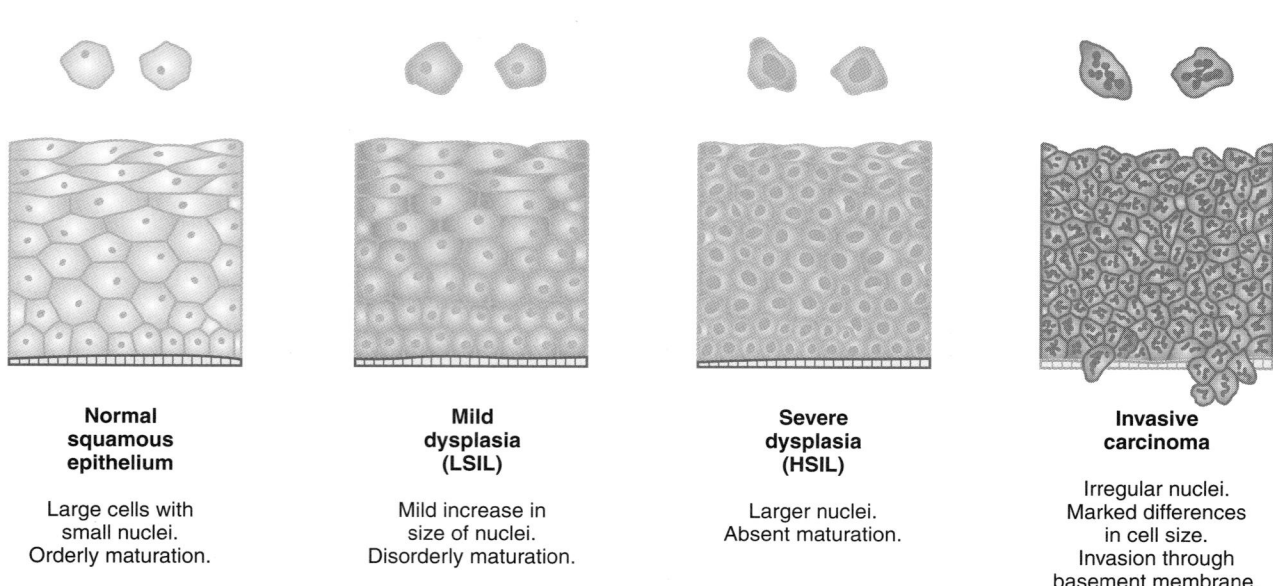

Normal squamous epithelium	**Mild dysplasia (LSIL)**	**Severe dysplasia (HSIL)**	**Invasive carcinoma**
Large cells with small nuclei. Orderly maturation.	Mild increase in size of nuclei. Disorderly maturation.	Larger nuclei. Absent maturation.	Irregular nuclei. Marked differences in cell size. Invasion through basement membrane.

FIG. 64-12 Cervical dysplasia. (From Matteson PS: *Women's health during the childbearing years: A community-based approach.* St. Louis, 2001, Mosby.)

the endometrial cavity; invasion of lymph nodes and blood vessels results in metastases to distant parts of the body. Table 64-3 lists the stages of cervical carcinoma with their associated 5-year survival rates.

No signs or symptoms are specific for cancer of the cervix. Preinvasive cervical carcinoma produces no symptoms, but early invasive carcinoma can cause a vaginal discharge or vaginal bleeding. Although bleeding is the only significant sign, it does not necessarily occur early, thus cancers can be far advanced before they are discovered. The most common type of vaginal bleeding is postcoital or intermenstrual spotting. Any discharge will be serosanguineous or purulent. As the tumor grows, late symptoms include low back or leg pain resulting from compression of lumbosacral nerves, urinary frequency, urgency, hematuria, or rectal bleeding.

Evaluation for cervical carcinoma includes examination by inspection or palpation, biochemical profile (liver and renal functions), chest x-ray film, cystoscopy, proctosigmoidoscopy, and CT scan. Use of the CT scan is increasing because evaluation of findings in several studies is correlated with surgical-pathologic findings that are 97% specific in patients with advanced disease. Treatment of invasive carcinoma of the cervix is determined by clinical and surgical evaluation. Treatment modalities include surgical excision, irradiation therapy, chemotherapy, or combinations of these modalities.

Carcinoma of the Ovary

Epithelial carcinoma of the ovary is one of the most common gynecologic cancers and the fifth most frequent cause of cancer death in women (CancerNet, 2001). A definitive cause of carcinoma of the ovary is unknown but is multifactorial. The risk of developing ovarian cancer is related to environmental, endocrine, and genetic factors. Environmental factors that are related to epithelial ovarian cancer are the subject of continuing debate and study. The highest incidence is in industrialized Western countries. Dietary habits, coffee and tobacco use, presence of asbestos in the environment, and use of talc have all been considered as possible cancer causes. No link between these factors and development of ovarian cancer has been found. Endocrine risk factors for ovarian cancer includes women who are nulliparous, have early menarche, late menopause, late first pregnancy, and have never breast-fed. Women with breast cancer have a twofold greater risk for developing ovarian cancer. Use of oral contraceptives does not increase the risk and may be protective. Estrogen replacement therapy (ERT) postmenopausally for 10 or more years is associated with an increased risk of mortality from ovarian cancer (Rodriguez et al, 2001). The tumor suppressor genes, BRCA-1 and BRCA-2, have been shown to play a role in some families. Hereditary ovarian cancer that is autosomal dominant with variable penetrance has been documented in familial ovarian cancer registries. If two or more first-degree relatives have ovarian cancer, a woman has a 50% chance of developing it. Some physicians recommend a prophylactic oophorectomy at age 35 for women in this high-risk group.

More than 30 types of ovarian neoplasms have been identified. Ovarian tumors are grouped into three broad categories: (1) epithelial tumors, (2) gonadal stromal tumors, and (3) germ cell tumors. Epithelial tumors make up 60% of all ovarian neoplasms and are classified as benign, borderline malignant, and malignant. Malignant forms of epithelial neoplasms make up 90% of all ovarian cancers. The most common epithelial malignancy is the serous adenocarcinoma.

Most neoplasms of epithelial origin develop from the surface epithelium, or serosa, of the ovary. In the embryo, the gonadal ridge (ovaries) and the müllerian ducts (fallopian tubes, uterus, and vagina) have a common mesodermal origin. Therefore epithelial neoplasms of the ovary reflect cell types of müllerian differentiations: that is, serous, resembling fallopian tube, 46%; mucinous, resembling endocervix, 36%; endometrioid, resembling endometrium, 8%; and clear cell, resembling endometrial glands in pregnancy, 3%. Other tumors are of urothelial cell type, mixed carcinomas, and undifferentiated carcinomas.

Ovarian cancer metastasizes by direct invasion of adjacent structures of the abdomen and pelvis and by cells seeding the abdominal and pelvic cavities. These cells follow the natural circulation of peritoneal fluid so that implantation and subsequent malignant growth can occur on all intraperitoneal surfaces. The lymphatics that drain the ovary are also a route for spread of malignant cells. All nodes of the pelvis and abdominal cavities will eventually be affected. Initial spread of ovarian cancer by the intraperitoneal and lymphatic routes occur without specific signs or symptoms. Vague symptoms that will develop with time are feelings of pelvic heaviness, urinary frequency and dysuria, and changes in gastrointestinal functioning, such as sensations of fullness, nausea, indigestion, early satiety, and constipation. Some women may have abnormal vaginal bleeding secondary to endometrial hyperplasia if the tumor is estrogen producing; some tumors produce testosterone and cause virilization. Symptoms of an acute condition in the abdomen can occur suddenly if there is hemorrhage into the tumor, rupture, or ovarian torsion. However, ovarian tumors are most often detected during routine pelvic examination.

In premenopausal women, most palpable adnexal masses are not malignant but are follicular or corpus luteum cysts. These functional cysts resolve in one to three menstrual cycles. If on pelvic examination the mass is believed to be less than 8 cm in size in a premenopausal woman, waiting and watching constitute an appropriate approach. The pelvic examination should be repeated within 1 to 2 months to reevaluate mass size and changes. However, in women who are premenarchal or postmenopausal, with any size mass, further immediate evaluation and perhaps surgical exploration are indicated. Because of a long asymptomatic period, diagnosis in 75% to 85% of women with epithelial ovarian cancer is not made until the tumor is well established throughout the peritoneal cavity. Although laparotomy is the primary procedure used to establish the diagnosis, less invasive studies (e.g., abdominal CT scans, abdominal and pelvic sonography) can often aid in defining the staging and extent of spread.

The surgical intervention for ovarian cancer is a total abdominal hysterectomy, bilateral salpingo-oophorectomy with omentectomy, a complete abdominal exploration, and multiple biopsies of peritoneum, aortic nodes, and pelvic nodes. The 5-year survival rate is about 30% but varies with tumor involvement in other structures and the amount of disease that could not be removed by surgery. Other therapeutic measures include chemotherapy, radiation therapy, or a combination of these. Table 64-3 lists the stages of ovarian cancer and the associated 5-year survival rates.

Prophylactic oophorectomy may be done for some women in families with documented transmission of familial ovarian cancer, but this procedure is not protective for all these high-risk women. Disseminated intraabdominal carcinomas that are histopathologically the same as ovarian carcinoma have occurred in some of these women after oophorectomy. The tissues at risk for carcinoma include those that develop from the same type of tissue from which the ovaries develop in the embryo.

Five percent of all ovarian neoplasms are gonadal stromal tumors; 2% of these account for 2% of ovarian malignancies. The World Health Organization (WHO) classifies ovarian neoplasms into five types with multiple subtypes.

There are three major categories of germ cell tumors: (1) benign tumors (dermoid cysts), (2) malignant tumors (constituents of dermoid cysts), and (3) primitive malignant germ cell tumors (embryonic and extraembryonic cells) that the WHO classifies into seven types with multiple subtypes. Dermoid cysts make up 25% to 33% of all ovarian neoplasms; 1% of ovarian cancers develop from constituents of dermoid cysts. Two to three percent of ovarian cancers are primitive malignant germ cell tumors. Accurate diagnosis of tumor type is important. Surgical excision is the primary treatment for all these ovarian tumors, with appropriate follow-up of any tumor determined to be malignant.

Carcinoma of the Fallopian Tubes

Primary cancer of the fallopian tubes is rare, accounting for the smallest number of primary malignant tumors of the female genital tract, namely, 0.5% to 1.0% of all gynecologic malignancies. Most malignant tumors that occur in the fallopian tubes are extensions from uterine or ovarian cancers. Therefore criteria exist to define any tumor as being a primary cancer of the fallopian tube. The cancer must be located within the tube, and the uterus and ovary must not contain carcinoma; if either site contains cancer, the tumor in the fallopian tube clearly must be histologically different.

The most common primary malignant tumors of the fallopian tube are adenocarcinoma. Other tumors can be sarcomas such as leiomyosarcomas, chondrosarcomas, mixed mesodermal tumors, lymphomas, and choriocarcinomas. All of these types of malignancies in fallopian tubes are quite rare. Malignant tumors of the fallopian tubes metastasize by lymph vessels to regional nodes and spread by migration into the pelvic or abdominal cavities, or they may penetrate the serosa and shed cells directly into the pelvic or abdominal cavities. Signs and symptoms, if present at all, include vaginal discharge, abnormal vaginal bleeding or discharge, menstrual irregularities, and pain. Diagnosis of fallopian tube malignancy is usually made with exploratory laparotomy. Noting an adnexal mass during pelvic examination makes an indication of a problem. Pain is probably caused by tubal distention and therefore is similar to that caused by a tubal pregnancy. The pain may be intermittent and colicky or dull and aching. Prognosis depends on the depth of invasion of the carcinoma in the tube and whether the tumor has spread beyond the tube. Bilateral involvement has a poorer prognosis than unilateral disease.

Treatment is total abdominal hysterectomy, bilateral salpingo-oophorectomy, and resection of as much gross disease as possible. Multiple biopsies of the peritoneum diaphragm and pelvic and paraaortic nodes are done. It is important to evaluate the lymph nodes. Postoperative adjuvant therapy with radiation, chemotherapy, or both has been shown to improve prognosis.

Carcinoma of the Vulva

Carcinoma of the vulva comprises 3% to 4% of all primary genital cancers in women. Ninety percent of the vulvar carcinomas are squamous cell cancer, and the remaining 10% are malignant melanoma, basal cell carcinoma, and adenocarcinoma of Bartholin's and Skene's glands. The classification of vulvar cancer ranges from carcinoma in situ to microinvasive carcinoma to invasive vulvar carcinoma. The median age for women with carcinoma in situ is 44 years; for microinvasive carcinoma, 58 years; and for frankly invasive carcinoma, 61 years. Sexually transmitted diseases are associated with vulvar carcinoma. These diseases include granulomatous venereal disease, syphilis, herpes hominis type II, condylomata acuminata, and infection from human papillomavirus (HPV). The most common sites of primary vulvar carcinoma are the labia, occurring three times more frequently on the labia majora than it does the labia minora, and the clitoris. Metastasis is spread by direct invasion of the surrounding organs to the inguinal lymph nodes and then to the pelvic nodes. Malignant melanoma is the only vulvar carcinoma that is spread by the bloodstream.

The gross appearance of the lesions of cancer of the vulva is flat or raised and maculopapular or verrucous. The lesions can be hyperpigmented (brown), red, or white. The various lesion patterns are referred to as Bowen's disease, erythroplasia of Queyrat, carcinoma simplex, and Paget's disease.

The initial signs and symptoms most frequently reported by the patient are a growth or mass on the vulva and pruritus. However, it is important to note that approximately 20% of women are asymptomatic, and small lesions are often undetected or ignored. This factor may result in delayed diagnosis and treatment, and the tumor may spread to secondary sites. Health care professionals must be suspicious about any lesion and obtain a biopsy for diagnosis. Any evaluation for metastasis is necessary whenever invasive carcinoma is evident on biopsy. This evaluation includes careful inspection of the vagina and cervix, a Pap smear of the cervix, a bimanual examination, cystoscopy, proctoscopy, chest x-ray examination, CT scan, and biochemical profile. A barium enema examination of the rectum and descending colon may also be necessary.

Radical vulvectomy and inguinal node and pelvic node dissection were considered the most effective treatment. However, over the last 5 years, less destructive procedures are being used that are contingent on the stage of disease. The depth of local invasion rather than the tumor size is related to the degree of spread. For example, carcinoma in situ of the vulva is treated with wide local excision of the tumor. Frequent follow-up examinations are necessary to check for recurrences. Tumors less than 2 cm in diameter with any degree of local invasion except the anus, vagina, or urethra may have lymph node metastasis. If the nodes are positive, radical vulvectomy and bilateral complete groin dissections are necessary; if negative, wide local excision of the lesion is done. With an invasion of 5 cm or more, a modified radical vulvectomy or hemivulvectomy with inguinofemoral lymphadenectomy is done. The treatment for more advanced stages involves radical vulvectomy, bilateral inguinal lymphadenectomy, and removal of a portion of the distal urethra or vagina or a portion of the rectum with postoperative pelvic irradiation. Tumors of the bladder or upper urethra require radical vulvectomy, inguinal node dissections, and possibly anterior exenteration. If the lesion involves the rectum, posterior exenteration may be done. If the tumor is fixed to bone or there are distant metastases, treatment is usually palliative and consists of irradiation and chemotherapy.

Treatment of other vulvar tumors such as malignant melanoma, basal cell carcinoma, and verrucous carcinoma of Bartholin's gland is managed by local excision; for deep melanomas, ipsilateral lymph node dissection may be done. Bartholin's gland carcinoma is usually treated by radical vulvectomy and bilateral inguinal node dissection.

Carcinoma of the Vagina

Primary vaginal carcinomas not involving the cervix or vulva are usually squamous cell cancers. Squamous cell carcinoma may appear as ulcerations, endophytic tumors, or exophytic tumors that may be manifested as dysplasia, carcinoma in situ, and invasion. This is not a common lesion and accounts for only 1% to 2% of all gynecologic cancers. The median age for carcinoma in situ is early in the fifth decade, whereas the median age for invasive carcinoma is in the middle of the sixth decade. Vaginal tumors that are secondary to tumors of other genital areas occur by direct extension or metastasis, especially from the cervix or rectum.

Significant risk factors for primary carcinoma of the vagina include (1) history of HPV infection, (2) hysterectomy before menopause, (3) history of an abnormal Pap smear, and (4) prior radiation for other carcinomas. The time between radiation therapy and development of vaginal carcinoma has been reported to be from 7 to 20 years. One percent to three percent of women with squamous cell carcinoma of the cervix also develop squamous cell carcinoma of the vagina. Carcinoma in situ of the vagina has been reported to occur from less than 2 years to 17 years after carcinoma in situ of the cervix.

In 1971 an increase was noted in the incidence of clear cell carcinoma of the vagina in young women who were exposed to diethylstilbestrol (DES) in utero. Clear cell adenocarcinoma in these women occurs most frequently in the upper third of the anterior vaginal wall. The risk that a DES-exposed woman will develop carcinoma is slight—0.4 to 1.4 per 1000 women, or less than 0.1%. The incidence stopped rising in the mid-1970s and continues to decline each year. As DES-exposed women approach menopause, it will be important to monitor their status closely because it is unknown what the effects of ERT or HRT will have. It is recommended that DES-exposed daughters have a yearly pelvic examination, which includes inspection and palpation of the entire vaginal canal and cervix, a bimanual examination of the uterus, tubes, and ovaries, and taking separate smears for a Pap test of the cervix, as well as the upper vaginal wall.

Other malignant lesions that may occur in the vagina are malignant melanoma, which is the second most common primary cancer of the vagina (2% to 3% incidence), verrucous carcinoma, small cell carcinoma, and sarcomas (2% incidence, usually in the fifth and sixth decades). Sarcoma botryoides is rare but is the most common tumor of the genital tract in female children between 2 and 3 years old.

Carcinomas of the vagina can spread by direct extension to paracolpial, parametrial, and pararectal tissues and to the pelvic sidewalls or by the lymphatics to regional lymph nodes. Clear cell carcinoma frequently spreads to supraclavicular nodes or lungs.

Preinvasive lesions of the vagina are asymptomatic, and lesions can be undetected. Therefore careful inspection during routine physical examination is important for early detection of these lesions. Examination of the vagina by colposcopy is recommended for all women with abnormal cervical cytology. Vaginal discharge and abnormal postmenopausal, postcoital, or intermenstrual vaginal bleeding are the most common signs. Pain or bladder and rectum problems usually occur with advanced disease. Diagnosis of invasive vaginal carcinoma is made by inspection, palpation, and biopsy. In addition, chest x-ray examination, biochemical profile, CT scan of the abdomen and pelvis, barium enema, cystoscopy, and proctoscopy are necessary for the diagnostic workup.

The primary treatment for vaginal squamous cell carcinoma is radiation therapy. Surgical excision is difficult because of the closeness of the bladder and rectum to the vagina. The thickness of the vesicovaginal and rectovaginal septa is usually only millimeters, making exenterative procedures necessary to allow adequate surgical margins around the tumor or tumors. Early lesions in clear cell carcinoma can be treated with surgery or radiation therapy; more advanced invasive lesions should be treated with surgery. Surgical procedures for any stage of the disease include radical hysterectomy, vaginectomy, and radical lymph node dissection.

BREAST

Anatomy and Physiology

The mammary gland is developmentally and structurally related to the integument. A major function is to secrete milk for nourishment of the infant. This function is directed and mediated by the same hormones that regulate the functions of the reproductive system. Therefore the mammary gland is considered an accessory of the reproductive system. The mammary gland reaches its full developmental potential with menarche in women; in the infant, child, and in men, it is present only in rudimentary form (Fig. 64-13).

The breasts are composed of glandular, fibrous, and adipose tissue. Connective tissue separates the breast from the chest wall muscles, the pectoral, and anterior serratus. Just a little below center of each mature breast is

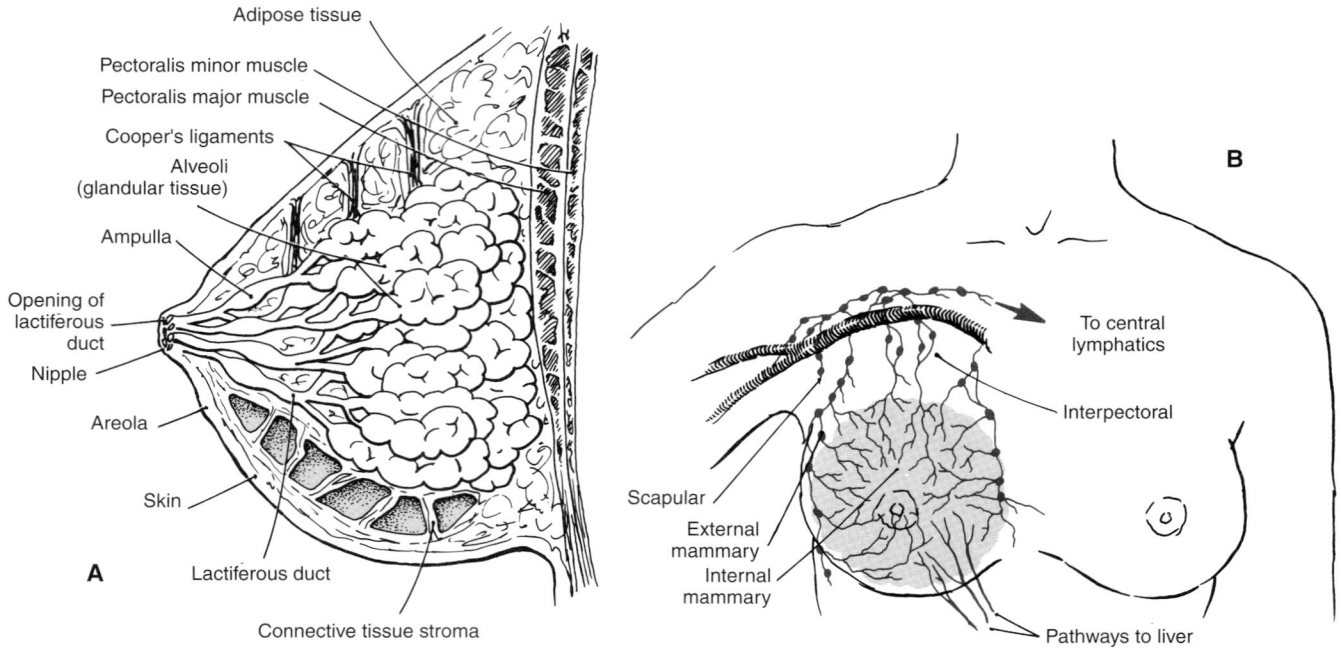

FIG. 64-13 Mature breast. **A,** Anatomy. **B,** Lymphatic drainage.

the nipple (mammary papilla), a pigmented projection surrounded by the areola. The nipple is perforated at the tip by several minute openings, the apertures of the lactiferous ducts. Montgomery's tubercles are sebaceous glands on the surface of the areola.

The glandular tissue forms 15 to 25 lobes arranged radially about the nipple and is separated by variable amounts of adipose tissue that surrounds the connective tissue (stroma) between the lobes. Each lobe is distinct so that disease that affects one lobe does not necessarily affect another. The lobes drain into the lactiferous sinuses, which then open into collecting ducts that open onto the nipple. The connective stroma in many places is concentrated into fibrous bands that course vertically through the substance of the breast, attaching the deep layer of the subcutaneous fascia to the dermis. These bands, *Cooper's ligaments,* are suspensory ligaments of the breast.

Changes during the Life Cycle

Breast development is sequential and the stages of growth predictable. At puberty, the breasts enlarge principally because of an increase in glandular tissue and a deposit of adipose tissue. With each menstrual cycle, there are typical changes of vascular engorgement, enlargement of the glands in the premenstrual phase followed by glandular regression in the postmenstrual phase. During late pregnancy and after parturition, the breasts secrete colostrum, a thin, yellowish fluid, until about 3 to 4 days postpartum, when secretion of milk begins in response to the stimulation of the infant's suckling. With suckling, oxytocin is released from the posterior pituitary gland, which then triggers the milk "let-down" reflex. Milk is then released from the nipple during the process of nursing. After weaning, the gland gradually regresses by loss of glandular tissue. At menopause, the adipose tissue regresses more slowly, compared with glandular tissue, but it eventually disappears, leaving the breasts pendulous and small.

Benign Conditions
Infections
Bacterial infections (mastitis) commonly occur postpartum during early lactation when organisms gain access to breast tissue by fissures in the nipple. The organisms most commonly involved are *Staphylococcus aureus* or streptococci. The breast becomes reddened, hot to touch, swollen, and tender. Symptoms are high fever, chills, and malaise. The treatment is local heat, antipyretics and mild analgesics, periodic emptying of the breast by continued breastfeeding or pumping, and oral antibiotic therapy. If an abscess occurs, hospitalization for administering intravenous antibiotics, aspiration, or incision and drainage may be necessary. Any aspirated material is sent for histologic evaluation to rule out malignancy.

Trauma
The most common injury to the breast is contusion. These injuries heal spontaneously but sometimes result in a fat necrosis, which is a mass that feels firm and irregular and occasionally causes skin retraction. For these reasons, it is necessary to rule out carcinoma when this lesion occurs.

Fibroadenoma
Fibroadenomas are benign tumors and are well circumscribed with a firm, rubbery consistency. The treatment for fibroadenomas is surgical removal of the tumor. The specimen is examined to rule out malignancy. A cystosarcoma phyllodes is a type of benign fibroadenoma that can recur if not completely removed.

Intraductal Papilloma
Papillomas that occur in the nipple ducts usually are too small to palpate but often cause a serosanguineous or bloody nipple discharge. The cause of any kind of abnormal nipple discharge, especially if sanguineous, must be determined and malignancy ruled out. Treatment is surgical excision of the involved ducts.

Fibrocystic Disease of the Breast

A number of changes of breast tissue are associated with fibrocystic disease. Included is cyst formation, ductal epithelial proliferation, diffuse papillomatosis, and ductal adenosis with formation of fibrous tissue. Clinically, these changes can result in palpable nodules, masses, and nipple discharge. Fibrocystic breast disease occurs during the childbearing years; the cause is most likely related to a relative excess of estrogen and a deficiency of progesterone during the luteal phase of the menstrual cycle. Approximately 50% of women have fibrocystic breast disease. The condition is usually bilateral.

About 30% of women with biopsy-proven fibrocystic disease have proliferative hyperplasia; this is important because this type of change is associated with an increased risk of later development of carcinoma. For patients who have *simple epithelial hyperplasia* (about 25% of all cases of fibrocystic disease), the risk of subsequent development of carcinoma is twofold. In other cases, abnormalities in cell cytology and architecture have some, but not all, of the features of carcinoma in situ, in which instances the term *atypical hyperplasia* is used. For women with atypical hyperplasia (about 5% of cases), the risk of subsequently developing a carcinoma increases fivefold.

Symptoms include swelling and tenderness of the breasts just before menstrual periods. Signs are palpable masses that move freely in the breast, a feeling of granularity of the breast tissue, and occasionally nonbloody nipple discharge. Many women are asymptomatic and seek medical care when they feel a palpable mass.

Treatment for symptomatic relief of tenderness is by use of mild analgesics and local heat. Improvement may result by avoiding coffee, tea, colas, and chocolate (with methylxanthines); cheese, wine, nuts, mushrooms, and bananas (with tyramines); and tobacco (with nicotine). About 30% of women with biopsy-proven fibrocystic disease have proliferative hyperplasia, which increases their risk for breast cancer by three times the general risk. The major problem for clinicians is distinguishing masses caused by fibrocystic disease and malignancy.

Carcinoma of the Breast

Breast cancer represents a malignant proliferation of epithelial cells lining the ducts or lobules of the breast. Initially there is hyperplasia of the cells with development of atypical cells. These cells progress to carcinoma in situ and then to stromal invasion. A cancer takes about 7 years to grow from a single cell to a mass large enough to palpate (about 1 cm in diameter). At that size, about 25% of breast cancers have already metastasized.

Breast cancer is the most common cancer in women (excluding skin cancer), although it is quite rare in men. Breast cancer is the second leading cause of cancer deaths in women (after lung cancer) in the United States. From 1973 to 1991, the incidence of invasive breast cancer in the United States increased 25.8% in Caucasians and 30.3% in African Americans, or roughly 2% per year. The reason for this increase is not clearly understood, but may be explained, in part, by a 75% increase in the use of mammography, because most of the increase has been for the lowest stage tumors. Although the incidence of breast cancer has been rising, the mortality rate fell sig-

TABLE 64-4   ■ ■ ■

Age and Risk of Breast Cancer

Age (Years)	Risk (Related to Total Female Population)
30-40	1:257
40-50	1:67
50-60	1:36
60-70	1:28
70-80	1:24
85	1:8 (Total lifetime cumulative risk)

Source: National Cancer Institute Surveillance, Epidemiology, and End Results Program, 1997.

nificantly from 1992 to 1996 because of early detection and better treatment (SEER, 2001; American Cancer Society, 2001).

Breast cancer may occur at any age outside childhood, but has a low incidence during the first three decades, rising steeply thereafter (Table 64-4). Overall, a woman's lifetime risk of developing breast cancer is one in eight (SEER, 2001). This figure is general for all women based on a lifetime to 85 years; it does not take into account the factors that will influence the individual risk for a particular woman.

The cause of breast cancer is uncertain but there are several defined risk factors, both environmental and genetic (Table 64-5). Factors associated with increased risk of breast cancer include residence in a developed western country, low socioeconomic status, race, history of proliferative breast disease, early onset of menarche, late birth of first child, late menopause, nulliparous state, exogenous hormone therapy, radiation exposure, and dietary factors (obesity and high alcohol intake).

If either a woman's mother or sister has breast cancer, the woman's risk increases two or three times. Having both a mother and a sister with breast cancer increases a woman's risk up to six times. Of the families with a strong history of breast cancer, many women have a mutation in the *breast cancer gene*, termed *BRCA-1*, on chromosome 17; it is estimated that 86% of these women will develop breast cancer by age 70. The inheritance pattern is autosomal dominant and can be inherited through both the maternal and paternal lines. The BRCA-1 gene is also associated with the development of cancer of the ovary and prostate. Another familial breast cancer syndrome is associated with a gene on chromosome 13, termed *BRCA-2*. However, only between 5% and 10% of all breast cancers seem to be attributable to an inherited genetic mutation. Other breast cancer genes are being actively sought. Through detection of these abnormal genes, it is now possible to use molecular genetic techniques to identify individuals at risk of developing breast cancer, although the best way to manage these patients clinically is uncertain.

Most breast tumors are adenocarcinomas. There are two main histologic types of breast adenocarcinoma, which arise from the terminal ducts and lobular units. *Noninvasive breast carcinoma in situ* (i.e., ductal carcinoma in situ [DCIS] or lobular carcinoma in situ [LCIS]) is within the lumen of the ducts or lobules. Radiologic screening can identify most intraduct and intralobular breast carcinomas. The significance of these noninvasive early carcinomas is that there is high risk for later development into invasive breast cancer.

TABLE 64-5

Risk Factors and Incidence for Breast Cancer

Risk Factor	High Incidence	Low Incidence
Age	30-50 yr of age Rises sharply	Levels off at menopause Rises at $1/6$ the earlier rate
Geographic location	Western Europe and North America: more than 6-10 times	Japan, most of Asia, Africa
Race	American-born, African-American women before 40 yr of age	Caucasian women before 40 yr of age
Socioeconomic status	Upper socioeconomic group	Lower socioeconomic group
Marital status	Single women 50% more likely to develop breast cancer	Married women
Parity	Nulliparous First birth after 30 yr of age Spontaneous abortions before first birth	Parous (decreases with each birth) High parity (four or more births) First birth before 20 yr of age
Menstrual history	Early age at menarche Late menopause: after 50 yr of age	Risk decreases 20% for each year delayed Natural onset of menopause before 45 yr of age Oophorectomy before 35 yr of age
Family history	First-degree female relatives (maternal or paternal families) of women with breast cancer: 2-3 times more likely to develop breast cancer Mother and sister, or 2 sisters have breast cancer: 6 times more likely to develop breast cancer	
Body habitus	Obesity (per 10-kg increment): 80% more likely to develop breast cancer	
Other breast disease	Ductal and lobular hyperplasia with atypia: 8 times more likely to develop breast cancer	
Radiation exposure	Increasing risk for each rad in young women and children; manifested after 30 yr of age; minimum latency period: 10-15 yr	
Second primary cancer	With primary ovarian cancer, risk of breast cancer 3-4 times greater With primary endometrial cancer, risk of breast cancer 2 times greater With colorectal cancer, risk of breast cancer 2 times greater	

Invasive or infiltrating carcinomas have spread into the stroma of the breast and there is the possibility of metastatic spread. *Invasive ductal carcinoma* is the most common type of breast cancer, comprising about 80% to 85% of all breast cancer. Invasive ductal carcinoma is stony hard, as is appreciated both on clinical palpation and when the resected specimen is cut. The old term applied to such a cancer is *scirrhous,* a Greek term meaning "hard." Distant metastasis sites are bone, lung, liver, or brain.

Invasive lobular carcinoma is the second most common type of breast cancer (about 10%). Importantly, tumor is often multifocal within the breast, and this type is associated with a high frequency of bilateral breast involvement compared with other types. Characteristically, tumor cells are compressed into narrow cords, which may present as an area of ill-defined thickening with palpation (rather than as a lump). With invasive lobular carcinoma, distant metastasis is usually to meningeal and serosal surfaces. Although uncommon (< 10%) certain specialized histologic types of invasive breast cancer (e.g., tubular, mucoid, medullary) are associated with a better prognosis than the ductal and lobular types.

Paget's disease of the nipple is an outward-growing malignancy along the nipple ducts from a deeper ductal or invasive ductal cancer with itching, burning, oozing, bleeding, or a combination of these, of the nipple. The underlying carcinoma is palpable in only 50% to 60% of patients. The malignant cells (Paget's cells) from the deeper tumor invade the epidermis of the nipple, causing a crusting, eczematoid appearance.

Inflammatory carcinoma is a rapidly growing tumor that is widespread dermal lymphatic invasion of carcinoma. The symptoms resemble an acute breast infection. The skin becomes reddened, hot, edematous, indurated, and painful. This type of cancer occurs in about 1% to 2% of women with breast cancer. Because the initial appearance is the same as that in infection, diagnosis of cancer may be delayed. The prognosis of patients with inflammatory breast cancer is poor, even with early diagnosis.

The spread of cancer through the breast occurs by direct invasion of the breast parenchyma, along mammary ducts, in overlying skin, and through the extensive breast lymphatic network. Regional lymph node involvement includes the axillary, internal mammary, and supraclavicular nodes. Lymph node involvement must be determined histologically rather than by clinical examination.

Clinical breast examination (CBE) by an experienced health professional and mammography are the main methods for early detection of breast cancer. The screening mammogram is used in an asymptomatic woman to detect any abnormality in a preclinical stage before invasion or axillary lymph node involvement when the rate of cure is high. The survival rate is directly related to tumor size and axillary lymph node status, making early diagnosis of prime importance. However, breast cancers are frequently first found by the woman herself during self-breast examination (SBE) after the mass is palpable (about 1 cm). Current recommendations for mammography from the American Cancer Society guidelines are listed in Table 64-6.

Detection and diagnosis of breast cancer (Box 64-3) begin with obtaining a thorough family and personal his-

TABLE 64-6   ▪▪▪

American Cancer Society (2001) Recommendations for the Early Detection of Breast Cancer

Age	Screening Examination
≥20 years	BSE monthly
20-39 years	CBE every 3 years
≥40 years	CBE and mammogram yearly

BSE, Breast self-examination; *CBE,* clinical breast examination.

▪ BOX 64-3

▪ Detection and Diagnosis of Breast Carcinoma

Breast self-examination
Medical history
Clinical breast examination
   Visual examination
   Palpation
Mammography
Tissue sampling
   Fine-needle aspiration
   Core needle biopsy
   Open biopsy
      Incisional
      Excisional

TABLE 64-7   ▪▪▪

TNM Classification of Breast Cancer and Survival*

PRIMARY TUMOR (T)
T0   No evidence of primary tumor
Tis Carcinoma in situ
T1   Tumor ≤2 cm
T2   Tumor >2 cm but ≤5 cm
T3   Tumor >5 cm
T4   Extension to chest wall, inflammation

REGIONAL LYMPH NODES (N)
N0 No tumor in regional lymph nodes
N1 Metastasis to movable ipsilateral nodes
N2 Metastasis to matted or fixed ipsilateral nodes
N3 Metastasis to ipsilateral internal mammary nodes

DISTANT METASTASIS (M)
M0 No distant metastasis
M1 Distant metastasis (includes spread to ipsilateral
     supraclavicular nodes)

Stage Grouping				5-Year Survival (% of Patients)**
Stage 0	Tis	N0	M0	99%
Stage 1	T1	N0	M0	92%
Stage IIA	T0	N1	M0	82%
	T1	N1	M0	
	T2	N0	M0	
Stage IIB	T2	N1	M0	65%
	T3	N0	M0	
Stage IIIA	T0	N2	M0	47%
	T1	N2	M0	
	T2	N2	M0	
	T3	N1, N2	M0	
Stage IIIB	T4	Any N	M0	44%
	Any T	N3	M0	
Stage IV	Any T	Any N	M1	14%

*American Joint Committee on Cancer, 1997
**National Cancer Institute—Surveillance, Epidemiology, and End Results (SEER), 2001.

tory of pertinent facts related to breast pathophysiology and a physical examination of the breasts. Mammography, which is a soft tissue radiograph, is an important adjunct to the CBE. Mammography can provide information during a diagnostic workup for an abnormality, as well as screen asymptomatic healthy women. Mammography can also detect masses too small to be felt and in many instances reveal the probable nature of a palpable mass. Tissue-sampling procedures done to obtain specimens for microscopic examination for diagnostic purposes include fine-needle aspiration, core needle biopsy, and open biopsy—either excisional (entire mass is removed) or incisional (some part of the mass is removed). If the specimen is malignant, further evaluation is necessary.

The prognosis and most appropriate treatment for breast cancer depend on several variables. The stage of the tumor is widely regarded as the most powerful prognostic factor (Table 64-7). The tumor nodes metastasis (TNM) classification system of breast cancer is most widely used and depends on tumor size spread to regional lymph nodes and the presence or absence of distal metastasis. Overall, the absence of axillary node metastasis is the best prognostic sign, but as the number of positive nodes increases beyond four, mortality increases dramatically. Other prognostic variables include *estrogen and progesterone receptor status* and *histologic grade of tumor* and *type of tumor.* Tumors that lack either or both estrogen and progesterone receptors are more likely to recur than tumors that have them. Histologic grade of tumor is based on parameters such as aneuploidy and presence of many nuclei—the higher the grade, the more aggressive the tumor, and the poorer the prognosis. As stated previously, if the histologic type of breast carcinoma is of the medullary, mucoid, or tubular types, the

prognosis is more favorable than it is for the more common ductal or lobular types.

Table 64-8 lists the treatment modalities for breast cancer. Surgical therapy varies from partial mastectomy (lumpectomy) to extended radical mastectomy. Since 1985, the management of breast cancer that is apparently localized to the breast or regional lymph nodes has changed to more breast-conserving surgery, with about one third now having a lumpectomy. Clinical research has shown that lumpectomy with or without irradiation results in a 10-year survival rate that is as good as is more extensive surgery.

Primary surgical treatment of breast cancer, including lumpectomy and total mastectomy with axillary node dissection, sets the stage for referral to the oncologist for adjuvant treatment. These treatments consist of irradiation, chemotherapy, and endocrine therapy (tamoxifen and ovarian ablation). The patient for whom the risk of recurrence is greatest is the most appropriate candidate for adjuvant therapy, such as nodal involvement, tumor size greater than 2 cm, or in whom unfavorable histologic characteristics have been discovered on microscopic examination. Studies suggest that premenopausal (younger)

TABLE 64-8

TABLE 64-8

Treatment for Breast Cancer

Treatment	Description
SURGICAL	
Partial mastectomy	Ranges from tylectomy (lumpectomy) to segmental removal (wide tissue removal with overlying skin) to quadrantectomy (removal of one quadrant of the breast); removal or sample of axillary lymph nodes for staging
Total mastectomy with low axillary dissection	Excision of entire breast, all lymph nodes lateral to pectoralis minor muscle
Modified radical mastectomy	Excision of entire breast, all or most of axillary tissue
Radical mastectomy	Excision of entire breast, underlying pectoralis major and minor muscles; entire axillary contents
Extended radical mastectomy	Same as radical mastectomy with the addition of the internal mammary lymph nodes
NONSURGICAL	
Irradiation	To breast and other chest areas as local adjuvant after surgical procedure; to breast and regional lymph nodes for unresectable advanced cancers, to bony metastases, to axillary lymph node metastases, to local or regional recurrence of tumor after prior treatment
Chemotherapy	Systemic adjuvant after surgery; palliation for advanced disease
Endocrine and hormone therapy	Disseminated cancer-using estrogens, androgens, progesterones, antiestrogens, oophorectomy, adrenalectomy, hypophysectomy

women respond better to combination chemotherapy agents, such as cyclophosphamide, methotrexate, fluorouracil, and doxorubicin, and postmenopausal (older) women respond better to antiestrogen agents, such as tamoxifen. Hormonal therapy (tamoxifen) is only used in the case of estrogen receptor–positive disease. Overall, adjuvant therapy may reduce the risk of recurrence by 30%. Recurrent breast cancer carries a dismal prognosis with as few as 3% achieving long-term remission after treatment. Clinical trials are now ongoing in the use of tamoxifen for the prevention of primary disease in high-risk women.

KEY CONCEPTS

- *The primitive gonad is neither ovary nor testis.* Unless a Y chromosome encoding a testis-determining factor is present, the indifferent gonad will inevitably become an ovary (the default).
- *Differentiation of the embryo into a male or female phenotype* is affected by the *genetic configuration*, as well as by *hormones*. Chromosomal sex (i.e., presence or absence of a Y chromosome) determines the gonadal sex and the type of gonad (i.e., presence or absence of dihydrotestosterone) and, in turn, is the principle factor in determining whether an individual has a male or female phenotype.
- *Menarche,* the onset of menstruation, usually begins between 12 and 13 years of age, with a range of 9.1 to 17.7 years.
- The *internal organs of the female reproductive system* include the ovaries, fallopian tubes, uterus, and vagina.
- *External genitalia in the female* include the mons pubis, labia majora, labia minora, clitoris, and vestibule or introitus of the vagina.
- The *menstrual cycle* averages about 28 days, and its purpose is to produce a mature ovum and to prepare and maintain an environment for conception and gestation by means of complex hormonal interactions.
- Events that take place within the pituitary, ovaries, and endometrium are precisely synchronized during the

normal menstrual cycle: **A,** *menstruation* (days 1 through 5) or the sloughing off of the endometrial lining of the uterus; **B,** *proliferative phase of the endometrium* (days 6 through 14): the ovarian follicles are stimulated by pituitary FSH, which, in turn, produce estrogen. Estrogen stimulates the endometrium to proliferate. At the midpoint of the cycle (day 14), a burst of pituitary FSH and LH stimulate ovulation; **C,** *secretory phase of the endometrium* (days 14 through 28): after ovulation the ruptured follicle changes into a corpus luteum that secretes estrogen and progesterone that causes the endometrium to become thick and velvetlike. If pregnancy does not occur, the corpus luteum degenerates, resulting in a sharp drop in serum progesterone and estrogen levels, with a sloughing off of the endometrium lining again to complete the cycle.
- The *normal sexual response* is composed of four phases: excitement, plateau, orgasm, and resolution.
- *Menopause,* the cessation of ovulation and menstrual cycles, usually occurs between the ages of 45 to 52 years. Estrogen levels fall (resulting in vascular instability and hot flushes), and decreased negative feedback to the hypothalamic-pituitary-gonadal axis causes increased secretion of FSH and LH.
- *Primary amenorrhea* is defined as the failure of menarche by age 17, regardless of the presence or

absence of secondary sexual characteristics; an endocrine disorder or structural disorder of the reproductive tract is the usual cause.
- Breast development and pubic hair are evaluated according to the *Tanner developmental scale.*
- *Secondary amenorrhea* is the cessation of menses for 3 months or longer in a (nonpregnant, nonmenopausal) woman with previous periodic menses. Causes include disorders of ovarian function (e.g., ovarian tumors), disorders of the anterior pituitary (e.g., pituitary adenoma), disruption of the hypothalamic-pituitary-gonadal axis (e.g., anorexia nervosa, intense exercise, tumor of the hypothalamus or adrenal), androgen excess, and iatrogenic factors (e.g., oral contraceptives, cytotoxic agents).
- *Premenstrual syndrome (PMS)* is the cyclic recurrence of distressing physical and psychologic manifestations during the luteal phase of the menstrual cycle.
- *Dysmenorrhea* is painful menstruation associated with uterine muscle cramping severe enough to limit activity; it may be primary or secondary.
- *Primary dysmenorrhea* is caused by excessive amounts of prostaglandin $F_{2\alpha}$ in menstrual blood, which stimulates uterine hyperactivity; it is effectively treated with nonsteroidal antiinflammatory drugs (NSAIDs), which block prostaglandin synthesis.
- *Secondary dysmenorrhea* occurs as a result of pelvic disorders, such as endometriosis, uterine polyps, pelvic inflammatory disease (PID), cervical stenosis, or leiomyoma.
- *Dysfunctional uterine bleeding* is defined as abnormal bleeding in the presence of a functional disturbance rather than an organic lesion of the endometrium or uterus.
- In most instances, *dysfunctional uterine bleeding* is caused by *anovulatory cycles,* which result in prolonged and excessive estrogen stimulation without the development of the progestational phase that normally follows ovulation. Dysfunctional uterine bleeding is most common in adolescents and perimenopausal women.
- *Abnormal uterine bleeding* is uterine bleeding that differs from the expected frequency, duration, and quantity of normal menstrual bleeding.
- *Abnormal uterine bleeding* may be related to pregnancy complications, benign or malignant gynecologic neoplasms, inflammation, systemic disease, and hormonal imbalances (anovulatory cycles).
- A large number of organisms can infect the female genital tract and, in total, account for considerable suffering and morbidity. Many of these infections are sexually transmitted and are discussed in Chapter 66.
- *Daughters of women who took diethylstilbestrol (DES)* during pregnancy to prevent threatened spontaneous abortion are at risk for vaginal adenosis, a precursor lesion for vaginal adenocarcinoma.
- Abnormalities along the pathway to genital development can result in *ambiguous genitalis* or *intersex conditions.* Common types of intersex problems include congenital adrenal hyperplasia, Turner syn-

drome, androgen insensitivity syndrome, and gonadal dysgenesis.
- Females with *congenital adrenal hyperplasia (CAH)* or *female pseudohermaphroditism* have a normal 46, XX karyotype with normal ovaries and internal genitalia but with masculinized or ambiguous external genitalia caused by exposure to androgen excess in utero.
- Most often, the *cause of CAH* is a congenital *deficiency of the enzyme, 21-hydroylase,* blocking the pathway to cortisol synthesis. The decrease in cortisol production causes an increase in ACTH production in response to the negative feedback of pituitary function. ACTH stimulates the adrenal cortex, causing the precursors of cortisol to be shunted to the biosynthesis of androgens.
- *Turner syndrome* results from the absence of one X chromosome (45, X0), causing gonadal dysgenesis, in which gonads are represented by fibrous streaks.
- *Androgen insensitive syndrome (AIS)* occurs when a genetic male *(46,XY)* fails to respond to androgen during fetal development because of an abnormal androgen receptor. Androgen resistance during embryogenesis prevents masculinization of the external genitalia and differentiation of the wolffian duct, resulting in female-appearing external genitalia.
- *Displacement disorders of the female genital tract* include anteflexion, retroflexion, and prolapse of the uterus.
- *A cystocele* (herniation of bladder into the vaginal canal) or *rectocele* (herniation of the rectum into the vaginal canal) caused by weakened vaginal wall muscles are common conditions often resulting from childbirth injury and aging.
- *Female genital mutilation (FGM)* (also called female circumcision [FC]) is the partial or complete excision of the external genitalia with infibulation (narrowing the vaginal opening by stitching it). FGM is a common practice in African and Middle Eastern countries and results in many gynecologic and childbirth complications. There is a movement among women's health professionals and advocates of women's rights to put an end to this practice.
- *Endometrial hyperplasia* (overgrowth of endometrium) is caused by excessive stimulation by estrogen. The most common cause is anovulatory cycles.
- *Leiomyomas (uterine fibroids)* are the most common benign tumors of the uterus, affecting 25% of women over the age of 35 years. Clinically, these tumors are associated with abnormal bleeding or infertility. Leiomyomas depend on the trophic action of estrogen for maintenance of size, and tumors usually shrink after the menopause.
- *Endometrial carcinoma* is the most common cancer of the female genital tract, and the majority is associated with excess estrogen (endogenous or exogenous) and endometrial hyperplasia.
- *Risk factors for endometrial carcinoma* include unopposed estrogen therapy, obesity (caused by endogenous production of estrogen in adipose tissue), early menarche and late menopause, nulliparity, hereditary nonpolyposis colorectal cancer (HNPCC), diabetes mellitus, and hypertension.

- *Endometrial polyps* are benign lesions, most common during the perimenopausal period, protruding into the uterine cavity. These polyps are caused by abnormal hormone production and are a common cause of dysfunctional uterine bleeding.
- *Cervical polyps* are common, small (1 to 2 cm), non-neoplastic masses derived from the endocervix and protrude from the cervix through the external os. Cervical polyps probably result from chronic inflammation and may cause intermenstrual bleeding.
- *Human papillomavirus (HPV) infection* (especially types 16, 18, and 31), transmitted sexually, is the principal etiologic agent in the development of *carcinoma of the cervix.*
- The vast majority of *carcinomas of the cervix* are *squamous cell carcinomas*, arising from the *squamocolumnar junction* or *transformation zone of the cervix.*
- *Cervical intraepithelial neoplasia (CIN)* ranging from mild dysplasia to carcinoma in situ is an important precursor of invasive cervical carcinoma and may be diagnosed with the Pap test.
- *Prognosis of squamous cell carcinoma of the cervix* is related to stage at diagnosis. Widespread *Pap smear test screening for CIN* (which is preinvasive and curable) has dramatically reduced the death rate from cervical cancer in the United States.
- *Carcinoma of the ovary* has a high mortality rate because it is usually diagnosed after it has metastasized. Risk factors include long-term postmenopausal HRT, personal history of breast cancer, and genetic factors (e.g., BRCA-1 or BRCA-2, two or more first-degree relatives with ovarian cancer).
- The most important malignant tumor of the *vulva* is *squamous cell carcinoma*, occurring most often in elderly women. Sexually transmitted diseases are associated with vulvar carcinoma.
- *Primary malignancies of the vagina or fallopian tubes are rare.* Clear cell carcinoma of the vagina is seen in women exposed in utero to the synthetic estrogen, diethylstilbestrol (DES).
- *Mastitis and breast abscesses* are seen as a complication of lactation. The common infecting organisms are *Staphylococcus aureus* and streptococci.
- *Fat necrosis* may follow *breast trauma* and can clinically mimic neoplastic disease.

- An important and common breast lump in young women is the well-circumscribed, mobile, rubbery-textured *fibroadenoma*, which contains both epithelial and fibrous elements. The lump is treated by surgical excision and examined histologically to rule out carcinoma.
- *Fibrocystic change* is the most common disorder of the female breast and is characterized by hyperplastic overgrowth of components of the mammary unit (i.e., lobules, ductules, stroma). As its name implies, a cystic component is frequent in this condition, which is the most common cause of a fluctuating cystic breast lump.
- *Fibrocystic disease* is believed to be caused by a relative excess of estrogen and deficiency of progesterone during the luteal phase of the menstrual cycle.
- The presence of epithelial hyperplasia, especially *atypical hyperplasia* in fibrocystic disease, is associated with an *increased risk of the subsequent development of breast carcinoma.*
- Carcinoma of the breast affects one in eight women during a life span of 85 years and is the second leading cause of cancer deaths (after lung cancer) in the United States.
- *Invasive ductal carcinoma* followed by *invasive lobular carcinoma* are the most common types of invasive breast cancer.
- One of the *most important prognostic indicators in breast cancer* is the presence or absence of axillary lymph node metastasis.
- *Surgical treatment of breast cancer* includes varying degrees of excision followed by *adjuvant therapy* (irradiation, chemotherapy, or hormonal therapy) when there is high risk of recurrence.
- Regular, periodic self-breast examination (SBE), clinical breast examination (CBE) by a trained health care professional, and mammography are important measures for the *early detection of breast cancer.*
- *Factors associated with an increased risk of breast cancer* include geographic location, familial breast cancer (especially having the BRCA-1 or BRCA-2 gene), proliferative breast disease, early onset of menarche, late birth of first child, late menopause, nulliparous state, exogenous hormones, and dietary factors (obesity and high alcohol intake).

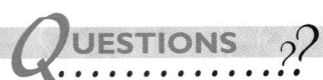

QUESTIONS ??

A sampling of review questions for this chapter appears here. Visit http://www.mosby.com/MERLIN/PriceWilson/ for additional questions.

Answer the following on a separate sheet of paper.

1. What are the functions of the ovary in the adult female?
2. What hormonal and ovarian changes occur during the climacteric and menopause?
3. Describe the rationale for the treatment of the amenorrheic patient.
4. Describe the changes that occur in the ovaries and uterus during the menstrual cycle.
5. Explain how the position of the internal reproductive organs of the female is associated with the infectious process.
6. Describe the high-risk factors and prophylactic treatment associated with developing ovarian cancer.
7. Describe the breast tissue changes and cause of fibrocystic disease of the breast.
8. Explain the pathologic changes associated with the development of carcinoma of the breast.
9. Describe the process for the detection and diagnosis of breast cancer.

CHAPTER

65

Male Reproductive System Disorders

LORRAINE M. WILSON AND KATHLEEN BRANSON HILLEGAS

ANATOMY AND PHYSIOLOGY

The male reproductive structures are the penis; the testis (plural, testes) in the scrotal sac; the duct system, which includes the epididymis (plural, epididymides), the vas deferens (plural, vasa deferens), the ejaculatory ducts, and the urethra; and the accessory glands, which include the seminal vesicles, the prostate, and the bulbourethral glands (Fig. 65-1).

The testes are divided internally into lobules that contain the seminiferous tubules, Sertoli's cells, and Leydig's cells (Fig. 65-2). Sperm production, or spermatogenesis, takes place in the seminiferous tubules. Leydig's cells secrete testosterone. On the posterior portion of each testis is a coiled duct called the *epididymis*. The head is connected with the seminiferous tubule (out-flowing duct) of the testis, and the tail is continuous with the vas deferens. The *vas deferens* is the excretory duct of the testis and extends to the duct of the seminal vesicle, which it joins to form the ejaculatory duct. The ejaculatory duct joins the urethra, which is the common passageway to outside the body for both sperm and urine. The accessory glands communicate with the duct system. The prostate surrounds the neck of the bladder and the upper urethra. The glandular ducts of the prostate open into the urethra. The bulbourethral glands (Cowper's glands) are located near the urethral meatus. The penis is composed of three elongated cylindric masses of erectile tissue, which makes up the shaft of the penis. An inner mass is the *corpus spongiosum*, which contains the urethra, and two outer parallel masses, the *corpus cavernosa*. The distal end of the penis, known as the glans, is covered by the *prepuce* (foreskin). The prepuce may be removed surgically (circumcision).

FUNCTIONS OF THE MALE REPRODUCTIVE SYSTEM

The primary functions of the male reproductive system are to produce mature spermatozoa and deposit sperm in the female reproductive tract with coitus. The testes serve the exocrine function of spermatogenesis and the en-

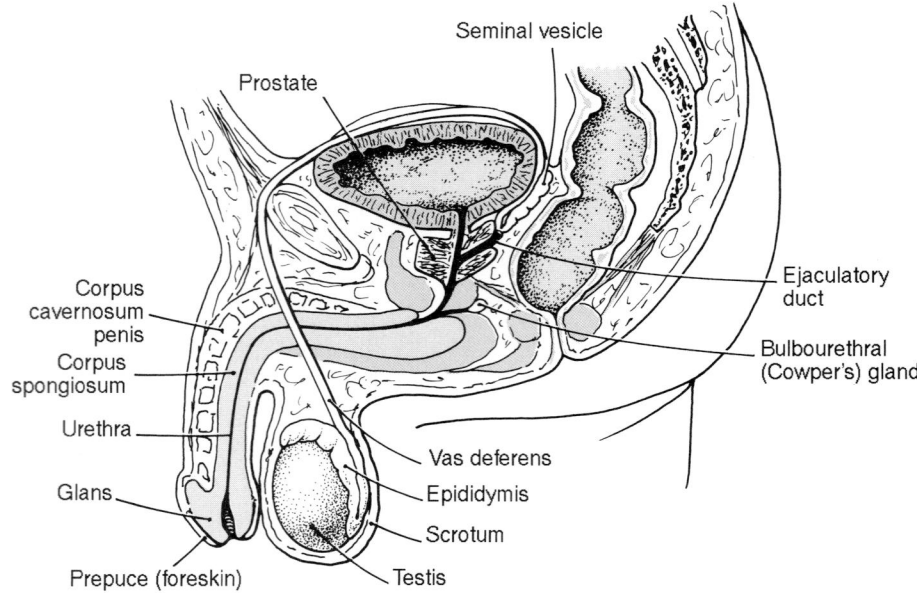

FIG. 65-1 Male reproductive system.

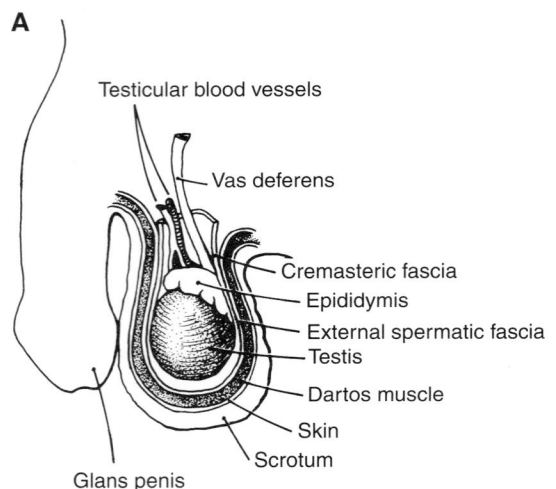

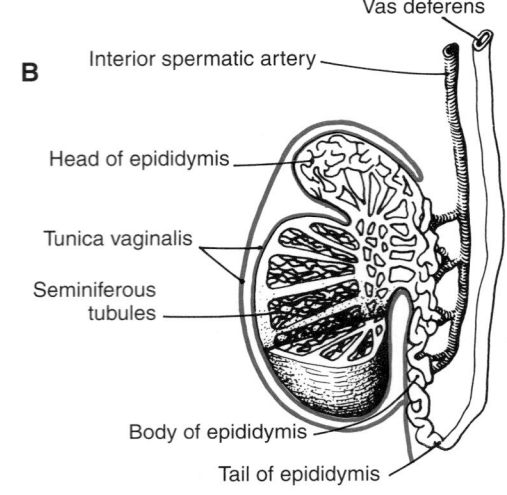

FIG. 65-2 The testes. **A**, External view. **B**, Sagittal section.

docrine function of secretion of sex hormones that control sexual development and function. All of the functions of the male reproductive system are regulated by means of complex hormonal interactions.

Hormonal Functions

The center of hormonal control of the reproductive system is the hypothalamic-pituitary axis (Fig. 65-3). Under the influence of various elements, such as heredity, environment, psychogenic stimuli, and circulating hormone levels, the hypothalamus produces gonadotropic hormone–releasing hormones (GnRH). These hormones are follicle-stimulating hormone–releasing hormone (FSHRH) and luteinizing hormone–releasing hormone (LHRH). These hormones are carried to the anterior pituitary to stimulate secretion of follicle-stimulating hormone (FSH), and luteinizing hormone (LH), more commonly called interstitial cell–stimulating hormone (ICSH) in men. Gonadotropins are secreted at a steady rate in men.

Testosterone directs and regulates characteristics of the masculine body, that is, development of the testes and male genitalia, descent of testes from the abdominal cavity to the scrotum during the fetal period, development of primary and secondary sexual characteristics, and spermatogenesis.

Testosterone production by the interstitial Leydig's cells in males increases greatly at the start of puberty. Increasing ICSH levels, which is produced at first during sleep, marks the onset of puberty. The high levels early in puberty result in high levels of testosterone production by the testes. Estrone and estradiol are also produced and are derived from conversion of testosterone produced by the adrenals and testes and from androstenedione. Sex hormone–binding globulin levels fall during puberty, resulting in more free testosterone in the circulation. A

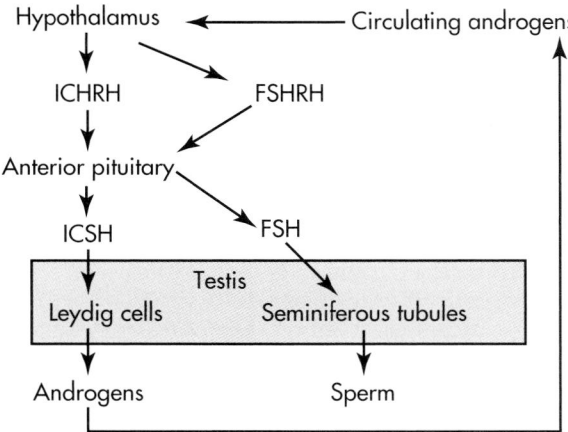

FIG. 65-3 Hypothalamic-pituitary-testicular hormone axis. *ICHRH,* Interstitial cell-hormone–releasing hormone; *FSHRH,* follicle-stimulating hormone–releasing hormone; *ICSH,* interstitial cell–stimulating hormone; *FSH,* follicle-stimulating hormone.

growth spurt occurs in every organ system in the body except the central nervous system and the lymphatic system. Alterations in height, weight, and secondary sexual characteristics are the most prominent changes. The peak of the growth spurt occurs at about 14 years of age. The usual rate of growth at the 50th percentile is 5 inches from 12.0 to 14.5 years plus another 3 inches by 16 years; weight gain peaks at 14 years, with about a 50% increase between the ages of 12 and 16 years, mostly as new muscle.

The earliest secondary sexual characteristic to appear is an increase in size of first the testes and scrotum and then the penis. Growth of the testes is caused by growth and development of the seminiferous tubules and the number of Leydig's and Sertoli's cells. Development of the genitalia to adult size and shape takes about 5 to 6 years. The primary sexual characteristics are then structurally at a level of full reproductive maturity. To achieve this goal, however, the male must produce viable sperm.

Spermatogenesis

Spermatogenesis begins with puberty, at about 13 years of age, and continues throughout life. In the seminiferous tubules, primary germ cells, the spermatogonia, begin to proliferate (mitosis). Some of the daughter cells remain spermatogonia, and others move to the lumen of the seminiferous tubule and enlarge into primary spermatocytes. The primary spermatocytes undergo meiotic division to form two secondary spermatocytes. Each secondary spermatocyte undergoes a second meiotic division, which results in two spermatids. Thus one spermatogonia produces four sperm. No further division occurs, and each spermatid undergoes a maturation and differentiation process to develop the head, neck, body, and tail of the mature sperm. Spermatogenesis takes place continuously throughout life after puberty. Sperm are stored in the epididymides and vasa deferens and retain their fertility for as long as 42 days. In the absence of emission or ejaculation, spermatozoa are thought to be absorbed by the body. During sexual intercourse, sperm are deposited in the female vagina. After ejaculation the

maximum life span of sperm at body temperature is 24 to 72 hours. At lowered temperatures semen may be stored for years.

Testicular Function

In the embryo, H-Y antigen produced by the Y chromosome induces differentiation of Sertoli's cells. These cells then direct the distribution of germ cells in the developing embryo-fetus and secrete müllerian-inhibiting substance (MIS). MIS causes regression of the müllerian duct system (which normally gives rise to female reproductive structures). Fetal Leydig's cells mature under the influence of the Y chromosome and, stimulated by ICSH, secrete testosterone. Testosterone causes differentiation of the vasa deferens and seminal vesicles; its metabolite, dihydrotestosterone (DHT), causes differentiation of the prostate and external genitalia.

During the first 6 months of life, Leydig's cells continue to produce low levels of testosterone but then regress until puberty. At puberty, FSH causes tubular and testicular growth and the testes begin the functions of the mature individual. ICSH stimulates Leydig's cells to produce testosterone, DHT, and estradiol; FSH binds to Sertoli's cells and influences sperm production. Simultaneous presence of a small amount of FSH potentiates the effect of ICSH. Testosterone must also be present in sufficient amount to complete the process of spermatogenesis. Thus the anterior pituitary must secrete both FSH and ICSH for spermatogenesis to occur. Testosterone, DHT, estradiol, and a tubular secretion, inhibin, in turn, inhibit the secretion of ICSH and FSH by the anterior pituitary, thereby regulating circulating blood levels of testosterone by a negative feedback system.

CHANGES WITH AGING

The male climacteric is the term applied to that time when physiologic reproductive function declines related to increased chronologic age. It is difficult to separate the decline of reproductive function from the decline in physical fitness that occurs with advancing age, and it is possible that the decline in physical fitness is responsible for the decline in reproductive function. The decline is more gradual in men than it is in women; thus the male reproductive system retains enough of its function to allow for continued reproduction late in life. The seminiferous tubules of the testes continue to produce sperm, although in fewer numbers with advancing age. Ten percent of the seminiferous tubules have stopped producing sperm by 40 years of age, 50% by 50 years, and 90% by 80 years. Testosterone levels decrease gradually. The number of Leydig's cells may decrease, as well as the ability of the remaining cells to produce testosterone.

Failure to attain or maintain erection of the penis (impotence) is more common in aging men. Causes of this condition are not always identifiable; however, psychologic factors are thought to be involved in some cases. Physiologically, the veins and arteries that supply the erectile tissue of the penis are subject to the same sclerosis caused by aging as other blood vessels in the body, which may contribute to impotence.

DISORDERS OF THE MALE REPRODUCTIVE SYSTEM

Hypogonadism

Hypogonadism may be either primary, caused by dysfunction of Leydig's cells, or secondary, caused by dysfunction of the hypothalamic-pituitary unit. Secondary hypogonadism may be further divided into hypothalamic dysfunction and pituitary dysfunction. Hypothalamic or pituitary dysfunction will then result in Leydig's cell hypofunction.

Hypogonadism in the male is a condition characterized by an abnormal decrease in functional activity of the testes and is the most common disorder of testicular function encountered in clinical practice. The androgens, testosterone and DHT, are essential for male development, beginning with embryogenesis and for continuing male development at puberty and reproductive system functioning throughout life. Interruption of the complex hormonal interactions at any level is the cause of a great many syndromes and disorders that have common consequences, including infertility, impotence, or complete lack of maleness (male pseudohermaphroditism) (Table 65-1).

The specific outcome of male hypogonadism varies with (1) the time of onset of testosterone deficiency (i.e., during embryogenesis, before puberty, after puberty), (2) the focus of the problem (i.e., a testicular defect or a hypothalamic-pituitary defect), and (3) the functioning status of the testes (i.e., low testosterone production followed by impairment of spermatogenesis, normal testosterone production with isolated impairment of spermatogenesis). In some cases, hypogonadism can be treated, but in other cases, the condition is irreversible.

Hypogonadism may be caused by congenital or developmental disorders, acquired disorders, or systemic disorders. Lack of testosterone that causes primary hypogonadism results in increased production of GnRH and gonadotropins to stimulate testicular production of androgens. This type is called *hypergonadotropic hypogonadism*. Included in this category are Klinefelter's syndrome, Reifenstein's syndrome, male Turner's syndrome, Sertoli-cell–only syndrome, anorchism, orchitis, and sequelae of irradiation. Lack of testosterone in secondary hypogonadism results from decreased levels of GnRH from the hypothalamus or decreased levels of gonadotropins from the pituitary. This type is called *hypo-*

TABLE 65-1

Causes of Male Hypogonadism

	Primary	Secondary	Androgen Resistance Syndromes
DEFICIENCY OF SPERM AND ANDROGEN PRODUCTION			
Congenital or developmental disorders	Klinefelter's syndrome and variants Functional prepubertal castrate syndrome Noonan's syndrome Myotonic dystrophy Polyglandular autoimmune disease Complex genetic disorders ? Normal aging	Hypogonadotropic eunuchoidism (Kallmann's syndrome) Hemochromatosis Complex genetic syndromes	Reifenstein's syndrome Idiopathic oligospermia or azoospermia
Acquired disorders	Orchitis (mumps, Hansen's disease) Surgical or traumatic castration Drugs (spironolactone, ketoconazole, alcohol, digitalis, cytotoxics) Irradiation	Hypopituitarism Hyperprolactinemia Estrogen excess Progestins Opiate-like drugs	
Systemic disorders	Chronic liver disease Chronic renal disease Sickle cell disease Paraplegia	Glucocorticoid excess (Cushing's syndrome) Acute stress or illness Nutritional deficiency Chronic illness Massive obesity	
ISOLATED DEFICIENCY OF SPERM PRODUCTION			

Congenital or developmental disorders	Germinal cell aplasia
	Cryptorchidism
	Varicocele
	Immotile cilia syndrome
	Myotonic dystrophy
		Androgen excess
		  Congenital adrenal hyperplasia
		  Androgenic anabolic steroids
		  Androgen-secreting tumors
		Hyperprolactemia
		Isolated FSH deficiency	

Acquired disorders	Orchitis Thermal trauma Irradiation Cytotoxic drugs Environmental toxins		
Systemic disorders	Acute febrile illness Paraplegia		
Idiopathic	Oligospermia or azoospermia		

FSH, Follicle-stimulating hormone.

gonadotropic hypogonadism. Included in this category are hypopituitarism, isolated FSH deficiency, Kallmann's syndrome, and Prader-Willi syndrome.

Clinical Presentation

Absence or decrease of testosterone in the developing XY chromosome complement embryo/fetus will result in development of female external genitalia or ambiguous external genitalia. In the late fetal period, the testes descend from the abdomen to the scrotum under the influence of testosterone. Without adequate levels of testosterone, the testes fail to descend. This condition, *cryptorchidism*, is associated with potential morbidity later in life. Abnormalities of the levels of testosterone in the prepubertal and pubertal periods result in delayed closure of epiphyses and eunuchoidal skeletal proportions of arm span 2 inches or more greater than height, and heel-to-pubic-bone length 2 inches or more greater than pubic-bone-to-crown length. In addition, other changes under the influence of testosterone such as deepening of voice; growth of pubic and axillary hair; growth of beard; testes, penis, and prostate size; and development of male body habitus will not occur. Hypogonadism before puberty results in *eunuchoidism*. Absence or impairment of testicular functions after puberty results in loss of libido, lessening volume of semen ejaculate, possible hot flushes, and some regression of coarse sexual hair. In the adult mature male, testosterone is responsible for maintenance of male sexual characteristics, but loss of testosterone is usually not apparent clinically. However, inadequate testosterone during this period of life results in poor sexual functioning (i.e., impotence, loss of libido) and low sperm quality and quantity (i.e., infertility). Loss of libido and impotence are caused by hypogonadism in approximately 15% to 20% of men with that diagnosis. The normal sperm count in a healthy young man ranges from 20 million to 200 million/ml. About 6% of men in the reproductive age group are infertile, as defined by a sperm count less than 20 million/ml. In 90% of cases, sperm count is reduced as the result of hypogonadism, 80% to 90% of which are idiopathic oligospermia with normal testosterone levels.

Assessment of Hypogonadism

A thorough history and physical examination, with attention to altered hormonal states, are essential first steps in the clinical evaluation. Laboratory evaluation of hypogonadism includes obtaining serum testosterone levels, serum gonadotropin levels, and karyotype and performing a clomiphene stimulation test, GnRH stimulation test, human chorionic gonadotropin (hCG) stimulation test, and semen analysis for sperm quantity and quality.

The normal range of serum testosterone levels is wide (3 to 10 ng/ml). Elevated serum gonadotropin levels indicate testicular disease; elevated FSH indicates severe, irreversible tubular disease.

Clomiphene is a nonsteroidal weak estrogen agonist that stimulates the release of gonadotropins. A clomiphene stimulation or GnRH stimulation test should be performed if gonadotropin level is low in association with low serum testosterone level. In men with low levels of testosterone and gonadotropins, clomiphene should cause

a 50% increase in ICSH. If ICSH does not increase, the clomiphene stimulation test indicates a hypothalamic-pituitary insufficiency. This test requires 100 mg clomiphene daily for 7 days.

Administering 100 μg of GnRH should cause a peak level three times the control of LH in 20 minutes. With hypothalamic dysfunction, a response may not occur until several injections are given over several days. An exaggerated response indicates a reduced feedback response secondary to low levels of testosterone and estradiol.

If there is no ambiguity of the male genitalia, a buccal smear is obtained to investigate for the presence of a Barr body, which would be diagnostic for Klinefelter's syndrome. Rarely a karyotype may be necessary.

Human chorionic gonadotropin (hCG) stimulates production of testosterone. An hCG stimulation test may be performed to determine Leydig's cell response of changes in production of testosterone. A 50% increase in serum testosterone in 1 to 3 days indicates normal functioning.

Treatment of Hypogonadism

Therapy undertaken for hypogonadism completely depends on the cause, diagnosis, underlying pathologic condition, and patient age. Testosterone deficiency from hypogonadism is treated with androgen replacement therapy. The goal of any therapy is to achieve normal physiologic effects of testosterone for that individual. Gonadotropin and LHRH therapy are used to stimulate spermatogenesis and establish or restore fertility. Once established, spermatogenesis can be maintained with use of hCG.

Cryptorchidism

At about 32 weeks gestation, the testes descend from the abdomen into the scrotum under the influence of testosterone. Cryptorchidism is the arrest of one testis or both testes in the normal path of descent. Unilateral cryptorchidism is the most common type, occurring in 30% of preterm infants, 3% to 4% of term infants, and 0.3% to 0.4% of 1-year-old boys. Spontaneous descent may occur by 1 year of age but is rare after 1 year. Most cases result from hypogonadism or mechanical obstruction. An ectopic testis fails to follow the normal path of descent and becomes lodged in an abnormal place. The common sites for an ectopic testis are the inguinal canal, the perineum, the thigh, the femoral area, or the base of the penis.

The undescended testis is usually smaller than is normal, does not produce sperm well, and is susceptible to malignant change at some time in the individual's life. In some cases of a nonpalpable testis, there is testicular agenesis.

An undescended testis in the newborn may descend spontaneously by 1 year of age under the influence of endogenous testosterone secreted by the neonatal testes. Possible therapy after 1 year of age is administration of hCG to stimulate testosterone production. If there is no descent with hCG, the testis is surgically brought down into the scrotum through the inguinal canal and attached to the scrotum (orchidopexy). Intervention, whether medical or surgical, is carried out at about 1 to 2 years of age.

Diethylstilbestrol Exposure

Between 1946 and 1971, 2 to 3 million women took diethylstilbestrol (DES) between the eighth and sixteenth weeks of pregnancy as treatment to prevent threatened spontaneous abortion. Men (the youngest of whom are now in their mid-30s) whose mothers took DES have sequelae that correspond with the time of embryologic development during which the drug was used. Abnormalities noted in boys and men whose mothers took DES during pregnancy are urethral meatal stenosis, hypospadias, epididymal cysts, varicoceles, increased incidence of cryptorchidism, and decreased fertility. The incidence of reproductive carcinoma in men as a result of DES exposure in utero or whether they are at risk for development of problems as they grow older is unknown.

Hypospadias

Hypospadias occurs in 1 in 300 male births and is the most common anomaly of the penis. Urethral development begins in utero at approximately 8 weeks and is complete by 15 weeks. The urethra is formed by the fusion of the urethral folds along the ventral surface of the penis. The glandular urethra is formed by canalization of an ectodermal cord that has grown through the glans to communicate with the fused urethral folds. Hypospadias results when midline fusion of the urethral folds is incomplete so that the urethral meatus opens on the ventral side of the penis (Fig. 65-4). There can be a spectrum of severity described as glandular (displacement of the meatus on the glans), coronal (at the coronal sulcus), penile (anywhere along the shaft of the penis), penoscrotal (at the ventral junction of the penis and scrotum), and perineal (on the perineum). The prepuce is absent on the ventral side and resembles a hood over the dorsal side of the glans. A band of fibrous tissue, called *chordee*, on the ventral side causes ventral curvature of the penis.

No physical problems are related to hypospadias in newborns or young children. However, in adults, chordee will prevent sexual intercourse; infertility can occur in perineal or penoscrotal hypospadias; meatal stenosis may be present, causing difficulty in directing the urinary stream; and cryptorchidism is more common.

Treatment of hypospadias with chordee involves releasing the chordee and surgically restructuring the meatal opening. Repair should be done before the age of learning to stand to void, which is usually about 2 years. The foreskin is used in the reconstructive process; therefore an infant with hypospadias should not be circumcised. Chordee can occur without hypospadias and is treated by releasing the fibrous tissue to improve the function and appearance of the penis.

Epispadias

Epispadias is a congenital anomaly in which the urethral meatus is located on the dorsal surface of the penis (see Fig. 65-4). The incidence of complete epispadias is approximately 1 in 120,000 males. This condition does not usually occur independently, but rather, with other urinary tract anomalies. Epispadias is classified according to the placement of the urinary meatus along the penile shaft: glandular (on the dorsal glans), penile (between the pubic symphysis and the coronal sulcus), and penopubic (at the junction of the penis and pubis). The urethral meatus is broad, and a dorsal groove extends from the meatus placement down through the glans. The prepuce hangs from the ventral side of the penis. The penis is flattened and small and may be curved dorsally because of chordee. Urinary incontinence occurs with penopubic (95%) and penile (75%) epispadias because of maldevelopment of urinary sphincters. Surgical repair is undertaken to correct the incontinence, remove the chordee, and extend the urethra to the glans. The foreskin is used in the reconstructive process; therefore an infant with epispadias should not be circumcised.

Testicular Torsion

A testis can twist within the scrotal sac (torsion) as a result of abnormal development of the tunica vaginalis and spermatic cord in the fetal period. An abnormally high insertion of the tunica vaginalis on the cord structures exists, which allows the testis mobility similar to a bell clapper within a bell and results in lack of the normal attachment of the testis to the visceral tunica vaginalis. The testis easily rotates and twists the spermatic cord. This type of torsion is called *intravaginal spermatic cord torsion* (Fig. 65-5). The incidence is higher in adolescents and young adults. Trauma may be a precipitating factor; in

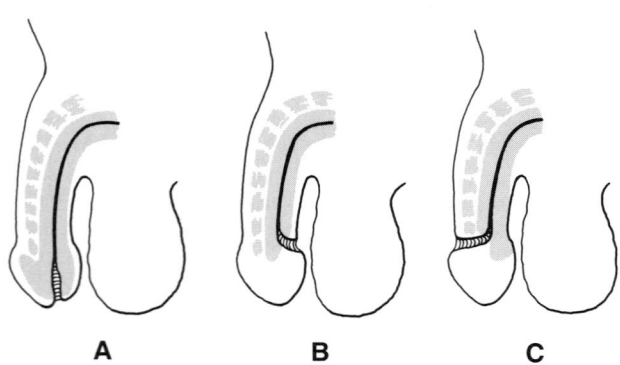

FIG. 65-4 **A**, Normal male urethral opening. **B**, Hypospadias and **C**, Epispadias developmental malformations.

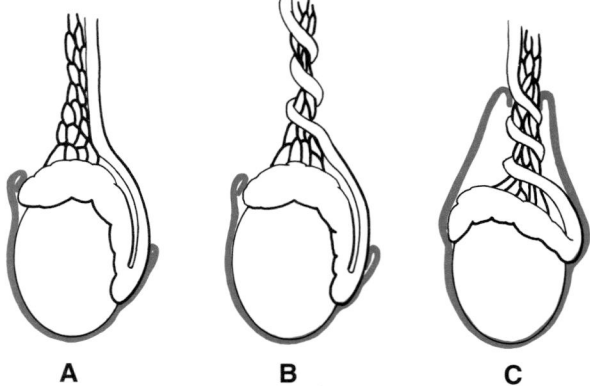

FIG. 65-5 Testicular torsion. **A**, Normal tunica vaginalis insertion. **B**, Extravaginal torsion. **C**, Intravaginal torsion with abnormally high vaginal insertion.

about 50% of patients, the occurrence of torsion is while the individual is asleep because of spasm of the cremaster muscle. Contraction of this muscle causes the left testis to rotate counterclockwise and the right testis to rotate clockwise. Blood supply is cut off, and edema forms; both events result in ischemia of the testis.

Symptoms are sudden onset of severe scrotal pain, low abdominal pain, nausea, and vomiting. Physical findings on examination are scrotal edema, erythema, tenderness, fever, new hydrocele, and loss of cremasteric reflex.

The epididymis will be palpated in an abnormal position if the examination is done before severe edema develops. Color Doppler sonography can show arterial flow rate. In torsion, blood flow is absent, and the twisted testis is avascular.

This condition requires prompt surgical intervention because ischemia and necrosis with permanent damage to the testis occur in a short time. Testicular salvage is more likely when surgery is performed within 6 hours from onset of torsion. The salvage rate is about 70% during the 6 to 12 hours after torsion and drops to 20% at 12 hours after the event. In surgery, detorsion of the testis is done and orchidopexy is performed on both testes as a prophylactic measure. Orchidectomy is not performed unless the testis is completely destroyed.

Torsion of the spermatic cord and testis can also occur in the fetus or neonate in utero or during birth. Twisting occurs in the inguinal portion of the cord above the insertion of the tunica vaginalis and is called extravaginal spermatic cord torsion (see Fig. 65-5). Extravaginal torsion occurs only in neonates; it is generally asymptomatic and is most often found during the initial newborn physical examination as a firm, scrotal mass accompanied by a blue-colored area in the scrotal skin covering the mass (blue dot sign). Often the testis is completely necrotic. Orchidectomy is performed on the necrotic testis, and orchidopexy is performed on the contralateral testis.

Hydrocele

A hydrocele is a collection of fluid in the potential space between the two membrane layers of the tunica vaginalis. Congenital hydrocele occurs because of a patent processus vaginalis (a communication between the scrotal sac and the peritoneal cavity) so that peritoneal fluids can collect in the scrotum. An inguinal hernia is also often present. Because the fluid will reabsorb and the patency will close, no intervention is required. If an inguinal hernia is diagnosed and bowel is present in the sac, surgical repair is performed to avoid strangulation of the bowel.

In adults, a hydrocele is noncommunicating with the peritoneal cavity; an acute onset of fluid collection is seen in response to infection, tumor, or trauma caused by either overproduction of fluid by the testis or obstruction of lymphatic or venous drainage in the spermatic cord. Chronic hydrocele usually occurs in men over 40 years of age. Fluid collects, and the resultant mass may be soft, cystic, or tense. The signs and symptoms are scrotal enlargement and a feeling of heaviness; a hydrocele is usually painless unless it is caused by an acute epididymal infection or testicular torsion. Diagnosis is aided by transillumination (a tumor does not transilluminate) and an

ultrasound of the scrotum to visualize the testis and determine whether a tumor is present.

Active therapy is not always necessary. In an adult, a tense hydrocele that impedes blood circulation or causes pain needs to be treated. The hydrocele in a neonate will usually resolve spontaneously. The processus vaginalis closes, and the fluid resorbs. When necessary, in a communicating hydrocele in a child, the processus vaginalis is ligated and the fluid drained. For a noncommunicating hydrocele, surgical drainage is done along with any indicated therapy for underlying causes.

Varicocele

A varicocele is an abnormal dilation (varicosity) of the pampiniform plexus of veins that drain each testis; it is more common on the left side compared with the right side. A varicocele on the right side may be a sign of obstruction caused by a tumor. A varicocele is palpable in 10% of men in the general population and 30% of men with infertility. Sperm concentration and motility are significantly decreased in 65% to 75% of men who have a varicocele. The mechanism for the relationship to infertility is unknown but may relate to testicular temperature increase because one of the functions of the pampiniform plexus is to keep the testes 1° to 2° F cooler than body temperature for optimal conditions for sperm production.

Usually no symptoms are associated with the presence of a varicocele, although some men describe a feeling of heaviness on the involved side and tenderness when it is palpated with examination. On physical examination, a mass that feels like a "bag of worms" is palpable when the patient is in the upright position; when the patient is recumbent, the mass drains and cannot be felt. The sudden development of a varicocele in an older man is sometimes a late sign of renal tumor. Pressure from metastasized tumor mass in the renal vein will interfere with blood flow in the spermatic vein on the right side. Testicular atrophy may occur because of reduced blood flow. Surgical repair of the varicosities by ligation of the internal spermatic veins at the internal inguinal ring has been reported to improve sperm quality. Chronic pain can be helped with scrotal support.

Hyperplasia of the Prostate

Benign prostatic hyperplasia (BPH) is a disease of advancing age. Clinical evidence of BPH usually occurs in more than 50% of men over the age of 50 years. Prostatic hyperplasia is growth of multiple fibroadenomatous nodules in the prostate; it begins in the periurethral region as a localized proliferation and progresses to compress the remaining normal gland. The hyperplastic tissue is mostly glandular, with varying amounts of fibrous stroma and smooth muscle. The prostate surrounds the urethra, and enlargement of the periurethral region of the prostate causes obstruction of the bladder neck and prostatic urethra, which decreases urine outflow from the bladder. The cause of BPH is probably related to aging and the accompanying hormone changes. With aging, as serum testosterone levels decline, serum estrogen levels increase. It is theorized that the resulting higher estrogen/androgen ratio stimulates hyperplasia of prostate tissues.

Common signs and symptoms that occur in various combinations and severity are urinary frequency, nocturia, urgency, urgency incontinence, hesitancy, diminished force of the urinary stream, a feeling of incomplete emptying, overflow incontinence, and postvoid dribbling. A distended bladder may be felt on abdominal examination, and suprapubic pressure on a distended bladder causes a sense of urgency. The prostate is palpated during rectal examination to assess the size of the gland.

Diagnostic tests include an abdominal ultrasound to look for hydronephrosis or renal masses and to measure volume of postvoid residual urine and prostatic size. Cystoscopy is done to rule out bladder diverticula, stones, and tumors. Measurement of urinary flow rate and a retrograde urethrogram may also be done.

Obstruction of the bladder neck causing decreased or absent outflow of urine requires intervention to reestablish a patent outlet for urine. Possible procedures include partial prostatectomy, either transurethral resection of the prostate (TUR) or open incision prostatectomy, to remove the hyperplastic periurethral tissue; transurethral incision through muscle fibers of the bladder neck to enlarge the opening; balloon dilation of the prostate to enlarge the urethral lumen; and antiandrogen therapy to cause prostatic atrophy. Indwelling urethral stents placed in the prostatic urethra are a recently developed nonsurgical method of treatment.

REPRODUCTIVE ORGAN INFECTIOUS PROCESSES

Infections of the genital organs occur in men from venereal transmission, as a manifestation of systemic disease, or as a result of instrumentation (catheterization, surgery). Men seek medical care because of a variety of symptoms such as urethral discharge, dysuria, frequency, scrotal tenderness or pain, genital skin eruptions, dyspareunia, and low back and perineal pain.

Balanitis

Balanitis is an inflammation of the glans; *balanoposthitis* is inflammation of the glans and prepuce in the uncircumcised male. The inflammation can be caused by gonorrhea, trichomoniasis, syphilis, *Candida albicans*, tinea, or coliform organisms; as a complication of a dermatitis such as psoriasis; or by a contact dermatitis caused by clothing, use of condoms, or contraceptive jellies.

Balanoposthitis is also associated with a tight prepuce or poor hygiene. Normal secretions from under the foreskin become infected with anaerobic bacteria, causing inflammation and necrosis. Symptoms and signs are irritation, soreness, and a foul-smelling discharge; edema may cause phimosis. Ulceration can occur, causing enlargement and tenderness of the inguinal lymph nodes.

Culture of any discharge should be performed for identification of causative organisms or of secondary bacterial infection. Treatment includes saline irrigation several times daily and antibiotics. Circumcision may need to be considered if phimosis is present after the infection subsides.

Urethritis

Urethritis is inflammation of the urethra from any cause and is a common syndrome in males. Infectious urethritis is classified as either gonococcal or nongonococcal (NGU), depending on the causative organism. The most common organisms are *Neisseria gonorrhoeae*, *Chlamydia trachomatis*, *Ureaplasma urealyticum*, *Trichomonas vaginalis*, herpes simplex viruses (both HSV types 1 and 2), and human papillomavirus (HPV). These organisms are commonly transmitted by sexual activities. The classic signs and symptoms are a urethral discharge; inflammation of the meatus; and burning, itching sensation, frequency, and urgency with urination.

Acute urethritis is the most common finding in men with gonorrhea, although some men with gonorrhea never develop overt signs or symptoms of urethritis. The discharge is a purulent, profuse discharge with a malodor with voiding. The incubation period for gonorrhea is 2 to 6 days.

The two most common organisms that cause NGU are *C. trachomatis* (30% to 50%) and *U. urealyticum* (25% to 35%). NGU may cause signs and symptoms similar to those of gonococcal urethritis, including urethral discharge, dysuria, and itching, but these are not as severe as those with gonococcal infection. The usual incubation period for NGU is 1 to 5 weeks. *T. vaginalis* usually does not cause symptomatic disease in men and is often self-limiting. This organism is probably killed rapidly by components of prostatic secretions. Herpesvirus genital infections are sexually transmitted during periods of both symptomatic and asymptomatic viral shedding by the partner. An outbreak of lesions can cause meatal inflammation and dysuria. Vesicles may be present on urethral mucosa. Some HVP genotypes have been found to increase risk for malignancy. Intraurethral warts can cause urethral discharge, dysuria, bloody discharge, or hematuria. Intraurethral spread of warts can involve the bladder and ureters. Urethritis is not the presenting complaint in patients with HSV or HVP infections but occurs after the infection is evident and the characteristic lesions are present.

Prostatitis

Prostatitis is inflammation of the prostate; it can be acute or chronic, and the cause can be either bacterial or nonbacterial. About 50% of men experience symptoms of prostatic inflammation during adult life, and only about 5% of these cases are caused by bacterial infection. Most bacterial infections of the prostate are caused by gram-negative organisms; the most common organism is *Escherichia coli*. Other causative organisms are enterococci, staphylococci, streptococci, *Chlamydia trachomatis*, *Ureaplasma urealyticum*, and *Neisseria gonorrhoeae*. Bacterial prostatic infections can be the result of a previous or concurrent urethral infection with direct ascent of bacteria from the urethra through the prostatic ducts into the prostate, reflux of urine from an infected bladder, or direct lymphatic or hematogenous spread.

Acute bacterial prostatitis occurs most often in men between the ages of 20 and 40 years; it causes fever as high as 39° to 40° C, chills, malaise, low back pain, perineal pain, dysuria, urethral spasm, and marked suprapubic tenderness. With rectal examination, the prostate is found to be tender, swollen, warm, and firm. Palpation of the prostate should be done very carefully. Vigorous massage, in addition to being very painful for the patient, can cause secondary epididymitis or septicemia because of a shower of bacteria being released systemically. Because there is usually also a cystitis, a urinalysis and a urine culture will often identify the organism.

Treatment of bacterial prostatitis is with antibacterial agents specific for the causative organism. Supportive therapy includes bed rest, hydration, analgesics, antipyretics, and stool softeners.

Chronic bacterial prostatitis is a major cause of recurrent urinary tract infections (UTIs) in men. Symptoms are dysuria, urgency, frequency, and nocturia. Pain may occur in the back, perineal area, penis, scrotum, and suprapubic area. Palpation of the prostate gland by rectal examination may be negative. Often the individual is asymptomatic until a significant bacteriuria develops. Frequently there is recurrent symptomatic cystitis. When treated with antibiotics, these symptoms resolve, and the urine culture becomes negative. However, the organism persists in the prostate, and the individual may continue to have recurrent infections once antibiotics have been discontinued. Suppressive antimicrobial therapy usually results in complete symptomatic relief and reduces the risk of serious illness. Nonbacterial prostatitis causes the same symptoms as does chronic prostatitis, but there is no UTI, and no organism can be found. Occasionally the individual will notice mucous filaments in the urine. There is no specific treatment or cure.

Epididymitis

Epididymitis is an inflammatory response of the epididymis from infection or trauma. Infection spreads from an established urethritis or prostatitis, and it may be unilateral or bilateral. Chronic or recurring bacterial epididymitis is secondary to chronic infection in these sites or to the presence of a continuous indwelling urethral catheter. Abscess formation may also occur. Hematogenous spread from other sites is not common but does occur. Organisms from the pharynx and tuberculosis infection of the lungs are transmitted through the bloodstream.

The most common sign of epididymitis is scrotal pain and swelling with erythema; a hydrocele may form. A urethral discharge, dysuria, frequency, and urgency are usual symptoms. The onset may occur acutely over 1 to 2 days or develop more gradually. Laboratory tests done to identify the organism are a urethral smear, urinalysis, urine culture, blood culture, and cultures for sexually transmitted diseases.

Epididymitis is classified as nonspecific bacterial epididymitis and sexually transmitted epididymitis. Nonspecific bacterial epididymitis is caused by *E. coli*, streptococci, and staphylococci and is associated with an underlying urologic pathologic condition. Sexually transmitted epididymitis is caused by gonorrhea, *Chlamydia*, *Treponema pallidum*, and *T. vaginalis*. Identification of organisms and antibacterial treatment should begin immediately because sterility or infertility as a result of mechanical obstruction from scarring is a threat. Treatment is with antibiotic therapy, depending on the sensitivity of

organisms identified. Supportive symptomatic therapy is bed rest, scrotal support, ice packs, and analgesics. In the case of chronic inflammation secondary to urethritis, prostatitis, or an indwelling catheter, vasectomy can be considered to avoid continuing spread of the organisms through the vas deferens.

Orchitis

Orchitis is inflammation of the testis; in combination with epididymitis it is called epididymoorchitis and is a serious complication of epididymitis. Orchitis differs from other infections of the genital tract in two ways: the major route of infection is hematogenous, and viruses are the most common organisms to cause orchitis. The infection is classified as viral orchitis, pyogenic bacterial orchitis, or granulomatous orchitis.

Viruses cause the most cases of orchitis. Mumps orchitis is the most common viral infection seen, although immunization against mumps in childhood has decreased the incidence. Twenty percent to thirty percent of mumps cases in adults are complicated by orchitis; it is bilateral in about 15% of men with mumps orchitis. In the pubertal or adult male, there usually is seminiferous tubule damage with risk for infertility and, in some cases, damage to Leydig's cells with resultant testosterone deficiency hypogonadism. Mumps orchitis rarely occurs in prepubertal males, but when it does, complete recovery can be expected without subsequent testicular dysfunction.

Signs and symptoms range from mild testicular discomfort and edema to severe testicular pain and marked edema in about 4 to 6 days after onset of the disease with high fever, nausea, and vomiting. Epididymitis and funiculitis (infection of the vas deferens) are possible complications.

Treatment for mumps orchitis is bed rest and scrotal support and elevation. Mild cases resolve in 4 to 5 days; severe cases resolve in 3 to 4 weeks.

Other viruses that can cause orchitis and present the same clinical picture are Coxsackie B virus, varicella, and mononucleosis.

Pyogenic bacterial orchitis is caused by bacteria (*Escherichia coli*, *Klebsiella pneumoniae*, *Pseudomonas aeruginosa*) and occasionally rickettsial or parasitic infections (malaria, filariasis, schistosomiasis, amebiasis) by spread from an epididymitis. Systemic diseases such as diphtheria, typhoid fever, paratyphoid fever, and scarlet fever may be transmitted by the bloodstream. The individual with pyogenic orchitis is acutely ill with high fever, edema, acute inflammatory hydrocele, and marked scrotal pain that radiates to the inguinal canal. Complications include testicular infarction, abscess, and pyocele of the scrotum.

Granulomatous orchitis may be caused by syphilis, mycobacterial diseases, actinomycosis, fungal diseases, *Mycobacterium tuberculosis*, and *Mycobacterium leprae*. Genital tuberculosis that spreads hematogenously usually starts unilaterally in the lower pole of an epididymis. Infection may spread through the spermatic cord to the testis. Further spread involves the contralateral epididymis and testis, the bladder, and the kidneys.

Urine and blood cultures are done, as well as direct cultures of the infected testis to identify the causative organism. Treatment for these infections is with antibiotics specific for the organism causing the infection. Comfort measures are bed rest, scrotal support, ice packs, and analgesics.

A rare cause of unilateral testicular enlargement, occurring predominantly in middle-aged men, is a nontuberculosis, *chronic granulomatous (autoimmune) orchitis.* The origin is unclear, although an autoimmune basis is suspected. A history of preceding trauma is often obtained, but it is not known whether this is causally related to the testicular inflammation. Chronic granulomatous orchitis is characterized by a nodular, often quite painless, enlargement of the testes, which feels quite firm. These physical findings are important because this form of orchitis must be distinguished from a testicular tumor, which it mimics. Histologically, the orchitis is distinguished by epithelioid granulomas, which appear to have seminiferous tubules at their centers.

MALIGNANT TUMORS OF THE MALE GENITAL TRACT

Carcinoma of the Prostate

Cancer of the prostate is the second most common malignancy in men in the United States and the third most common cause of cancer deaths in men over 55 years of age, after lung and colorectal cancer. In the United States, the incidence of prostatic cancer is 50% higher in African-American men compared with Caucasian men. The highest incidence is in North America and the Caribbean, and the lowest in China and Japan. The cause of prostatic cancer is unknown. As with nodular hyperplasia of the prostate, androgens are believed to play a role in the pathogenesis. Adenocarcinoma accounts for 95% of all prostate cancers; the remainder of neoplasms are transitional cell carcinomas, squamous cell carcinomas, and sarcomas. Adenocarcinoma of the prostate commonly develops in the periphery of the organ or in the periurethral tissue where benign prostatic hypertrophy occurs. No relationship exists between benign prostatic hyperplasia and the development of malignancy in the prostate.

As the tumor develops and progresses, there is direct extension to the urethra, bladder neck, and seminal vesicles. Prostatic cancer also spreads by lymphatic or hematogenous routes. The most common sites of metastases are to the pelvic lymph nodes and skeleton. Skeletal metastases are to bones of the pelvis, lumbar spine, femur, thoracic spine, and ribs, in that order. Organ metastases occur later and are commonly to liver and lung. Prostatic cancer is unpredictable in the course it will take. The cancer can progress very slowly in some men; in others it grows and metastasizes rapidly and causes death early in the course of the disease. Therefore most clinicians treat patients with prostate cancer aggressively.

Symptoms are not present or are nonspecific early in the course of the disease, and men with advanced disease can also be asymptomatic. Common symptoms are dysuria, difficulty in voiding, urinary frequency, urinary retention, back pain, and hematuria; with increasing obstruction, the patient may develop uremia. Signs of a pathologic condition are most often discovered during routine digital rectal examination.

Screening for prostatic cancer includes *digital rectal examination (DRE)* and serum *prostate-specific antigen (PSA),* and their combined use allows detection of more than 60% of the cases while the tumor is still localized. PSA is a serine protease produced by the prostate epithelium and periurethral glands in the male. PSA is the single test with the highest predictive value for cancer. Normal PSA values are <4 ng/ml; 4 to 10 ng/ml levels are equivocal and occur normally or often with prostatitis benign prostatic hyperplasia; values >10 ng/ml are highly correlated with the diagnosis of prostate adenocarcinoma. The American Cancer Society recommends a yearly DRE for all men over the age of 40 years. An annual PSA level is also recommended beginning at age 40 for men who are African American or have a family history of prostate cancer and all men over the age of 50 years. If the DRE is abnormal (palpation of a hard, irregular nodule) or if the PSA is elevated (>10 ng/ml) suggesting prostatic cancer, *transrectal ultrasound (TRUS)* is used to detect suspicious areas and to direct a needle biopsy. Biopsy of the prostate is essential for establishing the diagnosis.

After the diagnosis of adenocarcinoma of the prostate has been histologically confirmed, an accurate assessment of the stage—or extent—of the disease should be made. The goals in the staging of prostate cancer are twofold: (1) to evaluate prognosis and (2) to direct therapy rationally based on extent of disease. The methods in common use for assessing the extent of the prostate cancer include DRE for determination of the T (tumor size) stage, serum tumor markers (PSA and less commonly *prostatic acid phosphatase [PAP]*), Gleason histologic grading, radiologic imaging, and surgical lymphadenectomy. The staging accuracy can be significantly enhanced by combining the parameters of local disease extent (T stage), serum PSA level, and the Gleason grade from the prostate biopsy specimen. The status of pelvic lymph nodes provides important information with respect to management because a curative approach has a low probability of success in the setting of lymph node metastasis. The prevalence of lymph node metastasis correlates directly with T stage, serum PSA levels, and histologic grade.

Two systems are in common use for the staging of prostate cancer. The older Whitmore-Jewett system (stages A through D) was first described in 1975 and later modified. In 1997 the American Joint Committee on Cancer (AJCC) and the International Union Against Cancer adopted a revised tumor node metastasis (TNM) system, which employs the same broad T categories as does the Whitmore-Jewett system but includes subcategories of T stage, including a stage to describe patients diagnosed through PSA screening. The revised TNM system more precisely stratifies newly diagnosed patients into four stages, I to IV (roughly corresponding to the Whitmore-Jewett A to D stages). Table 65-2 presents a comparison of clinical stage by the revised TNM classification system and the older Whitmore-Jewett staging system.

The treatment of prostatic carcinoma depends on the size (volume) of the tumor or tumors and the extent or stage of the disease. Four major stages of prostate cancer are used, designated I to IV in the TNM classification system and A to D in the Whitmore-Jewett classification sys-

TABLE 65-2

Prostate Cancer: Comparison of Clinical Stage by TNM Classification with Whitmore-Jewett Staging System

TNM Stage	Description	Whitmore-Jewett Stage	Description	Comments
T1a	Nonpalpable, with 5% or less of resected tissue with cancer	A1	Well-differentiated on a few chips from 1 lobe	Early stage, clinically inapparent; incidental finding at prostate surgery for BPH
T1b	Nonpalpable, with >5% of resected tissue with cancer	A2	Involvement more diffuse	
T1c	Nonpalpable, detected by needle biopsy due to elevated PSA			
T2a	Palpable, half of one lobe or less	BIN	Palpable, <1 lobe surrounded by normal tissue	Confined to prostate (intracapsular)
T2b	Palpable, >half of one lobe	B1	Palpable, <1 lobe	
T2c	Palpable, both lobes	B2	Palpable, one entire lobe or both	
T3a	Palpable, unilateral extracapsular extension	C1	Palpable, outside capsule, not into seminal vesicles	Spread outside prostate to nearby tissues
T3b	Palpable, bilateral extracapsular extension			
T3c	Tumor invades seminal vesicles	C2	Palpable, extracapsular—bladder outlet or ureteral obstruction	
T4	Tumor fixed or invades adjacent structures other than seminal vesicles			
M	Distant metastasis	D	Metastatic disease	Spread to lymph nodes outside true pelvis, bone, or other sites

Data from American Joint Committee on Cancer: *Prostate: AJCC cancer staging manual,* ed 5, Philadelphia, 1997, Lippincott.

tem. The first stage (I or A) refers to clinically undetectable tumors confined to the prostate gland and an incidental finding at prostatic surgery, usually for benign prostatic hyperplasia (BPH). These tumors are small and nonpalpable. The second stage (II or B) refers to tumors that are palpable on rectal examination and are confined to the prostate gland. The third stage (III or C) refers to tumors that extend beyond the prostatic capsule and may involve the seminal vesicles, but are contained within the pelvis. The fourth stage (IV or D) refers to tumors that are metastatic, including regional lymph nodes, distant lymph nodes, bone, or visceral organs.

On rectal examination of the prostate, the tumor feels harder than is the normal or hyperplastic prostate as a firm mass within the substance of the gland. The diagnosis of prostate cancer is confirmed by either a transperineal or transrectal needle biopsy of the prostate or a transrectal fine-needle aspiration for a cytologic diagnosis. Also, TRUS and measurement of serum PSA are done as part of the diagnostic workup. The TRUS can provide some information regarding location and size of any mass, and PSA is elevated in the presence of prostate malignancy.

Evaluation of a stage includes measurement of serum acid phosphatase, which is elevated with metastatic disease, a bone scan to look for bony metastases, and a pelvic lymphadenectomy to determine node metastases. Removal of lymph nodes has no bearing on the course of prostate carcinoma, but presence of metastases in lymph nodes can spare the patient from a radical prostatectomy.

Treatment in stage I or A disease is variable and depends on the age and medical condition of the patient.

Although the malignancy was probably removed in the first surgery, about 16% of these men will develop metastatic disease within 10 years. Therefore most physicians carry out aggressive therapy and close follow-up is done, especially in men under the age of 65 years. Stage II or B disease is treated with either radical prostatectomy (removal of entire prostate and the seminal vesicles) or radiation therapy (external beam radiation or implanted interstitial radioactive seeds). Radical prostatectomy has an excellent cure rate of 15-year survival when the disease is localized in the gland. Serious complications are refractory incontinence and impotence. Radiation therapy is done less often but may be appropriate for men who do not want to undergo surgery or whose age or medical condition makes them unsuitable surgery candidates. Major complications of radiation therapy are proctitis and urethritis with possible stenosis.

Stage III or C prostatic cancer is treated with radiation therapy as just described. The extent of the tumor in this stage and beyond is not curable surgically.

Stage IV or D prostatic cancer is treated with hormonal therapy. The object is to deprive the tumor of circulating androgens and thus achieve regression of the tumors, both prostatic and metastatic, to provide palliation. This goal can be accomplished surgically with castration or pharmacologically with use of estrogens (diethylstilbestrol), antiandrogens (flutamide), or LH-releasing analogs (leuprolide acetate). Survival after hormone therapy is variable; 10% survive less than 6 months, and 50% survive less than 3 years.

Carcinoma of the Testes

Testicular cancer is a relatively rare form of cancer. Although it accounts for only 1% of cancers in men, testicular cancer is the most common solid malignancy in young men. The peak age for testicular cancer is 15 to 35 years. The incidence has slowly increased over the past 40 years. In 1995 there were 7000 new cases in the United States, resulting in 400 deaths. Testicular cancer is four to five times more common in Caucasians than it is in African Americans. Testicular cancer is highly treatable with cure rates exceeding 90% for all types.

There are two main groups of testicular tumors: (1) *germ cell tumors (GCTs)* originate in the sperm-producing cells lining the seminiferous tubules and comprise 95%; and (2) *sex cord tumors* are derived from specialized and nonspecialized support cells of the testis and make up less than 5%. GCTs are broadly divided into *seminoma* and *nonseminoma* subtypes for treatment planning because seminomas are more sensitive to radiation therapy. Seminomas are the most common type of GCT (50%), tend to be slower growing, and occur in the fourth decade of life. Nonseminomas are generally more aggressive than are seminomas and occur more often when men are in their thirties. Approximately 75% of seminomas are limited to the testes when first diagnosed, although approximately 75% of nonseminomas have already spread to the lymph nodes when diagnosed. There are four subtypes of nonseminoma: *teratoma, embryonal carcinoma, yolk sac carcinoma, choriocarcinoma*, and various mixtures of these cell types. Risk of metastasis is lowest for teratoma and highest for choriocarcinoma, with other cell types being intermediate. These cells secrete alpha-fetoprotein (AFP) and human chorionic gonadotropin (hCG), which can serve as tumor markers.

The cause of GCTs is unknown; however, there are several notable risk factors. Failure of a testis to descend into the scrotum (cryptorchidism or undescended testicle) increases the risk of developing testicular cancer several fold. Similarly, men whose testes descend after the age of 6 years have a greater risk of testicular cancer. An undescended testicle in the abdomen has a higher risk for testicular cancer than one arrested in the inguinal canal. Klinefelter's syndrome, a condition characterized by small testicles, is also associated with an increased risk of developing GCT. An isochromosome on the short arm of the chromosome 12 is pathognomic for GCT of all cell types although the gene on 12p involved in the pathogenesis has not yet been defined (Bosl, 1997; Motzer, Bosl, 2001).

The most common sign of testicular cancer is a painless swelling or lump in one testis. About a third of the time, a man may experience a dull ache or a feeling of heaviness in the lower abdomen, groin, or scrotum area. All men should be familiar with the size and feeling of their testicles so they can detect any type of change. The American Cancer Society recommends monthly testicular self-examination (TSE) for all men over the age of 15. A TSE is best done after a warm bath or shower when the skin of the scrotum is relaxed. Early misdiagnosis (e.g., epididymitis, orchitis) or a delay in diagnosis because of patient fear or embarrassment results in advanced disease at diagnosis and a reduced survival rate. The origin of scrotal masses must be determined because most masses growing in or from the testes are malignant while extratesticular masses are usually benign. Scrotal ultrasound can differentiate between extratesticular and testicular masses. Radical inguinal orchidectomy is the procedure of choice in diagnostically evaluating a testicular mass, as well as the first step in treating testicular cancer. Transscrotal biopsy is not recommended because of the risk of local dissemination of tumor into the scrotum or spread to inguinal lymph nodes.

The staging evaluation of GCT includes measurement of the serum level of the tumor markers, AFP and hCG, as well as lactase dehydrogenase (LDH), both before and after orchidectomy. Other procedures to determine the extent of disease include chest x-ray, computed tomography (CT) scan of the abdomen and pelvis, intravenous (IV) pyelograms, and lymphangiograms. The AJCC (1997) has designated staging by TNM classification and serum tumor markers. There are three stages of GCT based on the AJCC criteria, which help to determine prognosis and guide treatment. Stage I testicular cancer is limited to the testis, epididymis, or spermatic cord. Stage II disease involves the testis and is limited to the retroperitoneal (regional) lymph nodes. The number of nodes involved and the size of the nodes further characterize retroperitoneal lymph node involvement. The risk of recurrence is increased if more than 5 nodes are involved and if the size of one or more of the involved nodes is larger than 2 cm; recurrence risk is even greater if the size of the involved nodes is larger than 5 cm. Stage III disease implies spread outside the retroperitoneum, involving supradiaphragmatic nodal sites (supraclavicular, mediastinum, lung) or viscera.

The treatment of GCT depends on the stage and the type of tumor, whether seminoma or nonseminoma (Table 65-3). Careful monitoring of serum tumor markers (AFP, hCG, and LDH) is important following radical orchidectomy. A rise in levels of the tumor markers or failure to decline after treatment indicates persistent or recurrent tumor. Retroperitoneal radiation therapy is the treatment of choice following inguinal orchidectomy for patients with Stage I and II seminoma, which is very radiosensitive. Stage III and bulky Stage II disease is treated with combination chemotherapy (cisplatin/bleomycin/etoposide). Patients with Stage I and II nonseminoma GTC are managed by either a retroperitoneal lymph node dissection (RPLND) or close surveillance. Nearly all patients with stage II nonseminoma GCT will undergo RPLND, and those with large volume disease will also be treated by combination chemotherapy. The cure rate for stage I and II seminomas is 98% and 90%, respectively, and more that 80% with stage III disease are cured with chemotherapy. Stages I and II nonseminomas are highly curable (> 95%), and stage III is usually curable (70%) with standard chemotherapy. The 30% of patients who are not cured usually have widespread visceral metastases, high tumor markers, or mediastinal tumors at presentation.

Sex cord tumors are derived from the nongerm cell components of the testis and are much less common than germ cell tumors. *Leydig cell tumors* most often occur in adults but may also occur in children. These tumors are usually benign; however, it is hard to predict their potential for malignancy. These tumors commonly appear as

TABLE 65-3

Germ Cell Testicular Cancer Staging and Treatment

| Stage | Disease Extent | Treatment and Prognosis/Remission Rate (%) | |
		Seminoma	Nonseminoma
I	Limited to testis	Irradiation (98%)	RPLND or observation (>95%)
II	Involves testis and retroperitoneal lymph nodes	Irradiation (90%)	RPLND (>95%)
IIa	Nodes <2 cm	Irradiation	RPLND or chemotherapy; often by RPLND
IIb	Nodes 2-5 cm	Irradiation	RPLND ± chemotherapy or chemotherapy followed by RPNLD
IIc	Nodes >5 cm	Chemotherapy	Chemotherapy
III	Distant metastasis	Chemotherapy (>80%)	Chemotherapy (70%)

RPLND, Retroperitoneal lymph node dissection.

testicular swelling. They may secrete androgens or estrogens, resulting in precocious puberty in a male child or gynecomastia. *Sertoli cell tumors* may arise at any age, including infancy, but have a peak incidence in the fourth decade. These tumors are usually benign but occasionally (10%) behave in a malignant fashion. Either androgens or estrogens may be elaborated but not sufficiently to cause precocious masculinization or feminization. Treatment for these tumors is orchidectomy.

Carcinoma of the Scrotum

Carcinoma of the scrotum is rare; the most common carcinoma involving the scrotum is squamous cell carcinoma. Other lesions include liposarcoma, leiomyosarcoma, basal cell carcinoma, extramammary Paget's disease, malignant melanoma, and metastatic lesions. In the 1940s the incidence of squamous cell carcinoma was thought to be related to the type of work the individual does, with laborers being at higher risk compared with white-collar workers. Laborers were thought to be more exposed to industrial environmental irritants, mechanical irritation, and trauma. Carcinoma of the scrotum occurs more often in Caucasian men than it does in African-American men and in urban populations than in rural populations. Squamous cell carcinoma of the scrotum occurs most often in men 50 to 70 years of age. It begins as a solitary, slowly growing nodule that often goes undetected or ignored. Ulceration occurs after about 6 months of growth. Delay in medical assistance means that nearly 50% of men have palpable inguinal adenopathy with an advanced tumor stage when first seen by a physician and the diagnosis is made. Excision of the lesion is done for evaluation by histologic examination for determining the depth of invasion. Palpable inguinal lymph nodes potentially can be caused by inflammation, so frequently a 6-week course of antibiotic therapy is prescribed. Enlarged pelvic or periaortic lymph nodes are aspirated for biopsy and a CT scan of the abdomen and pelvis is done for staging. Wide local excision of the tumor with at least 2-cm margins and excision of the skin and underlying dartos muscle are done as treatment of early stage disease. Alternatively, laser therapy and Mohs' micrographic surgery are used. Radiation therapy and chemotherapy are not effective. If inguinal lymph nodes are not palpable, biopsy is done to determine whether metastasis has occurred. If the inguinal lymph nodes are

palpable after antibiotic therapy or the biopsy specimen is positive for malignancy, bilateral ilioinguinal lymphadenectomy is done.

The long-term survival rate is 70% if diagnosed and treated before metastases to the inguinal lymph nodes. Survival rates are significantly lower after metastases occur and with worsening stage of disease.

Basal cell carcinoma, extramammary Paget's disease, and sarcomas are all treated with wide excision of local disease with appropriate follow-up and further treatment for advanced disease, the same as for squamous cell carcinoma. Metastatic lesions to the scrotum are usually adenocarcinomas from primary tumors of the rectum, colon, and stomach.

Carcinoma of the Penis

Carcinoma of the penis occurs most commonly in men from 60 to 80 years of age but also is seen in men from 40 to 60 years of age. The incidence has been linked to the hygienic standards and differences in cultural and religious practices. Carcinoma of the penis is more common in uncircumcised men than it is in circumcised males. Neonatal circumcision has been said to eliminate the occurrence of penile carcinoma. Cervical carcinoma in sexual partners increases the risk of men developing penile cancer; and deoxyribonucleic acid (DNA) sequences of the sexually transmitted human papillomavirus have been identified in cases of penile cancer. Most malignancies of the penis are low-grade squamous cell carcinoma. Extent of metastasis to nodes indicates prognosis.

Carcinoma of the penis begins with a small lesion that begins beneath the prepuce or in the coronal region and gradually extends to involve the entire glans, prepuce, corona, and shaft. Carcinoma in situ (intraepithelial neoplasia) is also known as Bowen's disease of the penis or erythroplasia of Queyrat. This noninvasive form progresses to invasive carcinoma; it extends locally and first spreads through the lymphatic system to the inguinal lymph nodes. Metastatic enlargement of the regional inguinal lymph nodes eventually leads to skin necrosis, chronic infection, or hemorrhage from erosion into the femoral vessels. If penile carcinoma is untreated, death occurs within 2 years. Biopsies are necessary to determine extent of the tumor so that treatment can be planned. Small and noninvasive lesions are removed by wedge excision, or Mohs' micrographic surgery may be used for excision; if the prepuce is involved, circumcision is done. Radiation therapy has also been successful for noninvasive lesions, as has topical application of 5-fluorouracil. Carbon dioxide (CO_2) laser therapy and cryosurgery are other treatment options. Invasive tumors are treated by partial penectomy with a 2-cm margin around the tumor or by total penectomy with perineal urethrostomy. With advanced tumors, more extensive surgery such as hemipelvectomy may be necessary. Chemotherapy may be used in combination with surgery.

BREAST

Benign Conditions of the Breast

Gynecomastia is hypertrophy of the breast and may be unilateral or bilateral. In boys during puberty, gynecomastia is usually bilateral, but in men over 50 years of age, it is usually unilateral. Gynecomastia is a discoid enlargement beneath the areola. It is often physiologic and will resolve spontaneously in 6 to 12 months. Other causes include conditions resulting in increased estrogen levels such as testicular tumors, pituitary tumors, some hypogonadism syndromes, cirrhosis of the liver, thera-peutic use of estrogens for prostatic carcinoma, and use of steroidal preparations. Occasionally resection of extra breast tissue is performed for psychologic reasons, or biopsy is performed to rule out malignancy.

Malignant Conditions of the Breast

The incidence of cancer of the breast in men is about 1% of that in women, but clinically both are similar. The primary cause is thought to be excess estrogen synthesis, and many tumors are estrogen-receptor positive. Risk factors are similar to those in women, including living in a Western country, first-degree relatives with breast cancer, infertility, obesity, and exposure to ionizing radiation. Male breast cancer is strongly associated with the BRCA2 gene but not with the BRCA1 gene (Donegan, 1996). Lesions fall into the same spectrum as those seen in the female breast, with the exception of lobular carcinoma in situ (because the male breast contains no lobular tissue). Axillary lymph node involvement is present in about one half the cases at the time of diagnosis and distant metastases are common. Male breast cancer is best treated by modified radical mastectomy followed by radiation therapy when there is locally advanced disease or positive lymph nodes. The sites of relapse and response to chemotherapy are similar in men and women.

KEY CONCEPTS

- The *male reproductive system* is composed of the gonads (testes), seminal excretory ducts (epididymis and vas deferens), accessory glands (seminal vesicles and prostate), and copulatory organ (penis).
- The testes are composed of *seminiferous tubules* and include the hormone-secreting *Leydig's cells* (mostly testosterone) and the sperm-producing *Sertoli's cells*.
- The primary functions of the male reproductive system are to produce mature spermatozoa and deposit sperm in the female reproductive tract during coitus.
- Testicular function is under the control of the *hypothalamic-pituitary-gonadal axis*. Hypothalamic GnRH causes the release of pituitary FSH and LH. LH stimulates testosterone secretion and FSH and testosterone together stimulate spermatogenesis. Testosterone is also responsible for male secondary sex characteristics.
- Because the reproductive and urinary systems are structurally integrated in males, most disorders affect both systems. The most important disorders of the male reproductive system are infertility, infections, and tumors.
- The decline in *reproductive capability* is more gradual in men than in women, allowing continued reproduction capacity until late in life. However, failure to maintain an erection (impotence) is more common in aging men.
- *Male hypogonadism* is characterized by an abnormal decrease in testicular function. It may be primary, (involve Leydig's cell dysfunction) or secondary (involve dysfunction of the hypothalamic-pituitary-gonadal axis).
- *Causes of male hypogonadism* are many including congenital or developmental disorders (e.g., Klinefelter's syndrome, androgen resistance syndrome), acquired disorders (e.g., mumps orchitis, hypopituitarism), or systemic disorders (e.g., paraplegia, chronic illness). The specific outcome (complete lack of maleness, infertility, impotence) depends on age of onset, focus of problem (testicular or hypothalamic-pituitary defect) and the functional status of the testes.
- Maldescent of the testes gives rise to *cryptorchidism*, which is associated with infertility and an increased risk of testicular cancer, whether treated or untreated.
- Congenital malformation of the urethral groove and urethral canal may create abnormal openings on the ventral surface of the penis (*hypospadias*) or on the dorsal surface (*epispadias*). The treatment is surgical reconstruction.
- *Testicular torsion* occurs when the testis twists on its pedicle obstructing venous return and, if not corrected within 6 hours, results in infarction.
- The most common disorder of the tunica vaginalis is *hydrocele*. Congenital patency of the processus vaginalis may be a cause in a child, other causes being inflammatory and neoplastic disorders of the testis or epididymis.
- A *varicocele* is an abnormal dilation of the veins within the spermatic cord (more commonly on the left side) caused either by congenital absence of

- valves in the internal spermatic vein or acquired valvular incompetence.
- The main diseases of the prostate are inflammatory disorders, hyperplasia, and carcinoma.
- *Prostatitis* (inflammation of the prostate) may be acute or chronic, bacterial or nonbacterial in type. Bacterial prostatitis is mainly caused by infections that gain access from the urethra or bladder.
- Chronic bacterial prostatitis is a major cause of recurrent urinary tract infections in men.
- *Benign prostatic hyperplasia* affects most males over the age of 70 years. The cause is not known, but it is believed to be the result of androgen-estrogen imbalance. Clinically it presents with difficulty in micturition, caused by compression of the prostatic urethra by the enlarging prostate gland.
- A *mumps viral orchitis* (inflammation of the testes) occurs in 20% to 30% of male patients who acquire the infection. Complications of orchitis include hydrocele and testicular atrophy.
- *Epididymitis*, inflammation of the epididymis, may be caused by trauma or infection, resulting in scrotal pain, swelling, and infertility from scarring and stricture if not treated promptly. Infection is classified as nonspecific bacterial (e.g., spread from a UTI or prostatitis) and as sexually transmitted epididymitis (e.g., gonorrhea, *Chlamydia*).
- *Balanitis* is an inflammation of the glans penis and usually occurs in conjunction with inflammation of the prepuce (*balanoposthitis*) in the uncircumcised male. Balanitis is associated with a tight prepuce and inadequate cleansing under the foreskin, skin irritation, and infections.
- *Carcinoma of the prostate* is the second most common type of cancer in men in the United States and the third leading cause of cancer death in men over 55 years of age (after lung and colon cancer).
- Because *carcinoma of the prostate* originates in the periphery of the gland, it is often well-established before the patient develops symptoms of difficulty with micturition resulting from urethral obstruction.
- *Carcinoma of the prostate* metastasizes to bone (most commonly the pelvis and lumbar spine) and pelvic lymph nodes and invades the bladder base.
- The combined use of prostate-specific antigen (PSA) and digital rectal examination (DRE) allows *early detection of prostate carcinoma* while it is still localized. The diagnosis is confirmed by needle biopsy and transrectal ultrasound (TRUS).
- *Testicular malignancies* are common in early adult life (age 15 to 35 years). Although the cause is unknown, risk factors include history of cryptorchidism and chromosomal abnormalities (e.g., Klinefelter's syndrome).
- Primary germ-cell tumors, arising from the multipotential germs cells of the testis, comprise 95% of testicular cancers. Nongerm-cell tumors are derived from the specialized and nonspecialized support tissues (interstitial Leydig's cells and Sertoli's cells) or are lymphomas.
- Careful monitoring of alfa fetoprotein (AFP) and human chorionic gonadotropin (hCG) is essential in the management of patients with *germ cell testicular cancer* because these tumor markers are important in diagnosis, prognosis, and monitoring treatment response.
- *Carcinoma of the penis* is rare and is more common in uncircumcised men from 60 to 80 years.
- Although uncommon, *carcinoma of the breast in men* accounts for about 1% of breast cancers. Because of delay in seeking treatment, the tumor tends to be more advanced at the time of diagnosis and therefore the prognosis is poor.

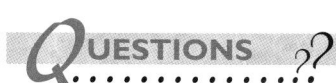

QUESTIONS

A sampling of review questions for this chapter appears here. Visit http://www.mosby.com/MERLIN/PriceWilson/ for additional questions.

Answer the following on a separate sheet of paper.

1. What are the primary functions of the male reproductive system?
2. Explain the process of spermatogenesis.
3. In the assessment of hypogonadism, explain the rationale for performing the clomiphene or GnRH stimulation test.
4. What hormonal and physiologic changes of the reproductive organs are associated with aging in the male?
5. Explain the causative factors responsible for genital tract infections of the male reproductive system.
6. Trace the pathway of metastasis of adenocarcinoma of the prostate.

Match the pathologic process in column B with the appropriate item in column A.

Column A
7. _____ Hypospadias
8. _____ Testicular torsion
9. _____ Benign prostatic hyperplasia
10. _____ Varicocele
11. _____ Hydrocele

Column B
a. Abnormally high insertion of the tunica vaginalis on the spermatic cord
b. Collection of fluid in the potential space between the membrane layers of the tunica vaginalis
c. Urethral meatus opening on the ventral side of the penis
d. Abnormal dilation of the pampiniform plexus of veins that drain the testes
e. Growth of multiple fibroadenomatous nodules in the prostate

CHAPTER

66

Infections of the Genital Tract

NANCY A. PRINCE

OVERVIEW

There are more than 25 infectious organisms that target the genital tract, and most are spread through sexual activity. This chapter will cover the most frequently encountered genital infections in the United States with the exception of the human immunodeficiency virus (HIV) that causes acquired immunodeficiency syndrome (AIDS) and is covered in Chapter 15. It is important to keep in mind while studying these infections, however, that the risk of acquiring or being infected with HIV is much greater in persons already infected with another genital infection. Infections of the genital tract are typical of infections elsewhere in the body once the first line of defense, the skin and mucous membranes, is broken. Depending on the nature of the invading organism, each infection will cause a fairly predictable immune or inflammatory response as described in Chapter 6. An understanding of each organism, and the symptoms generated by the body's response to it, provides important clues for identifying infective agents. Thus, as with other infections, a thorough history of exposure and symptoms often provides a high degree of suspicion as to the cause of an infection before the actual examination and laboratory testing are done. This investigation requires a sensitive exploration of sexual orientation and practices to ensure a thorough examination and collection of specimens for laboratory analysis.

Explicit sexual activity on television and in the movies, early onset of sexual relationships, and multiple sex partners give the impression that people are generally knowledgeable and comfortable with sexuality. The falseness of this assumption is demonstrated in cultural taboos, lack of communication with clinicians, and embarrassment attached to sexual issues. Anxiety and fear related to possible infections of the genital tract contribute significantly to delays in the diagnosis and treatment of infections. Infection and fear of infection of the genital tract is one of the most frequent reasons for young adults to seek medical care. Many, but certainly not all, infections of the reproductive tract are communicated through sexual activity.

Infections of the genital tract are unique compared with most other infections in the embarrassment and shame they produce in people. This observation is true even in individuals with genital infections who are not sexually active. Indeed, it is not just the patient that is uneasy about discussing sexual issues. A 1990 survey of physicians showed embarrassment as a major reason why physicians do not take sexual histories (Merrill, 1990). This embarrassment can be easily and unintentionally communicated to patients with concerns about sexuality and fear of genital infections. Infections that are acquired through sexual activity involve another person and an added emotional dimension. Infections often result in feelings of betrayal, distrust, and anger.

The culture in the United States places a high value on sexual privacy. There is frequently a reluctance to seek treatment for symptoms of genital infections from family physicians, practitioners, and community clinics for fear of a loss of anonymity. These facts together with the concentration of infections in teens who may be reluctant to confide their concern to a parent and young adults without insurance result in frequent delays in seeking or obtaining treatment. Delays contribute to complications and the spread of infection to partners. These delays are much more detrimental to women who are more likely to develop pelvic inflammatory infections (PID) and related complications as described later in this chapter.

Sexually transmitted infections (STIs), often called *sexually transmitted diseases (STDs)*, are at epidemic levels despite the fact that there are effective preventative practices and treatments that can contain or cure most of these infections. Table 66-1 provides a summary of the incidence and prevalence of the most frequent genital infections. An estimated 15 million new cases of STIs occur annually in the United States at an estimated cost of $17 billion (CDC, 2000). STIs are of interest to local, state, and national governments because many have a serious impact on the health of the individual and the community. Some are associated with long-term sequelae, including central nervous system (CNS) disease, cancer, and death. In addition, some genital infections may be transmitted to the fetus prenatally or to the neonate at birth. These infections may result in severe disability or death of the infant. Historically, the incidence of STIs, formerly called *venereal diseases*, was compiled by the U.S. Army and focused on gonorrhea and syphilis. Genital infections were considered more of a male problem, with rates of syphilis and gonorrhea doubling or tripling during times of war. Today, the U.S. Department of Health and Human Services Center for Disease Control and Prevention (CDC) compiles statistics on infectious diseases, including those transmitted sexually. Statistics often indicate higher levels of STIs among poor and minority populations (CDC, 2000). These reports must be examined critically. The most thorough reporting of STIs comes from health departments. Health departments frequently serve poverty and below poverty level individuals and higher numbers of minority populations, which may inflate the statistics for these groups. The statistics also may reflect a lack of access to quality health care and preventative services that accompany poverty.

The CDC publishes guidelines for the treatment, prevention, and counseling of individuals with or exposed to STIs. The 1998 Guidelines for the Treatment of Sexually Transmitted Diseases and treatment updates are available on the Internet at *www.cdc.gov* and should be accessed for the latest information. The guidelines also include treatment protocols for infections that are not or not exclusively transmitted sexually, such as vulvovaginal candidiasis, bacterial vaginosis, scabies, pediculosis, and hepatitis A and B. All states require that cases of syphilis, gonorrhea, and AIDS be reported. Reporting of other cases of STIs varies by state, and health care providers need to be familiar with the local and state reporting requirements. Identification of sexual contacts of infected persons is important to contain the spread of infection. Contact identification requires the cooperation of the infected individuals and may involve simply requesting that they contact persons they have had sexual relations with, advising them to get treatment, or letters sent from the health department to exposed individuals requesting that they seek treatment. Many counties provide free diagnosis and treatment services to individuals with STIs and their partners. STIs that are diagnosed in children or in adults with mental, emotional, or developmental disability, which prevent them from giving informed consent, must be reported to state protective service agencies.

Control of STIs and their consequences requires comprehensive treatment programs, education about transmission and prevention, and counseling about healthy responsible sexual behavior. The financing and support of research to identify effective treatment and prevention strategies is critical to controlling this epidemic.

▌▌ BACTERIAL INFECTIONS

Chlamydia

Chlamydia trachomatis is one of four species of the genus chlamydia that are specialized bacteria that live as intracellular parasites. *C. trachomatis* is the most common sexually transmitted bacterial infection in the United States

---

TABLE 66-1   ▪▪▪

The Incidence and Prevalence of Sexually Transmitted Diseases (STDs) in the United States

STD	Incidence (Estimated Number of New Cases Every Year)	Prevalence* (Estimated Number of People Currently Infected)
Chlamydia	3 million	2 million
Gonorrhea	650,000	Not available
Syphilis	70,000	Not available
Herpes	1 million	45 million
Human papillomavirus (HPV)	5.5 million	20 million
Hepatitis B	120,000	417,000
Trichomoniasis	5 million	Not available
Bacterial vaginosis**	Not available	Not available

*No recent surveys on national prevalence for gonorrhea, syphilis, trichomoniasis, or bacterial vaginosis have been conducted.
**Bacterial vaginosis is a genital infection that is not sexually transmitted but is associated with sexual intercourse.
Data from Cates W et al: Estimates of the incidence and prevalence of sexually transmitted diseases in the United States, *Sex Trans Dis* 26(suppl):S2-S7, 1999.

and is found worldwide. *C. trachomatis* is dimorphic; that is, it exists in two forms. In the infectious form, *C. trachomatis* are tiny, metabolically inactive, deoxyribonucleic acid (DNA)– and ribonucleic acid (RNA)–containing spheroids, called elementary bodies (EB). These spheroids gain access to host cells by endocytosis and, once inside, convert to metabolically active organisms that compete with their host cell for nutrients. The organisms initiate a cycle of replication and, condensing back into EB until the host cell bursts, release hundreds of EB to infect adjacent cells. *C. Trachomatis* has an affinity for the epithelium of the urethra, the cervix, and the conjunctiva of the eye. In men, urethritis, epididymitis, and prostatitis are the most common manifestations of infection. In women, cervicitis is most common, followed by urethritis, bartholinitis, and finally pelvic inflammatory disease (PID). *C. trachomatis* may infect the pharynx and rectum in persons engaging in oral and anal-receptive intercourse. Infants can be infected during the birth process and develop conjunctivitis and pneumonia. Infection with *C. trachomatis* does not confer immunity against future infection.

Young people between the ages of 15 and 19 years account for 40% of the reported cases of chlamydia (CDC, 2000). Rates are highest in sexually active females, with rates ranging from 5% to as high as 13% in screening programs, depending on the site and region. A total of 13,204 female military recruits were screened for chlamydia in 1996 and 1997 in an attempt to identify risk factors that were to be used to target populations for screening. Results revealed a chlamydia prevalence of 9.2%, with a peak of 12.2% among 17-year-old recruits (Gaydos, 1998). The higher rate of chlamydia in females is the result of greater susceptibility and greater screening efforts. Women are at twice the risk of contracting chlamydia after exposure because of the concentration of infected ejaculate held in the vagina, which prolongs exposure. In addition, screening efforts have focused on women because of the severe consequences of chlamydial infection in women, including PID, infertility, cervical cancer, and increased risk of becoming infected with HIV (CDC, 2000; Anttila, 2001; Zenilman, 2001). Chlamydia is a curable disease, and, although on the increase nationally, areas with active screening and treatment programs are showing a decline in infection (CDC, 2000).

Signs and Symptoms

The major signs of chlamydia infection in women are a mucopurulent cervical discharge and cervical ectopy, edema and friability, and, in men, urethritis with or without discharge. Dysuria may occur with urethral infections in men or women but is much more common in men than it is in women. *Proctitis*, an inflammation of the rectum, may be present in individuals engaging in anal intercourse. Unfortunately, up to 50% of men and 75% of women have no symptoms (Anttila, 2001). These large groups of asymptomatic, infectious individuals sustain transmission and support the case for mounting large-scale screening programs for high-risk populations. Asymptomatic infections also reinforce the importance of good sexual histories to ensure adequate testing and diagnosis of *C. trachomatis* infections.

Forty percent of women with untreated chlamydia infections will develop PID. *C. trachomatis* infections tend to extend upward from the endocervix to the endometrium, fallopian tubes, and finally out into the peritoneal cavity. Symptoms progress from mild cervical, uterine, and adnexal pain to severe abdominal pain that finally brings the woman in for treatment. By the time treatment is initiated, many women have scarring, adhesions, and occlusion of their fallopian tubes. Seventeen percent of women treated for PID will become infertile, and an equal number will experience chronic pelvic pain, and 10% of those who do conceive will have an ectopic pregnancy.

More than one half of men with chlamydia infection remain asymptomatic or have only mild symptoms. The urethra is the most common site of infection caused by *C. trachomatis* in men. *C. trachomatis* is the cause of 30% to 50% of cases of *nongonococcal urethritis (NGU)* and is found to coexist with gonococcal urethritis in about 20% of men. The most common complaint of men with urethral infection is dysuria and discharges that range from clear to grossly purulent. Symptoms typically begin 7 to 10 days after sexual contact with an infected partner. *C. trachomatis* infections usually remain localized to the urethra but may ascend the urogenital tract and cause epididymis or prostatitis. *Epididymitis*, an acute inflammation of the epididymis that causes swelling, testicular pain, fever and chills, occurs in about 5% of untreated men with chlamydia. Burning, frequency, and urgency of urination characterize *prostatitis*, an acute or chronic infection of the prostate. Progression of the infection causes scarring and tissue damage to the spermatic duct system in men, which can lead to infertility.

An infant born to a woman with a chlamydia infection of the endocervix has about a 70% chance of being infected. About 30% of infants born to infected women develop neonatal inclusion conjunctivitis, and 15% develop pneumonia. *C. trachomatis* is the most common cause of pneumonia in infants under 6 months of age (Morse, 1996).

Diagnostic Testing

Chlamydia can be diagnosed by culture of epithelial cells obtained from suspected infected sites and not just from secretions, because *C. trachomatis* is an intracellular parasite. Testing requires culture techniques similar to those used to isolate viruses, which makes chlamydia cultures more difficult and expensive than other bacterial cultures. Culture is the gold standard for testing and should be used in all cases of or suspected sexual assault and abuse. Antigen detection by *direct immunofluorescence antibody (DFA)* staining of smears and *enzyme immunosorbent assay (EIA)* are cost effective and are the most frequently used tests. EIA and DFA tests have sensitivity greater than 79% and specificity greater than 95% (Wallach, 2000). DNA amplification such as *ligase chain reaction (LCR)* and *polymerase chain reaction (PCR)* are DNA amplification methods that can isolate chlamydia from urine and vaginal swabs with minute amounts of the organism; they have higher sensitivity (95%) and specificity (99.5%) than DFA or EIA (Hooton, 2000). LCR and PCR are quickly becoming the gold standard for diagnosing chlamydia. Experimentation with self-administered vaginal swabs and tampons, as well as urine testing, makes large-scale screening for chlamydia increasingly feasible because it can be done in nonclinical settings (Cohon, 2000; Hooton, 2000). There are no reliable serologic tests for *C. trachomatis*.

Treatment

Single-dose treatment with azithromycin or a 7-day treatment regimen with doxycycline is the recommended CDC treatment protocol for *C. trachomatis* infections. The recommended drug treatment for *C. trachomatis* is highly efficacious and posttreatment testing (test of cure) is not necessary. Reoccurrence of chlamydia after treatment is most likely a result of reinfection or failure to complete the treatment regimen. Azithromycin is the preferred therapy because it involves a single dose and can be dispensed and taken under supervision in most STD clinics. Erythromycin is not teratogenic and is the treatment of choice for pregnant women and neonates. Erythromycin is less efficacious than are azithromycin and doxycycline, and should be followed with a test of cure after completion of the regimen.

Gonorrhea

Gonorrhea is the oldest described STI, dating back to reports in the Bible, Hindu literature, and Egyptian papyruses. Gonorrhea is caused by the invasion of the gram-negative diplococcal bacterium, *Neisseria gonorrhoeae*, that was first discovered by and named for the Polish dermatologist, Albert Neisseria. These bacteria act by attaching to and destroying the cell membrane of the epithelial cells lining the mucus membranes, especially those lining the endocervical canal and urethra. Extragenital infections of the pharynx, anus, and rectum may be found in both sexes. Direct mucosal-to-mucosal contact is necessary for transmission. Not everyone exposed to gonorrhea acquires the disease, and the risk of transmission from male to female is higher than is the risk of female-to-male transmission largely because of the female's greater mucous membrane surface exposure and vaginal harboring of exudate. Once inoculated, the infection can spread to the prostate, vas deferens, seminal vesicles, epididymis, and testes in men and to the urethra, Skene's glands, Bartholin's glands, endometrium, fallopian tubes, and peritoneal cavity, causing *PID* in women. PID is a major cause of infertility in women. Gonococcal infections can spread to and through the bloodstream, causing a systemic gonococcal bacteremia. Bacteremia can occur in both men and women but is much more prevalent in women by comparison. Women are at greatest risk during menstruation for the spread of infection. Perinatal transmission to the infant at birth, through an infected cervical os, may result in conjunctivitis and eventual blindness in the infant if not recognized or treated.

Gonorrhea rates in the United States are higher than they are in any other industrialized country, with estimated rates 50 times that of Sweden and 8 times that of Canada (CDC, 2000). Natural immunity does not occur after an infection with *N. gonorrhoeae*, so infection can be acquired more than once. Gonorrhea rates in the United States had shown a steady decline from the mid-1970s until 1997, when there was an increase of 9% between 1997 and 1999. Rates are highest in the young, with the highest rates in females 15 to 19 years of age and males 20 to 24 years of age, and in men who have sex with men.

A rapid local inflammatory response with cell destruction causes a characteristic purulent greenish-yellow discharge from the urethra in males and from the cervical os in females. Signs and symptoms in males can start as early as 2 days after exposure and begin with urethritis, followed by a purulent discharge, dysuria, and frequency of urination and malaise. Most men will become symptomatic within 2 weeks of inoculation with the organism. Although most men are symptomatic, up to 10% are not, but they remain infectious and capable of transmitting the infection. In most cases, men will seek treatment early in the disease because of bothersome symptoms. Because the infection is usually caught and treated early, few men develop prostatitis, epididymitis, or bacteremia. Local gonococcal infections, in men who are asymptomatic or men who are not treated, will usually be halted by the body's natural defenses in a few weeks to months.

In women, signs and symptoms develop in 7 to 21 days, beginning with vaginal discharge. On examination, the infected cervix is edematous and friable with mucopurulent drainage from the os. *N. gonorrhoeae* infections are asymptomatic or present minimal symptoms in as many as 25% to 50% of women. Women who develop no or minimal symptoms become a main source for the spread of infection and are at risk for developing complications. If untreated, the signs that infection is spreading will usually start to occur within 10 to 14 days. The most frequent site of spread in women is to the urethra, with symptoms of urethritis, dysuria, and frequency of urination and to Bartholin's and Skene's glands, causing swelling and pain. Infections that spread to the endometrium and fallopian tubes result in abnormal vaginal bleeding, pelvic and abdominal pain, and progressive symptoms of PID if untreated.

Extragenital infections that are either primary or secondary are more frequently encountered because of changing sexual practices. Gonococcal infections of the pharynx are frequently asymptomatic but may cause pharyngitis with a mucopurulent exudate, fever, and cervical lymphadenopathy. Perianal and rectal gonococcal infections may be asymptomatic, cause mild itching and discomfort, or cause perianal excoriation and pain, and mucopurulent discharge that coats the stool and lining of the rectal wall. Bacteremia from disseminated gonococcal infection is quite rare. Signs and symptoms are papular and pustular skin lesions on the hands and feet, polyarthritis, and painful inflammation of the tendons of the hands and feet.

Gonorrhea may be diagnosed quickly by gram staining a smear of exudes taken from an infected site. The smear is positive if intracellular gram negative diplococci are found. Unfortunately, stains are not reliable in diagnosing gonorrhea in women, asymptomatic persons, and for rectal or pharyngeal infections. A culture from all possible sites of infection should be obtained to confirm the diagnosis. Cultures take 48 to 96 hours to grow, and antibiotic therapy is usually started before obtaining results based on history and symptoms, or exposure. The polymerase chain reaction (PCR) and ligase chain reaction (LCR) DNA-amplification tests are more sensitive than cultures of the bacteria and can be used with vaginal and cervical secretions or urine. For men with urethral infections, DNA-amplification tests that can be done on voided urine specimens avoid uncomfortable swabbing of the sensitive urethra. Unfortunately, voided specimens are not as sensitive in women with urethral infections. Coexistent chlamydia infections that frequently accompany gonorrhea infection can be diagnosed with the same specimen. DNA-amplification tests are becoming more available and popular because of high sensitivity and ease in the handing and transporting of specimens. Nonculture tests such as antigen detection by direct immunofluorescence antibody (DFA) and enzyme immunosorbent assay (EIA) are not well developed and not frequently used.

Treatment

Gonorrhea was successfully treated with penicillin beginning in the 1940s; however, many penicillin-resistant strains of *N. gonorrhoeae* have developed. The current recommended treatment is either a cephalosporin or a fluoroquinolone (CDC, 1998). Unfortunately, fluoroquinolone-resistant *N. gonorrhoeae* (QRNG) infections have been reported in many parts of the world. Because of the threat of *N. gonorrhoeae*-resistant stains, susceptibility testing is recommended for all treatment failure. Because of the high incidence of coinfection with *C. trachomatis* in individuals with gonorrhea, concurrent treatment is recommended. Specific treatment regimens for gonorrhea, gonorrhea and chlamydia, pharyngeal and rectal gonorrhea, gonorrhea infections in pregnant women, gonorrhea in HIV-infected individuals can be found in the CDC guidelines (CDC, 1998). All sexual contacts of infected individuals should be evaluated and offered prophylactic treatment.

Syphilis

Syphilis is a highly contagious infection caused by the anaerobic spiral-shaped bacterium, *Treponema pallidum*. Except for neonatal transmission, syphilis occurs almost exclusively through sexual contact with an infected person; however, the *T. pallidum* spirochete can cross the placental barrier and infect the neonate. Spirochetes gain access through direct contact between a moist, infected lesion and any break, even microscopic, in the skin or mucosa of a host. Syphilis is curable in the early stages of infection, but, left untreated, it may become a chronic systemic infection. Syphilis is divided into three phases of infection: primary; secondary, including early and late latent syphilis; and tertiary. Each phase has its own distinct signs and symptoms.

Rates of syphilis in the United States have been steadily dropping since 1990. The CDC reported only 2.5 cases of syphilis per 100,000 people in 1999, and these cases were concentrated in specific large cities and counties. The rate of infants born with syphilis has dropped by 51% since 1997. According to the CDC, in 2000 there were only 529 cases of congenital syphilis in the United States (CDC, 2001). Although syphilis rates in the United States are low, it is still prevalent in Africa and Central and South America.

Signs and Symptoms
Primary syphilis

Typically, the first clinical manifestation of syphilis is a solitary, small, papule at the site of invasion, between 10 and 90 days after exposure. Over a period of one to several weeks, this papule progresses to form a red, painless, well-demarcated ulcer called a *chancre* that swarms with spirochetes (see color plate 39). These highly contagious chancres vary in size from a few millimeters to more than 2 centimeters. Chancres may be found anywhere but are most frequently found on the penis, anus, and rectum in men and the vulva, perineum, and cervix in women. Nontender lymphadenopathy ipsilateral to the chancre is common during primary syphilis. Extragenital chancres are most commonly found on the oral cavity, fingers, and breasts. Chancres heal spontaneously in 4 to 6 weeks.

Secondary Syphilis

If untreated, early signs of secondary syphilis begin to appear between 2 and 6 months after exposure. Secondary syphilis is a systemic disease in which the spirochetes spread from the chancre and lymph nodes into the blood stream and throughout the body, resulting in a multitude of symptoms far removed from the original local infection. The systems most commonly involved are the skin, lymphatic, gastrointestinal tract, bones, kidneys, eyes, and CNS. The most frequent sign of secondary syphilis is a cutaneous maculopapular rash that occurs in 80% of cases. Lesions are usually symmetric, nonitchy, and may be widespread; lesions of the palms and soles are most characteristic (see color plates 40 and 41).

Other lesions may appear as superficial ulcers of the oral and genital mucosa and as *condylomata lata*, a flat, wartlike lesion of the genitalia. All lesions of secondary syphilis are contagious and may be spread on contact. Additional signs and symptoms of secondary syphilis include lymphadenopathy, uveitis, malaise, low-grade fevers, headaches, anorexia and weight loss, alopecia, and bone and joint pain. The lesions of secondary syphilis heal spontaneously within 2 to 6 weeks, and a period of latency begins.

Latency is the stage in which the person tests serologically positive for syphilis but is clinically asymptomatic, and cerebrospinal fluid (CSF) laboratory tests are normal. The *early latent syphilis* period is demarcated as the time from the resolving of secondary signs and symptoms of syphilis to 1 year after the initial infection. During the early latent period, infectious relapses of secondary syphilis can occur. These relapses may continue to occur as long as 5 years after infection in 25% of patients. Eighty five percent of relapses involve the appearance of mucocutaneous lesions. The *late latent syphilis* period is from 1 year postinfection or until the symptoms of tertiary syphilis begin to appear. The classification of early or late latency is significant for treatment purposes.

Tertiary Syphilis

Years to decades after the initial infection, three forms of tertiary syphilis can appear: benign tertiary syphilis of the skin, bone, and viscera; cardiovascular syphilis; and neu-

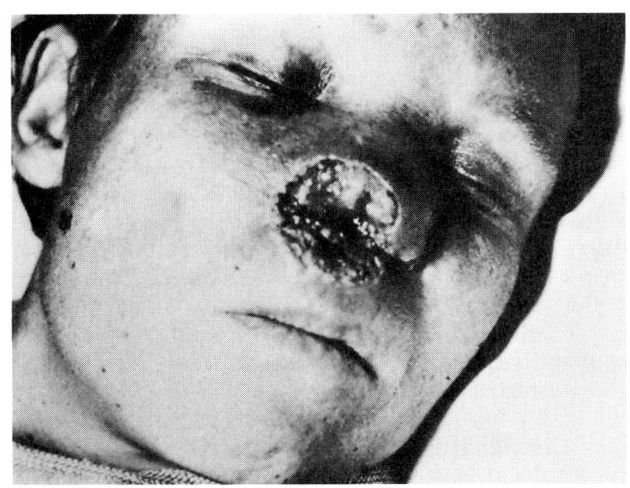

FIG. 66-1 Cutaneous gumma presenting as an ulcer over the nose. (Courtesy of Marek A. Stawiski, MD, Associate Clinical Professor of Internal Medicine, Michigan State University).

rosyphilis. About 30% of individuals with untreated primary and secondary syphilis will develop tertiary syphilis. *Benign tertiary syphilis* is characterized by the appearance of *gummas*, which are small nodular masses of granulation tissue with necrotic centers surrounded by a small margin of inflammation. Gummas may develop anywhere on the body, including the skin, bone, mucous membranes, eyes, viscera, and CNS (Fig. 66-1). Usually, there is simultaneous active inflammation with formation of new lesions and scars in one or more areas.

There are three major forms of symptomatic *cardiovascular syphilis*: aortic valvular insufficiency, aortic aneurysm, and coronary ostia stenosis. Symptoms appear from 10 to 40 years after infection. In the preantibiotic era, symptomatic cardiovascular complications developed in about 10% of persons with late untreated syphilis. Chapters 32 and 34 describe the pathology of these cardiovascular conditions.

Neurosyphilis is fundamentally a chronic meningitis that initially may be asymptomatic. The major clinical categories of symptomatic neurosyphilis include meningeal, meningovascular, and parenchymatous syphilis (the last of which includes general paresis and tabes dorsalis). The average time from infection to onset of symptoms for meningeal syphilis is usually less than 1 year, 7 years for meningovascular syphilis, 20 years for general paresis, and 25 to 30 years for tabes dorsalis. *Meningeal syphilis* may involve the brain or spinal cord, and patients may present with headache, dizziness, loss of memory, personality changes, aphasia, and seizures. *Meningovascular syphilis* reflects diffuse inflammation of the pia and arachnoid with evidence of focal or widespread involvement of brain vessels—the most common presentation is a stroke syndrome involving the middle cerebral artery preceded by encephalitic symptoms of headache, vertigo, insomnia, and psychologic disturbances. The *Parenchymatous neurosyphilis syndrome* reflects widespread damage to the brain parenchyma (general paresis) and abnormalities corresponding to the pneumonic PARESIS: Personality, Affect (emotional instability, irritability), Reflexes (hyperactive), Eye (Argyll Robertson pupils), Sensorium (hallucinations, illusions, delusions), Intel-

lect (deterioration of recent memory and capacity for orientation, calculations, and judgment), and Speech. *Tabes dorsalis* presents with signs and symptoms of demyelination of the posterior columns, dorsal roots, and dorsal root ganglia, resulting in truncal ataxia with a wide-based gait, loss of position, and foot-slapping; bladder dysfunction and impotence, areflexia, severe visceral pain, and paresthesias also occur. Optic atrophy often occurs in association with tabes, causing blindness. The small, irregular *Argyll Robertson pupil*, a feature of general paresis and tabes dorsalis, reacts to light but not to accommodation. Fortunately, tertiary syphilis is rare since the advent of penicillin.

Congenital Syphilis

Treponema pallidum can cross the placenta from the mother, infecting the fetus with congenitally acquired syphilis. Many infants with congenital syphilis have no obvious evidence of infection and are diagnosed based on maternal history and by serologic examination. Symptomatic congenital syphilis in infants is analogous in many respects to the secondary stage of syphilis. Clinical manifestations that appear in the first 2 years of life are designated as early, and those appearing after 2 years of age are designated as late. Signs and symptoms of *early congenital syphilis* include snuffles, mucous patches, and maculopapular rashes and condylomata lata. Bony lesions of early congenital syphilis are seen on radiographic examination. When infections are severe, visceral involvement and CNS and hematologic abnormalities may occur. Serologic tests can be nonreactive among infants infected late during their mother's pregnancy. Manifestations of *late congenital syphilis* include interstitial keratitis, *Hutchinson's teeth* (pegged lateral incisors and notched central incisors), deafness, osteitis, bone deformities, gummas, and neurosyphilis. If untreated, up to 40% of infants with congenital syphilis will die.

Diagnostic Testing

Diagnosis with darkfield microscopy of exudate from the chancres of primary syphilis and the mucocutaneous lesions of secondary syphilis and direct fluorescent antibody tests are the definitive methods for diagnosing syphilis. However, serologic tests are more convenient, economical, and the most frequently performed. There are two types: (1) *nontreponemal tests*, including the Venereal Disease Research Laboratory (VDRL) and rapid plasma reagin (RPR) tests, and (2) *treponemal tests*, including the fluorescent treponemal antibody-absorbed (FTA-ABS) test and microhemagglutination assay for antibody to *T. pallidum* (MHA-TP). The nontreponemal tests, VDRL and RPR, are nonspecific tests that measure *anticardiolipin antibodies*, sometimes referred to as *nontreponemal antibodies*, in serum. These antibodies are formed in response to changes in mammalian cells infected by *T. pallidum*. Nontreponemal tests are economical, easy to perform, and widely used for premarital testing, primary screening in pregnancy, military recruits, and individuals being incarcerated, as well as in clinics and offices for cases of suspected syphilis. The tests are also used for serial measurements of nontreponemal antibody titers to assess disease activity after therapy and are reported quantitatively. A nontreponemal test must demonstrate a fourfold change in titer, equivalent to a change of two dilutions (e.g., from 1:16 to 1:4 or from 1:32 to 1:8) to show a significant change in antibody activity, indicating response to treatment if falling or relapse if rising. Disadvantages of the nontreponemal tests are: (1) they do not become reactive until 4 to 6 weeks after infection; (2) they are nonreactive in about 25% of individuals with primary, late latent and tertiary disease; and (3) they have a false positive rate of up to 20%. A biologic false positive (BFP) can occur with a number of diseases, including acute viral illnesses, malaria, leprosy, malignancy, AIDS, and intravenous drug abuse, to name a few. This instance is why all reactive nontreponemal tests must be confirmed with a treponemal-specific test.

Treponemal tests are done to confirm that reactive nontreponemal serology is the result of *T. pallidum* infection. Falsely reactive treponemal tests occur in only about 1% of the general population. A person who has a reactive treponemal test will usually have it for life, unlike the nontreponemal tests that usually become negative within 2 years of treatment in primary and secondary syphilis. Treponemal test antibodies do no correlate with disease activity and should not be used to assess response to treatment.

Diagnosis of tertiary syphilis is based on a combination of serologic and other tests. These tests and results vary, depending on the manifestations of tertiary syphilis, whether it is benign tertiary syphilis of the skin, bone, and viscera, or whether it is cardiovascular syphilis or neurosyphilis. In general, VDRL is highly positive in the presence of gummatous lesions. VDRL is generally high in blood and cerebral spinal fluid (CSF) samples in neurosyphilis and variable in cardiovascular syphilis.

Treatment

Parenteral penicillin G is the drug of choice for therapy of all stages of syphilis. The susceptibility of *T. pallidum* to penicillin has not diminished since it was introduced for treatment in 1943. The dosage and length of treatment depend on the stage and clinical manifestations of disease. Penicillin G is the only therapy with documented efficacy for neurosyphilis or for syphilis during pregnancy. Persons in these two situations who report penicillin allergy should almost always undergo desensitization and be treated with penicillin. An acute febrile reaction accompanied by headache, myalgia, chills, tachycardia, and flushing, called *Jarisch-Herxheimer reaction*, may occur within the first 24 hours of the treatment of syphilis. Patients should be warned of this reaction when therapy is initiated. Sexual transmission of syphilis only occurs when lesions are present; however, generally, all sex partners of individuals with syphilis are treated presumptively. The most up-to-date information on treatment guidelines, including treatment in utero and penicillin dosages, is available in the CDC 1998 Guidelines for the Treatment of Sexually Transmitted Diseases and on the Internet at *www.cdc.gov*.

Bacterial Vaginosis

Bacterial vaginosis (BV) is a disturbance in the flora of the vaginal tract causing a thin, gray-white malodorous discharge. BV only affects women, and currently there is no evidence that it is transmitted sexually between heterosexual partners. BV is, however, associated with having multiple sex partners and has been cultured from the urethra of male partners of infected women. Lesbian partners have been shown to develop concordant vaginal secretion, and in the case of BV, this probably reflects sexual transmission in this group (Berger, 1995).

BV is caused by factors that alter the normal acidic environment of the vagina to an alkaline state that favors the overgrowth of alkaline-producing bacteria. *Lactobacilli acidophilus* are gram positive, rod-shaped bacteria that produce lactic acid from carbohydrates. Lactobacilli are the predominant bacteria of the vagina and help maintain the normal acidic pH of vaginal secretions. Factors that alter the pH through an alkalizing effect include cervical mucus, semen, menses, douching, antibiotic use, STIs, and hormonal changes of pregnancy and menopause (Keene, 1999). These factors may favor an overgrowth of *Gardnerella vaginalis*, *Mycoplasma hominis*, and anaerobic bacteria. Anaerobic bacterial metabolism results in an alkaline environment that inhibits the growth of lactobacillus and favors the other bacteria. BV has been associated with PID in infected women who underwent invasive procedures, such as endometrial biopsy, intrauterine device (IUD) insertion, and uterine curettage, while infected. BV has been clearly linked to preterm labor, preterm birth, and low birth weight.

Signs and Symptoms

Clinical presentation of BV includes the presence of a thin, white to gray malodorous discharge that adheres to the vaginal walls and introitus. There is no associated inflammation hence BV is a vaginosis rather than a vaginitis. BV is more of a disturbance in the vaginal environment than it is a true infection. Symptomatic women report a bad odor and often a mild itch and burning. Recurrent infections are common.

Diagnostic Testing

Diagnosis of BV is most often made based on clinical assessment and examination of vaginal fluids. Table 66-2 presents the Amsel criteria for the differential diagnosis of vaginal infections. The presence of three of the following four Amsel criteria are necessary for diagnosis: (1) a homogeneous, white, noninflammatory discharge coating the vaginal walls; (2) saline wet mount shows the presence of clue cells (Fig. 66-2, A); (3) vaginal fluid pH above 4.5; and (4) a positive "whiff test" (a fishy odor to vaginal fluids after the addition of 10% potassium hydroxide [KOH]). Because BV is not inflammatory, there is no increase in leukocytes on microscopic examination. Gram stain of vaginal fluids may be carried out with a diagnosis of BV based on the finding of a change from predominantly lactobacilli to a predominance of Gardnerella and anaerobic bacteria. Culture is not specific enough for diagnosis.

Treatment

Metronidazole and clindamycin, administered either orally or vaginally, are effective for the treatment of symptomatic BV. A 7-day regimen of oral metronidazole is more effective than single-dose therapy and is the preferred treatment. Treatment of sexual partners is not recommended because there is no data showing treatment reduces recurrence of infection (CDC, 1998). Treatment of asymptomatic women is controversial because up to

TABLE 66-2

Differential Diagnosis of Vaginal Infections

Diagnostic Criteria	Normal	Vulvovaginal Candidiasis	Bacterial Vaginosis	Trichomoniasis
Client Symptoms-Complaints	None	Itching, burning, discharge, dysuria	Foul odor, pruritus, discharge	Yellow-green discharge, odor, pruritus
Discharge	White, clear, flocculent	White, cottage cheese-like, increased	Thin, gray-white, increased	Frothy, yellow-green
Vaginal pH	3.8-4.2	<4.5	>4.5	>4.5
Amine odor	Absent	Absent	Bad, "fishy"	May have bad or "fishy" odor
Wet prep	Epithelial cells	Pseudohypha	Clue cells	Trichomonads
	Lactobacilli	Yeast buds	Positive whiff	May have positive whiff
	Few WBCs	Positive WBCs	Few WBCs	Positive WBCs

WBCs, White blood cells.

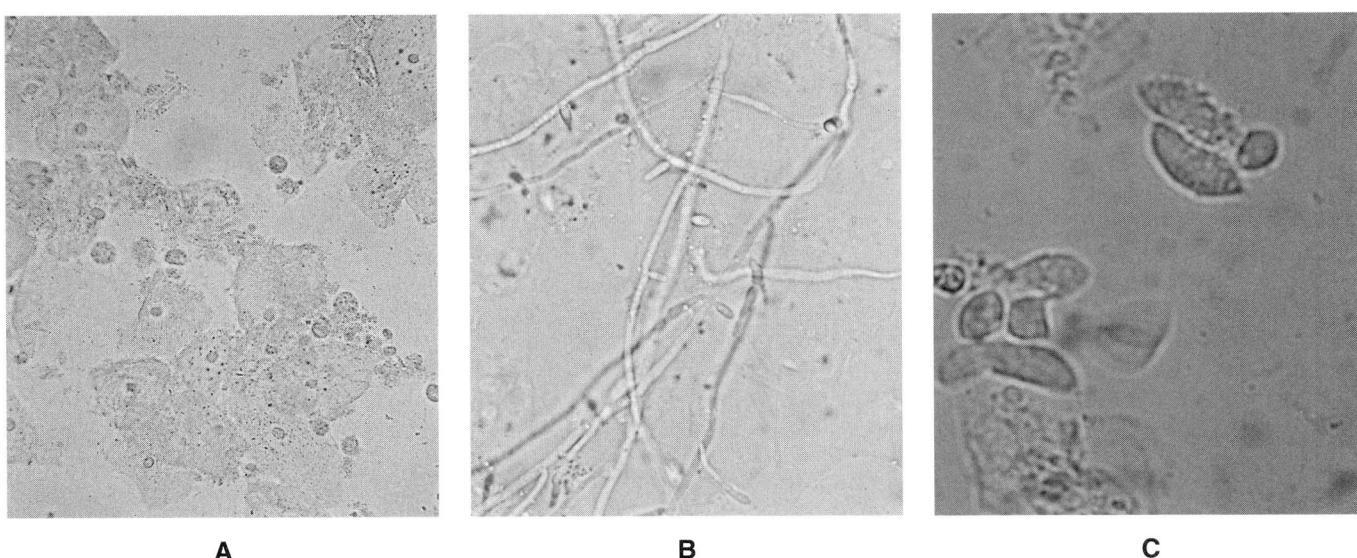

A   B   C

FIG. 66-2   Microscopic appearance of vaginal microorganisms. **A,** Bacterial vaginosis: "clue cells." **B,** Candida vulvovaginitis: "budding, branching hyphae." **C,** Trichomoniasis: "motile trichomonads." (From Zitelli BJ, Davis HW: *Atlas of pediatric physical diagnosis,* ed 4, St Louis, 2002, Mosby.)

70% of women develop recurrent BV infections within 3 months of therapy (Sobel, 1993). Schwebke (2000) found a low response rate to treatment in asymptomatic women and a 21% incidence of vaginal candidiasis after treatment of BV in asymptomatic women in the study group. Thus many women were trading an asymptomatic condition for a symptomatic infection. BV has been associated with preterm labor and birth; therefore treatment is usually recommended for pregnant women at high risk for these conditions. Clindamycin vaginal cream has been associated with preterm birth and is not recommended for use in pregnancy (Joesoef, 1999).

Lymphogranuloma Venereum, Chancroid, and Granuloma Inguinale

Lymphogranuloma venereum, chancroid, and granuloma inguinale infections are uncommon in the United States but, with global travel, need to be kept in mind when confronted with a genital ulcer. All of these infections cause ulcerative lesions that need to be differentiated from the more familiar ulcers caused by syphilis and herpes simplex virus. Treatment options for these conditions are available in the CDC 1998 Guidelines for Treatment of Sexually Transmitted Diseases.

Lymphogranuloma venereum (LGV) is caused by serovars of *C. trachomatis.* LGV is also known as *Durand-Nicolas-Favre disease, tropical bubo,* and *lymphogranuloma inguinale.* LGV occurs in most areas of the world, but most cases are concentrated in tropical and subtropical areas. Local epidemics and sporadic cases number between 200 and 400 annually in the United States. *C. trachomatis* cannot penetrate intact skin or mucus membranes but gains access through minor lacerations or abrasions. The primary lesion is a small, painless herpetiform vesicle or ulcer, usually on the posterior vaginal wall in women and on the coronal sulcus of the penis in men. The lesion is present for only a few days and heals without scarring. The infection is then carried through the lymphatics to the regional lymph nodes. The nodes swell and form exquisitely tender masses from which abscesses develop that may erode through the skin to form sinus tracts. Infections last from weeks to months and may be severe enough to cause obstruction of lymph vessels, resulting in chronic edema.

LGV presents with highly variable symptoms from mild to severe infections. The most common clinical manifestation of LGV among heterosexuals is tender, unilateral inguinal lymphadenopathy. Anal-receptive intercourse can cause proctocolitis and inflammatory involvement of perirectal or perianal lymphatic tissues, resulting in fistulas and strictures. Spontaneous remission of symptoms is common. Diagnosis of LGV is made serologically and by exclusion of other causes of genital ulcers and inguinal lymphadenopathy.

The gram-negative bacillus *Haemophilus ducreyi* is the most common cause of genital ulcer disease in developing countries; it also occurs as isolated cases in industrialized societies and is spread by people who have traveled to endemic areas. *H. ducreyi* causes a *chancroid (soft chancre)* beginning 4 to 10 days after exposure. The classic chancroidal ulcer begins as a small, tender, erythematous papule that ulcerates within 24 hours. The ulcer is characterized by a purulent dirty gray base and moderate to severe painful inguinal lymphadenopathy (Ronald, 1999). Diagnosis can be made by identifying *H. ducreyi* grown on a special culture medium not readily available commercially. A probable diagnosis can be made based on the following criteria: (1) the presence of one or more painful genital ulcers; (2) no evidence of *T. pallidum* by darkfield examination or serologic testing after onset of ulcers; and (3) appearance of genital ulcers and regional lymphadenopathy typical for chancroid (CDC, 1998). Serologic and PCR tests are not presently available.

Granuloma inguinale, also known as *donovanosis*, is a progressive inflammatory disease of the genital, inguinal, and perianal regions with low infectivity and morbidity. Most cases are sexually transmitted. The causative organism is *Calymmatobacterium granulomatis*, a gram-negative intracellular bacterium. The incidence is low in developed countries, but it is seen in the southeastern United States. Granuloma inguinale begins as one or more small, firm, indurated papules at the site of contact, which, over several days to weeks, ulcerates. Primary ulcers are bright, beefy-red, painless, and noninflammatory and involve no lymphadenopathy. Pain, exudate, and inguinal lymphadenopathy characterize secondary infections. The most common sites for lesions in women are the labia minora and fourchette and, in men, the foreskin and glans penis. Identifying Donovan bodies (the bacillus found in mononuclear cells) in smears or biopsy confirms the diagnosis.

VIRAL INFECTIONS

Herpes Simplex Virus

Herpes simplex virus (HSV) is an infectious viral disease with an affinity for the skin, mucus membranes and nervous system. HSV-1 and HSV-2 are two of the eight herpes viruses that infect humans and of the approximately 100 herpes viruses that have been identified (Pertel, 1999). HSV-1 typically infects the oropharyngeal area, causing facial, oral, and lip lesions, although it may be the cause of primary genital herpes. HSV-2 is the usual cause of genital herpes infections, causing most of the lesions in the genital area. HSV is not curable. Infections are usually mild and self-limiting in immunocompetent individuals. In immunocompromised individuals and newborns, however, HSV infections can be fatal. A primary HSV-2 infection in the first half of pregnancy is associated with spontaneous abortion and congenital defects.

HSV is spread through direct contact of the virus with the mucosa or any break in the skin. The herpes virus cannot live outside a moist environment and spread of infection other than by direct contact is unlikely. HSV has the ability to invade a wide range of cells by direct fusion with the cell membrane. Endocytosis of the virus is not required for entry (Pertel, 1999). HSV-1 and HSV-2 are chronic infections characterized by periods of active infection and latency. In primary active infections, viruses invade host cells and rapidly replicate, destroying the host cells and releasing more virions to infect adjacent cells. The virus spreads via the lymphatics to regional lymph nodes in primary infections, causing lymphadenopathy. The body mounts a cell-mediated and humoral immune response that contains the primary infection but does not prevent recurrence of active infection. After the initial infection, a period of latency begins. During this time, the virus enters the sensory nerve cells that supply the infected area and migrate along their axons to settle in the dorsal root ganglia where they exist without cytotoxicity or symptoms in their human host (Pertel, 1999). It is important to note that infective virions can be shed during latent periods and during active phases.

It is estimated that 45 million people in the United States are infected with HSV of the genital tract and an additional 1 million people become infected each year. Because HSV cannot be cured, the percentage of people infected increases with age. Approximately 1 of 4 women and 1 of 5 men are infected with genital herpes (CDC, 2000). Susceptibility to herpes infections varies. HSV is more common in women than with men, probably because of the larger mucosal area of the female genital tract and the occurrence of micro tears in the mucosa during sexual intercourse. Compared with the general population, people infected with HIV are more susceptible to HSV infections and more infectious to others once the virus is acquired. HSV-1 seropositive individuals appear to have some protection from acquisition of HSV-2 (Boardman, 2000). Because HSV infections are not life threatening and are often mild or asymptomatic, many people are unaware of the magnitude of this disease.

Signs and Symptoms

HSV infections are classified as initial primary, initial nonprimary, recurrent and asymptomatic, or unrecognized. Initial primary infections typically begin 2 to 7 days following intimate contact with an infected individual. Systemic symptoms, including fever, malaise, and headache, usually precede the outbreak of lesions by several days and occur in about two thirds of women and one third of men. HSV lesions begin as small, grouped erythematous papules that progress from clear fluid-filled vesicles, to pustules, to painful ulcerations. The most common sites are the labia and mons in women and the penile glans and shaft in men (see color plates 42 and 43). Contiguous skin sites can be involved, particularly on the buttocks, thighs, urethra, and perianal areas, or these may be the only sites involved. Herpes lesions cause localized severe pain in most people, and more than one half have accompanying dysuria. Dysuria may be caused by urine contacting ulcers within the urethra or from contact with external lesions. Crusting and reepithelization of lesions occur over a period of 2 to 6 weeks. Tender, bilateral inguinal lymphadenopathy occurs in most primary infections of the genital tract.

Other manifestations of primary herpes infections include cervicitis, proctitis, and pharyngitis. Herpes-induced cervicitis occurs in most women, resulting in complaints of vaginal discharge and intermittent bleeding. A red, friable, ulcerated cervix is observed on examination. Vaginal mucosal lesions occur in less than 10% of cases. Cervical and vaginal lesions may easily go unrecognized by a woman. Herpetic proctitis is more common in men who engage in rectal intercourse. The infection may be present with or without other genital herpes lesions. Severe pain, bloody or mucopurulent discharge, constipation, fever, and malaise are the chief signs and symptoms. Herpetic pharyngitis may be present in up to 20% of cases of primary genital herpes. Pain and a red, erythematous pharynx with ulceration and sometimes white exudate characterize the infection. Herpetic pharyngitis can be easily misdiagnosed as streptococcal pharyngitis on observation. Autoinoculation may result in involvement of remote areas, such as the fingers, and is believed to be the cause of most extragenital lesions.

Initial nonprimary genital herpes is a primary HSV-2 infection in persons who are seropositive for HSV-1 antibodies. Prior infection with HSV-1 has been shown to confer partial immunity to HSV-2. Symptoms of initial nonprimary genital herpes are much milder and shorter in duration compared with primary infections.

Recurrent episodes of genital herpes vary based on severity of the primary infection, sex, age, strain (HSV-1 or HSV-2), and a mix of other individual factors. If HSV-1 is the cause of symptomatic primary genital infections, 40% to 50% of people have recurrence within 1 year; with HSV-2, the recurrence rate is over 90% during the first year (Benedetti, 1999). Women experience more recurrences than do men. Typically, infected individuals will have five to eight episodes per year. Occasionally, a person will have symptoms with their primary infection and then never again. The more severe the primary infection is, the greater the frequency and severity of recurrent infections will be (Pertel, 1999). Recurrence has been associated with menses, sexual activity, and stress.

Recurrent herpes episodes are milder and shorter (5 to 10 days) than are primary infections. About one half of the people with recurrences will experience a prodrome of burning or itching at the site of developing lesions. Recurrent vesicles and ulcers are infectious, and two thirds of people with prodromal symptoms will shed infectious virus even if no lesions develop. Systemic symptoms are usually absent, and lesions, which tend to occur unilaterally in the same areas, are fewer and smaller compared

with primary infections. Dysuria occurs in 25% of women and 10% of men. Recurrent infections decrease over time in most individuals but one third of infected people will experience no decrease in recurrence rates (Benedetti, 1999; Corey, 2000).

Most individuals recognize the infective nature of herpes lesions but are not aware that viral shedding occurs without symptoms. Studies have shown that individuals infected with HSV-2, even in the absence of lesions or symptoms, will shed virions on 3% to 30% of days (DiCarlo, 1999; Johnson, 2000). In addition, most HSV-2 infections are subclinical, with less than one fifth of persons infected with HSV-2 reporting symptoms that would be recognized as HSV (Johnson, 2000). Most asymptomatic infections are discovered when a recurrent infection presents during physical examination or through antibody titer screening. With symptom education, many asymptomatic individuals will be able to identify recurrent infections. Some individuals, however, have no symptoms or such mild symptoms or atypical lesions that infection cannot be identified except through antibody titer. Nearly 80% of HSV transmission occurs during asymptomatic shedding of the virus (Boardman, 2000).

Diagnostic Testing

In most cases, genital herpes can be diagnosed clinically during acute and recurrent infections. Viral culture of vesicles or pustules was the gold standard for diagnosis before DNA-amplification testing became available. Cultures taken from crusted lesions and recurrent infections were less sensitive, resulting in frequent false-negative tests. DNA amplification is more accurate, virus-specific, and expensive compared with cultures. Antigen detection by EIA or direct fluorescence tests is available, rapid, and economical. Serum antibody tests are not useful because they cannot reliably distinguish type, and there is not a significant change in titers between acute and chronic states. Genital herpes is associated with abnormalities in Papanicolaou (Pap) smears, although they are not diagnostic. The frequency of asymptomatic and nontypical infections makes screening of high-risk groups desirable.

Treatment

Because HSV infections are not curable, treatment is aimed at symptom control and decreasing viral shedding. Nucleoside analogue antiviral medications are the recommended treatment. These drugs act by deactivating or antagonizing HSV DNA polymerase, which, in turn, stops DNA synthesis and viral replication. The three antiviral medications that are recommended by the 1998 CDC guidelines are acyclovir, famciclovir, and valacyclovir. Antiviral medications need to be started at the first sign of recurrence to decrease and shorten symptoms. If medication is delayed until skin lesions appear, symptoms are shortened by only 1 day. People with 6 or more recurrences per year should be offered daily suppressive therapy that can reduce the frequency of recurrences by about 75% (CDC, 1998). Suppressive therapy reduces but does not eliminate asymptomatic viral shedding. Topical treatment with antiviral creams or ointments has not proven to be effective. Suppressive or prophylaxis therapy has been recommended to reduce the risk of perinatal infection and the need for cesarean section in HSV-positive women (Boardman, 2000). Vaccines for the prevention of HSV-2 are being tested.

Human Papillomavirus

The *human papillomavirus (HPV)* is a small DNA pathogen that induces a variety of benign tumors (warts) and several premalignant and malignant lesions. Little is known about the life cycle of the HPVs because they have not been sufficiently propagated in tissue culture. Over 100 HPV subtypes have been identified, 33 of which are known to infect the anogenital tract (Richart, 2000). These viruses are able to bind with a wide range of cells, and various subtypes show preference for particular anatomic sites. HPV infections can lead to cervical, penile, and anal cancers. Most cervical cancers can be linked to HPV. HPV types 6 and 11 cause the majority of genital warts and are not associated with malignancy. HPV types 16, 18, 31, 33, 35, 51, 52, and 58 are associated with *cervical intraepithelial neoplasia (CIN)* and present an intermediate risk for cervical cancer. HPV-16 and HPV-18 are highly oncogenic (Lombard, 1998).

HPV is highly contagious and is the most common STI in the United States. An estimated 5.5 million people become infected every year, and an estimated 75% of people will be infected with genital HPV during their lifetime (CDC, 2000). Transmission of genital HPV is almost exclusively through sexual contact, although autoinoculation and fomite transmission is possible. Infection can be transmitted to the neonate during birth. The greatest risk factor for developing HPV is the number of sex partners. Smoking, use of oral contraceptives (OCs), and pregnancy appears to increase susceptibility to HPV infection. Most HPV infections will resolve and become undetectable within 2 years. It is unclear whether the virus is eliminated or just subclinical. Regardless, immunity appears to be type-specific, thus the individual is still susceptible to infection with other types of HPV.

Signs and Symptoms

Most HPV infections are subclinical and therefore go undetected. Only about 5% of infected people develop genital warts. The 1998 American Medical Association consensus conference identified four morphologic types of genital warts: (1) *condylomata acuminata* are soft, cauliflowerlike exophytic lesions found most often on moist, partially keratinized epithelium (see color plates 44 and 45); (2) papular warts are dome-shaped lesions found on fully keratinized skin; (3) keratotic warts have a thick horny layer, resemble common skin warts, and appear on keratinized skin; and (4) flat-topped papules that appear macular to slightly raised on fully or partially keratinized skin. Genital warts are usually painless and cause no problems for the infected individual other than being unsightly and embarrassing. Lack of uncomfortable symptoms unfortunately masks the serious aspects of the infection. In women, external lesions typically appear on the introitus, vulva, and perineum and, in men, on the penis, scrotum, and urinary meatus; both sexes are affected perianally. Internal lesions can be found on the vaginal wall and cervix in women and in both sexes within the rectum after anoreceptive intercourse. Laryn-

geal papillomatosis can occur with ororeceptive intercourse. Lesions are frequently found in several locations at one time and with other genital infections. The actual appearances of warts, if they occur, can vary from weeks to months after exposure.

Individuals who are immunocompromised, on chronic immunosuppressive therapy, or pregnant tend to develop very large wart clusters. Cesarean section is not recommended for HPV infected women unless the birth canal is obstructed; however, laryngeal papillomatosis may develop in 2% to 5% of exposed infants (Boardman, 2000; Thomas, 2001).

The vast majority of individuals with HPV infections have no symptoms. Disease may be found by colposcopy and cytology in women and by biopsy in either sex. The routine Pap smear is one of the most frequent means of discovering asymptomatic infections in women.

Diagnostic Testing

Most symptomatic HPV infections, those causing warts, can be diagnosed clinically. Asymptomatic HPV is suspected in the presence of characteristic koilocytic changes on Pap smears and cervical biopsy. DNA hybridization detects HPV DNA in endocervical or urethral swabs and tissues in most cases of genital warts and HPV causing cervical cancers. Liquid-based cytology allows screening for cervical dysplasia and cancer and later use of the same specimen for HPV testing. Liquid-based cytology is more expensive and accurate for detection of cervical dysplasia than is the traditional Pap smear. Routine screening for HPV at the time of Pap smear would decrease unnecessary colposcopy and biopsy, as well as the human worry and uncertainty associated with cervical abnormalities of undetermined significance. If this screening technique becomes the standard of care, then it will be included in health insurance programs.

Treatment

Warts caused by HPV may be treated topically and by surgical excision, cryotherapy, and intralesional interferon injections. The most common topical preparations are podophyllin resin, podofilox, imiquimod, and trichloroacetic acid (TCA). Podofilox and imiquimod have the advantage in that they can be self-administered. TCA treatment can be painful and cause scarring; however, it is cheap and can be used during pregnancy. Surgery is a good choice for individuals who want immediate removal, have very large lesions, or have lesions that have not responded to topical treatment. Cryotherapy with liquid nitrogen or nitrous oxide can cause pain and may require more than one treatment. Interferon injections are not usually used because of systemic side effects and the need for frequent visits to a provider (Riehart, 2000). Clearance rates are similar for most of the usual treatment options; however, actual rates are hard to determine because the definition of recurrence varies widely (Koutsky, 1999).

Treatment education should include the following points: (1) treatment may remove warts but does not ensure that the person is not infectious; (2) condoms reduce but do not eliminate the risk of HPV transmission because the virus can live on adjacent skin surfaces; (3) smoking decreases immune function and contributes to

HPV-associated cervical cancer; and (4) lifestyle practices that enhance an individual's immune system decrease the risk of cancer from HPV (Thomas, 2001). Currently, abstinence and a lifelong mutually monogamous relationship are the best protection against HPV infection.

FUNGAL INFECTIONS

Candida Albicans

Candida albicans is a species of candidiasis found normally in the mouth, throat, intestine, and skin of healthy men and women and commonly in the vagina of asymptomatic women. *C. albicans* is the causative species in over 80% of genital candidiasis infections. An overgrowth of *C. albicans* is the most frequent cause of vaginitis and vulvovaginitis in women. *C. glabrata* and *C. tropicalis* are two other species associated with vulvovaginitis in women. Up to 75% of women can expect to have at least one vulvovaginal candidiasis in their lifetime, and 40% to 45% will have recurrent infections (CDC, 1998). Candidiasis is not strictly speaking considered to be transmitted sexually; however, *C. albicans* can be cultured from the penis of 20% of male partners of women with recurrent candidiasis vulvovaginitis (Sobel, 1999).

Symptomatic infections occur when there is a change in host resistance or local bacterial flora. Predisposing factors in women are pregnancy, menstruation, diabetes mellitus, contraceptive use, and antibiotic therapy. Tight, constrictive, synthetic underclothing that creates a warm, moist environment for colonization, has been implicated in recurrent infections. Hypersensitive reactions to products such as douches, deodorant sprays, and scented and colored toilet tissue may also contribute to colonization in some individuals (Faro, 1997). Most commonly, women become infected secondary to one of the predisposing factors that cause organism overgrowth. Men most commonly acquire infection from sexual contact with women who have vaginal candidiasis. In both sexes, immunodeficiency diseases and immunosuppressive drugs greatly increase the risk of colony overgrowth in all areas that harbor candidiasis. Individuals with persistent intractable episodes of candidiasis should be tested for HIV infection.

Signs and Symptoms

The most prominent symptom of yeast vulvovaginitis in women is intense vulvar and vaginal pruritus and irritation. Vulvar edema, erythema, and fissures may occur, with dysuria secondary to inflamed tissue (external dysuria). A curdlike, "cottage cheese" vaginal discharge is often present. Internal pelvic examination reveals a dry, bright red vagina with adherent white plaques.

Men harboring *C. albicans* are often asymptomatic. When symptoms occur, the most common signs are an erythematous, "glazed skin" appearance on the penis and erosions of the glans or inner surface of the prepuce. Symptomatic infections in men cause varying degrees of balanoposthitis, resulting in itching, burning, and irritation of the glans and prepuce. Lesions appear crusted and adherent, and white cheesy patches may appear on the glans. Occasionally, the scrotal skin has scaling, pruritic

lesions. *Phimosis*, stenosis of the preputial orifice so that the foreskin cannot be pushed back over the glans penis, is a complication of candidal balanoposthitis. Candidiasis infections are more virulent in immunocompromised men.

Diagnostic Testing

History and clinical findings in conjunction with microscopic assessment is sufficient for diagnosis of candidiasis in most individuals (see Table 66-2). Microscopic examination of vaginal discharge in a 10% KOH solution will show the branching hyphae and budding characteristic of candidiasis (see Fig. 66-2, *B*). This test is diagnostic in 65% to 85% of symptomatic women (Sobel, 1999). The vagina maintains a normal pH of 4.0 to 4.5 during candidiasis infections. Vaginal cultures should be performed on symptomatic women when microscopy results are negative and on all women with recurrent candidiasis. A positive culture in asymptomatic women, however, should not lead to treatment because *C. albicans* is commensal in the vagina in many women.

Treatment

Genital candidiasis may be treated with topical or oral therapy. Azole drugs are 80% to 90% effective in patients that complete therapy (CDC, 1998). Topical agents effective against *C. albicans* can be purchased over the counter (OTC). A study by Ferris et al (1996), however, showed that only 35% of women previously diagnosed with genital candidiasis were able to correctly diagnose classic symptoms, and they were more likely to use OTC products inappropriately. This method can prove dangerous if it causes a delay in treatment of serious infections. Recurrent infections may be treated with combinations of topical and oral preparations. Recurrent vulvovaginal candidiasis is defined as four or more symptomatic infections within a year. Treatment of male partners of women with recurrent infection has shown no benefit in reducing recurrent infections (Sobel, 1999). Some success has also been reported in women taking oral yogurt daily and hyposensitization with *C. albicans* antigen preparations (Hilton, 1992; Rigg, 1990).

PROTOZOAN INFECTIONS

Trichomoniasis Vaginalis

Trichomoniasis is caused by the protozoan parasite *Trichomonas vaginalis*. The trichomonads of *T. vaginalis* are oval flagellated organisms about the size of a leukocyte (see Fig. 66-2, *C*). The organisms are propelled by flagella moving erratically in a twitching motion. Trichomonads bind to and eventually kill host epithelial cells, causing a humoral and secretory immune response that is not protective against repeated infection. Trichomonads are dependent on direct contact with erythrocytes for survival, and this may explain why women are more susceptible to infection then are men. *T. vaginalis* grows best between a pH of 4.9 and 7.5; therefore conditions that raise vaginal pH, such as menses, pregnancy, use of oral contraceptives, and frequent douching, predispose women to trichomoniasis. Female infants born to infected mothers may develop *T. vaginalis* infections. Female infants are susceptible because of the influence of maternal hormones on the epithelium of the infant's vagina. Over several weeks, as maternal hormones are metabolized, the infant's vaginal epithelium becomes resistant to *T. vaginalis*, and infections resolve even without treatment (Krieger, 1999).

It is estimated that there are 5 million cases of *T. vaginalis* infections annually in the United States. *T. vaginalis* infections are transmitted almost exclusively by sexual intercourse. Although trichomonads have been known to survive up to 45 minutes on fomites, this mode of transmission is extremely rare. Risk for *T. vaginalis* infection increases with number of sex partners and years of sexual activity.

Signs and Symptoms

Symptoms of trichomoniasis typically occur 5 to 28 days after inoculation in women and as early as 1 day in men. *T. vaginalis* produces symptomatic infections in 20% to 50% of women. The most common symptoms in women are a frothy yellow-green vaginal discharge that may be profuse and foul smelling, perineal pruritus, postcoital bleeding, and dyspareunia. Pelvic examination is characterized by discharge, marked inflammation of the vaginal epithelium, and cervical petechiae, commonly referred to as a strawberry cervix. If untreated, symptoms may resolve, but infections may persist subclinically. Most male sexual partners of women infected with *T. vaginalis* will carry the organism in the urethra. Males are more likely to become symptomatic soon after inoculation with signs of mild to severe urethritis characterized by discharge, dysuria, and urinary frequency. Symptoms in males are more often transient, probably because of the protective presence of antitrichomonal substances in prostatic secretions (Krieger, 1999). There is no evidence of severe complications or long-term sequelae from untreated *T. vaginalis* infections.

Diagnostic Testing

The presence of elevated vaginal pH, amine odor, and yellow-green frothy vaginal discharge is highly suspicious for *T. vaginalis* in women (see Table 66-2). Diagnosis based on symptoms alone, however, is not reliable because of the variety of symptoms and asymptomatic infections. In men, symptoms do not vary significantly from other organisms causing urethritis. Observation of trichomonads in saline wet mounts on microscopic examination of secretions can rule in but not rule out infection. Likewise, Pap smear–detected *T. vaginalis* is not reliable because of a high percentage of false-positive and false-negative reports. Culture is the gold standard for diagnosis; however, treatment is frequently instituted based on clinical findings.

Treatment

Metronidazole taken orally is highly effective in eradicating *T. vaginalis* from all sites and is the only oral medication available in the United States for the treatment of trichomoniasis (CDC, 1998). Pregnant women can be treated with metronidazole in a single dose. All sexual partners should be treated before intercourse is resumed.

NONSPECIFIC INFLAMMATORY INFECTIONS OF THE GENITAL TRACT

Infections can occur in any of the reproductive organs and structures. Inflammatory infections of the genital tract are diagnosed in general terms adding "itis" to the organ or structure until a specific infectious agent is identified. Infections in both men and women follow a normal ascent from lower to upper structures. Infections that reach the peritoneal cavity in women and the epididymis in men usually have infected the other structures along the way. Women with peritonitis will usually have cervicitis, endometritis, and salpingo-oophoritis. Men with infectious epididymitis will often have urethritis and prostatitis.

Cervicitis

Cervicitis, which is an inflammatory condition of the cervix, is divided into two distinct syndromes. *Endocervicitis* is an inflammation of the mucous membranes of the cervical canal most frequently caused by *C. trachomatis* and *N. gonorrhoeae*. *Ectocervicitis* is inflammation of the stratified epithelium of the cervix and is most often caused by *T. vaginalis*, *C. albicans*, and human papillomavirus. Cervicitis alone is usually asymptomatic for women. Other symptoms of the specific infectious organism causing the cervicitis would bring a woman in for treatment, for example, the pruritus associated with *C. albicans* infections. Clinical examination of the cervix shows an erythematous, friable cervix, with or without discharge. The presence of mucopurulent discharge at the os is more suggestive of *C. trachomatis*- and *N. gonorrhoeae*-caused cervicitis. *Cervical motion tenderness (CMT)* on palpation is a classic sign for not only cervicitis, but PID as well. Cervicitis must be carefully differentiated from PID, a much more serious infection. Diagnosis and treatment are based on clinical and laboratory findings. If there were a strong suspicion of a particular STI being the cause, treatment would be started before the laboratory data is completed.

Pelvic Inflammatory Disease

PID is a general term used for inflammatory disorders of the upper female genital tract. More precisely, PID includes any combination of endometritis, salpingitis, tubo-ovarian abscess and pelvic peritonitis (CDC, 1998). PID is caused almost exclusively by *N. gonorrhea* and *C. trachomatis*; however, other organisms that are part of the normal vaginal flora have been implicated. It is believed that these organisms are contributory rather than causative (Hemsel, 2001). Infections with *N. gonorrhoeae*, *C. trachomatis*, or both disrupt the normal defenses, allowing the ascent of a variety of infective agents, resulting in an endogenous superinfection (Hemsel, 2001). PID is a serious potentially life-threatening disease and a frequent cause of infertility, pelvic pain, and ectopic pregnancy. About 20% of women become infertile and 10% of those who do conceive have an ectopic pregnancy, and 20% of women develop chronic pain (Ross, 2001).

There are approximately 1 million cases of PID diagnosed annually. Adolescents are at special risk for PID be-

CDC Diagnostic Criteria for PID

MINIMAL CRITERIA (ALL MUST BE PRESENT)
- Lower abdominal tenderness
- Adnexal tenderness
- Cervical motion tenderness

SUPPORTIVE CRITERIA
- Fever greater than 101° F (38.3° C)
- Elevated erythrocyte sedimentation rate
- Elevated C-reactive protein
- Laboratory documented cervical infection with *N. gonor-rhoeae* or *C. trachomatis*

DEFINITIVE CRITERIA
- Histopathologic evidence of endometritis on endometrial biopsy
- Test showing thickened fluid-filled tubes or tubo-ovarian abscess (or both)
- Laparoscopic abnormalities consistent with PID

CDC and I-IDSOG-USA Criteria for Hospitalization for Treatment of PID

- Possible surgical emergencies cannot be ruled out
- Pregnancy
- Failure to respond to outpatient treatment within 48 hours
- Known or suspected inability to comply with treatment
- Severe illness with nausea and vomiting and/or fever greater than 38.5° C
- Intrauterine device
- Tubo-ovarian or pelvic abscess
- Immunodeficiency
- Adolescent

cause of the concentration of chlamydia infections and delays in treatment in this age group. Other risk factors include prior history of STIs and PID, multiple sexual partners, coitus during menses, cigarette smoking, and use of an IUD. The ascent of the causative organisms occurs most readily during menses.

Signs and symptoms of PID vary widely. The most common presenting symptoms are lower abdominal pain with guarding, abnormal bleeding or discharge, and dyspareunia. Pelvic examination reveals abdominal tenderness, cervical and uterine motion tenderness, mucopurulent cervical discharge, and adnexal tenderness. It must be remembered that many cases of PID remain mild and undetected until severe infection has occurred with resultant inflammation and scarring.

Box 66-1 summarizes the CDC diagnostic criteria for PID. Minimum criteria for a diagnosis of PID include lower abdominal tenderness, adnexal tenderness, and cervical motion tenderness. Other causes of symptoms, such as ectopic pregnancy, ovarian cysts, and appendicitis, must be ruled out. Despite the potential severity and the serious sequelae of PID, many women present with vague symptoms, making a clear-cut diagnosis difficult.

Broad-spectrum antibiotic therapy should be instituted promptly to reduce serious sequelae. Therapy should be effective against all of the most likely pathogens, *N. gonorrhoeae*, *C. trachomatis*, anaerobes, gram-negative facultative bacteria, and streptococci. The International-Infectious Disease Society for Obstetrics and Gynecology-USA (I-IDSOG-USA) recommends hospitalization for all infected adolescents and a more precise treatment plan based on a four-level staging criteria (Hemsel, 2001). Box 66-2 summaries the CDC and I-IDSOG-USA recommended guidelines for hospitalization for the treatment of PID.

Urethritis

Urethritis is an inflammation of the urethra from any cause and is much more common in males than in females. Urethritis is most frequently caused by an infectious organism but can also be caused by allergic reactions to substances such as latex and lotions. Urethritis and dysuria are frequent secondary symptoms in persons with HSV and HPV infections.

Infectious urethritis is classified as either gonococcal urethritis or nongonococcal urethritis (NGU) depending on the causative organism. Gonococcal urethritis is caused by *N. gonorrhoeae* and is characterized by dysuria and mucopurulent discharge. Any number of organisms, most frequently *C. trachomatis*, *Ureaplasma urealyticum*, Mycoplasma genitalium, and *T. vaginalis* may cause NGU. NGU infections are less invasive and symptoms less severe than is gonococcal urethritis. Individuals may be asymptomatic or have mild dysuria and discharge. All at-risk individuals with urethritis should be tested for gonorrhea and chlamydia infection and presumptive treatment initiated. If symptoms do not resolve with treatment, investigation of less frequent causes should be pursued.

Prostatitis

Prostatitis, which is inflammation of the prostate, can be acute or chronic, and the cause can be either bacterial or nonbacterial. Most bacterial infections of the prostate are caused by gram-negative organisms, most commonly *E. coli*. Other causative organisms are enterococci, staphylococci, streptococci, *C. trachomatis*, *U. uralyticum*, and *N. gonorrhoeae*. Bacterial prostatic infections can be the result of previous or concurrent urethral infection with direct ascent of bacteria from the urethra through the prostatic ducts in the prostate, reflux of urine from an infected bladder, or hematogenous spread.

Acute bacterial prostatitis causes fevers as high as 39° to 40° C, chills, malaise, low back pain, perineal pain, dysuria, urethral spasm, and marked suprapubic tenderness. Rectal examination will find the prostate tender, swollen, warm, and boggy. Massage of the prostate should be avoided during rectal examination because pain and the risk of spread of infection to the epididymis by expressed fluid. Severe acute prostatitis warrants hospitalization.

Chronic bacterial prostatitis is a major cause of recurrent urinary tract infections in men. Symptoms are dysuria, urgency, frequency, and pain in the back, perineal, and suprapubic area. Palpation of the prostate gland by rectal examination may be normal. Often the individual is asymptomatic until significant bacteriuria develops. Frequently there is recurrent symptomatic cystitis, which resolves with treatment but then reoccurs. This characteristic is caused by the persistence of the organism in the prostate resulting from poor penetration to the area by oral antibiotics. Suppressive antimicrobial therapy may result in complete symptomatic relief, but cure rates are inconsistent. Local injection of antimicrobials is no more effective than is oral or parenteral treatment (Stern, 2001). Chronic nonbacterial prostatitis causes similar symptoms, but no causative organism can be found. Therapy is aimed at symptom relief in the case of chronic bacterial prostatitis that does not respond to antibiotics and for chronic nonbacterial prostatitis.

Epididymitis

Epididymitis is an inflammatory response of the epididymis to infection or trauma. Infections are classified as *nonspecific bacterial epididymitis* or *sexually transmitted epididymitis*. Infection spreads from an established urethritis or prostatitis to the epididymitis. Among sexually active men less than 35 years of age, *C. trachomatis* or *N. gonorrhoeae* most often causes epididymitis. *E. Coli* is a common cause of infection in men who practice anal intercourse with same-sex or heterosexual partners. Nonspecific bacterial epididymitis occurs more frequently in men over 35 years of age who have an underlying pathologic condition, such as urinary tract infections, anatomical anomalies, or recent instrumentation or surgery. Epididymitis may occur with testicular cancer, therefore this rare but possible cause must not be overlooked.

The most common sign of epididymitis is scrotal pain, erythema, and swelling. Symptoms are usually unilateral but may be bilateral. Hydrocele, urethral discharge, dysuria, frequency, and urgency are frequent accompanying symptoms. Testicular torsion may occur and is a surgical emergency. Symptoms may occur over 1 to 2 days or develop more gradually. Both testicular torsion and testicular cancer are rare in men over 40 years of age.

Laboratory tests to identify the causative organism include (1) gram-stained smear of urethral exudate for urethritis and presumptive gonorrhea, (2) culture of urethral exudate or first-void urine for chlamydia and gonorrhea, and (3) urinalysis for detection of bacteria. Transillumination of the testicle may be helpful in determining whether swelling is the result of a solid mass or fluid. Cysts and hydroceles associated with epididymitis transilluminate.

Antibiotic treatment should be initiated before the return of cultures. When chlamydia or gonorrhea is the most likely cause of infection, the CDC recommends initiating treatment for both infections. Supportive symptomatic therapy is bed rest, scrotal support, ice packs, and analgesics.

Orchitis

Orchitis is inflammation of the testes; in combination with epididymitis, it is called *epididymoorchitis* and is a serious complication of epididymitis. Orchitis differs from other infections of the genital tract in two ways: (1) the major route of infection is hematogenous, and (2) viruses are the most common organisms to cause orchitis. Mumps orchitis is the most common viral infection encountered, although the incidence of mumps orchitis has decreased with mumps immunization. Twenty to thirty percent of mumps cases in adults are complicated by orchitis. In pubertal and adult males, there is usually seminiferous tubule damage with risk for infertility and, in some cases, damage to Leydig's cells with resultant testosterone deficiency and hypogonadism. Mumps orchitis rarely occurs in prepubertal males, but when it does, testicular dysfunction is rare. Other causes of viral orchitis are Coxsackie B virus, varicella, and mononucleosis.

Signs and symptoms of orchitis range from mild testicular pain and edema to severe testicular pain and marked edema about 4 to 6 days after the onset of infection. Epididymitis and *funiculitis* (infection of the vas deferens) are possible complications. Treatment is bed rest, scrotal support, and elevation. Symptoms resolve in days to weeks.

PREVENTION OF GENITAL INFECTIONS

The CDC has established five strategies for the prevention and control of STIs. First and foremost is health education. Adolescents and adults need accurate accessible information about STIs. Parents and teachers, as well as providers of health care, need assistance in talking about a variety of sexual concerns and issues. Knowledge of the high incidence of STIs and asymptomatic infections encourage safer sexual practices. Adolescents frequently underestimate their risk for infection. Information needs to target risky behaviors and ways to reduce transmission of infection. Other than abstinence, use of condoms provides the best protection against STIs at this time. A second prevention strategy is the detection of asymptomatic individuals and persons who are unlikely to seek diagnosis and treatment. Affordable or free centers for the diagnosis and treatment of STIs must be available in high-risk areas, such as school campuses. Innovative programs for voluntary screening, such as those that allow client specimen collection and drop off, need to be supported. Third is the effective diagnosis and treatment of infected persons. Primary care centers need to be staffed with individuals who are knowledgeable in the diagnosis of genital infection and who are comfortable in discussing sexual issues. Promoting healthy sexual behaviors should be part of routine health maintenance testing and screening. Fourth is the need for the evaluation, treatment, and counseling of sex partners of persons with genital infections. Fifth is preexposure vaccination of persons at risk for vaccine-preventable STIs. The only vaccine available at this writing is the Hepatitis B vaccine. Research in this area needs to continue and escalate. The STI epidemic needs to become a priority for local, state, and national government and for all health care professionals.

KEY CONCEPTS

- Infections of the genital tract are unique in the embarrassment they generate, which leads to delays in treatment, complications, and further spread of disease.
- *Sexually transmitted infections (STIs)* are at epidemic levels in the United States, costing billions of dollars in treatment and lost wages.
- *Chlamydia* is the most common sexually transmitted bacterial infection in the United States. Often asymptomatic, chlamydia is a major cause of PID and infertility in women.
- The incidence of *gonorrhea* is low, but the development of antibiotic resistant strains is of concern all around the world.
- *Syphilis* presents in three stages and may be contracted in utero from an infected mother. Undetected and untreated syphilis can result in severe cardiovascular and neurologic sequelae.
- *Herpes simplex virus (HSV)* is an incurable infection affecting an estimated 45 million people in the United States. Although usually a mild self-limiting infection, HSV can be fatal to newborns and immunocompromised individuals.
- *Human papillomavirus (HPV)* is highly contagious and the most common STI in the United States. HPV is frequently asymptomatic and is the *cause of most cervical cancers.*
- *Trichomoniasis*, a protozoan infection that may be present in the vagina or urethra, is transmitted sexually.
- *Bacterial vaginosis* and *candida infections* are usually specific to women and not usually transmitted sexually. These infections are frequent, self-limiting infections of the lower genital tract caused by a disruption of the normal balance in the vaginal flora.
- *Pelvic inflammatory disease (PID)* is an infection caused by the spread of an untreated lower genital tract infection that spreads to the upper genital tract. PID is severe, painful, and a threat to female fertility.
- *Epididymitis* is an inflammatory response of the epididymis to infection or trauma. In young men, *epididymitis* represents the progression of an untreated lower genital tract infection and can result in infertility.
- Most infections of the genital tract are preventable and curable. *Education regarding prevention*, early treatment, affordable and assessable treatment centers, research for vaccines, and new treatment remedies are essential to control this epidemic.

QUESTIONS

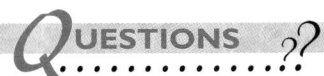
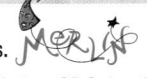

A sampling of review questions for this chapter appears here. Visit http://www.mosby.com/MERLIN/PriceWilson/ for additional questions.

Answer the following on a separate sheet of paper.

1. Discuss the reasons why people delay seeking treatment for genital tract infections.
2. What are some of the economic and social consequences of STIs?
3. Discuss issues related to partner notifications.
4. List three activities of the CDC in the fight to control STIs.
5. What are the potential sequelae of HPV infections?

BIBLIOGRAPHY ■ PART ELEVEN

American Academy of Pediatrics: Evaluation of the newborn with developmental anomalies of the external genitalia, *Pediatrics* 106:138-142, 2000a.

American Academy of Pediatrics: Technical report: congenital adrenal hyperplasia, *Pediatrics* 106:1511-1518, 2000b.

American Cancer Society: *American cancer society guidelines on testing for early detection of endometrial cancer—update 2001*, 2001. Retrieved November 19, 2001. *http://www.cancer.org/eprise/main/docroot/cri/cri_2_3x?dt=33*

American Cancer Society: *Cancer reference information—breast cancer*, 2001. Retrieved November 19, 2001. *http://www.cancer.org/eprise/main/docroot/cri/cri_0*

American Cancer Society: *HPV testing for cervical cancer: studies assess HPV testing as cervical cancer screening*, Atlanta, 2001, American Cancer Society.

American Cancer Society: *Ovarian cancer*, 2001. Retrieved November 19, 2001. *http://www.cancer.org/eprise/main/docroot/cri/cri_2_3x?dt=33*

American Joint Committee on Cancer: *Cancer staging manual*, ed 5, Philadelphia, 1997, Lippincott.

Anttila T et al: Serotypes of Chlamydia trachomatis and risk for development of cervical squamous cell carcinoma, *JAMA* 285(1):47-51, 2001.

Benedetti JK et al: Clinical reactivation of genital herpes simplex virus infection decreases in frequency over time, *Ann Intern Med* 131(1):14-20, 1999.

Berger BJ et al: Bacterial vaginosis in lesbians: a sexually transmitted disease, *Clin Infect Dis* 21:1402-1405, 1995.

Boardman LA: Managing genital herpes simplex virus infections, *Women's Health in Primary Care* 3(11):793-798, 1999.

Bosl GJ: Testicular germ cell cancer, *N Engl J Med* 337:242, 1997.

CancerNet: *Cervical cancer: treatment-health professionals*, 2001. Retrieved August 27, 2001: *http://www.cancer.gov/cervix*

CancerNet: *Endometrial cancer: treatment-health professionals*, 2001. Retrieved August 27, 2001: *http://www.cancer.gov/cancer_information/cancer_type/endometrial/*

CancerNet: *Prostate cancer: treatment-health professionals*, 2001. Retrieved December 14, 2001: *http://www.cancer.gov/cancer_information/cancer_type/prostate/*

CancerNet: *Testicular cancer: treatment-health professionals,* 2001. Retrieved December 14, 2001: *http://www.cancer.gov/cancer_ information/cancer_type/testicular/*

CancerNet: *Vaginal cancer: treatment-health professionals,* 2001. Retrieved August 27, 2001: *http://www.cancer.gov/cancer_ information/cancer_type/vaginal/*

CancerNet: *Vulvar cancer: treatment-health professionals,* 2001. Retrieved August 27, 2001: *http://www.cancer.gov/cancer_ information/cancer_type/vulvar/*

Cates W et al: Estimates of the incidence and prevalence of sexually transmitted diseases in the United States, *Sex Trans Dis* 26(suppl):S2-S7, 1999.

Centers for Disease Control and Prevention: 1998 guidelines for treatment of sexually transmitted disease, *MMWR* 47(RR-1):1-111, 1998.

Centers for Disease Control and Prevention: Syphilis among infants down more than half in three years, *MMWR,* July 13, 2001. *http://www.cdc.gov/std/press/presscsyph7-2001.htm*

Centers for Disease Control and Prevention: *Tracking the hidden epidemics: trends in STDs in the United States 2000,* Atlanta, 2000, National Prevention Information Network (NPIN).

Cohen M: *STDs: forgotten but not gone.* Program and abstracts of the 40th Interscience Conference on Antimicrobial Agents and Chemotherapy, Toronto, Ontario, Canada; September 17-20, 2000. *http://www.medscape.com*

Corey L et al: Recombinant glycoprotein vaccine for the prevention of genital HSV-2 infection: two randomized controlled trials, *JAMA* 282(4):331-341, 1999.

Corey L, Handsfield HH: Genital herpes and public health: addressing a global problem, *JAMA* 283(1):791-794, 2000.

Cox CE: Ten best readings on breast cancer, *Cancer Control* 8(5):452-453, 2001.

Cuzick J: Human papillomavirus testing for primary cervical cancer screening, *JAMA* 283: 108-109, 2000.

DiCarlo RP: *Preventing genital HSV infections on a large scale.* Presentation at the Thirteenth Meeting of the International Society for Sexually Transmitted Diseases Research, Denver, Colorado; July 11-14, 1999. *http://www.medscape.com*

Donegan WL, Redlich PN: Breast cancer in men, *Surg Clin N Am* 76:343, 1996.

Epstein RM et al: Awkward moments in patient-physician communication about HIV risk, *Ann Intern Med* 128(6):435-442, 1998.

Faro S et al: Treatment considerations in vulvovaginal candidiasis, *Female Patient* 2(3):39-54, 1997.

Ferris DG, Dekle C, Litaker MS: Women's use of over-the-counter antifungal medications for gynecologic symptoms, *J Fam Pract* 42:595-600, 1996.

Gaydos CA et al: Chlamydia trachomatis infection in female military recruits, *N Engl J Med* 339(11):739-744 1998.

Gunn GA et al: The changing paradigm of sexually transmitted disease control in the era of managed health care, *JAMA* 279:680-684, 1998.

Herman-Giddens ME, Slora EJ, Wasserman RC et al: Secondary sexual characteristics and menses in young girls seen in office practice: a study from the pediatric research in office setting networks. *Pediatrics* 99(4):505-512, 1997.

Hilton E et al: Ingestion of yogurt containing Lactobacillus acidophilus as prophylaxis for candidal vaginitis, *Ann Int Med* 116(5):353-357, 1992.

Hooton TM: *STDs: testing.* Program and abstracts of the 38th Annual Meeting of the Infectious Diseases Society of America, September 7-10, 2000; New Orleans, Louisiana. *http://www. medscape.com*

Institute of Medicine (IOM): *The hidden epidemic: confronting sexually transmitted diseases,* Washington, DC, 1997, National Academy Press.

Joesoef MR et al: Bacterial vaginosis: review of treatment options and potential clinical indications for therapy, *Clin Infect Dis* 28(suppl 1):S57-S65, 1999.

Johnson RA: Diagnosis and treatment of common sexually transmitted diseases in women, *Clinical Cornerstone* 3(1):1-11, 2000.

Keene GF: Office gynecology: common reproductive tract disorders, *Clinician Reviews* 9(1):58-78, 1999.

Koutsky LA, Kiviat NB: Genital human papillomavirus. In Holmes KK et al, editors: *Sexually transmitted diseases,* ed 3, New York, 1999, McGraw-Hill.

Lawson HW et al: Implementing recommendations for the early detection of breast and cervical cancer among low-income women, *MMWR Recommendations and Reports* 49(RR-2):37-55, 2000.

Manos MM et al: Identifying women with cervical neoplasia: using human papillomavirus DNA testing for equivocal Papanicolaou results, *JAMA* 281(17):1605-1610, 1999.

Merrill JM, Laux LF, Thornby JI: Why doctors have difficulty with sex histories, *South Med J* 83(6):113-117, 1990.

Morse SA, Moreland AA, Holmes KK, editors: *Atlas of sexually transmitted diseases and AIDS,* ed 2, London, 1996, Mosby-Wolfe.

Motzer RJ, Bosl GJ: Testicular cancer. In Braunwald E et al, editors: *Harrison's principles of internal medicine,* ed 15, New York, 2001, McGraw-Hill.

National Cancer Institute: *SEER cancer statistics review 1973–1999,* 2001. Retrieved August 27, 2001. *http://seer.cancer.gov/ CSR/1973_1998/sections.html*

National Institute of Allergy and Infectious Diseases (NIAID): Fact sheet: antimicrobial resistance, 2000, US Department of Health and Human Services. *http://www.niaid.nih.gov/factsheets/ antimicro.htm*

National Institutes of Health: Cervical cancer, Screening for cervical cancer. Screening/detection–health professionals, 1996, *NIH Consensus Statement* 14(1):1-38.

Pertel PE, Spear PG: Biology of herpes viruses. In Holmes KK et al, editors: *Sexually transmitted diseases,* ed 3, New York, 1999, McGraw-Hill.

Richart RM: Genital warts: the clinical challenge, *Medical Economics* (Fall suppl):4-14, 2000.

Rigg D et al: Recurrent allergic vulvovaginitis treatment with Candida albicans allergen immunotherapy, *Am J Obstet Gynecol* 162:332-336, 1990.

Ronald AR, Albritton W: Chancroid and Haemophilus ducreyi. In Holmes KK et al, editors: *Sexually transmitted diseases,* ed 3, New York, 1999, McGraw-Hill.

Ross J: Pelvic inflammatory disease. In *Clinical evidence,* issue 5, London, 2001, British Medical Journal Publishing Group.

Schairer C et al: Menopausal estrogen and estrogen-progestin replacement therapy and breast cancer risk, *JAMA* 283(4):485-491, 2000.

Schiffman M et al: HPV DNA testing in cervical cancer screening, *JAMA* 283(1):87-93, 2001.

Schwebke JR: Asymptomatic bacterial vaginosis: response to therapy, *Am J Obstet Gynecol* 183:1434-1439, 2000.

Seidel HM et al: *Mosby's guide to physical examination,* ed 4, St Louis, 1999, Mosby.

Sobel JD: Vulvoanal candidiasis. In Holmes KK et al, editors: *Sexually transmitted diseases,* ed 3, New York, 1999, McGraw-Hill.

Stern J, Schaeffer A: Chronic prostatitis. In *Clinical evidence,* issue 5: 1123-1127, London, 2001, British Medical Journal Publishing Group.

Tanagho EA et al: *Smith's general urology,* ed 15, New York, 2000, McGraw-Hill.

Teichman JMH: *20 common problems: urology*, New York, 2000, McGraw-Hill.

Thomas DJ: Sexually transmitted viral infections: epidemiology and treatment, *J Obstet Gynecol Neonatal Nurs* 30(3):316-323, 2001.

Toubla N: *Caring for women with circumcision*, New York, 1999, RAINBO. *http://www.rainbo.org*

Wallach J: *Interpretation of diagnostic tests*, ed 7, Philadelphia, 2000, Lippincott–Williams and Wilkins.

Willett WC, Colditz G, Stampfer M: Postmenopausal estrogens–opposed, unopposed, or none of the above, *JAMA* 283(4):534-535, 2000.

Wright TC et al: HPV DNA testing of self-collected vaginal samples compared with cytologic screening to detect cervical cancer, *JAMA* 283(1):81-86, 2000.

Zenilman JM: Chlamydia and cervical cancer: a real association? *JAMA* 285(1):81-82, 2001.

MUSCULOSKELETAL SYSTEM AND CONNECTIVE TISSUE DISORDERS

The diverse tissues and organs of the musculoskeletal system can develop a variety of disorders. Some disorders develop primarily within the system itself, whereas others may develop elsewhere but affect the musculoskeletal system. The major hallmarks of musculoskeletal disorders are pain and discomfort, which can range from mild to exceedingly severe.

This part presents a generalized discussion of various orthopedic and rheumatologic disorders. Because all conditions cannot be included, selected conditions are discussed because of their frequency of occurrence or because they provide a good example of similar types of conditions. The focus is to provide an understanding of the alterations in the physiology of the musculoskeletal system that can lead to disease and to use this understanding as the rationale for developing a treatment plan for the condition.

Anatomy and Physiology of Bones and Joints

MICHAEL A. CARTER

𝒯he musculoskeletal system provides the body's supporting framework and is responsible for movement. The major component of the musculoskeletal system is connective tissue. The system consists of the bones, the joints, skeletal muscles, tendons, ligaments, bursae, and the specialized tissues that connect these structures.

BONES

Bones form the supporting and protecting framework of the body and provide the areas for attachments of the muscles that move the skeleton. The central cavity of certain bones contains hematopoietic tissues, which form the various blood cells (see Chapter 16). Bones are the primary site for the storage and regulation of calcium and phosphate (see Chapter 21).

The major noncellular components of bone tissue are minerals and organic matrix (collagen and proteoglycans). Calcium and phosphate form a crystalline salt (hydroxyapatite), which is deposited in the collagen and proteoglycan matrix. These minerals provide the compressional strength of bone. The organic matrix of bone is referred to as *osteoid*. About 70% of the osteoid is type I collagen, which is rigid and gives bone its high tensile strength. The rest of the organic material in bone consists of proteoglycans such as hyaluronic acid.

Most bones are hollow tubes. This kind of structure maximizes the structural strength of bones while using the least amount of weight. Additional strength is provided by the arrangement of collagen and minerals within the bone tissues. Bone tissue can be either woven or lamellar. Woven bone is seen with rapid growth, such as during fetal development or after a fracture, in which it is subsequently replaced by mature, lamellar bone. In adults, woven bone is also found at ligament or tendon insertions. Osteogenic sarcoma tumors consist of woven bone. Lamellar bone is found throughout the body of an adult. Lamellar bone is constructed of highly organized mineralized plates, rather than being a solid crystalline mass. This pattern of organization provides bone's substantial strength.

Fig. 67-1 illustrates the parts of a typical long bone. The *diaphysis*, or *shaft*, is the cylindric midportion of the bone. This area is composed of cortical bone, which has great strength. The *metaphysis* is the flared region near the end of the shaft. This region is mostly trabecular or spongy bone and contains red marrow, which is composed of hematopoietic cells. Red bone marrow is also found in the *epiphysis* and diaphysis of the bone. In children, red marrow fills most of the interior portion of long bones, but it is replaced by yellow marrow as people mature. In adults, most of the hematopoietic activity is restricted to the sternum and iliac crest, although other bones retain the potential to become active once again if needed. The yellow bone marrow found in the shaft of adult bones is composed mainly of fat cells.

The metaphysis also supports the joint and provides appropriate areas for epiphyseal attachment of tendons and ligaments. The epiphyseal plate is the region of longitudinal growth in children, which disappears at skeletal maturity. The epiphysis directly adjacent to the joint of the long bone fuses to the metaphysis, causing the bone to stop growing in length. The entire bone is covered with a fibrous layer, the *periosteum*, which contains the proliferating cells that contribute to the long bone's transverse growth. Most long bones have specific nutrient arteries. The location and patency of these arteries may govern the success of bone healing after fracture.

The specific histology of the *epiphyseal plate*, or *growth plate*, is pertinent to understanding injuries in children (Fig. 67-2). The uppermost layer of cells near the epiphysis is the *area of resting cells.* The next layer is the *zone of proliferation.* In this zone, active cell division occurs and growth of long bones begins. The active cells are pushed toward the shaft and into the *area of hypertrophy,* where they swell and become weak and metabolically inactive. Epiphyseal fracture separations in children frequently occur in this region, and the injury may extend into the area of provisional calcification. In the *area of provisional calcification,* the extracellular matrix hardens as minerals are deposited on the collagen and proteoglycans. Damage to the proliferating zone may cause growth arrest with either retardation of the longitudinal growth of the limb or

progressive deformity if only a portion of the plate is seriously damaged.

Bone is a dynamic tissue formed by three types of cells: osteoblasts, osteocytes, and osteoclasts. *Osteoblasts* build bone by forming type I collagen and proteoglycans, which construct the bone matrix or osteoid tissue by a process called *ossification.* When they are actively producing osteoid tissue, osteoblasts secrete large quantities of alkaline phosphatase, which plays an important role in the deposition of calcium and phosphate in the bone matrix. Part of the alkaline phosphatase moves into the bloodstream, making the blood level of alkaline phosphatase a good indicator of the rate of bone formation after a fracture or after cancer metastasis to bone.

Osteocytes are mature bone cells that act as a pathway for chemical exchange through the dense bone.

Osteoclasts are large, multinuclear cells that enable the minerals and matrix of the bone to be absorbed. Unlike osteoblasts and osteocytes, osteoclasts move over the bone. These cells produce proteolytic enzymes that break down the matrix and several acids that cause bone minerals to dissolve, thus releasing calcium and phosphate into the bloodstream.

Bone normally undergoes deposition and absorption at a constant rate, except during childhood growth, when there is more deposition than there is absorption. The continual turnover is important for the normal function of bone and allows bone to respond to increased stress and to prevent fracture. The bone's shape can be adjusted to support increased mechanical forces. The turnover also helps maintain bone strength during aging. Aging organic matrix degenerates, making bone relatively weak and brittle. The formation of new bone requires new organic matrix, adding to the strength of bone.

Several hormones regulate bone metabolism. An increased level of *parathyroid hormone (PTH)* has a direct and immediate effect on the bone mineral, causing calcium and phosphate to be absorbed and moved into the serum. Also, an increased level of PTH causes a slow increase in the number and activity of osteoclasts, leading

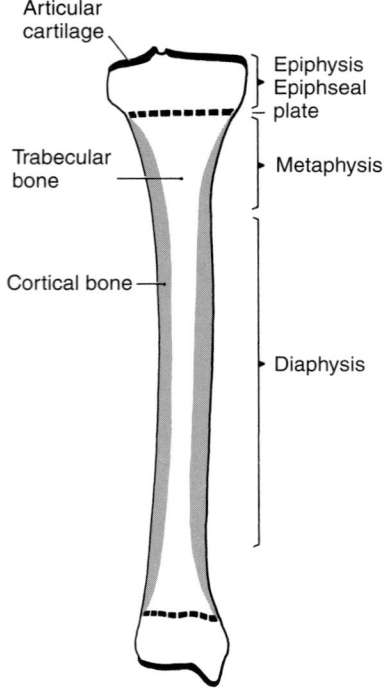

FIG. 67-1 Anatomy of a long bone.

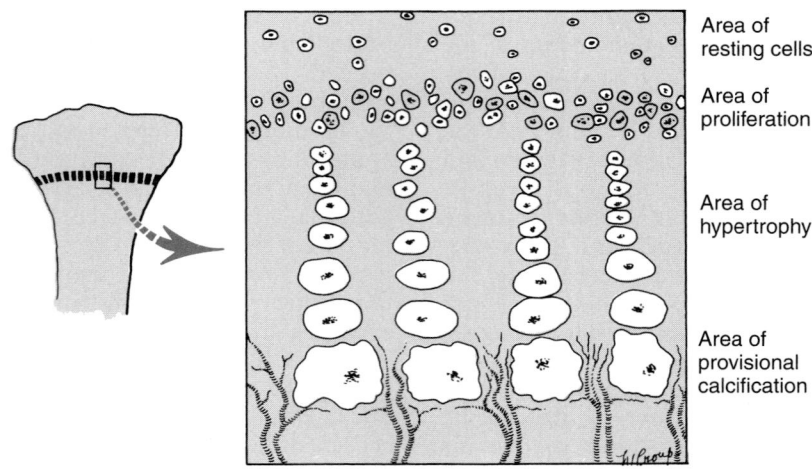

FIG. 67-2 Growth of a normal bone.

to demineralization. The increased serum calcium level in hyperparathyroidism can also lead to the formation of kidney stones.

Vitamin D affects bone deposition and absorption. Large quantities of vitamin D cause bone absorption similar to that seen with high levels of PTH. If no vitamin D is present, PTH will not cause bone absorption. Small quantities of vitamin D promote bone calcification, partly by increasing the absorption of calcium and phosphate from the intestines.

Osteoporosis is a reduction in bone mass and is caused by an increase of bone resorption over bone formation. The two most important causes of this imbalance are loss of gonadal function and normal aging. Postmenopausal osteoporosis (type I) is caused by a loss of estrogen production, which occurs with loss of ovary function in women and with castration in men. *Estrogen* stimulates the osteoblasts, and loss of estrogen decreases osteoblastic activity. This decrease leads to a decrease in the organic matrix of bone. There is also an increase in the number of osteoclasts in trabecular bone, meaning that the most typical fractures associated with type I osteoporosis are seen in the vertebra and the forearm (Colles' fracture).

Age-related osteoporosis (type II) is caused by a decrease in the amount of bone being formed during each remodeling cycle. This form of osteoporosis occurs equally in men and women after age 65 and is caused by a decrease in the overall number of osteoblasts in relation to the number needed. Fractures associated with type II osteoporosis are seen in cortical bone, including the hip, proximal femur, humerus, ribs, pelvis, and vertebral bodies.

Osteoblastic function is also suppressed when large doses of *glucocorticoids* are administered. This excess of glucocorticoids can lead to osteoporosis from the failure of the osteoblasts to form new bone matrix.

JOINTS

Joints are the areas where two or more bones meet. These bones are held together by various means, such as joint capsules, fibrous bands, ligaments, tendons, fasciae, or muscles. The three types of joints are as follows:

1. Fibrous (synarthrodial) joints, which allow no movement
2. Cartilaginous (amphiarthrodial) joints, which have only minimal movement
3. Synovial (diarthrodial) joints, which are freely movable

Fibrous Joints

Fibrous joints do not have a cartilaginous lining, and the bones are joined by fibrous connective tissue. There are two types of fibrous joints: (1) the sutures between the bones in the cranium and (2) a *syndesmosis*, which consists of an interosseous membrane or a ligament between the bones. These fibers permit a slight "give" but no real movement. The attachment in the distal tibiofibular joint is an example of this type of fibrous joint.

Cartilaginous Joints

Cartilaginous joints are those in which the ends of the bones are covered by hyaline cartilage, supported by ligaments, and have only slight movement. There are two types of cartilaginous joints. *Synchondroses* are those in which the entire joint is covered by hyaline cartilage. The costochondral joints are an example of synchondroses. *Symphyses* are joints that have a fibrocartilage connection between the bones and a thin layer of hyaline cartilage covering articular surfaces. The pubic symphysis and the joints between the bodies of the vertebrae are examples of symphyses.

Synovial Joints

Synovial joints are the movable joints in the body. These areas have a joint cavity and hyaline cartilage over the articular surfaces of the bones (Fig. 67-3).

The *joint capsule* is made up of a dense fibrous outer covering, an inner layer of highly vascularized connective tissue, and synovium, which forms a sac that lines the entire joint and covers the tendons that pass through the joint. The *synovium* does not extend across to the articular surface of the joint; rather, it is folded to allow full joint motion. The linings of the bursae throughout the body resemble synovium. The periosteum does not extend into the joint capsule.

The synovium produces a highly viscous liquid that lubricates the joint surfaces. Normal *synovial fluid* is clear, nonclotting, and either colorless or straw colored. Relatively small amounts (1 to 3 ml) are found in normal joints. The white blood cell count of the fluid is normally less than 200 cells/ml and is composed primarily of mononuclear cells. Hyaluronic acid is responsible for the viscosity of synovial fluid and is synthesized by synovial lining cells. The liquid component of the synovial fluid is thought to be a transudate from plasma. Synovial fluid also serves as a source of nutrition for the articular cartilage.

Hyaline cartilage covers the load-bearing portions of the bones in synovial joints. This cartilage serves an important role in distributing weight loads. Articular carti-

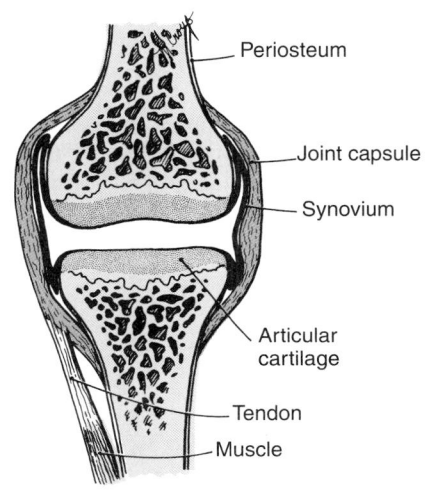

FIG. 67-3 Normal joint.

lage is made up of few cells and a large amount of ground substance. This ground substance consists of type II collagen and proteoglycans produced by the cartilage cells. The proteoglycans found in articular cartilage are very hydrophilic, which enables them to resist wear with heavy joint use.

Articular cartilage in the adult does not have any blood supply, lymphatic channels, or nerves. The synovial fluid that bathes the cartilage carries oxygen and other necessary products for metabolism. Alterations may occur in collagen and proteoglycan synthesis after injury or with increasing age. Some of the new collagen produced at this time begins to resemble type I collagen and is much more fibrous. The proteoglycans can lose some of their hydrophilic abilities. These changes mean that the cartilage can lose its ability to resist wear with heavy usage.

The joint is lubricated by synovial fluid and by hydrostatic changes in the interstitial fluid of the cartilage. Pressure on the cartilage causes fluid to move from the cartilage to an area of less pressure. As the joint glides forward, this weeping fluid moves ahead of the load. The fluid moves back into the portions of the cartilage from which the pressure is relieved. The articular cartilage and the bones of the joint are normally held apart during action by the film of fluid. The articular cartilage cannot be worn out by excessive use as long as an adequate film of fluid is present.

The blood supply to the joint is richest in the synovium. The vessels arise from the subchondral bone at the level of the margin of the capsule. The capillary network is particularly thick in the portions of the synovium immediately adjacent to the joint space. This characteristic allows products from the plasma to diffuse easily into the joint space. The inflammatory process can be especially pronounced in the synovium, because there is such a rich supply of blood vessels, as well as the presence of a large number of mast cells and other cells and chemicals that dynamically interact to stimulate and amplify the inflammatory response.

Autonomic and sensory nerves are widely distributed in the ligaments, joint capsule, and synovium. These nerves account for the sensitivity of these structures to position and movement. Nerve endings in the capsule, ligaments, and adventitia of blood vessels are particularly sensitive to stretching or twisting. Pain that arises from the joint capsule or synovium tends to be diffuse rather than localized. Peripheral nerves that cross the articulation innervate the joints, which means that pain from one joint may be reported as coming from another; for example, pain arising in the hip may be felt as knee pain.

CONNECTIVE TISSUE

The tissues found in the joints and adjoining areas are primarily connective tissues composed of cells and ground substance. The two types of cells found in connective tissue include cells that permanently remain in or do not develop in connective tissue, such as mast cells, plasma cells, lymphocytes, monocytes, and polymorphonuclear leukocytes. These cells play an important role in the inflammatory and immune reactions seen in the rheumatic disorders. The second type of cells found in connective tissue includes those permanently located there, such as fibroblasts, chondrocytes, and osteoblasts. These cells synthesize the various fibers and proteoglycans of the ground substance and give each type of connective tissue its unique properties.

The fibers found in the ground substance include collagen and elastin. At least 14 forms of collagen can be classified by their molecular chain structure, location, and function. *Collagen* can be broken down by the action of collagenases. These proteolytic enzymes cleave the stable molecule so that it becomes unstable at physiologic temperatures and is hydrolyzed by other proteases. Alterations in the synthesis of cartilage collagen are seen with increasing age. Increased collagenase activity is seen in immune-mediated forms of rheumatic disorders such as rheumatoid arthritis.

Elastin fibers have a unique cross-linking property that provides important elastic properties. These fibers are found in the ligaments, the walls of the larger blood vessels, and the skin. Enzymes called *elastases* break down elastin. Elastases may be important in the development of arteriosclerosis and emphysema. Some evidence suggests that changes in the cardiovascular system because of aging may result from increased breakdown of elastin fibers.

Proteoglycans are the other important product found in the ground substance along with the fibers. Proteoglycans are large molecules made up of long polysaccharide chains attached to polypeptide cores. Proteoglycans in articular cartilage cushion the joints to withstand great physical forces. The relationship of the proteoglycans to the inflammatory and immunologic processes is complex. Lymphokines can induce connective tissue cells to produce new proteoglycans, inhibit their production, or increase their breakdown. Proteoglycans can become the focus of autoimmune action in disorders such as rheumatoid arthritis. Increasing age changes the proteoglycans in cartilage; they become less able to aggregate with each other and interact with collagen. The major structural and functional changes that are a part of the normal aging process result from changes in the biochemistry of the connective tissues and occur primarily in the fibers and proteoglycans.

EVALUATION OF SYNOVIAL FLUID

The synovial fluid may be affected differently by each of the rheumatic disorders. Table 67-1 compares normal synovial fluid with the changes seen in some of the more common disorders. The *mucin clot test* is performed by adding acetic acid to the synovial fluid. This forms a precipitate by interaction with hyaluronic acid. The mucin clot has poor results with the more inflammatory fluids, since the hyaluronic acid has been broken down by the lysosomal enzymes and therefore is not available to precipitate when the fluid is treated with acetic acid. The clarity of normal synovial fluid is diminished by an increase in the cells and protein, as seen in some pathologic conditions.

TABLE 67-1

Synovial Fluid

	Normal	Degenerative Joint Disease	Systemic Lupus Erythematosus (SLE)*	Gout†	Rheumatoid Arthritis	Reiter's Syndrome	Infectious Arthritis‡
Color and clarity	Straw colored; clear	Straw colored; clear	Straw colored; clear	Straw colored or white; cloudy	Straw colored or light yellow; cloudy	Opaque	Gray, purulent; cloudy
Mucin clot	Good	Usually good	Fair to good	Poor	Poor	Poor	Poor
White blood cell count (average)	200/mm³	1000/mm³	5000/mm³	10,000 to 20,000/mm³	15,000 to 20,000/mm³	20,000/mm³	50,000 to 75,000/mm³

*LE cells may be present.
†Uric acid crystals are present.
‡Bacteria can be cultured.

KEY CONCEPTS

- Diverse tissues and organs of the musculoskeletal system can develop a variety of disorders that develop primarily within the system itself or elsewhere but affect the musculoskeletal system.
- Major hallmarks of musculoskeletal disorders are pain and discomfort, which can range from mild to exceedingly severe.
- The musculoskeletal system provides the body's supporting framework and is responsible for movement.
- The major component of the musculoskeletal system is *connective tissue*, which consists of bones, the joints, skeletal muscles, tendons, ligaments, bursae, and the specialized tissues that connect these structures.
- *Bones* form the supporting and protecting framework of the body and provide the areas for attachments of the muscles that move the skeleton.
- Major noncellular components of bone tissue are minerals and organic matrix (collagen and proteoglycans, calcium, and phosphate form a crystalline salt [hydroxyapatite]), which is deposited in the collagen and proteoglycan matrix, which provide the compressional strength of bone.
- The organic matrix of bone is *osteoid* that is about 70% type I collagen, which is rigid and gives bone its high tensile strength. The rest of the organic material in bone consists of proteoglycans such as hyaluronic acid.
- Most bones are hollow tubes which maximizes the structural strength of bones while using the least amount of weight.
- Bone tissue can be either woven or lamellar bone, which is found throughout the body of an adult.
- The parts of the bone include the following: (1) the diaphysis, or shaft, is the cylindric midportion of the bone and is composed of cortical bone, which has great strength; and (2) the metaphysis is the flared region near the end of the shaft and is mostly trabecular or spongy bone and contains red marrow that is also found in the epiphysis and diaphysis of

the bone of adult bones. The metaphysis is composed mainly of fat cells.
- The *epiphyseal plate* is the region of longitudinal growth in children and is pertinent to understanding injuries in children.
- Three types of bone cells are *osteoblasts, osteocytes,* and *osteoclasts*. Osteoblasts build bone by forming type I collagen and proteoglycans, which construct the bone matrix or osteoid tissue by a process called *ossification*.
- Bone normally undergoes deposition and absorption at a constant rate, except during childhood growth, when there is more deposition than there is absorption.
- Vitamin D affects bone deposition and absorption.
- *Osteoporosis* is a reduction in bone mass and is caused by an increase of bone resorption over bone formation. The two most important causes of this imbalance are loss of gonadal function and normal aging.
- Age-related osteoporosis (type II) is caused by a decrease in the amount of bone being formed during each remodeling cycle and occurs equally in men and women after age 65 and is caused by a decrease in the overall number of osteoblasts in relation to the number needed.
- Fractures associated with type II osteoporosis are seen in cortical bone, including the hip, proximal femur, humerus, ribs, pelvis, and vertebral bodies.
- *Joints* are the areas where two or more bones meet and are held together by various means, such as joint capsules, fibrous bands, ligaments, tendons, fasciae, or muscles.
- The three types of joints are as follows: (1) fibrous (synarthrodial) joints that do not have a cartilaginous lining, and are joined by fibrous connective tissue, which allow no movement; (2) cartilaginous (amphiarthrodial) joints where the ends of bones are covered by hyaline cartilage, supported by liga-

ments, and have only minimal movement; and (3) synovial (diarthrodial) joints that have a joint cavity and hyaline cartilage over the articular surfaces of the bones, which are freely movable.

■ Joint capsule consists of a dense fibrous outer covering, an inner layer of highly vascularized connective tissue, and synovium, which produces a highly viscous liquid that lubricates the joint surfaces. The capillary network is particularly thick in the portions of the synovium immediately adjacent to the joint space.

■ Tissues found in the joints and adjoining areas are primarily connective tissues composed of cells and ground substance. These cells, found in connective cells, are mast cells, plasma cells, lymphocytes, monocytes, and polymorphonuclear leukocytes and play an important role in the inflammatory and immune reactions seen in rheumatic disorders.

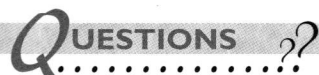

QUESTIONS ??

A sampling of review questions for this chapter appears here. Visit http://www.mosby.com/MERLIN/PriceWilson/ for additional questions.

Answer the following on a separate sheet of paper.

1. List the structures of the musculoskeletal system.
2. What are the characteristics of woven bone as compared with lamellar bone?
3. List the various means by which joints are held together.

4. Explain the process by which a joint is lubricated.
5. What is the role of osteoclasts in the process of bone resorption?
6. What is the relationship of osteoid (organic matrix of bone) to the formation of new bone?

7. Why is it significant that some joints are innervated by peripheral nerves that cross the articulation?
8. Label the parts of the long bone in Fig. 67-4.

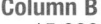

Match the conditions in column A with the synovial fluid white cell counts in column B.

Column A		Column B
9._____	Normal joint	a. 15,000 to 20,000/mm³
10._____	Rheumatoid arthritis	b. 5000/mm³
11._____	Infectious arthritis	c. 200/mm³
12._____	Systemic lupus erythematosus	d. 50,000 to 75,000/mm³

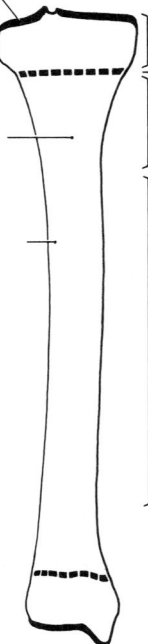

FIG. 67-4 Anatomy of a long bone.

CHAPTER
68

Fractures and Dislocations

MICHAEL A. CARTER

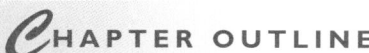

FRACTURES

Classification of Fractures

A fracture is a break in a bone, usually caused by trauma or physical forces. The strength and angle of the force, the underlying condition of the bone, and surrounding soft tissue determine whether the fracture is complete or incomplete. Complete fractures result when a break extends completely through the bone, whereas incomplete fractures do not extend through the entire thickness of the bone. Several terms are used to describe fractures.

Angle of Break

Transverse fractures proceed directly across the bone. When the broken segments of such a transversely fractured bone are repositioned, or reduced, back to their original location, they are stable and usually easy to control with casts (Fig. 68-1, *A*). *Oblique fractures* proceed at an angle across the bone. These fractures are unstable and difficult to control (see Fig. 68-1, *B*). *Spiral fractures* are the result of torsion of a limb. Of interest, these low-energy fractures are associated with little soft-tissue damage, and these fractures tend to heal readily with external immobilization (see Fig. 68-1, *C*).

Multiple Fractures in One Bone

Segmental fractures are two adjacent fractures that isolate a central segment from its blood supply. These fractures

are difficult to treat. The fracture at one end of the avascular segment often fails to heal, and this situation may require surgical treatment (Fig. 68-2, *A*). *Comminuted fractures* are splinters or disruptions in continuity of tissue in which there are more than two fracture fragments.

Impaction Fractures

Compression fractures occur when two bones crush (by impaction) a third bone between them, such as a vertebra between two other vertebrae. These fractures of the vertebral bodies are diagnosed by their radiographic appearance. Lateral views of the spine show a decrease in vertical height and a mild angulation at one or a few vertebrae. In young people, a compression fracture may

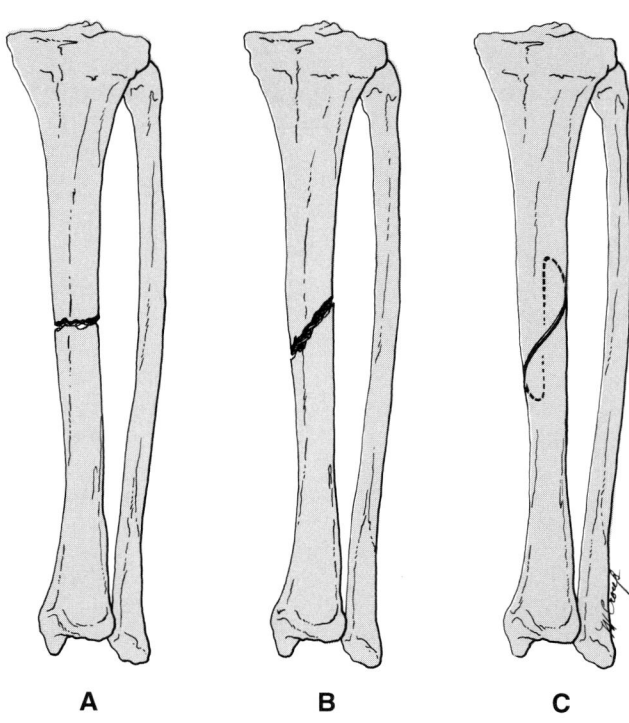

A   **B**   **C**

FIG. 68-1   Classification of fractures. **A,** Transverse. **B,** Oblique. **C,** Spiral.

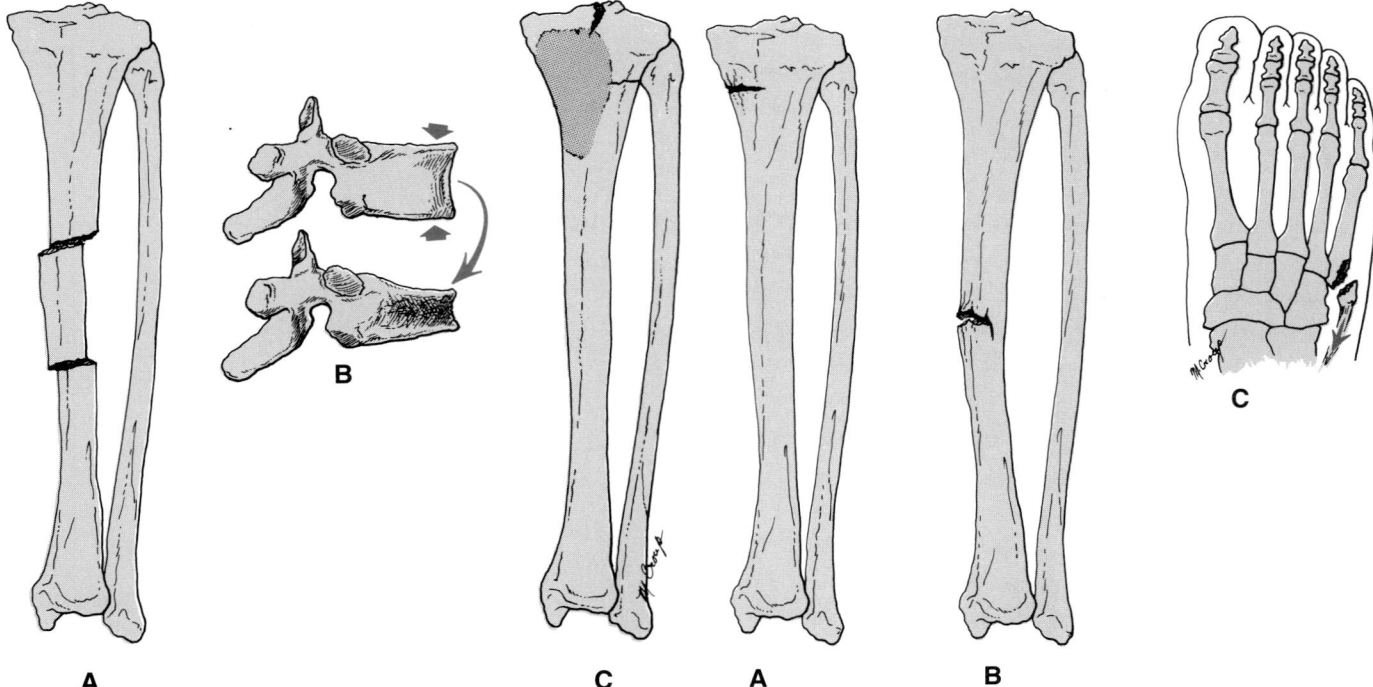

FIG. 68-2 Types of fractures. **A**, Segmental. **B**, Compression. **C**, Pathologic.

FIG. 68-3 Other fractures. **A**, Stress (fatigue). **B**, Greenstick. **C**, Avulsion.

be associated with considerable retroperitoneal hemorrhage. As in pelvic fractures, the patient may rapidly develop hypovolemic shock and die if repeated accurate assessments of the pulse, blood pressure, and respiration are not obtained during the first 24 to 48 postinjury hours. Ileus and urinary retention may also result from these injuries (see Fig. 68-2, *B*).

Pathologic Fractures
Pathologic fractures occur through regions of bone that have been weakened by a tumor or some other pathologic process. The adjacent bone often shows decreased bone density. The most frequent cause of these fractures is a primary or metastatic tumor (see Fig. 68-2, *C*).

Other Stress (Fatigue) Fractures
Stress, or fatigue, fractures occur in individuals who have recently increased their activity level, such as recruits in the army in basic training or persons who have recently taken up jogging. With the onset of symptoms, the radiographs may not demonstrate the fracture. However, usually after 2 weeks, linear radiopaque lines appear perpendicular to the long axis of the bone. These fractures heal well if the bone is immobilized for a few weeks. However, if the fractures are not diagnosed, the bones can become displaced and fail to heal properly. Thus any patient with severe extremity pain after a recent increase in activity may have this type of lesion and should be protected by the use of crutches or an appropriate cast. After 2 weeks, radiographs should be obtained (Fig. 68-3, *A*).

Greenstick Fractures
Greenstick fractures are incomplete fractures and are frequently seen in children. The cortex is partially intact, as

is the periosteum. Greenstick fractures will heal readily and rapidly remodel back to a normal shape and function (see Fig. 68-3, *B*).

Avulsion Fractures
Avulsion fractures separate a fragment of bone at a site of tendon or ligament insertion. Usually, no specific treatment is required. However, if joint instability or another cause of disability is expected to result from such a fracture, the displaced fragment may be surgically excised or realigned in most cases (see Fig. 68-3, *C*).

Joint Fractures
Specific note should be made of fractures that involve joints, particularly if the joint geometry is significantly disturbed by displacement of these fragments. Unless adequately treated, this type of injury may lead to a progressive posttraumatic osteoarthritis of the injured joint (Fig. 68-4).

Description of Fractures
Angulation and opposition are two terms frequently used in the description of long-bone fractures. The degree and direction of *angulation* from the normal position of a long bone may indicate the degree of fracture severity and the type of treatment program. Angulation is described by estimating the degrees of deviation of the distal fragment from the normal longitudinal axis, indicating the direction of the apex of the angle (Fig. 68-5, *A*). *Opposition* refers to the extent of displacement of the fracture surfaces and is used to describe what proportion of the fractured portion of one fragment touches its mate (see Fig. 68-5, *B*).

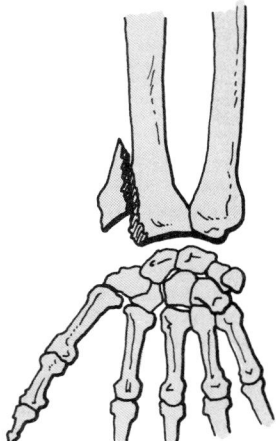

FIG. 68-4 Fracture of the distal radius with extension into the wrist joint.

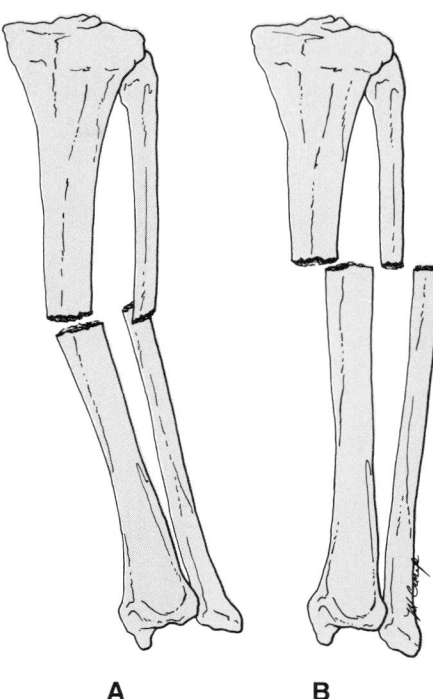

A   **B**

FIG. 68-5 Description of fractures. **A**, Angulation. **B**, Opposition.

Exposure to Environment

Closed (simple) and open (compound) are terms commonly used in fracture description. A *closed*, or *simple, fracture* is one in which the skin is not perforated, so the fracture site is not exposed to the environment.

Technically, an *open*, or *compound, fracture* is one in which the skin on the involved limb has been penetrated. The important concept is whether the contaminated outside environment has come into contact with the fracture site. A fracture fragment may perforate the skin at the time of injury, become contaminated, and then return to near its normal position. Under these conditions, operative irrigation, débridement, and administration of intravenous antibiotics may be necessary to prevent osteomyelitis. In general, open fractures should have operative irrigation and débridement within 6 hours of the time of injury for the best chance of preventing infection.

Fracture Healing

When a bone is fractured, the adjacent soft tissues are damaged, the periosteum is separated from the bone, and considerable bleeding takes place. A blood clot develops in the area. The clot forms granulation tissue within which the primitive bone-forming (osteogenic) cells differentiate into chondroblasts and osteoblasts. The chondroblasts secrete phosphate, which stimulates the deposition of calcium. A thickened band (callus) forms around the fracture site. The band continues to thicken and expand across the fracture site and converges with the band from the opposite fragment and fuses with it. Fusion of the two fragments (fracture healing) progresses as osteoblasts form trabeculae, which adhere to the bone and extend across the fracture site. This provisional bony union undergoes metaplastic transformation to become stronger and more organized. The bone callus remodels to assume the shape of intact bone as osteoblasts form new bone and osteoclasts remove the damaged and temporary bone (Fig. 68-6).

HEALING POTENTIAL OF CHILDREN'S FRACTURES

Children's fractures usually heal rapidly and well. The active periosteal sleeve around the tubular bones in children is strong. Because this area is rarely completely ruptured, fracture fragments tend to be maintained in an acceptable position after fracture. Children's bones have great potential for corrective remodeling. Thus a considerable postreduction angular deformity may be accepted with confidence that the mature bone will be straight without evidence of injury. In addition, the injured limb tends to grow faster than the normal one. *Bayonet apposition* is often preferable to an end-on-end reduction to achieve equal adult limb lengths (Fig. 68-7). Although angular deformities do rapidly correct, there is no similar tendency for rotational deformities to resolve spontaneously. Normal rotational position during healing should be maintained.

Most fractures in children are appropriately treated by closed reduction and external immobilization with casts or traction. Only a few children's fractures are optimally treated surgically. An example is a fracture of the lateral condyle of the humerus that extends into the joint and may also involve an injury to the epiphyseal growth plate. Failure to accurately reduce the fragment back to its normal anatomic position may lead to a reduction of elbow function and growth arrest of the limb, which may result in gross deformity developing with increasing maturity. Fractures of the head of the radius and of the hip in children also frequently demand surgical treatment. In general, fractures that extend into joints or that pass

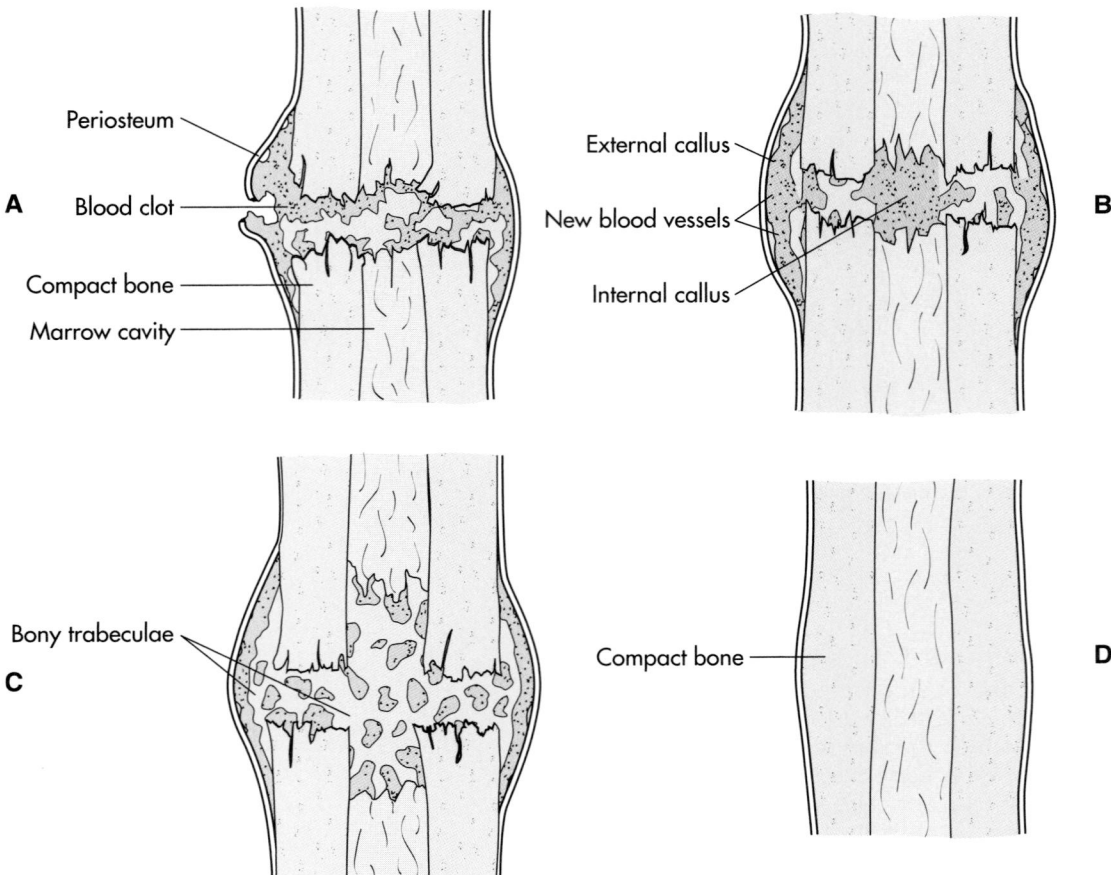

FIG. 68-6   **A**, In a fracture, usually the periosteum is torn, blood vessels are damaged, and bone fragments are separated. **B**, Rapid division of bone-forming and cartilage-forming cells in the region of the break forms a thickened band composed of an internal callus and an external callus. **C**, Osteoblasts form trabeculae, which adhere to existing bone and extend across the break. **D**, The break is bridged by compact bone, and the contour of the new, intact bone is remodeled.

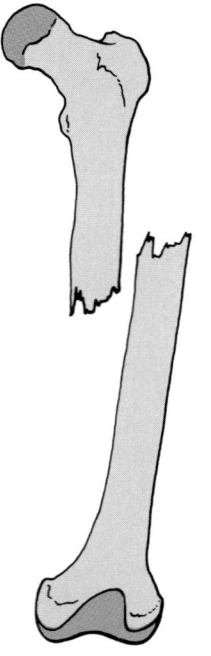

FIG. 68-7   Bayonet apposition.

across or through growth plates are the ones most likely to require surgery.

DISLOCATION AND SUBLUXATION

The articular cartilage-bearing surfaces of normal joints fit one another with considerable accuracy (Fig. 68-8). *Subluxation* refers to any deviation from the normal relationship in which the articular cartilage is still touching any portion of its mating cartilage. If no portion of its articular cartilage touches the usual mate, the joint is said to be *dislocated*. Early recognition and reduction of all dislocations are essential for a satisfactory end result.

Shoulder dislocations are most common in young people and usually result from a traumatic exaggerated abduction, extension, and external rotation position of the upper extremity (Fig. 68-9). The cocked position for throwing a ball is an example of the position that most frequently, if exaggerated, may cause dislocation. The humeral head is generally displaced anteriorly and inferiorly through a traumatic rent in the shoulder capsule. Characteristically, the patient is seen sitting bent over, supporting the injured limb in a flexed position away

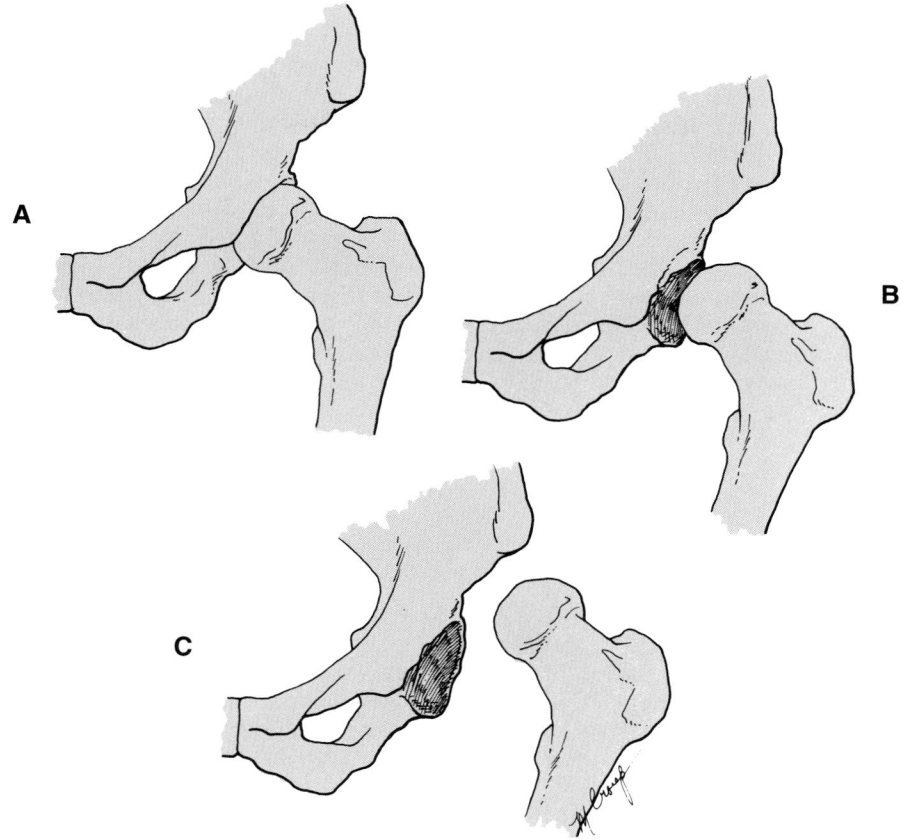

FIG. 68-8   **A**, Normal joint. **B**, Subluxation. **C**, Dislocation.

from the chest or the side. The humeral head may be easily palpated in the anterior axilla. There is a palpable depression beneath the central origin of the deltoid at the acromion.

During the initial evaluation, the neurovascular status of the limb is examined by testing the sensation in the area of the insertion of the deltoid on the humerus. This area is uniquely served by the sensory fibers of the axillary nerve. Local circumscribed anesthesia indicates the likelihood of an axillary nerve injury. Similarly, the patient's ability to minimally tense the deltoid in a voluntary attempt to initiate abduction also allows an estimate of the function of the axillary nerve. Axillary nerve function is necessary for shoulder abduction so that the patient may functionally position the arm. This nerve is frequently injured by the trauma of dislocation.

Ulnar nerve deficit occurs with nearly the same frequency as axillary nerve injury in shoulder dislocations. Ulnar nerve palsy has a severe effect on hand function.

Sustained anterior traction is the safest and most dependable method of reducing a dislocated shoulder. With this type of traction, the patient is given an analgesic, generally a narcotic, and is put in a prone position on an examination table or cart with the affected limb hanging over the side. Slow, gentle, sustained traction toward the floor is applied. Most patients can feel the reduction as a "clunk." This method of reduction is extremely successful and virtually without complications. A

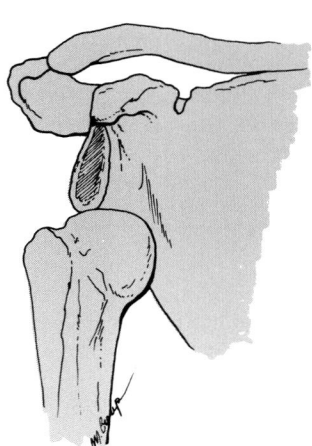

FIG. 68-9   Shoulder dislocation.

postreduction radiograph should demonstrate normal anatomy.

Dislocation of the hip is one of the few orthopedic emergencies. If a dislocated hip is not reduced within a few hours of the injury, the probability of the patient's developing aseptic necrosis is extremely great. Hip dislocation is recognized usually by gluteal, groin, and thigh pain in association with a rigid position of the limb in adduction, internal rotation, and flexion.

OSTEOMYELITIS

Osteomyelitis is infection of bone tissue and may be acute or chronic. The acute form is characterized by rapid onset of fever with systemic and local manifestations. In children, infections of bone develop as a complication of infection from other sites, such as the pharynx (pharyngitis), ear (otitis media), and skin (impetigo). The bacteria (*Staphylococcus aureus, Streptococcus, Haemophilus influenzae*) travel via the bloodstream to the metaphysis near the growth plates, where the blood flows into sinusoids. With bacterial proliferation and tissue necrosis, the localized area of inflammation is tender and painful.

Osteomyelitis, especially in children, must be diagnosed early so that appropriate antibiotic and surgical treatment can be administered to prevent the local spread of infection and crippling destruction of the entire bone. In adults, osteomyelitis may also be initiated by blood-borne bacteria but usually is the result of tissue contamination at the time of injury or surgery.

Chronic osteomyelitis results from inadequately treated acute osteomyelitis. Osteomyelitis is extremely resistant to antibiotic therapy. It is theorized that this resistance is partially because of the avascular nature of cortical bone. Appropriate quantities of antibodies may never reach the infected tissue. Bone infections are extremely difficult to eradicate, and even treatment by surgical drainage and débridement with appropriate antibiotic therapy are often insufficient to eliminate the disease.

KEY CONCEPTS

- A *fracture* is a break in a bone, usually caused by trauma or physical forces.
- The strength and angle of the force, the underlying condition of the bone, and surrounding soft tissue determine whether the fracture is complete (break extends completely through the bone) or incomplete (fractures do not extend through the entire thickness of the bone).
- *Transverse fractures* proceed directly across the bone, whereas oblique fractures proceed at an angle across the bone; spiral fractures are the result of torsion of a limb.
- *Segmental fractures* are two adjacent fractures that isolate a central segment from its blood supply, and *comminuted fractures* are splinters or disruptions in continuity of tissue in which there are more than two fracture fragments.
- *Compression fractures* occur when two bones crush (by impaction) a third bone between them, such as a vertebra between two other vertebrae; *pathologic fractures* occur through regions of bone that have been weakened by a tumor or some other pathologic process.
- *Stress*, or *fatigue*, *fractures* occur in individuals who have recently increased their activity level.
- *Greenstick fractures* are incomplete fractures and are frequently seen in children in which the cortex is partially intact, as is the periosteum.
- *Avulsion fractures* separate a fragment of bone at a site of tendon or ligament insertion.
- Specific note should be made of fractures that involve joints, particularly if the joint geometry is significantly disturbed by displacement of these fragments.
- *Angulation* and *opposition* are two terms used in the description of long-bone fractures that are described by estimating the degrees of deviation of the distal fragment from the normal longitudinal axis, indicating the direction of the apex of the angle.

- *Opposition* refers to the extent of displacement of the fracture surfaces and is used to describe what proportion of the fractured portion of one fragment touches its mate.
- *Closed*, or *simple*, *fracture* is one in which the skin is not perforated, thus the fracture site is not exposed to the environment, whereas an *open*, or *compound*, *fracture* is one in which the skin on the involved limb has been penetrated.
- When a bone is fractured, the adjacent soft tissues are damaged; periosteum is separated from the bone, bleeding occurs, and a blood clot develops, which forms granulation tissue; the osteogenic cells differentiate into chondroblasts and osteoblasts. A thickened band (callus) forms around the fracture site; bone callus remodels to assume the shape of intact bone.
- Children's fractures usually heal rapidly and well because the active periosteal sleeve around the tubular bones in children is strong.
- *Shoulder dislocations* are most common in young people and usually result from a traumatic exaggerated abduction, extension, and external rotation position of the upper extremity.
- Dislocation of the hip is one of the few orthopedic emergencies. If a dislocated hip is not reduced within a few hours of the injury, the probability of the patient developing aseptic necrosis is extremely great.
- *Osteomyelitis* is infection of bone tissue and may be acute or chronic.
- *Osteomyelitis*, especially in children, must be diagnosed early so that appropriate antibiotic and surgical treatment can be administered to prevent the local spread of infection and crippling destruction of the entire bone. In adults, osteomyelitis may also be initiated by blood-borne bacteria but usually is the result of tissue contamination at the time of injury or surgery.

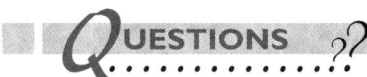

QUESTIONS ??

A sampling of review questions for this chapter appears here. Visit http://www.mosby.com/MERLIN/PriceWilson/ for additional questions.

Circle the letter preceding each item that correctly answers the question or completes the statement. More than one answer may be correct.

1. Which of the following fractures is illustrated in Fig. 68-10, *A*?
   a. Segmental
   b. Compression
   c. Greenstick
   d. Transverse
2. Which type of fracture is illustrated in Fig. 68-10, *B*?
   a. Oblique
   b. Greenstick
   c. Stress (fatigue)
   d. Avulsion

Answer the following on a separate sheet of paper.

3. Explain the changes that occur in the process of fracture healing.
4. Why is it important to diagnose osteomyelitis early, especially in children?
5. Explain why children's fractures usually heal rapidly and well.
6. Why is bayonet apposition often preferable in reduction of children's fractures?

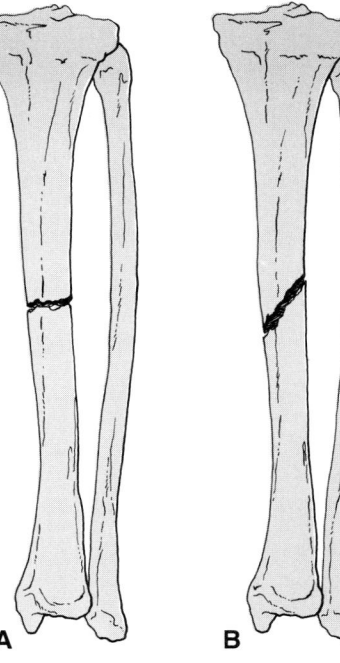

A   B

FIG. 68-10   Fractures.

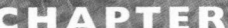

Tumors of the Musculoskeletal System

MICHAEL A. CARTER

𝒜 number of types of neoplasms can occur in bone tissue. These neoplasms may originate in the bone tissue itself or may spread to the bone from other primary sites.

Bone tumor cells produce factors that stimulate osteoclast function, leading to bone resorption that can be seen radiographically. Some tumors cause increased osteoblast activity with an increased density that also can be seen radiographically. Generally, bone tumors are recognized because of a mass in the soft tissues around the bone, deformity of the bone, pain and tenderness, or pathologic fractures.

Primary bone tumors can be benign or malignant. Benign tumors are much more common compared with malignant tumors, and malignant tumors are often fatal. Malignant tumors tend to grow rapidly, spread, and invade irregularly. These tumors are seen most often in adolescents and young adults.

A number of neoplasms that originate in other tissues can spread to bone by way of the bloodstream. The most common primary sites of these neoplasms are prostate, breast, lung, thyroid, kidney, and bladder. The most common bones affected are the vertebrae, proximal femur, pelvis, ribs, sternum, and proximal humerus.

BENIGN TUMORS

Osteoma

Osteomas are benign bone lesions characterized by an abnormal outgrowth of bone. The classic osteoma presents as a slowly growing, painless, hard bump. Radiographically, peripheral osteomas present as radiopaque lesions that extend from the surface of bone; central osteomas are seen as well-delineated sclerotic masses inside the bone. Surgical excision of the osteoma is the preferred treatment when the lesion is symptomatic, enlarging, or causing disability. Removal is also done for diagnostic purposes for large lesions. Excision usually produces curative results.

Chondroblastoma

Chondroblastoma is a rare, usually benign tumor that occurs most frequently in adolescent males. This tumor is uniquely found in the epiphysis. The most common site of occurrence is the humerus. The most frequent symptom is joint pain arising from cartilaginous tissue. Treatment consists of surgical excision. Recurrence is treated with surgical excision, cryosurgery, or radiotherapy.

Enchondroma

Enchondroma, or *central chondroma*, is a benign tumor of dysplastic cartilage cells occurring in the metaphysis of tubular bones, particularly of the hands and feet. Radiographically, spotty calcification in the circumscribed, enlarged, rarefied lesion is characteristic of this tumor. The tumor is believed to develop during the growth period in children and adolescents. This condition increases the likelihood of pathologic fractures. Surgical curettage and bone grafting are usually the treatments of choice for this lesion.

Giant-Cell Tumor

A characteristic feature of a giant-cell tumor is the vascular and cellular stroma make up of oval-shaped cells containing small, elongated, darkly staining nuclei. The giant cell is large and has pink-staining cytoplasm; it contains

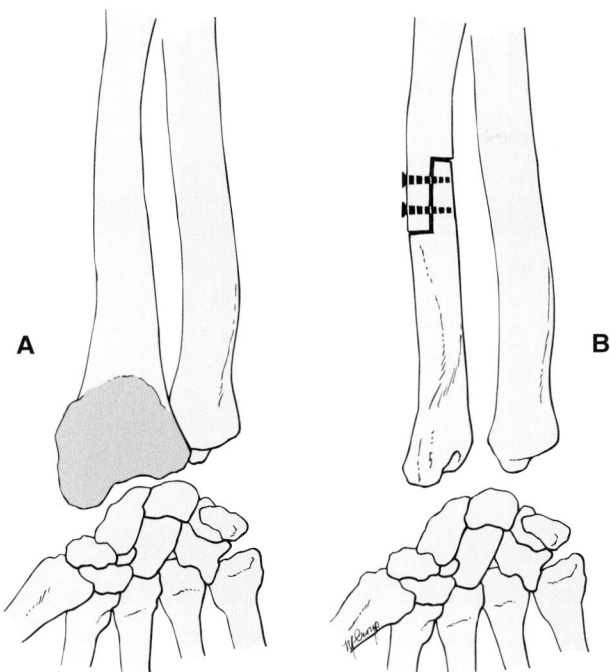

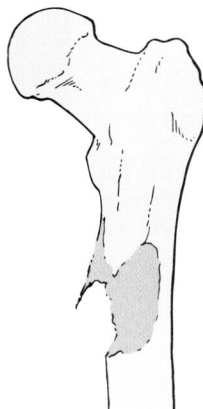

FIG. 69-2   Osteogenic sarcoma with Codman's triangle.

FIG. 69-1   **A**, Giant-cell tumor of the distal radius. **B**, Use of a bone transplant to reconstruct the limb after total excision of a giant-cell tumor.

numerous nuclei, which are vesicular and appear similar to stromal cells. Although this tumor is usually considered benign, there are varying degrees of malignancy, depending on the sarcomatous nature of the stroma. In the malignant types, the tumor becomes anaplastic and has areas of necrosis and hemorrhage.

Giant-cell tumors occur chiefly in young adults and occur more frequently in women than they do in men. The common sites are the ends of the long bones, especially at the knee and the lower end of the radius. The most common symptom is pain. Joint motion limitation and weakness may also be seen. After biopsy identification, this type of tumor usually requires a definitive gross local excision, including removal of a safe border of normal tissue. This tumor tends to be locally recurrent (probably 60% or greater) and of increasingly malignant character after incomplete excision. With prior biopsy, diagnosis, and gross local removal, an immediate reconstruction of the area may be possible. In the case of a large giant-cell tumor of the distal radius (Fig. 69-1, *A*), the patient's proximal fibula can be substituted to reconstruct the forearm (Fig. 69-1, *B*).

MALIGNANT TUMORS

Multiple Myeloma

The most common malignant bone tumor is multiple myeloma, which is caused by a malignant proliferation of plasma cells. Multiple myeloma is rarely seen in individuals younger than age 40 years. Men are more often affected than are women, and African Americans have twice the incidence of Caucasians.

Bone pain is the most common symptom, and the back and rib areas are the most common sites of this pain. Palpable bone lesions may occur, especially in the skull and clavicles. Lesions in the back can lead to vertebral collapse and occasionally spinal cord compression. Treatment involves a number of activities, because multiple myeloma affects many organs. Long-term survival depends on the stage of the illness at diagnosis (see Chapter 18).

Osteogenic Sarcoma

Osteogenic sarcoma, or *osteosarcoma*, is a malignant primary neoplasm of bone. The tumor arises in the metaphysis of the bone. The most common sites are at the ends of the long bones, especially at the knee. The incidence of osteogenic sarcoma is greatest in adolescents and young adults, but it may also affect people with Paget's disease who are over 50 years of age. Severe pain associated with bone destruction and erosion is a usual symptom of this condition.

The gross appearance of osteogenic sarcoma is variable. The neoplasm may be (1) osteolytic, in which case the bone is destroyed, and the soft tissue is invaded by the lesion, or (2) osteoblastic as a result of the formation of new sclerotic bone. Periosteal new bone may be deposited adjacent to the lesion itself, appearing as a triangle on radiographs (Fig. 69-2). Although this bone deposit is seen with many malignancies of bone, it is characteristic of osteogenic sarcoma; the tumor itself may produce a somewhat abortive form of bone. The radiographic appearance of this type of lesion is referred to as a "sunburst," as depicted in Fig. 69-3.

Chondrosarcoma

Chondrosarcoma is a malignant tumor composed of anaplastic chondrocytes and may occur as a central or peripheral bone tumor. The tumor occurs most often in men over 35 years of age. A painless mass of long duration is the most frequent presenting symptom. For example, peripheral lesions are often asymptomatic for long periods, presenting with only minor discomfort and palpable enlargement. However, rapid aggressive growth may occur. The pelvis, femur, ribs, shoulder girdle, and craniofacial bones are the most frequent sites of the lesion.

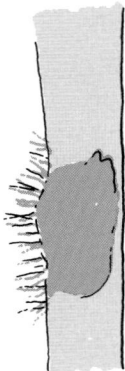

FIG. 69-3 Radiographic "sunburst" appearance seen in osteogenic sarcoma.

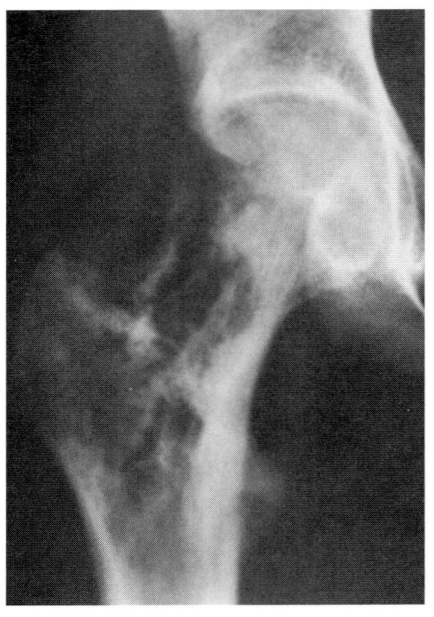

A

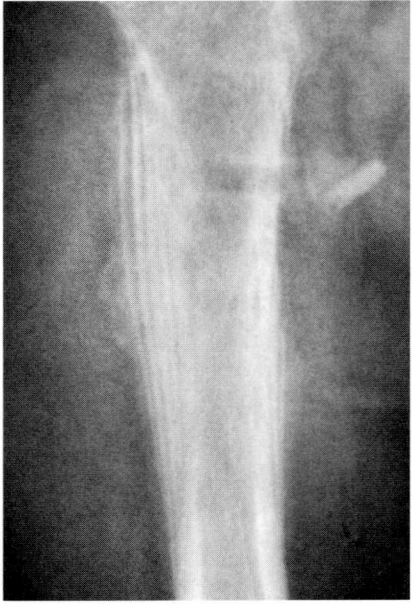

FIG. 69-4 Radiographic "onionskin" appearance seen in Ewing's sarcoma. (Courtesy of William Martel, MD.)

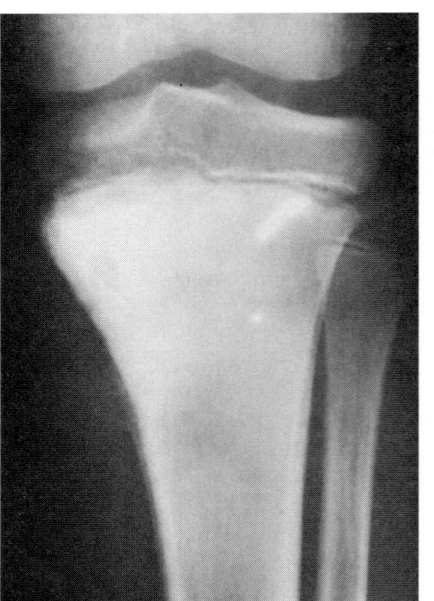

B

FIG. 69-5 Radiographic appearance of a malignant tumor. **A**, Femur. **B**, Tibia. (Courtesy of William Martel, MD.)

Chondrosarcomas appear as radiolucent areas with stippled and blotchy calcification of radiographs. Radical surgical excision is the treatment preferred; however, cryosurgery, radiotherapy, and chemotherapy may also be used. For large, aggressive, or recurrent lesions, amputation may be an appropriate treatment.

Ewing's Sarcoma

Ewing's sarcoma is most often seen in teenaged children, and the most common site is the shaft of long bones. The gross appearance is a soft, gray tumor arising into the bone marrow reticulum that erodes bone cortex from within. Under the periosteum, layers of new bone are deposited parallel to the shaft, producing an onionskin ef-

fect (Fig. 69-4). The typical signs and symptoms are pain, tender swelling, fever (38° to 40° C), and leukocytosis (20,000 to 40,000 leukocytes/mm^3).

DIAGNOSTIC MEASURES

As a general rule, the radiographic appearance of a lesion may help determine its relative malignancy. For example, a lesion with discrete rounded margins tends to be benign. This type of lesion frequently has a sclerotic margin, indicating that the bone has had the time and ability to respond to the mass. The lack of a definable margin indicates invasion of the tumor into adjacent bone (Fig. 69-5, *A*). This lesion grows rapidly, and the

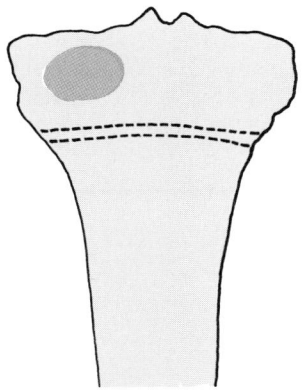

FIG. 69-6   Chondroblastoma.

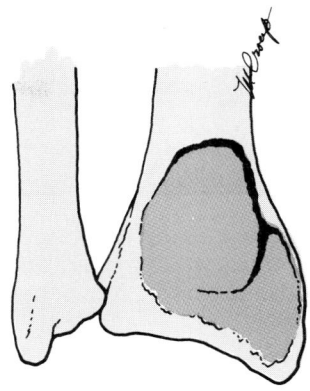

FIG. 69-7   Unicameral bone cyst.

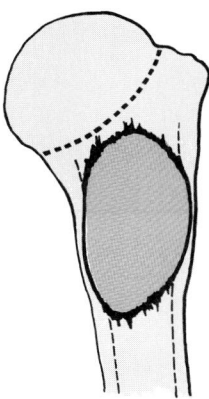

FIG. 69-8   Giant-cell tumor.

bone does not have sufficient time or a defense response to react against it. Extension of the lesion through the cortex of the bone is typical of a malignancy. When the tumor penetrates the cortex, the periosteum may be lifted off. The bone may respond by depositing a thin layer of reactive bone, which is then lifted off, and the periosteal reaction begins again. As mentioned previously, this produces an onionskin effect typical of Ewing's sarcoma (see Fig. 69-5, *B*).

Although the previous signs indicate the degree of malignancy of a lesion, other specific radiologic signs lead to a more definitive diagnosis. For example, a radiolucent lesion located within the epiphysis of a growing bone is apt to be a chondroblastoma (Fig. 69-6). A sclerotic marginated cystic lesion in the metaphysis of a long bone near an active growth plate is likely to be a benign unicameral bone cyst (Fig. 69-7). A radiolucent lesion in an adult in the metaphysis near the old growth plate is likely to be a giant-cell tumor (Fig. 69-8).

A large, destructive lesion penetrating the cortex of the metaphysis of a long bone of an adolescent or young adult is indicative of osteogenic sarcoma. A reticulated, spotty, and extensive radiolucent cortical lesion in a child

is likely to be Ewing's sarcoma. A "target" or "bull's-eye" lesion, sclerotic bone around a radiolucent area surrounding a central dense nucleus, in an individual with night pain that responds to salicylates, is nearly always an osteoid osteoma.

KEY CONCEPTS

- *Neoplasms* can occur in *bone tissue* and may originate in the bone tissue itself or may spread to the bone from other primary sites.
- *Bone tumor cells* produce factors that stimulate osteoclast function, leading to bone resorption that can be seen radiographically.
- *Primary bone tumors* can be benign or malignant. Benign tumors are much more common than are malignant tumors, and malignant tumors tend to grow rapidly, spread, and invade irregularly.
- A number of neoplasms that originate in other tissues can spread to bone by way of the bloodstream (most common sites are the prostate, breast, lung, thyroid, kidney, and bladder). The most common bones affected are the vertebrae, proximal femur, pelvis, ribs, sternum, and proximal humerus.
- *Osteomas* are benign bone lesions characterized by an abnormal outgrowth of bone.
- *Chondroblastoma* is a rare, usually benign tumor, which occurs most frequently in adolescent males.
- *Enchondroma,* or central chondroma, is a benign tumor of dysplastic cartilage cells occurring in the metaphysis of tubular bones, particularly of the hands and feet.
- A characteristic feature of a *giant-cell tumor* is the vascular and cellular stroma make up of oval-shaped cells containing small, elongated, darkly staining nuclei. These tumors occur chiefly in young adults, and they occur more frequently in women than they do in men.
- The most common malignant bone tumor is *multiple myeloma,* which is caused by a malignant prolifera-

tion of plasma cells and it is rarely seen in individuals younger than 40 years of age.

■ *Osteogenic sarcoma*, or *osteosarcoma*, is a malignant primary neoplasm of bone and it arises in the metaphysis of the bone. Severe pain associated with bone destruction and erosion is a usual symptom of this condition.

■ *Chondrosarcoma* is a malignant tumor composed of anaplastic chondrocytes and may occur as a central or peripheral bone tumor. Chondrosarcoma occurs most often in men over 35 years of age. However, rapid aggressive growth may occur.

■ *Ewing's sarcoma* is most often seen in teenaged children, and the most common site is the shaft of long bones. A "target" or "bull's-eye" lesion, sclerotic bone around a radiolucent area surrounding a central dense nucleus, in an individual with night pain that responds to salicylates, is nearly always an osteoid osteoma.

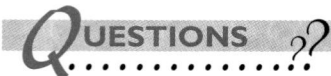

A sampling of review questions for this chapter appears here. Visit http://www.mosby.com/MERLIN/PriceWilson/ for additional questions.

Answer the following on a separate sheet of paper.

1. What is the rationale for treatment of a lesion that is benign rather than a lesion that is less certainly benign?

2. What is the relationship of osteoclast activity to the formation of bone tumors?

3. Differentiate between benign and malignant tumors as to incidence, growth, and invasiveness.

4. What are the most common primary sites of bone neoplasms?

5. List the bones most frequently affected by neoplasms.

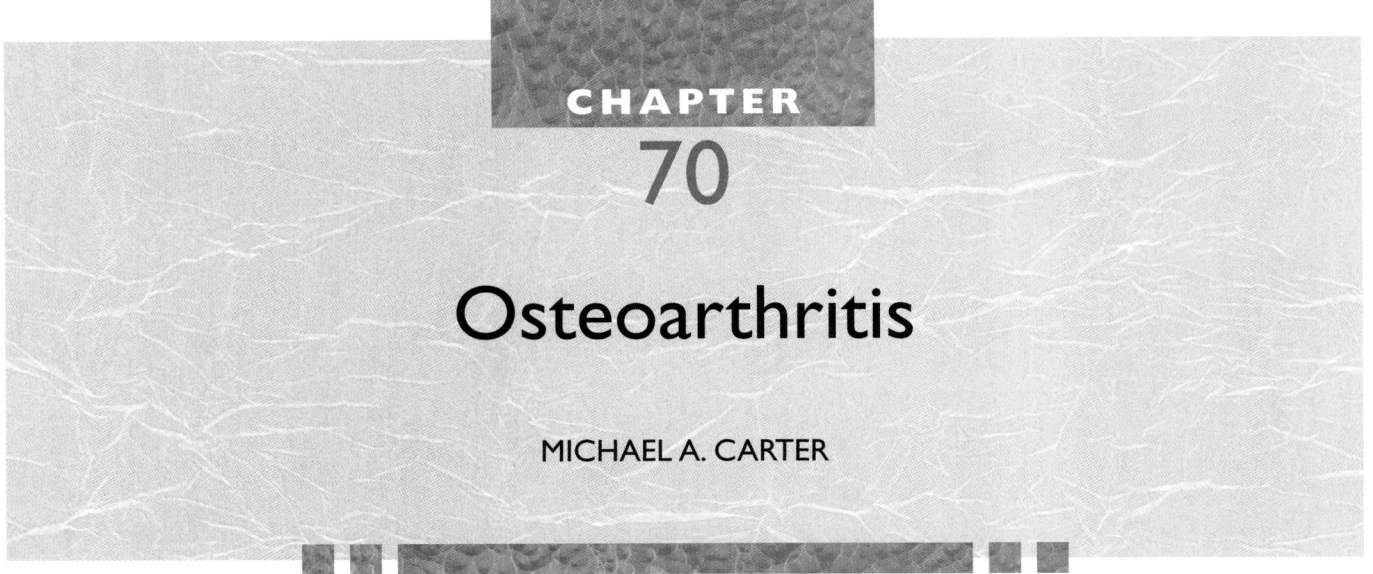

CHAPTER
70

Osteoarthritis

MICHAEL A. CARTER

*O*steoarthritis is a disorder of movable joints. The disease is chronic, slowly progressive, noninflammatory, and characterized by the deterioration and abrasion of articular cartilage and the formation of new bone at the articular surface.

Osteoarthritis, the most common form of arthritis, constitutes slightly more than one half of all cases of arthritis. The disorder is more common in women than in men and is found primarily in persons over age 45. This disorder was once thought to be a normal consequence of the aging process, because the incidence increases with age. Osteoarthritis was given the name of "wear and tear" arthritis, based on the idea that the joint wore out with age. However, newer findings of the biochemistry and biomechanics of the joint have disproved this theory.

Chondrocytes are the cells responsible for the formation of the proteoglycans and collagen in the articular cartilage. For unknown reasons, the synthesis of proteoglycans and collagen is greatly increased in osteoarthritis. However, these substances are degraded at an even more rapid rate, resulting in a net loss over time. As small amounts of type I cartilage replace the normal type II, changes in the collagen fiber diameters and orientation occur that alter the biomechanics of the cartilage. The articular cartilage then loses its unique compressibility. Although the actual cause of osteoarthritis remains unknown, it appears that the aging process is related to changes in chondrocyte functioning, causing the composition of the articular cartilage to alter and leading to the development of osteoarthritis.

Genetic factors play a role in some forms of osteoarthritis. The development of osteoarthritis of the distal interphalangeal joints of the hands (Heberden's nodes) is gender influenced and dominant in females. Women develop Heberden's nodes 10 times more often than men.

Sex hormones and other hormonal factors seem to be related to the development of osteoarthritis. The relationship between estrogens and bone formation and the prevalence of osteoarthritis in women both strongly suggest that hormones play an active part in the disease's development and progression.

The joints most often affected in osteoarthritis are the weight-bearing joints, including the knees, hips, lumbar and cervical spine, and the phalangeal joints. A distinguishing feature of osteoarthritis is that the proximal and distal phalangeal joints are often affected, whereas the metacarpophalangeal joints are usually unaffected. In rheumatoid arthritis, however, the proximal phalangeal joints and the metacarpal joints are affected, and the distal interphalangeal joints are spared.

Osteoarthritis primarily involves biochemical and biomechanical changes within the joint; it is not an inflammatory disorder. Synovitis frequently accompanies the changes seen in the joint, however, and causes pain and discomfort.

In addition to the common form of osteoarthritis, there are several variants. *Primary generalized osteoarthritis* is different in that there is an increase in the number and severity of the joints involved. *Erosive inflammatory osteoarthritis* primarily affects the finger joints and is associated with acute inflammatory episodes that lead to deformities and ankylosis. *Ankylosis hyperostosis* involves ossification of the vertebrae. *Secondary osteoarthritis* develops as a consequence of some other illness, such as rheumatoid arthritis or gout.

CLINICAL FEATURES

The most common feature of osteoarthritis is pain in the joint, especially with movement or weight bearing. This dull, aching pain is relieved by rest and exacerbated by motion or weight bearing. The patient may have stiffness after resting, but this goes away with motion. Morning stiffness, if present, usually lasts only a few minutes, as

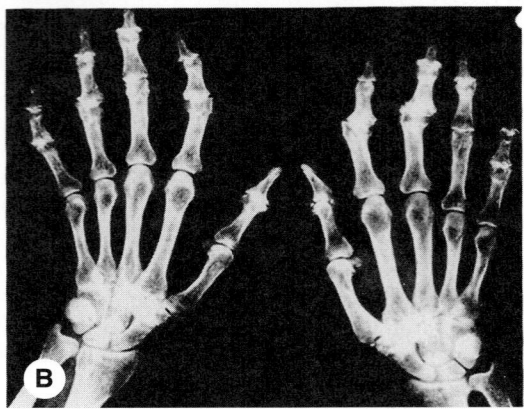

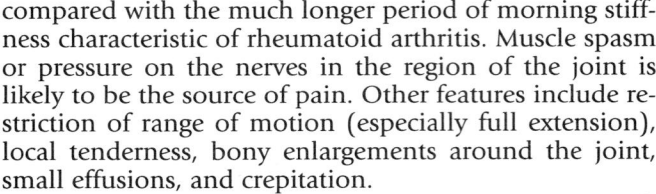

FIG. 70-1 Osteoarthritis. **A**, Primary osteoarthritis of the hands with marked proximal interphalangeal involvement (Bouchard's nodes) along with distal interphalangeal joint involvement. **B**, Radiograph of the same hands. (From Hollander JL, editor: *Arthritis and allied conditions: a textbook of rheumatology*, ed 8, Philadelphia, 1972, Lea & Febiger.)

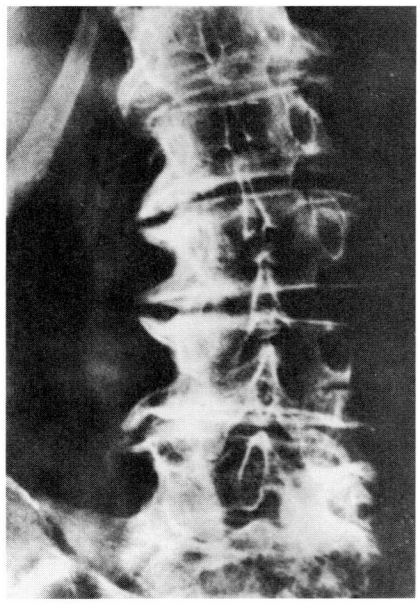

FIG. 70-2 Spine radiograph of osteoarthritis. This anteroposterior projection of the lumbar spine shows scoliosis and narrowing of the intervertebral spaces on the concave side, where extensive osteophyte formation is present. The osteophytes are not continuous, as is seen in ankylosing spondylitis. Adjacent bony margins are sclerosed. (Reproduced from the Arthritis Foundation, New York, 1972.)

compared with the much longer period of morning stiffness characteristic of rheumatoid arthritis. Muscle spasm or pressure on the nerves in the region of the joint is likely to be the source of pain. Other features include restriction of range of motion (especially full extension), local tenderness, bony enlargements around the joint, small effusions, and crepitation.

Characteristic changes occur in the hands. Heberden's nodes, or bony enlargements of the distal interphalangeal joints, are frequently seen. Less common are Bouchard's nodes (Fig. 70-1), which are bony enlargements of the proximal interphalangeal joints.

Characteristic changes are also seen in the spine, which becomes painful, stiff, and limited in range of motion (ROM). Bony overgrowths or spurs may irritate the nerve roots as they pass through the vertebrae. This irritation results in neuromuscular changes, such as pain, stiffness, and limited ROM. Some people complain of headaches that are a direct result of osteoarthritis of the cervical spine.

LABORATORY FINDINGS

Osteoarthritis is a local arthritic disorder, so no specific blood tests are used in the diagnosis. Laboratory tests are sometimes used to exclude other forms of arthritis. Rheumatoid factor may be present in the serum, because it normally increases in frequency with aging. The erythrocyte sedimentation rate may be slightly elevated if there is extensive synovitis.

RADIOLOGIC FINDINGS

A common radiographic characteristic of osteoarthritis is narrowing of the joint space, which happens because of loss of cartilage. In the knee, the joint space may be narrowed in only one compartment. In addition to narrowing, bone density is increased around the joint. *Osteophytes* (spurs) can be seen at the marginal aspects of the joint (Fig. 70-2). Cystic changes of various sizes are sometimes seen.

The extent of the change in the joints noted radiographically may not be related to the presence of symptoms. Radiologic evidence of osteoarthritis can be demonstrated in as many as 85% of persons over age 75, although a much lower percentage of individuals actually complain of pain and stiffness.

Specialized radiographs may help evaluate osteoarthritis. Weight-bearing radiographs of the knees may give a better picture of the effects of the illness than non-weight-bearing views. Osteoarthritis is not a symmetric disorder, so views of the contralateral joint can be helpful.

TREATMENT

The treatment of osteoarthritis is multifocal and consists of an individualized plan. The goals of treatment are to prevent or retard further damage to the joint, to manage pain and stiffness, and to maintain mobility.

Protecting the joints from additional trauma is important in slowing the progression of the disorder. Evaluating work patterns and activities of daily living assists in eliminating the specific activities that increase the load-bearing strain to an affected joint. Canes and walkers can significantly decrease the weight load on knees and hips. Reducing weight, if the person is overweight, can greatly decrease the load placed on knees and hips.

Physical therapy measures are important for relieving pain and preserving muscle strength and ROM. The use of ice or heat on the involved joints may provide temporary relief of pain. ROM exercises may help maintain full ROM of involved joints. Isometric exercises help build the muscles that support the joints. Isotonic exercises should not be used with resistance, because this can further stress the joint.

Drug therapy is designed to control the pain in the joint and any synovitis. Over-the-counter analgesic drugs such as acetaminophen, aspirin, and ibuprofen are usually adequate for pain relief. Aspirin and ibuprofen have the added advantage of controlling the synovitis. Other nonsteroidal antiinflammatory drugs are frequently used for pain and synovitis control. Adverse effects of these drugs are generally more common in older persons; drug therapy should be considered carefully in this age group, because so many have osteoarthritis.

Disease-modifying antirheumatic drugs are not used in the treatment of osteoarthritis because synovitis is not a systemic disorder. Oral corticosteroids are usually contraindicated. These agents are generally ineffective in improving symptoms, and their toxic potential makes their use risky. Intraarticular injections can provide relief of synovitis. If used too frequently, the agents deplete the normal ground substance of the cartilage and can accelerate the arthritic progression.

Surgical treatment of osteoarthritis is designed to remove loose bodies, repair damaged supporting tissues, or replace the entire joint. Arthroscopic surgery allows a variety of surgical procedures to be performed with much less morbidity than that associated with open surgeries. Particles of cartilage can be removed as efficiently as can those in other surgical procedures.

Another form of surgery used in osteoarthritis is angulation osteotomy. This procedure is used to treat osteoarthritis of the knee that affects only one compartment. Pain is relieved in the joint by correcting the varus or valgus deformity and bringing healthy articular cartilage into contact with other healthy articular cartilage.

Total joint replacements for hips and knees have been successful in maintaining near-normal function for many people with osteoarthritis. Osteoarthritis is a hypertrophic form of arthritis, which means that the bone adjacent to the artificial joint is strong, forming an excellent base for attachment. Various complications can occur with joint replacement, and these are weighed against the acquired benefits. Long-term evaluation studies of total prostheses for finger and other joints are still underway.

Joint fusions may be necessary for the relief of pain in advanced cases of osteoarthritis. The cervical spine is an area in which joint fusion can provide dramatic pain relief.

PROGNOSIS

Osteoarthritis generally progresses slowly. The major problems encountered are pain on the use of a joint and increasing instability with weight bearing, particularly in the knee. These problems mean that the person usually must develop a new lifestyle. This new lifestyle often includes altering lifelong patterns of eating and exercise, manipulating complex drug regimens, and using adaptive and assisting devices.

KEY CONCEPTS

- *Osteoarthritis* is a disorder of movable joints and is chronic, slowly progressive, noninflammatory, and characterized by the deterioration and abrasion of articular cartilage and the formation of new bone at the articular surface.
- Osteoarthritis, the most common form of arthritis, constitutes slightly more than one half of all cases of arthritis. Osteoarthritis is more common in women than it is in men and is found primarily in persons over age 45 and was called "wear and tear" arthritis, based on the idea that the joint wore out with age. Newer findings of the biochemistry and biomechanics of the joint have disproved this theory.
- *Chondrocytes* are the cells responsible for the formation of the proteoglycans and collagen in the articular cartilage. For unknown reasons, the synthesis of proteoglycans and collagen is greatly increased in osteoarthritis.
- As *small amounts of type I cartilage replace the normal type II*, changes in the collagen fiber diameters and orientation occur that alter the biomechanics of the cartilage, and the articular cartilage then loses its unique compressibility.

- The *cause of osteoarthritis* remains unknown, although the aging process is related to changes in chondrocyte functioning, causing the composition of the articular cartilage to alter and leading to the development of osteoarthritis.
- The development of osteoarthritis of the distal interphalangeal joints of the hands (*Heberden's nodes*) is gender influenced and dominant in females.
- Sex hormones and other hormonal factors seem to be related to the development of osteoarthritis.
- The relationship between estrogens and bone formation and the prevalence of osteoarthritis in women strongly suggest that hormones play an active part in the disease's development and progression.
- The joints most often affected in osteoarthritis are the weight-bearing joints, including the knees, hips, lumbar and cervical spine, and the phalangeal joints.
- A distinguishing feature of osteoarthritis is that the *proximal* and *distal phalangeal joints* are often affected.
- Osteoarthritis primarily involves biochemical and biomechanical changes within the joint; *synovitis* frequently accompanies the changes seen in the joint and causes pain and discomfort.

- There are several variants of osteoarthritis, such as *primary generalized osteoarthritis, erosive inflammatory, ankylosis hyperostosis,* and *secondary osteoarthritis.*
- The most common feature of osteoarthritis is pain in the joint, especially with movement or weight bearing.
- Characteristic changes occur in the hands. *Heberden's nodes,* or bony enlargements of the distal interphalangeal joints, are frequently seen. Characteristic changes are also seen in the spine, which becomes painful, stiff, and limited in range of motion (ROM).
- Osteoarthritis is a local arthritic disorder, so no specific blood tests are used in the diagnosis.
- A common radiographic characteristic of osteoarthritis is narrowing of the joint space.
- The treatment of osteoarthritis is multifocal and consists of an individualized plan.

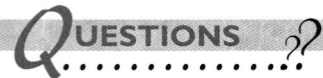

QUESTIONS ??

A sampling of review questions for this chapter appears here. Visit http://www.mosby.com/MERLIN/PriceWilson/ for additional questions.

Answer the following on a separate sheet of paper.

1. Define osteoarthritis.
2. Describe the synthesis of proteoglycans and collagen in osteoarthritis.
3. Explain why the aging process seems to be related to the development of osteoarthritis.
4. Explain the rationale for total joint replacements for hips and knees in osteoarthritis.
5. Explain the radiologic findings for osteoarthritis.
6. Identify the goals of treatment of osteoarthritis.

CHAPTER
71

Rheumatoid Arthritis

MICHAEL A. CARTER

Rheumatoid arthritis is a chronic disorder that affects multiple organ systems. This disorder is one of a group of diffuse connective tissue diseases that are immune mediated and of unknown cause. Patients usually have progressive joint destruction, although the episodes of joint inflammation may have periods of remission (Fig. 71-1).

Rheumatoid arthritis affects women about $2\frac{1}{2}$ times more frequently than it does men. The incidence increases with age, especially in women. The peak incidence is between 40 and 60 years of age. The disease is seen worldwide in all racial groups. About 1% of all adults have definite rheumatoid arthritis, and about 750 new cases per million are reported each year in the United States.

The causes of rheumatoid arthritis are still unknown, even though much is known about the pathogenesis. The disorder cannot be shown to have a definite genetic link. There is an association with the genetic markers of the human leukocyte antigen HLA-Dw4 and HLA-DR5 in Caucasians. Only an association with HLA-Dw4 has been shown in African Americans, Japanese, and Chippewa Indians.

Destruction of the tissues in the joint occurs in two ways. First, a digestive destruction is brought about by the production of proteases, collagenases, and other hydrolytic enzymes. These enzymes break down the cartilage, ligaments, tendons, and bones in the joints and are released along with oxygen radicals and arachidonic acid metabolites by polymorphonuclear leukocytes in the synovial fluid. The process is thought to be part of an autoimmune response to locally produced antigens.

Tissue destruction also occurs through the action of rheumatoid pannus, a vascular granulation tissue that

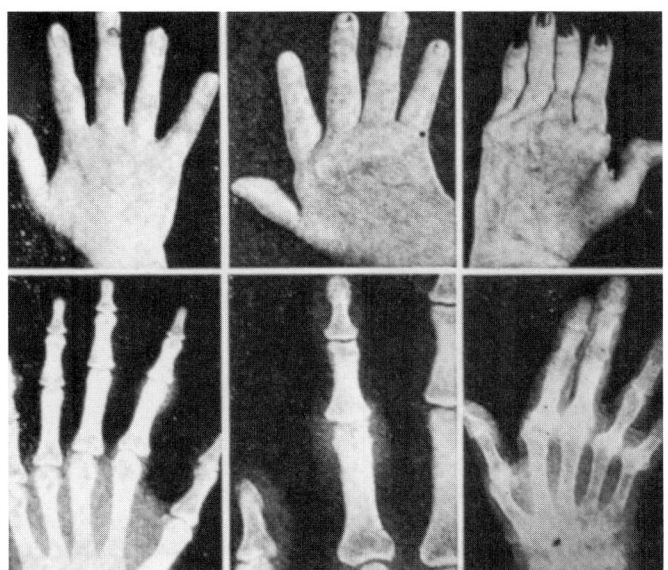

FIG. 71-1 Early, moderate, and advanced rheumatoid arthritis in the hands. Note the swelling of the second proximal interphalangeal (PIP) joint as part of the early changes. In the moderate stage, swelling of the metacarpophalangeal (MCP) joints occurs. The advanced stage shows subluxation of the MCP joints. (From Ensign DC: *Mod Med*, March 1, 1955, p 128, copyright Harcourt Brace Jovanovich.)

forms from the inflamed synovium and later extends into the joint. Along the edge of the pannus, destruction of collagen and proteoglycans occurs through the production of enzymes by cells in the pannus.

CLINICAL FEATURES

Several common clinical features are seen in persons with rheumatoid arthritis and are listed next. These may not all be present at one time in any particular individual, because the disorder is so variable.

1. *Constitutional symptoms:* these include fatigue, anorexia, weight loss, and fever. At times, the fatigue can be disabling.

2. *Symmetric polyarthritis,* primarily of peripheral joints: this includes the joints of the hands, usually sparing the distal interphalangeal joints. Almost any diarthrodial joint can be affected.

3. *Morning stiffness* greater than 1 hour: this may be generalized stiffness but primarily involves the joints. This stiffness is different from the stiffness seen in osteoarthritis, which usually lasts only a few minutes and always less than an hour.

4. *Erosive arthritis:* radiologic characteristic of this disorder. The chronic inflammatory response results in loss of the marginal aspects of the bones (Fig. 71-2).

5. *Deformity:* destruction of the supportive structures of the joints occurs as the disease progresses. Ulnar drift or deviation of the fingers, subluxation of the metacarpophalangeal joints, and boutonniere and swan neck deformities (Fig. 71-3) are some of the common deformities of the hands. There is a protrusion of the metatarsal heads secondary to metatarsal subluxation in the feet. Large joints may also be involved and have decreased range of motion, primarily in extension.

6. *Rheumatoid nodules:* subcutaneous masses occurring in about one third of adults with rheumatoid arthritis. The most common site for these is in the olecranon bursa (elbow) or along the extensor surface of the forearm; however, they can occur elsewhere. The presence of these nodules is usually indicative of an active or more severe disease (Fig. 71-4).

7. *Extraarticular manifestations:* rheumatoid arthritis may involve organs other than the joints. The heart (pericarditis), lungs (pleuritis), eyes, and blood vessels can be damaged. Box 71-1 outlines extraarticular manifestations of this disorder.

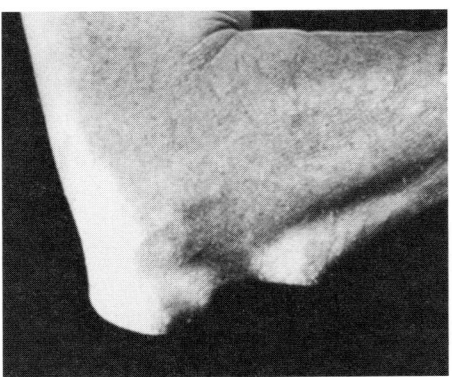

FIG. 71-4 Rheumatoid nodules in the elbow. Two large subcutaneous nodules are located about the elbow. One is in the olecranon bursa, and the other is on the extensor surface of the forearm. Nodules may be fixed or movable and are usually tender. They occur most frequently at the elbow but may also be found elsewhere, as on the feet, fingers, occiput, heels, and buttocks. Nodules occur in about 20% of patients with rheumatoid arthritis, may fluctuate in size, and are usually associated with high titers of rheumatoid factor. (From the Arthritis Foundation, New York, 1972.)

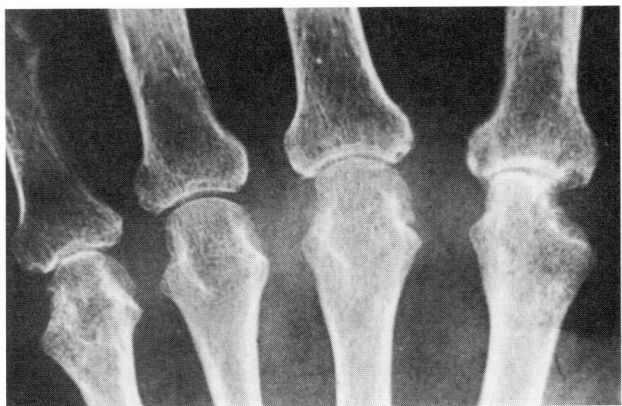

FIG. 71-2 Radiograph of a rheumatoid hand. Note the erosion of the second metacarpal head and early erosion of the third metacarpal head. The cortex of the fourth metacarpal head remains indistinct. Compare this with the well-defined cortex of the fifth metacarpal head. (From the Canadian Arthritis and Rheumatism Society, JB Houpt, editor.)

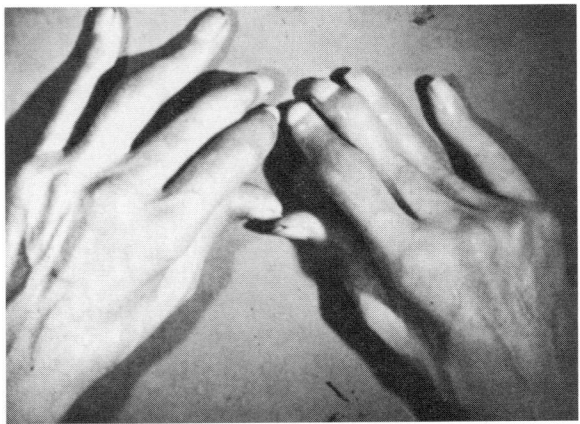

FIG. 71-3 Rheumatoid hand with boutonniere and swan neck deformities. Polyarthritis of the joints of the hands is seen. Among the advanced deforming changes is the muscle wasting in the anatomic snuffbox (between thumb and forefinger). Boutonniere deformity affects the left fourth digit, and swan neck deformity involves the right third and fourth digits. (From the Arthritis Division, University Hospital, University of Michigan.)

BOX 71-1

Extraarticular Manifestations of Rheumatoid Arthritis

Skin	Subcutaneous nodules
	Vasculitis, causing brown spots
	Ecchymotic lesions
Heart	Pericarditis
	Pericardial tamponade (rare)
	Inflammatory lesions in myocardium and valves
Lungs	Pleurisy, with or without effusion
	Pulmonary inflammatory lesions
Eyes	Scleritis
Nervous system	Peripheral neuropathy
	Peripheral compression syndromes, including carpal tunnel syndrome, ulnar nerve neuropathy, peroneal palsy, and cervical spine abnormalities
Systemic	Anemia (common)
	Generalized osteoporosis
	Felty's syndrome
	Sjögren's syndrome (keratoconjunctivitis sicca)
	Amyloidosis (rare)

LABORATORY FINDINGS

Several laboratory tests are used to diagnose rheumatoid arthritis. *Rheumatoid factor* is found in the serum of about 85% of the individuals who have rheumatoid arthritis. This autoantibody is an anti–gamma globulin factor, immunoglobulin M (IgM), that reacts against altered IgG. Higher titers, greater than 1:160, are usually associated with rheumatoid nodules, severe disease, vasculitis, and a poor prognosis. Rheumatoid factor is a helpful diagnostic indicator, but it is not an exclusive test for rheumatoid arthritis. A positive test can indicate other connective tissue disorders, such as systemic lupus erythematosus, progressive systemic sclerosis, and dermatomyositis. Furthermore, about 5% of normal people have a positive test. The incidence of positive rheumatoid factor in the normal population increases with age. As many as 20% of people over 60 years of age may have positive factors with low titers.

The erythrocyte sedimentation rate (ESR) is a nonspecific index of inflammation. Patients with rheumatoid arthritis may have high values (100 mm/hour or higher). This observation means that the ESR may be useful for monitoring disease activity.

Rheumatoid arthritis can cause a normocytic normochromic anemia by acting on the bone marrow. This anemia does not respond to the usual forms of therapy and can make the person feel fatigued. Iron deficiency anemia often occurs as a consequence of drug therapy for the illness. This form of anemia may respond to iron replacement.

Normal synovial fluid is a clear, light-yellow fluid with a white blood cell (WBC) count of less than 200/mm³. In rheumatoid arthritis, the synovial fluid loses its viscosity, and the WBC count is increased to 15,000 to 20,000/mm³, making the fluid turbid. The fluid may clot, but the clot is usually poor and friable.

RADIOLOGIC FEATURES

In the early stages of the illness, no radiologic findings other than soft tissue swelling may be seen. As the joint damage progresses, narrowing of the joint space may occur because of the loss of articular cartilage. Bone erosions at the margin of the joint and decreased bone density occur. These changes are not usually reversible.

DIAGNOSTIC CRITERIA

The diagnosis of rheumatoid arthritis can be a complex process. In the early stages, there may be only a few or no positive laboratory tests, the joint changes can be minor, and the symptoms can be transitory. The diagnosis does not rest on any single characteristic but is based on the evaluation of a number of signs and symptoms. The diagnostic criteria are as follows:

1. Morning stiffness (lasting at least 1 hour)
2. Arthritis of three or more joint areas
3. Arthritis of hand joints
4. Symmetric arthritis
5. Rheumatoid nodules
6. Serum rheumatoid factor
7. Radiographic changes (erosions or bony decalcification)

Rheumatoid arthritis is said to be present if at least four of the seven criteria are met. The first four criteria must be present for at least 6 weeks.

TREATMENT

The treatment of rheumatoid arthritis is based on an understanding of the pathophysiology of the disorder. In addition, attention needs to be directed toward the psychophysiologic manifestations and the attendant psychosocial disruptions caused by the chronic, fluctuating course of the problem. Making an accurate diagnosis may take years, but treatment is initiated early.

The overall goals of the therapeutic program are as follows:

1. To relieve pain and inflammation
2. To maintain joint function and maximum functional capacity of the person
3. To prevent and correct joint deformities

There are a number of therapeutic prescriptions designed to achieve these goals: education, rest, exercise and thermotherapy, nutrition, and medication.

The first step of the therapeutic program is to provide an adequate *education* about the illness to the patient, the family, and those with whom the patient comes into contact. This education includes an understanding of the pathophysiology, causes, and prognosis of the illness and all the components of the management program, including the complex drug regimen, sources of assistance for coping with the illness, and effective methods of management offered by the health care team. The educational process is a constant one. Patient clubs, community agencies, and other people with rheumatoid arthritis and their families can provide assistance.

Rest is important because rheumatoid arthritis usually is accompanied by profound fatigue. Although the person may have some fatigue each day, at times, the person will be better or worse. Stiffness and discomfort may worsen with rest, meaning that the person can frequently awaken at night with pain. Methods of decreasing nighttime pain should be advised, such as long-acting antiinflammatory drugs and analgesia. In addition, the treatment plan should cover activity pacing. The person should break each day into periods of activity followed by rest. If a particularly heavy activity is planned, such as a party, the rest period should be before that activity.

Specific *exercises* are useful in maintenance of joint function. These include active and passive range of motion to all affected joints at least twice a day. Pain medications may be necessary before beginning these exercises. *Heat* applications to painful and swollen joints may decrease pain. Special temperature-regulated paraffin baths and contrast baths of heat and cold can be used at home. The exercise and thermotherapy program is best prescribed by a health care provider who has special training, such as a physical therapist or an occupational therapist. Overuse of exercise can tear supporting structures of the joint that are already weakened by the illness.

Adaptive and assistive equipment may be necessary for the person to perform activities of daily living. The Arthritis Foundation or one of its many local chapters can provide materials that show how to use these devices and where to purchase them.

No specific nutritional prescription exists for rheumatoid arthritis. There are many unproven claims about various types of dietary interventions. The general principle is that a well-balanced diet is important. The illness may affect the temporomandibular joint, making chewing difficult at times. A number of the medications used to treat the illness can cause stomach discomfort and decrease adequate nutrition. Keeping the body weight in the proper limits is important. Weight can be easily gained, because activity levels usually are low. This increased weight can place additional stress on hip, knee, and foot joints. Referral to a registered dietitian may be of assistance.

Medication therapy is an important part of the overall treatment program. Medications are prescribed to reduce pain, decrease the inflammation of the illness, and attempt to modify the course of the illness. Different drugs may be used for each of these goals.

Pain is a constant part of rheumatoid arthritis, which means that the use of dependency-causing drugs should be kept to a minimum. Therapeutic measures such as heat and exercise can do much to diminish pain.

The mainstay of drug therapy in rheumatoid arthritis is the use of *nonsteroidal antiinflammatory drugs (NSAIDs)*. This class of drugs reduces inflammation by interrupting the cascade of production of inflammatory mediators. Specifically, NSAIDs inhibit either cyclooxygenase or prostaglandin synthetase. These enzymes convert the endogenous systemic fatty acid arachidonic acid to prostaglandins, prostacyclins, thromboxanes, and oxygen radicals. The historical standard drug in this class is aspirin, and all other NSAIDs are considered equally effective as is aspirin at appropriate doses of each drug.

Additional drug therapy is indicated when the NSAIDs do not control the rheumatoid arthritis. These medications include a group of diverse, slow-acting drugs such as gold compounds, antimalarials, penicillamine, azathioprine, and methotrexate. Several of these do not have U.S. Food and Drug Administration approval for the treatment of rheumatoid arthritis. The goals of treatment with slow-acting drugs are to control the clinical manifestations and to arrest or slow the progression of the illness. The onset of response to these drugs is often gradual and can take as long as 3 to 6 months. Maximum response usually occurs after 1 year of therapy.

At least four indications exist for the use of corticosteroid therapy. Chronic oral therapy is used in persons with rheumatoid arthritis who do not respond to NSAIDs and slow-acting drugs. The second indication is for the control of symptoms during the waiting period before the onset of action of slow-acting drugs. Third, intraartic-ular injections are indicated for acute exacerbations of synovitis in single joints in which mobility is significantly impaired. The fourth indication is high-dose oral therapy for short periods for severe attacks. The mechanism of action of these agents is twofold through antiinflammatory and immunosuppressive properties. Inflammation is reduced by blockage of prostaglandin formation, inhibition of leukocyte and monocyte chemotaxis and phagocytosis, stabilization of lysosomal enzymes, and prevention of changes in capillary membranes. Immunosuppression is caused by decreased reticuloendothelial, or monocyte-macrophage, procession of antigens, and altered functions of lymphocytes. Many adverse effects occur from the use of these drugs, particularly with chronic use. The effects of these drugs disturb almost all organ systems.

JUVENILE RHEUMATOID ARTHRITIS

Children can develop rheumatoid arthritis similar to the disease in adults. In the United States, 13.9 per 100,000 children will develop this illness. There are three subtypes of juvenile rheumatoid arthritis based on the onset of the symptoms.

Systemic onset (Still's disease) accounts for about 20% of all cases. Boys and girls are equally affected, and this form can occur at any age. As the name implies, there is systemic involvement of multiple organ systems in addition to a chronic polyarthritis. This subtype has the poorest prognosis of the three types and can lead to growth retardation.

Polyarticular onset accounts for about 40% of all cases. Girls are affected at a 2:1 ratio over boys, and this form can occur at any age as well. Five or more joints are involved at one time, but generally with only moderate extraarticular involvement. This form has a better prognosis than systemic onset but can also cause growth retardation.

Pauciarticular onset accounts for about 40% of all cases. Girls are affected 6:1 over boys. This form usually occurs before age 6. No more than four joints are involved, generally with few, if any, extraarticular involvements. This form has the best prognosis of the three forms.

Treatment of juvenile rheumatoid arthritis is similar to the treatment in adults, but with some important differences. Several of the drugs used in adults are not approved for use in children. Systemic corticosteroids can lead to growth retardation, osteoporosis, and cataracts. Some of the immunosuppressive agents can cause bone marrow suppression, sterility, and malignancy in children.

KEY CONCEPTS

- *Rheumatoid arthritis* is a chronic disorder that affects multiple organ systems that is one of a group of diffuse connective tissue diseases that are immune mediated and of unknown etiology.
- Rheumatoid arthritis affects women about $2\frac{1}{2}$ times more frequently than men. The incidence increases with age, especially in women, with the peak incidence between 40 and 60 years of age.
- The *cause of rheumatoid arthritis* is still unknown, even though much is known about the pathogenesis.
- There is an association with the *genetic markers* of HLA-Dw4 and HLA-DR5 in Caucasians. Only an association with HLA-Dw4 has been shown in African Americans, Japanese, and Chippewa Indians.
- Destruction of the tissues in the joint occurs in two ways. First, a digestive destruction is brought about by the production of proteases, collagenases, and other hydrolytic enzymes. Tissue destruction also occurs through the action of rheumatoid pannus.
- Several *common clinical features* include (1) fatigue, anorexia, weight loss, and fever; (2) symmetric polyarthritis, primarily of peripheral joints, and morning stiffness greater than 1 hour; (3) erosive arthritis and deformity as destruction of the supportive structures of the joints occurs; (4) rheumatoid nodules, which are subcutaneous masses; and (5) extraarticular

- manifestations that may involve organs (e.g., heart, lungs, eyes, blood vessels).
- Several *laboratory tests* are used for *diagnosis of rheumatoid arthritis*. For example, rheumatoid factor is found in the serum of about 85% of the individuals who have rheumatoid arthritis.
- *Diagnostic criteria* are as follows: (1) morning stiffness (lasting at least 1 hour), (2) arthritis of three or more joint areas, (3) arthritis of hand joints, (4) symmetric arthritis, (5) rheumatoid nodules, (6) serum rheumatoid factor, and (7) radiographic changes (erosions or bony decalcification). Rheumatoid arthritis is said to be present if at least four of the seven criteria are met.
- The *treatment of rheumatoid arthritis* is based on an understanding of the pathophysiology of the disorder, and attention needs to be directed toward the psychophysiologic manifestations and the attendant psychosocial disruptions caused by the chronic, fluctuating course of the problem.
- The overall *goals of the therapeutic program* are as follows: (1) to relieve pain and inflammation, (2) to maintain joint function and maximum functional capacity of the person, and (3) to prevent and correct joint deformities.

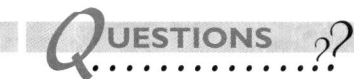

QUESTIONS

A sampling of review questions for this chapter appears here. Visit http://www.mosby.com/MERLIN/PriceWilson/ for additional questions.

Answer the following on a separate sheet of paper.

1. Define rheumatoid arthritis.
2. What is the association between the genetic markers HLA-Dw4 and HLA-DR5 and the development of rheumatoid arthritis?
3. Describe the two ways in which destruction of tissues in the joint occurs in rheumatoid arthritis.

4. List the seven diagnostic criteria for rheumatoid arthritis.
5. What are the overall goals of the therapeutic program for rheumatoid arthritis?
6. Describe the mechanism by which NSAIDs reduce inflammation.
7. Cite the four indications for the use of corticosteroid therapy in persons with rheumatoid arthritis.

8. What is the mechanism of action of these corticosteroid drugs?
9. Discuss two of the systemic organ involvements that may be seen in rheumatoid arthritis.

Systemic Lupus Erythematosus

MICHAEL A. CARTER

*S*ystemic lupus erythematosus (SLE) is a multisystem, chronic autoimmune disease. The signs and symptoms of this disorder can be diverse, transitory, and difficult to diagnose. Therefore the exact number of people with the disorder is difficult to obtain. SLE affects women about eight times as often as men. The disorder frequently begins in late adolescence or early adulthood. In the United States, African-American women are affected about three times more often than Caucasian women. The disorder is usually milder and more easily controlled if SLE develops after age 60.

SLE was originally described as a skin disorder in the 1800s and given the name lupus because of the characteristic "butterfly rash" across the bridge of the nose and the cheeks that resembles the bite of a wolf (*lupus* is the Latin word for wolf). *Discoid lupus* is the name now given to the disorder when it is limited to cutaneous involvement.

SLE is one of a group of diffuse connective tissue disorders of unknown origin. These disorders include SLE, scleroderma, polymyositis, rheumatoid arthritis, and Sjögren's syndrome. These disorders frequently have overlapping symptoms and may be present at the same time, making an accurate diagnosis difficult. SLE can vary from a mild disorder to one that is rapidly fulminating and fatal. The most common situation, however, is one of exacerbations and near remissions that can last for long periods. Early identification and treatment of SLE usually lead to a more favorable prognosis.

CLINICAL FEATURES

The clinical picture of SLE can be confusing, particularly in the early stages of the disorder. The most common symptom is a symmetric arthritis or arthralgia that is present 90% of the time, often as an initial manifestation. The most frequently affected joints are the proximal joints of the hands, wrists, elbows, shoulders, knees, and ankles. The polyarthritis of SLE differs from that of rheumatoid arthritis in that it is rarely erosive or deforming. Also, subcutaneous nodules are rarely seen in SLE.

Constitutional symptoms of fever, fatigue, weakness, and weight loss generally occur early and may recur throughout the course of the disorder. Fatigue and weakness may be secondary to a mild anemia that is caused by SLE.

Skin manifestations include an erythematous rash that may appear on the face (Fig. 72-1), neck, extremities, or trunk. About 40% of individuals with SLE have

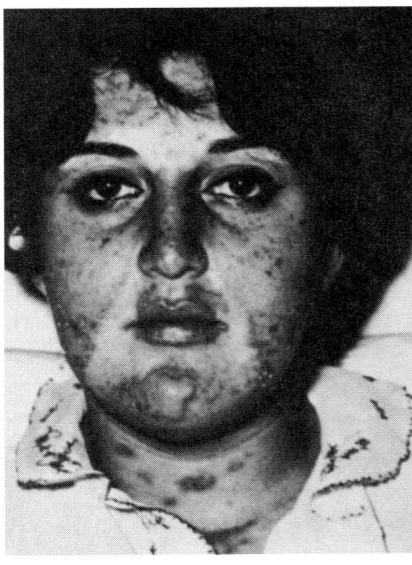

FIG. 72-1   Systemic lupus erythematous (SLE). Widespread discrete and confluent erythematous lesions are present on the face and neck. Typical peeling is noted on the chin and cheeks. (From the Arthritis Foundation, New York, 1972.)

the characteristic butterfly rash. Exposure to sunlight may aggravate this rash. Alopecia (hair loss) can develop and can sometimes be severe. Hair growth usually returns without major problems. Small ulcerations of the oral or nasopharyngeal mucous membranes can occur.

Pleurisy (chest pain) may occur as a result of the chronic inflammatory process of SLE. SLE can also cause carditis involving the myocardium, endocardium, or pericardium.

Raynaud's phenomenon occurs in about 40% of individuals with SLE. Some cases may be so severe that gangrene of the digits occurs. Vasculitis may affect all sizes of arteries and veins.

Lupus nephritis occurs as the antinuclear antibody (anti–deoxyribonucleic acid [DNA]) attaches to its antigen (DNA) and is deposited in the renal glomerulus. DNA is not normally antigenic in humans but becomes so in SLE. Complement is fixed to this immune complex, and the inflammatory process begins. Renal inflammation, tissue damage, and scarring may result.

About 65% of persons with SLE develop some renal involvement. Only 25%, however, develop severe problems. Lupus nephritis is detected by examining the urine for protein, red blood cells (RBCs), or casts. A kidney biopsy may be necessary for an accurate diagnosis (see Chapter 46).

SLE may affect the central or peripheral nervous system. Symptoms include behavioral changes (depression, psychosis), convulsions, cranial nerve disorders, and peripheral neuropathies. Central nervous system (CNS) changes are often associated with severe forms of the disorder and are frequently fatal.

Antibodies to double-stranded DNA (dsDNA) and to an ribonucleic acid (RNA)–protein complex termed Sm are found only in SLE patients. Other rheumatologic disorders can cause a positive antinuclear antibody (ANA), but anti-dsDNA and anti-Sm are rarely found except in SLE.

DIAGNOSIS

The American Rheumatism Association has developed revised criteria for the classification of SLE. The presence of four or more of the following 11 criteria, either serially or simultaneously is considered diagnostic:

1. Malar rash
2. Discoid rash
3. Photosensitivity
4. Oral ulcers
5. Arthritis: nonerosive, of two or more peripheral joints
6. Serositis: pleuritis or pericarditis
7. Renal disorder: persistent proteinuria with greater than 0.5 g/day, or cellular casts
8. Neurologic disorder: seizures or psychosis
9. Hematologic disorder: hemolytic anemia, leukopenia, lymphopenia, or thrombocytopenia
10. Immunologic disorder: positive lupus erythematosus (LE) cells, anti-DNA, anti-Sm, or a false-positive serologic test for syphilis
11. Antinuclear antibody (ANA)

DRUG-INDUCED SYSTEMIC LUPUS ERYTHEMATOSUS

A number of drugs can induce in susceptible individuals a syndrome that is similar to SLE. This syndrome includes most of the symptoms of SLE, including positive tests for ANA, but renal and CNS effects rarely occur. The SLE symptoms begin to disappear within a few weeks after the discontinuation of these drugs. The positive ANA test reverts to negative after several months. Hydralazine and procainamide are two of the more common drugs that can cause this reaction. A number of other drugs are capable of producing a positive ANA, including penicillamine, isoniazid, chlorpromazine, and anticonvulsants such as barbiturates, phenytoin, ethosuximide, methsuximide, and primidone. Some drugs can cause an exacerbation of SLE in patients who are in a remission. These drugs include sulfonamides, penicillin, and oral contraceptives.

LABORATORY TESTS

ANAs are positive in more than 95% of individuals with SLE. This test indicates whether there are antibodies capable of destroying the nucleus of one's own body cells. In addition to the presence of ANA, the ANA pattern and the specific antibodies are evaluated. The pattern refers to the appearance of the slide when viewed under ultraviolet light. A differential evaluation of the specific types of ANA is now available and is useful in differentiating SLE from other types of disorders. Antibodies to dsDNA is a specific test for SLE. Other rheumatologic disorders can cause a positive ANA, but anti-DNA antibodies are rarely found except in SLE.

The erythrocyte sedimentation rate is usually elevated in SLE. This test is a nonspecific test that measures inflammation and does not relate to the level of disease involvement in SLE.

A laboratory test that was previously used and may occasionally be used today is the LE factor. The LE cell is formed by damaging some of the person's white blood cells (WBCs) so that they will release their nucleoprotein. This protein reacts with immunoglobulin G (IgG), and the complex is phagocytosed by the remaining WBCs. The resulting cell is easily identified (Fig. 72-2). This factor can usually be demonstrated at some time in the course of the disorder if enough tests are done. LE cells

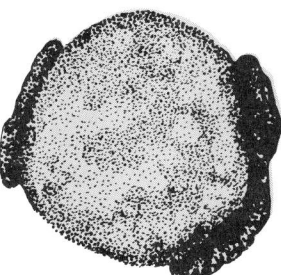

FIG. 72-2   SLE:LE cell; a neutrophil containing homogeneous material, the LE body. The nucleus is pushed to one side and flattened around the mass.

can be demonstrated in other immune-mediated systemic forms of rheumatic disorders.

Urine is examined for the presence of protein, WBCs, RBCs, and casts. These tests are used both to determine the presence of renal complications of SLE and to monitor the progression of the illness.

TREATMENT

The treatment of the person with SLE is multifaceted and includes counseling, complex drug therapy, and preventive measures. The most frequent onset period of SLE is during late adolescence and early adulthood for women. Because these are the prime reproductive years, much counseling is needed to assist in making the decision concerning having children. Pregnancy may cause a flare of SLE, which can be dangerous for women with renal damage. Cytotoxic drugs may be necessary to control the illness, and these can potentially affect the fetus. Contraceptive methods cannot usually include oral contraceptives because these may aggravate SLE. The intrauterine device can be a problem for women taking systemic corticosteroids because of the potential for infection.

Drug therapy for SLE includes nonsteroidal antiinflammatory drugs (NSAIDs), corticosteroids, antimalarials, and immunosuppressive agents. The selection of appropriate drug therapy depends on the specific organs affected by the illness. NSAIDs are used to control the arthritis and arthralgia. Aspirin is used less frequently now because it produces the highest incidence of hepatotoxicity and some patients with SLE have hepatic involvement. Persons with SLE are at a higher risk of the cutaneous, hepatic, and renal adverse effects of NSAIDs and should be monitored closely.

Antimalarial therapy is sometimes effective if the NSAIDs cannot control the symptoms of SLE. Antimalarials are usually given at an initially high dose to achieve a remission. The clearance of skin lesions offers a monitoring parameter to use in dose adjustment. Immunosuppressive therapy (cyclophosphamide or azathioprine) can be used to suppress the autoimmune activity of SLE. These drugs are usually prescribed when there is (1) a well-established diagnosis, (2) the presence of severe, life-threatening symptoms, (3) failure of other therapeutic measures, such as a failure to respond to steroids or the need for reduction of steroids because of the adverse effects, and (4) the absence of infection, pregnancy, and neoplasm.

Acute flares of SLE, especially in individuals with interstitial nephritis, are treated with high-dose oral corticosteroids for short periods. These drugs are then gradually reduced in dose over the next several weeks. Both SLE and systemic corticosteroids can produce behavioral changes, and the cause can be difficult to distinguish.

An important aspect of the prevention of flares of SLE is avoidance of exposure to ultraviolet (UV) light. Just how the sun causes SLE to flare is not fully understood. One explanation is that DNA exposed to UV light normally becomes antigenic, which leads to the flares seen after sun exposure. Patients with SLE should be encouraged to use umbrellas, hats, and long-sleeved shirts when outdoors. There may be problems getting adolescents to follow these suggestions. A sunscreen with a protection factor of 15 should be used to block the UV light exposure. The sunscreen should be reapplied after swimming or heavy exercise. The person should receive a list of drugs that can cause exacerbations so that this type of flare can be avoided.

PROGNOSIS

The prognosis for SLE varies and depends on the severity of the symptoms, the organs involved, and the length of time remissions may be maintained. No cure exists for SLE, and treatment is focused on the management of the symptoms. The prognosis is related to how well the symptoms are managed.

KEY CONCEPTS

- *Systemic lupus erythematosus (SLE)* is a multisystem, chronic autoimmune disease, the signs and symptoms of which can be diverse, transitory, and difficult to diagnose.
- The disorder frequently begins in late adolescence or early adulthood. In the United States, African-American women are affected about three times more often than Caucasian women.
- SLE was originally described as a skin disorder in the 1800s and given the name lupus because of the characteristic "butterfly rash" across the bridge of the nose and the cheeks that resembles the bite of a wolf.
- SLE is one of a group of diffuse connective tissue disorders of unknown origin. SLE can vary from a mild disorder to one that is rapidly fulminating and fatal. The most common situation is one of exacerbations and near remissions that can last for long periods.

- Early identification and treatment of SLE usually lead to a more favorable prognosis.
- The most common symptom is a symmetric arthritis or arthralgia, and the most frequently affected joints are the proximal joints of the hands, wrists, elbows, shoulders, knees, and ankles.
- *Skin manifestations* include an erythematous rash that may appear on the face neck, extremities, or trunk. About 40% of individuals with SLE have the characteristic butterfly rash. Exposure to sunlight may aggravate this rash.
- *Pleurisy* may occur as a result of the chronic inflammatory process of SLE, and carditis involving the myocardium, endocardium, or pericardium can also occur.
- *Raynaud's phenomenon* occurs in about 40% of individuals with SLE; inflammation, tissue damage, and scarring may result.

- About 65% of persons with *SLE* develop some *renal involvement*, and it may also affect the central or peripheral nervous system.
- The presence of *four or more* of the following 11 *criteria* either serially or simultaneously is considered *diagnostic of SLE*: malar rash; discoid rash; photosensitivity; oral ulcers; arthritis—nonerosive; serositis—pleuritis or pericarditis; renal disorder; neurologic disorder— seizures or psychosis; hematologic disorder—hemolytic anemia, leukopenia, lymphopenia, or thrombocytopenia; immunologic disorder—positive LE cells, anti-DNA, anti-Sm, or a false-positive serologic test for syphilis; and ANA.
- The *treatment* of the person with SLE is multifaceted and includes counseling, complex drug therapy, and preventive measures.

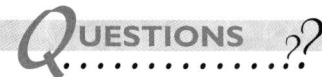

QUESTIONS ??

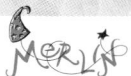

A sampling of review questions for this chapter appears here. Visit http://www.mosby.com/MERLIN/PriceWilson/ for additional questions.

Answer the following on a separate sheet of paper.

1. Formulate a definition of SLE.
2. Contrast the ANA test with the LE factor test.
3. Discuss the importance of counseling females of childbearing age regarding SLE.
4. Explain the rationale in SLE for avoidance of exposure to the sun.
5. What is the rationale for the selection of drugs used in the treatment of SLE?

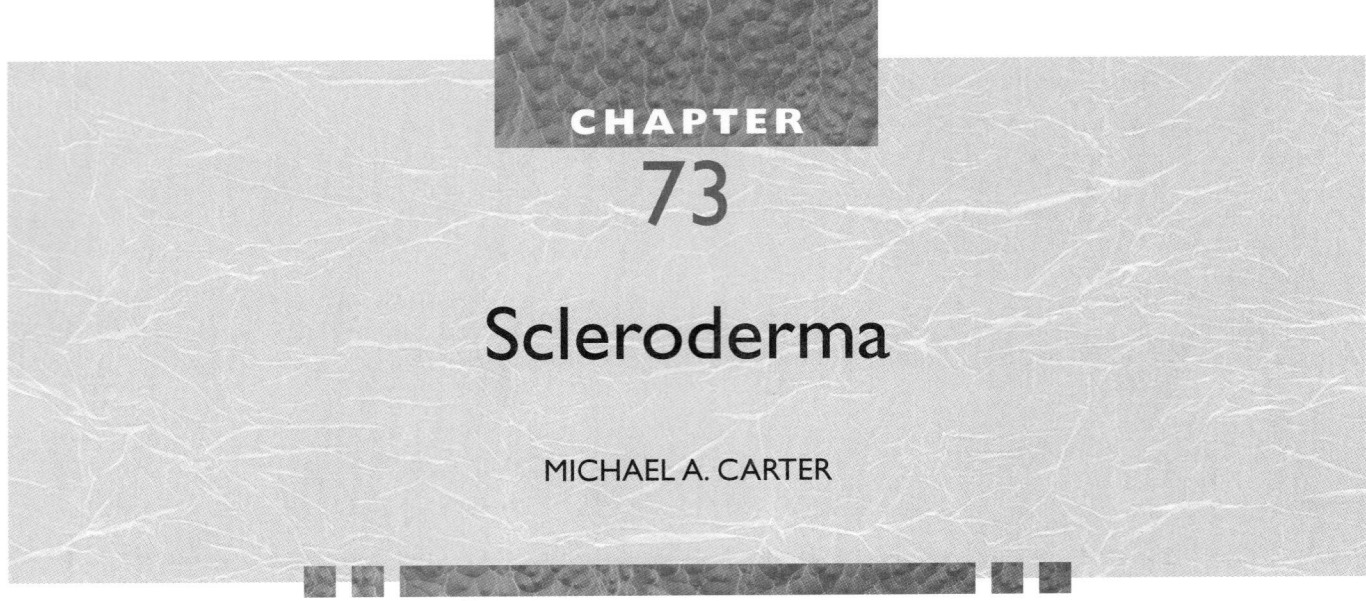

Scleroderma

MICHAEL A. CARTER

𝒮cleroderma, or *systemic sclerosis*, is an uncommon connective tissue disorder characterized by fibrosis of the skin and other organs. Scleroderma can be classified into one of three groups based on the extent of the skin disease. *Generalized scleroderma* (systemic sclerosis) can be one of two types: (1) diffuse cutaneous systemic sclerosis with truncal skin involvement, widespread visceral disease, and rapid progression or (2) limited cutaneous systemic sclerosis, including the CREST variant (see Clinical Features). *Localized scleroderma* usually affects only limited skin areas and does not affect visceral organs. *Occupational and environmental scleroderma-like syndromes* can be seen after exposure to agents such as vinyl chloride, bleomycin, and rapeseed oil.

Systemic sclerosis leads to fibrosis and degenerative changes in the synovium, digital arteries, and parenchyma and small arteries of the esophagus, intestine, lungs, heart, kidney, and thyroid gland. The cause of progressive systemic sclerosis is not known, although a number of serologic and cellular immune reaction abnormalities exist, indicating that an immunologic mechanism is involved.

The disorder is seen worldwide in all races. Women are affected three times more often than are men. The disease onset is usually in the third to fifth decades of life; only rarely does the disorder affect children. The disease occurs with particularly high frequency in coal miners, leading to the suggestion that silicosis is a predisposing factor.

Scleroderma is similar to other connective tissue disorders in that remissions and exacerbations may occur, with a generally slow progression that allows for a reasonably long life. The disorder may be rapidly progressive, however, and lead to an early death when vital organs are affected and damaged. Renal failure is the leading cause of death for persons with systemic sclerosis (see Chapter 46).

The changes seen in the skin and other organs are the result of the overproduction of collagen. The reason for the overproduction is not known. The changes in the blood vessels are similar. The lesions that develop in the small arteries and arterioles begin as proliferations on the intimal side of the internal elastic membrane. A medial thinning then occurs, and finally the deposit of a connective tissue cuff rich in collagen proceeds. All these changes are thought to be brought on by alterations in B cell and T cell activity.

CLINICAL FEATURES

Raynaud's phenomenon (Fig. 73-1) is the most common manifestation seen in persons with systemic sclerosis. *Raynaud's phenomenon* is a paroxysmal vasospastic disorder in which an abnormal spasm of the arteries of the hand occurs in response to cold temperatures or extreme emotions. This reaction causes the digits to become white (vasospasm), then blue (cyanosis), and then red (reactive hyperemia). Other common symptoms are swelling and puffiness of the hands and gradual thickening and tightening of the skin of the fingers and other body parts. The fingers develop a sausagelike appearance. The skin slowly thickens and becomes taut, shiny, and tightly bound to the underlying subcutaneous tissue. This process progresses proximally, involving the arms, chest, and face. The face becomes taut (Fig. 73-2), the oral orifice becomes wrinkled, and the opening of the orifice is restricted. The forehead loses its normal wrinkles. Polyarthralgia, joint stiffness, and polyarthritis are also seen.

One form of systemic sclerosis is the *CREST* variant. This mnemonic stands for the first letter in calcinosis, Raynaud's phenomenon, esophageal dysmotility, sclerodactyly, and telangiectasia (Fig. 73-3).

The colon may be affected, which results in diarrhea or constipation, cramping, malabsorption, and, in a few patients, perforation.

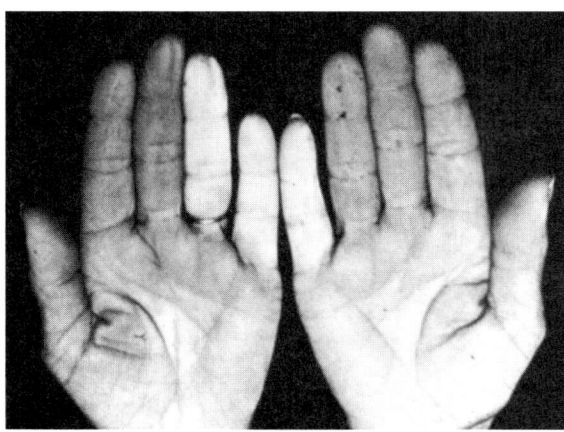

FIG. 73-1   Scleroderma: Raynaud's phenomenon. The marked pallor of the fourth and fifth digits of the left hand and the fifth digit of the right hand is characteristic of Raynaud's phenomenon. Vasospastic changes are common in systemic sclerosis. (From the Arthritis Foundation, New York, 1972.)

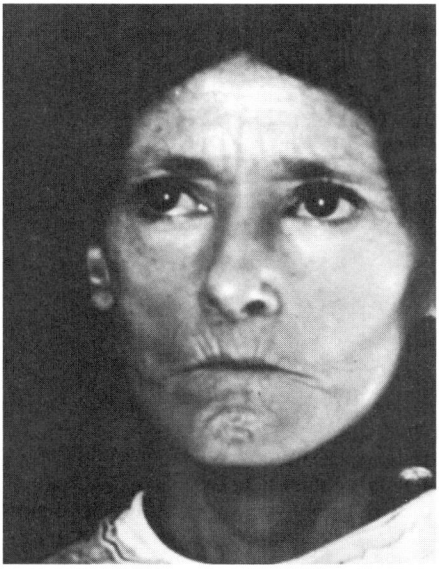

FIG. 73-2   Scleroderma: skin changes. This young woman demonstrates many features of systemic sclerosis: drawn, pursed lips, shiny skin over the cheeks and forehead, and atrophy of muscles of the temple, face, and neck. Such facial changes are known as *Mauskopf* ("mouse head"). (From the Arthritis Foundation, New York, 1972.)

Exertional dyspnea is usually the first sign of pulmonary involvement. Pulmonary function studies may show alteration in the gas exchange, that is, a decrease in breathing capacity and an increase in residual air. Pericarditis, dysrhythmias, and electrocardiogram changes may occur with cardiac involvement.

Renal involvement, exhibited as proteinuria, microscopic hematuria, and hypertension, may rapidly deteriorate to renal failure. Any vital organ involvement, especially when rapidly deteriorating, indicates a poor prognosis.

LABORATORY AND RADIOLOGIC FINDINGS

The erythrocyte sedimentation rate may be elevated in patients with scleroderma. A small group of patients may demonstrate rheumatoid factor in their serum. A positive reaction to antinuclear antibody and hypergammaglobulinemia may be demonstrated. Skin biopsies are the most specific way of making the diagnosis but are usually not necessary because of the striking clinical picture.

Radiologic examination may demonstrate subcutaneous calcifications of the digits of the hand (Fig. 73-4). Esophageal and intestinal abnormalities may also be detected.

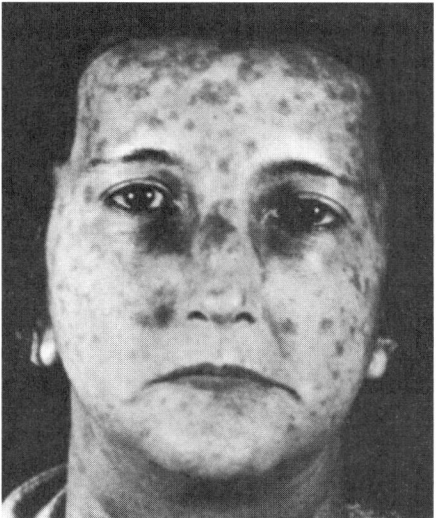

FIG. 73-3   Scleroderma: telangiectasia. Multiple telangiectases are present on the face and blanch with pressure. Telangiectasia occurs frequently in scleroderma, at times leading to confusion in differentiation from hereditary hemorrhagic telangiectasia. (From the Arthritis Foundation, New York, 1972.)

TREATMENT

Currently, no effective therapy will reverse the fibrosis of scleroderma. A variety of drugs are used to help manage symptoms. Penicillamine, dimethyl sulfoxide (DMSO), immunosuppressive drugs, and alkylating agents are sometimes used.

Protection of the hands to help avoid Raynaud's phenomenon is an important part of the management plan. Grasping a cold glass can initiate an attack. Gloves may be necessary most of the time. The person should stop using all tobacco products because of the adverse effects of nicotine on the blood vessels. Vasodilators are sometimes of benefit in treatment of Raynaud's phenomenon.

Low doses of corticosteroids may relieve joint complaints but are usually not of great benefit for treatment of systemic sclerosis. Nonsteroidal antiinflammatory agents can be used to decrease discomfort.

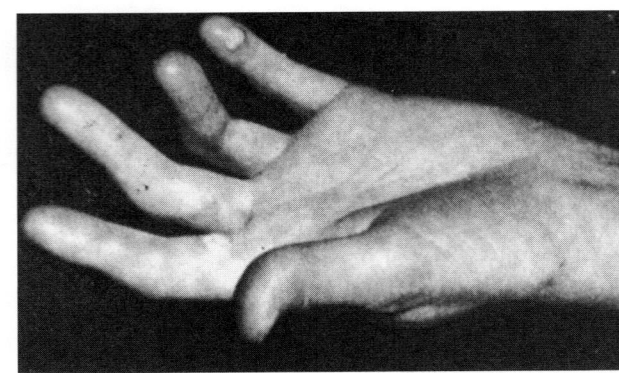

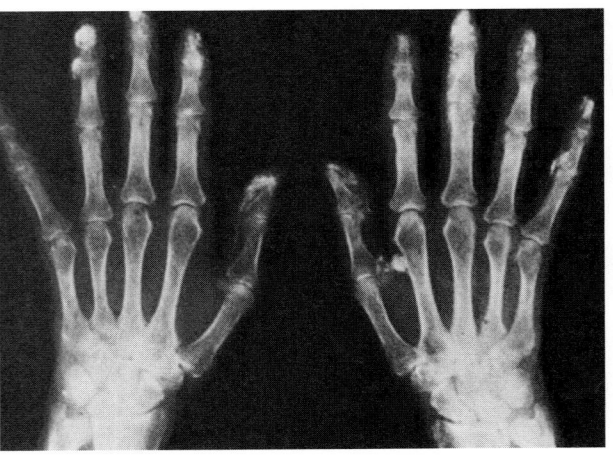

FIG. 73-4   Scleroderma: subcutaneous calcification. **A**, Hand of an adolescent girl with systemic sclerosis. Note the circumscribed lesions of calcinosis in the skin of the volar surface of the proximal portion of the second digit and the distal portion of the fifth digit. **B**, Radiograph of the hands of a woman with systemic sclerosis, as depicted by the extensive subcutaneous calcinosis in the fingers and near the joint of the right hand. (From Hollander JR, editor: *Arthritis and allied conditions: a textbook of rheumatology,* ed 8, Philadelphia, 1972, Lea & Febiger.)

Antibiotics have been used with some success in the treatment of small-bowel involvement. The hypomotility of the bowel allows for an overgrowth of microorganisms, and these interfere with absorption. Treatment with antibiotics reduces the overgrowth.

Physical therapy is an important component of therapy. The characteristic restriction of the opening of the mouth can interfere with the person's ability to eat. Mouth function can be greatly improved through stretching and muscle strengthening.

KEY CONCEPTS

- *Scleroderma*, or *systemic sclerosis*, is an uncommon connective tissue disorder characterized by fibrosis of the skin and other organs.
- Scleroderma can be classified into one of the following three groups based on the extent of the skin disease: (1) generalized scleroderma (systemic sclerosis), (2) limited cutaneous systemic sclerosis, and (3) localized scleroderma.
- Systemic sclerosis leads to fibrosis and degenerative changes in the synovium, digital arteries, and parenchyma and small arteries of the esophagus, intestine, lungs, heart, kidney, and thyroid gland.
- The etiology of progressive systemic sclerosis is unknown, although a number of serologic and cellular immune reaction abnormalities exist, indicating that an immunologic mechanism is involved.
- Women are affected three times more often than men. The disease onset is usually in the third to fifth decades of life; only rarely does the disorder affect children.
- Scleroderma is similar to other connective tissue disorders in that remissions and exacerbations may occur, with a generally slow progression that allows for a reasonably long life.
- The changes seen in the skin and other organs are the result of the overproduction of collagen, and changes in the blood vessels are similar.
- *Raynaud's phenomenon* is the most common manifestation seen in persons with systemic sclerosis.

- Other symptoms are swelling and puffiness of the hands and gradual thickening and tightening of the skin of the fingers and other body parts. The skin slowly thickens and becomes taut, shiny, and tightly bound to the underlying subcutaneous tissue; the face becomes taut, the oral orifice becomes wrinkled, and the opening of the orifice is restricted.
- Polyarthralgia, joint stiffness, and polyarthritis are also seen. The colon may be affected. Exertional dyspnea is usually the first sign of pulmonary involvement.
- Pulmonary function studies may show alteration in the gas exchange, that is, a decrease in breathing capacity and an increase in residual air. Pericarditis, dysrhythmias, and electrocardiogram changes may occur with cardiac involvement.
- *Renal involvement*, manifested as proteinuria, microscopic hematuria, and hypertension, may rapidly deteriorate to *renal failure*. Any vital organ involvement, especially when rapidly deteriorating, indicates a poor prognosis.
- Radiologic examination may demonstrate subcutaneous calcifications of the digits of the hand. Esophageal and intestinal abnormalities may also be detected.
- Currently, no effective therapy will reverse the fibrosis of scleroderma. A variety of drugs are used to help manage symptoms. Penicillamine, DMSO, immunosuppressive drugs, and alkylating agents are sometimes used.

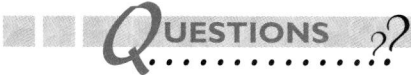

QUESTIONS

A sampling of review questions for this chapter appears here. Visit http://www.mosby.com/MERLIN/PriceWilson/ for additional questions.

Answer the following on a separate sheet of paper.

1. Differentiate among generalized scleroderma, localized scleroderma, and occupational and environmental scleroderma-like syndromes as to the extent of the skin disease.

2. Describe the changes in skin and other organs in scleroderma.

3. Describe the CREST variant of scleroderma.

4. Identify the therapeutic measures used for patients with scleroderma.

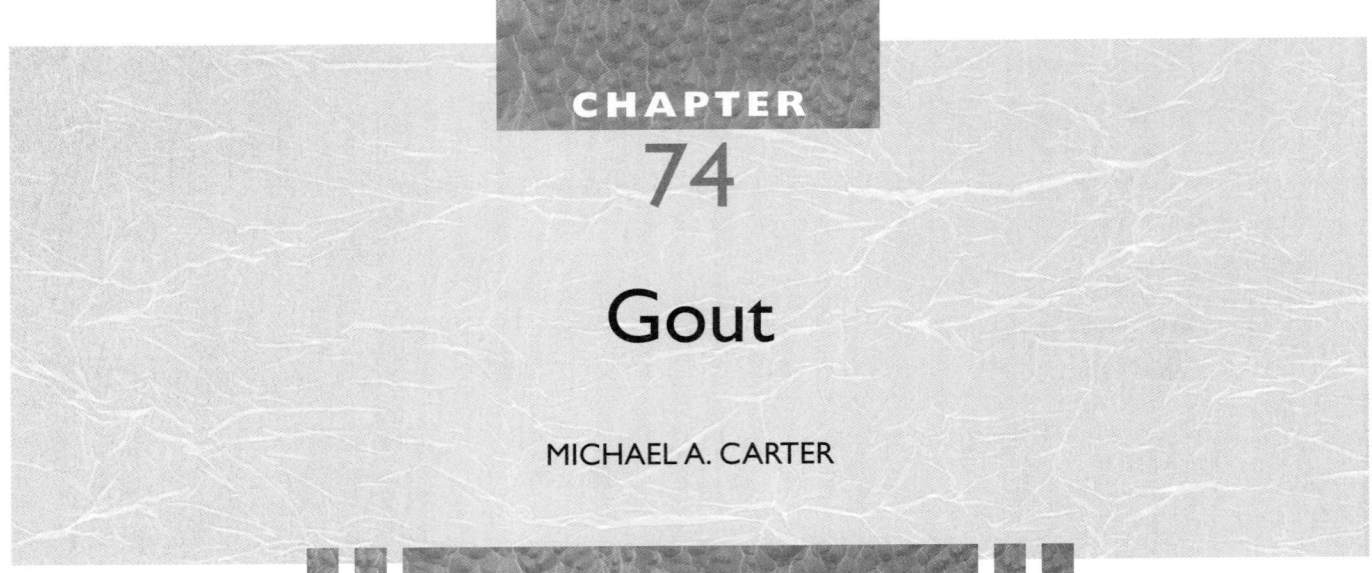

CHAPTER
74

Gout

MICHAEL A. CARTER

*G*out is a metabolic disorder that was described by Hippocrates in ancient Greece. Early theories indicated that gout was a problem only of the elite social class and was caused by overindulgence in food, wine, and sex. Many etiologic and therapeutic theories have been proposed over the ages, but today, much is known about gout, and treatment has a high success rate.

Gout is a term used for a group of at least nine metabolic disorders characterized by an elevation in the serum uric acid concentration *(hyperuricemia)*. Gout may be primary or secondary. *Primary gout* is the direct result of the body's overproduction or decreased excretion of uric acid. *Secondary gout* occurs when the overproduction or decreased excretion of uric acid is secondary to another disease process or medication.

The problem develops when crystals of monosodium urate monohydrate form in the joints and surrounding tissues. These needlelike crystals are responsible for the acute inflammatory reaction that develops, resulting in the severe pain typically associated with an acute gouty attack. These crystal deposits can lead to extensive joint and soft tissue damage if untreated.

CLINICAL FEATURES

The serum urate level in men normally begins to increase after puberty. The urate level does not increase in women until after menopause, since estrogens increase the renal excretion of uric acid. After menopause the serum urate levels of women begin to rise to those of men.

Gout is seldom seen in women. Men account for almost 95% of the cases. Gout is seen worldwide in all racial groups. A familial prevalence suggests a genetic basis. A number of factors likely influence the expression of the illness, however, including diet, body weight, and lifestyle.

There are four stages in the clinical progression of untreated gout. The first stage is *asymptomatic hyperuricemia*. The normal value of serum uric acid in men is 5.1 ± 1.0 mg/dl, and in women the value is 4.0 ± 1.0 mg/dl. These levels rise to an average of 9 to 10 mg/dl in persons with gout. At this stage, the person has no symptoms other than an elevated serum uric acid. Only 20% of the people with asymptomatic hyperuricemia develop an acute gouty attack.

The second stage is *acute gouty arthritis*. At this stage, the person has a sudden onset of exquisitely painful swelling and tenderness, usually of the great toe and metatarsophalangeal joint (Fig. 74-1). The arthritis is monarticular and shows signs of local inflammation. The person may have fever and an elevated white blood cell count. Surgery, trauma, drugs, alcohol, or emotional stress may precipitate the attack. This stage usually leads the person to seek prompt medical attention. Other joints can be affected, including the finger joints, knees, ankles, wrists, and elbows. Acute gouty attacks usually resolve if untreated but may take 10 to 14 days to do so.

The development of the acute attack of gout generally follows a set sequence of events. First, a supersaturation of urate occurs in the plasma and body fluids, followed by a deposition into and around the joints. The mechanism of the crystallization of urates out of the serum is not clearly understood. Gouty attacks frequently follow local trauma or the rupture of *tophi* (deposits of sodium urate), which accounts for a rapid increase in local concentrations of uric acid. The body may not be able to handle this increase appropriately, resulting in the precipitation of uric acid out of the serum. Crystallization and deposition of the uric acid then trigger the gouty attack. These uric acid crystals initiate a phagocytic response by leukocytes, and as the leukocytes ingest the urate crystals, the responses of other inflammatory mechanisms are triggered. The site and magnitude of uric acid crystal deposition may influence the inflammatory response. The inflammatory reaction may become self-propagating and self-enhancing because of the deposition of additional crystals from the serum.

The third stage, which follows the acute gouty attack, is the *intercritical stage.* There are no symptoms during this period, which may last for months to years. Most people have a repeat gouty attack in less than 1 year if they are untreated.

The fourth stage is the *chronic gout stage,* in which the urate pool continues to expand over years if treatment is not begun. Chronic inflammation from the presence of urate crystals results in the development of pain, aching, and stiffness, as well as large and nodular joint swelling. Acute attacks of gouty arthritis may occur during this stage. Tophi develop in chronic gout because of the relative insolubility of urates (Fig. 74-2). The onset and the size of tophi may be proportionally related to the level of serum urate. The olecranon bursa, Achilles tendon, extensor surface of the forearm, infrapatellar bursa, and helix of the ear (Fig. 74-3) are the most common sites for tophi. These tophi may be difficult to distinguish clinically from rheumatoid nodules. Tophi are rarely seen today and will resolve with appropriate therapy.

Gout can damage the kidneys, leading to even poorer excretion of uric acid. Uric acid crystals can form in the medullary interstitium, papillae, and pyramids, leading to proteinuria and mild hypertension. Uric acid kidney stones can also occur secondary to gout. These stones are usually small and round and do not show up on radiographs.

DIAGNOSTIC CRITERIA

Gout should be considered in men who develop monarticular arthritis, particularly of the great toe, that is acute in onset. An elevated serum uric acid is helpful in making the diagnosis but not specific, because a number of drugs can elevate the serum uric acid level. Also, a fairly large number of people have asymptomatic hyperuricemia.

Another test used to diagnose gout is the response of the joint symptoms to colchicine. *Colchicine* is a drug that

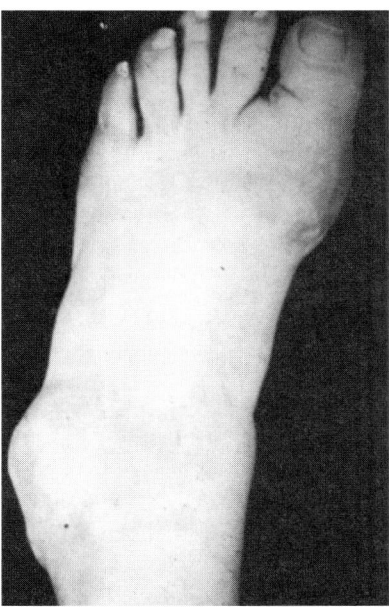

FIG. 74-1 Typical inflammatory response of gout involving the great toe. This is the most common site of acute gout. (From the Arthritis Division, University Hospital, University of Michigan.)

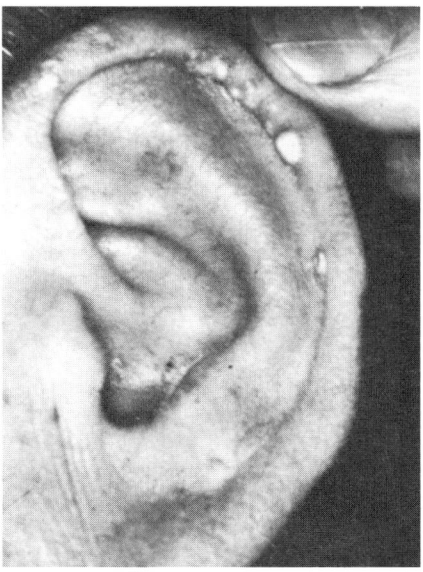

FIG. 74-3 In this patient with gout, small tophi can be seen on the helix of the ear, having a typical whitish appearance as a result of urate deposition. Small cartilaginous nodules are usually present in the ears of normal individuals and can be mistaken for tophi. A tophus characteristically stands out as a discrete white nodule when pressed by the examiner's fingers; in contrast, the cartilaginous nodule blanches out and blends with the rest of the ear. Transillumination reveals an opaque center in the tophus but not in the cartilaginous nodule. (From the Arthritis Foundation, New York, 1972.)

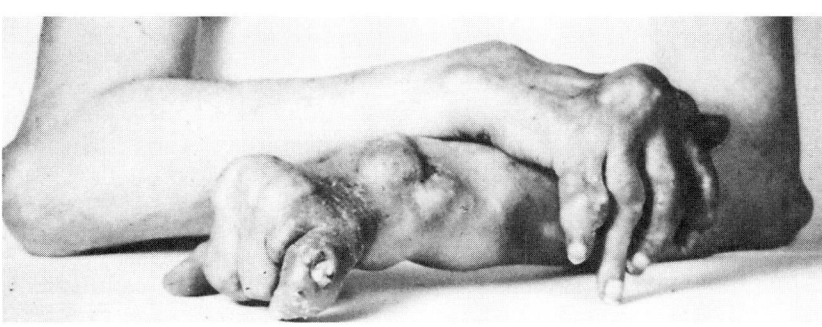

FIG. 74-2 Many tophi are present on the hands of this patient with gout. One asymmetrically shaped tophus on the little finger has ulcerated. Tophi are also present in both olecranon bursae; these are common sites for tophi. Swelling of some joints as a result of synovitis is also present. (From the Arthritis Foundation, New York, 1972.)

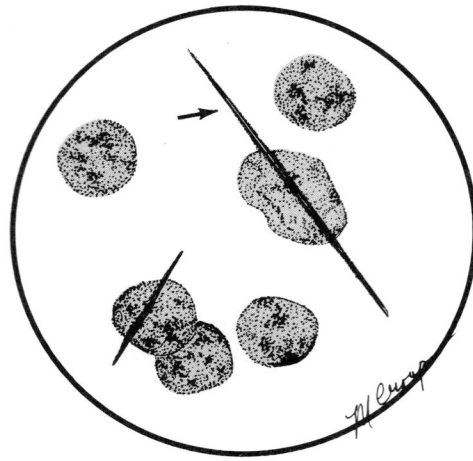

FIG. 74-4 Gout: one uric acid crystal in a white blood cell in synovial fluid.

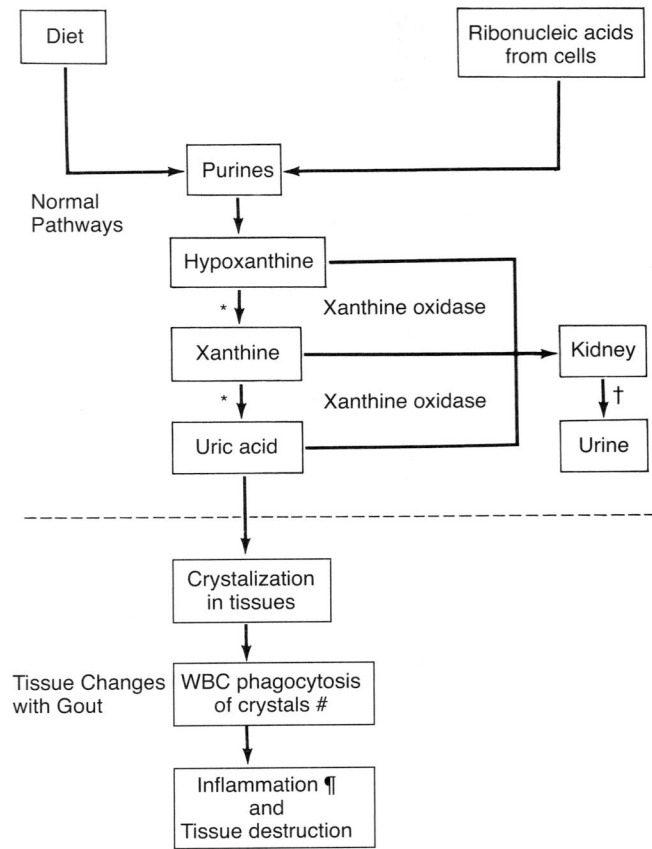

Sites for the drugs' mechanisms of action.

* Allopurinol
† Probenecid and sulfinpyrazone
# Colchicine
¶ NSAIDS

FIG. 74-5 Gout pathophysiology and drug actions. (From Weiner MB, Pepper GA: *Clinical pharmacology and therapeutics in nursing,* ed 2, New York, 1985, McGraw-Hill.)

inhibits phagocytic leukocytes and thereby produces a dramatic and rapid relief of symptoms. Radiologic changes other than soft tissue swelling are usually not present in the early stages of gout. The demonstration of urate crystals in the synovial fluid of an involved joint is considered diagnostic (Fig. 74-4).

CONTRIBUTING FACTORS

The factors that contribute to the development of gout depend on the cause of the hyperuricemia. A diet high in purines can trigger a gouty attack in a person with one of the inborn errors of purine metabolism that cause an overproduction of uric acid. A low-purine diet, however, will not usually lower the serum urate level to any great extent.

The ingestion of alcohol can bring on a gouty attack because alcohol increases urate production. Blood lactate levels increase as a by-product of the normal metabolism of alcohol. Lactic acid blocks the renal excretion of uric acid with a concomitant rise in serum levels.

A number of drugs can block the renal excretion of uric acid and lead to a gouty attack. These drugs include aspirin in low doses (less than 1 to 2 g/day), most diuretics, levodopa, diazoxide, nicotinic acid, acetazolamide, and ethambutol.

TREATMENT

The treatment of gout depends on the stage. Asymptomatic hyperuricemia usually requires no treatment. The acute attack of gouty arthritis is treated by the use of nonsteroidal antiinflammatory drugs or colchicine. These drugs are given in high doses or in loading doses to reduce the acute inflammation of the joint. The dose is then decreased gradually over the next few days.

The treatment of chronic gout is based on decreasing the production of uric acid or on increasing the renal excretion of uric acid. The drug allopurinol blocks the formation of uric acid from its precursors (xanthine and hy-

poxanthine) by inhibiting the enzyme xanthine oxidase. This drug can be given in a convenient once-a-day dose.

Uricosuric agents enhance the excretion of uric acid by blocking renal tubular reabsorption. Adequate kidney function is necessary for uricosuric agents to be effective. The creatinine clearance is evaluated to determine kidney function (normal is 115 to 120 ml/minute). Probenecid and sulfinpyrazone are two widely used uricosuric agents. Fluid intake of at least 1500 ml/day is needed to promote the excretion of uric acid while a patient is taking a uricosuric agent. All aspirin products should be avoided because they block the uricosuric action of these drugs. Fig. 74-5 depicts gout pathophysiology and drug actions.

Strict dietary modifications are not usually necessary in the treatment of gout. The person can be helped to avoid those factors that precipitate an attack, but this is usually determined by trial and error for each person. Obviously, products high in purines may be problematic. These products include organ meats such as liver, kidneys, sweetbreads, and brains, as well as a number of luncheon meats. Excessive use of alcohol can also precipitate an attack.

KEY CONCEPTS

- *Gout* is a metabolic disorder that was first described by Hippocrates in ancient Greece.
- Gout comprises at least nine metabolic disorders characterized by an elevation in the serum uric acid concentration (hyperuricemia).
- Gout may be primary (direct result of the body's overproduction or decreased excretion of uric acid) or secondary (occurs when the overproduction or decreased excretion of uric acid is secondary to another disease process or medication).
- Crystals of monosodium urate monohydrate form in the joints and surrounding tissues and are responsible for the acute inflammatory reaction that develops, resulting in the severe pain typically associated with an acute gouty attack.
- The serum urate level in men normally begins to increase after puberty, whereas the urate level does not increase in women until after menopause. Men account for almost 95% of the cases.
- There are *four stages* in the clinical progression of *untreated gout*. The *first stage* is asymptomatic hyperuricemia in which the serum uric acid in men rises; the person has no symptoms other than an elevated serum uric acid.
- The *second stage* is *acute gouty arthritis* with sudden onset of exquisitely painful swelling and tenderness, usually of the great toe and metatarsophalangeal joint. This stage usually leads the person to seek prompt medical attention.
- The *third stage*, which follows the acute gouty attack, is the *intercritical stage*. There are no symptoms during this period, which may last for months to years, and most people have a repeat gouty attack in less than 1 year if they are untreated.
- The *fourth stage* is the *chronic gout stage*, in which the urate pool continues to expand over years if treatment is not begun. Chronic inflammation from the presence of urate crystals results in the development of pain, aching, and stiffness, as well as large and nodular joint swelling.
- Gout should be considered in men who develop monarticular arthritis, particularly of the great toe, that is acute in onset; an elevated serum uric acid is helpful in making the diagnosis but not specific, because a number of drugs can elevate the serum uric acid level.
- Another test used to diagnose gout is the response of the joint symptoms to colchicine.
- The treatment of gout depends on the stage. Asymptomatic hyperuricemia usually requires no treatment. The acute attack of gouty arthritis is treated with nonsteroidal antiinflammatory drugs or colchicine.
- The treatment of chronic gout is based on decreasing the production of uric acid or on increasing the renal excretion of uric acid.

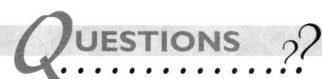 UESTIONS

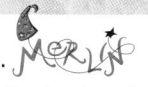

A sampling of review questions for this chapter appears here. Visit http://www.mosby.com/MERLIN/PriceWilson/ for additional questions.

Answer the following on a separate sheet of paper.

1. Formulate a definition for gout.
2. Differentiate between the causes of primary and secondary gout.
3. Explain the rapid response to colchicine in gout.
4. Discuss the contributing factors that result in development of gout.
5. State the rationale for the treatment of chronic gout.
6. Explain why gout can damage the kidneys.

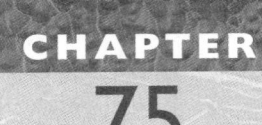

Seronegative Spondyloarthropathies

MICHAEL A. CARTER

*S*eronegative spondyloarthropathies are a group of related disorders that include ankylosing spondylitis, psoriatic arthritis, and Reiter's syndrome. These disorders are called *seronegative* because rheumatoid factor is lacking in the serum. In addition, these disorders are associated with the human leukocyte antigen HLA-B27. These arthropathies are distinct in that they involve the sacroiliac and peripheral joints and usually have a higher incidence in men than in women.

ANKYLOSING SPONDYLITIS

Ankylosing spondylitis is a chronic inflammatory disease that can be progressive. The illness usually involves the sacroiliac joints and the spinal articulations. The hips and costovertebral articulations can be affected as the disease progresses. Ankylosing spondylitis was once thought to be a variant of rheumatoid arthritis. This belief is no longer the case, based on the criteria of negative rheumatoid factor,

the absence of rheumatoid nodules, and the differences in the bone changes in the spine. The 9:1 male/female ratio of the illness is no longer believed accurate now that better criteria for diagnosis have been established. Men tend to have a more progressive spinal disease and are more likely to be diagnosed as having ankylosing spondylitis than women, giving a clinical ratio of about three men for each woman with spinal involvement. Ankylosing spondylitis occurs less frequently in Japanese and African Americans but more frequently in Pima Indians.

Ankylosing spondylitis affects the cartilaginous and fibrocartilaginous joints of the spine and paravertebral ligaments. Calcification of the joints and articular structures occurs when intervertebral disks become invaded by vascular and fibrous tissue and later become calcified. Calcified soft tissue bridges one vertebra to another. The synovial tissue around the joints involved becomes inflamed. Heart disease can also occur with ankylosing spondylitis.

The causes of ankylosing spondylitis are still unknown. A genetic factor appears to be involved. Approximately 90% of persons diagnosed as having ankylosing spondylitis have a positive HLA-B27 antigen.

Clinical Features

Ankylosing spondylitis has an insidious onset, beginning with feelings of fatigue and intermittent lower back or hip pain. Morning stiffness relieved by mild activity may occur. The symptoms can be so mild and unprogressive that many people are never diagnosed. In addition, the symptoms of ankylosing spondylitis can be confused with those of mechanical back problems.

The evaluation indicates a basically healthy person who has a history of persistent back pain with insidious onset. The person is usually under 40 years of age. The back pain improves with exercise and worsens with rest and has diffuse radiation throughout the lower back and buttock. The physical examination shows no scoliosis, a symmetric decrease in range of motion, diffuse tenderness, and a negative straight-leg-raising test. The peripheral neurologic system is usually unchanged. As the illness progresses, there is a loss of normal lumbar lordosis, fusion of the dorsal spine into kyphosis, and restriction

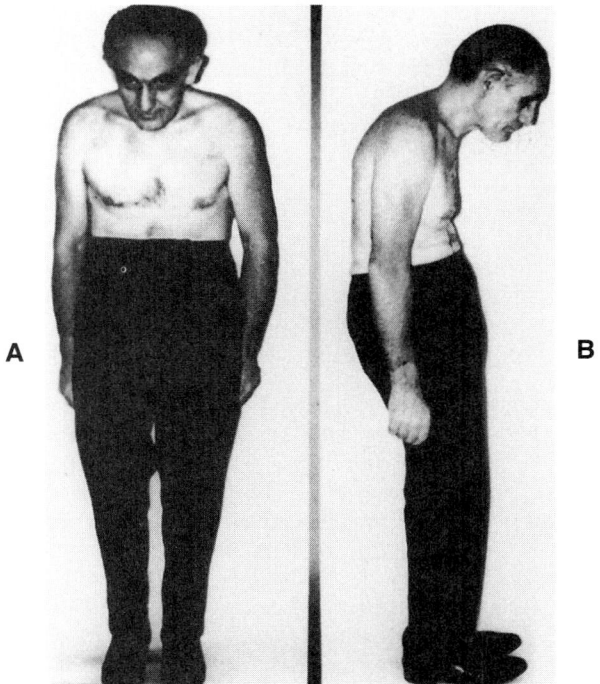

FIG. 75-1   Ankylosing spondylitis. **A**, Frontal view demonstrates the characteristic upward gaze of the eyes when they look straight ahead, necessitated by the flexion deformity of the neck. **B**, Lateral view demonstrates forward protrusion of the head, flattening of the anterior chest wall, thoracic kyphosis, protrusion of the abdomen, and flattening of the lumbar lordotic curvature. Slight flexion of the hip is also present because of hip involvement. (From the *Revised clinical slide collection on the rheumatic diseases,* New York, 1981, Arthritis Foundation.)

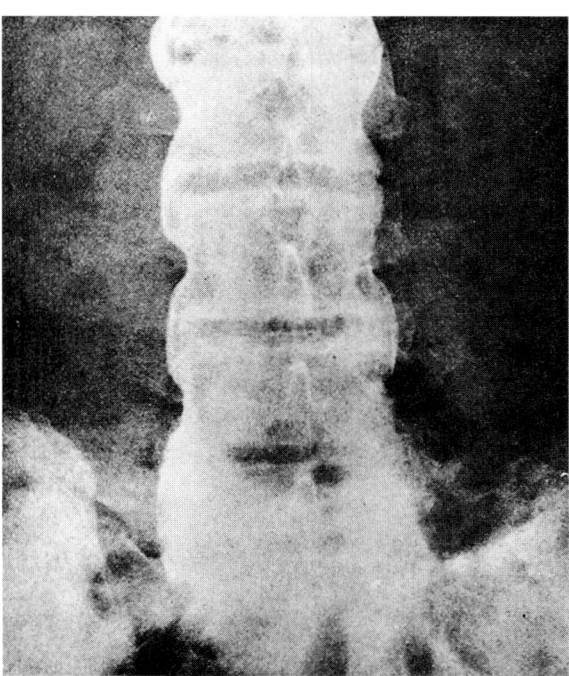

FIG. 75-2   Radiograph depicting advanced ankylosing spondylitis of the lumbar spine. There is generalized symmetric osseous bridging between the vertebrae (syndesmophytes). The apophyseal and sacroiliac joints are fused. (From Hollander JL, editor: *Arthritis and allied conditions: a textbook of rheumatology,* ed 8, Philadelphia, 1972, Lea & Febiger.)

of thoracic excursion. In the late stages of the illness, fusion of the spine can result in hip flexion contractures, and the patient uses flexed knees to maintain an erect position (Fig. 75-1). Pain is usually diminished after ankylosis is complete, and synovitis is markedly decreased.

Laboratory Findings

No specific laboratory tests are used in diagnosing ankylosing spondylitis. The erythrocyte sedimentation rate (ESR) is usually elevated during active phases of the illness. The rheumatoid factor is usually negative. The antigen HLA-B27 is likely to be positive, but this is not specific to ankylosing spondylitis.

Radiologic Findings

Characteristic radiologic changes occur in ankylosing spondylitis. In the early stages of the illness, there may be only blurring of the sacroiliac joint and diffuse osteoporosis of the spine. As the illness progresses, joint erosion, squaring of the vertebrae, and narrowing of the disk spaces are seen. In the last stages of the illness, calcification of the disks and paravertebral ligaments occurs. Vertical bony growths, called *syndesmophytes,* can be demonstrated bridging the gaps between the vertebrae (Fig. 75-2). About 25% of patients with ankylosing spondylitis have complete fusing of the spine, including the cervical spine.

Treatment

Treatment of ankylosing spondylitis is multifocal and related to the stage of the illness. A focused intervention is aimed at increasing the patient's and family's understanding of the illness. Changes in work patterns may be necessary, because bending, lifting, and prolonged static positions are difficult. Medication therapy is aimed at decreasing the synovitis and resulting pain. Nonsteroidal antiinflammatory drugs (NSAIDs) are used for this purpose, particularly those with high prostaglandin-blocking ability and a long half-life. Indomethacin is frequently the drug of choice. Corticosteroids, slow-acting drugs, and muscle relaxants are of limited value. An active program of physical therapy is often helpful, focusing on breathing exercises, muscle strengthening, maintaining or improving posture, and range of motion exercises. Braces and splints may be used for limited times to decrease muscle spasm and pain.

Prognosis

About 20% of people with ankylosing spondylitis develop the disabling stages of the illness. About one half of people have a slow, extended course that can last for decades. A number of the remaining persons can be successfully treated with a focused program of education, drug therapy, and physical therapy. These individuals can develop a fulfilling lifestyle within the confines of their illness. Less than 5% develop fatal manifestations of their illness.

PSORIATIC ARTHRITIS

About 7% of persons with psoriasis (see Chapter 79) develop inflammatory joint disease. Usually the arthritis occurs after the appearance of the skin lesions, but it can occur before or at the same time as the skin lesions. The male/female ratio of this illness is nearly equal.

Clinical Features

Psoriatic arthritis most often occurs as an asymmetric inflammation involving only a few peripheral joints at a certain time. The distal joints of the hands and feet are the ones usually affected (Fig. 75-3), but other joints that can become affected include all joints of the hands, feet, knees, and hips. The activity of the arthritis tends to vary with the psoriasis, particularly the nail involvement of psoriasis. Psoriatic arthritis can present as a symmetric arthritis resembling rheumatoid arthritis; as arthritis mutilans, in which the entire joint is completely resorbed; or as spondylitis similar to that of ankylosing spondylitis. Psoriatic arthritis generally tends to be much less debilitating than rheumatoid arthritis.

Laboratory and Radiologic Findings

No specific laboratory tests exist for psoriatic arthritis. The ESR can be elevated during acute phases of the illness. The antigen HLA-B27 is positive about 20% of the time. This level increases to a 50% positive rate if the person has sacroiliac inflammation with the illness.

Radiographs in the early stages of the illness are usually normal. A characteristic finding in later stages is the "pencil-in-cup" sign. The distal end of the proximal phalanx erodes to a rather sharp point, with a concomitant bony overgrowth of the proximal end of the distal phalanx where the tendons insert.

Treatment

The treatment for psoriatic arthritis is appropriate doses of aspirin or other NSAIDs. These measures are combined with treatment of the skin lesions. Corticosteroids are not generally used because such large doses are required, and the adverse effects are beyond acceptable levels. Other drug therapies include gold and immunosuppressive agents. These drugs are usually reserved for patients with severe illness who do not respond to other forms of therapy.

The long-term treatment involves a multifocal approach that includes physical therapy, alterations in activities of daily living, and occasionally hospitalization and surgery. Most people with psoriatic arthritis, however, do not require extensive medical intervention; they have frequent periods of remission that last for several months.

REITER'S SYNDROME

Reiter's syndrome is one of the leading causes of arthritis in young men. The syndrome is named for Hans Reiter, who described the clinical picture of nongonococcal urethritis, arthritis, and conjunctivitis in 1916. This syndrome rarely occurs in women, children, or older persons. In the United States, the syndrome begins suddenly, usually following venereal exposure to *Chlamydia trachomatis*. In other parts of the world, the syndrome follows an infection with *Shigella flexneri*, salmonella, or campylobacter.

Reiter's syndrome is accompanied by a triad of symptoms: urethritis, arthritis, and conjunctivitis. Oral mucocutaneous lesions, keratoderma blennorrhagicum (a characteristic dermatitis; Fig. 75-4), and balanitis circinata are also seen.

The causes are unknown. An association exists between HLA-B27 and the development of Reiter's syndrome. Psoriatic arthritis and Reiter's syndrome may be nearly the same disease, because the dermatitis and nail changes are very similar in the two. A history of sexual ex-

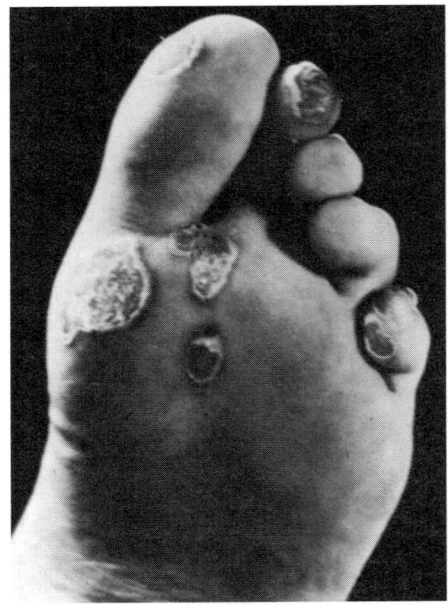

FIG. 75-4 Discrete, circinate, scaly, and plaquelike lesions on the foot (keratoderma blennorrhagicum) are caused by Reiter's syndrome and resemble secondary syphilis and psoriasis. Note two small lesions in an early phase of keratoderma. (From the Arthritis Foundation, New York, 1972.)

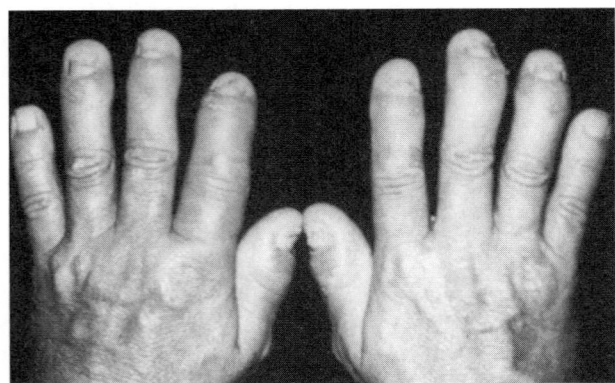

FIG. 75-3 Psoriatic arthritis. Swelling and deformity of distal interphalangeal joints are present, together with typical psoriatic involvement of the skin and nails. Several digits, including the left thumb and index finger, are diffusely swollen, suggesting a sausage-like appearance. (From the *Revised clinical slide collection on the rheumatic diseases*, New York, 1981, Arthritis Foundation.)

posure or dysentery leads to the suspicion that these illnesses are immune responses to some infectious agent.

Clinical Features

Constitutional symptoms, weight loss, and fever may occur at the onset of Reiter's syndrome. A purulent or watery urethritis that the person may think is a venereal disease is often the factor that prompts a visit to seek health care.

Articular manifestations most often involve the joints of the feet and ankles, the knees, and the sacroiliac joints. Heel pain is fairly common. Conjunctivitis can occur with a purulent discharge and photophobia. The oral and penile lesions are usually painless. A few patients have electrocardiographic changes and aortic valve involvement.

The course of the illness is unpredictable. Reiter's syndrome can be acute, subacute, or chronic. Most people recover from the first attack in several months, but most have one or two more attacks within 2 years. Thirty percent of people develop long-term disability or permanent sequelae, including residual joint damage after severe joint involvement and long-term back pain after sacroiliac involvement.

Laboratory and Radiologic Findings

No specific laboratory tests exist for Reiter's syndrome. Ninety percent of patients with Reiter's syndrome have a positive antigen HLA-B27, but the frequency of positive rheumatoid factor is equal to that in the general population. Synovial fluid is inflammatory, with 15,000 to 20,000 white blood cells/mm³.

There are radiographic changes specific for Reiter's syndrome, including a tendency for joints of the lower extremities to be involved, isolated osteoporosis, articular erosive changes, periostitis at the insertion of the Achilles tendon, calcaneal spurs, sacroiliac inflammations, and nonmarginal spurs along the vertebral column.

Treatment

The treatment of Reiter's syndrome is primarily symptomatic. Therapeutic doses of NSAIDs are used to relieve the inflammation and pain. The use of corticosteroids systemically or locally is controversial. Antibiotics are not of proven value.

ENTEROPATHIC ARTHRITIS

Arthritis occurs in about 20% of persons who have ulcerative colitis and Crohn's disease. This arthritis is similar to the other spondyloarthropathies in that the peripheral joints are affected. The arthritis activity reflects the activity of the inflammatory bowel disease. Effective treatment of the bowel disease usually causes the arthritis to resolve.

KEY CONCEPTS

- *Seronegative spondyloarthropathies* are a group of related disorders that include ankylosing spondylitis, psoriatic arthritis, and Reiter's syndrome.
- These disorders are called *seronegative* because rheumatoid factor is lacking in the serum, and these disorders are associated with the HLA-B27.
- These arthropathies involve the sacroiliac and peripheral joints and usually have a higher incidence in men than women.
- Men tend to have a more progressive spinal disease and are more likely to be diagnosed as having ankylosing spondylitis than do women, which gives a clinical ratio of about three men for each woman with spinal involvement.
- *Ankylosing spondylitis* affects the cartilaginous and fibrocartilaginous joints of the spine and paravertebral ligaments.
- The causes of ankylosing spondylitis are still unknown, although a genetic factor appears to be involved.
- Ankylosing spondylitis has an insidious onset, beginning with feelings of fatigue and intermittent lower back or hip pain.
- Characteristic radiologic changes occur in ankylosing spondylitis as evidenced by only a blurring of the sacroiliac joint and diffuse osteoporosis of the spine.
- Treatment of ankylosing spondylitis is multifocal and related to the stage of the illness.
- *Psoriatic arthritis* most often occurs as an asymmetric inflammation involving only a few peripheral joints at a certain time, with the distal joints of the hands and feet being the ones usually affected. Other joints that can become affected include all joints of the hands, feet, knees, and hips.
- No specific laboratory tests exist for psoriatic arthritis. Radiographs in the early stages of the illness are usually normal.
- The treatment for psoriatic arthritis is appropriate doses of aspirin or other NSAIDs. The long-term treatment involves a multifocal approach that includes physical therapy, alterations in activities of daily living, and occasionally hospitalization and surgery.
- *Reiter's syndrome* is one of the leading causes of arthritis in young men. In the United States, the syndrome begins suddenly, usually following venereal exposure.
- Reiter's syndrome is accompanied by a triad of symptoms: urethritis, arthritis, and conjunctivitis. The causes of Reiter's syndrome are unknown, but an association exists between HLA-B27 and the development of Reiter's syndrome.
- Articular manifestations most often involve the joints of the feet and ankles, the knees, and the sacroiliac joints. Heel pain is fairly common. Conjunctivitis can occur with a purulent discharge and photophobia.
- No specific laboratory tests exist for Reiter's syndrome; however, 90% of patients with Reiter's syndrome have a positive antigen HLA-B27.
- The treatment of Reiter's syndrome is primarily symptomatic. Therapeutic doses of NSAIDs are used to relieve the inflammation and pain.

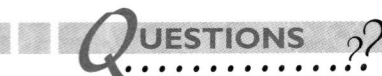

Answer the following on a separate sheet of paper.

1. Explain the goals of the treatment measures and the prognosis for ankylosing spondylitis.
2. What is the relationship between psoriasis and psoriatic arthritis?
3. What are the components of the treatment program for Reiter's syndrome?

Circle "T" if the statement is true and "F" if it is false. Correct any false statements.

4. T F The psoriasis usually precedes the arthritis in psoriatic arthritis.
5. T F Reiter's syndrome is characterized by a triad of symptoms: urethritis, arthritis, and conjunctivitis.
6. T F About 35% of individuals with ankylosing spondylitis develop disabling stages of the illness.
7. T F In the United States, Reiter's syndrome begins suddenly, usually following venereal exposure to syphilis or gonorrhea.

BIBLIOGRAPHY ■ PART TWELVE

Canale TS, editor: *Campbell's operative orthopedics*, ed 9, St Louis, 1998, Mosby.

Carter MA et al: Immune and inflammatory disorders. In Weiner MB, Pepper GA, editors: *Clinical pharmacology and therapeutics in nursing*, New York, 1985, McGraw-Hill.

Guyton AC: *Textbook of physiology*, ed 10, Philadelphia, 1990, WB Saunders.

Kelley WN et al, editors: *Textbook of rheumatology*, ed 5, Philadelphia, 1997, WB Saunders.

Klippel JH, editor: *Primer on the rheumatic diseases*, ed 11, Atlanta, 1997, Arthritis Foundation.

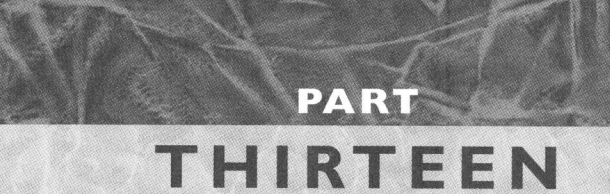

DERMATOLOGIC SYSTEM DISORDERS

Dermatology is concerned with the structure, function, and diseases of the skin. The skin forms a protective barrier around the entire body and has a role in body thermoregulation, glandular secretion, and sensory communication with the external environment. Any structure of the skin has a potential for disease. A skin disorder may be restricted to cutaneous involvement or be indicative of a systemic disease.

This section includes a review of skin anatomy and physiology. Selected cutaneous diseases and their etiology, pathogenesis, and treatment are also discussed.

Anatomy and Physiology of the Skin

MAREK A. STAWISKI

DERMATOLOGIC VOCABULARY

annular lesion A ring-shaped lesion with an active margin and often a clear center; *example:* ringworm (see Fig. 80-12).

atrophy A loss of epidermal and dermal substance; *example:* atrophy after treatment with topical steroids (see Fig. 78-3).

burrow A linear trail produced by a parasite; *example:* scabies (see Fig. 82-2).

circinate lesion An arcuate lesion; *example:* urticaria (see color plate 52).

comedo A plugged pilosebaceous opening; *example:* acne vulgaris (see Fig. 77-3).

confluent Blending into adjacent lesions; *example:* tinea versicolor (see color plate 59).

crust An excessive accumulation of serum and cellular, bacterial, and squamous debris; *example:* impetigo (see color plate 61).

eczematoid lesion An inflammatory lesion with scale, vesiculation, crust, and weeping; *example:* poison ivy (see color plate 50).

erosion A loss of epidermis only; *example:* impetigo (see color plate 61).

excoriations A linear erosion; frequently, self-inducement is implied; *example:* neurotic excoriation (see Fig. 78-2).

fissure A crack in the skin extending to the dermis; *example:* hand eczema (see color plate 51).

herpetiform Having groups of vesicles; *example:* herpes simplex (see Fig. 80-5).

hyperkeratosis A lesion with excessive scales; *example:* psoriasis (see color plate 54).

iris or target lesion Two or three concentric circles that form an irislike lesion; *example:* erythema multiforme (see Fig. 78-9).

Koebner's phenomenon Lesions that form in areas of previous trauma of the skin; *example:* psoriasis.

lichenification An area of accentuated skin markings associated with a thickening of the skin caused by scratching and rubbing; *example:* neurodermatitis (see Fig. 78-1).

macule A nonpalpable circumscribed area usually demarcated by a change of color; *example:* tinea versicolor (see color plate 59).

morbilliform lesions A small confluent maculopapular lesion; *example:* a viral exanthem.

nodule, tumor A palpable lesion usually larger than 5 mm; *example:* basal cell carcinoma (see color plate 63).

nummular lesion A coin-shaped lesion; *example:* nummular eczema.

papule An elevated palpable lesion usually smaller than 5 mm; *example:* a blue nevus (see color plate 68).

photodistribution Distribution in areas exposed to sunlight; *example:* sunburn.

plaque A palpable lesion that has a greater dimension in area than in thickness; *example:* psoriasis (see color plate 54).

pustule A lesion that contains pus; *example:* acne vulgaris (see Fig. 77-4).

scale An excessive accumulation of keratin; *example:* psoriasis (see color plate 54).

telangiectasis A dilation of superficial vessels; *example:* dilated vessels in a basal cell carcinoma (see color plate 63).

verrucous Wartlike; *example:* verruca vulgaris (see Fig. 80-1).

vesicle, bulla A fluid-filled, elevated lesion; *example:* a vesicle of herpes simplex (see Fig. 80-5).

wheal A transitory palpable lesion; *example:* urticaria (hives) (see color plate 52).

zosteriform Having a linear dermatomal distribution; *example:* herpes zoster (shingles) (see color plate 57).

The skin, which is the largest organ of the human body, envelops the muscles and internal organs. The skin is an endless network of blood vessels, nerves, and glands, all of which have a potential for disease. Because the number of cutaneous diseases is extensive, only the most frequently encountered are discussed in this section. The most common dermatologic condition, acne, and new advances in its treatment are described. Another frequently seen disease is eczema, which can be inherited or caused by allergens. Psoriasis is thought to be the most economically ravaging skin disease. Most dermatologic hospital admissions are caused by severe exacerbations of psoriasis.

Cutaneous infections with viruses, causing warts and herpes simplex, have captured the attention of not only the health care community, but also the press and public. Fungal infections are responsible for ringworm, athlete's foot, and jock itch. Presentation and treatment of these fungal infections and bacterial skin infections are included.

Neoplasms of the skin are the most common of the cancers encountered in humans. Neoplasms range from nonmetastatic basal cell carcinomas to aggressive and frequently fatal melanomas. Description of diagnostic features and causes of these tumors should help the reader diagnose and prevent these malignancies. Diagnosis, prevention, and treatment of Lyme disease and infestation with scabies and lice are discussed. These conditions can be a considerable challenge to nurses, especially public health, community health, or school nurses. However, before the various skin diseases are considered, this chapter summarizes the basic structure and functions of the skin.

FUNCTIONS OF SKIN

The skin protects the body from trauma and shields it from bacterial, viral, and fungal infections. Heat loss and conservation are regulated by cutaneous vasodilation or secretion by the sweat glands. After complete loss of skin, essential body fluids evaporate, and electrolytes are lost within hours; an example of this is seen in burn patients. The pleasant or unpleasant odors of the skin serve as social and sexual signs of acceptability or rejection. Epidermal appendages of the skin, such as nails and hair, have their well-established cosmetic values unique to specific cultures. The skin also provides the sensations of touch, pressure, temperature, pain, and pleasure by an intricate network of nerve endings.

SKIN STRUCTURE

Microscopically the skin consists of three layers: epidermis, dermis, and subcutaneous fat (Fig. 76-1). The *epidermis,* the outermost portion of the skin, is divided into two main layers: a stratum of anucleated cornified cells (the *stratum corneum,* or horny layer) and the inner, malpighian layer, from which the surface cornified cells arise by differentiation. The *malpighian layer* is subdivided into the (1) stratum granulosum, (2) basal

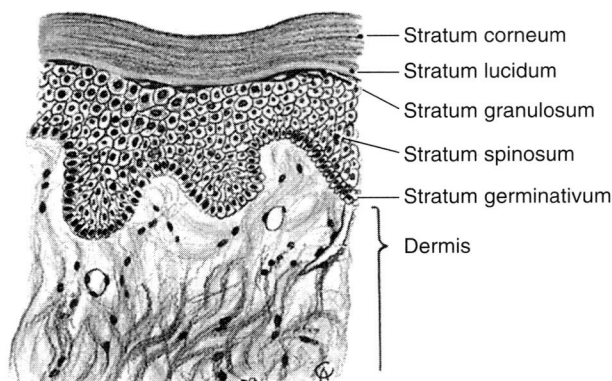

FIG. 76-1 Epidermis and upper layer of the dermis. Superficial capillaries are seen in the upper dermis. Subcutaneous layer is below the dermal layer. (From Jacob SW, Francone CA: *Elements of anatomy and physiology,* ed 2, Philadelphia, 1989, WB Saunders.)

cell layer (or stratum germinativum), and (3) stratum spinosum.

The *basal layer* consists largely of undifferentiated epidermal cells that undergo constant mitosis, renewing the epidermis. When this type of cell undergoes mitosis, one of the daughter cells remains in the basal layer to divide again while the other cell migrates outward toward the stratum spinosum.

The major differentiating cell of the *stratum spinosum* is the *keratinocyte,* which produces keratin, a fibrous protein. As keratinocytes leave the stratum spinosum and move upward, they undergo changes in shape, orientation, cytoplasmic structure, and composition. This change leads to the transformation of viable, actively synthesizing cells into the dead, cornified cells of the stratum corneum, a process termed *keratinization.* The *stratum granulosum* lies just below the stratum corneum and has an important function in the production of stratum corneum proteins and chemical bonds. Keratinocytes of the basal layer are cylindric in shape; they become polyhedral in the stratum spinosum, flatter in the granular layer, and scaly in the stratum corneum. Important changes also occur in their cytoplasmic constituents, the nucleus, and the cell membranes. The keratinocytes synthesize tonofilaments, or filamentous proteins. In the stratum germinativum, the tonofilaments are arranged in bundles that surround the nucleus of the cell. In the stratum spinosum, synthesis continues, and these tonofilament bundles become more compact, forming an interlacing network extending through the cytoplasm. As they move through the stratum granulosum, keratohyalin granules appear within these cells, deposited within and around the tonofilament bundles. In the stratum corneum, the granules appear tightly packed. *Keratohyalin* is not sufficiently defined chemically, and its final role in the keratinization process is not clear. Keratohyalin does appear to contribute to the amorphous, electron-dense matrix of the cornified cells.

It appears that, during differentiation, keratinocytes pass through a synthetic phase in which tonofilaments, keratohyalin, lamellar bodies, and other cell constituents are formed. Finally, keratinocytes enter a transition

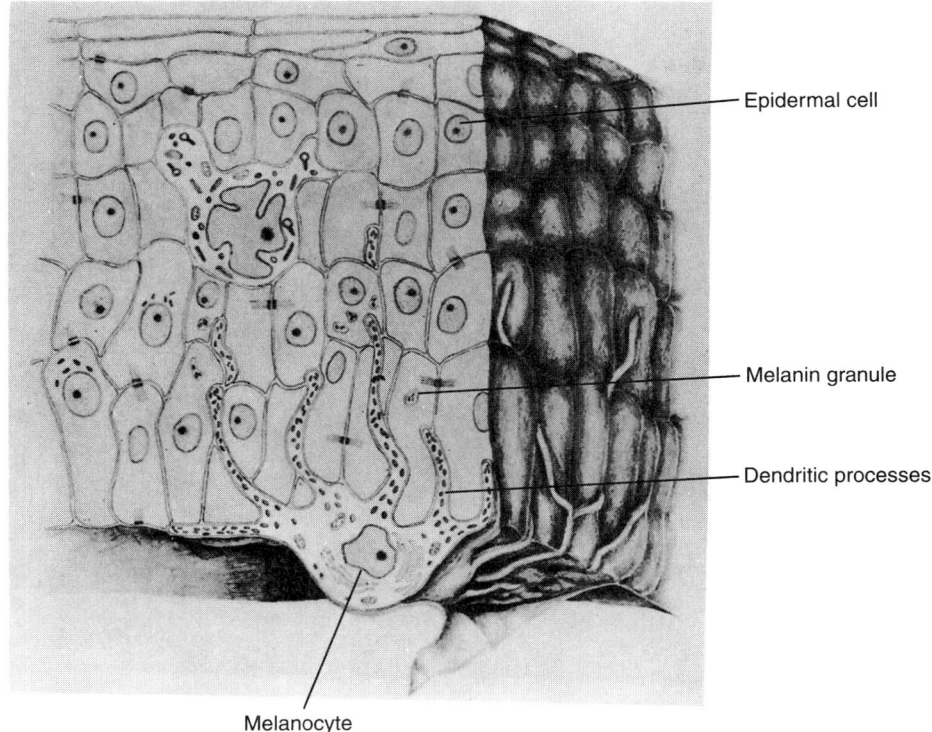

FIG. 76-2 The epidermal melanin unit. Relationship of a single melanocyte to multiple epidermal cells is well illustrated. (From Fitzpatrick TB et al, editors: *Dermatology in general medicine*, ed 2, New York, 1979, McGraw-Hill.)

phase, in which the cytoplasmic components are dissociated and degraded. The remaining cell constituents form a fibrous, amorphous complex surrounded by a reinforced impermeable membrane, the horny cell. This programmed process of epidermal cell migration normally takes about 28 days.

The second major cell of the epidermis (after keratinocytes) is the *melanocyte,* found in the basal layer. The ratio of basal cells to melanocytes is 10:1. Within the melanocyte, pigment granules called *melanosomes* are synthesized. Melanosomes contain brown biochrome called *melanin.* The melanosomes are transferred to keratinocytes through long dendritic processes. Each melanocyte is connected through these projections, and about 36 keratinocytes form what is referred to as the *epidermal melanin unit* (Fig. 76-2). Melanosomes are hydrolyzed at varying rates by enzymes. The amount of melanin within the keratinocyte determines the color of the skin. Melanin protects the skin from harmful effects of the sun. Paradoxically, the sun's rays increase the production of melanosomes and melanin. African Americans and Caucasians each have the same number of melanocytes. African Americans have large melanosomes that resist destruction by the hydrolyzing enzymes, whereas Caucasians have smaller melanosomes that are more readily destroyed.

The *dermis* is located immediately below the epidermis and is composed of collagen fibers, elastin, and reticulin embedded in a ground substance. The dermal matrix contains blood vessels and nerves, which provide support and nourishment to the growing epidermis. Surrounding the small blood vessels are lymphocytes, histi-

ocytes, mast cells, and polymorphonuclear neutrophils (PMNs), which protect the body from infections and foreign body invasion. Specialized collagen fibers anchor the epidermal basal cells into the dermis.

Underlying the dermis is the third layer of skin, the *subcutaneous fat.* This layer provides a cushion for the skin, insulation to maintain body heat, and a store of energy. Cosmetically, subcutaneous fat influences the attractiveness of either gender.

Sweat (eccrine) glands are present almost everywhere on the skin except in the ears and on the lips. These glands produce a hypotonic solution that is clear and watery and has a high content of urea and lactate. Sweat glands help maintain the appropriate body temperature.

Sebaceous glands are lobulated structures that consist of lipid-filled cells. The lipid oily substance referred to as *sebum* is passed to the central duct and drained to the pilosebaceous ducts of the hair follicles (Fig. 76-3). Sebaceous glands are concentrated over the face, chest, back, and proximal arms. The activity of these glands is hormonally regulated primarily by androgenic hormones.

The *apocrine glands* are found primarily in the axilla, in the genital skin, around the nipples, and in the perianal area. The apocrine duct empties into the hair follicle above the entrance of the sebaceous duct (Fig. 76-4). The apocrine secretions do not serve any useful function in humans but contribute to the axillary odor when apocrine secretions are decomposed by bacteria. Apocrine glands produce a milky, viscous substance that results from a high content of organic components. These glands begin their secretory activity at puberty.

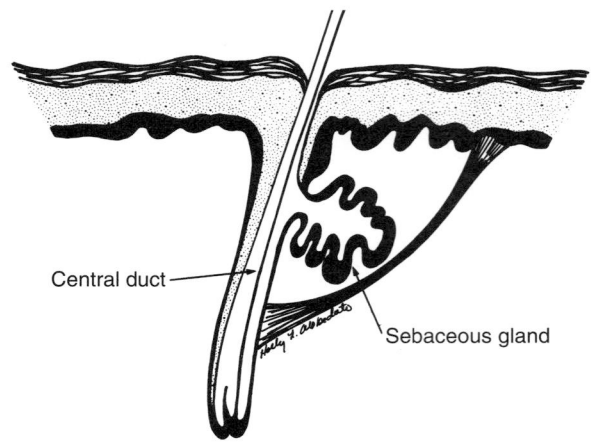

FIG. 76-3 Sebaceous gland opens into the central duct. (From the Biomedical Media Production Unit, University of Michigan Medical Center.)

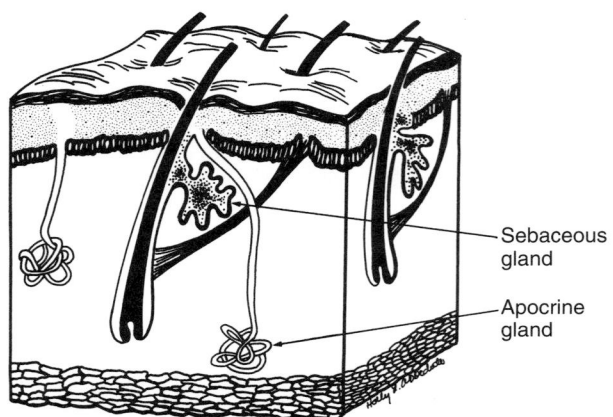

FIG. 76-4 Apocrine gland empties above the entrance of the sebaceous duct. (From the Biomedical Media Production Unit, University of Michigan Medical Center.)

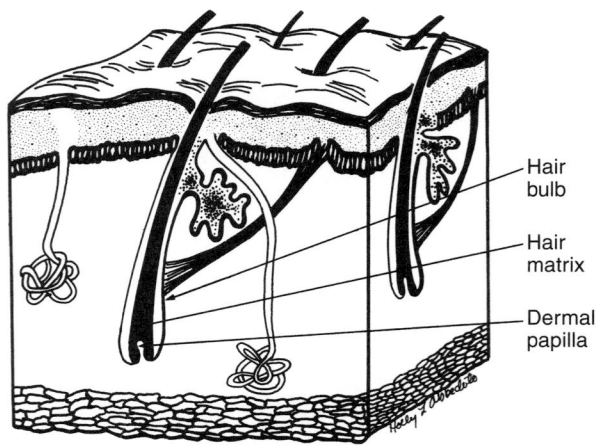

FIG. 76-5 Hair matrix is supported by a dermal papilla and differentiates into hair. (From the Biomedical Media Production Unit, University of Michigan Medical Center.)

Hair is formed from keratin. By a predetermined differentiating process, certain epidermal cells form the hair follicle. The hair follicle is supported by dermal matrix and differentiates into the hair (Fig. 76-5). An epithelial canal is formed, through which the hair passes to the surface. Hair is dead keratin just as is a scale, and it is formed at a predetermined rate. Cystine and methionine, sulfur-containing amino acids, contribute strong covalent bonds, giving strength to hair. On the scalp, the rate of the growth of hair is usually 3 mm/day. Each hair follicle goes through a cycle of growth *(anagen hair)*, intermediate stage *(catagen hair)*, and involution *(telogen hair)*. The anagen stage on the scalp lasts about 5 years, and the telogen stage lasts only about 3 months. Once the hair follicle reaches the telogen stage, the hair falls out. Eventually, the hair follicle regenerates into the anagen stage, and a new hair is produced. This cycle of activity for hair follicles is independent for each hair follicle. The mosaic pattern prevents the occurrence of temporary baldness of the scalp. When the process stops, the person becomes permanently bald. Various commercial preparations ad-

vertised to strengthen hair are of questionable value. Protein shampoos affect only the dead keratin and not the hair follicle and therefore cannot prevent hair loss. Recent developments have shown that male and female patterns of baldness can sometimes be treated with topical 2% minoxidil (Rogaine).

The *nail* is a dead keratin plate produced by epidermal cells of nail matrix (Fig. 76-6). The nail matrix is located beneath the proximal portion of the nail plate in the dermis and is visible as a white area, called the *lunula*, which is covered by the nail fold and cuticle. Because both nail and hair are dead keratin structures, they have no nerve endings and no blood supply.

SKIN EXAMINATION

Skin should be examined in a well-illuminated room, preferably in natural daylight. A dimly illuminated hospital room is the least desirable place to inspect the skin, and examination there may lead to serious errors in diagnosis. The color of the skin should be recorded. Purplish, cyanotic discoloration of the toes or fingers can provide a useful clue to the presence of internal diseases. Pallor can be a sign of anemia (see Chapter 17). Skin has turgor and elasticity on palpation. Excessive dryness causes this organ to be scaly and wrinkled, which may indicate dehydration or thyroid disease. Skin ridges are visible over the palms and feet and are also present over the entire body surface. Skin ridges are called *dermatoglyphics* and form the pattern unique for every individual and species. The dermatoglyphics over the volar aspects of the fingers are used for fingerprinting, which are useful in criminology; however, health care professionals are also interested in the presence of these whorls. The disappearance of dermatoglyphics over fingertips can be a first sign of vascular insufficiency, as in systemic sclerosis (scleroderma; see Chapter 73).

There is an expected pattern of hair distribution in males and females. In many men, and some women, temporal and occipital scalp hair thinning becomes evident with advancing age. However, a sudden hair loss

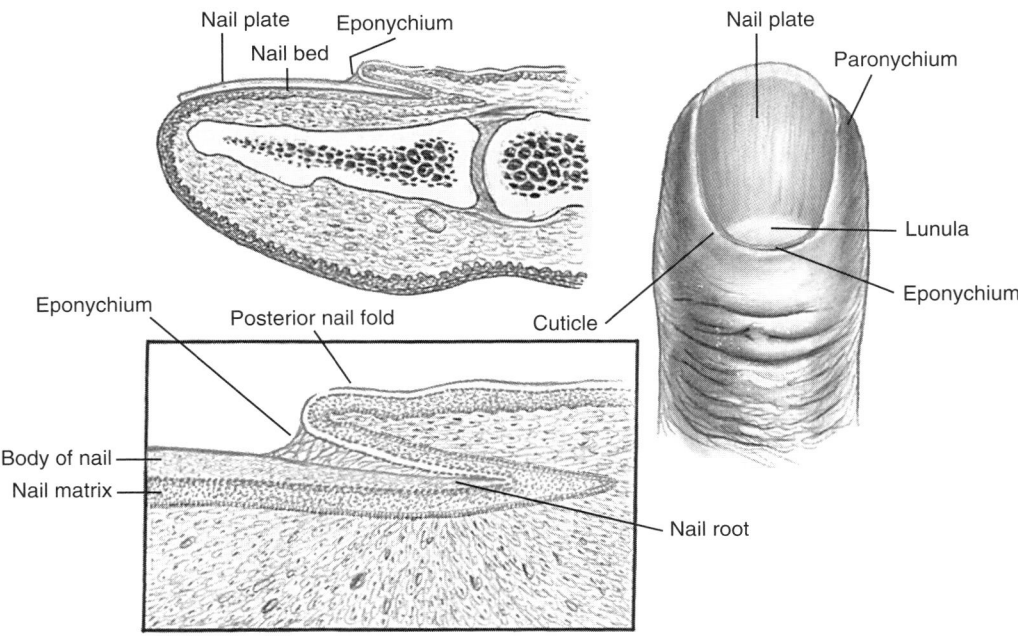

FIG. 76-6 Diagrammatic drawing of normal adult fingernails. (From Thompson JM et al: *Mosby's clinical nursing,* ed 5, St Louis, 2002, Mosby.)

over the scalp or even the entire body may indicate possible thyroid abnormalities (see Chapter 60). The lack of hair over distal extremities can be the first sign of vascular insufficiency, whereas abnormal hair growth over the face, especially in females, should be investigated for a hormone-producing tumor.

Nails can be damaged and thinned in many diseases, such as psoriasis, fungal infections, and thyroid abnormalities. Excessive sweat production can be a sign of anxiety or an underlying internal illness.

KEY CONCEPTS

- *Dermatology* is concerned with the structure, function, and diseases of the skin.
- The skin forms a protective barrier around the entire body and has a role in body thermoregulation, glandular secretion, and sensory communication with the external environment.
- The skin is the largest organ of the human body that envelops the muscles and internal organs and has an endless network of blood vessels, nerves, and glands, all of which have a potential for disease.
- The skin consists of three layers: epidermis, dermis, and subcutaneous fat.
- The *epidermis,* the outermost portion of the skin, is divided into two main layers: a stratum of anucleated cornified cells (the *stratum corneum,* or horny layer) and the inner, *malpighian layer,* from which the surface cornified cells arise by differentiation. The malpighian layer is subdivided into the (1) stratum granulosum, (2) basal cell layer (or stratum germinativum), and (3) stratum spinosum.
- The *basal layer* consists largely of undifferentiated epidermal cells that undergo constant mitosis, renewing the epidermis as one of the daughter cells remains in the basal layer to divide again while the other cell migrates outward toward the stratum spinosum.

- The major differentiating cell of the *stratum spinosum* is the keratinocyte, which produces keratin, a fibrous protein.
- The second major cell of the epidermis is the *melanocyte,* found in the basal layer. The ratio of basal cells to melanocytes is 10:1.
- The *dermis* is located immediately below the epidermis and is composed of collagen fibers, elastin, and reticulin embedded in a ground substance.
- Underlying the dermis is the third layer of skin, the subcutaneous fat that provides a cushion for the skin, insulation to maintain body heat, and a store of energy.
- *Sweat (eccrine) glands* are present almost everywhere on the skin except in the ears and on the lips. These glands aid in maintaining the appropriate body temperature.
- *Sebaceous glands* are lobulated structures that consist of lipid-filled cells, and primarily androgenic hormones hormonally regulate their activity.
- The *apocrine glands* are found primarily in the axilla, in the genital skin, around the nipples, and in the perianal area; they contribute to the axillary odor when apocrine bacteria decompose secretions.
- *Hair* is formed from keratin. By a predetermined differentiating process, certain epidermal cells form the

hair follicle, which is supported by dermal matrix and differentiates into the hair.

- The *nail* is a dead keratin plate produced by epidermal cells of nail matrix and is located beneath the proximal portion of the nail plate in the dermis.
- Skin should be examined in a well-illuminated room, preferably in natural daylight. Skin has turgor and elasticity on palpation.

- *Dermatoglyphics* are skin ridges that are visible over the palms and feet and are also present over the entire body surface. They form the pattern unique for every individual and species.
- The dermatoglyphics over the volar aspects of the fingers are used for fingerprinting.

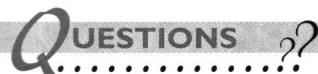

QUESTIONS ??

A sampling of review questions for this chapter appears here. Visit http://www.mosby.com/MERLIN/PriceWilson/ for additional questions.

Answer the following on a separate sheet of paper.

1. Explain the skin proliferation process by identifying the layer of the skin that produces new cells and the direction of movement of the new cells.
2. List the function of the two adnexal structures of the skin: eccrine (sweat) glands and sebaceous glands.
3. Describe the essential elements of a skin examination.
4. What is the function of the subcutaneous fat layer of the skin?
5. In Fig. 76-7, label the three layers of the skin: epidermis, dermis, and subcutaneous fat.

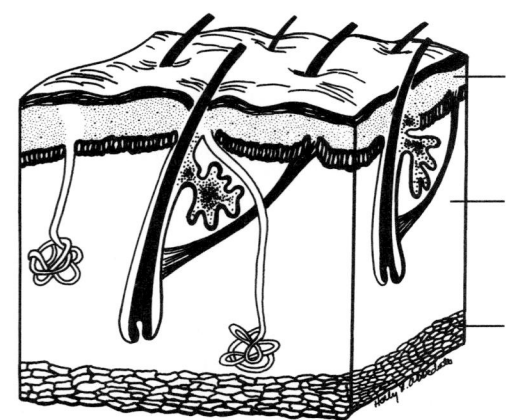

FIG. 76-7

CHAPTER
77

Acne and Related Conditions

MAREK A. STAWISKI

ACNE VULGARIS

Acne is an acute or chronic inflammatory process of sebaceous glands. The disease can be minor with only comedones or inflammatory with multiple pustules or cysts. Acne generally occurs among most adolescents and young adults and usually spontaneously resolves about 20 to 30 years of age. However, many middle-age adults experience acne eruptions. Acne is usually associated with a high rate of sebum secretion. Androgens are known stimulants of sebum secretion, and estrogen reduces sebum production. Without androgens, sebaceous glands remain small. Acne is not observed in males castrated before puberty or in oophorectomized women.

A sudden onset of severe acne associated with hirsutism or menstrual abnormalities may indicate an endocrine disorder in a female patient. Acne in women in their 20s, 30s, and 40s is frequently caused by comedo-producing oil-based cosmetics and moisturizers. Mechanical factors, such as rubbing, friction, pressure, and stretching of the skin rich in sebaceous glands, can make the existing acne worse. The more common mechanical causes include football helmets, surgical tape, and shirt collars. Comedogenic agents such as petrolatum and greasy cosmetics can also exacerbate acne.

Medications can also precipitate the onset of acne. Chronic oral corticosteroids used for treatment of other conditions (e.g., systemic lupus erythematosus, renal transplants) can trigger superficial pustules over the face, chest, and back. Oral contraceptives usually are helpful in acne treatment because of their estrogen content. In some women, however, oral contraceptives can exacerbate the condition. Other drugs known to aggravate or

precipitate acne are bromides, iodides, diphenytoin, lithium, or isonicotinic acid hydrazide. Industrial workers may be exposed to chlorinated hydrocarbons, which are acnegenic.

Management of acne patients requires a careful history to rule out acnegenic factors and more serious endocrine abnormalities. Most acne patients have a family history of acne.

The distribution of acne corresponds to the areas of sebaceous glands and occurs over the face, neck, chest, back, and shoulders (Fig. 77-1). The earliest lesion to appear in the skin is the *comedo*. *White comedones*, or closed comedones, are more likely to progress to inflammatory papules and pustules of acne. *Black comedones*, or open comedones, have a dark, horny material plugging up dilated pilosebaceous ducts. These comedones obstruct the flow of sebum to the surface. Patients with only comedones have noninflammatory acne. The sebum, bacteria *(Propionibacterium acnes)*, and fatty acids are thought to be responsible for the development of inflammation around the pilosebaceous ducts and sebaceous glands.

Once the flow of sebum to the surface is obstructed by comedones, *P. acnes* produces lipases that break down sebum triglycerides into free fatty acids. These acids, in combination with bacteria, produce an inflammatory response in the dermis. This inflammation leads to formation of erythematous papules, inflammatory pustules, and inflammatory cysts (Fig. 77-2). The pustules and cysts drain and heal over time. Deeper papules and cysts can leave permanent scars, whereas mild acne resolves without scarring. The tendency to scar varies among individuals and increases when the person attempts to empty the lesions. All scarring, except the keloidal type and pitted scars, generally improves with time.

Acne is classified as comedonal (black and white comedones) (Fig. 77-3), papulopustular (papules and pustules) (Fig. 77-4; see color plate 46), or cystic (see color plate 47). Comedonal and papulopustular acne are given numeric grades. Grade I acne has less than 10 comedones, papules, or pustules on one side of the face (see Fig. 77-3); grade II, 10 to 20 comedones, papules, or pustules; grade III, 25 to 50; and grade IV, more than 50 (see color plate 47).

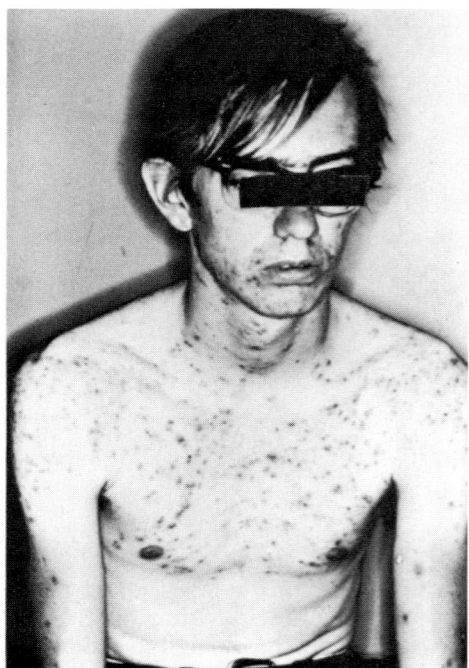

FIG. 77-1 Characteristic distribution of acne pustules over the face, chest, and shoulders.

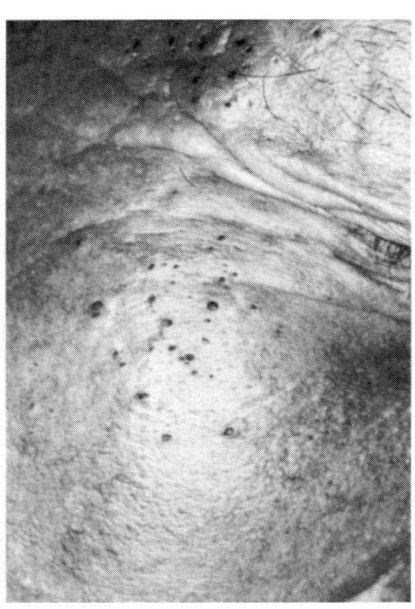

FIG. 77-3 Multiple comedones in a superficial comedonal acne.

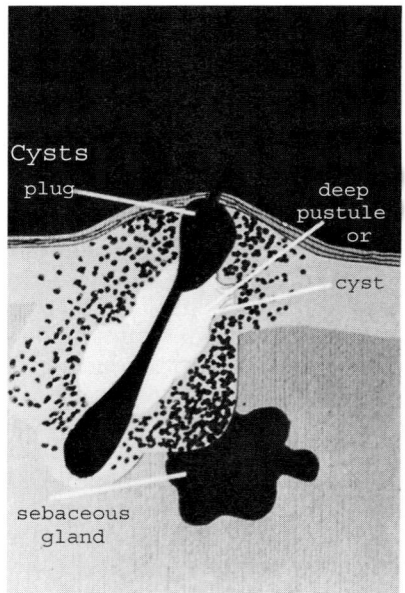

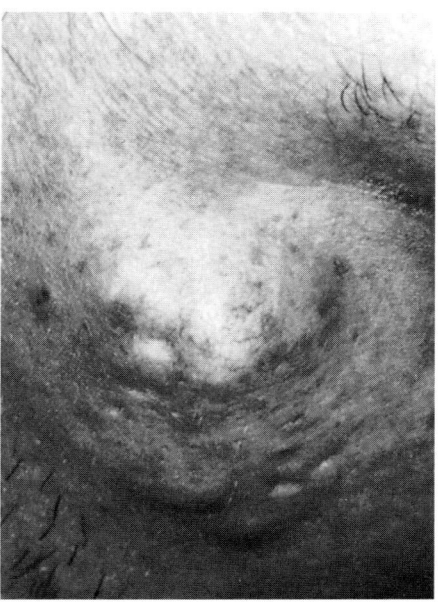

FIG. 77-2 Inflammation around the pilosebaceous glands that leads to formation of papules, pustules, and cysts.

VARIANTS OF ACNE

Several variants of acne should be recognized. *Excoriated acne* occurs in individuals who obsessively manipulate the acne lesions; this action can cause extreme scarring. *Conglobate acne*, or *acne conglobata*, is the most severe cys-

tic acne, with deep cysts, multiple comedones, and marked scarring. This form of acne can be associated with malaise and fever and may even require hospitalization (see Fig. 77-4 and color plate 47). Individuals with *acne keloidalis* have multiple scars and keloids in the areas where acne lesions were present (Fig. 77-5).

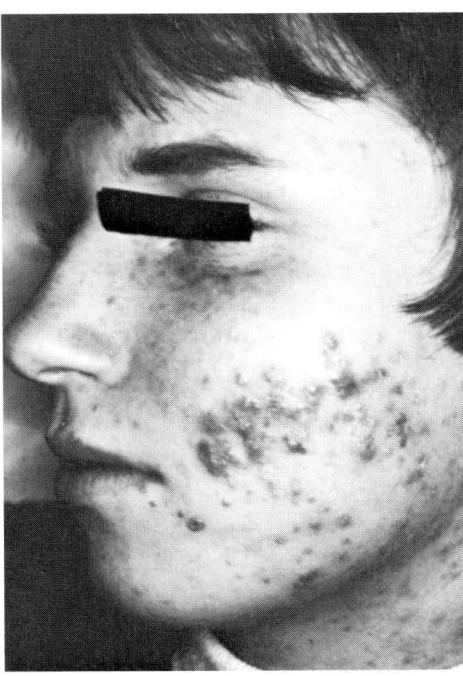

FIG. 77-4   Severe scarring can follow obsessive manipulation of acne papules and pustules.

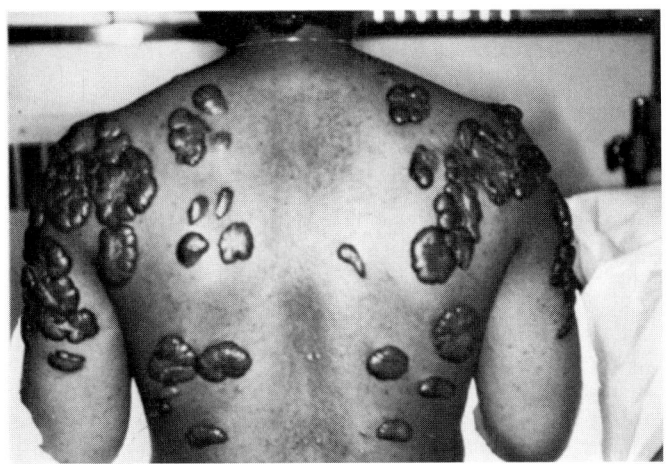

FIG. 77-5   Keloids can complicate a course of acne vulgaris.

TREATMENT OF ACNE

The goal of acne therapy is to decrease the inflammatory process of pilosebaceous glands until spontaneous remission occurs. Treatment of acne and related conditions improves the patient's cosmetic appearance and self-image and prevents scars related to acne.

Acne treatment includes halting the use of all exacerbating factors such as oil-based makeup and moisturizing creams. Dietary restrictions are usually not required or effective.

Cleaning and scrubbing the face with soap removes the surface oil and dislodges some comedones. The affected areas should be washed twice daily. Soaps such as Dial, Pernox, Fostex, Neutrogena, Desquam-X Wash, and benzoyl peroxide (Brevoxyl Cleansing Lotion) are recommended. A keratolytic agent such as benzoyl peroxide at a concentration of 3% to 10% is used daily. Benzoyl peroxide is now available over the counter. Many patients have tried this on their own, developing excessive dryness and irritation. Tretinoin gel microsphere (Retin-A micro), Retin-A gel (0.01%, 0.025%), and Retin-A cream (0.025%, 0.05%, 0.1%) are useful because of their keratolytic effect on superficial comedones. However, Retin-A derivatives can enhance skin irritability from exposure to the wind, sunlight, or cold weather. Recently, topical tretinoin emollient cream 0.05% (Renova) has received much attention from its antiwrinkle properties. Tretinoin should be used with caution because it can cause irritant dermatitis. Other popular compounds used for their anti-acne and antiwrinkle effects are glycolic acids; no reliable studies support their popularity.

Topical antibiotics used to treat superficial acne papules and pustules include clindamycin (1% Cleocin-T gel, solution, or lotion), erythromycin (A.T.S. solution and cream, 2% Emgel, 2% Erycette solution). Azelaic acid (Azelex), topical adapalene retinoid-like compound (Differin), and benzoyl peroxide (Triaz) are also effective topical acne medications. Topical antibiotics are frequently used in the morning and benzoyl peroxides or Retin-A compounds at bedtime.

Systemic antibiotics remain the principle mode of therapy for deep pustular and deep papular acne. Patients are usually treated with tetracycline, erythromycin, or minocycline. For superficial pustular acne, the dose of tetracycline is 250 to 500 mg daily. For severe, deep papulopustular or cystic acne, 1000 mg of tetracycline is administered daily. Long-term tetracycline therapy has been shown to be safe. Children under 12 are not treated with tetracycline because permanent staining of the teeth can occur. Tetracycline is not given to pregnant women, because enamel hypoplasia and permanent discoloration of the teeth may occur in newborns. Some patients may develop photosensitivity, nausea, and candidiasis while receiving tetracycline. Oral tetracycline can make oral contraceptives less effective, and women can become pregnant. This characteristic is especially true if a patient has breakthrough bleeding while taking tetracycline and oral contraceptives together.

A derivative of tetracycline, minocycline, at a dose of 50 to 100 mg daily, is the most effective antibiotic for acne. Minocycline is a more expensive antibiotic than tetracycline and can also cause dizziness and a reversible bluish discoloration of the skin at higher doses. The pharmacologic action of tetracycline and minocycline on acne is not completely understood. The antibiotics decrease the population of *P. acnes* in the pilosebaceous gland. This bacterium produces lipases that hydrolyze sebum to fatty acids. Fatty acids may be responsible for inflammation of the pilosebaceous duct. Tetracycline and minocycline also inhibit these lipases.

Erythromycin is less effective in treatment of acne. This antibiotic is used at a dose of 250 to 500 mg daily. Patients can develop gastrointestinal irritation while taking erythromycin.

An oral drug, *isotretinoin* (Accutane), was approved by the U.S. Food and Drug Administration for treatment of severe, antibiotic-resistant cystic-conglobate acne. A single 20-week course of 0.5 mg/kg/day or 1.0 mg/kg/day results in remission of the disease in about 80% to 90% of patients. In many of these patients, remission appears to be permanent, even after a 3-year follow-up. Truncal acne and acne in young adolescents relapse more frequently. Some patients require a second course of isoretinoin therapy. Isoretinoin, if used in the early course of acne, can prevent most of the scarring caused by deep papules and pustules.

The exact mechanism of isotretinoin is unknown. Chemically, isotretinoin is related to vitamin A. In contrast to vitamin A, however, isotretinoin is not stored in the liver but is rapidly excreted; the half-life of oral isotretinoin is approximately 10 to 20 hours. Consequently, the drug has fewer side effects than does vitamin A. Isotretinoin inhibits sebaceous gland function, and this presumably is its mechanism of action in acne.

Because isotretinoin is a known teratogen, *it must not be used in women who are pregnant or who intend to become pregnant* while undergoing therapy or soon after completion of therapy. Before isotretinoin is administered to women of childbearing age, a pregnancy test should be performed, and an effective method of contraception should be used for 2 weeks before therapy, throughout the therapy, and for 2 months after therapy is discontinued. Isoretinoin can cause depression and rarely suicidal attempts. The drug must be stopped immediately when depression occurs. Cheilitis, xerosis, conjunctivitis, and drying of nasal mucosa with nosebleeds are the most common side effects, which are reversible after isotretinoin is discontinued. Other side effects include myalgias, transient arthralgias, and thinning of scalp hair. Rare but serious side effects include increased intracranial pressure with papilledema, nausea, vomiting, headaches, and visual disturbances. Because ingestion has been associated with inflammatory bowel diseases, isotretinoin should not be used in patients with inflammatory bowel diseases. If signs of increased intracranial pressure or severe diarrhea develop, isotretinoin must be stopped immediately. Transient elevation of triglycerides has been observed in 25% of patients. Furthermore, elevation of uric acid and liver enzyme levels and minor depression of red blood cell and white blood cell counts have been reported. Patients receiving isotretinoin should have blood lipid determinations, white blood cell counts, red blood cell counts, and levels of platelets, alkaline phosphatase, serum aspartate and alanine aminotransferases (AST, ALT; formerly SGOT, SGPT), and lactate dehydrogenase (LDH) obtained before and at intervals throughout therapy.

Much optimism surrounds the potential role of isotretinoin in the treatment of severe acne. The use of isotretinoin should be restricted to short-term, low-dose therapy of patients with antibiotic-resistant cystic acne. Patients who are obese, diabetic, alcoholic, or those who have high triglyceride levels, and women planning families in the near future should not be treated with this medication. Furthermore, only physicians who are experienced or trained in its use should prescribe isotretinoin.

Outpatient therapy for acne includes acne surgery, which consists of removal of comedones and opening and draining of pustules. Self-manipulation of acne lesions usually results in more scar formation and should be discouraged. The benefit of ultraviolet light is minimal, and home sunlamps are not recommended. Cryotherapy has been sometimes effective in the treatment of superficial pustules and cysts.

Dermabrasion is used to smooth and plane the scars and pits that develop as a result of acne. However, as a procedure that usually requires long surgery, dermabrasion is reserved for more severe cases of scarring. Patients with broad-based scars obtain a better cosmetic result than those with deep pitted lesions. The procedure involves the use of a high-speed metal brush to plane the skin to various levels. Improvement occurs in about 50% of patients. Scarring, hyperpigmentation, and hypopigmentation are the main complications. Only a dermatologist well trained in this procedure, or a plastic surgeon, should perform this technique on carefully screened patients. This surgical procedure has been replaced by the use of carbon dioxide resurfacing laser, which is safer and more effective than dermabrasion. Hyperpigmentation, hypopigmentation, and scarring are most frequently seen complications of this new modality.

RELATED CONDITIONS

Acne rosacea is a separate disease entity that usually occurs in persons between ages 40 and 60. Acne rosacea presents with pronounced erythema and superficial pustules and papules over the central portion of the face. A large, multilobulated rhinophyma is rare but can result from this acne as the sebaceous glands become larger (Fig. 77-6; see color plate 48).

Blepharitis can complicate acne rosacea. The predisposing factors of acne rosacea are not known, but there is frequently a family history of acne rosacea and of ruddy complexion. Acne rosacea patients have an increased number of sebaceous glands over the face associated with erythema and multiple, small telangiectases. The acne rosacea patient should avoid excessive amounts of alcohol and spicy foods. The main therapeutic modality is oral tetracycline, which is usually started at doses of 500 to 1000 mg daily. As the pustules and papules decrease in number, tetracycline is gradually tapered. Minocycline, 50 to 100 mg daily, can also be used. The topical antibiotic metronidazole (MetroGel, MetroCream, Metrolo-

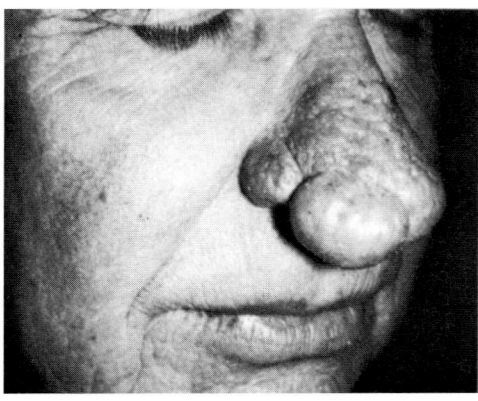

FIG. 77-6 Large rhinophyma of the nose in a patient with acne rosacea. The skin is erythematous, and multiple pustules are present.

tion, Noritate) is helpful in the management of this type of acne. A 1% hydrocortisone cream, with or without 1% or 2% precipitated sulfur, can help treat the erythema and superficial pustules. Acne rosacea is a chronic disease that may have to be treated for a prolonged period. Telangiectases can be treated with a pulse dye laser, copper vapor laser, or electrodesiccation. Rhinophyma can be removed with a carbon dioxide laser.

Women in their 20s and 30s can develop superficial pustules, papules, and erythematous, greasy, scaly patches in perioral distribution (Fig. 77-7). This disorder is called *perioral dermatitis*, or *perioral acne*, and is the acne most frequently seen in adult women. Perioral acne spares the skin immediately adjacent to the lips. These patients frequently report a previous use of strong fluorinated steroid creams on the face. However, the cause of this condition is unknown. In treating this condition, all strong topical steroid creams should be stopped. A 1% hydrocortisone cream helps treat erythema and prevents exacerbation of this acne when stronger topical steroids are stopped. Oral tetracycline, 250 to 500 mg daily, is usually effective. The antibiotic is gradually tapered over a few months. Frequently, resolution of perioral acne occurs within 4 months.

Pseudofolliculitis barbae occurs predominantly in bearded areas of African-American men. Curved, stiff beard hairs, when shaved close to the skin surface, reenter the skin and cause foreign body granulomas. The patients develop perifollicular inflammatory papules and pustules (Fig. 77-8). Scars and keloids frequently form secondary to these foreign body granulomas. The condition starts at the time when individuals begin shaving, and the most practical way to treat it is to grow a beard. Because this treatment method is not always acceptable, as in the armed forces and some places of employment, other remedies are used. Depilatories (e.g., Magic Shave) are helpful but can cause severe irritation of the skin. Using a toothbrush to comb and remove the ingrown hairs from the skin is helpful. Patients are instructed not to shave close in the skin by using a single-edged blade razor or electric shaver.

A chronic inflammation of the apocrine glands results in *hidradenitis suppurativa*. Painful nodules, cysts, scars, and

sinus tracts form in the axillae, groin, perianal area, and breasts where the apocrine glands are present (Fig. 77-9). Frequently, there is a history of cystic acne in the family, and patients have cystic acne over the face, chest, and back. However, the etiology of hidradenitis suppurativa is unknown. Cysts are frequently sterile or grow a common epi-

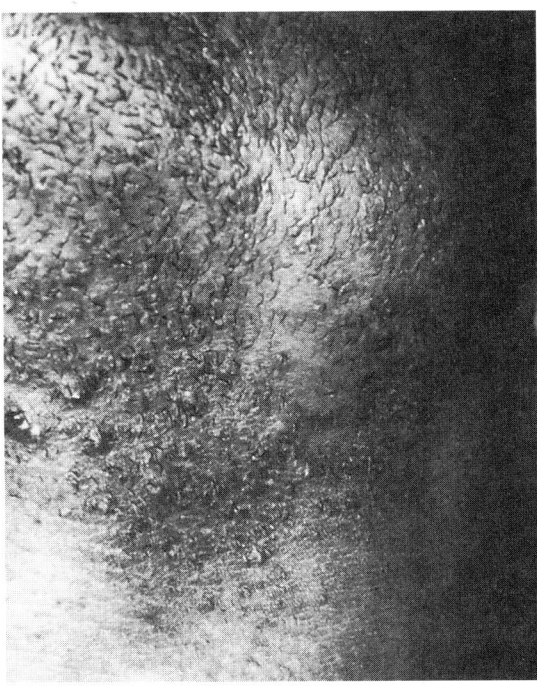

FIG. 77-8 Multiple papules and pustules in perifollicular distribution over the neck of a patient with pseudofolliculitis barbae.

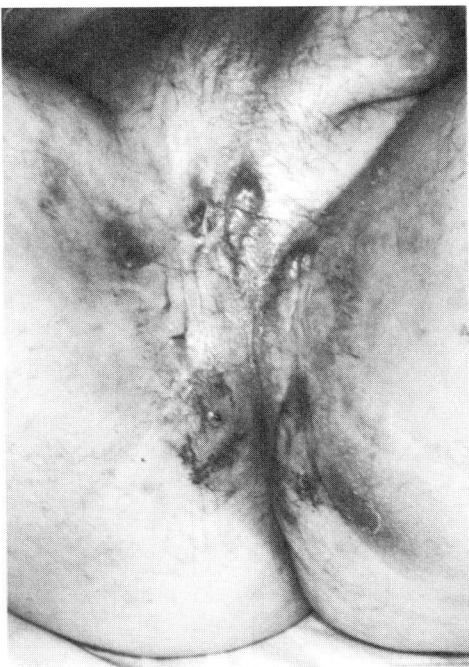

FIG. 77-9 Painful nodules, cysts, and sinus tracts in hidradenitis suppurativa of the groin.

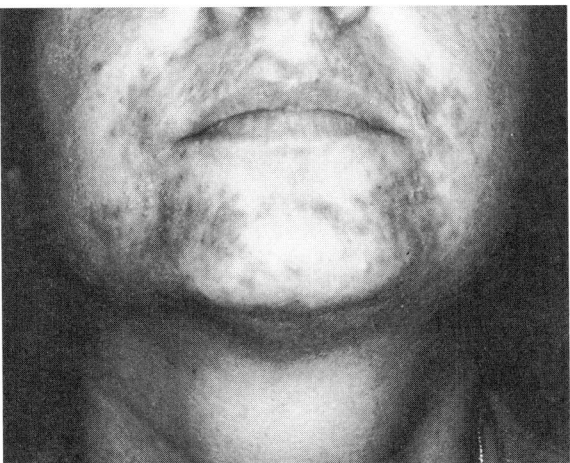

FIG. 77-7 Erythema, papules, and scaliness in perioral distribution are characteristic of perioral dermatitis.

dermal contaminant, *Staphylococcus epidermidis.* The inflammatory process of the apocrine glands may be secondary to bacteria or their breakdown products. In treating this condition, drainage of the cysts is helpful. Systemic tetracycline, minocycline, or erythromycin is useful in conservative management of inflamed, painful cysts. Patients are instructed to lose weight and clean the area of involvement with antibacterial soaps (e.g., pHisoHex). In chronic, refractory cases of hidradenitis suppurativa, surgical resection of the affected area is sometimes indicated.

KEY CONCEPTS

- *Acne* is an acute or chronic inflammatory process of sebaceous glands.
- Acne occurs among adolescents and young adults and usually spontaneously resolves by about 20 to 30 years of age; many middle-age adults experience acne eruptions.
- Acne is usually associated with a high rate of sebum secretion. Androgens are known stimulants of sebum secretion, and estrogen reduces sebum production.
- Medications can also precipitate the onset of acne, such as chronic oral corticosteroids used for treatment of other conditions (e.g., systemic lupus erythematosus, renal transplants), and can trigger superficial pustules over the face, chest, and back.
- Management of acne patients requires a careful history to rule out acnegenic factors and more serious endocrine abnormalities.
- The distribution of acne corresponds to the areas of sebaceous glands and occurs over the face, neck, chest, back, and shoulders.
- The earliest lesion to appear in the skin is the comedo.
- White comedones, or closed comedones, are more likely to progress to inflammatory papules and pustules of acne. Black comedones, or open comedones, have a dark, horny material plugging up dilated pilosebaceous ducts.
- These comedones obstruct the flow of sebum to the surface.

- Acne is classified as *comedonal* (black and white comedones), *papulopustular* (papules and pustules), or *cystic.* Comedonal and papulopustular acne are given numeric grades.
- Several variants of acne should be recognized, such as excoriated acne, which occurs in individuals who obsessively manipulate the acne lesions; this action can cause extreme scarring.
- The goal of acne therapy is to decrease the inflammatory process of pilosebaceous glands until spontaneous remission occurs. Treatment of acne and related conditions improves the patient's cosmetic appearance and self-image and prevents scars related to acne.
- Acne treatment includes halting the use of all exacerbating factors such as oil-based makeup and moisturizing creams. Topical antibiotics are used to treat superficial acne papules and pustules. Systemic antibiotics are the principle mode of therapy for deep pustular and deep papular acne.
- *Acne rosacea* is a separate disease entity that usually occurs in persons between ages 40 and 60; it presents with pronounced erythema and superficial pustules and papules over the central portion of the face.
- *Pseudofolliculitis barbae* occurs predominantly in bearded areas of African-American men.

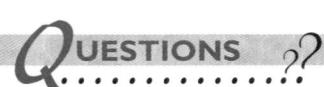 UESTIONS ??

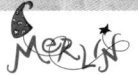

A sampling of review questions for this chapter appears here. Visit http://www.mosby.com/MERLIN/PriceWilson/ for additional questions.

Answer the following on a separate sheet of paper.
1. Define acne.
2. Which age groups have the highest incidence rates of acne?
3. Describe the formation of acne lesions.

4. Explain the purpose of each of the following treatments for acne:
   a. Proper cleansing of the skin
   b. Antibiotic therapy with tetracycline

Eczema and Vascular Disorders

MAREK A. STAWISKI

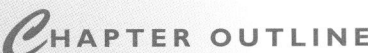

ECZEMA

Eczema encompasses all types of red, blistering, weeping, scaly, thickened, itchy skin lesions. *Acute eczema* presents with vesicles, bullae, erythema, weeping, and crusting. *Chronic eczema* has thickened, scaly, pruritic patches and plaques. Examples of eczema include the following:

1. Atopic eczema, characterized by weeping, crusted, dry, scaly, pruritic patches on the faces of infants and in the folds of skin found in the antecubital and popliteal fossae in adolescents and adults
2. Allergic contact eczema, characterized by pruritic vesicles, erythema, and patches in areas where patients have touched allergens such as poison ivy, poison sumac, cosmetics, rubber, and cement, among many others
3. Hand eczema characterized by erythematous, scaly, fissured patches over the hands
4. Neurodermatitis, characterized by excoriated patches and lines secondary to compulsive scratching of the skin
5. Seborrheic dermatitis, characterized by yellow-red-brown, greasy, scaly patches over the scalp and face
6. Stasis eczema, characterized by stasis edema, hyperpigmentation, and scaliness of the lower legs

Atopic Eczema

Atopic eczema, or *atopic dermatitis,* is a hereditary chronic skin disease that can appear at any age (see Chapter 9). There is often a family history of this eczema and associated allergic rhinitis or extrinsic asthma. Some children outgrow the cutaneous eczema only to develop hay fever or extrinsic asthma in later years. Infantile atopic eczema frequently presents with weeping, eroded, erythematous patches in the diaper area and on the cheeks and scalp (see color plate 49). Because the eruptions are pruritic, the infant is irritable. Secondary infections with bacteria are common. In some infants, the eczema disappears spontaneously. In some infants, the condition can progress into childhood or adult forms. Pruritus is the universal complaint of all these patients. The eroded patches of eczema in the groin and under the breasts can be painful.

In children or adults, the areas of involvement include the popliteal spaces, the antecubital fossae, the neck areas, and other flexural surfaces (Fig. 78-1). In adults, eczematous skin changes can become generalized over the entire body. Spontaneous remission of adulthood eczema occurs infrequently. Patients have erythematous, excoriated, thickened skin over the face, trunk, and extremities (Fig. 78-2). Changes in the weather and irritation from wool clothing, soap, and water frequently exacerbate the disease. Upper respiratory infections and bacterial skin infections can also aggravate the skin condition. Atopic eczema patients should not be vaccinated against smallpox because disseminated vaccinia can develop. Exposure to herpes virus can result in disseminated herpetic infection of the skin.

The causes of atopic eczema are unknown. Hereditary factors definitely play a role. When two parents have atopic eczema, the child has about an 80% chance of developing the same skin condition. Irritation of the skin with wool, water, harsh soaps, climate changes, stress, and infection frequently result in clinical exacerbations. Many of the patients have abnormal levels of serum immunoglobulin E (IgE). Some investigators have demonstrated IgE on the surface of epidermal Langerhans cells in atopic eczema patients. Blood eosinophils are also elevated in this disease. The number of thymus-derived lymphocytes is decreased in some patients. Some investi-

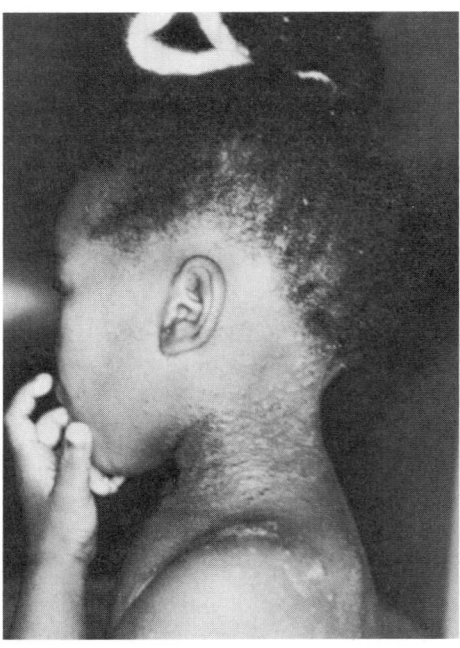

FIG. 78-1 Lichenified, thickened, scaly skin over the neck area in childhood atopic eczema.

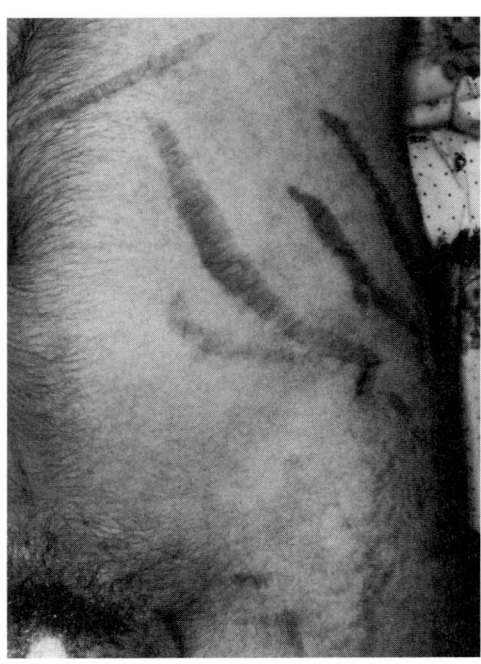

FIG. 78-3 Atrophy of skin causing striae after prolonged use of high-strength steroids.

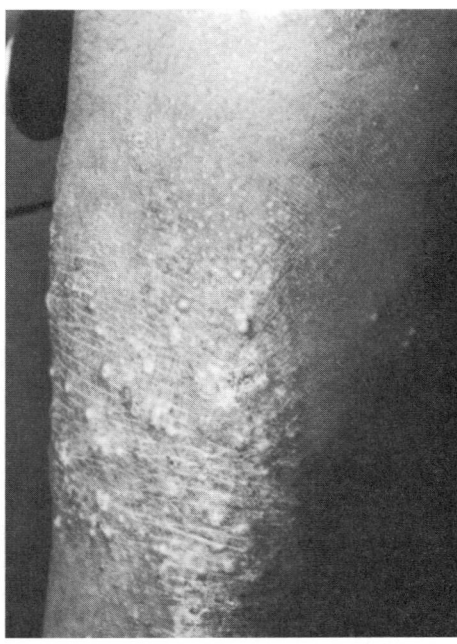

FIG. 78-2 Thickened skin with multiple excoriated papules of chronic eczema.

gators have postulated an abnormality in the receptors responsible for production of cyclic adenosine monophosphate (cAMP) nucleotides. How these abnormalities produce an extremely pruritic, eczematous skin is not understood.

Therapy of atopic eczema focuses on hydration, prevention, and treatment. All possible exacerbating factors must be avoided or eliminated. Superfatted soaps and lubricating creams are recommended. In infants, dietary restrictions may be helpful (e.g., cow's milk, wheat, eggs), but they are not useful with older children and adults. Moisturizers such as Eucerin, Moisturel, and Aquaphor are applied to dry skin. Antibiotics are used to treat secondary bacterial infections. Pruritus is controlled with antihistaminics such as diphenhydramine (Benadryl), hydroxyzine (Atarax), cyproheptadine (Periactin), or cetirizine (Zyrtec). Newer, nonsedating antihistaminics such as loratadine (Claritin) or fexofenadine (Allegra) are frequently used but are less effective in controlling pruritus than the antihistaminics previously listed. Topical corticosteroids in the weakest possible strength are used for children. Topical 2.5% hydrocortisone is usually prescribed for infants, whereas 0.025% triamcinolone cream is given to adults. A 0.05% desonide, 2.5% hydrocortisone cream, or 0.05% alclometasone (Aclovate) are used to treat eczema of the face, groin, and axillae in adults. Other medium- or high-strength topical steroids used in adults include clobetasol dipropionate (Temovate), betamethasone (Diprolene), halcinonide (Halog), fluocinonide (Lidex), fluticasone (Cutivate), and mometasone (Elocon). Medium- or high-strength topical steroids used for a prolonged time can cause skin atrophy (Fig. 78-3), depigmentation, and acne formation. Ultraviolet light B (UVB) and oral psoralens combined with ultraviolet light A (PUVA) can be useful in treatment of recalcitrant chronic atopic eczema. A new immunosuppressive ointment, tacrolimus (Protopic), appears to have great efficacy in treatment of atopic eczema when applied topically. The drug blocks release of cytokines by T lymphocytes. Hyposensitization immunotherapy may exacerbate, benefit, or have no effect on atopic eczema and is therefore not indicated in this form of eczema.

Allergic Contact Eczema

Allergic contact eczema is common and occurs in localized areas where an allergen comes into contact with the skin. The skin reaction to the oil of poison ivy, *Rhus* dermatitis, is best known. Linear areas of vesiculation, weeping, and erythema occur in the places where the skin has touched the poison ivy, poison sumac, or poison oak plant (Fig. 78-4; see color plate 50). The oil can be carried in many ways: on a pet's fur, on clothing, on shoes, or on fingernails. Once the oil is washed off, the dermatitis does not spread. *Rhus* dermatitis is not transmitted from person to person through the blister fluid.

Another frequent cause of contact eczema is nickel. This metal is found in virtually all jewelry, metal eyeglass frames, and coins. A patient sensitive to nickel has crusted, well-defined patches of eczema at the site of exposure (e.g., neck, ears, wrists, abdomen). Patients allergic to potassium dichromate develop eczema when exposed to the compound in cement or leather shoes. Shoes can also contain rubber, which is a frequent cause of shoe-contact eczema. The medications neomycin and benzocaine and the preservative ethylenediamine are common causes of allergic eczema. In *photodermatitis*, topical agents (e.g., halogenated salicylamides in soaps) or an oral medication (e.g., tetracycline) in combination with sunlight can cause erythema, edema, and occasionally vesiculation. Photodermatitis usually occurs on sunlight-exposed areas of the face, neck, and forearms.

Allergic contact eczema is mediated through a cellular type IV delayed hypersensitivity (see Chapter 12). After primary exposure, a second contact with the allergen is required to produce eczema. Patch-testing the patient in whom the allergy is suspected can produce this type of eczema. A careful history is required for selection of appropriate allergens to be tested. Patch testing is usually performed on the patient's back after the eczema is under control.

Therapy necessitates the removal of offending allergens. Patients must learn how to identify *Rhus* plants. Cosmetics, jewelry, and other objects that contain the allergen responsible for eczema should be avoided. Topical care of acute allergic eczema includes soaks and corticosteroid creams and gels. Frequently, severe allergic eczema, such as poison ivy, is treated with systemic steroids. A short treatment with systemic prednisone at the initial dosage of 40 to 60 mg/day is tapered over 7 to 14 days.

Hand Eczema

Hand eczema most often occurs in persons who must wash their hands frequently or who wear gloves in their occupation. Often, a family history of eczema is present in these patients. Small vesicles appear on the lateral aspects of fingers, toes, and feet. Pruritus accompanies the appearance of vesicles. The small blisters develop into scaly, eczematous patches over the palms and soles (see color plate 51). The condition can be a chronic problem that is extremely difficult to control. When exposure to an industrial chemical exacerbates hand eczema, patch testing is required to rule out allergic eczema. In the absence of positive allergic test irritants, heredity may play an important role in hand eczema.

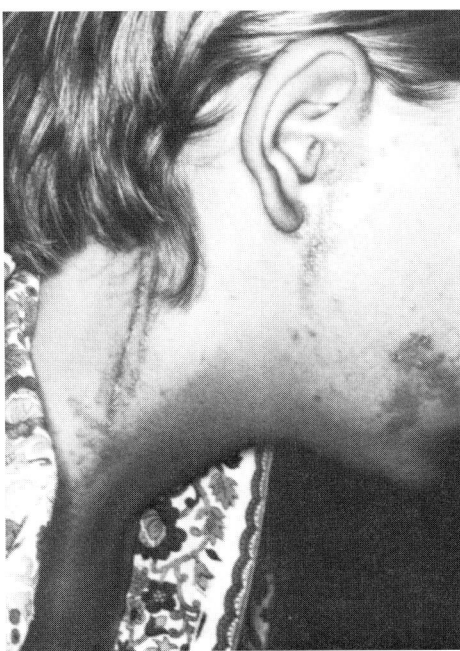

FIG. 78-4   Grouped and linear vesicular eruptions are characteristic of poison ivy dermatitis.

Hand eczema is sometimes prevented through avoiding harsh soaps and wearing protective gloves. Oral antihistamines and strong, fluorinated topical corticosteroids (Lidex, Halog) are used to suppress this form of eczema. Occasionally, a short course of a systemic corticosteroid is required, such as prednisone at a dosage of 30 to 40 mg/day initially, tapered daily over 6 to 8 days. Secondary bacterial infections are treated with appropriate systemic antibiotics.

Immediate IgE-mediated hypersensitivity to latex has become a major cause of contact dermatitis of the hands in health care professionals and patients with a history of multiple surgeries and atopic eczema. Patients report itching, burning, swelling of the hands when they wear latex containing gloves. Respiratory symptoms can be mild to severe, even fatal. To confirm the diagnosis, an antilatex IgE radioallergosorbent test (RAST) can be performed. Skin testing with latex allergen is difficult and can be accompanied by severe reactions. Individuals who have latex allergy should wear vinyl gloves. Patients with latex allergy should inform their dentists and physicians about their allergy.

Neurodermatitis

Neurodermatitis is caused by compulsive scratching of pruritic skin. The condition can be localized to the neck, scrotum, or anywhere on the body. Linear, thickened, dry patches of eczema result from persistent scratching.

Generalized neurodermatitis frequently occurs during the cold, dry winter months in older patients who have dry, pruritic skin. Compulsive scratching can result in factitious ulcers (Fig. 78-5). These self-induced ulcers have

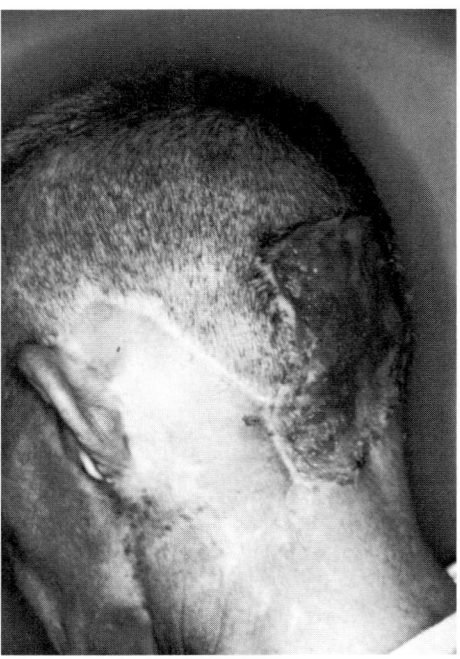

FIG. 78-5 Neurodermatitis. Compulsive scratching can result in factitious ulcers associated with hair loss.

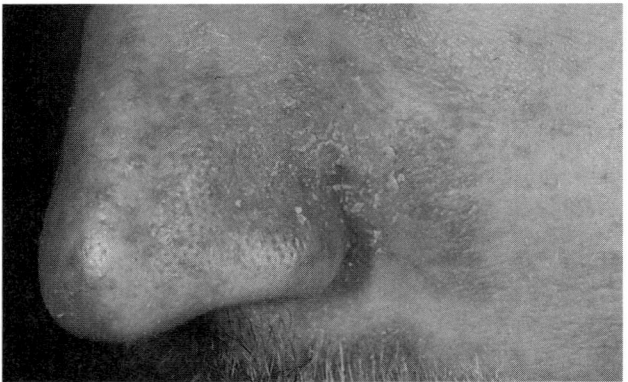

FIG. 78-6 Seborrheic dermatitis. The lesions appear as scaly, white, or yellowish inflammatory plaques with mild pruritus. (Courtesy Department of Dermatology, School of Medicine, University of Utah.)

odd angles and square borders, which should alert the examiner to this diagnosis. However, scabies, atopic eczema, systemic lymphoma, hypothyroidism, diabetes mellitus, cirrhosis, and severe uremia can also cause diffuse pruritus and scratching. These conditions must be carefully ruled out before the diagnosis of neurodermatitis is made.

Treatment of this condition consists of lubrication and application of topical corticosteroids to the skin. Older patients with generalized neurodermatitis should be treated only with emollients (Eucerin) or low-potency topical corticosteroids (2.5% hydrocortisone) or medium-potency topical corticosteroids (Kenalog 0.25% cream or Elocon cream). The skin of older persons is thin from ag-

ing, and stronger topical steroids can lead to further atrophy and excessive bruising. Systemic antihistaminic agents (Benadryl, Atarax, Sinequan, Zyrtec) may be useful in controlling pruritus. Topical doxepin cream (Zonalon) can be used for a limited time of about 8 days to the areas of neurodermatitis. Older patients must use systemic antihistamines with caution because excessive drowsiness or even paradoxical restlessness may occur. Nonsedating antihistamine (Claritin, Allegra, Zyrtec) can be tried. Localized neurodermatitis in younger patients may require stronger topical corticosteroids. Psychotherapy may be required in treating severe neurodermatitis, especially if the face is affected.

Seborrheic Dermatitis

Seborrheic dermatitis typically involves the scalp, eyebrows, nasolabial folds, ears, and anterior chest. Erythematous, scaly patches appear intermittently (Fig. 78-6). The condition may begin any time from infancy to old age and may be slightly pruritic. The cause is unknown, but genetic factors seem to play an important part. Recently, *Pityrosporum ovale* has been implicated as playing a role in the pathogenesis of seborrheic dermatitis.

Therapy of scalp seborrheic dermatitis includes shampoos that contain selenium sulfide (Selsun), ketoconazole (Nizoral), tar (Tegrin, Sebutone), salicylic acid (Sebulex), and peyrithioneyine (Head & Shoulders). Topical corticosteroid sprays or solutions are useful. Weak topical corticosteroids (1% hydrocortisone) combined with precipitated sulfur (0.5% to 1%) are used to treat seborrheic dermatitis of the face and the chest. Topical antifungal agents (ketoconazole) are helpful additions to the therapy. Fluocinolone acetonide in peanut oil base (Derma-smoothe/FS) can be applied under a shower cap to resistant seborrheic dermatitis of the scalp.

Stasis Eczema

Stasis eczema is localized to the areas of venous stasis and edema on the lower legs. Crusted, scaly, weeping erythematous patches appear (Fig. 78-7). The eruptions are pruritic and can lead to secondary excoriations, erosions, and ulcers.

Therapy requires removal of edema fluid and improvement of circulation. The legs are elevated; wraps and Jobst stockings are frequently recommended. Eczema is treated with weak- or intermediate-strength topical corticosteroids (1% hydrocortisone, 0.025% triamcinolone). Ulcers are soaked, cleansed, and débrided. An occlusive dressing (Duoderm) can be used to treat venous stasis ulcers. Patients apply the occlusive dressing every 3 days.

VASCULAR DISORDERS

Urticaria

Urticaria *(hives)* is the most common cutaneous reaction in which edema and erythema result (Fig. 78-8; see color plate 52) (see Chapter 11). Within a few hours after onset, lesions disappear. These transient skin eruptions ap-

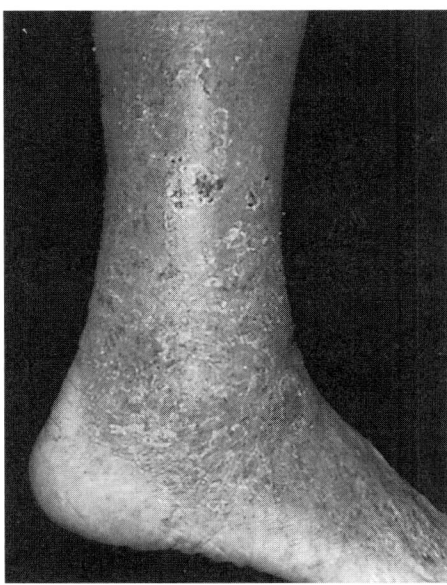

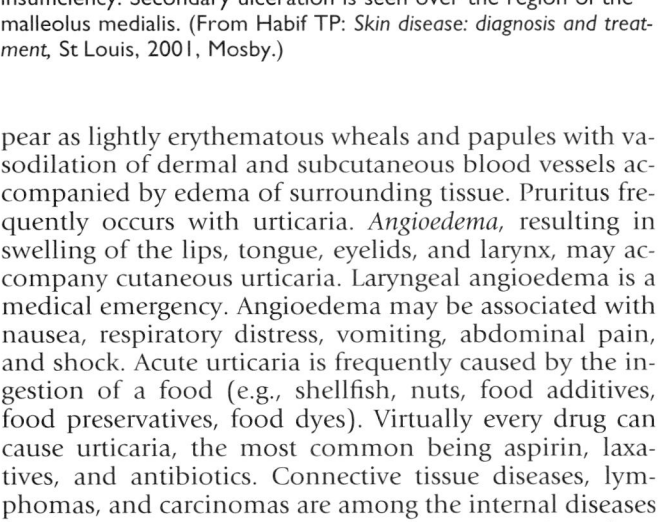

FIG. 78-7 Stasis eczema localized to the area of chronic venous insufficiency. Secondary ulceration is seen over the region of the malleolus medialis. (From Habif TP: *Skin disease: diagnosis and treatment,* St Louis, 2001, Mosby.)

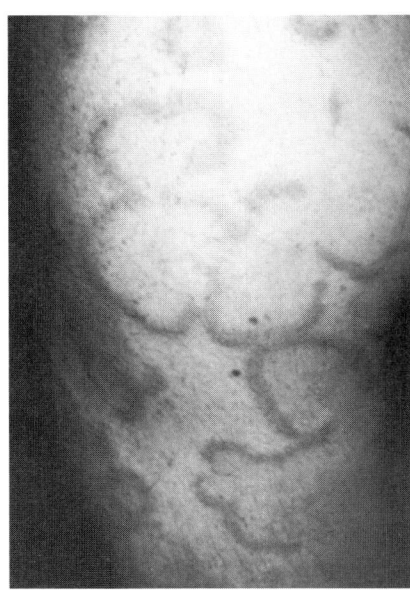

FIG. 78-8 Edema, erythema, and pruritus are the clinical features of urticarial welts.

pear as lightly erythematous wheals and papules with vasodilation of dermal and subcutaneous blood vessels accompanied by edema of surrounding tissue. Pruritus frequently occurs with urticaria. *Angioedema,* resulting in swelling of the lips, tongue, eyelids, and larynx, may accompany cutaneous urticaria. Laryngeal angioedema is a medical emergency. Angioedema may be associated with nausea, respiratory distress, vomiting, abdominal pain, and shock. Acute urticaria is frequently caused by the ingestion of a food (e.g., shellfish, nuts, food additives, food preservatives, food dyes). Virtually every drug can cause urticaria, the most common being aspirin, laxatives, and antibiotics. Connective tissue diseases, lymphomas, and carcinomas are among the internal diseases causing urticaria. Insect bites can cause papules of urticaria. Pregnant women can develop pruritic urticarial papules and plaques.

Chronic urticaria is idiopathic in 75% to 90% of all patients but may be caused by food preservatives, collagen, vascular diseases, medications, or infections. Occasionally, cold temperatures, sunlight, exercise, stress, or alcohol can trigger urticaria. Urticaria results from release of histamines, serotonins, bradykinins, and other mediators. These mediators result in vasodilation and edema in the dermis and subcutaneous layers. Because so many mediators of inflammation are involved in formation of urticarial lesions, treatment can be difficult. The search for an underlying cause can also be extremely difficult. Patients with chronic urticaria are evaluated by a complete history, physical examination, and blood tests, including tests for differential leukocyte count, sedimentation rate, and antinuclear factor. Blood tests should also include liver tests such as those for serum aspartate and alanine aminotransferases (AST, ALT; formerly SGOT, SGPT), lactate dehydrogenase (LDH), alkaline phosphatase, and bilirubin. Search for the infectious agent in-

cludes examination of the stool for ova and parasites, chest radiographs, sinus radiographs, and a dental checkup. Skin testing with antigens is of little merit in the evaluation of urticaria. Hereditary angioedema is associated with a deficiency of the inhibitor of the first complement component. Stroking of the skin, applying ice cubes, exercising, light testing, and water testing can sometimes trigger the skin lesions.

In therapy, all precipitating factors (medications, dyes, food) should be eliminated. Elimination diets avoiding chocolate, azo dyes, cheeses, shellfish, nuts, eggs, milk, tomatoes, and fresh berries can be tried. Urticaria is treated symptomatically. Acute urticaria with angioedema is treated with subcutaneous epinephrine. Less severe urticaria is treated with oral H_1-receptor antihistamines, such as diphenhydramine, hydroxyzine, cyproheptadine, and cetirizine. These medications can cause severe drowsiness and sleepiness; patients should be advised about these potentially dangerous side effects. Nonsedating H_1-receptor antihistamines include fexofenadine and loratadine and are slightly less effective but can be used in the morning and during the day. A tricyclic antidepressant such as doxepin can be used in patients resistant to therapy. H_2-receptor antihistamines such as cimetidine are also useful. Prophylaxis of hereditary angioedema can be achieved with antifibrinolytic agents (E-aminocaproic acid) and androgens (danazol).

Erythema Multiforme

Patients with erythema multiforme present with macules, papules, and vesicles. The characteristic lesion has the central "target" discoloration or necrosis (Fig. 78-9). The lesions are symmetric and frequently involve the palms of the hands. Erythema multiforme is usually asymptomatic but can be painful and pruritic.

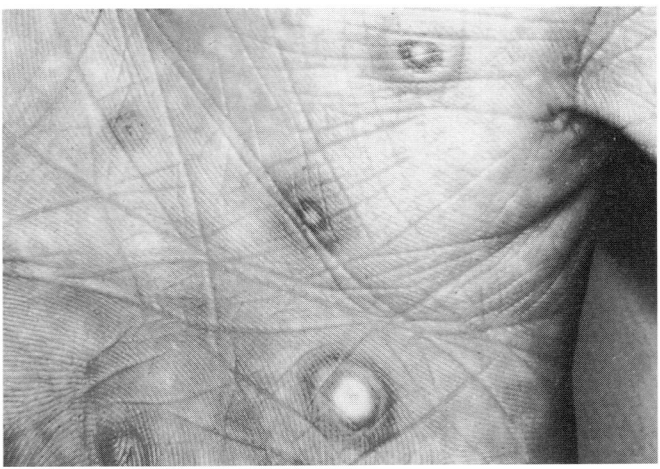

FIG. 78-9 Targetlike lesions are seen in erythema multiforme.

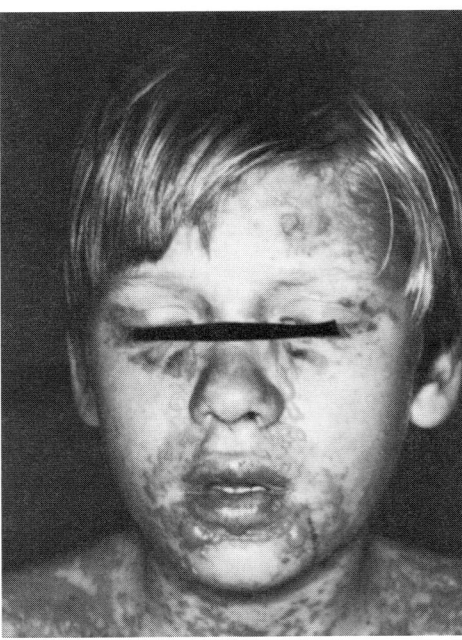

FIG. 78-10 Erosions of the lips and conjunctiva associated with fever in this boy with Stevens-Johnson syndrome.

When the mucous membranes of the lips, mouth, genitalia, and conjunctiva are involved, erythema multiforme is called *Stevens-Johnson syndrome* (Fig. 78-10). These patients are toxic and febrile. Corneal scarring can result. Maculopapular lesions can become confluent, forming large areas of bullae and necrosis. This condition is called *toxic epidermal necrolysis;* death occurs in about 50% of these patients. Complications of erythema multiforme include postinflammatory hyperpigmentation, keratitis with visual impairment, and pneumonia. The causes of erythema multiform include drugs (sulfa, penicillin, barbiturates, diphenylhydantoin) and infections (herpes simplex, *Mycoplasma*). However, in more than 50% of patients, the cause is idiopathic. Severe erythema multiforme, or Stevens-Johnson syndrome, is treated with systemic corticosteroids.

Erythema Nodosum

Patients with erythema nodosum present with painful, erythematous nodules usually localized to the anterior aspect of the lower legs. This condition is more common in women than in men. Fever, arthritis, and arthralgia accompany the eruptions. Specific causes can be determined in only about 20% to 30% of patients. These causes include streptococcal infections, sarcoidosis, drug ingestion, and inflammatory bowel disease. Resolution of the disease occurs in 3 to 6 weeks. Chest radiography, complete blood count, throat culture, and antistreptolysin O titer are obtained to elucidate underlying causes of erythema nodosum. Patients are usually treated with bedrest and aspirin and occasionally with oral corticosteroids.

Cutaneous Vasculitis

In cutaneous vasculitis, persistent palpable urticarial lesions, hemorrhagic macules, papules, ulcers, and purpura are observed (see color plate 53). The lesions are usually found over the distal extremities. Cutaneous vasculitis can be associated with systemic vasculitis of the kidney, gastrointestinal tract, and other organs. Therefore a patient may have fever, arthralgia, gastrointestinal bleeding, or hematuria. The causes of vasculitis include drugs, infections (particularly streptococcal), collagen vascular diseases (rheumatoid arthritis, systemic lupus erythematosus), and hepatitis type B virus. In most patients, the cause is idiopathic. Patients with clinical lesions of cutaneous vasculitis require skin biopsy to confirm this diagnosis. The biopsy reveals infiltrates of polymorphonuclear leukocytes, which are associated with necrosis of the blood vessel walls. Once the diagnosis is established, patients are evaluated for systemic involvement through urinalysis, creatinine clearance, and tests for the presence of cryoglobulins, antinuclear factor, rheumatoid factor, and hepatitis B antigen. Therapy is based on the severity of cutaneous involvement and on systemic involvement. Systemic corticosteroids usually help in resolution of the process. Cyclophosphamide and colchicine may also be used.

KEY CONCEPTS

- *Eczema* encompasses all types of red, blistering, weeping, scaly, thickened, itchy skin lesions.
- *Acute eczema* presents with vesicles, bullae, erythema, weeping, and crusting, whereas *chronic eczema* has thickened, scaly, pruritic patches and plaques. Examples of eczema include atopic eczema or atopic dermatitis and infantile atopic eczema.
- *Atopic eczema*, or *atopic dermatitis*, is a hereditary chronic skin disease that can appear at any age. The cause of this condition is unknown.
- *Infantile atopic eczema* frequently presents with weeping, eroded, erythematous patches in the diaper area and on the cheeks and scalp.
- Therapy of atopic eczema focuses on hydration, prevention, and treatment. All possible exacerbating factors must be avoided or eliminated.
- *Allergic contact eczema* is common and occurs in localized areas where an allergen comes into contact with the skin. The skin reaction to the oil of poison ivy, Rhus dermatitis, is best known.
- Therapy of allergic contact eczema necessitates the removal of offending allergens.
- *Hand eczema* most often occurs in persons who must wash their hands frequently or wear gloves in their occupation. Small vesicles appear on the lateral aspects of fingers, toes, and feet and pruritus accompanies the appearance of vesicles.
- *Neurodermatitis* is caused by compulsive scratching of pruritic skin and can be localized to the neck, scrotum, or anywhere on the body.
- Generalized neurodermatitis frequently occurs during the cold, dry winter months in older patients who have dry, pruritic skin.
- Treatment of neurodermatitis consists of lubrication and application of topical corticosteroids to the skin.
- *Seborrheic dermatitis* typically involves the scalp, eyebrows, nasolabial folds, ears, and anterior chest. The cause is unknown, but genetic factors seem to play an important part. Recently, *Pityrosporum ovale* has been implicated as playing a role in the pathogenesis of seborrheic dermatitis.
- *Stasis eczema* is localized to the areas of venous stasis and edema on the lower legs. Crusted, scaly, weeping erythematous patches appear. Therapy requires removal of edema fluid and improvement of circulation.
- *Urticaria (hives)* is the most common cutaneous reaction in which edema and erythema result. These transient skin eruptions appear as lightly erythematous wheals and papules with vasodilation of dermal and subcutaneous blood vessels accompanied by edema of surrounding tissue.
- *Chronic urticaria* is idiopathic in 75% to 90% of all patients but may be caused by food preservatives, collagen vascular diseases, medications, or infections. In therapy, all precipitating factors (medications, dyes, food) should be eliminated.
- Patients with *erythema multiforme* present with macules, papules, and vesicles. The characteristic lesion has the central "target" discoloration or necrosis.
- *Severe erythema multiforme*, or *Stevens-Johnson syndrome*, is treated with systemic corticosteroids.
- Patients with *erythema nodosum* present with painful, erythematous nodules usually localized to the anterior aspect of the lower legs.
- In *cutaneous vasculitis*, persistent palpable urticarial lesions, hemorrhagic macules, papules, ulcers, and purpura are observed. Therapy is based on the severity of cutaneous involvement and on systemic involvement.

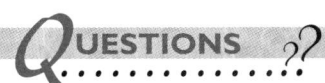
QUESTIONS ??

A sampling of review questions for this chapter appears here. Visit http://www.mosby.com/MERLIN/PriceWilson/ for additional questions.

Answer the following on a separate sheet of paper.
1. Describe the characteristic lesions of acute and chronic eczema.
2. List five of the causes of allergic contact eczema.
3. What are the most frequent causes and treatments of hand eczema?
4. List the drugs most often used in the treatment of acute urticaria.

Psoriasis and Pityriasis Rosea

MAREK A. STAWISKI

𝒟isorders of the skin characterized by the presence of plaques, patches, and scales are called *papulosquamous diseases*. These disorders include psoriasis and pityriasis rosea.

PSORIASIS

Psoriasis is reported in 2 to 5 million Americans and appears as thick, erythematous plaques and papules covered by a silvery white scale. The plaques are usually located over the knees, elbows, and scalp (Fig. 79-1; see color plate 54). However, the skin eruptions can affect any part of the body, with the exception of the mucous membranes. The nails frequently appear thickened, with yellowish discoloration, multiple pits, and separation from the nail bed. Arthritis can also accompany this skin disease and classically involves the distal interphalangeal joints. In these patients, the rheumatoid factor is not present. Arthritis does not always correlate with severity of the psoriasis. Psoriasis is usually not pruritic.

Psoriasis is a chronic disease that can occur at any age. Fluctuations mark the natural course of this condition. For example, sunlight, relaxation, and the summer season are usually beneficial to psoriasis patients. An upper respiratory tract infection can trigger an acute exacerbation of psoriasis, as evidenced by eruptions of multiple small papules over the trunk (Fig. 79-2). Medications (lithium, beta blockers, corticosteroids, antimalarials) and sunburn can also exacerbate psoriasis. Generalized psoriasis, as characterized by multiple pustules with inflammatory plaques, is called *pustular psoriasis*. Chills,

high temperature, and electrolyte imbalances can accompany this condition. Pustular psoriasis is a medical emergency that can be fatal and frequently requires hospitalization.

Psoriasis is an inherited disease, although the mode of inheritance is not well understood. A family history of psoriasis is found in 66% of psoriasis patients. Histocompatibility human leukocyte antigens HLA-B13, HLA-B17, and HLA-Cw6 are increased fourfold in those with psoriasis. Environmental factors also play a significant role in the disease. Trauma to the skin can produce new lesions of psoriasis, especially in the area where the skin is punctured, scraped, or cut.

Histopathologic examination of a psoriatic skin biopsy reveals thickened epidermis and stratum corneum and dilated upper dermal blood vessels. The number of basal cells undergoing mitosis is markedly increased. These fast-dividing cells move rapidly to the surface of the thickened epidermis. This rapid proliferation and migration of epidermal cells result in thick epidermis covered by a thick keratin (silvery scale). Abnormal levels of cyclic nucleotides, especially cyclic adenosine monophosphate (cAMP) and cyclic guanosine monophosphate (cGMP), may be partially responsible for this rapid mitosis rate of epidermal cells. Prostaglandins and polyamines are also abnormal in the disease. The exact role of these abnormalities in influencing the formation of a psoriatic plaque is not clearly understood. Numerous neutrophils are attracted to the epidermis. Promoters of this neutrophil chemotaxis (complements, peptides, leukotrienes) may be abnormal in psoriasis. Epidermal proteinases that activate complement and attract neutrophils are also elevated. T lymphocytes are also important in the pathogenesis of psoriasis. The efficacy of cyclosporin in treatment of psoriasis and infiltration of psoriatic plaques with activated T cells seem to support the autoimmune cause of the disease.

Treatment

Therapy of chronic psoriasis requires knowledge of various treatment modalities, patience, and an experienced physician or nurse practitioner. Localized disease is treated with

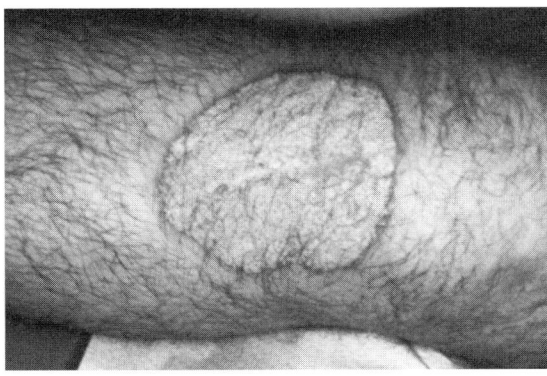

FIG. 79-1   Thick psoriatic plaques with a white silvery scale as seen in the psoriatic patient.

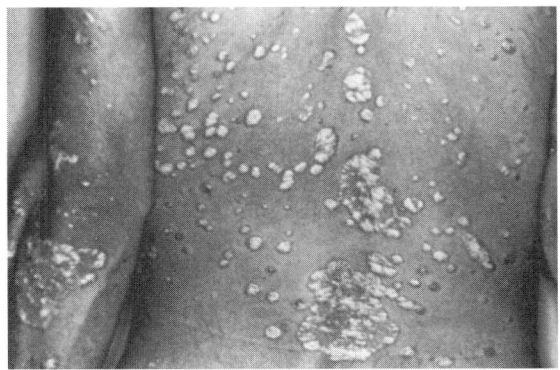

FIG. 79-2   Multiple small psoriatic papules can erupt after an upper respiratory infection. This form of psoriasis is termed *guttate psoriasis*.

topical corticosteroids over the face and intertriginous areas; in children, weak steroids such as 1.5% hydrocortisone are used. Other weak steroids are alclometasone (Aclovate) and desonide (DesOwen). Over the trunk, extremities, and scalp, intermediate-strength steroids such as triamcinolone (Aristocort), mometasone (Elocon), betamethasone valerate (Valisone), and fluticasone (Cultivate) are recommended. The strong steroids—fluocinonide (Lidex), halcinonide (Halog), clobetasol (Temovate), halobetasol (Ultravate), and betamethasone dipropionate (Diprolene)—are reserved for localized, resistant plaques. Stronger topical steroids are more effective than intermediate-strength steroids but can cause irreversible skin atrophy and suppression of the hypothalamic-pituitary adrenal axis. Treatment with strong topical steroids beyond 2 weeks is not recommended, and the total dose should not exceed 50 gm of cream per week.

A tar preparation of cream or shampoo is frequently used. A bath oil with tar (Balnetar) is also helpful. All these medications result in decreased cell proliferation, which makes the epidermis thinner and causes the plaques and scales of psoriasis to disappear. A new vitamin-D derivative, 1,25-dihydroxy vitamin D_3 (Dovonex) ointment, can be used with great efficacy in about 30% of patients who have plaque psoriasis. Frequently, Dovonex is used 3 to 4 times a week in combination with stronger topical steroids, which are applied 3 to 4 times per week. A derivative of retinoid (Tazorac) is used as a topical gel for thick localized plaques of psoriasis. The medication can cause local irritation and should not be used in women who can become pregnant during the therapy.

Severe generalized psoriasis requires hospitalization for intensive topical steroid, tar, and ultraviolet light therapy. Unfortunately, relapses of psoriasis often occur 3 to 6 months after hospitalization. Severe psoriasis can now be managed on an outpatient basis by the treatment that combines the use of psoralen, an oral photosensitizing medication, with psoralens with long ultraviolet light (PUVA). Long ultraviolet light (UVA) is not effective unless it is used in combination with psoralen. This treatment is not indicated in patients with a previous history of x-ray irradiation, skin cancer, or cataracts. This therapy can result in squamous cell carcinoma, especially over the scrotum. Shorter ultraviolet light (UVB) is used successfully in the treatment of severe psoriasis. A modification of the UVB light allows the physician to treat the patient with the extremely narrow band of UVB, which is more effective than conventional UVB light. An oral antineoplastic medication, methotrexate, may be useful in treating patients with severe plaque-type psoriasis, pustular psoriasis, or debilitating arthritis. However, this oral agent may cause irreversible cirrhosis of the liver or bone marrow suppression. Chronic therapy with methotrexate requires frequent monitoring of liver enzymes, white blood cell counts, and red blood cell counts. Liver biopsy is usually obtained when a cumulative dose of methotrexate reaches 1 gm.

A new treatment modality for psoriasis is oral etretinate (Tegison). This new oral aromatic retinoid is excellent for treatment of pustular and erythrodermic psoriasis and is useful for recalcitrant plaque psoriasis. The drug should not be given to women who are of childbearing age because it is a powerful teratogen. Oral etretinate also elevates liver enzymes, cholesterol, and triglyceride levels. Side effects include dryness of skin and mucous membranes, hair loss, headaches, diarrhea, myalgia, and arthralgias. If used for longer than 12 months, radiographic studies of the bones should be obtained to check for calcium deposits in the joints.

Oral acitretin (Soriatane) is a retinoid indicated for the treatment of severe psoriasis, including the erythrodermic and pustular types. Women who are pregnant or who intend to get pregnant for at least 3 years following discontinuation of therapy should not use oral acitretin. Side effects and the necessity to monitor liver enzymes and cholesterol are identical to oral etretinate.

PITYRIASIS ROSEA

In contrast to psoriasis, pityriasis rosea is an acute, self-limited eruption seen in young adults and adolescents. Pityriasis rosea begins with an oval, scaly lesion called the "herald patch." Within a week, multiple, pale-red, oval patches with a fine scale around the periphery appear over the neck, trunk, and proximal extremities (Figs. 79-3 and 79-4; see color plate 55). Obtaining an adequate

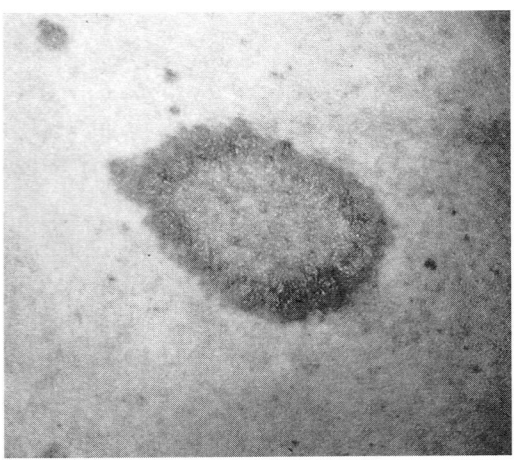

FIG. 79-3 Oval-shaped, scaly lesion of pityriasis rosea; a so-called "herald patch" with typical peripheral scale.

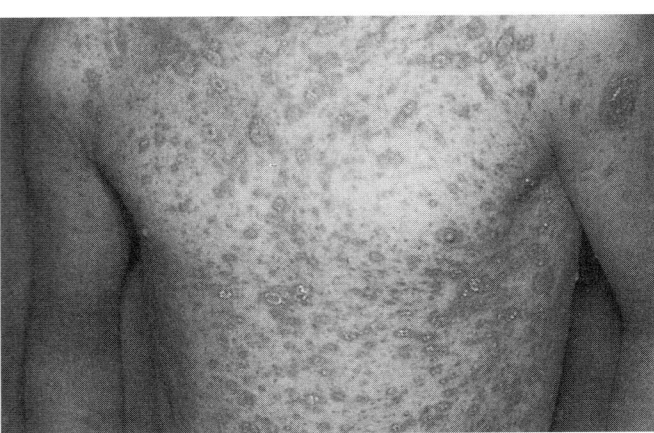

FIG. 79-4 Oval-shaped papules and patches in pityriasis rosea showing the dermatome-type pattern. (From Cohen BA: *Atlas of pediatric dermatology*, London, 1993, Wolfe.)

history is necessary to rule out drug eruptions and viral exanthems. Syphilis can mimic pityriasis rosea thus serology is required (see Chapter 66). Pruritus is usually not severe and may not occur at all. Lesions of pityriasis rosea usually do not occur on the face, palms, and soles, in contrast to secondary syphilis. The cutaneous eruptions, which can be accompanied by malaise and fever, persist for 4 to 8 weeks and rarely recur. The cause of this common disease is unknown; however, viral agents have been suspected. If present, pruritus is treated with antihistaminics. Exposure to sunlight usually results in faster disappearance of the lesions.

KEY CONCEPTS

- *Papulosquamous diseases* are disorders of the skin characterized by the presence of plaques, patches, and scales. These diseases include psoriasis and pityriasis rosea.
- Psoriasis is a chronic disease that can occur at any age and is reported in 2 to 5 million Americans.
- Psoriasis is an inherited disease, although the mode of inheritance is not well understood.
- *Psoriasis* appears as thick, erythematous plaques and papules covered by a silvery white scale. The plaques are usually located over the knees, elbows, and scalp.
- Histopathologic examination of a psoriatic skin biopsy reveals thickened epidermis and stratum corneum and dilated upper dermal blood vessels.
- The number of basal cells undergoing mitosis is markedly increased. These fast-dividing cells move rapidly to the surface of the thickened epidermis. This rapid proliferation and migration of epidermal cells result in thick epidermis covered by a thick keratin (silvery scale).
- Therapy of chronic psoriasis requires knowledge of various treatment modalities, patience, and an experienced physician or nurse practitioner. The treatment must be flexible, and alternative therapy must be administered if the patient fails to respond to the original program of treatment.
- Localized disease is treated with topical corticosteroids over the face and intertriginous areas; in children, weak steroids are used. A tar preparation of cream or shampoo is frequently used.
- Severe generalized psoriasis requires hospitalization for intensive topical steroid, tar, and ultraviolet light therapy.
- *Pityriasis rosea* is an acute, self-limited eruption seen in young adults and adolescents. Pityriasis rosea begins with an oval, scaly lesion called the "herald patch."

QUESTIONS ??

A sampling of review questions for this chapter appears here. Visit http://www.mosby.com/MERLIN/PriceWilson/ for additional questions.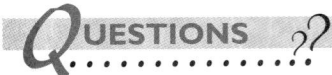

Answer the following on a separate sheet of paper.

1. What is the new oral treatment modality for psoriasis? What are contraindications for its use?

2. What is the latest topical treatment modality for psoriasis?

3. Describe the histopathologic examination of a psoriatic skin biopsy and the clinical appearance and distribution of psoriasis.

Cutaneous Infections

MAREK A. STAWISKI AND SYLVIA A. PRICE

WARTS

Verrucae vulgaris, or *warts,* are caused by the human papillomavirus (HPV). The virus replicates in the epidermal cells and is transmitted from person to person. Warts also disseminate to the patient's self by autoinoculation. The virus is contagious to specific individuals who lack the virus-specific immunity in the skin. The immunity to warts is not well understood. Verrucae appear as rough, warty nodules over the trunk, legs, hands, arms, feet, genitalia, and even mucous membranes of the mouth (Fig. 80-1). Flat warts are more prevalent on the face than on the rest of the body. Plantar warts grow into the thick stratum corneum of the foot and have small black dots within, which represent infarcted capillaries. In the genitalia and the mucous membranes of the vagina, rectum, and urethra, the verrucae are called *condylomata acuminata.* These warts appear as verrucous, moist nodules that may occur in large numbers (Fig. 80-2; see color plates 44 and 45). Condyloma acuminata has been associated with cervical squamous cell cancer in women and premalignant bowenoid papulosis in men. Eighty-five percent of cervical squamous cell cancers are associated with HPV types 16 and 18. The warts usually resolve sponta-

neously within 2 years when immunity against the virus develops. However, the development of this immune response can be delayed for many years.

Verrucae are usually removed by cryosurgery or curettage combined with electrodesiccation. Large numbers of verrucae that occur in children are removed with preparations of salicylic acid (Occlusal-HP) or Duofilm. Salicylic acid preparations are preferred in treatment of plantar warts (Sal-Acid Plaster). A podophyllin derivative (Condylox) is usually applied to condylomata acuminata. An immune response modifier (Aldara) can be effective in the treatment of extreme genital and perianal warts. Treatment of warts is often difficult, prolonged, and frustrating and can be painful. Recalcitrant warts of the feet, groin, and periungual areas are frequently treated with a carbon dioxide laser. If genital warts are present, sexual partners should be examined and treated. Abstinence or condoms should be used until the warts are eradicated from both partners. Perianal warts in children can be signs of sexual abuse.

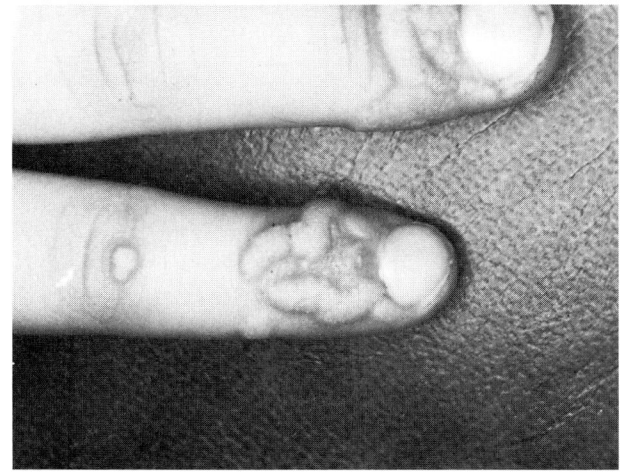

FIG. 80-1   Rough nodules of verrucae vulgaris (warts) over the fingers.

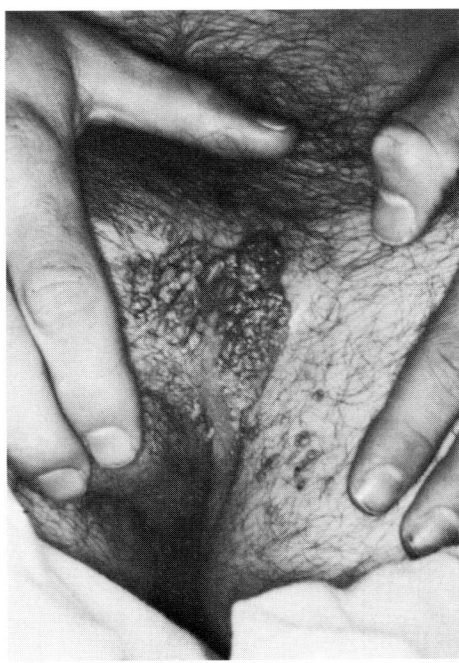

FIG. 80-2 Moist verrucous nodules of condyloma acuminatum in the groin area.

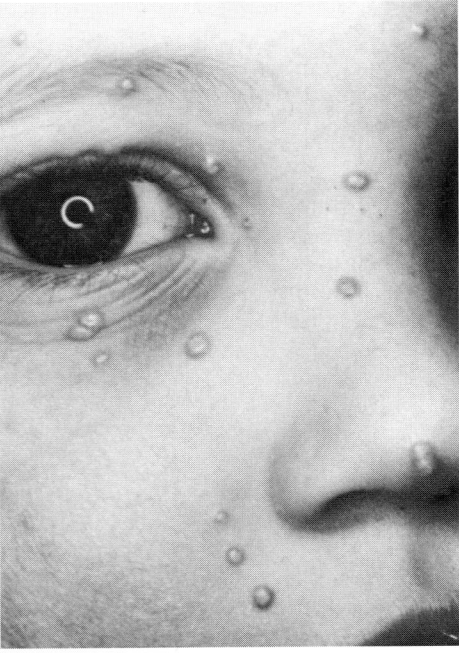

FIG. 80-3 Smooth, umbilicated, dome-shaped nodules of molluscum contagiosum over the face of a child.

MOLLUSCUM CONTAGIOSUM

Molluscum contagiosum is a dome-shaped, smooth, umbilicated nodule (Fig. 80-3) that is caused by a deoxyribonucleic acid (DNA) virus of the pox family. Molluscum contagiosum is transmitted from person to person. The virus is contagious to people who lack immunity to this specific virus. Most often, the lesions occur in children, frequently on the head and trunk. In young adults, the nodules usually appear in the groin area. The preferred modes of treatment are cantharidin solution in children and gentle curettage or liquid nitrogen cryosurgery in adults. In both adults and children, spontaneous resolution occurs in about 2 years. Widespread molluscum lesions in children are usually followed without therapy. The lesions disappear spontaneously without leaving any scarring.

HERPES SIMPLEX

Herpes simplex infection is caused by a DNA virus. An infectious DNA particle enters the nucleus of the cell and uses the reproductive machinery of the cell for its own replication. It is estimated that more than 25 million persons have or have had the infection today. Herpes labialis of the lip is even more common. There are two types of herpes: type I and type II. *Type I* usually affects the lips, mouth, nose, and cheeks. This form of herpes is acquired from close contact with an infected family member or friend in a nonsexual manner. The infection is transmitted by kissing, touching, and the use of common towels. *Type II* herpes simplex virus usually infects the genital areas and frequently follows a sexual encounter, but not necessarily. It is estimated that as many as 20% of sexually active persons in the United States have or have had herpes type II.

Multiple, grouped, painful vesicles appear after primary exposure of the patient to the virus. Primary infections occur anywhere on a person's skin, although they usually occur around the mouth and nose, causing gingivostomatitis; around the eyes, causing conjunctivitis; the fingers, causing herpetic whitlow; and the buttocks and genitals, causing vulvovaginitis. Primary infections cause intense skin edema, extensive vesiculation, and exquisite pain (Fig. 80-4). Nurses frequently develop extremely painful edematous vesicles on their fingers. This herpetic whitlow follows exposure to a patient with herpetic infection. This primary infection lasts for as long as 6 weeks, and the nurse should not have contact with surgical, debilitated, or immunosuppressed patients during this time. During the primary infection, the virus ascends via peripheral nerves to dorsal root ganglia, where it is present in the dormant stage. Some patients are subject to recurrent activations of the latent virus. Most patients do not experience recurrent infections. Recurrent infections are usually less painful than primary infections and are frequently localized to the lips and genitals. Recurrences can be triggered by fever, sunlight, or trauma. Grouped vesicles (Fig. 80-5) become pustules within a few days and usually resolve spontaneously within 2 weeks.

Herpes progenitalis has been the most prominent sexually transmitted disease in the United States during the last 10 years. Recurrent herpes progenitalis causes painful vesicles and ulcers. The recurrent herpetic infection can follow primary infection within weeks, months, or years. Because the initial herpetic infection can be mild, a patient may not realize that she or he has had the primary infection. Years later, when a recurrent infection appears, mistaken accusations of infidelity by a partner can arise.

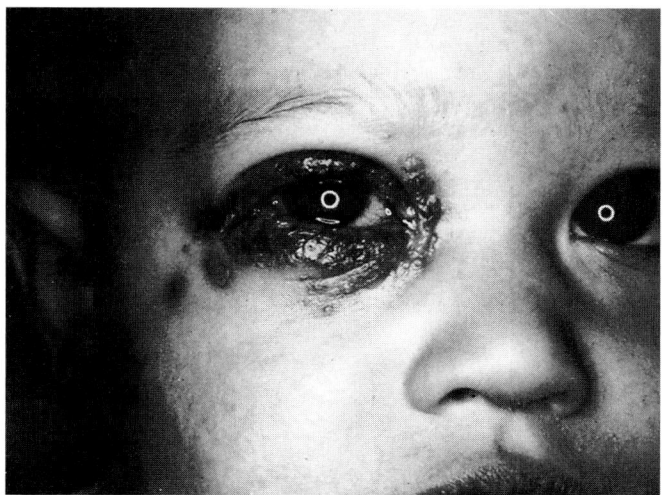

FIG. 80-4 Multiple vesicles, edema, and erythema in a primary herpetic infection causing conjunctivitis.

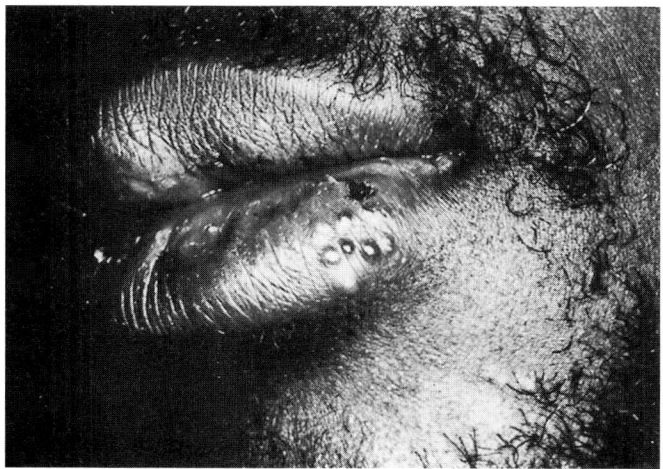

FIG. 80-5 Grouped, localized, painful vesicles of recurrent herpes simplex of the lips.

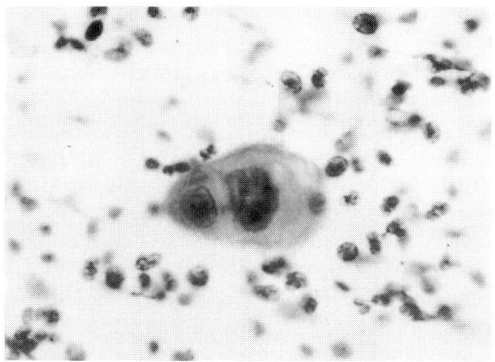

FIG. 80-6 Giant cells seen in vesicles of a patient with herpes simplex. The cells are surrounded by neutrophils. Slide is stained with 1% toluidine blue.

In humans, only 14% of patients with type I herpes acquire recurrent herpes, whereas 60% of herpes type II infections become recurrent. Type II virus causes 98% of recurrent genital herpes. Many factors affect recurrence; it can be triggered by fever, emotional stress, fatigue, ovulation, and physical trauma.

Herpes infection has serious implications if the infection occurs in the eye, around the cervix, in newborns, or in immunosuppressed individuals. The herpes infection of the eye may lead to herpetic keratitis. Scarring of the cornea, and even corneal perforation, can result. A pregnant woman with active genital herpes at the time of delivery can transmit the virus to the baby as it passes through the birth canal. Severe encephalitis in a newborn can result in death or mental retardation. Cesarean section is indicated in women who have genital herpes at the time of delivery. Similarly, if the mother or a person working in the nursery has active vesicles of herpes on the lips or the hands, the baby can become infected. Infection with herpes type I can result in the same severe condition as can type II herpes infection. Herpes infection in seriously ill or immunosuppressed patients can result in chronic, nonhealing ulcers (see color plate 56), dissemination, and encephalitis.

The diagnosis of herpes is usually made on the basis of history and clinical appearance. The diagnosis can be confirmed by a herpetic culture, which is positive in about 80% of the patients with herpes. The *Tzanck test* is positive in 50% to 80% of patients with herpes. In this test, the material from the vesicle is placed on a glass slide and stained with 1% toluidine blue. Large multinucleated giant cells can be seen in smears taken from a patient with herpes simplex (Fig. 80-6). The Tzanck test takes only a few minutes to perform and is much less expensive than a herpes culture, but it is less accurate.

No adequate treatment exists for cutaneous herpes infections. No vaccine has been developed to prevent these infections from recurring. Using opaque sunscreens or avoiding excessive sun exposure can sometimes prevent recurrent episodes of herpes of the lips. Sexual spread of genital herpes is frequently avoided by use of rubber condoms when vesicles are present and for 7 days afterward. Sexual abstinence when vesicles are present is an alternative method of prevention. Furthermore, towels, underclothing, and swimming suits should not be shared. Acyclovir is the treatment of choice in herpes simplex infections. This drug, administered in tablets or intravenous fluids, is effective in treating cutaneous herpes infections. The drug is an inhibitor of herpes simplex virus DNA synthesis. Acyclovir ointment does not prevent recurrence or shorten the duration of the herpetic eruption in otherwise healthy individuals. Usually, patients with primary herpes are treated symptomatically, using soaks, topical antibiotics, pain medication, and oral acyclovir, 200 mg five times a day for 5 to 10 days. Recurrent herpetic infections are treated with acyclovir, 200 mg orally five times a day for 5 days. Acyclovir, 400 mg orally three times a day, helps suppress frequent attacks of recurrent herpes simplex. Long-term suppression up to 1 year appears safe and free of side effects. Oral valacyclovir (Valtrex) is the salt of L-Valyl ester of acyclovir, which is converted to acyclovir as it passes through intestines and is readily absorbed from the gastrointestinal tract. Valtrex is indicated for treatment of primary herpes (1 g twice daily for 10 days) and recurrent herpes (500 mg twice a day for 5 days). Suppressive therapy of recurrent herpes (500 mg daily) appears to be safe for at least 1 year of therapy. Oral Famvir, which contains famciclovir, is also effective against herpes virus. The drug is used for recurrent herpes simplex (125 mg twice daily for 5 days) and suppression of recurrent herpes simplex (250 mg twice daily) for up to 1 year.

CHICKENPOX (VARICELLA) AND HERPES ZOSTER

The virus that causes varicella is a DNA virus. When the disease is active, it is highly contagious. The incubation period is 14 to 21 days. The infection usually occurs in school-age children but occasionally affects young adults. Varicella is characterized by malaise and fever, followed by the eruption of multiple small erythematous macules, papules, and vesicles.

The vesicles become purulent and crusted and heal spontaneously, usually within 1 week. Characteristically, multiple stages of the lesions are present. The lesions initially appear on the trunk and face and spread peripherally to the extremities. Adults can develop varicella pneumonitis or encephalitis. In immunosuppressed children, complications from varicella infection include pneumonitis and encephalitis, both of which can be fatal. Acyclovir, 800 mg five times daily for 7 days, helps shorten the severity and duration of the infection.

The same herpes virus that causes varicella, or chickenpox, also causes herpes zoster. After the primary varicella infection, the virus apparently persists in the dorsal root ganglia. Herpes zoster, or *shingles*, usually occurs in older individuals. The dormant varicella virus is activated, and inflammatory vesicles appear unilaterally along a single dermatome. The adjacent skin is edematous and hemorrhagic (Fig. 80-7; see color plate 57). This condition is usually preceded or accompanied by intense pain or burning or both. Even though any nerve can be involved, the thoracic, lumbar, and cranial nerves are most often affected. Herpes zoster persists for about 3 weeks. The pain that may follow an attack of herpes zoster is referred to as *postherpetic neuralgia* and frequently may persist for several months or, rarely, many years. Postherpetic neuralgia is more common in older individuals than in the younger population. Dissemination of herpes zoster to the entire body surface, lungs, and brain can be fatal. This dissemination is usually seen in patients with lymphoma or leukemia. Thus any patient who develops disseminated herpes zoster should be evaluated for a possible underlying malignancy.

Treatment of localized herpes zoster is symptomatic with soaks and pain medication. If the ophthalmic branch of the trigeminal nerve is affected, an ophthalmologist should also be consulted because corneal perforations may result from the infection. Early administration of systemic corticosteroids may be helpful in the prevention of postherpetic neuralgia. Oral acyclovir, 800 mg five times daily for 10 days, can shorten the duration of herpes zoster infection. This drug decreases pain, reduces new lesion formation, and shortens time of healing. Oral famciclovir (Famvir) at the dosages of 500 mg three times daily for 7 days and valacyclovir (Valtrex) at

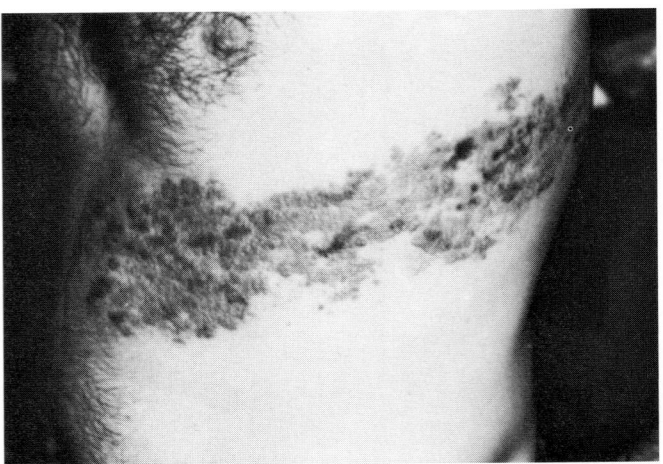

FIG. 80-7 Inflammatory vesicles appear along a single dermatome on edematous and hemorrhagic skin of herpes zoster.

1 g three times a day for 7 days can shorten the duration of herpes zoster infection.

Persistent postherpetic neuralgia can be treated with topical capsaicin (Zostrix) but usually requires stronger analgesics (Tylenol #3, Vicodin). Amitriptyline and tricyclic antidepressants can also be useful, but patients with severe pain are usually referred to pain clinics.

VIRAL EXANTHEMS

Rubeola, or measles, is caused by a ribonucleic acid (RNA) myxovirus. About 2 weeks after exposure, the patient develops fever, cough, headache, and conjunctivitis. The exanthem appears on the face, trunk, and proximal extremities and consists of brightly erythematous, confluent macules. Over the buccal mucosa or the upper palate, mottled bright spots called *Koplik's spots* appear. Pneumonia and otitis media are present in many patients. Atypical measles occurs in individuals immunized with a killed-virus vaccine. Atypical measles usually presents without the Koplik's spots. In this type of measles, a polymorphous rash appears on the distal extremities, and the incidence of pneumonia is very high. Typical measles eruptions last 5 to 10 days. Treatment of this infection is symptomatic. Administration of the rubeola vaccine has substantially decreased the incidence of the disease.

Rubella, or German measles, is also caused by an RNA myxovirus. The disease occurs 2 to 3 weeks after exposure and is associated with malaise and a mild fever. Pale red macules appear over the face and within a day spread to the trunk. The exanthem fades within a few days. Painful postauricular and suboccipital enlarged lymph nodes are usually present. The diagnosis is confirmed by rising antibody titers of rubella-specific immunoglobulin M (IgM) molecules. If the infection occurs in the first trimester of pregnancy, congenital defects (cataracts, mental retardation, heart defects, deafness) are common. Therapy is symptomatic; vaccination of school-age children and women of childbearing age with low rubella titers is advisable.

Erythema infectiosum, also called *fifth disease*, is a viral disease usually seen in children and is caused by a

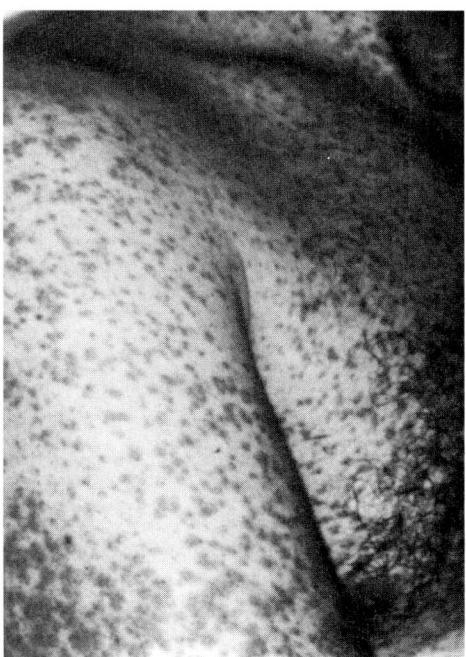

FIG. 80-8   Confluent, bright, erythematous macules after administration of ampicillin to a patient with infectious mononucleosis.

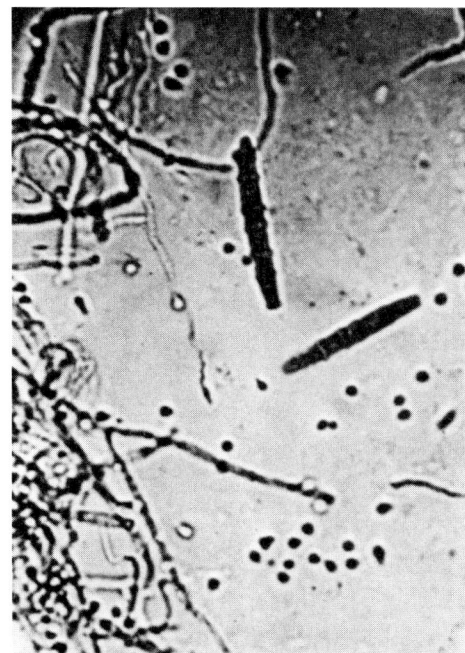

FIG. 80-9   Multiple hyphae and spores can be seen on microscopic examination of skin scrapings from a patient with superficial fungal infection of the skin.

parvovirus. Pale, reticulated macules appear over the cheeks and extremities, sometimes accompanied by a low-grade fever, malaise, and pruritus of skin eruptions. The infection persists for 1 to 2 weeks, and no treatment is necessary.

Infectious mononucleosis is caused by the Epstein-Barr virus. The infection presents with malaise, fever, exudative pharyngitis, postauricular adenopathy, and hepatosplenomegaly. The cutaneous eruptions occur over the trunk as erythematous macules and papulovesicles. Patients with mononucleosis who receive ampicillin invariably develop erythematous, confluent, hemorrhagic macules, and therefore this therapy is contraindicated (Fig. 80-8).

An interesting infection caused by coxsackievirus A16 or enterovirus 71 is *hand-foot-and-mouth disease.* Multiple oval-shaped vesicles surrounded by erythema appear on the palms, fingers, soles, and mucous membranes of the mouth. The infection can be associated with low-grade fever, sore mouth and throat, and malaise. The infection resolves in 7 days. Only symptomatic therapy with oral acetaminophen-diphenhydramine elixir and topical lidocaine (Xylocaine Viscous) is given to patients.

FUNGAL SKIN INFECTIONS

Superficial fungal infections can involve the skin, hair, and nails. Fungal infections of the scalp and the skin are known as *ringworm infections.*

Most fungal infections in humans are caused by three genera of fungi: *Microsporum, Trichophyton,* and *Epidermophyton.* The fungi are transmitted from human to human (anthropophilic), from animal to human (zoophilic), or from soil to human (geophilic). A suspected fungal infection can be confirmed by microscopic examination of

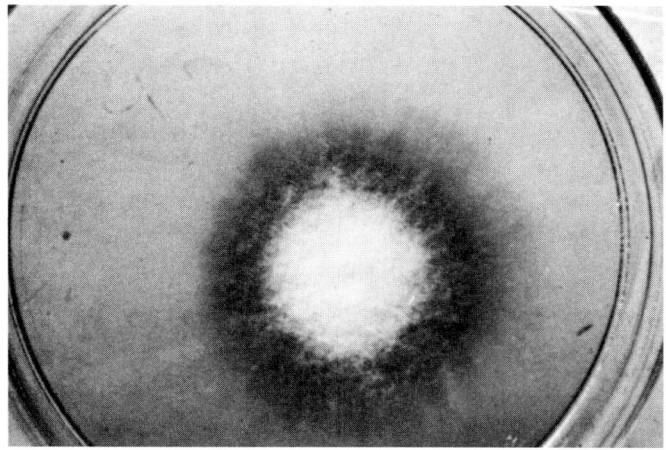

FIG. 80-10   *Trichophyton rubrum,* the most common cause of superficial fungal skin infection, as seen on fungal culture grown at room temperature.

skin scrapings in a solution of potassium hydroxide (Fig. 80-9). Multiple hyphae can be found on microscopic examination of the skin scrapings of a patient with a fungus infection.

A fungal culture is done to identify the fungus responsible for the infection, to confirm a diagnosis, and to suggest a mode of transmission (Fig. 80-10).

Tinea capitis, or fungal infection of the scalp, is usually caused by *Trichophyton tonsurans* or *Microsporum canis. T. tonsurans* is transmitted by child-to-child contact and results in oval patches of hair loss. Individual hairs are broken at various lengths, and the scalp surface is scaly and crusted with discrete papules (Fig. 80-11). *M. canis* is usually transmitted from young kittens to children and

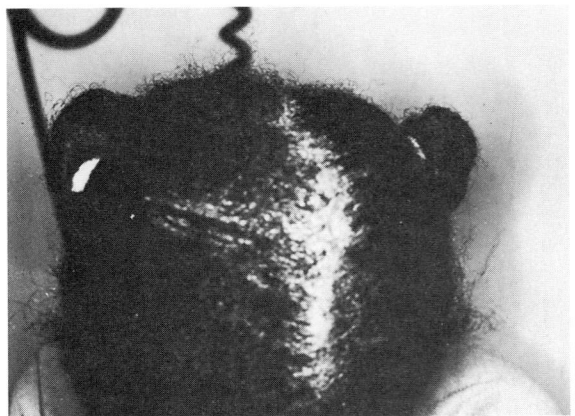

FIG. 80-11 Scaly patches of hair loss in a young child with tinea capitis.

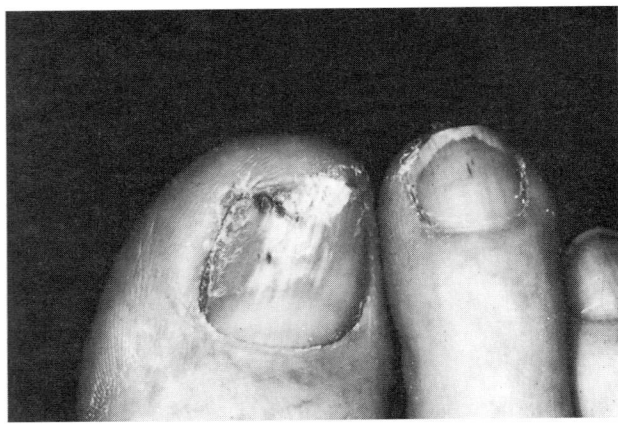

FIG. 80-13 Subungual hyperkeratosis and discoloration of the nail plate seen in onychomycosis.

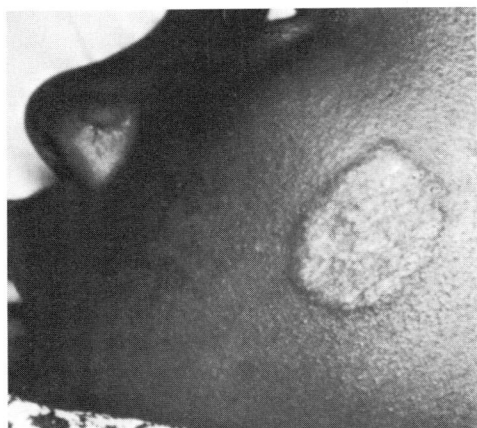

FIG. 80-12 Tinea corporis of the face, with peripheral scale and ringlike shape.

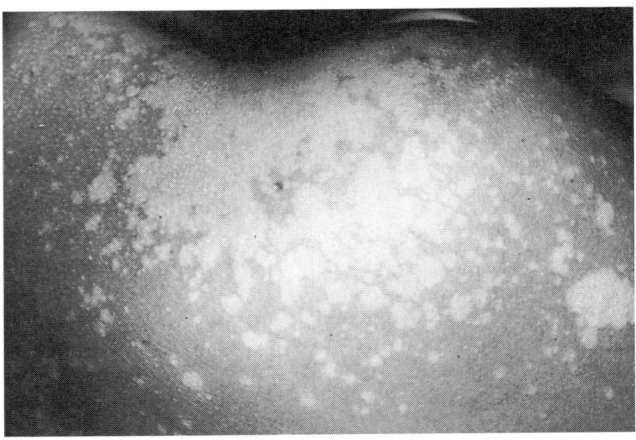

FIG. 80-14 Sharply marginated, scaly, hypopigmented patches of tinea versicolor are usually seen over the back.

causes inflammatory, purulent patches of hair loss. The patch is frequently crusted with multiple pustules and can result in permanent alopecia. Every patch of hair loss associated with scaly, crusted scalp should be suspected for a possible fungal infection. Inflammatory lesions can form large, tender, boggy masses called *kerions*. To confirm the diagnosis of *tinea capitis* infection, hairs are plucked, examined under a microscope after potassium hydroxide treatment, and cultured.

Tinea corporis is a fungal infection of the skin over the face, trunk, and extremities. Frequently, a peripheral scale associated with erythema and pustules appears with a ringlike shape (Fig. 80-12). This infection can be contracted from animals with *M. canis* or *Trichophyton mentagrophytes* and from humans with *Trichophyton rubrum*. The diagnosis is confirmed by potassium hydroxide examination and fungal culture.

Tinea cruris is a fungal infection of the groin. The infection occurs more frequently in males than in females and is associated with severe pruritus and annular or arclike lesions with peripheral erythema and scale that frequently extends to the thighs. The scrotum is usually not involved. A common term for this infection is jock itch (see color plate 58).

Tinea pedis and *tinea manuum*, fungal infections of the feet and hands, are probably the most common fungal

infections. *T. rubrum* causes scaly, erythematous patches on the soles and palms. Both feet and only one hand are frequently involved. *T. mentagrophytes* causes inflammatory, crusty, pustular eruptions on the feet. *Tinea pedis*, *manuum*, and *cruris* are confirmed by microscopic examination of potassium hydroxide–treated skin scrapings and fungal cultures.

Tinea barbae presents with scaly, crusted patches associated with pustules over the beard area. Large, verrucous nodules can appear, resembling kerion infection of the scalp. The infection usually results from exposure to cattle and is caused by *T. mentagrophytes*.

Fungal infection of the nails, *onychomycosis*, presents with dystrophic nails. The patient has subungual hyperkeratosis and separation of the nail plate from the nail bed (Fig. 80-13). The diagnosis is confirmed by fungal cultures and potassium hydroxide examination. This common fungal infection is extremely resistant to therapy and frequently recurs when treatment is discontinued.

Tinea versicolor is caused by *Pityrosporum orbiculare*. Sharply marginated, scaly, white or brownish patches appear over the trunk, neck, and extremities (Fig. 80-14; see color plate 59). The infection is more apparent in the summer than in other times of the year. Microscopic examination of potassium hydroxide–treated scales confirms the diagnosis. Multiple short hyphae and spores are present.

Treatment

The usual treatment of *tinea pedis, tinea cruris,* and *tinea corporis* is with topical antifungal agents, which include econazole (Spectazole), clotrimazole (Mycelex), ciclopirox olamine (Loprox), terbinaphine (Lamisil), oxiconazole (Oxistat), haloprogin (Halotex), and ketoconazole (Nizoral). These agents are used twice daily, generally for 1 month. Patients are also instructed in proper foot hygiene and told to wear loose-fitting cotton underwear and nonocclusive shoes. For prevention of infections, the useful agents available include undecylenic acid (Desenex) and tolnaftate (Tinactin).

Resistant infections of the feet and pruritic infections of the groin can also be treated with oral griseofulvin, an effective antifungal agent. Oral griseofulvin is also used for infections of the scalp. The treatment is continued until the organisms are eradicated. *Tinea capitis* infection usually requires 4 to 6 weeks of 250 to 500 mg of griseofulvin daily; *tinea corporis,* 2 to 4 weeks; *tinea pedis,* 4 to 8 weeks. It is important to note that this drug is phototoxic and interferes with the activity of medications such as warfarin and barbiturates. Bone marrow and liver toxicity occur extremely infrequently in patients who have no preexisting liver disease. The most common side effects from griseofulvin are headaches and gastrointestinal symptoms.

Severe infections of the nails are treated with oral terbinafine (Lamisil), 250 mg daily for 2 to 3 months. Liver enzyme abnormalities have been reported and must be monitored 6 weeks after initiation of therapy. Oral itraconazole (Sporanox) is used for treatment of onychomycosis at the dose of 200 mg twice daily for 1 week (so-called pulse therapy). Usually, two to three of these pulses are separated by a 3-week period without medication. Because itraconazole is an inhibitor of the cytochrome P450, it can interfere with metabolism of interferon, terfenadine, and benzodiazepines, among others. Neither Sporanox nor Lamisil have been approved by the U.S. Food and Drug Administration for treatment of fungal infections of hair or skin.

Tinea versicolor is treated with selenium sulfide (Selsun shampoo) or ketoconazole (Nizoral shampoo), which is applied twice weekly to the affected areas for at least 60 minutes. Pigmentary changes secondary to tinea versicolor may persist for several months. Localized patches of tinea versicolor can be treated with topical Loprox, Mycelex, or Nizoral creams.

CANDIDIASIS

Candidiasis, a type of yeast infection, is caused by *Candida albicans.* The organism is normally present in the gastrointestinal tract, but it can cause an opportunistic infection (see Chapters 5, 6 and 15). Persons who are obese, have diabetes mellitus, or are taking broad-spectrum antibiotics (tetracycline) or corticosteroids can develop the cutaneous infection. In the groin and intertriginous areas, candidiasis presents with erythema, whitish pseudomembrane, and peripheral papules and pustules (Fig. 80-15; see color plates 57 and 60). The infection frequently occurs in infants and obese patients. *Candida* infection of the paronychial area causes swelling, erythema, and pus formation. *Candida* of the mouth, or

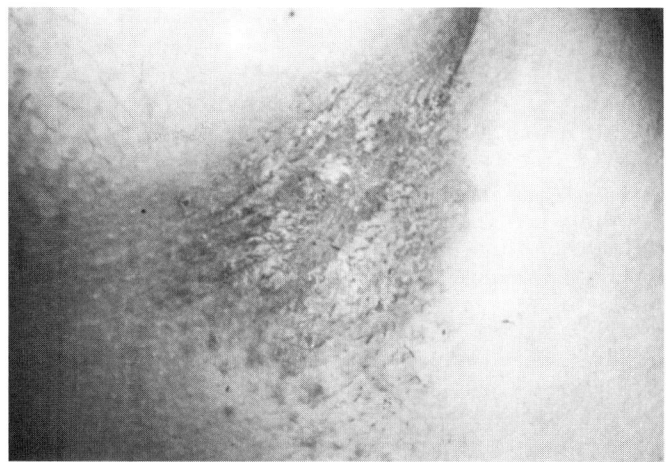

FIG. 80-15 Plaque of candidiasis in the axilla with a whitish pseudomembrane and peripheral papules.

thrush, presents with a white coating of the tongue and occasional macerated, fissured patches in the corner of the mouth. Disseminated candidiasis can be a life-threatening infection in immunocompromised patients with leukemia, cancer, or acquired immunodeficiency syndrome (AIDS). This systemic candidiasis can cause candidal meningitis, endocarditis, or septicemia. Diagnosis of *Candida* infection is confirmed by a microscopic examination of a potassium hydroxide–treated skin scraping and culture.

Treatment consists of removing predisposing factors. Cutaneous *Candida* infections are treated with oral or topical nystatin, topical miconazole, topical clotrimazole, or amphotericin cream. These medications are also used for vaginal candidiasis. Fluconazole (Diflucan) 150 mg in a single dose is a convenient way to treat vaginal infections. Systemic infection is treated by intravenous amphotericin B. An oral medication, ketoconazole (Nizoral), is also effective in treatment of systemic candidiasis.

CUTANEOUS BACTERIAL INFECTIONS

Impetigo is the most common bacterial infection of the skin and is caused by streptococci and staphylococci. The infection is frequently transferred by human-to-human contact, usually among children. Hot, humid temperatures and poor hygiene predispose the individuals to this infection. Cuts, insect bites, and abrasions are sometimes complicated by impetigo. Patients with eczema occasionally develop impetigo secondary to excoriations of pruritic skin lesions. Impetigo begins as a purulent vesicle. As the lesion spreads, it becomes eroded and a golden crust develops on the surface (Fig. 80-16; see color plate 61). The infection usually starts on the face and extremities but can spread to any surface of the body. In less than 1% of cases, poststreptococcal glomerulonephritis can develop.

Treatment should include instructions in proper hygienic techniques to control spread of the infection. Topical antibiotics (polymyxin, neomycin, bacitracin) and antiseptics (Betadine) are used. Mupirocin (Bactroban) ointment used topically three times a day is the most effective topical agent for impetigo now available. Oral penicillin or erythromycin therapy is indicated when large or multiple lesions are present. This approach can prevent the incidence of poststreptococcal glomerular nephritis, especially in children. Impetigo usually heals without scar formation.

Cellulitis is a streptococcal infection that presents with spreading areas of erythema, fever, and lymphangitis. Oral penicillin is the treatment of choice.

Erysipelas is a serious, toxic, streptococcal infection of the skin. The lesions are brightly erythematous, sharply marginated, and tender. Bullae are hemorrhaged and may be seen within the inflamed skin (see color plate 62). The lesions frequently occur over the face or extremities. The patient has high fever and malaise and is toxic. Regional lymph nodes are enlarged. Complications such as endocarditis and septicemia may result. Patients with erysipelas are usually hospitalized and treated with intravenous penicillin. Occasionally, prolonged treatment is required to eradicate the infection. Repeated episodes of erysipelas may produce lymphedema and predispose the individual to further infections.

Erythrasma causes erythematous, dry, scaly patches in the intertriginous areas and is caused by *Corynebacterium*

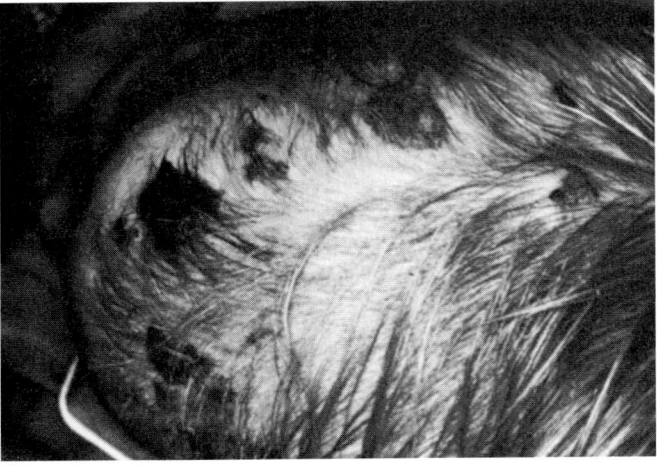

FIG. 80-16 Crusted, eroded patches of impetigo on the scalp.

minutissimum. The infection is most often seen in obese individuals and can be confirmed by a characteristic coral-red fluorescence under a Wood's light examination. Erythrasma is usually treated with topical antibiotics (clindamycin), but systemic erythromycin is also effective.

Trichomycosis axillaris is an infection of the axillary hair and, rarely, the pubic hair. Yellow, red, or black concretions form on the hair (Fig. 80-17). The infection is asymptomatic and not contagious. Patients report an abnormal coloring of sweat and possibly an axillary odor. *Corynebacterium* species isolated from these infections can be treated by topical applications of antibiotics (e.g., erythromycin) or by shaving the hair from the affected areas.

Superficial folliculitis, caused by staphylococci, presents with small pustules surrounded by erythema found at the opening of hair follicles. The scalp and extremities are the usual sites. Poor hygiene practices, maceration, and excoriations are the predisposing factors of this infection. Treatment is with antibacterial soaps (e.g., pHisoHex) and, occasionally, systemic antibiotics. *Recurrent chronic folliculitis* can be difficult to eradicate and may require systemic antibiotics after specimens for appropriate bacterial cultures and sensitivity studies are obtained.

Hot tub folliculitis is seen in patients exposed to inadequately disinfected whirlpools and hot tubs. These eruptions are usually localized to bathing trunk areas and are caused by *Pseudomonas aeruginosa.* Ciprofloxacin (Cipro) is effective treatment of this infection. Deep staphylococcal infections are responsible for furuncles (boils) and carbuncles (multiple confluent furuncles). Deep-seated, erythematous, tender nodules frequently occur over the buttocks, neck, and axillae. The nodules become fluctuant in a few days and discharge a purulent, necrotic material. Furuncles can be painful when located in the nasal area, axillae, or ears. Furuncles are treated with surgical draining; hot, wet dressings; and appropriate systemic antibiotics. The antibiotics are selected after aerobic and anaerobic cultures and sensitivity studies are performed.

Infection of the nail fold with staphylococci and streptococci can lead to a painful infection called *paronychia.* The infection can follow a hangnail and is common among individuals whose hands are frequently immersed in water. The nail folds are erythematous, swollen, and painful in this infection (Fig. 80-18). Be-

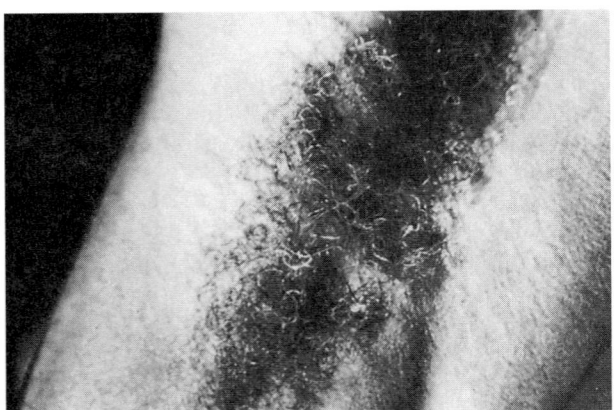

FIG. 80-17 Trichomycosis axillaris with yellow concretions on the hair.

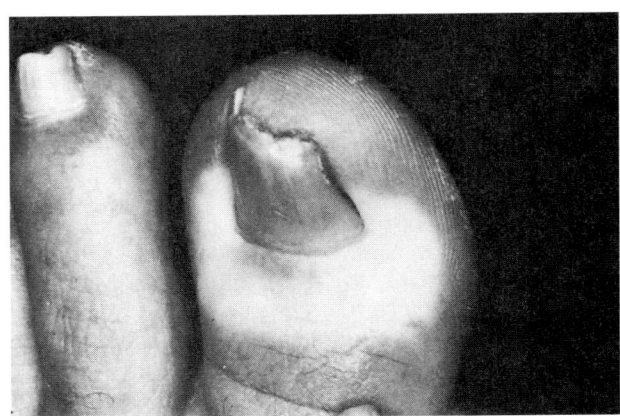

FIG. 80-18 Swollen, painful toe secondary to bacterial paronychia. The whitish area contains purulent material.

cause paronychia can also be caused by *Candida*, fungal cultures are required to confirm the disease. Acute bacterial paronychia is treated with systemic antibiotics, and localized pus is drained. Chronic paronychia is treated by avoidance of prolonged exposure to water. Broad-spectrum topical antibacterial and antifungal solutions such as clotrimazole (Mycelex) or mupirocin (Bactroban) can be used.

KEY CONCEPTS

- *Verrucae vulgaris*, or *warts*, are caused by human papillomavirus (HPV). The virus replicates in the epidermal cells and is transmitted from person to person.
- *Plantar warts* grow into the thick stratum corneum of the foot and have small black dots within, which represent infarcted capillaries.
- *Verrucae* are usually removed by cryosurgery or curettage combined with electrodesiccation.
- *Molluscum contagiosum* is a dome-shaped, smooth, umbilicated nodule.
- A DNA virus causes *herpes simplex infection*. Two types of herpes are type I and type II. Type I usually affects the lips, mouth, nose, and cheeks. Type II herpes simplex virus usually infects the genital areas.
- *Herpes progenitalis* has been the most prominent sexually transmitted disease in the United States during the last 10 years.
- No adequate treatment exists for cutaneous herpes infections. Acyclovir is the treatment of choice in herpes simplex infections.
- The virus that causes *chickenpox (varicella)* is a DNA virus. No adequate treatment exists for cutaneous herpes infections.
- When the chickenpox (varicella) disease is active, it is highly contagious.
- *Varicella* is characterized by malaise and fever, followed by the eruption of multiple small erythematous macules, papules, and vesicles.
- *Herpes zoster* is caused by the same herpes virus as varicella, or chickenpox. After the primary varicella infection, the virus apparently persists in the dorsal root ganglia.
- Herpes zoster, or shingles, usually occurs in older individuals. The dormant varicella virus is activated, and inflammatory vesicles appear unilaterally along a single dermatome.
- Treatment of localized herpes zoster is symptomatic with soaks and pain medication. Oral acyclovir, can shorten the duration of herpes zoster infection.
- *Rubeola*, or *measles*, is caused by an RNA myxovirus. Rubella, or German measles, is also caused by an RNA myxovirus.
- *Erythema infectiosum*, also called fifth disease, is a viral disease usually seen in children that is caused by a parvovirus.
- *Infectious mononucleosis* is caused by the Epstein-Barr virus. The infection presents with malaise, fever, exudative pharyngitis, postauricular adenopathy, and hepatosplenomegaly.
- Fungal infections of the scalp and the skin are known as *ringworm infections*.
- *Tinea capitis*, or fungal infection of the scalp, is usually caused by *Trichophyton tonsurans* or *Microsporum canis*.
- *T. tonsurans* is transmitted by child-to-child contact and results in oval patches of hair loss.
- *M. canis* is usually transmitted from young kittens to children and causes inflammatory, purulent patches of hair loss.
- *Tinea corporis* is a fungal infection of the skin over the face, trunk, and extremities. Frequently a peripheral scale associated with erythema and pustules appears with a ringlike shape.
- *Tinea cruris* is a fungal infection of the groin.
- *Tinea pedis* and *tinea manuum*, fungal infections of the feet and hands, are probably the most common fungal infections.
- *Tinea barbae* presents with scaly, crusted patches associated with pustules over the beard area.
- Fungal infection of the nails, *onychomycosis*, presents with dystrophic nails. The patient has subungual hyperkeratosis and separation of the nail plate from the nail bed.
- *Tinea versicolor* is caused by *Pityrosporum orbiculare*. Sharply marginated, scaly, white or brownish patches appear over the trunk, neck, and extremities.
- The usual treatment of *tinea pedis, tinea cruris*, and *tinea corporis* is with topical antifungal agents.
- *Candidiasis*, a type of yeast infection, is caused by *Candida albicans*. Treatment consists of removing predisposing factors.
- *Impetigo*, which is the most common bacterial infection of the skin, is caused by streptococci and staphylococci. Treatment should include instructions in proper hygienic techniques to control spread of the infection.
- *Cellulitis* is a streptococcal infection that presents with spreading areas of erythema, fever, and lymphangitis. Oral penicillin is the treatment of choice.
- *Erysipelas* is a serious, toxic, streptococcal infection of the skin.
- *Erythrasma* causes erythematous, dry, scaly patches in the intertriginous areas.
- *Trichomycosis axillaris* is an infection of the axillary hair and rarely the pubic hair.
- *Superficial folliculitis*, caused by staphylococci, presents with small pustules surrounded by erythema found at the opening of hair follicles.
- *Hot tub folliculitis* is seen in patients exposed to inadequately disinfected whirlpools and hot tubs.

A sampling of review questions for this chapter appears here. Visit http://www.mosby.com/MERLIN/PriceWilson/ for additional questions.

Answer the following on a separate sheet of paper.

1. Describe the two tests used to attempt to confirm the diagnosis of herpes simplex.

2. What are the therapeutic measures that can be used in an attempt to prevent recurrent infections of cutaneous herpes infections?

3. Describe the serious complications associated with herpes simplex infection of the eye.

4. Describe the lesion characteristic of impetigo.

5. Contrast impetigo and erysipelas as to etiologic agent and pathogenesis.

6. State the predisposing factors associated with superficial folliculitis.

7. Describe the treatment for herpes zoster.

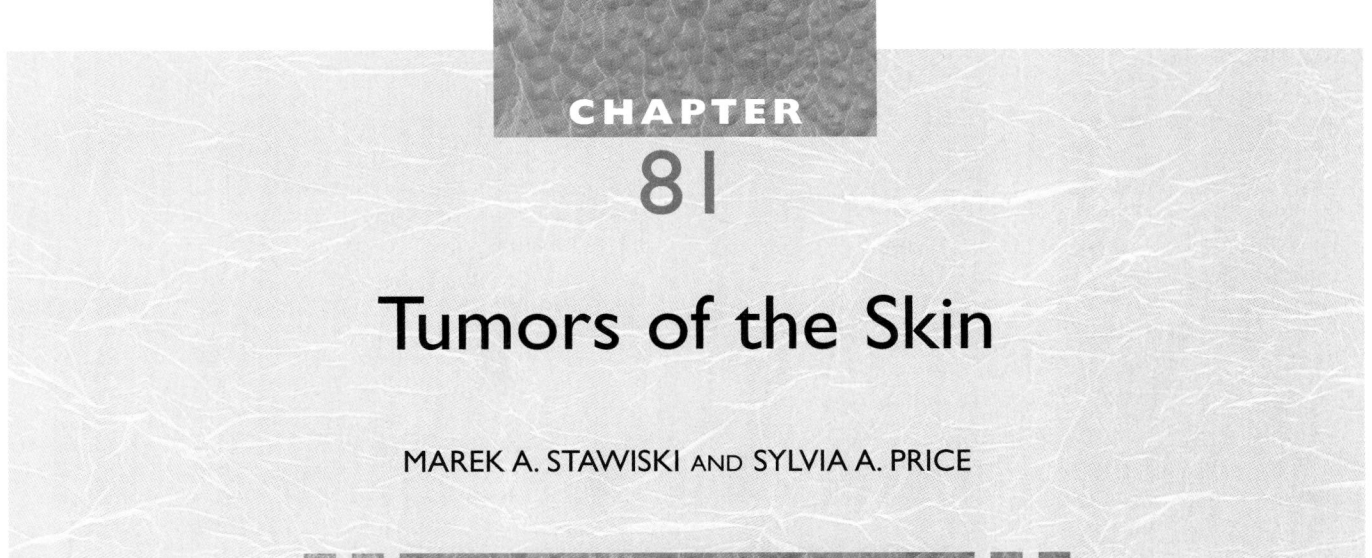

Tumors of the Skin

MAREK A. STAWISKI AND SYLVIA A. PRICE

𝒞utaneous tumors can derive from various cell types in the skin, such as epidermal cells and melanocytes. These tumors can be benign or malignant and either localized in the epidermis or invasive to the dermis and subcutaneous tissue.

MALIGNANT SKIN TUMORS

Basal Cell Carcinoma

Basal cell carcinoma is the most common malignant tumor of the skin. Approximately 500,000 new cases are diagnosed in the United States each year. Basal cell carcinoma arises from epidermal cells along the basal layer of the epidermis. The incidence of basal cell carcinoma is directly proportional to the age of the patient and inversely proportional to the amount of melanin pigment in the epidermis. A direct correlation also exists between this condition and the total lifetime exposure to sunlight. About 80% of basal cell cancers occur on the sunlight-exposed areas of the face, head, and neck. Fortunately, the tumor rarely metastasizes. However, a patient with a single basal cell cancer is likely to develop future skin cancers and must be followed indefinitely on an annual basis.

The carcinogenic range in the solar spectrum lies primarily between 280 and 320 nm. This spectrum is primarily responsible for burning of the skin exposed to the sunlight. Sunscreens, sun blocks, and avoidance of excessive sunlight exposure are recommended for patients with a family history of skin cancer and for fair-skinned individuals who have a tendency to sunburn easily. Also, patients with a history of basal cell carcinoma should use sunscreens or protective clothing to avoid the sun's carcinogenic rays. Most sunscreens contain *para-aminobenzoic acid (PABA)*, which absorbs the carcinogenic rays. PABA was the first chemical sunscreen but has potential to cause allergic reactions. PABA esters (padimate cinnamates [Parsol mcx]) are the most commonly used sunscreens that block ultraviolet light B (UVB). Benzophenone (Parsol 1789) mainly blocks longer wavelength light (ultraviolet A [UVA]).

Other causes of basal cell carcinoma include previous radiologic therapy of other skin disorders, contact with arsenic, and rare genetic disorders (xeroderma pigmentosum, nevoid basal cell carcinoma syndrome). The long ultraviolet light (UVA) in suntanning booths also damages the epidermis and is considered to be carcinogenic.

The tumor is characterized by an erythematous, smooth, pearly nodule (Fig. 81-1). The borders are frequently elevated and have telangiectatic vessels on the surface. Central ulceration and bleeding are frequently observed (Fig. 81-2; see color plate 63). The tumor bleeds frequently, invades the dermis, and destroys normal tissue.

Basal cell carcinoma should be treated promptly. Treatments include curettage with electrodesiccation, scalpel surgery, irradiation, chemosurgery, and cryosurgery. A small basal cell cancer less than 2 cm in diameter is usually treated with scalpel excision or electrodessication and curettage after biopsy is obtained to confirm the diagnosis. The cure rate is about 95%. Roentgen therapy may be used in patients over age 60 to 70 years who have very large tumors around the eyelids, earlobes, or lips. Mohs' chemosurgery is useful in the treatment of large, infiltrating, and recurrent cancers, especially around the ears, nasolabial folds, and eyes. In chemosurgery, the mi-

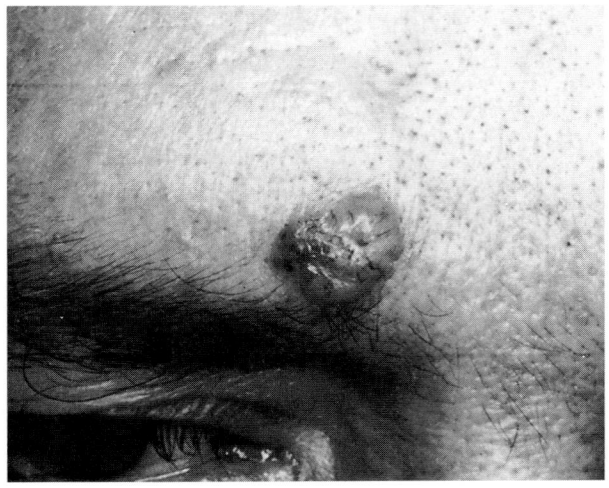

FIG. 81-1 A smooth, pearly nodule of early basal cell carcinoma.

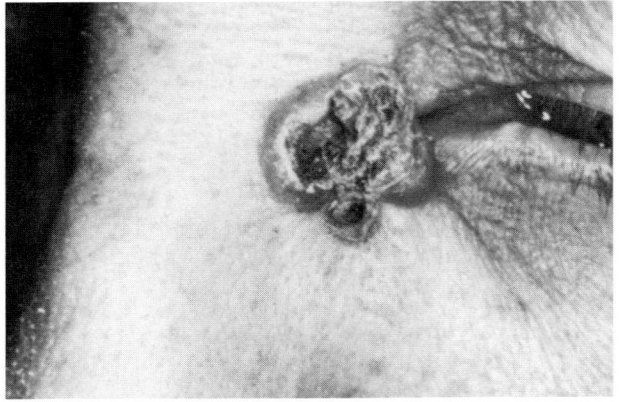

FIG. 81-2 Ulcerated tumor with elevated smooth borders in a patient with advanced basal cell carcinoma.

croscopic excision of the tumor is accomplished by removing layer by layer with a scalpel; frozen sections are prepared, and a map of the tumor is constructed; then the undersurface of each removed frozen section is examined for evidence of basal cell cancer. This technique is the most tedious, effective, and expensive, but it has a cure rate of more than 97%. Cryosurgery uses liquid nitrogen, and the cure rate is similar to that for electrodesiccation and curettage.

Squamous Cell Carcinoma

Squamous cell carcinoma is a malignant neoplasm of keratinocytes that arises from more differentiated cells of epidermis (keratinocytes). Frequently, the tumor is seen in older, fair-skinned individuals. Squamous cell carcinoma typically arises on sun-damaged skin with multiple actinic keratoses present. Sunlight is the main etiologic factor causing squamous cell carcinoma of the skin. As in basal cell carcinoma, sunlight in the ultraviolet (UV) light spectrum between 280 and 320 nm (UVB spectrum) is responsible. However, recent cooperative studies on

the use of long UV light, between 320 and 400 nm (UVA spectrum), combined with oral psoralen in treatment of psoriasis have demonstrated that prolonged, chronic exposure to UVA with psoralen can also produce squamous cell carcinoma.

Fair-skinned persons of Celtic origin who are chronically exposed to the sunlight (e.g., farmers, sailors) have a high incidence of squamous cell carcinomas. Both basal cell carcinomas and squamous cell carcinomas are much more common in sunbelt areas of the United States than in the Midwest or Northeast areas. The incidence of skin squamous cell carcinoma and basal cell carcinoma in African Americans is extremely low.

Other causes of squamous cell carcinoma include ingestion of arsenic, x-ray irradiation, burns, scars, and genetic susceptibility. Patients who were treated for acne or hemangiomas with radiologic therapy many years ago can develop basal cell cancers and squamous cell cancers. Individuals who were treated with arsenic for psoriasis or asthma 50 years ago, who ingested arsenic in their drinking water, or who inhaled it in smelting plants have a tendency to develop squamous cell carcinomas. A few rare genetic diseases (albinism, xeroderma pigmentosum) also predispose individuals to these cancers. Excessive use of suntanning booths will likely lead to an increased incidence of squamous cell carcinoma in future years.

Squamous cell carcinomas that arise in sunlight-damaged skin usually do not metastasize and rarely cause death. Squamous cell cancers arising on areas not exposed to the sun (lips, buttocks, groin), after ingestion of arsenic, or on an old scar have the greatest risk of metastasis. Squamous cell carcinoma that occurs on areas not exposed to sunlight can be a cutaneous marker of internal malignancy. Once squamous cell carcinoma is diagnosed, a thorough history and physical examination are required.

A variant of squamous cell carcinoma is localized to the epidermis and is called *Bowen's disease*. Bowen's disease is usually caused by chronic sunlight exposure; it can also be caused by ingestion of arsenic. Some sources believe that there is an increased incidence of internal malignancies with this tumor. Patients with Bowen's disease should undergo a workup, including a complete history and physical examination, if this cancer occurs on areas not exposed to sunlight.

Squamous cell carcinoma presents with an ulcerated, scaly, thickened nodule or tumor that bleeds occasionally (Fig. 81-3; see color plate 64). The nodules usually arise on sunlight-damaged skin of the face, scalp, ears, neck, hands, or forearms. Frequently these nodules are surrounded by multiple actinic keratoses, many of which, if untreated, may degenerate into squamous cell cancers. Bowen's disease presents as an erythematous plaque with undulating borders, scaliness, and frequently central erosion. Squamous cell carcinoma can be indistinguishable from eczema or psoriasis (Fig. 81-4; see color plate 65). A longstanding lesion of psoriasis or eczema unresponsive to appropriate therapy should therefore be biopsied.

The treatment of squamous cell carcinoma and its variant, Bowen's disease, is primarily surgical excision. Radiation therapy, cryosurgery, and chemosurgery have

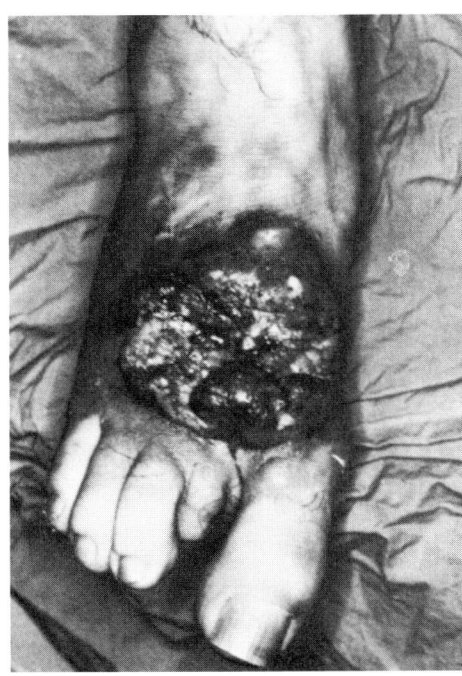

FIG. 81-3   Verrucous, ulcerated tumor of squamous cell carcinoma after radiographic therapy to the foot.

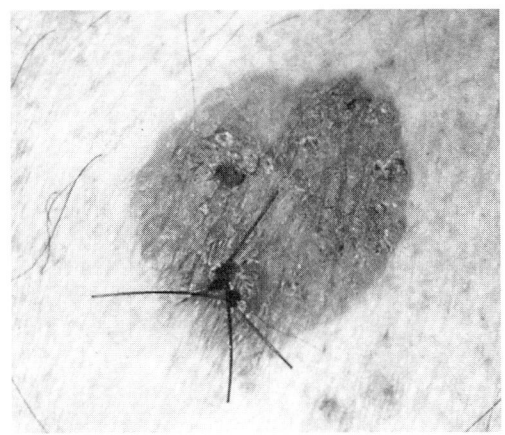

FIG. 81-4   Undulating borders and central erosion of a plaque in Bowen's disease.

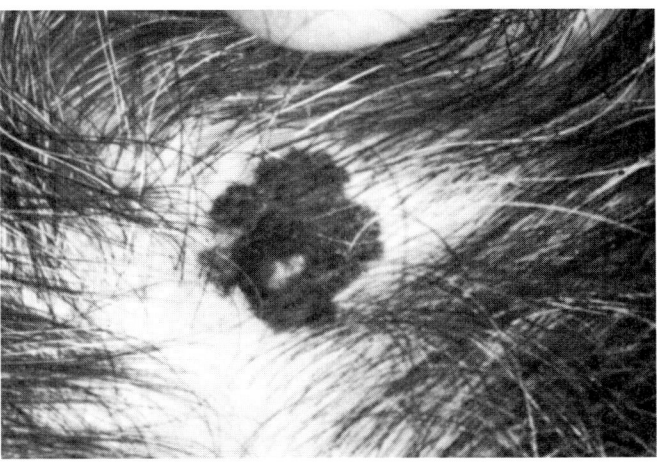

FIG. 81-5   Irregular borders, uneven pigmentation, and ulceration in a superficial, spreading malignant melanoma.

cure rates of 95% to 98%. The lymph nodes are not removed if they are clinically negative, but they should be carefully palpated during the surgical procedure. Metastatic lesions of squamous cell carcinoma do not respond well to chemotherapy. As with patients with basal cell carcinoma, those with squamous cell carcinomas must be monitored indefinitely, because there is a high risk for development of new squamous cell carcinomas. The lymph nodes are palpated during these follow-up visits. Of these patients, 20% to 50% with one squamous cell carcinoma eventually develop another squamous cell carcinoma or basal cell carcinoma.

Melanoma

Malignant melanoma makes up only 3% of all primary cutaneous malignancies but is responsible for almost all the deaths secondary to skin cancers. Furthermore, the incidence of melanoma is increasing. Early diagnosis and surgical treatment are the only ways to ensure long-term survival and even cure. Unless recognized and treated early, melanomas invade deeper layers of the dermis and the subcutaneous tissues and metastasize to distant sites. Most melanomas occur in the 40- to 70-year age group, but the number of cases has increased among the 20- to 40-year age group. One of the explanations for this increased incidence is a greater sunlight exposure secondary to recreation and attire changes. The number of severe sunburns is believed to be an important risk factor for developing cutaneous melanomas. Further evidence for the role of UV light in causing melanomas is the increased frequency of this tumor in sunbelt states. The mode of inheritance of melanomas is undetermined, and only a small percentage of melanoma patients have a family history of melanoma. However, an experienced dermatologist should examine all family members for atypical nevi. Atypical nevi in individuals with a family history of melanomas should be removed, because atypical nevi can degenerate to malignant melanomas. These persons have a 15% risk to develop a cutaneous melanoma. Large congenital nevi give rise to malignant melanomas in 2% to 13% of patients, and these melanomas should be surgically excised.

Diagnosis is based on the change in shape, color, size, and configuration of a pigmented lesion. Clinical manifestations of early melanoma can be remembered by four rules of appearance of this tumor: A, asymmetry of lesion; B, border irregularity; C, color variegation; and D, diameter greater than 6 mm.

Irregular pigmentation with shades of blue, purple, red, and brown should alert the examiner. The borders of this tumor are irregular, and the surface is frequently ulcerated (Fig. 81-5). The lesion is asymmetric and is frequently greater than 6 mm in diameter. Satellite lesions

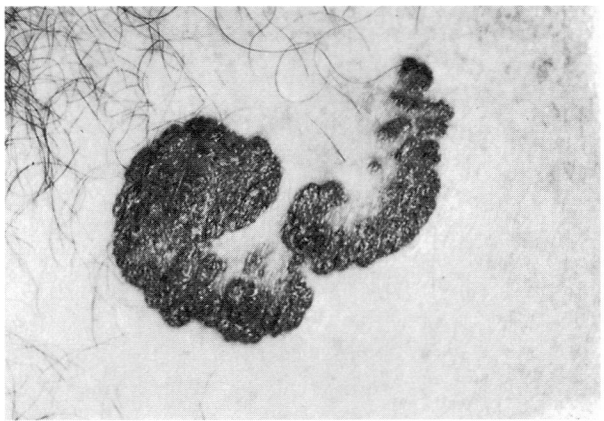

FIG. 81-6 Irregular borders in a superficial, spreading malignant melanoma.

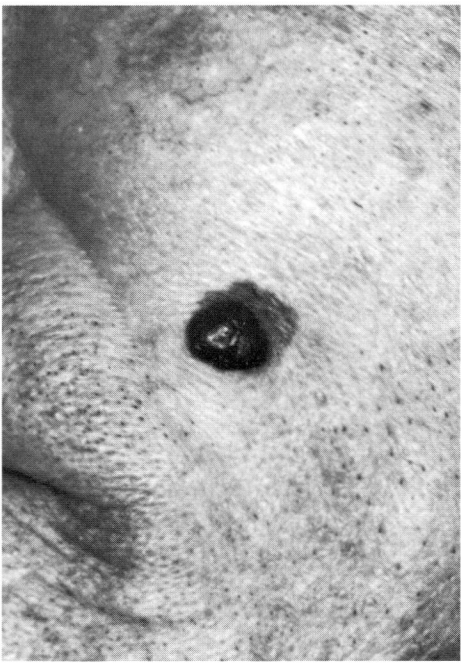

FIG. 81-7 Nodule with diffusion of pigment in nodular malignant melanoma.

and diffusion of pigment into the surrounding skin are also observed (Fig. 81-6; see color plate 66).

The superficial spreading melanoma is the most common type (60% to 80%) and has the best prognosis. This type of melanoma presents as a flat growth with bizarre colors and configuration (see Fig. 81-6). The nodular melanoma is less common (20%) and presents as a tumor (Fig. 81-7). This variant has the worst prognosis. The lentigo maligna melanoma arises on a preexisting, irregularly pigmented, brown patch (lentigo maligna) (see color plate 67). This tumor is even less common (5% to 10%) and, if detected early, has a good prognosis.

The prognosis for patients with malignant melanoma is not as poor as once thought. The great majority of pa-

tients survive for 5 years or more, and many are cured. Early diagnosis and surgical treatment are responsible for these improved statistics. Several factors determine the survival of melanoma patients. Patients with superficial spreading melanoma have the best prognosis, followed by lentigo maligna melanoma; nodular melanoma has the worst prognosis. Lesions located over the head, neck, trunk, hands, and feet in patients over age 50 and in males have a worse prognosis. Clinical ulceration of the tumor carries a poor prognosis. Histologic levels of primary malignant melanoma invasion of the dermis, as defined by Clark, determine the prognosis: the best survival rates are seen with levels I and II melanomas, confined to the epidermis and upper dermis; intermediate survival rates are seen with levels III and IV, extending to the lower dermis; and the worst rates are seen with level V, invading the subcutaneous tissue. Breslow was able to correlate vertical tumor thickness with prognosis of malignant melanomas; melanomas less than 1 mm in thickness do not usually metastasize if removed locally, melanomas between 1 and 2 mm in thickness can develop metastasis, and tumors greater than 2 mm are likely to metastasize.

The treatment of malignant melanoma is primarily surgical. Controversy exists over whether levels I, II, and III melanomas should be widely excised. Many authorities believe that a narrow excision with 1 to 2 cm margins is adequate. Levels IV and V melanomas should receive a wide excision and possible elective regional lymph node dissection, if feasible. Sentinel node biopsy is an alternative to regional lymph node dissection. The blue dye is used to identify the sentinel node, which is removed and examined microscopically. This procedure is usually performed when melanoma is 1 mm or greater in thickness. Patients with disseminated melanomas receive chemotherapy using dacarbazine (DTIC) with alpha-interferons or antimelanoma vaccination. Intensive melphalan or carmustine therapy combined with autologous bone marrow transplantation can sometimes result in remission. Immunotherapy using interleukin-2 to expand T cells with antitumor reactivity may induce response of the tumor. Unfortunately, disseminated melanoma has a 1-year mortality as high as 83%. The most effective treatments of melanoma remain early detection and aggressive surgical removal.

BENIGN SKIN TUMORS

Acquired nevi, or *moles*, are the most common tumors derived from the melanocyte. The melanin pigment produces a uniform brown, dark-brown, light-brown, or blue color in flat or elevated nevi (Fig. 81-8; see color plate 68). Flat nevi do not infiltrate the dermis and can occur anywhere on the body. Nevi are rarely excised unless they become irritated, bleed, grow rapidly, or change in appearance. Acquired nevi appear between the ages of childhood and 25 years. The lesions become flatter with age and disappear in older age (80 to 90 years).

The *compound nevus* and derma nevus are elevated nodules usually brown in color. The compound nevus is elevated because melanocytes are found in the dermis.

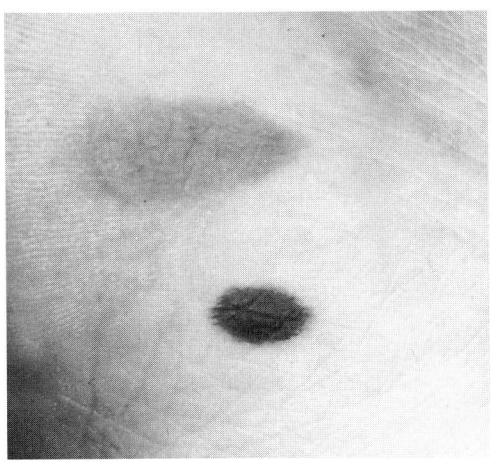

FIG. 81-8   Dark-brown, flat macules with uniform pigment; no skin ulceration; and no history of recent change are typical of benign junctional nevi.

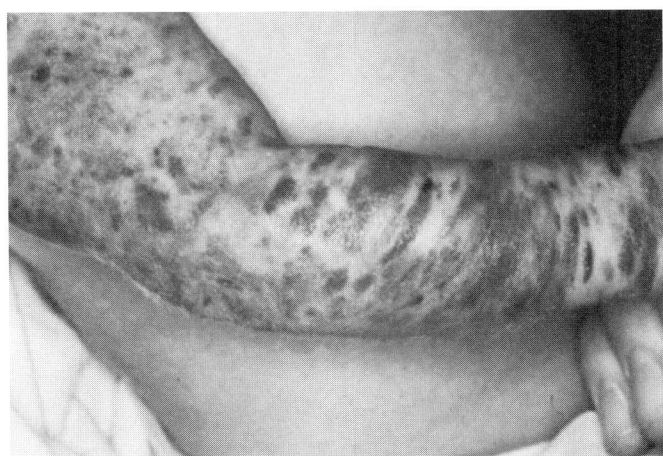

FIG. 81-10   Giant pigmented nevus present at birth has an increased incidence of progression to a melanoma.

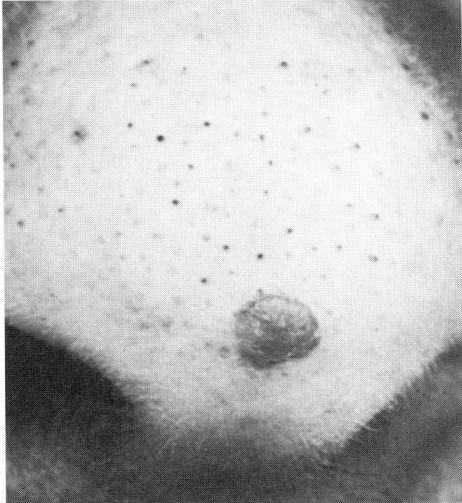

FIG. 81-9   Brownish, elevated papule with uniform color and no history of recent change is typical of a benign compound nevus.

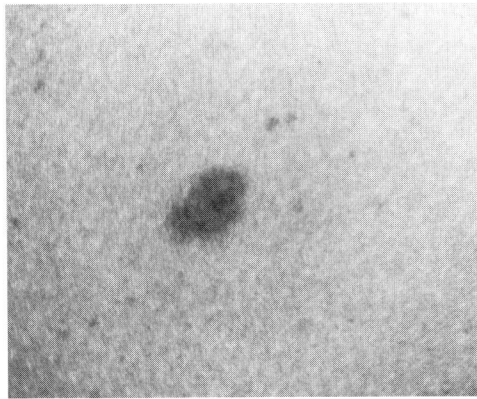

FIG. 81-11   A large nevus with irregular surface, color, and configuration typical of dysplastic nevus.

These nodules are also composed of melanocytes in the epidermis and can occur anywhere on the body. Surgical excision is not necessary unless the area is irritated by clothing or is cosmetically unattractive (Fig. 81-9).

Large nevi present at birth are called *giant congenital nevi* (Fig. 81-10). Because melanomas can arise in giant congenital nevi, they should be excised by surgical removal down to the layer of subcutaneous fat. Regrowth of the nevus will occur if this procedure is not done. The skin should be replaced with grafts if necessary.

Large nevi greater than 6 mm in diameter with irregular color, borders, configuration, and atypical histologic appearance are called *dysplastic nevi* (Fig. 81-11). An individual who has this type of nevi and a family history of melanoma is at high risk for developing melanoma. He or she should be examined by a physician every 6 months, avoid sunlight exposure, use sunscreens when playing or working outside, and self-examine the skin every few weeks. At least some of these nevi with atypical colors, borders, configuration and large size should be biopsied. Nevi in patients with dysplastic nevi and a family history of melanoma should be biopsied if a change in color, shape, or size is noted.

Seborrheic Keratosis

Seborrheic keratosis manifests as a verrucous, brown growth that appears to be glued to the surface of the epidermis (Fig. 81-12). The cause of this benign tumor is unknown. The tumor cells are derived from small basal cells localized in the epidermis. Older patients develop multiple seborrheic keratoses over the trunk, face, and upper extremities. Treatment is not necessary except for cosmetic or diagnostic reasons.

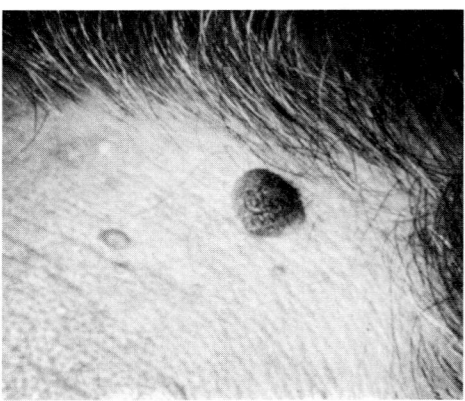

FIG. 81-12 Verrucous, superficial nodule of seborrheic keratosis, which appears to be glued to the surface.

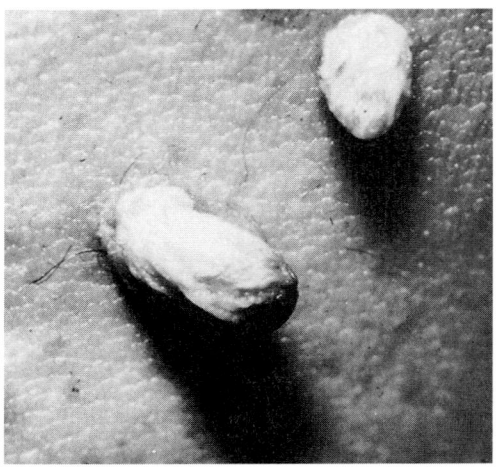

FIG. 81-14 Pedunculated, filiform lesions of acrochordons over the neck.

Keratoacanthoma

Keratoacanthoma is a dome-shaped tumor with a central keratotic crater or ulceration (Fig. 81-13). The tumor grows rapidly over a few months and usually occurs in fair-skinned, older persons. The tumor is benign and may undergo spontaneous involution. Because the tumor can resemble squamous cell carcinoma, it should be excised and examined by a histopathologist.

Dermatofibroma, Acrochordon, and Keloid

Four common benign tumors are dermatofibromas, acrochordons (skin tags), keloids, and sebaceous hyperplasias. *Dermatofibroma* is a brown nodule usually found on the legs, the trunk, or the arms. On palpation, the tumor has a hard buttonlike consistency. The tumor is excised only for cosmetic or diagnostic reasons, because it is benign. *Skin tags (acrochordons)* are common over the neck, axilla, and groin of middle-age and older persons (Fig. 81-14). Acrochordons are more common in obese patients and in pregnant women than in the general population. The lesions are removed if associated with pain and for cosmetic reasons. *Keloids* are caused by an abnormal scar formation after even a minor injury (see Fig. 77-5). Keloids are more common in African Americans than Caucasians, and the tendency to form them is genetic. Surgical excision of keloids may be attempted for cosmetic reasons. Excision of keloids in combination with injection of corticosteroids into the lesions is frequently an effective treatment.

Sebaceous hyperplasia begins as yellow, well-developed lobules with central umbilication. These tumors can resemble basal cell cancers, but there is no skin ulceration. Sebaceous hyperplasia is usually found on the forehead, cheeks, and nose.

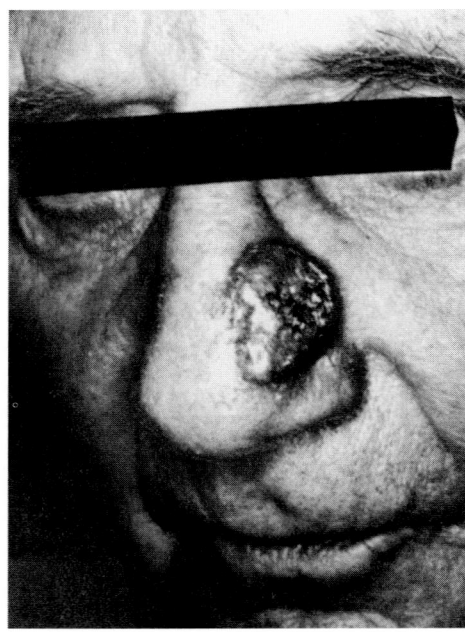

FIG. 81-13 Rapidly growing, dome-shaped tumor with central keratotic crater is a benign keratoacanthoma.

Actinic Keratosis

Actinic keratosis usually occurs on the sunlight-exposed areas of the face, neck, scalp, and extremities. The affected area appears as an erythematous, scaly, rough surface lesion (see color plate 69). The lesion is caused by chronic exposure to sunlight, particularly in older patients. This premalignant growth can develop into squamous cell carcinoma and should be treated. Treatment measures include electrodesiccation with curettage or cryosurgery. Patients are warned about future exposure to sunlight and instructed in the use of sunscreens. Sunscreens that block UV_1B and UVA light with a protection factor of 15 or 30 are recommended (Presun, Solbar, Sundown, Bain de Soleil).

Benign Tumors of Blood Vessels

Among the numerous tumors of blood vessels of the skin, the most frequently encountered are nevus flammeus, strawberry angioma, cherry angioma, spider angioma, and pyogenic granuloma.

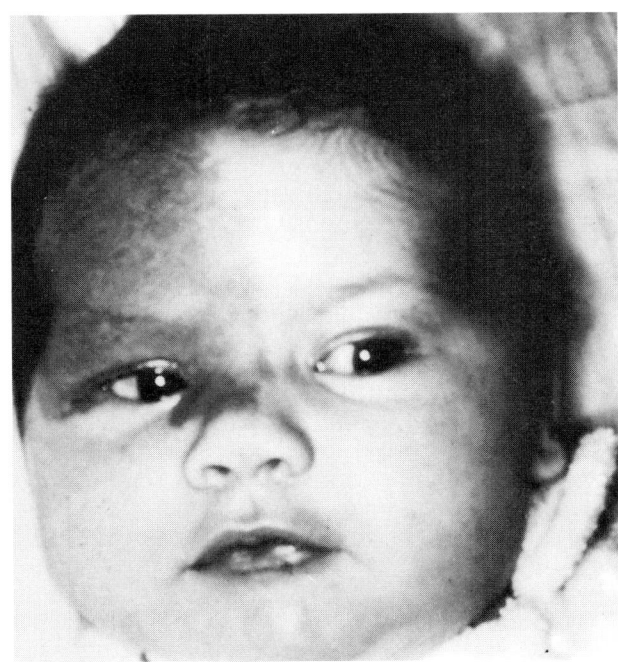

FIG. 81-15   Proliferation of capillaries causes a pink skin discoloration known as *nevus flammeus* or *capillary hemangioma*.

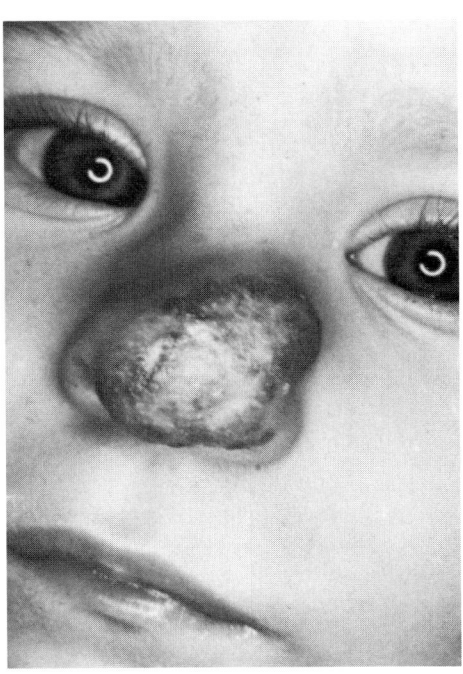

FIG. 81-16   Strawberry angioma presents with an elevated, erythematous tumor, shown here over the nose.

Proliferation of mature capillaries producing a pink discoloration of the skin on newborns is called *nevus flammeus* (Fig. 81-15). When the capillaries follow a branch of the trigeminal nerve, the condition has been associated with angioma of the ipsilateral eye and the central nervous system *(Sturge-Weber syndrome)*. This condition can lead to glaucoma and contralateral seizures. Nevus flammeus can fade or persist indefinitely. If the lesion persists, a cover-up makeup (e.g., Covermark, DermaBlend) is recommended. The pulsed, tunable dye laser has been useful in treatment of these hemangiomas.

Strawberry angioma arises after birth and involutes spontaneously by age 7 in 70% to 95% of cases. Proliferating capillaries in the dermis cause an elevated bluish red nodule (Fig. 81-16; see color plate 70), usually on the head or upper trunk, but it can occur anywhere on the body's surface. Because most of these tumors involute spontaneously, no treatment is usually required.

Cherry angiomas are red, slightly elevated papules over the trunk and extremities of middle-age and older persons (Fig. 81-17). Cherry angiomas are asymptomatic and benign, and treatment is not necessary.

Spider angiomas appear in women during pregnancy, in alcoholics, and also in children. A central arteriole feeds multiple small branches of this tumor. Multiple spider angiomas can be associated with liver disease such as cirrhosis. Most spider angiomas in children and pregnant women resolve spontaneously. Persistent spider angiomas can be electrodesiccated or treated with a pulsed dye laser.

Pyogenic granuloma is caused by an abnormal proliferation of granulation tissue. The tumor occurs after trauma to the site. A red or purple, pedunculated, moist nodule appears (Fig. 81-18). This benign tumor bleeds occasionally and is treated by surgical removal.

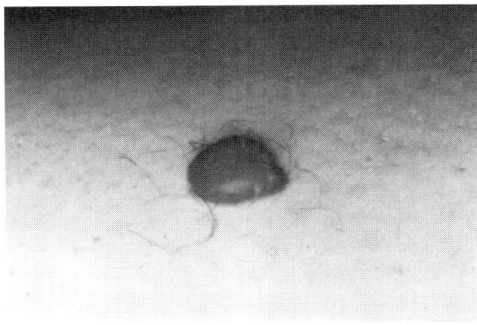

FIG. 81-17   Elevated, erythematous papule of cherry angioma.

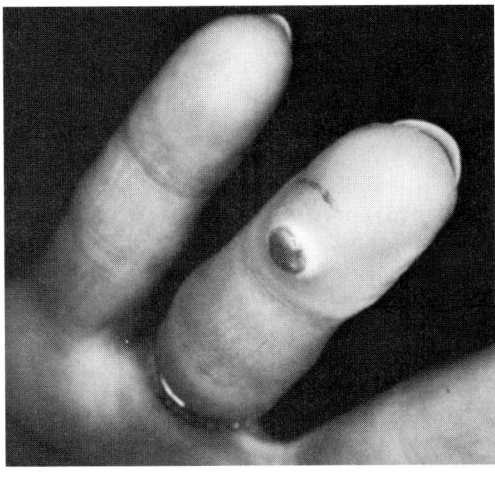

FIG. 81-18   Pedunculated, red, moist nodule of pyogenic granuloma of the finger.

KEY CONCEPTS

■ Cutaneous tumors can derive from various cell types in the skin, such as epidermal cells and melanocytes.

■ *Basal cell carcinoma,* which is the most common malignant tumor of the skin, arises from epidermal cells along the basal layer of the epidermis.

■ The incidence of basal cell carcinoma is directly proportional to the age of the patient and inversely proportional to the amount of melanin pigment in the epidermis.

■ Patients with a history of basal cell carcinoma should use sunscreens or protective clothing to avoid the sun's carcinogenic rays.

■ The tumor is characterized by an erythematous, smooth, pearly nodule.

■ Basal cell carcinoma should be treated promptly. Treatments include curettage with electrodesiccation, scalpel surgery, irradiation, chemosurgery, and cryosurgery.

■ *Squamous cell carcinoma* is a malignant neoplasm of keratinocytes that arises from more differentiated cells of epidermis (keratinocytes).

■ Typically it arises on sunlight-damaged skin with multiple actinic keratoses present. Sunlight is the main etiologic factor causing squamous cell carcinoma of the skin. Other causes of squamous cell carcinoma include ingestion of arsenic, x-ray irradiation, burns, scars, and genetic susceptibility.

■ Squamous cell carcinomas that arise in sunlight-damaged skin usually do not metastasize and rarely cause death; however, areas not exposed to sunlight, after ingestion of arsenic or on an old scar, have the greatest risk of metastasis.

■ A variant of squamous cell carcinoma is localized to the epidermis and is called *Bowen's disease,* which is usually caused by chronic sunlight exposure.

■ Squamous cell carcinoma presents with an ulcerated, scaly, thickened nodule or tumor that bleeds occasionally and usually arises on sunlight-damaged skin of the face, scalp, ears, neck, hands, or forearms.

■ The treatment of squamous cell carcinoma and its variant, Bowen's disease, is primarily surgical excision.

■ *Malignant melanoma* makes up only 3% of all primary cutaneous malignancies but is responsible for almost all the deaths secondary to skin cancers.

■ Most melanomas occur in the 40- to 70-year age group, but the number of cases has increased among the 20- to 40-year age group. One of the explanations for this increased incidence is a greater sunlight exposure secondary to recreation and attire changes.

■ Diagnosis is based on the change in shape, color, size, and configuration of a pigmented lesion.

■ The *superficial spreading melanoma* is the most common type (60% to 80%) and has the best prognosis.

■ The great majority of patients survive for 5 years or more, and many are cured. Early diagnosis and surgical treatment are responsible for these improved statistics.

■ The treatment of malignant melanoma is primarily surgical. Patients with disseminated melanomas receive chemotherapy.

■ Acquired *nevi,* or *moles,* are the most common tumors derived from the melanocyte.

■ The *compound nevus* and *derma nevus* are elevated nodules, usually brown in color.

■ Large nevi present at birth are called *giant congenital nevi.*

■ *Seborrheic keratosis* manifests as a verrucous, brown growth that appears to be glued to the surface of the epidermis.

■ *Actinic keratosis* usually occurs on the sunlight-exposed areas of the face, neck, scalp, and extremities.

■ *Keratoacanthoma* is a dome-shaped tumor with a central keratotic crater or ulceration.

■ Four common benign tumors are dermatofibromas, acrochordons (skin tags), keloids, and sebaceous hyperplasias.

■ *Dermatofibroma* is a brown nodule usually found on the legs, the trunk, or the arms. *Acrochordons* are more common in obese patients and in pregnant women.

■ *Keloids* are caused by an abnormal scar formation after even a minor injury.

■ *Sebaceous hyperplasia* begin as yellow, well-defined lobules with central umbilication.

■ The most frequently encountered *tumors of blood vessels of the skin* are nevus flammeus, strawberry angioma, cherry angioma, spider angioma, and pyogenic granuloma.

■ Proliferation of mature capillaries producing a pink discoloration of the skin on newborns is called *nevus flammeus.*

■ *Strawberry angioma* arises after birth and involutes spontaneously by age 7 in 70% to 95% of cases.

■ *Cherry angiomas* are red, slightly elevated papules over the trunk and extremities of middle-age and older persons.

■ *Spider angiomas* appear in women during pregnancy, in alcoholics, and also in children.

■ *Pyogenic granuloma* is caused by an abnormal proliferation of granulation tissue. The tumor occurs after trauma to the site.

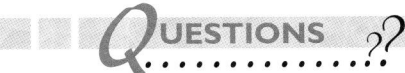

QUESTIONS

A sampling of review questions for this chapter appears here. Visit http://www.mosby.com/MERLIN/PriceWilson/ for additional questions.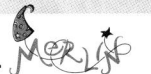

Answer the following on a separate sheet of paper.

1. Describe the characteristic appearance of malignant melanoma.
2. What are the predisposing factors and common sites of occurrence of basal cell carcinoma?
3. Discuss the preventive measures recommended for patients with a family history of melanoma or dysplastic nevi and for fair-skinned individuals.
4. What is the usual treatment of basal cell carcinoma?
5. Describe the causes, pathogenesis, type of lesion, and treatment of squamous cell carcinoma.

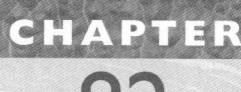
Lyme Disease and Infestations

MAREK A. STAWISKI AND SYLVIA A. PRICE

LYME DISEASE

Lyme disease is the most common arthropod-borne infection in the United States. The disease is caused by the spirochete *Borrelia burgdorferi*. The spirochetes are found in the guts of the tick *Ixodes dammini*. It appears that white-tailed deer and white-footed mice are the main reservoirs of this disease-causing spirochete. The spirochete is injected into the bloodstream through saliva and regurgitated contents from the gut of infected ticks. Lyme disease seems to be endemic and occurs chiefly in the United States along northeastern, mid-Atlantic, and north central states (i.e., Connecticut, Rhode Island, New York, Pennsylvania, Delaware, New Jersey, Maryland, Massachusetts, Wisconsin).

The disease has three clinical stages. *Stage I* usually occurs in the summer and early fall with single or multiple lesions of *erythema chronicum migrans (ECM)* and is frequently accompanied by influenza-like symptoms (fatigue, headache, chills, fever, sore throat, stiff neck, nausea, myalgias, arthralgias). ECM begins as an erythematous papule where the tick bite occurred. The papule expands with central clearing, measuring up to 25 to 50 mm in diameter (Fig. 82-1). The lesion usually disappears spontaneously without therapy within 1 month. The lesion may itch, sting, or burn. The thighs, groin, and axillae are particularly common sites of involvement.

ECM is the most characteristic early sign of the disease and occurs in 80% of patients. A history of a tick bite is obtained in only 60% of patients.

Patients who are not treated can enter stage II of the disease. *Stage II* Lyme disease occurs weeks to months later and is characterized by the triad of meningitis, cranial nerve palsies, and peripheral neuropathy. Fewer than 10% of patients experience cardiac manifestations.

In *stage III, oligoarticular arthritis* occurs from 6 weeks to several years after the tick bite. About 50% of patients who are not treated in stages I and II will evolve to this stage. Recurrences are common, and patients may develop a chronic erosive arthritis.

Laboratory diagnosis is not completely accurate in the diagnosis of Lyme disease. *B. burgdorferi* cannot be readily isolated from blood or skin biopsies. The diagnosis can be confirmed by two serologic tests: indirect immunofluorescence assay (IFA) or enzyme-linked immunosorbent assay (ELISA). Both tests are poorly standardized, and false-negative and false-positive results can occur.

Early Lyme disease is treated with doxycycline or amoxicillin or erythromycin for 10 to 21 days. Neurologic disease, arthritis, or cardiac disease is treated with doxycycline or amoxicillin for 1 month or intravenous penicillin for 10 to 14 days.

Lyme disease caused by the spirochete *B. burgdorferi* causes a multisystem disease affecting the skin, nervous system, heart, and musculoskeletal system. Early recognition of the symptoms and characteristic lesions of ECM should lead to early treatment and cure.

INFECTIONS AND BITES

Scabies is a common infestation caused by the mite *Sarcoptes scabiei* and transmitted by close human contact. The infection is especially common among children and sexually active adults. The incubation period may vary from 3 days to 3 weeks. Pruritus is the chief complaint of these patients. Excoriated linear papules and vesicles are classically found between the fingers and over the elbows, wrists, breasts, and genitalia (Fig. 82-2). Scabies must be suspected if one or more family members develop nocturnal pruritus. The diagnosis is confirmed by microscopic demonstration of the female mite or hatching larvae from a skin scraping (Fig. 82-3). Occasionally, the microscopic examination is negative for scabies. Treatment consists of application of gamma benzene hexachloride (Kwell) or 5% permethrin cream (Elimite) for two 12-hour periods. Secondary irritant eczema can

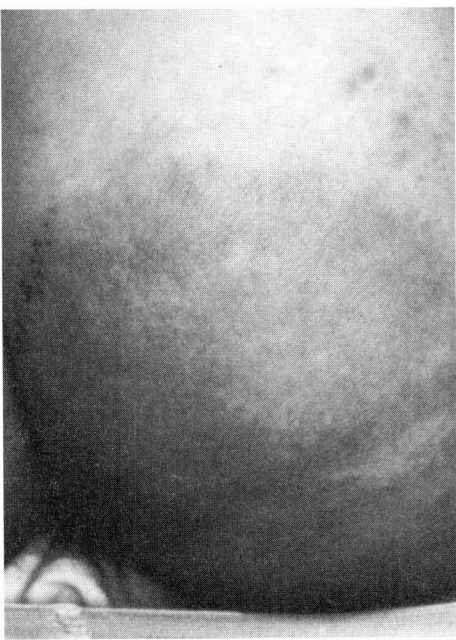

FIG. 82-1 An enlarging erythematous patch with central clearing, typical of erythema chronicum migrans.

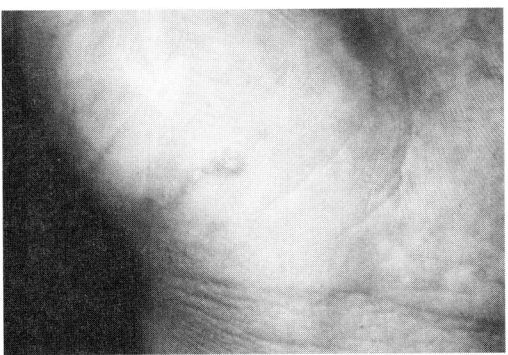

FIG. 82-2 Linear, pruritic papules of scabies on the wrist with a typical linear burrow.

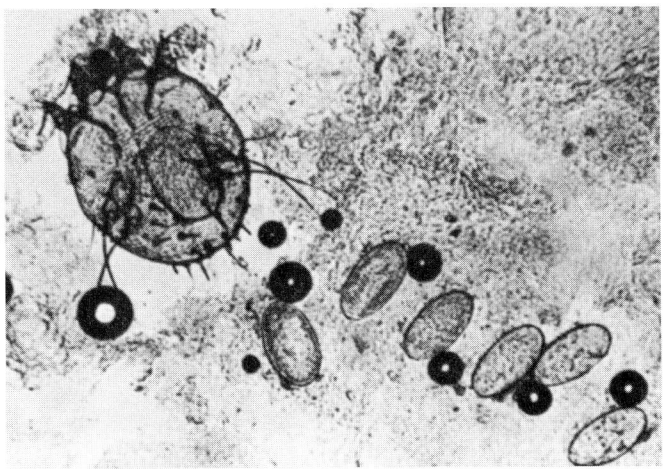

FIG. 82-3 Microscopic examination of scraped scabies reveals a mite and multiple eggs.

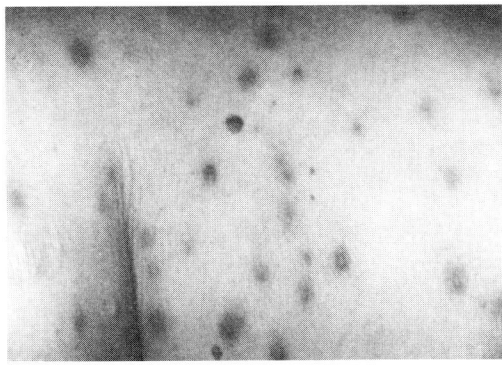

FIG. 82-4 Multiple pubic lice located in the suprapubic area.

complicate the treatment and result in persistence of pruritus. All family members must be treated prophylactically overnight with gamma benzene hexachloride or permethrin, even if they present no evidence of scabietic lesions or pruritus.

Treatment of patients with human immunodeficiency virus (HIV) infection, elderly patients in nursing homes, and occasional patients resistant to Kwell and Elimite can be unsuccessful. These patients are treated with the antihelmintic agent Ivermectin, 6 mg given in a single oral dose.

Pediculosis pubis (pubic crabs) is a frequent infection of the pubic hair and skin. The infection is transmitted by human contact. Lice and nits, which attach to the pubic hair and can be seen with the naked eye, cause intense pruritus (Fig. 82-4). *Pediculosis capitis* (head lice) is caused by lice transmitted from person to person and can often cause epidemics, particularly in schools. Pruritus

usually is the only complaint. Kwell shampoo or pyrethrins (RID) shampoo is the treatment of choice for both types of louse infestations. Patients are instructed to apply the shampoo two times. Nits may also be removed with a fine-toothed comb soaked in vinegar.

Animal fleas that live on pets and in homes cause *fleabites*. A flea bites a person and then leaves the skin; the usual result is a group of erythematous papules with central puncta that are localized to the lower extremities (Fig. 82-5). Only some family members may react with pruritus and clinical lesions, even though all members are bitten. Household furniture (e.g., carpeting) must be treated with an appropriate insecticide to eliminate the fleas. Bites are treated symptomatically with topical steroids and oral antihistamine agents.

Chigger bites are caused by a venomous harvest mite. The bites are usually seen in warm months of July through September. The bites usually occur in lines under tight-fitting clothing. Multiple pruritic, erythematous papules or vesicles with central puncta are observed (Fig. 82-6). Symptomatic relief from these bites with antipruritics and topical corticosteroids is usually helpful. Repellents containing permethrin can also be used.

Bedbugs live in wood surfaces near beds or in bedding. Bites occur during the night and characteristically appear

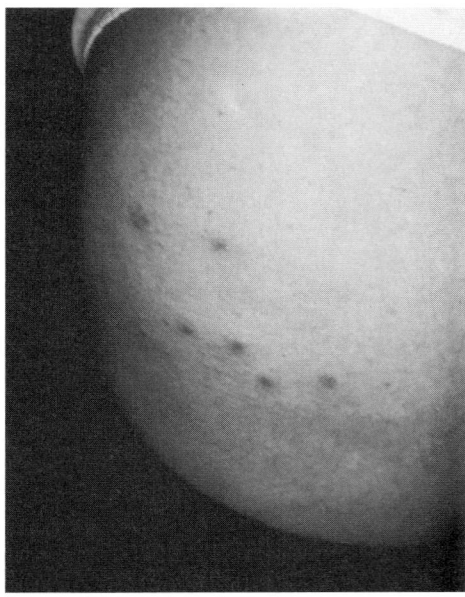

FIG. 82-5 Grouped erythematous papules secondary to flea bites over the knee area.

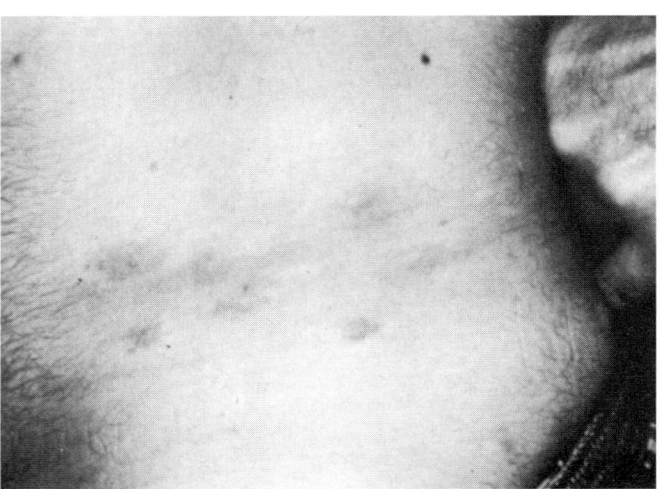

FIG. 82-6 Erythematous, urticarial papules secondary to chigger bites over the trunk.

as grouped vesicles and erythematous papules. Extermination of the bedbugs is required, and clinical lesions are treated symptomatically.

Ticks live in forests, in grass, and on animals. Once attached to the skin, the tick will engorge itself with blood and remain attached; it can be removed with a forceps. Ticks can transmit viral encephalitis, Rocky Mountain spotted fever, and Lyme disease. When visiting certain areas, people should be warned about the possibility of developing Rocky Mountain spotted fever.

*K*EY CONCEPTS

- *Lyme disease* is the most common arthropod-borne infection in the United States.
- The disease is caused by the spirochete *Borrelia burgdorferi*. The spirochetes are found in the guts of the tick *Ixodes dammini*.
- The disease has three clinical stages. Stage I usually occurs in the summer and early fall with single or multiple lesions of ECM and is frequently accompanied by influenza-like symptoms (e.g., fatigue, headache, chills, fever, sore throat, stiff neck, nausea, myalgias, arthralgias).
- *Erythema chronicum migrans (ECM)* begins as an erythematous papule where the tick bite occurred. ECM is the most characteristic early sign of the disease and occurs in 80% of patients. A history of a tick bite is obtained in only 60% of patients.
- Patients who are not treated can enter stage II of the disease. Stage II Lyme disease occurs weeks to months later and is characterized by the triad of meningitis, cranial nerve palsies, and peripheral neuropathy.
- In stage III, *oligoarticular arthritis* occurs from 6 weeks to several years after the tick bite.
- Laboratory diagnosis is not completely accurate in diagnosis of Lyme disease. *B. burgdorferi* cannot be readily isolated from blood or skin biopsies.

- The diagnosis can be confirmed by two serologic tests: IFA or ELISA. Both tests are poorly standardized, and false-negative and false-positive results can occur.
- Early Lyme disease is treated with doxycycline or amoxicillin or erythromycin for 10 to 21 days.
- Lyme disease caused by the spirochete *B. burgdorferi* causes a multisystem disease affecting the skin, nervous system, heart, and musculoskeletal system.
- *Scabies* is a common infestation caused by the mite *Sarcoptes scabiei* and is transmitted by close human contact. Pruritus is the chief complaint of these patients.
- Treatment consists of application of gamma benzene hexachloride (Kwell) or 5% permethrin cream (Elimite).
- *Pediculosis pubis (pubic crabs)* is a frequent infection of the pubic hair and skin. The infection is transmitted by human contact. Lice and nits, which attach to the pubic hair and can be seen with the naked eye, cause intense pruritus.
- *Pediculosis capitis (head lice)* is caused by lice transmitted from person to person and can often cause epidemics, particularly in schools. Pruritus usually is the only complaint.
- *Fleabites* are caused by animal fleas that live on pets and in homes. A flea bites a person and then leaves the skin.

■ *Chigger bites* are caused by a venomous harvest mite. The bites usually occur in lines under tight-fitting clothing.

■ *Bedbugs* live in wood surfaces near beds or in bedding. Bites occur during the night and characteristically appear as grouped vesicles and erythematous papules.

■ *Ticks* live in forests, in grass, and on animals. Once attached to the skin, the tick will engorge itself with blood and remain attached; it can be removed with a forceps.

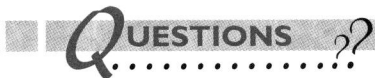 **UESTIONS**

A sampling of review questions for this chapter appears here. Visit http://www.mosby.com/MERLIN/PriceWilson/ for additional questions.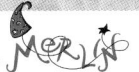

Answer the following on a separate sheet of paper.

1. Describe the appearance of erythema chronicum migrans (ECM) and other early symptoms of Lyme disease.
2. Describe the etiology, signs and symptoms, and treatment for scabies and pediculosis pubis.

Circle the letter preceding each item below that correctly completes the statement. More than one answer may be correct.

3. Mr. M., a 35-year-old man who likes to go hunting in Rhode Island, developed a lesion of ECM over his buttock. The way to confirm the diagnosis is:
   a. Influenzalike symptoms are present during the first 2 months after the bite.
   b. History of a tick bite is found in 100% of patients.
   c. Serologic tests are positive but can sometimes be negative.
   d. If not treated, he has 50% chance of developing arthritis 6 weeks to several years later.

BIBLIOGRAPHY ■ PART THIRTEEN

Akers WA, Allen AN, Botkus D: Isotretinoin versus placebo in the treatment of cystic acne, *J Am Acad Dermatol* 6:737-745, 1982

Anderson G et al: Systemic treatment for advanced cutaneous melanoma, *Oncology* 9:1149, 1995.

Anderson TF: Psoriasis, *Med Clin North Am* 66(4):769-794, 1982.

Arndt KA: *A manual of dermatological therapeutics*, ed 5, Boston, 1995, Little, Brown.

Balch CM et al: Efficacy of an elective regional lymph node dissection of 1 to 4 mm thick melanomas for patients 60 years of age and younger, *Ann Surg* 224(3):255-263, 1996.

Champion RH et al, editors: *Rook Wilkson Ebling textbook of dermatology*, ed 6, Oxford, 1998, Osney Mead Blackwell Science.

Freedberg IM et al, editors: *Dermatology in general medicine*, ed 5, New York, 1999, McGraw Hill.

George SA et al: Narrow band (TL-01) UVB air-conditioned phototherapy for chronic severe adult atopic dermatitis, *Br J Dermatol* 128(15):49-56, 1993.

Gough A: Minocycline induced autoimmune hepatitis and systemic lupus erythematosus-like syndrome, *BMJ* 312(7024):169-172, 1996.

Gupta AK et al: Current management of onychomycosis, *Dermatol Clin* 15:121, 1997.

Habif TP: *Clinical dermatology*, ed 3, St Louis, 1996, Mosby.

Harper J, Orange A, Prose N, editors: *Textbook of pediatric dermatology*, Oxford, 2000, Osney Mead Blackwell Science.

Hassan W: Methotrexate and liver toxicity: role of surveillance liver biopsy: conflict between guidelines for rheumatologists and dermatologists, *Ann Rheum Dis* 55(5):273-275, 1996.

Ho VC, Sober AJ: Therapy for cutaneous melanoma: an update, *J Am Acad Dermatol* 22(2, pt 1):159-176, 1990.

Kay JM et al: The prevalence of childhood atopic eczema in a general population, *J Am Acad Dermatol* 30(1):35-39, 1994.

Kliigman AM, Plegwig G: Classification of acne, *Cutis* 17(3):520-522, 1976.

Kraemer KH, Greene MH: Dysplastic nevus syndrome: familial and sporadic precursors of cutaneous melanoma, *Dermatol Clin* 3(2):225-237, 1985.

Langley RGB, Sober AJ: A clinical review of the evidence for the role of ultraviolet radiation in the etiology of cutaneous melanoma, *Cancer Invest* 15:561, 1987.

Melanby K: *Scabies*, ed 2, Oxfordshire, Engl, 1943, Classey.

Menter MA et al: Proceedings of the Psoriasis Combination and Rotation Therapy Conference, Dear Valley, Utah, October 7-9, 1994, *J Am Acad Dermatology* 34:315, 1996.

Morton DL et al: Technical details of intraoperative lymphatic mapping for early stage melanoma, *Arch Surg* 127(4):392-399, 1992.

Rietschell RL, fowler YF: *Fisher's contact dermatitis*, Philadelphia, 2001, Lippincott–Williams & Wilkins.

Rigel DS et al: Dysplastic nevi: markers for increased risk for melanoma, *Cancer* 63(2):386-389, 1989.

Roberts DJ: Oral terbinafine in the treatment of fungal infections of the skin and nails, *Dermatology* 194(supp 1):37, 1997.

Ruzicka T et al: A short trial of tacrolimus ointment for atopic dermatitis, European Tacrolimus Multicenter Atopic Dermatitis Study Group, *N Engl J Med* 337(12):816-821, 1997.

Shalita AR et al: Isotretinoin treatment of acne and related disorders: an update, *J Am Acad Dermatol* 9(4):621-638, 1983.

Stechenberg BW: Lyme disease: the latest great imitator, *Pediatr Infect Dis J* 7(6):402-409, 1988.

Stern RS et al: Malignant melanoma in patients treated for psoriasis with methoxsalen (Psoralen) and ultraviolet A radiation (PUVA), the PUVA follow-up study, *N Engl J Med* 336(15):1041-1045, 1997.

Stern RS et al: Isotretinoin and pregnancy, *J Am Acad Dermatol* 10(5, pt 1):851-854, 1984.

CHAPTER 1

1. *Pathology* is the science or study of disease. It includes the study of the pathogenesis of disease and structural and functional alterations that result from disease. Pathology is literally abnormal biology, the study of biologic processes gone awry and of individuals who are ill or have disorders. *Pathophysiology* studies the dynamic aspects of disease processes. It is concerned with the disruption of normal physiology; with the alterations, derangements, and mechanisms involved in disruption and how they are expressed as signs and symptoms; and with their expression in physical and laboratory findings. Pathophysiology provides the basic link among the sciences of anatomy, physiology, and chemistry and their applications to clinical practice.

2. *Anatomic pathology* is the study of the morphology of cells, organs, and tissues in disease. *Clinical pathology* refers to the application of laboratory techniques to the study of disease. Examples of anatomic pathology include surgical pathology, exfoliative cytology, and autopsy pathology. Examples of clinical pathology include clinical chemistry, microbiology, hematology, immunology, and immunohematology.

3. *Pathogenesis* is the way disease unfolds, the mechanism of its development.

4. The concept of *normalcy* is complex and difficult to define succinctly. Selecting any parameter that might be applied to an individual or group, the concept of *normal* involves some average value for that parameter. For example, average values for height and weight are derived from observations of many individuals. A certain amount of variation from the average is implicitly accepted as being permissible or normal. The usual concept of normalcy involves an average value and a range of variation either above or below that value.

5. A given disease is a dynamic phenomenon with a rhythm and pattern of its own. Each disease has a natural history, a typical pattern of evolution, an effect, and a duration, unless the disease is successfully modified by some intervention.

CHAPTER 2

1. *Mitosis* is the process by which a somatic cell splits into two new daughter cells. After each chromosome has been replicated to form the two chromatids, mitosis follows. All 46 pairs of chromatids are separated, forming two separate sets of 46 daughter chromosomes, which are identical to the mother cell. No genetic information is lost in this process. *Meiosis* is a type of cell division of germ cells (sperm or ova) in which two successive divisions of the nucleus produce cells that contain one half the number of chromosomes present in somatic cells. When fertilization occurs, the nuclei of the sperm and ovum fuse and produce a zygote with the full chromosome complement.

2. Because nearly all DNA is located in the nucleus of the cell, yet most of the functions of the cell are carried out in the cytoplasm, the genes must have a means of controlling the chemical reactions in the cytoplasm. This goal is achieved through an intermediary, RNA, which is controlled by the DNA in the cell nucleus. This process is accomplished through *transcription* in which DNA transfers its code to RNA. The RNA then diffuses from the nucleus into the cytoplasm, where it controls protein synthesis. During the synthesis of RNA, the two strands of DNA separate temporarily; one of the strands is then used as a template for constructing the RNA molecule. The code triplets in the DNA cause the formation of complementary code triplets called *codons* in the RNA; these codons, in turn, control the sequence of amino acids in a protein to be synthesized later in the cytoplasm, a process called *translation*. The transcription process is under the influence of an enzyme called *RNA polymerase*, which interacts with promoter and terminator sites on the DNA to initiate and stop the process.

3. A trait is *dominant* when it is observable in the heterozygote and may be expressed by all individuals with that allele. A *recessive* trait is observable only in the *homozygote*; an individual who is *heterozygous* for the allele would be a carrier but not express the trait.

4.

	B	b
B	BB	Bb
b	Bb	bb

25% of the offspring will be normal (BB); 50% will be carriers (Bb); and 25% will have the disease (bb).

5. Because females are homozygous for the sex chromosomes and 50% of their X chromosomes are inactivated at random, if a female inherits an X-linked disorder, then only part of the cells express the disorder, while other cells are totally unaffected *(mosaics)*. Thus the clinical symptoms depend on the percentage of cells inactivating the normal allele for each tissue. Because of mosaicism, an X-linked disorder is likely to be milder in the female than it is in the hemizygous male.

6. Translocations are often associated with hematologic malignancies, because many genes expressed by cells of the immune system normally require structural changes to become functional. During this normal process, pathologic translocations may occur, resulting in a malignancy.

7. The advantages of chorionic villus sampling compared with amniocentesis are that it can be performed earlier in the pregnancy and that it is faster; the disadvantage is that a nonrepresentative sample may result, because the sample is obtained from the placenta and not the fetus.

8. Dominant genetic disorders are associated with the overproduction of a protein or the production of an abnormal protein. Using an antisense gene to cause down-regulation can control overproduction of the gene. When the antisense gene is expressed, it makes the complement (antisense) of the mRNA for the defective gene, blocking the ability of the ribosome to bind to the mRNA. Consequently, the protein coded by the defective gene cannot be made. Thus antisense genes limit the expression of the defective gene by controlling its translation.

9. b
10. d
11. a
12. d
13. c
14. c
15. c
16. d
17. c
18. c
19. b
20. a

CHAPTER 3

1. Biochemical; functional; anatomic
2. Central nervous; brain
3. Dystrophic; metastatic
4. Rigor mortis
5. d
6. f
7. b
8. e
9. a

10. c
11. b
12. a
13. b
14. a
15. b
16. b
17. a

CHAPTER 4

1. b
2. e
3. a
4. d
5. c
6. Abscess
7. Ulcer
8. Empyema
9. Fistula
10. -itis
11. Margination
12. Emigration
13. Resolution
14. Repair
15. Lymphadenitis
16. a, b, e, d, c

CHAPTER 5

1. c
2. d
3. a
4. b
5. e
6. c
7. b
8. d
9. a
10. Components of the immune system include the bone marrow, thymus, spleen, lymphoid organs, and mononuclear phagocyte cells scattered throughout the body. The immune system functions to provide immunity, the collection of physiologic mechanisms that provide the organism with the ability to recognize and destroy foreign or non-self materials that enter the body. Three functions of the immune system are (1) *defense* (destruction of external harmful non-self agents, such as viruses or bacteria to prevent infection by foreign pathogens); (2) *homeostasis* (ridding the body of dysfunctional or damaged cells, thus preventing cellular debris from posing a threat); and (3) *surveillance* (recognition and destruction of mutated cells, such as cancer cells).
11. Immunoglobulins are a group of serum protein molecules formed in response to antigens. They are produced by activated B cells (plasma cells) and have the ability to react with a specific antigen. IgG is the most abundant immunoglobulin in plasma, can cross the placenta, constitutes the primary defense against pyogenic bacteria, fixes complement,

and is responsible for the secondary immune response. IgA protects the body surfaces and mucous membranes. IgM is the first immunoglobulin produced in the primary immune response, fixes complement, and is responsible for ABO antibody-antigen reactions. IgD assists B cell differentiation but its actions are uncertain. IgE is a cytophilic molecule bound to mast cells and basophils and is involved in type I hypersensitivity reactions.

12. *Humoral immunity.* B lymphocytes, attacks simple protein antigens, indirect attack by antibodies, can fix complement, and reaction mainly confined to circulating blood
    Cellular immunity. T lymphocytes, attacks complex protein antigens, direct attack by cytotoxic T cells, does not fix complement, and more able to react in sequestered areas of the body (cellular).
13. Immunodeficiency disorders (primary and secondary), hypersensitivity disorders, and autoimmune disorders
14. Types I, II, and III hypersensitivity are mediated by the humoral immune system, Type IV by the cellular immune system. Type I (anaphylactic) hypersensitivity involves IgE mechanisms and is exemplified by an allergic reaction to a bee sting or penicillin or the various atopic disorders. Type II (cytotoxic) hypersensitivity reactions involve IgG or IgM mechanisms exemplified by ABO and Rh blood transfusion incompatibilities. Serum sickness is an example of type III (immune complex) hypersensitivity and also involves IgG or IgM mechanisms. Allergic eczematous contact dermatitis, a positive tuberculin skin reaction, and organ transplant rejection are examples of type IV (delayed hypersensitivity) reactions and antibodies are not involved.

CHAPTER 6

1. *Infection* is present if a microbial agent has been able to adhere to the body surface or to colonize and invade the tissues of the host and then grow and multiply. The presence of infection, however, indicates only the relationship of the parasite to the host; its presence does not necessarily indicate disease. Infectious disease is usually evident by clinical illness. Infection may be totally asymptomatic.
2. *Skin* (especially if traumatized). Ordinarily, the multilayered epithelium, dry keratin layer, and shedding of cells provide a mechanical barrier to infection. The chemical properties of sweat and sebaceous secretions have a

mild bactericidal effect, and the normal flora provides a biologic barrier.
   Mouth, pharynx, and gastrointestinal tract. The entire alimentary canal is lined with a mucous membrane, which, along with the protective layer of mucus, provides a mechanical barrier to invasion by microbes. The flow of saliva mechanically washes away many microbes. Rapid peristalsis in the stomach and especially in the small intestine provides another mechanical barrier. The high acidity of the stomach provides an excellent chemical barrier. Finally, the normal flora of the mouth, throat, and especially the large intestine provides a biologic barrier to microbial proliferation and invasion. The gastrointestinal mucus contains antibodies that provide an immunologic defense.
   Respiratory tract. A mechanical barrier is provided by a layer of mucus that covers the surface and by the constant action of the cilia, which move the secretions toward the exterior of the body. Antibodies are present in respiratory secretions, and motile macrophages in the alveoli engulf and destroy microbes.
   Urinary tract. Defense is provided by the multilayered epithelium and the flushing action of urine flow.
   Eyes. The flow of tears is a defense; antibodies are also present in tears.
   The defenses of the body surfaces against microbial invasion are mechanical, chemical, biologic (normal flora of each surface area), and immunologic.
3. The microorganisms may spread locally along fascial planes or tubular structures, such as a bronchus or an ureter. The organisms may be passively carried by the fluid currents of the body. They may spread via the lymphatic system, ultimately infecting the lymph nodes, or they may be transferred to another location by a phagocyte, if it does not kill the ingested organism. The next step is systemic spread of the microorganisms via the circulating blood. Organisms may even enter blood vessels directly in the local area of initial invasion.
4. If an infectious agent is not locally contained by either the inflammatory response or by the regional lymph nodes, the microorganisms may enter the systemic blood (bacteremia) and possibly disseminate throughout the body. The phagocytic cells of the monocyte-macrophage system, chiefly in the liver and spleen, cleanse the blood of the microorganisms.
5. An infectious disease is produced in a debilitated host by an organism ordinarily harmless to a healthy individual with intact defenses.

6. *Antimicrobial therapy,* which would suppress part of the normal flora and allow a normal resident organism to overgrow, might cause the treated person to become susceptible to an exogenous invader.

Adrenocorticosteroids, which would affect inflammatory and immunologic mechanisms, might allow overgrowth of bacteria that would ordinarily be held in check.

Radiation therapy or chemotherapy, which might depress the bone marrow and lymphoid tissue, could possibly result in severe infection.

Immunosuppressive therapy (used to prevent rejection of a transplanted organ) causes a depression of immune defenses against microbes.

Unavoidable situations in patients who are hospitalized, such as anesthesia, shock, and burns, will lower many defenses.

Primary disease conditions, such as a viral infection of the upper respiratory tract might be followed by bacterial pneumonia.

Environmental factors, such as overcrowding, famine, or weather, might cause a depression of immune defenses.
7. Bacterial flora modifies the surface on which it grows and, by competitive or direct inhibition, prevents others potentially more pathogenic microorganisms from establishing residence.
8. Some pathogenic organisms may damage tissue by immunologic means, producing cellular hypersensitivity (tuberculosis), or they may produce circulating antigen-antibody complexes (poststreptococcal glomerulonephritis). Others may produce exotoxins or endotoxins. Viruses act as intracellular parasites, altering cellular metabolism and synthetic activity.
9. c
10. b
11. a
12. d
13. b
14. a
15. c

CHAPTER 7

1. In *active congestion,* more blood than usual is actively flowing into the area. This increased local blood flow is accomplished by dilation of arterioles, which behave as valves that govern the blood flow into the local microcirculation. In *passive congestion,* some impairment of drainage of blood from the area occurs. Anything that compresses the venules and veins, which will drain a tissue or otherwise hinder flow, may produce passive congestion.
2. When the heart fails in its pumping action, impaired venous drainage re-

sults. For example, if the left side of the heart fails in its pumping action, the flow of blood returning to the heart from the lung will be adversely affected. The blood will be dammed back into the lung, producing passive congestion of the pulmonary vasculature.
3. If the passive congestion is short-lived, no effects on the involved tissue will occur. In chronic passive congestion, however, permanent effects on the tissue may occur, because in a passively congested area, if the change in blood flow is severe enough, an element of tissue hypoxia may lead to shrinkage or to a loss of cells of the involved tissue. Additionally, in many areas a local breakdown of red blood cells is evident, which results in the deposition of certain pigments within the tissues. Fibrosis may also ensue.
4. Edema is an accumulation of excess fluid among the cells of the body or within the various body cavities (or, according to some, within cells).
5. The most common cause of hemorrhage is loss of integrity of vascular walls, permitting the escape of blood. Hemorrhage most often the result of external trauma, as with injuries accompanied by bruising.
6. *Blood platelet system.* With a small hole in the blood vessel, the blood platelets may aggregate over the hole and simply plug it up.

Blood-clotting system. A fibrin clot is formed by the activation of a series of clotting factors in the blood.
7. The local effects of hemorrhage are related to the presence of extravasated blood in the tissues and can range from trivial to lethal. The most trivial local effect is perhaps a bruise, which may be of only cosmetic importance, whereas a small volume of hemorrhage in a vital area of the brain can produce death. Systemic effects depend on two factors: (1) rate of loss, and (2) volume of blood extravasated. If blood loss is rapid, the patient may actually die or may go into hemorrhagic shock. With survival and the passage of time, the patient may develop blood-loss anemia.
8. Thrombosis may (1) result in obstruction of an artery or vein, with possible ischemia or congestion, respectively, and (2) may provide a source of possible emboli.
9. Thrombus in an artery, narrowing of an atherosclerotic artery, embolus in an artery, tumor pressing on a vessel
10. Functional disturbance (pain, such as angina); atrophy of ischemic tissue; infarction of ischemic tissue

CHAPTER 8

1. c
2. d
3. f
4. e
5. a
6. g
7. b
8. Ischemia; advancing age related to decreasing hormone production (e.g., breast tissue); disuse (e.g., cast)
9. The ability to invade normal tissue; the ability to form metastases
10. Lymphatic channels; direct "transplantation," such as across serosal cavities (or, in fact, into incisions via surgical instruments); bloodstream
11. Neoplasms can produce a variety of local mechanical symptoms by impinging on normal structures, producing obstruction of passages, and destroying vital functions. Neoplasms may ulcerate, become secondarily infected, or give rise to hemorrhages. Neoplasms may also have endocrine function and produce signs and symptoms on that basis. Advanced malignant growths may produce cachexia.
12. The most important criterion used in the classification of neoplasms is the distinction between benign and malignant biologic behavior. That is, if a neoplasm has invaded neighboring nonneoplastic tissue or has produced metastases, it is malignant. When neither invasion nor metastasis is evident, a neoplasm can still be classified as malignant if its potential for malignant behavior can be predicted by its microscopic appearance alone; untreated neoplasms of certain types will invade and metastasize. Both the cell type of origin of the neoplasm and the organ of origin of the neoplasm are also criteria.
13. CIN III is severe dysplasia and is tantamount to preinvasive cancer. Destruction of foci of cervical dysplasia can prevent invasive cancer.
14. The significance of tumor cachexia is likely related to the effects of cytokines generated within the tumor or part of the response to the tumor.
15. Transformation or carcinogenesis is not completely understood at present. It is thought that the behavior of cancer cells is "antisocial" with regard to normal cells of the body. Malignant cells disobey the usual territorial rules and grow in inappropriate locations. Evidence is beginning to accumulate indicating that the important abnormalities of cancer cells seem to lie within the cell membrane. On the cell membrane, homeostatic signals are received from other cells and from other points in the body and are transmitted to the interior of the

cell. Abnormalities in this membrane may result in abnormal reception of control signals or abnormal responses to them. Evidence also indicates that events at the cell membrane are important in controlling cellular proliferation. The antigenic structure of cell membranes is important with regard to the immunologic interactions of the cell with its surroundings.

16. Ultraviolet radiation (sunlight); ionizing radiation (gamma rays, x-rays, atomic particles); many chemicals, most of which have mutagenic capabilities; aromatic hydrocarbons; amines, nitrosamines, azo dyes; certain viruses

17. The classic explanation of phenotypic expression of malignancy is somatic mutation, which suggests that the basic carcinogenic event involves a chemical change in the DNA of a cell(mutation). Somatic mutation involves a nongerm cell or somatic cell. Once a cell is transformed into a neoplastic cell, its characteristics breed true, giving rise to an expanding clone of cells with similar properties, determined by the mutated DNA.

    Another explanation for the expression of malignant behavior is the "addition" of genetic information to the cell by viral infection, with the "new" genetic information expressed as abnormal cellular behavior.

    Finally, some evidence indicates that malignancy may be a matter of abnormal differentiation; that is, an abnormal and inappropriate expression of genetic information is always present in each cell of the body, but they are usually kept repressed except, for instance, in embryonic life.

18. T refers to the primary tumor (T_1 is smaller than T_4); N is the status of regional lymph nodes (N_0 designates absence of nodal metastases, and N_1, N_2, and N_3 indicate increasing metastatic involvement); M refers to distant metastasis with appropriate adscripts.

19. It is becoming evident that some genetic abnormalities may be inherited, yielding a predisposition for the development of a tumor in a given family. Molecular methods of analysis identify specific genes and gene products involved in familial cancer syndromes. Individuals at higher-than-normal risk of developing tumors can be identified, and preventive or intervention strategies can be designed and implemented.

20. The means used to establish a diagnosis include the confirmation of the neoplasm's presence by physical examination and by radiographic, ultrasonographic, and/or endoscopic means. A final step in determining the diagnosis of neoplasm involves morphologic examination based on microscopic features of the tissue. Decisions about treatment are related to the clinical stage of the cancer. The concept of staging is based on a given type of cancer being likely to follow a certain progression. Several different modalities of cancer treatment exist, including extirpation of the cancerous tissue surgically, radiotherapy, application of ionizing radiation to the neoplasm, chemotherapy (based on the differential sensitivity of proliferating cancer cells and normal cells to a variety of cytotoxic chemical agents), and immunotherapy. The selected approach is not limited to the use of a single treatment modality; rather, it is based on the needs of the individual patient and the particular neoplasm at its given clinical stage.

CHAPTER 9

1. *Hypersensitivity* denotes the immunologic capacity acquired through contact with a specific, chemically characterizable agent to hyperreact to that agent. The cellular events that follow exposure and establish a capacity for responses of hypersensitivity are termed *sensitization*.

2. *Angioedema* reflects a localized inflammatory increase in vascular permeability without an evident injury to small veins and capillaries, usually reversible within a short period, whereas *lymphedema* results from abnormal pressures (caused by an obstruction to flow upstream) that promote passage of fluid out into tissues.

3. Evidence suggests that clinical anaphylaxis in both animals and humans involves a sudden multifocal reaction of allergen with mast cell–bound, specific IgE followed by widespread tissue response to the mediator substances (e.g., histamine, leukotrienes) released.

4. This generally requires the injection of potent allergens, although certain gastrointestinal and respiratory parasites also elicit prominent IgE responses. Many persons also make specific IgE responses to mucosal contact with innocuous materials, including foods, pollens, and animal emanations (danders). In addition, individual capacities to overproduce IgE and to respond immunologically to specific antigens also seem to be involved.

5. Exercise-induced anaphylaxis presents the typical syndrome evoked *inconsistently* by exertion. No premedication has been useful, and affected individuals *must* rest when symptoms occur and carry epinephrine. It is advisable to exercise with another individual.

6. Efforts to reduce allergen (and irritant) exposure; suppressive medications to mitigate symptom severity nonspecifically; specific hyposensitization to reduce responsiveness to unavoidable challenge

7. Measures taken to reduce the risk of an anaphylactic reaction include (a) avoidance of known offenders (allergens), which is critical in reducing the risk of anaphylaxis, and (b) susceptible individuals being urged to carry commercially prepared, preloaded syringes of epinephrine whenever possible.

CHAPTER 10

1. *Bronchial asthma* is a clinically defined condition marked by recurrent, discrete episodes of reversible bronchial narrowing, separated by periods in which ventilation approaches normal. These events occur in asthma-prone subjects in response to a variety of stimuli; bronchial asthma denotes a state of bronchial hyperreactivity. Allergic factors are evident determinants in some asthmatic individuals but absent in others despite exhaustive study.

2. Bronchial narrowing produces an increased resistance to airflow, which underlies an inability to achieve normal rates of flow during respiration, especially expiration. This results in uneven lung aeration and a loss of the normal spatial matching of ventilation and pulmonary blood flow. These defects, depending on their severity, may produce no symptoms or merely a sense of tracheal irritation; alternatively, respiratory distress may be intolerable.

3. Although atopy is implicated in many instances of bronchial asthma, in a substantial number of asthmatic individuals, no allergic factors are demonstrated even after exhaustive study. These persons are often said to have "intrinsic" asthma, although their problem is more properly idiopathic. In addition, many allergic (atopic) asthmatic individuals also adversely respond to nonallergic factors.

4. Asthmatic airways behave as if their beta-adrenergic innervation are incompetent, and, at least functionally, partial beta blockage seems to exist. Without adequate bronchodilator tone, bronchoconstrictor influences, known to be mediated normally by parasympathetic (cholinergic) and alpha-adrenergic pathways, will tend to predominate. In clinical practice the bronchial lability of asthmatic patients may be confirmed by demonstrating their ready airway obstructive

responses to extremely low concentrations of inhaled histamine and methacholine.

5. Because invading organisms frequently destroy ciliated epithelium and localize agents of inflammation in labile bronchi, their adverse effects on asthma is predictable. In addition, animal studies suggest that microbial substances may further weaken beta-adrenergic activity.

6. (a) The overall severity of impairment from asthma differs widely among individuals and typically varies with time in any affected person; (b) treatment programs of increasing potency (and complexity) are appropriate to control asthma of mounting severity (i.e., a "stepped" approach); (c) anti-inflammatory drugs are fundamental in the treatment for all but the most minimal asthma; (d) increasing symptom intensity should prompt a *preplanned* set of remedial behaviors designed to improve the individual's functional status; (e) patient education and informed compliance are essential for favorable outcomes.

7. The effectiveness of these agents is thought to reflect direct stimulation of the enzyme, adenyl cyclase, which promotes the synthesis of cyclic AMP. Cyclic AMP–induced effects (e.g., relaxation of bronchial smooth muscle and inhibition of mediator release from mast cells and basophils) are promoted both by beta-adrenergic agents and by theophylline; additive effects of these two groups of drugs often result.

8. Faulty inhalation techniques include (1) failure to synchronize inhalation and nebulizer discharge; (2) inadequate time allowed before passive exhalation occurs to permit aerosol mixing and deposition in the airways; and (3) interception and effective loss of rapidly moving particles by oropharyngeal baffles (e.g., teeth, tongue). Many of these deficiencies are reduced when metered-dose inhalers (MDIs) are used with spacers. Such devices are essential for children and many adult users to increase substantial lung deposition of drug.

9. Steroid-dependent asthmatic individuals require regular oral corticosteroid treatment to maintain acceptable function. Symptoms are controlled with the lowest possible daily dose of a rapidly metabolized agent such as prednisone. Administration of moderate doses on alternate days may also be effective while reducing systemic side effects and suppressing hypothalamic-pituitary-adrenal function. The latter treatment benefits must reflect brief periods (longer than 36 hours after

dosing) when no drug effect remains, because the required alternate-day doses are often more than twice those necessary in daily administration.

10. b, d
11. a, c
12. e

CHAPTER 11

1. Anaphylactic reaction and urticaria can result from IgE-mediated responses to protein allergens. In both situations the implicated agents are usually (a) ingestants, such as egg, fish, shellfish, and nuts, including peanuts; or (b) drugs or drug metabolites that are capable of stable bonding to proteins (e.g., penicillins) or that are themselves complete antigens. Many drugs also appear to cause urticaria, although not typically anaphylaxis, by mechanisms exclusive of IgE (e.g., aspirin).

2. Since bouts of hives are generally self-limited and vary in duration and severity, the value of treatment measures for affected individuals is often difficult to discern. Epinephrine has demonstrated effectiveness in speeding resolution. Agents such as diphenhydramine and hydroxyzine also are acknowledged to have value in the treatment of this condition. Adrenal corticosteroids have been beneficial in treating severe acute hives. Hydroxyzine is often the most valuable agent in chronic urticaria.

3. Hives (urticaria) probably affect at least 25% of the population at some time.

4. Treatment modalities for urticaria are difficult to evaluate, because bouts of hives tend to be self-limiting and vary in duration and severity.

5. Individuals who develop atopic (allergic) disorders tend to have high serum IgE levels and show positive reactions to multiple allergens with skin testing.

6. The lesions of atopic dermatitis and AECD are difficult to distinguish because their appearance and symptoms are very similar (itching, weeping vesicles, scaling, cracking). AECD, however, is caused by an allergen that contacts the skin and is mediated by sensitized T lymphocytes, a type IV hypersensitivity reaction. On the other hand, atopic dermatitis is classified as a type I hypersensitivity reaction because it tends to occur in individuals with other atopic conditions, such as allergic rhinitis and asthma, although it is rare to identify an allergen with flare-ups.

7. Low threshold for itching perception, dry skin, deficient delivery of sweat and oil to skin, and tendency to lichenify (thicken)

8. Interrupt the scratch-itch cycle with Benadryl and padded mittens for infants and young children at bedtime; avoid excess bathing and drying of skin, with minimal use of soap; use topical lubricants and corticosteroids and antibiotics for secondary infection.

CHAPTER 12

1. The appearance of *autoantibodies* (antibodies that react with autologous tissue components) provides valuable diagnostic markers. However, these serum factors seldom inflict direct tissue injury. Their appearance implies either an acquired mutation among immunocompetent cells or the reactivation of cells that had been suppressed but not eliminated. Several mechanisms may result in autoimmunity.

2. In certain instances the inciting antigens are normally sequestered and may remain "foreign" even to mature tissue. These responses (i.e., "altered self") arise after subtle injury incident to microbial invasion. The possibility that infecting bacteria and viruses may produce limited changes in host tissue components, rendering them foreign to immune surveillance, has been proposed. Antibodies (or sensitized lymphocytes) resulting from this process might have specificities broad enough to permit reaction with native and altered tissue determinants. Autoimmune phenomena could arise if an invading organism and host tissues share an antigen or closely similar antigenic groups as a result of parallel evolution. Mutant ("forbidden") clones of lymphoid cells programmed to recognize normal host components as foreign could be involved as well. Such cells might be antigen-specific or nonspecific T_H (helper-promoter lymphocytes) that foster the immune responses of both T and B lymphocytes. Alternatively, a decline of suppressor (T_S) lymphocytes that normally inhibit these responses might be implicated.

3. Circulating antibodies, which are reactive with glomerular and alveolar basement membrane glycoproteins, especially type 4 collagen, are usually present; and along with complement components, they form linear deposits at these sites. The associated tissue damage is thought to reflect, in part, complement-mediated cytotoxicity and local effects of recruited neutrophils.

4. The signs and symptoms of transfusion reactions include chills, fever, and low back pain, occasionally preceded by urticaria or flushing, uneasiness, and air hunger. When cell lysis is massive, the resulting debris may trigger widespread intravascular clotting with depletion of coagulation

factors and bleeding from wounds and venipuncture sites.

5. All the following measures must be used to prevent or mitigate hemolytic transfusion reactions:
   a. The source and proper recipient of blood products must be identified.
   b. Continual surveillance of individuals receiving blood is a must, especially those whose mobility or awareness is impaired.
   c. If any suggestion of an incipient reaction should occur, the subject infusion should be discontinued immediately, IV access should be maintained, and careful clinical observation should be sustained.
   d. A carefully drawn venous sample from the recipient should be checked for serum hemoglobin, a sign of intravascular red cell breakdown, and the compatibility of donor and recipient should be reconfirmed.
   e. All materials used for transfusion must be saved to facilitate serologic and microbiologic testing.
   f. Special precautions to monitor urine output are essential, and examination of serial centrifuged urine specimens for hemoglobin is desirable, because clearance of serum hemoglobin is rapid.
   g. Maintenance of adequate hydration and urine flow are important considerations in all survivors, and osmotic diuresis with cautiously administered IV mannitol may help in achieving this goal.
   h. Safe fluid therapy demands precise and regular evaluation of cardiopulmonary and renal function. Measures to combat shock, pulmonary edema, acute renal failure, or defibrination with bleeding may be required.

6. Recipients of leukoagglutinins have developed fever, cough, shortness of breath, and lung shadows on chest radiograph films; several days have been required for full resolution.

7. b
8. a
9. d
10. c

CHAPTER 13
1. e
2. a, c
3. b, c, d
4. f
5. b, d
6. c
7. Initially, complexes of host IgG or IgM and drug (or drug protein conjugate) become attached to one or more types of blood cells. Complement components are localized to the cell surface, and their interaction

results in discrete membrane lesions or enhanced removal of affected cells from the circulation, the formed elements being injured as "innocent bystanders" rather than direct participants. After fixation of complement factors, the immune complexes often dissociate from affected membranes.

8. The probable mechanisms of reactions associated with the administration of local anesthetics include syncope, hypotension, cardiac rhythm disturbances, and, at times, convulsions. These reactions are probably a direct toxic effect of the large drug doses required for local infiltration.

9. a. An effective approach to the prevention of adverse drug reactions requires knowledge of the potential complications of medication and a willingness to consider adverse drug reactions as a possible cause of any unexpected clinical event.
   b. Since adverse responses usually occur with reexposure, no drug should be given without first assessing the individual's history with that agent. The clinical database requires no less than a comprehensive assessment of past drug reactivity. Health care personnel must also be prepared to accept, at face value, reports of past problems arising from medication until these reactions have been conclusively disproved.
   c. Close surveillance can reveal the earliest stigmata of drug reactions, facilitating prompt withdrawal of the offender and often abbreviating morbidity. Once recognized, adverse reactivity must be clearly indicated in the clinical record and, if possible, made clear to the patient or responsible family members. Documentation and recall are both aided if the patient carries a card, bracelet, or medallion indicating medication(s) to be avoided. Careful instruction is necessary when a risk of reaction from related agents exists or when the offender has many readily available, poorly identified sources.

CHAPTER 14
1. Three methods are used to evaluate antigen-specific antibody activity associated with one or more Ig classes: (1) *Determining naturally occurring (IgM) antibodies to ABO blood group substances absent from the subject's red cells.* Normal persons consistently demonstrate such isohemagglutins by age 1 year. (2) *Schick testing individuals previously immunized with diphtheria toxoid.* If adequate levels of (IgG) specific antibody have been

produced, tissue breakdown at the site of toxin injection is prevented. (3) *Determining antibody titers before and after administering nonviable immunizing materials such as tetanus toxoid and typhoid vaccine.*

2. Reactivity to DTH skin tests provides a readily available indicator of cellular immune competence measuring both antigen processing and cellular response. Intradermal injections are performed with 0.1 ml portions of substances that elicit DTH and to which a previous sensitizing exposure may be assumed. Commonly used materials include PPD (of the tubercle bacillus) and streptokinase and streptodornase (enzymes of beta-hemolytic streptococci). Test sites are observed and palpated after 48 hours, and an indurated area with a diameter of 10 mm or larger is generally regarded as a positive reaction. Using a battery of such materials, at least one positive test should be evident in the vast majority of normal individuals (excluding infants). For nonreactors, the next step is determining B- and T-cell categories using monoclonal antibodies to tag their cell membrane components. Automated approaches to such assays (by flow cytometry) can estimate levels of helper/inducer, suppressor/cytotoxic, and null cells and functional subcomponents within these groups.

3. Two laboratory tests reflect lymphocyte function. (1) Response of lymphocytes in short-term tissue culture respond to antigens and nonspecific agents, which stimulates cell division and associated nucleic acid synthesis. An increase in the incorporation of thymidine tagged with tritium is normally observed in response to these agents. (2) Assays of lymphokines are produced in response to appropriate antigens added to lymphocyte preparations. Currently available monoclonal antibodies provide an expanding variety of specific reagents.

4. The numbers and functional state of T lymphocytes also affect antibody secretion, because antigen recognition by T cells must precede most antibody (humoral) responses.

5. Signs of immunodeficiency disorders primarily include recurrent infections, chronic infections, unusual infections (with opportunistic infecting agents), and poor or slow response to antimicrobial treatment.

6. Primary immunodeficiency disorders are generally inherited and may involve B-cell deficiency (e.g., X-linked agammaglobulinemia), selective IgA deficiency, T-cell deficiency (e.g., DiGeorge syndrome, chronic mucocutaneous candidiasis), or combined B-

and T-cell deficiency (e.g., severe combined immunodeficiency). Secondary or acquired immunodeficiency may result from corticosteroid or cytotoxic drug therapy, radiation therapy, immunosuppressive therapy to prevent organ transplant rejection, or HIV infection, or it may be associated with chronic diseases such as malignancy, liver cirrhosis, or renal failure.

7. Selective IgA deficiency is the most common primary immunodeficiency and occurs in 1 out of every 500 to 1000 persons. Some individuals so afflicted may be asymptomatic, while some may have recurrent paranasal sinus and respiratory infections, autoimmune disease, GI disease, allergies, and malignancies. Individuals with IgA deficiency must receive IgA-deficient transfustion blood because anaphylactic sensititivty may be induced by the infusion of the missing IgA (which is recognized as a foreign antigen).

CHAPTER 15
1. c
2. d
3. b
4. a
5. e
6. c
7. a
8. e
9. b
10. d
11. f

CHAPTER 16
1. A science involving the study of blood, its nature, function, and disease and blood-forming tissues
2. The hematologic system, which includes blood and blood-forming tissues and monocyte-macrophage system located throughout the body (spleen, liver, lymph nodes, bone marrow), phagocytizes foreign materials (microorganisms to dying RBCs). Disorders arising from these systems are called *blood dyscrasias.*
3. RBCs (erythrocytes or red corpuscles), WBCs (leukocytes or white corpuscles), and platelets (or thrombocytes)
4. Because RBCs, WBCs, and platelets have a finite life span, a constant optimal production is necessary to maintain levels required meeting tissue needs. In adults, this production, called *hematopoiesis* (formation and maturation of blood cells), takes place in the bone marrow of the skull, vertebrae, pelvis, sternum, ribs, and proximal epiphyses of the long bones. However, during periods of increased demand (e.g., hemorrhage, cell destruction), production may resume in all the bones, as is normal in

children. The stem cell can differentiate into lymphoid and hematopoietic stem cells that become progenitor cells. Progenitor cells differentiate along a single pathway. Through a series of divisions and maturational changes, these cells become specific mature cells in the circulating blood.

5. Daughters of stem cells can differentiate into lymphoid or myeloid stem cells, which become progenitor cells. Differentiation occurs in the presence of colon stimulating factors such as erythropoietin for RCB production and G-CSF for WBC production. Progenitor cells differentiate along a single pathway. Through a series of divisions and maturational changes, these cells become specific mature cells in the circulating blood.

6. A complete history or profile (including past and current illnesses, drug exposure, bleeding tendencies, nutritional habits, and family history), physical assessment, and selective diagnostic studies. These studies attempt to quantify the various constituents of blood and bone marrow.

7. d
8. a
9. g
10. b
11. e
12. i
13. c
14. j
15. h
16. f

CHAPTER 17
1. The major component of the RBC is the protein hemoglobin (Hb), which transports O_2 and CO_2 and maintains the normal pH through a series of intercellular buffers. The Hb molecule consists of two pairs of polypeptide chains (globin) and four heme groups, each one containing an atom of ferrous iron. This configuration allows the most expedient exchange of gases.
2. RBC production is stimulated by a glycoprotein, *erythropoietin,* believed to originate in the kidney, with 10% coming from liver hepatocytes. Theories suggest that erythropoietin production is influenced by tissue hypoxia resulting from factors such as changes in atmospheric O_2, decreased O_2 content of arterial blood, and decreased Hb concentration. The stem cells committed to erythrocyte production appear to be the targets of erythropoietin and initiate proliferation and maturation of RBCs.
3. *Anemia* is a reduction below the normal level in the number of RBCs, the quantity of Hb, and the volume of packed RBCs (hematocrit) per deciliter of blood.

4. Pallor (nail beds, palms, mucous membranes of the mouth and conjunctivae), tachycardia, shortness of breath, dyspnea, headache, dizziness, faintness, tinnitus
5. (1) Increased RBC loss: direct loss from the circulation through bleeding. Bleeding from trauma or ulcers, polyps in the colon, malignant growth, hemorrhoids, and menstruation. (2) Destruction of RBCs in the circulation (hemolysis). Hemoglobinopathies (inherited abnormal Hb): sickle cell disease, impaired globin synthesis, thalassemia; RBC membrane defects: hereditary spherocytosis and elliptocytosis; enzyme deficiencies: G6PD deficiency and pyruvate kinase deficiency.
6. (1) Normocytic, normochromic anemia: RBCs are of normal size and shape, contain the normal amount of Hb (MCV and MCHC are normal or low normal). Examples are acute blood loss, hemolysis, renal disease, and metastatic infiltrative diseases of the bone marrow. (2) Macrocytic, normochromic anemia: RBCs are larger than is normal but are normochromic because the Hb concentration is normal (MCV is increased; MCHC is normal). Examples are deficiency states of vitamin B_{12} or folic acid or both; cancer chemotherapy. (3) Microcytic, hypochromic anemia: microcytic means small cell, hypochromic means decreased coloration. Because the hue comes from hemoglobulin, these cells contain less than the normal amount of Hb (MCV and MCHC are decreased). Examples are iron deficiency anemia, chronic blood loss, and thalassemia.
7. (1) Treatment necessitates identification of the cause of the anemia. (2) When possible, resolve the underlying cause. (3) Start specific treatment only when indicated.
8. Excess *(poly-)* of all cell lines *(-cythemia)*, but generally used for conditions in which the RBC mass exceeds normal
9. Polycythemia may be classified as primary or secondary. (1) *Primary polycythemia* or *polycythemia vera:* in polycythemia vera the pluripotential stem cell is abnormal. A marked erythrocytosis, leukocytosis, and thrombocytosis are present. (2) *Secondary polycythemia:* occurs when the volume of circulating plasma is decreased (hemoconcentrated) but the total volume of circulating RBCs is normal. Hemocrit in men rises to about 57% and 54% in women; the most likely cause is dehydration.
10. Refer to Figure 17-1.
11. Erythrocytes containing Hb S traverse the microcirculation more slowly than

do normal erythrocytes, resulting in deoxygenation. Hb S erythrocytes adhere to endothelium, retarding blood flow. Increased deoxygenation may take the abnormal RBCs below a critical point, causing sickling within the microvasculature.

12. Life-threatening disorder of the stem cell in the bone marrow in which an insufficient number of blood cells are produced. May be congenital, idiopathic, or secondary. Deficient in all types of blood cells (pancytopenia).

13. Systematic lupus erythematosus-autoimmune basis, antineoplastic or cytotoxic agents; radiation therapy; certain antibiotics; miscellaneous drugs (e.g., anticonvulsants, thyroid medications, gold compounds, phenylbutazone); chemicals (e.g., benzene, organic solvents insecticides, agents thought to damage directly), viral diseases, aplastic anemia following vial hepatitis.

14. Allogenic stem cell transplantation with compatible donors (e.g., siblings with matching HLA antigens). Success rate exceeds 80% in previously untransfused patients.

15. Normocytic, normochromic

16. Visceral sequestration crisis with sickling and pooling of blood, particularly in the chest.

CHAPTER 18

1. CSFs are glycoproteins that are part of a group of WBC regulators known as *cytokines*. CSFs are continuously synthesized by cells (e.g., lymphocyte-macrophage system, fibroblasts, endothelial cells in the bone marrow). CSFs are believed to circulate fully and attach themselves to specific receptors on the cell surface of hematopoietic precursors, committing them to differentiation, which, in the case of the WBCs, to the neutrophil and monocyte cell lines.

2. Morphologic classification is based on differentiation and maturation of the predominant leukemic cells in the bone marrow, as well as cytochemical studies.

3. Familial leukemia is rare, but siblings of affected children appear to have a higher incidence of leukemia, with the incidence increasing to 20% in monozygotic (identical) twins. People with chromosomal abnormalities appear to have a twenty-fold increase in the incidence of acute leukemia. Chemicals are being implicated with increased frequency, particularly the alkylating agents. A likelihood exists of increased incidence of leukemia in patients treated with both radiation and chemotherapy.

4. Therapy is directed toward elimination of the abnormal cell line; 65% of patients, with resumption of normal hematopoiesis, achieve remission of disease. Attaining a complete molecular remission with reversal of all cytogenic abnormalities is imperative for long-term remission or cure.

5. Neoplastic plasma dyscrasias arising from a single clone (monoclonal) of plasma cells, manifested by the uncontrolled proliferation of immature and mature plasma cells in the bone marrow.

6. Younger patients: nontender, "rubbery" enlarged lymph node in the low cervical or supraclavicular area or a nonproductive cough secondary to hilar adenopathy; older patients: unexplained fever or night sweats or both. Constitutional symptoms such as anorexia, cachexia, weight loss, and fatigue are present in disseminated disease.

7. Multiple myeloma: treatment is aimed at reducing the tumor burden (malignant plasma cells and immunoglobulins); preventing and controlling complications such as infections, anemia, hypercalcemia, pathologic fractures; and pain management. Waldenström's macroglobulinemia: treatment is aimed at decreasing the IgM plasma load and bone marrow infiltration and lymphoid tissues.

8. Leukemia

9. Reed-Sternberg cells

10. Leukopenia

11. Chronic granulocytic leukemia

12. 80

13. a. Neutrophils (neutrophilia)
    b. Eosinophils (eosinophilia)
    c. Basophils (basophilia)

CHAPTER 19

1. Platelets are derived from a noncommitted pluripotential stem cell, which, on demand and in the presence of thrombopoietin, differentiates into the committed stem cell pool to form the *megakaryoblast*. This cell, through a maturation sequence, becomes a megakaryocyte. The cell cytoplasm eventually breaks up into individual platelets.

2. Vasoconstriction is an immediate response to the injury, followed by adhesion of platelets to collagen in the vessel wall exposed by the injury. ADP is released by the platelets, causing them to aggregate. Minute amounts of thrombin stimulate platelet aggregation. Platelet factor III also accelerates plasma clotting. In this way, a platelet plug forms. Platelets also play a role in the formation of fibrin and in clot retraction.

3. Factors V and X

4. After the platelet level reaches a certain peak level, spontaneous aggregates of platelets occur. In the large vessels, this action has little effect, but the platelets plug the tiny capillaries. In the process, the capillary wall is damaged and bleeding occurs into the tissues. Examples of primary thrombocytosis are polycythemia vera and chronic granulocytic leukemia. Examples of secondary thrombocytosis are those occurring temporarily after stress or exercise with storage pool release from the spleen or accompanying increased bone marrow demand states (hemorrhage or hemolytic anemia).

5. von Willebrand's disease is the most common inherited coagulation disorder. Most common subtype is type I. Except for types II and III, which are autosomal recessive, all types are inherited as an autosomal dominant trait. von Willebrand's factor facilitates platelet adhesion to components in the vascular subendothelium under conditions of high flow and shear stress. von Willebrand's is also the intravascular carrier for factor VIII to sites of active hemorrhage.

6. Treatment options: cryoprecipitate, factor VIII concentrates, desmopressin (DDAVP), fresh-frozen plasma, and estrogens. The goal is to increase availability of von Willebrand's factor.

7. Treatment dictates prophylactic infusions beginning at 1 to 2 years of age in severely deficient children to prevent chronic joint disease. Intervention at the earliest signs of bleeding, as well as preoperative factor replacement in preparation for surgical procedures, is essential. Treatment is aimed at increasing the deficient factor or activity to a normal level and preventing complications.

8. DIC refers to a multifaceted complex syndrome in which a normally homeostatic and physiologic system of maintaining fluidity of blood becomes a pathologic system, leading to diffuse fibrin thrombi occluding the microvasculature of the body. DIC is initiated by the introduction of a procoagulant material or activity into the circulating blood.

9. The role of heparin is to neutralize thrombin activity inhibiting the consumption of the coagulation factors and fibrin deposition. Increasing the concentration of clotting factors and platelets with infusions of plasma and platelets should then inhibit the bleeding diathesis.

10. Improved donor screening, HIV testing of blood, development of virucidal methods, and recombinant (genetically engineered) factor preparations (factors VIII and IX)

11. INR was developed comparing local reagents against an International Reagent and assigning a relative value (In-

ternational Sensitivity Index), which results in a normalized value across all laboratories. INR has become the standard for monitoring patients on oral anticoagulant therapy. Oral anticoagulant doses are adjusted to maintain a specific INR, depending on the individual's condition requiring oral anticoagulant therapy.

CHAPTER 20

1. Intracellular, intravascular, and interstitial
2. Refer to Box 20-3 for a review.
3. Blood buffers, kidneys, and lungs
4. False. Active transport
5. True
6. True
7. True
8. False. Causes sodium reabsorption
9. True
10. True
11. False. 2 L
12. False. Requires data from history and clinical observations
13. False. Only when the ion valence is one
14. True

CHAPTER 21

1. a; b and c are nonspecific; d is less sensitive and specific; serum sodium reflects osmotic concentration, not volume changes.
2. a, c, e
3. b; because the patient is hypovolemic and hypokalemic
4. d; BSA of 70 kg man = 1.76 m²; fluid loss moderate; 1.76×2400 ml = 4200 ml, or according to 4 kg weight loss, fluid loss = 4 L
5. (a) The effective circulating blood volume would decrease; (b) and (c) plasma osmolality and Na^+ concentration would not change, because the fluid loss is isotonic with equal amounts of sodium and water lost; (d) ADH secretion would increase because of ECF volume depletion; (e) and (f) urine osmolality and thirst would increase because of the increased ADH secretion; (g) blood pressure would decrease because of hypovolemia.
6. Hyponatremia and hypoosmolality would occur.
7. (a) Two thirds of pure water losses would come from the ICF, whereas one third would come from the ECF because these compartments make up 40% and 20% of the fluid, respectively, of the 60% of the body weight that is fluid. Isotonic fluid loss, on the other hand, comes from the ECF entirely. Therefore a greater decrease is present in the ECF volume and in the blood pressure with isotonic fluid losses; (b) the plasma osmolality will increase as a result of the loss of pure water but will not change with isotonic losses; (c) the brain cells will shrink and become dehydrated with pure water losses, but the volume does not change with isotonic losses.
8. Normal (isotonic) saline remains in the ECF and is effective in restoring the effective circulating blood volume and tissue perfusion. The 5% dextrose in water (D_5W) is metabolized to pure water; only one third remains in the ECF, whereas two thirds enters the ICF. Therefore D_5W has less effect on restoring the ECF volume and tissue perfusion. Additionally, the D_5W would cause a dilutional hyponatremia.
9. All are correct.
10. c, d; because the patient has both a fluid volume deficit and hyponatremia as well as hypokalemia
11. a, b, d
12. a, c, e

CHAPTER 22

1. Cellular enzymes that maintain the life processes can function only within a narrow pH range. Cardiac function, in particular, is adversely affected by a pH that is less than 7.25 or greater than 7.55. Contractility is depressed, and dysrhythmias may occur.
2. pH is the negative log of the $[H^+]$ concentration and has an inverse relationship to the actual $[H^+]$. An *acid* is a compound that releases a H^+ when in a solution with water (proton donor). A *base* is a H^+ acceptor; that is, it incorporates H^+ into its molecular structure by removing it from solution. The pK of a buffer system is the pH at which the buffer is 50% dissociated and has its maximal buffering capacity. The carbonic acid-bicarbonate buffer system would be more effective as a blood buffer if its pK were 7.4 rather than 6.1. A *buffer* system consists of a weak acid, and its salt (or a weak base and its salt) and is only partially dissociated in solution. A buffer acts as a chemical sponge by soaking up extra H^+ or releasing them to prevent fluctuations in the pH.
3. A volatile acid (carbonic acid) is one that can change from a liquid to a gas ($CO_2 + H_2O$) and is excreted by the lungs. Nonvolatile acids or fixed acids (e.g., phosphoric acid, sulfuric acid, lactic acid, ketoacids) cannot be excreted by the lungs but must be excreted by the kidneys.
4. The bicarbonate-carbonic acid system is the major buffer system of the ECF. The phosphate, hemoglobin, and protein buffer systems are primarily intracellular.
5. The kidney tubules excrete excess H^+ in combination with phosphate and ammonia buffers. The H^+ is excreted in exchange for Na^+. The kidneys restore the bicarbonate level in the blood by absorbing HCO_3^- and Na^+.
6. The lungs excrete CO_2, which is the anhydride of carbonic acid (minus a water molecule), and thus help to regulate $[H^+]$ in the blood. Hyperventilation means that CO_2 is being excreted by the lungs (blown off) faster than it is produced in the body, as indicated by a low $Paco_2$. Hyperventilation cannot be identified accurately by observing an increased rate and depth of breathing. The rate might be normal. Hypoventilation means that the lungs are deficient in eliminating CO_2 thus the $Paco_2$ is increased.
7. The anion gap is actually a calculation of anions in the body that are unmeasured, such as organic acids and is calculated by subtracting the sum of the concentration of the major ECF anions from the cations. The normal value is 8 to 16, with a mean of 12. $Na^+ - (Cl^- + HCO_3^-)$. The anion gap helps to identify the type of metabolic acidosis.
8. *The isohydric principle* states that all buffer systems in a solution are in equilibrium with the same H^+. Thus one only needs to measure and analyze one buffer system. Clinically, we need only measure the $Paco_2$ and HCO_3^- to assess the acid-base status in the body.
9. The CO_2 content measures the alkali reserve of the body, which is primarily bicarbonate but also contains the carbonic acid component (which is small). CO_2 content is measured using venous blood. The CO_2 content should not be confused with the $Paco_2$, which is a measure of the pressure (tension) of dissolved CO_2 gas in arterial blood and is influenced by the lungs. The standard bicarbonate is measured after the blood specimen is equilibrated with CO_2 at a $Paco_2$ of 40 mm Hg, thus "eliminating" the effect of respiration on the bicarbonate concentration, and is therefore said to represent only metabolic changes in acid-base balance. In reality, the standard bicarbonate is no more accurate in estimating the bicarbonate concentration than the CO_2 content measure. The base excess (BE) is a method of identifying and assessing the severity of acid-base disorders. A positive value ($>+2$) means an excess of alkali (metabolic alkalosis), and a negative value (<-2) means a deficit of alkali (metabolic acidosis). Some authorities have criticized the BE, in particular, as misleading. Normal values: CO_2 content = 21 to 29 mEq/L; $Paco_2$ = 40 mm Hg; standard HCO_3^- = 22 to 26 mEq/L.

10. a. Examine the clinical history for potential causes.
    b. Note clinical signs and symptoms, which might indicate an acid-base imbalance.
    c. Examine laboratory data of electrolytes and other data for disease processes associated with acid-base disorders.
    d. Examine pH.
    e. Examine the $Paco_2$ and HCO_3^- in relationship to the pH and make a tentative decision about the primary disorder.
    f. Estimate the expected compensatory response to the primary acid-base disturbance.
    g. Calculate the anion gap and compare its change to the change in the bicarbonate concentration.
    h. Make the final interpretation

11. A value greater than or less than expected suggests a mixed acid-base disturbance.

12. (a) $NaHCO_3$ administration can shut off the respiratory drive, because the pH of the CSF may be increased; (b) it may cause postacidosis respiratory alkalosis as a result of persistent hyperventilation; (c) a complicating respiratory alkalosis may cause tissue hypoxia, because the oxyhemoglobin dissociation curve is shifted to the left; (d) metabolic alkalosis may result if $NaHCO_3$ is given to a patient with DKA; (e) a serious metabolic alkalosis may result in the treatment of cardiopulmonary arrest; (f) tetany and convulsions may occur in a patient with renal failure; (g) it may cause hypervolemia and pulmonary edema, particularly in patients with congestive heart failure or renal failure.

13. H^+; HCO_3^-

14. H^+; HCO_3^-

15. Hyperventilation or blowing off CO_2

16. Hypoventilation or CO_2 retention

17. a. The diarrhea suggests possible metabolic acidosis.
    b. Physical assessment data (orthostatic hypotension, weakness, poor skin turgor, dry mucus membranes) suggest an ECF volume deficit and is supported by the low urinary sodium. She may even have a K^+ deficit, since it is normal and not elevated in the presence of an acidosis.
    c. The pH shows an acidemia. The HCO_3 and $Paco_2$ are both decreased (change in the same direction) suggesting a compensated metabolic acidosis.
    d. For every 1 mEq decrease in HCO_3, expect a 1.2 mm Hg drop in the $Paco_2$; change in $HCO_3 = 12 (24 - 12)$; expected change in $Paco_2 = 25.6 (40 - [12 \times 1.2])$; actual $Paco_2 = 28$ mm Hg. Thus it

represents a simple compensated metabolic acidosis.
    e. $AG = 142 - (118 + 12) = 12$ mEq/L; normal anion gap
    f. Conclusion: normal anion gap, compensated metabolic acidosis

18. a. History suggests probable metabolic acidosis, an expected chronic disturbance with this condition.
    b. The creatinine and BUN indicate severe renal insufficiency.
    c. pH reveals acidemia. The HCO_3 and $Paco_2$ change in the same direction, showing respiratory compensation. The HCO_3 of 8 mEq/L indicates a moderately severe metabolic acidosis.
    d. The acid-base values fall within the metabolic acidosis confidence band on the acid-base nomogram, thus the disorder is probably not a mixed disorder. Change in $HCO_3^- = 16 (24 - 8)$. Expected drop in $Paco_2 = 20.8 (40 - [16 \times 1.2])$. Actual $Paco_2 = 24$ mm Hg. Might be a small amount of respiratory acidosis from fluid overload and wet lungs (data unavailable).
    e. $AG = 137 - (102 + 8) = 27$ mEq/L; increased anion gap common in renal failure because of the retention of fixed acids: sulphates, phosphates
    f. Conclusion: high anion gap, partly compensated metabolic acidosis

19. a. History suggests possible metabolic acidosis.
    b. Physical assessment and chest radiograph suggest acute respiratory acidosis.
    c. pH shows acidemia; the $Paco_2$ and HCO_3 have changed in opposite directions, suggesting a mixed disorder. Increase in the $Paco_2$ is much greater than is the decrease in the HCO_3, thus perhaps the respiratory acidosis is primary.
    d. Expected rise in $HCO_3 = 1$ mEq/L for every 10 mm Hg rise in the $Paco_2$; change in $Paco_2 = +20 (60 - 40) = 2 \times 10$. Expected $HCO_3 = 24 + (2 \times 1) = 26$ mEq/L; actual $= 15$ mEq/L; rise less than expected suggests mixed disorder.
    e. No data available
    f. Conclusion: acute respiratory acidosis superimposed on chronic metabolic acidosis

20. Acute respiratory acidosis secondary to probable pulmonary infection; no data are available to state whether man also has COPD in addition to probable pulmonary edema from CHF.

21. Chronic respiratory acidosis; kidneys are retaining HCO_3.

22. The patient has developed metabolic alkalosis secondary to diuretic therapy.

23. *Posthypercapneic metabolic alkalosis.* This condition is related to chloride

deficiency, which occurred during the development of chronic respiratory acidosis and was worsened by the administration of diuretics.

24. See answers 20 to 23 for probable causes.

CHAPTER 23

1. Transportation of ingested material from the pharynx to the stomach

2. Regurgitation is the backflow or welling up of gastric or esophageal contents into the oral cavity. Regurgitation is different from vomiting in that it is effortless and not accompanied by nausea.

3. The first symptom of esophageal tumor is usually dysphagia; it does not occur until the tumor involves the entire circumference of the esophagus, which is the main reason for the poor prognosis.

4. An *esophagomyotomy* is a surgical procedure on the lower esophagus to enlarge the opening into the stomach. A *pyloroplasty* is a procedure to repair the pylorus, particularly to enlarge the gastric outlet. These procedures are often used to treat achalasia and are often combined, because incompetence of the LES and reflux esophagitis may follow the myotomy. Enlarging the gastric outlet helps to prevent gastric reflux into the esophagus.

5. a. Avoid hot, cold, or spicy foods; eat bland foods.
    b. Eat slowly and chew food thoroughly before swallowing.
    c. Sleep with head of bed elevated.
    d. Take antacids.
    e. Avoid eating immediately before going to bed.
    f. Avoid tight clothes.
    g. Lose weight, if overweight.
    h. Avoid stooping and bending.
    i. Avoid straining to have a bowel movement (stool softeners may be necessary).
    j. Eat in a quiet, relaxed environment.
    k. Avoid alcohol and tobacco.

6. Refer to Figure 23-5. The most important mechanism preventing reflux is the zone of high pressure between the esophagus and stomach (physiologic LES). The acute gastroesophageal angle produces a flap-valve effect. The phrenoesophageal ligament produces a pinchcock-valve effect.

7. Chronic reflux esophagitis causes esophageal inflammation, ulcer formation, bleeding, and eventually scarring and stricture.

8. Because these patients often aspirate esophageal or gastric contents into the lungs, particularly during sleep

9. The symptom of pyrosis, or heartburn, is poorly correlated with the presence or absence of esophagitis.

Some patients with heartburn do not have evidence of esophagitis, and some patients with esophagitis caused by reflux may not have symptoms until the condition is advanced. The acid perfusion test is the best method of identifying esophagitis.

10. c
11. e
12. d
13. a
14. b
15. f
16. b
17. c, e
18. a, d

CHAPTER 24

1. Refer to Figure 24-1.
2. The outer layer of the stomach consists of peritoneum, which is reflected off the lesser curvature as the lesser omentum and off the greater curvature as the greater omentum.
3. Mucosal folds that allow for expansion of the stomach.
4. Pepsinogen is converted to pepsin in the presence of a low pH. Pepsin and HCl begin the process of protein digestion.
5. The extrinsic nerve supply of the stomach is entirely from the autonomic nervous system. Parasympathetic fibers travel via the vagus nerve and control gastric motor and secretory activity. Sympathetic fibers travel via the greater splanchnic nerves. Sympathetic stimulation inhibits gastric secretion and motility, which is opposite to the effect of vagal stimulation. Auerbach's and Meissner's nerve plexuses are involved in local reflexes and help to coordinate peristalsis. These plexuses constitute the intrinsic gastric innervation.
6. Celiac artery comes off the aorta; right and left gastric and gastroepiploic arteries supply most of the stomach.
7. Because posterior wall duodenal ulcers frequently erode into the gastroduodenal and pancreaticoduodenal arteries located immediately behind the duodenum
8. Reservoir function, mixing function, and emptying function
9. Barium radiologic studies; gastric analysis; endoscopy with a gastroscope; urea breath test
10. Intrinsic factor combines with vitamin B_{12} and is necessary for its absorption in the ileum. Vitamin B_{12} is necessary for the normal maturation of RBCs.
11. The peristaltic activity of the stomach has a basic intrinsic rhythm that is modified by nervous and hormonal factors. Gastrin stimulates gastric motility, as does parasympathetic stimulation, whereas sympathetic stimulation inhibits motility. Gastric

emptying is also controlled by nervous and hormonal factors elicited by distention of the duodenum and the physical and chemical state of the chyme as it enters the duodenum.
12. The gastric mucus forms a protective coat for the gastric mucosa against mechanical and chemical injury (Hollander). The mucus in the columnar epithelial cells and the tight junctions between the epithelial cells prevent back diffusion of H^+ (Davenport). Aspirin, alcohol, and bile salts are the most common substances causing disruption of the gastric mucosal barrier. The result is increased back diffusion of H^+, mucosal injury, and ulceration caused by the action of gastric acid and pepsin. The duodenum is protected by secretion of a highly alkaline, viscid mucus that neutralizes the acid chyme from the stomach. Brunner's glands in the duodenum produce the mucus.
13. Increases closure strength of the LES, thus preventing gastric reflux into the esophagus during gastric mixing; increases pyloric sphincter tone, thus preventing gastric emptying until mixing is completed; stimulates the secretion of acid and pepsin in the stomach so that protein digestion may begin; promotes receptive relaxation of the stomach thus filling can occur without an increase in intragastric pressure; stimulates gastric and intestinal motility thus mixing and propulsion of chyme is promoted; stimulates secretion of insulin, bile, and pancreatic juice.
14. Superficial inflammation of the gastric mucosa. If you have ever had "food poisoning" or "intestinal flu" with nausea, vomiting, or diarrhea, you no doubt have had acute superficial gastritis.
15. a. *Cephalic phase:* sight, smell, or thought of food is mediated through parasympathetic fibers of the vagus nerve, which stimulates gastric acid secretion.
    b. *Gastric phase:* antral distention is the prime stimulus to release of the hormone gastrin, which stimulates gastric acid secretion.
    c. *Intestinal phase:* of little importance in stimulating gastric acid secretion; influence is mainly inhibitory.
16. a
17. b
18. a, b, d
19. a, b, e, f

CHAPTER 25

1. Cytotoxic drugs interfere with the metabolism of all rapidly proliferating cells (cancer and leukemic cells). Because hair cells and the epithelial cells of the GI mucosa are the most rapidly proliferating cells in the body, they

are especially vulnerable to the effects of these drugs. Cell division is inhibited, resulting in atrophy of both the villi and the crypts of Lieberkühn, and ulceration and bleeding of the mucosa occur occasionally.
2. The secretion of bile from the liver aids the digestive process by emulsifying fats so that a greater surface area is presented for pancreatic action. Bile salts act as detergents solubilizing fatty acids, glycerides, and fat-soluble vitamins by the formation of micelles. These substances are thus held in solution until absorption takes place.
3. *Maldigestion* means that digestion of a particular nutrient failed to take place at some instance in the stepwise process of food breakdown into the simplest products that can be absorbed. Maldigestion can be caused by general lack of a secretion containing enzymes (pancreatic insufficiency) or lack of a specific enzyme (lactase insufficiency). Other causes of maldigestion are lack of mechanical breakdown of food particles, so that digestive enzymes cannot reach all the food substances, or a transit time through the intestine that is too rapid to allow time for hydrolysis by enzymes. Maldigestion always results in malabsorption, because nutrients cannot be absorbed until they have been hydrolyzed into the simplest substances.

    Malabsorption refers to lack of transport of a substance across the intestinal mucosa.
4. The stool is pale, large in volume, greasy, frothy, tends to float, tends to stick to the side of the toilet, and is difficult to flush away.
5. The lesion is granulomatous and similar to the lesion of tuberculosis. Because the tubercular lesion represents a hypersensitivity reaction (cellular immune mechanism), medical scientists have looked for an infectious agent and autoantibodies but have not been successful in identifying either.
6. Valvulae conniventes, villi, and microvilli
7. (a) Inadequate digestion as a result of rapid emptying of stomach and poor mixing; (b) insufficient stimulation of CCK release (which stimulates pancreatic secretion) caused by bypass of duodenum in Billroth II gastrectomy; (c) deconjugation of bile salts by abnormal bacterial proliferation in blind loop after Billroth II; (d) loss of reservoir function, resulting in dumping of stomach contents into small bowel, with rapid transit time.
8. When the small bowel is obstructed either mechanically or functionally, it loses its absorptive and forward propulsive capacity, thus GI secretions pool within the lumen. The re-

sulting ischemia of the intestinal wall from the distention further compromises the absorptive and motile function of the bowel, thus a vicious cycle of degeneration develops. The pooling of fluids in the gut depletes the ECF volume, resulting in hypovolemic shock. Bacterial proliferation occurs in the pooled fluids, and increased permeability of the ischemic mucosa allows absorption of bacteria and their toxins into the circulation, causing septicemia and toxemia.

9. Superior mesenteric
10. Pyloric; ileocecal
11. Mesentery
12. Greater omentum; infection
13. Ligament of Treitz
14. Valvulae conniventes
15. Villi
16. Crypts of Lieberkühn
17. Lacteal
18. Umbilicus; iliac; appendix

CHAPTER 26

1. Refer to Figure 26-1.
2. The absorption of water and the elimination of the wastes of digestion
3. The large intestine is one half as long as is the small intestine, with a diameter more than twice that of the small intestine. The external anal sphincter is under voluntary control, whereas the sphincters at each end of the small intestine are under autonomic control. The large intestine has no villi, its longitudinal muscle layer is incomplete throughout most of its length, and the mucosa contains more goblet cells than that of the small intestine. These structural differences between the small and large intestine are in keeping with their primary functions. The villi, large volume of secretions, and active motility pattern of the small intestine serve well its primary function of digestion and absorption. In contrast, the large intestine is much less motile, and although one of its main functions is absorption of water, it only absorbs about 1/13 the amount absorbed by the small intestine. The decreased motility allows more time for absorption, because its ability to absorb is lessened by its lack of villi. One of the functions of the large intestine is to act as a reservoir until elimination can take place. The increased number of goblet cells and increased mucus secretion are important because the feces are semisolid in the large intestine and lubrication is more necessary for propulsion of the fecal mass.
4. *Haustral churning* refers to back-and-forth pendular movements that are especially prominent in the transverse colon, caused by annular contractions of short segments of the bowel, particularly the circular muscles. These movements allow time for the absorption of water. *Mass peristalsis* is a contraction involving a long segment of the large intestine that propels a large amount of fecal material forward. Feces are frequently moved into the rectum by mass peristalsis, and the defecation reflex is initiated.
5. Hemorrhoids, constipation, cancer of the rectum, anorectal abscesses, fissures, and fistulas
6. a. *Palpation of abdomen:* presence of mass, tenderness
   b. *Rectal digital examination:* palpation of tumors, hemorrhoids
   c. *Proctosigmoidoscopic examination:* direct visualization of tumors, internal hemorrhoids, ulcerated or hyperemic mucosa; biopsy or cell washings may also be obtained for histologic study (lower 25 cm of bowel observed)
   d. *Colonoscopy:* direct visualization of entire large bowel with same information obtained as above
   e. *Barium enema radiography:* neoplasms, strictures, diverticula, and polyps may all be visualized.
   f. *Stool examination:* blood, parasites, shape, and size may give clues to many disorders of the GI tract.
7. Only a small percentage of the patients with diverticulitis require surgery. Surgery is indicated when disease or complications such as perforation is severe and extensive. During an attack of acute diverticulitis, the medical treatment usually consists of bedrest, liquid diet, stool softeners, and antibiotics.
8. Ulcerative colitis of more than 10 years' duration; certain types of colonic polyps; eating a diet low in fiber and high in refined carbohydrates
9. Burkitt proposed that slow transit with low-fiber diets permits bacterial action on bile acids or other normal bowel constituents to produce carcinogens, which then act on the colonic mucosa.
10. Because the superior hemorrhoidal vein is connected to the portal system, increased portal pressure may cause backflow into these veins and hemorrhoids.
11. A *fissure in ano* is a persistent crack in the perianal skin. A *fistula in ano* is an abnormal granulation-lined tract connecting two epithelial surfaces—in this region running between the anal canal and the skin of the perianal area. A fistula in ano is the consequence of anorectal abscess that has been inadequately treated. Any of these conditions may be a complication of hemorrhoids. Crohn's disease of the colon is especially likely to be associated with anorectal fistulas.
12. Diverticulosis; diverticulitis
13. Pedunculated; juvenile; villous; familial polyposis
14. Annular; polypoid
15. Direct extension to adjacent structure; metastasis via lymph nodes; metastasis via bloodstream
16. Superior; middle; inside; inferior
17. Bleeding; thrombosis; strangulation

CHAPTER 27

1. Blood circulation through the liver is unusual because a mixture of portal venous blood and arterial blood flows through the liver sinusoids. The portal blood contains many nutrients absorbed from the intestines that are metabolized in the liver.
2. The *gallbladder* is a pear-shaped hollow muscular bag that has a capacity of about 45 ml; its primary function is to concentrate hepatic bile transported to the gallbladder via the cystic duct. Bile is stored in the gallbladder and released as needed for digestion of fats in the intestine. Cholecystokinin-pancreozymin stimulates the gallbladder to contract and release bile. The *pancreas* is about 6 inches in length and $1^{1}/_{2}$ inches wide and resembles a bunch of grapes. The main pancreatic duct runs through the entire length of the organ and opens into the duodenum. An accessory pancreatic duct (duct of Santorini) may also open into the duodenum at a different point. The pancreas has an exocrine secretion, pancreatic juice from the acini, and endocrine secretions, glucagon and insulin, produced by the alpha and beta cells in the islands of Langerhans. The release of pancreatic juice is controlled by CCK and secretin.
3. a. Formation and excretion of bile; carbohydrate metabolism, including synthesis, storage, and release of glucose to maintain proper blood level; protein metabolism, including synthesis of most proteins, urea formation, and storage of amino acids; fat metabolism, including cholesterol synthesis and fat storage; storage of many vitamins and minerals; metabolism of steroid hormones; detoxification of both endogenous and exogenous substances that are potentially harmful; acting as flood chamber and filter
   b. The liver is called an organ of defense because of its large concentration of phagocytic Kupffer cells lining the sinusoids. These cells are actually part of the monocyte-macrophage (reticuloendothelial) defense system.
   c. The liver is capable of holding a liter or more of blood and holds a strategic position between the in-

testinal and general circulation; it can serve as a reservoir (flood chamber) when blood backs up, as in right ventricular failure. Sudden release of the blood from the reservoir can cause circulatory overload and pulmonary congestion.

d. The liver detoxifies drugs and other potentially harmful chemicals by oxidation, reduction, hydrolysis, or conjugation so that they become physiologically inactive. Conjugation with glucuronic acid, for example, makes the substance water soluble thus it may be excreted in the urine.

e. The liver is the central chemical laboratory for the metabolism of carbohydrates, fats, and proteins, and this role alone makes the liver essential for life; it plays a major role in the regulation of blood glucose, serum lipids, serum proteins, and coagulation factors.

4. Excess production of bilirubin exceeding the processing ability of the liver; impaired uptake of unconjugated bilirubin; impaired conjugation; and impaired excretion of bilirubin

5. *Kernicterus* is the deposition of bilirubin in lipid-rich brain, particularly the basal ganglia, causing damage to the cells by its toxic action. Kernicterus occurs when levels of unconjugated bilirubin (lipid-soluble) in the blood are high.

6. The jaundice is physiologic because the immaturity of the liver leads to relative deficiency of the glucuronyl transferase, which conjugates free bilirubin with glucuronic acid. The acceptor proteins may also be inadequate, thus uptake by the hepatocyte is also deficient.

7. No; it is useful only in helping to prevent hepatitis in exposed individuals, particularly hepatitis A.

8. a. *Community:* safe and inspected water supply and sewage disposal; inspection of all wells and septic tanks; restaurant inspection; inspection of public swimming pools and beaches for safety of water

b. *Home:* good general sanitary habits—hand washing, separate drinking glasses and eating utensils, adequate dish washing and sterilization

c. *Clinical unit:* use of disposable syringes, needles, and catheters; screening of blood for hepatitis B antigen; careful disposal of urine and feces from infected patients; hand washing; avoidance of needle puncture; isolation of infected patients in a private room with separate bathroom facilities, disposable dishes, and gowns and gloves worn by workers attending patient

9. About 90% removal or destruction of the liver is still compatible with life. Complete removal results in death in about 10 hours.

10. (a) Triangular, 1500, right upper; (b) kidney, gallbladder; (c) stomach, pancreas; (d) falciform; (e) capsule of Glisson

11. (a) Bile, hepatic, hepatic; (b) cystic, bile; (c) pancreatic, Vater; (d) Oddi

12. (a) Hepatic portal, hepatic, vena cava; (b) portal; (c) hepatic; (d) spleen, esophageal, rectal

13. (a) Lobule; (b) sinusoids, Kupffer; (c) canaliculi

14. *Alcoholic hepatitis* is a lesion characterized by hepatocellular necrosis and infiltration with inflammatory cells; it is associated with alcohol ingestion and is believed to be the critical lesion in the development of Laënnec's cirrhosis.

15. Because cirrhosis is generally silent until far advanced, when major signs and symptoms appear. Early symptoms are vague and nonspecific, thus patients do not seek medical help.

16. *Portal hypertension* is a sustained elevation of the portal venous pressure above the normal 6 to 12 cm H_2O. The primary mechanism causing portal hypertension is increased resistance to blood flow through the liver. Portal hypertension can occur in cirrhosis, congestive heart failure (backup of blood from right atrium), and hepatic vein thrombosis. Increased inflow through the splanchnic arteries in cirrhosis also contributes to portal hypertension.

17. Compression of varices by esophageal and gastric balloons (Sengstaken-Blakemore tube); vasopressin infusion. Removing the blood from the GI tract is important because large amounts of ammonia may be produced from the action of gut bacteria on the blood protein. The ammonia may reach the systemic circulation, causing hepatic encephalopathy by interfering with cerebral metabolism. Reducing the pressure and blood flow through the varices by creating a surgical shunt between the portal and systemic circulation may prevent recurrent bleeding from esophageal varices. Flow through the esophageal veins is reduced, but ammonia and other protein metabolites may pass directly into the systemic circulation, causing hepatic encephalopathy.

18. a. *Hepatic encephalopathy* is a form of cerebral intoxication caused by ammonia or other protein metabolites or both. Hepatic encephalopathy is demonstrated clinically by a neuropsychiatric syndrome characterized by mental clouding and neu-

romuscular dysfunction progressing to coma.

b. Hepatic encephalopathy occurs when more ammonia is presented to the liver than the failing cells can synthesize into urea or when the ammonia bypasses the liver through shunts and enters the systemic circulation.

c. Detecting hepatic encephalopathy during the early stages is important because prompt treatment may be successful in reversing the process. The mortality is high if the condition progresses to an advanced stage.

19. *Asterixis* is a peripheral manifestation of impaired cerebral metabolism characterized by a peculiar flapping tremor of the wrists and metacarpophalangeal joints; it is tested by having the patient extend both arms out with fingers spread.

20. *Constructional apraxia* is the inability to construct simple diagrams or to write legibly in the absence of paralysis or motor weakness. Deterioration in the ability to perform purposeful, skilled construction or to write reflects the progress of the encephalopathy, and a serial record can be kept in the patient's records.

21. a. *Stage I:* slowness of mentation and affect, untidiness, slurred speech, personality change, inappropriate behavior, disordered sleep rhythm

b. *Stage II:* accentuation of stage I, inappropriate behavior, lethargy, asterixis, muscle tremor

c. *Stage III:* sleeps most of time but can be aroused; marked confusion, may be abusive and violent; abnormal EEG pattern

d. *Stage IV:* comatose, positive Babinski's sign, hyperactive reflexes, abnormal EEG, hepatic fetor sometimes detected

22. In *acute cholecystitis,* the patient has a sudden onset of severe pain in the right upper quadrant that may last for several hours and is often associated with the passage of a gallstone through the cystic or common bile duct. Tenderness over the gallbladder may be present. *Chronic cholecystitis* is characterized by symptoms that are much milder. Episodes of mild pain in the right upper quadrant and a long history of dyspepsia, flatulence, heartburn, and fat intolerance may be present.

23. Because the liver acts as a filter, with about one third of the cardiac output traversing it each minute. Malignant cells transported from the intestines, stomach, or pancreas through the portal vein are readily trapped in the liver capillary bed.

24. a. The primary mechanism causing *ascites* is resistance to blood flow

through the liver resulting in portal hypertension. Portal hypertension raises the hydrostatic pressure in the intestinal vascular bed, which favors the transudation of fluid from the intravascular space to the interstitial space, resulting in ascites. Other mechanisms contributing to the development of ascites include hypoalbuminemia (decreased liver synthesis), which causes decreased colloid osmotic pressure (COP), favoring transudation; increased production and flow of hepatic lymph (caused by the portal hypertension), which "weeps" a high-protein fluid into the ascitic fluid in the peritoneal cavity and raises the COP in ascitic fluid, which favors more transudation; and retention of Na$^+$ and water because of increased aldosterone (because less is inactivated by the failing liver cells).

b. Signs and symptoms of ascites include increased abdominal girth, bulging flanks, and shortness of breath when the volume is large.

c. Treatment consists of a low-sodium diet and the judicious use of diuretics. Paracentesis should be used only when the volume of fluid is great enough to cause respiratory distress and for diagnostic purposes.

CHAPTER 28

1. Venae cavae → right atrium → pulmonary artery → lung capillaries → pulmonary veins → left atrium → left ventricle → aorta → systemic arteries → arterioles → capillaries → venules → systemic veins

2. The AV node delays the wave of electrical excitation to allow time for ventricular filling during atrial contraction before ventricular contraction: it also prevents an excessive number of electrical impulses from reaching the ventricles.

3. The thickness of the right ventricle is only one third that of the left ventricle. These differences in muscular size reflect their respective pumping functions in the circulatory system. The right ventricle pumps blood through the low-pressure, low-resistance pulmonary circuit. The workload of the left ventricle is much greater than that of the right, because it must generate about five times as much pressure to overcome the high resistance of the systemic circulation.

4. To support the AV valves during ventricular contraction and prevent leaflet eversion into the atria

5. Three; aortic valves; sinuses of Valsalva; to protect the coronary orifices

from occlusion by the aortic valve cusps during ventricular ejection

6. The visceral and parietal pericardium; this small space contains a small amount of lubricating fluid that functions as protection against friction.

7. Lymph is propelled by muscle compression of the lymph vessels. Flow is aided by lymphatic peristalsis.

8. Sympathetic stimulation of the alpha receptors causes vasoconstriction, whereas stimulation of beta receptors causes vasodilation. This vasodilatory effect is produced by beta$_2$ receptors. In contrast, the beta$_1$ receptors produce cardiac effects of increased heart rate, force of contraction, and velocity of AV conduction.

9. Automaticity; excitability; conductivity; rhythmicity

10. Valves

11. Collateral

12. Right coronary; left anterior descending

13. 60 to 100; 40 to 60; 15 to 40

14. Smooth muscle cells; resistance

CHAPTER 29

1. Systole and diastole represent the mechanical activity of the heart. *Systole* is the period during which the heart muscle contracts; *diastole* indicates the resting period of the heart during which the muscles relax. The terms *systole* and *diastole* are typically used in referring to ventricular activity. The ECG represents a body surface recording of the summated electrical activity of all the myocardial cells. An action potential is an intracellular recording of the electrical activity of a single cell. Electrical activity stimulates mechanical activity.

2. The Frank-Starling mechanism states that, within limits, the force of contraction is a function of the length of muscle fibers, that is, their end-diastolic length. Thus the horizontal axis of the ventricular function curve represents the stretching of the myocardium. As the degree of stretch and EDV increases, the SV, or ventricular performance, increases (vertical axis). However, where the curve flattens, no increase in performance occurs as EDV increases. Then, with further EDV increases, dyspnea and finally pulmonary edema develop. The position of the ventricular function curve represents the degree of contractility. When the curve is shifted to the left (increased contractility caused by influence of norepinephrine or Ca^{++}), greater increase in ventricular performance or SV occurs at a given EDV or degree of muscle fiber length (the curve is steeper). A shift of the curve to the right represents myocardial depression and decreased contractility, thus a

smaller increase in SV occurs for increments in stretch or EDV. The ejection fraction (EF) (SV ÷ EDV) is a good index of contractility. A steeper curve indicates greater contractility . From these relationships, it can be seen that contractility has a greater influence on ventricular performance than does the Starling mechanism (increasing EDV to increase performance).

3. *Ohm's law,* stated in terms of the circulation, says that the volume of blood circulated per minute is directly related to the systemic blood pressure gradient and inversely related to the resistance ($Q = \Delta P/R$). The systemic blood pressure gradient is calculated by subtracting pressures at the arterial and venous end of the circulation (i.e., mean arterial pressure – central venous pressure).

4. SV = EDV – ESV = 100 ml – 30 ml = 70 ml (which is in the normal range). CI = CO ÷ body surface area = 4.5 L/minute ÷ 1.5 m^2 = 3.0 (which is also in the normal range). EF = SV ÷ EDV = 70 ÷ 100 = 0.70 (the EF should be 2/3, or 0.67; thus it is normal).

5. d

6. c

7. a

8. e

9. b

10. f

11. Absolute refractory; relative refractory

12. Negatively; potassium; sodium

13. Open; closed

14. Closed; open

15. AV node

16. Atrial contraction; atrial kick

17. b

18. c

19. a

20. d, f

21. e

CHAPTER 30

1. Class III

2. The left carotid may be partially occluded, possibly because of an atherosclerotic plaque. Her MAP is about 126 mm Hg. MAP = diastolic blood pressure + pulse pressure/3 = 100 + 78/3 = 126.

3. The *hepatojugular test* is performed by manually applying pressure over the right upper quadrant of the abdomen for 30 to 60 seconds and simultaneously observing the jugular veins. A rise in the level of the venous pressure head in the neck veins indicates a positive test. A positive test signifies that the right side of the heart was unable to accept the increased venous return (main source, venous reservoir in the liver, which is being compressed), which might result from right ventricular failure.

4. The *hexaxial reference system* is a representation of all the limb leads of the electrocardiogram (ECG). The system is formed by moving the bipolar limb leads centrally so that these lines intersect. The position of the heart may be pictured at the center of this electrical reference system. When the unipolar limb leads are added to the reference system, the hexaxial reference system is produced. Using this reference system, the summation vector, or electrical axis, for the P, QRS, and T waves can be derived. An analysis of deviations of the electrical axis from the various leads assists in diagnosing conditions such as conduction abnormalities and chamber enlargement.

5. Pressures in the various cardiac chambers and great vessels may be recorded and the waveforms of the pressure tracings analyzed to detect valvular stenosis and regurgitation. The injection of radiopaque material into the various cardiac chambers allows visualization of chamber size and wall movement so that deviations from normal may be detected. Cardiac output may also be determined. Sampling of oxygen content in the right and left sides of the heart allows detection of right-to-left shunts, as from a ruptured septum. Selective coronary artery angiography allows detection of lesions in these vessels.

6. Indications for coronary angiography: (a) to determine the feasibility of coronary bypass surgery; (b) to evaluate atypical angina; and (c) to evaluate the results of coronary revascularization surgery.

7. c
8. d
9. b
10. f
11. a
12. e
13. a
14. d
15. c
16. c
17. b
18. c
19. a
20. b
21. d
22. e
23. b
24. c
25. a
26. f
27. Regurgitation
28. 5 mm Hg; aortic stenosis
29. Turbulent

CHAPTER 31

1. Oxygen demand is greater for the left ventricle than it is for the right because of its greater workload and larger muscle mass. Oxygen supply is more restricted because little coronary perfusion of the left ventricle occurs during systole. The firm compression of blood vessels by the thick muscular wall limits perfusion during systole. On the other hand, the thinner-walled right ventricle continues to have some perfusion during systole.

2. Atherosclerotic lesions tend to occur in the epicardial proximal segments of the right and left coronary arteries and at points of abrupt curvature, as where the left coronary artery branches into the left anterior descending.

3. Size and location of the infarct; function of the uninvolved myocardium; collateral circulation; cardiovascular compensatory mechanisms

4. A *vasovagal response* is a reflex parasympathetic response resulting from pain or stimulation of parasympathetic ganglia in the myocardium. The effect is to slow the heart rate and reduce the blood pressure and cardiac output. Thus the response has an adverse effect in myocardial infarction, because sympathetic support of the compromised circulation is needed.

5. Severe, prolonged chest pain; elevated serum cardiac enzymes; ECG changes in leads overlying the area of necrosis (deep Q waves, ST segment elevation, inverted T waves)

6. Because cardiac output is a function of heart rate and stroke volume, a slow heart rate can reduce the total volume ejected in a given time by lowering the frequency of ejection. A rapid rate reduces ventricular filling time, thus less blood is ejected per beat. Tachycardia also reduces the length of diastole, thus perfusion time of the myocardium is limited. Oxygen supply is therefore reduced at the same time that demand is increased because of the increased cardiac work.

7. Heart rate, force of contraction, and arterial pressure (a determinant of wall tension)

8. Silent ischemia is the absence of a normal anginal warning system in that no painful angina is perceived. Rather, many patients experience an anginal equivalent, such as shortness of breath; silent ischemia is prevalent in patients with diabetes and theorized to be the result of autonomic neuropathy.

9. CK and CK-MB and the troponins, cTnT and cTnI

10. ACE inhibitors prevent the conversion of angiotensin I to angiotensin II, thereby decreasing preload and afterload. Less circulating angiotensin II (a powerful vasoconstrictor), translates into lower systolic blood pressure and afterload.

Decreased aldosterone secretion, resulting in less sodium and water retention, occurs with less circulating angiotensin II ultimately reducing preload.

11. The patient needs individualized guidance and teaching to achieve maximal functional ability. Both psychologic and physical variables are involved.

12. Ischemia
13. Increases
14. b, d, a, c
15. a
16. b
17. b
18. a
19. b
20. a
21. a
22. a
23. b
24. d
25. a
26. c
27. b

CHAPTER 32

1. a. Recurrent attacks of rheumatic fever: most common cause
   b. Subacute bacterial endocarditis: most infections in patients with rheumatic or congenital heart deformities
   c. Papillary muscle dysfunction or rupture: may be a complication of myocardial infarction
   d. Congenital malformations
   e. Inborn defects of connective tissue

2. Functional AV regurgitation is regurgitation secondary to chamber enlargement. As a result of ventricular chamber enlargement, the papillary muscles and chordae tendineae are unable to anchor the valve leaflets securely. The valvular annulus may also enlarge.

3. Prophylactic antibiotics are necessary to reduce the risk of bacterial endocarditis in susceptible patients, including those with a history of rheumatic carditis and those with cardiac deformities. Even minor procedures such as dental work and urinary catheterization may cause a transient bacteremia and the implantation of organisms on the endocardial surface.

4. a. Pulmonary congestion: diuretics to decrease blood volume; digitalis to increase heart contractility
   b. Atrial fibrillation: antidysrhythmic drugs
   c. Systemic emboli: anticoagulant drugs

5. Splitting of fused valvular commissures by the surgical introduction of an instrument to dilate them by blunt pressure or by inflating a balloon

6. The *Jones criteria* consist of a list of major and minor manifestations used to help establish a diagnosis of rheumatic fever. If evidence indicates that the sub-

ject has had a preceding streptococcal infection (positive throat culture (ASO titer) and also has two major manifestations or one major and two minor manifestations, a diagnosis of rheumatic fever is made. Major manifestations include carditis, polyarthritis, erythema marginatum, and subcutaneous nodules. Minor manifestations are fever, arthralgia, elevated ESR or CRP and prolonged PR interval.

7. a, c, e, f
8. b, d, f

CHAPTER 33

1. Circulatory; pump
2. Left atrial pressure; pulmonary venous; pulmonary edema
3. Heart failure
4. 40
5. Patient; reservoir
6. Venae cavae; oxygenator; aorta; femoral artery
7. 3, 5, 1, 7, 2, 4, 6
8. Concentric; eccentric; dilation
9. b, e, f
10. a, c, d
11. b
12. e
13. f
14. a
15. c
16. d
17. c
18. a
19. b
20. a
21. c
22. b
23. a

CHAPTER 34

1. a. 4; b. 3; c. 6; d. 2; e. 5; f. 8; g. 1; h. 7
2. *Varicose veins* are dilated, tortuous veins generally present in the lower extremities. Pathogenic factors include inflammatory destruction of valves, weak vein walls, and increased venous pressure (as in pregnancy), all of which cause varying degrees of valvular incompetence and regurgitation. The two major complications of varicosities are thrombosis and venous ulcer, both of which result from venous stasis. A *varicosity* differs from an aneurysm in that the vessel is affected throughout a significant segment of its length, whereas an aneurysm generally involves a short segment of a blood vessel.
3. DVT is more serious because of the potential complication of pulmonary embolus. The superficial veins may become distended as a result of impaired deep venous drainage.
4. Early ambulation, leg exercises, oral anticoagulants, external intermittent compression, elastic stockings, and elevation of the lower extremities to

promote deep venous drainage are all methods of preventing DVT.
5. An *aneurysm* is a localized dilation of the arterial wall, resulting from degeneration and weakening of the medial layer of the artery. Aneurysms are frequently asymptomatic. The first sign of disease may be a serious, potentially life-threatening complication, such as rupture, acute thrombosis, or embolization.
6. The deposition of the products of red blood cell destruction such as hemosiderin, caused by venous stasis with subsequent capillary destruction, results in the brownish skin discoloration present in patients with chronic venous insufficiency (CVI).
7. Stasis of blood flow, endothelial injury, and hypercoagulability
8. Thrombophlebitis; phlebothrombosis
9. Thromboangiitis obliterans
10. b
11. a
12. c
13. d
14. c
15. b
16. a

CHAPTER 35

1. Infections, malignant diseases, and chronic bronchitis and emphysema
2. *Respiration* is the combined activity of the various mechanisms that supply O_2 to the body cells and remove CO_2.
3. The blanket of mucus serves to trap dust and bacteria, which are then moved by ciliary action to the pharynx, where they are swallowed or expectorated. Inspired air is also humidified and warmed by the mucus blanket and underlying vascular network.
4. The right main stem bronchus compared with the left mainstream bronchus is larger and runs a more vertical course from the trachea.
5. The lung would collapse (atelectasis).
6. The lung has a dual blood supply: the bronchial and the pulmonary circulation. (Did you remember to include the bronchial circulation?) The pulmonary circulation is a low-pressure, low- resistance system (the mean pulmonary artery pressure, at 15 mm Hg, is only approximately one sixth that of the systemic circulation, at approximately 90 mm Hg).
7. Yes; a net pressure of 10 mm Hg occurs in the direction of the alveolus.
8. Larynx or glottis
9. Surfactant; surface tension
10. Ventilation; respiratory bellows; diaphragm
11. Hering-Breuer
12. Pons and medulla
13. a. 6; b. 3; c. 1; d. 5; e. 7; f. 8; g. 9; h. 4; i. 10; j. 2; k. 12; l. 11
14. a. 4; b. 5; c. 2; d. 1; e. 7; f. 6; g. 3

15. Because of dilution with water vapor and other gases in the anatomic dead space
16. The volume of anatomic dead space is equal to 1 ml/lb of body weight; if you weigh 120 pounds, your anatomic dead space is approximately 120 ml.
17. Diffusion; the driving force is the pressure gradient between the partial pressure of the gas in the alveolus and in the pulmonary capillary.
18. No; perfusion increases going from the apex to the base of the lungs because of the effect of gravity in the low-pressure, low-resistance pulmonary circulation. The overall $\dot{V}/\dot{Q}$ is 0.8, which is less than unity.
19. $\dot{V}/\dot{Q} = 3$ L/min $\div 6$ L/min $= 0.5$. This value would represent wasted perfusion and would be present in a shunt-producing disease.
20. More O_2 could be transported to the tissues in physical solution, which might make the critical difference in cases where there is very little hemoglobin (Hb) available to transport O_2 to the tissue cells.
21. No; an increased concentration of O_2 in the inspired air will be wasted, because the blood is already 97% to 98% saturated when it leaves the lungs and the O_2 content is normal. An examination of the HbO_2 dissociation curve (flat upper portion) shows that little if any advantage could be gained.
22. The **S** shape of the HbO_2 dissociation curve indicates that under normal environmental conditions, large changes of Po_2 of the inspired air cause only small changes in HbO_2 saturation. Even at a Po_2 of 50 mm Hg in the alveoli, Hb is 80% to 85% saturated with O_2, which is sufficient to meet tissue demands for O_2 under most conditions.
23. The Bohr effect is the slight shift to the right of the HbO_2 dissociation curve caused by the increase in acidity as a result of the effect of CO_2 being released from the tissues. The rightward shift in the curve causes O_2 to be more easily released from its association with Hb and thus facilitates tissue uptake of O_2.
24. Although alveolar Po_2 may be increased slightly by hyperventilation, this does not significantly increase the O_2 content of the arterial blood, because of the sigmoid shape of the O_2 dissociation curve and because blood leaving normally ventilated alveoli is already almost fully saturated with O_2. The CO_2 dissociation curve, however, is linear in shape, indicating that the CO_2 content of the blood is directly related to the alveolar Pco_2. When CO_2 is "washed out" of the lungs during hyperventilation, the CO_2 content of the blood is similarly reduced.

25. If diffusion were impaired enough to affect CO_2 transport, the patient would be dead. CO_2 diffuses more readily than O_2 does at the same pressure gradient. Even a minute pressure gradient (less than 1 mm Hg) is enough to ensure elimination of all the CO_2 produced at rest.

26. No; knowledge of the blood gases does not give information about the extent to which the tissues are being perfused, the quantity of O_2 that is being delivered to the tissues, and the PO_2 in the tissue cells. Data must be available on Hb concentration and adequacy of cardiac function and other clinical observations must be made to assess the adequacy of respiratory function. All data must be correlated, and the final judgment is a clinical one.

27. All the following are examples of altered mechanisms or conditions that may interfere with normal respiration: (1) low PO_2 of inspired air: high altitudes; (2) depression of respiratory center: barbiturate overdose; (3) alveolar hypoventilation from inadequate bellows function: obesity, deformed chest cage, weak respiratory muscles; (4) impaired diffusion of gases at the alveolocapillary membrane: pulmonary edema or fibrosis; (5) $\dot{V}/\dot{Q}$ imbalance: pneumonia or pulmonary embolism; (6) impaired transport of blood gases by systemic circulation: anemia, CO poisoning, inadequate cardiac output or shunting by tissues as in shock; (7) impairment of gas diffusion at tissue level: edema.

28. Stage 1 is *ventilation:* flow of air into and out of the lungs effected by the respiratory bellows.

    Stage 2 is *transportation:* includes the diffusion of gases between the alveolus and the pulmonary blood and between the tissue cells and the systemic blood. Transportation also includes the distribution of the pulmonary and systemic blood and the distribution of air in the lungs.

    Stage 3 is *cell respiration:* oxidation of cell metabolites with the production of energy, water, and CO_2.

29. Normal inspiration is principally caused by contraction of the diaphragm and the muscles elevating the rib cage (sternocleidomastoids, serrati, scalene, scapular elevators). Activity in these muscles during forceful inspiration is increased. Expiration involves the relaxation of these muscles and is largely passive. The internal intercostal and abdominal muscles are more active during forced expiration.

30. 201 ml/min (12 g/dl × 1.34 ml/g × 5000 ml/min × 0.25)

31. Mixed venous blood containing reduced Hb from the bronchial circulation is mixed with oxygenated pulmonary blood leaving the lungs, thus accounting for the slight reduction in Hb saturation.

32. Decreases; increases (alkalosis); shifts to the left; thus Hb is reluctant to release O_2 to the tissues

33. 42 mm Hg ([247 − 47] × 0.21); no, a PO_2 of 42 mm Hg would barely be able to supply tissue O_2 requirements at rest. The climber might be expected to pass out unless he uses cylinder O_2 supply.

34. Increase; decrease; less; into

35. Ascends; decreasing

36. Increase; more; out of

37. Normal; low; low

38. Decrease; increase; alkalosis

39. Right; decreased

CHAPTER 36

1. Routine chest radiography, CT, MRI, ultrasound, angiography, lung scans

2. (a) Status of the thoracic cage, including the ribs, pleura, and contour of the diaphragm and of the upper airway as it enters the chest; (b) the size, contour, and position of the mediastinum and hilus of the lung, including the heart, aorta, lymph nodes, and root of the bronchial tree; (c) the texture and degree of aeration of the lung parenchyma; (d) the size, shape, number, and location of pulmonary lesions, including cavitation, fibrous markings, and zones of consolidation

3. b

4. a

5. c

6. h

7. d

8. e

9. i

10. f

11. g

12. The chief value of ventilatory function tests is that quantitative data are provided to assess the degree of pulmonary disability, follow the progress of the disability, and assess response to treatment. Generally, ventilatory function test data are not specifically diagnostic, although patterns of disordered pulmonary function may be discerned. Blood gas measurements, as well as ventilatory function tests, provide quantitative data to assess the degree of respiratory insufficiency and are particularly helpful in guiding O_2 therapy, but these data do not provide all the information necessary to assess total respiratory function.

13. Alveolar ventilation takes into account the amount of air wasted in ventilating the dead space.

14. Measurements of the change in volume at different degrees of lung inflation and the change in alveolar or intrapleural pressure measured by means of an esophageal balloon are made simultaneously. Compliance is then calculated by the following formula:

$$\text{Compliance} = \frac{\Delta \text{ volume}}{\Delta \text{ pressure}}$$

15. Causes of decreased lung compliance include pulmonary fibrosis, pulmonary edema, pneumonia, and deficiency of surfactant. Causes of decreased thoracic cage compliance include obesity, abdominal distention, and skeletal deformities of the chest cage.

16. The emphysema patient whose main problem is increased airways resistance caused by premature collapse of the airways during expiration adopts a slow, deep pattern of respiration to minimize the work of breathing. Airflow is less turbulent with slow, deep respirations.

17. The chief problem for a patient with stiff lungs is an increase in the elastic resistance. The work of breathing is minimized by a rapid, shallow pattern of respiration.

18. The radial artery is usually chosen for the arterial puncture because of its easy access. The wrist is extended (positioned over a rolled towel) and the artery is stabilized with two fingers of one hand, while the arterial puncture is made with the other hand using a heparinized syringe. Air is displaced from the blood specimen. Finally, the specimen is placed on ice and taken to the blood gas laboratory.

19. *Hyperventilation* can occur as a result of anxiety, brain injury, and pneumonia; it may also be secondary to metabolic acidosis occurring as compensation. Causes of *hypoventilation* include narcotic or barbiturate overdose and increased physiologic dead space; it may also occur as a compensation for metabolic alkalosis.

20. *Hypoxemia* is caused by ventilation/perfusion imbalance, alveolar hypoventilation, impaired diffusion, and intrapulmonary anatomic shunts. Hypoxemia caused by intrapulmonary anatomic shunting is not corrected by O_2 administration because the blood bypasses the pulmonary unit.

21. Refer to Table 36-5 and text.

CHAPTER 37

1. c

2. f

3. g

4. b

5. a

6. e

7. d

8. *Digital clubbing* refers to a loss of the base angle of the nail thus this angle is greater than the normal 160 degrees; bulbous changes in the digital

tips are also indicative of clubbing. Loss of the base angle is the earliest sign of digital clubbing, whereas the bulbous change is a late sign. Digital clubbing is important to detect because it is frequently associated with pulmonary disease (particularly bronchogenic carcinoma), cardiovascular disease, and GI disease.

9. Inspection of the buccal mucosa, particularly under the tongue, is the most reliable method of detecting central cyanosis in African-American and Caucasian patients. The lighting must be good, preferably daylight.

CHAPTER 38

1. An increased resistance to airflow
2. All three diseases may exist in the pure form, although it is more common for patients to show aspects of all these diseases. It is especially common for patients to have features of chronic bronchitis and emphysema at the same time. This overlap and difficulty in separating the diseases are the reason for the label COPD.
3. An asthmatic attack is characterized by orthopnea (having to sit up to breathe), dyspnea, fear of suffocation, prolonged wheezing expirations, and subsequent cough and sputum production. Treatment consists of bronchodilator drugs and oxygen, if the blood gases are abnormal. Corticosteroid drugs are used occasionally for severe attacks. Long-term therapy consists of desensitization and avoidance of known allergens. Status asthmaticus is a prolonged, severe attack of asthma that may cause ventilatory insufficiency so severe that death results.

4.

Feature	CLE	PLE
Sex prevalence	More common in males	Equal sex distribution
Etiology	Associated with smoking	Possible genetic factor
Pathologic anatomy	Respiratory bronchioles primarily affected	Entire acinus affected
Part of lung affected	Uneven distribution; upper lobes may be more severely affected	Uniform in distribution; basal lung more severely affected
Type of associated COPD	Chronic bronchitis	Primary emphysema; chronic bronchitis; aging

5. Measures to relieve obstruction of the small airways; cessation of smoking; avoidance of air pollutants; prompt treatment of infection; administration of bronchodilator drugs, continuous low flow O_2 therapy, breathing exercises, exercise program
6. Excessive production of mucus, chronic cough; 3 months per year for 2 consecutive years
7. Abnormal enlargement of the alveoli and alveolar ducts and destruction of the alveolar walls
8. Blebs; ruptured alveoli
9. Bullae; check valve obstruction of the bronchiole
10. In asthma, hypersensitivity of the tracheobronchial tree to various stimuli occurs, demonstrated by periodic, reversible airway narrowing caused by bronchospasm.
11. Chronic inflammation causes weakening of the bronchial walls; consequently, they become dilated. The dilated areas may be cylindric or saccular in shape. The dilated areas serve as a reservoir for the collection of sputum. The stagnant sputum collection may, in turn, lead to chronic reinfection; thus progressive destruction and persistence of the process occur. Precipitating factors include whooping cough, measles, pneumonia, aspiration of a foreign body, and bronchial obstruction from a tumor.
12. Chronic loose cough, expectoration of a large amount (up to 200 ml/day) of foul-smelling sputum, malnutrition, digital clubbing, cor pulmonale, and right ventricular failure
13. Daily bronchial hygiene with postural drainage and antibiotics
14. Removal of the obstructing bronchial secretions
15. b
16. a
17. c
18. b, e
19. a, c
20. d, e

CHAPTER 39

1. Alveolar hypoventilation and an inability to maintain normal blood gas tensions
2. *Traumatic:* penetrating wound to the chest (knife or gunshot wound)
   Spontaneous: rupture of blebs and bullae in emphysema, pneumonia, neoplasm
3. Airtight seal is placed over the wound immediately.
4. Air gains access to the pleural cavity through the defect.
5. A large pneumothorax (more than 20% lung collapse) is treated by closed (water-sealed) chest tube drainage. A large pleural effusion may be removed

by thoracentesis. If a pleural effusion is an exudate, then it is treated by closed chest tube drainage to prevent fibrothorax.
6. Pleural effusion
7. Pulmonary venous pressure
8. An exudate
9. A transudate
10. (a) Invasion by bacteria, viruses, fungi, malignant cells—infection and destruction of lung tissue; (b) inhalation of irritating dusts—inflammation and pulmonary fibrosis; (c) inhalation of irritating gases—inflammation and pulmonary fibrosis; (d) damage to the alveolocapillary endothelium—edema; (e) deficiency of pulmonary surfactant—atelectasis.
11.

	Absorption Atelectasis	**Compression Atelectasis**
Common cause	Intrinsic obstruction of airway by mucus plug	Extrinsic pressure on lung from pleural effusion, hemothorax, pyothorax, or pneumothorax
Mechanism	Obstruction prevents air from entering alveoli distal to obstruction; air in alveoli is gradually absorbed into bloodstream; alveoli collapse	External pressure from fluid or air causes compression collapse of alveoli

12. These small pores (between the alveoli) provide a path for collateral ventilation between alveoli and whole segments of the lung in case the normal airway is obstructed. Deep inspiration is effective in opening the pores and providing ventilation to adjacent obstructed alveoli. Collapse caused by absorption of gases into the bloodstream is thus prevented. (After collapse occurs, reexpansion is much more difficult.) During expiration the pores close and pressure builds, aiding in the expulsion of the mucus plug.
13. *Engorgement* (4 to 12 hours): serous exudate from leaking blood vessels pours into alveoli.
   Red hepatization (next 48 hours): lung is red and granular in appearance (red blood cells, polymorphonuclear neutrophils, and fibrin fill the alveoli).
   Gray hepatization (3 to 8 days): lung has grayish appearance (leukocytes and fibrin consolidate in the alveoli).

Resolution (7 to 11 days): lysis and resorption of exudate by macrophages and restoration of tissue to normal.

14. Administration of antibiotic effective against the specific infecting organism, O_2 therapy for hypoxemia, and treatment of complications

15. *Size of dust particles:* those 1 to 5 mm can easily reach alveoli.

    Concentration and length of exposure: high concentration and long exposure generally are needed to produce adverse affects.

    Nature of the dusts: some organic dusts produce an allergic alveolitis; the chemical nature of inorganic dusts is important; some are harmless and inert, whereas others harm macrophages, by which they are phagocytized and form fibrotic nodules.

16. Histoplasmosis, coccidioidomycosis, and blastomycosis

17. Decreased lung compliance; interference with the gas diffusion pathway

18. Restrictive lung disease

19. Interstitial

20. Parenchyma; lung abscess, empyema; poor

21. c

22. a

23. b

24. c, g, j

25. d, h, i

26. a, f

27. b, e

CHAPTER 40

1. Local injury to the vascular wall; stasis of blood flow; hypercoagulability

2. COPD

3. Increased hydrostatic pressure within the pulmonary capillaries, decrease in the colloid osmotic pressure (as in nephritis), damage to the capillary wall (as when noxious gases are inhaled), left ventricular heart failure

4. It is the name given to attacks of dyspnea caused by pulmonary edema at night. The increased hydrostatic pressure in the lungs is caused by the horizontal position in patients with chronic passive congestion of the lungs resulting from left ventricular failure.

5. It is the condition in which hypertrophy and dilation of the right ventricle develop from disease affecting the structure and function of the lung. (Congenital and left heart disease are not included.)

6. When the left ventricle fails while the right ventricle continues to pump blood, the pulmonary hydrostatic pressure rises until pulmonary edema results. Yes.

7. Prevent the recurrence of PE; relieve symptoms resulting from the embolism; fibrinolytic therapy

8. To improve the underlying pulmonary disorder and correct the hypoxemia

9. Two mechanisms leading to increased pulmonary vascular resistance are (a) anatomic alterations in the pulmonary blood vessels leading to a reduction of the pulmonary vascular bed and (b) hypoxic vasoconstriction.

10. Embolism

11. Pulmonary hypertension

CHAPTER 41

1. *Respiratory insufficiency* refers to an impairment of the normal ability to oxygenate arterial blood and eliminate CO_2, meaning an inability to maintain normal arterial blood gas levels under conditions of increased demand such as increased activity or exercise.

2. Chronic obstructive pulmonary disease (COPD)

3. Hypoxemia without hypercapnia (hypoxemic respiratory failure, or oxygenation failure); hypoxemia with hypercapnia (hypercapnic respiratory failure, or ventilatory failure)

4. High concentrations of O_2 will reduce the hypoxic drive for breathing (on which patients with this condition depend) and may aggravate hypoventilation and CO_2 retention.

5. PaO_2 approximately 40 mm Hg; $PaCO_2$ 60 to 70 mm Hg

6. Liquefy and remove secretions by adequate hydration and administration of expectorants and aerosols; supervise patient's coughing; use suctioning, percussion, vibration, and postural drainage; treat respiratory infection with the appropriate antibiotic.

7. Ensure that hypoxemia, acidosis, and hypercapnia do not reach hazardous levels.

8. Retained respiratory tract secretions, infection, and bronchospasm, which are all related. For example, bronchospasm can be a response to inflammation and infection or to the inhalation of irritants, such as smoke or allergens. Injudicious administration of sedatives or narcotics or inhalation of high O_2 concentration are important iatrogenic factors. Refer to Box 41-2 for a list of other common factors.

9. A $\dot{V}/\dot{Q}$ mismatch means that some regions of the lung have high $\dot{V}/\dot{Q}$ ratios, whereas others have low $\dot{V}/\dot{Q}$ ratios. The high $\dot{V}/\dot{Q}$ gas–exchanging units compensate for the units with a low $\dot{V}/\dot{Q}$ in the case of CO_2 because of the linear relationship between CO_2 content and $PaCO_2$; consequently the $PaCO_2$ does not rise. The $PaCO_2$ is a function of overall alveolar ventilation and CO_2 production. In the case of the PaO_2, the high $\dot{V}/\dot{Q}$ units cannot compensate for the low $\dot{V}/\dot{Q}$ units because O_2 content increases little even when the increase in ventilation is large (flat part of oxy-

hemoglobin dissociation curve). Thus the PaO_2 is greatly affected by regional $\dot{V}/\dot{Q}$ imbalance, but the $PaCO_2$ is not.

10. $PaO_2 = PiO_2 - (PaCO_2 \div R)$
    $PiO_2 = FiO_2 \times (PB - PH_2O)$
    $PiO_2 = 0.21 \times (760 - 47) =$
    149.7 mm Hg (breathing air)
    $PiO_2 = 0.50 \times (760 - 47) =$
    356.5 mm Hg (breathing 50% O_2)
    $PAO_2 = 149.7 - (80 \div 0.8) =$
    49.7 mm Hg (predicted breathing air)
    $PAO_2 = 356.5 - (80 \div 0.8) =$
    256.5 mm Hg (predicted breathing 50% O_2)
    $P(A - a)O_2 = 49.7 - 50 =$ essentially 0 (breathing air)
    $P(A - a)O_2 = 256.5 - 246 =$
    10.2 mm Hg (breathing 50% O_2)

    The hypoxemia is caused by pure hypoventilation, because his $(A - a)$ gradient breathing air is essentially zero (normal, less than 20, allowing for some measurement error). The depression of the PaO_2 is accounted for by the increase in $PaCO_2$ in the situation when he is breathing air and when he is breathing 50% O_2. Of particular note is that his hypoxemia was corrected by O_2 therapy but that his $PaCO_2$ was not, which is because overall alveolar ventilation is reduced because of depression of the respiratory center by the narcotic. He may eventually need to be mechanically ventilated.

11. $PAO_2 = 0.21 \times (747 - 47) - (55 \div 0.8) = 78.25$ mm Hg (predicted on admission)
    $P(A - a)O_2 = 78.25 - 35 = 43.25$ mm Hg (on admission)
    $PAO_2 = 0.24 \times (747 - 47) - (40 \div 0.8) = 111.75$ (predicted 2 days later)
    $P(A - a)O_2 = 111.75 - 50 = 61.75$ mm Hg (2 days later)

    Because $(A - a)$ gradient breathing air on admission is greater than 20, he probably has $\dot{V}/\dot{Q}$ imbalance in addition to hypoventilation. Two days later, on 24% O_2, his condition appears to be deteriorating (even though his PaO_2 has increased) because the $(A - a)$ gradient has increased. He is not hypoventilating because $PaCO_2$ is now normal, but his $\dot{V}/\dot{Q}$ imbalance has probably become worse.

12. c, d, e, g

13. a, b, f

14. f

15. a

16. c

17. e

18. b

19. d

20. Hypoxemia

21. Hypoventilation

22. 5.73 mm Hg; yes

$$P_{AO_2} = F_{IO_2} \times (P_B - 47 \text{ mm Hg}) - P_{aCO_2} \div 0.8$$
$$= 0.21 \times (760 - 47) - 84 \div 0.8$$
$$= 149.73 - 105$$
$$= 44.73 \text{ mm Hg}$$
$$P(A - a)O_2 = P_{AO_2} - P_{aO_2}$$
$$= 44.73 - 39$$
$$= 5.73 \text{ mm Hg}$$

23. 10.08 ml O_2/dl; NO (normal, 18 to 20 ml/dl blood)

$$C_{aO_2} = S_{aO_2} \times Hb \text{ (g/dl)} \times 1.34 \text{ (ml } O_2/\text{g Hb)} + (P_{aO_2} \times 0.0031)$$
$$= 0.62 \times 12\text{g/dl} \times 1.34$$
$$= 0.12$$
$$= 9.96 \text{ ml } O_2/\text{dl} + 0.12$$
$$= 10.08 \text{ ml } O_2/\text{dl}$$

24. b
25. b
26. b
27. a

CHAPTER 42

1. The *carcinoid syndrome* is a symptom complex characterized by attacks of anxiety, tremulousness, hypotension, flushing, dyspnea, and cyanosis resulting from bronchoconstriction. The carcinoid syndrome is caused by the elaboration of serotonin and other biologically active substances secreted by a carcinoid type of bronchial adenoma.
2. Cough, chest pain, sputum expectoration, mild dyspnea, digital clubbing, and hemoptysis are common, but symptoms may be minimal. Diagnosis on the basis of symptoms is difficult, because the onset may be insidious and the symptoms are not specific. Lung cancer may imitate a number of other lung disorders.
3. *Radiology:* "coin lesion" seen on radiograph
   Bronchoscopy: direct visualization of tumor and biopsy identification of malignant cells
   Cytology: examination of sputum, bronchial washings, or pleural fluid for malignant cells
4. a, f, i
5. a, e, h, j
6. b, c, g, i
7. b, d, i

CHAPTER 43

1. In the United States, about 10% of people infected with TB will develop clinical TB during their lifetime, but the risk is higher for immunosuppressed individuals, especially those with HIV infection. CDC 1996 data indicates that the rate of TB disease among HIV-infected TB skin test positive persons is 200 to 800 times greater than the rate of TB for the overall U.S. population.
2. (a) Risk of acquiring the infection and (b) risk of developing clinically active disease after infection has occurred. The risk of acquiring the infection and developing disease depend on the existence of infection in the population, especially among persons infected with HIV, immigration of persons from areas of high prevalence of TB, high-risk racial and ethnic minority groups (e.g., African Americans, Native Americans, Alaskan natives, Asians, Pacific Islanders, Hispanics), and transmission of TB within high-risk environments (e.g., correctional facilities, homeless shelters, hospitals, nursing homes).
3. At least two drugs are used in treatment of TB because of the possibility of drug resistance, For example, a 6-month drug regimen consisting of INH, rifampin, and pyrazinamide given for 2 months followed by INH and rifampin for 4 months is recommended for the initial therapy of TB for patients with fully susceptible organisms who adhere to treatment. A 4-month regimen of INH and rifampin, preferably with pyrazinamide for the first 2 months, is recommended for adults who have active TB and who are smear and culture negative, if minimal possibility of drug resistance exists.
4. Principles on which treatment for TB is based include (a) regimens must include multiple drugs to which the organisms are susceptible, (b) the drugs must be taken regularly, and (c) drug therapy must continue for a sufficient period to provide the safest and most effective therapy in the shortest time.
5. Isoniazid, 300 mg/day for adults for 9 months is the recommended treatment for LTBI in HIV-infected persons.
6. BCG vaccination is not generally recommended against TB in the United States because of the low risk of infection and the variable effectiveness of the vaccine. Health care providers considering BCG vaccination for their patients are encouraged to discuss this characteristic with their local health department TB control staff.
7. The purpose of DOT therapy is to foster adherence and ensure that patients take the TB drugs as prescribed.
8. Risk factors for MDR-TB in patients with no previous history of TB treatment include exposure to a patient who has drug-resistant TB, being from a country with a high prevalence of drug resistance, and greater than 4% primary resistance to isoniazid in the community.
9. TB eradication involves a combination of effective chemotherapy, prompt case and contact identification and follow-up, management of persons exposed to patients with infectious MDR TB, and targeted tuberculin testing and treatment of high-risk population groups with LTBI.
10. c, d, g, l, n
11. k, m, n
12. d, g, j
13. a, n
14. f, l
15. b, k, g, n

CHAPTER 44

1. 1, Left kidney; 2, right kidney; 3, ureter; 4, bladder; 5, urethra; 6, urinary meatus
2. 1, Eleventh rib; 2, twelfth rib; 3, transversus abdominus muscle; 4, psoas major muscle
3. 1, Fibrous capsule; 2, cortex; 3 medulla; 4, column of Bertin; 5, papilla; 6, pyramid; 7, minor calyx; 8, major calyx; 9, renal pelvis; 10, ureter
4. 1, Proximal convoluted tubule; 2, glomerular capillary tuft; 3, Bowman's capsule; 4, efferent arteriole; 5, JG cells; 6, afferent arteriole; 7, macula densa; 8, loop of Henle; 9, distal convoluted tubule; 10, collecting duct
5. Check your drawing with Fig. 44-1. The hilus of each kidney should be at about the level of the second lumbar vertebra. The superior pole of the left kidney is at about the level of the lower border of the eleventh rib, while the right is at about the level of the twelfth rib.
6. (a) Bowman's capsule; (b) proximal convoluted tubule; (c) distal convoluted tubule; (d) collecting ducts; (e) papillary ducts of Bellini; (f) minor calyces; (g) major calyces; (h) renal pelvis; (i) ureter; (j) bladder
7. (a) Abdominal aorta; (b) renal artery; (c) interlobar arteries; (d) arcuate arteries; (e) interlobular arterioles; (f) afferent arterioles; (g) glomerular capillaries; (h) efferent arterioles; (i) peritubular capillaries; (j) interlobular veins; (k) arcuate veins; (l) interlobar veins; (m) renal vein; (n) inferior vena cava
8. More than 25% of the population has more than one renal artery supplying a kidney, which may cause technical difficulties for the surgeon. Some difficulties presented by aberrant blood vessels may be insurmountable.
9. A decrease in the hydrostatic pressure of the blood flowing through the afferent arteriole sensed by the JG cells or a decrease in Na^+ concentration in the distal tubule filtrate sensed by the macula densa cells causes the release of renin from the JG cells. This action results in the conversion of angiotensinogen to angiotensin I and finally to the active form, angiotensin II. Angiotensin II increases arterial blood pressure by causing peripheral vasoconstriction and stimulates the

secretion of aldosterone. Increased aldosterone levels cause increased Na^+ reabsorption in the distal tubule. More water is then reabsorbed, resulting in an increase in plasma volume. Both vasoconstriction and increased plasma volume help to elevate blood pressure. An increase in the blood pressure in the afferent arteriole has the opposite effect. An increase in the Na^+ concentration of the distal tubule, however, does not affect renin output.

10. A severe blunt impact over the back, flank, or even the abdomen can cause trauma to the kidney. This situation is common in motor vehicle accidents. The most common trauma in such cases results from the kidney being pushed against a transverse process or being punctured by a fractured twelfth rib. The resulting injury can vary from a simple bruise to a shattering of the renal parenchyma. Complete transection of a kidney by the twelfth rib may occur in severe cases.

11. It is called *ultrafiltration* because the glomerular filtrate has the same composition as does plasma, with the absence of proteins—almost everything is filtered through and at a high flow rate.

12. The differences in pressure between the glomerulus and Bowman's capsule tend to force fluid into the capsule. Net filtration pressure = P_{gc} – oncotic pressure of the blood – intracapsular hydrostatic pressure.

13. The GFR is the rate of appearance of glomerular filtrate from filtration of the blood at the glomerulus. The average GFR in men is 125 ml/min; in women, it is 110 ml/min.

14. To measure the GFR, a substance must be used that is freely filtered by the glomerulus but is neither secreted nor reabsorbed along the tubules. A substance that was cleared by both filtration and secretion along the tubule would cause the apparent GFR to be higher than the true GFR. A substance that was both filtered and reabsorbed would cause the apparent GFR to be lower than the true GFR.

15.

$$GFR = \frac{UV}{P}$$

$$= \frac{500 \text{ mg/dl} \times 2 \text{ ml/min}}{25 \text{ mg/dl}}$$

$$= 40 \text{ ml/min}$$

A GFR of 40 ml/min indicates that this patient has moderately severe impairment of renal function. The calculated value is normally corrected for body surface area (BSA) by means of a nomogram. The standard BSA is 1.73 m² (BSA of an average man).

The final result is then reported in milliliters per minute per 1.73 m².

16. Regulation of water and acid-base balance. Water is reabsorbed in the presence of ADH. Acid-base balance is regulated by regeneration of HCO_3^- and H^+ excretion in combination with $HPO_4^=$ and NH_3.

17. The lungs control the excretion of CO_2, and the kidneys control the reabsorption of HCO_3^-, both important components of the bicarbonate–carbonic acid buffer system in the blood. The ratio of these two components is important in maintaining a normal blood pH.

18. H^+ is excreted in the urine by combining with $HPO_4^=$ to form $H_2PO_4^-$ and by combining with NH_3 to form NH_4^+.

19. (a) Maintains plasma osmolality at 285 mOsm by varying water excretion; (b) maintains ECF volume and tissue perfusion by varying Na^+ excretion; (c) maintains plasma pH near 7.4 by regulating acid-base balance; (d) maintains concentration of each individual electrolyte within the normal range; (e) excretory route for most drugs; (f) excretes nitrogenous end products; (g) secretes or activates certain hormones: erythropoietin, prostaglandins, 1,25-dihydroxyvitamin D_3; (h) degradation of polypeptide hormones, especially insulin.

20. (a) Vapor pressure is lowered; (b) boiling point is elevated; (c) freezing point is lowered; (d) osmotic pressure is increased. Osmotic pressure refers to the external pressure that would have to be applied to a solution with a greater number of particles to prevent water from diffusing across a semipermeable membrane from a solution with a lesser number of particles. Osmotic pressure is a measure of water concentration; there are no real physical pressures present in the solutions—the pressure is that used to characterize the system. Adding particles to water lowers its chemical potential (molar free energy), and water always flows from an area of higher potential (more dilute) to an area of lower potential (more concentrated). The attainment of equilibrium by the application of pressure to the more concentrated solution is because its chemical potential is raised so that it is equal to the water in the more dilute solution on the other side of the membrane. The application of pressure prevents an increase in volume in the more concentrated solution because of water diffusion.

21. The osmometer is an apparatus for measuring the freezing point of a solution. The freezing point depression

below that of pure water can then be used to calculate accurately the osmotic concentration of the solution, because it depends only on the number of particles in solution. The urinometer actually measures the density or specific gravity of a solution and does not measure true concentration, which depends on the number of particles in solution. Therefore the osmometer is more accurate in estimating the concentration of a solution.

22.
$$\text{Osmolality} = \frac{\Delta T}{K_f} = \frac{-0.53}{-1.86}$$
$$\times 1000 = 285 \text{ mOsm}$$

The result is multiplied by 1000 to convert to milliosmols.

23. Check your drawing with Fig. 44-15. Cortical glomeruli should be located high in the cortex, with relatively short loops of Henle, which extend slightly into the medullary area. Juxtamedullary glomeruli should be located deep in the cortex next to the medulla, and the loops of Henle should be relatively long, extending deep into the medulla.

24. The vasa recta are medullary blood vessels that form hairpin loops beside the juxtamedullary loop of Henle. The vasa recta help maintain the concentration gradient of the medullary interstitial fluid.

25. The purpose of the countercurrent mechanism is the conservation of water (or the concentration of urine) by the kidney. The two basic processes involved are the loop of Henle acting as a countercurrent multiplier of concentration to build up the concentration gradient in the medulla and the vasa recta acting as a countercurrent exchanger to prevent washing out the hyperosmolality built up by the loop of Henle.

26. a
27. a
28. b
29. a
30. a
31. a
32. a
33. b
34. c
35. c

CHAPTER 45

1. A normal healthy adult may excrete up to 150 mg of protein in the urine per day. The amounts in excess of 150 mg/day are considered pathologic and occur most frequently in renal disease, particularly glomerulonephritis. Patients with the nephrotic syndrome excrete more than 3.5 g of protein/day and may excrete as much as 20 to 30 g.

2. The direct cause of proteinuria is always an increase in glomerular permeability usually a result of the loss of the size or charge barrier.

3. When urine stands for a period, urea breaks down to ammonia and the urine becomes more alkaline.

4. Uric acid is derived principally from the catabolism of nucleoproteins in the cells. Cytotoxic drugs cause increased degradation of the rapidly proliferating cells, and thus uric acid production is increased. Two thirds of the uric acid is normally excreted by the kidneys. The uric acid may crystallize and obstruct the tubules under conditions of acid urine.

5. (a) Infection with urea-splitting organisms producing alkaline urine; (b) hypercalciuria caused by prolonged immobilization; (c) urinary stasis as a result of low fluid intake. All three of these conditions are often present in patients with chronic illness who are confined to bed, thus favoring the formation of urinary calculi, which form in alkaline urine. Calcium salts are mobilized from bone, and precipitation is favored by highly concentrated, alkaline urine.

6. High fluid intake

7. (a) Check the accuracy of the urinometer using distilled water; (b) gently mix urine to ensure a uniform solution; (c) avoid errors of surface tensions; (d) read the calibrated units from top to bottom at eye level; (e) correct for temperature.

8. Creatinine is a nitrogenous end product of muscle metabolism. The normal plasma level is 0.7 to 1.5 mg/dl. The plasma level is constant in the healthy person and depends on muscle mass.

9. A substance that is filtered by the glomerulus and that is neither secreted nor reabsorbed by the tubules is required for a true measurement of GFR. Creatinine is secreted by the tubules, and there is an error inherent in the laboratory method of measuring the plasma level. These two large errors nearly cancel each other out so that C_{cr} approximately equals GFR.

10. GFR decreases with increasing age. After age 30 it decreases at the rate of about 1 ml/min each year.

11. The PAH excretion test is the most accurate test of effective renal plasma flow (RPF).

12. The P_{cr} level, because its production rate in the body is constant; it depends on muscle mass, which changes very little. Urea production varies with dietary protein intake and catabolism of body protein. Azotemia means that there is an increase in nitrogenous substances in the blood.

This increase occurs when the kidneys are not able to excrete these substances as rapidly as they are produced.

13. (a) The correct interpretation of a trace reading must take into account the concentration of the urine specimen and the time of day it is collected. A trace reading in an early-morning concentrated specimen is probably within normal limits. If the urine is collected later in the day and is dilute, a trace response might indicate excessive proteinuria; (b) contamination by vaginal secretions in the female (contain protein).

14. Albumin; Tamm-Horsfall

15. 6

16. a, alkaline

17. b, c, nocturnal acid

18. 285

19. 1.001, 1.040; to maintain the osmolality of the ECF at a constant value

20. 28%; this is the minimum for normal renal function; average excretion is 35%.

21. 1.025, 1.003

22. Urine acidification or ammonium chloride; 5.3

23. Sodium conservation; a

24. RBCs, WBCs, casts, bacteria

25. A bacterial count of 10^5 (100,000) CFU/ml of urine is considered significant and is an indication of urinary tract infection (more than three or four WBCs per high-power field during microscopic examination of the urine sediment suggests significant bacteriuria and indicates that a bacterial count should be done). However, the urine must not have been contaminated by bacteria from other sources, as from the container or from the genitalia. Therefore the genitalia must be cleansed with soap and water before voiding into the sterile specimen bottle, and care must be taken to avoid contamination of the urine by the labia or vaginal secretions in the woman ("sterile-voided"). Catheterization gives greater insurance that the specimen is "sterile." The urine must be examined immediately or a preservative should be added and the specimen refrigerated to avoid bacterial growth.

26. An IVP is accomplished by injecting into a vein radiologic contrast medium, which is then excreted by the kidneys; while in the retrograde pyelogram, a catheter is passed up a ureter and contrast medium is injected directly into the renal pelvis.

The purpose of an IVP is to visualize the cortex, calyces, renal pelvis, ureters, and bladder. The adequacy of filling of the calyces and renal pelvis may also be determined. The purpose of the retrograde pyelogram is to ob-

tain better visualization when the IVP is not clear and to investigate a non-functioning kidney.

27. (a) Hypertension: may be caused by renal artery stenosis or other obstruction; (b) possible neoplasm: blood vessels of tumor can be visualized; (c) transplant: to visualize the precise vascular supply before surgery; (d) to visualize the blood supply to the cortex: may have patchy appearance indicating ischemia.

28. The GFR is probably low and the dye will not be excreted well; the pyelogram will be difficult to visualize.

29. The entry site should be checked periodically for signs of hematoma or inflammation. Vital signs are checked every 15 minutes until stable and then every 4 hours for 24 hours. Peripheral pulses (in the leg when the femoral artery is used as the entry site) should be checked for diminished strength at the same time intervals as above to detect occlusion of blood flow as a result of thrombus or embolus formation. Color and skin temperature are other signs that should be observed to detect occlusion.

30. The patient should lie prone with a sandbag under the abdomen for 30 minutes after a renal biopsy. Firm pressure with 4×4-inch sponges is applied over the biopsy site for 10 minutes, followed by application of a pressure dressing. The patient should be kept in bed and as quiet as possible for 24 hours. Vital signs are checked and the abdomen observed for swelling during this period. The urine should also be observed for gross and occult blood.

31. (a) Microscopic; (b) bacteriologic; (c) radiology; (d) biopsy

32. Tamm-Horsfall; distal

33. Cylindruria, protein

34. Culture and sensitivity

35. Clubbing (also may be seen in some other forms of chronic renal disease)

CHAPTER 46

1. The period of development of the disease condition; chronic renal failure is a progressive, slow process over a period of years, whereas acute renal failure develops over a few days to weeks. In both cases, the kidneys lose their ability to keep the internal environment of the body normal.

2. Stage I, decreased renal reserve: up to 75% of nephron mass destroyed. Stage II, renal insufficiency: 75% to 90% nephron mass destroyed. Stage III, uremia or end-stage renal failure (ESRF): 90% or more of the nephron mass destroyed.

3. First stage: BUN and plasma creatinine levels both normal; second stage: BUN and plasma creatinine

levels rising just above normal, unstable; third stage: BUN and plasma creatinine levels both rising sharply with each decrement of GFR.

4. The creatinine clearance progresses toward zero as nephrons are progressively destroyed by the renal disease process (creatinine clearance rate gives a fairly good estimate of the true GFR in the middle range but is much less accurate at either high or low filtration rates).

5. Polyuria means an increase in the volume of urine, whereas oliguria is just the opposite—urine output is decreased below the normal range. (Do not confuse polyuria and frequency, a common mistake made by students. Frequency means an increase in the number of voidings, but there is not necessarily an increase in the volume. With moderate polyuria, there is not necessarily an increase in frequency.) Nocturia means that a person has to get up more than once to void during normal sleeping hours or output is 700 ml or more during the night.

6. Polyuria and nocturia occur because of the solute diuresis and inability to concentrate the urine. Both symptoms occur early in the course of progressive renal failure and are compensatory. When most of the nephrons are destroyed, the patient becomes oliguric because the total net filtration rate is low (because there are few nephrons), even though the GFR for each individual intact nephron may be high (decompensation stage). Primary lesions of the medulla may interfere with the chloride pump, the countercurrent mechanism, and tubular secretion and reabsorption, whereas lesions of the glomerulus may prevent glomerular filtration from occurring or cause the loss of protein and formed elements into the urine.

7. An increased solute load may be induced in a normal person by ingestion of a high-protein diet or by giving mannitol intravenously. The usual solute load of the kidneys is thus extended many times. Each normal nephron is undergoing an osmotic diuresis, which results in an obligatory loss of water. The kidney loses its flexibility to either concentrate or dilute the urine from the plasma osmolality of 285 mOsm under the stress of water deprivation or overload. Identical principles are involved in progressive renal failure, and both conditions are explained by the intact nephron hypothesis.

8. The remaining intact nephrons compensate by hypertrophying. Filtration

rate, solute load, and tubular reabsorption per nephron are all increased, and glomerular-tubular balance is maintained until most of the renal nephrons are destroyed.

9. The renal disease may not be diagnosed until it is far advanced, when functional and morphologic characteristics may be similar for a number of chronic renal diseases.

10. a. Obstruction of urinary outflow of any cause, such as urethral valves or stricture, calculi, or tumors, usually results in UTI if the obstruction is partial or acute renal failure if the obstruction is complete.
    b. Females are at greater risk for UTI presumably because of their short urethra and proximity of the urinary meatus to the anus; males have the greater risk for UTI during infancy because of congenital structural defects of the urinary tract and during old age because of obstruction from prostatic hypertrophy.
    c. The regurgitation of infected urine into the renal pelvis and interstitium in severe VUR predisposes to UTI and the development of chronic PN.
    d. Instrumentation of the urinary tract, especially the use of indwelling catheter, is associated with a high incidence of UTI.
    e. UTI and ESRD is common in patients with neurogenic bladder (e.g., diabetes, paraplegics) because urinary drainage is impaired.
    f. UTI is typically associated with analgesic nephropathy.
    g. UTI is a common complication in ESRD probably because of defective immunity and damaged kidneys are more susceptible to infection.
    h. Metabolic disturbances such as gout, diabetes, and hypercalcemia are frequently associated with UTI.

11. School-aged girls with significant bacteriuria (whether symptomatic or asymptomatic) are more likely to have recurrent UTI during their childbearing years. All children with significant bacteriuria should be screened for VUR (especially boys), because boys may have a correctable structural defect of the urinary tract that, if treated, may prevent the development of progressive renal disease.

12. VUR, intrarenal reflux, and infection

13. According to this theory, progressive renal failure continues when a critical mass of nephrons has been destroyed, even in the absence of the original destructive factor (e.g., reflux or infection), because of compensatory intrarenal hypertension in the

remaining healthy nephrons. If this theory is correct, lowering intraglomerular pressure by restricting dietary protein and administering antihypertensive drugs (especially ACE inhibitors) would slow down the progression to renal failure.

14. Acute, rapidly progressive, and chronic glomerulonephritis (GN) are the three clinical types of renal disease that initially and primarily cause diffuse inflammation of the glomeruli. The classic case of acute GN follows a beta-hemolytic streptococcal infection of the throat, typically in a child, causing hematuria, albuminuria, hypertension, and edema. More than 90% of patients have a complete recovery, death occurs in a few, and the remainder may develop RPGN or CGN. RPGN refers to a type of GN with a fulminant course and progression to ESRD within a few months. Goodpasture's syndrome is a good example of this type. CGN is characterized by slow destruction of nephrons from longstanding GN until ESRD is reached (2 to 30 years). A number of systemic diseases can cause CGN, and often the cause is unknown. In most cases, CGN has no known relationship to acute GN or RPGN. However, an acute nephritic syndrome may occur during the course of CGN.

15. c
16. b
17. a
18. b, c, g
19. a, d, e, f, h
20. c, d
21. b, e
22. a, e
23. b, f
24. b, g
25. b, c, d, i, j
26. b, c, i
27. a, b
28. b, h
29. d
30. e
31. PMNs; tubules; lymphocytes; plasma
32. a, Atrophied tubule with cast; b, normal tubule; c, area of interstitial fibrosis; d, hypertrophied tubule with atrophy of epithelial cells; e, PMNs

CHAPTER 47

1. The uremic syndrome refers to a symptom complex that results from or is associated with retention of nitrogenous metabolites related to renal failure.

2. The first group of symptoms relates to deranged regulatory and excretory functions (such as fluid and electrolyte disturbances, acid-base imbalances). The second group of symptoms refers to cardiovascular, neuromuscular, GI, and other system

abnormalities. The middle molecular hypothesis postulates that molecules of intermediate size present in uremia (guanidines, indican, phenols, amines, etc.) may act as toxins and may be responsible, in part, for the multifarious systemic manifestations of the uremic syndrome. The theory also implies that a treatment method allowing effective removal of middle molecules will reduce the symptoms of the uremic syndrome.

3. Because the total number of nephrons is decreased, not because of a tubular transport problem.

4. H^+ is probably being buffered by calcium carbonate from the bones. No doubt this process contributes to the dissolution of bone, although it is not as important as are the increased parathormone levels.

5. Because of the increased solute load of each intact nephron. The osmotic diuresis results in obligatory salt losses.

6. Milk of magnesia and magnesium citrate

7. A fixed urine specific gravity of 1.010 means that the patient has severe renal failure with no ability to either concentrate or dilute the urine. Consequently, there is little ability to regulate the fluid balance in the body, and fluid intake must be carefully prescribed.

8. When the GFR falls to about 5 ml/min in terminal renal failure, both men and women lose their libido and are generally sterile. Men are generally impotent, and women cease to menstruate.

9. Poor nutrition, overhydration, indwelling catheters and cannulas, immunosuppressive drugs

10. White-skinned person—waxy yellow (bronze) cast to the skin; brown-skinned person—yellowish brown coloration; black-skinned person—ashen gray with yellow tones. All these skin color changes are caused by the anemia and retention of urochrome pigments in the uremic patient. Skin color changes in dark-skinned persons are caused by a loss of the red undertones that give the dark skin a "look-alive" appearance. Yellow tones are more evident in the conjunctiva and on the palms and soles.

11. • GI bleeding → hypotension → ↓ renal perfusion → ↓ GFR
    • GI bleeding → digestion of blood protein → ↑ BUN
    • Vomiting → dehydration → hypovolemia → ↓ renal perfusion → ↓ GFR
    • Diarrhea → loss of HCO_3^- → aggravation of acidosis

12. You might expect the patient to complain of tiring easily, of not being able to work long without resting, and of being unable to sleep at night or being lethargic during the day. You might observe that the patient's affect seemed flat, and the patient had difficulty following a complex train of thought. Muscular weakness and muscular twitching might be complaints. The untreated patient in terminal renal failure will eventually become confused and comatose and may have convulsions, especially if severely hypertensive.

13. *Stage I:* nerve conduction test reveals decreased velocity of nerve conduction. Patient may complain of needing to walk or move the legs (restless leg syndrome). *Stage II:* sensory nerve changes. Patient complains of burning sensation on the soles of the feet and numbness or prickling sensation moving up legs in stockinglike fashion; the patient may also have paresthesias of the hands. *Stage III:* the patient may have motor nerve involvement. Loss of motor function usually is first observed as foot drop and may progress to paraplegia.

14. Check your illustration with the radiograph of the hand in Fig. 47-2. The radial aspect of the bone is eroded and has a jagged appearance.

15. See Fig. 47-3 if you have forgotten this sequence of events. Bone disorders associated with secondary hyperparathyroidism might include "honeycombing" demineralization of the bone, especially notable on skull radiograph, and subperiosteal bone resorption, giving the phalanges a ragged border. Pathologic fractures of the long bones and ribs may result. Ca^{++} salts may be deposited in the soft tissues of the body, around joints, in the arteries, and in the eyes.

16. This patient has a calcium-phosphate cross product of $8 \times 10 = 80$, which exceeds the solubility product of Ca^{++} and phosphate by a large margin. Soft tissue deposition of calcium phosphate would certainly be expected.

17. Check your illustration with Fig. 47-4. Irritation from the Ca^{++} salts deposited in the eye may cause conjunctivitis, called "uremic red eye" from its appearance.

18. c
19. a, d
20. b, e

CHAPTER 48

1. When the patient becomes azotemic. Four causes of sudden deterioration of renal function include (a) ECF volume depletion; (b) urinary tract obstruction; (c) infection, especially of the urinary tract; and (d) severe or malignant hypertension. The principles of conservative treatment are based on regulating individual solute and fluids to achieve as normal an internal milieu as possible in view of the kidney's decreased ability to adapt to a variable intake. Dietary phosphate restriction and phosphate-binding medications should be given early in the course of CRF.

2. Dialysis, renal transplantation, or death in terminal renal failure

3. Approximately 500 ml + 500 ml = 1000 ml

4. Chronic intermittent dialysis and renal transplantation. Dialysis may be used for long-term maintenance of the patient with end-stage renal failure. Even if the patient chooses renal transplantation as the mode of therapy, dialysis will undoubtedly play a role in treatment. Dialysis can be used to restore and maintain an optimal physical state in the uremic patient before the transplanted kidney is available and as a backup treatment modality should the transplanted kidney fail. The patient who has chosen maintenance home or satellite-center dialysis may also opt for a transplant at a later date.

5. *Dialysis* is the process by which water and low–molecular-weight solutes pass through a semipermeable membrane from one fluid compartment to another and achieve equilibrium.

6. An artificial shunt is a device for diverting arterial blood to a vein; the pressure and flow are therefore great enough to allow hemodialysis and provide for easy blood access. With an *external shunt* or cannula system, an external silicone rubber tubing directs or shunts blood from artery to vein. An *internal shunt* can be created by anastomosing an artery to a nearby vein (AV fistula) or using a graft of bovine carotid artery.

7. a, b, d, i
8. g
9. e, k
10. h
11. f
12. j
13. c
14. b
15. a
16. d
17. c
18. (a) Rapid serologic testing for HLA-DR antigens is highly predictive of success rate. Thus when a cadaver becomes available, there is sufficient time to find the best match with the aid of a national computer bank of potential recipients. If the cadaver graft success rate improves sufficiently, it may be possible to solicit nonrelated living donors; and (b) cyclosporin A has greatly increased cadaver graft survival.

19. HFHE dialysis, hemodiafiltration, and CAPD. All are supposedly more successful in removing middle molecules.

CHAPTER 49

1. Because the fumes of CCl_4 (and other organic solvents) inhaled and the ingested ethyl alcohol react chemically in the body to produce a potent nephrotoxin, which may produce acute tubular necrosis

2. Nephrotoxic injury and renal ischemia

3. ARF is superimposed on chronic renal insufficiency because of intrinsic renal disease. Precipitating causes include nausea, vomiting, and infections.

4. Two basic types of lesion are involved in ATN, though in some cases they may be mixed. The less serious lesion results in necrosis of the tubular epithelium only. This lesion commonly results from mild doses of CCl_4 or $HgCl_2$. When only epithelial damage takes place, complete healing of the lesion commonly occurs in 3 to 4 weeks. In the second type of lesion, there is necrosis of the epithelium and also the basement membrane. This is commonly associated with severe renal ischemia. The prognosis of this type of lesion depends on the extent of the damage. When the basement membrane is disrupted, epithelial regeneration occurs in a haphazard manner, frequently leading to obstruction of the nephron at the site of necrosis.

5. Acute cortical necrosis means that the entire nephron is infarcted. It is commonly associated with pregnancy complications such as postpartum hemorrhage, premature separation of the placenta, eclampsia, and septic abortion. The prognosis is generally poor. If the patient survives the acute phase of illness, calcification and permanent renal damage often occur in the area of cortical necrosis. Glycol (antifreeze) poisoning may also cause this lesion.

6. Infection

7. This classification stresses the identification of extrarenal causes (prerenal, postrenal) and the prevention of progression to intrinsic ARF. The categories provide a systematic diagnostic approach, because the diagnosis of ARF is made on the basis of exclusion of extrarenal (immediately reversible) causes.

8. Bladder outlet obstruction: benign or malignant prostatic hypertrophy; cancer of cervix or rectum. Bilateral ureteral obstruction: cellular debris from necrotizing papillitis in a person with diabetes mellitus; obstruction of the ureter by a calculus in a patient with one functioning kidney; trauma or accidental ligation during extensive pelvic surgery. Intrarenal obstruction: uric acid crystallization in the renal collecting ducts in a leukemic patient receiving chemotherapy; obstruction of the renal tubules with Bence Jones protein in a patient with multiple myeloma (see also Chapter 18). Inadequate hydration and hypovolemia are important predisposing factors in both cited examples of renal tubule obstruction.

9. Penicillin: methicillin; aminoglycosides: neomycin, gentamicin, kanamycin, tobramycin. Chronic renal insufficiency and advanced age (>60 years) are characteristics of patients at high risk for drug-induced ARF.

10. All the theories concerning the pathogenesis of ARF attempt to explain the severe reduction in the GFR. Suggested mechanisms include the following:
    a. Mechanical obstruction of the renal tubule lumina by necrotic tubular cells that have sloughed off; cellular swelling may also collapse the tubules, blocking them off.
    b. Backleak of filtrate into the peritubular circulation through damaged tubular cells.
    c. Impermeability or reduction in surface area of the glomerular filtration membrane.
    d. Intrarenal vascular dysfunction, with redistribution of blood from cortex to medulla maintained by the release of renin from the juxtaglomerular cells, activation of angiotensin II, and consequent vasoconstriction of the afferent arterioles. Inhibition of prostaglandin synthesis may also play a role in the intrarenal vascular dysfunction.
    e. Stimulation of renin-angiotensin, with consequent vasoconstriction of the afferent arterioles through the tubuloglomerular feedback mechanism.

11. Fractional excretion of sodium (FE_{Na}); it is actually the ratio of the renal clearance of sodium to that of creatinine ($C_{Na} \div C_{cr} \times 100\%$). Formula for calculation:

$$FE_{Na} = \frac{U_{Na} \times P_{cr}}{P_{Na} \times U_{cr}} \times 100\%$$

The measurement should be done before a diuretic is given, and only fresh urine should be used. Intermittent urinary tract obstruction and preexisting chronic renal insufficiency cause problems in interpretation. These factors are hazards in the use of renal indices to differentiate prerenal azotemia from ATN. Because the laboratory tests are simple, they should be repeated several times.

12. Mannitol and furosemide

CHAPTER 50

1. True
2. False; nerves do not exist in the CNS; cranial nerves are part of the PNS, although their nuclei are located in the CNS.
3. True
4. True
5. False; it forms the craniosacral outflow.
6. True
7. True
8. False; they are bipolar.
9. False; transmission of impulses between neurons can occur only at synapses, and the transmission is unidirectional from presynaptic terminal to postsynaptic membrane (called the law of Bell-Magendie).
10. True
11. False; it covers nerve fibers only in the PNS.
12. False; they are properly called fiber tracts or nerve fiber tracts to distinguish them from nerves that exist in the PNS.
13. False; they are CNS tracts.
14. d
15. e
16. a
17. c
18. b
19. c, d, e
20. a, b, f
21. Anatomic components of the extrapyramidal system (although difficult to define anatomically) probably include the basal ganglia and their connections to the cerebral cortex, cerebellum, reticular formation, and certain thalamic nuclei. The substantia nigra, red nucleus, and subthalamic nucleus in the brainstem are also considered part of the extrapyramidal system. The main function of this system is to provide coarse control of voluntary muscular movement.

| Caudate nucleus | | Corpus striatum (some authors include part of adjacent internal capsule) |
| Lenticular nucleus | Putamen / Globus pallidus | |

| Amygdaloid nucleus Claustrum Red nucleus Substantia nigra Subthalamic nucleus (corpus Luysii) | Structures closely associated with basal ganglia |

The basal ganglia function in some way to prevent oscillation and after-discharge in motor systems, probably by direct action on the midbrain centers and in part as inhibitory feedback to the motor cortex. They are also involved in the control of stretch reflexes and in the generation of mannerisms and automatic activity.

CHAPTER 51

1. Neurologic illness is usually well defined, and a clear history will provide clues that will assist in an accurate assessment of the patient's condition.
2. Examination of the motor system (e.g., testing the gait, voluntary muscle strength, muscle tone)
   Sensory examination (e.g., pain, temperature, vibration sense, examination of the reflexes)
   Coordination of arms and legs
   Examination of mental status and speech
   Examination of cranial nerves
   Examination of reflex status
3. (a) Superficial tactile sense; (b) proprioceptive (motion or position) sense; (c) vibratory sense; (d) cortical sensory function
4. Romberg
5. L5 to S1
6. d
7. i
8. f
9. g
10. j
11. b
12. e
13. h
14. a

CHAPTER 52

1. b
2. b
3. a
4. a
5. a
6. b
7. b
8. b
9. c
10. a
11. a, c
12. c
13. b
14. a
15. a
16. c
17. d
18. Location; onset; pattern (timing, frequency, duration); aggravating or relieving factors; quality; intensity; associated symptoms; effects on lifestyle; methods of relief
19. Observation of patient's verbal and nonverbal behavior that may indicate pain (e.g., abnormal posture or gait, muscle guarding, moaning, expressions of anger); autonomic hyperactivity, such as increased blood pressure or heart rate; tenderness or muscle guarding on palpation
20. The major function of the pain sensory system is to prevent injury. Individuals who have a congenital insensitivity to pain (very rare) do not react to or avoid noxious stimuli and are not particularly disturbed by them. These persons repeatedly injure themselves by failing to avoid high temperatures, intense pressure, extreme twisting, or corrosive substances. They may be totally unaware of internal diseases that would be painful to a normal person. These individuals typically have pressure sores, missing digits, and damaged joints. Although lack of pain sensitivity might seem to be an advantage on superficial examination, the multiple injuries present in persons with this "advantage" attest to its disadvantage.
21. Questions need to be asked concerning the onset, frequency, duration, location, precipitating or relieving factors; whether there are prodromal symptoms or associated symptoms such as dizziness, nausea, vomiting, or blurred vision; type of pain and whether it is incapacitating; whether other members of the family have a headache problem; and whether there has been head injury in the past. Medical conditions must be considered in relation to the headache pattern.
22. Anterior; trigeminal
23. Posterior; upper cervical
24. b, c, e, i, j
25. a, c, h, j
26. d, f, a, k

CHAPTER 53

1. Stroke is a focal brain dysfunction resulting from ischemia. The ischemia may arise from atherosclerotic narrowing of a blood vessel, from an embolus, or from other causes.
2. *Thrombotic strokes* (the most common type) may have a gradual, stuttering, or step-wise onset rather than an abrupt instantaneous onset. The cause is generally atherosclerosis, which generally affects large vessels. The large vessel involvement explains why thrombotic strokes tend to cause considerable neurologic deficit. More than one half are preceded by TIAs. *Embolic strokes* are most often cardiogenic in origin and associated with an underlying cardiac disease, such as valvular heart disease, atrial fibrillation, or mural thrombus. They tend to be abrupt in onset with more rapid resolution and tend to cause smaller neurologic deficits than does thrombotic stroke. Because an embolus will travel in the arterial stream until it reaches a blood vessel of sufficiently small caliber to occlude, it often travels all the way to the cortex. Cortical deficits, such as aphasia, are thus characteristic of embolic strokes.
3. Lacunar strokes are very small, discrete infarcts, less than 1 cc in size, occurring deep within the brain or brain stem (lacune means little lake). These strokes are caused by occlusion of tiny penetrating arterioles that supply the deep brain substance, usually in the region of the basal ganglia, thalamus, or internal capsule. The brain stem is the other common location for lacunar infarcts. Because these strokes are so small, they cause discrete clinical symptoms, such as pure motor stroke (hemiparesis without any sensory loss) or pure sensory stroke.
4. Intracerebral bleeds into the parenchyma, causing stroke, have an abrupt onset and are usually accompanied by a significant headache and other signs of increased ICP, such as nausea, vomiting, and a diminished mental status. These bleeds are often devastating events with a poor prognosis. Bleeds tend to occur in the same deep locations as lacunar strokes, namely the basal ganglia and brainstem.
5. Antiplatelet agents, specifically aspirin, have been advocated for the secondary prevention of stroke. Patients with TIAs are often treated with aspirin, usually 325 mg/day, to prevent further episodes of cerebrovascular ischemia.
6. The person with cardiac disease that has caused embolization will probably benefit from anticoagulation therapy. The usual settings in which this occurs are atrial fibrillation, mural thrombus after myocardial infarction, thrombosis on abnormal valves (as in rheumatic mitral valve disease), or prosthetic heart valves.
7. It is common practice to perform carotid endarterectomy on otherwise healthy, good surgical candidates who have experienced a TIA in the carotid distribution and who have angiographic evidence of a significant appropriate carotid lesion, defined as either a 70% stenosis or deep ulceration.
8. To prevent recurrent hemorrhage

CHAPTER 54

1. Basal ganglia; slow degeneration of nerve cells; below the cortex (subcortical)
2. Extrapyramidal motor nerve tract; it regulates semiautomatic movements, such as coordination of hand movements and swallowing.
3. *Parkinson's syndrome* is a chronic disorder of the CNS characterized by a specific group of symptoms that become progressively worse until the patient is unable to perform the activities of daily living and becomes bedridden. Parkinson's syndrome may be idiopathic, postencephalitic, or drug induced (the last a type of pseudoparkinsonism).
4. *Parkinson's disease (PD)* results from a loss of dopaminergic neurons in the substantia nigra and other pigmented nuclei. As a result, deficiency of dopamine (a neurotransmitter)

within the nigrostriatal pathway running from the substantia nigra to the basal ganglia occurs. This deficiency leads to an imbalance between dopamine (inhibitory) and acetylcholine (excitatory) neurotransmitters and underlies most of the symptoms of PD. PD is best treated by a combination of L-dopa plus carbidopa (Sinemet). Dopamine cannot be given directly, because it does not cross the blood-brain barrier.

5. (a) *Resting tremor:* fine or coarse rhythmic alternating contraction of opposing muscle groups, occurring at rest in disease of the basal ganglia and decreasing with voluntary motion; (b) *choreiform movement:* rapid, irregular, jerky, purposeless contractions of random muscle groups followed by prompt relaxation; (c) *athetoid movement:* continuous slow, writhing movements that may be tonic avoiding or grasping reactions; (d) *dystonia:* slow, powerful movements, such as bending a lead pipe; (e) *hemiballism:* flailing, intense violent movements involving one side of the body

6. Phenothiazine, *Rauwolfia* agents

7. Hyperactive glabellar reflex; resting tremor (pill-rolling); expressionless face; festinating gait; micrographia; monotone voice; plastic or cogwheel rigidity

8. Acute disseminated encephalomyelitis, in which patchy areas of demyelinization occur in the brain and spinal cord. Routine measles vaccination, discontinuation of routine smallpox vaccination, and use of the newer killed-duck embryo rabies vaccine (free of nerve tissue) when necessary has greatly reduced the incidence.

9. There are widespread patches of myelin destruction and gliosis in the CNS. If the patient reported a temporary blurring of vision in one eye or blindness or an episode of weakness or tingling in an extremity, this would be grounds for suspicion.

10. Major morphologic changes include neurofibrillary tangles (consisting of twisted abnormal tau protein) and senile plaque (composed of amyloid-beta). Biochemical changes include depletion of somatostatin and acetylcholinesterase (an enzyme that normally breaks down acetylcholine).

CHAPTER 55

1. *Epilepsy* is a paroxysmal disorder of the nervous system characterized by recurrent attacks of loss or alteration of consciousness with or without motor convulsive phenomena. The condition is usually caused by excessive, uncontrolled local discharges of a group of cerebral neurons, usually in the cortex.

2. The incidence is estimated to be about 0.3% or slightly higher. The in-

cidence in the offspring of epileptic persons is higher than that in the general population.

3. Head injury, hypoglycemia, vitamin B_6 deficiency, alcohol withdrawal, encephalitis, brain tumors

4. Midbrain, thalamus, cerebral cortex

5. Current theory postulates epileptic neurons that have lower thresholds for firing abnormal discharges. A deafferented neuron has been identified in some focal lesions. These neurons are hypersensitive and in a chronic state of depolarization. The cytoplasmic membranes exhibit increased permeability, making them susceptible to activation by various factors (hypoxia, hyperthermia) and circumstances (repeated sensory stimuli).

6. Metabolic needs are increased during convulsions; the electrical discharges of motor nerve cells may be increased to 1000/sec. Cerebral blood flow is increased, and there is some increase in respiration and glycolysis. Acetylcholine appears in the CSF during and after seizures. Glutamic acid may be depleted during seizure activity.

7. Convulsive status epilepticus is overt seizure activity lasting 20 minutes or longer. In nonconvulsive status epilepticus the patient continues to seize without overt clinical evidence of seizure activity.

CHAPTER 56

1. Normal intracranial pressure (ICP) is about 4 to 15 mm Hg. The basic cause of increased ICP is an expanding mass within the rigid, bony cranium that allows very little room for expansion (about 5 cm³) before pressure starts to increase. Normally the cranial contents consist of tissue, blood, and cerebrospinal fluid (CSF). An increase in ICP can be caused by increased tissue (as from a growing tumor), blood (hematoma secondary to rupture of a blood vessel), blockage of the flow of CSF and its accumulation, and cerebral edema (typically associated with cerebral trauma). Increased ICP is dangerous because it causes cerebral ischemia, hypoxia, compression of the cortex, and herniation of the brain stem through the foramen magnum. This compression causes cessation of function of the vital regulatory centers within the brain stem and death.

2. Compression of cortex: hemiparesis is caused by compression of motor cortex; seizures may result from local cortical disruption; mental dysfunction occurs because cortex is involved in higher thought processes.

   Displacement of brain stem down into foramen magnum, causing its compression: reticular formation in brain stem is involved in level of con-

sciousness; systolic blood pressure increases thus it will be higher than ICP, and cerebral circulation will be maintained; this also causes decerebrate rigidity from removal of normal influence of higher centers on muscle tone.

   Compression of the oculomotor nerve by herniated uncus causes ipsilateral dilated pupil.

3. (a) Local tissue damage from direct force (penetration or compression by missiles or bone fragments or damage as a result of displacement of cranial contents in rapid acceleration or deceleration); (b) cerebral ischemia caused by lack of autoregulation secondary to increasing ICP

4. Forceful thrusting of the brain contents against the inner surface of the skull on the side opposite the impact. The areas most likely to be damaged in a decelerating motor vehicle accident are the anterior portion of the frontal and temporal lobes and the upper section of the midbrain.

5. The most common sites are those at which a relatively mobile portion of the vertebral column meets a relatively fixed segment. These sites occur between the lower cervical and upper thoracic spine, between the lower thoracic and upper lumbar spine, and between the lower lumbar spine and the sacrum.

6. Stabilize the spinal column to prevent contusion, laceration, and further damage to the spinal cord from bony fragments and foreign bodies.

7. *Epidural hematomas* usually result from a tear in the middle meningeal artery. The bleeding occurs between the dura mater and the skull, usually in the temporal area. The development of clinical symptoms and the course are rapid and proceed to completion within a few hours, because the bleeding is arterial. On the other hand, *subdural hematomas* usually result from the tearing of veins that pass from the surface of the brain to one of the major dural sinuses. Blood escapes between the dura and the arachnoid. Because bleeding is under venous low pressure, the accumulation of blood may be much more prolonged and the clinical course much more protracted.

8. c, e
9. a, d
10. b

CHAPTER 57

1. b
2. d
3. a
4. c
5. c
6. d
7. b
8. a

9. e
10. It is difficult because the symptoms are diverse and depend on the location and size of the growth. However, the symptoms tend to progress. The most common general symptoms are headache, vomiting, and papilledema, all a result of increased ICP from the expanding mass.
11. a
12. b
13. c
14. d
15. c
16. b

CHAPTER 58

1. One mechanism by which hormones work on cells is the adenylate cyclase system. In this case the polypeptide hormones interact with a specific membrane receptor. As a result of this interaction, adenylate cyclase is activated and ATP is converted to cyclic AMP. Cyclic AMP binds to the regulatory subunit of a protein kinase, liberating a catalytic subunit of the enzyme. This action, in turn, initiates the phosphorylation of certain enzymes that either activate or inactivate the biologic potency of these enzymes.

   A second mechanism by which hormones work on target cells is exemplified by steroid hormones, which work directly inside the cell by entering the cell across the cell membrane and binding to cytosol receptor proteins. The steroid receptor complex then is translocated to the nucleus of the cell, where it binds specifically to its locus on the chromatin, activating RNA polymerase with ultimate synthesis of one or several specific mRNAs. These products travel from the nucleus to the ribosome, where they direct the synthesis of proteins. By changing mRNA, steroids can modify the way protein is synthesized.

2.

Type of Hormone	Location of Production	Examples
Proteins (polypeptides, glycoproteins)	Posterior pituitary gland	Pitressin
	Beta cells of islets of Langerhans	Insulin
	Thyroid gland	Thyroxine
	Parathyroid gland	Parathyroid hormone
	Anterior pituitary	Tropic hormones
Steroids (lipids)	Adrenal cortex	Cortisol
	Gonads	Estrogen Progesterone

3. A decrease in the pressure of the blood flowing through the afferent arteriole of the renal glomerulus is sensed by JG cells, causing release of renin. This action results in the following sequence of events:

   Renin → Renin substrate
   ↓
   Angiotensin I
   ↓
   Angiotensin II
   ↓
   Adrenal cortex
   ↓
   Aldosterone

4. The hypothalamus possesses a variety of nuclei made up of neurons having a secretory function. These neurons manufacture proteins, called releasing hormones, secreted through axons into blood vessels. The hypothalamus receives fibers from other areas of the brain that influence hypothalamic neuronal function.
5. This anatomic mechanism permits the movement of neurostimuli from the hypothalamus to the pituitary gland; this is the mechanism by which the CNS influences the pituitary gland.
6. Any neurostimuli reaching the corticotropin-releasing center causes release of CRH into the portal system. CRH causes release of ACTH by cells in the anterior pituitary gland. ACTH stimulates the adrenal cortex to produce cortisol, which affects the rate and amount of CRH-ACTH secreted by the hypothalamic-pituitary axis.
7. ACTH production typically exhibits a cyclic pattern throughout the 24-hour period. The levels usually go up early in the day, go down later in the day, and go up again during the night, to reach a peak level by the next morning.
8. The two postulated mechanisms for endocrine disorders are (1) those in which the hormone concentrations are primarily disturbed and (2) those in which the receptors are primarily defective. Most endocrine disorders can be understood conceptually in terms of the metabolic action of the hormones involved.
9. If a disease arises from excessive production of a hormone, the problem may be treated surgically by removing the gland or part of the gland that produces the hormone. This procedure is followed by replacement with normal amounts of the hormone. If a disease is caused by hormone deficit, the treatment is replacement of the hormones that are not being produced.

CHAPTER 59

1. b
2. a

3. a
4. c
5. d
6. e
7. g
8. a
9. c
10. b
11. h
12. f
13. Medical treatment using a somatostatin analog is currently being tested. This analog can induce sustained suppression of GH and somatomedin C levels, decrease in tumor size, and marked clinical improvements.
14. It is produced by recombinant DNA techniques.
15. (a) Pituitary tumor that destroys normal pituitary cells; (b) vascular thrombosis leading to necrosis of the normal pituitary gland; (c) infiltrative granulomatous diseases that destroy the pituitary; (d) idiopathic or possible autoimmune destruction of pituitary cells
16. Their urine specific gravity fails to increase, and urine osmolality remains low. Thirst may become intense, and they may develop orthostatic hypotension and experience significant weight loss. Rationale for administration of aqueous pitressin: urine volume decreases; specific gravity increases.
17. Treatment of SIADH is based on water restriction to less than 1000 ml/day; administration of 3% to 5% sodium chloride solutions with furosemide. Diuretic induces loss of water and sodium chloride, which is restored in hypertonic form. Demeclocycline can be used effectively to reverse the hypoosmolality associated with SIADH.

CHAPTER 60

1. The thyroid gland located below the cricoid cartilage in the neck is made up of nodules of tiny follicles. These follicles are lined by cuboidal epithelium, and their lumen is filled with colloid. The follicular epithelial cells initiate the synthesis of thyroid hormones and activate their release into the circulation. The thyroid hormones produced by the follicles are T_4 and T_3.
2. The process of biosynthesis of thyroid hormones is as follows: (a) Trapping of iodine by the thyroid follicular cells. The thyroid takes up and concentrates large amounts of iodine from the circulating iodide pool. (b) Oxidation of iodide to iodine. The thyroid plasma gradient is 20 to 30:1 at a wide range of plasma inorganic iodide concentrations. Iodide is catalyzed by an iodide perox-

idase enzyme and converted to iodine. (c) Organification of iodine into monoiodotyrosine. Iodine is incorporated into a tyrosine molecule, which occurs at the cell-colloid interphase. (d) Coupling of iodinated precursors. The resulting compounds, monoiodotyrosine and diiodotyrosine, are coupled as follows: two molecules of diiodotyrosine make T_4, and one molecule of diiodotyrosine and one molecule of monoiodotyrosine make T_3. (e) Storage. The coupling of these compounds and the storage of the resulting hormones take place within thyroglobulin. (f) Hormone release from storage. This release occurs by incorporation of colloid droplets into the follicular cells by a process called pinocytosis. Thyroglobulin is hydrolyzed, and the hormones are released into the circulation.

3. Tests presently used in the diagnosis of thyroid disease are (a) serum T_4 and T_3, (b) free T_4, (c) serum TSH levels, and (d) radioisotope thyroid uptake.

4. The significance of elevated serum thyroglobulin in patients with metastatic disease is indicative of recurring disease.

5. 20 to 30

6. 5

7. 4 to 11; 80 to 160

8. Graves' disease; toxic nodular goiter

CHAPTER 61

1. The catabolic effect of glucocorticoid excess causes a decrease in the ability of protein-forming cells to synthesize protein from amino acids.

2. Interferes with the action of insulin in the peripheral cells, which results in the impairment of the ability of the receptor cells to metabolize glucose.

3. Stress causes the CNS to activate the corticotropin-releasing center, causing CRH and ACTH to be released. Increased ACTH leads to an increase in cortisol release. The important concept is that stress causes an increased secretion of cortisol by the adrenal gland.

4. 9Alpha-fluorocortisol has a fluorine group in the 9alpha-position of the cortisol molecule. Prednisolone has a double bond between carbons 1 and 2 of this molecule. The metabolic effects of these compounds are different from those of the parent compound. For example, prednisolone, compared with cortisol, has less sodium-retaining activity and more antiinflammatory activity per milligram. 9Alpha-fluorocortisol has much greater sodium-retaining activity than cortisol.

5. Pituitary irradiation, removal of a pituitary tumor, and adrenalectomy. The excess cortisol is eliminated if the procedure is successful.

6. Surgical removal of the neoplasm

7. In congestive heart failure, patients are unable to pump blood normally and cardiac output decreases. The renal afferent arteriole experiences a change in perfusion pressure, causing increased production of renin, which activates synthesis of angiotensin. This action stimulates aldosterone production, causing resorption of sodium and water and volume expansion.

CHAPTER 62

1. The most common cause of primary adrenal insufficiency (Addison's disease) is autoimmune destruction of the adrenal gland; less commonly, adrenal gland destruction is a result of infection, infarction, malignancy, or bilateral adrenalectomy. Secondary adrenal insufficiency may be caused by hypothalamic-pituitary disease or sudden withdrawal of exogenous corticosteroid drug therapy. ACTH levels are elevated in primary adrenal insufficiency and depressed in secondary adrenal insufficiency.

2. (a) Hypersecretion of ACTH and, consequently, increased MSH causes the characteristic hyperpigmentation of the skin in Addison's disease. (b, c) Aldosterone deficiency results in renal K^+ retention, loss of Na^+, and water in the urine, thus resulting in hyperkalemia, hyponatremia, ECF volume depletion, and, consequently, orthostatic hypotension. (d) Glucocorticoid deficiency results in fasting hypoglycemia. (e) Scant pubic and axillary hair results from decreased adrenal secretion of androgens.

3. Hormone replacement therapy—cortisol 20 to 30 mg/day in divided doses and 9-alpha-fluorocortisol (aldosterone analogue) if necessary.

4. Prolonged high-dose corticosteroid therapy leads to suppression of normal endogenous steroid production by the adrenal cortex through negative feedback. In this circumstance, sudden cessation of the exogenous steroid produces acute adrenocortical failure (a medical emergency). Tapering the exogenous drug allows time for adrenocortical function to recover.

CHAPTER 63

1. FPG is measured to check the function of the regulating mechanisms that control carbohydrate metabolism. This measurement can help evaluate the integrity of the mechanism regulating plasma glucose. In general, these levels become abnormal only in the advanced state of a disease; therefore it does not provide information about early abnormalities in glucose metabolism.

2. Insulin. In people without diabetes, a rise in blood glucose stimulates release of insulin, which triggers disposal of excess glucose.

3. This system assists diabetics in managing their own diets. The food exchange lists help patients identify food alternatives.

4. The newer, second-generation sulfonylureas have advantages over the first-generation compounds in that they have little or no antidiuretic effect.

5. The recognition of individuals at risk for developing type 1 diabetes may lead to early detection of the autoimmune process causing destruction of beta cells and treatment with specific immunosuppressive agents. Once the disease has developed, pancreatic transplantation may restore insulin-secreting capacity. In type 2 diabetes patients, a better understanding of the molecular mechanism of insulin resistance may lead to the development of pharmacologic agents that could specifically enhance insulin action.

6. c
7. d
8. a
9. b
10. b
11. a
12. c
13. a
14. b
15. c
16. c
17. a, b

CHAPTER 64

1. The development and release of ova (oogenesis) and the production of steroid hormones (estrogens, E_1, E_2, E_3, androgens, progesterone)

2. During menopause, estradiol levels decrease and the ovary decreases in size and is virtually devoid of follicles. The decrease in circulating estradiol levels increases, by negative feedback, pituitary gonadotropin secretion.

3. Treatment of amenorrhea is often based on the underlying disorder causing the problem. For example, patients with prolactin-secreting pituitary adenomas should be treated with either transsphenoidal resection of the pituitary tumor or suppression of prolactin secretion with bromocriptine. Patients with hypothalamic-pituitary or ovarian deficiency should receive replacement therapy with estrogens and progesterone administered cyclically.

4. During the years of reproductive maturity, cyclic changes occur in the ovaries and uterus that serve the purpose of preparing the ovum and endometrium each month for a pregnancy. These cyclic changes are regulated by hormones of the hypothalamic-pituitary-gonadal axis. The following outline presents a simplified summary of these changes.
   A. Normal menstrual cycle: average length of cycle = 28 days
   B. Ovarian cycle
      1. Follicular phase
         a. FSH levels rise on day 1 of 28-day cycle, peaks on day 7, and declines thereafter
         b. FSH initiates maturation of several ovarian follicles (ovum and surrounding cells)
         c. FSH stimulates follicles to secrete estrogens
      2. Luteal phase
         a. LH levels rises on about day 9 of 28-day cycle, peaks at day 14 (ovulation), and gradually decreases during premenstrual phase
         b. LH induces ovulation (approximately day 14 but variable) of maturing ovum and formation of corpus luteum
         c. Corpus luteum secretes increasing amounts of progesterone and small amounts of estrogen
   C. Endometrial or menstrual cycle
      1. Proliferative or postmenstrual (preovulatory) phase
         a. Days 6 to 14 of 28-day cycle
         b. Rising estrogens levels stimulate proliferation and thickening of endometrium
      2. Ovulation (approximately day 14)
      3. Secretory of premenstrual phase
         a. Days 15 to 28 of 28-day cycle
         b. Increasing progesterone levels produced by corpus luteum stimulate endometrium to become vascular, edematous, and with a thicker mucosa capable of implanting a fertilized ovum
      4. Menstrual phase
         a. If ovum unfertilized, corpus luteum begins to regress on day 23 or 24 of 28-day cycle
         b. As luteal function degenerates, progesterone and estrogen levels decline, causing degeneration of uterine endometrium and initiation of menstruation
         c. Superficial endometrial lining is sloughed, accompanied with menstrual bleeding lasting about 5 days (day 1 to day 5 of 28-day cycle).

5. The anatomic structure of the female reproductive system, with access from outside the body to internal structures, allows ascent of organisms from the lower tract to the upper tract and potentially the perineal cavity, as well as descent from the upper tract, where there is hematogenous spread of the organism from a primary site of infection elsewhere in the body.

6. High-risk factors for ovarian cancer are early menarche, late menopause, nulliparous, or first pregnancy late; and if two or more first-degree relatives have ovarian cancer, a woman has a 50% chance of developing ovarian cancer. Some physicians recommend prophylactic oophorectomy at age 35 years for women in the latter high-risk group.

7. The breast changes are cystic formation, ductal epithelial proliferation, diffuse papillomatosis, and ductal adenosis with formation of fibrous tissue. Fibrocystic breast disease occurs during childbearing years; the cause is likely a relative excess of estrogen and a deficiency of progesterone during the luteal phase of the menstrual cycle.

8. Breast cancers develop from epithelial tissues, with most being in the duct system. Initially there is hyperplasia of the cells with development of atypical cells that progress to carcinoma in situ and then to stromal invasion. A cancer takes about 7 years to grow from a single cell to a mass large enough to palpate (about 1 cm in diameter). At that size, about one fourth of breast cancers have already metastasized.

9. Detection and diagnosis begin with obtaining a thorough history of pertinent information related to the breasts and a physical examination of the breasts. Mammography is essential because it can detect masses too small to be felt and in many instances reveals the probable nature of a palpable mass. Tissue-sampling procedures done to obtain specimens for microscopic examination include fine-needle aspiration, core needle biopsy, and open biopsy. If the specimen is malignant, further evaluation is needed.

CHAPTER 65

1. Primary functions are to produce mature spermatozoa and to deposit sperm in the female reproductive tract with coitus.

2. Spermatogenesis begins with puberty (about age 13) and continues throughout life. In the seminiferous tubules, spermatogonia begin to proliferate. Some of the daughter cells remain spermatogonia, and others move to the lumen of the seminiferous tubule and enlarge into primary spermatocytes. These cells undergo meiotic division to form two secondary spermatocytes. Each secondary spermatocyte undergoes a second meiotic division, resulting in two spermatids. One spermatogonium produces four sperm. Each spermatid undergoes a maturation and differentiation process to develop the head, neck, body, and tail of the mature sperm. This process takes place continuously throughout life. Sperm are stored in the epididymides and vasa deferens and retain their fertility for as long as 42 days.

3. A clomiphene or GnRH stimulation test should be done if low gonadotropins are present with low serum testosterone. In this case, clomiphene should cause a 50% increase in the ICSH. If ICSH does not increase, the test indicates a hypothalamic-pituitary insufficiency. However, administering GnRH should cause a peak level three times the control of LH within minutes. With hypothalamic dysfunction, a response may not occur until repeated injections are given over several days. An exaggerated response indicates a reduced feedback response secondary to low levels of testosterone and estradiol.

4. It is difficult to separate the decline of reproductive function with the decline in physical fitness that occurs with advancing age; the latter decline may be responsible for the decrease in reproductive function. The seminiferous tubules of the testes continue to produce sperm but in less numbers with advancing age. Testosterone levels gradually decrease. The number of Leydig's cells may decrease as the ability of the remaining cells to produce testosterone decreases. Failure to attain or maintain erection of the penis (impotence) is more common with advanced age. Psychologic and physiologic factors are involved, such as veins and arteries that supply the erectile tissue of the penis being subject to sclerosis.

5. The factors responsible for infections of the genital organs in men are venereal transmission, a manifestation of systemic disease, or a result of instrumentation (catheterization or surgery).

6. As the tumor progresses, there can be direct extension to the urethra, bladder neck, and seminal vesicles. The tumor can also spread via lymphatic or hematogenous routes. Most common site of metastasis is by the

hematogenous route to the bones of the pelvis, lumbar spine, femur, thoracic spine, and ribs. Organ metastases are to the liver and lung.

7. c
8. a
9. e
10. d
11. b

CHAPTER 66

1. Lack of knowledge and comfort with personal sexuality; cultural taboos related to sexual issues; fear and embarrassment about having a STI; fear of a loss of anonymity; poor communication and embarrassment of health care providers when discussing issues related to sexuality; lack of health insurance.
2. Spread of infection causing more people to be hurt; more infections increase treatment expense; infertility
3. Requires cooperation of infected individual; increases risk or may require loss of anonymity; raises issues of blame and accusations; may result in termination of relationships.
4. Education, treatment programs, counseling about sexually responsible behavior, research
5. Cervical, penile or anal cancers; neonatal infection

CHAPTER 67

1. The structures of the musculoskeletal system include bones, joints, skeletal muscles, tendons, ligaments, bursae, and the specialized tissues that connect these structures.
2. *Woven bone* is a type of bone seen with rapid growth (e.g., in fetal development or after a fracture; in adults it is found at ligament or tendon insertions). *Lamella bone* is mature bone found throughout the body of adults. The structure of lamella bone is highly organized, mineralized plates rather than a solid, crystalline mass, which provides substantial strength for bone.
3. Joints are held together by joint capsules, fibrous bands, ligaments, tendons, fasciae, or muscles.
4. The joint is lubricated by synovial fluid and by hydrostatic changes in the interstitial fluid of the cartilage. Pressure on the cartilages causes fluid to move to an area of less pressure. As the joint glides forward, this weeping fluid moves ahead to the load. The fluid moves back into the portions of the cartilage from which the pressure is relieved. Articular cartilage and the bones of the joint are normally held apart during action by the film of the fluid.
5. The process of bone resorption occurs because the osteoclasts produce proteolytic enzymes that break down matrix and several acids that cause dissolution of the bone minerals. Calcium and phosphorus are released into the bloodstream during this process.
6. Osteoid is the organic matrix of bone that is about 70% type I collagen. This type of collagen is rigid, giving bone its high tensile strength.
7. The significance of joints innervated by peripheral nerves crossing the articulation is that pain from one joint may be reported as coming from another (e.g., pain arising in the hip can be felt by the person as knee pain).
8. Refer to Fig. 67-1.
9. c
10. a
11. d
12. b

CHAPTER 68

1. d
2. a
3. When a fracture occurs, the periosteum is generally torn, blood vessels are damaged, and bone fragments are separated. A blood clot forms, and granulation tissue develops within which osteogenic cells differentiate into chondroblasts and osteoblasts. A band (callus) forms around a fragment at the fracture site and continues to thicken and expand, converging with the band from the opposite fragment and fusing with it. Fusion of the two fragments and fracture healing progress as osteoblasts to form trabeculae, which adhere to the bone and extend across the fracture site. The bony callus remodels to assume the shape of intact bone, as osteoblasts form, new bone and osteoclasts remove the damaged and temporary bone.
4. Early diagnosis of osteomyelitis, especially in children, is important so that appropriate antibiotic and surgical treatment can be administered to prevent the local spread of infection and crippling destruction of the entire bone.
5. In children, the periosteal sleeve around the tubular bones is strong and active, allowing for rapid healing.
6. Children's limbs grow quickly; bayonet apposition is often used to achieve equal length by adulthood.

CHAPTER 69

1. When a lesion is definitely diagnosed as benign and self-limiting, no further diagnostic studies are generally needed. However, when a lesion is diagnosed as benign with a lesser degree of certainty, the patient should be reexamined at regular intervals with repeat radiographs. If over several months there is no change in the lesion or in the patient's condition, follow-up visits may be discontinued. The patient must be instructed to return for further examination if any changes occur. It is important to assess whether the patient and the family are responsible and will follow through with the repeated examination.
2. Bone tumor cells produce factors that stimulate osteoclast activity, which leads to bone resorption. Some tumors cause increased osteoblast activity and increased density.
3. Benign tumors are much more common, although malignant tumors are often fatal. Malignant tumors tend to grow rapidly and spread and invade irregularly; most often, they occur in adolescents and young adults.
4. The most common primary sites of bone neoplasms are the prostrate, breast, lung, thyroid, kidney, and bladder.
5. The most common bones affected by neoplasms are vertebrae, proximal femur, pelvis, ribs, sternum, and proximal humerus.

CHAPTER 70

1. *Osteoarthritis* is a disorder of the movable joints. The disorder is chronic, slowly progressive, and noninflammatory and is characterized by the deterioration and abrasion of articular cartilage and the formation of new bone at the articular surface.
2. The synthesis of proteoglycans and collagen in the joint is greatly increased in osteoarthritis. There is a net loss of proteoglycans and collagen over time because degradation is even more rapid.
3. The aging process seems to be related to the development and progression of osteoarthritis through changes in chondrocyte functioning. Chondrocytes are the cells responsible for the formation of the proteoglycans and collagen in the articular cartilage. The aging chondrocytes may lose their ability to function appropriately.
4. Total joint replacements for hips and knees have been successful in maintaining near-normal function for many people with osteoarthritis. Osteoarthritis is a hypertrophic form of arthritis; that is, the bone adjacent to the joint is strong, forming an excellent base for attachment of the artificial joint. A number of complications can occur with joint replacement, and these must be weighed against the benefits.
5. Narrowing of the joint space is typically seen in osteoarthritis because of loss of cartilage. Radiologic findings also reveal an increase in bone density around the joint. Cystic changes of various sizes are some-

times seen. Osteophytes (spurs) can be seen at the marginal aspects of the joint.

6. The goals of the treatment of osteoarthritis are retardation or prevention of further damage to the joint and management of pain and stiffness to maintain mobility.

CHAPTER 71

1. *Rheumatoid arthritis* is a chronic disorder that affects multiple organ systems and is one of a group of diffuse connective tissue diseases that are immune mediated and of unknown cause. There is usually progressive joint destruction, although the episodes of joint inflammation may alternate with periods of remission.

2. There is an association of the genetic markers HLA-Dw4 and HLA-DR5 with the development of rheumatoid arthritis in Caucasians.

3. Destruction of the tissues in the joints occurs in the following ways. (a) There is a digestive destruction caused by the production of proteases, collagenases, and other hydrolytic enzymes. These enzymes break down the cartilage, ligaments, tendons, and bones in the joints and are released along with oxygen radicals and arachidonic acid metabolites by PMNs in the synovial fluid. (b) Destruction of tissue appears to take place through the action of rheumatoid pannus. Along the edge of the pannus, there is destruction of collagen and proteoglycans through the production of enzymes of cells in the pannus.

4. The diagnostic criteria are (a) morning stiffness (at least 1 hour), (b) arthritis of three or more joint areas, (c) arthritis of hand joints, (d) symmetric arthritis, (e) rheumatoid nodules, (f) serum rheumatoid factor, and (g) radiographic changes (erosions of bony decalcification).

5. The overall goals of the therapeutic program for rheumatoid arthritis are to relieve pain and inflammation, maintain joint function and the patient's maximum functional capacity, and prevent and/or correct joint deformities.

6. NSAIDs reduce inflammation by interrupting the cascade of production of inflammatory mediators; they act by inhibiting either cyclooxygenase or prostaglandin synthetase. These enzymes are responsible for the conversion of the endogenous systemic fatty acid arachidonic acid to prostaglandins, prostacyclins, thromboxanes, and oxygen radicals.

7. The indications for corticosteroid therapy are as follows: (a) Chronic oral therapy is used in those persons with rheumatoid arthritis who do not respond to NSAIDs and slow-acting drugs. (b) Corticosteroid therapy is used for control of symptoms while awaiting the onset of action by slow-acting drug therapy. (c) Intraarticular injections are indicated for acute exacerbations of synovitis in single joints where mobility is significantly impaired. (d) High-dose oral therapy is used for short periods for a severe attack.

8. Corticosteroid agents act through their antiinflammatory and immunosuppressive properties. Inflammation is reduced by blocking prostaglandin formation, inhibiting leukocyte and monocyte chemotaxis and phagocytosis, stabilizing lysosomal enzymes, and preventing changes in capillary membranes. Immunosuppression results from the decreased reticuloendothelial, or monocyte-macrophage, procession of antigens, and the altered function of lymphocytes.

9. Rheumatoid arthritis may involve the heart (pericarditis), lungs (pleuritis), eyes, and blood vessels. Refer to Box 71-1.

CHAPTER 72

1. SLE is a multisystem, chronic, autoimmune disease. The signs and symptoms of this disorder can be diverse and transitory.

2. The ANA test indicates whether there are antibodies capable of destroying the nucleus of the subject's own body cells. In addition to the presence of ANA, the ANA pattern and the specific antibodies are evaluated. The LE factor test may occasionally be used today to identify the LE factor. The LE cell is formed by damage to some of a person's WBCs, causing release of their nucleoprotein, which reacts with IgG; this complex is phagocytosed by the remaining WBCs. The resulting cell is easily identified.

3. The onset of SLE occurs most frequently during late adolescence and early adulthood in women. Counseling is needed to assist persons affected regarding the decision about having children. Pregnancy may cause a flare-up of SLE, which can be dangerous for women with renal damage. Cytotoxic drugs may be necessary to control the illness, and these can affect the fetus. Contraceptives, including birth control pills, cannot be prescribed, because they may aggravate SLE.

4. Just how sunlight causes SLE to flare up is not fully understood. One explanation is that DNA exposed to ultraviolet light normally becomes antigenic, and this leads to the flares seen after sunlight exposure.

5. The selection of appropriate drug therapy depends on the specific organs affected by the illness. NSAIDs are used to control the arthritis and arthralgia. Aspirin is used less frequently because it produces the highest incidence of hepatotoxicity, and some people with SLE have hepatic involvement.

CHAPTER 73

1. *Generalized* scleroderma (systemic sclerosis) can be diffuse cutaneous systemic sclerosis with truncal involvement, widespread visceral disease, or limited cutaneous systemic sclerosis including the CREST variant; *localized* scleroderma usually affects only limited skin areas and does not affect visceral organs; *occupational and environmental* scleroderma-like syndromes can be seen after exposure to substances such as chloride, bleomycin, and rapeseed oil.

2. The skin and other organ changes in scleroderma are the result of the overproduction of collagen. Lesions that develop in the small arteries and arterioles begin as proliferations on the intimal side of the internal elastic membrane. A medial thinning then occurs, and finally, a connective tissue cuff rich in collagen is deposited.

3. One form of systemic sclerosis is the CREST variant. The colon may be affected, which results in diarrhea or constipation, cramping, and malabsorption. Exertional dyspnea is usually the first sign of pulmonary involvement; pulmonary function studies may show alterations in gas exchange (decrease in breathing capacity and increase in residual air); pericarditis; dysrhythmias; electrocardiogram changes with cardiac involvement; renal involvement exhibited as proteinuria, microscopic hematuria, and hypertension may rapidly deteriorate to renal failure.

4. Drugs such as penicillamine, DMSO, immunosuppressive drugs, and alkylating agents are sometimes used to manage symptoms. Protection of the hands to help avoid Raynaud's phenomenon is an important part of the management plan. NSAIDs can be used to decrease discomfort. Physical therapy is an important component of the treatment plan.

CHAPTER 74

1. *Gout* is a term used for a group of at least nine metabolic disorders that are characterized by an elevation in the serum uric acid concentration (hyperuricemia).

2. Primary gout is the direct result of the body's overproduction or decreased

excretion of uric acid. Secondary gout occurs when the overproduction or decreased excretion of uric acid is secondary to another disease process or to medication.

3. Colchicine is a drug that inhibits phagocytic leukocytes and produces a dramatic and rapid relief of the symptoms of gout.

4. The factors that contribute to the development of gout depend on the cause of the hyperuricemia. For example, a diet high in purines can trigger a gouty attack in a person with one of the inborn errors of purine metabolism. The ingestion of alcohol can produce a gouty attack because blood lactate levels increase as a by-product of the normal metabolism of alcohol. Lactic acid blocks the renal excretion of uric acid, with a concomitant rise in serum levels.

5. The treatment of chronic gout is based on decreasing the production of uric acid or increasing the renal excretion of uric acid.

6. Gout can damage the kidneys, leading to an even poorer excretion of uric acid. These uric acid crystals can form in the medullary interstitium, papillae, and pyramids, leading to proteinuria and mild hypertension. Uric acid kidney stones can also occur secondary to gout.

CHAPTER 75

1. The goals of the treatment of ankylosing spondylitis are multifocal and relate to the stage of the illness. There is a focused intervention aimed at increasing the understanding of the illness by the patient and the family. Changes in work patterns may be necessary, because bending, lifting, and prolonged static positions will be difficult. Medication is aimed at decreasing the synovitis and pain. An active exercise program is often focused on breathing exercises, muscle strengthening, and reducing limitations in range of motion.

2. About 7% of people with psoriasis develop inflammatory joint disease (psoriatic arthritis). Usually the arthritis occurs after the appearance of the skin lesions, but it can occur before or at the same time as the skin lesions occur.

3. The treatment of Reiter's syndrome is primarily symptomatic. Therapeutic doses of NSAIDs are used to relieve the inflammation and pain. Antibiotics are not of proven value.

4. True

5. True

6. False. About 20% of individuals with ankylosing spondylitis develop disabling stages of the illness.

7. True

CHAPTER 76

1. The basal layer consists largely of undifferentiated cells that undergo constant mitoses, renewing the epidermis. One of the daughter cells migrates outward toward the stratum spinosum. These undifferentiated basal-layer cells are precursors of keratinocytes. Keratinocytes migrate upward through the stratum granulosum to the stratum corneum to form a fibrous-amorphous complex surrounded by a reinforced impermeable membrane, the horny cell.

2. Eccrine (sweat) glands produce a hypotonic solution and allow excess heat to be eliminated from the body, which aids in maintaining appropriate body temperature. Sebaceous glands produce sebum, which lubricates the epidermis.

3. (a) Skin should be examined in a well-illuminated room, preferably in natural daylight. (b) Color should be recorded (e.g., purplish, cyanotic discoloration, pallor). (c) Skin characteristics such as turgor and elasticity on palpation should be noted. (d) Hair distribution and condition of nails should be recorded.

4. The subcutaneous layer provides a cushion for the skin, insulation to maintain body heat, and a store of energy.

5. Refer to the following figure.

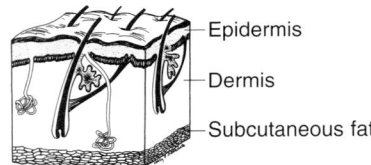

Epidermis
Dermis
Subcutaneous fat

CHAPTER 77

1. Acne is an acute or chronic inflammatory disease of the pilosebaceous glands that results in the formation of comedones, papules, pustules, and cysts.

2. Acne generally occurs among adolescents and young adults and spontaneously resolves by 20 to 30 years of age.

3. The earliest lesion is the comedo. White comedones are likely to progress to the inflammatory papules and pustules of acne. Black comedones obstruct the flow of sebum to the surface. The sebum, bacteria, and fatty acids are thought to be responsible for the development of inflammation around the pilosebaceous ducts and sebaceous glands. This inflammation leads to the formation of papules, inflammatory pustules, and cysts. The cysts open in time, drain, and heal. Deeper papules and cysts can leave permanent scars, whereas mild acne resolves without scarring.

4. (a) To remove the surface oil and to dislodge some comedones. (b) Tetracycline. This antibiotic eliminates *Propionibacterium acnes* in the sebaceous gland. Tetracycline has an inhibitory effect on the enzyme lipase, thus preventing breakdown of fat into fatty acids.

CHAPTER 78

1. The characteristic lesions of eczema are pruritic, erythematous, crusty, weepy, and scaly eruptions. Acute eczema presents with many vesicles and bullae and with erythema, weeping, and crusting, whereas chronic eczema presents with thickened (lichenified), scaly, pruritic patches and plaques.

2. (a) Skin reaction to the oil of poison ivy; (b) nickel sensitivity; (c) allergic reaction to potassium and dichromate; (d) allergic reaction to shoes that contain rubber; (e) allergic reaction to medications such as neomycin or benzocaine

3. Dyshidrotic hand eczema occurs in persons who must wash their hands frequently or are under stress. In the absence of positive allergic tests, heredity and irritants play an important role in the cause of hand eczema.

4. Acute urticaria with angioedema is treated with subcutaneous epinephrine. Less severe urticaria is treated with oral antihistamines, such as diphenhydramine, hydroxyzine, cyproheptadine, cetirizine, loratadine, and fexofenadine.

CHAPTER 79

1. The new treatment modalities for psoriasis are oral etretinate (Tegison) and oral acitretin (Soriatane). These oral aromatic retinoids are excellent for the treatment of pustular and erythrodermic psoriasis and are useful for recalcitrant plaque psoriasis. These drugs should not be given to women of childbearing age because they are a powerful teratogen; they also elevate liver enzymes, cholesterol, and triglycerides. Side effects include dryness, hair loss, headaches, diarrhea, myalgia, and arthralgias. If used longer than 6 months, radiographic studies of the bones should be done to check for calcium deposits in the joints.

2. A vitamin D derivative, 1,25-dihydroxy vitamin D_3, can be used for psoriasis.

3. A psoriatic skin biopsy reveals thickened epidermis and stratum corneum and dilated upper dermal blood vessels. The number of basal cells undergoing mitosis is increased. These fast-dividing cells move rapidly to the surface of thickened epidermis. This rapid proliferation and migration of epidermal cells result in thick epider-

mis covered by a thick keratin (silvery scale) over the trunk. Abnormal levels of cyclic nucleotides, especially cAMP and cGMP, may be partially responsible for this rapid mitosis of epidermal cells. Prostaglandins and polyamines are also possibly abnormal in the disease. The role of these abnormalities in influencing the formation of a psoriatic plaque is not clearly understood.

CHAPTER 80

1. The diagnosis of herpes can be confirmed by a positive herpetic culture in about 80% of patients. Another test is the Tzanck test, which is positive in 50% to 80% of patients with herpes. In this test, the material from the vesicle is placed on a glass slide and stained with 1% toluidine blue. Large, multinucleated giant cells can be seen in patients with herpes. This test can be performed in a few minutes; it is cheaper than is a herpetic culture but is less reliable.

2. At present, there is no vaccine to prevent herpes infections from recurring. Using opaque sunscreens or avoiding sunlight exposure can sometimes prevent recurrent episodes of herpes of the lips. Oral acyclovir (Zovirax) 400 mg twice daily, Voltrax 500 mg daily, or famciclovir (Famvir) 250 mg twice daily frequently prevents recurrent eruptions of herpes simplex. Sexual spread of genital herpes is frequently aborted by use of rubber condoms when vesicles are present and for 7 days afterward. Sexual abstinence when vesicles are present is an alternative method of prevention. Towels, underclothing, and swimming suits should not be shared.

3. A primary herpes simplex infection can cause severe conjunctivitis and even blindness.

4. Impetigo first appears as a purulent lesion. As the lesion spreads, it becomes eroded, and a golden crust develops on the surface.

5. Streptococci and staphylococci cause impetigo. The infection is transferred by human-to-human contact, usually among children. Heat, humidity, and poor hygiene predispose to this infection. Erysipelas, on the other hand, is a serious toxic infection of the skin.

The patient has a high fever and malaise and is toxic. Streptococci causes the infection.

6. Poor hygiene and excoriations; exposure to inadequately disinfected hot tubs.

7. Treatment of localized herpes zoster is symptomatic with soaks and pain medication. If the ophthalmic branch of the trigeminal nerve is affected, an ophthalmologist should also be consulted because corneal perforations may result from the infection. Early administration of systemic corticosteroids may be helpful in the prevention of postherpetic neuralgia. Oral acyclovir at the dosage of 800 mg 5 times daily for 7 days, Valtrex 1 g 3 times daily for 7 days, or Famvir 500 mg 3 times daily for 7 days can shorten the duration of herpes zoster infection.

CHAPTER 81

1. Characteristic of malignant melanoma is an irregular pigmented lesion with shades of blue, purple, red, and brown. The borders of the tumor are irregular, and the surface is frequently ulcerated. Satellite lesions and diffusion of pigment into the surrounding skin are also observed.

2. Basal cell carcinoma is derived from epidermal cells in the skin. This tumor rarely metastasizes. The most common sites of occurrence are on the sunlight-exposed areas of the face, head, and neck.

3. The preventive measures for patients with a history of melanoma and for fair-skinned individuals are sunscreens, sun blocks, and avoidance of excess sunlight. Any individual who has dysplastic nevi and a family history of melanoma is at high risk for developing melanoma. He or she should be examined by a physician every 6 months, should avoid sunlight exposure, should use sunscreens when outside, and should self-examine the skin every few weeks.

4. Treatment includes curettage with electrodesiccation, scalpel surgery, irradiation, or cryosurgery.

5. Squamous cell carcinoma is a tumor that arises from keratinocytes in the epidermis. This tumor develops in older, fair-skinned persons. The tumor

usually presents as an ulcerated, hyperkeratotic nodule with evidence of dermal invasion on palpation. Squamous cell carcinoma of the skin arising in sunlight-exposed areas rarely metastasizes. This cancer is treated with scalpel surgery or irradiation.

CHAPTER 82

1. ECM begins as an erythematous papule where the tick bite occurred. The papule expands with central clearing, measuring up to 25 to 50 mm in diameter and usually disappears spontaneously without therapy within 1 month. The lesion may itch, sting, or burn. The thighs, groin, and axillae are common sites of involvement. Other symptoms occur weeks to months later in patients who are not treated. A triad of meningitis, cranial nerve palsies, and peripheral neuropathy characterize these symptoms. Fewer than 10% of patients experience cardiac manifestations.

2. The mite *Sarcoptes scabiei* cause *scabies*. Close human contact, especially among children and sexually active adults, transmits the infection. Pruritus is the chief complaint. Excoriated linear papules and vesicles are classically found between the fingers, over the elbows, and on the wrists, breasts, and genitalia. Treatment consists of application of gamma benzene hexachloride (Kwell) for two 24-hour periods. Children under 5 years of age are treated for a limited time with 5% permethrin Elimite. Secondary irritant eczema can complicate treatment and result in persistence of pruritus. All family members must be treated prophylactically overnight with gamma benzene hexachloride or permethrin, even if they present no evidence of scabietic lesions or pruritus. *Pediculosis pubis* (pubic crabs) is a frequent infection of the pubic hair and skin and is transmitted by human contact. Lice and nits, which attach to the pubic hair, can be seen with the naked eye and cause intense pruritus. Kwell shampoo is the treatment of choice and should be applied twice. Nits may also be removed with a fine-toothed comb soaked in vinegar.

3. a, c, d

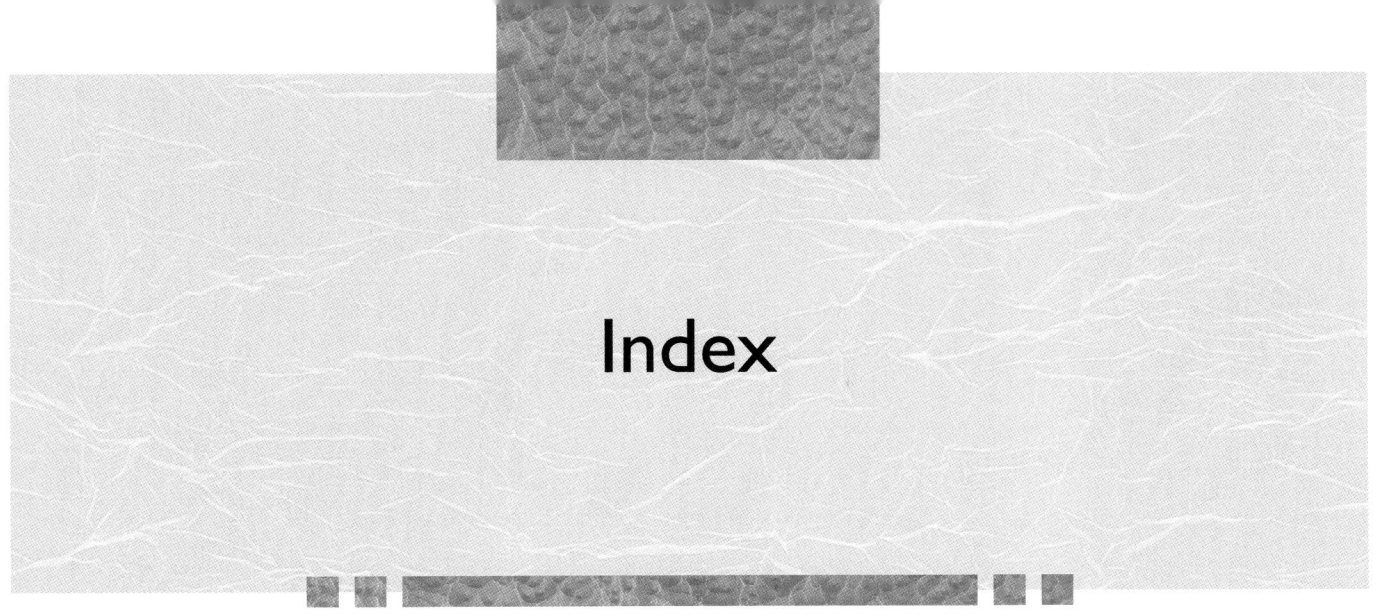

Index

A

Abacavir (Ziagen), 185, 185*t*
Abciximab (ReoPro), 473, 473*t*
Abdomen, 374*t*, 749*t*
Abdominal aorta, 513
Abdominal aortic aneurysms, 523, 524, 524*f*
Abducens nerve (cranial nerve VI)
    function of, 768, 768*t*
    functional examination of, 780-781
A-beta (A-β) primary afferent fibers, 792
ABGs. *See* Arterial blood gases
AbioCor Replacement Heart, 507-508, 508*f*
ABO blood group system, 726-727, 727*t*
Abscesses, 61
    anorectal, 365, 365*f*, 367
    brain, 53-54, 54*f*, 859
    breast, 982
    pancreatic, 394
Absence (petit mal) seizures, 867
Absorption, 344
    sites of, 344, 344*f*
    of vitamin B$_{12}$, 346
Absorption atelectasis, 593, 593*f*, 600
Absorptive cells, 342
Abuse, analgesic, 699-700
Acarbose, 951
Accessory nerve (cranial nerve XI)
    function of, 768, 768*t*
    functional examination of, 783
Accutane. *See* Isotretinoin
Acetaminophen (Tylenol), 807, 820, 1090
Acetazolamide (Diamox), 664, 866
Acetylcholine, 413
Acetylsalicylic acid (Colsalide), 202*t*
Achalasia, 323-324
    esophageal, 320-321, 320*f*
    primary, 320, 323
    secondary, 320, 323-324
Achlorhydria, 329
Acid hydrolases, 129-130, 130*t*
Acid perfusion test, 319-320
Acid reflux tests, 319-320
Acid-base disorders, 292-312, 296*t*
    arterial blood parameters, 297, 298*t*
    assessment of, 296-299, 297*b*
        tests for, 616, 616*t*
    expected compensatory responses, 297, 298*t*
    nomogram for, 297, 299*f*, 614-615, 614*f*
    overview of, 295, 295*f*

Acidemia, 294, 840
Acidosis
    acid-base changes in, 565, 565*t*
    diabetic ketoacidosis, 948, 951
    dilutional, 299
    metabolic, 295, 296*t*, 299-301, 300*b*, 300*f*
        acid-base changes in, 565, 565*t*
        compensatory responses to, 298*t*, 300, 565
        oxyhemoglobin dissociation curve in, 550-551
        with respiratory acidosis, 306
        with respiratory alkalosis, 307
        in uremia, 704-705, 712
    renal tubular, 695-696, 701
    respiratory, 295, 296*t*, 303-304, 303*b*
        acid-base changes in, 565, 565*t*
        acute, 298*t*, 304
        acute-on-chronic, 307
        chronic, 298*t*, 304
        compensatory responses to, 298*t*
        with metabolic acidosis, 306
        with metabolic alkalosis, 307
    in uremia, 717-718
Acids, 293
    nonvolatile or fixed, 293, 650
    volatile, 293
Acinus(i), 372, 542, 542*f*, 552
Acitretin (Soriatane), 1085
Aclovate. *See* Alclometasone
Acne, 1071-1076
    comedonal, 1071, 1072*f*, 1076
    conglobate, 1072, 1073*f*
    papulopustular, 1071, 1073*f*, 1076
Acne conglobata, 1072, 1073*f*
Acne keloidalis, 1072, 1073*f*
Acne rosacea, 1074, 1074*f*, 1076
Acne vulgaris, 1071, 1072*f*
Acquired immunity, 80
Acquired immunodeficiency syndrome, 173-189
    CDC surveillance case definition for, 175, 176*b*
    distribution of, 173, 174*f*
    epidemiology of, 173-175, 174*f*
    expanded surveillance case definition for, 174-175, 175*t*
Acrochordons, 1102, 1102*f*
Acromegaly, 908-910, 909*f*, 910*f*, 913
Actin, 419

Actinic keratosis, 1102, 1104
Action potential, 416-419, 418*f*, 754-755
Activated partial thromboplastin time, 232, 233*t*
Activation gates, 417
Active immunity, 80
Active transport, 246
Acupressure, 809
Acupuncture, 809
Acute nephritic syndrome, 686*t*, 688, 701
Acute (adult) respiratory distress syndrome, 617-618, 617*b*, 620
ADA. *See* Adenosine deaminase
Adapalene retinoidlike compound (Differin), 1073
Adaptive and assistive equipment, 1043
Adaptive plasticity, 838
Addiction, 808
Addisonian crisis, 940
Addison's disease, 938, 939-940
A-delta (A-δ) primary afferent fibers, 792, 819
Adenine, 9
Adenocarcinoma, 116, 125
    of colon and rectum, 363-364
    of gallbladder, 396
    of lung, 624, 627
    well-differentiated, 115, 115*f*
Adenohypophysis, 906, 912
Adenoma
    adrenocortical
        aldosterone-secreting, 928, 929*f*
        Cushing's syndrome secondary to, 927, 927*f*
    basophil, 883
    bronchial, 625
    eosinophilic, 883
    fibroadenoma, 976
    pedunculated, 363, 366
    polypoid, 363
    sessile, 363
    somatotrope, 913
    villous, 363, 366
Adenomatous polyps, 363
Adenosine deaminase deficiency, 27, 28*f*
Adhesions, 62
    intestinal, 342
Adipose tissue, 749*t*
Adnexal tumors, 884
Adrenal carcinoma, 936

Page references followed by *f, b, n* or *t* indicate figures, boxes, notes, or tables, respectively.

NORMAL VALUES OF COMMON LABORATORY AND FUNCTION TESTS

These tables list some of the most common laboratory tests and their normal values.
Laboratory values may vary with different techniques or different laboratories.

Serum Normal Values

Acetoacetate	0.3-2.0 mg/dl	Immunoglobulin, quantitation	
Acid phosphatase	0-0.8 U/ml	IgG	700-1500 mg/dl
Acid phosphatase, prostatic	2.5-12.0 IU/L	IaA	70-400 mg/dl
Albumin	3.0-5.5 g/dl	IgM	
Aldolase	1-6 IU/L	Female	30-300 mg/dl
Alkaline phosphatase		Male	30-250 mg/dl
15-20 years	40-200 IU/L	IgD	0-40 mg/dl
20-101 years	35-125 IU/L	Insulin, fasting	6-20 μU/ml
Alpha-1 antitrypsin	200-500 mg/dl	Iron-binding capacity	250-400 μg/dl
ALT	0-40 IU/L	Iron, total, serum	40-150 μg/dl
Ammonia	11-35 μmol/L	Lactic acid	0.6-1.8 mEq/L
Amylase, serum	2-20 U/L	LDH, serum	20-220 IU/L
Anion gap	8-12 mEq/L (mmol/L)	LDH isoenzymes	
Ascorbic acid	0.4-1.5 mg/dl	LDH_1	20%-34%
AST	5-40 IU/L	LDH_2	28%-41%
Bilirubin		LDH_3	15%-25%
Total	0.2-1.2 mg/dl	LDH_4	3%-12%
Direct	0-0.4 mg/dl	LDH_5	6%-15%
Calcium, serum	8.7-10.6 mg/dl	Leucine aminopeptidase (LAP)	30-55 IU/L
Carbon dioxide, total	18-30 mEq/L (mmol/L)	Lipase	4-24 IU/dl
Carcinoembryonic antigen, serum	<2.5 μg/L	Magnesium, serum	1.5-2.5 mEq/L
Carotene (carotenoids)	50-300 μg/dl	5'-Nucleotidase	0.3-3.2 Bodansky units
C3 complement	55-120 mg/dl	Osmolality, serum	278-305 mOsm/kg serum water
C4 complement	14-51 mg/dl	Phenylalanine	3 mg/dl
Ceruloplasmin	15-60 mg/dl	Phosphorus, inorganic, serum	2.0-4.3 mg/dl
Chloride, serum	95-105 mEq/L (mmol/L)	Potassium, plasma	3.1-4.3 mEq/L
Cholesterol, total		Potassium, serum	3.5-5.2 mEq/L
12-19 years	120-230 mg/dl	Protein, total, serum	
20-29 years	120-240 mg/dl	2-55 years	5.0-8.0 g/dl
30-39 years	140-270 mg/dl	55-101 years	6.0-8.3 g/dl
40-49 years	150-310 mg/dl	Protein electrophoresis, serum	
50-59 years	160-330 mg/dl	Albumin	3.2-5.2 g/dl
Copper	100-200 μg/dl	Alpha-1	0.6-1.0 g/dl
Creatine kinase, total	20-200 IU/L	Alpha-2	0.6-1.0 g/dl
Creatine kinase, isoenzymes		Beta	0.6-1.2 g/dl
MM fraction	94%-95%	Gamma	0.7-1.5 g/dl
MB fraction	0%-5%	Sodium, serum	135-145 mEq/L
BB fraction	0%-2%	Sulfate	0.5-1.5 mg/dl
Normal values in		T_3 uptake	25%-45%
Heart	80% MM, 20% MB	T_4	4-11 μg/dl
Brain	100% BB	Triglycerides	
Skeletal muscle	95% MM, 2% MB	2-29 years	10-140 mg/dl
Creatinine, serum		30-39 years	20-150 mg/dl
Female adult	0.5-1.3 mg/dl	40-49 years	20-160 mg/dl
Male adult	0.7-1.5 mg/dl	50-59 years	20-190 mg/dl
Delta-aminolevulinic acid (ALA)	<200 μg/dl	60-101 years	20-200 mg/dl
α-Fetoprotein, serum	<40 μg/L	Urea nitrogen, serum	
Folate, serum	1.9-14.0 ng/ml	2-65 years	5-22 mg/dl
Gamma glutamyl transpeptidase		Female	8-26 mg/dl
Female	9-31 IU/L	Male	10-38 mg/dl
Male	12-38 IU/L	Uric acid	
Gastrin	150 pg/ml	10-59 years	
Glucose, serum (fasting)	70-115 mg/dl	Female	2.0-8.0 mg/dl
Glucose-6-phosphate dehydrogenase	5-10 IU/g Hb	Male	2.5-9.0 mg/dl
G6PD screen, qualitative	Negative	60-101 years	
Haptoglobin	100-300 mg/dl	Female	2.5-9.0 mg/dl
Hemoglobin A_2	0%-4% of total Hb	Male	2.5-9.0 mg/dl
Hemoglobin F	0%-2% of total Hb	Viscosity	1.4-1.8 (serum compared to H_2O)
		Vitamin A	0.15-0.60 μg/ml
		Vitamin B_{12}	200-850 pg/ml

Cerebrospinal Fluid Normal Values

Bilirubin	0	Protein, lumbar	15-45 mg/dl
Cells	0-5/mm³, all lymphocytes	Albumin	58%
Chloride	110-129 mEq/L	α_1-Globulins	9%
Glucose	48-86 mg/dl or $\geq$60% of serum glucose	α_2-Globulins	8%
pH	7.34-7.43	β-Globulins	10%
Pressure	7-20 cm water	γ-Globulins	10% (5%-12%)
		Protein, cisternal	15-25 mg/dl
		Protein, ventricular	5-15 mg/dl